The Practice of

GENERAL
SURGERY

The Practice of
GENERAL SURGERY

EDITOR

Kirby I. Bland, M.D.

ASSOCIATE EDITOR

Michael G. Sarr, M.D.

SECTION EDITORS

William G. Cioffi, M.D.
Orlo H. Clark, M.D.
Richard L. Gamelli, M.D.
Edward E. Partridge, M.D.
James M. Seeger, M.D.
Jatin P. Shah, M.D.
H. Hank Simms, M.D.
Thomas F. Tracy, M.D.

W.B. SAUNDERS COMPANY
A Harcourt Health Sciences Company
Philadelphia   London   New York   St. Louis   Sydney   Toronto

W.B. SAUNDERS COMPANY
A Harcourt Health Sciences Company

The Curtis Center
Independence Square West
Philadelphia, Pennsylvania 19106

BS

Library of Congress Cataloging-in-Publication Data

The practice of general surgery / edited by Kirby I. Bland—1st ed.

p.   cm.

ISBN 0–7216–8476–9

1. Surgery, Operative.   2. Surgery.   I. Bland, K. I.
  [DNLM: 1. Surgical Procedures, Operative—methods. WO 500 P8956 2002]

RD32.P665   2002   617′.91—dc21

DNLM/DLC   2001020111

Editor-in-Chief: Richard Lampert
Acquisitions Editor: Lisette Bralow
Developmental Editor: Hazel Hacker
Copyediting Supervisor: Gina Scala
Production Manager: Mary Stermel
Illustration Specialist: Rita Martello
Book Designer: Marie Gardocky-Clifton

THE PRACTICE OF GENERAL SURGERY   ISBN 0–7216–8476–9

Printed in the United States of America.

Last digit is the print number: 9   8   7   6   5   4   3   2   1

5·20·03

To the surgical residents and practicing general surgeons
with whom we have had the privilege of teaching
the art and science of surgery

Contributors

Herand Abcarian, M.D.

Turi Josefsen Professor and Head, Department of Surgery, University of Illinois at Chicago College of Medicine; Chief of Service, Department of Surgery, University of Illinois–Chicago Medical Center, Chicago, Illinois

Anal Fissure and Fistula

Syed A. Ahmad, M.D.

Junior Faculty Associate, University of Texas–Houston Medical School, M.D. Anderson Cancer Center, Houston, Texas

Lymphoma of the Small Bowel

Steven A. Ahrendt, M.D.

Associate Professor, Department of Surgery, University of Rochester School of Medicine; Attending Physician and Director of Gastrointestinal Malignancies Program, Strong Memorial Hospital, Rochester, New York

Primary Sclerosing Cholangitis

Michele Aizenberg, M.D.

Resident, Department of Neurological Surgery, George Washington University Hospital, Washington, District of Columbia

Status Epilepticus

Amjad Ali, M.D.

Assistant Professor and Director of Laparoscopic Surgery, Truman Medical Center, University of Missouri–Columbia School of Medicine, Kansas City, Missouri

Achalasia

John Alverdy, M.D., F.A.C.S.

Associate Professor, Department of Surgery, University of Chicago Pritzker School of Medicine; Co-Director of Critical Care, University of Chicago Hospitals, Chicago, Illinois

Nutritional Support in the Surgical Patient

Gordon Anderson, M.D.

Neurosurgery Resident, Department of Clinical Neuroscience, Brown University School of Medicine, Providence, Rhode Island

Coma: Diagnosis of Brain Death

Peter Angelos, M.D., Ph.D.

Assistant Professor of Surgery and of Medical Ethics and Humanities, Department of Surgery, Northwestern University Medical School, Chicago, Illinois

Papillary Thyroid Cancer

Gerard V. Aranha, M.D., F.R.C.S.(C.), F.A.C.S.

Professor, Loyola University Stritch School of Medicine, Maywood; Chief, General Surgery and Surgical Oncology Sections, Hines Veterans Administration Hospital, Hines, Illinois

Pancreatic Pseudocyst

Martin R. Back, M.D., M.S., R.V.T.

Assistant Professor, Department of Surgery, Division of Vascular Surgery, University of South Florida College of Medicine; Chief, Division of Vascular Surgery, James A. Haley Veterans Hospital, Tampa, Florida

Management of Complications of Vascular Surgery: Infected Vascular Grafts, Aortoenteric Fistulas, and Pseudoaneurysms

Charles M. Balch, M.D.

Professor, Departments of Surgery and Oncology, Johns Hopkins University School of Medicine, Baltimore, Maryland; Executive Vice-President and CEO, American Society of Clinical Oncology, Alexandria, Virginia

Staging and Selection of Treatment Options for Melanoma

Garth H. Ballantyne, M.D.

Professor, Department of Surgery, University of Medicine and Dentistry of New Jersey–New Jersey Medical School, Newark; Director, Minimally Invasive Surgery, Hackensack University Medical Center, Hackensack, New Jersey

Colonic Volvulus

Dennis F. Bandyk, M.D.

Professor, Department of Surgery, and Director, Division of Vascular Surgery, University of South Florida College of Medicine, Tampa, Florida

Management of Complications of Vascular Surgery: Infected Vascular Grafts, Aortoenteric Fistulas, and Pseudoaneurysms

Paul E. Bankey, M.D., Ph.D.

Visiting Associate Professor, Department of Surgery, University of Rochester Medical School; Chief of Trauma and Surgical Critical Care, University of Rochester Medical Center, Rochester, New York

Acute Renal Failure

Michael P. Bannon, M.D.

Assistant Professor, Department of Surgery, Mayo Medical School; Consultant, Division of Gastroenterologic and General Surgery, Mayo Clinic, Rochester, Minnesota

Appendicitis

Adrian Barbul, M.D.
Professor, Johns Hopkins University School of Medicine; Chairman, Department of Surgery, Sinai Hospital, Baltimore, Maryland
> Adrenal Insufficiency

Philip S. Barie, M.D.
Associate Professor, Department of Surgery, Cornell University Joan and Sanford I. Weill Medical College and Graduate School of Medical Sciences; Chief, Division of Trauma and Critical Care, and Director, Anne and Max A. Cohen Surgical Intensive Care Unit, New York-Presbyterian Hospital, New York Weill Cornell Campus, New York, New York
> Monitoring Respiratory Function and Weaning from the Ventilator

Felix D. Battistella, M.D.
Associate Professor, Department of Surgery, University of California, Davis, School of Medicine; Attending Physician, University of California, Davis Health System, Sacramento, California
> Vascular Trauma: Extremity Vascular Trauma

Robert W. Beart, Jr., M.D.
Charles W. and Carolyn Costello Professor of Surgery, Department of Surgery, Division of Colon and Rectal Surgery, Keck School of Medicine of the University of Southern California, Los Angeles, California
> Colon Cancer

David E. Beck, M.D.
Chairman, Department of Colon and Rectal Surgery, Ochsner Clinic, New Orleans, Louisiana
> Pilonidal Disease

James M. Becker, M.D.
James Utley Professor, Boston University School of Medicine; Chairman of Surgery and Surgeon-in-Chief, Boston Medical Center, Boston, Massachusetts
> Chronic Ulcerative Colitis

Samuel W. Beenken, M.D.
Associate Professor, Department of Surgery, University of Alabama School of Medicine; Scientist, UAB Comprehensive Cancer Center, Birmingham, Alabama
> Advanced Breast Carcinoma (Stages IIIa and IIIb)

Bruce M. Belin, M.D.
Staff Surgeon, Department of Colorectal Surgery, St. Joseph's Hospital, Lexington, Kentucky
> Crohn's Disease of the Small Bowel: Crohn's Disease of the Colon

Claudia Berman, M.D.
Chief, Department of Radiology, Moffitt Cancer Center, University of South Florida College of Medicine, Tampa, Florida
> Technique and Application of Sentinel Lymph Node Biopsy in Melanoma and Breast Cancer

Carina G. Biggs, M.D.
Assistant Professor, Department of Surgery, University of Illinois at Chicago College of Medicine; Senior Attending Surgeon, Cook County Hospital; Rush-Presbyterian-St. Luke's Medical Center, Chicago, Illinois
> Massive Upper Gastrointestinal Hemorrhage

Malcolm M. Bilimoria, M.D.
Assistant Professor, Department of Surgery, General Surgeon, Evanston Hospital, Evanston, Illinois
> Stromal Tumors of the Stomach and Small Bowel

Kirby I. Bland, M.D.
Professor and Chairman, Department of Surgery, University of Alabama School of Medicine; Deputy Director, UAB Comprehensive Cancer Center, Birmingham, Alabama
> Cancer of the Rectum; In Situ Carcinoma of the Breast: Ductal and Lobular Origin; Advanced Breast Carcinoma (Stage IIIA and IIIB); Editor, Section 7: Oncology

Leslie H. Blumgart, M.D., D.Sc.(Hon.), F.A.C.S., F.R.C.S.(Engl., Glas., Edinb.)
Professor, Department of Surgery, Cornell University Joan and Sanford I. Weill Medical College and Graduate School of Medical Sciences; Attending Surgeon and Chief, Hepatobiliary Service, and Enid A. Haupt Chair in Surgery, Memorial Sloan-Kettering Cancer Center, New York, New York
> Cholangiocarcinoma

Matthew Borst, M.D.
Clinical Assistant Professor, University of Arizona College of Medicine, Tucson; Director of Gynecology, Good Samaritan Regional Medical Center, Phoenix, Arizona
> Ovarian (Adnexal) Neoplasm, Benign

Jay O. Boyle, M.D.
Assistant Professor, Department of Surgery, Joan and Sanford I. Weill Medical College and Graduate School of Medical Sciences; Assistant Attending Surgeon, Head and Neck Service, Memorial Sloan-Kettering Cancer Center, New York, New York
> Oral Cavity and Oropharynx

Christopher K. Breuer, M.D.
Assistant Professor, University of Texas Medical School at San Antonio; Chief, Pediatric Surgery, Wilford Hall USAF Medical Center, San Antonio, Texas
> Anomalies of Bowel Rotation: Malrotation and Midgut Volvulus; Meckel's Diverticulum

Lunzy D. Britt, M.D., M.P.H.
Brickhouse Professor and Chairman, Department of Surgery, Eastern Virginia Medical School; Attending Physician, Sentara Hospitals, Norfolk, Virginia
> Management of Penetrating Trauma: Neck, Thorax, and Abdomen; Acute Systemic Hypertension

Dan W. Brock, Ph.D.
Director, Center for Biomedical Ethics, Department of Philosophy, Brown University, Providence, Rhode Island
> Do Not Resuscitate, Do Not Treat

Robert E. Brolin, M.D.
Professor, Department of Surgery, St. Peter's University Medical Center, New Brunswick, New Jersey
> Small Bowel Obstruction

David L. Brown, M.D.
Chief Resident, Section of Plastic and Reconstructive Surgery, University of Michigan Medical Center, Ann Arbor, Michigan
> General Evaluation and Biopsy of Cutaneous Lesions

Joseph F. Buell, M.D.
Assistant Professor, Department of Surgery, University of Cincinnati College of Medicine, Cincinnati, Ohio
Neuroendocrine Tumors of the Pancreas

Gregory B. Bulkley, M.D., F.A.C.S., Dr. Med.(Hon.) Uppsala
Ravitch Professor, Department of Surgery, Johns Hopkins University School of Medicine; Active Staff, Johns Hopkins Hospital, Baltimore, Maryland
The Thymus

Jon M. Burch, M.D.
Professor, Department of Surgery, University of Colorado School of Medicine; Chief, General and Vascular Surgery, Denver Health Medical Center, Denver, Colorado
Vascular Trauma: Thoracic Vascular Trauma

Kenneth Burchard, M.D.
Professor, Department of Surgery, Dartmouth Medical School; Surgeon, Division of General Surgery, Dartmouth–Hitchcock Medical Center, Lebanon, New Hampshire
Multisystem Organ Dysfunction and Failure: The Systemic Response to Critical Surgical Illness

Joseph Califano, M.D.
Assistant Professor, Department of Otolaryngology–Head and Neck, Johns Hopkins University School of Medicine, Baltimore, Maryland
Salivary Glands

Mark P. Callery, M.D., F.A.C.S.
Associate Professor, Departments of Surgery and Cell Biology, and Chief, Division of General Surgery, University of Massachusetts Medical School, Worcester, Massachusetts
Benign Hepatic Neoplasm

John L. Cameron, M.D.
William Stewart Halsted Professor and Chairman, Department of Surgery, Johns Hopkins University School of Medicine; Chief of Surgery, Johns Hopkins Hospital, Baltimore, Maryland
Budd-Chiari Syndrome

William G. Cance, M.D.
Professor, Department of Surgery, and Chief of Surgical Oncology, University of North Carolina School of Medicine, Chapel Hill, North Carolina
Malignant Diseases of the Spleen

John F. Carew, M.D.
Assistant Professor, Cornell University Joan and Sanford I. Weill Medical College and Graduate School of Medical Sciences; Associate Professor, Department of Otorhinolaryngology, New York Presbyterian Hospital–Cornell and Columbia Medical Centers, New York, New York
Larynx and Hypopharynx

Susan W. Caro, M.S.N., R.N.C.
Adjunct Faculty, Vanderbilt University School of Nursing; Director, Family Cancer Risk Service, Vanderbilt-Ingram Cancer Center, Vanderbilt University Medical Center, Nashville, Tennessee
High-Risk Indicators: Microscopic Lesions, Personal and Family History, Assessment, and Management

Robert J. Cerfolio, M.D., F.A.C.S., F.C.C.P.
Associate Professor, University of Alabama School of Medicine; Chief of Thoracic Surgery, Veterans Administration Hospital, Birmingham, Alabama
Hemoptysis in Benign Disease

Craig G. Chang, M.D.
Chief Resident in General Surgery, University of Missouri–Kansas City School of Medicine, Kansas City, Missouri
Laparoscopic Common Bile Duct Exploration

Ravi S. Chari, M.D.
Associate Professor, Department of Surgery, Division of Liver Transplantation and Hepatobiliary Surgery, Vanderbilt University School of Medicine, Nashville, Tennessee
Benign Hepatic Neoplasm

William G. Cheadle, M.D.
Professor, Department of Surgery, University of Louisville School of Medicine; ACOS for Research and Development, Veterans Affairs Medical Center, Louisville, Kentucky
Basic and Advanced Mechanical Ventilation

Herbert Chen, M.D.
Assistant Professor, Department of Surgery, University of Wisconsin Medical School, Madison, Wisconsin
Follicular, Hürthle Cell, and Anaplastic Thyroid Cancer

Seine Chiang, M.D.
Assistant Professor, Department of Obstetrics and Gynecology, Division of Medical and Surgical Gynecology, University of Alabama School of Medicine, Birmingham, Alabama
Surgical Management of Pelvic Inflammatory Disease

Lori L. Cindrick, M.D.
Senior Vascular Surgery Fellow, Temple University Hospital, Philadelphia, Pennsylvania
Management of Venous and Lymphatic Disease

William G. Cioffi, M.D.
Professor, Department of Surgery, Brown University School of Medicine; Chief, Division of Trauma and Burns, Department of Surgery, Rhode Island Hospital, Providence, Rhode Island
Editor, Section 2: Trauma and Burns

Orlo H. Clark, M.D.
Professor and Vice-Chairman, Department of Surgery, University of California, San Francisco, School of Medicine; Chief, Department of Surgery, The Medical Center at the University of California, San Francisco, San Francisco, California
Hyperparathyroidism; Editor, Section 8: Endocrine

John Mitchell Clarke, M.D.
Active Staff, Palms of Pasadena Hospital, Saint Anthony's Hospital, and Edward H. White Hospital, St. Petersburg, Florida
Incisional Hernia

Rhonda A. Cole, M.D.
Assistant Professor, Baylor College of Medicine; Chief, Gastrointestinal Endoscopy, Veterans Affairs Medical Center, Houston, Texas
  Peptic Ulcer Disease and *Helicobacter pylori*

Lisa Colletti, M.D.
Associate Professor, Department of Surgery, and Associate Chair for Education, University of Michigan Medical School, Ann Arbor, Michigan
  Pseudomembranous Enterocolitis

Anthony J. Comerota, M.D.
Professor, Department of Surgery, Temple University School of Medicine; Chief, Vascular Surgery, Temple University Hospital, Philadelphia, Pennsylvania
  Management of Venous and Lymphatic Disease

Kevin C. Conlon, M.D., M.B.A., M.Ch., F.A.C.S., F.R.C.S.I.
Associate Chairman, Department of Minimally Invasive Surgery, Memorial Sloan-Kettering Cancer Center, New York, New York
  Gastric Adenocarcinoma

Edward M. Copeland, III, M.D.
Professor and Chairman, Department of Surgery, University of Florida College of Medicine, Shands Hospital, Gainesville, Florida
  Breast Carcinoma: Stages I and II

Charles Cox, M.D.
Professor, Department of Surgery, University of South Florida College of Medicine; Program Leader, Comprehensive Breast Cancer Program, Moffitt Cancer Center, Tampa, Florida
  Technique and Application of Sentinel Lymph Node Biopsy in Melanoma and Breast Cancer

Martin A. Croce, M.D.
Professor, Department of Surgery, University of Tennessee Health Science Center, Memphis, Tennessee
  Management of Blunt Abdominal Injuries

Daniel C. Cullinane, M.D.
Assistant Professor, Department of Surgery, Mayo Medical School; Consultant, Division of Gastroenterologic and General Surgery, Mayo Clinic, Rochester, Minnesota
  Appendicitis

Jennifer R. Curry, M.D.
Surgical Resident, Northwestern Memorial Hospital, Chicago, Illinois
  Choledochal Cyst

Rory R. Dalton, M.D.
Associate Professor, Department of Surgery, Medical College of Georgia, Augusta, Georgia
  Pseudomyxoma Peritonei

Kimberly A. Davis, M.D.
Assistant Professor, Department of Surgery, Division of Trauma, Critical Care and Burns, Loyola University of Chicago Stritch School of Medicine, Maywood, Illinois
  Fluids and Electrolytes

Neil A. Davis, Pharm.D.
Clinical Assistant Professor, Department of Surgery, Eastern Virginia Medical School of the Medical College of Hampton Roads; Clinical Pharmacy Specialist, Critical Care, Sentara Health System, Norfolk, Virginia
  Acute Systemic Hypertension

Malcolm M. DeCamp, Jr., M.D.
Director, Lung Transplant Program, Department of Thoracic and Cardiovascular Surgery, The Cleveland Clinic Foundation, Cleveland, Ohio
  Mediastinal Masses

Alberto L. de Hoyos, M.D.
Chief Resident, Department of Surgery, University of Nevada School of Medicine, Las Vegas, Nevada
  Infections of the Pleural Cavity

Daniel T. Dempsey, M.D., F.A.C.S.
Professor of Surgery, University of Pennsylvania School of Medicine; Chairman of Surgery, Pennsylvania Hospital, Philadelphia, Pennsylvania
  Peptic Ulcer Disease: Obstruction

James W. Dennis, M.D., F.A.C.S.
Professor, Department of Surgery, University of Florida College of Medicine; Chief, Division of Vascular Surgery, University of Florida Health Science Center, Jacksonville, Florida
  Management of Vascular Trauma

Claude Deschamps, M.D.
Associate Professor of Surgery, Department of Surgery, Mayo Medical School; Consultant, Division of General Thoracic Surgery, Mayo Clinic, Rochester, Minnesota
  Spontaneous Pneumothorax and Lung Volume Reduction Surgery

Clifford S. Deutschman, M.D., F.C.C.M.
Professor, Department of Anesthesia and Surgery, University of Pennsylvania School of Medicine; Attending Physician, Surgical Intensive Care Units, Hospital of the University of Pennsylvania, Philadelphia, Pennsylvania
  Hepatic Failure

Curtis Doberstein, M.D.
Assistant Professor of Neurosurgery, Department of Clinical Neuroscience, and Director, Cerebrovascular Surgery, Brown University School of Medicine; Staff Neurosurgeon, Rhode Island Hospital, Providence, Rhode Island
  Coma: Diagnosis of Brain Death; Status Epilepticus

Elvis S. Donaldson, Jr., M.D.
Clinical Professor, Department of Obstetrics and Gynecology, University of Kentucky College of Medicine; Medical Director of Cancer Services, Central Baptist Hospital, Lexington, Kentucky
  Malignant Ovarian Neoplasms

Philip E. Donahue, M.D.
Professor, Department of Surgery, University of Illinois at Chicago College of Medicine; Chairman, Division of General Surgery, Cook County Hospital, Chicago, Illinois
  Massive Upper Gastrointestinal Hemorrhage

John H. Donohue, M.D.

Professor, Department of Surgery, Mayo Medical School;
Consultant in Surgery, Mayo Clinic, Rochester, Minnesota

Gastric Lymphoma

James M. Doty, M.D.

Surgery Resident, Virginia Commonwealth University School
of Medicine, Richmond, Virginia

Compartment Syndrome: Abdominal Compartment Syndrome

Eric J. Dozois, M.D.

Fellow, Colon and Rectal Surgery, Mayo Graduate School of
Medicine, Rochester, Minnesota

Polyposis Syndromes of the Colon

Roger R. Dozois, M.D., F.R.C.S.(Glasg.)(Hon.)

Professor, Department of Surgery, Mayo Medical School;
Consultant in Surgery, Mayo Clinic and Mayo Foundation,
Rochester, Minnesota

Polyposis Syndromes of the Colon

Quan-Yang Duh, M.D.

Professor, Department of Surgery, University of California, San
Francisco, School of Medicine; Surgical Service, Veterans
Administration Medical Center, San Francisco, California

Functioning and Nonfunctioning Adrenal Tumors

Nadine L. Duhan, M.D.

Instructor, Department of General Surgery, Rush Medical
College, Chicago, Illinois

Lower Gastrointestinal Bleeding

Troy M. Duininck, M.D.

Resident, Mayo Clinic, Rochester, Minnesota

Advanced Gastrointestinal Laparoscopic Procedures

Mark D. Duncan, M.D.

Associate Professor, Department of Surgery, Johns Hopkins
University School of Medicine, Baltimore, Maryland

Gastrointestinal Bleeding of Obscure Origin

Soumitra R. Eachempati, M.D.

Assistant Professor, Department of Surgery, Cornell University
Joan and Sanford I. Weill Medical College and Graduate
School of Medical Sciences; Assistant Attending Surgeon, New
York Presbyterian Hospital, New York Hospital–Weill Cornell
Medical Center, New York, New York

Monitoring Respiratory Function and Weaning from the Ventilator

David T. Efron, M.D.

Surgical Resident, Johns Hopkins Medical Institutions,
Baltimore, Maryland

Adrenal Insufficiency

Gershon Efron, M.D., F.R.C.S., F.A.C.S.

Professor, Department of Surgery, Johns Hopkins University
School of Medicine; Surgeon-in-Chief Emeritus, Sinai Hospital
of Baltimore, Baltimore, Maryland

Adrenal Insufficiency

Lee M. Ellis, M.D.

Associate Professor of Surgery and Cancer Biology, University
of Texas–Houston Medical School; M.D. Anderson Cancer
Center, Houston, Texas

Lymphoma of the Small Bowel

Said Elshihabi, M.D.

Resident in Neurosurgery, University of Arkansas Medical
Center, Little Rock, Arkansas

Nonfunctional Islet Cell Neoplasms

Michael Englesbee, M.D.

Surgical Resident, Department of Surgery, University of
Michigan Medical Center, Ann Arbor, Michigan

Pseudomembranous Enterocolitis

Stephen E. Ettinghausen, M.D.

Assistant Professor, Department of Surgery, University of
Rochester School of Medicine and Dentistry; Associate
Attending Surgeon, Rochester General Hospital, Rochester,
New York

Pseudomyxoma Peritonei

Douglas B. Evans, M.D.

Professor, Department of Surgery, University of
Texas–Houston Medical School, Houston, Texas

Pancreatic Carcinoma

B. Mark Evers, M.D.

Professor and Robertson-Poth Distinguished Chair in General
Surgery, Department of Surgery, The University of Texas
Medical Branch, University of Texas Medical School at
Galveston, Galveston, Texas

Adenocarcinoma of the Small Bowel

Goodluck Eze, M.D.

Research Fellow, Department of Colorectal Surgery, Cleveland
Clinic Florida, Fort Lauderdale, Florida

Laparoscopic Small Bowel Resection

David R. Farley, M.D.

Associate Professor, Department of Surgery, Mayo Medical
School; Consultant in Surgery, Mayo Clinic, Rochester,
Minnesota

Carcinoid of the Small Bowel

Mark K. Ferguson, M.D.

Professor, University of Chicago Pritzker School of Medicine;
Chief, Thoracic Surgery Service, University of Chicago
Medical Center, Chicago, Illinois

Esophageal Cancer: Transthoracic Resection

Mitchell P. Fink, M.D.

Chief, Critical Care Medicine, University of Pittsburgh
Medical Center System, Pittsburgh, Pennsylvania

General Principles of Sepsis

Timothy C. Flynn, M.D.

Professor, Department of Surgery, University of Florida
College of Medicine; Vice President for Medical Affairs,
Shands Health Care, Gainesville, Florida

Amputations

Yuman Fong, M.D.

Professor of Surgery, Cornell University Joan and Sanford I. Weill Medical College and Graduate School of Medical Sciences; Attending Surgeon, Memorial Sloan-Kettering Cancer Center, New York, New York

Cancer of the Gallbladder

Robert R. Franklin, M.D.

Clinical Associate Professor, Baylor College of Medicine; Medical Staff, The Woman's Hospital of Texas, Houston, Texas

Endometriosis

Dana Frazer, M.D.

Chief Resident Instructor, Wright State University School of Medicine; Chief Surgical Resident, Miami Valley Hospital, Dayton, Ohio

Abnormal Bleeding and Coagulopathies

Gerhard M. Friehs, M.D.

Assistant Professor, Department of Neurosurgery, Brown University School of Medicine, Providence, Rhode Island

Neurologic Physiology: The Brain and Its Response to Injury

Donald E. Fry, M.D.

Professor and Chairman, Department of Surgery, University of New Mexico School of Medicine, Albuquerque, New Mexico

Cyst and Abscess of the Spleen

Robert Fry, M.D.

Professor, Department of Surgery, and Director, Division of Colon and Rectal Surgery, Jefferson Medical College of Thomas Jefferson University; Attending Surgeon, Thomas Jefferson University Hospital, Philadelphia, Pennsylvania

Polyps of the Colon and Rectum

Thomas R. Gadacz, M.D.

Moretz-Mansberger Professor and Chairman, Department of Surgery, Medical College of Georgia, Augusta, Georgia

Stromal Tumors of the Small Bowel

Henning A. Gaissert, M.D.

Assistant Professor, Department of Surgery, Harvard Medical School; Thoracic Surgeon, Massachusetts General Hospital, Boston, Massachusetts

Lung Abscess

Richard L. Gamelli, M.D., F.A.C.S.

Robert J. Freeark Professor and Chairman, Department of Surgery, Loyola University of Chicago Stritch School of Medicine; Director, Burn and Shock Trauma Institute, and Chief, Burn Center, Loyola University Medical Center, Maywood, Illinois

Fluids and Electrolytes; Editor, Section 1: General Principles

Rose B. Ganim, M.D.

Research Fellow in Surgery, University of California, San Francisco, School of Medicine, San Francisco; Resident, Department of Surgery, University of California, Davis–East Bay, Davis, California

Carcinoid Tumors

Paul M. Gardner, M.D.

Assistant Professor, Department of Surgery, Division of Plastic Surgery, University of Alabama School of Medicine, Birmingham, Alabama

Breast Reconstruction

Glenn W. Geelhoed, M.D., M.P.H., D.T.M.H., Ph.D.

Professor, Departments of Surgery, International Medical Education, and Microbiology and Tropical Medicine, George Washington University School of Medicine and Health Sciences; Attending Physician, George Washington University Medical Center, Washington, District of Columbia

Thyroid Abnormalities Encountered in Surgical Critical Care

Thomas Genuit, M.D.

Assistant Professor, Department of Surgery, University of Maryland School of Medicine; Attending Physician, University of Maryland Medical Center, Veterans Administration Maryland Healthcare System, and R. Adams Cowley Shock Trauma Center, Baltimore, Maryland

Gastrointestinal Failure

Jeffrey E. Gershenwald, M.D.

Assistant Professor, Department of Surgical Oncology, University of Texas–Houston Medical School; The University of Texas M.D. Anderson Cancer Center, Houston, Texas

Staging and Selection of Treatment Options for Melanoma

Rosemary Giuliano, A.R.N.P.

Research Coordinator, Moffitt Cancer Center, University of South Florida College of Medicine, Tampa, Florida

Technique and Application of Sentinel Lymph Node Biopsy in Melanoma and Breast Cancer

Virginia L. Glen, Pharm.D.

Clinical Assistant, University of Minnesota College of Pharmacy; Pain Management Specialist, Pain Management Center, Fairview-University Medical Center, Minneapolis, Minnesota

Basic Pharmacokinetics, Pharmacodynamics, and Important Drug Interactions

Jessica E. Gosnell, M.D.

Chief Resident, University of California, Davis, School of Medicine, Oakland, California

Human Immunodeficiency Virus Infection

David Y. Graham, M.D.

Professor, Departments of Medicine, Molecular Virology, and Microbiology and Immunology, Baylor College of Medicine; Chief of Gastroenterology, Veterans Administration Medical Center, Houston, Texas

Peptic Ulcer Disease and *Helicobacter pylori*

Ana M. Grau, M.D.

Surgical Oncology Fellow, The University of Texas M.D. Anderson Cancer Center, Houston, Texas

Management of Soft Tissue Sarcomas: Extremity and Chest Wall

Theresa A. Graves, M.D., F.A.C.S.

Assistant Professor, Department of Surgery, Brown University School of Medicine; Assistant Professor, Department of Surgery, Rhode Island Hospital, Providence, Rhode Island

In Situ Carcinoma of the Breast: Ductal and Lobular Origin

Kathleen Graziano, M.D.

Senior Resident, Department of General Surgery, University of Michigan Medical Center, Ann Arbor, Michigan

Gastric Ulcer

A. Gerson Greenburg, M.D., Ph.D.

Professor of Surgery, Brown University School of Medicine; Surgeon-in-Chief, The Miriam Hospital, Providence, Rhode Island

Inguinal Hernias

Steven C. Gross, M.D.

Senior Resident in General Surgery, Lineberger Comprehensive Cancer Center, Chapel Hill, North Carolina

Malignant Diseases of the Spleen

David T. Harrington, M.D.

Assistant Professor, Department of Surgery, Brown University School of Medicine, Providence, Rhode Island

Spinal Trauma: Evaluation and Initial Treatment

J. Frederick Harrington, M.D.

Assistant Professor of Surgery, Brown University School of Medicine, Providence, Rhode Island

Spinal Trauma: Evaluation and Initial Treatment

Hobart W. Harris, M.D., M.P.H.

Associate Professor, University of California, San Francisco, School of Medicine; Chief, Department of Gastrointestinal Surgery, San Francisco General Hospital, San Francisco, California

Human Immunodeficiency Virus Infection

Heitham T. Hassoun, M.D.

Fellow, Trauma Research Center, Department of Surgery, The University of Texas–Houston Medical School; General Surgery Resident, General Surgery Training Program, The University of Texas–Houston Medical School and Affiliated Hospitals, Houston, Texas

Pericardial Tamponade

Richard F. Heitmiller, M.D., F.A.C.S.

Associate Professor, Department of Surgery and Oncology, Johns Hopkins University School of Medicine; Chief, Division of Thoracic Surgery, Johns Hopkins Medical Institutions, Baltimore, Maryland

Esophageal Cancer: Transhiatal Resection

Martin J. Heslin, M.D.

Assistant Professor, Department of Surgery, University of Alabama School of Medicine; Associate Scientist, UAB Comprehensive Cancer Center, Birmingham, Alabama

Cancer of the Rectum

Oscar Joseph Hines, M.D.

Assistant Professor, Department of Surgery, University of California, Los Angeles, UCLA School of Medicine, Los Angeles, California

Acute Pancreatitis

Mark Hiraoka, M.D.

Chief Resident, Department of Obstetrics and Gynecology, Good Samaritan Regional Medical Center, Phoenix, Arizona

Ovarian (Adnexal) Neoplasm, Benign

Richard Hodin, M.D.

Associate Professor, Department of Surgery, Harvard Medical School; Consultant Surgeon, General Surgery, Massachusetts General Hospital, Boston, Massachusetts

Laparoscopic Appendectomy

Robert L. Holley, M.D.

Clinical Assistant Professor, Department of Obstetrics and Gynecology, Division of Medical and Surgical Gynecology, University of Alabama School of Medicine, Birmingham, Alabama

Surgical Management of Pelvic Inflammatory Disease

Gabriel N. Hortobagyi, M.D.

Professor, Department of Medicine, The University of Texas–Houston Medical School; Chairman, Department of Breast Medical Oncology, The University of Texas M.D. Anderson Cancer Center, Houston, Texas

Metastatic Carcinoma of the Breast (Stage IV)

Thomas S. Huber, M.D., Ph.D.

Associate Professor, Department of Surgery, University of Florida College of Medicine; Staff Surgeon, Shands Teaching Hospital of The University of Florida, Gainesville, Florida

Visceral Artery Occlusive Disease

Steven J. Hughes, M.D.

Assistant Professor of Surgery, University of Pittsburgh School of Medicine; Attending Physician, Oakland Veterans Affairs Medical Center, Pittsburgh, Pennsylvania

Large Bowel Obstruction

Kelly K. Hunt, M.D.

Associate Professor, Department of Surgery, The University of Texas–Houston Medical School; Chief, Surgical Breast Section, The University of Texas M. D. Anderson Cancer Center, Houston, Texas

Stromal Tumors of the Stomach and Small Bowel

Matthew M. Hutter, M.D.

Surgical Resident, Department of Surgery, Massachusetts General Hospital, Boston, Massachusetts

Postgastrectomy and Postvagotomy Syndromes

Nuhad K. Ibrahim, M.D.

Associate Professor, Department of Medicine, The University of Texas–Houston Medical School, Houston, Texas

Metastatic Carcinoma of the Breast (Stage IV)

Kamal M. F. Itani, M.D.

Associate Professor, Michael E. DeBakey Department of Surgery, Baylor College of Medicine; Chief of General Surgery, Veterans Administration Medical Center, Houston, Texas

Uncommon Abdominal Wall Hernias

Rao R. Ivatury, M.D.

Professor, Departments of Surgery, Emergency Medicine, and Physiology, and Director of Trauma and Critical Care, Virginia Commonwealth University School of Medicine, Richmond, Virginia

Compartment Syndrome: Abdominal Compartment Syndrome

Jay Jan, M.D.
Surgical Resident, University of California, San Francisco, Surgical Research Laboratory at San Francisco General Hospital, San Francisco, California
Human Immunodeficiency Virus Infection

Marina E. Jean, M.D.
Fellow, Department of Surgical Oncology, University of Texas M.D. Anderson Cancer Center, Houston, Texas
Pancreatic Carcinoma

W. Scott Jellish, M.D., Ph.D.
Professor and Chair, Department of Anesthesiology, Loyola University of Chicago Stritch School of Medicine; Attending Physician, Loyola University Medical Center and Foster G. McGaw Hospital, Maywood, Illinois
Anesthesia and Risk Assessment

Roger L. Jenkins, M.D.
Professor, Department of Surgery, Tufts University School of Medicine, Boston; Chief of Hepatobiliary Surgery, Lahey Clinic Medical Center, Burlington, Massachusetts
Hepatocellular Carcinoma

Raymond J. Joehl, M.D.
James R. Hines Professor of Surgery, Department of Surgery, Northwestern University Medical School; Chief, Surgical Services, Veterans Administration Chicago-Lakeside, and Chief, Surgical Services, Northwestern Memorial Hospital, Chicago, Illinois
Choledochal Cyst

Daniel B. Jones, M.D., F.A.C.S.
Assistant Professor, Department of Surgery, University of Texas Southwestern Medical Center; Director, Southwestern Center for Minimally Invasive Surgery, Dallas, Texas
Asymptomatic Gallstones

Fernando E. Kafie
Vascular Surgeon, Baptist Hospital, Pensacola, Florida
Management of Cerebrovascular Disease

Steven A. Kagan, M.D.
Assistant Professor, Department of Surgery, Temple University School of Medicine; Staff Surgeon, Temple University Hospital, Philadelphia, Pennsylvania
Management of Venous and Lymphatic Disease

Andreas M. Kaiser, M.D.
Clinical Instructor, Department of Surgery, Division of Colon and Rectal Surgery, Keck School of Medicine of the University of Southern California, Los Angeles, California
Colon Cancer

Edwin L. Kaplan, M.D.
Professor, Department of Surgery, University of Chicago Pritzker School of Medicine, Chicago, Illinois
Neuroendocrine Tumors of the Pancreas

Constantine P. Karakousis, M.D., Ph.D.
Professor, Department of Surgery, State University of New York at Buffalo School of Medicine and Biomedical Sciences; Chief, Department of Surgical Oncology, Kaleida Health, Buffalo, New York
Surgical Treatment of Malignant Melanoma

Howard S. Kaufman, M.D.
Associate Professor of Surgery, Gynecology, and Obstetrics, The Johns Hopkins University School of Medicine; Active Staff, The Johns Hopkins Hospital, Baltimore, Maryland
Diverticulitis

Paul A. Kedeshian, M.D.
Visiting Assistant Professor, Division of Head and Neck Surgery, University of California, Los Angeles, UCLA School of Medicine, Los Angeles, California
Sinuses and Skull Base

Christina Kim, M.D.
Fellow in Surgical Oncology, H. Lee Moffitt Cancer Center, University of South Florida, Tampa, Florida
Stromal Tumors of the Small Bowel

Patrick K. Kim, M.D.
Fellow, Trauma and Critical Care Medicine, Department of Surgery, University of Pennsylvania School of Medicine, Philadelphia, Pennsylvania
Hepatic Failure

Kimberly S. Kirkwood, M.D.
Associate Professor, Department of Surgery, University of California, San Francisco, School of Medicine, San Francisco, California
Upper Gastrointestinal Hemorrhage: Diagnosis and Treatment

Andrew S. Klein, M.D.
Professor, Department of Surgery, The Johns Hopkins University School of Medicine; Chief, Division of Transplantation, and Director, Comprehensive Transplant Center, The Johns Hopkins Hospital, Baltimore, Maryland
Budd-Chiari Syndrome

V. Suzanne Klimberg, M.D.
Professor, Department of Surgery, University of Arkansas for Medical Sciences; Chief, Division of Breast Surgical Oncology, Arkansas Cancer Research Center, Little Rock, Arkansas
Diagnosis and Assessment of Benign and Malignant Breast Diseases

Stuart J. Knechtle, M.D.
Professor, Department of Surgery, University of Wisconsin Medical School; Professor of Surgery, University of Wisconsin Hospital and Clinics, Madison, Wisconsin
Portal Hypertension

M. Margaret Knudson, M.D.
Professor, Department of Surgery, University of California, San Francisco, School of Medicine; Director, San Francisco Injury Center for Research and Prevention, San Francisco, California
Blood Transfusions and Alternative Therapies

Jonathan B. Koea, M.D., F.R.A.C.S.
Hepatobiliary Surgeon, HBP/Upper GI Surgical Unit, Auckland Hospital, Auckland, New Zealand
Cholangiocarcinoma

Maha Lakshmana Rao Koka, M.D.
Professor Emeritus, Gunter Medical College, Andhra Pradesh, India
Neuroendocrine Tumors of the Pancreas

Thomas Kossmann, M.D.
Associate Professor of Surgery, Division of Trauma Surgery, Department of Surgery, University Hospital of Zurich, Zurich, Switzerland
Closed Head Injury

Sonya Krolik, M.D.
Resident, General Surgery, George Washington University School of Medicine and Health Sciences, Washington, District of Columbia
Toxic Megacolon

David Krusch, M.D.
Associate Professor, Department of Surgery, University of Rochester School of Medicine and Dentistry, Rochester, New York
Femoral Hernia

Ni Ni Ku, M.D.
Cutaneous Oncology and Comprehensive Breast Cancer Programs, H. Lee Moffitt Cancer Center, University of South Florida College of Medicine, Tampa, Florida
Technique and Application of Sentinel Lymph Node Biopsy in Melanoma and Breast Cancer

Arlet G. Kurkchubasche, M.D.
Assistant Professor, Departments of Surgery and Pediatrics, Brown University School of Medicine; Pediatric Surgeon, Hasbro Children's Hospital, Providence, Rhode Island
Intussusception

Karen L. Kwong, M.D.
Assistant Professor, Department of Surgery, University of Texas–Houston Medical School; Staff Surgeon, LBJ General Hospital, Houston, Texas
Postcholecystectomy Syndrome

Anne L. Lally, M.D.
Liver Transplant Fellow, Lahey Clinic, Burlington, Massachusetts
Hepatocellular Carcinoma

Jeffrey T. Landers, M.D.
Resident, General Surgery, University of Rochester School of Medicine, Rochester, New York
Femoral Hernia

Lorrie A. Langdale, M.D.
Associate Professor of Surgery, University of Washington School of Medicine; VA Puget Sound Health Care System, Seattle, Washington
Pulmonary Embolism

Julie R. Lange, M.D., Sc.M.
Assistant Professor, Department of Surgery, Johns Hopkins University School of Medicine, Baltimore, Maryland
Staging and Selection of Treatment Options for Melanoma

Rifat Latifi, M.D.
Assistant Professor, Department of Surgery, Virginia Commonwealth University School of Medicine, Richmond, Virginia
Bariatric Surgery

W. Anthony Lee, M.D.
Assistant Professor, Department of Surgery, Division of Vascular Surgery, University of Florida College of Medicine, Gainesville, Florida
Management of Thoracic, Abdominal, Peripheral, and Visceral Aneurysmal Disease

Karen D. Libsch, M.D.
Resident in General Surgery, Mayo Clinic, Rochester, Minnesota
Necrotizing Pancreatitis

Alex G. Little, M.D.
Professor and Chairman, Department of Surgery, University of Nevada School of Medicine, Las Vegas, Nevada
Infections of the Pleural Cavity

David H. Livingston, M.D.
Professor, Department of Surgery, Chief, Section of Trauma Surgery, University of Medicine and Dentistry of New Jersey Robert Wood Johnson Medical School, Newark, New Jersey
Right Ventricular Failure and Cardiogenic Shock

Reginald V. N. Lord, M.D.
Assistant Professor, Department of Surgery, Keck School of Medicine of the University of Southern California, Los Angeles, California
Motility Disorders of the Small Bowel

Ann C. Lowry, M.D., F.A.C.S.
Clinical Associate Professor, Department of Surgery, Division of Colon and Rectal Surgery, University of Minnesota Medical School, Minneapolis, Minnesota
Rectovaginal Fistulas

François I. Luks, M.D., Ph.D.
Associate Professor, Department of Surgery and Pediatrics, Brown Medical School; Pediatric Surgeon, Hasbro Children's Hospital/Rhode Island Hospital, Providence, Rhode Island
Pyloric Stenosis

John Maa, M.D.
General Surgical Resident, Department of General Surgery, University of California, San Francisco, School of Medicine, San Francisco, California
Upper Gastrointestinal Hemorrhage: Diagnosis and Treatment

Thomas H. Magnuson, M.D.
Associate Professor, Department of Surgery, Johns Hopkins University School of Medicine, Baltimore, Maryland
Gastrointestinal Bleeding of Obscure Origin

Nora Malaisrie, B.S.
Student, Johns Hopkins Hospital, Baltimore, Maryland
The Thymus

Mark A. Malangoni, M.D.
Professor and Vice Chairman, Department of Surgery, Case Western Reserve University School of Medicine; Chairperson, Department of Surgery, MetroHealth Medical Center, Cleveland, Ohio
Nosocomial Pneumonia

Sandeep Malhotra, M.D.

Surgical Fellow, Memorial Sloan-Kettering Cancer Center, New York, New York

Cancer of the Gallbladder

Michael S. Malian, M.D.

Instructor, Department of Surgery, Mayo Medical School; Consultant, Division of Gastroenterologic and General Surgery, Mayo Clinic, Rochester, Minnesota

Appendicitis

Rakesh K. Mangal, M.D.

Clinical Instructor, Baylor College of Medicine; Medical Staff, The Woman's Hospital of Texas, Houston, Texas

Endometriosis

John B. Martinie, M.D.

Major, United States Air Force, Kirtland Air Force Base, Albuquerque, New Mexico

Inguinal Hernias

Mary C. McCarthy, M.D.

Professor, Department of Surgery, Wright State University School of Medicine; Director of Trauma, Miami Valley Hospital, Dayton, Ohio

Abnormal Bleeding and Coagulopathies

Christopher R. McHenry, M.D., F.A.C.S., F.A.C.E.

Associate Professor, Department of Surgery, Case Western Reserve University School of Medicine; Director, Division of General Surgery, MetroHealth Medical Center, Cleveland, Ohio

Goiter and Nontoxic Benign Thyroid Conditions

David S. McKindley, Pharm.D.

Adjunct Associate Professor, Department of Pharmacy Practice, University of Rhode Island College of Pharmacy, Kingston, Rhode Island; Scientific Manager, Aventir Pharma, Parsippany, New Jersey

Basic Pharmacokinetics, Pharmacodynamics, and Important Drug Interactions

Leonard A. Mermel, D.O., Sc.M., A.M.(Hon.)

Associate Professor, Department of Medicine, Brown University School of Medicine; Medical Director, Department of Infection Control, and Attending Physician, Division of Infectious Diseases, Rhode Island Hospital, Providence, Rhode Island

Lung Abscess

Alexander R. Miller, M.D.

Assistant Professor, Department of Surgery, University of Texas Health Science Center at San Antonio, San Antonio, Texas

Nonfunctional Islet Cell Neoplasms

Daniel L. Miller, M.D.

Associate Professor, Department of Surgery, Mayo Medical School; Consultant, Division of General Thoracic Surgery, Mayo Clinic and Foundation, Rochester, Minnesota

Esophageal Perforation

Preston R. Miller, M.D.

Instructor, Department of Surgery, University of Tennessee Health Sciences Center, Memphis, Tennessee

Management of Blunt Abdominal Injuries

Mark A. Mittler, M.D.

Long Island Neurosurgical Associates, P.C., and Division of Neurosurgery, Department of Surgery, North Shore University Hospital, Manhasset; and the Long Island Jewish Medical Center, New Hyde Park, New York

Coma: Coma and Altered Mental Status in the Surgical Critical Care Setting

Frank G. Moody, M.D.

Professor, Department of Surgery, University of Texas–Houston Medical School; Staff Surgeon, Memorial Hermann Hospital, Houston, Texas

Postcholecystectomy Syndrome

Ernest E. Moore, M.D.

Professor and Vice Chairman, Department of Surgery, University of Colorado Health Sciences Center; Chief, Department of Surgery, Denver Health Medical Center, Denver, Colorado

Vascular Trauma: Thoracic Vascular Trauma

Frederick A. Moore, M.D.

James H. "Red" Duke Professor and Vice Chairman, Department of Surgery, and Chief, General Surgery and Trauma and Critical Care, University of Texas–Houston Medical School; Medical Director, Trauma, Memorial Hermann Hospital, Houston, Texas

Pericardial Tamponade

Wesley S. Moore, M.D.

Professor, Division of Vascular Surgery, University of California, Los Angeles, UCLA School of Medicine, Los Angeles, California

Management of Cerebrovascular Disease

Donald L. Morton, M.D., F.A.C.S.

Professor and Chief, Emeritus, Departments of Surgery and Oncology, University of California, Los Angeles, UCLA School of Medicine, Los Angeles; Medical Director and Surgeon-in-Chief, John Wayne Cancer Institute at Saint John's Health Center, Santa Monica, California

Management of Regional and Systemic Metastases of Melanoma

David W. Mozingo, M.D.

Associate Professor, Departments of Surgery and Anesthesiology, University of Florida College of Medicine; Director, Shands Burn Center at the University of Florida Shands Hospital, Gainesville, Florida

Thermal Injury

Sean J. Mulvihill, M.D.

Professor, Department of Surgery, and Chief, Division of General Surgery, University of California, San Francisco, School of Medicine, San Francisco, California

Postgastrectomy and Postvagotomy Syndromes

Sudish C. Murthy, M.D., Ph.D.

Associate Staff, Department of Thoracic and Cardiovascular Surgery, The Cleveland Clinic Foundation, Cleveland, Ohio

Mediastinal Masses

Gordon K. Nakata, M.D.

Resident, Department of Clinical Neurosciences, Rhode Island Hospital, Providence, Rhode Island

Neurologic Physiology: The Brain and Its Response to Injury

Attila Nakeeb, M.D.

Assistant Professor, Department of Surgery, Medical College of Wisconsin, Milwaukee, Wisconsin

Choledocholithiasis

Lena M. Napolitano, M.D.

Associate Professor, Department of Surgery, University of Maryland School of Medicine; Director, Surgical Critical Care, University of Maryland Medical Center, Veterans Administration Maryland Healthcare System, Baltimore, Maryland

Gastrointestinal Failure

Heidi Nelson, M.D., F.A.C.S.

Professor, Department of Surgery, Mayo Medical School; Chair, Division of Colon and Rectal Surgery, Mayo Clinic and Mayo Foundation, Rochester, Minnesota

Laparoscopic Colectomy

Hannah Ngoc-Ha, M.D.

University of California, San Diego, School of Medicine; Kaiser Foundation Hospital, San Diego, California

Rectal Prolapse

Santhat Nivatvongs, M.D.

Professor, Department of Surgery, Mayo Medical School; Consultant in Colon and Rectal Surgery, Mayo Clinic, Rochester, Minnesota

Pruritus Ani

Jeffrey A. Norton, M.D.

Vice Chairman, Department of Surgery, University of California, San Francisco, School of Medicine; Chief, Department of Surgery, San Francisco Veterans Affairs Medical Center, San Francisco, California

Carcinoid Tumors

Bruce A. Orkin, M.D.

Associate Professor, and Director, Division of Colon and Rectal Surgery, The George Washington University School of Medicine and Health Sciences, Washington, District of Columbia

Toxic Megacolon

James W. Orr, Jr., M.D., F.A.C.S., F.A.C.O.G.

Clinical Professor, Department of Obstetrics and Gynecology, University of South Florida College of Medicine, Tampa; Director, Gynecologic Oncology and Gynecologic Oncology Research, Lee Cancer Care, Fort Myers, Florida

Cervical Cancer

Mary F. Otterson, M.D.

Associate Professor, Zablocki Veterans Administration Medical Center, Milwaukee, Wisconsin

Radiation Enteropathy

Kenneth Ouriel, M.D.

Chairman, Department of Vascular Surgery, The Cleveland Clinic Foundation, Cleveland, Ohio

Management of Acute Adrenal Occlusions

C. Keith Ozaki, M.D.

Assistant Professor, Department of Surgery, University of Florida College of Medicine, Gainesville, Florida

Vascular Access for Hemodialysis

David L. Page, M.D.

Professor, Departments of Pathology and Epidemiology, Vanderbilt University Medical School, Nashville, Tennessee

High-Risk Indicators: Microscopic Lesions, Personal and Family History, Assessment, and Management (Oncology: Breast)

Sareh Parangi, M.D.

Instructor in Surgery, Harvard Medical School; Staff Surgeon, Beth Israel Deaconess Medical Center, Boston, Massachusetts

Laparoscopic Appendectomy

Edward E. Partridge, M.D.

Professor and Vice Chairman, Department of Obstetrics and Gynecology, and Director, Division of Gynecologic Oncology, University of Alabama School of Medicine, Birmingham, Alabama

Editor, Section 9: Gynecology

Pankaj H. Patel, M.D.

Fellow in Trauma and Critical Care, Department of Surgery, University of Medicine and Dentistry of New Jersey Robert Wood Johnson Medical School, Newark, New Jersey

Right Ventricular Failure and Cardiogenic Shock

Snehal G. Patel, M.S., F.R.C.S.

Fellow, Head and Neck Service, Memorial Sloan-Kettering Cancer Center, New York, New York

Neurovascular and Soft Tissue Tumors of the Head and Neck

Gustav Paumgartner, M.D., F.R.C.P.

Professor, Department of Medicine, University of Munich–Grosshadern; Attending Physician, Clinic of the University of Munich-Grosshadern, Munich, Germany

Lithotripsy of Gallstones

Carlos A. Pellegrini, M.D.

Professor and Chairman, Department of Surgery, University of Washington School of Medicine; Attending Surgeon, University Hospital, Seattle, Washington

Achalasia

Stephen G. Pereira, M.D.

Clinical Assistant Professor, Department of Surgery, University of Medicine and Dentistry of New Jersey–New Jersey Medical School; Attending Surgeon, Hackensack University Medical Center, Hackensack, New Jersey

Colonic Volvulus

Jon Perlstein, M.D.

Assistant Clinical Professor, Department of Surgery, University of California, Davis, School of Medicine, Sacramento; Attending Physician, David Grant Medical Center, Travis Air Force Base, California

Vascular Trauma: Extremity Vascular Trauma

Nancy D. Perrier, M.D.

Assistant Professor, Department of General Surgery, Wake Forest University School of Medicine, Winston-Salem, North Carolina

Hyperparathyroidism

Jeffrey H. Peters, M.D., F.A.C.S.

Professor of Surgery, University of Southern California School of Medicine; Chief, Section of General Surgery, USC University Hospital, Los Angeles, California

Barrett's Esophagus

Henry A. Pitt, M.D.

Professor and Chairman, Department of Surgery, Medical College of Wisconsin; Chief, Department of Surgery, Froedtert Memorial Hospital, Milwaukee, Wisconsin

Primary Sclerosing Cholangitis

Hiram C. Polk, Jr., M.D.

Ben A. Reid, Sr., Professor and Chairman, Department of Surgery, University of Louisville School of Medicine, Louisville, Kentucky

Hepatic Abscess

Raphael E. Pollock, M.D., Ph.D.

Professor, Department of Cancer Biology, The University of Texas–Houston Medical School; M.D. Anderson Cancer Center, Houston, Texas

Management of Soft Tissue Sarcomas: Extremity and Chest Wall

Fabio M. Potenti, M.D.

Assistant Professor, Department of Surgery, Brown University School of Medicine; Active Staff, Department of Surgery, Rhode Island Hospital; Medical Staff, Department of Surgery, Women and Infants Hospital and Fatima Hospital, Providence, Rhode Island

Fecal Incontinence

John J. Poterucha, M.D.

Associate Professor, Department of Medicine, Mayo Medical School; Education Chair, Division of Gastroenterology and Hepatology, Mayo Clinic and Foundation, Rochester, Minnesota

Hepatitis

Ourania A. Preventza

Cardiothoracic Fellow, Albert Einstein College of Medicine, Montefiore Medical Center, New York, New York

Ischemic Colitis

Timothy L. Pruett, M.D.

Professor, Department of Surgery, University of Virginia School of Medicine, Charlottesville, Virginia

Diabetes Mellitus and Diabetes Insipidus

Terri B. Pustilnik, M.D.

Assistant Professor, Department of Obstetrics and Gynecology, Division of Gynecologic Oncology, University of Alabama School of Medicine, Birmingham, Alabama

Endometrial Cancer

Florencia G. Que, M.D.

Assistant Professor, Department of Surgery, Mayo Medical School; Surgeon, Mayo Clinic, Rochester, Minnesota

Cystic Diseases of the Liver

Thomas E. Read, M.D.

Assistant Professor, Department of Surgery, Washington University School of Medicine; Attending Surgeon, Barnes-Jewish Hospital, St. Louis, Missouri

Rectal Prolapse

Howard A. Reber, M.D.

Professor, Department of Surgery, University of California, Los Angeles, UCLA School of Medicine, Los Angeles, California

Acute Pancreatitis

R. Lawrence Reed, II, M.D.

Professor, Department of Surgery, Loyola University of Chicago Stritch School of Medicine; Chief, Division of Trauma, Surgical Critical Care and Burns, Loyola University Medical Center, Maywood, Illinois

Circulatory Monitoring

Robert V. Rege, M.D.

Professor and Chairman, Department of Surgery, University of Texas Southwestern Medical School, Dallas, Texas

Asymptomatic Gallstones

Donald A. Reiff, M.D.

Research Fellow, Center for Injury Sciences at UAB, and Senior Surgical Resident, The University of Alabama Medical Center, Birmingham, Alabama

Initial Evaluation of the Trauma Patient

Douglas Reintgen, M.D.

Professor, Department of Surgery, University of South Florida College of Medicine; Program Leader, Cutaneous Oncology, H. Lee Moffitt Cancer Center, Tampa, Florida

Technique and Application of Sentinel Lymph Node Biopsy in Melanoma and Breast Cancer

Harry M. Richter, III, M.D.

Associate Professor, Department of Surgery, Rush Medical College; Senior Attending Surgeon, Cook County Hospital, Chicago, Illinois

Peptic Ulcer Disease: Perforation

Holly E. Richter, Ph.D., M.D.

Associate Professor, Department of Obstetrics and Gynecology, Division of Medical Surgical Gynecology, University of Alabama School of Medicine, Birmingham, Alabama

Surgical Management of Pelvic Inflammatory Disease

Layton F. Rikkers, M.D.

A. R. Curreri Professor of Surgery, University of Wisconsin Medical School; Chairman, Department of Surgery, University of Wisconsin Hospital and Clinics, Madison, Wisconsin

Portal Hypertension

Jorge E. Romaguera, M.D.

Associate Professor, University of Texas–Houston Medical School; M.D. Anderson Cancer Center, Houston, Texas

Lymphoma of the Small Bowel

Stephen A. Rowe, M.D.
Surgical Resident, Department of General Surgery, University of Louisville School of Medicine, Louisville, Kentucky

Basic and Advanced Mechanical Ventilation

Loring W. Rue, III, M.D., F.A.C.S.
Professor, Department of Surgery, University of Alabama School of Medicine; Chief, Section of Trauma, Burns and Surgical Critical Care, and Director, Center for Injury Sciences at UAB, The University of Alabama Medical Center, Birmingham, Alabama

Initial Evaluation of the Trauma Patient

Theodore J. Saclarides, M.D.
Professor, Department of General Surgery, Section of Colon and Rectal Surgery, Rush-Presbyterian-St. Luke's Medical Center, Chicago, Illinois

Lower Gastrointestinal Bleeding

George H. Sakorafas, M.D., Ph.D.
Consultant, Department of Surgery, Hellenic Airforce (HAF) Hospital, Athens, Greece

Cystic Neoplasms of the Pancreas

Timur P. Sarac, M.D.
Surgeon, Department of Vascular Surgery, The Cleveland Clinic Foundation, Cleveland, Ohio

Management of Acute Arterial Occlusions

Juan M. Sarmiento, M.D.
Gastrointestinal Surgical Scholar, Mayo Clinic, Rochester, Minnesota

Carcinoid of the Small Bowel

George A. Sarosi, Jr., M.D.
Assistant Professor, Department of Surgery, University of Texas Southwestern Medical School; Staff Surgeon, North Texas Veterans Affairs Medical Center, Dallas, Texas

Small Intestinal Diverticular Disease

Michael G. Sarr, M.D.
Professor, Department of Surgery, Mayo Medical School; Chair, Division of Gastroenterologic and General Surgery, Mayo Clinic, Rochester, Minnesota

Splanchnic Venous Thrombosis; Necrotizing Pancreatitis; Acute Pancreatitis; Cystic Neoplasms of the Pancreas; Advanced Gastrointestinal Laparoscopic Procedures; Editor, Section 5: Gastrointestinal

Mark D. Sawyer, M.D.
Assistant Professor, Department of Surgery, Mayo Medical School; Consultant in Surgery, Mayo Clinic, Rochester, Minnesota

Ischemic Colitis

William P. Schecter, M.D.
Professor of Clinical Surgery, University of California, San Francisco, School of Medicine; Chief of Surgery, San Francisco General Hospital, San Francisco, California

Human Immunodeficiency Virus Infection

Scott R. Schell, M.D., Ph.D.
Assistant Professor, Departments of Surgery and Molecular Genetics and Microbiology, University of Florida College of Medicine; Staff Surgeon, Malcolm Randall Veterans Affairs Medical Center, Gainesville, Florida

Breast Carcinoma: Stages I and II

Richard T. Schlinkert, M.D.
Professor, Department of Surgery, Mayo Graduate School of Medicine, Rochester, Minnesota; Consultant in Surgery, Mayo Clinic Scottsdale, Scottsdale, Arizona

Splenectomy

Leon Schlossberg, M.D.*
Associate Professor of Art as Applied to Medicine, Johns Hopkins University School of Medicine, Baltimore, Maryland

The Thymus

*Deceased.

James M. Seeger, M.D.
Professor, Division of Vascular Surgery, and Associate Chairman, Department of Surgery, University of Florida College of Medicine; Chief, Division of Vascular Surgery, Malcolm Randall Veterans Affairs Medical Center, Gainesville, Florida

Diagnosis and Management of Chronic Peripheral Arterial Occlusive Disease; Editor, Section 10: Vascular

Jatin P. Shah, M.D., F.A.C.S.
Professor, Department of Surgery, Cornell University Joan and Sanford I. Weill Medical College and Graduate School of Medical Sciences; Chief, Head and Neck Surgery, and Elliot Strong Chair, Head and Neck Oncology, Memorial Sloan-Kettering Cancer Center, New York, New York

Incidence, Etiology, Diagnosis, and Staging of Head and Neck Cancer; Salivary Glands; Neurovascular and Soft Tissue Tumors of the Head and Neck; Editor, Section 4: Head and Neck

Lelan F. Sillin, M.D.
Professor of Clinical Surgery, Keck School of Medicine of the University of Southern California; Attending Surgeon, USC University Hospital/LAC-USC Medical Center, Los Angeles, California

Motility Disorders of the Small Bowel

Diane M. Simeone, M.D.
Assistant Professor, Department of General Surgery, University of Michigan Medical School, Ann Arbor, Michigan

Gastric Ulcer

H. Hank Simms, M.D.
John D. Mountain Professor and Chairman, Department of Surgery, North Shore/Long Island Jewish Health System, Surgeon-in-Chief, North Shore University Hospital, Long Island Jewish Medical Center, Manhasset, New York

Editor, Section 3: Critical Care

Bhuvanesh Singh, M.D.
Assistant Professor, Department of Surgery, Cornell University Joan and Sanford I. Weill Medical College and Graduate School of Medical Sciences; Assistant Attending Surgeon and Director, Laboratory of Epithelial Cancer Biology, Memorial Sloan-Kettering Cancer Center, New York, New York

Cervical Lymph Nodes and Unknown Primary Tumor

James V. Sitzmann, M.D.
Chair, Department of Surgery, University of Rochester School of Medicine and Dentistry, Rochester, New York
Hemangioma

C. Daniel Smith, M.D.
Associate Professor and Chief, General and Gastrointestinal Surgery, Emory University School of Medicine, Atlanta, Georgia
Gastroesophageal Reflux Disease (GERD)

David J. Smith, Jr., M.D.
Professor and Head, Section of Plastic and Reconstructive Surgery, University of Michigan Medical School, Ann Arbor, Michigan
General Evaluation and Biopsy of Cutaneous Lesions

LaNette F. Smith, M.D.
Instructor, Department of Surgery, Division of Surgical Oncology, and Virginia Clinton Kelley Breast Fellow, University of Arkansas for Medical Sciences, Little Rock, Arkansas
Diagnosis and Assessment of Benign and Malignant Breast Diseases

Christopher J. Sonnenday, M.D.
Senior Resident, Department of Surgery, Johns Hopkins Hospital, Baltimore, Maryland
Diverticulitis

Donald L. Sorrells, M.D.
Assistant Professor, University of Texas Medical School at San Antonio; Staff Surgeon, Pediatric Surgery, Wilford Hall Medical Center, San Antonio, Texas
Anomalies of Bowel Rotation: Malrotation and Midgut Volvulus; Meckel's Diverticulum

Michael P. Spencer, M.D.
Clinical Assistant Professor, Department of Surgery, Division of Colon and Rectal Surgery, University of Minnesota Medical School, Minneapolis; Chief of Surgery, Unity Hospital, Fridley, and Section Chief, Colon and Rectal Surgery, Veterans Affairs Medical Center, Minneapolis, Minnesota
Anal Cancer

Philip F. Stahel, M.D.
Division of Trauma Surgery, Department of Surgery, University Hospital Zurich, Zurich, Switzerland
Closed Head Injury

Catherine L. Stanfield, M.S.N., C.R.N.P.
Adjunct Instructor, Johns Hopkins University School of Nursing; Acute Care Nurse Practitioner, Department of Surgery, Johns Hopkins Hospital, Baltimore, Maryland
Cholecystolithiasis

Scott A. Strong, M.D.
Staff Surgeon, Department of Colorectal Surgery, The Cleveland Clinic Foundation, Cleveland, Ohio
Crohn's Disease of the Small Bowel: Crohn's Disease of the Small Bowel

Harvey J. Sugerman, M.D.
David M. Hume Professor of Surgery; Chief, General and Trauma Surgery Division; Vice-Chairman, Department of Surgery, Virginia Commonwealth University School of Medicine, Richmond, Virginia
Compartment Syndrome: Abdominal Compartment Syndrome; Bariatric Surgery

Sonia L. Sugg, M.D.
Assistant Professor, Department of Surgery, University of Chicago Pritzker School of Medicine, Chicago, Illinois
Neuroendocrine Tumors of the Pancreas

W. Jay Suggs, M.D.
Resident, Department of General Surgery, Mayo Clinic, Rochester, Minnesota
Pseudo-obstruction of the Colon

Mark A. Talamini, M.D.
Associate Professor, Department of Surgery, and Director of Minimally Invasive Surgery, Johns Hopkins University School of Medicine, Baltimore, Maryland
Cholecystolithiasis

Benjamin D. Tanner, M.D.
Administrative Chief Resident, Department of Surgery, University of Louisville School of Medicine, Louisville, Kentucky
Hepatic Abscess

Geoffrey B. Thompson, M.D.
Associate Professor, Department of Surgery, Mayo Medical School; Consultant, Department of Surgery, Mayo Clinic and Foundation, Rochester, Minnesota
Medullary Thyroid Carcinoma

Jon S. Thompson, M.D.
Professor, Department of Surgery, University of Nebraska College of Medicine; Vice-Chair, Department of Surgery, and Chairman, Department of General Surgery, University of Nebraska Medical Center, Omaha, Nebraska
Short Bowel Syndrome

M. Bulent Tirnaksiz
Clinical Fellow, Division of General Thoracic Surgery, Mayo Clinic and Foundation, Rochester, Minnesota
Spontaneous Pneumothorax and Lung Volume Reduction Surgery

Bernardo Tisminezky, M.D.
Research Collaborator, Division of Colon and Rectal Surgery, Mayo Clinic; General Surgeon, Centro Quirurgico Valencia, Valencia, Venezuela
Laparoscopic Colectomy

James Toouli, M.B.B.S., Ph.D., F.R.C.A.S.
Professor, Department of Surgery, Flinders University; Head, General and Digestive Surgery Department, Flinders Medical Centre, Adelaide, SA, Australia
Biliary Dyskinesia

Thomas F. Tracy, Jr., M.D.
Professor, Departments of Surgery and Pediatrics, Brown University School of Medicine; Pediatric Surgeon-in-Chief, Hasbro Children's Hospital, Providence, Rhode Island

Neonatal Bowel Obstruction; Anomalies of Bowel Rotation: Malrotation and Midgut Volvulus; Abdominal Wall Defects: Omphalocele and Gastroschisis; Meckel's Diverticulum; Editor, Section 6: Pediatric

Peter G. Trafton, M.D.
Professor and Vice Chairman, Department of Orthopaedic Surgery, Brown University School of Medicine; Surgeon-in-Charge, Orthopaedic Trauma, Rhode Island Hospital, Providence, Rhode Island

Compartment Syndrome: Extremity Compartment Syndrome

L. William Traverso, M.D.
Clinical Professor, Department of Surgery, University of Washington School of Medicine; Attending Surgeon, Virginia Mason Medical Center, Seattle, Washington

Chronic Pancreatitis: Endotherapy First, Then Surgery

Gregory G. Tsiotos, M.D.
Assistant Professor, Department of Surgery, Athens Medical School, Athens; Director, Hepatobiliary and Pancreatic Surgery, Athens Medical Center, Marousi, Greece

Obstructive Jaundice: Preoperative Evaluation; Laparoscopic Common Bile Duct Exploration

George Tsioulias, M.D., D.M.Sc.
Senior Fellow, Department of Surgical Oncology, John Wayne Cancer Institute at Saint John's Health Center, Santa Monica, California

Management of Regional and Systemic Metastases of Melanoma

Richard H. Turnage, M.D.
Associate Professor and Vice Chairman, Department of Surgery, University of Texas Southwestern Medical School; Chief, Surgical Service, Dallas Veterans Administration Medical Center, Dallas, Texas

Small Intestinal Diverticular Disease

Robert Udelsman, M.D., M.B.A., F.A.C.S.
Lampman Professor of Surgery and Oncology and Chair, Department of Surgery, Yale University School of Medicine; Chief, Surgery Service, Yale–New Haven Hospital, New Haven, Connecticut

Follicular, Hürthle Cell, and Anaplastic Thyroid Cancer

Giampaolo Ugolini, M.D.
Staff Surgeon, Department of Surgery, Policlinico S. Orsola–Malpighi, University of Bologna, Bologna, Italy

Fecal Incontinence

Marshall M. Urist, M.D.
Professor, Department of Surgery, University of Alabama School of Medicine, Birmingham, Alabama

Advanced Breast Carcinoma (Stages IIIa and IIIb)

Madhulika G. Varma, M.D.
Assistant Professor, Department of Surgery, University of California, San Francisco, School of Medicine, San Francisco, California

Rectovaginal Fistulas

R. Edward Varner, M.D.
Professor, Department of Obstetrics and Gynecology, Division of Medical and Surgical Gynecology, University of Alabama School of Medicine, Birmingham, Alabama

Surgical Management of Pelvic Inflammatory Disease

Luis O. Vasconez, M.D.
Professor and Chief, Department of Plastic Surgery, and Director, Residency Training, Plastic Surgery, University of Alabama School of Medicine, Birmingham, Alabama

Breast Reconstruction

Jean-Nicolas Vauthey, M.D.
Associate Professor, Department of Surgery, Department of Surgical Oncology, The University of Texas–Houston Medical School; Chief, Liver Service, The University of Texas M. D. Anderson Cancer Center, Houston, Texas

Metastatic Cancer of the Liver

Antonio L. Visbal, M.D.
Clinical Fellow, Division of General Thoracic Surgery, Mayo Clinic and Foundation, Rochester, Minnesota

Spontaneous Pneumothorax and Lung Volume Reduction Surgery

Andrew L. Warshaw, M.D.
W. Gerard Austen Professor of Surgery, Harvard Medical School; Surgeon-in-Chief and Chairman, Department of Surgery, Massachusetts General Hospital, Boston, Massachusetts

Pancreas Divisum

Jeffrey D. Wayne, M.D.
Junior Faculty Associate, Department of Surgical Oncology, University of Texas–Houston Medical School; Fellow, Department of Surgical Oncology, University of Texas M. D. Anderson Cancer Center, Houston, Texas

Metastatic Cancer of the Liver

Martin R. Weiser, M.D.
Assistant Professor, Cornell University Joan and Sanford I. Weill Medical College and Graduate School of Medical Sciences; Assistant Surgeon, Memorial Sloan-Kettering Cancer Center, New York, New York

Gastric Adenocarcinoma

Michael A. West, M.D., Ph.D.
Professor, Department of Surgery, University of Minnesota Medical School–Minneapolis; Assistant Chief of Surgery and Director, Surgical Intensive Care Unit, Hennein County Medical Center, Minneapolis, Minnesota

Aspiration Pneumonitis

Steven D. Wexner, M.D.
Professor, Department of Surgery, The Cleveland Clinic Foundation Health Sciences Center of the Ohio State University, and Clinical Professor, Department of Surgery, Division of Surgery, University of South Florida College of Medicine; Chairman, Department of Colorectal Surgery, and Chief of Staff, Cleveland Clinic Florida, Fort Lauderdale, Florida

Crohn's Disease of the Small Bowel: Crohn's Disease of the Colon; Laparoscopic Small Bowel Resection

Kirsten Bass Wilkins, M.D.
Chief Resident, General Surgery, Duke University Medical Center, Durham, North Carolina
The Thymus

Ronald Witteles, M.D.
Resident, Department of Medicine, Stanford University School of Medicine, Stanford, California
Neuroendocrine Tumors of the Pancreas

Richard J. Wong, M.D.
Head and Neck Fellow, Memorial Sloan-Kettering Cancer Center, New York, New York
Incidence, Etiology, Diagnosis, and Staging of Head and Neck Cancer

Douglas E. Wood, M.D.
Associate Professor, Department of Surgery, and Endowed Chair in Lung Cancer Research, University of Washington School of Medicine; Chief, General Thoracic Surgery, Division of Cardiothoracic Surgery, University of Washington Medical Center, Seattle, Washington
Esophageal Diverticula

Byron E. Wright, M.D.
Surgical Fellow, Hennepin County Medical Center, Minneapolis, Minnesota
Aspiration Pneumonitis

Karen A. Yeh, M.D.
Associate Professor, Department of Surgery, Medical College of Georgia School of Medicine, Augusta, Georgia
Stromal Tumors of the Small Bowel

Tonia M. Young-Fadok, M.D., F.A.C.S.
Associate Professor, Department of Surgery, Mayo Medical School; Consultant, Division of Colon and Rectal Surgery, Mayo Clinic, Rochester, Minnesota
Pseudo-obstruction of the Colon; Advanced Gastrointestinal Laparoscopic Procedures

Christopher K. Zarins, M.D.
Chidester Professor of Surgery and Chief, Division of Vascular Surgery, Stanford University School of Medicine, Stanford, California
Management of Thoracic, Abdominal, Peripheral, and Visceral Aneurysmal Disease

Nicholas J. Zyromski, M.D.
Research Fellow, Department of Surgery and Gastrointestinal Research Unit, Mayo Clinic, Rochester, Minnesota
Splanchnic Venous Thrombosis

Preface

The Editors acknowledge the importance to the practicing general surgeon and resident-in-training of a readable and concise state-of-the-art volume containing the evolutionary principles of the practice of surgery. We further acknowledge the physical, psychological, and socioeconomic importance of surgical diseases and their impact on society. The scientific community has witnessed extraordinary advances in the therapy for both benign and malignant surgical diseases at various organ sites, in particular over the past decade. Implicit in these advances are new concepts and techniques of management that integrate medicine and surgery with pharmacology, immunology, biostatistics, pathology, medical and radiation oncology, and diagnostic radiology and imaging. Further, each of these major disciplines contributes only a small component of the diagnostic and therapeutic approaches to clinical care; hence, comprehensive planning and integration of patient care throughout the preoperative, intraoperative, and postoperative phases are essential for successful surgical management.

The goal of this work is to provide an illustrative, instructive, and comprehensive text that depicts the rationale for the basic operative principles essential to surgical therapy. Many treatises are currently available that integrate scientific rationale, clinical trials, multidisciplinary approaches, and anatomical and technical maneuvers for the management of surgical diseases. In organizing this volume, we have chosen authors renowned in their disciplines for informing, illustrating, and explaining surgical treatments involving metabolic, infectious, endocrine, and neoplastic derangements in adult and pediatric patients. While we consider this text to be inclusive regarding the technical and operative considerations for preoperative, intraoperative, and postoperative care, it is not intended to replace standard textbooks of surgery, nor should it be considered complete with regard to the discussion of various pathophysiologic disorders. Rather, this volume is organized to familiarize residents, fellows, and practicing surgeons with the state-of-the-art surgical principles and techniques essential to contemporary sugical practice. This work was developed to coexist with other major surgical reference texts dedicated to the treatment of individual organs and systemic diseases.

Every chapter includes a condensed bibliography of carefully selected journal articles, reviews, and texts, which we hope will enhance the education of the reader about accepted surgical principles involved in patient care. Moreover, we have sought to provide a counterviewpoint for the selection of therapy by presenting, at the end of each chapter, a table of *"Pearls and Pitfalls"* that highlights particular concerns.

This volume is organized into ten sections, each representing an important branch of surgical science: General Principles, Trauma and Burns, Critical Care, Head and Neck, Gastrointestinal, Pediatric, Oncology, Endocrine, Gynecology, and Vascular. In most chapters, the pertinent anatomy and physiology are summarized, a history of the surgical illness is described, and the stages of the operative procedure are outlined, with technical considerations and complications extensively reviewed. The text is amply supported by line drawings and photographs that depict relevant anatomical or technical principles. Although some overlap exists among related chapters, the Editors have made every effort to minimize repetition, except when controversial or state-of-the-art issues are presented. We have made every attempt to ensure that accurate presentations and illustrations properly document the most complex problems confronting the general surgeon.

This work has been organized to address advanced and contemporary concepts for the conduct of expeditious, safe, and anatomically accurate operations that incorporate standard as well as evolving surgical principles and techniques. The text is organized with the specific goal of documenting the basic surgical tenets for the management of various surgical diseases in adults and children. These principles have been tested in the field of valid scientific knowledge and are well supported by insights gained in clinical practice. The Editors are grateful for having had the opportunity to respond to the challenge of developing this text, and we are hopeful that our readers will find this book to be a repository of valuable, useful, and timely information.

KIRBY I. BLAND, M.D.

Acknowledgments

I am grateful to have been entrusted with the responsibility of developing this text. To organize and publish it required the knowledge and assistance of many people.

To our residents in surgery and research fellows, at both Brown University and the University of Alabama in Birmingham, the Editors acknowledge an intellectual debt. We are grateful for their questions and for their encouragement.

I would like to thank each of the Section Editors for the many hours of additional work that went into the management of the separate surgical sections of this book. I would also like to acknowledge the help of their assistants Ellen Tetrault (Dr. Cioffi); Kate Poole (Dr. Clark); Ross C. Duchene (Dr. Gamelli); Kristin Scherr (Dr. Seeger); Jayne Scorpio (Dr. Tracy); Patti Reicher (Dr. Partridge); Stacey Moya (Dr. Shah); and Jane Pariseault (Dr. Simms).

I deeply appreciate the assistance of Michael G. Sarr, M.D., who edited the entire gastrointestinal section. His editorial advice, review, and assistance were indispensable to the book as a whole. Dr. Sarr's assistant, Deborah Frank, managed and coordinated the work from Dr. Sarr's office in Rochester with superlative grace and efficiency. I also thank my UAB assistant, Caryl Johnston, for encouraging authors, seeing that chapters were submitted in a timely fashion, and attending to many details of fact and style. From the publishing firm of W.B. Saunders, Catherine Carroll and Hazel Hacker, in-house editors; Judy Gandy, the off-site editor who assembled the book; and Lisette Bralow, Executive Editor, all provided invaluable advice and insight.

KIRBY I. BLAND, M.D.

Contents

THREE
CRITICAL CARE

FOUR
HEAD AND NECK

FIVE
GASTROINTESTINAL

SIX

PEDIATRIC

SEVEN

ONCOLOGY

EIGHT
ENDOCRINE

NINE
GYNECOLOGY

TEN
VASCULAR

GENERAL PRINCIPLES

Chapter 1
Anesthesia and Risk Assessment
W. Scott Jellish

Risk assessment by the anesthesiologist is a complex task that incorporates the consideration of numerous physical and laboratory findings. The patient's physical status and ability to withstand the stress of the surgical procedure must be determined. The practitioner's assessment of risk is based on a knowledge of the prevalence rates of untoward consequences in population groups sharing the same characteristics or risk factors. Important in the preoperative interview with patients is their own perception of risk, which is the subjective interpretation of their attempt to estimate risk. The complex mental process that comprises the cognitive interaction between the patient's perceptions of risk and benefit, and his or her acceptance of that risk, is influenced by factors such as familiarity with the procedure, sense of control, perceived potential for catastrophe, and level of knowledge regarding the pathology and the treatment. Most of the medical counseling done by the practitioner during the presurgical assessment deals with how the patient can handle the uncertainty inherent in the practice of medicine. Relieving the patient's anxiety and establishing mutual trust between patient and practitioner are important goals in the preoperative preparation for surgery.

Risk management involves the identification of risk and either avoidance of the condition predisposing the patient to that risk or development of a means of altering the consequences of an action or event that usually leads to an adverse outcome. Factors that affect risk include the nature and duration of the illness that necessitates the operation, comorbidities, age of the patient, and nutritional status of the patient as well as the type of operation considered. It is the task of the anesthesiologist to assess risk and formulate an acceptable plan that anticipates potential problems, increases patient safety, produces an acceptable operating field, and provides a stable postoperative environment in which the patient's pain can be controlled.

PREOPERATIVE RISK ASSESSMENT

The preoperative risk assessment should be based on a thorough and efficient fact-finding process. The preoperative evaluation should address three key points. (1) Does the physical status of the patient increase the risk of mortality and morbidity during the perioperative period? (2) What concurrent disease processes and medications might influence the intraoperative and postoperative courses? (3) Which immediate medical actions would be most beneficial to the patient and increase the chances for a successful outcome? This assessment includes decisions for noninvasive testing to better estimate risk and identify the patients who might benefit from specific preoperative procedures. When anesthesiologists assess surgical risk, the fact-finding methods include an adequate history, physical examination, and, finally, as directed by the history and physical examination, confirmatory laboratory tests. The medical history gives the greatest amount of information concerning the patient and his or her ability to undergo the surgical procedure. It has been demonstrated that the history gives primary information concerning the patient's physical state in approximately 60% of cases. A prospective study of preoperative patients concluded that a comprehensive review of medical systems gave positive information of some interest in about 80% of the patients examined. Practitioners ask basic questions to determine patient vitality, mobility, and fitness; they also perform a review of systems focusing on chronic disease, cardiopulmonary dysfunction, gastrointestinal disorders, and recent upper airway or genitourinary infections.

AGE-RELATED RISK

A major factor that is always considered in the patient undergoing surgery is age. Although much of the increased morbidity related to age is appropriately attributable to comorbidity and the extent of the existing disease, a patient older than 80 years of age will have a reduced physiologic reserve. The decision to recommend surgery ultimately relies on the assumption that the elderly patient undergoing the procedure will live long enough to obtain an important benefit if the operation is successful. Numerous studies have found a significant increase in mortality after surgery beginning at the age of 70. Other investigators have found that the highest rate of anesthetic complications occurs in the older-than-75 age group and among those with the greatest number of comorbidities. A total of 36% of patients older than 70 had nonfatal complications after surgery. Sixty-five percent of this group also had three or more preoperative abnormalities. It has also been determined that age is a preoperative risk for cardiovascular and pulmonary complications. In patients undergoing vascular procedures, the single best predictor of death, pulmonary edema, cardiac arrest, or myocardial infarction was age greater than 70.

Age-related physiologic changes that impact intraoperative care include arterial wall stiffening, resulting in afterload increases and left ventricular hypertrophy. The elderly patient has diminished cardiac reserve and a higher incidence of atrial fibrillation secondary to degenerative changes in the conduction system. Depression, dementia, and other neurologic disorders are also associated with advanced age. Questions directed toward neurologic impairment, loss of vision, or changes in vision should be asked of elderly patients. Their answers may provide evidence of poor cerebral blood flow, transient ischemic attacks, or ischemic encephalopathy. A preoperative assessment of the patient's mental status subsequently helps determine when a confused postoperative patient has returned to baseline and directs practitioners' attention to the patients who may be at increased risk for postoperative delirium.

The elderly patient has a diminished respiratory reserve. Lung tissue tends to lose elasticity because of loss of alveolar septa, and subsequent atelectasis. Vital capacity and forced expiratory volume at 1 second (FEV_1) decrease roughly 1% per year. Effective gas exchange also deteriorates because of a diminution in capillary surface area and a dropout of pulmonary capillaries. Elderly patients may also have decreased airway protective reflexes, may chronically aspirate, and may have underlying pneumonia. These physiologic changes, coupled with the comorbidity induced by chronic cigarette smoking, job-related lung injury, and chronic infection, produce postoperative pulmonary complication rates as high as 40% of overall morbidity and approximately 20% of total mortality. Questions concerning cough or sputum production, hemoptysis, recent pneumonias, shortness of breath or chest pain, and reduced physical activity may point to changes in either cardiac or respiratory status that need to be further evaluated before surgery.

Age also affects kidney and liver function. Glomerular filtration rate declines linearly from 80 mL/min per m^2 at age 30 to 58 mL/min per m^2 by age 80. By age 65, blood flow to the kidneys is half that of a young adult. This diminution may result in a decreased ability to concentrate urine and an inability to regulate electrolytes. Comorbidity involving prostatic hypertrophy may also be exacerbated by anesthetic agents, leading to urinary retention. Liver function and blood flow to the liver may be reduced, and the nutritional status of the patient may be questionable. Drug clearance and metabolism may be reduced and serum albumin may be low, producing an increase in the free fraction of highly protein-bound drugs. The history obtained by the anesthesiologist should focus on eating habits, bowel and bladder function, and nutrition in general. Nutrition and serum albumin levels are so important for good wound healing and decreased morbidity that several surgical risk assessment profiles include albumin concentration as an important determinant of good outcome.

THE PHYSICAL EXAMINATION

To assess operative risk, the anesthesiologist must also include a physical examination of the patient. In most instances, pertinent physical findings have already been established by the primary care or general medicine physician. However, there are some instances in which the anesthesiologist discovers a previously undiagnosed finding (e.g., murmur, bruit) that may require further investigation. A few physical features that are important to the anesthesiologist directly affect intraoperative risk; namely, the anatomy of the airway and the body habitus of the patient as it pertains to the anatomic features that could increase the difficulty of administering a regional anesthetic.

The ability to intubate and ventilate a patient for a surgical procedure is of primary importance to the anesthesiologist and weighs heavily in the assessment of risk criteria. Closed claims analysis reveals that 85% of airway-related incidents involve brain damage or death and as many as one third of deaths attributable solely to anesthesia have been related to the inability to maintain a patent airway. Numerous complications and morbidities are associated with endotracheal intubation (Table 1–1). The identification of a patient with a difficult airway is vital in planning the anesthetic management and the assessment of risk that the patient will assume. Several clinical criteria are routinely assessed prior to the surgical procedure to obtain an idea of the difficulty of intubation. Malformations of the face, acromegaly, cervical spondylosis, occipital-atlanto-axial disease, tumors of the airway, and long-term diabetes producing stiff joint syndrome carry added risk. Head movement and the ability to hyperextend the neck producing a thyromental distance of more than 6.5 cm would be consistent with a normal airway and easy mask ventilation. The ability of the patient to protrude the jaw to a prognathous position and an interincisor gap

Table 1–1 Complications of Endotracheal Intubation

During Intubation
Laryngospasm
Laceration, bruising of lips, tongue, and pharynx
Fracture, chipping, dislodgement of teeth or dental appliances
Perforation of trachea or esophagus
Retropharyngeal dissection
Fracture or dislocation of cervical spine
Trauma to eyes
Hemorrhage
Bacteremia
Aspiration of gastric contents or foreign bodies
Endobronchial or esophageal intubation
Dislocation of arytenoid cartilages or mandible
Hypoxemia, hypercapnia
Bradycardia, tachycardia
Hypertension
Increased intracranial or intraocular pressure
With Tube in Situ
Accidental extubation
Endobronchial intubation
Obstruction or kinking
Bronchospasm
Ignition of tube by laser device
Aspiration
Sinusitis
Excoriation of nose or mouth
Evident after Extubation
Laryngospasm
Aspiration of secretions, gastric contents, blood, or foreign bodies
Glottic, subglottic, or uvular edema
Dysphonia, aphonia
Paralysis of vocal cords or hypoglossal, lingual nerves
Sore throat
Noncardiogenic pulmonary edema
Laryngeal incompetence
Soreness, dislocation of jaw
Tracheomalacia
Glottic, subglottic, or tracheal stenosis
Vocal cord granulomas or synechiae

From Stehling LC: Management of the airway. In Barash PG, Cullen BF, Stoelting RF (eds): Clinical Anesthesia. Philadelphia, JB Lippincott, 1982, p 700.

of more than 5 cm would provide evidence of a large mouth opening, which is suggestive of an easy laryngoscopy. A small mouth opening would be characterized by an interincisor gap of less than 3.5 cm, with the inability to protrude the jaw to a prognathous position. Tooth morphology, especially buck teeth, may make the intubation extremely difficult. Loose teeth should also be identified, as they could easily become dislodged and aspirated during intubation, adding considerable morbidity to the surgical procedure.

The visibility of the oropharnygeal structures is assessed in the sitting position without phonation. The Mallampati classification is the set of criteria most often used for achieving ease of intubation and minimizing risk in obtaining a patent airway. A class I designation is made when faucial pillars, soft palate, and uvula are visualized. This classification would be consistent with a normal-appearing airway and is assigned a low risk. Visualization of the faucial pillars and soft palate, with a view of the uvula obstructed by the base of the tongue, is consistent with a class II airway. This designation is also considered low risk, with minimal problems associated with laryngoscopy and intubation. The class III airway is characterized by visualization of the soft palate only, and carries a higher risk of a difficult intubation. The class IV airway is considered the most difficult to intubate and carries the highest risk of perioperative morbidity.

Dyspnea related to airway compression, dysphagia, and sleep apnea (as documented by test or a case of snoring associated with two other major symptoms, including sudden arousal with choking, excessive daytime sleepiness, or nonrefreshing sleep) may be indicative of a problematic airway.

The ideal method for preoperative airway assessment should have high sensitivity and specificity and result in minimal false-positive and false-negative predictions. While false-positive outcome may result in a greater time expenditure and inconvenience, the outcome of a false-negative difficult airway analysis could be catastrophic. Using a composite airway risk index determined from the combination of multiple factors listed previously, in addition to body weight and history of difficult intubation in the past, El-Ganzouri and colleagues developed a simplified airway risk index that correlates well with difficulty in intubation as derived from class III and IV groups. The application of this mutivariate composite airway risk index stratified the degree of difficulty encountered in visualizing the laryngeal structures better than any of the individual airway assessment criteria used to derive it. In contrast to the Mallampati classification, the multivariate model had a much greater ability to distinguish the actual occurrence of laryngeal grade IV with a higher positive predictive value. Despite the better prediction values of this risk index, especially at the higher airway scores, it has not surpassed the Mallampati classification's ease of use and overall universal acceptance among anesthesiologists.

CARDIOVASCULAR-ASSOCIATED RISK

The next major anesthetic assessment of perioperative risk involves the cardiovascular system and the patient's fitness to undergo the procedure without major morbidity and mortality. The type and duration of surgery affect risk; in particular, the major surgical procedures with the greatest potential for complications are those that carry a risk of a large blood loss, volume shifts, or violation of visceral cavities, and vascular procedures (Table 1–2). In addition, certain timing factors may influence the risk of the surgical procedure. Several major studies have determined that cardiac complications are two to five times more likely to occur in the emergency setting than during elective surgery. Patients presenting for cardiac procedures (e.g., bypass, valve replacement) assume a higher risk of cardiac-related morbidity and mortality by the nature of their surgery. In most instances, the anesthesiologist will have additional studies performed (stress tests, angiograms, ventriculograms) to help determine the suitability of the patient for surgery.

The patient who presents for noncardiac surgery represents the biggest challenge for the practitioner in the assessment of fitness to undergo a surgical procedure. History-taking alone often provides enough information to determine a patient's risk of complications for the proposed surgery. The patient's ability to exercise or walk up a flight of stairs may be an important estimate of cardiac reserve. Questions directed toward the occurrence of any previous myocardial infarction and the presence and frequency of any precipitating or potentiating factors involving any chest discomfort may yield an indication of ischemia. Questions should also be directed toward symptoms of heart failure (orthopnea, paroxysmal nocturnal dyspnea, and dyspnea on exertion) and the results of previous cardiac tests. The physical examination should include the measurement of vital signs and the search for evidence of peripheral vascular disease (carotid or femoral bruits or diminished pulses). The lung fields should be examined for decreased breath sounds, rales, or rhonchi. The patient with a suspicious history who has symptoms or physical evidence of unstable angina,

Table 1–2 Cardiac Risk Stratification for Noncardiac Surgical Procedures*

High (reported cardiac risk often >5%)
  Emergent major operations, particularly in the elderly
  Aortic and other major vascular
  Peripheral vascular
  Anticipated prolonged surgical procedures associated with large fluid shifts and/or blood loss
Intermediate (reported cardiac risk generally <5%)
  Carotid endarterectomy
  Head and neck
  Intraperitoneal and intrathoracic
  Orthopedic
  Prostate
Low** (reported cardiac risk generally <1%)
  Endoscopic procedures
  Superficial procedure
  Cataract
  Breast

*Cardiac risk signifies combined incidence of cardiac death and nonfatal myocardial infarction.
**Does not generally require further preoperative testing.
From Belzberg H, Rivkind AI: Preoperative cardiac preparation. Chest 1999;115:86S.

congestive heart failure, or rhythm disturbances is at high risk for a myocardial event. The preoperative evaluation attempts to categorize patients as being low, intermediate, or high risk. Additional tests add little information to the estimates obtained from the clinical evaluation in low-risk patients. However, high-risk cardiac patients, as assessed from the history and physical examination, need further investigation to determine functional status or whether the degree of myocardial ischemia will be altered by subsequent therapy. The additional diagnostic procedures performed in high- or intermediate-risk patients help the anesthesiologist determine the amount of intraoperative monitoring, the anesthetic plan, and whether the procedure is warranted or is to be avoided altogether.

An electrocardiogram (ECG) sometimes uncovers occult disease in older adults, but it rarely shows clinically important abnormalities in younger, asymptomatic patients who do not have cardiac risk factors. Routine ECGs are not indicated in asymptomatic women younger than 50 years of age and men younger than 40. Further cardiac studies for stratifying risk may be most beneficial in patients who, according to the history or findings on physical examination, are considered to be at intermediate risk for cardiac complications. These tests may also be indicated in patients with known or suspected coronary artery disease who are undergoing high-risk procedures and in whom functional status and stability of ischemia are difficult to assess. The threshold for ordering these tests should reflect the cardiac risk of the planned procedure. The ECG exercise treadmill test is useful in patients who can exercise but is rarely appropriate in patients with ischemic lower extremities. Studies have demonstrated that standard exercise stress test results were falsely positive for significant coronary artery disease in 40% of patients and falsely negative in 15%. Many times, the patient cannot achieve the maximal predicted heart rate because of dyspnea or claudication. Thus, in a population with a high prevalence of coronary artery disease, a positive result on exercise stress testing only slightly increases the likelihood of coronary artery disease and a negative test result correlates poorly with the absence of heart disease.

Pharmacologic stress testing should be considered for patients with an abnormal ECG (including left and, possibly, right bundle branch block and a history of myocardial infarction). It should also be considered for those taking digoxin and in those who cannot exercise to acceptable levels. Studies of cardiac risk using dipyridamole thallium scans (DTS) suggest that patients with normal studies have a low risk of cardiac complications (good negative predictive value); however, the prognostic implications of an abnormal scan are less well established. Prospective studies for determining the efficacy of DTS in predicting intraoperative myocardial ischemia or infarct suggest a close relationship between reversible defects and adverse cardiac outcome. However, recent reports demonstrate no correlation between redistribution defects and adverse cardiac outcome or risk of perioperative ischemia. Thus, routine DTS screening is not recommended for the determination of adverse cardiac outcome.

Holter monitoring for asymptomatic ischemia is not widely used, but its findings may correlate well with those of exercise testing and DTS in predicting adverse cardiac events. The ST segment changes indicative of ischemia (1-mm ST depression for at least 1 minute) often can be seen at heart rates below those obtained by conventional stress testing. Several studies have concluded that ischemia detected during Holter monitoring was the most reliable predictor of postoperative cardiac events, even after all other risk factors were controlled. Comparisons of exercise tolerance tests, Holter monitoring, and cardiac catheterization in patients with stable angina revealed that patients with positive Holter monitoring results had a greater likelihood of having multivessel coronary artery disease. The advantages of Holter monitoring in identifying patients at high risk for cardiac complications include its availability, ease of interpretation, and low cost. It is of no value in patients with preexisting ECG abnormalities that obfuscate determinations of ST segment depression.

Radionuclide ventriculography (RNVG) and assessment of left ventricle function and ejection fraction can predict perioperative cardiac morbidity in patients undergoing vascular procedures. In addition to determining ejection fraction, the scan can show ventricular wall motion abnormalities and systolic and diastolic dysfunction. Pasternack and associates demonstrated that a calculated ejection fraction of less than 35% was associated with a preoperative incidence of myocardial infarction greater than 75%. Although not all studies have substantiated the accuracy of RNVG in predicting postoperative cardiac mortality, measurement of ejection fraction with the use of this technique is one of the strongest predictors of overall and late survival after vascular surgery.

Coronary angiography is not recommended for risk assessment in patients scheduled for noncardiac surgery unless they have clinical evidence of coronary artery disease and are undergoing moderate- to high-risk surgical procedures. If coronary artery disease or cardiac dysfunction is severe enough to necessitate coronary angiography, the anesthesiologist presumes the risk to be high and the patient in question will undergo a cardiac event during surgery. The anesthesiologist also presumes that a coronary artery bypass graft (CABG) or percutaneous transluminal coronary angioplasty (PTCA) will be performed if appropriate lesions are found. A Cleveland Clinic study revealed that severe correctable coronary artery disease was present in 34% of patients with clinical evidence of the disease. The presence of significant coronary stenosis does not always indicate that a myocardial infarction is unavoidable or that invasive monitoring is required because the involved artery may supply nonfunctioning myocardial tissue, or its stenosis may be compensated by collaterals. The use of coronary angiography to assess the risk of perioperative morbidity and mortality is not supported at present, and studies to evaluate its use are ongoing.

The widespread need for and potential complexity of the preoperative evaluation of cardiac risk is apparent. Numerous algorithms have been devised to assess perioperative myocardial risk (Fig. 1–1). The criteria of Goldman and colleagues are possibly the best and most widely used, but they are antiquated and do not account for the information obtained from newer invasive tests or

Perioperative morbidity seems to be significantly lower in
patients who quit smoking at least 1 to 2 months before surgery.

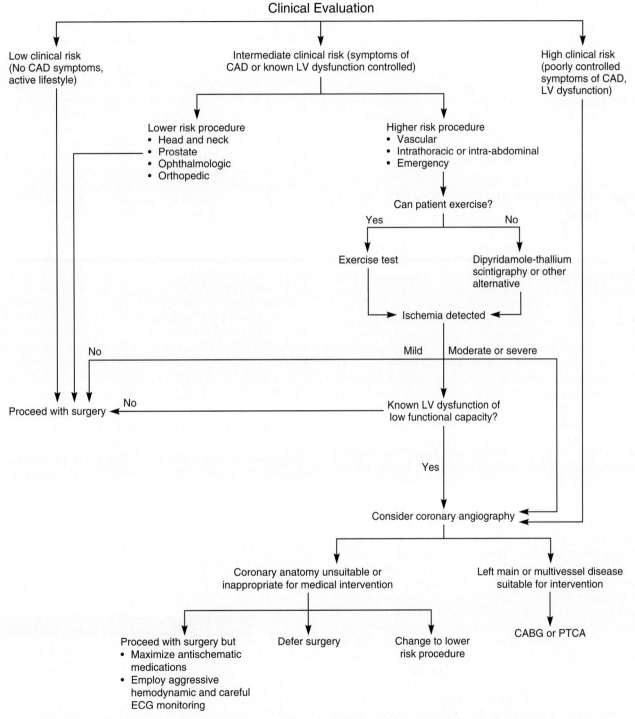

Figure 1–1. Algorithm for the assessment of cardiac risk before noncardiac surgery. CABG, coronary artery bypass graft; CAD, coronary artery disease; ECG, electrocardiogram; LV, left ventricular; PTCA, percutaneous transluminal coronary angioplasty. (From Almany SL, Mileto L, Kahn JK: Preoperative cardiac evaluation. Postgrad Med 1995;98:131. © 1995, The McGraw-Hill Companies.)

advances in the medical treatment of coronary artery disease. Eagle and colleagues used multivariate predictors, including age of at least 70, history of angina, q waves on ECG, ventricular ectopic activity, and diabetes, and divided patients into groups according to clinical variables. The patients with no clinical risk factors had a 3.1% incidence of myocardial events, whereas those who had three or more factors had a 50% incidence of perioperative myocardial events. Patients who had one or two variables and had been subjected to DTS with negative results were found to have a 3.2% incidence of cardiac events, whereas the patients with positive DTS results had a 29.6% incidence of perioperative cardiac complications. Thus, the incorporation of invasive tests along with known cardiac risk factors improved the positive predictive value of knowledge of the risk factors when the occurrence of adverse myocardial events was not totally predictable from preoperative cardiac complaints.

RISK ASSESSMENT AND PULMONARY FUNCTION

The evaluation of pulmonary function is also important in assessing the risk of surgery in patients. The clinical factors useful in determining the risk of pulmonary complications include a history of cigarette smoking, chronic bronchitis, airflow obstructive disease, obesity, and a prolonged preoperative hospital stay. Pulmonary complications are the most common form of postoperative morbidity manifested by patients who undergo abdominal and thoracic procedures. In addition to pneumonia, postoperative pulmonary complications include massive lobar collapse due to mucus plugging, pneumonitis, atelectasis, and a combination of one or more of these common problems. The high incidence of these complications and their associated costs make it imperative that the patients at increased risk be identified and pulmonary function optimized prior to the surgical procedure. Abdominal and thoracotomy procedures cause large reductions in vital capacity and smaller but important reductions in functional residual capacity (FRC). The incidence of postoperative pulmonary complications after thoracotomy and lung resection is about 30% and is related not only to removal of lung tissue but also to alterations in chest wall mechanics. The anesthesiologist may request pulmonary function tests to assess risk prior to intrathoracic procedures to determine whether the patient can tolerate loss of functional lung units. The calculation of percent predicted volume has increased the accuracy of spirometry as a preoperative tool for evaluating pulmonary risk. The risk assessment by the anesthesiologist also includes methods for reducing pain and techniques for preserving viable lung function postoperatively.

Abdominal procedures also produce a 30% incidence of pulmonary complications. In addition to dysfunction of the abdominal musculature, abdominal surgery impairs diaphragmatic function, which further reduces FRC. The preoperative evaluation of pulmonary risk in the patient undergoing abdominal surgery should include age, general health, weight, coexisting pulmonary morbidity, the type of operation, and the approach for the surgery. Spirometry is indicated in patients in whom severe pulmonary dysfunction is evident, as a means of assessing whether the patient may need pulmonary rehabilitation prior to surgery.

RISK ASSOCIATED WITH ANEMIA

Anemia in the surgical patient produces additional stresses during and after surgery that could place the patient at additional risk for cardiac morbidity. Cardiac output and tissue perfusion can increase five fold in patients with normal heart function in the presence of anemia. The increase in cardiac output is mediated by an increase in heart rate, stroke volume, and contractility. If heart function is not compromised, normal blood flow can be maintained at hemoglobin levels as low as 5 g/dL. In the patient with coronary artery disease, however, hemoglobin levels of less than 10 g/dL may be detrimental to ventricular function. Coronary artery disease and congestive heart failure reduce the body's ability to compensate for anemia. An inadequate oxygen supply may precipitate angina and impair left ventricular function. If cardiac or pulmonary disease is confirmed, interventions for anemia should be considered at a level higher than the level at which intervention occurs in the absence of cardiac or pulmonary disease (Table 1–3). Few studies have considered the effect of preoperative anemia on mortality. However, an inverse relationship exists between the preoperative hemoglobin level and the percent mortality in Jehovah's Witness patients. The morbidity associated with transfusion, especially the risk of infection or human error during inappropriate administration of blood, must also be factored into the risk of undergoing elective surgery.

OVERALL ASSESSMENT OF RISK

The numerous factors that are considered in the perioperative assessment of risk make exchange of information difficult. A generalized scoring system of risk allows groups of patients to be stratified according to the severity of their illness before treatment is begun and facilitates better analysis of morbidity and mortality for these groups. A risk scoring system should have several essential features: (1) simplicity of use, (2) applicability to most general surgery cases, (3) effectiveness for both elective

Table 1–3	Transfusion Recommendations	
	HIGHER Hb (≥ 10 g/dL)	**LOWER Hb** (7–10 g/dL)
	Coronary artery disease	↓ Age
	Congestive heart failure	↑ Life
	Chronic obstructive pulmonary disease	expectancy
	Peripheral vascular disease	Otherwise healthy
	Stroke	
	Use of beta-blockers	
	↑ Blood loss	
	↑ Age	
	↓ Life expectancy	

From Carson JL: Morbidity risk assessment in the surgically anemic patient. Am J Surg 1995;170(6A suppl):32S. With permission from Excerpta Medica Inc.

and emergency procedures, and (4) universal acceptance for use in assessing both morbidity and mortality. The scoring system most often used by anesthesiologists to assess risk is the American Society of Anesthesiologists (ASA) Physical Status classification. Patients are allocated to one of five categories, based on the medical history and physical examination without the use of any specific tests. A physical status I (PS I) designates a normal healthy patient, while a PS II indicates a patient who has mild systemic disease. PS III patients have moderate systemic disease that is controlled and not incapacitating. PS IV individuals have incapacitating disease that limits lifestyle and is a threat to life. PS V patients are moribund and not expected to survive more than 24 hours. Additional tests may be ordered by the anesthesiologist and are used to adjust the designation of patients to a more or less severe state, depending on the results. An "E" designation is added to denote an emergency procedure with an associated increase in risk. Postoperative morbidity and mortality rise with increased ASA grade, and if age is added as a covariable the scoring system has an even better predictive potential. A variant of the ASA scoring system has been developed by Klotz and colleagues in which patients are assigned to one of three risk groups on the basis of a score obtained from a combination of four variables: (1) severity of the operation, (2) ASA grade, (3) presence of malignancy, and (4) symptoms of respiratory disease. This scoring system provides a more accurate assessment of risk but has not been widely used or accepted at present.

The Goldman Cardiac Risk Index was designed to predict the risk of cardiac complications following noncardiac surgery. Nine factors are considered to give a total score of 0 to 53. Scores are then grouped into four risk classes. Originally Goldman criticized the ASA classification system as being poorly defined and subjective, but it has proved to be as good as the more cumbersome Goldman classification, which is not routinely used today by anesthesiologists. Other classification systems such as The Pulmonary Complication Risk and The Prognostic Nutritional Risk scoring systems are used to determine operative risk based on prolonged preoperative hospitalizations of debilitated patients. A number of other systems have also been developed based on the physiologic response to illness but are specifically used for assessment of the seriously ill or debilitated patient. These scoring systems are too wide-ranging and are not specific enough to be used as the basis for individual decision-making concerning the patient who is about to undergo surgery; thus, the tests are rarely used by anesthesiologists.

PREOPERATIVE "TUNE-UP"

Once the assessment of operative risk has been determined, the anesthesiologist should also make specific recommendations for strategies for reducing risk in preparation for surgery. The preoperative "tune-up" can be done on an outpatient basis before surgery or in the hospital if the patient is seriously ill but is not in a life-threatening situation. Dehydration due to overzealous diuresis or prolonged periods during which the patient has not eaten must be avoided and corrected prior to surgery. Patients

with pulmonary disease should be evaluated, and their preoperative regimens maximized. Bronchodilator use should be enhanced and incentive spirometry begun before surgery to maximize recruitment of lung units in the preoperative period.

Diabetic patients have been noted to have an increased risk of perioperative complications; these sequelae can be reduced by tight glucose control. Oral hypoglycemics should be withheld on the morning of surgery, while insulin-dependant diabetics should use half of their dose of long-acting insulin on the morning of surgery. An intravenous solution of 5% dextrose can be started if necessary, and blood sugar should be monitored every 2 to 3 hours during the procedure, with additional insulin administered if necessary. Cardiac patients should be allowed to continue their medications during the preoperative period. Antiarrhythmics can be temporarily switched to intravenous forms, and sublingual medication such as nifedipine should be administered to control hypertension prior to the placement of an intravenous line.

The final portion of the preoperative tune-up is the evaluation of NPO (nothing by mouth) status and reduction of aspiration risk. Metoclopramide, ranitidine, and sodium citrate may be given prior to the scheduled surgery to reduce the risk of aspiration, especially if the patient has a condition that predisposes him or her to passive reflux of stomach contents (hiatal hernia, gastroesophageal reflux disease). If the airway is judged acceptable for proceeding with direct laryngoscopy, cricoid pressure is used and a rapid-sequence induction performed to obtain a patent airway. These procedures, correctly done, will reduce the risk of aspiration and the accompanying increase in morbidity and mortality associated with such an occurrence.

RISK AND THE HUMAN FACTOR

The overall fitness of the anesthesiologist, although not assessed at the time of the preoperative visit, may affect the risk of the surgical procedure. Human errors affect patient safety in two ways: (1) they increase the probability of accident occurrence; (2) they increase the probability of a failure to properly respond to a problem. Anesthesiologists can experience a number of potential problems that could affect patient outcome. Fatigue and sleep deprivation affect vigilance and the recognition of problems as they occur during the operation. Cognitive problems may occur in which individuals cannot process all of the information presented to them at a particular time. In addition, individuals may try to cut corners or may be careless. Distractions in the operating room could also increase risk to the patient. Social conversations, noise, and concerns about upcoming cases may distract the anesthesiologist from events that occur during the surgical procedure that may lead to increased morbidity. Aging also affects the operating team; with age, the abilities of both the surgeon and the anesthesiologist decline. Lack of continuing education and unfamiliarity with new techniques puts the older anesthesiologist at a distinct disadvantage when dangerous situations arise. These human factors could ultimately increase the risk of a particular surgical procedure more than what would be predicted

Pearls and Pitfalls

PEARLS

- Preoperative medical assessment has four goals:
  1. Obtaining pertinent information about patient's medical conditions to assess risk
  2. Education of the patient and establishment of a relationship of trust between patient and practitioner
  3. Choice of a care plan and discussion of risk with the patient
  4. Obtaining informed consent from patient

- An adequate review of systems is key to determining the patient's physical health and assessing perioperative risk. A few extra minutes spent in obtaining an adequate history will reduce cost by avoiding unnecessary tests.
- The physical characteristics most important in determining anesthetic risk are airway anatomy and body habitus.
- The Mallampati classification of airway assessment is still the best and most widely accepted predictor of a difficult intubation.
- A patient's emotional and psychiatric needs are as important as his or her physical status in the assessment of perioperative risk and postoperative outcome. These variables should be thoroughly evaluated.

PITFALLS

- Avoid the technology trap. Nonselective batteries of tests will
  1. Fail to uncover pathologic conditions
  2. Detect abnormalities that do not necessarily improve outcome
  3. Increase medicolegal liability because of poor follow-up

by the risk assessments obtained from the medical history and laboratory testing.

RISK EXPLANATION AND ACCEPTANCE

The final portion of the preoperative assessment involves the explanation of risk to patients and their acceptance of the perceived risk. This explanation also includes discussion of the anesthetic plan and the reaching of an agreement between the patient and the practitioner to use that plan. The assessment of surgical risk is the best guess of what might happen from a combination of past clinical experiences, cohort data from groups of patients with similar problems, and the patient's own comorbidities. Medical counseling and decision-making are largely about handling these risks. However simple the awaited surgical procedure, it is a very important event in the patient's life. Though small, a certain level of risk is associated with the most simple surgical interventions, and the patient has a legal right to secure information, including risk factors that are specific to his or her particular case. The patient's agreement to undergo the surgical procedure, utilizing the anesthetic technique discussed, is perceived as a contract between physician and patient that is governed by the mutual trust established during the preoperative visit. At a time when the patient's right to decide his or her own medical management is becoming more prevalent, the preoperative assessment and the estimate of operative risk plays a vital role in the informed consent process and is the cornerstone of successful surgical outcome.

SELECTED READINGS

Almany SL, Mileto L, Kahn JK: Preoperative cardiac evaluation: Assessing risk before noncardiac surgery. Postgrad Med 1995;98:171.

Arne J, Descoins P, Fusciardi J, et al: Preoperative aassessment for difficult intubation in general and ENT surgery: Predictive value of a clinical multivariate risk index. Br J Anaesth 1998;80:140.

Arvidsson S: Preparation of the adult patient for anaesthesia and surgery. Acta Anaesthesiol Scand 1996;40:962.

Belzberg H, Rivkind AI: Preoperative cardiac preparation. Chest 115:82S, 1999.

Carson JL: Morbidity risk assessment in the surgically anemic patient. Am J Surg 1995;170(6A suppl):32S.

Chung OY, Beattie C, Friesinger GC: Assessment of cardiovascular risks and overall risks for noncardiac surgery. Cardiol Clin 1999;17:197.

Eagle KA, Coley CM, Newell JB, et al: Combining clinical and thallium data optimizes preoperative assessment of cardiac risk before major vascular surgery. Ann Intern Med 1989;110:859.

El-Ganzouri AR, McCarthy RJ, Tuman KJ, et al: Preoperative airway assessment: Predictive value of a multivariate risk index. Anesth Analg 1996;82:1197.

Ferguson MK: Preoperative assessment of pulmonary risk. Chest 1999;115:58S.

Pasternak PF, Imparato AM, Bear G, et al: The value of radionuclide angiography as a predictor of perioperative myocardial infarction in patients undergoing abdominal aortic aneurysm resection. J Vasc Surg 1984;1:320.

Pate-Cornell ME, Lakats LM, Murphy DM, Gaba DM: Anesthesia patient risk: A quantitative approach to organizational factors and risk management options. Risk Anal 1997;17:511.

Chapter 2
Fluids and Electrolytes
Kimberly A. Davis and Richard L. Gamelli

The great French physiologist Claude Bernard was the first to recognize that humans live in two very different environments: the external environment, and that which he described as the *milieu intérieur*, in which the tissues live. Another 50 years passed before it was known that this internal environment is closely protected by several intrinsic mechanisms. The end result of these protective mechanisms was termed *homeostasis* by Walter Cannon, a professor of physiology at Harvard. Essential to this *milieu intérieur* is the maintenance of normal fluid and electrolyte balance.

Preservation of an adequate volume of body water by the administration of replacement fluid and electrolytes is a fundamental component of the surgeon's practice. An understanding of the complex mechanisms of homeostasis is necessary, as most diseases and many injuries, including operative trauma, significantly alter the physiology of fluids and the balance of electrolytes within the body. Redistribution of body fluids from one compartment to another, as is seen in inflammation and infection as well as in response to traumatic injury, usually results in a decrease in the volume of circulating extracellular fluid, and subsequent hypoperfusion, or "shock." It is in the resuscitation of patients from shock that a knowledge of normal body fluids and electrolytes is of paramount importance to surgeons, so that they can rapidly restore circulating volume and thus prevent the untoward sequelae of systemic inflammatory response syndrome (SIRS) and multiple organ system failure (MOSF).

DISTRIBUTION OF BODY FLUIDS

Approximately 60% of body mass is made up of water, although this percentage varies with age and gender. The total percentage of body water decreases with increasing age, and women tend to have a lower percentage of body water than do men. Body water is classically divided into two fluid compartments: the intracellular compartment (two thirds, or 40% of total body water) and the extracellular compartment (one third, or 20% total body water) (Fig. 2–1). The intracellular space is represented predominantly by muscle mass, in which the major cations are magnesium and potassium, buffered by bicarbonate and negatively charged proteins. The extracellular space has sodium and chloride as its main ions, and is further subdivided into the plasma (one quarter, or 5% of total body water) and the interstitium (three quarters, or 15% of total body water). Water is freely diffusible across semipermeable membranes, keeping osmotic forces in balance. The forces that drive fluid movement are the relative Starling forces between the intracellular and the extracellular fluid compartments.

REGULATION OF NORMAL HOMEOSTASIS

Fluid and Electrolyte Balance

In order to maintain a balance of fluid and electrolytes, water input must equal output. When input exceeds output, the term *positive balance* is employed. Conversely, in patients in whom output exceeds input, the term *negative balance* is applied. Under normal circumstances, this balance between input and output is usually controlled by the kidneys and the neuroendocrine system.

Most of the water taken in by humans is in the form of liquid, while a third is derived from solids. Output is usually classified as either *sensible* or *insensible*. Sensible water losses are measurable and include urine (800 to 1500 mL), feces (150 mL), and sweat (200 to 1000 mL). Insensible water losses are nonmeasurable, including those that occur via evaporation of water from the lungs and diffusion of water through the skin. There may be insensible water losses of as much as 8 to 12 mL/kg through the skin and respiratory tract in the normal human. Although this amount is fairly fixed, insensible water loss can vary with body temperature, ambient temperature, physical activity, and daily fluid intake.

The Kidney

Although the type and quantity of water input is important, the composition of the *milieu intérieur* is maintained more by what is retained and what is excreted; thus, the kidney is viewed as the primary organ for maintaining the constancy of the internal environment. By varying the glomerular filtration rate, the kidney is able to respond appropriately and rapidly to changes in the volume, solute content, and composition of body fluids.

Normal kidney function results in the filtration of ap-

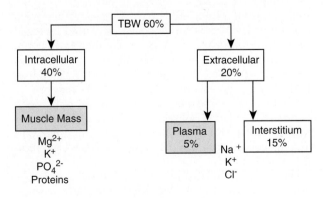

Figure 2–1. Body water distribution.

proximately 180 L of plasma per day. Sodium is preferentially resorbed in the proximal tubule, in conjunction with bicarbonate, and other divalent cations. The loop of Henle is responsible predominantly for the resorption of water, and sodium in conjunction with chloride. In the distal tubule, active sodium transport is coupled with excretion of potassium and hydrogen ion, under the control of aldosterone. In the collecting duct, under the control of ADH (antidiuretic hormone, or arginine vasopressin), water is resorbed and urine is concentrated. Thus, the maintenance of normal fluid and electrolyte balance is dependent on the formation of a large quantity of glomerular filtrate that is almost completely resorbed from the renal tubules prior to excretion.

Neuroendocrine Control of Renal Function

Changes in the fluid and electrolyte balance and renal function occur daily, as the result of injury, illness, or normal variations in intake and output. Both the volume and the composition of body fluids are monitored continuously by receptors, and their signals transduced via the neuroendocrine system to changes in renal handling of water and electrolytes.

Effective circulating volume is continuously monitored by arterial and renal baroreceptors and by atrial stretch receptors. When effective circulating volume decreases, the activity from these receptors decreases, releasing tonic inhibitions of the neuroendocrine system. This results in increased secretion of adrenocorticotropic hormone (ACTH) through central pathways, and increased secretion of renin and catecholamines through the peripheral autonomic nervous system. The aforementioned changes lead to increased formation of angiotensin by renin, and stimulation of aldosterone secretion.

The mineralocorticoid aldosterone is synthesized, stored, and secreted by the zona glomerulosa of the adrenal gland. Secretion is stimulated in response to ACTH, angiotensin II, and elevated serum potassium levels. Aldosterone increases sodium and chloride resorption in the early distal tubule of the kidney, as well as promoting sodium resorption and potassium excretion in the distal tubule and collecting system.

Renin secretion is stimulated from myoepithelial cells of the glomerulus, when the baroreceptors of the juxtaglomerular cells sense a decrease in blood pressure and renal perfusion. Renin then converts angiotensinogen to angiotensin I, which is subsequently converted by angiotensin-converting enzyme (ACE) in the lung to angiotensin II. In addition to being a potent vasoconstrictor and myocardial stimulant, angiotensin stimulates the release of ADH and augments the release of aldosterone.

ADH is released from the pituitary in response to decreased circulating volumes and increased plasma osmolarity. ADH stimulates the resorption of free water from the collecting duct of the kidney by increasing tubular permeability.

The net effect of the aforementioned neuroendocrine pathways is to restore circulating volume and maintain normal body fluid and electrolyte balance.

MAINTENANCE OF NORMAL FLUID BALANCE

Baseline fluid requirements for healthy humans must account for insensible losses of approximately 750 mL of pure water, through evaporation via the skin and lungs, and the sensible loss of hypotonic fluids of approximately 100 mL of sweat and 250 mL of stool. Additionally, a normal person must excrete approximately 600 mOsm per day via the urine to maintain normal body composition. The volume of urine necessary for accomplishing this varies widely, based on the ability of the kidney to concentrate the urine, but approximates 500 to 800 mL per day. Therefore, the average 70-kg male requires between 2000 and 2500 mL of fluid per day, or about 25 mL/kg body weight per day (Table 2–1).

The healthy human also requires a minimal amount of salt in order to maintain a normal balance. Although humans conserve sodium almost absolutely, they do so at the expense of potassium owing to increased aldosterone secretion. Approximately 60 to 100 mEq of sodium per day are necessary to prevent excess potassium loss, or approximately 1 mEq/kg body weight. With adequate maintenance doses of sodium, urinary potassium loss will be about 30 to 60 mEq per day, or approximately 0.5 mEq/kg body weight per day.

CONDITIONS OF ABNORMAL FLUID LOSS

Any abnormal fluid losses must be added to the daily fluid and electrolyte requirements described earlier. Most represent losses of transcellular fluids, with varied electrolyte compositions. Normal concentrations found in several body fluids are listed in Table 2–2. Abnormally high secretion of any of these fluids, particularly those from the gastrointestinal system, is a major cause of fluid and electrolyte disturbances in surgical patients. Knowledge of the electrolyte composition of the fluid lost, as well as the volume lost, is vital in the determination of replacement therapy. The electrolyte compositions of commonly available replacement fluids are listed in Table 2–3. Common metabolic disturbances from fluid loss and suggested volume replacement are listed in Table 2–4.

A practical way of thinking about abnormal fluid and electrolyte losses divides the types of loss into alterations in volume, concentration, composition, and/or distribution.

Table 2–1	Maintenance Fluid Requirements	
BODY WEIGHT	**FLUID REQUIREMENT**	
For 0–10 kg	100 mL/kg/day	
For 10–20 kg	50 mL/kg/day	
For >20 kg	20 mL/kg/day	
For 70-kg adult	2500 mL/day	

Table 2–2	**Electrolyte Compositions of Body Fluids**				
	Na$^+$	K$^+$	Cl$^-$	HCO$_3^-$	VOLUME (mL)
Saliva	10	26	10	30	1000
Stomach	60	10	130	0	1500
Duodenum	140	5	80	0	1500
Ileum	140	5	104	30	3000
Colon	60	35	40	0	750
Pancreas	145	5	75	115	1000
Bile	145	5	100	35	1000
Sweat	50	5	55	0	500
Blood	140	5	100	24	5000

Alterations in Volume

If an isotonic salt solution is added to or subtracted from body fluids, the volume of extracellular fluid is changed. Sudden loss of an isotonic fluid, such as an intestinal fluid, results in an acute decrease in extracellular fluid volume without changing intracellular fluid volume. As long as the osmolarities of the two compartments remain identical, no net movement of fluid from the intracellular to the extracellular space will occur.

The sudden loss of circulating blood volume is different from the loss of an isotonic salt solution. Hemorrhage results in decreased cardiac output, and resultant total body ischemia, which cannot be corrected until blood volume is restored. In the absence of transfusion therapy, this correction requires the movement of fluid and protein from the interstitium to the plasma, or "transcapillary plasma refill." Initially triggered by a fall in capillary hydrostatic pressure, this mechanism results in the movement of protein-free fluid from the interstitium to the plasma. A second phase involves the movement of protein into the plasma space in support of plasma oncotic pressure. This results in the restoration of plasma volume and protein concentration, with reduced oxygen-carrying capacity due to a decrease in total red blood cell mass, i.e., a normovolemic anemia. Transcapillary refill is capable of sustaining a relatively fixed level of plasma volume, equal to approximately two thirds of the initial plasma volume, irrespective of the rate of bleeding. Laboratory studies have demonstrated that plasma refill reaches 33% by 0.5 hour after hemorrhage, and 50% by 3 hours, allowing fairly rapid restoration of circulating blood volume.

Volume deficit or excess is a clinical diagnosis. *Volume deficit* is the most common fluid disorder in the surgical patient. Common disorders resulting in a loss of fluid that is isotonic with respect to extracellular fluid include vomiting, diarrhea, nasogastric suctioning, and gastrointestinal fistulae. Other causes include sequestration of fluids in soft tissue injuries and infections, intra-abdominal and retroperitoneal inflammation, intestinal obstruction, and burns. The signs and symptoms of volume deficit include, but are not limited to, altered mental status, hypotension, tachycardia, decreased skin turgor, and hypothermia. Oliguria secondary to renal hypoperfusion is also seen.

Volume excess may be iatrogenic or secondary to cirrhosis, renal failure, or congestive heart failure. Both plasma and interstitial volumes are increased. Signs include pulmonary edema and peripheral edema.

Alterations in Concentration

If water is added to or lost from the extracellular space, the concentration of osmotically active particles will change. Sodium represents approximately 90% of the osmotically active particles in the extracellular fluid. Therefore, changes in total body water are reflected by the sodium concentration. A change in the concentration of osmotically active particles will necessitate the movement of water from one compartment to another, so as to restore osmotic balance across membranes.

HYPONATREMIA. Hyponatremia (sodium <130 mEq/L) is associated with free water excess. Hyponatremia includes central nervous system signs of acutely increased intracranial pressure, and tissue edema. It is important to recognize that severe hyponatremia may be associated with oliguric renal failure, which may not be reversible if therapy is delayed. In the surgical patient, acute hyponatremia usually reflects one of two iatrogenic errors. The first is infusion or ingestion of a large volume of free water

Table 2–3	**Electrolyte Composition of Replacement Fluids**					
SOLUTION	pH	Na$^+$	Cl$^-$	K$^+$	Ca^{2+}	OTHER COMPONENTS
Lactate Ringer's (LR)	5	130	109	4	3	Lactate 28 mEq/L
NS	4	154	154	0	0	
D$_5$LR	5	130	109	4	3	Dextrose 50 g/L, lactate 28 mEq/L
D$_5$NS	4	154	154	0	0	Dextrose 50 g/L
D$_5$0.45NS	4	77	77	0	0	Dextrose 50 g/L
D$_5$0.25NS	4	34	34	0	0	Dextrose 50 g/L

Table
2–4 | **Replacement Fluids for the Management of Common Metabolic Disturbances**

SOURCE OF FLUID	METABOLIC DISTURBANCE	SUGGESTED REPLACEMENT
Gastric	Hypochloremic, hypokalemic metabolic alkalosis	D$_5$0.45NS with 20 mEq/L KCl
Pancreatic	Acidemia, hypoproteinemia	LR (bicarbonate may be supplemented in D$_5$ water)
Small bowel	Hypovolemia	LR
Colon (diarrhea)	Hypokalemic metabolic acidosis	D$_5$0.45NS with 20 mEq/L KCl

at a time when high levels of ADH inhibit compensatory diuresis. This is most common early in the postoperative period when there may be a high level of ADH in response to pain and anxiety. The second error is the use of hypotonic fluids to replace isotonic fluid losses. In the trauma patient with a head injury, hyponatremia may herald the development of SIADH, or the *syndrome of inappropriate ADH secretion*. The need for therapy depends on the severity of associated symptoms. Free water restriction can return sodium concentrations to normal. However, in selected cases, free water restriction is not adequate, and supplementation with salt-containing solutions is necessary to return serum sodium levels to normal.

HYPERNATREMIA. Hypernatremia (sodium >145 mEq/L) represents excessive free water loss, which can be extrarenal or renal in nature. Extrarenal free water loss can result from an increase in metabolism from any cause, particularly fever. Evaporative water loss, either through open wounds or through the administration of nonhumidified oxygen to hyperventilating patients (particularly those with a tracheostomy), can also result in dehydration and resultant hypernatremia. Hypernatremia can also be the result of increased renal water loss. High-output renal failure due to ischemia-reperfusion damage to the distal tubules and collecting ducts impairs water resorption. Additionally, the loss of central nervous system stimulation of ADH secretion, such as that which occurs following some severe head injuries, can impair water resorption (diabetes insipidus). Finally, high osmotic loads, due to the iatrogenic administration of mannitol, glycosuria from poorly controlled diabetes, or excess urea from high-nitrogen diets can result in osmotically driven diuresis and subsequent free water loss.

The treatment of hypernatremia is directed toward restoring normal osmolality of body fluids, but caution must be observed, because the central nervous system poorly tolerates overly vigorous adjustments in sodium concentration. The volume of free water needed to replace a patient's deficit should be calculated from the following formula, and then replaced over 2 to 3 days.

$$\text{Free water deficit} = (\text{total body water}) \times ([\text{Na}^+_{\text{patient}}] / [\text{Na}^+_{\text{normal}}]) - (\text{total body water})$$

Alterations in Composition

The concentration of most other ions in the extracellular space can change without affecting osmolarity. These rep-

resent changes only in composition, and do not cause fluid shifts. Of particular importance are the concentration changes that affect potassium and hydrogen ions, or the acid-base balance.

The normal intake of potassium per day is approximately 50 to 100 mEq, and in the absence of hypokalemia most of this intake is secreted in the urine. Approximately 98% of the potassium in the body is located in the intracellular compartment, at a concentration of 150 mEq/L. Although the amount of extracellular potassium is relatively small, normal potassium concentrations are critical for myocardial and neuromuscular functioning.

HYPOKALEMIA. Hypokalemia (<3.5 mEq/L) is one of the most common electrolyte abnormalities seen in postsurgical patients. This condition occurs via several mechanisms, including excessive renal secretion, movement of potassium intracellularly, prolonged administration of potassium-free intravenous solutions and nutrition with ongoing obligatory renal losses, and loss via increased gastrointestinal secretions, particularly colonic (i.e., diarrhea). Renal tubular excretion of potassium is increased when large volumes of sodium ions are available for resorption, via the normal cation exchange mechanisms of the kidney. After large isotonic volume replacement, potassium requirements are increased, probably through the aforementioned mechanism. Additionally, potassium is important in acid-base balance, as movement of potassium in or out of the cell occurs in response to the hydrogen ion concentration in the blood. There is net movement of potassium out of cells in alkalotic patients. Severe metabolic alkalosis may exacerbate hypokalemia, as the kidney will respond by increasing hydrogen ion resorption at the expense of potassium. Finally, excessive loss of gastrointestinal fluid can result in profound hypokalemia (see Table 2–1).

Signs and symptoms of hypokalemia include muscle weakness, paralytic ileus, and, if severe, cardiac dysrhythmias. Treatment of hypokalemia involves potassium replacement, although no more than 40 mEq/L of potassium may be added to intravenous fluids in the absence of electrocardiographic monitoring. Potassium replacement must be undertaken cautiously in patients with acute or chronic renal insufficiency.

HYPERKALEMIA. Hyperkalemia (>5.0 mEq/L) is rarely encountered in patients with normal renal function. Most factors in surgical patients that tend to affect potassium metabolism result in excess secretion and a tendency toward hypokalemia, except in the patient with abnormal renal function. Signs and symptoms of hyperkalemia include nausea, vomiting, intestinal colic, and diarrhea. Electrocardiographic abnormalities of mild to moderate hyperkalemia include peaked T waves. Cardiac dysrhythmias occur at concentrations of more than 7 mEq/L, and include atrial asystole, with subsequent ventricular tachycardia and/or fibrillation. Temporary suppression of myocardial irritation can be accomplished with the administration of 1 g of 10% calcium gluconate intravenously, as well as by the concomitant administration of glucose and insulin (50 g of glucose with 10 U of insulin intravenously), which will drive potassium intracellularly. Definitive treatment involves the use of cation exchange resins (Kayexalate) or hemodialysis, to remove potassium from the patient.

ACID-BASE BALANCE. The pH of normal body fluids is maintained within a narrow range of 7.37 to 7.42, which is necessary for maintenance of normal body functions. This regulation of pH occurs in the setting of a large daily production of both organic and inorganic acids by normal metabolism. The three regulatory mechanisms of acid-base metabolism are rapid buffering of acids by salts of weak acids (the bicarbonate buffer system), rapid elimination of acids via the lungs (expired CO_2), and slow elimination of acids by the kidneys (renal compensation).

The Henderson-Hasselbalch equation defines the pH of the extracellular space as a function of the ratio of bicarbonate salt to carbonic acid (which, in turn, is related to the partial pressure of carbon dioxide [PCO_2]). In simple terms, a ratio of 20:1 between bicarbonate and PCO_2 will result in a normal pH. This results in an efficient system of buffering. For example, when an acid is added to the system (metabolic acidosis), the concentration of bicarbonate decreases, lowering the numerator of the Henderson-Hasselbalch equation. Respiration will then rapidly increase, eliminating larger amounts of CO_2 with a subsequent decrease in the denominator of the equation, returning the ratio to 20:1. The reverse will occur if an alkali is added to the system. On the other hand, respiratory acidosis and alkalosis are produced by disturbances in ventilation, resulting in a 0.08 change in pH from normal values for each 10 mm Hg change in PCO_2. Compensation is primarily renal. In respiratory acidosis ($PCO_2 > 45$ mm Hg), chronic renal compensation results in a 3.5 mEq increase in HCO_3^- for each 10 mm Hg increase in PCO_2. Similarly, in respiratory alkalosis ($PCO_2 < 35$ mm Hg), renal compensation yields a 5.0 mEq decrease in HCO_3^- for each 10 mm Hg decrease in PCO_2.

Common abnormalities of acid-base metabolism and their causes are shown in Table 2–5.

Alterations in Distribution

Of particular importance is the decrease in circulating volume due to "third space" losses. Third space loss refers to fluid that extravasates into a compartment other than the intracellular or extracellular compartments. Classically, it is generally considered only in relation to patients with massive ascites, burns, bowel obstruction, peritonitis, and crush injuries. Inflammatory conditions of the abdomen and retroperitoneum, including pancreatitis, result in significant intraperitoneal fluid and bowel wall edema. However, the magnitude of fluid loss from these conditions can be difficult to appreciate without the realization that the peritoneum alone has a 1 m² surface area, so that a slight increase in thickness due to peritonitis will result in a functional loss of several liters of fluid. Similar large-volume losses occur with massive infections of the soft tissue, including necrotizing fasciitis, with burn wounds, and with severe crush injuries. Finally, systemic sepsis or SIRS can cause a diffuse capillary leak, with a resultant significant loss of intravascular volume into the interstitium. In all cases, volume resuscitation is the therapy of choice for restoring intravascular volume.

FLUID REPLACEMENT THERAPY

In surgical patients, fluids are used for either maintenance or resuscitation. Since the therapeutic goals of these two types of fluid are different, the composition of the fluids used for maintenance or resuscitation and the approaches to their administration are fundamentally different. Maintenance fluids supply the ongoing fluid and electrolyte requirements of the patient. These needs were covered in the section entitled Maintenance of Normal Fluid Balance. Resuscitative fluids, on the other hand, are administered to patients in hypovolemic shock and are used to replace existing fluid deficits, or ongoing abnormal fluid losses. Initial resuscitative fluids should be isotonic crystalloid solutions, including normal saline and/or lactated Ringer's. They should be administered in bolus form, starting with approximately 30 mL/kg or 2000 mL in an average-sized adult, or 20 mL/kg in a child.

Hypovolemia, or the loss of intravascular volume, re-

Table 2–5	Common Abnormalities of Acid-Base Metabolism			
ACID-BASE DISORDER	DEFECT	COMMON CAUSE	$HCO_3^{2-} = 20$ $H_2CO_3 = 1$	COMPENSATION
Metabolic acidosis	Acid gain or base loss	Lactate, diabetes, diarrhea, fistulae, azotemia	Decreased	Pulmonary (rapid)
Metabolic alkalosis	Base gain or acid loss	Vomiting, NG suction, diuretics	Increased	Pulmonary (rapid)
Respiratory acidosis	CO_2 retention (hypoventilation)	Sedation, COPD	Decreased	Renal (slow)
Respiratory alkalosis	Excessive CO_2 loss (hyperventilation)	Pain, agitation, mechanical ventilation	Increased	Renal (slow)

sults in inadequate perfusion to the tissues of the body, with a resultant inability of the patient's system to meet metabolic demands and remove metabolic wastes. The primary goal of resuscitation therefore is the restoration of normal tissue perfusion in the most expeditious way, through volume expansion. When one plans resuscitation, it is important to realize that administration of fluids containing glucose will result in hyperglycemia, with a resultant osmotic diuresis, and exacerbation of hypovolemia. Furthermore, as one often uses urine output as a measure of adequacy of visceral perfusion, an osmotic diuresis might be incorrectly viewed as adequate resuscitation, thereby prolonging the shock period. Therefore, isotonic crystalloid solutions without dextrose are the initial resuscitation fluid of choice.

Lactated Ringer's solution (LR) is isotonic, readily available, and inexpensive. Its administration does not aggravate any preexisting electrolyte abnormalities. Studies have demonstrated that LR administration does not worsen the lactic acidosis normally present in shock. As volume is restored, lactate is mobilized to the liver and metabolized into bicarbonate. Therefore, a mild metabolic alkalosis may occur 1 to 2 days following massive resuscitation with LR. Additionally, mild to moderate hyponatremia may be seen after resuscitation with LR, as LR has only 130 mEq/L of sodium.

Normal saline (NS) is also an effective resuscitation fluid, particularly in patients with head injuries in whom hyponatremia must be avoided. Hypernatremic, hyperchloremic metabolic acidosis is possible after massive resuscitation with NS, particularly in children and in patients with large burns or severe trauma.

Resuscitation with hypotonic fluids will dilute the intravascular space, resulting in a relatively higher osmotic pressure in the interstitial space. Because water diffuses freely across membranes, it is drawn into the interstitium. The goal of intravascular volume restoration will then be lost as interstitial edema results.

Inadequate restoration of circulating volume can lead to a cascade of related complications, including persistent acidosis, SIRS, multiple organ dysfunction syndrome (MODS), multiple organ failure syndrome (MOFS), and eventual death. The traditional resuscitation endpoints were the normalization of hemodynamic parameters, the restoration of adequate urine output (0.5 mL/kg per hour), and the return of a normal mental status. However, with the knowledge that hypoperfusion could exist with normotension, better markers of perfusion have been sought. Pulmonary artery catheter monitoring, and optimization of oxygen delivery and mixed venous oxygen saturations, have been demonstrated to improve outcome after major surgical procedures. Rapid normalization of base deficits in the patient during resuscitation from trauma has been associated with improved survival. Finally, as the splanchnic bed is the region earliest affected by hypoperfusion, measuring intramucosal pH with tonometry has gained popularity, with studies demonstra-

---

Pearls and Pitfalls

PEARLS

- Volume deficit is the most common fluid disorder in the surgical patient.
- Isotonic fluid losses are commonly due to vomiting, diarrhea, nasogastric suctioning, gastrointestinal fistulae, and sequestration of fluids in soft tissue injuries and infections.
- Following hemorrhage, there is movement of fluid and protein from the interstitium to the plasma, or "transcapillary plasma refill." This results in restoration of plasma volume and protein concentration, with reduced oxygen-carrying capacity due to a decrease in total red blood cell mass, i.e., normovolemic anemia.
- The primary goal of resuscitation therefore is the restoration of normal tissue perfusion in the most expeditious way, through volume expansion.

PITFALLS

- Inadequate restoration of circulating volume can lead to a cascade of related complications, including persistent acidosis, SIRS, MODS, MOFS, and eventual death.

---

ting improved outcome after restoration to a normal gastric pH. The ideal marker of adequate resuscitation remains elusive, but trends toward monitoring specific end-organ perfusion in the future may further improve resuscitative efforts.

Summary

The management of fluids and electrolytes remains vital to the maintenance of normal homeostasis. Disruption of homeostasis, whether by surgery, trauma, inflammation, or infection, requires early correction to prevent cell injury and death. Volume losses, particularly those of an acute nature, need to be replaced rapidly, so as to restore adequate perfusion. During resuscitation, it is necessary to monitor serum levels of important electrolytes, as they can change rapidly.

SELECTED READINGS

Drucker WR, Chadwick CDJ, Gann DS: Transcapillary refill in hemorrhage and shock. Arch Surg 116:1344, 1981.

Elliot DC: An evaluation of endpoints of resuscitation. J Am Coll Surg 187:536, 1998.

Henry S, Scalea TM: Resuscitation in the new millennium. Surg Clin North Am 79:1259, 1999.

Maynard N, Bihari D, Beale R, et al: Assessment of splanchnic oxygenation by gastric tonometry in patients with acute circulatory failure. JAMA 270:1203, 1993.

Porter JM, Ivatury RR: In search of the optimal end points of resuscitation in trauma patients: A review. J Trauma 44:908, 1998.

Shoemaker WC, Kram HB, Appel PL: Therapy of shock based on pathophysiology, monitoring and outcome prediction. Crit Care Med 18:S19, 1990.

Chapter 3

Nutritional Support in the Surgical Patient

John Alverdy

Nutritional management of the surgical patient requires a basic understanding of the balance between nutritional biochemistry and the body's response to injury and infection. While the care of the surgical patient is often a planned event that takes place in the monitored arena of the operating room, the victim of trauma or a postoperative complication is subject to a tissue-destroying, sudden stress complicated by microbial contamination. Although access to medical care and early detection of cancer have made the incidence of nutritional deficiencies attributable to chronic disease a less frequent occurrence, the decision to operate on a severely malnourished patient requires careful risk assessment. The safe practice of surgery requires a keen clinical sense of how the nutritional status of the patient may change rapidly through the course of surgical intervention, as well as the potential for surgical complications and infection to affect the chances of a good outcome. Although predictive equations and compulsory nutritional support have been used to compensate for the fallibility of the clinical nutritional assessment, there is little consensus on which patients should receive perioperative nutritional support. Lack of a clear demonstration of improved clinical outcome is the main reason that nutritional support is not advocated in all circumstances involving complex surgical procedures. Confounding the impact of nutritional support on outcome is the rapid development of techniques that reduce operative trauma, pain, and infection. As little as 15 years ago, a typical time to oral nutrition following a major pancreatic resection was 10 to 12 days, with mandatory nasogastric decompression until bowel function completely returned (i.e., flatus or bowel movement). Today, major pancreatic resections are performed without nasogastric tubes and patients are orally fed before the development of overt evidence of bowel function. As nutritional therapies have become more tailored to support the metabolic response to stress and infection, complicated operations are being performed with less stress to the host. While complex operations are performed with less tissue trauma and a faster recovery time, an aging population and more resistant bacteria continue to complicate these procedures. Therefore, a better understanding of the basic biology of surgical stress and its effects on the nutritional biochemistry of the host, coupled with new concepts of surgical nutrition, will permit a more rational approach to prescribing nutritional support to patients following major operative intervention, injury, or infection.

BODY COMPOSITION

The nonaqueous body mass is composed of bone, tendons, mineral mass, and adipose tissue. The remaining cellular mass, muscle, chest and abdominal organs, and skin and blood cells, together with the interstitial and intravascular volumes, make up the aqueous portion of the remaining body mass. Within the total cellular mass, total body water constitutes 55% to 60% of the total body mass. Total body water is distributed in the intracellular and extracellular spaces. The intracellular space makes up one third of the total body water, while the extracellular space constitutes the remaining two thirds. Following surgery, injury, or infection, fluid shifts from the extracellular space to the intracellular space as the result of dysregulation of, and energy deficits in, the Na^+,K^+-ATPase pump. Fluids accumulate in the skeletal muscle, adipose tissue, and skin from stress-induced fluid sequestration. Although this is often referred to as the "third space" phenomenon, there is no defined third space in the body. The transcellular space, cerebrospinal fluid, aqueous humor of the eyes, peritoneal and pleural fluid, joint space fluid, and bile are part of the extracellular space and, even following traumatic stress, make up only 3% to 5% of the extracellular fluid. Following injury or surgery, body mass dramatically changes and is determined by extent of injury, expansion of total body fluids, loss of fat mass, and loss of lean body mass. Thus, while total weight is increased, the functional metabolic unit of the body is decreased.

ENERGY METABOLISM

The metabolic machinery of the human body can sustain itself by using readily available fuel reserves. Fat, the largest fuel reserve in the body, contains 9 kcal/g, while protein, the next largest fuel reserve, has only 4 kcal/g. Fortunately, loss of fat mass has little immediate functional consequence to the host, while erosion of body protein from stress-induced proteolysis can result in a harmful loss of muscle function. Glycogen stores in the liver can provide glucose substrate immediately following starvation; however, only 1200 kcal are available before this reserve is depleted. Muscle glycogen is not immediately available because of a lack of enzymes that permit its mobilization. Carbohydrate (glucose), protein (amino acids), and lipids (fatty acids) are oxidized to provide energy, and their metabolism does this, however with the inefficient byproduct of heat. At least 50% of the work performed following oxidation of body fuels is lost as heat. When this occurs during an acute surgical problem, such as injury or infection, excess heat may be produced as thermoregulatory mechanisms are reset and body temperature rises. When injury and infection are combined, heat production is significant and may be beneficial. As endogenous body fuels are oxidized, fever acts to induce the expression of a number of cytoprotective proteins. It has been demonstrated that heat shock proteins protect intestinal epithelial cells from injury and aid in maintaining their barrier function. Similarly, inducible forms of heat shock proteins maintain endothelial cell integrity. Experiments in animals clearly demonstrate that exposure of animals to high temperatures, which induce heat shock protein expression, protects the animals from subsequent infection-related insults. Thus, the production of heat, which is metabolically expensive, may be an essential component of the response to surgical stress. On the other hand, the failure to account for heat production and loss may lead to an underestimation of the actual ongoing erosion of lean body mass, and the delivery of inadequate calories.

Mobilization of body fuel sources following surgical stress is an orchestrated process initiated and driven by the counter-regulatory hormone response characteristic of acute catabolic stress. The release of epinephrine, cortisol, and glucagon in response to surgical stress serves to mobilize fuels from their various sources to provide energy. If surgical stress is complicated by massive tissue necrosis or infection, the release of inflammatory cytokines is initiated. Glucagon promotes glycogenolysis and induces amino acids released from the breakdown of skeletal muscle to enter gluconeogenesis and produce glucose. Cortisol promotes the mobilization of amino acids from skeletal muscle and increased hepatic gluconeogenesis. Norepinephrine and epinephrine increase the metabolic rate and increase lipolysis. Epinephrine also activates hormone-sensitive lipase, which mediates fat mobilization from adipose tissue. Glucose oxidation, proteolysis, gluconeogenesis, and free fatty acid mobilization all are increased and driven by the magnitude of the hormonal response. At the same time, a paradoxical decrease in fuel utilization and clearance from the bloodstream can occur. Driven by the inflammatory arm of the catabolic response to stress, lipoprotein lipase expression in endothelial cells may be decreased and lipid clearance impaired. Hyperglycemia, as a result of epinephrine-induced insulin resistance, can occur. Negative nitrogen balance can become worse despite nitrogen and calorie loading. These same metabolic derangements can be produced in human volunteers following infusion of stress levels of counter-regulatory hormones. Human trials using the cytokine interleukin-2 (IL-2) as an antineoplastic agent demonstrate severe metabolic perturbations similar to those seen following injury and infection. While the catabolic effects of the counter-regulatory response may appear designed to mitigate against a successful outcome following injury and infection, extreme pathophysiologic states of stress can be successfully treated when properly supported by surgery, infection eradication, and nutritional support. Although the counter-regulatory response will continue to erode lean body mass and hence muscle function, the duration and magnitude of this response are attenuated and ultimately eliminated by the combination of surgical débridement, antibiotics, provision of exogenous nutrients, and host recovery.

CYTOKINES AND THE HOST RESPONSE TO SURGERY

Cytokines differ from classic hormones because, unlike hormones, they are not secreted as preformed molecules but, rather, are released after stimulation of gene transcription and translation. While specific hormonal mediators initiate the response to injury and infection in surgical patients via their release into the circulation and remote cellular effects, cytokines can function in classic autocrine and paracrine fashion and allow cell-to-cell communication.

Injury, be it elective surgery or traumatic injury, exerts a suppressive effect on immune function. Attenuation of the production of specific cytokines, such as those produced by T_H1 helper T lymphocytes, following surgery play a direct role in this observation. Impairment of the production of cytokines following surgery may predispose patients to infectious complications due to impaired cell-mediated immunity or macrophage function. Alternatively, overexpression of the cytokine response can result in sustained and inappropriate inflammation leading to multiple organ failure and death. Type 1 (T_H1) and type 2 (T_H2) helper T cells make up the repertoire of cytokine-mediated immunity against tissue trauma and microbial infection. A T_H1 response is observed in smaller injuries where cell-mediated and opsonizing antibody responses remain intact. A T_H2 response is seen with more severe injury and is less effective against microbial infection. Significant crosstalk between these cells occurs, as injury and infection require varying degrees of stimulation and attenuation of the response. Injury severity and microbial infection may act together or independently to activate the cytokine response. Each cytokine has been defined as having specific dependent and interdependent effects on the immune response. The responses can be cell-specific or can affect a number of cellular arms of immunity.

The counter-regulatory hormones can affect release of cytokines and in this way may play a significant role in their global regulation. For example, glucocorticoids stimulate the T_H2 response and decrease tumor necrosis factor-alpha (TNF-α) and IL-1. In healthy subjects, glucocorticoid administration can attenuate the cytokine response to infused endotoxin, resulting in dampening of the systemic inflammatory response. This effect may be mediated in part by the stimulation of IL-10 release. The administration of IL-10 to rats reduces the mortality from septic peritonitis. In this context, glucocorticoids may dampen systemic inflammation, yet their administration to septic patients may be ill advised, since they are associated with infectious complications in the long term. Attenuating inflammation with IL-10 in the short term, however, may offer some benefit to patients in whom the inflammatory response is causing end-organ damage, such as acute respiratory distress syndrome (ARDS), myocardial depression, hepatic insufficiency, and renal dysfunction. Whether the body maintains appropriate homeostasis through the course of critical illness depends not only on the nature and duration of the initiating insult but also on the development of intercurrent infection and the maintenance of appropriate nutritional therapy. Despite a large and growing list of studies that have measured plasma cytokines following surgical stress, there is no cytokine profile predictive of outcome. The finding that many cytokines have circulating soluble receptors that can bind to the cytokine agonist and counter-regulate their response, adds to the poor predictive value of plasma cytokines. Theses same soluble receptors can also function to transport the circulating cytokine to a remote cellular target, where the response can be amplified. Thus, plasma cytokine measurements alone may belie the plasma and tissue activity of these substances.

A critical question in the nutritional management of the critically ill therefore remains: Have nutritional strategies been developed that affect the cytokine network in a way that better supports homeostatic mechanisms and thus leads to improved outcome? Although no consensus on the "appropriate" cytokine response exists, certain nutrients and growth factors show promise in delivering such an effect. For example, the production of three cytokines, TNF-α, IL-1β, and IL-6, was greater for lipopolysaccharide-stimulated macrophages from mice fed a glutamine-enriched diet. Glutamine, a well-studied nutrient, has been shown to positively affect outcome in both animal experiments and human trials. Many of these cytokine responses have been demonstrated to be depressed following major surgical stress; thus, it is presumed that their increased production in response to specific nutrient manipulation is beneficial. Despite some compelling studies, the causal relationship between specific nutrient-enhanced cytokine responses and improved outcome remains undefined.

Arginine and fish oils have also been shown to increase the production of a number of cytokines in vitro and in vivo. Diets rich in glutamine, arginine, and fish oils administered to critically ill patients have been shown to result in improved outcome compared to more standard diets. While these studies remain controversial, the precise mechanism of their beneficial effects will require further study. Many of these nutrients, especially glutamine, have profound positive effects on nitrogen economy, and thus may be beneficial by their effects on the maintenance of nitrogen balance.

As mentioned, the catabolic response to stress is characterized by erosion of lean body mass and net negative nitrogen balance. If left untreated, this effect will necessarily negatively affect organ function. An alternative strategy for developing an opposing effect on the catabolic hormone response is via the use of anabolic hormones to abrogate negative nitrogen balance. The most potent of these agents, growth hormone, has been shown to be of significant benefit in animals models of sepsis and injury. The effects of growth hormone appear to act through the release of insulin-like growth factor type I (IGF-I). In parenterally fed animals, the co-administration of IGF-I resulted in increased protein synthesis and better nitrogen economy following catabolic stress. Yet, a recent prospective, placebo-controlled, double-blind, randomized trial of recombinant human growth hormone (rhGH) administered to critically ill patients demonstrated an *increase* (39% versus 20%) in mortality in patients receiving rhGH. These findings force a rethinking of our ability to pharmacologically manipulate the catabolic hormone response as opposed to the accepted approach of its support with exogenous nutrients.

INTESTINAL EPITHELIAL BARRIER DYSFUNCTION AND THE STRESS RESPONSE

As critical illness is prolonged and the intestinal microflora change from commensal to pathogenic, the intestinal tract may participate in the hypermetabolic response to stress by its failure to contain whole bacteria or their cytotoxic products. This state of enterogenic inflammation driven by the intestinal microflora may further accentuate the systemic inflammatory response. The factors that promote this process may include alterations in the intestinal microcirculation, ischemia-reperfusion injury to the intestine, bacterial overgrowth resulting from alterations in diet, intestinal stasis, antibiotic use, and finally alterations in local mucosal defense that occur from immunosuppressive pharmacotherapies, protein depletion, or total parenteral nutrition. Currently, it is postulated that the cumulative effects of these therapies alter intestinal epithelial barrier function significantly enough to permit bacteria or their proinflammatory macromolecular products to enter the systemic immune compartment and provoke inflammation. Most of the current support measures for critically ill patients (total parenteral nutrition, antibiotics, vasoactive pressor use, immunosuppression) have been shown to alter the function of the intestinal barrier to a wide variety of paracellular probes in animal models of injury and infection. Alterations in intestinal permeability correlate with the development of multiple organ failure and systemic inflammatory responses following traumatic injury. Whether loss of gut barrier function during catabolic stress is a cause or consequence of this process remains to be clarified.

NUTRITIONAL SUPPORT FOR PATIENTS UNDERGOING ELECTIVE SURGERY

The majority of patients undergoing elective surgery are adequately nourished. Operations that do not interfere with the normal consumption of food postoperatively do not require nutritional support. Operations that impose a period of no oral nutrition, such as major intestinal procedures, can be successfully managed for as long as 7 days with patients receiving 5% dextrose only. Even following major operations such as pancreatic resection, recent studies suggest that neither enteral nor parenteral nutrition administered postoperatively improves outcome compared with 5% dextrose alone. In fact, patients administered parenteral nutrition postoperatively had an infectious complication rate higher than that of the patients who received 5% dextrose alone. Many of the patients in this study required as many as 10 days before oral nutrition was adequate. Therefore, improvements in operative technique and patient care may obviate the need for postoperative nutritional support, even in the circumstance of major operations.

The decision to provide preoperative nutrition should

be considered only in patients in whom severe malnutrition is evident. The category of severe malnutrition includes patients who present with a decrease in body weight of at least 15% below their norm. Nutritional assessment parameters, such as transferrin, albumin, and cell-mediated immunity measured by skin reactivity to microbial antigens, may aid in determining whether preoperative nutritional support is necessary. A thorough history and physical examination incorporating skinfold thickness to estimate fat mass, a 24-hour urine collection to determine the creatinine-height index for estimating muscle mass, and skin hypersensitivity tests all aid in determining the body mass and immunologic reserve of the patient. Several prognostic nutritional indices incorporating these nutritional parameters have been developed and have been shown to be useful tools for predicting postoperative complications.

A logical progression to preoperative "normalization" of clinical nutritional assessment parameters using enteral or parenteral nutrition, however, has not been associated with improved outcome. The causes of this are multifactorial. First, enteral and parenteral nutrition interventions are costly, may require an invasive procedure, and are associated with infectious complications. The placement of feeding tubes can result in aspiration, small bowel obstruction, and infection. Parenteral nutrition requires a central venous catheter, which carries a significant risk of catheter-related sepsis. Furthermore, the use of chemically defined diets or parenteral nutrition does not maintain local mucosal or systemic immune function to the same degree as does the ingestion of regular food; therefore, the former may be less desirable. Finally, the delay of definitive surgical intervention may offset the benefits of preoperative nutritional therapies. Preoperative nutritional support in cancer patients may be somewhat problematic in those with a resectable malignancy, as nutritional therapy may benefit the tumor more than the host. Although animal studies do not substantiate the claim that tumors are "sinks" for certain exogenously administered nutrients, preoperative nutritional support in cancer patients should be reserved for extreme cases of malnutrition.

The total energy required postoperatively in elective surgery patients ranges from 25 to 30 kcal/kg body weight per day. A patient's total energy requirement is based on the basal metabolic rate (BMR), the degree of imposed stress from the surgical intervention, the underlying disease process (e.g., infection, tumor), and the amount of physical activity. Standard charts for age, sex, weight, and height are available. Nitrogen requirements range from 0.8 to 1.5 g/kg body weight per day in most cases. Nutritional support can be given 48 hours following operative intervention, since this represents a time in which the catabolic response to injury is most likely attenuated and exogenous nutrients are better utilized and preferred over endogenous fuel and protein sources. The goal of therapy should be positive nitrogen balance, not necessarily weight gain. Since fat can still be mobilized and utilized for energy, the goal of therapy should be to err on the side of lower amounts of total calories, rather than excess calories. Excess calories in the form of glucose can lead to hyperglycemia and excess carbon dioxide production, which may complicate postoperative recovery. Hyperglycemia can also result in the glycosylation of circulating immunoglobulins, thereby impairing their ability to bind complement and opsonize bacteria. Although it has been proposed that intravenous long-chain fatty acid administration is immunosuppressive, this hypothesis has yet to be definitively proved. Excessive fat administration, however, has the potential to result in lipidemia and thus could impair white blood cell function. Therefore, although the goal of nutritional therapy is to meet the energy and protein requirements of the body during accelerated nitrogen loss, as estimated by the global nutritional assessment, overfeeding has inherent harmful effects. The practice of underfeeding may, in fact, have some physiologic basis during the course of catabolic stress. Experiments performed in animals with experimental burn wound sepsis randomly assigned to receive 30% fewer calories or protein relative to their actual estimated requirements found a better survival rate than that of their normal-fed cohorts. Since the hallmark of catabolic stress is anorexia and erosion of lean body mass, slight underfeeding may be a more rational target than overfeeding when caloric needs are confounded by the complexity of a critically ill patient. Because permissive underfeeding is a provocative topic in the nutritional management of the critically ill, this strategy remains experimental at this time.

The route for feeding a postoperative patient is dictated by the functioning state of the gastrointestinal tract. Enteral alimentation is always the preferred route. Elemental diets, which require minimal digestive function, are nearly completely absorbed within the first few feet of small intestine. Therefore, enteral nutrition may be delivered in the postoperative patient with limited absorptive surface. Enteral access must be planned, and the techniques described include feeding jejunostomies, gastrojejunal tubes, and needle catheter jejunostomies. Since enteral nutrition can increase intestinal blood flow by as much as 40%, caution should be employed when one attempts to enterally feed patients with intestinal ischemia.

A rare phenomenon of jejunostomy feeding–induced intestinal necrosis has been described. The etiopathogenesis of this problem remains unclear. However, aggressive enteral nutrition given directly into the jejunum of elderly patients following major surgery of the upper intestinal tract may be complicated by full-thickness intestinal necrosis a few feet beyond the feeding point. This phenomenon is believed to be due not to arterial insufficiency but, rather, to a combination of bacterial overgrowth, local mucosal defense impairment, and alterations in the mucosal microcirculation.

When use of the enteral route is not possible, total parenteral nutrition (TPN) is used. Central venous feedings consisting of hypertonic glucose and amino acid solutions are administered through a catheter placed in the superior vena cava.

NUTRITIONAL MANAGEMENT OF THE PATIENT WITH TRAUMA, SEPSIS, OR BURN INJURY

Accumulating lines of evidence continue to emphasize the importance of early nutritional intervention in the patient following major traumatic injury, infection, and burn injury. Trauma and burn injury can be transformed from a surgically treatable disease to a complicated life-threatening problem when infection develops. The goal of early and aggressive nutritional intervention in trauma and burn injury is to preserve organ function and maintain immune homeostasis. The ultimate goal is to provide the patient with nutrients to heal injured tissue and resist microbial infection. Inappropriate nutritional therapies have the potential to adversely affect outcome if their nutrient composition is inadequate for maintenance of a functional immune system. Injury and infection present the greatest challenge to the clinician and necessitate that significant attention be dedicated to the composition and delivery of nutritional support. The delivery of such nutritional support may be particularly difficult, as the physiologic complexity of this patient population often results in the inability to deliver fuel sources (i.e., due to hyperglycemia-lipidemia), or numerous intervention and access issues that lead to the interruption of nutritional support.

The metabolic response to injury or infection is unique in that it has evolved as a orchestrated physiologic survival response with no expectation of exogenous nutrition. The metabolic pathways following injury or infection are intensely energy-demanding and favor the function of selected tissues while starving others. The metabolic response to injury is characterized by severe proteolysis of skeletal muscle, anorexia, splanchnic vasoconstriction, decreased intestinal absorption, catabolism of serum proteins of low biologic priority, and fever. Some nutrients such as iron are decreased in order to deprive iron-dependent bacteria (siderophores) and thus impede their proliferation. This effect is achieved in the acute phase by protein transferrin, which acts to bind free iron. Following a 50% burn injury, patients can have resting metabolic rates twice their basal values, and since many of these calories are mobilized by the breakdown of skeletal muscle, severe erosion of lean body mass and muscle dysfunction can occur.

The release of skeletal muscle protein following traumatic stress involves the efflux of two biologically important amino acids, alanine and glutamine. These two amino acids alone constitute one third of the amino acids released during traumatic stress. In addition to providing interorgan transfer of nitrogen, they also serve as oxidative fuels for the liver and intestinal tract. Glutamine is the preferred oxidative fuel for the intestinal epithelial cells and submucosal immune cells. Skeletal muscle release of glutamine results in its rapid uptake into the gastrointestinal tract, where it is converted to alanine and ammonia. Alanine is released into the portal system and participates in acute phase protein synthesis as well as acting as a gluconeogenic precursor. Glutamine uptake by the intestinal tract may be important for the maintenance of gut metabolism, immune function of the intestinal tract, and function of the epithelial barrier against bacteria and their toxins. Nutritional support enriched with glutamine maintains intestinal immune and barrier functions to a much greater degree than do standard solutions. Another important destination for skeletal muscle glutamine is the renal bed. Here, glutamine is deaminated and ammonium can accept protons to treat the imposed acid load of hypercatabolism.

The accelerated glutamine and alanine efflux from skeletal muscle due to surgical stress appears to be influenced by glucocorticoid release. As glutamine and alanine are consumed, the end result is the production of ammonia and urea. Nitrogen loss, the net effect of lost urea and ammonia, is the hallmark of the catabolic response to injury. The provision of amino acid formulations high in alanine and glutamine is nitrogen-sparing. The mechanisms of this effect may lie beyond their nitrogen content alone, and may result from the unique ability of these amino acids to preserve immune function and organ performance.

Catabolic stress may also dramatically affect fat metabolism. While fat stores may be abundant, lipolysis alone cannot meet the energy demands of tissue repair. In addition, gluconeogenesis continues despite fat mobilization or administration of exogenous fat. Therefore, proteolysis will continue even if fat mobilization and glucose administration are adequate, as long as the hormonal milieu of catabolism persists. The morbidly obese patient (>100 pounds above ideal body weight; body mass index > 40 kg/m^2) presents a more complicated problem.

General Formula for Nutritional Support of the Catabolically Stressed Patient

1. Determine the basal metabolic rate (BMR) using the Harris-Benedict equation normalized for age, sex, and body surface area, or assess BMR using indirect calorimetry that measures oxygen consumption per unit of time ($\dot{V}o_2$) and carbon dioxide consumption per unit of time ($\dot{V}co_2$).
2. Multiply the BMR by 1.25 to account for an increase in physical activity.
3. Multiply the BMR in step 2 by a factor commensurate with the severity of the catabolic stress: that is, major surgery, 0.1 to 0.25; multiple fractures, 0.15 to 0.30; sepsis, 0.5 to 0.6; major burns, up to 1.
4. Estimate protein needs by assuming that most patients need 1 to 2 g/kg per day.
5. Make the nutritional formulation so that the calorie-to-nitrogen ratio is 150:1.
6. Provide 70% of the calories as glucose and 30% as fat.
7. Evaluate calorie and nitrogen needs twice weekly by performing indirect calorimetry and calculating the nitrogen balance.
8. If the patient continues to erode lean body mass and has no appreciable change in visceral protein status (retinol-binding protein, transferrin, prealbumin), consider assessing nitrogen losses through wounds, fistula outputs, nasogastric tubes, and so forth.

CASE EXAMPLE

A 65-year-old obese (wt, 308 lb; ht, 5'2"; BMI, 56 kg/m^2), insulin-dependent diabetic female is brought to the emergency department with the acute onset of abdominal pain, fever, anorexia, and dyspnea. Vital signs on admission are pulse 124, respiratory rate 26, blood pressure 100/60, and temperature 39°C. Computed tomography (CT) of the abdomen reveals free-air and a large phlegmon in the sigmoid colon. Surgical exploration reveals a perforated diverticular abscess of the sigmoid colon with frank fecal peritonitis. The small intestine appears markedly dilated and inflamed, with serositis of the intestinal wall and exudate throughout segmental areas of the small bowel. Sigmoid resection is carried out, with oversewing of the distal rectal stump and an end-colostomy of the transverse colon (Hartmann's procedure). Because of the patient's marked obesity and the inflamed small intestine, there is reluctance to place a feeding jejunostomy. Instead, a gastrostomy is performed with a gastrojejunal tube fed into the proximal small bowel. The patient is periodically hypotensive during the procedure and requires vasoactive pharmacologic support to maintain her blood pressure. At the conclusion of the procedure, a central venous line for total parenteral nutrition is placed. Over the next 48 hours, intravenous fluids, vasoactive agents, and blood transfusions resuscitate the patient to a hemodynamically stable condition. Serum creatinine was 2.8 g/dL and the bilirubin was 7.2 mg/dL. The patient, however, was persistently tachycardic and febrile. Dopamine was necessary to maintain a blood pressure of 110/60. The abdomen was distended, and bowel sounds were absent.

Nutritional Support. At 48 hours postoperatively, a nutritional assessment was made. The history and physical examination demonstrated a severely stressed and ill-appearing female. A significant period of catabolic stress was anticipated, as was an indeterminate period of pressor and ventilator dependence. Using several estimates of energy expenditure and taking into account the adjusted body weight (80 kg), the practitioner estimated the energy expenditure to be 2800 kcal/day (Table 3–1). With the use of the ideal body weight for calculating protein, 120 g/day was calculated (2.0 g/kg per day). One third of the nonprotein calories were given as fat. The patient was fed via the parenteral route for the first

---

Table 3–1 | Predictive Equations for Estimating Energy Expenditure

Harris-Benedict

Men: 66.47 + 13.75 (W) + 5.0 (H) − 6.75 (A)
Women: 65.51 + 9.56 (W) + 1.85 (H) − 4.68 (A)
  W, weight (kg); H, height (cm); A, age (yr)

Ireton-Jones

  EEE (v) =
        1925 − 10 (A) + 5 (W) + 281 (S) + 292 (T) + 851 (B)

  EEE (s) = 629 − 11 (A) + 25 (W) − 609 (O)

v, ventilator; s, spontaneous breather; A, age (yr); W, weight (kg); S, sex (male = 1, female = 0); T, trauma (present = 1, absent = 0); B, burns (present = 1, absent = 0); O, obesity (present = 1, absent = 0); EEE, estimated energy expenditure.

Amato

  Energy expenditure = 21 kcal/kg (kg in actual weight)

Adjustment of Body Weight for Obesity

  Adjusted body weight =
        [(actual weight − ideal weight) × 0.25) + ideal weight]

Pearls and Pitfalls

Goals of Nutritional Support

PEARLS

- Identify patients early in the course of their illness who are at risk for postoperative malnutrition.
- Obtain appropriate enteral or parenteral access for nutritional support. Keep in mind that nasoenteric feeding tubes are often dislodged in patients on ventilatory support, and at best, only 60% of the daily goals of nutritional support are met when enteral access is not secure. Secure and sterilely placed central venous lines should be established for nutrition only.
- Use calculation of nitrogen balance and indirect calorimetry to evaluate the adequacy of nutritional support.
- Use the enteral route when possible.
- Dynamically assess visceral protein parameters (transferrin, retinol binding protein, prealbumin) and determine the efficacy of nutritional support.
- Consider specialized formulations of nutritional support rich in alanine, glutamine, or fish oils when nitrogen losses are excessive.

---

5 days, and thereafter 30 mL/hr of an elemental diet was administered via the jejunal portion of the gastrojejunostomy tube. At this time, the patient was no longer receiving any vasoactive agents, and a CT scan was performed and a pelvic abscess percutaneously drained. Over the next 5 days, the colostomy began to put out fluid, gas, and stool, and the patient's enteral feeding slowly replaced the parenteral nutrition.

Comment. Estimating the caloric needs of a catabolically stressed, morbidly obese patient can present a formidable challenge even to the experienced clinician. Indirect calorimetry is especially useful in this population, as formulary estimates are often imprecise. The perceived risk of underestimating caloric need, however, may be unwarranted. It should be noted that when obese, catabolically stressed patients are fed a hypocaloric diet, good outcome, wound healing, and improved plasma proteins can be achieved. Of course, this assumes adequate intake of nitrogen and micronutrients. These "protein-sparing modified fasts" promote the utilization of endogenous fat stores for energy while maintaining nitrogen balance. Although this approach is traditionally used in weight loss clinics, it is now being applied to morbidly obese hospitalized patients. This nutritional strategy can be especially useful when type 2 diabetes and hyperglycemia complicate nutritional management.

Enteral nutrition has been proposed as the preferred route of nutrition because of its well-documented enhancing effect on systemic and mucosal immunity. Animals randomized to enteral versus parenteral nutrition have a greater survival following 80% hepatectomy, intraperitoneal *Escherichia coli* challenge, steroid administration, and endotoxin challenge. Animals fed enterally also resist mucosal colonization, invasion, and translocation with commensal and pathogenic strains of bacteria. Experiments in animals suggest that the enteral presentation of nutrients stimulates the release of gut hormones that directly signal immune cells. This elaborate neuroendocrine immune system is most evolved in the intestinal tract, where the greatest numbers of endocrine and immune cells are found in the body. Parenteral nutrition does not stimulate these cells to function normally. However, "minimal enteral nutrition" can result in the release of these hormones, and so this partial measure may be beneficial when full enteral nutrition is not possible. Therefore, stimulating the gastrointestinal tract with minimal enteral nutrition may be important with regard to maintaining immune function in the critically ill. Caution should be used, however, when one aggressively attempts to feed a critically ill patient whose splanchnic circulation may be compromised by stasis, ischemia, or the use of vasoactive pressors. A syndrome of nonocclusive bowel necrosis due to jejunal feeding has been reported and occurs in the absence of any reliable clinical signs that signal its development. The incidence of this finding may be as high as 8.5% in some series. This problem is similar to necrotizing enterocolitis in newborns, and its etiology is probably due to a microvascular perfusion defect, an increased demand imposed by the prokinetic and blood flow effects of intraluminal nutrition, and luminal bacteria and toxins. Therefore, in critically ill patients with major cardiopulmonary instability, enteral nutrition should be cautiously initiated and slowly advanced.

SELECTED READINGS

Alverdy J, Stern E, Poticha S, et al: Cholecystokinin modulates mucosal immunoglobulin A function. Surgery 122:386, 1997.

Bessey PQ, Watters JM, Aoki TT, Wilmore DW: Combined hormonal infusion stimulates the metabolic response to injury. Ann Surg 200:264, 1984.

Bower RH, Cerra FB, Bershadsky B, et al: Early enteral administration of a formula (Impact) supplemented with arginine, nucleotides, and fish oil in intensive care unit patients: Results of a multicenter, prospective, randomized, clinical trial. Crit Care Med 23:436, 1995.

Brennan MF, Pisters PW, Posner M, et al: A prospective randomized trial of total parenteral nutrition after major pancreatic resection for malignancy. Ann Surg 220:436, 1994.

Choban PS, Burge JC, Scales D, Flancbaum L: Hypoenergetic nutrition support in hospitalized obese patients: A simplified method for clinical application. Am J Clin Nutr 66:546, 1997.

Dickerson R, Rosato E, Mullen J: Net protein anabolism with hypocaloric parenteral nutrition in obese stressed patients. Am J Clin Nutr 44:747, 1986.

Faries PL, Simon RJ, Martella AT, et al: Intestinal permeability correlates with severity of injury in trauma patients. J Trauma 44:1031, 1998.

Kudsk KA: Early enteral nutrition in surgical patients. Nutrition 14:541, 1998.

Lin E, Calvano SE, Lowry SF: Inflammatory cytokines and cell responses in surgery. Surgery 127:117, 2000.

Lucas A, Bloom SR, Aybskey-Greeb A: Gut hormones and "minimal enteral feeding." Act Pediatr Scand 75:719, 1986.

Marvin RG, McKinley BA, McQuiggan M, et al: Nonocclusive bowel necrosis occurring in critically ill trauma patients receiving enteral nutrition manifests no reliable clinical signs for early detection. Am J Surg 179:7, 2000.

Ribeiro SP, Villar J, Downey GP, et al: Sodium arsenite induces heat shock protein-72 kilodalton expression in the lungs and protects rats against sepsis. Crit Care Med 22:922, 1994.

Takala J, Ruokonen E, Webster NR, et al: Increased mortality associated with growth hormone treatment in critically ill adults. N Engl J Med 341:785, 1999.

Van der Poll T, Marchant A, Buurman WA, et al: Endogenous IL-10 protects mice from death during septic peritonitis. J Immunol 155:5397, 1995.

Chapter 4
Abnormal Bleeding and Coagulopathies

Dana Frazer and Mary C. McCarthy

Hemostasis is the process by which the body repairs vascular injuries, stops bleeding, and yet maintains blood in the fluid state within the vascular compartment. Hemostasis must be maintained. Any disturbance of this balance, either congenital or acquired, can lead to excessive bleeding or vascular thrombosis. It is important to the practicing general surgeon to have an understanding of these processes and to be able to evaluate patients with disruption of the normal hemostatic process.

NORMAL HEMOSTATIC PROCESS

The major systems involved in maintaining hemostasis include the vascular system, platelets, the coagulation system, and the fibrinolytic system. The minor systems include the kinin system, the serine protease inhibitors, and the complement system. These systems are intimately involved with one another in the maintenance of normal hemostasis.

The normal vascular response to injury includes vasoconstriction, diversion of blood flow around damaged areas, and contact activation of platelets followed by platelet aggregation. Normally, the smooth endothelial lining of the vascular system is inert and does not interact with platelets or coagulation factors. In the setting of injury, there is a disruption of the endothelial lining and exposure of the basement membrane and collagen. Interaction of the subendothelium and collagen with substances circulating in the bloodstream leads to activation of platelets and the coagulation system. Substances involved in this process include adenosine diphosphate, tissue thromboplastin, fibronectin, laminin, and von Willebrand factor. Coagulation factors then interact to form a fibrin clot. The purpose of the fibrin clot (secondary hemostasis) is to reinforce the platelet plug (primary hemostasis). This cascade of biochemical reactions can be segregated into intrinsic and extrinsic activation pathways, which share a common final pathway that leads to the generation of the enzyme thrombin, which converts fibrinogen to fibrin.

The coagulation system is in balance with the fibrinolytic system. Fibrinolysis represents enzymatic cleavage of the fibrin to soluble fragments, which are removed by reticuloendothelial system macrophages, reestablishing blood flow in occluded vessels.

PREOPERATIVE EVALUATION OF THE SURGICAL PATIENT

When one plans an operative procedure, an assessment of the risk of bleeding or thrombosis is essential. If an abnormality is found during the preoperative evaluation, appropriate treatment can be initiated.

The first step is a detailed past medical history. Questions should address easy bruising, prolonged bleeding after minor cuts or dental work, and any history of a bleeding disorder. The patient should also be asked about any history of vascular thrombosis. In women, the history of pregnancies and deliveries is important. A review of the family history is also pertinent, as many coagulation abnormalities are inherited. Drug history is another important aspect; a list of prescription and over-the-counter medications should be obtained. Herbal supplements and vitamins should also be explored. Aspirin use should be specifically addressed, as many patients do not consider this a drug, and it may significantly alter coagulation. If a patient is receiving anticoagulants or receiving a medication that would interfere with the normal hemostatic mechanisms, it may be necessary to discontinue these prior to the procedure.

A thorough physical examination should also be performed. Attention should be paid to stigmata of bleeding disorders, such as petechiae, mucocutaneous bleeding, and abnormal unexplained areas of ecchymosis.

Routine preoperative laboratory testing has declined as its cost-effectiveness has been questioned. If a bleeding disorder is suspected, testing should include a complete blood count (CBC), protime (PT), activated partial thromboplastin time (APTT), thrombin time (TT), platelet count, and a template bleeding time (TBT). The CBC may reveal anemia or may demonstrate an abnormality in red blood cell morphology. A platelet count is usually included in a CBC, and therefore quantitative platelet abnormalities will be detected. The PT measures the function of the extrinsic pathway of coagulation. The APTT is a test of the intrinsic pathway. Both the PT and the APTT will be prolonged with an abnormality of the shared factors of the common pathway. Thrombin time is a measure of the ability of thrombin to convert fibrinogen to fibrin. A TBT should be performed if abnormal platelet function is suspected. Interpretation of coagulation tests involves the identification of a pattern of abnormal studies and correlation with a disorder that could account for them.

If a coagulation disorder is suspected after the initial evaluation, more specific tests are indicated. These may include qualitative or quantitative testing for a factor deficiency and testing for inhibitors of clotting factors. Specific abnormalities of platelets can be assessed by a platelet aggregation study.

EVALUATION OF A BLEEDING PATIENT

Evaluation

A quick review of the patient's past and current medical history and family history is vital when bleeding is encountered in the operating room or when one is caring for a patient. It is also important to review local factors that may contribute to problems with hemostasis. These include patient temperature, medications, invasive devices, and nutrition.

When one performs a physical examination in a bleeding patient, attention should be turned to the nature of the bleeding as well as the location, the temporal sequence, and the relationship to any procedures or transfusions. The body temperature is crucial to maintenance of normal coagulation and hemostasis. The nature of the bleeding should be evaluated. Focal intraoperative bleeding may be addressed by mechanical means, whereas diffuse oozing from multiple sites is indicative of a defect in the hemostatic process.

Laboratory testing should include CBC with platelet count and morphology, PT, PTT, TT, and TBT. An interpretation scheme for evaluation of coagulation test results is presented in Table 4–1. If a bleeding disorder appears to be secondary to a specific factor, an assay for that factor should be performed.

Disorders of Hemostasis

There are many different congenital and acquired disorders of hemostasis. A disturbance of normal hemostasis may be attributed to vascular disorders, abnormalities in

Table 4–1	Interpretation of Coagulation Test Results	
TEST	**RESULTS**	**POSSIBLE CAUSE**
APTT	Abnormal	Vitamin K defect
PT	Abnormal	Liver disease
TT	Normal	Inhibitor present
		Factor deficiency in common pathway (X, V, II)
APTT	Abnormal	Factor deficiency in the intrinsic pathway (XII, XI, IX, VIII Fletcher, Fitzgerald)
PT	Normal	Lupus anticoagulant
		Specific factor inhibitor
APTT	Normal	Factor deficiency in the extrinsic pathway (VII)
PT	Abnormal	Specific factor inhibitor
APTT	Abnormal	Factor deficiency (I)
PT	Abnormal	Severe liver disease
TT	Abnormal	DIC
		Potent inhibitor
		Hypofibrinogenemia or dysfibrinogenemia
APTT	Abnormal	Factor deficiency (XIII)
PT	Normal	Specific factor inhibitor
TT	Normal	Normal patient or laboratory error

PT, prothrombin time; APTT, activated partial thromboplastin time; TT, thrombin time; DIC, disseminated intravascular coagulation.

Adapted from Harmening DM: Introduction to hemostasis. *In* Clinical Hematology and Fundamentals of Hemostasis, 3rd ed. Philadelphia, FA Davis, 1997.

platelet function, or a deficiency of or defect in specific coagulation factors.

Vascular System

The vascular system acts to prevent bleeding by vasoconstriction and activation of the coagulation system. Abnormalities in the structure or functional ability of the vasculature can lead to abnormal hemostasis. These problems can also be congenital or acquired. The congenital disorders are not common and are characterized by abnormalities in connective tissue and vessel wall matrix. The disorders in this class include hereditary hemorrhagic telangiectasia, Ehlers-Danlos syndrome, Marfan's syndrome, and osteogenesis imperfecta. The acquired disorders are characterized by the deposition of abnormal complexes on the endothelial surface, leading to impaired vascular function and increased permeability. These acquired disorders include paraproteinemias, amyloidosis, autoimmune disorders, presence of drugs, and infection. Treatment is aimed at the underlying disorder, with supportive care provided as necessary.

Platelets

Platelet disorders can be congenital or acquired. Congenital disorders of platelet function can be classified according to the mechanism of impaired function. These include disorders of adhesion, aggregation, and secretion. The most common disorder of adhesion is von Willebrand's disease. Von Willebrand's disease is an autosomal dominant disorder that is characterized by mucocutaneous bleeding. There can be qualitative or quantitative abnormalities. The primary biologic activity of von Willebrand's factor is platelet adhesion to the vessel wall. It is also a carrier protein for factor VIII:C. The clinical presentation of a patient with von Willebrand's disease can be varied, ranging from a vague history of easy bruising to a substantial history of unexplained bleeding. All subclassifications are characterized by an abnormal bleeding time. Treatment consists of replacement of von Willebrand's factor, which may be accomplished by the administration of Factor VIII concentrates, cryoprecipitate, or von Willebrand factor concentrates. Other congenital disorders of platelet function are seen less commonly and include disorders of platelet adhesion (Bernard-Soulier syndrome), disorders of platelet aggregation (Glanzmann's thrombasthenia and congenital afibrinogenemia), and disorders of platelet secretion, such as those seen in storage pool deficiencies.

Acquired platelet defects can be quantitative or qualitative. Thrombocytopenia may be secondary to decreased production, ineffective thrombopoiesis, increased destruction, or abnormal distribution. Qualitative defects, or impairment in platelet function, may be due to a number of disease states (Table 4–2).

Coagulation Factors

Coagulation factor deficiencies can be the result of decreased synthesis, production of abnormal molecules that

Table 4–2	**Acquired Disorders of Platelet Function**

Uremia
Dysproteinemias
Myeloproliferative disorders
Collagen vascular diseases
Acute leukemia and malignancy
Cardiopulmonary bypass
Liver disease
Acquired storage pool deficiencies
Disseminated intravascular coagulation
Drug therapy
Platelet antibodies

interfere with normal function of the coagulation cascade, loss or consumption of the coagulation factors, or inactivation of the factors by antibodies or inhibitors. The physiologic consequences of factor deficiencies may be a slowing of the coagulation process, delay in subsequent reaction steps, or prolongation of clot formation.

Malnutrition with vitamin K deficiency, hepatic failure with an inability to synthesize the normal coagulation factors, and impaired renal function with nephrotic syndrome and increased proteinuria all may result in coagulation problems. Treatment of the underlying condition as well as supportive care and replacement therapy will help restore normal hemostasis.

Congenital factor deficiencies can be varied in their mode of inheritance and presentation. Coagulation factor deficiencies are delineated in Table 4–3. The most common hereditary factor deficiency is factor VIII deficiency, hemophilia A. This is a sex-linked recessive disorder. The percentage of functionally active factor VIII determines the severity of the clinical presentation. The clinical manifestations include hemarthrosis, hematuria, intracranial bleeding, hematomas, and unexplained spontaneous hemorrhage. Treatment is directed at providing the patient with a functional level of factor VIII. This can be done by the administration of factor VIII concentrates or cryoprecipitate. Other congenital factor deficiencies are less common.

Disseminated Intravascular Coagulation

Disseminated intravascular coagulation (DIC) is a disease process characterized by an imbalance in the normal hemostatic and coagulation systems. In this disorder, the coagulation system is activated and the normal inhibitory mechanisms are overwhelmed and unable to keep the coagulation system in check. Consumption of clotting factors and platelets occurs, leading to microvascular thrombus formation. Once this system has been activated, secondary activation of the fibrinolytic system occurs, resulting in an imbalance in normal homeostatic mechanisms. DIC can be manifested as diffuse hemorrhage or vascular occlusion, or a mixture of both.

The stimulus for activation of this abnormal process is through one of three possible mechanisms: the first is release of tissue thromboplastin and subsequent activation of the extrinsic coagulation pathway (trauma, fat emboli, sepsis, hemolysis, placental abruption); the second is activation of the intrinsic pathway and factor XIIa formation (immune complex disease, hemolysis, liver disease, sepsis, burns, anoxia, vasculitis, acidosis); and the third is direct activation of factor II or X (snake venom, pancreatitis, liver disease, fat emboli syndrome).

The diagnosis of DIC can be difficult, as the presentation is variable. Once the condition is suspected, prompt diagnosis and treatment are imperative. Laboratory tests that may aid in the diagnosis include a prolonged PT, PTT, and TT, and decreased platelets and fibrinogen. Increased fibrin degradation products and D-dimers, as well as decreased levels of factors V and VIII, may also be seen.

The treatment of DIC should be directed at correction of the underlying cause and at provision of supportive care with blood component replacement therapy. This includes transfusion of packed red blood cells, platelet concentrates, fresh-frozen plasma, and cryoprecipitate.

Massive Transfusion

Coagulopathy is responsible for the majority of early trauma deaths. A vicious cycle develops with hemorrhage, multiple transfusions, core hypothermia, progressive metabolic acidosis, and the inability to establish hemostasis. The most common laboratory abnormality in patients receiving massive transfusion is thrombocytopenia. Prolonged PT and APTT are also typical findings. Prevention and early recognition are key in the prevention of further deterioration. Procedures should be terminated with correction of the underlying physiologic abnormalities and delayed definitive repair of injuries. Presumptive replacement of blood components, and practitioner recognition of ongoing coagulation factor dilution and consumption, is important.

EVALUATION OF THE PATIENT WITH THROMBOSIS

Evaluation

Evaluation of the patient with recurrent thrombosis should include a detailed medical history and evaluation of risk factors in addition to a detailed personal and family history of any thrombotic events. A general physical examination with detailed inspection of the extremities should be performed. Laboratory testing immediately following an acute thrombotic event is minimal. A baseline CBC, PT, and APTT should be obtained prior to initiating treatment of the thrombosis.

Congenital thrombotic disorders cannot be evaluated when the patient is suffering from an acute event. Recent pregnancy (within 1 to 2 months) or estrogen use also precludes testing. Warfarin must be discontinued 10 days prior to laboratory studies. Once all of these conditions have been met, more extensive evaluation can be completed. Appropriate laboratory testing would include a CBC, including platelet count and morphology, PT, PTT, activated protein C resistance levels, antigenic and functional levels of proteins C and S, and antithrombin III levels.

| Table 4–3 | **Factor Deficiencies** | | | |

FACTOR	DEFICIENCY	LABORATORY ABNORMALITY	CLINICAL ABNORMALITY
I	Afibrinogenemia (rare), autosomal recessive-homozygous	No clot formation, abnormal PT, APTT, TT; no fibrinogen	Umbilical stump bleeding, easy bruising, ecchymosis, gingival oozing, hematuria, poor wound healing
	Hypofibrinogenemia, autosomal recessive-heterozygous	Abnormal PT, APTT, TT; low fibrinogen	Mild bleeding, thrombotic episodes
	Dysfibrinogenemia, variable inheritance	Fibrinogen qualitative abnormal, quantitative normal	Possible hemorrhage, possible thrombosis, possible normal
II	Hypoprothrombinemia, autosomal recessive, very rare	Abnormal PT, APTT	Postoperative bleeding, epistaxis, menorrhagia, easy bruising
V	Parahemophilia, autosomal recessive	Abnormal PT, APTT, TBT	Epistaxis, menorrhagia, easy bruising
VII	Hypoproconvertinemia, incomplete autosomal recessive	Abnormal PT, normal APTT	Epistaxis, menorrhagia, cerebral hemorrhage
VIII	Hemophilia A (classic hemophilia), sex-linked, recessive	Abnormal APTT, normal PT, TBT	May be severe, moderate, mild spontaneous hemorrhage
Hemarthroses, crippling muscle hemorrhage, post-traumatic postoperative bleeding
	Von Willebrand's syndrome, variable inheritance, autosomal dominant, variable penetrance	Variable results, platelet studies, BT, APTT	Mucous membrane bleeding; superficial wound bleeding variable—depending on level of factor VIII:C
IX	Hemophilia B (Christmas disease), sex-linked recessive	Abnormal APTT, normal PT	Clinical picture similar to hemophilia A
X	Stuart-Prower defect, autosomal recessive	Abnormal PT, APTT	Menorrhagia, ecchymosis, CNS bleeding, excessive bleeding after childbirth
XI	Hemophilia C, incomplete autosomal recessive	Abnormal APTT, normal PT	Mild bleeding, bruising, epistaxis, retinal hemorrhage, menorrhagia
XII	Hageman trait (rare), autosomal recessive	Abnormal APTT, normal PT	Asymptomatic, rarely bleed, thrombosis
XIII	Factor XIII deficiency, autosomal recessive	Normal PT, APTT, clot soluble in urea	Umbilical cord bleeding, delayed wound healing
Minor injuries causing prolonged bleeding, fetal wastage, excessive fibrinolysis, male sterility, intracranial hemorrhage
PK	Prekallikrein (Fletcher factor), autosomal recessive	Abnormal APTT	Asymptomatic
HMWK	Fitzgerald factor deficiency (rare) Autosomal recessive	Abnormal APTT	Asymptomatic

PT, prothrombin time; APTT, activated partial thromboplastin time; TT, thrombin time; TBT, template bleeding time; DIC, disseminated intravascular coagulation.
Adapted from Pittiglio DH: Hemostasis overview. In Pittiglio DH, McMillan K, Otter J, Wright NE (eds): Treating Hemostatic Disorders: A Problem-Oriented Approach. Arlington, VA: American Association of Blood Banks, 1984, pp 28–29.

Hereditary Disorders of Thrombosis

Hereditary Antithrombin III Deficiency

Antithrombin III (AT III) is a naturally occurring inhibitor-regulator of coagulation. It is an α2-glycoprotein synthesized in the liver and endothelial cells. It acts by inactivating thrombin and other serine proteases (IXa, Xa, XIa, and XIIa). It is usually weakly reactive, but activation by heparin makes it a much stronger and more effective inhibitor. A deficiency in AT III can be either inherited or acquired.

Congenital AT III deficiency is an autosomal dominant disorder that can result in a quantitative or qualitative deficiency. Congenital deficiency of AT III is seen in 0.01% to 0.05% of the general population and 2% to 4%

of patients who present with venous thrombosis and no known risk factor. The deficiency is characterized by lower extremity venous thrombosis starting in the teenage years. Patients are initially treated with heparin, followed by long-term coumadin anticoagulation. The disorder should be suspected in patients who appear to be "heparin resistant." Adequate levels of AT III must be present for heparin to be effective. Administration of AT III or fresh-frozen plasma allows heparin therapy to be effective at normal doses.

The acquired form of AT III deficiency is seen most often with disorders of consumption (acute thrombosis and DIC) and in illnesses such as liver disease and nephrotic syndrome. In these instances, the deficiency can be attributed to depletion of normal AT III, decreased production and excess excretion. The treatment of these acquired deficiencies is best aimed at treatment of the underlying disorder.

Protein C Deficiency

Protein C is a vitamin K–dependent protein that is involved in the regulation and inhibition of the coagulation system. It is synthesized in the hepatocyte. It exerts its primary inhibitory activity by inactivating factors V and VIII:C. These are the two cofactors necessary for thrombin and factor Xa activation. The activity of protein C is inhibited by antithrombin and enhanced by protein S. There are congenital and acquired deficiencies of protein C. The congenital deficiency of protein C is an autosomal dominant disorder. It can be a quantitative or qualitative deficiency. Recurrent deep venous thrombosis or pulmonary embolism, most often beginning in the late teenage years, characterizes the disorder. As many as 75% of affected individuals have one or more thrombotic events. Treatment of patients with acute thrombosis is indicated, with initial anticoagulation with heparin and subsequent treatment with coumadin.

The acquired disorders are generally disorders of consumption, such as DIC, pulmonary embolism, and deep vein thrombosis. Protein C deficiency can also be seen in patients with liver disease and other systemic illnesses.

Activated Protein C Resistance—Factor V Leiden

Activated protein C resistance is the most common risk factor for venous thrombosis. The defect is due to a single point mutation in the factor V gene. The mutation causes synthesis of an abnormal molecule of factor V in which there is a substitution of glutamine for arginine (factor V Leiden). The result of this mutation is the impaired inactivation of factor V, and thus impaired inactivation of coagulation. The condition is usually characterized by venous thrombosis, but it can also be manifested as arterial thrombosis. The prevalence of the factor V Leiden mutation has been estimated to be as high as 15% in a general white population. It is relatively uncommon in other populations. Treatment of thrombosis with systemic anticoagulation is indicated.

Protein S Deficiency

Protein S is a vitamin K–dependent protein that is also involved in the regulation and inhibition of the coagulation system. It is synthesized in the hepatocyte and megakaryocyte. It exerts its primary inhibitory activity by acting as a cofactor for inactivation of plasma factor V and platelet factor V. It also serves as a cofactor for protein C enhancement. There are congenital and acquired deficiencies of protein S. The congenital deficiency of protein S is an autosomal dominant disorder. It can be a quantitative or qualitative deficiency. Its clinical manifestations are similar to those seen with deficiency of AT III and protein C. It can also precipitate warfarin-induced skin and fat necrosis. Acquired deficiencies are seen in pa-

tients placed on warfarin therapy. Therapy is directed at treatment of the thrombotic event.

Acquired Disorders of Thrombosis

Acquired disorders of thrombosis are varied. They can be associated with malignancy, pregnancy, major trauma, or drugs. They may also be secondary to antiphospholipid antibody syndrome. Antiphospholipid antibody syndrome is characterized by at least two of the following clinical problems: deep vein thrombosis, arterial occlusion, thrombocytopenia, hemolytic anemia, recurrent fetal loss, leg ulcers, and livedo reticularis in the absence of systemic lupus erythematosus or other connective tissue disorders. Laboratory evaluation of antiphospholipid antibody syndrome includes a coagulation test to identify a phospholipid dependent inhibitor of fibrin formation and a highly specific enzyme-linked immunosorbent assay (ELISA) for antiphospholipid antibody.

Heparin-Induced Thrombocytopenia

Heparin-induced thrombocytopenia (HIT) can be classified into two types. Type I is seen early after administration of heparin, usually within 48 hours. It produces mild thrombocytopenia (rarely $<100,000$ mm^3), and usually resolves completely even with continuation of heparin therapy. There are no documented major adverse effects. Type II is an immune-mediated disease characterized by clinical symptoms and heparin antibodies. It is characterized by a severe thrombocytopenia (usually $<100,000$ mm^3), typically occurring 4 to 14 delays after initiation of heparin therapy. It can even occur in patients receiving only low-dose heparin. The platelet count will not recover

---

Pearls and Pitfalls

PEARLS

- Effective hemostasis relies on the interaction of the vascular system, platelets, the coagulation system, and the fibrinolytic system.
- Aspirin use should always be specifically addressed in the patient's medical history.
- If a bleeding disorder is suspected, the preoperative laboratory evaluation should include a complete blood count (CBC) with platelet count, protime (PT), activated partial thromboplastin time (APTT), thrombin time (TT), and a template bleeding time (TBT).
- The most common disorder of platelet adhesion is von Willebrand's disease.
- Prevention and early recognition of coagulopathy in major trauma are key in preventing further deterioration.
- Thrombotic disorders should be assessed by ordering a CBC, including platelet count and morphology, PT, PTT, activated protein C resistance levels, antigenic and functional levels of protein C and S, and antithrombin III levels.
- Platelet counts should be monitored in all patients receiving heparin therapy.

unless heparin therapy is discontinued. A platelet antibody interacts with platelet factor IV and complexes with heparin, resulting in platelet activation, thromboxane synthesis, and release of platelet granules with platelet aggregation and thrombosis. The clinical diagnosis of HIT is based on the occurrence of thrombocytopenia during heparin therapy, resolution of thrombocytopenia after cessation of heparin, and exclusion of other causes. Major sequelae associated with HIT include venous thrombosis and arterial thrombosis. Laboratory diagnosis of HIT can be confirmed via a functional assay or an immunoassay.

Treatment consists of discontinuation of all heparin therapy, with the administration of an antithrombin compound. Recombinant hirudin, a medicinal leech–derived antithrombin, is the only currently approved treatment for HIT in the United States. It acts by inactivating thrombin. It is also capable of inactivating fibrin clot-bound thrombin, aiding in the dissolution of already formed clot.

SELECTED READINGS

Aiach M, Borgel D, Gaussem P, et al: Protein C and protein S deficiencies. Semin Hematol 34:205, 1997.

Bick RL, Kaplan H: Syndromes of thrombosis and hypercoagulability: Congenital and acquired causes of thrombosis. Med Clin North Am 82:409, 1998.

Caruana CC, Schwartz SL: Disorders of plasma clotting factors. In Harmening DM (ed): Clinical Hematology and Fundamentals of Hemostasis. Philadelphia, FA Davis, 1997, pp 531–546.

Chong BH, Eisbacher M: Pathophysiology and laboratory testing of heparin-induced thrombocytopenia. Semin Hematol 35:3, 1998.

Cosgriff N, Moore EE, Sauaia A, et al: Predicting life-threatening coagulopathy in the massively transfused trauma patient: Hypothermia and acidoses revisited. J Trauma 42:857, 1997.

Green RM: Treatment of heparin-induced thrombocytopenia and thrombosis. Semin Vasc Surg 9:284, 1996.

Harmening DM, Lemery LD: Introduction to hemostasis. In Harmening DM (ed): Clinical Hematology and Fundamentals of Hemostasis. Philadelphia, FA Davis, 1997, pp 481–507.

Jackson MR, Krishnamurti C, Aylesworth CA, Alving BM: Diagnosis of heparin-induced thrombocytopenia in the vascular surgery patient. Surgery 121:419, 1997.

Kelton JG: The clinical management of heparin-induced thrombocytopenia. Semin Hematol 36:17, 1999.

Lazarchick J, Kizer J: Interaction of the fibrinolytic, coagulation, and kinin systems and related pathology. In Harmening DM (ed): Clinical Hematology and Fundamentals of Hemostasis. Philadelphia, FA Davis, 1997, pp 554–564.

Thomas DP, Roberts HR: Hypercoagulablity in venous and arterial thrombosis. Ann Intern Med 126:638, 1997.

Van Cott EM, Laposata M: Laboratory evaluation of hypercoagulable states. Hematol Oncol Clin North Am 12:1141, 1998.

Warkentin TE: Clinical presentation of heparin induced thrombocytopenia. Semin Hematol 35:9, 1998.

Wyrick-Glatzel J: Quantitative and qualitative vascular and platelet disorders, both congenital and acquired. In Harmening DM (ed): Clinical Hematology and Fundamentals of Hemostasis. Philadelphia, FA Davis, 1997, pp 509–525.

Wyrick-Glatzel J: Quantitative and qualitative vascular and platelet disorders, both congenital and acquired. In Harmening DM (ed): Clinical Hematology and Fundamentals of Hemostasis. Philadelphia, FA Davis, 1997, pp 525–529.

Chapter 5

Blood Transfusions and Alternative Therapies

M. Margaret Knudson

Jean Baptiste Denis and his surgical colleague, Emmerez, are credited with performing the first transfusion into a human. In 1667, these two physicians transfused blood from a sheep into a 15-year-old boy who had been made anemic by several bleeds performed as treatment for fever. While this patient ultimately improved, two subsequent deaths were associated with transfusions between animals and humans, and criminal charges were brought against Denis. In April 1668, further transfusions in humans were forbidden unless approved by the Faculty of Medicine in Paris. The potential use of human blood transfusions was not considered until the 19th century. The blood groups were described by Landsteiner and others in 1900, but it took until World War II for blood transfusions to become a common practice. The ability to administer blood and blood products greatly expanded the scope of surgery, especially in the areas of trauma and cardiovascular surgery. It is estimated that 12.2 million red-cell units were transfused in the United States in 1986. Since that time, however, there has been a steady decrease in transfusion rates (11.4 million U in 1997), despite a growing and aging population. Among the many therapeutic factors contributing to this decline are auto-transfusion, hemodilution, erythropoietin, and asanguinous resuscitation fluids. Fears of disease transmission and subsequent blood shortages have reinforced the need for transfusion practices based on outcome measures and have resulted in a lowering of the "transfusion trigger." Finally, exciting new oxygen-carrying solutions are just entering the clinical arena, which will allow for safe and cost-effective transfusion practices in various settings, while reducing the need for blood collection centers, refrigerated storage units, and crossmatching.

INDICATIONS FOR BLOOD TRANSFUSIONS

Red Blood Cells

Although it is obvious that the patient who is bleeding rapidly requires resuscitation with red blood cells and other blood products until hemostasis can be obtained, other indications for transfusion in surgical patients are less clearly defined. In 1998, the Development Task Force of the College of American Pathologists published practice parameters for the use of red blood cell transfusions. These parameters were prepared to assist physicians in the use of red blood cells in the treatment of patients requiring an increase in oxygen delivery. Thus, the ideal method of detecting the patients in need of

transfusion would be to monitor systemic oxygen delivery–extraction ratios, systemic lactate production, or, even better, the partial pressure of oxygen in the tissue bed of interest. If these data are unavailable, heart rate and blood pressure measurements, coupled with the nature of the bleeding (active, controlled, uncontrolled), should guide transfusion therapy. In stable patients, a hemoglobin of 4.0 g/dL or less leads to significant lactate production and an oxygen extraction ratio of more than 50%. Therefore, the minimal hemoglobin level that should prompt transfusion in an otherwise stable patient is 6.0 g/dL. In patients undergoing surgery without risk factors for ischemia, a level of 8.0 g/dL seems to be a reasonable goal. However, because the risk of perioperative myocardial infarction increases significantly in elderly patients undergoing noncardiac surgery with hematocrits (Hcts) below 28%, the threshold of 10 g/dL may be more appropriate in these higher risk patients.

The need for careful evaluation of red-cell transfusion practices was brought to light in a recent report from the Canadian Critical Care Trials Group. In a prospective trial, 838 critically ill patients were randomly assigned to a restrictive transfusion policy (no transfusion unless the hemoglobin dropped below 7.0 g/dL) or to a more liberal protocol, where transfusions were given to maintain a hemoglobin level of 10.0 to 12.0 g/dL. This restrictive strategy leads to a relative decrease in the number of transfusions by 54%. While the overall 30-day mortalities in the two groups were similar, the mortality rate during hospitalization was significantly lower in the restrictive-strategy group. It is apparent, then, that the indications for transfusion must be individualized, and that there is no universal "trigger" which should prompt the call to the blood bank. In addition to the hemoglobin level, the physiologic status of the patient, including evidence of tissue hypoxia and symptoms of anemia, must also be considered. Several investigators have demonstrated that hospital-wide education programs, including monitoring of transfusion request forms for the indications for transfusion, can improve transfusion practices.

Component Therapy

The majority of surgical patients will require either no transfusions or a limited number of packed red blood cells only. However, for patients undergoing massive transfusion, plasma proteins and platelets must also be transfused, in order to maintain hemostasis. Ideally, the patient who is bleeding should receive fresh, warm, whole blood, but this is seldom available in the emergency situation. Instead, the majority of blood is collected with anticoagulant and rapidly separated into its components: packed red blood cells, platelets, plasma, cryoprecipitate, white blood cells, and concentrated clotting factors. Preoperative administration of concentrated clotting factors, cryoprecipitate, or platelets may be indicated in patients with inherited coagulation disorders (e.g., hemophilia A or B, von Willebrand's disease). In contrast, in patients with acquired coagulopathy, which typically involves multiple factor deficiencies as well as thrombocytopenia and platelet dysfunction, component therapy should be guided by *measured or observed defects* in clotting and platelet function. The properties of the various blood products are summarized as follows.

WHOLE BLOOD. Whole blood contains all the components of normal blood, including red cells, white cells, platelets, and plasma proteins. However, with cold storage, approximately 50% of the activity of labile factors V and VIII are lost within the first week, and platelet function is impaired within just 1 day. While whole blood is ideal for transfusion in patients with massive hemorrhage, the quantities of this substance are extremely limited in most blood banks. Recipients must be ABO identical.

RED BLOOD CELLS. Packed red blood cells are derived from a unit of fresh whole blood from which the platelets and plasma have been removed. The volume is usually 250 to 300 mL and the Hct 60% to 75%. ABO compatibility is required for each unit transfused.

PLATELETS. One unit of platelets is derived from a unit of fresh whole blood by centrifugation; platelets can be stored for up to 5 days at 24°C. Each unit provides 5×10^{10} platelets in 50 mL of plasma. For an average adult, 1 U of platelets provides an increase of 5 to 6×10^9/L. More typically, the platelets are collected from a single donor by plateletpheresis (thrombocytapheresis), yielding 300 mL of product. Transfusion of this platelet "sixpack" offers the advantage of single-donor exposure and results in a rise in platelet count of 30,000 to 60,000/μL. The typical lifespan of a platelet is 7 days, but longevity is dependent on a number factors, including consumption and splenic function. No crossmatch is required.

FRESH-FROZEN PLASMA. Fresh-frozen plasma (FFP) is collected from a unit of whole blood after the red cells and platelets have been removed; if the plasma is frozen within 6 hours of collection, it can be stored for as long as 1 year. The volume of each unit is 200 to 250 mL. Although all the clotting factors are contained in each unit, they are not concentrated. Therefore, restoration of a particular clotting factor with FFP alone will be limited to 20% to 30% of normal circulating levels. A typical initial dose is 10 to 15 mL/kg, with subsequent dosing guided by point-of-care monitoring of prothrombin time (PT) and partial thromboplastin time (PTT). Ideally, FFP should be ABO compatible. Thawing requires 30 to 45 minutes, so the need for FFP should be anticipated and the blood bank alerted early for patients requiring massive transfusion (e.g., one blood volume transfusion over 24 hours, or 10 U of blood).

CRYOPRECIPITATE. Cryoprecipitate is prepared by thawing a unit of FFP at 4°C. The precipitate contains high levels of fibrinogen, factor VIII, von Willebrand's factor, and factor XIII, making it the product of choice for the treatment of hypofibrinogenemia or of factor XIII deficiency. Because factor VIII concentrates undergo viral inactivation, these concentrates are preferred over cryoprecipitate for hemophilia A and von Willebrand's disease. Each unit of cryoprecipitate should increase the fibrinogen concentration by 5 to 7 mg/dL. No crossmatch is required. The guidelines for transfusion of cryoprecipitate and other blood products are summarized in Table 5–1.

Hemostatic Drugs

A number of agents have been introduced as therapy in patients with bleeding disorders and anemia, in order to decrease transfusion requirements. *Epsilon-aminocaproic acid (EACA)* is an analogue of lysine that is capable of inhibiting fibrinolysis by blocking the conversion of plasminogen to plasmin. This, in turn, will prolong the life of a formed clot. Patients undergoing cardiopulmonary bypass may be candidates for treatment with EACA, as postpump bleeding has been attributed to increased plasminogen activity. EACA has also been used in patients with von Willebrand's disease and with hemophilia who are undergoing minor surgical procedures. The dose is 4 to 5 g to load, followed by 1 g/hr. *Desmopressin acetate (DDAVP)* is an analogue of vasopressin that causes the release of von Willebrand's factor from vascular endothelial cells. Although facial flushing may occur, this synthetic preparation lacks vasoconstrictor activity. DDAVP is indicated in patients with mild hemophilia A, von Willebrand's disease, and other disorders of platelet function, such as uremia. The dose of 0.3 μg/kg can be given as a nasal spray or intravenously, but when given too rapidly can produce hypotension. *Estrogens* have been demon-

Table 5–1	Blood Component Therapy	
AGENT	**INDICATIONS**	
FFP	Active bleeding and PT >16 sec	
	Active bleeding and APTT >55 sec	
	Massive transfusion	
	Reverse warfarin anticoagulation	
	Liver disease	
Platelets	Count <50,000, and active bleeding	
	Prolonged bleeding time	
	Uremia–platelet dysfunction	
Cryoprecipitate	Fibrinogen levels <100 mg/dL	
	Von Willebrand's disease	
	Uremia	
Factor concentrates	VIII and IX (hemophilia A and B)	
DDAVP	Von Willebrand's disease (type I)	
	Factor VIII deficiency	
	Uremia	
EACA	Minor factor VIII deficiency	
	Thrombocytopenia	
Protamine	Reverse heparin	
Vitamin K	Reverse warfarin	
Estrogens	Uremia	
Aprotonin	Blood loss after cardiac surgery	

APTT, activated partial thromboplastin time; DDAVP, 1-deamino(8-D-arginine) vasopressin; EACA, epsilon-aminocaproic acid; FFP, fresh-frozen plasma; PT, prothrombin time.

strated to improve hemostasis in women with von Wille-brand's disease who were also taking oral contraceptives, and they have been observed to shorten bleeding time when administered to uremic patients. While the precise mechanism of action has not been clarified, estrogens can be given for a short period of time with few serious side effects. *Vitamin K* is essential for the function of clotting factors produced in the liver, particularly factors II, VII, IX, and X. Hospitalized patients who are poorly nour-ished, or patients receiving prolonged antibiotic therapy, are frequently vitamin K deficient. Administration of vita-min K partially reverses Coumadin-induced anticoagula-tion within 6 hours, and is the mainstay in the treatment of the coagulopathy produced by severe liver disease. A dose of 5 to 10 mg should be given intravenously slowly, in order to avoid hypotension.

Aprotinin is a serine protease inhibitor derived from bovine pancreas that acts to inhibit kallikrein and plasmin. Aprotinin also preserves platelet adhesion receptors, mak-ing it useful for bleeding patients who routinely take aspirin. The recommended test dose is 1 mL, followed by a loading dose of 200 mL administered over 20 minutes. Complications with the use of aprotinin include hypoten-sion during infusion, renal damage, and high cost. Its primary use among surgery patients is in the prevention of platelet dysfunction that is associated with cardiopul-monary bypass. When administered intraoperatively, this drug has been shown to reduce erythrocyte and platelet transfusion requirements in cardiac surgery patients.

Erythropoietin, a naturally occurring hormone synthe-sized in the kidneys, is a potent stimulus of red blood cell production. Recombinant human erythropoietin has been used to treat anemia in patients undergoing dialysis, and with cancer and human immunodeficiency virus (HIV) disease. More recently, it has been approved for use in the United States for patients donating blood preopera-tively. As such, it has been shown to be an effective alternative to allogeneic red-cell transfusion in patients undergoing orthopedic, urologic, cardiac, gynecologic, and colorectal surgery. The patients who appear to benefit the most are those whose initial Hct is 33% to 39% and who are anticipated to lose 1000 to 3000 mL during surgery. The recommended regimen is the administration of four weekly subcutaneous doses of erythropoietin, starting at 100 U/kg with an increase of as much as 600 U/kg as needed to produce a reticulocyte response. In general, stimulation of erythropoiesis is seen as an in-crease in the reticulocyte count by day 3 of treatment and the equivalent of 1 U of blood produced by day 7. Some authors have recommended adding iron therapy for maximal effect. The thrombotic events described with renal failure have not been seen with erythropoietin ther-apy in the surgical setting. Erythropoietin therapy may be most cost-effective when combined with the procurement of autologous blood by methods such as normovolemic hemodilution (see later).

RISKS OF BLOOD TRANSFUSIONS

The dangers of transfusions can be related either to the *quantity* of the blood transfused or to the *rate* of infusion.

The risks of disease transmission and immunosuppression are related to the volume of transfusion or, more cor-rectly, to the number of donors. On the other hand, overloading with citrate or potassium is related to the rate of infusion. Because the potentially fatal complica-tions that can result from a transfusion are numerous (Table 5–2), with the administration of *each unit* of blood or blood product, the surgeon must carefully consider the risks versus potential benefits to the patient.

Disease Transmission

The potential risks of disease transmission with each unit of blood are listed in Table 5–3. Patients are most fearful of contracting the HIV virus through transfusions, but surgeons know that the risk of getting hepatitis C is actually much greater. In actuality, the estimated risks of transfusion-transmitted diseases are lower now than ever before, owing to the intense screening of blood donors. The labeling of blood from paid donors beginning in 1972 and the implementation of third-generation screening tests for hepatitis B surface antigen in 1975 have resulted in a marked reduction in transfusion-transmitted hepatitis B virus (HBV) infection. Currently, HBV accounts for only about 10% of all cases of post-transfusion hepatitis. With the widespread vaccination programs that are now in effect, there will probably be a further reduction in hepatitis B. Similarly, although there is no vaccine for hepatitis C (non-A, non-B), when patients with risk fac-tors for HIV disease were excluded from the donor pool, particularly those with elevated alanine aminotransferase levels, the risk of contracting hepatitis C through transfu-sions was reduced. Still, each unit may carry a risk as high as 1/30,000. The seriousness of hepatitis C infection is appreciated when one considers that 85% of those infected will become chronic, 20% will develop cirrhosis, and 1% to 5% will develop hepatocellular carcinoma. The combined mortality from cirrhosis and hepatocellular carcinoma approaches 15%.

Since the implementation of HIV-antibody testing in March of 1985, only about 5 cases of transfusion-related HIV infection are reported to the Centers for Disease Control and Prevention (CDC) each year (as compared to 714 cases in 1984). In late 1995, blood banks began to test donors for p24 antigen as well. In screening 6 million potential donors for p24 antigens, only 2 people were identified who were p24 antigen positive while HIV-anti-

Table 5–2	**Complications of Transfusions**
	Disease transmission
	Transfusion reactions
	Immunomodulation
	Citrate toxicity
	Acid-base disturbances
	Electrolyte imbalance
	Hypothermia
	Pulmonary dysfunction
	Absorption of plasticizers
	Adenine toxicity
	Acute lung injury

Table 5–3	Risks of Blood Transfusions	
	RISKS OF CONTRACTING/PER UNIT	**DEATHS/MILLION UNITS**
Hepatitis A	1/1,000,000	0
Hepatitis B	1/30,000–1/250,000	0–0.14
Hepatitis C	1/30,000–1/150,000	0.5–17
HIV	1/200,000–1/2,000,000	0.5–5
HTLV-I and -II	1/250,000–1/2,000,000	0
Bacterial contamination		
Red cells	1/500,000	0.1–0.25
Platelets	1/12,000	21
Acute hemolytic reaction	1/250,000–1/1,000,000	0.67
Delayed reaction	1/1,000	0.4
Acute lung injury	1/5000	0.2

Adapted from Goodnough LT, Brecher ME, Kanter MH, AuBuchon JP: Transfusion medicine. N Engl J Med 340:438, 1999. Copyright 1999 Massachusetts Medical Society. All rights reserved.

body negative. Thus, the current risk of contracting HIV from a single unit of blood is estimated to be between 1/200,000 and 1/2,000,000!

Other organisms that are known to be transmitted via transfusion include cytomegalovirus (CMV), Epstein-Barr virus, and the human T-cell lymphotropic virus (HTLV-I and -II). Infection will develop in 20% to 60% of recipients of blood infected by HTLV-I or -II. Infection appears to be related to the length of time that the blood has been stored and to the number of white cells in the unit. Those infected can develop myelopathy, and one case of adult T-cell leukemia was reported after transfusion-acquired disease. Tests are now available for detecting both HTLV-I and HTLV-II in the blood of potential donors. In fact, the ability to detect viral contamination in donors has advanced to the point that death is as likely to occur after other transfusion-related complications (bacterial contamination, transfusion reactions, acute lung injury) as it is from a viral disease transmitted through transfusion.

Transfusion Reactions

Acute hemolytic transfusion reactions are the most common cause of death associated with a transfusion. Hemolytic reactions occur in the range of 1 in 250,000 to 1 in 1 million transfusions and result from the interaction of antibodies in the plasma of the recipient with antigens in the red cells of the donor. Approximately half of all deaths from acute hemolytic reactions are caused by ABO incompatibility as the result of administrative errors, and these errors almost always occur outside of the blood bank. Acute hemolytic transfusion reactions are manifested by the acute onset of fever, chills, flank pain, tachycardia, hypotension, rash or flush, and jaundice. Bleeding from intravenous or surgical sites may also occur. Oliguria and hemoglobinuria are also common. These signs and symptoms typically occur just after the transfusion has begun, but many of the signs may be masked by anesthesia. The treatment of a suspected acute hemolytic transfusion reaction is to immediately cease the transfusion and initiate resuscitation with crystalloid solutions. The bag of blood and all tubing, as well as a fresh sample of the patient's blood and urine, should be sent directly

to the blood bank for testing. A positive reaction to a direct antiglobulin (Coombs') test confirms a hemolytic reaction. In addition to fluid resuscitation, a forced diuresis may be induced with either furosemide or mannitol, and the urine alkalinized. The patient should be followed carefully for disorders in renal function, coagulation, and hemoglobin metabolism. The severity of the reaction is directly related to the amount of mismatched blood transfused.

Approximately 1 in 1000 patients has clinical manifestations of a delayed reaction to transfusion and 1 in 260,000 patients has an overt hemolytic reaction. A delayed transfusion reaction is also related to red blood cell antibodies, but these antibodies are typically not detected at the time of crossmatching. These types of reactions are more likely to occur in patients who have undergone a previous transfusion. The antibody titer develops over a course of hours or days after the transfusion, leading to the delayed development of fever, anemia, disseminated intravascular coagulation (DIC), jaundice, and renal failure. The diagnosis of delayed hemolytic transfusion reaction can be confirmed by repeat compatibility testing in conjunction with a positive direct antiglobulin test (Coombs'). While many of these delayed reactions will be mild, approximately 10% of all deaths due to red-cell transfusion are from delayed reactions.

Allergic reactions occur at a rate of 1 in every 100 U of blood transfused. Most of these reactions are mild and are manifested by pruritus, hives, or bronchospasm and are a reaction to infused plasma proteins. Treatment is symptomatic, and may include the administration of antihistamine. Febrile reactions are also common and usually mild. If fever develops following transfusion, a hemolytic reaction must be ruled out. Most febrile reactions result from bacterial contamination of the blood or from a reaction to transfused white blood cells contained in the unit of blood. Washing or filtering the red blood cell product may prevent febrile reactions.

Contamination of Blood Products

Yersinia enterocolitica is the organism most responsible for contamination of red blood cells, but other gram-negative organisms have also been implicated. The risk of bacterial contamination is directly related to the length of storage of the blood prior to infusion. Over a 9-year period, 20 recipients of *Yersinia*-infected blood were reported to the CDC and 12 of these patients died. The symptoms began during the transfusion and death occurred within 25 hours. When a recipient experiences fever, chills, or hypotension during a transfusion, the possibility of contamination should be considered. The patient's blood, the blood bag, and the filter should be cultured, and broad-spectrum antibiotics initiated. Contamination with *Yersinia* should also be considered when the color of the blood in the bag is darker than that in the tubing, owing to hemolysis and decreased oxygen supply. Platelets may also be contaminated, and the risk of infection is obviously greater when a patient receives pooled platelets from multiple donors, rather than a unit obtained by apheresis from a single donor. Organisms that have been responsible for deaths from contamination of platelets include *Staphylococcus aureus*, *Klebsiella pneumoniae*, *Serratia marcescens*, and *Staphylococcus epidermidis*. The clinical manifestations may be mild (e.g., fever only), but acute septic shock may also occur. Currently, there is no method of identifying contaminated blood products. However, in the future, the treatment of blood products with psoralens and ultraviolet light may render the products both sterile (including HIV virus free) and nonimmunogenic.

Metabolic Disturbances

When large volumes of blood are administered quickly (e.g., >12 U/24 hr or 1 U every 5 minutes), a number of metabolic disturbances may occur. The most common complication observed in patients receiving massive transfusions is hypothermia. Hypothermia may contribute to coagulopathy and can render the heart unresponsive to resuscitative measures. Red blood cells are stored at 1°C to 6°C, and should be warmed before infusions. However, warming above 45°C will cause hemolysis. To warm cells to the desired temperature of 37°C, infusion devices that expose the cells to a large surface of warming coil (e.g., Level I Technologies [Rockland, Mass]) should be utilized. Additionally, the patient's environment and other solutions must also be warmed.

Potassium tends to leak from red cells during storage, and at the end of allowable storage time each unit of blood carries an extra 4 to 8 mEq of potassium. Rapid transfusion of old blood into cold, acidotic patients can lead to hyperkalemia and even fatal cardiac arrest. Hypokalemia has also been reported following large-volume infusions. Therefore, both the electrocardiogram (ECG) and the potassium levels must be monitored in patients undergoing transfusion. Stored blood also becomes acidotic over time. However, most patients who are being rapidly transfused are actually more likely to be alkalotic, owing to the metabolism of citrate. Similarly, while hyperphosphatemia is a potential complication following massive transfusion, owing to the storage of red cells in phosphate solutions, most patients receiving large volumes of blood or fluids are actually more likely to have low serum phosphate levels. Ammonia levels also increase

in red cells during storage, and this ammonia load may be problematic in patients with liver failure.

Adenine is added to red cell preservative solutions in order to promote adenosine triphosphate (ATP) formation and thus increase the acceptable shelf-life of blood. After the blood is transfused, adenine is converted to uric acid, a potential renal toxin. Blood also contains a number of powerful inflammatory substances that normally remain inactivated. However, should activation occur during storage, transfused blood could produce further harm in an already compromised patient. Partial activation of some component of the coagulation, fibrinolytic, kallikrein, or complement system has been discovered in citrated plasma and in platelet concentrates. Interference with blood clotting and immunocompromise are potential complications that result from the infusion of these vasoactive substances.

Citrate is used as an anticoagulant during storage of red blood cells. For prevention of coagulation during storage, citrate concentrations must be high enough to bind almost all of the ionized calcium in the unit of blood. As a result, infusion of a unit of blood provides a solution that is calcium poor and gives a load of citrate that will readily bind to the ionized calcium in the recipient's serum. Animal studies have demonstrated that it is possible to infuse citrate rapidly enough to kill the recipient by lowering calcium below the critical level. The cardiac manifestations of hypocalcemia include ventricular fibrillation and decreased contractility. In order to maintain normal serum calcium levels, the recipient must be able to both metabolize citrate and mobilize calcium from other stores in the body. The rate of metabolism and excretion of citrate from the body is related to perfusion, body temperature, acid-base balance, and hepatic function, whereas restoration of serum calcium levels from skeletal stores requires the action of parathyroid hormone. The effects of parathyroid hormone are also related to perfusion, acid-base balance, and temperature. A warm, well-perfused adult can tolerate an infusion of 1 U of whole blood every 5 minutes without developing major problems with calcium. However, in patients given transfusions of blood at higher rates or who are cold or hypotensive, or have hepatic dysfunction, calcium levels must be carefully monitored, and replacement initiated when ionized calcium falls below 4.0 mg/dL (1 mmol/L).

Acute Lung Injury

Transfusion-related acute lung injury is manifested by dyspnea, hypoxia, and noncardiogenic pulmonary edema that occurs within 4 hours after transfusion. It is estimated to occur at least once in every 5000 transfusions, but it is likely to be underappreciated in critically ill or injured patients who already have some degree of pulmonary dysfunction. Pulmonary failure following massive transfusion was originally thought to be caused by the introduction of microemboli from the stored blood. However, the addition of a micropore filter to trap this microemboli was shown to have no effect on the incidence of pulmonary failure after transfusion, and instead it just prolongs the transfusion. More recently, reactive lipid products from donor blood-cell membranes that arise during storage have been implicated as the cause of transfusion-related acute lung injury. Such substances are capable of neutrophil priming, which in turn damages the endothelium of the pulmonary capillary beds. Another potential cause of this acute lung injury is the presence of antibodies from the donor interacting with host neutrophils and resulting in excessive permeability in the pulmonary microcirculation. Whatever the cause, with prompt recognition and early pulmonary support, most patients recover from transfusion-induced pulmonary dysfunction.

Immunosuppression

Transplant surgeons were among the first to recognize that blood transfusion leads to a persistent form of immunosuppression. Kidney transplant patients who were given blood transfusions prior to transplantation had improved graft survival compared to those who received no transfusions. Other studies suggested that oncology patients who were transfused during their surgical resection had worse outcomes than those patients not requiring blood products. Patients who had received transfusions had a higher than expected rate of cancer recurrence and a higher rate of postoperative infections. Similar studies in trauma and burn patients have demonstrated an association between the development of infection and multiorgan failure and the use of blood transfusions. The immunosuppressive effects have been attributed to the presence of leukocytes in the transfused products, with subsequent sensitization. Although the mechanism and the overall importance of transfusion-associated immunomodulation is still hotly debated, as always, it is prudent to avoid transfusion whenever possible.

ALTERNATIVES TO ALLOGENEIC TRANSFUSION

Autotransfusion

Given all the potential complications associated with allogeneic transfusion, a search for safer methods of transfusion is a high priority. A pamphlet distributed to preoperative patients in the state of California clearly states that, "The safest blood is your own. Use it whenever possible." The methods of autotransfusion can be conveniently divided into preoperative, intraoperative, and postoperative donations. Patients undergoing elective surgical procedures may choose to donate their own blood preoperatively. These patients must have baseline hemoglobin of 11 g/dL or higher and be free from contraindications such as coronary artery disease, pregnancy, and the extremes of age. A unit of blood can be donated every 4 to 7 days, with the last unit taken 3 days before the planned operative procedure. The latest data indicate that 1 of every 12 units in the United States is now donated before the surgical procedure. Unfortunately, as much as half of the predonated blood that is collected is discarded, primarily owing to overestimation of how much blood would be required for the individual patient. In addition, the process is costly: if the unit is not used, it must be discarded,

as the patient is not required to go through a "voluntary donor screening." Increasing pressures to decrease medical costs, the lack of reimbursement for preoperative autologous donations from some insurers, and the decreased likelihood of the transmission of viruses by the transfusion of allogeneic blood has led to a reevaluation of autologous donation. It has recently been shown that the risk of a transfusion-related complication is 12 times higher in patients receiving autologous blood than in those receiving voluntary donations by healthy individuals. The risk of ABO incompatibility (iatrogenic errors), hemolysis, and bacterial contamination are common to all transfusions, including autologous blood. Some ischemic events have been reported, and the patient who has been now rendered anemic may actual require more blood than he or she might have if preoperative collections were not performed. In one study, the preoperative donation of 2 U of blood before coronary artery bypass grafting was estimated to cost $500,000 per quality-adjusted life year (QALY). By comparison, most accepted medical and surgical interventions cost less than $50,000 per QALY. Taking all of these problems into consideration, autologous blood donation cannot be looked on as the best method of restoring oxygen-carrying capacity in the surgical patient.

Acute normovolemic hemodilution is a method of intraoperative autotransfusion. Just before the surgery begins, whole blood (approximately 1 L) is withdrawn from the patient and stored in standard blood bags in the operating room. The lost volume is replaced with asanguinous crystalloid or colloid solutions at a ratio of 3:1. After the major blood loss is over, the collected blood is re-infused. The value of hemodilution is that lowering of Hct reduces the loss of red blood cell volume during the procedure. Currently available data suggest that hemodilution compares favorably with autologous blood donation in patients undergoing total joint arthroplasty or radical prostatectomy. The advantages of hemodilution compared to preoperative autologous blood donation include a reduction in cost, in patient time invested, and in the potential for mistakes, as the blood does not leave the operating room.

Blood that is rapidly collected from the chest or abdomen during surgery can be processed and returned quickly to the patient. A number of re-infusion devices are available, but all involve anticoagulation, washing, concentrating, and storing blood for re-infusion. Some devices can return 3 U of blood within 9 minutes, and the returned blood is virtually free from plasma, clotting factors, and anticoagulant. Many of the higher-end machines require the presence of a technician for setup and collection, but the net savings of units of banked blood rapidly offset cost. This method of transfusion, however, is not free from complications (Table 5–4). The development of DIC from the re-infusion of activated products of coagulation and fibrinolysis rapidly offsets the benefits. This complication is more likely to occur if more than 1500 mL of blood is re-infused. Thrombocytopenia and hypofibrinogenemia also contribute to the coagulopathy associated with these devices. Deaths have been directly attributed to intraoperative blood recovery and re-infusion. Two studies performed in vascular patients found

Table 5–4	Complications Associated with Intraoperative Blood Salvage Techniques

Thrombocytopenia
Hypofibrinogenemia
Disseminated intravascular coagulation
Increased levels of plasma free hemoglobin
Sepsis
Air emboli
Tumor embolization
Particulate microemboli

Pearls and Pitfalls

PEARLS

- A risk-benefit analysis should be performed each time a transfusion of blood or a blood component is considered.
- Current methods of autotransfusion offer little benefit over allogeneic transfusion.
- Surgeons should be familiar with the various hemostatic drugs that can be utilized in surgical patients to decrease bleeding.
- The use of manufactured oxygen-carrying solutions will likely be most beneficial in the early management of the patient in shock.

that autotransfusion did not reduce the need for allogeneic blood transfusions. This method of transfusion may have its greatest value when blood supplies are limited (i.e., a difficult crossmatch), when blood is needed immediately, during mass casualties, or in patients who refuse allogeneic transfusions.

Blood collected from chest tubes after cardiothoracic surgery is the only situation where re-infusion of collected blood is practical in the postoperative setting. While authors disagree as to the effectiveness of this practice, what is clear is that the blood that is returned is defibrinated and partially hemolyzed. This sets the stage for the development of DIC. In trauma patients, it is the practice at UCSF to limit the re-infusion of chest-tube blood to no more than 2 L, to avoid coagulopathy.

Hypertonic Saline

Saline solutions containing 1.8% to 10% sodium chloride, usually combined with dextran or other anions, are collectively referred to as hypertonic saline solutions. The major advantage of hypertonic solutions is that the administration of a small volume can have the same hemodynamic effects as infusion of larger amounts of standard crystalloid solutions containing 0.9% NaCl. These solutions have been shown to improve cardiac function (a direct inotropic effect) and lower vascular resistance when used intraoperatively in patients undergoing aortic surgery. They have been used effectively in resuscitating burn patients and have been shown to decrease intracranial pressure. Prehospital administration of 250 mL of 7.5% sodium chloride in 6% dextran 70 hypertonic saline dextran (HSD) has been shown to be safe and effective in restoring blood pressure in injured patients, but a survival

benefit in these patients compared with patients resuscitated with the same volume of crystalloid solution could not be established. In a review of eight double-blind, randomized controlled trials of HSD, there appeared to be a trend toward improved survival in seven of the eight trials when 250 mL of HSD was administered in the prehospital setting to trauma patients. Further research in this area will probably define the patient most likely to benefit from hypertonic resuscitation.

HEMOGLOBIN-BASED OXYGEN CARRIERS

The ideal resuscitation fluid would be immediately available, universally compatible, capable of providing simultaneous replacement of both volume and oxygen-carrying capacity, and free from adverse effects such as transfusion reactions and disease transmission. While no such fluid is yet available for widespread clinical use, several hemoglobin-based oxygen carriers, which meet all the criteria of the ideal fluid, are now entering clinical trials.

The first attempt to provide a substitute for blood dates back to the 17th century, when Wren gave wine intravenously in an attempt to revive a dog! However, it was not until World War II, when it was realized that plasma expansion alone was not an adequate replacement for blood in the treatment of hemorrhagic shock, that the active search for a blood substitute was begun. Early efforts to administer a hemoglobin solution derived from the human red blood cell were fraught with unacceptable adverse effects, including the development of fever, gastrointestinal symptoms, flank pain, hypertension, and re-

Table 5–5	Characteristics of Currently Available HBOCs			
	NAME	**SOURCE**	**CLINICAL TRIALS**	**TOXICITY**
	DCLHb/Baxter	Expired human blood	Trauma/surgery	Vasoconstriction/GI
	RHb1.1/Somatogen	Recombinant engineered	Cardiac surgery	Vasoconstriction/GI
	HBOC-201/Biopure	Polymerized bovine Hb	Surgery/sickle crisis	Vasoconstriction
	Polyheme/Northfield	Expired human blood	Trauma/surgery	None?

GI, gastrointestinal; HBOCs, hemoglobin-based oxygen carriers.
Adapted from Ketcham EM, Cairns CB: Hemoglobin-based oxygen carriers: Development and clinical potential. Ann Emerg Med 33:326, 1999.

nal dysfunction. These side effects were eventually attributed to the dissociable tetrameric hemoglobin and the interaction of free hemoglobin with nitric oxide. More recently, several solutions have been developed that polymerize or cross-link hemoglobin derived from human or bovine sources, in order to both avoid the toxicity of the tetramer and decrease the oxygen affinity of these cell-free solutions. Additionally, polymerization increases the half-life of these solutions and reduces the glomerular filtration of the dissociated fragments of the hemoglobin (Hb) tetramer, thus essentially eliminating renal toxicity. Nonetheless, vasoactivity persists in many of these solutions, and this fact may limit the amount that can be transfused. The characteristics of the various hemoglobin-based oxygen-carrying (HBOC) solutions are summarized in Table 5–5.

SELECTED READINGS

Goodnough LT, Monk TG, Andriole GL: Erythropoietin therapy. N Engl J Med 336:933, 1997.

Goodnough LT, Brecher ME, Kanter MH, AuBuchon JP: Transfusion medicine (two parts). N Engl J Med 340:438–447 and 525–533, 1999.

Gould SA, Moore EE, Hoyt DB, et al: The first randomized trial of human polymerized hemoglobin as a blood substitute in acute trauma and emergent surgery. J Am Coll Surg 187:113, 1998.

Hebert PC, Wells G, Blajchman MA, et al: A multicenter, randomized, controlled clinical trial of transfusion requirements in critical care. N Engl J Med 340:409, 1999.

Humphries JE: Transfusion therapy in acquired coagulopathies. Hematol Oncol Clin North Am 8:1181, 1994.

Ketcham EM, Cairns CB: Hemoglobin-based oxygen carriers: Development and clinical potential. Ann Emerg Med 33:326, 1999.

Simon TL, Alverson DC, AuBuchon JP, et al: Practice parameters for the use of red blood cell transfusions: Developed by the Red Blood Cell Administration Practice Guideline Development Task Force of the College of American Pathologists. Arch Pathol Lab Med 122:130, 1998.

Chapter 6
Human Immunodeficiency Virus Infection

Jessica E. Gosnell, H.W. Harris, J. Jan, and William P. Schecter

INTRODUCTION

The surgical treatment of patients infected with human immunodeficiency virus (HIV) evokes powerful issues of science, ethics, and human behavior, largely because HIV infection confers a progressively debilitating and usually fatal illness on its victims. In the early stages of the acquired immunodeficiency syndrome (AIDS) epidemic, many surgical procedures (lymph node biopsy, exploratory laparotomy, open lung biopsy, brain biopsy) were performed for diagnostic purposes. As our understanding of the molecular virology and clinical manifestations of HIV infection improved, noninvasive and minimally invasive diagnostic procedures (helical computed tomography [CT] scans, fine-needle aspiration cytology, bronchoalveolar lavage, and transbronchial biopsy) reduced the necessity for open surgical procedures. The introduction of highly active antiretroviral therapy (HAART) in the mid-1990s, consisting of various combinations of protease inhibitors, combined with the routine use of sophisticated molecular biology techniques for measuring and serially monitoring the HIV viral load, has dramatically altered the efficacy of treatment of HIV. These strategies have converted AIDS from a devastating progressive illness with a usually lethal prognosis to a chronic disease, especially for patients with access to care by physicians experienced in the management of HIV.

Over the course of time, the epidemic, which was initially confined to the gay male population and patients receiving transfusion of blood products (hemophiliacs), has spread to heterosexuals, women of color, and parenteral drug users, challenging public health prevention measures and efforts to provide effective treatment to all patients. Worldwide, AIDS remains a devastating epidemic, particularly in developing countries. Most affected patients in the developing world have absolutely no access to effective treatment.

The following HIV-related issues affect the daily practice of surgery: (1) diagnostic evaluation of HIV-related opportunistic infections and neoplasia; (2) surgical treatment of the complications of HIV-related opportunistic infections and neoplasia; (3) provision of vascular access for long-term chemotherapy and/or hemodialysis in HIV-infected patients; (4) diagnostic evaluation and/or treatment of diseases or injuries in HIV-infected patients that are not related to the underlying HIV infection; (5) risk reduction strategies for perioperative transmission of HIV and other blood-borne infections; (6) treatment of health care workers who have had parenteral exposure to HIV-infected blood or body fluids; (7) assessment of operative risk in HIV-infected patients; and (8) the moral impera-

tive for physicians and surgeons to treat all patients, regardless of HIV infection status.

In this chapter, the authors discuss the evaluation and management of patients with abdominal pain and anorectal disease, and requirements for vascular access (issues 1 to 4), because general surgeons commonly encounter HIV-infected patients for these reasons. Then, issues 5 to 8 are discussed separately. Trauma is another common reason for the practitioner's encountering HIV-infected patients. Most of the issues relating to trauma are covered in the discussion of risk reduction strategies for perioperative HIV transmission.

ACUTE ABDOMINAL PAIN

CLINICAL PRESENTATION. Abdominal pain is a common complaint, with an estimated 30% to 90% of all patients with HIV disease reporting this symptom at some point during the course of their illness. Consequently, a large number of patients infected with HIV are evaluated by health care professionals for acute abdominal pain. In the majority of cases, the patients are not suffering from a surgical disease even though the pain can be quite severe and may be associated with mild peritonitis. Understanding the natural history of acute abdominal pain in patients with HIV disease is one of many critical elements necessary for their optimal management. LaRaja and colleagues' review (1989) of several published reports, involving a total of more than 2000 patients with AIDS, revealed that approximately 2% to 3% of these patients required emergent abdominal surgery.

Patients with HIV disease are subject to conditions that are either coincident with or unique to HIV infection. Consequently, when the clinician evaluates acute abdominal pain in an AIDS patient, the differential diagnosis must include not only common diseases such as acute appendicitis, peptic ulcers, diverticulitis, and adhesive obstruction of the small bowel, but also opportunistic enteric infection, ileus, organomegaly, pancreatitis, and retroperitoneal lymphadenopathy. For example, cytomegalovirus (CMV) infection of the intestinal tract may produce perforations of the small bowel and colon. Kaposi's sarcoma and lymphoma of the intestine can present as perforation, hemorrhage, or obstruction. To make an accurate and timely diagnosis, the surgeon must be methodical, thorough, and thoughtful; more than 95% of patients with abdominal pain will not require surgical therapy.

The history and physical examination are critical elements in the evaluation. A history of previous abdominal pain, diarrhea, fever, failure to thrive, prior opportunistic infections, or neoplasms, and knowledge of the patient's entire medical regimen, all must be incorporated into the evaluation process. A history of chronic diarrhea mixed with blood and mucus could indicate colitis. These symptoms, combined with abdominal pain and cramps, on the other hand, may suggest colitis with perforation. Signs and symptoms of gastrointestinal bleeding, such as hematemesis or melena, may be caused by ulceration or neoplasms (Kaposi's sarcoma). Earlier in the epidemic, a common cause of upper gastrointestinal bleeding with or without abdominal pain was Kaposi's sarcoma. Since the introduction of HAART, however, the number of cases of Kaposi's sarcoma have dramatically declined. Right upper quadrant pain (RUQP), associated with dark-colored urine and jaundice, suggests extrahepatic biliary tract obstruction. A history of shaking chills may indicate ascending cholangitis. Biliary stones might be the cause, but AIDS cholangiopathy resulting from CMV or cryptosporidiosis must also be considered. Other typically important components of the patient history may be less relevant in the patient with AIDS. Chronic anorexia, weight loss, nausea, and vomiting all may result from immunocompromise and/or medications. While the presence of fever is a classic sign of an acute abdomen, it may not be particularly helpful because many AIDS patients are chronically febrile.

The abdominal examination is undoubtedly the single most informative aspect of the physical examination. Even though the initial examination may not yield a definitive conclusion regarding the need for laparotomy, serial examinations in patients with HIV are invaluable to the experienced clinician. The performance of serial abdominal examinations, with the examiner searching for the presence and character of localized tenderness, guarding, direct and referred rebound tenderness, and shifting pain,

allows the surgeon to effectively monitor the evolution of the intra-abdominal process. This is important since regardless of the exact diagnosis, surgical diseases reliably progress, their physiologic manifestations intensifying, whereas nonsurgical diseases tend to remain static over time, if they do not resolve altogether. In addition, physical findings may guide further diagnostic modalities (Fig. 6–1). The presence of organomegaly must not be overlooked, as it may suggest a nonsurgical cause of the pain, presumably owing to the organ's increased volume stretching the overlying capsule. Definitive evidence of peritonitis, however, should be considered an absolute indication for at least exploratory laparoscopy, if not laparotomy. The patient cannot afford to have this frequently life-threatening finding dismissed as the result of his or her underlying chronic condition.

The use of laboratory tests in the evaluation of acute abdominal pain in patients with HIV disease must be, just as the patient's physical examination, tempered by an appreciation for the complexity of the viral infection. A complete blood count (CBC) and liver function tests are a routine part of the evaluation of the acute abdomen. While these tests are often helpful, the surgeon must recognize that HIV-infected patients with acute surgical conditions can have relatively low white blood cell counts, probably reflecting immune suppression. The kidney, ureter, and bladder (KUB) and upright chest x-ray examinations are also important components of the evaluation. If an abdominal film reveals the presence of free intraperitoneal air, this finding, like the presence of frank peritoneal signs, should be considered an absolute indication for an invasive investigation of the abdomen. In addition, the chest x-ray film may reveal pulmonary infection or neoplasia that can be manifested as abdominal symptoms and signs. In general, in the absence of definitive signs of

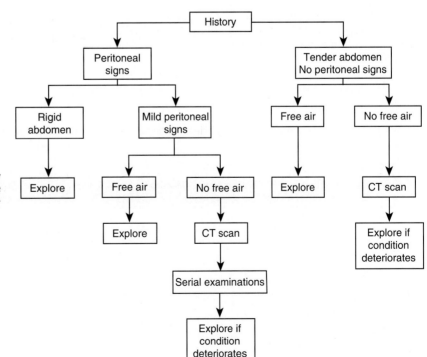

Figure 6–1. Evaluation of hemodynamically stable patients who have HIV disease with acute abdominal pain. Most AIDS patients with abdominal complaints do not require surgery.

peritonitis, hemorrhage, or free air under the diaphragm, few AIDS patients should be taken directly to the operating room until further radiographic evidence has been obtained.

ROLE OF CT SCAN. In patients with HIV disease, CT scan evaluation of the acute abdomen is extremely useful, especially when the history or physical examination are inconclusive. The CT scan often identifies the pathology, and may lead to the diagnosis of a nonsurgical etiology of abdominal pain, thus avoiding an unnecessary celiotomy. Provided that the patient is physiologically stable, this radiographic modality can be used to identify and characterize the pathology and to guide therapy (see Fig. 6–1). Compared with sonography or contrast-enhanced studies, CT is clearly the noninvasive examination of choice because it yields information regarding the entire abdomen and pelvis, including the viscera, vasculature, retroperitoneum, and lymph nodes. Intestinal perforation, bowel obstruction, and intra-abdominal abscess are conditions that present as an acute abdomen. Each of these entities, regardless of etiology, can be accurately diagnosed by CT scan. Plain films of the abdomen and lower chest are the usual tests performed to identify free air within the peritoneal cavity. However, CT is superior to plain films in this regard because it (1) is a more sensitive technique, capable of detecting much smaller collections of air than plain films; (2) can simultaneously demonstrate associated abscess formation or phlegmonous response to the diseased area; (3) can identify additional signs of intraperitoneal pathology, such as pneumatosis intestinalis, portal venous air, or peri-intestinal mass lesions; (4) can identify the presence, level, and cause of bowel obstructions; and (5) provides specific anatomic localization of the pathology, which is information that can direct both open and percutaneous surgical intervention.

In addition to providing data to confirm the need for surgery, abdominal CT can also identify nonsurgical conditions and thus prevent unnecessary laparotomy. For example, approximately 10% of patients with AIDS nationwide are also infected with tuberculosis. It is estimated that more than 70% of these patients have disseminated and extrapulmonary disease, including gastrointestinal tuberculosis. Since 90% of mycobacterial infections of the intestine involve the ileocecal region, this medically treatable condition can readily masquerade as acute appendicitis or colitis and thus precipitate unnecessary surgery.

PERIOPERATIVE MANAGEMENT AND RESULTS OF SURGERY. The pathologic conditions that require emergency laparotomy generally present with evidence of peritonitis, perforation, obstruction, or hemorrhage. The benefit of early diagnosis and treatment is relevant for all patients with surgical disease regardless of HIV infection. However, immunocompromised patients frequently present with fewer and less dramatic physical findings, often contributing to a delay in diagnosis. Numerous studies have shown that emergency surgery is associated with more complications and a higher mortality rate than are elective procedures, further highlighting the value of early versus late intervention. Therefore, expedient evaluation and decision making is of vital importance in the management of surgical problems in patients with HIV disease.

The authors recently reviewed the collected data from six published series on emergency surgery in patients with AIDS to better determine these patients' (1) clinical presentation, (2) most frequent diagnoses at surgery, and (3) overall morbidity and mortality rates following surgical intervention. The data in Tables 6–1 and 6–2 summarize the results of surgery in a total of 165 patients (147 men) reported between 1989 and 1995. More than one third of patients who underwent emergency surgery were thought to have acute appendicitis (35%), with intestinal perforation (13%) and peritonitis (13%) the next most frequent indications for laparotomy. As discussed, the presence of localized or diffuse peritoneal findings on examination or pneumoperitoneum were sufficient indications for surgery. Acute appendicitis (29%) was diagnosed at surgery in approximately one third of cases. Complications from lymphoma, Kaposi's sarcoma, CMV infection, and mycobacterial involvement of the intestine accounted for another one third of cases, presenting as pain, perforation, hemorrhage, or obstruction. The remaining patients suffered from peptic ulcer disease (6%), cholecystitis (3%), and a cornucopia of less frequent diagnoses, such as ruptured ovarian cysts, intestinal volvulus, and pancreatitis. Three percent of patients underwent a negative exploratory laparotomy.

ANORECTAL SURGERY

CLINICAL PRESENTATION. Anorectal disease in HIV-infected patients is common. In Burke and colleagues' review (1991) of seropositive patients, 33% had anal and rectal complaints. Miles and associates' review (1990)

Table 6–1	Clinical Presentation for Patients with AIDS Who Underwent Emergency Laparotomy		
CLINICAL DIAGNOSIS/ REASON TO OPERATE	**RANK ORDER**	**NO. OF CASES**	**% OF TOTAL CASES**
Acute appendicitis	1	58	35.2
Intestinal perforation	2	22	13.3
Peritonitis	3	21	12.7
Bowel obstruction	4	16	9.7
Hemorrhage	5	15	9.1
RUQ abdominal pain	5	15	9.1
Unknown	7	11	6.7
Toxic megacolon	8	7	4.2
TOTALS		165	100

Table 6–2	Pathologic Diagnoses, Morbidity, and Mortality in Patients with AIDS Who Underwent Emergency Laparotomy

PATHOLOGIC DIAGNOSIS	RANK ORDER	NO. OF CASES	% OF TOTAL CASES	MORBIDITY	MORTALITY
Acute appendicitis	1	48	29.1	—	—
Other	2	39°	23.6	—	—
Intestinal lymphoma or Kaposi's sarcoma	3	19	11.5	—	—
Colitis	4	16	9.7	—	—
Intestinal perforation	5	13	7.9	—	—
Mycobacterial infection	6	11	6.7	—	—
Peptic ulcer disease	7	9	5.5	—	—
Negative laparotomy	8	5	3.0	—	—
Cholecystitis	8	5	3.0	—	—
TOTALS		165	100	56/133 (42.1%)	42/165 (25.5%)

°Includes two or less cases of ruptured ovarian cysts, abdominal traumas, intestinal volvulus, adenocarcinoma of the small bowel, pancreatitis, diverticulitis, and so forth.

reported anorectal disease as the most common reason for surgical referral, accounting for 5.9% of the 1090 HIV-infected patients seen for management of their HIV disease. Patients most commonly present with anorectal pain, mucopurulent discharge, diarrhea, bleeding, or masses. Of symptomatic patients, Wexner and co-workers (1986) estimated that 50% to 80% will require surgery. Common diagnoses range from indolent, minimally symptomatic lesions, such as hemorrhoids and anal fissures, to rapidly growing, debilitating neoplasms of the anal canal. While the management of many common anorectal problems can be straightforward, there are several factors that must be taken into consideration in patients with HIV. First, the perianal region is often at increased risk for local trauma in individuals practicing anoreceptive intercourse, leading to a decrease in normal protective barriers of the perianal region, and subsequent increased susceptibility to infectious pathogens. Second, it is critical to remember that patients with AIDS are at significant risk for the development of anorectal cancer. Sexually transmitted human papillomavirus infection (HPV) of the anorectum is very common in gay men. HPV presents as a spectrum of disease ranging from asymptomatic dysplasia to condylomas, carcinoma in situ, and invasive squamous cell carcinoma. All gay men practicing anoreceptive intercourse should be screened for anorectal HPV and followed carefully to promote the timely detection and treatment of squamous cell carcinoma.

The evaluation of HIV-infected patients with complaints referable to the anorectum can be complex, as the differential diagnosis must include the entities responsible for anorectal problems in uninfected patients, such as fistulas and hemorrhoids, in addition to the entities unique to those infected with HIV, such as Kaposi's sarcoma and lymphoma. Again, a careful history is a critical component of the initial evaluation. A history of chronic diarrhea mixed with blood and mucus could indicate colitis, proctitis, or disruption of the sphincter mechanism. Anorectal pain or tenesmus often suggests the presence of an anal fissure. Perianal masses can be attributed to hemorrhoids, anal condyloma, lymphoma, Kaposi's sar-

coma, or cancer of the anal canal. Signs and symptoms of systemic infection may indicate an infectious etiology.

Careful physical examination, anoscopy, and sigmoidoscopy can correctly diagnose most anorectal diseases. Rectal swabs are also important, as they can identify bacteria, viruses, and ova or parasites. The importance of biopsy in the work-up for anorectal disease cannot be overemphasized. Referral to a general surgeon for hemorrhoids or for anal condylomas can instigate knee-jerk treatment regimens, when in fact the patient may be harboring a malignancy or indolent infection. In general terms, long-term treatment for a presumably benign condition should be undertaken only when the diagnosis has been certified by histologic examination.

PERIOPERATIVE MANAGEMENT. Management guidelines for anorectal problems are predicated on the specific diagnosis and the functional status of the patient. In general, suggested guidelines are similar to those employed in seronegative individuals. It should be noted, however, that for both HIV-infected and non–HIV-infected individuals, there are few randomized, prospective data with which to standardize treatment.

Most commonly encountered diseases of the anorectum can be managed in the outpatient clinic. For example, fistula in ano can generally be managed conservatively, with sitz baths, bulk laxatives, or stool softeners. Likewise, grade I and II hemorrhoids are also initially treated conservatively, although occasionally formal surgical intervention is warranted if medical treatment is unsuccessful. Grade III and IV hemorrhoids (prolapsed) are also thought to benefit from early surgical treatment. Several early series in the literature reported prohibitively high morbidity and mortality rates after traditional surgical procedures for hemorrhoidal disease (e.g., hemorrhoidal banding and hemorrhoidectomy) in patients with HIV; however, newer data suggest that HIV status should not alter the indications for surgical management (Hewitt, 1998). Ulcerations of the anal and perianal region can be difficult to eradicate. They are frequently associated with a variety of infectious organisms and may not respond to appropriate antibiotic or antifungal therapy. Excision of the ulcer with the patient under general anesthesia is the definitive therapy if medical treatment fails. Anal fissures, after a brief trial of conservative therapy, also appear to benefit from lateral sphincterotomy or simple excision. With respect to the operative handling of the anal sphincter mechanism, care must always be taken to avoid overly aggressive muscle division, leading to functional collapse of an already potentially marginal sphincter.

Anal condylomas are a common disorder in patients with HIV disease. Treatment is often straightforward, but it must be undertaken with the knowledge that affected patients are at increased risk for harboring malignancy. Treatment depends on the appearance, size, and location of the lesion or lesions. Anal condylomas often appear as relatively small (<1 cm), well-circumscribed, raised lesions in the perianal region, although they can also present as large, cauliflower-like masses. Lesions associated with ulceration or inflammation, or larger lesions (>1.5 to 2 cm), should be biopsied. Smaller lesions can generally be managed by the topical application of podophyllum solution, Bichloracetic Acid (dichloroacetic acid), or imiquimod (Aldara) cream. These compounds are caustic; therefore, it is imperative to protect the uninvolved skin with petroleum jelly, and to remove the applied agent from the affected areas after several hours. For larger or more extensive warts in the perianal area or in the anal canal, or condylomas located proximal to the dentate line, the authors generally recommend surgical excision or electrodesiccation. Patients usually require repeat visits to the clinic, as topical therapy is time dependent, and the recurrence rate for anal condylomas can be high. Again, as discussed by Lee and colleagues (1986), biopsy of large (>2 cm) or ulcerating anal warts should be obtained to exclude the diagnosis of squamous cell carcinoma or malignant perianal lesions, such as Kaposi's sarcoma, lymphoma, or squamous cell carcinoma, which are treated by chemotherapy with or without adjuvant radiation.

HIV AND VASCULAR ACCESS

Patients with HIV and AIDS frequently require long-term venous access, and the general surgeon is integral to both the insertion and the management of these vascular access devices. Although the need for chronic venous access catheters has declined since the introduction of protease inhibitors in the HAART protocol, the placement of central venous access catheters remains one of the more common surgical procedures performed on patients with HIV infection or AIDS. Currently, the most common indications for venous access include long-term antibiotic therapy for opportunistic infection, chemotherapy for HIV- or non–HIV-related neoplasms, and hemodialysis for renal failure, including HIV-associated nephropathy (HIVAN). Numerous retrospective studies, including those of Dega and associates (1996) and Azarow and co-workers (1992), have examined the complication rates for venous access devices. Infection is the most common long-term complication, with an incidence of 0.13 to 0.4 infections per 100 days of line insertion, depending on the type of catheter used, the patient's stage of HIV infection, and the specific indication for long-term venous access. While there appears to be a slightly increased incidence of infection in HIV patients compared with non-HIV patients, central venous access catheters can be safely placed in patients with HIV infection, and with reasonable durability. There are currently no prospective trials examining the relative safety of individual types of catheters (nontunneled catheter, percutaneous indwelling catheter, and totally implanted catheter).

Hemodialysis is often required in patients with HIV disease, frequently due to HIVAN. The complications of hemodialysis access in this population have been poorly defined. Prior studies evaluating the influence of HIV infection on hemodialysis have shown that prosthetic graft infection rates were increased, and patency rates were decreased in patients with HIV, thus leading to the recommendation that prosthetic graft be avoided in this patient population. The authors disagree with this recommendation. We recently reviewed our experience with hemodialysis access procedures in HIV-infected patients at San Francisco General Hospital over the 10-year period from 1985 to 1995. A total of 54 seropositive patients underwent 150 hemodialysis access procedures (123 surgical; 27 interventional radiology). There were 31 prosthetic and 22 autogenous primary access procedures performed, with an average follow-up of 16 months. Infection and patency rates were calculated and compared with a group of age- and sex-matched HIV-negative patients. There were no statistically significant differences in the rates of graft infection (13.8% vs. 20%; $P < 0.05$) or in primary patency (46.0% vs. 51.6%; $P < 0.05$) between HIV-negative and HIV-positive patients. Furthermore, there was no significant difference in the graft infection rate in HIV-negative or HIV-positive patients when stratified for prosthetic versus autogenous grafts. As a result of these data, it is our recommendation that patients with HIV be offered long-term hemodialysis access, with both prosthetic and autogenous graft materials as acceptable alternatives.

RISK ASSESSMENT IN PATIENTS

The current practice at the San Francisco General Hospital is to evaluate the risk of surgery in patients with HIV infection with the use of the same basic tools and guidelines as those applied to the uninfected (see also Schecter, 1994). In our experience, the best predictors of surgical morbidity and mortality stem from a careful and accurate assessment of the patient's physiologic status, including cardiopulmonary, renal, endocrine, and nutritional reserve. We do not consider HIV infection to be a significant, independent risk factor for major surgical procedures. Instead, we evaluate the clinical stage of the patient's disease, with a focus on the overall level of organ system function. While HIV disease offers a unique constellation of diagnoses and challenges to the health care provider, *physiology is function and function is predictive.* We, along with others, have shown that (1) an active opportunistic infection, (2) a serum albumin < 2.5 g/dL, and (3) the presence of concurrent organ failure are highly predictive of a poor prognosis in patients with AIDS, just as these findings are in any immunocompromised, malnourished patient. Therefore, a thorough understanding and familiarity with the clinical spectrum of HIV disease is essential to the adequate evaluation of the HIV-infected patient for an invasive surgical procedure. We believe that the poor early experience with surgery in patients with HIV disease resulted from a number of factors. First, most of the patients were in the advanced or terminal stages of the disease and thus had a very short life expectancy regardless of surgery. Second, the HIV epidemic was in its infancy, and thus the decision to operate was often delayed, thereby increasing the risk of surgery. Third, our overall ability to diagnose and treat specific AIDS-related infections was poor, therefore severely hampering the effectiveness of the perioperative care of these patients.

HIV disease, of which AIDS is the seemingly inevitable conclusion, represents a broad clinical spectrum of medical conditions. While there is no widely accepted standard system for staging HIV disease, some systems have been suggested. In 1994, Cohen and Volberding presented a system for the clinical staging of HIV disease that utilizes molecular or immunologic tests along with clinical manifestations of disease. This system reduces the spectrum of HIV disease to early, middle, and advanced stages (Table 6–3). On *initial infection,* there may be few or no clinical signs to betray the viral inoculation, but if they are present they are nonspecific and constitutional in nature. The signs of primary HIV infection can include fever, malaise, fatigue, arthralgias, myalgias, anorexia, headache, and lymphadenopathy. Patients in this stage of the disease are virtually indistinguishable from uninfected people. Short of directly measuring the virus in the blood, these patients appear well or to be suffering from a mild viral illness.

Early- and middle-stage HIV disease begin after the initial host response, generally within 6 months of the primary infection, and ends with the development of a severely compromised immune system. Most patients infected with HIV are in this stage of the disease, which lasts an average of 10 years. It is during this period that the patient's helper T-cell (CD4) count falls from the normal range of 500 to 1250 cells/mm^3 to 200 to 300 cells/mm^3. Early on, the patients are essentially healthy but experience self-limited illnesses such as skin and nail infections (folliculitis, fungal intertrigo, paronychia), thrush, herpes zoster, and bacterial infections (sinusitis, pneumonia, bronchitis). Central nervous system (CNS) changes can occur, including peripheral neuropathy and mild HIV dementia. As the disease progresses, the CD4 count continues to decrease and the patients develop more frequent non–HIV-associated infections that still respond to standard therapies. Isolated, non-CNS malignancies, such as Kaposi's sarcoma and non-Hodgkin's lymphoma can appear in patients with middle-stage disease.

Advanced-stage HIV disease is associated with a CD4 count of less than 200 cells/mm^3 and overt clinical signs of a severely immunocompromised condition. By this stage, the disease clearly meets the definition of AIDS put forward by the Centers for Disease Control and Prevention (CDC). These patients experience opportunistic and uncommon infections that often present in an unusual manner and incompletely respond to therapy. Reactivation of mycobacterial or fungal infections is not uncommon. The late or terminal stage of HIV disease is frequently characterized by a CD4 count of fewer than 50 cells/mm^3 and evidence of organ failure. It is at this time that patients develop debilitating and intractable pulmonary, CNS, and gastrointestinal infections with pathogens including *Pneumocystis,* atypical mycobacteria, *Toxoplasma, Cryptococcus,* CMV, and *Candida.* Life expectancy is measured in weeks to months, with the patients succumbing to organ failure, profound wasting, and severe metabolic abnormalities.

COMPLICATIONS OF ABDOMINAL SURGERY. Complication and mortality rates for abdominal surgery in HIV-infected individuals are far from prohibitive. The data seen previously in Table 6–2 represent the collected data from six published series on emergency surgery in patients with HIV or AIDS in a total of 165 patients, reported between 1989 and 1995. Complications occurred in 42% of patients, with an overall 30-day mortality rate of 26% (Flum and Wallack, 1999). There were considerable variations in the morbidity and mortality rates reported

Table 6–3	Clinical Staging of HIV Disease and Surgical Mortality						
STAGE OF HIV DISEASE	CDC CLASS (1993)	CD4 COUNT (cells/mm³)	CLINICAL MANIFESTATIONS	VIRAL BURDEN	LIFE EXPECTANCY (mos)	LEAN MUSCLE MASS	ESTIMATED SURGICAL MORTALITY (30 days)
Early	A	>500	Fevers, zoster, thrush, pneumonia, skin and nail infections, mild CNS	Variable	120–132	WNL	0%–3%°
Middle	B	200–300	More frequent infections, isolated Kaposi's sarcoma, NHL, early HIV dementia	Low	48–60	↓ <10%	3%–5%
Advanced (terminal)	C	<200 (<50)	Opportunistic infections, immunocompromised, reactivation of infections, severe weight loss	High	2–3	↓ >10%	11%–23%

°Same as uninfected individual, mortality related to specific operative procedure.
CNS, central nervous system; NHL, non-Hodgkin's lymphoma; WNL, within normal limits.

from different institutions, with the values ranging from 23% to 60% and 11% to 70%, respectively. In 1995, the authors reported the single largest series in the literature regarding emergency surgery in patients with AIDS, with a morbidity rate of 35% and mortality rate of 12% (Whitney et al, 1994) and consider these values more representative than those from earlier reports. Most perioperative complications were infectious in nature, undoubtedly related to the patients' immunocompromised condition, and death generally followed multiorgan failure.While the AIDS diagnosis must temper the clinical evaluation of the acute abdomen, the indications for surgery are nearly identical to those of uninfected patients, and the frequencies of common diagnoses and unusual diagnoses are approximately equal. Yet, further analysis of the literature also confirms the fact that the presence of AIDS-related pathology as the cause for emergency abdominal surgery increases the operative mortality rate approximately threefold compared with other unrelated etiologies (Whitney et al, 1994). This information is of prognostic, but little clinical, value to the surgeon initially evaluating the patient with abdominal pain, since both coincident and AIDS-related diagnoses can present in an identical manner.

COMPLICATIONS OF ANORECTAL SURGERY. Historically, wound healing has been a concern following anorectal surgery in HIV-infected patients. In a study published in 1986 by Wexner and colleagues, in 52 patients with AIDS who underwent 73 anorectal procedures (23 biopsies, 16 incision and drainage procedures, 14 fistulotomies, 8 sphincterotomies, 8 excisions, 3 colostomies, and 1 hemorrhoidectomy), 88% of the cases were associated with poor wound healing. A more recent study by Burke and co-workers done at our institution subgrouped HIV-infected patients based on the CDC classification for HIV disease progression, with more promising results. Fifty-two HIV-infected patients were available for analysis. Twenty-four operations were performed in asymptomatic HIV-infected patients, 19 in HIV-infected patients with persistent lymphadenopathy, and 37 in patients with AIDS. Anorectal surgical wounds healed in 94% of all the patients. While patients with constitutional symptoms associated with HIV healed more slowly than asymptomatic patients or those with lymphadenopathy, this difference did not reach statistical significance. The mortality rate 30 days after surgery was 2%, and there were no major complications. The mean survival time of HIV-infected patients after surgery was 15 months, compared with 7.4 months in the Wexner series, probably related to improved antiretroviral treatment. Our conclusions are that patients with uncomfortable or debilitating anorectal disease, especially those who are physically active and have normal laboratory profiles, should be considered good surgical candidates and undergo appropriate surgical treatment.

RISK MANAGEMENT FOR SURGICAL PROVIDERS

Although the extent of risk of HIV transmission to surgical personnel can vary, there are sufficient data to permit some estimates. Published data are derived primarily from studies of single needlestick or mucocutaneous blood exposures. Unfortunately, surgeons are likely to have multiple exposures during the course of a career. There are no data to guide risk assessment of occupational HIV transmission with multiple parenteral exposures, although cumulative risk almost certainly depends on the size of the inoculum, the depth of the injection, and host immunity. Chambers has developed a mathematical model to predict the risk of HIV transmission with multiple exposures based on the seroprevalence of HIV in the patient population and an assumed seroconversion rate of 0.2%. With the use of this model, the risk of seroconversion approaches 1 in 500 for 10 needlesticks (Gerberding et al, 1987). The risk is 1 in 63 for 100 needlesticks. Although this is a predictive model, and not a method based on empirical data, the authors believe that the principle is valid. The higher the prevalence rates of HIV in the patient population served and the higher the number of needlestick exposures, the greater the risk of HIV transmission to the surgeon. For example, surgeons who care for trauma victims, particularly inner-city trauma victims, are treating a patient population with a high prevalence of HIV infection. In a study of 203 critically ill or severely injured emergency patients, only trauma (particularly penetrating trauma) patients between the ages of 25 and 34 years were associated with HIV infection. The prevalence of HIV-infected trauma patients at the Johns Hopkins Hospital was 6%. Despite the lack of published data for surgeons over the course of their career, seroconversion virtually guarantees the future development of AIDS. There is no effective cure for HIV infection at present; thus, surgeons as well as all health care workers must assume responsibility for and adopt a leadership role in the prevention of HIV transmission as the result of occupational exposure.

In order to minimize the risk of HIV transmission to members of the surgical and operating room teams, parenteral and mucocutaneous exposure to the patient's blood and body fluids must be kept to an absolute minimum. There are two basic principles that must be accepted by all members of the surgical team in order to achieve effective infection control (Fauci et al, 1984): Every patient is considered to be infected with HIV and it is unacceptable to have the patient's blood or other body fluids in contact with the health care provider's skin or mucous membranes (LaRaja et al, 1984). The infection control guidelines must be accepted and strictly enforced from the top leadership down. If the most senior members of the surgical team do not respect and follow these principles in their daily work, both their trainees and the nursing and support staffs are unlikely to maintain the appropriate level of vigilance. The younger members of the team are likely to have numerous exposures to HIV-infected blood and secretions as part of the routine care of acutely ill surgical patients; for example, when they are obtaining venous access. Therefore, all personnel on the surgical team should receive formal training in infection control precautions. Adequate equipment for protection of health care providers should be available in the emergency department, the operating room, and on the ward.

The CDC developed the infection-control system

termed *The Universal Blood and Body Fluid Precautions* (Table 6–4) to prevent exposure to infectious blood and body fluids. The so-called universal precautions were designed to allow health care workers to avoid exposure to blood-borne pathogens, and these rules should be followed routinely when one treats all patients and handles all specimens. Contemporary data indicate poor compliance with the recommended precautions by health professionals. Gloves should be used when one touches the blood, body fluids, mucous membranes, or nonintact skin of patients. Gowns, masks, and protective eyewear are mandatory when one engages in any activity likely to expose one to infected fluids or secretions, such as vascular access procedures (venipuncture, arterial blood gas sampling), inspection of wounds, changing of dressings, or placement of tubes and drains (nasogastric tube, Foley catheter). The authors firmly believe that double gloves should be worn as a precaution against cutaneous blood exposure due to damaged or defective gloves if prolonged exposure is anticipated, such as in the operating room. Once the task is completed, gloves should be removed and the hands thoroughly washed. Hands and other skin surfaces should be washed immediately with detergent if accidental exposure occurs. Although the CDC (1988) has stated that universal precautions do not apply to feces, nasal secretions, sputum, sweat, tears, urine, and vomitus, health care workers should not be directly exposed to these fluids.

None of these precautions will prevent needlestick inoculation of HIV-infected blood, which is the primary mechanism of occupational HIV transmission. Obviously, extreme care should be taken at all times to avoid needlesticks. Needles should never be recapped, bent, or broken. Needles and other disposable sharp instruments should be placed in rigid, puncture-resistant containers for disposal immediately after use. Despite these precau-

Table 6–4	**Universal Blood and Body Fluid Precautions**

Take care to prevent injuries when using needles, scalpels, and other sharp instruments or devices; when handling sharp instruments after procedures; when cleaning used instruments; and when disposing of needles. Do not recap used needles by hand; do not remove used needles from disposable syringes by hand; and do not bend, break, or otherwise manipulate used needles by hand. Place used disposable syringes in puncture-resistant containers for disposal.
Use protective barriers to prevent exposure to blood, body fluids containing visible blood, and other body fluids.
Immediately and thoroughly wash hands and other skin surfaces that are contaminated with blood or body fluids containing visible blood.
Use gloves for performing phlebotomy.
Use sterile gloves for procedures involving contact with normally sterile areas of the body.
Use examination gloves for procedures involving contact with mucous membranes.
Change gloves between patient contacts.
Do not wash or disinfect surgical or examination gloves for reuse. Washing with surfactants may cause "wicking," i.e., the enhanced penetration of liquids through undetected holes in the gloves. Disinfecting agents may cause deterioration.
Use general-purpose utility gloves for housekeeping chores involving potential blood contact and for instrument cleaning and decontamination procedures.

tions, needlesticks and other injuries that violate the skin and mucous membranes of health care workers will occur. In a study conducted by the CDC, injuries were sustained in approximately 6.9% of surgical procedures, a figure in close agreement with the results of our prospective observational study (Tokars et al, 1992). Approximately one third of the injuries resulted from practitioners using fingers to either hold tissue or feel a needle tip. In virtually all exposures, a sharp edge or needle passed through glove material. The highest risk of injury occurs during procedures lasting more than 3 hours, especially if the blood loss is greater than 300 mL, and during intra-abdominal gynecologic surgery, vaginal hysterectomies, and major vascular procedures. While gloves rarely prevent a percutaneous injury, the practice of double-gloving does significantly reduce exposure to blood during surgery. The use of double gloves should be routine in the operating room, as it reduces inner-glove perforation rates by 50% to 80%. A glove that is a half-size larger than normal should be worn underneath the normal-size glove. This technique prevents the double gloves from being too constrictive and reduces hand contamination with blood by up to 50%.

Precautions in the operating room must be strict. No one should work in an active operating room without protective eyewear. If aerosolization of fluid or solid material such as bone is expected, a face shield should be worn. Frequently during operations, especially trauma cases, the surgeon must stand in a pool of blood during an attempt to control major hemorrhage. The surgeon's shoes, socks, scrub suits, and undergarments are often soaked with the patient's blood. This practice is no longer acceptable. Impermeable shoe covers or rubber boots should be worn in all cases. The sterile gowns currently available are not impermeable to blood or other body fluids. An impermeable, disposable cystoscopy apron can be worn under the sterile gown for added protection. This apron hangs down over calf-high rubber boots and prevents blood that has soaked through the sterile gown from contacting the surgeon's skin. Surgeons wearing the apron often become uncomfortably warm. However, the cystoscopy apron represents an effective and affordable mechanical barrier. Extra sleeves may be worn so that there is a double layer of protection for the arms. Soiled attire should be changed during procedures to decrease the possibility of exposure to infected blood. State-of-the-art operating room gowns made of Gore-Tex are now available. While these are lightweight, impermeable to fluids, and comfortable to wear, they are expensive to clean and require special handling.

The use or manipulation of sharp instruments or objects in the operating room must be viewed as a high-risk activity since it is the source of many percutaneous exposures and injuries. The use of one's hands and fingers to retract or suture tissues together should be avoided. Self-retaining and hand-held retractors, blunt suture needles, and specific "no-touch" surgical techniques should dramatically reduce the risk inherent to the operating room environment. Passing needles and scalpels between members of the team represents another high-risk activity that can also be avoided. Placing sharp instruments on a sterile Mayo stand or in an emesis basin allows the surgical and nursing staff to transfer sharps between one another with minimal risk of accidental injury.

TREATMENT OF HEALTH CARE WORKERS WITH PARENTERAL OCCUPATIONAL EXPOSURE TO HIV.

Occupational exposure to HIV remains an important problem. Even in settings where health care workers use the most up-to-date safety devices available and adhere to strict infection control precautions, the risk of HIV exposure and transmission is never zero. Therefore, having a program in place that is designed to respond to the medical and psychological needs of the occupationally exposed health care worker is essential.

In brief, the steps we recommend after an occupational exposure are as follows. First, as soon as it is medically safe for the patient, the exposure site should be vigorously washed with soap and water. There is no evidence to prove that antiseptics are of any added benefit in decontaminating the exposed skin or wound, but their use is not contraindicated. Exposed mucous membranes should be flushed with copious quantities of clean water or pH-balanced saline, especially for use in the eyes. If the exposure involves a bite or a wound requiring suturing, prophylactic antibiotics may be appropriate.

Second, the exposure must be reported to the appropriate occupational or employee health agency. At the San Francisco General Hospital, health care workers are encouraged to report occupational exposures to a "Needlestick Hotline" that operates 24 hours a day, 7 days a week. This agency provides expert advice, triage services where indicated, postexposure HIV and hepatitis care, confidential counseling, follow-up testing, and documentation. An informed and immediate response to a provider's occupational exposure helps to significantly reduce the stress and anxiety that such an event understandably generates.

Third, the involved health care worker should obtain postexposure follow-up regarding possible HIV and hepatitis seroconversion. In 1995, a CDC case-control study of occupational exposure to HIV demonstrated an 80-fold reduction in the risk of HIV seroconversion if zidovudine was prophylactically administered. In May of 1998, the CDC published updated provisional recommendations for chemoprophylaxis after occupational exposure to HIV, reflecting the introduction of multiple-drug, antiretroviral chemotherapy including protease inhibitors. Health care workers with parenteral exposure to blood from high-risk patients should be offered chemoprophylaxis. Zidovudine and lamivudine (3TC) should be appropriate for most HIV exposures, while an "expanded" regimen of indinavir or nelfinavir in addition to the "basic" regimen should be used for exposures that pose an increased risk of transmission or where resistance to one or more agents is known or suspected (Table 6–5).

Exposed health care workers should be tested for HIV infection at once, with retesting at 6 weeks and periodically thereafter for 6 months, provided that they remain seronegative. Screening for HIV-antibody after an occupational exposure (1) identifies infected individuals as early in the course of their HIV disease as possible, (2) documents the infection for both medical and legal reasons, and (3) ameliorates unnecessary fear and anxiety.

Table 6–5	**Basic and Expanded Postexposure Prophylaxis Regimens**	
REGIMEN CATEGORY	APPLICATION	DRUG REGIMEN
Basic	Occupational HIV exposure for which there is a recognized transmission risk	4 weeks (28 days) of both zidovudine, 600 mg every day in divided doses, *and* lamivudine, 150 mg twice a day
Expanded	Occupational HIV exposures that pose an increased risk of transmission (e.g., larger volume of blood and/or higher virus titer in blood)	Basic regimen plus *either* indinavir, 800 mg every 8 hours, *or* nelfinavir, 750 mg three times a day

MORAL IMPERATIVE. Although a legitimate debate occurred early in the HIV epidemic concerning the risks of surgery for both the HIV-infected patient and the surgical team, the issue is now resolved. If after weighing the known risks and benefits of a surgical procedure for a given patient with HIV or AIDS the surgeon concludes that the operation is likely to have a positive effect on the patient's life, that patient deserves surgery. There is a small but real risk of perioperative transmission of HIV and other blood-borne infections (hepatitis B and C) to the surgical team if parenteral exposure to blood or body fluids occurs. Every effort must be made to reduce the risk of exposure. However, the refusal to operate on HIV-infected patients, for the sole reason of avoiding this risk, is not acceptable behavior for a practicing surgeon.

Summary

In summary, there will continue to be a role for surgery in the care of patients with HIV and AIDS. Aside from venous access, gastrointestinal procedures are the most commonly performed. Acute abdominal and anorectal pain are very common complaints in patients with HIV disease, yet the need for surgery is relatively infrequent. However, when indicated, surgery in patients with AIDS can be performed with acceptable morbidity and mortality rates. In fact, the patients suffering from non–AIDS-related pathology will greatly benefit from rapid and aggressive surgical intervention. Evaluation of the gastrointestinal tract in this patient population is made all the more challenging by numerous factors, including the need to entertain an expanded list of potential diagnoses. Although neoplastic, viral, and mycobacterial involvement of the intestinal tract are frequent etiologies of abdominal emergencies in patients with full-blown AIDS, the etiology of the patient's problem is just as likely to be unrelated to their viral infection. A thorough history, careful physical examination, routine laboratory tests, and plain radiographs remain the foundation of the patient evaluation. The abdominal CT scan can prove an invaluable tool for the accurate diagnosis of the acute abdomen, especially under circumstances of clinical uncertainty. For the

Pearls and Pitfalls

Abdominal Pain

PEARLS

- While 30% to 90% of HIV-infected patients present for evaluation of their abdominal pain, only approximately 2% to 3% will require emergency surgery.
- The CT scan is an extremely useful tool for the evaluation of the abdomen and pelvis, including the viscera, vasculature, retroperitoneum, and lymph nodes.
- Laparoscopy can be used as a diagnostic and therapeutic tool in patients with peritonitis of unclear etiology.
- Immunosuppressed patients may present with less dramatic physical findings (i.e., fever).

PITFALLS

- Failure to consider entities both coincident with and unique to HIV infection
- Use of normal laboratory profile (especially WBC count) to exclude acute surgical conditions
- Failure to perform serial abdominal examinations to monitor the evolution of an intra-abdominal process
- Failure to consider aggressive surgical therapy in the patient with HIV disease and peritonitis

Anorectal Disease

PEARLS

- Approximately one third of HIV-infected patients have anorectal complaints.
- The perianal region may be at increased risk for local trauma in individuals practicing anoreceptive intercourse.
- HPV is very common in gay men with HIV disease, and presents as a spectrum from dysplasia to condylomas to carcinoma (SCCA, squamous cell carcinoma).
- HIV status does not alter wound healing following hemorrhoidectomy and thus should not alter indications for the surgical management of hemorrhoidal disease.

PITFALLS

- Failure to establish histologic diagnosis by biopsy
- Failure to surgically treat patients with debilitating anorectal disease
- Acceptance of referral diagnosis, without histologic or laboratory evidence supporting that diagnosis
- Overly aggressive anal sphincter division in the treatment of hemorrhoidal or anal fissure disease

surgery in this population is not unlike that for other immunocompromised or malnourished patients.

We believe that health professionals who are privileged to be members of the surgical team have a professional, moral, and ethical responsibility to provide the highest possible quality of compassionate care for their patients, regardless of their HIV status. If after weighing the risks and benefits to the patient the surgeon believes the procedure will have a positive effect on the patient's life, he or she must offer surgical treatment. To do less would be a disservice to the patient, the provider, and the profession as a whole.

SELECTED READINGS

Azarow KS, Molloy M, Kavolius J, et al: Perioperative complications of long-term central venous catheters in high-risk patients: Predictors versus myths. South Med J 85:498, 1992.

Bizer L, Pettorino R, Ashikari A: Emergency abdominal operations in the patient with acquired immunodeficiency syndrome. J Am Coll Surg 180:205, 1995.

Burke EC, Orloff SL, Freise CE, et al: Wound healing after anorectal surgery in human immunodeficiency virus–infected patients. Arch Surg 126:1267–1270; discussion 1270–1271, 1991.

CDC: Update: Universal precautions for prevention of HIV transmission in health-care settings. MMWR Morb Mortal Wkly Rep 37:377, 1988.

CDC: Case-control study of HIV seroconversion in health-care workers after percutaneous exposure to HIV-infected blood—France, United Kingdom, and United States, January 1988–August 1994. MMWR Morb Mortal Wkly Rep 44:928, 1995.

CDC: Public Health Service Guidelines for the Management of Health-Care Worker Exposures to HIV and Recommendations for Postexposure Prophylaxis. MMWR Morb Mortal Wkly Rep 47:14, 1998.

Cohen P, Volberding P: Clinical spectrum of HIV disease. In Cohen P, Sande M, Volberding P (eds): The AIDS Knowledge Base. Boston, Little, Brown, 1994, pp 4.1–1 to 4.1–15.

Davidson T, Allen-Marsh T, Miles A, et al: Emergency laparotomy in patients with AIDS. Br J Surg 78:924, 1991.

Dega H, Eliaszewicz M, Gisselbrecht M, et al: Infections associated with totally implantable venous access devices (TIVAD) in human immunodeficiency virus–infected patients. J Acquir Immune Defic Syndr 13:146, 1996.

Fauci A, Macher A, Longo D, et al: NIH Conference. Acquired immunodeficiency syndrome: Epidemiologic, clinical, immunologic, and therapeutic consideration. Ann Intern Med 100:92, 1984.

Flum D, Wallack M: The Role of Surgery in AIDS: An Outcomes-Based Approach. Philadelphia, Lippincott–Williams & Wilkins, 1999.

Gerberding JL, Bryant-LeBlanc CE, Nelson K, et al: Risk of transmitting the human immunodeficiency virus, cytomegalovirus, and hepatitis B virus to health care workers exposed to patients with AIDS and AIDS-related conditions. J Infect Dis 156:1, 1987.

Hewitt W: Should HIV status alter indications for hemorrhoidectomy? Dis Colon Rectum 39:615, 1998.

LaRaja RD, Rothenberg RE, Nadkarni PP: The acute abdomen in the HIV patient. In Wilson SE, Williams RA (eds): Surgical Problems in the AIDS Patient. New York, Igaku-Shoin, 1984, pp 43–63.

LaRaja R, Rothenberg R, Odom J, Mueller S: The incidence of intra-abdominal surgery in acquired immunodeficiency syndrome: A statistical review of 904 patients. Surgery 105:175, 1989.

Lee M, Waxman M, Gillooley J: Primary malignant lymphoma of the anorectum in homosexual men. Dis Colon Rectum 29:423, 1986.

Miles AJ, Mellor CH, Gazzard B, et al: Surgical management of anorectal disease in HIV-positive homosexuals. Br J Surg 77:869, 1990.

Schecter W: Surgery in HIV-infected patients. In Cohen P, Sande M, Volberding P (eds): The AIDS Knowledge Base. Boston, Little, Brown, 1994, pp 4.12–13 to 14.12–15.

Tokars J, Bell D, Culver D, et al: Percutaneous injuries during surgical procedures. JAMA 267:2899, 1992.

Wexner SD, Smithy WB, Milsom JW, Dailey TH: The surgical management of anorectal diseases in AIDS and pre-AIDS patients. Dis Colon Rectum 29:719, 1986.

Whitney T, Macho J, Russell T, et al: Appendicitis in acquired immunodeficiency syndrome. Am J Surg 164:467, 1992.

Whitney T, Brunel W, Russell T, et al: Emergent abdominal surgery in AIDS: Experience in San Francisco. Am J Surg 168:239, 1994.

Yii M, Saunder A, Scott D: Abdominal surgery in HIV/AIDS patients: Indications, operative management, pathology and outcome. Aust N Z J Surg 65:320, 1995.

anorectal region, anoscopy, sigmoidoscopy, and biopsy are the cornerstones of evaluation.

In practice, we evaluate the risk of surgery in patients with HIV infection using the same basic tools and guidelines applied to the uninfected, with the best predictors of surgical morbidity and mortality stemming from a careful and accurate assessment of the patient's cardiopulmonary, renal, endocrine, and nutritional reserve. While HIV disease provides a unique constellation of diagnoses and challenges to the health care provider, the risk of major

Chapter 7
Circulatory Monitoring

R. Lawrence Reed

Circulatory failure and insufficiency are responsible for much of the organ failure and insufficiency that can develop in critically ill and injured patients. Hence, circulatory monitoring provides a mechanism for determining the presence, nature, and degree of any circulatory insufficiency. It also enables titration of therapeutic maneuvers. While hemodynamics are important, circulatory performance is measured by more than hemodynamics alone. Fundamentally, hemodynamics deals with the interrelationships of pressures and flows. As the circulation is responsible for delivery of fuel to meet the demands of the various organs and tissues, circulatory monitoring also incorporates concepts relevant to energy supply.

The discussion in this chapter describes the concepts involved in the various hemodynamic measurements and calculations. The actual calculations and normal ranges are presented in Table 7–1.

CLINICAL PRESENTATION

A variety of conditions can suggest a potential problem with the circulation (Table 7–2). While each of these entities can be highly suggestive of the presence of circulatory insufficiency, they are not confirmatory. Hypotension is the clinical finding clinicians most commonly identify with a potential circulatory problem. However, the severity of the circulatory problem is best assessed by evaluating its impact on organ and tissue metabolism (e.g., base deficit, mixed venous oxygen saturation, gastrointestinal tonometry, creatinine clearance). Moreover, the specific etiology of the hypotension can be determined only through an accurate assessment of hemodynamic parameters (Table 7–3). Currently, this information is best obtained invasively, through the use of a pulmonary artery flotation catheter.

The pulmonary artery catheter balloon promotes flotation of the catheter tip to wedge in a distal branch of the pulmonary arterial tree. When thus wedged, the catheter occludes the influence of pressures generated by the right ventricle and selectively reflects the more passive pressure of the capillary bed downstream. In the unwedged position, the catheter can monitor the pulmonary systolic and diastolic pressures. Several modifications of the original pulmonary artery catheter have been added to the device, enhancing the quantity of information provided. A thermistor on the tip of the catheter senses changes in temperature of the blood flowing past it, enabling determination of cardiac output with the use of indicator dilution technology.

HEMODYNAMICS

Hemodynamics represents the hydraulic relationships involved in circulatory performance. As with other hydraulic systems, the parameters involved are pressures, flows, and volumes. The variability in body sizes among humans necessitates that the interpretation of abnormalities related to volumes and flows be standardized. Standardization is accomplished by indexing the various parameters to body surface area. Body surface area, in turn, can be determined from nomograms or calculations based on height or weight. In several textbook chapters on the subject of hemodynamics, all parameters have been indiscriminately indexed. However, indexing is appropriate and useful only for those parameters representing volumes and flows. Parameters such as systemic vascular resistance are not benefited by indexing. Indeed, when indexed, systemic vascular resistance provides a *wider* range of normal values, owing to the nature of the calculation, rather than narrowing the normal range, as is desired when indexing is performed.

Pressure Monitoring

Traditional hemodynamics are derived from the oldest measurements of circulatory performance: systemic arterial blood pressure and heart rate. Invasive measurements of central venous pressures and pulmonary arterial pressures can be determined from the insertion of a central venous catheter and pulmonary artery catheter, respectively. This pulmonary capillary wedge pressure corresponds well with left atrial pressure under most circumstances.

Pressures in the vessels and heart chambers have been used as stand-ins for measurements of volume. This substitution has occurred because of the relative ease of pressure measurements compared with volume measurements. Pressure and volume are related in a positive manner through the concept of compliance ($\Delta V/\Delta P$), although this relationship is curvilinear and variable. Because of this nonlinearity, a large change in filling pressure could represent a small change in filling volume, and vice versa. Moreover, the variability of the contractile state between different patients and even within the same patient at different points in time impairs the accuracy and reliability of the relationship. Nevertheless, most clinicians treat changes in filling pressures as reflecting circulating volumes; in most instances, such is likely the case.

Volume Monitoring

Recent technologic innovations have enabled a more precise assessment of filling volumes. Modifications to the design of pulmonary artery catheters incorporating a fast-responding thermistor allow for the determination of the

Table 7–1	Circulatory Measurements, Calculations, Normal Ranges, and Units

PARAMETER	ABBREVIATION	HOW DETERMINED	NORMAL RANGE AND UNITS
Heart rate	HR	Measured	60–100 beats/min
Systolic/diastolic systemic arterial blood pressure	SBP/DBP	Measured	100–140/60–90 mm Hg
Mean systemic arterial blood pressure	MAP	$DBP + \dfrac{SBP - DBP}{3}$	70–105 mm Hg
Systolic/diastolic pulmonary arterial pressure	PSP/PDP	Measured	15–30/4–12 mm Hg
Mean pulmonary arterial pressure	MPAP	$PDP + \dfrac{PSP - PDP}{3}$	9–16 mm Hg
Right ventricular systolic pressure	RVSP	Measured	15–30 mm Hg
Right ventricular end-diastolic pressure	RVEDP	Measured	0–8 mm Hg
Cardiac output	CO	Measured (using thermodilution)	3.0–7.0 L/min
Body surface area	BSA	Calculated/nomogram	N/A
Cardiac index	CI	CO/BSA	2.8–4.2 L/min/m²
Central venous pressure	CVP	Measured	2–5 mm Hg
Pulmonary capillary wedge pressure	PCWP	Measured	5–10 mm Hg
Stroke volume	SV	CO/HR	40–115 mL
Stroke volume index	SVI	CI/BSA	30–50 mL/m²
Left ventricular stroke work index	LVSWI	$(MAP - PCWP) \times SVI \times 0.0136$	40–60 g-m/m²
Right ventricular stroke work index	RVSWI	$(MPAP - CVP) \times SVI \times 0.0136$	7–12 g-m/m²
Systemic vascular resistance	SVR	$\dfrac{MAP - CVP}{CO} \times 79.9$	800–1200 dyne-sec/cm⁵
Pulmonary vascular resistance	PVR	$\dfrac{MPAP - PCWP}{CO} \times 79.9$	150–250 dyne-sec/cm⁵
Arterial oxygen tension	PaO_2	Measured	60–100 mm Hg
Arterial oxygen saturation	SaO_2	Measured	93%–100%
Arterial oxygen content	CaO_2	$([Hgb][SaO_2/100\%][1.39]) + ([PaO_2][0.0032])$	16–22 mL O_2/dL blood
Mixed venous oxygen tension	$P\bar{v}O_2$	Measured	36–42 mm Hg
Mixed venous oxygen saturation	$S\bar{v}O_2$	Measured	72%–78%
Mixed venous oxygen content	$C\bar{v}O_2$	$([Hgb][S\bar{v}O_2/100\%][1.39]) + ([P\bar{v}O_2][0.0032])$	12–17 mL O_2/dL blood
Arteriovenous oxygen content difference	$C(a-v)O_2$	$CaO_2 - C\bar{v}O_2$	3–5 mL O_2/dL blood
Oxygen delivery	$\dot{D}O_2$	$CaO_2 \times CO \times 10$	640–1400 mL O_2/min
Oxygen consumption	$\dot{V}O_2$	$(CaO_2 - C\bar{v}O_2) \times CO \times 10$	180–250 mL O_2/min
Oxygen delivery index	$\dot{D}O_2\,I$	$\dot{D}O_2/BSA$	350–760 mL O_2/min/m²
Oxygen consumption index	$\dot{V}O_2\,I$	$\dot{V}O_2/BSA$	100–140 mL O_2/min/m²
Oxygen extraction ratio	O_2ER	$\dfrac{\dot{V}O_2}{\dot{D}O_2}$	0.22–0.28
Creatinine clearance	C_{cr}	$\dfrac{U_{cr} \times V}{P_{cr} \times T}$	110–125 mL/min (age-dependent)
Fractional excretion of sodium	Fe_{Na}	$\dfrac{U_{Na^+} \times P_{cr}}{P_{Na^+} \times U_{cr}} \times 100\%$	< 1%

50 GENERAL PRINCIPLES

Table 7–2	Conditions Suggesting Circulatory Insufficiency or Failure

Hypotension
Tachycardia or bradycardia
Oliguria
Decreased skin temperature
Decreased skin turgor
Clammy skin
Decreased capillary refill
Thirst
Decreased cardiac output
Increased or decreased PCWP
Decreased creatinine clearance
Decreased S$\bar{v}O_2$
Confusion
Tachypnea
Pallor
Thready pulse
Distended neck veins
Elevated serum lactate
Negative base excess (elevated base deficit)
Low intramural gastric pH (pH$_i$)
High gastric luminal PCO_2 (P$_r$CO$_2$)

actual ejection fraction of each heartbeat. From this, the actual end-diastolic volume index can be derived. The stroke volume (SV) represents the difference between the end-diastolic volume (EDV) and the end-systolic volume (ESV). Thus, EDV is determined by the sum of SV and ESV. The ejection fraction (EF) represents the ratio of SV to EDV. Because the right heart ejection fraction is directly measured through the volumetric pulmonary artery catheter and the stroke volume is calculated by the cardiac output divided by the heart rate, the end-diastolic volume can be determined by SV/EF. (An assumption is made that right ventricular and left-ventricular end-diastolic volumes are equivalent.)

The goals in resuscitating a failed circulation are to ensure that the circulating volume is adequate, but not excessive, and that the heart is contracting as optimally as possible. Accurate determination of circulating volume is critical and usually takes precedence. Volume restoration is the initial goal because it is difficult to assess the pump's intrinsic function in the presence of an abnormal circulating volume, and because abnormal circulating volumes are counterproductive to effective pumping. Circulatory volume optimization improves circulatory performance through two fundamental mechanisms: improved cardiac output from an adequate stroke volume, and improved cardiac work through the Frank-Starling mechanism. As previously mentioned, cardiac output is the

product of stroke volume times heart rate. As circulating volume increases, stroke volume typically increases, regardless of the ejection fraction.

Frank-Starling Relationship

Optimization of cardiac performance can also be produced through the use of the Frank-Starling relationship. Through this mechanism, as ventricular filling volumes are increased, cardiac work is improved. Preload affects sarcomere length: progressive increases in sarcomere length increase the work produced by the muscle's contraction. However, excessive stretching is associated with progressive deterioration in muscle work.

In clinical practice, several assumptions are made in the application of the Frank-Starling principle (Fig. 7–1). First, sarcomere length in the left ventricle is assumed to be proportional to left ventricular volume, which would actually be true only if the ventricle were a perfect sphere. Maximal stretch during the cardiac cycle exists at the end of diastole, represented by the left ventricular end-diastolic volume (LVEDV). This volume and left ventricular end-diastolic pressure (LVEDP) are proportional to each other, related by the property of the ventricle's compliance. In the absence of mitral stenosis, LVEDP is proportional to left atrial end-diastolic pressure (LAEDP). Finally, as no valves or other gradients are normally present in the pulmonary circulation, the pulmonary capillary wedge pressure (PCWP) corresponds to the LAEDP. However, this relationship deteriorates in the setting of elevated alveolar pressures, such as seen with positive end-expiratory pressure (PEEP).

In common clinical practice, cardiac output is assessed as PCWP is progressively increased. However, in the Frank-Starling relationship, the parameter influenced by filling volume is actually cardiac work. Work (W) is defined as the product of force (F) times distance (d): $W = F \times d$. In hemodynamic terms, pressure (P) is equivalent to force per unit area (A): $P = F/A$. Hence, force is equal to the product of pressure and area: $F = P \times A$. Thus, work will equal the product of pressure times area times distance. Area times distance, in turn, results in a measurement of volume. Thus, work is equivalent to pressure times volume.

The pressure involved in the development of cardiac work is the change in pressure produced by the heart's contraction. Thus, work for the left ventricle will be equivalent to the mean systemic arterial pressure (MAP) minus the pressure existing prior to the initiation of ventricular contraction; that is, the left ventricular end-dia-

| Table 7–3 | Hemodynamic Discrimination of Etiology of Hypotension |

HEMODYNAMIC PARAMETER	TYPE OF HYPOTENSION			
	Hypovolemic	Cardiogenic	Neurogenic/Vasogenic	Septic
PCWP	↓	↑	↓	Variable
Cardiac output	↓	↓	Normal or variable	↑
S$\bar{v}O_2$	↓	↓	Normal	↑

PCWP, pulmonary capillary wedge pressure; S$\bar{v}O_2$, mixed venous oxygen saturation.

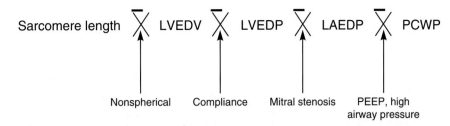

Figure 7–1. Assumptions made in using the pulmonary capillary wedge pressure to assess cardiac performance relative to changes in circulating volume and the common situations that violate those assumptions. LVEDV, left ventricular end-diastolic volume; LVEDP, left ventricular end-diastolic pressure; LAEDP, left atrial end-diastolic pressure; PCWP, pulmonary capillary wedge pressure.

stolic pressure (LVEDP). The clinical approximation for LVEDP is, as previously described, the pulmonary capillary wedge pressure (PCWP). The volume employed in the determination of cardiac work is the cardiac output. The ventricular stroke work assesses the work associated with each heartbeat; hence, the stroke volume is the volume used in the calculation.

Resistance

For at least a century, physiologists have employed a concept inherent in electrical circuits: resistance. Resistance was originally described by Ohm to explain the continuous relationship between voltage gradient and current as $\Delta V = IR$. The circulatory application of Ohm's law employs the parameters of pressure gradient and flow (or cardiac output [CO]), so that $R = \Delta P/CO$. For systemic vascular resistance, the pressure gradient across the circuit is represented by the difference between the mean arterial pressure and the central venous pressure. The calculation for pulmonary vascular resistance employs the gradient between the mean pulmonary artery pressure and the pulmonary capillary wedge pressure.

Unfortunately, Ohm's law is misapplied to the circulation. In electrical circuits, there is no y-intercept in the relationship $V = IR$. However, in studies of the relationships between pressure and flow in the circulation, there is an inherent critical opening pressure (P_c) that must be overcome for flow to initiate through blood vessels. Thus, the circulatory version of Ohm's law should be written $\Delta P = (CO \times R) + P_c$, although P_c cannot be determined in current clinical practice. The actual parameters that affect resistance directly, derived from Poiseuille's law, are the length and radii of the vessels constituting the circulation and the blood viscosity. Of these parameters, only viscosity can actually be measured, although it is not a routine part of common clinical practice.

The inability to assess the variables actually controlling resistance results in clinicians often resorting to the use of calculation based on pressure gradient and cardiac output. However, most ignore the fact that both of these parameters can change independently. This oversight often leads to misinterpretation of vascular resistance. While many assume that a change in the calculated systemic vascular resistance represents a change in vascular tone, it is often the case that an alteration in cardiac output has been responsible for the change in resistance.

The calculation involves a simple ratio of variables, rather than measurement of the parameters directly responsible for resistance to flow. Indeed, of the two basic variables in the resistance calculation, only the pressure gradient is directly related to flow resistance; cardiac output is influenced by resistance but is not, itself, an influencer of resistance. Therefore, when practitioners use a calculation that employs cardiac output in the denominator, there will always be a risk of misinterpretation if a primary change in cardiac output occurs. For example, a patient with a mean arterial pressure of 90 mm Hg, a central venous pressure of 10 mm Hg, and a cardiac output of 2 L/min would have an elevated calculated systemic vascular resistance of 3200. However, appropriate therapy for such a condition is unlikely to be vasodilation; it would usually be more important to directly improve cardiac output through volume replacement or the administration of inotropic agents.

To effectively use systemic vascular resistance in clinical practice, therefore, it is important to analyze which component—either the numerator or the denominator—is responsible for any abnormality. It is usually a simple process first to substitute a normal pressure gradient for the actual pressure gradient and recalculate the resistance. Next, replace the actual pressure gradient, substitute a normal cardiac output for the actual cardiac output, and recalculate yet again. The substitution that brings the calculated resistance closest to normal indicates which variable is most responsible for the abnormality; this knowledge therefore directs therapy.

Clinical Scenarios and Pitfalls

Six hours after the performance of an abdominal aortic aneurysmorrhaphy, a 64-year-old man develops oliguria. His arterial blood gas determination indicates a base deficit of -8. In the context of the history, the most likely etiology for his apparent circulatory dysfunction is hypovolemia. Therefore, a fluid challenge of 500 mL of lactated Ringer's solution is infused rapidly. When the patient's urine output fails to improve, a second fluid challenge of 500 mL is administered. He fails to respond, and ultimately a total of 2 L of lactated Ringer's solution is infused, without success.

A common pitfall in this circumstance is to administer a diuretic such as furosemide, with the goal of increasing the urine output. Even if the urine output is increased by the inhibitory effect on renal tubular function provided by the diuretic, the patient is not usually benefited by this trial. Clinicians faced with this dilemma are responding to conflicting concerns: They believe the patient is severely hypovolemic, but they are concerned about blindly giving too much volume. If the patient's metabolic acidosis and oliguria are, in fact, due to a primary cardiac process (a common condition in vascular patients), then excess volume could aggravate congestive heart failure. Hence, a diuretic could be beneficial in such a circumstance. Yet, if the patient were still severely hypovolemic despite the volume already administered, the diuretic would more likely be harmful.

This situation indicates confusion regarding the volume status of the circulation. The confusion can be eliminated by insertion of a pulmonary artery catheter and determination of the patient's hemodynamics. A low cardiac index (i.e., <2.8 L/min per m²) confirms the presence of circulatory insufficiency. A low PCWP (i.e., <10 cm H_2O) indicates that hypovolemia is responsible, while a higher PCWP suggests that primary cardiac dysfunction is the primary problem. This distinction dictates subsequent treatment in a much more defined manner.

In another patient, a 70-kg man with a body surface area of 1.83 m², the blood pressure is 120/80 mm Hg, the heart rate is 60 beats/min, the cardiac output is 5 L/min per m² (cardiac index 2.7 L/min per m²), the central venous pressure is 2 mm Hg, and the pulmonary capillary wedge pressure is 20 mm Hg. The low CVP suggests hypovolemia, while the high PCWP indicates hypervolemia. This apparent paradox is not uncommonly encountered. It is important to realize, however, that patients with poor ventricular reserve often demonstrate poor correlations between the filling pressures of the right and left heart. Also, if the patient happens to be tachypneic or in respiratory distress, the excessively negative intrathoracic pressures can artifactually lower measurements of the central venous pressure. The same phenomenon can influence PCWP readings; however, with the online tracing capabilities and wave analysis provided for interpretation of PCWP, this error is often avoided by determining the PCWP at end-expiration.

Therefore, because of the high PCWP, it appears that the patient's volume status is adequate. Inotropic support would thus be of benefit to help the patient's ailing heart. A point of confusion can often develop in such situations because of a calculation that reveals a systemic vascular resistance of 1460 dyne-sec/cm⁵. Because this is relatively high, clinicians are often uncertain at this point, believing that it represents vasoconstriction; the use of a catecholamine inotropic agent has the potential of worsening the vasoconstriction. However, simple calculations reveal that the primary abnormality producing the high calculated resistance is the cardiac output. Even though a cardiac output of 5 L/min seems normal enough, it actually produces a low cardiac index. Correction of the cardiac output to 7 L/min (producing a normal cardiac index of 3.8 L/min per m²) would produce a systemic vascular resistance of 1043 dyne-sec/cm⁵, well within the normal range. On the other hand, the other component of the resistance equation, the systemic pressure gradient, needs no correction toward normal, as it is already within a normal range. Thus, the elevated systemic vascular resistance reflects the low cardiac output, and not vasoconstriction. The use of a vasodilator would be inappropriate, but the use of an inotropic agent would be quite reasonable.

The use of a volumetric pulmonary artery catheter can often provide further refinement in the analysis. Rarely, there are some patients who may have a relatively high PCWP but still be experiencing hypovolemia because of their poor ventricular compliance. In such circumstances, the presence of a relatively low end-diastolic volume can indicate the need for further volume administration despite the presence of a relatively high PCWP.

OXYGEN DELIVERY MONITORING

The circulation is primarily responsible for fuel delivery to living tissues and organs; thus, it is important to monitor the quality of oxygen delivery, especially in the critically ill or injured patient. Oxygen delivery (DO_2) is provided by hemoglobin-based transport of oxygen conducted by the cardiac output. Thus, it is determined by the product of cardiac output (in L blood/min) and the oxygen content of arterial blood (in mL O_2/dL blood). Oxygen content, in turn, represents the sum of hemoglobin-bound oxygen and dissolved oxygen. Hemoglobin-bound oxygen is the product of the hemoglobin concentration in g Hgb/dL blood, the hemoglobin saturation, and the hemoglobin binding coefficient for oxygen in mL O_2/g Hgb. Dissolved oxygen is the product of the partial pressure of oxygen in mm Hg and the solubility coefficient for oxygen in blood in units of mL O_2/dL blood/mm Hg. Because the solubility of oxygen in blood is very poor (at 0.0032 mL O_2/dL blood/mm Hg), the primary influences on oxygen delivery are cardiac output, hemoglobin concentration, and hemoglobin saturation. Although commonly monitored in clinical practice, the arterial partial pressure of oxygen (PaO_2) contributes very little to oxygen transport to the tissues. However, at the capillary level, the partial pressure of oxygen is the major driving force for diffusion of oxygen toward the mitochondria. Clinically, this driving force is represented more accurately by the amount of oxygen in mixed venous blood (see later) than by the arterial partial pressure.

Oxygen Consumption

In 1870, Adolphus Fick described the important relationship between cardiac output, the oxygen content of blood, and oxygen consumption ($\dot{V}O_2$). Simply put, arteriovenous oxygen content difference multiplied by the cardiac output is equivalent to the body's oxygen consumption. The relationship between oxygen consumption and oxygen delivery is biphasic (Fig. 7–2). Oxygen consumption ideally depends on metabolic rate, but in the critically ill or injured patient it may become supply-dependent. In such situations, some tissues are forced to depend on anaerobic metabolism, as the level of oxygen delivery places consumption below the anaerobic threshold. The inferior efficiency of anaerobic metabolism means that prolonged existence at this level of metabolism can lead to the

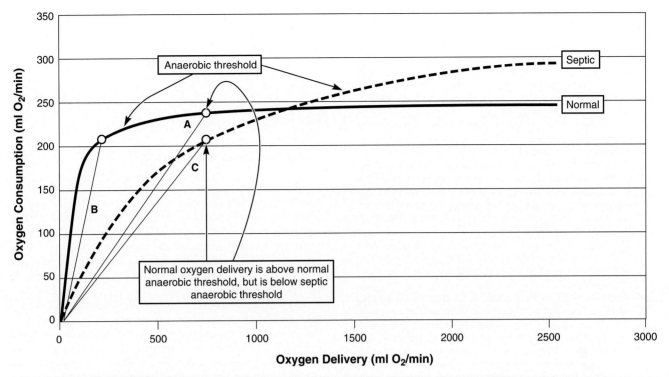

Figure 7–2. Relationship between oxygen delivery and oxygen consumption. The normal relationship provides an extraction ratio of 0.25 *(line A)*. During hypovolemic and cardiogenic shock, oxygen delivery declines so that oxygen consumption becomes supply-dependent and drops below the anaerobic threshold *(line B)*, resulting in an increased extraction ratio *(line B)*. In septic shock, the anaerobic threshold shifts to the right and the maximal rate of oxygen consumption typically increases (as is seen with febrile states). As a result, a normal rate of oxygen delivery places oxygen consumption below the anaerobic threshold with a lower extraction ratio *(line C)*. A hyperdynamic circulation has a better chance of satisfying tissue oxygen demands if oxygen delivery can bring oxygen consumption over the anaerobic threshold.

failure of cells, tissues, and organs to perform their normal functions and, potentially, to survive.

Oxygen Extraction Ratio

The relationship between oxygen consumption and delivery is often expressed as the oxygen extraction ratio:

$$O_2ER = \frac{\dot{V}O_2}{\dot{D}O_2} \qquad (1)$$

This works as a demand-supply relationship for the circulation's task of providing energy to the body's tissues. Normally, 25% of the delivered oxygen is consumed. If the extraction ratio increases, it indicates that consumption has increased or delivery has dropped, or both. The shared components in the relationship and the fact that most patients in intensive care units have an arterial saturation in excess of 90% means that the oxygen extraction ratio can usually be approximated by $1 - S\bar{v}O_2$. The benefit of this approximation is that it enables continuous on-line monitoring of the demand-supply relationship for the circulation's performance at fuel delivery through the use of the indwelling oximetry technology.

In hypovolemic and cardiogenic shock conditions, the oxygen extraction ratio increases, as indicated by a declining $S\bar{v}O_2$. However, in early septic shock, the anaerobic threshold appears to shift to the right and the maximal $\dot{V}O_2$ increases, such that the extraction ratio decreases (and $S\bar{v}O_2$ rises).

Clinical Scenarios and Pitfalls

The previously described patient who recently underwent abdominal aortic aneurysmorrhaphy receives inotropic support in the form of a dobutamine infusion. With that, his cardiac output improves, and his $S\bar{v}O_2$ increases from 52% to 64%. All too often, this result is considered adequate. However, this still indicates an increased extraction ratio, meaning that the tissues are required to extract more oxygen than normal off the circulating hemoglobin because the oxygen delivery is still inadequate to meet the demand. Analysis of the components of oxygen delivery reveals that the patient has a hemoglobin of 8.2 g/dL. Although adequate in a normal healthy individual, this degree of anemia in a stressed vasculopathic individual is very worrisome, potentially setting the stage for acute myocardial ischemia. Judicious transfusion to correct the anemia should progressively improve the patient's hemoglobin, oxygen delivery, and $S\bar{v}O_2$.

As the patient recovers, it is noted that his $S\bar{v}O_2$ reaches 81%. While this could certainly suggest a septic condition, other parameters that indicate infection (e.g., fever, leukocytosis) are absent. Moreover, the patient is still receiv-

Pearls and Pitfalls

PEARLS

- Use of end-organ functional measures (i.e., urine output or, even better, 2-hour creatinine clearance) or indicators of anaerobic metabolism (i.e., base deficit) as end-points of resuscitation
- Interpreting flows and volumes can be benefited by indexing to body surface area in order to assess the parameter's degree of normality or abnormality
- Observe the different responses of pressures (i.e., PCWP, CVP, and MAP), volume (i.e., RVEDV), and flow (i.e., cardiac output) to therapeutic interventions, especially with an eye to improving an end-point reflective of energy supply (i.e., $S\bar{v}O_2$, base deficit, 2-hour creatinine clearance)
- Optimize cardiac performance first by ensuring that volume and hemoglobin levels are adequate before attempting to stimulate cardiac inotropic activity chemically
- Interpret changes in vascular resistance by observing whether the cardiac output has changed, as a change in cardiac output will produce a change in calculated resistance with no change in microvascular tone
- Determine whether there is a circulatory abnormality (i.e., hypovolemia, poor cardiac function, sepsis) responsible for oliguria—using invasive hemodynamic measurements if necessary—and correct the specific abnormalities found; determination of a 2-hour creatinine clearance is also a useful tool and monitor for helping detect renal dysfunction at an early stage

PITFALLS

- Use of hemodynamic parameters (i.e., PCWP, cardiac output, blood pressure) as end-points of resuscitation
- Indexing pressures and pressure-based parameters (e.g., vascular resistance) to body surface area
- Assumption that a particular pressure measurement, such as a PCWP, directly reflects volume or flow
- Use of inotropic agents (i.e., catecholamines) without ensuring that circulating volume is adequate
- Assuming that a change in the calculated vascular resistance represents only a change in microvascular tone
- Administering a loop diuretic to an oliguric patient

ing inotropic support that may now be unnecessary. To help make this distinction, the oxygen consumption before and after abrupt discontinuation of the dobutamine should be determined. Oxygen delivery will more than likely drop as the result of the discontinuation. If oxygen consumption also drops, it may be the case that the patient is experiencing supply-dependent oxygen consumption and could, in fact, be septic. However, the more probable result is that oxygen consumption will not change appreciably, indicating that excessive oxygen delivery was being provided, thereby accounting for the reduced extraction ratio.

ORGAN-SPECIFIC MONITORING

The growing realization that multiple organ failure results at least in part from inadequate circulatory energy supply has focused greater attention on the actual monitoring of organ fuel supply and function as an indicator of circulatory performance. There is an expanding list of devices and techniques that allow the intensive care physician the opportunity to dynamically assess organ oxygen delivery and function. Which of these will ultimately emerge as essential and standard to the care of the critically ill or injured patient remains to be seen.

Renal Function Monitoring

Clinical determination of the glomerular filtration rate can be accurately assessed with the use of the creatinine clearance calculation. One of the oldest techniques, determination of creatinine clearance is also one of the most sensitive for the potential development of acute renal failure. This is useful because the kidneys, in turn, are among the organs most sensitive to any downturn in circulatory performance.

Creatinine clearance is defined as the amount of creatinine produced in urine over a period of time relative to the existing plasma concentration. In fact, the basic equation (UV/PT) can be employed for determining the renal clearance of any substance from plasma. Three quarters of the variables used in the equation are routinely obtained on virtually every critically ill patient: the urine flow rate (V/T) is typically obtained on an hourly basis, and the plasma creatinine concentration is often obtained at least daily. The only measurement needed to complete the calculation is the urine creatinine concentration, which usually costs very little for the laboratory to determine. In contrast to the plasma creatinine value, the urine creatinine concentration can change rapidly from hour to hour as the result of dynamic changes in the glomerular filtration rate.

Renal tubular function is critical to renal performance, and the development of acute tubular necrosis portends a grim prognosis for the critically ill or injured patient. The fractional excretion of sodium (Fe_{Na}) provides an accurate method of determining the adequacy of renal tubular performance. It calculates the amount of sodium excreted in the urine relative to the amount filtered into the tubular lumens.

$$Fe_{Na} = \frac{\text{Sodium excreted}}{\text{Sodium filtered}} = \frac{U_{Na^+} \times V/T}{P_{Na^+} \times GFR} \quad [2]$$

$$= \frac{U_{Na^+} \times V/T}{P_{Na^+} = C_{cr}} \times \frac{\dfrac{U_{Na^+} \times V}{T}}{\dfrac{P_{Na^+} \times U_{cr} \times V}{P_{cr} \times T}} =$$

$$\frac{\dfrac{U_{Na^+} \times V}{P_{Na^+} \times T}}{\dfrac{U_{cr} \times V}{P_{cr} \times T}} = \frac{C_{Na^+}}{Ccr}$$

$$Fe_{Na} = \frac{\dfrac{U_{Na^+}}{P_{Na^+}}}{\dfrac{U_{cr}}{P_{cr}}} \times \frac{U_{Na^+} \times P_{cr}}{U_{cr^+} \times P_{Na^+}} \times 100\%$$

Note that the equation can produce a derivation that makes the Fe_{Na} equivalent to the sodium clearance divided by the creatinine clearance. Also, the result is usually expressed as a percentage to keep the expression from having excessive leading zeros following the decimal, as the normal fractional excretion of sodium is less than 1%.

Gastrointestinal Tonometry

Gastric tonometry employs a measurement of the partial pressure of carbon dioxide in the gastric lumen. The device is a modified nasogastric tube that contains a distal balloon allowing for gas sampling from the balloon. Carbon dioxide from the gastric lumen diffuses freely with the gas in the balloon. As the circulation is responsible for removing carbon dioxide from the surrounding tissue, an accumulation of the regional Pco_2 (P_rco_2) represents circulatory insufficiency to the stomach. Also, through the use of the Henderson-Hasselbalch equation, an arterial bicarbonate determination, and some assumptions, the pH of the gastric wall (pH_i) can be approximated. As the circulation deteriorates, the intramural pH will correspondingly decline. A similar device can be used to assess perfusion to the sigmoid colon.

Cutaneous Perfusion Monitoring

The skin continuously exhales oxygen at a rate proportional to the partial pressure of oxygen in the tissue and the blood flow. This Po_2 can be monitored transcutaneously with the use of a modified Clark polarographic electrode. Correlation with arterial Po_2 is improved through a built-in heater unit on the transcutaneous electrode.

Another technology for evaluating cutaneous perfusion involves laser Doppler velocimetry. Laser light is targeted at the skin, penetrating and reflecting to a distance of a few millimeters. Through the use of the Doppler shift effect on reflected frequencies, the average velocity of blood cells moving through the dermal vessels can be determined.

Both of these technologies allow for dynamic monitoring of cutaneous perfusion. They have found clinical applications in monitoring perfusion to pedicled and free flaps in plastic surgery and in monitoring the cutaneous perfusion of threatened extremities in vascular surgery. The skin is relatively sensitive to the presence of an inadequate circulation. Thus, monitoring skin perfusion also makes sense in the critically ill or injured patient, especially because these techniques are noninvasive. However, such clinical application has not yet been widely accepted.

Near-Infrared Spectroscopy

Near-infrared spectroscopy employs light waves in the wavelengths between 700 and 1000 nm, which can pass through tissues such as bone, skin, and muscle. Chromophoric molecules such as hemoglobin, myoglobin, and cytochrome aa_3 absorb the light variably along a spectrum, allowing for the determination of their relative concentrations. With this technique, continuous monitoring of local blood flow and tissue oxidation state is theoretically possible, and some clinical experience has indicated that it is useful in noninvasive monitoring of extremities for compartment syndrome. Its ultimate utility in the critically ill or injured patient appears to be promising, but more experience is necessary.

SELECTED READINGS

Berne RM, Levy MN: Cardiovascular Physiology. St. Louis, CV Mosby, 1972.

Espinel CH: The FENa test: Use in the differential diagnosis of acute renal failure. JAMA 236:579, 1976.

Hamilton WF, Richards DW: The output of the heart. In Fishman AP, Richards DW (eds): Circulation of the Blood: Men and Ideas. Baltimore, Waverly Press, 1982, pp 95–97.

Mythen MG, Woolf R, Noone RB: Gastric mucosal tonometry: Towards new methods and applications. Anasthesiol Intensivmed Notfallmed Schmerzther 33(suppl 2):S85, 1998.

Nelson LD: The new pulmonary artery catheters: Right ventricular ejection fraction and continuous cardiac output. Crit Care Clin 12:795, 1996.

Reed RL, Maier RV, Landicho D, et al: Correlation of hemodynamic variables with transcutaneous PO₂ measurements in critically ill adult patients. J Trauma 25:1045, 1985.

Reed RL: Oxygen consumption and delivery. Curr Opin Anaesth 6:329, 1993.

Schabauer AM, Rooke TW: Cutaneous laser Doppler flowmetry: Applications and findings. Mayo Clin Proc 69:564, 1994.

Shin B, Mackenzie CF, Helrich M: Creatinine clearance of early detection of post-traumatic renal dysfunction. Anesthesiology 64:605, 1986.

Simonson SG, Piantadosi CA: Near-infrared spectroscopy: Clinical applications. Crit Care Clin 12:1019, 1996.

TRAUMA AND BURNS

Chapter 8

Initial Evaluation of the Trauma Patient

Donald A. Reiff and Loring W. Rue, III

Documentation of the approach to the injured patient predates the ancient Egyptian era, but no record is as important as the Edwin Smith papyrus. Believed to be a copy of an earlier text created in 3000 BC, the Smith papyrus (circa 1600 BC) describes 48 patients with traumatic injuries and their surgical management. Injury remains the leading cause of death for the first four decades of life and results in more than 300,000 permanent disabilities each year. The first 60 minutes after trauma has occurred is often termed the *golden hour*, and outcomes for injured patients are enhanced by expeditious and appropriate surgical care rendered soon after injury. With the development of the Advanced Trauma Life Support (ATLS) protocols designed by the American College of Surgeons in 1978, a system for care of the acutely injured patient was developed. Using this template, physicians have guidelines for rapidly evaluating and treating critically injured patients.

INITIAL APPROACH TO THE INJURED PATIENT

On arrival of the injured patient to the resuscitation suite, a member of the trauma team should obtain, preferably from the prehospital personnel, the mechanism of injury and other pertinent clinical data in rapid and organized fashion. The victim, if alert, can provide much of this information. The trauma team can quickly obtain baseline information essential to both the immediate and long-term care of the injured patient with the use of the mnemonic AMPLE:

A = Allergies
M = Medications
P = Past illness and surgeries
L = Last meal
E = Events related to injury

Simultaneously, the "primary survey," focusing on life-sustaining physiologic functions, is conducted while monitoring devices are placed on the patient. As the primary survey is underway, life-threatening injuries are treated when identified. Following completion of this initial survey, the "secondary survey," which consists of the traditional head-to-toe physical examination, is performed, radiographic studies are obtained, and a definitive management plan is formulated for the patient. The resuscitation of the patient with multiple injuries can be a chaotic event, but when the trauma team has focused responsibilities and pays close attention to detail, the evaluation and concomitant resuscitation can proceed rapidly, with reduced chances of missing injuries. To enhance efficiency, a "command" physician should be designated for each resuscitation. This concept of a team leader for the resuscitation has demonstrated greater adherence to ATLS protocols, more orderly completion of primary and secondary surveys, and more rapid formulation of definitive management plans. The senior surgeon in attendance should assume this role and accept final responsibility for the patient's overall care.

PRIMARY SURVEY

Airway

The initial evaluation of the polytrauma patient begins with an assessment of airway adequacy. The clinician should seek signs of compromise in the primary survey by using the "look, listen, and feel" approach. Alert and conversant patients who respond with a normal-sounding voice suggest no immediate problem with airway patency, whereas those appearing agitated may be hypoxic or under the influence of alcohol and/or drugs, unable to protect their airways. Patients who are minimally responsive or obtunded may be hypercapnic or also may suffer from alcohol and/or drug intoxication. Abnormal sounds such as gurgling, snoring, hoarseness, and stridor all are signs of a compromised airway. The use of the accessory muscles of respiration is also suggestive of airway compromise.

The most common cause of upper airway obstruction is the tongue. The obtunded or unconscious patient experiences a generalized reduction in muscular tone; when the patient is placed supine, the tongue is displaced posteriorly, thereby occluding the airway. Other common causes of obstruction include foreign bodies, blood, teeth, and vomitus. The oropharynx should be assessed and cleared of such material early in the patient's evaluation.

A quick and effective technique for establishing a patient's airway is the chin-lift and jaw-thrust maneuver; this maneuver is particularly helpful when the tongue is the obstructing agent. These actions displace the soft tissue anteriorly, opening the upper airway and allowing for air passage. Other techniques include the placement of an oropharyngeal or nasopharyngeal airway. The oropharyngeal airway should be restricted to obtunded patients, as this device is not tolerated by conscious patients. Nasopharyngeal airways are less likely to induce vomiting but should be avoided if facial or basilar skull fractures are suspected. If these measures are unsuccessful, the patient will require more definitive control of the airway by insertion of either an orotracheal or a nasotracheal tube or, in certain circumstances, creation of a surgical airway.

All trauma patients are treated as "full stomachs" and a rapid-sequence method for intubation is recommended. This technique begins with preoxygenation of the patient while the induction and paralytic agents are being administered. Yankour suction should be available to clear the oropharynx and supraglottic region of all secretions. Instruments necessary for a surgical airway should be available in the event that intubation is unsuccessful. Induction agents include thiopental, ketamine, or etomidate, and the preferred paralytic agent is succinylcholine. As these drugs are administered, pressure should be applied firmly over the cricoid ring. Properly applied cricoid pressure minimizes the risk of aspirating regurgitated gastric contents during mask ventilation. Of importance, patients in shock should not receive any form of induction, as most of these drugs will worsen the existing hypotension. Furthermore, patients who are unresponsive typically do not require pharmacologic paralysis. Succinylcholine should be withheld from patients at risk for hyperkalemia, as this depolarizing agent results in a rapid release of intracellular potassium, which may precipitate cardiac dysrhythmias. Patients particularly at risk include those with extensive soft tissue injury and burn patients 4 to 6 hours after injury. Under direct laryngoscopic visualization or with the use of a bronchoscope, the cuff of the endotracheal tube is positioned distal to the vocal cords. Correct placement of the endotracheal tube is confirmed with the use of an end-tidal carbon dioxide detection device, auscultation of the chest, and a chest radiograph.

Controlled comparisons have demonstrated that blind nasotracheal intubations have a higher rate of complication than do rapid-sequence orotracheal intubations. Further, orotracheal intubation can be safely performed on patients with cervical spine injury, as long as in-line stabilization is carefully maintained. Nasotracheal intubation requires spontaneous ventilation and can cause significant epistaxis, aggravating airway compromise. Consequently, nasotracheal intubations have a limited role in the care of injured patients.

If attempts at intubation fail or the oral and nasal routes are contraindicated because of maxillofacial injuries or anatomic distortion, a surgical airway is mandated. The needle cricothyroidotomy with jet insufflation can be used as a temporizing measure, but the surgical cricothyroidotomy remains the preferred technique in these emergency situations. When properly performed, the cricothyroidotomy can be undertaken faster and has a lower complication rate than does tracheostomy. Further, cricothyroidotomy is tolerated quite well for up to 7 days before tracheostomy is necessary to avoid the complication of subglottic stenosis.

Breathing and Ventilation

Once the airway is adequately addressed, oxygenation and ventilation must be ensured. Oxygenation can be assessed with the noninvasive pulse oximeter and confirmed with an arterial blood gas measurement. Satisfactory ventilation can be evaluated by inspection, palpation, percussion, and auscultation of the chest. If inadequate ventilation is detected, the airway should be reassessed to ensure that the esophagus has not been intubated inadvertently. If ventilation remains inadequate, life-threatening chest injuries that impede ventilation must be considered. These conditions include a tension pneumothorax, massive hemothorax, open pneumothorax, and flail chest.

A *tension pneumothorax* can result from either blunt or penetrating trauma to the lung, bronchi, or trachea, allowing air to continually leak into the pleural space. This differs from a simple pneumothorax in that the lung parenchymal injury remains patent and no chest wall defect is produced to allow venting of the progressively accumulating pleural air. Consequently, with each breath, the patient generates negative intrathoracic pressure, which progressively accumulates air into the pleural space and results in collapse of the ipsilateral lung. The resultant increased pleural pressure will ultimately shift the mediastinum to the contralateral side. This mediastinal distortion causes decreased venous return to the heart, resulting in depressed cardiac output and hemodynamic instability. Patients appear anxious with tachycardia, hypotension, marked respiratory distress, absent ipsilateral breath sounds, tracheal deviation to the contralateral side, and neck vein distention. Consequently, *tension pneumothorax* is a clinical diagnosis. It is quickly treated by placing a large-bore angiocatheter into the second intercostal space along the midclavicular line so as to decompress the pleural space. Definitive treatment requires the placement of a tube thoracostomy attached to 20 cm of water suction.

A *massive hemothorax* can occur as the consequence of either blunt or penetrating trauma due to an injury to an intercostal or hilar vessel. Massive hemothorax is defined as 1500 mL of blood loss into the hemithorax, with subsequent compression of the lung. The diagnosis is established when shock is identified in concert with absent breath sounds and dullness to percussion on one side of the chest. The injury is treated by simultaneous restoration of the intravascular space with crystalloids and blood products and decompression of the pleural space with a large-tube (38- or 40-French) thoracostomy. A chest radiograph should be obtained following placement of the chest tube to ensure that the hemothorax has been completely evacuated, so as to minimize the risk of a subsequent fibrothorax or empyema. If more than 1500 mL of blood is initially evacuated or if blood loss exceeds 200 mL/hr for the next 2 to 3 hours, a thoracotomy may be required.

An *open pneumothorax,* or "sucking chest wound," results from a defect in the chest wall that exceeds two thirds of the diameter of the trachea. Following the injury, which is typically penetrating trauma, the intrathoracic pressure will equate with the atmospheric pressure. With each subsequent inspiratory effort, air will preferentially follow the path of least resistance through the thoracic defect and into the pleural space. The injury can be initially controlled with placement of an occlusive dressing over the wound and the securing of the dressing on three sides. This creates a flap valve where air is permitted to escape from the pleural space during expiration but no air is allowed to enter during inspiration. Tube thoracostomy should be performed at a site remote from the injury. Frequently, definitive surgical closure of the chest wall defect is required.

A *flail chest* is defined as a fracture of three or more consecutive ribs in two or more places, with or without sternal involvement, allowing for paradoxical respiratory motion. Frequently, a *flail chest* will have an associated hemothorax or pneumothorax and will require the placement of a chest tube. Although there is a severe disruption of normal chest wall movement associated with the flail segment, the resulting physiologic derangement is the consequence of the underlying pulmonary contusion and poor respiratory mechanics related to chest wall pain. Treatment is directed at providing physiologic support of the gas exchange abnormalities and alleviating pain.

Parenteral analgesics, particularly with patient-controlled analgesia, are the mainstay of therapy and should be employed liberally. Some patients benefit from early placement of thoracic epidural catheters. This patient population includes those with three or more rib fractures, age greater than 65, and sternal fractures, as well as patients with poor pulmonary mechanics or inadequate pulmonary toilet despite parenteral analgesics. Thoracic epidural analgesia for *flail chest* has been demonstrated to improve the patient's maximal inspiratory effort, tidal volumes, and vital capacity (Mackersie et al, 1987). In the event that pulmonary toilet and ventilation are still suboptimal with epidural analgesia, mechanical ventilatory support is required. Ventilator support is best implemented early, as this has been demonstrated to reduce overall duration of ventilatory support as well as mortality.

Circulation

With the airway secured and ventilation deemed adequate, the circulatory system is the next priority. Shock is best defined as inadequate delivery of oxygen to meet the metabolic demands of peripheral tissue. The most common etiology of shock for the trauma patient remains hemorrhagic shock, but other sources including cardiogenic (cardiac tamponade or tension pneumothorax) and neurogenic (spinal injury) must be considered. Following blunt trauma, hypovolemic shock is most often due to intraperitoneal blood loss, pelvic fractures, musculoskeletal injuries, and/or thoracic trauma. Hemorrhagic shock associated with penetrating trauma can result from a laceration of any major blood vessel, causing external exsanguination through the wound or internal exsanguination into any of the major corporeal compartments.

The treatment of shock begins first with its recognition. The hallmark clinical signs of shock include tachycardia, hypotension, narrowing of the pulse pressure, cutaneous vasoconstriction, oliguria, and mental status changes that comprise the spectrum from apprehension to obtundation. Hemorrhagic shock has been classically divided into four categories, each signifying an increasing volume of blood loss. Class I shock represents a 10% to 15% loss of total blood volume, or about 500 to 750 mL. Minimal clinical signs are present, perhaps only manifested by a mild elevation in heart rate. As blood loss continues and 750 to 1500 mL, or 20% to 30% of the total blood volume,

is lost, patients will demonstrate further tachycardia and a drop in pulse pressure, but systolic blood pressure will remain largely unaffected. These signs result from an increased concentration of circulating catecholamines, which compensates for the blood loss by increasing the heart rate and systemic vascular resistance. Consequently, systolic blood pressure is maintained and diastolic blood pressure is increased, thereby reducing the pulse pressure. When blood loss reaches 1500 to 2000 mL, approximately 30% to 40% of the total blood volume, the classic signs of shock are present, with patients demonstrating tachycardia, oliguria, hypotension, and altered mental status exhibited as confusion or agitation. Blood loss in excess of 2000 mL is an immediate life-threatening situation, and patients present with marked tachycardia, systolic hypotension, absent diastolic pressure, anuria, and obtundation.

Following the recognition of shock, initial management includes gaining access to the vascular system and stanching obvious external hemorrhage. Intravenous (IV) access is obtained by placing two large-bore short angiocatheters in peripheral veins. According to Poiseuille's law, the rate of fluid movement through a conduit is directly proportional to the radius of the channel raised to the fourth power and is inversely proportional to its length. Thus, a peripheral 14-gauge angiocatheter is a superior choice to any central line and will allow for more rapid fluid administration. Once intravenous access is obtained, phlebotomy can be performed for basic laboratory studies and for blood typing and cross-matching. Initial volume expansion is achieved with a 2-L bolus of warmed lactated Ringer's solution. Crystalloid solution resuscitations, compared with colloid-based trauma resuscitations, have been demonstrated to be superior both physiologically and in terms of patient survival. Dogs bled into shock and then treated with shed blood and lactated Ringer's solution exhibited a return of extracellular fluid volume to control levels and an increased survival rate compared with those treated with shed blood and colloid infusion (Shires et al, 1964). A meta-analysis of previously published work (Velanovich, 1989) demonstrates resuscitation with crystalloid provided a 12.3% reduced mortality rate over resuscitation with colloid solutions for trauma patients.

The volume required for the resuscitation of a patient is difficult to predict, but the "3 for 1 rule" can provide a rough approximation of a patient's initial fluid needs. This estimate assumes that a patient will need 3 mL of crystalloid for every milliliter of blood loss. Patients in class III or IV shock, or those who do not respond to their initial bolus of lactated Ringer's solution, should receive additional crystalloid boluses and early administration of blood products. The goal of any resuscitation strategy is the reversal of the shock state, and aggressive resuscitation should continue until adequate end-organ perfusion and tissue oxygenation have been achieved. Traditionally, the end-points of shock resuscitation have been the restoration of normal blood pressure and heart rate and adequate urinary output. Unfortunately, the use of these measures alone as a guide for adequate resuscitation may leave as many as 50% to 85% of trauma patients in "compensated" shock. In these situations, a patient's hemodynamic indices may be normal, but there may still be evidence of suboptimal tissue perfusion, as demonstrated by the persistence of systemic acidemia, elevated lactate levels, and low mixed venous oxygen saturations. This situation can occur as blood flow and oxygen delivery are redistributed from the splanchnic bed to other critical organs, such as the brain and heart. Resuscitation data (Porter and Ivatury, 1998) suggest that in addition to restoring normal hemodynamic indices and urinary output, correction of the base deficit and restoration of lactate levels to normal will result in significantly reduced mortality.

While fluid resuscitation is ongoing, the source of the circulatory collapse must be identified. Blood loss must first be excluded and may be as obvious as external hemorrhage, or it can occur occultly and find its way into any one or a combination of spaces, including the abdomen, thorax, retroperitoneum, or extremities. In the past, diagnostic peritoneal lavage (DPL) was the preferred technique used in the emergency department to exclude hemoperitoneum as a potential cause of hemodynamic instability. DPL remains a reliable study, with reported sensitivities ranging from 90% to 96% and specificities from 99% to 100% (Fabian et al, 1986; Meyer et al, 1989), but it is an invasive procedure performed with the use of the open, semiopen, or closed technique. Regardless of the approach, prior to beginning the procedure, the patient should have the stomach and bladder decompressed with a nasogastric (NG) tube and Foley catheter. Patients who have sustained an associated pelvic fracture should have their DPL performed in the supraumbilical location because of the potential for retroperitoneal hematoma, whereas other DPLs are performed infraumbilically. For all techniques, once peritoneal access is obtained, aspiration of peritoneal fluid is first attempted. If gross blood is returned, the study is positive; if no blood is returned, 1 L of sterile crystalloid is instilled into the abdomen. Before the bag is emptied, it should be lowered to the floor to create a siphon action in the tubing, thereby removing peritoneal fluid for laboratory analysis. Criteria for a positive study include a lavage with more than 100,000 red blood cells (RBCs) or 500 white blood cells (WBCs) per mL, the presence of particulate matter, and elevated concentrations of amylase or bilirubin. This technique has been replaced in many centers by the focused abdominal sonogram for trauma (FAST) evaluation. FAST is a technique that surgeons can quickly master and is proving to be a dependable, rapid, and noninvasive technique. FAST is highly sensitive in detecting solid-organ injury and is very reliable in the identification of hemoperitoneum, with some studies demonstrating a sensitivity approaching 95% (Yoshii et al, 1998).

Pelvic fractures are an underappreciated source of blood loss in the polytrauma patient, and blood loss can be of arterial, venous, or osseous origin. The patient can essentially exsanguinate from a pelvic fracture, with the potential for several liters of blood to be sequestered in the retroperitoneum. Therapy begins with immobilization of the pelvis by external fixation or the application of a pneumatic antishock garment. This approach aligns the cancellous bone fragments and reduces the volume of the pelvis, thus allowing for a tamponade effect to arrest the venous and osseous hemorrhage. Failure to control

hemorrhage in these circumstances is probably due to an arterial injury and may require angiography and therapeutic embolization. Femur fractures can be associated with 1500 mL of blood loss and, similar to pelvic fractures, require immobilization as the initial treatment priority.

One of the greatest challenges faced by the surgeon in the setting of blunt trauma with a known pelvic fracture is deciding whether the peritoneal cavity or the pelvis is the source of the blood loss. Patients who remain hemodynamically stable are evaluated, preferably with computed tomography (CT) scanning. Hemodynamically unstable patients should first be evaluated with a DPL or FAST study. Although FAST is highly sensitive in detecting hemoperitoneum, recent data (Ballard et al, 1999) suggest that this study is associated with a high false-negative rate in that a significant number of intra-abdominal injuries are missed in patients with concomitant pelvic fractures. Further, DPL remains reliable in the setting of a pelvic fracture, with a reported sensitivity and specificity of 94% and 99%, respectively (Mendez et al, 1994).

Neurologic Deficit and Exposure

The final aspect of the primary survey consists of identifying any gross neurologic deficit and exposing the patient completely. An assessment of gross neurologic function is accomplished by evaluating a patient's response to stimuli using the mnemonic AVPU:

A = Alert
V = Responds to verbal stimulus
P = Responds to painful stimulus
U = Unresponsive

The Glasgow Coma Scale (GCS) is a more detailed evaluation of function and an alternative measure for evaluating the neurologic status of injured patients. The Glasgow Coma score is the sum of the three components of assessment, found in Table 8–1. Pupillary size, symmetry, and reaction to light are also assessed during the

Table 8–1	Glasgow Coma Scale	
PARAMETER		**SCORE**
Best Motor Response		
Normal		6
Localizes		5
Withdraws		4
Flexion		3
Extension		2
None		1
Best Verbal Response		
Oriented		5
Confused		4
Verbalizes		3
Vocalizes		2
None/intubated		1
Eye Opening		
Spontaneous		4
To command		3
To pain		2
None		1

Minor injury: 13–15; moderate injury: 9–12; severe injury: 8 or below.

primary survey. These evaluations should occur early in the resuscitation process, with frequent re-evaluations to document either patient improvement or deterioration. A worsening examination will prompt the decision for additional therapy or diagnostic studies.

To allow completion of the primary survey, the patient must be completely disrobed so that any obvious external injury will not be overlooked. The most expedient and safest means for exposure is to simply cut the clothing off the patient and remove any metal objects that will interfere with radiographs. After logrolling the patient, the back, perineum, and axillae are examined and a rectal examination is performed. Afterward, warm blankets are placed over the patient to minimize the risk of hypothermia. Other measures for preserving body temperature include heating the room, warming IV fluids and the inspired air in the ventilator circuit, and using environmental heaters such as the Bair Hugger. Hypothermia induces patient shivering to generate heat. This results in an increase in oxygen demand and a worsening of the shock state. Hypothermia can also impair both the primary and the secondary hemostatic mechanisms. Temperatures below 35°C induce platelet dysfunction as demonstrated by alterations of adherence, loss of shape, and impaired production and secretion of thromboxane A_2, a potent vasoconstrictor. Secondary hemostasis involves activation of the proteolytic enzymes of the coagulation cascade. All enzyme activity slows with decreasing body temperature, and thus formation of the stable fibrin clot is impaired.

Before beginning the secondary survey, the patient's clinical status should be reassessed by quickly reviewing all components of the primary survey. Additionally, basic radiographic and laboratory studies are performed. A minimum of three radiographic studies are performed for the trauma patient, including an anteroposterior view of the chest and pelvis as well as a cross-table lateral view of the cervical spine. The information yielded from these studies is helpful in piecing together the clinical picture. Laboratory studies are frequently acquired when intravenous access is obtained. Additionally, an arterial blood gas should be drawn, usually from the femoral artery, to determine the extent of base deficit suggesting the degree of shock.

All severely injured patients should have a Foley catheter placed during their resuscitation. The only contraindication for Foley placement is a urethral injury, which should be suspected with complex pelvic fractures, blood noted at the penile meatus, or a high-riding prostate detected during the rectal examination. If a urethral injury is suspected, a retrograde urethrogram is performed prior to the placement of the catheter.

An NG is placed to decompress the stomach so as to reduce the risk of aspiration for intubated patients and those who are unable to protect their airways adequately because of depression of the central nervous system. The NG tube serves as a route for administering oral contrast medium prior to CT studies. Patients with midface instability or evidence of basilar skull fractures should have orogastric tubes placed, instead of using the transnasal route, to prevent potential iatrogenic injury.

SECONDARY SURVEY

The *secondary survey* consists of a review of the information regarding the injury mechanism, the patient's past medical history, and a complete head-to-toe physical examination. This portion of the evaluation should not begin until the primary survey has been completed, all lifesaving interventions have been performed, and a satisfactory response to resuscitation has been observed. The physical examination needs to be performed in an organized and thorough manner, beginning with the scalp and systematically moving caudally to the feet. Once this examination has been completed, and based on physical examination findings, the remainder of necessary diagnostic studies are obtained, including radiographs of potential fractures, CT scans, and arteriograms.

Physical Examination

Central Nervous System

As noted earlier, a brief neurologic examination is conducted during the primary survey. During the secondary survey, a more complete examination is performed, with the examination of the cranial nerves, motor strength of all extremities, spinal reflexes, and loss of sensation to pain, temperature, and proprioception from head to toe. Abnormalities identified in the physical examination should prompt further evaluation with a head CT or magnetic resonance imaging (MRI) scan, as well as consultation with a neurosurgeon. Hyperventilation, previously employed for the head-injured patient, is currently contraindicated because it results in cerebral vasoconstriction and decreased cerebral perfusion, thus potentially worsening the brain injury. Further, recent studies have demonstrated no beneficial effects of steroid use in the treatment of closed head injury.

Blunt trauma patients should be assumed to have sustained a vertebral column injury until proved otherwise by an unequivocal physical examination and radiographic survey. Based on the mechanism of injury or physical examination findings, clinicians should have a low threshold for obtaining thoracic and lumbar spine radiographs. Patients under the influence of alcohol and/or drugs and those with an abnormal Glasgow Coma score should remain in rigid cervical collars until their mental status has improved and a normal examination is demonstrated. Alert patients, with normal cervical spine films, who complain of neck tenderness should have flexion and extension radiographs of their cervical spine obtained. For this study, the rigid cervical collar is removed by a physician who then maintains in-line alignment of the cervical spine and allows the patient to flex and extend their neck. These views help identify malalignment due to ligamentous instability, which cannot be visualized with the static cross-table lateral or anteroposterior radiographs of the cervical spine. Patients without confirmed injury, but in whom clinical suspicion is high based on the history or physical examination, should have a CT of the cervical spine with thin cuts through the suspicious region. Patients with identified spinal cord injuries have been shown to have improved long-term outcomes when intravenous steroids are administered within 8 hours of the damage. Initially, Solu-Medrol (methylprednisolone sodium succinate) is delivered as a bolus and then administered at a continuous rate over a 24-hour period.

Head

Because of the abundant blood supply to the head, lacerations of the scalp and face can bleed briskly and are usually controlled during the primary survey with direct pressure or quick placement of temporary sutures. During the secondary survey, these injuries should be débrided, adequately cleansed with a surgical soap, and primarily closed. Extraocular motion should be assessed, and the face should be closely examined for any asymmetry. Most facial fractures can be detected by palpation of the bony prominences, while fractures of the midface can be detected by inserting a finger into the mouth and examining for instability of the hard palate or incisors. Maxillary or mandibular fractures are suggested by malocclusion. The tympanic membranes and external auditory canals are inspected with an otoscope. The presence of a hemotympanum or cerebrospinal fluid otorrhea is diagnostic of a basilar skull fracture. Further evidence of a basilar skull fracture is suggested by bruising around the eyes and behind the ears, so-called Battle's sign. If facial or basilar skull fractures are suspected, a CT scan of the face should be performed to confirm the diagnosis and better define the injury.

Neck

The neck is typically divided into three zones. Zone I extends from the clavicles to the base of the cricoid cartilage; zone II extends from the cricoid to the angle of the mandible; and zone III spans the region from the angle of the mandible to the base of the skull. These zones are of particular importance in managing the patient with penetrating trauma. Unstable patients require surgical exploration. Hemodynamically stable patients with penetrating injury to zone I or III, because of the inherent anatomic inaccessibility of these areas, are best approached with a diagnostic evaluation that may include arteriography, bronchoscopy, rigid esophagoscopy, and a barium swallow. A great deal of debate continues regarding management of zone II injuries, with some authors advocating diagnostic evaluation as with zone I and III injuries. Alternatively, patients with wounds that penetrate the platysma often undergo surgical exploration because of the ease of accessibility and exposure, as well as the high incidence of serious injuries in this unprotected region.

Chest

The chest should be reevaluated in the secondary survey by inspection, palpation, percussion, and auscultation. The chest radiograph should be closely examined for rib fractures, soft tissue injury, pneumothorax, hemothorax,

subcutaneous emphysema, deviation of the trachea or esophagus, and shifted or widened mediastinum. Following blunt trauma, the diagnosis of a diaphragmatic rupture is suggested by an elevated left hemidiaphragm, loculated hydropneumothorax, or visualization of the NG tube in the left hemithorax.

A transected thoracic aorta is commonly associated with a deceleration injury and is frequently fatal at the scene. Clinicians having a high index of suspicion based on the mechanism of injury and appreciating the hallmark signs seen on chest radiographs can identify these injuries early in the resuscitation. Radiographic findings consistent with a transected aorta include a mediastinal width greater than 8 cm, fracture of the first or second rib, obliteration of the aortic knob, deviation of the trachea and esophagus to the right, pleural cap, elevation and rightward shift of the right mainstem bronchus, and depression of the left mainstem bronchus. Suspicion of injury should lead to a helical CT of the chest with IV contrast. These new-generation scanners are proving to be effective at identifying aortic injury accurately with few missed injuries (Agee et al, 1992; Tello et al, 1998). Aortography is then reserved for patients with an equivocal study or as a preoperative study for confirmed transection. Patients will require surgical repair through a posterolateral thoracotomy. Timing of surgery is dependent on the patient's overall condition. Patients with hemodynamic instability require immediate surgery, whereas the condition of stable patients can be medically optimized in the intensive care unit prior to surgical repair.

Abdomen

The abdomen encompasses the pelvis, the retroperitoneum, and the peritoneal cavity. During the secondary survey, a thorough examination of the abdomen is conducted with the use of the traditional approach of inspection, palpation, and percussion. Visual examination of the abdomen should reveal any penetrating injuries, lacerations, or contusions. The flank and back are examined during the *exposure* portion of the primary survey when the patient is carefully logrolled. Palpation of the abdomen may reveal localized or generalized tenderness, voluntary guarding, or rebound tenderness, all signs that would raise suspicion of intra-abdominal injury. These findings prompt the need for further evaluation with an IV or oral contrast-enhanced CT scan of the abdomen, or surgical exploration. The abdominal examination is completed by rocking the pelvis to assess for instability and pain. Patients with unreliable examinations due to alcohol and/or drug intoxication or central nervous system trauma should have a CT scan of their abdomen with contrast enhancement to evaluate for possible occult injury.

Penetrating injuries to the abdomen deserve special attention. It should be remembered that the diaphragm ascends to the level of the fourth intercostal space, and thus any penetrating injury affecting the lower chest wall can potentially injure the intra-abdominal viscera. All gunshot wounds to the abdomen and lower chest should be explored. A stab wound to the anterior abdominal wall

Pearls and Pitfalls

PEARLS

- Based on the mechanism of trauma, all possible injuries should be excluded through the pursuit of appropriate examinations and diagnostic studies to reduce the risk of unrecognized occult injury.
- Uncooperative and combative patients should be assumed to be hypoxic or under the influence of drugs and/or alcohol or to have suffered significant head injury.
- When in doubt, definitively control the airway using an endotracheal tube; the tube can always be removed.
- Use an end-tidal carbon dioxide detection device followed by auscultation to determine whether the tube has been adequately placed.
- If the esophagus is inadvertently intubated while one is attempting airway control, leave the tube in place. This will protect the airway from gastric contents and eliminate the chance for subsequent esophageal intubation.
- Large, persistent pleural air leaks may be caused by a disrupted mainstem bronchus. This injury will likely require a second tube thoracostomy, selective intubation of the uninjured bronchus by experienced personnel, and surgical repair.
- Proximal-extremity injuries should have intravenous access obtained in the contralateral uninjured limb.
- A worsening base deficit is probably caused by unrecognized blood loss or inadequate volume resuscitation.
- DPL should be performed above the umbilicus for patients with pelvic fractures or a gravid uterus.
- Following blunt trauma, maintain spine precautions until the possibility of injury has been ruled out, and apply cervical spine protection devices to patients who arrive in the emergency room without them.

PITFALLS

- Failure to follow the ABCs of the primary survey for the multiply injured patient. Initial attention should not be directed toward the most dramatically obvious injury, such as a mangled extremity.
- Failure to expose and examine the entire patient, including the axillae, back, and perineum.
- Failure to perform a rectal examination and vaginal examination when appropriate.
- Failure to identify early signs of shock, which include tachycardia, falling pulse pressure, and poor capillary refill. Compensatory mechanisms can maintain a normal systolic pressure until more than 20% to 30% of the blood volume is lost.
- Placement of a subclavian central line on the uninjured side of a patient with thoracic trauma.
- Normal spine radiographs do not ensure the absence of osseous, ligamentous, or spinal injury. These diagnostic studies should be followed by a physical examination and comprehensive neurologic assessment when the patient is not under the influence of intoxicating agents to complete the evaluation.
- Failure to obtain appropriate and adequate radiographs in a timely fashion.

should be explored locally for the presence or absence of fascial penetration. If exploration reveals that the posterior fascia has been violated or if the exploration is indeterminate, the patient should undergo exploratory celiotomy. Penetrating wounds to the flank have the potential to cause occult intra-abdominal injury and mandate, at a minimum, evaluation with a triple contrast-enhanced CT study and serial examinations.

Extremities

The extremities should be examined for obvious fractures and lacerations. Suspected fractures should be radiographed and obvious fractures splinted as soon as possible. Assessment of the neurovascular status is of paramount importance. Hard signs of vascular trauma include active hemorrhage, distal pulse deficit, distal ischemia, and large or expanding hematomas. If detected on physical examination, surgical exploration is mandated (Frykberg et al, 1991). Penetrating trauma in proximity to the major vascular structures without the "hard signs" of injury should be evaluated with either color-flow Doppler imaging or arteriography. Motor or sensory deficits found during the physical examination can result from either spinal cord injury, local peripheral nerve injury, or vascu-

lar injury with ischemia. Once vascular injury is excluded and the probable source of neurologic impairment is identified, appropriate consultation should be obtained.

Summary

A rapid and complete primary survey with early correction of life-threatening injuries has been shown to enhance patient survival and improve eventual outcomes. Delayed or inadequate resuscitation and unrecognized injuries ultimately increase the patient's chance of developing multisystem organ dysfunction. Physicians who will care for acutely injured patients need to rehearse the steps of the primary and secondary surveys until the steps become second nature, to ensure that the "golden hour" is not wasted.

SELECTED READINGS

Agee CK, Metzler MH, Churchill RJ, Mitchell FL: Computed tomographic evaluation to exclude traumatic aortic disruption. J Trauma 1992;33:876.
Ballard RB, Rozycki GS, Newman PG, et al: An algorithm to reduce the incidence of false-negative FAST examinations in patients at high risk for occult injury: Focused Assessment for the Sonographic Examination of the Trauma patient. J Am Coll Surg 1999;189:145.
Brantigan CO, Grow JB: Cricothyroidotomy: Elective use in respiratory problems requiring tracheotomy. J Thorac Cardiovasc Surg 1976;71:72.

Dronen SC, Merigian KS, Hedges JR, et al: A comparison of blind nasotracheal and succinylcholine-assisted intubation in the poisoned patient. Ann Emerg Med 1987;16:650.

Fabian TC, Mangiante EC, White TJ, et al: A prospective study of 91 patients undergoing both computed tomography and peritoneal lavage following blunt abdominal trauma. J Trauma 1986;26:602.

Freedland M, Wilson RF, Bender JS, Levison MA: The management of flail chest injury: Factors affecting outcome. J Trauma 1990;30:1460.

Frykberg ER, Dennis JW, Bishop K, et al: The reliability of physical examination in the evaluation of penetrating extremity trauma for vascular injury: Results at one year. J Trauma 1991;31:502.

Knudson MM, Lewis FR, Atkinson K, Neuhaus A: The role of duplex ultrasound arterial imaging in patients with penetrating extremity trauma. Arch Surg 1993;128:1033.

Mackersie RC, Shackford SR, Hoyt DB, Karagianes TG: Continuous epidural fentanyl analgesia: Ventilatory function improvement with routine use in treatment of blunt chest injury. J Trauma 1987;27:1207.

Mendez C, Gubler KD, Maier RV: Diagnostic accuracy of peritoneal lavage in patients with pelvic fractures. Arch Surg 1994;129:477.

Meyer DM, Thal ER, Weigett JA, Redman HC: Evaluation of computed tomography and diagnostic peritoneal lavage in blunt abdominal trauma. J Trauma 1989;29:1168.

Porter JM, Ivatury RR: In search of the optimal end points of resuscitation in trauma patients: A review. J Trauma 1998;44:908.

Scannell G, Waxman K, Tominaga G, et al: Orotracheal intubation in trauma patients with cervical fractures. Arch Surg 1993;128:903.

Shires T, Coln D, Carrico J, Lightfoot S: Fluid therapy in hemorrhagic shock. Arch Surg 1964;88:688.

Tello R, Munden RF, Hooten S, et al: Value of spiral CT in hemodynamically stable patients following blunt chest trauma. Comput Med Imaging Graph 1998;22:447.

Velanovich V: Crystalloid versus colloid fluid resuscitation: A meta-analysis of mortality. Surgery 1989;105:65.

Yoshii H, Sato M, Yamamoto S, et al: Usefulness and limitation of ultrasound in the initial evaluation of blunt abdominal trauma. J Trauma 1998;45:45.

Chapter 9

Management of Blunt Abdominal Injuries

Preston R. Miller and Martin A. Croce

Despite advances in trauma care, the diagnosis and treatment of blunt abdominal injury remains a significant challenge. Concomitant brain or spinal cord injury, as well as the presence of alcohol or drug intoxication, may make physical examination unreliable or impossible to assess. The severe multisystem injuries frequently seen with blunt abdominal trauma may cloud the issues surrounding diagnosis and make priorities in injury evaluation difficult to establish. Although diagnosis may be problematic, its importance is underscored by the fact that several authors have found abdominal injury to be the most common cause of preventable death from blunt trauma. Delay in the diagnosis of hollow-viscus injury is a major contributor to morbidity and mortality in several series. It is because of these factors that multiple methods of evaluation of the abdomen have been developed over time, and understanding the strengths and weaknesses of each will allow logical interpretation of test results and timely diagnosis of intra-abdominal injury. This chapter provides an overview of the use of physical examination, diagnostic peritoneal lavage (DPL), ultrasonography (US), and computed tomography (CT) in the evaluation of blunt abdominal trauma. These discussions are followed by a review of specific injuries and their management.

PHYSICAL EXAMINATION

Physical examination is an important although sometimes confusing method of initial evaluation for blunt abdominal injury. As with all trauma patients, the evaluation of patients with suspected abdominal injury should begin with assessment of the airway, breathing, and adequacy of circulation. Following these steps, the abdomen is evaluated during the secondary survey. Patients with frank peritonitis should undergo laparotomy, and no further diagnostic work-up of the abdomen is indicated. Patients with these signs and symptoms, however, are few. Frequently repeated physical examination of the abdomen may be needed to determine the improvement or worsening of symptoms. Patients under the influence of drugs or alcohol may have altered pain perception, leading to false-negative physical examination. This population of patients approaches 50% in most urban trauma centers. In addition, patients with significant brain injury, or spinal cord injury, may have a benign abdominal examination in the setting of significant pathology. Patients frequently have significant hemoperitoneum with no obvious change in abdominal girth or tenderness on physical examination. Conversely, patients with hemoperitoneum may exhibit varying degrees of peritoneal irritation in the setting of

solid-organ injury, which can be successfully managed without laparotomy. It is for these reasons that physical examination is often combined with other methods of evaluation to determine the presence of intra-abdominal injury and the need for laparotomy.

DIAGNOSTIC PERITONEAL LAVAGE

DPL is a highly sensitive method of determining the presence of hemoperitoneum or hollow-viscus injury. This technique requires passing a catheter into the pelvis via either an open or a percutaneous technique and should be performed only after both a urinary catheter and a nasogastric tube are in place to decompress the bladder and stomach. An open technique should be used in pregnant patients or patients who have had previous abdominal surgery. The catheter may be passed above, below, or through the umbilicus; however, the supraumbilical position is preferred in the setting of pelvic fracture so as to avoid accessing the pelvic hematoma. After insertion, the catheter is aspirated. Ten milliliters of blood obtained on aspiration has long been considered an indication for laparotomy. If no blood is obtained, 1 L of warm crystalloid is infused into the abdomen and allowed to return via siphon. The fluid is then sent for analysis. A DPL is considered positive in blunt trauma victims if it contains $\geq 100,000$ RBCs/mm^3, ≥ 500 WBCs/mm^3, bile, or fibers. Using these cutoff values, DPL has a sensitivity of 98% in determining the presence of intra-abdominal injury. Its specificity is poor, however, as DPL provides little information about the specific organ injured. As the ability to successfully manage solid-organ injuries nonoperatively has grown, it has become clear that hemoperitoneum leading to a grossly positive DPL in a hemodynamically stable patient may not necessarily signify an injury best managed by laparotomy. In addition, only 30 mL of free blood in the peritoneal cavity is required to yield an RBC count of 100,000/mm^3, and clearly it is possible to have this small amount of blood in the abdomen and not require operation. It is for these reasons that the role of DPL, once considered the mainstay of evaluation of blunt abdominal injury, is being redefined. DPL is currently most useful in the rapid search for occult hemorrhage in the hemodynamically unstable patient, and for determining the presence of hollow-viscus injury. The abdomen is one of the few places into which patients can exsanguinate without an obvious show of blood. DPL in the hemodynamically unstable patient with an equivocal abdominal ultrasound study provides a method of rapid assessment of the abdomen as a source of hemorrhage. With the widespread use of CT in trauma evaluation, it is recognized that hollow-viscus injuries may be difficult to detect, leading to diagnostic delay. In patients with free peritoneal fluid on CT without solid-organ injury, or in patients with abdominal tenderness seemingly out of proportion to documented solid-organ injury, DPL for WBC count provides a reliable method of evaluating for hollow-viscus injury. It should be noted that patients undergoing DPL shortly after injury may have negative studies despite the presence of injury because adequate migration of WBCs in response to injury has not yet occurred. Patients in whom a high suspicion of hollow-viscus injury exists may benefit from a second DPL several hours later after leukosequestration has occurred. Although DPL has good accuracy in diagnosing hollow-viscus injury, significant injuries to retroperitoneal structures such as the pancreas or duodenum may be missed by this modality, and other studies such as CT may be needed in patients who are suspected of having these injuries.

Complications of DPL are uncommon, occurring in approximately 1% of patients undergoing the procedure. These range from local bleeding or infection to intestinal or vascular injury.

ULTRASONOGRAPHY

Abdominal ultrasonography (US) is beginning to supplant DPL in the evaluation of the abdomen in blunt trauma for several reasons. With the advent of portable, user-friendly ultrasound machines, US can be rapidly performed in the resuscitation area. It is easily repeatable and noninvasive. While detailed interpretation of US images requires significant training, it is possible to acquire proficiency in the diagnosis of hemoperitoneum with only a modicum of experience. The sensitivity of US for detecting peritoneum is 93% to 95%, a sensitivity similar to that of DPL. In addition, surgeons have been shown to perform a focused abdominal sonogram for trauma (FAST) with accuracy similar to that of formally trained radiologists. Finally, the cost of US is relatively low, making it even more attractive as an evaluation tool.

The FAST includes evaluation of the pericardium, Morison's pouch, the splenorenal recess, and the pelvis. The rapidity and sensitivity of the test make it very helpful in the rapid search for a source of hemorrhage, especially in the hemodynamically unstable trauma patient. Training programs designed to teach surgeons the FAST are currently in place in most trauma centers, which helps to ensure consistent training and experience.

Drawbacks to US, as with DPL, include its low specificity as well as the limitations in image quality seen in obese patients or those with significant subcutaneous emphysema. While some practitioners are using US for evaluation of specific organs, it is clear that there is a learning-curve phenomenon to such use. Its major role currently remains the evaluation for hemoperitoneum.

COMPUTED TOMOGRAPHY

Abdominal CT is the most versatile and probably the most common screening tool used in the evaluation of blunt abdominal injury today. This modality has a combination of sensitivity, specificity, and versatility not found in other methods of diagnosis. There have been concerns in the past with the greater time required for CT, but with the newer generation of helical scanners the actual scan time is about 5 minutes, and improved image quality has enhanced the specificity of the examination. With increasing evidence that nonoperative management of many injuries is desirable, the abilities to accurately define which intra-abdominal organs are injured and the extent of damage have become more important. Computed tomography scanning detects both the presence of hemorrhage and, usually, the source of bleeding. In addition to the information concerning injuries in the peritoneal cavity, CT yields important information about retroperitoneal structures, such as the pancreas, duodenum, and genitourinary system. In short, this technique has excellent sensitivity and good specificity for most organ injuries and is essential to the ability of the practitioner to successfully manage major solid-organ injury nonoperatively.

Although CT is quite useful, it is important to recognize its drawbacks and limitations. Perhaps most importantly, it requires transport from the resuscitation area and thus is not suitable for hemodynamically unstable patients. In addition, although sensitivity is good for liver and spleen injuries, it is less for diaphragm, hollow-viscus, or pancreas injuries. Thus, it is important to combine repeated physical examination and laboratory examination with CT in patients at risk for these injuries. CT scans for the evaluation of the trauma patient are usually done with intravenous contrast enhancement to increase diagnostic accuracy, and this carries with it a small but real risk of nephrotoxicity. Such toxicity is usually self-limited and can be improved with aggressive crystalloid hydration. Contrast reaction occurs in 1 per 1000 patients or less with nonionic contrast. Fatal reactions are seen in 0.9 per 100,000 patients.

While the indications for operation following penetrating abdominal trauma are relatively straightforward and have remained constant, the indications for laparotomy following blunt injury continue to evolve. In the unstable patient, DPL or US are the diagnostic methods of choice. In the situation of an unstable patient and a microscopically positive DPL for RBCs ($>100,000$ mm^3), it is unlikely that the patient is suffering from exsanguinating abdominal hemorrhage, and a quick search for other sites of hemorrhage should ensue.

In the hemodynamically stable patient with an unevaluable abdomen, CT scanning provides the most information about abdominal injuries. It also will allow for quantitation of the severity of injury (Fig. 9–1). The American Association for the Surgery of Trauma (AAST) has devised organ injury scales in an attempt to quantitate injury severity. In addition, evaluation of the retroperitoneal organs is possible. With the information provided by the CT, and the overall status of the patient, a rational decision for operative or nonoperative management may be made.

OPERATIVE MANAGEMENT

While there may be debate about whether to operate following some blunt solid-organ injuries, there is no

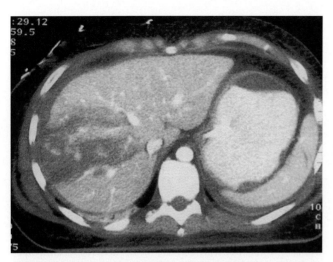

Figure 9–1. Computed tomography demonstration of AAST grade V liver laceration extending to the inferior vena cava.

debate about hollow-organ injuries. The diagnosis is usually straightforward in patients with normal sensorium and no distracting injuries. These patients typically exhibit signs of peritoneal irritation, and physical examination is usually sufficient for diagnosis. However, the patient with altered sensorium requires additional diagnostic evaluation. Diagnostic peritoneal lavage has historically been the test of choice to exclude hollow-organ injury, since earlier reports using CT demonstrated low sensitivity and specificity. However, advances in image quality and helical technology have substantially improved its diagnostic accuracy. A major advantage involves the diagnosis of duodenal injuries. The presence of fluid in the retroperitoneum around the duodenum, which may not be accessible by DPL, is suggestive of injury and may require laparotomy.

Other abdominal injuries that require operation are pancreatic and intraperitoneal bladder wounds. Bladder injuries may be closed primarily, and bladder drainage should be maintained approximately 1 week. Pancreatic injuries may be subtle, and their diagnosis can be difficult. Rising or persistent elevations of serum amylase or lipase are suggestive, but not diagnostic. Abdominal CT may identify unexplained fluid in the lesser sac. Other diagnostic tests, such as US or DPL, are generally not helpful for definitive diagnosis, since they do not adequately evaluate the retroperitoneum. Endoscopic retrograde cholangiopancreatography adds very little and should not be performed routinely. If the pancreas is transected or if there is an injury to the main duct in the body or tail, distal resection is the preferred procedure. If the patient is stable, splenic preservation may be attempted. For pancreatic head injuries, excellent results may be expected with simple drainage of the wound. Pancreaticoduodenectomy should be reserved for destructive wounds (primarily following penetrating injury) in which most of the dissection was accomplished by the trauma itself. After definitive management, the pancreas should be drained with a soft closed-suction drain to minimize the chances of abdominal abscess. Pancreatic fistula may occur up to 10 days postoperatively, so the drain should be left in place for the duration.

Optimal management of duodenal injuries is somewhat controversial, and should be individualized to the injury type. Most blunt wounds can be closed primarily. The authors' preferred drainage method is with afferent tube jejunostomy and gastric decompression (nasogastric tube for patients without associated brain injury, gastrostomy for those with brain injury), with placement of an efferent jejunostomy tube for enteral feeding. More destructive injuries, especially combined pancreaticoduodenal wounds, may require diversion. This can be accomplished by oversewing the pylorus from within, then performing gastrojejunostomy at the gastrotomy site. The pylorus should reopen within 2 to 4 weeks, since only the mucosa was approximated. Vagotomy is usually not necessary. An alternative approach is to use a noncutting stapling device to close the pylorus and then perform gastrojejunostomy. Vagotomy should be considered because the stapled pylorus may not open and gastrojejunostomy is ulcerogenic.

Operative treatment for liver injuries should be reserved for hemodynamically unstable patients. In this instance, significant hemorrhage from the liver is the expected finding. This can usually be controlled with direct pressure and manual compression, which allows for adequate resuscitation of the patient. It is important to adequately mobilize the liver. This requires division of the triangular ligament and the coronary ligaments as well as the posterior peritoneal attachments so that the right lobe may be delivered from its recess. The only exception may be the situation in which there is a hematoma dissecting in the coronary and/or triangular ligaments, suggestive of a suprahepatic caval injury, which may best be managed by gauze packing. Bleeding lacerations may be gently explored to expose the vessels responsible so that they may be ligated. If the major hemorrhage is then controlled, the use of viable omental pack will stop the low-pressure venous oozing from the raw surface. This omental tongue should be mobilized on its vascular pedicle and secured with a running monofilament suture. Blind, deep mattress sutures are not advisable, since they do not address the source of bleeding and predispose to hepatic artery pseudoaneurysm formation with hemobilia. For patients with exsanguinating hemorrhage, gauze packing should be used before the patient becomes too acidotic and coagulopathic. These packs should be removed within 48 hours to lessen the chance for abdominal abscess.

The operative management of splenic injuries is relatively straightforward. As with liver injuries, operation should be reserved for unstable patients. In addition, selected patients with high-grade injuries may benefit from operation even if they are hemodynamically stable. High-grade splenic injuries have higher failure rates with nonoperative therapy because arterial injuries are far more likely in the spleen than in the liver, where bleeding is more often due to low-pressure venous wounds. In the setting of continuing hemorrhage or a laceration extending into the hilum, splenectomy is the best option. Care must be taken not to injure the pancreatic tail. For patients with a laceration that has stopped bleeding, splenorrhaphy is a consideration. Pledgeted sutures or splenic wrap with absorbable mesh are options. As with the liver, mobilization is imperative. The lateral peritoneal attachments, splenic flexure, and short gastric vessels all must be divided if splenorrhaphy is attempted.

The majority of blunt renal injuries may be managed nonoperatively, with exceptions due primarily to hemodynamic instability. Occasionally, partial nephrectomy may be performed, but usually nephrectomy is required in the unstable patient. For patients with blunt renal artery injuries, the management is controversial. Some authors advocate revascularization, others prefer observation. In these authors' experience, approximately one third will eventually require nephrectomy owing to hypertension. It seems prudent to observe these patients initially, and if operation is required it may be performed on an elective basis. Revascularization may be attempted in instances in which the diagnosis is made promptly after injury, as prolonged ischemic time is detrimental to functional outcome.

Two groups of patients deserve special mention: those with diaphragm injuries and those with fluid or hemoperitoneum without solid-organ injury. Patients with diaphragm injuries present a diagnostic dilemma at times because no test is very accurate for diagnosis. Chest radiograph is probably the most helpful, and it is diagnostic when abdominal viscera are seen in the chest. However, the deviated hemidiaphragm is difficult to evaluate. Ultrasonography is not very helpful, and CT is likewise undiagnostic. One CT finding suggestive of injury is thickening of the diaphragm close to the midline. Laparoscopy is diagnostic for most diaphragm injuries, and laparotomy may be required to unequivocally diagnose the injury. For patients with peritoneal fluid and no obvious injury, DPL may be performed to rule out a hollow-viscus injury. Patients with significant hemoperitoneum without solid-organ injury are at high risk for mesenteric injury, which requires laparotomy. The bleeding mesenteric vessels may be ligated and the defect closed to prevent internal hernias. In addition, assessment of bowel viability may be done, and the bowel may require resection if it is compromised.

NONOPERATIVE MANAGEMENT

Based on the success of nonoperative therapy for liver and spleen injuries in the pediatric population, the concept has expanded to include adults. Abdominal CT scanning allows for grading of injury, which then allows for valid comparisons of management schemes between different institutions. It should be emphasized that nonoperative management should be considered only in hemodynamically stable patients.

A number of retrospective reviews demonstrated that selected patients with low-grade hepatic injuries may be successfully managed without operation. However, these data are difficult to interpret, since different grading systems were used. With the advent of the AAST organ injury scales, there is more uniformity in reporting. The main point of these studies is that all patients remained hemodynamically stable, and all transfusions (primarily from associated injuries) must be explained. A prospective study was then reported in which all patients with blunt liver injury who were hemodynamically stable and had no

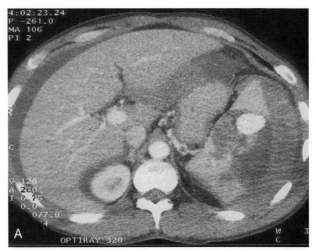
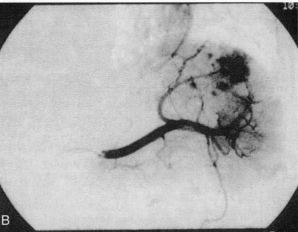
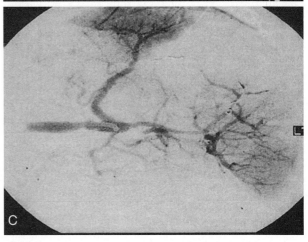

Figure 9–2. *A,* Computed tomography demonstrating splenic injury with a large pseudoaneurysm. *B,* Angiogram demonstrating an intraparenchymal pseudoaneurysm. *C,* Embolization of a pseudoaneurysm.

other indication for laparotomy were managed nonoperatively regardless of their grade of injury. Of the 136 patients studied, 82% were initially managed nonoperatively with only a 5% liver-related failure rate. A follow-up study illustrated the paradigm shift from operative to nonoperative therapy for blunt hepatic injury. It clearly demonstrated that abdominal infections, transfusion requirements, and lengths of hospital stays all were decreased with nonoperative management without any change in mortality. Thus, for the hemodynamically stable patient with blunt liver injury, nonoperative management is the treatment of choice.

Nonoperative management of splenic injuries has been increasing in recent years. As with liver injuries, it cannot be overemphasized that this treatment is only for hemodynamically stable patients. While some authors advocate routine angiography for splenic wounds, we have reported more than 90% success rates for nonoperative management with the use of selective angiography. Angiography with embolization for patients with a vascular blush (Fig. 9–2) indicative of intraparenchymal splenic artery pseudoaneurysm has significantly decreased the failure rate to

6%. Embolization is not always successful, however. In those instances, the prudent choice is to perform splenectomy if the patient's general condition permits, since the pseudoaneurysm is significantly associated with failure of nonoperative management.

Summary

The evaluation and management of patients with blunt abdominal trauma continue to evolve as advances are made in technology and patient care. Since the diagnostic measures and care of the patients differ depending on the hemodynamic stability of the patient, separate algorithms may be made for stable and unstable patients (Fig. 9–3). The algorithms allow for successful management of

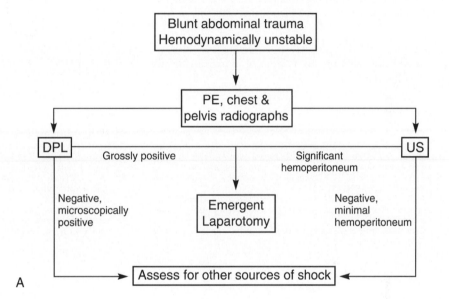

Figure 9–3. Treatment algorithms for blunt abdominal trauma. *A,* Hemodynamically unstable patient. *B,* Hemodynamically stable patient. PE, physical examination.

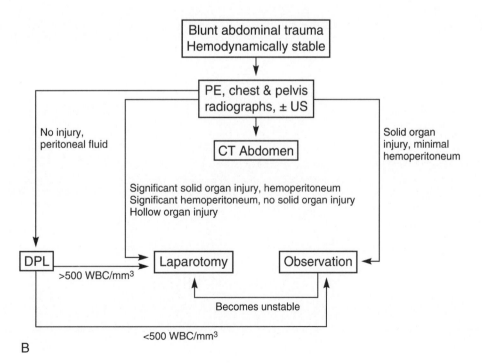

Pearls and Pitfalls

PEARLS

- Drugs, alcohol, or neurologic injury may make physical examination of the patient unreliable, and adjunctive measures such as US and CT should be used for patient evaluation in this setting.
- *CT scanning should be reserved only for hemodynamically stable patients.* Ultrasonography or DPL is helpful in the rapid evaluation for a source of abdominal hemorrhage in unstable patients.
- It is unlikely that unstable patients with a microscopically positive DPL have significant intra-abdominal bleeding. A search for other sources of hemorrhage must be performed in this situation.
- Patients with a small amount of intra-abdominal fluid on CT without solid-organ injury may have hollow-viscus injury, which can be diagnosed with DPL.

- Patients with large volumes of intraperitoneal fluid in the absence of solid-organ injury usually have mesenteric injuries and require laparotomy.
- Although it is safe and even preferable to manage many solid-organ injuries nonoperatively, this concept should not be seen as an ironclad rule. The safest place for patients in whom there is a question of ongoing bleeding from solid-organ injury is in the operating room.
- Serial US may be helpful in distinguishing between this continued blood loss from solid-organ injury and blood loss from other sources, such as long bone fracture.

---

the majority of patients, but are not a substitute for clinical judgment.

SELECTED READINGS

Croce MA, Fabian TC, Menke PG, et al: Nonoperative management of blunt hepatic trauma is the treatment of choice for hemodynamically stable patients: Results of a prospective trial. Ann Surg 1995;221:744.

Davis KA, Brody JM, Cioffi WG: Computed tomography in blunt hepatic trauma. Arch Surg 1996;131:225.

Davis KA, Fabian TC, Croce MA, et al: Improved success in nonoperative management of blunt splenic artery pseudoaneurysms. J Trauma 1998;44:1008.

Feliciano DV: Diagnostic modalities in abdominal trauma: Peritoneal lavage, ultrasonography, computed tomography scanning, and arteriography. Surg Clin North Am 1991;71:241.

Malhotra AK, Fabian TC, Croce MA, et al: Blunt hepatic injury: A paradigm shift from operative to nonoperative management in the 1990's. Ann Surg 2000;231:804.

Malhotra AK, Fabian TC, Katsis S, et al: Blunt bowel and mesenteric injury: The role of screening CT. J Trauma 2000;48:991.

Moore EE, Cogbill TH, Jurkovich GJ, et al: Organ injury scaling: Spleen and liver (1994 revision). J Trauma 1995;38:323.

Root HD, Hauser CW, McKinley CR, et al: Diagnostic peritoneal lavage. Surgery 1965;57:633.

Rozycki GS, Ochsner MG, Jaffin JH, et al: Prospective evaluation of surgeons' use of ultrasound in the evaluation of trauma patients. J Trauma 1993;34:516.

Rozycki GS, Ochsner MG, Schmidt JA, et al: A prospective study of surgeon-performed ultrasound as the primary adjuvant modality for injured patient assessment. J Trauma 1995;38:492.

Chapter 10

Management of Penetrating Trauma: Neck, Thorax, and Abdomen

Lunzy D. Britt

Although the initial management of any trauma patient closely follows a very systematic format, which is highlighted in the Advanced Traumatic Support Protocol, the specific management of penetrating trauma has changed significantly over the last two decades in practically every category, including penetrating injuries to the neck, thorax, and abdomen. These evolving management paradigms have not occurred, however, without significant challenges and controversies. Even with evidence-based data supporting the advantage of a particular approach, management is often ultimately institution-dependent. A more resource-intense medical facility (i.e., with technology and personnel) is more capable of advocating a nonoperative or selective approach to a patient who has sustained penetrating trauma to the neck or torso than is a facility that has limited resources with regard to medical personnel and diagnostic modalities.

CLINICAL PRESENTATION

The most crucial aspect of the presentation of penetrating trauma of the neck, thorax, and abdomen is the hemodynamic status of the patient. Significant hemodynamic lability will probably obviate the need for any time-consuming diagnostic work-up or imaging studies, particularly if the patient remains unstable after initial resuscitation. For example, a person who sustains an isolated penetrating injury to the neck and who is hemodynamically unstable mandates operative intervention, regardless of the mechanism or specific anatomic area. The same is true for a penetrating injury to the abdomen or the chest, depending on the extent of hemodynamic compromise. However, diagnostic imaging does play a pivotal role in many of the penetrating injuries of the neck and torso in the hemodynamically stable patient. Laboratory studies should be done in an expeditious and cost-effective manner. The basic tests should include hemoglobin (Hb), hemotocrit (Hct), blood ethanol (ETOH) level, and urine dipstick for blood, and human chorionic gonadotropin (hCG) in women of childbearing age.

PREOPERATIVE MANAGEMENT

Adequate airway, ventilation, and resuscitation (large-bore intravenous catheters) and determination of any severe neurologic deficits are essential to the optimal preoperative management of any patient. This initial priority should always be followed, regardless of the mechanism of injury or hemodynamic status.

Neck

With penetrating neck injuries, some form of diagnostic work-up is still advocated prior to definitive operative interventions. There is little, if any, controversy related to the need for immediate exploration in patients who present with exsanguinating hemorrhage, hemodynamic lability, expanding or pulsatile hematoma, air bubbling from the wound, or stridor.

In general, a more selective approach is taken for zones I and III because of the inherent difficulty in examining and operatively exposing these areas (Fig. 10–1). For example, a penetrating zone I injury could neces-

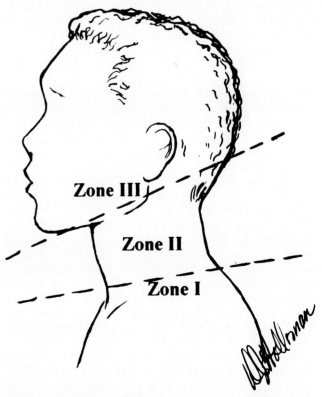

Figure 10–1. Anatomic zones of the neck, lateral view. (From Britt LD, Peyser MB. In Moore EE, Mattox KL, Feliciano DV [eds]: Trauma, 4th ed. Stamford, Conn, Appleton & Lange, 1999, p 438.)

sitate a thoracotomy (median sternotomy or anterolateral approach) to optimally manage a vascular injury. Also, disarticulation of the mandible, resection of the angle of the mandible, resection of the styloid, or other maneuvers may be required to obtain adequate exposure with zone III penetrating injuries.

The paramount controversy centers around patients who present as hemodynamically stable with penetrating neck wounds in zone II and no findings suggestive of injury to a vital structure. While many factors must be considered and treatment individualized, there is an ongoing debate over how this particular subset of patients should be managed. In the past, there have been two basic management options for penetrating zone II injuries: (1) mandatory operative intervention for any injury that penetrates the platysma, and (2) selective management that involves panendoscopy (laryngoscopy, tracheoscopy, bronchoscopy, and esophagoscopy), esophagography, and arteriography with the selective management approach. Only when a vital structure is noted to be injured is a neck exploration performed with the selective management approach.

The concept of mandatory neck exploration is deeply rooted in experience during military campaigns. In pre–World War II military campaigns a lack of necessary skills, equipment, and ancillary support for operative intervention resulted in penetrating neck wounds being frequently treated nonoperatively, which resulted in a complicated course and a relatively high mortality. A more aggressive operative approach, along with better surgical skills and equipment, was adopted in subsequent military campaigns, with a corresponding decline in mortality. As a result, mandatory exploration was also embraced in civilian practice because of a relatively high negative exploration rate. Mandatory exploration has lost widespread support. A more selective approach for this subset of patients has been adopted by most surgeons. Although each decision should be based on the resources of the hospital, the experience of the surgeon, and the compliance and cooperation of the patient, selective management of zone II injuries is the approach of choice in most tertiary care medical centers today. There is an emerging camp, however, that has challenged the necessity of various diagnostic modalities used in selective management. Fryberg and colleagues have advocated a strictly nondiagnostic, nonoperative approach to zone II penetrating injuries when there is no "hard" clinical finding of a vascular injury. Even though some of their preliminary data are encouraging, this expectant management schema, in which no diagnostic modalities are utilized, needs to be carefully examined. Historically, it was the unacceptable morbidity and mortality of the nondiagnostic, nonoperative approach that prompted surgeons to embrace an operative or more selective management paradigm. Currently, a nonoperative, nondiagnostic approach in penetrating zone II neck injuries is not standard management. Which diagnostic modalities are essential in the selective management of penetrating zone II injuries when there are no physical or clinical findings suggestive of an injury? The gold standard in selective management determines whether there is an arterial, esophageal, or laryngotracheal injury; the armamentarium of diagnostic modalities

Table 10–1	Diagnostic Modalities	
Arteriography	Esophagoscopy	
Doppler flow studies	Esophagogram	
Laryngoscopy	Computed tomography	
Bronchoscopy		

is listed in Table 10–1. The specific procedure required for each patient depends on the mechanism of injury, hospital resources, and the physician's experience.

In regard to gunshot injuries in zone II, there are advocates for a selective approach. In general, however, if the missile clearly traverses the neck, operative intervention is the preferred and safest approach. Demetriades and co-workers advocate that a careful clinical examination with appropriate diagnostic investigations can result in safe, nonoperative management of the majority of injuries. If the patient is hemodynamically stable, diagnostic studies such as angiography might be helpful in delineating an injury. However, operative management is still the treatment of choice for zone II injuries in this cohort of patients. Also, under no circumstances should a high-velocity missile wound be managed nonoperatively in a viable patient. Close-range shotgun blasts can cause significant tissue destruction and should be managed in a manner similar to that for a high-velocity missile injury. Figure 10–2 offers some guidance in the management of penetrating neck injuries.

Chest

In all penetrating chest trauma and in most major trauma cases, the chest radiograph (frontal anteroposterior) is essential in the preoperative management. Significant information can be obtained from plain radiography, including pneumothorax, hemothorax, and abnormalities of the mediastinum and traumatic diaphragmatic herniations. Although chest radiography is essential, it should not supplant good clinical acumen and physical examination. For example, a diagnosis of tension pneumothorax should never be made based on a chest radiograph. If, however, a diagnosis was made on such grounds, it should be considered an inappropriately delayed diagnosis. Fortunately, the majority of penetrating injuries to the chest—particularly penetrating chest wounds above the nipple—do not require operative intervention. A resulting pneumothorax or hemothorax, or both, can be optimally managed by the insertion of a chest tube. The indications for operative intervention (thoracotomy or sternotomy) include acute deterioration; massive hemothorax (≥ 1500 mL of blood initially evacuated with chest tube insertion or ongoing bleeding with >200 mL/hr for 3 hours or more); cardiac tamponade; massive air leak or a documented tracheobronchial injury; documented esophageal injury; impaled object to the chest; and radiographic evidence of a great vessel injury or a thoracic outlet vascular injury with associated hemodynamic lability.

A transmediastinal penetrating injury requires expeditious evaluation, especially in the unstable patient who is likely to require a thoracotomy or sternotomy. In the

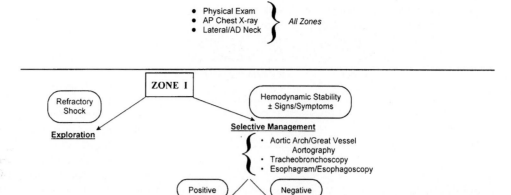

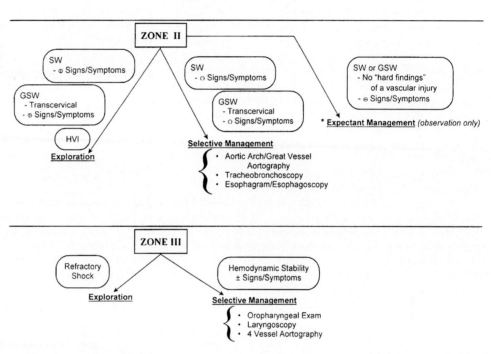

Figure 10–2. Penetrating neck injuries, management guideline. (From Britt LD, Peyser MB. In Moore EE, Mattox KL, Feliciano DV [eds]: Trauma, 4th ed. Stamford, Conn, Appleton & Lange, 1999, p 443.)

stable patient, bilateral chest tubes are required for documented pneumothoraces. If a cardiac injury is suspected, ultrasonography, echocardiography, or performing pericardial window would be necessary to definitively exclude such an injury.

The lower chest or the thoracoabdominal region (from the nipple level to the costal margin) is the ultimate "blind spot" with respect to penetrating torso wounds and associated diaphragmatic perforation. Unfortunately, there is no predictable timetable for the possible development of traumatic diaphragmatic hernia. With the abdominal cavity having persistent positive pressure, compared with the relative negative intrathoracic pressure, the potential for herniation through a diaphragmatic laceration is omnipresent. Emphasis is placed on left-sided diaphragmatic injuries and the likelihood of herniation; however, complications can occur as the result of right-sided diaphragmatic injuries, including the development of biliary-pleural fistulas and possible hepatic herniation. Because there is no set timetable for such a herniation, initial recognition and treatment of this injury is im-

portant in avoiding long-term sequelae. A plethora of diagnostic studies have been proposed for the detection of diaphragmatic rents and thus the determination of the need for operative intervention. Until recently, mandatory celiotomy was the only prudent diagnostic option for detecting a diaphragmatic laceration, since chest plain radiography, diagnostic peritoneal lavage, computed tomography (CT), magnetic resonance imaging (MRI), and ultrasonography evaluation all had been inconclusive. Although there are several potential indications for minimal invasive surgery in the trauma setting, laparoscopy (or thoracostomy) as a diagnostic modality has a pivotal role in the definitive evaluation of penetrating diaphragmatic injuries.

Abdomen

The anterior abdomen is defined by the following boundaries: below the costal margin, above the inguinal ligaments, and anterior to the midaxillary lines. Penetrating

Table 10–2	**Penetrating Anterior Abdominal Injury, Shock Trauma Center, Sentara Norfolk General Hospital**	
	TOTAL PATIENTS, 661	NONTHERAPEUTIC LAPAROTOMIES
Gunshot injuries	442	94 (21%)
Shotgun injuries	7	2 (29%)
Stab injuries	212	48 (23%)

injuries to the anterior abdomen with associated hemodynamic lability of the patient should dictate an emergency celiotomy. Currently, the most raging controversy in penetrating trauma deals with gunshot wounds to the abdomen in the hemodynamically stable patient and the role of nonoperative or selective management, as opposed to mandatory exploration. The concept of nonoperative management of patients with gunshot missiles penetrating and traversing the abdominal cavity highlights a major departure from what has been considered sound clinical judgment. With a greater than 95% risk of significant intra-abdominal injury and with gunshot wounds to the abdomen as reported by some authors, the role of nonoperative management in this setting is questionable. Even if the nontherapeutic or negative exploration rate is higher, mandatory laparotomy is still justified.

Selective or nonoperative management has been more widely accepted in the management of stab wounds to the anterior abdomen in the hemodynamically stable and examinable patient with no peritoneal signs, evisceration, or gross blood coming from any orifice. With this particular mechanism of injury, there are two basic management options: expectant management (observation) or selective management (local wound exploration for the determina-

tion of peritoneal penetration). Recent data analysis at the author's institution revealed that local exploration of stab wounds to confirm peritoneal penetration in a patient with no stigmata of an intra-abdominal injury demonstrated the unacceptably high nontherapeutic laparotomy rate of 23% (Table 10–2).

Although there is some interest in the selective management of gunshot wounds to the back and flank with no clinical or plain radiographic evidence of peritoneal penetration, the gold standard approach is still operative intervention. Selective management is the rule, however, when the mechanism is a stab wound to the back and flank of a patient who is hemodynamically stable and has no peritoneal signs or evisceration. A triple-contrast assessment (intravenous, oral, or rectal-colonic contrast-enhanced CT scan) is the selective management approach of choice, along with possible performance of a diagnostic peritoneal lavage.

INTRAOPERATIVE MANAGEMENT

The primary operative strategy is optimal and expeditious exposure. Inappropriately placed small incisions often jeopardize a favorable outcome for the patient.

Neck

The standard incisions for neck exploration in penetrating trauma are demonstrated in Figure 10–3. Operative exposure of zone I injuries may necessitate a supraclavicular incision with removal of the head of the clavicle or a "trapdoor" or "book" thoracotomy, which requires a supraclavicular incision, and a median sternotomy with an arterolateral extension. Optimal exposure of zone III injuries may necessitate cephalad extension of the incision

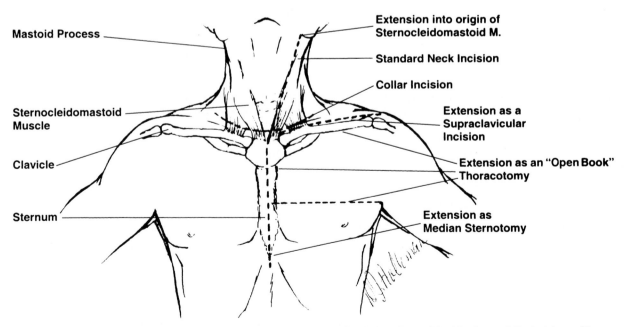

Figure 10–3. Incisions for operative exposure of penetrating neck injuries. (From Britt LD, Peyser MB. In Moore EE, Mattox KL, Feliciano DV [eds]: Trauma, 4th ed. Stamford, Conn, Appleton & Lange, 1999, p 438.)

at the anterior border of the sternocleidomastoid muscle and possible disarticulation, or partial resection of the mandible or performance of a craniotomy. For most penetrating zone II injuries that require operative intervention, an incision at the anterior border of the sternocleidomastoid muscle is the approach of choice. If there is suspicion or evidence that the projectile has traversed the cervical region, a collar incision would provide adequate access to both the left and right neck, therefore obviating the need for bilateral neck incisions. Either incision can be expeditiously extended into the chest should a sternotomy be required for better exposure and vascular control.

Chest

The location trajectory of the missile and the hemodynamic status of the patient determine the operative approach of choice. A left anterolateral thoracotomy allows rapid access to the chest for decompression of cardiac tamponade, repair of the heart, and access to the aorta for possible compression. This is the best approach for the patient with penetrating chest trauma who has significant hemodynamic instability. The contralateral chest can be entered by extending the incision into the right chest. Although it provides limited access to the descending aorta and esophagus, the median sternotomy is the best operative approach for exposing the heart and associated great vessels. There is very limited access, however, to the pulmonary hilum with this incision.

Abdomen

The midline vertical incision from the xiphoid to the symphysis pubis provides the most rapid access to and best exposure of possible intra-abdominal and retroperitoneal injuries resulting from penetrating trauma. Wide sterile preparation and draping on the abdomen allow for the establishment of ostomies, if required. Full exploration of the abdominal cavity is mandatory if operative intervention is indicated. This should include the evaluation of all quadrants and the lesser sac, along with a detailed assessment of the hollow viscera and solid organs. Meticulous evaluation of any retroperitoneal hematoma is imperative. Appropriate vascular control prior to the surgeon's entering a retroperitoneal hematoma is always prudent.

POSTOPERATIVE MANAGEMENT

With definitive management, regardless of the injury, the goals of postoperative management remain the same: restoration and maintenance of adequate tissue oxygenation; aggressive pulmonary toilet; maintenance of normothermia; correction of any coagulopathy; prevention of electrolyte disturbance; optimal prophylaxis to prevent stress ulcerations, deep venous thrombosis, pulmonary emboli, decubitus ulcers, and nosocomial infections; early mobilization; and enteral nutrition.

At times, special adjuncts are necessary. For example, when optimization of circulation is difficult to achieve,

pulmonary artery catheter monitoring might be necessary to ensure adequate intravascular volume resuscitation. Also, knowing when interventions and therapies should be initiated is crucial. The importance of early enteral nutritional support is well established. Hemodynamic instability is an absolute contraindication to tube feedings, even if the conduit is in a postpyloric position. The specific aspects of postoperative management depend on the type of injury and the interventions required (e.g., chest tubes, drains, delay closures).

COMPLICATIONS

Although complications can occur even when the patient has received optimal preoperative management, their frequency is significantly increased when strict adherence to the basic principles of surgical management is not present. The possible complications are numerous and cover the full spectrum of adverse sequelae, including wound infection, dehiscence, nosocomial pneumonia, catheter sepsis, deep cavity abscesses, deep renal thrombosis, pulmonary embolism, and myocardial infarction.

OUTCOMES

The overall outcomes in penetrating neck and torso injuries are influenced by multiple factors, including the hemodynamic status of the patient, the mechanism of injury, comorbid factors, and prehospital delays. The trauma surgeon obviously cannot directly control many of these and other factors, which can result in a poor outcome for the patient. Expeditious, definitive management is the only means of gaining a favorable patient outcome.

Pearls and Pitfalls

PEARLS

- Airway, breathing, and circulation have the same priority in the initial assessment, regardless of the mechanism of injury.
- There are several clear indications for operative intervention in penetrating neck and torso injuries, which include the following:
  Sustained hemodynamic instability
  Expanding hematoma or pulsatile mass of the neck
  Cardiac tamponade
  Diffuse peritoneal signs
  Evisceration
  Object impaled in a body cavity
- Operative intervention should be done expeditiously when there are clear indications for surgery.
- Thoracoabdominal penetrating injury, especially on the left side, necessitates laparoscopic (thoracoscopic) intervention or celiotomy to best evaluate a diaphragmatic rent and possible intra-abdominal injuries.
- In general, a hemodynamically labile patient should *not* be transported to a radiology suite unless therapeutic intervention can be done expeditiously.

SELECTED READINGS

Blaisdell FW, Trunkey DD (eds): Abdominal Trauma. New York, Thieme, 1993.
Britt LD, Peyser MB: Penetrating and blunt neck trauma. In Moore EE, Mattox KL, Feliciano DV (eds): Trauma, 4th ed. Stamford, Conn, Appleton & Lange, 1999.
Fabian TC, Croce MA: Abdominal trauma, including indications for celiotomy. In Feliciano DV, Moore EE, Mattox KL (eds): Trauma. Stamford, Conn, Appleton & Lange, 1996, pp 525–550.
Renz BM, Cava RA, Feliciano DV, Rozycki GS: Transmediastinal gunshot wounds: A prospective study. J Trauma 2000;48:416.
Rotondo MF, Schwab CW, McGonigal MD, et al: Damage control: An approach for improved survival in exsanguinating penetrating abdominal injury. J Trauma 1993;35:375.
Rozycki GS, Feliciano DV, Ochsner MG, et al: The role of ultrasound in patients with possible penetrating cardiac wounds: A prospective multicenter study. J Trauma 1999;46:543.

Chapter 11
Vascular Trauma

Jon Perlstein, Felix D. Battistella, Jon M. Burch, and Ernest E. Moore

Extremity Vascular Trauma

Jon Perlstein and Felix D. Battistella

Before World War I, the technology and experience required for vascular repair were known, but at that time vascular surgery techniques were used only for chronic vascular problems, such as arteriovenous fistula or pseudoaneurysms resulting from previous trauma. In the acute trauma setting, ligation was used to save life at the expense of a limb. Even as recently as World War II, amputation rates after vascular injury exceeded 50%. During the Vietnam War, helicopter evacuation dramatically decreased the morbidity and mortality associated with vascular trauma. Today, rapid transport remains a vital component of the treatment of serious vascular injuries. With improvements in rapid diagnosis and surgery, the amputation rate has steadily decreased from 13% during the Vietnam War to 5% to 10% in current civilian series.

Blood vessel injuries account for more than 100,000 accidental deaths per year in the United States. More than 75% of these injuries occur in the extremities. Approximately 55% of the extremity vascular injuries are secondary to gunshot or shotgun wounds; 35% are due to stab wounds; and 10% occur in victims of blunt injury.

CLINICAL PRESENTATION

After immediately life-threatening injuries have been treated, attention can be directed to the management of other injuries, such as extremity vascular injuries. Critical aspects of the history include the mechanism of injury, amount of blood loss, neurologic signs and symptoms (e.g., pain, paralysis, paresthesias, numbness), and whether there is a history of previous occlusive vascular disease. On physical examination, extremity wounds should be inspected for hematoma, active bleeding, neurologic function, and proximity to a major blood vessel. The pulse examination should include palpation of the pulses proximal and distal to the injury as well as auscultation for bruits and thrills. It is important to compare the pulse of the injured extremity with that of the noninjured extremity; a difference in caliber of the pulses should prompt further workup. The arterial pressure index (API), which is similar to the ankle-brachial index, should be used as an extension of the physical examination. The API is measured by dividing the systolic pressure in the affected limb by the systolic pressure in the unaffected

limb. The systolic pressure should be measured distal to the injury using a continuous-wave Doppler probe. Johansen and colleagues have shown that an API less than 0.9 has a 95% sensitivity and 97% specificity in identifying occult arterial injury. The authors therefore recommend that patients with an API less than 0.9 be evaluated with an arteriogram. Based on the history and physical examination, the authors classify extremity vascular injuries into one of four categories: pulseless extremity, hard signs, soft signs, or no signs of vascular injury.

The pulseless extremity requires prompt surgical intervention (Fig. 11–1). Further diagnostic studies that may delay reestablishment of perfusion are not necessary unless the location or extent of injury is uncertain. In patients with shotgun wounds who may have multiple injuries along the course of a vessel, patients with chronic vascular occlusive disease, or patients with extensive bone or soft tissue injury due to blunt injury, the authors perform on-table arteriography in the operating room to minimize warm ischemia time. Arteriograms of the lower extremities can be performed via percutaneous transfemoral arterial access. However, when vessels in the distal two thirds of the calf are in question, the images obtained with the use of percutaneous groin access are frequently suboptimal. The remedy for this is to cut down on the distal superficial femoral artery (just proximal to the adductor canal); a cutdown in this location adds little morbidity because the anatomy is straightforward and the vessel is easy to expose. Once the artery is exposed and cannulated, a standard intraoperative arteriogram with inflow occlusion can be performed. Images obtained with this technique have better resolution and ensure an accurate diagnosis.

Patients with hard signs of vascular injury (Table 11–1)

Table 11–1	Clinical Signs of Extremity Vascular Injuries
HARD SIGNS	**SOFT SIGNS**
Diminished pulse	Adjacent neurologic injury
Expanding hematoma	Small to moderate-sized hematoma
Active arterial bleeding	Large blood loss at the scene
Bruit or thrill	Unexplained hypotension
Arterial pressure index <0.9	Proximity to major blood vessel

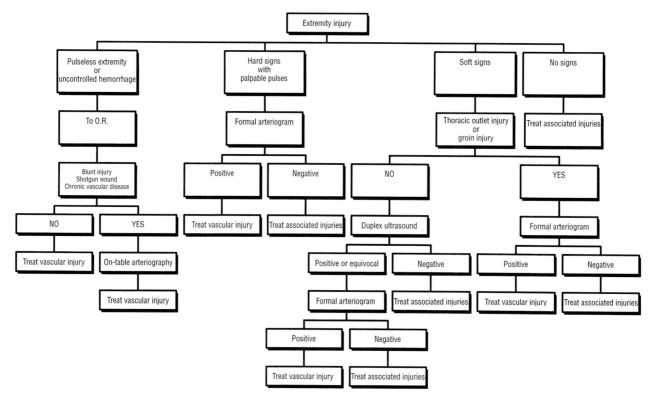

Figure 11–1. Algorithm for extremity vascular trauma.

but who have a palpable pulse distal to the injury should undergo formal arteriography to identify the location and character of the injury (see Fig. 11–1). The exception to this is when there is persistent active bleeding. In this case, patients should be taken directly to the operating room for exploration and vascular control.

Patients with soft signs of vascular injury (see Table 11–1) or proximity injuries should undergo further testing to exclude occult arterial injury (see Fig. 11–1). Before the 1970s, surgical exploration was performed to exclude occult vascular injury. By the 1980s, screening arteriography became the standard of care for proximity injuries. A less invasive test, duplex ultrasonography (US), has replaced arteriography for extremity injuries of this kind. Duplex US has a 95% sensitivity and 99% specificity. If the screening duplex US is positive or equivocal, arteriography should be performed to confirm and characterize the injury. The authors recommend proceeding directly to arteriography in patients with soft signs who have thoracic outlet or groin injuries because duplex US can miss injuries to vessels in these areas (Table 11–2). The

subclavian and axillary arteries are difficult to image with duplex US because of their location behind the clavicle. Missed injuries to these vessels may present with hemorrhagic shock due to intrapleural decompression. Iliac vessels are also difficult to visualize with duplex US, and missed injuries to these vessels can also be catastrophic.

PREOPERATIVE MANAGEMENT

Bleeding wounds are best controlled with direct digital compression. Tourniquets should be used only as a last resort because they will increase distal ischemia by occluding all collateral vessels or worsen bleeding if it is inadequately insufflated, thus acting as a venous tourniquet. Broad-spectrum antibiotics are administered as soon as possible, and tetanus prophylaxis is given as needed. If there are associated bony injuries, orthopedic surgeons should be consulted to assist with stabilization of the fractures.

NONOPERATIVE MANAGEMENT

Laboratory and clinical work have shown that some minimal arterial injuries can be managed nonoperatively. Most of these injuries are nonocclusive injuries that are usually diagnosed with arteriography. Frykberg and colleagues have published the largest series pertaining to observation of occult arterial injuries and have concluded that small intimal flaps, segmental stenoses, pseudoaneurysms, and arteriovenous fistulas are safe to manage nonsurgically.

The authors also manage minimal intimal injuries non-

Table 11–2	Indications for Formal Arteriography

Extremity injury in patients with a palpable distal pulse and one of the following:
   Hard signs of vascular injury
   Groin injury
   Thoracic outlet injury
   Extensive bone or soft tissue loss
   Equivocal duplex ultrasonography

operatively; however, we recommend a more aggressive approach to other occult injuries, such as pseudoaneurysms and arteriovenous fistulas because the failure rates with nonoperative management tend to be higher with these injuries. Nonoperative management requires serial physical examinations, noninvasive segmental pressure measurements, and imaging with duplex US to detect life- and limb-threatening progression of the injury.

Other nonoperative strategies include endovascular techniques in conjunction with diagnostic arteriography. Coil, Gelfoam, or balloon embolization can be used to treat branch vessel hemorrhage, pseudoaneurysms, and arteriovenous fistulas.

INTRAOPERATIVE MANAGEMENT

Extensive skin preparation and draping are used to ensure adequate proximal and distal exposure of the injured vessels (Fig. 11–2). An uninjured extremity should also be prepped in case an autogenous conduit, such as a saphenous or cephalic vein, is needed.

The first decision to be made is whether to revascu-

Table 11–3	Mangled Extremity Severity Score	
VARIABLE		**POINTS**
Skeletal and soft tissue injury		
Low-energy		1
Medium-energy		2
High-energy		3
Limb ischemia		
Pulse deficit but good perfusion		1
Pulseless, parethesias, pale		2
Cool, paralyzed, insensate		3
(°score doubles for ischemia >6 hr)		
Shock		
Systemic BP always >90 mm Hg		0
Transient hypotension		1
Persistent hypotension		2
Age		
<30		0
30–50		1
>50		2

From Johansen K, Daines M, Howey T, et al: Objective criteria accurately predict amputation following lower extremity trauma. J Trauma 1990;30:568, with permission.

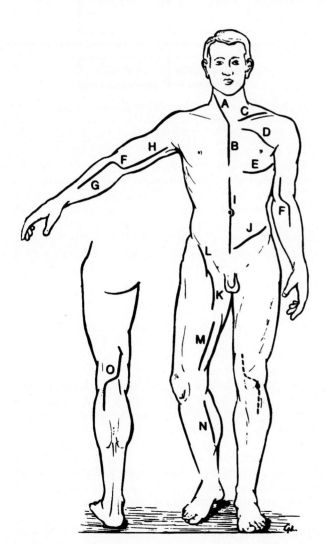

Figure 11–2. Incisions for vascular exposure and control. (From Rich NM, Spencer FC: Vascular Trauma. Philadelphia, WB Saunders, 1978, with permission.)

larize or amputate. There are two situations in which primary amputation is the best treatment option. The first is when a patient has had vascular occlusion for an extended period of time (>8 hours). In this situation a careful examination is performed to determine limb viability. If the limb is insensate and paralyzed, it should be deemed nonviable and an amputation should be performed. If the limb is potentially viable, revascularization should be attempted, but with the understanding that the reperfusion injury may be life-threatening and subsequent amputation may still be required. The second situation is the patient with a mangled extremity. Decisions in these cases can be extremely difficult. It is clear that some patients benefit from primary amputation because they will eventually end up with a nonfunctional limb requiring delayed amputation. In such cases, it is not worth incurring the risks of the reperfusion syndrome, which may prove lethal. Several scoring systems have been developed to aid in making the decision whether to revascularize or to amputate (Table 11–3). These scoring systems grade the extent of the vascular injury, neurologic deficit, and soft tissue and bone loss. Many surgeons have found that calculating these scores in the acute setting is cumbersome. The authors use a simpler algorithm as outlined in Figure 11–3. In the patient with a sciatic or tibial nerve deficit due to a transected nerve, a primary amputation should be performed because even if perfusion is reestablished, the result is a nonfunctional limb. If the nerves are intact or their integrity is unknown or equivocal and the limb has not been ischemic for an excessive period of time (>8 hours), salvage should be attempted. When revascularization and limb salvage are attempted in patients with mangled extremities, the 24-hour fluid balance is a key prognostic variable. A positive fluid balance greater than 3 L in the first 12 to 24 hours after repair signals the presence of life-threatening reperfusion injury, and secondary amputation should be considered to improve patient survival.

Once the decision to revascularize has been made,

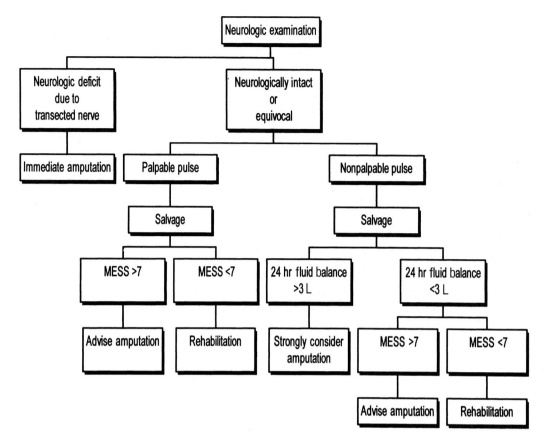

Figure 11–3. Algorithm for management of the mangled lower extremity. (From Roessker MS, Wisner DH, Holcroft JW: The mangled extremity: When to amputate? Arch Surg 1991;126:1243, with permission.)

obtaining proximal and distal control is a priority. This should be performed remote from the injury and hematoma via standard incisions along the course of the injured vessels (see Fig. 11–2). On occasion, staying away from the hematoma is not possible and, if necessary, temporary proximal and distal control can be obtained via balloon catheters placed through the injury. With bleeding controlled, proximal and distal dissection is performed and vascular clamps are placed. A tourniquet can be used for proximal control, if the injury is distal enough to permit its application. The use of a tourniquet avoids damage due to vascular clamps; however, the use of tourniquets should be avoided in polytrauma victims and patients with mangled extremities. The surgeon should also assess the vessel for distal embolism or thrombosis by back-bleeding the artery. If the back-bleeding is sluggish or absent, compression of the distal muscular bed is performed in order to milk back any clot. If there are no other injuries precluding anticoagulation, patients should be anticoagulated with 5000 U of heparin administered intravenously prior to occluding the vessels. If bleeding from associated injuries is a potential problem, a dilute solution of heparin is administered directly into the injured artery. Next, the injured arterial wall is débrided to healthy adventitia, media, and intima. With small punctures or lacerations, a lateral repair with interrupted sutures can be performed. If primary lateral arteriorrhaphy will result in stenosis of the vessel, a patch angioplasty can be employed with the use of autogenous vein graft.

When more extensive injury to the artery is encountered, segmental resection is required. If the arterial ends can be approximated without undue tension, the optimal reconstruction is a primary end-to-end anastomosis with fine interrupted polypropylene sutures. When a larger portion of the vessel requires resection, reconstruction is best preformed with an autogenous venous interposition graft using greater saphenous, lesser saphenous, or cephalic vein. It is important to harvest the autogenous conduit from an unaffected limb. If the deep venous system is injured in a given limb and one interrupts the superficial system by harvesting venous grafts, the patient may end up with severe, debilitating venous hypertension. When an autogenous conduit is not available or there is a large size discrepancy between the native artery and venous graft, a prosthetic graft (polytetrafluoroethylene [PTFE] or Dacron) should be used. Despite concerns about graft infections, the incidence appears to be reasonably low.

After the vascular reconstruction has been performed, completion arteriography should be performed in the operating room to assess the adequacy of the repair and the distal runoff and to verify that there are no other injuries or residual thrombus in the distal vessel.

VENOUS INJURIES

Isolated venous injuries are rarely recognized because they usually do not cause significant hemorrhage. Deep venous thrombosis may occur secondarily, resulting in valvular damage and long-term venous insufficiency. The majority of isolated venous injuries do not require operative intervention.

The correct management of venous injuries, when combined with arterial injuries, remains controversial. The Vietnam War demonstrated that patients with venous repair fared better than patients with venous ligation. Rich and colleagues showed the importance of venous repairs in the popliteal region and reported a decrease in the postoperative edema in the patients with repairs (51% vs. 13%). Aside from decreasing the incidence of edema, compartment syndrome, and postphlebitic syndrome, an additional theoretical advantage to repairing the venous injury is improving outflow for the associated arterial repair. As a result of the extensive work of Rich and others, the authors repair venous injuries whenever possible. The same principles of arterial repair apply to venous reconstructions: lateral venorrhaphy, if possible, followed by patch angioplasty, primary repair, or interposition graft with autogenous venous conduits. If the patient is moribund or the venous repair is so complex that it requires a panel graft, spiral graft, or prosthetics, the vein should be ligated. The authors' recommendation is to repair the arterial injury first to minimize warm ischemia time because the severity of reperfusion injury is directly proportional to the length of time the limb is without blood supply.

INTRALUMINAL SHUNTS

The use of intraluminal arterial shunts in patients with combined arterial and bony injuries has been shown to delay the arterial repair until after the bones have been stabilized. The authors' protocol with combined orthopedic and vascular injuries has been to repair the vascular injuries first, followed by orthopedic fixation. The authors have rarely witnessed disruption or thrombosis of the repair in this setting.

Intraluminal shunts have also been used in patients with associated life-threatening injuries and metabolic exhaustion manifested by hypothermia, acidosis, and coagulopathy. In this setting, shunts can be left in place for as long as 24 hours without significant risk of thrombosis. The authors use shunts in damage-control situations where the options for the arterial injury are to ligate or shunt. With the shunt, the authors have been able to save both life and limb in some patients who were too sick to have an arterial reconstruction performed during the initial operation.

FASCIOTOMY

Compartment syndrome can develop after extremity vascular injuries because of bleeding into the compartment or reperfusion induced edema. The authors do not perform routine fasciotomies for prolonged ischemia or venous injuries because the majority of these patients do not develop compartment syndrome. The authors monitor the extremities closely and measure compartment pressures. This can be done with a hand-held needle monitor or an 18-gauge needle connected to a continuous pressure monitor. Patients with compartment pressures higher than 30 mm Hg require fasciotomies.

For lower-leg compartment syndrome, the authors favor the one-incision fasciotomy technique. A long incision is made from the fibular head to the lateral malleolus down to fascia. Next, anterior and posterior flaps are created, followed by a transverse fascial incision to identify the anterior, lateral, and superficial, posterior compartments. These compartments are then decompressed with longitudinal fascial incisions. The deep posterior compartment is identified and decompressed via dissection posterior and medial to the fibula. Care must be taken to avoid injury to the peroneal vessels during this dissection. The key to the success of this technique is a long skin incision because a well-performed fasciotomy can fail as the result of inadequate dermal decompression. The fascial compartments of the thigh and arm rarely require decompression, but, when indicated, decompression is conducted via anterior and posterior longitudinal incisions.

POSTOPERATIVE MANAGEMENT

The keys to postoperative management of patients with vascular repairs are to maintain adequate intravascular volume and actively rewarm these patients. Blood products and crystalloid fluids are used to maintain normal blood pressure and urine output to ensure adequate flow through the vascular repair. Hypothermia, a common problem after vascular injuries, is associated with peripheral vasoconstriction. This in turn reduces the outflow bed of the arterial repair, which may result in early thrombosis.

Frequent evaluation of distal perfusion is paramount. Postoperatively, distal pulses may be absent owing to vasoconstriction. In this early postoperative phase, capillary refill and skin warmth and color are used to assess tissue perfusion until the pulse returns. Once the pulse returns, the new reference point is the palpable pulse. If there is a change and the pulse becomes weaker or absent, or distal perfusion deteriorates, the repair should be inspected and revised as needed.

Perioperative antibiotic administration for 24 hours is indicated because of the contaminated nature of the wounds. Elevation of the injured extremity is useful in reducing the edema seen with reperfusion. This is especially true with venous repairs and ligations. Compression stockings and bandages are helpful in further reducing the edema that comes with venous ligations.

There is no reason to routinely anticoagulate patients with arterial injuries because no improvement in patency will be realized and it carries a significant risk of postoperative hemorrhage. Postrepair bleeding can be especially profuse when fasciotomies have been performed. Conversely, if no associated injuries preclude heparin administration, venous repairs appear to benefit from short-term anticoagulation. Based on work by Smith and colleagues, the authors image all venous repairs at 72 hours after repair with duplex ultrasound. If the repairs are patent, heparin is discontinued. If the repair is occluded, the patient is then placed on anticoagulation for 3 months. The majority of these early occlusions will recanalize.

COMPLICATIONS

Early occlusion of the arterial repair occurs occasionally after arterial reconstruction. Thrombosis of the repair is usually due to a technical problem that requires revision of the repair. Loss of the pulse suggests occlusion at the anastomosis, and the patient should be immediately returned to the operating room for anastomotic revision. Frequent evaluations of distal perfusion are performed to identify problems promptly. Any delays in recognition or return to the operating room result in a higher incidence of limb loss.

Infection at the site of vascular repair can be a catastrophic complication that may lead to secondary amputation. Both prosthetic and autogenous tissue grafts can become infected, resulting in pseudoaneurysm formation, anastomotic breakdown, and possible hemorrhage. On occasion, these infections can be locally débrided with revision of the anastomosis. If the infection is drained and the repair preserved, it is imperative that the vascular repair is covered with a well-vascularized flap to ensure healing. When local treatment is not possible or is not safe, the artery should be ligated. In most cases, ligation will result in distal ischemia. Reconstruction can then be performed with the use of an extra-anatomic bypass (e.g., axillofemoral bypass, femoral-femoral bypass, obturator bypass).

Late complications include false aneurysms, arteriovenous fistulas, and anastomotic or graft stenosis. The key is to identify these lesions before they become a major problem. Periodic physical examination, segmental pressures, and noninvasive imaging play an important role in detecting late complications of vascular repairs. Another late complication is venous insufficiency in patients with venous repairs. The manifestations of this can be as mild as leg swelling, aching, and stasis dermatitis to severe ulcerations and tissue loss. Previous series have shown those patients with complex venous repairs or ligations combined with fasciotomies are associated with the most severe functional changes.

OUTCOMES

Improved trauma systems with rapid transport and improved surgical techniques account for the low mortality rate (0 to 3%) documented in patients with peripheral vascular injuries. The amputation rate continues to decline because of our better understanding of optimal treatment methods of these vascular injuries. A multitude of factors, such as delay in diagnosis, delay in reestablishing perfusion, severe bone and soft-tissue loss, nerve transection, and infection, contribute to the amputation rate after vascular injury. Prompt reperfusion of the non-perfused limb is critical in avoiding amputation and achieving optimal limb salvage.

PEARLS AND PITFALLS

PITFALLS

- Percutaneous on-table angiogram may not show tibial vessels well.
- Thoracic outlet injuries may have false-negative duplex US and present with exsanguinating hemothorax.
- Penetrating thigh wounds may yield a false-negative duplex US with interval swelling of the thigh.
- Occasionally, direct control of a bleeding vessel cannot be obtained owing to distorted anatomy.
- Determining appropriate incisions to expose subclavian–axillary artery injury.
- Tibial nerve transected.
- Patient in extremis.

PEARLS

- Perform angiogram by cutting down on distal superficial femoral artery.
- All proximity thoracic outlet injuries should be imaged with formal arteriography.
- Exclude profunda femoris artery injury with arteriography and possible endovascular treatment.
- Temporary control can be obtained with intraluminal balloon tamponade using Fogarty catheters.
- If injury is distal to the internal mammary artery, exposure can be obtained without entering the chest.
- Acute amputation.
- Ligate vessel and amputate extremity.

SELECTED READINGS

Ben-Menachem Y, Handel SF, Thaggard A III, et al: Therapeutic arterial embolization in trauma. J Trauma 1979;19:944.
DeBakey ME, Simeone FA: Battle injuries of the arteries in World War II: An analysis of 2,471 cases. Ann Surg 1946;123:534.
Feliciano DV, Mattox KL, Graham JM, et al: Five-year experience with PTFE grafts in vascular wounds. J Trauma 1985;25:71.
Feliciano DV, Herskowitz K, O'Gorman RB, et al: Management of vascular injuries in the lower extremities. J Trauma 1988;28:319.
Frykberg ER, Crump JM, Dennis JW, et al: Nonoperative observation of clinically occult arterial injuries: A prospective evaluation. Surgery 1991;109:85.
Johansen K, Daines M, Howey T, et al: Objective criteria accurately predict amputation following lower extremity trauma. J Trauma 1990;30:568.
Johansen K, Lynch K, Paul M, et al: Non-invasive vascular tests reliably exclude occult arterial trauma in injured extremities. J Trauma 1991;31:515.
Knudson MM, Lewis FR, Atkinson K, et al: The role of duplex ultrasound arterial imaging in patients with penetrating extremity trauma. Arch Surg 1993;128:1033.
Menzoin JO, Doyle JE, Cantelmo NL, et al: A comprehensive approach to extremity trauma. Arch Surg 1985;120:801.
Nichols JG, Svoboda JA, Parks SN: Use of temporary intraluminal shunts in selected peripheral arterial injuries. J Trauma 1986;26:1094.
Owings JT, Kennedy JP, Blaisdell FW: Injuries to the extremities. Sci Am pp 1-24.
Rich NM, Baugh JH, Hughes CW: Acute arterial injuries in Vietnam: 1,000 cases. J Trauma 1970;10:359.
Rich NM, Hobson RW, Collins Jr, GJ: The effect of acute popliteal venous interruption. Ann Surg 1976;183:365.
Roessler MS, Wisner DH, Holcroft JW: The mangled extremity: When to amputate? Arch Surg 1991;126:1243.
Smith LM, Block FJ, Buechter KJ, et al: The natural history of extremity venous repair performed for trauma. Am Surg 1999;65:116.

Thoracic Vascular Trauma

Jon M. Burch and Ernest E. Moore

INTRODUCTION

Thoracic vascular injuries are uncommon, yet often pose an immediate threat to the patient's life. These patients are usually cared for by general surgeons providing trauma care who usually do not have extensive ongoing thoracic vascular experience. Therefore, those who are obliged to care for these patients must be prepared with a knowledge of relevant anatomy, diagnostic maneuvers, and therapeutic options before the encounter occurs.

PREOPERATIVE EVALUATION

Thoracic vascular injuries occur with both blunt and penetrating injuries; however, the patterns of injury are distinctly different. Blunt trauma to the chest may involve the chest wall, thoracic spine, heart, lungs, thoracic aorta, great vessels, and rarely the esophagus. Most of these injuries are suspected by physical examination and plain chest radiograph. The most threatening occult injury in blunt trauma surgery is a tear of the descending thoracic aorta. Aortic tears occur when shearing forces are created in the chest, most often seen in high-energy transfer deceleration motor vehicle injuries with frontal or lateral impact. However, they may occur following recreational injury or fall. The tear usually occurs just distal to the left subclavian artery, where the aorta is tethered by the ligamentum arteriosum. In 2% to 5% of cases, the tear occurs in the ascending aorta, in the transverse arch, or at the diaphragm. Widening of the mediastinum on an AP chest radiograph strongly suggests this injury. The widening is caused by the formation of a hematoma around the injured aorta, which is temporarily contained by the endothoracic fascia and mediastinal pleura. Posterior rib fractures, laceration of small arteries, and mediastinal venous injuries can also produce similar hematomas. Should the hematoma rupture into the chest with an aortic injury, the patient will exsanguinate in seconds. Other findings suggestive of an aortic tear are listed in Table 11–4. However, it is well established that this injury can occur with an entirely normal chest radiograph; a recent AAST multicenter study suggests the incidence is approximately 7%. Because of the dire consequences of missing the diagnosis, CT and angiography are frequently performed based solely on mechanism of injury. Dynamic spiral CT is an excellent screening test. Positive findings are a hematoma contiguous with the aorta or changes in the aorta (Fig. 11–4). CT scanning is virtually 100% sensitive, but the specificity of finding an aortic injury in a patient with a periaortic hematoma is relatively low, approximately 50%. A clearly widened mediastinum on chest radiograph or abnormalities on CT are an absolute indication for emergent aortography. Computed tomography reconstruction may obviate the need for confirmatory aortography in certain cases.

Penetrating thoracic trauma is considerably easier to evaluate. Physical examination, plain posteroanterior and lateral chest radiographs with metallic markings of entrance and exit wounds, pericardial ultrasonography, and central venous pressure (CVP) measurement will disclose the vast majority of injuries. Injuries of the esophagus and trachea are exceptions. Based on the estimated trajectory of the missile or blade, esophagoscopy may be required to evaluate the esophagus, but injuries have been missed with this technique alone. Therefore, patients at risk should also undergo a soluble contrast-enhanced esophagogram looking for extravasation of contrast medium. If no extravasation is seen, a barium esophagogram should be performed for greater detail. Failure to identify

Table 11–4	**Findings on Chest X-Ray Suggestive of an Aortic Tear***

Widened mediastinum
Abnormal aortic contour
Tracheal shift
Nasogastric tube shift
Left apical cap
Left or right paraspinal stripe thickening
Depression of the left main bronchus
Obliteration of the aorticopulmonary window
Left pulmonary hilar hematoma

*Findings are listed in order of decreasing sensitivity.
From Burch JM, Francoise RJ, Moore EE: Trauma. In Schwartz SS (ed): Principles of Surgery. New York; McGraw-Hill, 1999, with permission.

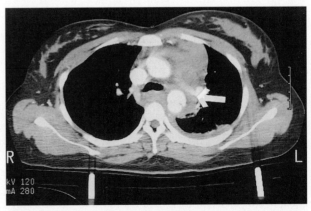

Figure 11–4. Spiral CT of a young woman with a widened mediastinum on anteroposterior chest radiograph who was a restrained driver suffering from a lateral impact motor vehicle accident on her side. The arrow points to a large pseudoaneurysm in continuity with the more posterior descending thoracic aorta. (From Burch JM, Francoise RJ, Moore EE: Trauma. In Schwartz SS [ed]: Principles of Surgery. New York, McGraw-Hill, 1999, with permission.)

esophageal injuries leads to fulminant mediastinitis, which is often fatal. Conversely, bronchoscopy is usually reserved for specific signs—that is, persistent air leak, mediastinal air, or hemoptysis. As in the neck, transmediastinal gunshot wounds frequently cause visceral or vascular injuries. Stable patients should be carefully evaluated for vascular, tracheal, and esophageal injuries, as outlined apreviously. Contrast-enhanceded CT scanning may permit more selective use of these invasive studies.

Penetrating injuries of the thoracic outlet (also referred to as zone I neck injuries) are considered a subset of thoracic injuries. Angiography is highly desirable because of the density of major vascular structures in the base of the neck, and because the incision employed is based on the specific vascular injury.

OPERATIVE MANAGEMENT

By far, the most common and versatile incision for trauma is an anterolateral thoracotomy with the patient in the supine position. Depending on findings, the incision can be extended across the sternum or even further for a bilateral anterolateral thoracotomy. The fifth interspace is usually preferred unless the surgeon has a precise knowledge of which organs are injured and that exposure would be enhanced by selecting a different interspace. The heart, lungs, aortic arch, great vessels, and esophagus are accessible with these incisions. Although it may seem obvious, care should be taken to ligate the internal thoracic artery and veins if they are transected. It is remarkable how often this step is overlooked, resulting in continuous blood loss, which obscures the field and endangers the patient.

Posterolateral thoracotomies are rarely used, since ventilation is impaired in the dependent lung, and the incision cannot be extended. There are two specific exceptions. Injuries of the posterior aspect of the trachea or mainstem bronchi near the carina are inaccessible from the left or from the front. The only possible approach is through the right chest, using a posterolateral thoracotomy. A tear of the descending thoracic aorta can be repaired only through a left posterolateral thoracotomy. Since the authors utilize left-heart bypass for these procedures, the patient's hips and legs are rotated toward the supine position to gain access to the left groin for femoral artery cannulation. It is also helpful for optimal exposure to transect the fourth rib posteriorly and enter the chest through the fourth intercostal space.

For patients with thoracic outlet injuries who are hemodynamically unstable and cannot undergo angiography, a reasonable approach can be inferred from the chest radiograph and the location of the wounds. If the patient has a left hemothorax, a left fourth interspace anterolateral thoracotomy should be performed because the proximal left subclavian artery may be injured. Hemorrhage can be controlled digitally until the vascular injury is delineated and clamps are applied. Additional incisions or extensions are often required. A fourth interspace right anterolateral thoracotomy may be used for thoracic outlet injury presenting with hemodynamic instability and a right hemothorax. A median sternotomy with a right su-

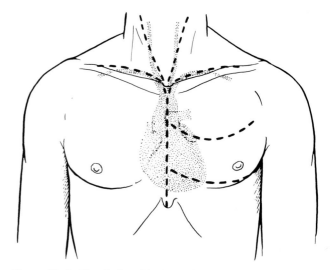

Figure 11–5. The choice of incisions for thoracic outlet injuries is based on the location of the underlying arterial injury and the urgency to obtain vascular control. See text. (From Burch JM, Francoise RJ, Moore EE: Trauma. In Schwartz SS [ed]: Principles of Surgery. New York, McGraw-Hill, 1999, with permission.)

praclavicular extension can also be used. Unstable patients with injuries near the sternal notch may have a large mediastinal hematoma, and these patients should be explored via a median sternotomy.

For stable patients with thoracic outlet injuries in whom angiography has identified an arterial injury, a more directed approach can be employed. Figure 11–5 shows the various incisions that are used, depending on the location of the arterial injury. A median sternotomy is used for exposure of the innominate, proximal right carotid, proximal right subclavian, and the proximal left carotid arteries. The proximal left subclavian artery presents a unique challenge. Because this vessel arises from the aortic arch far posteriorly, it is not readily approached via a median sternotomy. A posterolateral thoracotomy provides excellent exposure but severely limits access to other structures and, therefore, is not recommended. The best option is to create a full-thickness flap of the upper chest wall. This is accomplished with a fourth interspace anterolateral thoracotomy for proximal control, a supraclavicular incision, and a median sternotomy that links the two horizontal incisions. The ribs can be cut laterally, which allows the flap to be folded laterally for additional exposure. This incision has been referred to as a book or trapdoor thoracotomy for obvious reasons.

The midportion of either subclavian artery is accessible by removing the proximal third of either clavicle, with the skin incision made directly over the clavicle. Muscular attachments are stripped away and the clavicle is divided with a Gigli saw. The medial remnant of the clavicle is forcefully elevated, and the periosteum is dissected from the posterior aspect of the bone until the sternoclavicular joint is reached. The capsular attachments are cut with a heavy scissors or knife, and the bone is discarded. The periosteum and underlying fascia are very tough and must be sharply incised along the direction of the vessel. The subclavian vein is mobilized and the artery is directly underneath. The anterior scalene is divided for injuries just proximal to the thyrocervical trunk; the relatively small phrenic nerve must be identified on its anterior aspect and spared.

Vascular Repair

The initial control of vascular injuries should be accomplished digitally by applying just enough pressure directly on the bleeding site to stop the hemorrhage. Some bleeding vessels may need to be gently pinched between the thumb and the index finger. These maneuvers, along with suction, usually create a dry enough field to safely permit the dissection necessary for definition of the injury. In general, sharp dissection with fine scissors is preferable to blunt dissection, since the latter may aggravate the injury. Once a sufficient length of vessel is available, a vascular thumb forceps is used to grasp the vessel. If the vessel is not transected, forceps can be placed directly across the injury. This will minimize or eliminate bleeding while the dissection necessary for clamping is completed. If the vessel is transected (or nearly so), digital control is maintained on one side while the other side is occluded with a thumb forceps. The vessel is then sharply mobilized to allow an appropriate vascular clamp to be applied. When definitive control of all injuries is achieved, heparinized saline (50 U/mL) is injected into the proximal and distal ends of the injured vessel to prevent thrombosis. The exposed intima and media at the site of the injury is highly thrombogenic, and small clots often form. These clots should be removed to prevent thrombosis; otherwise, embolism may occur when the clamps are removed. The frequency with which embolism occurs necessitates routine balloon catheter exploration of the distal vessel. Ragged edges of the injury site should be judiciously débrided with the use of sharp dissection.

The great vessels are rather fragile and are easily torn during dissection or crushed with a clamp. For this reason, some authorities advocate oversewing proximal injuries of the artery on the side of the aortic arch and sewing a graft onto a new location on the arch. The graft is then sewn to the artery without tension. The authors have not found this to be necessary when the vessels are handled with care.

Injuries of the large veins, such as the superior vena cava and innominate, pose a special problem for hemostasis. Numerous large tributaries make adequate hemostasis difficult to achieve, and their thin walls render them susceptible to iatrogenic injury. When such an injury is encountered, tamponade with a folded laparotomy pad held directly over the bleeding site usually establishes hemostasis sufficient to prevent exsanguination. If hemostasis is not adequate for exposing the vessel proximal and distal to the injury, sponge sticks can be strategically placed on either side of the injury and carefully adjusted to improve hemostasis. This maneuver requires both skill and discipline to maintain a dry field. On occasion, the operative field will be sufficiently dry to delineate and repair the injury. However, it is often difficult or impossible for the assistant or assistants to maintain complete control of hemorrhage with sponge sticks. In this situation, the vessel can be exposed on either side of the

sponge sticks and a vascular clamp applied. The clamp can then be sequentially advanced toward the injury until hemostasis is complete.

Therapeutic options in the treatment of vascular injuries include lateral suture, end-to-end anastomosis, interposition grafting, and ligation. Some arteries and most veins can be ligated without significant sequelae. Arteries for which repair should always be attempted include the carotid, the innominate, and the aorta. Only the superior vena cava requires repair. The surgeon must keep in mind that there are few absolutes when one discusses the treatment of vascular injuries. If the alternative to ligation is exsanguination, the correct decision is obvious. On the other hand, ligation of some vessels may result in patient morbidity that is not life-threatening. Therefore, the authors attempt to repair all arteries larger than 3 mm and all veins larger than 10 mm in diameter, depending on the patient's physiologic condition.

Lateral suture is appropriate for arterial injuries with little or no loss of tissue. End-to-end anastomosis is used if the vessel is transected or almost transected. The severed ends of the vessel are mobilized, and small branches are ligated and divided as necessary to obtain the desired length. Arterial defects of 1 to 2 cm can usually be bridged. The surgeon should not be reluctant to divide small branches to obtain additional length, since most injured patients have normal vasculature and the preservation of potential collateral flow is not as important as it is in atherosclerotic surgery. To avoid postoperative stenosis, particularly in smaller arteries, some technique such as beveling or spatulation should be used so that the completed anastomosis is slightly larger in diameter than the native artery. The parachute technique for placement of initial suture is especially helpful in small vessels.

Interposition grafts are employed when end-to-end anastomosis cannot be accomplished without tension and despite mobilization. The great vessels of the chest must be bridged by arterial grafts. There is no place for the use of saphenous vein in these injuries.

Suture selection for arterial injuries is based on the diameter of the vessel being repaired. Double-needled polypropylene sutures are used almost exclusively. When performing anastomoses where the vessels are tethered (e.g., the thoracic aorta), the authors employ the parachute technique to ensure precision placement of the posterior suture line (Fig. 11–6). If this technique is used, traction on both ends of the suture must be maintained, or leakage from the posterior aspect of the suture line is probable. A single temporary suture, 180 degrees from the posterior row, may be used to maintain alignment.

Penetrating injuries often create wounds in adjacent structures; thus, it is likely that subsequent suture lines will contact one another. This does not seem to be a problem with adjacent arteries and veins. However, arterial-esophageal and arterial-tracheal fistulas can occur postoperatively; therefore, arterial and aerodigestive suture lines that may come into contact must be separated by viable tissue. For our purposes, this situation usually occurs in the thoracic outlet, where the innominate artery may contact the trachea. In this instance, a portion of the sternocleidomastoid muscle may be rotated down and interposed between these structures. Rarely, the esopha-

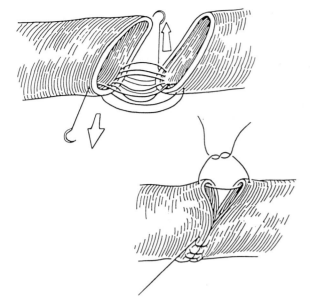

Figure 11–6. The parachute technique is used to precisely place the posterior sutures, especially when the injured artery is tethered—for example, the descending thoracic aorta. (From Burch JM, Francoise RJ, Moore EE: Trauma. In Schwartz SS [ed]: Principles of Surgery. New York, McGraw-Hill, 1999, with permission.)

gus and aorta may share adjacent suture lines. In this instance, avascularized intercostal muscle flap may be used.

Venous injuries are inherently more difficult to repair successfully because of their propensity to thrombose. Small injuries in which there has been loss of tissue can be treated with lateral suture. More complex repairs often fail. It should be noted that thrombosis does not occur acutely, but rather gradually over 1 to 2 weeks. Advantage can be taken of this fact because adequate collateral circulation, sufficient to avoid acute venous hypertensive complications, usually develops within several days.

There is one instance in which a more aggressive approach should be considered. Ligation of the superior vena cava has been associated with sudden blindness owing to compression of the optic nerve from venous hypertension. Artificial grafts have performed satisfactorily for injuries of the superior vena cava when lateral suture cannot be performed.

Management of the Torn Thoracic Aorta

The occurrence of paraplegia from ischemic injury of the spinal cord has been a concern in blunt injuries of the descending thoracic aorta. Conceptually, two techniques have been advocated. The simpler technique, often referred to as "clamp and sew," is accomplished with the application of vascular clamps proximal and distal to the injury and repair or replacement of the damaged portion of the aorta. This method results in transient hypoperfusion of the spinal cord distal to the clamps as well as all abdominal organs. Large doses of vasodilators are also required to reduce afterload and avoid acute left-heart failure. If the clamping time is short, less than 30 minutes, paraplegia has been uncommon. Longer clamping times,

however, have been associated with paraplegia in approximately 10% to 15% of patients. Unfortunately, clamping times of less than 30 minutes have been difficult to achieve for many cases requiring complex repair—that is, interposition grafting. The alternative approach has been to provide some method for maintaining a reasonable degree of perfusion for organs distal to the clamps. Two techniques have been used to accomplish this goal. The first is with the use of a shunt, a temporary extra-anatomic route around the clamps. A heparin-impregnated tube, the Gott shunt, has been specifically designed for this purpose. However, the volume of blood flow to the distal aorta with the passive technique is marginal. The second method has been to employ left-heart bypass. With this method, a volume of oxygenated blood is siphoned from the left heart and is actively pumped into the distal aorta. Flow rates of 2 to 3 L appear to provide adequate protection by maintaining a distal perfusion pressure greater than 65 mm Hg. The authors prefer this method. The left superior pulmonary vein is cannulated to remove blood from the heart, rather than the left atrium, because the vein is tougher and less prone to tearng. The left femoral artery is cannulated to return the blood to the distal aorta. A centrifugal pump is employed because it is not as thrombogenic as a roller pump, and, strictly speaking, heparinization is not required. This can be a significant benefit in a patient with multiple injuries, particularly in those with intracranial hemorrhage. However, occasional small cerebral infarcts have occurred, and 5000 to 10,000 U of heparin is usually administered unless contraindicated by associated injuries.

Once bypass is initiated, the proximal vascular clamp is usually applied between the left common carotid and the left subclavian artery and the distal clamp is placed just distal to the injury. The left subclavian artery is clamped separately. The hematoma is entered, and the injury evaluated. Primary repair without a graft is possible in many patients; 3-0 polypropylene suture is used for the anastomoses or suture lines. In patients requiring an interposition graft, a short gelatin-sealed Dacron graft is placed, usually 18 to 20 mm in diameter. Air and clot are flushed from the aorta between the clamps and the subclavian artery prior to completing the last anastomosis or suture line. Following completion of the repair, the clamps are removed and the patient is weaned from the pump. The cannulae are removed, and the vessels are repaired. A recent meta-analysis comparing clamp-and-sew with left-heart bypass revealed a significantly lower incidence of paraplegia when the pump is used.

Injuries of the transverse arch do occur from blunt trauma. In some instances, proximal control can be obtained by placing the clamp between the innominate and the left carotid arteries without cerebral infarction. However, the proximal clamp cannot be placed proximal to the innominate artery. A possible approach to injuries in which the clamps completely exclude the cerebral circulation is profound hypothermia with circulatory arrest.

Small intimal flaps of the thoracic aorta without hematomas can be treated nonoperatively. Intraluminal mediastinal stents may also provide a solution, but their role remains to be defined. Penetrating injuries of the thoracic aorta are rare and do not afford enough time to set up the pump. Therefore, there is no choice but to use the clamp-and-sew technique. Partial occlusion of the clamps should be performed if possible.

Postoperative Management

There is nothing unique about postoperative care for most patients with thoracic vascular injuries. Large chest tubes (36-French) are place prior to closure of thoracotomies. The tubes are removed when air leaks stop, the drainage fluid becomes clear, and its volume approaches 100 mL or less per day. Perioperative antibiotics are routinely employed. Cefazolin is used for most patients. A preoperative dose is administered at the induction of anesthesia and repeated every 3 hours during the operation. Many surgeons continue antibiotics until chest tubes and central venous lines are removed in patients with PTFE or Dacron arterial interposition grafts. The authors are more conservative and usually administer only a single postoperative dose. Despite the frequently emergent conditions, graft and wound infections have been rare. Nutritional support remains a critical adjunct. For patients who will not begin oral intake in 4 or 5 days, enteral feedings are initiated. Unless direct access to the stomach or proximal jejunum is available, the authors employ small-diameter nasojejunal feeding tubes placed with endoscopic assistance.

Another consideration is the use of thoracic epidural analgesia. The pain caused by thoracic incisions is severe and difficult to control with doses of parenteral narcotics that do not impair ventilation. Epidural analgesia reliably provides adequate analgesia without hyperventilation. However, serious complications can occur with epidurals, and vigilance must be maintained.

Blood loss and shock puts patients with thoracic vascular injuries at risk for multiple-organ failure. In these instances, lung-protective ventilation is employed to prevent microscopic barotrauma, which can cause or perpetuate acute respiratory distress syndrome (ARDS). This form of ventilation is characterized by low tidal volumes

---

Pearls and Pitfalls

Thoracic Vascular Injury

PEARLS

- Patients with thoracic vascular injuries who are breathing on their own can have precipitous deterioration because of persistent or recurrent hemorrhage aggravated by negative intrathoracic pressure and/or pneumothorax.
- While angiography is highly desirable for patients with injuries of the thoracic outlet, it should be reserved for hemodynamically stable patients.
- Blunt injury to the descending thoracic aorta may occur with an entirely normal chest radiograph.
- Patients with blunt injury of the descending thoracic aorta whose blood pressure is greater than 110 mm Hg systolic may benefit from short-acting beta-blocking agents to prevent rupture of the pseudoaneurysm during transport or following arrival in the emergency department.

(6 to 7 mL/kg), relatively high positive end-expiratory pressure (approximately 15 cm), and permissive hypercapnia. The efficacy of this strategy has been demonstrated in at least two prospective randomized studies.

Graft infections are uncommon following repair of thoracic vascular injuries, despite the frequently emergent conditions. Thoracic wall incisional infections are also rare.

SELECTED READINGS

Feliciano DV: Trauma to the aorta and major vessels. Chest Surg Clin North Am 1997;7:305.

Graham JM, Feliciano DV, Mattox KL, et al: Management of subclavian vascular injuries. J Trauma 1980;20:537.

Graham JM, Feliciano DV, Mattox KL: Innominate vascular injury. J Trauma 1982;22:647.

Mattox KL: Red River anthology. J Trauma 1997;42:353.

Read RA, Moore EE, Moore FA, Haenel JB: Partial left heart bypass for thoracic aortic repair. Arch Surg 1993;128:746.

Chapter 12
Thermal Injury

David W. Mozingo

The majority of burn injuries are of limited severity, with more than 80% of patients having burns that involve less than 20% total body surface area (TBSA) who can be cared for in an outpatient setting. The remainder will require hospital care owing to the extent of burn or complicating factors, such as associated injuries, preexisting disease, or extremes of age. Approximately one fourth of patients who require in-hospital care are classified as having major burn injury and are best cared for in burn centers, where specialized staff, equipment, and facilities ensure optimal treatment.

CLINICAL PRESENTATION

The first priority at the accident scene is to stop the burning process. Burning and smoldering clothing should be extinguished, and patients with electrical injury should be separated from points of electric contact. If the burn was caused by a chemical agent, all contaminated clothing should be removed and copious water lavage initiated.

As with all trauma patients, the primary concern during the initial assessment is maintenance of cardiopulmonary function. Airway patency and adequacy of ventilation must be maintained, and supplemental oxygen administered as necessary. Unconscious patients or those with associated mechanical trauma should be provided spinal immobilization during their initial care until a complete evaluation can be performed. In patients with suspected smoke inhalation injury, treatment of carbon monoxide poisoning should be initiated by delivering 100% oxygen by endotracheal tube or face mask. This treatment should be continued until carboxyhemoglobin measurements are obtained and are less than 5%.

On arrival of the patient in the emergency department, the patency of the airway and adequacy of breathing should be reassessed. Intravenous fluid resuscitation is initiated by infusing lactated Ringer's solution through a large-bore intravenous cannula. The order of preference for the intravenous site is a peripheral vein underlying unburned skin, a peripheral vein underlying burned skin, and, lastly, a central vein. A history should be obtained regarding the circumstances of the injury, the presence of preexisting diseases, allergies, and medications, and the use of alcohol or illicit drugs prior to injury. A complete physical examination should be performed, and associated injuries identified. Baseline laboratory data should include measurements of arterial blood gas, serum electrolytes, blood urea nitrogen (BUN) and creatine, glucose, and a complete blood count (CBC). Determination of oxygen saturation should be by transcutaneous pulse oximetry used in patients with suspected inhalation injury or extensive burns; however, it should be noted that the oxygen saturation may be falsely elevated in patients with carbon monoxide poisoning.

Fluid resuscitation is based on body weight and the percentage of the body that is burned. The patient should be weighed, and the depth and extent of burn estimated. The extent of body surface area burn can be estimated easily using the "rule of nines," which recognizes that specific anatomic regions represent 9% or 18% of the TBSA (Fig. 12–1). The surface area of irregularly shaped burns can be estimated more simply by considering the size of the patient's hand to represent 1% of the body surface area. Infants and children have a different body surface area distribution, with larger heads and smaller legs. When one estimates the body surface area for children younger than 10 years of age, the Lund and Browder burn diagram (Fig. 12–2) or other similar diagrams should be used to more precisely determine the body surface area burned.

The depth of burn is classified as partial-thickness or full-thickness with respect to the depth of dermal destruction by coagulation necrosis. First- and second-degree burns are considered partial-thickness injuries, and third-degree burns are categorized as full-thickness injuries. First-degree burns show erythema of the skin only, and there is no loss of epidermal integrity. Therefore, the extent of first-degree burn is not calculated in the determination for fluid resuscitation. Superficial partial-thickness burns heal spontaneously by epithelial migration from preserved dermal appendages. Full-thickness injuries have complete destruction of all epithelial elements and require skin grafting for wound closure. Deep partial-thickness burns may heal over a long period of time; however, grafting is frequently performed to decrease the time to wound closure, reduce scar formation, and improve functional outcome. Partial-thickness burns typically have a pink or mottled red appearance, and blisters or bullae are present. When the bullae are disrupted, the surface is moist and weeping and very painful. Conversely, third-degree or full-thickness burns have a pearly white, charged, or translucent parchment-like appearance. Thrombosed vessels may be visible beneath the surface of the wound. They are typically dry and inelastic and have an insensate surface.

Other interventions during the initial care phase include insertion of the urethral catheter in patients with burns involving more than 20% TBSA. The initial volume of urine should be discarded, and the urine volume measured and recorded hourly. Ileus is common in burn patients with a TBSA burn greater than 20%, and a nasogastric tube should be inserted to prevent gastric distention and emesis and decrease the risk of aspiration.

A booster dose of tetanus toxoid should be administered if the last dose was given within the past 5 years. Patients without prior active immunization should receive

Rule of Nines
(Adult)

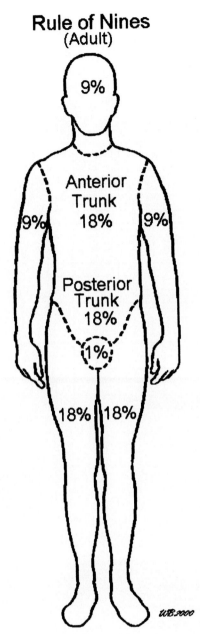

9%

Anterior
Trunk
18%

9%   9%

Posterior
Trunk
18%

1%

18%   18%

WB 2000

Figure 12–1. The rule of nines demonstrating that specific anatomic regions represent 9% or 18% of the total body surface area.

hyperimmune tetanus immune globulin in addition to the initial dose of tetanus toxoid. Active immunization is completed according to the routine dosage schedule.

Controlling pain during the early care of thermally injured patients is best accomplished by administration of small frequent doses of morphine sulfate. Doses of 3 to 5 mg may be administered to adults and repeated until pain relief is achieved. Subcutaneous and intramuscular injections should be avoided owing to the unpredictable absorption during wound edema formation.

Any gross contamination of the burn wound surface should be removed, and the wound covered with a clean dry sheet and blankets to prevent hypothermia. When the burn patient is to be transferred to another care facility, wound débridement and application of topical antimicro-

bial agents is unnecessary and this treatment should be deferred to the receiving hospital.

The American Burn Association has developed guidelines by which those patients requiring treatment in a burn center can be identified. These criteria use the extent, depth, and location of the burn; the mechanism of injury; and the presence of preexisting comorbid factors and associated injuries to guide personnel in the referral of patients requiring multispecialty burn care (Table 12–1).

PREOPERATIVE MANAGEMENT

Fluid Resuscitation

By knowing the extent of the burn, the patient's weight, and the time elapsed since the injury occurred, one can calculate the volume of resuscitation fluid required to initiate resuscitation in these patients. The various burn formulas in use today differ considerably with respect to the volume and composition of the resuscitation fluid; however, each formula has been found to be clinically effective when administered on the basis of the patient's physiologic response. A central theme is that the volume of fluid required is dependent on the patient's weight and the extent of the burn. It is recommended that half of the calculated requirement be infused over the first 8 hours following the injury (the time of maximal vascular permeability) and the remainder of the first 24-hour resuscitation volume delivered over the ensuing 16 hours.

The two most common formulas in use in the United States are the Modified Brooke formula and the Parkland formula. Both recommend the use of lactated Ringer's solution during the first 24 hours without the addition of colloid or electrolyte-free crystalloid solutions until the second 24 hours. Lactated Ringer's solution is the pre-

Table 12–1	**Burn Unit Referral Criteria**

Burn injuries that should be referred to a burn unit include the following:
   Partial-thickness burns constituting more than 10% of total body surface area (TBSA)
   Burns that involve the face, hands, feet, genitalia, perineum, or major joints
   Third-degree burns in any age group
   Electrical burns, including lightning injury
   Chemical burns
   Inhalation injury
   Burn injury in patients with preexisting medical disorders that could complicate management, prolong recovery, or affect mortality
   Any patients with burns and concomitant trauma (e.g., fractures) in which the burn injury poses the greatest risk of morbidity or mortality. In such cases, if the trauma poses the greater immediate risk, the patient may initially be stabilized in a trauma center before being transferred to a burn unit. Physician judgment will be necessary in such situations and should be in concert with the regional medical control plan and triage protocols.
   Burned children in hospitals without qualified personnel or equipment for the care of children
   Burn injury in patients who will require special social, emotional, or long-term rehabilitative intervention

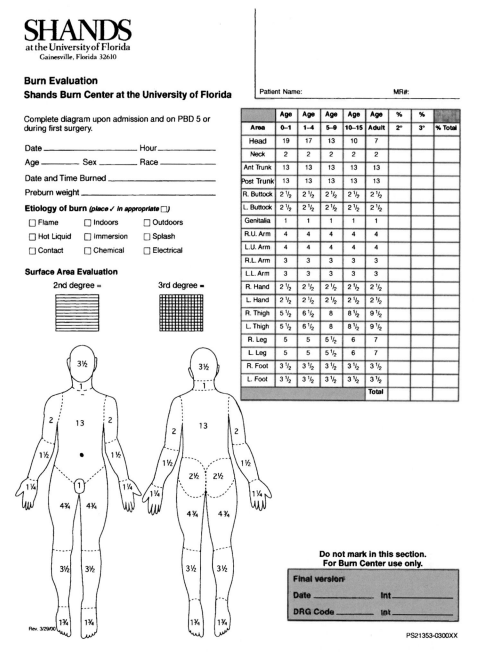

SHANDS
at the University of Florida
Gainesville, Florida 32610

Burn Evaluation
Shands Burn Center at the University of Florida

Patient Name: MR#:

Complete diagram upon admission and on PBD 5 or
during first surgery.

Date _____ Hour _____

Age _____ Sex _____ Race _____

Date and Time Burned _____

Preburn weight _____

Etiology of burn *(place ✓ in appropriate ☐)*

☐ Flame   ☐ Indoors   ☐ Outdoors

☐ Hot Liquid ☐ Immersion   ☐ Splash

☐ Contact   ☐ Chemical   ☐ Electrical

Surface Area Evaluation

2nd degree =   3rd degree =

Area	Age 0–1	Age 1–4	Age 5–9	Age 10–15	Age Adult	% 2°	% 3°	% Total
Head	19	17	13	10	7			
Neck	2	2	2	2	2			
Ant Trunk	13	13	13	13	13			
Post Trunk	13	13	13	13	13			
R. Buttock	2½	2½	2½	2½	2½			
L. Buttock	2½	2½	2½	2½	2½			
Genitalia	1	1	1	1	1			
R.U. Arm	4	4	4	4	4			
L.U. Arm	4	4	4	4	4			
R.L. Arm	3	3	3	3	3			
L.L. Arm	3	3	3	3	3			
R. Hand	2½	2½	2½	2½	2½			
L. Hand	2½	2½	2½	2½	2½			
R. Thigh	5½	6½	8	8½	9½			
L. Thigh	5½	6½	8	8½	9½			
R. Leg	5	5	5½	6	7			
L. Leg	5	5	5½	6	7			
R. Foot	3½	3½	3½	3½	3½			
L. Foot	3½	3½	3½	3½	3½			
					Total			

Rev. 3/29/00

Do not mark in this section.
For Burn Center use only.

Final version

Date _____ Int _____

DRG Code _____ Int _____

PS21353-0300XX

Figure 12–2. A more exact estimation of the extent of burn is possible with the use of a burn diagram. Note that the body surface area distribution changes with age, particularly the head and lower extremities.

ferred solution because the concentration of chloride ion is more physiologic compared with that of normal saline. Using the Modified Brooke formula, fluid needs in adults are estimated as 2 mL of lactated Ringer's solution per kilogram body weight per percent TBSA burn. The Parkland formula specifies twice that volume using 4 mL/kg/% TBSA burn. Both require one half of the calculated volume to be administered in the first 8 hours and the second half over the subsequent 16 hours post burn. When the initiation of fluid resuscitation is delayed, that amount of fluid calculated to be administered in the first 8 hours should be infused at a rate so that half of the estimated 24-hour fluid requirement will be given by

8 hours post burn. However, any resuscitation formula serves only to guide the initiation of fluid therapy, and the actual amount of resuscitation fluid delivered is guided by each patient's physiologic response. Frequent reassessment, on at least an hourly basis, and adjustment of the fluid infusion rate are essential to ensuring adequate tissue perfusion. Failure to reevaluate the patient's response to resuscitation on a scheduled basis may lead to either over-resuscitation or under-resuscitation. Inadequate fluid administration results in organ dysfunction or failure, while excessive administration of resuscitation fluids may cause pulmonary, cerebral, and/or excessive burn wound edema.

In the second 24 hours following injury, a solution of 5% albumin in physiologic saline is administered in an amount proportionate to preburn body weight and the extent of burn, to aid in correction of the plasma volume deficit. In burns involving less than 30% of the body surface, the plasma volume deficit is not profound and routine colloid replacement is unnecessary. The following formulas are used to estimate colloid replacement based on the extent of burn injury: 30% to 50% burn, 0.3 mL/kg body weight per percent burn; 50% to 70% burn, 0.4 mL/kg body weight per percent burn; more than 70% burn, 0.5 mL/ kg body weight per percent burn. These formulas calculate the total volume of 5% albumin solution to be infused at a constant rate over the second 24 hours following injury. Additionally, the lactated Ringer's infusion is discontinued and 5% dextrose in water (D_5W) is delivered to maintain urine output between 30 and 50 mL/hr during the second 24 hours.

Fluid Resuscitation in Children

Several important differences must be considered in the fluid resuscitation of the burned child. Children have a greater body surface area per unit of body mass and, thus, require more resuscitation fluid compared with adults. Fluid needs in children weighing less than 30 kg are estimated as 3 mL of lactated Ringer's solution/kg body weight per percent TBSA burn. The addition of supplemental intravenous fluid to account for metabolic water requirements in the form of 5% dextrose in 0.45% saline is also necessary. This is essential because in patients with small to moderate-sized burns the volume of fluid calculated on the basis of the extent of burn may not meet maintenance fluid requirements. As burn size increases, the contribution of the additional maintenance fluid to the overall resuscitation fluid volume becomes less significant. Also, the addition of dextrose in this maintenance fluid ensures that infants, who have limited hepatic glycogen reserves, do not become symptomatically hypoglycemic during the initial phase of resuscitation. During the second 24 hours following injury, the plasma volume deficit is replaced, with the use of the same calculations as those for adult patients. However, D_5 one-half normal saline is used instead of D_5W and titrated to maintain adequate urine output. The use of D_5W in pediatric burn victims should be avoided to prevent the occurrence of symptomatic hyponatremia, which may be accompanied by the rapid development of cerebral edema and profound neurologic sequelae, including brain death.

Monitoring Resuscitation

The best indicator of the adequacy of resuscitation is the hourly urinary output, which should be maintained between 30 and 50 mL/hr in patients weighing more than 30 kg and 1 mL/kg per hour in patients weighing less than 30 kg. Oliguria in the first 48 hours post burn is rarely caused by acute renal or cardiac failure and is initially treated with increasing fluid administration, and not by pharmacologically inducing a diuresis. Assessment of the hemodynamic response and the status of mental function indicating the adequacy of cerebral perfusion are also helpful in monitoring fluid resuscitation therapy. Patient anxiety, restlessness, and disorientation may be early signs of hypovolemia or hypoxemia that require immediate assessment and correction. A resting tachycardia between 100 and 120 beats per minute is common following burn injury, and heart rates above this level may reflect inadequate fluid resuscitation or inadequate pain control. Blood pressure measurements, even when obtained by an indwelling peripheral arterial cannula, may not be indicative of the true hydration status. The presence of circumferential burns on the extremities may impair arterial perfusion, resulting in blood pressure measurements not reflecting the true central arterial pressure. Additionally, markedly elevated circulating levels of catecholamines may cause vasospasm and compromise the utility of blood pressure monitoring to guide the adequacy of resuscitation. Invasive hemodynamic monitoring with a pulmonary artery catheter is reserved for patients who do not respond to fluid resuscitation as expected or whose fluid administration in the first 6 hours exceeds the volume that will result in a 6 mL/kg per percent burn resuscitation.

As blood flow to the burn wound increases following the resuscitative phase, the evaporative water loss from the wound increases and persists until the burn wound is healed or grafted. The insensible water losses that include the evaporative wound losses may be estimated according to the following formula: insensible water loss in milliliters per hour = (25 + % body surface area burn) × TBSA in meters.[2] This formula provides a useful estimation of the insensible loss; however, replacement of fluid losses in the postresuscitation phase should be guided by monitoring the patient's weight and serum sodium concentration.

Escharotomy and Fasciotomy

Circumferential full-thickness burns of the limbs may impair circulation to distal and underlying tissues. To prevent ischemic necrosis of these tissues, an escharotomy may be required to relieve the constriction caused by edema beneath the eschar. To identify the need for escharotomy, the adequacy of circulation should be assessed at hourly intervals. The detection of pulsatile arterial flow in the palmar arch and digital vessels of the fingers, and the pedal vessels in the feet, is made with a Doppler flowmeter. A progressive decrease in or the absence of pulsatile flow is an indication for escharotomy. Cyanosis, impaired capillary refilling, progressive paresthesias, and deep tissue pain are difficult to assess in an extensively burned extremity but may also indicate the need for escharotomy. The escharotomy procedure is performed at the patient's bedside without the need for anesthesia, since only insensate full-thickness burn tissue is incised. The first escharotomy incision is placed in the midlateral line of the involved extremity. If pulsatile flow is not detected within 5 to 10 minutes, a second escharotomy is made in the midmedial line of that limb. The escharotomy incision must be performed along the entire length of the full-thickness burn to provide adequate release of vascular and neural compression. The incision must be carried across the involved joints, where there is a relative lack of subcutaneous tissue, and compression of nerves and vessels occurs rapidly. The escharotomy incises just the eschar and immediate subjacent tissue to allow expansion of the edematous underlying tissue. Blood loss from the escharotomy incision is minimal and readily controlled by application of pressure or electrocoagulation when performed at this level. Deeper incisions often lead to excessive bleeding.

Patients with circumferential truncal burns may also require escharotomy along the anterior axillary lines to relieve restriction of chest wall movement and ensure effective ventilation. An incision along the costal margin may be required in patients with full-thickness burns extending onto the upper abdominal wall. In mechanically ventilated patients, a progressive rise in peak inspiratory pressure or increase in arterial carbon dioxide tension may indicate the need for chest escharotomy. In spontaneously breathing patients, the development of restlessness, agitation, or tachypnea may signal the need for chest escharotomy.

Fasciotomy is rarely necessary to restore circulation in a limb with typical thermal injury. However, in patients with extensive deep burns involving fascia and muscle, or in patients with associated traumatic injuries, fasciotomies may be required to ensure adequate tissue perfusion. Additionally, in patients with high-voltage electrical injury, fasciotomy is often required. The need for fasciotomy is evident when escharotomy fails to restore pulsatile arterial flow to an extremity in an otherwise successfully resuscitated patient.

Electrical Injury

Tissue damage from an electrical injury results from the heat generated by the passage of electric current through the body and direct thermal injury caused by flash burns or the ignition of clothing. High-voltage and low-voltage injuries are arbitrarily defined as those above or below 1000 V, respectively. The severity of injury is influenced by the voltage, the type of current, the duration of contact, and the path of current through the body.

The estimation of resuscitation fluid requirements in patients who have sustained electrical injury is difficult because of extensive subcutaneous or deep tissue involvement accompanied by limited areas of cutaneous injury. This "iceberg" effect often necessitates the performance of a fasciotomy, rather than an escharotomy, to ensure viability of the distal, uninjured extremity and to evaluate the underlying subcutaneous tissue and muscle. With extensive muscle necrosis, hemochromogens may be liberated, resulting in the production of pigmented urine. In this case, intravenous fluids are administered in the volume required to produce a urine output of 100 mL/hr. If the urinary pigments do not clear with this rate of urine output, additional treatments are indicated to prevent acute tubular necrosis. Sodium bicarbonate (50 mEq) should be added to each liter of intravenous fluid to alkalinize the urine and decrease pigment accumulation in

the renal tubules. An osmotic diuretic, such as mannitol, may be administered to force an increase in urine output if alkalization of the urine does not result in pigment clearing.

Patients with electrical injury are more likely to have associated injuries owing to falls or tetanic skeletal muscle contractions induced by the electric current. The patient's spine should be immobilized until cervical, thoracic, and lumbar radiographs and physical examination exclude spinal fractures. Cardiac dysrhythmias occur in a small percentage of patients with electrical injury. Thus, these patients should have continuous electrocardiographic monitoring for at least 24 hours, and dysrhythmias should be treated promptly, if they occur. Neurologic changes are common in patients with electrical injury, and a thorough neurologic examination must be performed on admission and at scheduled intervals in these patients. Neurologic changes may be early or late in onset. Early peripheral deficits due to the damaging effects of electric current may be irreversible; however, early deficits in a distribution where there is no clear tissue damage often resolve. Signs and symptoms of delayed onset, often resembling upper motor neuron disease, tend to be progressive and permanent.

About one third of patients with significant electrical injury of the extremities will require amputation. Conservative operations are performed according to the principles of limb salvage, and only obviously necrotic tissue is débrided. It is often difficult to distinguish nonviable from viable tissue with certainty during the initial débridement and patients with these injuries are frequently returned to the operating room at 24- to 48-hour intervals to reevaluate the extent of injury. Occasionally, unrelenting hyperkalemia, acidosis, or hemochromogenuria force early amputation to prevent systemic organ failure.

Chemical Burns

The depth and severity of chemical burns are related to the concentration of the chemical agent and the duration of contact with the tissues. The caustic agent must be thoroughly washed from the surface of the skin as soon as possible. All clothing, including shoes, must be removed, and the wounds copiously irrigated with water. When the chemical agent is present in the form of a dry powder, this should be brushed from the skin surface prior to water irrigation. If ocular injury is suspected, prompt and prolonged irrigation with saline or water should begin.

The amount of tissue damage incurred is dependent on the nature of the specific agent. Strong alkalis react with tissues to produce saponification and liquefaction necrosis, whereas acids are water-soluble and penetrate easily into subcutaneous tissues, causing coagulation necrosis soon after contact. Cutaneous absorption of certain chemical agents may cause systemic toxicity, which may complicate subsequent therapy; therefore, identification of the causative agent is required. Initial wound management is not dependent on the nature of the specific agent, and prompt and thorough water lavage is employed for all chemical exposures.

Assessing the depth of the injury in chemical burns is often difficult, since many agents produce a tanned or bronzed appearance of the skin. These wounds may remain pliable to the touch but actually represent extensive full-thickness tissue necrosis. With the exception of the initial attention given to the burn wound and possible systemic toxicity due to absorption of the causative agent, fluid resuscitation and later treatment of chemical injury follow that of thermal burns.

Management of the Burn Wound

Following the initial wound assessment and thorough cleansing and débridement, the burn wound should be treated with topical antimicrobial agents to limit bacterial proliferation on the wound surface and to prevent bacterial wound invasion. Three commonly employed topical agents, mafenide acetate cream, silver sulfadiazine cream, and 0.5% silver nitrate soaks have been used extensively in burn patients and are effective in controlling bacterial proliferation. Recently, a nanocrystalline preparation of elemental silver deposited on a polyurethane film (Acticoat, Westaim Biomedical, Exeter, NH) has been introduced for use in partial-thickness burns. The development and clinical use of the effective topical antimicrobial agents have significantly decreased the incidence of invasive burn wound infection and subsequent sepsis. Each agent has specific advantages and limitations with which the physician must be familiar to ensure optimal benefit and patient safety (Table 12–2). All of the agents are effective in the prevention of invasive burn wound infection; however, because of their lack of eschar penetration, silver sulfadiazine burn cream, silver nitrate soaks, and Acticoat are most effective when applied within 48 hours of injury. On the other hand, mafenide acetate readily penetrates the burn eschar, thus exerting its antimicrobial action at the wound surface, within the eschar, and at the viable-nonviable tissue interface.

Silver nitrate solution is delivered in multilayer occlusive gauze dressings. These are changed twice daily and moistened every 2 hours to limit evaporation, which may increase the silver nitrate concentration to cytotoxic levels within the dressings. Acticoat should be moistened with sterile water, placed on the burn wound, and covered with gauze dressings. These dressings must be moistened with water periodically to permit the silver to remain in aqueous suspension at the wound interface. These dressings require removal and replacement only every 48 hours. Patients with more than 30% TBSA burns should receive twice-daily applications of topical therapy, preferably mafenide acetate cream in the morning, and silver sulfadiazine cream in the evening. Mafenide acetate cream has a high osmolality; thus, its application causes pain in the areas of partial-thickness burn that persists for approximately 20 minutes. Therefore, daytime application is advised to limit patient discomfort prior to bedtime. Either cream is applied as a ⅛-inch-thick layer to the entire burn wound in an aseptic manner following initial débridement and reapplied at 12-hour intervals to ensure continuous topical chemotherapy. Once each day, all of the topical agent should be cleansed from the wounds with the use of a surgical detergent disinfectant solution.

Care of Partial-Thickness Burns

Partial-thickness burns reepithelialize from uninjured epidermal elements in hair follicles and sweat and sebaceous glands residing within the dermis. The healing of partial-thickness burns generally requires 2 to 3 weeks; however, deep partial-thickness injuries may require up to 6 weeks before epithelial coverage is complete. These deeper wounds are best managed by burn wound excision and split-thickness skin grafts, which hasten wound closure and decrease hospital stay. The rapidity with which partial-thickness burns heal is dependent not only on the depth of injury but also on the area involved, the general condition of the patient, and the density of the microbial flora. Daily wound cleansing and débridement of partial-thickness burns should be employed to remove the fibrinous coagulum that accumulates on the surface of these wounds. When the wound surface is free from exudate, a petrolatum-impregnated gauze may be applied to the wound surface and left in place until spontaneous healing is complete. At this point, the gauze may be sequentially trimmed as it separates from the healed wound surface. Alternatively, clean wounds may be covered in biologic dressings (see later), which markedly decrease pain and promote reepithelialization.

Table 12–2	**Properties of Topical Antimicrobial Agents**					
	ANTIMICROBIAL SPECTRUM					
	Gram-Positive	**Gram-Negative**	**ESCHAR PENETRATION**	**DRESSING REQUIREMENT**	**USE ON FULL-THICKNESS BURN**	**SYSTEMIC COMPLICATION**
Mafenide acetate	+ +	+ + +	Yes	Optional	Yes	Pain on application, carbonic anhydrase inhibition with metabolic acidosis
Silver sulfadiazine	+ + +	+	No	Optional	Yes	Neutropenia, dermatitis
Silver nitrate	+ + +	+ + +	No	Yes (kept moistened)	Yes	Electrolyte abnormalities
Acticoat	+ + +	+ + +	No	Yes (kept moistened)	No	None reported

Smoke Inhalation Injury

Smoke inhalation injury is frequently observed in patients with thermal injury and is present in one third of the patients admitted to burn centers. The inhalation of smoke or toxic gases may induce chemical damage to the respiratory epithelium. Although uncommon, direct thermal injury to the tracheobronchial tree, usually associated with the inhalation of steam, may occur. Additionally, inhalation of cytotoxic gases, such as carbon monoxide and cyanide, may produce systemic sequelae, rather than local injury.

The diagnosis of smoke inhalation should be considered in patients with a history of being burned in a closed space, or the presence of facial burns, singed facial hair, and nasal vibrissae, carbonaceous deposits in the oropharynx and intraoral burns, altered mental status, and signs of respiratory distress. The classic signs and symptoms of inhalation injury, however, have a poor predictive value in either excluding or ensuring the diagnosis. Fiberoptic bronchoscopic examination of the upper airway and tracheobronchial tree is the most commonly utilized and most accurate method of diagnosing inhalation injury. The presence of carbonaceous material, erythema, edema, or mucosal ulcerations below the level of the true vocal cords confirms the presence of smoke inhalation injury.

Patients with mild smoke inhalation injury require only administration of humidified oxygen-enriched air and noninvasive pulmonary physiotherapy. Those with copious secretions, severe smoke inhalation, or sloughing of the tracheobronchial mucosa may require endotracheal intubation for adequate pulmonary toilet. Mucolytic agents or bronchodilators may be useful in clearing secretions and relieving bronchospasm. Frequent flexible fiberoptic or rigid bronchoscopy to clear the airways of sloughed mucosal debris or inspissated secretions may be required in severe cases. The use of steroids in patients with inhalation injury should be avoided; this treatment is appropriate only in patients with unrelenting bronchospasm.

The use of high-frequency percussive mechanical ventilation has been shown to decrease the incidence of pneumonia and decrease the mortality associated with smoke inhalation injury. Although the exact mechanism by which high-frequency percussive ventilation exerts its beneficial effect is not known, the ability to maintain oxygenation and ventilation at lower peak airway pressures and inspired oxygen concentrations may reduce the iatrogenic injury associated with the use of volume-controlled ventilators. Also, the high-frequency percussive breaths improve clearance of secretions and mucosal debris.

Smoke inhalation may also be associated with carbon monoxide poisoning, which impairs tissue oxygenation. Mild carbon monoxide poisoning may be manifested by headache, whereas moderate exposure may cause restlessness and confusion. More severe exposure produces obtundation and coma. Carbon monoxide displaces oxygen from oxyhemoglobin-producing carboxyhemoglobin. In addition, carbon monoxide produces chemical alterations of the cytochrome oxidase system, further impairing tissue oxygenation. The amount of dissolved oxygen in the blood is not affected; thus, the arterial partial pressure of oxygen (Pao_2) will remain normal. However, saturation of hemoglobin by oxygen will be markedly reduced. Carbon monoxide poisoning is treated by the administration of 100% oxygen by nonrebreathing mask or endotracheal tube to accelerate the dissociation of carboxyhemoglobin. Patients with altered mental status or those who are comatose should be presumed to have carbon monoxide poisoning and should receive treatment with 100% oxygen until the measured level of carboxyhemoglobin is less than 5%.

INTRAOPERATIVE MANAGEMENT

Excision of burn tissues with the use of several techniques is frequently employed as a means of effecting early closure of the burn wound. Current operative management utilizes tangential excision, which entails sequential excision of thin layers of eschar until viable dermis is exposed, multiple applications of tangential excision technique to reach deeper viable tissue, or scalpel excision to the level of the investing muscle fascia for burn wound removal. These surgical procedures may be performed early in the postburn course once the patient is hemodynamically stable and resuscitation is complete. The depth of excision in tangential and sequential burn wound removal is governed by the appearance of healthy tissue and punctate bleeding from dermal or subcutaneous beds. Scalpel excision of burns involves removal of the wound and underlying subcutaneous tissue to the level of the investing muscle fascia. This is accomplished more rapidly and with significantly less blood loss than is the tangential or sequential wound excision. Careful anesthetic management is necessary to avoid hypotension and hypothermia. When a viable wound surface is obtained and hemostasis ensured, wound coverage is accomplished with split-thickness cutaneous autograft or biologic dressings.

Cutaneous autografts, 0.008- to 0.012-inch thick, are usually obtained with the use of an electric or compressed nitrogen–powered dermatome. As a general rule, the thinner the autograft, the more certain the take, and the thicker the graft, the better the cosmetic result. Thicker autografts result in slower donor site healing and a poorer cosmetic result at the donor site. Skin grafts may be applied as sheet grafts or meshed to provide expansion ratios ranging from 1.5:1 to 9:1. Expansion ratios of 4:1 or greater require prolonged time for interstitial closure and have a greater propensity for scar formation. Therefore, large expansion ratios are utilized only in patients with massive burns and limited donor sites. Following autografting, occlusive dressings moistened with topical antibacterial agents are usually applied. The wounds are kept moist to prevent desiccation until the interstices of the graph have epithelialized.

Skin Substitutes and Biologic Dressings

In the massively burned patient, the disparity between donor site availability and burn wound area requires that the surgeon use temporary skin substitutes or biologic dressings to accomplish temporary wound closure while awaiting donor site healing and subsequent donor site reharvesting. The application of biologic dressings to an excised wound bed prevents wound desiccation, reduces wound pain, facilitates patient movement, limits bacterial growth, functions as a barrier against bacterial contamination, and reduces evaporative water and heat losses from the wound surface. Additionally, application of these dressings to partial-thickness burns improves subsequent healing quality and permits prompt and orderly regeneration of the wound surface. Currently, the gold standard of biologic dressings is viable human cutaneous allograft, which derives a temporary blood supply through direct vessel-to-vessel connection from the underlying wound bed. Successful engraftment produces a temporarily healed burn wound until the allograft is lost to rejection, usually occurring in 2 to 3 weeks. At this point, the allograft may be replaced with autograft if available, or new allograft may be reapplied. Another less effective but commonly available biologic dressing is porcine xenograft. This biologic dressing does not become vascularized and adheres to the wound bed by fibrin bonding and partial penetration of the xenograft dermis by the fibrovascular tissue of the host. The underside of the graft is nourished by the plasmatic circulation. Desiccation and necrosis of the outer surface usually occur within 1 week.

Several synthetic skin substitutes have been developed in an attempt to avoid the problems of disease transmission and storage requirements common to biologic dressings. Bilayer membranes composed of a dermal and an epidermal analogue have been developed. The outer layer mimics the epidermis, allowing water vapor transmission and preventing bacterial contamination, whereas the inner dermal layer is designed to promote adherence and fibrovascular ingrowth from the wound bed. Biobrane, a commonly used synthetic skin substitute, is composed of an epidermal layer of pliable Silastic and a dermal component derived from porcine collagen. This product is removed in its entirety prior to subsequent autografting. Integra is a synthetic dermal substitute that is unique in that a neodermis is formed by fibrovascular ingrowth into a glycosaminoglycan-enriched collagen fibril dermal analogue. The epidermal component is also made of Silastic and is removed once the dermal analogue is vascularized, allowing definitive closure of the wound with ultrathin split-thickness skin grafts. Common problems encountered with all biologic dressings, in general, and synthetic skin substitutes, in particular, include incomplete adherence, submembrane suppuration, and technical problems with premature separation due to shearing or submembrane fluid collections.

Successful in vitro cultivation of human keratinocytes has led to recent evaluation of cultured autologous keratinocytes for coverage of wounds in massively burned patients. Current culture techniques require 3 or more weeks of preparation for a product six to eight epidermal cell layers in thickness. These grafts are quite fragile and susceptible to bacterial colonization of the recipient wound bed. Additionally, minimal shear forces may dislodge these cells from the wound surface. Application of cultured autologous keratinocytes has resulted in a disappointingly small average extent of body surface area closed in the larger reported series. The percent take is inversely proportional to the extent of burn, an unfortunate relationship. The lack of a transplantable dermis, the

3- to 4-week delay from skin biopsy to the availability of cultured skin, and the lack of long-term durability of skin that does engraft are also limiting features. This technology has the potential for providing timely coverage of large surface areas, and active research to improve engraftment is ongoing.

POSTOPERATIVE MANAGEMENT

Nutritional Support

Extensive thermal injury can increase the resting metabolic rate 1.5 to 2 times normal. The hypermetabolic response is related to the extent of burn, with the actual physiologic response influenced by environmental temperature, physical activity, pain and anxiety, the presence of infection, and the patient's age. Increased circulating levels of catecholamines, glucagon, and cortisol are the primary neurohumoral mediators of hypermetabolism, which result in increased oxygen consumption, a hyperdynamic circulation, wasting of lean body mass, increased core temperature, and increased urinary nitrogen excretion. The persistence of the hypermetabolic response in the flow phase of thermal injury may be caused, in part, by the presence of proinflammatory cytokines and other inflammatory mediators. Consequently, the provision of nutritional support to thermally injured patients is an essential element of patient care.

The delivery of nutritional support is best accomplished using the enteral route. Most patients tolerate enteral feeding beginning in the first week post burn, and their metabolic demands can be successfully met with nutritional supplementation provided through a nasoduodenal tube. The metabolic requirements of burn patients may be minimized through effective pain control with parenteral dosing of narcotics, nursing in a warm environment to prevent excessive thermogenesis, and timely treatment of infection. Many formulas exist for the estimation of caloric needs following burn injury. The more common ones are based on body size, age, gender, and extent of cutaneous burn. One such formula developed at the U.S. Army Institute of Surgical Research predicts resting energy expenditure (REE) as follows: REE (in kilocalories/m²/hr) equals BMR $(0.8914 + [0.01335 \times$ percent burn]), where BMR is the expected normal basal metabolic rate based on age, gender, and body surface area in noninjured humans. The resting energy expenditure can also be measured at the bedside by indirect calorimetry.

Careful monitoring of nutritional therapy is necessary if the high metabolic demand is to be met and adequate nutrition maintained throughout the hospital course. Serial body weight, calorie counts, nitrogen balance studies, and indirect calorimetry studies are used to evaluate the adequacy of nutritional support following burn.

Physical and Occupational Therapy

Functional rehabilitation of the burned patient begins on the day of admission. Burned limbs are elevated and actively exercised to minimize edema and reduce the need for escharotomy. When the patient becomes hemo-dynamically stable after resuscitation, a progressive program of ambulation and active exercise is begun. Initially, the patient may only tolerate chair sitting, but graded transition to the upright position can be achieved with the use of a tilt table and supported standing. Before the patient gets out of bed, the burned legs should be wrapped with elastic bandages to prevent venous stasis and edema. Active exercises are preferred if the patient's condition permits, because active movement helps maintain muscle mass and strength. Active assisted exercise is used to aid articulating movements in patients who cannot achieve full range of motion independently. Passive exercises must be used with great care because overzealous implementation may lead to tendon disruption, muscle tears (and later heterotopic ossification), and traumatic release of scar contractures. Because passive exercises are used most commonly in debilitated or comatose patients, therapists must rely on their own experience to gauge the limits of tissue extensibility. Finally, the patient must be encouraged to engage in the activities of daily living: Eating, dressing, grooming, and other customary activities should be carried out as independently as possible. Adaptive devices, such as eating utensils with built-up or extended handles, aid such actions. A sense of self-sufficiency reinforces patient well-being and compliance with therapy.

Duration of Hospital Care

Duration of hospital care of burn patients is related to burn depth, burn extent, preexisting disease, presence of associated injuries, and occurrence of complications. Partial-thickness burns that are other than deep dermal in character and remain infected characteristically heal within 3 weeks. Full-thickness burns require skin grafting for closure, and staged excision and grafting will be necessary in patients with extensive full-thickness injuries. Most burn injuries are of varying depth, with intermixed areas of partial-thickness and full-thickness skin damage. In patients with burns of more than 20% of the body surface, one can anticipate, in general, that the hospital stay will be equal in days to the extent of the burn expressed as a percentage of the total surface (e.g., 40 hospital days for a patient with a 40% burn). This "average" comprises patients with massive burns or burns complicated by associated injury who die early after the burn has occurred and those whose hospital stay far exceeds the average because of associated injury or supervening complication.

Multidisciplinary Team Approach to Burn Care

The complexity of care required in the management of patients with extensive thermal injury successfully requires the coordinated effort of a team of dedicated specialists spanning diverse disciplines. The concept of a multidisciplinary team was paramount in the development of a hierarchical regionalized system of burn centers throughout North America. The relatively prolonged acute hospitalization, compared with other forms of injury or illness, necessitates the input of specialists in nutrition, physical and occupational rehabilitation, respiratory therapy, clinical psychology and psychiatry, social work, anesthesiology, medical laboratory sciences, nursing, critical care, and surgery. Assessment and treatment by all team members begins on admission and continues throughout the acute hospitalization in preparation for the transition to the rehabilitative phase of burn care. This team approach to patient care and to the timely solution of clinical problems through effective clinical and basic science research has been responsible for the advancements in the care of thermally injured patients that have been realized over the past 40 years.

PREVENTION AND TREATMENT OF COMPLICATIONS

A strict infection control program can minimize the clinical impact of exposure to nosocomial pathogens during a prolonged hospital stay in an immunocompromised patient. Such a program could employ scheduled microbial surveillance, an actively functioning infection control committee, environmental monitoring procedures, biopsy monitoring of the burn wound, and cohort patient care as deemed necessary.

Cross-contamination is minimized by strict enforcement of hand washing, gowning, and gloving policies. The establishment of patient care teams to provide care for only one specific patient or a limited number of patients and restriction of the traffic of convalescing patients (often colonized with resistant organisms) are imperative in reducing cross-contamination and eradicating endemic microorganisms.

Bronchopneumonia remains the most common cause of morbidity in patients with inhalation injury. The daily chest radiograph should be carefully examined. Appropriate antimicrobial therapy, based on the presence of sputum leukocytosis, the detection of microorganisms on Gram stain, and the evolution of pulmonary infiltrates, should be initiated. Pneumonia occurring after inhalation injury is usually caused by gram-positive organisms; gram-negative pneumonia, which occurs infrequently, usually develops later in the hospital course.

Acute infective endocarditis is an infrequent but consistent source of morbidity and mortality in burn patients (1.3%) owing to the bacteremias associated with wound manipulation, prolonged intravenous cannulation, and septic thrombophlebitis. Preventive measures include effective topical antimicrobial therapy, timely excision and closure of the burn wound, and early discontinuation or frequent replacement of intravenous cannulae. *Staphylococcus aureus* is the most common causative organism, and the right side of the heart is most frequently affected. Recurrent staphylococcal bacteremia in a burn patient with sepsis and no other apparent identifiable source of infection should suggest the diagnosis.

The true incidence of sinusitis in burn patients is unclear, but patients requiring prolonged transnasal intubation of both the airway and the stomach are at increased risk. One study reported an incidence of 36% in transnasally intubated burn patients in the intensive care unit. Sinusitis is most often clinically undetectable and requires radiographic examination by plain films or computed tomography to establish the diagnosis. These studies help to direct sinus aspiration to differentiate between congestion and infection. Treatment involves topical mucosal vasoconstrictors to improve patency of the sinus ostia and removal of transnasal tubes. Appropriate systemic antibiotic therapy should be initiated. Surgical drainage is required in cases not responsive to these procedures. Tracheostomy or gastrostomy may be necessary if prolonged ventilatory support and enteral nutrition are required.

The presence of the avascular, nonviable eschar provides an excellent culture medium for microbial proliferation. When confined to the nonviable eschar, the bacteria merely colonize the burn wound, whereas invasion beneath the eschar into viable tissue constitutes bacterial burn wound infection. The early colonizing organisms are indigenous bacteria, usually gram-positive organisms. Gram-negative bacteria and fungi appear in the wound later in the postburn course.

The clinical signs of invasive burn wound infection are often indistinguishable from those observed in uninfected hypermetabolic burn patients or burn patients with other sources of infection. These signs include hyperthermia or hypothermia, tachycardia, tachypnea, glucose intolerance, ileus, and disorientation. The tinctorial and physical changes in the burn wound are more reliable signs of invasive infection and include focal, dark brown or black discoloration of the wound, rapid eschar separation, hemorrhagic discoloration of subcutaneous fat, erythema and edema of the wound margin, and the appearance of metastatic septic lesions in unburned tissue. The development of clinical signs and symptoms of sepsis in the thermally injured patients should prompt a thorough examination of the burn wound to identify areas of invasive infection.

Surface cultures of the burn wound do not differentiate colonization from invasive infection, and quantitative bacteriologic cultures of burn tissue correlate poorly with the presence of invasive burn wound infection. The most reliable means of diagnosing burn wound infection involves histologic examination of a biopsy of the burn wound and underlying viable tissue. When bacteria are present in the subjacent viable tissue, the diagnosis of burn wound infection can be made with certainty. If only colonization (the presence of bacteria in nonviable tissue) is present, no specific change in therapy is warranted.

When the diagnosis of invasive burn wound infection is made, changes in local wound treatment and the initiation of systemic antibiotic therapy are indicated. Twice-daily applications of mafenide acetate cream to the affected wounds is recommended owing to the superior ability of this agent to penetrate eschar. Systemic antibiotic therapy based on prior surface cultures or burn center organism prevalence is initiated, with further refinements in therapy based on biopsy, culture, and sensitivity results. Subeschar antibiotic clysis of the infected area with a broad-spectrum penicillin is performed at 12-hour intervals and immediately prior to operation to minimize the risk of precipitating florid septic shock at the time of eschar excision. Half of the daily dose of a broad-spectrum penicillin delivered in 1 L of normal saline is injected into the subeschar tissues with the use of a No. 20 spinal needle. The burn wound is thereafter excised to the level of the investing fascia to ensure removal of all nonviable tissue. The wound is usually treated with moist dressings, and the patient is returned to the operating room in 24 to 48 hours for wound inspection, repeat débridement if necessary, or split-thickness skin grafting.

Many gastrointestinal complications have been documented following thermal injury and include pancreatitis, acalculous cholecystitis, gastroduodenal stress ulceration, and Ogilvie's syndrome. Stress ulceration of the upper gastrointestinal tract has been effectively controlled with prophylactic antacid or H_2 histamine receptor antagonist therapy.

OUTCOMES

In the past half-century, substantial improvements in the field of burn care have been realized. In the United States, the incidence of burn injury has decreased from 2 million persons per year in the 1970s to 1.2 million persons per year in the 1990s. Deaths attributed to burns

---

Pearls and Pitfalls

Early Care

PITFALLS

- Overestimation of burn size leads to overresuscitation, congestive heart failure, pulmonary edema, and increased need for escharotomy; thus, the patient must be carefully examined with the use of the Lund-Browder diagram.
- Inadequate irrigation of chemical burn wounds leads to inadequate fluid resuscitation, and hypoglycemia in infants; thus, add D_5 0.5 NS maintenance fluid to resuscitation fluid estimate.
- Failure to include maintenance fluid in resuscitation of children results in muscle necrosis, and loss of digits, hands, feet, and limbs; therefore, check pulses by Doppler examination hourly, carry escharotomy incisions across joints, and continue to monitor pulses even after escharotomy.
- Failure to monitor peripheral circulation or perform adequate escharotomy or fasciotomy results in increased depth of burn, systemic toxicity, and blindness; thus, irrigate wound copiously until agent is removed, and irrigate eyes thoroughly if involved.

Burn Wound Management

PITFALLS

- Delay in surgical treatment results in burn wound infection and sepsis; thus, practitioner should perform prompt, complete excision of full-thickness burns (within 2 weeks of injury).
- Inadequate burn excision results in poor graft take, wound infection, lengthened hospital stay; therefore, excise wounds until punctate bleeding occurs or until subcutaneous tissues have normal color and texture.
- Inadequate postoperative splinting therapy results in deformity, the need for contracture release, and prolonged rehabilitation; therefore, splint should be in position of function, and aggressive therapy program should be maintained.

have decreased by 40% during this same time period. The LA_{50} defines the extent of burn that is associated with death in 50% of the patients having burns of that extent. In the mid-1940s the LA_{50} of young adults was 43% of the TBSA. Current estimates now reveal a LA_{50} of between 75% and 85% TBSA for this population. The decline in the incidence of major burns may be attributed to effective prevention strategies, including smoke detection and automated sprinkler systems. The improvement in survival reflects the effects of physiologically based fluid resuscitation, improvements in wound care and control of burn wound infection, better management of smoke inhalation injury, and improvements in critical care that have occurred during the last half-century.

SELECTED READINGS

Cancio LC, Mozingo DW, Pruitt BA: Strategies for diagnosing and treating asphyxiation and inhalation injuries. J Crit Ill 1997;12:217.
Herndon DW (ed): Total Burn Care. Philadelphia, WB Saunders, 1996.
Luterman A: Burns and metabolism. J Am Coll Surg 2000;190:104.
Mozingo DW, Smith AA, McManus WF, et al: Chemical burns. J Trauma 1988;28:642.
Mozingo DW, Barillo DJ, Pruitt BA Jr: Acute resuscitation and transfer management of burned and electrically injured patients. Trauma Q 1994;11:94.
Mozingo DW: Surgical management. In Carrougher GJ (ed): Burn Care and Therapy. St. Louis, Mosby, 1998, pp 233–248.
Pruitt BA Jr, Goodwin CW Jr, Pruitt SK: Burns: Including cold, chemical, and electric injuries. In Sabiston DC Jr (ed): Sabiston Textbook of Surgery: The Biological Basis of Modern Surgical Practice, 15th ed. Philadelphia, WB Saunders, 1997, pp 221–252.
Sheridan RL, Tompkins RG: Skin substitutes in burns. Burns 1999;25:97.
Yowler CJ, Fratianne RB: Current status of burn resuscitation. Clin Plast Surg 2000;27:1.

Chapter 13

Closed Head Injury

Thomas Kossmann and Philip F. Stahel

In Western countries, closed head injury represents the leading cause of mortality and morbidity in patients younger than 45 years of age. In the United States, approximately 500,000 patients are hospitalized for traumatic brain injury each year, of which about 80% can be classified as mild, 10% as moderate, and 10% as severe. About 50,000 head-injured patients die each year, and another 50,000 remain severely disabled. The extent of residual brain damage is determined by primary and secondary injuries. The primary injury results from mechanical forces applied to the skull and brain at the time of impact, leading to either focal or diffuse brain injury patterns. Focal brain injury is due to direct concussion or compression forces, while diffuse axonal shearing injuries are usually caused by indirect trauma mechanisms, such as sudden deceleration or rotational acceleration. Secondary brain injury occurs after the initial trauma and is a consequence of complicating processes initiated by the primary injury, such as ischemia-reperfusion, cerebral edema, intracranial hemorrhage, and intracranial hypertension. However, the main risk factors for developing secondary brain injury are hypoxemia and systemic hypotension, mostly due to hypovolemia. Evidence of secondary brain injury has been found at autopsy in 70% to 90% of all fatally head-injured patients.

The general surgeon who sees brain-injured patients first must be skilled in their initial assessment and resuscitation, as a neurosurgeon may not be immediately available. The maintenance of adequate systemic blood pressure and oxygenation are of paramount importance. The following chapter provides concise guidelines for the initial assessment and management of patients with traumatic brain injury.

CLINICAL PRESENTATION

The diagnosis of traumatic brain injury is established by the history of trauma, the clinical status, and imaging studies, such as radiographs and computed tomography (CT) scan. Efforts should be made to learn the details of the accident, including the mechanism of trauma: for example, blunt versus penetrating injury, force of the traumatic impact, condition of the vehicle, and presence of other injured or dead occupants. The condition of the vehicle's interior may reveal potential associated injury patterns; for example, a "bull's-eye" break of the windscreen suggesting direct skull impact with associated shear forces to brain tissue, or a bent steering wheel, which may indicate severe chest trauma leading to hypoxia. The likelihood of serious injuries is significantly increased in patients who have been ejected from the vehicle or in the case of death of another occupant in the same vehicle compartment. Furthermore, it is important to obtain information about the level of consciousness at the accident scene, the presence of impaired neurologic function, and changes in the level of consciousness up until the time the patient is admitted to the clinic. Of particular importance is the knowledge of the postresuscitation Glasgow Coma Scale (GCS) score, since this parameter represents an important predictor of outcome (see section on outcomes that follows). Other crucial information includes the presence of anoxia or hypoxia (compromised airways, chest trauma, delay in endotracheal intubation) and the approximate blood loss at the accident scene (massive external bleeding, hemorrhagic shock), as well as the therapy instituted before admission (secured airways, endotracheal intubation, adequate fluid resuscitation).

At the accident scene as well as on hospital admission, all head-injured patients must be systemically assessed and resuscitated according to the American College of Surgeons' "Advanced Trauma Life Support" (ATLS) protocol (see first selected reading). The algorithm for the initial management of head-trauma patients is shown in Table 13–1. After securing the airway and ensuring adequate oxygenation and fluid replacement, concomitant intra-abdominal injuries leading to exsanguinating hemorrhage must be excluded in all head-injured patients with an altered level of consciousness, either by diagnostic peritoneal lavage (DPL), ultrasonography, or CT scan. Furthermore, an associated cervical spine injury must be assumed in *all* head-injured patients until proven otherwise, since about 5% to 10% of head-injured patients have concomitant injuries of the cervical spine. The neurologic evaluation is initiated only after vital functions have been stabilized. The level of consciousness is rapidly assessed by the GCS score (Table 13–2) or by the "AVPU" method (Table 13–3), which represents a mnemonic for a quick estimation of the level of consciousness. When one assesses the GCS, the *best* response is used to calculate the score. It must be noted whether a patient is not able to complete a task because of external circumstances; for example, impaired opening of the eyes due to ocular hematoma or impaired speech in intubated patients. In addition to the level of consciousness, the neurologic examination should include the assessment of pupillary size and reactivity, and a brief evaluation of peripheral motor function. The clinical examination also includes inspection of the scalp for lacerations, palpation of the skull for impression fractures, and the search for indirect signs of basilar skull fractures, including periorbital ecchymosis ("raccoon eyes"), retroauricular ecchymosis ("Battle's sign"), rhinorrhea and/or otorrhea due to cerebrospinal fluid leakage, and seventh nerve palsy. Standard radiographs of the skull and cervical spine should be obtained in all patients with suspected head injury. The necessity of obtaining a CT scan is a given under the

Table 13–1	Initial Management of Head-Injured Patients*

Initial assessment and resuscitation according to the ATLS protocol (ABCDE). Secure airway and ensure adequate oxygenation and fluid replacement. Avoid hypoxemia and hypotension!

Exclude exsanguinating intra-abdominal injury (DPL, ultrasonography, CT scan) and other associated systemic injuries.

Screening radiographs of the skull and cervical spine in all head trauma patients.

Blood alcohol level and urine toxic screening in all patients.

History
  Mechanism and time of injury.
  Loss of consciousness.
  Amnesia (retrograde/anterograde).
  Postresuscitation level of consciousness (Glasgow Coma Scale [GCS]).
  Seizures.
  "AMPLE" history: *a*llergies, *m*edications, *p*ast illnesses/pregnancy, *l*ast meal, *e*vents/environment related to the injury.
  Presence of headache (mild, moderate, severe).

Brief Neurologic Examination
  Level of consciousness (GCS, AVPU mnemonic [see Table 13–3]).
  Pupillary size and reaction.
  Focal motor deficits.

Indications for CT Scan
  All patients with *moderate* to *severe* head injury (GCS <14).
  Mild head injury (GCS 14 and 15):
    Presence of skull fracture (clinically or radiograph).
    CSF leak (rhinorrhea, otorrhea).
    Alcohol/drug intoxication.
    Moderate to severe headache.
    Focal neurologic deficits, abnormal pupil size or reactivity.
    Deteriorating level of consciousness (GCS <14).
  Perform a control CT scan before discharge in all patients with *moderate* to *severe* head injury (GCS <14) and in cases of *mild* head injury (GCS 14 and 15) with pathologic initial CT scan.

Admission to Hospital
  All patients with GCS <15 (for at least 24 hr, with frequent neurologic examinations).
  All patients with open head injuries, CSF leak, skull fractures.
  Patients with GCS 15 and one of the following: (1) moderate to severe headache; (2) history of loss of consciousness; (3) amnesia; (4) significant alcohol/drug intoxication; (5) no reliable companion at home for observation; and (6) inability to return promptly in case of deterioration.

*See text for details and abbreviations.

Table 13–2	Glasgow Coma Scale (GCS)

CLINICAL PARAMETER	POINTS
Eye Opening (E)	
Spontaneous	4
To speech	3
To pain	2
None	1
BEST Motor Response (M)	
Obeys commands	6
Localizes pain	5
Normal flexion (withdrawal)	4
Abnormal flexion (decorticate)	3
Extension (decerebrate)	2
None (flaccid)	1
Verbal Response (V)	
Fully oriented	5
Disoriented/confused conversation	4
Inappropriate words	3
Incomprehensible words	2
None	1
GCS Score (E + M + V)	**3 (worst) to 15 (best)**

From Teasdale G, Jennett B: Assessment of coma and impaired consciousness: A practical scale. Lancet 1974;2:81–84. © by the Lancet Ltd., 1974.

following circumstances: (1) altered level of consciousness; (2) pathologic neurostatus; (3) differences in pupil size or reactivity; and (4) suspected skull fracture. Furthermore, the CT scan should be repeated whenever there is a deterioration in the patient's neurologic status.

Included in the *differential diagnosis* are other causes of coma or an altered state of consciousness that should be evaluated and may have contributed to the accident. Among these, alcohol intoxication represents one of the major risk factors for trauma. A complete drug screening (alcohol, opiates, cocaine, benzodiazepines, barbiturates, amphetamine) should be performed in all head-trauma patients. A metabolic cause of impaired consciousness is usually detected by serum laboratory analyses; for example, hypoglycemia or hyperglycemia, hyponatremia, and hypo-osmolarity or hyperosmolarity, as well as encephalopathies due to hepatic or renal failure. Importantly, an altered level of consciousness in the traumatized patient may represent an early sign of hemorrhagic shock due to

hypotension and cerebral hypoperfusion. Thus, significant internal or external bleeding sources must be excluded before the patient is further neurologically evaluated. Hypoxia should not represent a factor contributing to altered consciousness once the patient has been adequately resuscitated. However, the possibility of preexisting nontraumatic brain damage should be considered, including ischemic or hemorrhagic brain injury ("stroke," subarachnoidal bleeding, hypertensive intracranial bleeding) that may have occurred shortly before the accident. After trauma, these pathologies are often difficult to differentiate from trauma-induced brain damage on the CT scan. Epilepsy may represent a factor contributing to trauma, and post-traumatic electroencephalographic (EEG) abnormalities may be difficult to distinguish from preexisting pathology, unless medical records are available with regard to antiepileptic medications or preexisting neurologic examinations. Other causes of coma, such as basilar artery thrombosis, bacterial meningitis, brain abscess, or tumor are rarely associated with traumatic brain injury.

Closed head injury may be classified by either morphology or severity. The morphologic classification is based on findings in the CT scan according to the guide-

Table 13–3	"AVPU": Mnemonic for Rapid Assessment of the Level of Consciousness

A — **A**lert
V — Responds to **V**ocal stimuli
P — Responds only to **P**ainful stimuli
U — **U**nresponsive to all stimuli

From Advanced Trauma Life Support (ATLS). Chicago, IL, American College of Surgeons, Committee on Trauma, 1997, p. 444.

Table 13–4	Marshall Score*	

CATEGORY	DEFINITION
Diffuse injury I	No visible intracranial pathology in CT scan.
Diffuse injury II	Cisterns are present with midline shift 0–5 mm and/or:
	Lesion densities present.
	No high- or mixed-density lesion > 25 cc.
	May include bone fragments and foreign bodies.
Diffuse injury III	Cisterns compressed or absent with midline shift 0–5 mm, no high- or mixed-density lesion > 25 cc.
Diffuse injury IV	Midline shift > 5 mm, no high- or mixed-density lesion > 25 cc.
Evacuated mass lesion	Any lesion surgically evacuated.
Nonevacuated mass lesion	High- or mixed-density lesion > 25 cc, not surgically evacuated.

*Classification of intracranial pathology according to the computed tomography (CT) scan.

Adapted from Marshall LF, Bowers Marshall S, Klauber MR, et al: A new classification of head injury based on computerized tomography. J Neurosurg 1991;75:S14.

lines of Marshall and colleagues (Table 13–4). Intracranial lesions may be either focal (subdural, epidural, intracerebral bleeding; "evacuated" vs. "nonevacuated") or diffuse (grades I to IV).

The classification by severity according to the GCS score is clinically relevant, since the postresuscitation score has been shown to significantly correlate with the patients' outcome. Patients with *mild* head injury (GCS 14 or 15) represent about 80% of all head-trauma patients admitted to the emergency department. These patients usually suffer from a mild cerebral concussion that corresponds to diffuse brain injury with preserved consciousness but a certain degree of temporary neurologic dysfunction. In contrast, a "classic" cerebral concussion results in a reversible loss of consciousness, which is always accompanied by post-traumatic amnesia. It is important to keep in mind that approximately 3% of patients with *mild* head injury will have an intracranial hemorrhage. Thus, these patients should be admitted to the hospital according to the guidelines outlined in Table 13–1. The presence of a vault fracture is associated with a 400-fold increased risk of an intracranial hematoma. Crucial to management of closed head trauma is assessment to identify the patients who "talk and die," referring to the patients who have a GCS greater than 8 on admission and suddenly deteriorate as their course progresses; for example, because of an intracranial mass lesion such as an acute epidural hematoma.

Moderate head injury corresponds to a GCS score between 9 and 13 and is associated with an increased risk of intracranial pathology compared with patients with *mild head injury*. As outlined in Table 13–1, a CT scan should be performed in all patients with *moderate head injury*, and all of these patients should be admitted to the hospital for observation.

A GCS score of 8 points or less corresponds to a comatose patient, as defined by the inability to open the eyes, to obey commands, and to respond verbally. Thus,

severe head injury is defined as a GCS score of 3 to 8. The initial assessment and management of these patients is described in the following paragraph.

PREOPERATIVE MANAGEMENT

The immediate goal in the management of head-injured patients is the prevention of secondary brain damage by rapid correction of hypotension, hypoxemia, hypercapnia, and hypoglycemia. An oropharyngeal or nasopharyngeal airway may be adequate in drowsy patients with sufficient breathing, while endotracheal intubation ("rapid-sequence intubation") is indicated in comatose patients (GCS ≤8) or in cases of apnea, hypoventilation, risk of upper airway obstruction (maxillofacial fractures, laryngeal injury), and aspiration (vomiting, bleeding). Adequate volume resuscitation is crucial, including the control of external and internal hemorrhages. According to the ATLS guidelines, the initial fluid therapy should be an isotonic electrolyte solution, such as lactated Ringer's solution, with an initial volume of 1000 to 2000 mL in adults and 20 mL/kg in children. Measurement of the urinary output represents a "prime monitor" for the patients' response to resuscitation, and should be about 0.5 mL/kg per hour in adults and 1 to 2 mL/kg per hour in pediatric patients. *It is important to watch for increased urinary output in head-injured patients due to SIADH* (syndrome of inappropriate secretion of antidiuretic hormone; see section on complications, which follows). The neurologic evaluation will be initiated only after the vital systems have been stabilized. Furthermore, associated injuries should receive adequate attention; for example, a cervical spine injury.

The main priority in the early management of head trauma patients is the maintenance of an adequate cerebral perfusion pressure (CPP), which should be above 70 to 80 mm Hg.

Definition:
CPP = mean arterial blood pressure (MAP)
    − intracranial pressure (ICP)

Due to the relationship between CPP and MAP, an increased systemic blood pressure should not be therapeutically lowered in head-injured patients unless continuous ICP monitoring is available ("demand" hypertension!). According to the "Monro-Kellie doctrine" (Fig. 13–1), the total intracranial volume remains constant, implying that expanding mass lesions will result in a reduced CPP, thus contributing to secondary brain injury. Different therapeutic approaches are aimed at lowering the ICP in order to maintain an adequate CPP. Among the therapeutic modalities are the reduction of mass lesions by surgical evacuation of intracranial hematomas, the reduction of brain swelling with osmotic drugs (e.g., mannitol), and the therapeutic drainage of cerebrospinal fluid through intraventricular catheters.

Osmotic Therapy (Mannitol)

When given as a bolus, mannitol augments the intravascular volume, resulting in a transient increase in MAP and

MONRO-KELLIE DOCTRINE: THE TOTAL INTRACRANIAL VOLUME REMAINS CONSTANT

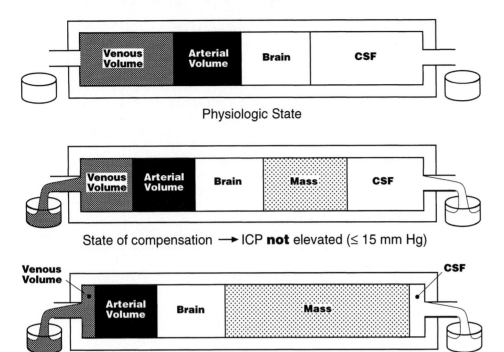

Figure 13–1. Monro-Kellie doctrine: The volume of the intracranial compartment remains constant. State of compensation: Despite the presence of expanding mass lesions, the ICP remains normal as long as an equal volume is drained (cerebrospinal fluid or blood). State of decompensation: Exponential increase in ICP after saturation of the drainage capacity. CSF, cerebrospinal fluid; ICP, intracranial pressure.

CPP. Mannitol also causes an increase in cerebral blood flow (CBF) in cases of impaired cerebrovascular autoregulation, where CBF is directly dependent on systemic arterial pressure. Mannitol can furthermore induce a cerebral vasoconstriction, resulting in a diminished intracranial volume.

Indications

The indications for osmotic therapy include the following:

- Clinical signs of transtentorial herniation (i.e., loss of consciousness, decerebrate rigidity, ipsilateral pupil dilatation, contralateral hemiparesis), or progressive neurologic deterioration, not attributable to systemic pathology
- Bilaterally dilated and nonreactive pupils

The therapeutic regimen is mannitol (20%), 0.25 to 1 g/kg IV in 5 minutes.

Indications for Operative Intervention or Evacuation of Intracranial Hematomas

- Generally, an intracranial hematoma causing neurologic deterioration or a midline shift of more than 5 mm as seen on CT scan should be evacuated as soon as possible!
- Evacuation of acute subdural hematomas (ASDH) of more than 3-mm thickness.
- Evacuation of ASDH of less than 3 mm in comatose

patients with severe parenchymal injuries and mass effect.
- For epidural hematomas (EDH), surgical evacuation is generally indicated, except for clinically stable patients with a small EDH and minimal pathologic findings (GCS 14 or 15).
- Evacuation of large intracranial hematomas (ICH) in patients with a depressed level of consciousness, focal neurologic deficit, and shift of midline structures in CT scan.
- Depressed skull fractures: Indication for operative elevation if the extent of depression is thicker than the adjacent skull (CT scan).
- All *open* head injuries.

Indications for Continuous ICP Monitoring

- Patients with severe head injury (postresuscitation GCS ≤8) and *abnormal* admission CT scan.
- Patients with severe head injury (GCS ≤8) and *normal* initial CT scan, but with a prolonged coma that has lasted more than 6 hours.
- Patients requiring evacuation of intracranial hematomas.
- Neurologic deterioration (GCS <9).
- Head-injured patients requiring prolonged mechanical ventilation; for example, due to operations for extracranial injuries, unless the initial CT scan is normal.

The use of *glucocorticoids* is not recommended for

improving outcome or reducing elevated ICP in patients with severe head injury. *Barbiturates* are effective in reducing ICP; however, their use is restricted to intensive care therapy with continuous EEG monitoring (see section on postoperative management, which follows).

Intraoperative Management

Craniotomy

One third of patients with severe closed head injury need immediate craniotomy for evacuation of mass lesions, most commonly for acute subdural hematoma (ASDH). The benefit of early evacuation of significant mass lesions has been demonstrated. In other patients with clinically mild or moderate TBI, craniotomy is performed for depressed skull fractures or for delayed hematomas on a less urgent basis. The timing of surgery depends on the clinical condition of the patient, in particular on the neurologic examination and CT findings. A comatose patient with a significant intracerebral hematoma causing brain shifting should be taken immediately to surgery.

Three types of intracranial hematomas are encountered as surgically removable mass lesions: an SDH from tearing of a bridging vein from the cortex to the venous sinuses or a cortical artery (Fig. 13–2), EDH from laceration of the middle meningeal artery or from the edges of a skull fracture (Fig. 13–3), and ICH within the brain parenchyma (Fig. 13–4). A standard craniotomy is performed with the patient supine and the head turned to the appropriate side and fixed in a Mayfield clamp. The incision is started just anterior to the ear and extended superiorly, 2 cm lateral and parallel to the midline, in the shape of a large question mark. A burr hole is made above the ear, which marks the bottom part of the temporal fossa, to allow immediate evacuation in case of EDH,

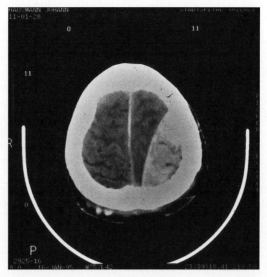

Figure 13–3. Axial CT scan demonstrating the typical form of an epidural hematoma.

or evacuation of SDH following incision of the dura. Additional burr holes have to be placed approximately 1.5 cm off the midline to avoid injury to major venous structures, such as the sinus sagittalis. Depending on the type of hematoma, a sufficient large bone flap is performed for adequate exposure. An EDH is removed after elevation of the bone flap, and the lacerated vessel has to be identified and cauterized. SDHs and ICHs can be approached after opening of the dura, which has to be lifted off the underlying cortex carefully. The hematoma is then gently evacuated by suction, irrigation, or other mechanical means. The origin of the hematoma must be identified and cauterized. If necessary, parts of contused brain can be débrided. Complete hemostasis must be achieved prior to closure of the dura. If this is not possible, tamponade may be obtained by collagen (e.g., Gelfoam, Surgicel) or by autologous muscle interponates. A Valsalva maneuver

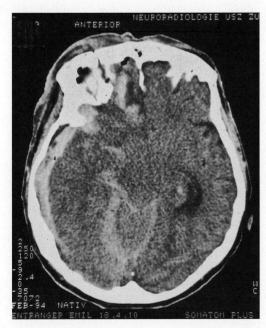

Figure 13–2. Axial CT scan showing a large subdural hematoma with midline shift greater than 5 mm.

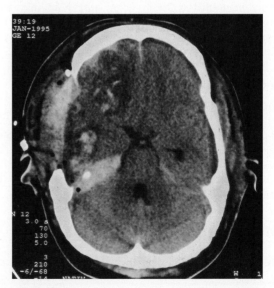

Figure 13–4. Axial CT scan after craniotomy showing substantial intracerebral contusions and intracerebral bleeding.

may be helpful for verification of secure hemostasis. The dura must be sealed tightly, which may be achieved by the use of an artificial dura patch. Dural tack-up sutures are placed around the periphery of the bony exposure and in the center of the flap. Epidural drains are put in place, whereafter the bone flap is replaced tightly. In cases of expected brain swelling, it is advisable to postpone the implantation of the bone flap to a later time. Under these circumstances, the bone flap may be stored safely at −80°C or else implanted subcutaneously into the abdominal wall of the patient. Finally, the temporal fascia, the galea, and the skin are closed.

Note. Small lesions in the temporal or the posterior fossa may cause compression to the brainstem and/or obstruction of the cerebrospinal fluid flow; therefore, early surgical intervention is warranted. For removal of hematomas in the posterior fossa, the patient is operated on in a prone position.

Emergency Burr Holes

In areas where neuroradiologic imaging (CT scan) or neurosurgical interventions are not readily available, general surgeons should have the ability to place cranial burr holes for the evacuation of intracranial hematomas. The indications include rapidly deteriorating neurologic status, unresponsive to osmotic therapy; for example, patients with suspected EDH whose level of consciousness or focal neurologic deficit is acutely worsening. The patient is positioned as for a craniotomy. A burr hole is placed on the side of the pupillary dilatation or contralateral to the side of the motor deficit. An incision anterior to the ear is taken down to the os zygomaticum, which marks the bottom of the temporal fossa. The hole may be enlarged for evacuation of an EDH or an SDH, the latter after incision of the dura. If necessary, a complete craniotomy can be performed as an enlargement of this approach.

The majority of comatose patients do *not* have intracranial hematomas! A burr hole may miss the hematoma or only inadequately drain it. A burr hole may itself induce intracranial bleeding. Placing a burr hole may consume as much time as transferring the patient to a center with neurosurgical capabilities.

ICP Monitoring Devices (Intraventricular, Subdural, and Parenchymal)

The patient is put in prone position, if possible. A sagittal incision is placed where the pupillary line crosses the coronal suture. Thereafter, a burr hole is made just 1.5 cm frontal to the coronal suture for installation of an ICP monitoring device.

Postoperative Management

Postoperatively, patients are transferred to the intensive care unit and are treated according to a standardized protocol (Stocker et al, 1995). The goals of ICU therapy are as follows:

Achievement and maintenance of adequate gas exchange and circulatory stability by means of intubation, mechanical ventilation, adequate volume resuscitation, and administration of vasoactive drugs, if necessary. Prevention of hypoxemia and hypercapnia. The goal is to keep an arterial partial pressure of oxygen (PaO_2) greater than 13 kPa and a $PaCO_2$ between 3.3 and 4.5 kPa. Prophylactic hyperventilation is not performed, owing to the risk of focal ischemia. Aggressive circulatory stabilization: MAP > 80 mm Hg, normovolemia, hematocrit ≥ 30%. *Note.* No antihypertensive therapy is given up to MAP of 130 mm Hg ("demand" hypertension!).

Repeated, scheduled CT scans for detection of delayed secondary intracranial pathology that may be surgically treatable.

Profound sedation and analgesia to avoid stress and pain, which may result in increases of ICP and the cerebral metabolic rate.

Achievement and maintenance of optimal CPP (>70 mm Hg) and cerebral oxygen balance, allowing recovery of damaged brain areas and prevention of secondary brain damage. Here, the monitoring tools include (1) frequent blood gas analyses, (2) continuous ICP registration, (3) jugular bulb oximetry, (4) assessment of arteriojugular difference in lactate concentrations, (5) transcranial Doppler sonography for assessment of cerebral blood flow and vasospasms, and (6) repeated or continuous EEG registration. Administration of nimodipine in patients with signs of vasospasm detected by Doppler sonography.

Avoidance of hyperthermia (>38°C).

Prevention of hyperglycemia and hyponatremia.

No routinely performed head elevation, due to lowered CPP.

Prevention of stress ulcers and maintenance of gut mucosal integrity by early administration of enteral nutrition.

Prophylaxis for complicating factors (e.g., pneumonia or meningitis), repeated bacteriologic sampling, including cerebrospinal fluid through ventricular catheters, and anti-infectious treatment, if necessary.

Therapy in case of elevated ICP (>15 mm Hg; >5 minutes), after exclusion of surgically removable intracranial mass lesions (step-by-step regimen):

1. Deepening of sedation, analgesia, muscle relaxation.
2. Cerebrospinal fluid drainage through ventricular catheters, where applicable.
3. Moderate hyperventilation, as long as (a) jugular bulb oxygenation is greater than 60%, (b) arteriojugular difference in lactate is less than 0.2 mmol/L, (c) an ICP-lowering effect can be achieved by hyperventilation.
4. Osmotherapy: mannitol (20%) bolus IV in steps of 25 to 50 to 100 mL, as long as serum osmolarity remains below 315 mOsm/L.
5. Moderate hypothermia (approx. 34°C).
6. Barbiturate coma (thiopental IV) under continuous EEG registration. *Goal:* burst-suppression pattern of 6 bursts per minute and a burst-suppression relationship of 1:1.

An alternative concept for the treatment of post-traumatic brain edema and elevated ICP is represented by the "Lund concept," as described elsewhere (Asgeirsson et al, 1994).

Complications

General Complications of Severe Head Injury

Cerebral edema. This condition may lead to supratentorial swelling and *herniation of the brain* through the dural hiatuses and the foramen magnum.
Ischemic brain injury, following brain herniation or focal cerebral vasospasm.
Post-traumatic immunosuppression. This condition leads to increased susceptibility to pulmonary infections, sepsis, and multiorgan failure.
Neurogenic pulmonary edema. Definition: Pulmonary edema after head injury in the absence of cardiac or pulmonary disorders or hypervolemia. It is essential to avoid fluid overload in brain-injured patients.
Syndrome of inappropriate ADH secretion (SIADH). This condition is characterized by hyponatremia, hypoosmolarity and urinary sodium above 25 mEq/L. After hemodynamic stabilization, these patients should be treated with restriction of fluid intake to about 800 to 1000 mL/day, with the use of isotonic intravenous fluids (e.g., lactated Ringer's solution).
Disseminated intravascular coagulation (DIC). The damaged brain tissue represents a powerful activator of the coagulation cascade and may cause a severe consumptive coagulopathy.
Gastrointestinal bleeding. Ulcers of the esophagus, stomach, and duodenum are frequent in comatose head trauma patients. Prophylaxis is early enteral nutrition and buffering of gastric acid.
Heterotopic ossification. Definition: Late complication of brain injury with unclear etiology, characterized by bone formation in tissues that do not normally ossify. The ossification has been reported in 10% to 86% of patients with severe head trauma or spinal cord injury, and represents a major source of morbidity and persisting disability in the course of rehabilitation.

Postoperative Complications

- Incomplete evacuation of intracranial mass lesions
- Recurrence of intracranial bleeding
- Surgical infections; for example, meningitis, meningoencephalitis, brain abscess

The complications of ICU therapy are as follows:

1. *Cerebral vasospasm* after therapeutic hyperventilation. Prophylaxis: Keep $Paco_2$ in constant range (3.3 to 4.5 kPa) and monitor arteriojugular lactate concentrations and perform jugular bulb oximetry and frequent transcranial Doppler ultrasonography.
2. Complications of *barbiturate coma:* Cardiovascular depression, hepatotoxicity, immunosuppression, and increased incidence of pulmonary infections.

Outcomes

The GCS, although originally not intended as a prognostic index, is a strong indicator of outcome after closed head injury. Prospective data from the Traumatic Coma Data Bank (TCDB) in the 1980s revealed that patients with *severe* head injury (GCS score ≤ 8) had an overall mortality rate of 36% at 6 months post injury. Among these, an initial GCS score of 3 was associated with the highest mortality (76%), compared with patients with a score of

---

Pearls and Pitfalls

Common Errors of Practice

PITFALLS

- Delayed resuscitation from hypotension and hypoxemia
- Delayed intubation in patients with a GCS score ≤ 8
- Inadequate attention to associated injuries (thoracic, abdominal, orthopedic)
- Underestimating patients with *mild* or *moderate* head injury, assuming there is no intracranial pathology (patients who "talk and die")
- Underestimating comatose patients with normal CT scan (diffuse axonal injury)
- Failures in awake patients: (1) inadequate frequency of neurologic examinations, and (2) not obtaining a CT scan on neurologic deterioration or change in pupil size or reactivity
- Therapeutically lowering elevated systemic blood pressure in brain-injured patients ("demand hypertension")
- Therapeutic reduction of ICP (≤ 15 mm Hg) without caring for the maintenance of an adequate CPP (>70 mm Hg) by means of therapeutic elevation of the MAP
- Therapeutic hyperventilation without keeping the $Paco_2$ in the constant range (3.3 to 4.7 kPa) and without bedside jugular bulb oximetry and sequential measurement of the arteriojugular differences in lactate concentrations
- Delay in transfer of severely head-injured patients to a facility with neurosurgical capabilities

Mannitol Therapy

PEARLS

- Hypovolemia should be avoided by adequate fluid replacement.
- Serum osmolarity should be kept <315 mOsm/L, since hyperosmolarity may induce acute renal failure.

Emergency Burr Hole Therapy

PEARLS

- The majority of comatose patients do not have intracranial hematomas!
- A burr hole may miss the hematoma or only inadequately drain it.
- A burr hole may itself induce intracranial bleeding.
- Placing a burr hole may consume as much time as transferring the patient to a center with neurosurgical capabilities.

| Table 13–5 | Glasgow Outcome Scale (GOS) | |

OUTCOME (3 OR 6 MONTHS AFTER HEAD INJURY)	CHARACTERISTICS	SCORE
Good recovery	Reintegrated	5
Moderate disability	Independent but disabled	4
Severe disability	Conscious but dependent	3
Persistent vegetative state	Wakefulness without awareness	2
Death		1

From Jennett B, Bond M: Assessment of outcome after severe brain damage. Lancet 1975;1:480–484. © by the Lancet Ltd., 1975.

6 to 8 (18%). Patients with *moderate head injury* (GCS score 9 to 13) are at particular risk for intracranial complications, and their overall mortality is about 7%. Interestingly, patients who "talk" at admission (GCS score >8) and then deteriorate have a significantly higher mortality than patients with an initial score of 6 to 8. While mortality represents a parameter of outcome that is easy to define, the residual impairment in terms of neurologic, cognitive, or behavioral deficits is more difficult to assess. Numerous tests and scores offer different approaches for determining the post-traumatic neurologic and neuropsychological impairment. For example, the Disability Rating Scale (DRS; Rappaport et al, 1982) and the Glasgow Outcome Scale (GOS; Jennett and Bond, 1975; Table 13–5) represent traditional measures of global outcome that provide a basis for comparing the results of treatment in different centers. When patients are analyzed using the GOS, only about 60% of patients with *moderate* head injury have an overall good recovery by 6 months after trauma (GOS score 5), whereas a moderate (GOS score 4) to severe disability (GOS score 3) is described in 26% and 7%, respectively. Analysis of the outcome after *mild*

head injury (GCS score 14 or 15) revealed that these patients frequently have post-traumatic neuropsychological sequelae. The likelihood of postconcussional symptoms 1 week after trauma ranged from 80% to 93%, and follow-up studies revealed that as many as 60% of patients had residual neurobehavioral deficits after 3 months. However, long-term neurological deficits are rare in patients with *mild* head injury.

SELECTED READINGS

Advanced Trauma Life Support (ATLS). Chicago, IL, American College of Surgeons, Committee on Trauma, 1997, p 444.

Asgeirsson B, Grände PO, Nordström CH: A new therapy for post-trauma brain oedema based on hemodynamic principles for brain volume regulation. Intensive Care Med 1994;20:260.

Bullock MR, Lyeth BG, Muizelaar JP: Current status of neuroprotection trials for traumatic brain injury: Lessons from animal models and clinical studies. Neurosurgery 1999;45:207.

Cooper PR (ed): Head Injury. Baltimore, Williams & Wilkins, 1993, p 590.

Gennarelli TA: Mechanisms of brain injury. J Emerg Med 1993;11:5.

Guidelines for the Management of Severe Head Injury. New York, The Brain Trauma Foundation, 1995.

Harrison-Felix C, Newton CN, Hall KM, Kreutzer JS: Descriptive findings from the traumatic brain injury model systems national data base. J Head Trauma Rehabil 1996;11:1.

Jennett B, Bond M: Assessment of outcome after severe brain damage. Lancet 1975;1:480.

Jennett B: Epidemiology of head injury. J Neurol Neurosurg Psychiatry 1996;60:362.

Marshall LF, Bowers Marshall S, Klauber MR, et al: A new classification of head injury based on computerized tomography. J Neurosurg 1991;75:S14.

Maxwell WL, Povlishock JT, Graham DL: A mechanistic analysis of nondisruptive axonal injury: A review. J Neurotrauma 1997;14:419.

Narayan RK, Wilberger JE Jr, Povlishock JT (eds): Neurotrauma. New York, McGraw-Hill, 1996, p 1558.

Rappaport M, Hall KM, Hopkins K, et al: Disability rating scale for severe head trauma: Coma to community. Arch Phys Med Rehabil 1982;63:118.

Stocker R, Bernays R, Kossmann T, Imhof HG: Monitoring and treatment of acute head injury. In Goris RJA, Trentz O (eds): The Integrated Approach to Trauma Care. Berlin, Springer, 1995, pp 196–210.

Teasdale G, Jennett B: Assessment of coma and impaired consciousness: A practical scale. Lancet 1974;2:81.

Chapter 14

Spinal Trauma: Evaluation and Initial Treatment

David T. Harrington and J. Frederick Harrington

INCIDENCE

In the trauma population, spinal cord injury is uncommon, occurring in only 1% to 2% of patients (Burney et al, 1993). The uncommon nature of this condition, 12,000 new cases per year, should not diminish its importance, for these injuries are associated with significant long-term morbidity and mortality and represent a cost to the government of 4 to 5 billion dollars annually. Loss of productivity of these patients is also significant, with a 27-year-old quadriplegic having a projected lifetime loss of income of almost 1 million dollars (Berkowitz, 1993).

Young male adults are the most frequently injured group. Spinal injury patients have an average age of 33 years and a male-to-female ratio of 4:1. Motor vehicle crashes (MVCs) are the most common cause of injury, with falls and gunshot wounds being the next two most common etiologies. In children, however, more than 75% of injuries are caused by falls or by the victim's being struck by vehicles. Spinal cord injuries are rarely an isolated injury, and more than 80% of patients present with other traumatic injuries. The cervical spine is the most common fractured region, accounting for 55% of spine fractures and also a majority of spinal cord injuries.

NORMAL ANATOMY

The spine supports the thoracic and abdominal cavities and protects the spinal cord, which carries the motor efferents from, and the sensory afferents to, the brain. It is composed of 29 vertebrae distributed in four regions: cervical (7), thoracic (12), lumbar (5), and sacral (5). The intervertebral discs are the joints of the spine and support the axial load of the body. The nucleus pulposus, the central component of the disc, shares the axial load with the surrounding annulus fibrosis of the disc. The degree of normal range of motion allowed by the spine is determined mostly by the paired posterior structures called facets. The quite mobile cervical spine has facets that are aligned 45 degrees to the endplate of the vertebral body, with relatively flat surfaces allowing for simultaneous rotation and lateral bending. The facets of the lumbar spine, which carry more of an axial load, are close to perpendicular to the endplates in the sagittal plane, allowing for less rotation and lateral bending. The thoracic facets have structure intermediate to these extremes. The thoracic cavity, ribs and muscles, buttress the upper thoracic spine and protect it from injury. At all spinal levels, the anterior and posterior longitudinal ligaments serve, to some degree, to limit extension and flexion of the spine. Together, the disc, facet joints, and bony structures maintain the stability of the spine.

Understanding when a spine is unstable is important in the avoidance of further injury to the spinal cord or spinal roots. Two models exist that suggest a potential for spinal instability, based on the stabilizing forces of the anterior longitudinal ligament, the vertebral body, the posterior longitudinal ligament, and the posterior structures of the facets, neural arch, and their ligamentous attachments (Table 14–1). In the two-column model of Holdsworth, disruption of one column creates an unstable spine, whereas the three-column model of Denis specifies that disruption of at least two columns creates an unstable spine. The spinal cord fills 35% of the spinal canal at the level of C1 and roughly 50% in the remainder of the cervical and thoracic canals. Because the canal is relatively smaller, injury in lower cervical and thoracic regions is more commonly associated with neurologic defects. Although cord injuries occur in 10% to 25% of vertebral fractures on average, spinal cord injury occurs in as many as 40% of middle and lower cervical spine fractures.

FRACTURES AND CORD INJURY SYNDROMES

The cervical spine can be injured by a variety of forces from extension, flexion, compression, and combinations of these. Atlanto-occipital fractures are highly unstable and are often fatal. The uncommon survivors are often left with an incomplete cord injury and require cervical stabilization. A C1 fracture (Jefferson's fracture) is often secondary to an axial load. Many of these fractures are stable and do not require operative fixation. C2 fractures constitute 20% of all acute cervical spine fractures and fall into three categories: hangman's fractures (23%), odontoid fractures (55%), and miscellaneous types (22%). Hangman's fracture is a bilateral fracture through the neural arches of C2 from a hyperextension injury. Odontoid fractures are classified by three types: type I involves the tip of the odontoid process; type II involves the base of the odontoid; and type III is a fracture within the body of C2 involving the odontoid. Odontoid fractures occurring with atlantoaxial instability, where the ligamentous connection between the odontoid and C1 ring is disrupted, are very unstable and require surgical fusion in most cases. The lower cervical spine (C3–T1) can be injured in several ways. Axial loading and flexion can cause compression fractures or the classic "teardrop" fracture of the vertebral body, which can be accompanied by posterior column disruption. Unilateral or bilateral

Table 14–1	**Models of Spine Stability**					
STABILIZER	ANTERIOR LONGITUDINAL LIGAMENT	ANTERIOR TWO THIRDS VERTEBRAL BODY	POSTERIOR ONE THIRD VERTEBRAL BODY	POSTERIOR LONGITUDINAL LIGAMENT	NEURAL ARCH	FACETS
2-Column	Anterior	Anterior	Anterior	Anterior	Post	Post
3-Column	Anterior	Anterior	Middle	Middle	Post	Post

The two-column model describes spine stability in terms of anterior and posterior columns. The three-column model divides this into anterior, middle, and posterior columns. The components of each of these columns are described in the table above.

jumped facets are caused predominantly by shearing forces significant enough to disrupt the anterior and posterior ligaments and facet capsules. With a unilateral facet injury, neurologic spinal cord injury occurs less than half the time, but with bilateral facet disruption spinal cord injury is usually found.

The thoracic and lumbar spines rarely suffer an extension injury, with most injuries occurring from flexion or translational injury (direct movement anteriorly, laterally, or posteriorly). Flexion injuries result in wedge fractures, which are generally stable fractures. However, wedge fractures involving more than 50% of the vertebral body or 25 degrees of angulation can be unstable, owing to the failure of the middle column. Axial loading, if severe enough, can create a burst fracture of the vertebral body that can send fragments into the spinal canal, potentially creating spinal cord and/or nerve root trauma. A special kind of injury created by flexion and distraction is the Chance fracture. The fracture occurs through the superior portion of the vertebral body through the pedicle and facet joint. These injuries, which are associated with the use of a lap belt restraint without shoulder harness, are unstable, but when they are detected they may be treated nonoperatively in a rigid brace.

In most young adults, spinal cord injury requires fracture or dislocation of the spine, but in the degenerated spine or in the spine with a congenitally narrow canal, spinal cord injury may occur without associated fracture or subluxation. Determination of a complete cord injury requires a careful examination to detect any sacral sparing, such as perianal sensation, rectal tone, or plantar flexion in the lower extremities. The presence of any of these physical findings implies an incomplete injury and a better prognosis for return of function.

Several partial spinal cord injury syndromes have been described. The central cord syndrome is caused by the increased sensitivity of spinal cord gray matter and more central portions of the spinal cord to the effects of injury. The somatotopic organization of the corticospinal (motor) and spinothalamic tracts (pain and temperature) is such that motor and sensory fiber tracts for the upper extremities are located relatively centrally. Motor and sensory changes are, therefore, more profound in the upper extremities, leaving lower extremity and sphincter function relatively spaced. Recovery from this syndrome is common. Anterior cord syndrome results from an injury to the anterior spinal artery, which supplies the anterior two thirds of the cord. Loss of corticospinal (motor) and spinal thalamic tracts (pain) with preservation of posterior column sensation (vibration, proprioception, touch) below

the level of injury occurs. The prognosis for recovery from this lesion is poor, with roughly 10% of patients regaining functional motor recovery. Brown-Séquard syndrome, first described in a patient with a spinal cord injury by a knife, is a functional hemitransection of the cord. Patients present with ipsilateral loss of motor function and dorsal column sensation (vibration, proprioception, touch) and contralateral loss of spinothalamic sensation (pain and temperature). The prognosis for recovery is intermediate between the anterior cord syndrome and the central cord syndrome. Spinal root injury may occur and is distinguished by involvement of a single limb, mixed motor and sensory defects in that limb, and significant pain on the affected side. An uncommon spinal cord injury is a cord concussion. This injury, which accounts for 3% to 4% of cord injuries, results in immediate loss of function but complete resolution in 48 hours.

Neurogenic shock occurs secondary to the loss of sympathetic outflow from the spinal cord in cervical and upper thoracic regions. Although sympathetic reflexes are physically intact, controlling descending influences from the brainstem are, to a great degree, lost. Over the first several weeks, the effects are significant, but a recalibration of the sympathetic reflex leads to improvement over time. Initially, the patient is hypotensive with widened pulse pressures. The skin appears well perfused, but patients may become dangerously hypotensive with even the most minimal changes in the position of the head of the bed. Although neurogenic shock may be suspected, all trauma patients should have hypovolemic shock considered as their most probable cause of hypotension, and common sites of hemorrhage should be investigated. Treatment should initially be volume support and then, as causes of hemorrhagic shock are eliminated, vasopressor therapy (dopamine, Levophed [norepinephrine bitartrate], and Neo-Synephrine [phenylephrine HCl]) can be instituted.

DIAGNOSIS

Every trauma patient should be considered at risk for a spinal injury. The clinician has many tools for accurately diagnosing spinal fractures from mechanism of injury and history, to physical examination, and to radiologic tests. No one test is definitive, and an accurate diagnosis often requires several complementary examinations. Initially, the clinician must ask: Is there a sufficient mechanism for causing an injury? Does the patient have a clear enough sensorium? Does the patient have distracting injuries that may compromise his or her reliability in reporting symptoms and responding to a physical examination?

The mechanism of injury can often give clues to the amount of energy imparted to the patient, and certain types of trauma, particularly falls from heights, have higher rates of associated spinal fracture. A critical portion of the history is the patient's complaint of pain along the spine or neurologic symptoms of paresthesias. In patients with a clear sensorium, neck pain, as a solitary screening evaluation, has an 86% sensitivity in patients with cervical fracture. Adding the elicitation of tenderness of the cervical spine on physical examination raises the sensitivity to 98.7% (Roberge and Wears, 1992). A thorough patient history also includes assessing the presence of pre-existing conditions, such as rheumatoid arthritis or ankylosing spondylitis, which can lead to a spine that can be rendered unstable by even minor trauma.

Critical in the evaluation of the patient with a potential spine fracture is the physical examination. This examination begins with an assessment of the patient's mental status to gauge the reliability of the physical findings. The incidence of spinal fractures is not any greater in the head-injured population (4.7% vs. 4.4%) than in the non–head-injured population, but the patient's inclination or ability to report pain and paresthesias or to experience tenderness elicited drops off significantly at a Glasgow Coma Scale score of less than 14, leading to the potential for missed spine injury. In patients with an unclear sensorium, radiologic studies must be used as an adjunct to the history and examination. Spine fractures occur at multiple, noncontiguous levels in 5% to 10% of patients with spinal fracture, making an evaluation of the entire spine imperative. Initially, the spine should be examined for alignment, ecchymosis, tenderness, muscle spasm, and bony stepoffs. While it is not critical to test each sensory column (pain, light touch–two point discrimination, proprioception, and motor function), a brief but inclusive examination should be performed. Motor function should be tested, both proximally and distally, on each extremity. The use of a standard spinal injury sheet is conducive to this goal (Fig. 14–1).

Patients with a mechanism of injury unlikely to cause a vertebral fracture and who are without pain or tenderness both on an examination at rest and through a full active range of motion have an extremely low rate of spine injury and do not routinely need radiographic examination of their spine (Zabel et al, 1997). Patients who have received a significant kinetic injury or patients with pain or tenderness on history or examination should have a screening test. Although multiple radiographic tests are available for evaluating the spine, plain radiographs remain the best initial evaluation, being inexpensive and reasonably sensitive screening devices for injury. Plain films usually involve a three-view series of lateral, anteroposterior, and open-mouth views, which will detect more than 98% of cervical spine fractures. Inability to obtain the open-mouth view should prompt computed tomography (CT) scan of C1–C2. Films should be read for any obvious fracture, jumped facets, or malalignment. Other signs of injury include prevertebral swelling or vertebral body angulation greater than 11% or subluxation at a single level. Of these three standard views the lateral view is the most important, with this film alone detecting 85% or more of cervical spine fractures. Some centers add two additional oblique films to the three-view plain radiograph series in the hope of detecting more subtle fractures of the facet joints. Screening of the cervical spine with CT scan or magnetic resonance imaging (MRI) has many proponents. Some centers use either or both of these tests routinely to evaluate patients with suspected spine injury and claim that they can detect as many as 99% of fractures. Whether the added interpretation time and expense of these tests justifies an additional increase in sensitivity of 1% depends on the degree of syptomatology or questions raised by the radiograph and clinical evaluation.

Two common clinical dilemmas exist in spine clearance, particularly in regard to the cervical spine. What should be the evaluation of choice in the patient with a normal three-view evaluation but continued pain or tenderness, and how is the cervical spine cleared in a patient with normal three views yet an unclear sensorium from intoxication or head injury? In the absence of a visible fracture but with continued pain or tenderness, patients can be evaluated by active flexion-extension films or by MRI. Flexion-extension films take x-rays at maximal active flexion and extension. Distraction of the spine during this test can sometimes uncover subtle instabilities not visible on conventional three-view series or detect ligamentous injury that will be manifested by subluxation. However, flexion-extension films poorly visualize the lower cervical spine (C5–C7) and, in the presence of neck pain, patients often will not perform a full range of motion. Patients with pain who have inadequate films need continued immobilization until the pain resolves and full flexion and extension films can be obtained, usually in 2 weeks. MRI is useful but may be overly sensitive, detecting signs of soft tissue and ligamentous changes in as many as 35% of patients with neck pain and without spine fracture (Benzel et al, 1996). This rate of injury is in excess of rates of ligamentous injury found by flexion-extension films and is incompatible with rates of ligamentous injury (0.1% of patients) previously reported in trauma patients.

TREATMENT

The first priorities of trauma are always as follows: Airway, Breathing, and Circulation. During this initial evaluation, the immobilization of the spine is the first treatment of potential spine fractures. All patients with mechanisms suggestive of spine fracture should be immobilized by a rigid cervical collar and long spine board in the field. Since rigid cervical collars have a limited ability to limit flexion and extension and poor ability to limit lateral motion and rotation, sandbags and a strap or tape across the forehead can provide additional necessary immobilization during transportation. To evaluate the back for injury during the primary and secondary trauma surveys, the patient should be logrolled with maximal spine support. It requires four points of coordinated control at the head, shoulders, hips, and feet to ensure that the patient is turned as a unit with minimal spine torsion.

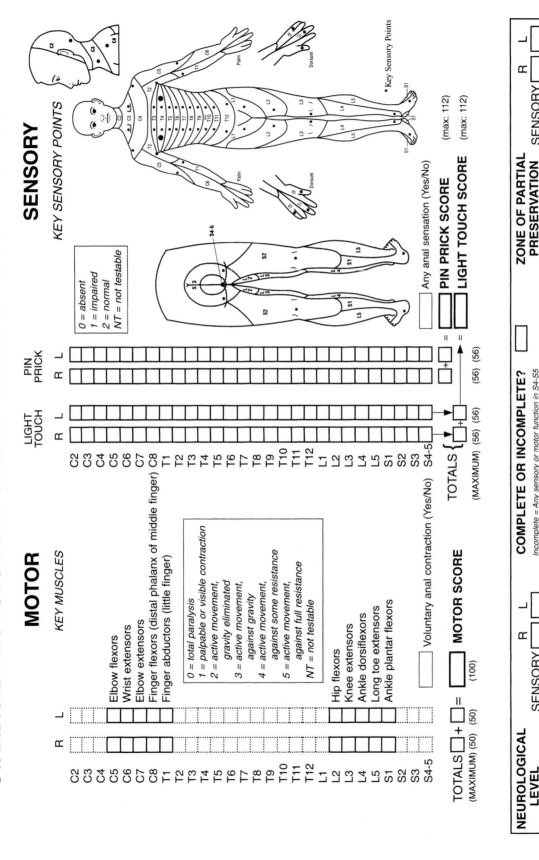

Figure 14–1. Neurologic scoring sheet. (From the American Spinal Injury Association.)

112

Unstable spine fractures usually require more definitive immobilization than can be delivered by either of the commonly used rigid collars, Philadelphia or Miami-J collars, which essentially limit only flexion and extension. Gardner-Well tongs and other traction devices are effective and can reduce fractures by the progressive addition of weight to the traction device. Such manipulations should be performed with caution, for overdistraction can result in spinal cord injury. Serial radiographs for assessing intervertebral widening, increasing traction in only 2.5- to 5-pound increments, and keeping a weight limit of 30 pounds for upper cervical spine and 60 pounds for lower cervical spine injuries will reduce these iatrogenic events. Traction devices are cumbersome and often do not allow for the treatment of other injuries. For these reasons, the traction is commonly changed to halo-vest immobilization following cervical fracture reduction. In the ambulatory or rehabilitative phase, the thermoplastic Minerva body jacket (TMBJ) offers similar immobilization and improved patient comfort over the halo-vest. Stable thoracic spine fractures are usually immobilized in a fitted thoracolumbosacral orthosis for several months.

The attention and concern shown in trauma centers for the detection and treatment of spine fractures and instability is based on the importance of preventing spinal cord injury or, if already present, at ameliorating its impact. Once the primary cord injury has occurred, a number of mediators can create a secondary injury secondary to the inflammatory response or continued cord ischemia. When cellular function deteriorates, large intracellular shifts of calcium occur, which can lead to further cell death. The neurotransmitters glutamate and aspartate are found at neurotoxic levels for 1 hour after injury (Liu et al., 1999). Activation of membrane phospholipases and increases in the products of the cyclo-oxygenase pathway, notably thromboxane A_2, may decrease blood flow to the injured tissue (Tempel and Martin, 1992). These pathways point to potential therapies. At this time, however, only methylprednisolone has shown any efficacy on double-blinded trials. Although GM-1 ganglioside was thought to have the potential for preservation and restoration of neurologic function, this tenet was not borne out in a multicenter trial. Pharmacologic doses of this methylprednisolone (30 mg/kg bolus over the first hour followed by a 23-hour infusion of 5.4 mg/kg per hour) has been shown in well powered, multi-institutional trials to improve sensory and motor scores for both complete and incomplete cord injuries in comparison to both placebo and naloxone. The improved neurologic scores remain stable for a period extending to a year in follow-up (Bracken et al, 1990). Other modifications of this regimen have shown that the best outcomes occur in patients treated within 3 hours of injury, and that if treatment is initiated within the 3- to 8-hour window after injury the steroid infusion should be continued up to 48 hours to maximize the neurologic outcome. Patients treated more than 8 hours after injury do not benefit from this regimen (Bracken et al, 1998). The presumed mechanism of methylprednisolone appears to be decreased membrane perioxidation and amelioration of the inflammatory cascade. This regimen increased infection and gastrointestinal bleeding rates in the treated groups, although not in a statistically significant manner. These complications, in addition to the inability of this regimen to improve the overall functional status of the patient, leave room for further innovations in the treatment of these devastating injuries.

Many factors influence the need for surgical fixation of a spine fracture, although there are some general guidelines that can guide therapy. Most Jefferson fractures (C1), unless associated with odontoid fractures or transverse ligament disruptions, are considered stable and can be managed in a rigid cervical collar or halo-vest. Hagman's fractures (C2) are usually unstable but can be treated with traction and then external immobilization. Type I and type III odontoid fractures are generally stable and can be managed with immobilization alone without surgery. Type II odontoid fractures with greater than 5 mm of displacement should be considered for surgical fixation. Although each presentation of a lower cervical spine fracture may require individualized therapy, in general terms treatment of these fractures is dependent on angulation of the vertebral bodies on lateral radiograph (or on flexion-extension films), on the presence of facet subluxation, and also on the presence of a neurologic deficit. Owing to the intrinsic added stability of the thoracic spine provided by the rib cage, many thoracic spine fractures can be managed with external immobilization alone. However, severe compressive fractures, burst fractures, and fractures associated with subluxation or neurologic deficit should be considered for operative decompression of the spinal canal and surgical immobilization. The need for surgical débridement and repair of penetrating spine injuries is controversial, although enteric contamination of penetrating spinal injuries should, at a minimum, be well drained surgically and treated with intravenous antibiotics (Kihtir et al, 1991).

COMPLICATIONS

The presence of a neurologic deficit can make evaluation of other injuries problematic. Reliance on diagnostic studies such as abdominal ultrasound and CT is often necessary in screening for abdominal trauma in the absence of a reliable physical examination. The diagnosis of compartment syndrome may necessitate frequent measurements of intracompartmental pressures to ensure timely diagnosis and prevent tissue loss. Physical examination findings that do not correlate with known head or spinal injuries should prompt an evaluation of brachial plexus or carotid and vertebral artery injuries. Although previously thought to be uncommon, occurring in fewer than 0.1% of trauma patients, recent screening programs have identified carotid and vertebral injuries in nearly 1% of trauma patients. Detection and treatment of these injuries is thought to improve outcome (Fabian et al, 1996).

Many injuries can develop secondary to spine fracture or the initial spinal cord injury. Delayed neurologic deterioration can occur secondary to syringomyelia, localized infection, or spinal cord tethering at the site of injury. Pulmonary complications account for a quarter of the mortality rate for spinal cord injuries (DeVivo et al, 1993). Low cervical (C5–7) and high thoracic level injuries result in respiratory embarrassment secondary to the loss of

Pearls and Pitfalls

PEARLS

- Every trauma patient should be considered at risk for a spinal injury.
- The first priorities of trauma are always as follows: Airway, Breathing, and Circulation. During this initial evaluation, immobilization of the spine is the first treatment of potential spine fractures.
- Spine fractures occur at multiple, noncontiguous levels in 5% to 10% of patients with spinal fracture.
- Unstable cervical spine fractures require more definitive immobilization than can be delivered by the rigid collars, which essentially limit only flexion and extension.
- Although neurogenic shock may be suspected, all trauma patients should have hypovolemic shock considered as their most probable cause of hypotension, and common sites of hemorrhage should be investigated.

PITFALLS

- Spinal cord injury usually requires fracture or dislocation of the spine, but in the degenerated spine or in the spine with a congenitally narrow canal spinal cord injury may occur without associated fracture or subluxation.
- The incidence of spine fractures is not more common in the head-injured population (4.7% vs. 4.4%) than in the non–head-injured population, but the patient's inclination or ability to report pain and paresthesias or to experience tenderness elicited drops off significantly at GCS less than 14, leading to the potential for missed spine injury.
- Although previously thought to be uncommon, screening programs have identified blunt carotid and vertebral injuries in nearly 1% of trauma patients.
- Even with history, physical examination, and radiologic tests, 5% of spine fractures still are missed at initial evaluation.

thoracic innervation and chest wall excursion. High cervical injuries (C1–4), above the level of phrenic nerve afferents (C3–5), additionally cause loss of diaphragmatic motion, and total respiratory collapse. These patients need good pulmonary toilet, and as many as 15% eventually require tracheostomies. Spinal cord injuries also carry the risk of bladder dysfunction. Initially, flaccidity predominates but 1 to 3 weeks after injury spasticity and urinary frequency develop. These patients should be monitored for bladder distention in the acute setting with either indwelling catheter or intermittent catheterization. Although intermittent catheterization is the preferred long-term management, this technique still carries a high risk of bladder infections (Larsen et al, 1997). Half or more of the patients with spinal cord injury will develop a thromboembolic complication during their initial inpatient or rehabilitative hospitalizations. Low-molecular-weight heparin is an effective prophylactic regimen for trauma patients, but it has been associated with epidural bleeding and may be contraindicated during the first 2 weeks after injury (Green et al, 1994). In patients with profound lower-extremity motor deficits, a combination of sequential compression devices and vena caval filters can be employed. Two other common, and potentially fatal complications of spinal cord injury, upper gastrointestinal bleeding and pressure ulcers, are most effectively treated by preventing their occurrence with proton-pump inhibitors and histamine receptor antagonists and meticulous skin care, respectively.

Even with a history, physical examination, and radiologic tests, 5% of spine fractures still are missed at initial evaluation (Davis et al, 1993). A majority of these cases are secondary to absent or inadequate screening films or misinterpretation. Delayed diagnoses are more common in the multiply injured, intoxicated, or head-injured patient. The occurrence of delayed neurologic deterioration is 10 times more common in patients with a delayed diagnosis of spinal fracture than in patients whose spinal fracture is diagnosed on admission, making accurate diagnosis of these injuries critically important.

PROGNOSIS

The return of neurologic function varies from patient to patient. Patients with complete spinal cord injuries with some activity at the level of injury improved neurologically within the first 4 to 6 months after injury, but patients without function at the level of injury had less return of function and took up to 2 years to show even modest gains. Patients with incomplete spinal cord injuries had a much better return of function than did patients with complete spinal cord injuries, so that in a C4 injury group 90% versus 70%, respectively, had return of biceps function (Ditunno et al, 2000).

Mortality can vary, depending on associated injuries and the patient's age and neurologic status. Overall mortality at 1 year after injury for isolated spinal cord trauma is 7%, but patients with spinal cord injury and associated injuries had an inpatient mortality approaching 20% (Burney et al, 1993). Younger patients, under 25 years of age, with incomplete spinal cord levels have a 12-year survival of 95%; however, patients older than the age of 50 years with complete injuries have a 12-year survival of only 18% (DeVivo et al, 1992).

SELECTED READINGS

Benzel EC, Hart BL, Ball PA, et al: Magnetic resonance imaging for the evaluation of patients with occult cervical spine injury. J Neurosurg 1996;85:824.
Berkowitz M: Assessing the socioeconomic impact of improved treatment of head and spinal cord injuries. J Emerg Med 1993;11(suppl 1):63.
Bracken MB, Shepard MJ, Collins WF Jr, et al: A randomized, controlled trial of methylprednisolone or naloxone in the treatment of acute spinal-cord injury. N Engl J Med 1990;322:1405.
Bracken MB, Shepard MJ, Holford TR, et al: Methylprednisolone or tirilazad mesylate administration after acute spinal cord injury: 1-year follow up.

Results of the Third National Acute Spinal Cord Injury Randomized Controlled Trial. J Neurosurg 1998;89:699.

Burney RE, Maio RD, Maynord F, Karunas R: Incidence, characteristics, and outcome of spinal cord injury at trauma centers in North America. Arch Surg 1993;128:596.

Davis JW, Phreaner DL, Hoyt DB, Mackersie RC: The etiology of missed cervical spine injuries. J Trauma 1993;34:342.

DeVivo MJ, Stover SL, Black KJ: Prognostic factors for 12-year survival after spinal cord injury. Arch Phys Med Rehabil 1992;73:152.

DeVivo MJ, Black KJ, Stover SL: Causes of death during the first 12 years after spinal cord injury. Arch Phys Med Rehabil 1993;74:248.

Ditunno JF Jr, Cohen ME, Hauck WW, et al: Recovery of upper-extremity strength in complete and incomplete tetraplegia: A multicenter study. Arch Phys Med Rehabil 2000;81:389.

Fabian TC, Patton JH Jr, Croce MA, et al: Blunt carotid injury: Importance of early diagnosis and anticoagulant therapy. Ann Surg 1996;223:522.

Green D, Chen DM, Chmiel JS, et al: Prevention of thromboembolism in spinal cord injury: Role of low molecular weight heparin. Arch Phys Med Rehabil 1994;75:290.

Kihtir T, Ivatury RR, Simon R, Stahl WM: Management of transperitoneal gunshot wounds of the spine. J Trauma 1991;31:1579.

Larsen LD, Chamberlin DA, Khonsari F, Ahlering TE: Retrospective analysis of urologic complications in male patients with spinal cord injury managed with and without indwelling urinary catheters. Urology 1997;50:418.

Liu D, Xu GY, Pan E, McAdoo DJ: Neurotoxicity of glucamate at the concentration released upon spinal cord injury. Neuroscience 1999;93:1383.

Roberge RJ, Wears RC: Evaluation of neck discomfort, neck tenderness, and neurologic deficits as indicators for radiography in blunt trauma victims. J Emerg Med 1992;10:539.

Tempel GE, Martin HD III: The beneficial effects of a thromboxane receptor antagonist on spinal cord perfusion following experimental cord injury. J Neurol Sci 1992;109:162.

Zabel DD, Tinkoff G, Wittenborn W, et al: Adequacy and efficacy of lateral cervical spine radiography in alert, high-risk blunt trauma patient. J Trauma 1997;43:952.

Chapter 15
Compartment Syndrome
Peter G. Trafton, James M. Doty, Rao R. Ivatury, and Harvey J. Sugerman

Extremity Compartment Syndrome
Peter G. Trafton

Acute compartment syndrome (CS) refers to the *progressive ischemic necrosis* of nerve and muscle due to elevated tissue pressure within a closed space, typically bounded by fascia and bone. When tissue pressure exceeds a level 30 to 40 mm Hg below diastolic pressure, intracompartmental capillary blood flow is blocked by venular occlusion. But further inflow produces increased swelling while ischemia-sensitive neuromuscular tissue develops irreversible changes over 4 to 8 hours (Fig. 15–1).

Acute compartment syndrome typically develops and/ or progresses in patients who are under medical care for injuries or other conditions. Untreated CS results in significant permanent functional deficits. Prompt and effective treatment, with release of constricting dressings and surgical fasciotomies, which are usually necessary, greatly improves patient outcome. Failure to provide this treatment frequently results in successful malpractice claims against the responsible physicians and surgeons. In the absence of timely treatment, patients are typically left with hypesthesia, dysesthesia, and contractures. Necrosis of involved muscles may release significant amounts of myoglobin, acidic metabolites, and potassium into the

circulation, resulting in acute renal failure or fatal arrhythmia. Necrotic tissue, particularly if exposed through tardy fasciotomy or another open wound, poses a serious risk of infection. Amputation or death are possible consequences.

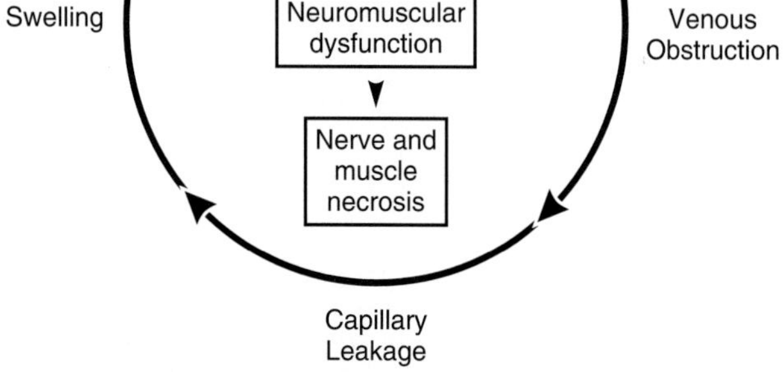

CLINICAL PRESENTATION

Differential diagnosis of CS includes all of the conditions with which it might be associated: fractures, contusions, hematomas, and myotendinous disruptions, as well as other causes of soft tissue swelling such as deep venous thrombosis, necrotizing fasciitis, cellulitis, clostridial myonecrosis (gas gangrene), and various envenomations, which are usually subcutaneous. Always to be considered, particularly when sensation and motor function are impaired, are arterial obstruction or injury and peripheral nerve injury, both of which may coexist with, or precede, CS.

The history, physical examination, and anteroposterior or lateral radiographs of the involved area are the essential tools for the diagnosis of CS. The typical patient with CS is a young male with a closed tibia fracture. More than two thirds of McQueen's series of 164 extremity compartment syndromes were associated with a fracture. Fractures of the distal radius and forearm are also frequent, but essentially any fracture can be associated with a CS. Blunt soft tissue injuries (23%) and crush syndrome (7.9%) without fractures were the causes of a sizable portion of their CSs. Despite their wounds, open fractures, including gunshot injuries, have a significant risk of CS. Patients with clotting disorders may develop intracompartmental hematomas that cause CS. Compression of a muscular region sustained for several hours or more is another important cause of CS. This may happen in disaster scenarios, when individuals are trapped under heavy debris, or to an unconscious patient, who lies on an unprotected extremity for a long time, or when a pneumatic antishock garment is left inflated for several hours. Extremity CSs occur after an acutely ischemic extremity is reperfused, as happens after repair of an arterial injury, or after lengthy operative procedures with several hours of leg elevation (lithotomy position, etc.), especially if exacerbated by periods of hypotension.

Extremity muscle groups, particularly in the forearm

Figure 15–1. Progressive, inexorable tissue loss results from untreated compartment syndrome. Enlarging the compartment's space (fasciotomy) is essential to break this vicious cycle.

and calf, are surrounded by noncompliant (i.e., does not stretch easily in response to increasing pressure of contents) investing fascia. In some regions, these fascial layers are moored to bone, which itself forms a portion of the walls surrounding a group of muscles. Typically, the muscles within a compartment share common functions—such as the ankle and toe dorsiflexors of the anterior tibial compartment. Within many important compartments travel peripheral nerves, arteries, and veins. Nerve involvement is an early finding in CS. Knowledge of peripheral nerve anatomy and function is thus a vital aid in the diagnosis of these conditions. One must systematically evaluate, by physical examination, the function of each compartmental muscle group, and each compartmental peripheral nerve.

Elevation of tissue pressure within an enclosed fascial compartment occurs either because of an increase in the compartment's contents, or a reduction in its size and/or compliance. Compartmental contents may increase because of hemorrhage, edema, fluid infusion, or (rarely) neoplasia. Acute blunt or penetrating injuries, with or without fractures, elective extremity surgery, and periods of ischemia with reperfusion edema are the usual causes. Reduction in compartmental volume is typically due to constricting casts, splints, or circumferential dressings, occasionally including pneumatic anti-shock garments (PASG, or medical antishock trousers [MAST]), and may also be caused by surgical closure of a compartmental fascial defect (Table 15–1).

The most important indicators of a CS are absent or unreliable in a patient who is unconscious or severely obtunded, or who has a peripheral nerve injury. The alert patient with a developing CS complains of increasing severe local pain, and perhaps tightness of any cast or dressing. The pain is increased by stretching the ischemic muscle in which it arises. For example, this is readily done by the examiner passively extending the fingers, which the patient with an anterior forearm CS prefers to keep flexed. As the duration of a CS increases, neuromuscular function becomes progressively impaired. The patient complains of paresthesia, dysesthesia, and then loss of sensation. Muscle strength wanes and then is lost. Distal pulses are usually present until late in the process, and the skin is well perfused, because these areas depend upon high-pressure arterial flow through the involved compartments, which is not compromised by pressure elevation that completely occludes neuromuscular capillaries. Swelling may be obvious, but not necessarily distal to the involved compartments, as subcutaneous veins are not occluded. Involved compartments are tightly swollen and are abnormally firm to palpation. In the unconscious patient, CS is suggested only by swelling, and a history consistent with injury, typically sustained compression of the swollen area.

Measurement of intracompartmental tissue pressure can be a very helpful adjunct for diagnosing CS in the patient whose neuromuscular evaluation is impaired. Confirmation of normal pressure can be reassuring when a patient with a limb at risk has significant swelling (for instance, from subcutaneous, rather than subfascial, hematoma) but does not have a neuromuscular deficit. However, the surgeon must remember that the diagnosis of CS is above all a clinical one. A firmly swollen muscle compartment with impaired or indeterminate neuromuscular function needs a fasciotomy, not pressure measurements. Various techniques have been described. That of Whitesides requires no special equipment. The pressure necessary to initiate movement of a column of saline solution along IV tubing toward an 18-gauge needle placed into a muscle compartment is read from an attached mercury manometer (Fig. 15–2). Direct reading of pressure with arterial line tubing connecting an 18-gauge needle to an electronic strain gauge is also possible, with the caution not to inject too much fluid. Pressure in a muscle compartment should respond to brief manual compression with a rapid rise and fall, if the measurement system is working properly. Pressure should be measured close to a fracture, if one is present, because it is highest there. Compartmental anatomy must be considered to ensure measurement of all potentially involved spaces; for example, the deep posterior compartment of the calf, which is almost entirely covered by the superficial compartment.

Normal tissue pressure is approximately 4 mm Hg. Absolute pressure is not a valid guide to the unequivocal presence of CS, since perfusion depends on whether arterial pressure is sufficient to overcome intracompartmental pressure. Furthermore, contused tissue is less able than normal to withstand elevated pressure. The duration of elevated pressure also plays a role, so that a lower pressure maintained for a longer time can produce as much injury as a higher pressure for a briefer period. Several researchers have offered different threshold pressures as indications for fasciotomy. Whitesides and colleagues recommend within 20 mm or less of the diastolic pressure. In a prospective study, McQueen found that a pressure within 30 mm Hg or less of diastolic identified all of the patients with CS. None of her patients with greater differential pressures developed sequelae of CS. Heppenstall referenced mean arterial pressure (diastolic

Table 15–1	**Causes of Compartment Syndrome**

Fractures, commonly of the tibia or radius and ulna, but any fracture, open or closed
Soft tissue injuries
Surgical procedures that cause intracompartmental swelling (e.g., osteotomies)
  May be masked by anesthesia or analgesia (postoperative epidural, etc.)
Intracompartmental hemorrhage
Ischemia-reperfusion
Arterial injuries
Prolonged limb elevation (e.g., lithotomy position in surgery)
Drug overdose—prolonged unconsciousness with postural limb compression
Burns
Crush syndrome, with sustained limb compression from fallen debris, etc.
Casts or other constrictive dressings
Intraosseous infusions during pediatric fluid resuscitation
Massive edema after fluid resuscitation of hypovolemic shock
Hemophilia or other bleeding dyscrasias, including anticoagulation
Arthroscopic fluid infusion

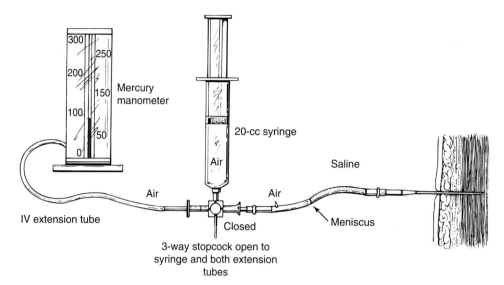

Figure 15–2. The needle-injection technique measures compartment tissue pressure by assessing the pressure required to initiate movement of the air-saline meniscus toward the patient. Pressure is increased by slowly advancing the syringe plunger while observing the meniscus for motion and reading the pressure from the mercury manometer. (Modified with permission from Amendola A, Twaddle BC: Compartment syndromes. In Browner BD, Jupiter JB, Levine AM, Trafton PG [eds]: Skeletal Trauma, 2nd ed. Philadelphia, WB Saunders, 1998, p 372. Redrawn from Whitesides TE Jr, Haney TC, Morimoto K, Hirada H: Clin Orthop 113:46, 1975.)

+ 1/3 pulse pressure) and recommended fasciotomy if tissue pressure was within 40 mm Hg of this value. Agreement among these recommendations is close. Note that they typically involve absolute tissue pressures much higher than the thresholds recommended initially by Hargens, Mubarak, and others—an *absolute pressure* of 30 mm Hg (which would have resulted in many unnecessary fasciotomies in McQueen's prospective study). No matter what pressures are measured, the patient with a tightly swollen muscle compartment and impaired sensorimotor function almost always is best treated with an urgent fasciotomy.

Since CS is an evolving phenomenon, it is essential for the surgeon to determine where a presenting patient is located in the evolutionary process. Ischemic nerve and muscle have the potential for full recovery during the first 2 to 4 hours of ischemia. Thereafter, progressively more irreversible damage occurs until, at 8 hours or so of total ischemia time, little if any salvageable muscle or nerve remain. Thus, for each patient with a CS that has persisted long enough, there reaches a point where fasciotomy is of no benefit—it exposes necrotic muscle to the risk of infection, but restores no function. In fact, by removing necrotic muscle that might otherwise become scar tissue that stabilizes an otherwise uncontrollable joint (as may happen with neglected anterior tibial CS), function might actually be impaired by a fasciotomy done too late. The clinical problem is that it is almost always impossible to be certain that partial necrosis has become complete, unless many hours have elapsed since the patient's neuromuscular function was clearly lost. In such cases, nonoperative acute management is the best advice. When in doubt about the possibility of viable nerve and muscle, however, the surgeon should proceed with emergency fasciotomy, but with the understanding that radical débridement of necrotic muscle may be required.

PREOPERATIVE MANAGEMENT

Significant volumes of acutely necrotic muscle result in a pathophysiologic process called crush syndrome, rhabdomyolysis, or myoglobinuria. Necrotic muscle releases myoglobin, potassium, and acidic breakdown products into the circulation, with the potential for multiple metabolic derangements, particularly arrhythmias and myoglobinuric renal failure. It is important to anticipate and identify these potentially life-threatening problems. Laboratory studies are key: Dark, heme-positive urine with no visible red cells strongly suggests myoglobin, which can be assayed directly in serum and urine. Serum creatine kinase level helps quantitate the volume of necrotic muscle: Values above 25,000 are significantly associated with acute renal failure. Electrolytes, blood urea nitrogen (BUN), creatinine, and arterial blood gases clarify the metabolic situation. Urine output must be measured. An electrocardiographic monitor is wise if electrolyte disturbances are anticipated. The unstable injured limb is splinted, without constricting bandages. When one observes a patient for possible CS, minimal elevation is advisable, to avoid interfering with limb arterial in-flow. Intravenous fluids are begun in large volume, along with alkalinization, in an attempt to avoid myoglobin precipitating in the renal tubules. There may be a role for mannitol, as well. Patients with open wounds should receive tetanus prophylaxis and intravenous antibiotics. Most important for adequate fasciotomies is emergency access to an operating room.

OPERATIVE MANAGEMENT

Fasciotomies are best done with general anesthesia. The supine position is usually appropriate, but location of the involved compartment, and any other necessary treatment must be considered. The entire involved limb should be prepared circumferentially, and draped free for optimal access. A tourniquet may be applied for use if necessary, but it should not be inflated routinely. Incisions are determined by the site of involvement. It is important that adequate decompression be achieved. This typically requires long incisions, extending from one end of the compartment to the other. Little subcutaneous dissection is required, but within each compartment fascial investments of individual muscle or muscle groups must be incised longitudinally to ensure that each muscle has adequately been released. Intraoperative measurement of tissue pressure can help determine the adequacy of decompression. If an open fracture is present, the usual thorough débridement and irrigation are mandatory. Carefully evaluate muscle viability, using Scully's criteria (contractility, capillary bleeding, consistency, and color). Nonviable muscle should be débrided. However, viability is often difficult to determine acutely, because necrosis may be patchy throughout the compartment. The wounds should be reassessed in the operating room in 48 to 72 hours, continuing débridement as necessary until all remaining tissue is viable. If a fracture is present, it should be stabilized at the time of fasciotomy. This can be done provisionally with an external fixator, even one that extends across joints from above to below the involved compartment. Definitive fixation should be determined by the treating surgeon, but typically involves an intramedullary nail for femoral or tibial shaft fractures, plates for humerus and forearm fractures, and specialized plates for metaphyseal or articular fractures.

LEG. Typically, all four calf compartments should be released for the patient with an acute CS, since involvement of both anterior and deep posterior compartments is relatively frequent. It is possible to decompress all four calf compartments with a perifibular approach using a single lateral incision, but this is more difficult, and probably more traumatic, than is the use of two incisions. These incisions should be placed midlateral and midmedial, with the medial posterior to the tibia's posteromedial border to ensure adequate width of the anterior skin flap (Fig. 15–3).

FOOT. Each of the medial, central, lateral, calcaneal, and interosseous compartments may need decompression. This can be done with two dorsal incisions over the second and fourth metatarsal shafts, with dissection around the bones into the plantar compartments, or, typically for hindfoot injuries, with a medial incision that is carried through the medial and calcaneal spaces to the lateral compartment, protecting plantar neurovascular structures. Both medial and dorsal incisions may be required.

THIGH. Each of the quadriceps, hamstring, and adductor compartments can be involved. A midlateral incision over the vastus lateralis, with extension posteriorly through the lateral intermuscular septum, releases both extensor and flexor compartments. A separate medial incision is required for the adductors.

FOREARM. The four major forearm compartments are the superficial and deep flexor spaces anteriorly and the extensor and mobile-wad posteriorly. Well-developed fascial investments around individual forearm muscles may require release, so that a thorough exploration from elbow to wrist is essential to ensuring adequate decompression. The flexor compartments are approached through Henry's midanterior incision, or McConnell's ulnar approach, with its incision more over muscle bellies than flexor tendons. Decompression of the carpal tunnel may be required as well, through distal extension of either incision. Typically, pressure elevation is most marked in the anterior compartments. After the posterior compartments have been adequately released, reassessment of them may reveal that their pressure has also fallen. If not, they should be released through a separate dorsal incision exposing both the mobile wad–brachialis and radial wrist extensors, and the deeper extensors of fingers and thumb.

HAND. Interossei are typically involved in this rare location for CS. Dorsal incisions over the second and fourth metacarpal shafts allow adequate release.

POSTOPERATIVE MANAGEMENT

Surgical fracture stabilization, with external fixation, plate, or intramedullary nail should be secure enough that any splint or cast can be loose, supportive of mobile joints and soft tissues, but not compressive. Injured soft tissue recovers best if it is immobilized. Functional positions (neutral foot and ankle, straight knee, slightly dorsiflexed wrist with finger MP joints flexed to 90 degrees) help prevent contractures. Fasciotomies for acute CS should be left open initially. An occlusive dressing, like the tobramycin bead-pouch described by Seligson, prevents tissue desiccation and probably reduces the risk of infection. Alternatives are Epigard, or a moist gauze dressing with overlying Xeroform or plastic vapor barrier. Changing fasciotomy wound dressings at the bedside is an invitation to contamination and infection, which should be avoided.

Planning for fasciotomy closure is important. (Closure involves skin and subcutaneous tissue only—the fascia should not be sutured closed, as this might precipitate a recurrent CS!) Wounds tend to contract, but this can be prevented with the use of elastic vessel loops laced through skin staples along the wound margin. Tightening the laces progressively with returns to the operating room facilitates delayed primary closure as swelling resolves. If tension-free delayed closure of the skin cannot be achieved in a reasonable time, split-thickness skin grafting of the fasciotomy defect can be done. It leaves both a donor site wound, and an unsightly fasciotomy scar. Although this can be excised and closed months later, waiting a bit longer to achieve delayed primary closure often yields better results with a shorter hospital stay. Patients with CS are usually kept hospitalized until wounds have been closed and any necessary period of enforced elevation, as might be advised after skin grafting, has elapsed. Typically, this is a week or two after injury.

As wound healing permits, range-of-motion and functional (activities of daily living, etc.) exercises are begun, with intermittent splinting if necessary to prevent contractures. If healing fractures or ligament injuries must

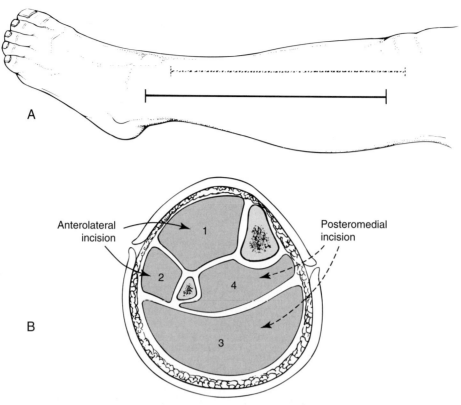

Figure 15–3. Double-incision technique for calf fasciotomies. *A,* The two incisions should be 180 degrees opposite each other. *B,* The medial incision, just posterior to the posteromedial border of the tibia, provides access to the deep (4) and superficial (3) posterior compartments. The fascia of the deep posterior compartment must be released from the tibia. The lateral incision allows decompression of the anterior and lateral compartments, with care taken to protect the superficial peroneal nerve. Both incisions must be long enough to release the entirety of the fascial spaces, from knee to ankle. (With permission from Amendola A, Twaddle BC: Compartment syndromes. In Browner BD, Jupiter JB, Levine AM, Trafton PG [eds]: Skeletal Trauma, 2nd ed. Philadelphia, WB Saunders, 1998, p 383.)

be protected, weightbearing or other forceful use of the injured extremity must be delayed. Once all tissues can withstand unrestricted use, progressive resistance exercises are begun in earnest. Typically, fracture healing, rather than recovery from CS, determines duration of the disability.

COMPLICATIONS

DELAYED DIAGNOSIS OF CS. Discussed previously. This is still the commonest problem of CS, and it must be prevented by maintained vigilance, pressure monitoring in patients at risk, and consideration of prophylactic fasciotomy for patients at significant risk.

MUSCLE NECROSIS. The result of damage from injury and/or tardy diagnosis. All necrotic muscle must be débrided to decrease the risk of infection. Fasciotomy wounds should be left open until adequate débridement is certain.

MYOGLOBINURIC RENAL FAILURE. Diagnosis and management discussed earlier.

INFECTION. This usually is caused by inadequate débridement of necrotic muscle. Patients at risk are typically those with delayed fasciotomy. Sterile management of open fasciotomy wounds and judicious use of antibiotics

perioperatively, or to treat a proven infection, help to minimize and to manage this problem. Established infections typically require further surgical débridement and operative cultures to confirm appropriate choice of antibiotics.

DIFFICULT WOUND CLOSURE. Discussed previously.

ISCHEMIC NEUROPATHY. Persisting pain may require analgesics, possibly supplemented by diphenylhydantoin (Dilantin), carbamazepine (Tegretol), and/or gabapentin (Neurontin). Multidisciplinary pain management should be considered. Muscle weakness may require functional bracing. Insensate skin must be protected from rubbing and pressure.

CONTRACTURES. Splint in a neutral position. Physical therapy for passive stretching should begin early.

OUTCOMES

Failure to identify and treat CS before nerve and muscle develop significant necrosis results in permanent functional impairment, the severity of which depends on the location and extent of myoneural necrosis. Neuropathic pain can be a problem, as well as impaired sensation, weakness, loss of passive motion, and joint contractures (fixed postures in dysfunctional positions). Sheridan and

Pearls and Pitfalls

PITFALLS

- **Failure to Diagnose.** Think about compartment syndrome whenever a patient has an extremity injury, a swollen limb, extremity ischemia and reperfusion, or weakness or numbness. If the patient cannot demonstrate normal strength and sensation, proceed with either pressure measurements or fasciotomy.
- **Pressure Measurement.** Tissue pressure elevation within 30 to 40 mm Hg of diastolic blood pressure is strongly associated with compartmental ischemia. If a clinically convincing CS is present, pressure measurement is unnecessary. It may be helpful for patients with atypical presentations because of nerve injury or obtundation, or in those with significant swelling and pain, but no signs of weakness or sensory neuropathy. Convincingly low pressures in such patients should indicate observation in lieu of fasciotomy.
- **Inadequate Fasciotomy Incisions.** Short incisions are often associated with inadequate muscle decompression. Fasciotomy incisions for acute compartment syndrome should extend from one end of the compartment to the other. Intracompartmental fascial spaces must also be released so that all muscles are soft.
- **Delayed Diagnosis.** From 8 to 12 hours after compartmental pressure rises above threshold level for CS, all intracompartmental tissue becomes nonviable. Fasciotomy does not salvage function, but incurs a serious risk of infection. If there is no chance of viable tissue remaining, fasciotomy should not be done.
- **Myoglobinuria.** Consider whenever there may be a significant volume of necrotic muscle. Hydrate, give sodium bicarbonate to alkalinize urine, give mannitol. If renal failure develops, dialysis is indicated, as renal function usually recovers.

- **Necrotic Muscle.** If you do encounter convincingly necrotic muscle, it should be completely excised. This may require repeated trips to the operating room but should be completed within a few days, because of the significant risk of infection. After radical débridement of dead muscle, suture closure is usually easy, and helps reduce the risk of infection.
- **Problems with Fasciotomy Closure.** Be prepared for repeated surgical attempts to close. Waiting for swelling to resolve, and use of elastic vessel loop lacing to prevent or correct flap contraction can help. Sometimes split-thickness grafting is the best alternative, but temporary skin graft alternatives can be helpful if closure must be delayed.
- **Long-Term Functional Deficits.** Rehabilitation, including delayed orthopaedic surgical reconstructive procedures, should be considered for all patients with residual functional deficits after CS.
- **Crush Syndrome.** Typically, patients given this diagnosis have significantly delayed treatment. Often, they have been injured in natural disasters, war, or other violent incidents. Usually, the opportunity for fasciotomy has long since passed, along with the chance of metabolic management, plus long-term functional rehabilitation and reconstruction.
- **Chronic (Exertional) Compartment Syndrome.** Some patients, typically endurance athletes or weightlifters, may have symptomatic neuromuscular ischemia due to transient exercise-induced elevation of compartmental pressure. Only very rarely do patients with this problem develop a superimposed acute CS. After proving that exercise-related pressure elevation is the cause of symptoms, fasciotomy may be needed to relieve them.

Matsen found residual defects in 7 of 22 extremity CS patients who had fasciotomies within 12 hours of onset. Only one was significant. A total of 22 of 24 such patients whose fasciotomies were done more than 12 hours after CS symptoms began had significant functional loss. Thirteen of these patients had complications. Five required amputation.

SELECTED READINGS

Asgari MM, Spinelli HM: The vessel loop shoelace technique for closure of fasciotomy wounds. Ann Plast Surg 2000;44:225.

Barnes M: Diagnosis and management of chronic compartment syndromes: A review of the literature. Br J Sports Med 1997;31:21.

Hargens AR, Mubarak SJ: Current concepts in the pathophysiology, evaluation, and diagnosis of compartment syndromes. Hand Clin 1998;14:371.

Heppenstall RB: An Update in Compartment Syndrome Investigation and Treatment (1997). *http://health.upenn.edu/ortho/oj/oj10sp97p49.html*

McQueen MM, Gaston P, Court-Brown CM: Acute compartment syndrome, who is at risk? J Bone Joint Surg 2000;82B:200.

McQueen MM, Court-Brown CM: Compartment monitoring in tibial fractures: The pressure threshold for decompression. J Bone Joint Surg 1996;78B:99.

Matsen FA 3d (ed): Compartmental Syndromes. University of Washington Bone and Joint Sources. Last Modified 04/24/2000 (ajl). Copyright © 2000 University of Washington. http://www.orthop.washington.edu/Bone%20and%20Joint%20Sources/yyccyyyy1_1.html

Ouellette EA: Compartment syndromes in obtunded patients. Hand Clin 1998;14:431.

Seybold EAS, Busconi BD: Traumatic popliteal artery thrombosis and compartment syndrome of the leg following blunt trauma to the knee: A discussion of treatment and complications. J Orthop Trauma 1996;10:138.

Sheridan GW, Matsen FA 3d: Fasciotomy in the treatment of the acute compartment syndrome. J Bone Joint Surg 1976;58A:112.

Shimazu T, Yoshioka T, Nakata Y, et al: Fluid resuscitation and systemic complications in crush syndrome: 14 Hanshin-Awaji earthquake patients. J Trauma 1997;42:641.

Tollens T, Janzing H, Broos P: The pathophysiology of the acute compartment syndrome. Acta Chir Belg 1998;98:171.

Whitesides TE Jr, Heckman MM: Acute compartment syndrome: Update on diagnosis and treatment. J Am Acad Orthop Surg 1996;4:209.

Williams AB, Luchette FA, Papaconstantinou HT, et al: The effect of early versus late fasciotomy in the management of extremity trauma. Surgery 1997;122:861.

Abdominal Compartment Syndrome

James M. Doty, Rao R. Ivatury, and Harvey J. Sugerman

The abdominal compartment syndrome (ACS) is a syndrome in which elevated intra-abdominal pressure (IAP) causes dysfunction of one or more organ systems. Although ACS is most commonly seen in trauma patients and in the surgical intensive care unit (ICU); however, it is not limited to these settings, occurring in multiple surgical and nonsurgical situations (Fig. 15–4). Among the organ systems affected are pulmonary, cardiovascular, renal, neurologic, abdominal wall, and splanchnic. Elevated IAP may develop acutely over a period of hours with severe morbidity or mortality, known as the acute abdominal compartment syndrome (AACS). Alternatively, it may develop over a period of years with chronic progressive morbidity, as seen in the morbidly obese, called the chronic abdominal compartment syndrome (CACS). The authors propose a subacute abdominal compartment syndrome that develops over a period of weeks to months, in the case of preeclampsia. Regardless of the etiology or the chronicity of its onset, ACS affects a significant por-

tion of the critically ill and can have high morbidity and mortality if not treated appropriately.

Historically, intra-abdominal hypertension (IAH) was first alluded to in the 1870s, when Marey and Burt described the respiratory effect of elevated IAP. In the 1890s, Heinricius noted that elevated IAP caused death in animal models. Several decades later, hemodynamic alterations and renal derangements were documented with elevated IAP by Emerson and Wendt, respectively. More recently, Kron coined the term ACS in describing a patient with elevated IAP due to a bleeding abdominal aortic aneurysm. ACS was first reported in a trauma patient in 1988. Currently, the term ACS is used to describe the phenomenon in which elevation of IAP has deleterious effects on one or more organ systems.

The national incidence of ACS is not known. Subpopulations where the prevalence is high have been studied. Meldrum and colleagues noted in a study of 145 severe abdominal trauma patients (ISS >15) that 21 (14%) de-

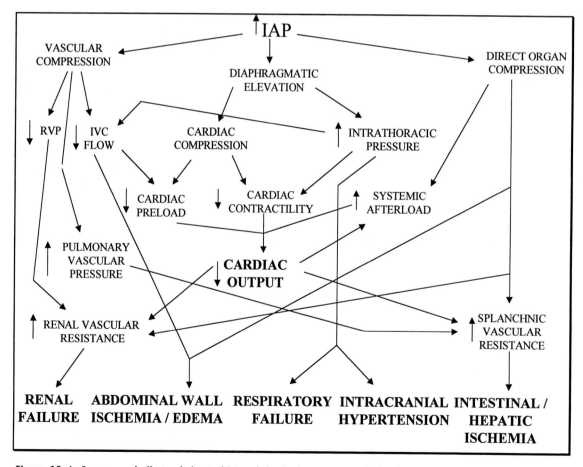

Figure 15–4. Summary of effects of elevated intra-abdominal pressure on the body. IAP, intra-abdominal pressure; IVC, inferior vena cava; RVP, renal venous pressure; PV, pulmonary vascular.

veloped ACS. The literature reports a prevalence of ACS among patients with severe abdominal trauma as high as 33%. The demographics appear to follow the trauma statistics, with ACS occurring primarily in young adult males.

CLINICAL PRESENTATION

The abdominal compartment syndrome occurs primarily in the critically ill. Its manifestations are those of organ failure with a tense distended abdomen. As there are multiple possible etiologies for organ failure in critically ill patients, one must have a high index of suspicion to identify an ACS. It is important to recognize that ACS is a clinical diagnosis, supported by bedside and laboratory measurements.

The acute abdominal compartment syndrome most often occurs in trauma patients with significant intra-abdominal injuries. Regardless of the etiology, the mechanisms of increased IAP are of two types. The first is from acute increases in intra-abdominal volume; for example, intra-abdominal hemorrhage, edema, bowel distention, mesenteric venous obstruction, abdominal packing, tense ascites, or tumor. In the second mechanism intra-abdominal volume is unchanged, but the abdomen is compressed such as in burn eschars, MAST trousers, tense abdominal closure, or repair of large abdominal wall defects.

According to a study by Ivatury and co-workers in the trauma patient, predictors of elevated IAP include injury severity score (ISS), base deficit, and amount of blood transfused in 24 hours. Their results were as follows ($\pm$SEM): ISS 21.8 ± 9.2, base deficit 12 ± 6.1, lactate 6.1 ± 3.8, and red blood cell (RBC) transfusion 13.4 ± 9.4 U.

Objective bedside measurements of IAP can be made by transvenous, nasogastric, or urinary catheterization. Measurement of urinary bladder pressures (UBPs) is the most common method and has been shown to accurately reflect IAP. Moore and Meldrum have developed a grading system for acute ACS based on UBP. In Grades I and II (UBP <25mm Hg), the patients most typically have mild organ compromise, and volume loading may be adequate to preserve organ perfusion. Grade III patients have UBPs between 26 and 35 mm Hg, and more severe organ compromise is present. These patients need some form of abdominal decompression. Finally, in grade IV (UBP >35) organ compromise is severe and laparotomy is necessary for patient salvage.

Essentially, when UBP is increased more than 20 to 25 mm Hg with evidence of organ system dysfunction, such as cardiovascular (Do_2I <600 mL O_2/min per m^2), pulmonary (airway pressure $\geq$45 cm H_2O $Paco_2$ $\geq$50), renal (urine output <0.5 mL/kg per minute, azotemia), and splanchnic (pHi decreased <7.3, lactic acidosis, dusky bowel), laparotomy is indicated. There is some evidence that refractory elevated ICP in the setting of increased IAP may be an indication for laparotomy as well. It is important to understand that the reliability of the UBP measurements may be affected by several factors so that elevated UBP by itself should not mandate laparotomy. For example, morbidly obese patients may have resting UBPs of 30 to 40 mm Hg without any immediate threat to their organ function. Other complicating factors include hypovolemia, and anesthetics.

ORGAN SYSTEM PROBLEMS WITH AACS

Cardiovascular

The manifestations of AACS on the cardiovascular system are those of shock. The AACS causes decreased preload, increased afterload, and decreased contractility. Preload is decreased (IAP approximately 20 mm Hg) owing to decreased inferior vena cava (IVC) and superior vena cava (SVC) flow. Increased pressure in the abdomen causes IVC compression (maximal at the diaphragm) and thus decreased flow. Elevated IAP is transmitted to the thorax, increasing intrathoracic pressure and decreasing superior vena cava (SVC) flow. With increased intrathoracic pressure, there is also some direct cardiac compression, which decreases contractility and limits end-diastolic volume. This mechanism becomes significant around IAP 30 mm Hg. Afterload is increased as the result of arteriolar compression in the abdomen and increased levels of the hormonal mediators angiotensin II (see section on renal system that follows) and vasopressin (released in response to decreased atrial stretch). The end result of these factors is movement of the Frank-Starling curve to the right and down.

Monitoring of cardiac filling pressures in the ACS may be misleading. Increased intrathoracic pressure causes elevated pressure in the great vessels so central venous pressure (CVP), pulmonary artery occlusion pressure (PAOP), and pulmonary artery pressure (PAP) are artificially elevated. Actual transmural pressures may be normal or decreased, misleading the practitioner into believing that preload is adequate when it is not. A final cardiac insult occurs secondary to the requirement for increased ventilatory pressures, which further affects cardiac function. Prompt decompression reverses these defects.

Renal

The renal derangements that occur in AACS are manifested clinically by oliguria (IAP 15 to 20 mm Hg), progressing to anuria (>30 mm Hg) with prerenal azotemia. The mechanism of these derangements is thought to be multifactorial, including decreased cardiac output, increased renal venous pressure, and renal parenchymal compression. Decreased cardiac output leads to decreased organ perfusion. Studies have shown that in the setting of an AACS, however, resuscitation to a normal cardiac output is insufficient to reverse the renal derangements. The role of renal venous pressure as a primary mediator of renal derangements in ACS is supported by recent animal studies. Renal compression has been studied in an animal model and has been shown to have minimal effects on renal function by itself. However, increased renal parenchymal pressure, in combination with elevated renal venous pressure, may have an additive or synergistic effect. Ureteral compression seems unlikely to play a role, as ureteral stenting has no effect on AACS-induced azotemia. Decreased renal perfusion causes reduced glomerular filtration rate (GFR) with decreased delivery of sodium to the distal nephron. As a result, there is activation of the renin-angiotensin-aldosterone system, causing increased afterload. Prompt abdominal decompression reverses AACS-mediated renal dysfunction and results in a brisk diuresis.

Pulmonary

The pulmonary derangements observed in AACS are consistent with respiratory failure. The elevated IAP causes limited diaphragmatic excursion and elevated intrathoracic pressures, which result in a decrease in static and dynamic compliance of the lung parenchyma and increased pulmonary vascular resistance (PVR). There is a reduction in total lung capacity, functional residual capacity, and residual lung volume. Ventilation-perfusion mismatch occurs with hypoxemia and hypercapnia, with both a metabolic and a respiratory acidosis. Hypoxemia exacerbates the elevated PVR. Clinically, there are increased airway pressures with progressive difficulty in ventilation as the AACS worsens. These changes are often completely and immediately reversible if the abdomen is decompressed in a timely fashion. Some authors report ventilatory insufficiency as the first sign of ACS; however, pHi and UBPs are probably more sensitive indicators.

Gastrointestinal

As with shock, the splanchnic bed is extremely sensitive to the effects of elevated IAP. The literature documents decreased blood flow secondary to AACS in the mesenteric, hepatic, and portal venous vessels as well as decreased intestinal mucosal blood flow. The mechanisms are not entirely clear; however, venous outflow obstruction, arteriolar compression (at high IAPs), and systemic hormones such as angiotensin II are thought to be involved. IAPs as low as 10 mm Hg have been shown to significantly affect portal blood flow and IAPs less than 20 mm Hg can cause decreased intestinal blood flow. Gastric tonometry (pHi) has been used to monitor altered splanchnic perfusion and may serve as an earlier indicator for abdominal decompression. When there is intestinal ischemia, there may be bacterial translocation, which may lead to sepsis and multiple-system organ failure (MSOF) in some patients. Laparoscopic animal studies with elevated IAP have shown an increase in free radical production in the liver, spleen, lung, and intestinal mucosa.

Abdominal computed tomographic findings of AACS have been reported in a small series of patients. Cited changes include (1) tense infiltration of the retroperitoneum out of proportion with peritoneal disease, (2) extrinsic compression of the IVC by retroperitoneal hemorrhage or exudates, and (3) massive abdominal distention with an increased anteroposterior to transverse abdominal diameter (positive round-belly sign).

Neurologic Derangements

Elevated intracranial pressure and decreased cerebral perfusion pressure (CPP) occur in the AACS. In non–head-injured animal models, IAPs of 25 mmHg have been shown to significantly decrease CPP. Elevation in ICP occurs owing to decreased cerebral venous (jugular) outflow as the result of increased intrathoracic pressure (transmitted from elevated IAP) and results presumably in cerebral venous engorgement and thus elevated ICP. Pleuropericardotomy in experimental animals with AACS has been shown to prevent the increase in ICP. Decreased cardiac output due to AACS cardiovascular effects exacerbates the CPP problem. A case report of a multisystem trauma patient with refractory elevated ICP (despite ventriculostomy) and AACS was shown to have significantly reduced ICP following abdominal decompression.

Abdominal Wall

Direct compression from elevated IAP results in decreased abdominal wall blood flow, which may decrease the distensibility of the abdominal wall exacerbating the IAP and increases the risk of both infectious (wound infections) and noninfectious (fascial necrosis, dehiscence) complications of laparotomy wound healing.

PREOPERATIVE MANAGEMENT

Once the diagnosis has been made, the first task is to identify the optimal time for operative management. In the setting of postoperative AACS in a trauma patient, there has been some debate in the literature. One school of thought is that once a patient is operated on, for damage control one should not reoperate until the patient's physiology has significantly recovered. However, a patient's physiology is unlikely to significantly improve in the setting of progressing AACS. This results in surgeons operating on patients in the more advanced stages of AACS and, thus, in a poorer survival (37.5%), as documented in a study by Morris and colleagues. The other school of thought focuses on early monitoring, recognition, and decompression of the AACS before it further insults the patient's physiology. A study by Meldrum and associates showed improved survival with this management scheme (71%) in a similar patient population.

If possible prior to laparotomy, correction of coagulopathy and hypothermia, reversal of acidosis, and volume loading should be accomplished. The importance of volume loading is controversial. Some authors advocate infusion of 2 L of 0.45% NS with 50 g of mannitol and 50 mEq of sodium bicarbonate, 1 L preoperatively and 1 L infused during decompression. The authors believe that the more severe the AACS, the greater the volume requirement to avoid hypotension and reperfusion injury when the abdomen is decompressed. Inotropic support should be used as needed once volume loading and adequate hemoglobin concentrations have been achieved. Invasive monitoring is essential but, as discussed previously, may be misleading with elevated intrathoracic pressures artificially elevating measurements of cardiac filling pressures. In AACS, one must resuscitate the patient to optimal cardiac output. Right ventricular end-diastolic volume, as measured with a volumetric right-

Pearls and Pitfalls

PEARLS

- ACS is a clinical diagnosis, supported by bedside and laboratory measurements.
- In trauma, predictors of elevated IAP include injury severity score (ISS), base deficit, and amount of blood transfused in 24 hours.
- UBP greater than 20 to 25 mm Hg with evidence of organ system dysfunction indicates the need for decompression.
- An elevated UBP by itself should not mandate laparotomy; morbidly obese patients may have resting UBPs of 30 to 40 mm Hg without any immediate threat to their organ function.
- Monitoring of cardiac filling pressures in the ACS may be misleading. Actual transmural pressures may be normal or decreased, misleading the practitioner into believing that preload is adequate when it is not.
- Prompt abdominal decompression will reverse AACS-mediated organ dysfunction.
- pHi and UBPs are probably the most sensitive indicators of early ACS.
- IAPs greater than 10 mm Hg have been shown to significantly affect portal blood flow, and IAPs less than 20 mm Hg can cause decreased intestinal blood flow.
- A patient's physiology is unlikely to significantly improve in the setting of progressing AACS; early operation for ACS improves survival.
- The goal of resuscitation is to resuscitate to an optimal cardiac output.

- In ACS, right ventricular end-diastolic volume, as measured with a volumetric right-heart catheter, is a better indicator of preload than is pulmonary artery occlusion pressure.
- Leave the abdomen open when there is hemodynamic or pulmonary compromise with closure, when there is massive bowel edema and fascial closure is tight, when reoperation is planned, or when packing is left in the peritoneal cavity.
- Intraoperative measurement of UBPs may be helpful in guiding the decision regarding abdominal closure.
- If the abdomen is left open, use of an absorbable polyglactin mesh allows leakage of fluid and can be used with a large redundancy should it need to be expanded to lower a rising IAP.
- Towel-clip closure may bring the skin edges together quickly but may further increase IAP in the edematous abdomen.
- High fluid volume requirements are typical with an open abdomen, often appearing in the first 24 hours.
- During abdominal wall closure, UBPs should be monitored regularly for recurrent AACS.
- Postoperatively, elevated UBPs and organ impairment is a sign of recurrent AACS and should be managed with further decompression.
- Re-exploration for ACS in the setting of coagulopathy has improved management in many patients.
- Avoid the reperfusion syndrome by volume loading and early decompression.

heart catheter, is a much better indicator of preload than pulmonary artery occlusion pressure.

INTRAOPERATIVE MANAGEMENT

Intraoperative management occurs in two settings. The first is in the severe abdominal trauma victim in whom AACS has not developed but one attempts to prevent it, and the second setting is where AACS has developed and the abdomen must be decompressed.

AACS Prevention

The gold standard of trauma care in the severely injured patient is damage control or the staged celiotomy. The purpose of this management scheme is to avoid the vicious cycle of acidosis, hypothermia, and coagulopathy. However, this same management scheme that helps manage severely injured patients puts them at increased risk for AACS.

After appropriate damage control measures have been taken, the decision that must be made is whether to close the abdomen or not. A survey of experienced trauma physicians in the United States reports that the majority of these doctors leave the abdomen open (1) when there is hemodynamic or pulmonary compromise with closure, (2) when there is massive bowel edema and fascial closure is tight, (3) when reoperation is planned, or (4) when

packing is left in the peritoneal cavity. It can be a difficult decision, as there is a balance between the pressure needed to stop nonsurgical bleeding and the pressure that causes organ impairment. Ultimately, the judgment is individualized on the basis of the patient's condition and the physician's experience. One advantage of leaving the abdomen open is the rapidity with which the procedure can be completed so the patient can be transferred to the ICU for resuscitation. Intraoperative measurement of UBPs may be helpful in guiding the decision regarding abdominal closure. If the abdomen is left open, an absorbable polyglactin mesh may be sutured to skin or fascia. The mesh allows leakage of fluid and can be used with a large redundancy should it need to be expanded to decrease a rising IAP. An alternative to the use of mesh is the "Bogata Bag." This method involves the use of a sterile, nonreactive material to bridge the gap between the skin edges of the wound, such as a Foley irrigation bag or nonsticky plastic drape (Via Drape), and has the benefit of visualization of bowel viability. Towel-clip closure may bring the skin edges together quickly but may further increase IAP in the edematous abdomen. Some nontrauma patients may also benefit from "damage control laparotomy," as may be seen with necrotizing pancreatitis or bacterial peritonitis.

AACS Treatment

Once the physician is committed to a decompressive laparotomy, the goal is to be as swift as possible. Many patients have a significantly reduced physiologic reserve and cannot tolerate long operations. In fact, many such laparotomies are performed at the bedside. Whether to perform the laparotomy in the ICU versus the operating room may depend on the safety of transporting a patient requiring high peak inspiratory pressures. Any immediate life-threatening problems should be corrected. For example, in the setting of trauma, the abdomen is decompressed, bleeding is controlled with sutures and/or packing, and any bowel injuries are stapled off. The abdomen is then closed in a noncompressive manner (as discussed earlier), and definitive repair delayed until the patient's status has improved.

POSTOPERATIVE MANAGEMENT

Postoperative care consists of standard ICU care with invasive monitoring (pulmonary artery catheter and arterial line). Goals of resuscitation include oxygen delivery index >600 mL/min per m², oxygen consumption index >150, lactate <2.5 mmol/L within 12 hours, core temp >35 degrees C, PT and PTT <1.25 normal, PLT >100,000/mm³, and fibrinogen >100 mg/dL. Oxygen delivery should be optimized with blood transfusions, volume replacement, and inotropes as needed. High-volume requirements are typical, with an open abdomen often in the first 24 hours. In addition, UBPs should be monitored regularly for recurrent AACS. Elevated UBPs and organ impairment are signs of recurrent AACS and should be managed with further decompression. Consistently increasing IAP in a trauma patient often means bleeding and indicates the need for laparotomy. Some think that reexploration in the setting of coagulopathy is poor judgment; however, improved management has been reported in many such patients.

When the patient's physiology has recovered sufficiently, definitive repair of injuries should be undertaken, and, if bowel and retroperitoneal edema have resolved, closure of the abdomen can be attempted. However, an increase in UBP may preclude primary closure. This may necessitate successive procedures for definitive closure. Often, primary closure is not possible owing to persistent edema, fascial retraction, or necrosis. In this situation, the abdomen must be allowed to granulate either over the viscera or, preferably, over an absorbable mesh with subsequent application of a split-thickness skin graft. These skin grafts may be easily excised in 6 to 12 months. Fascial closure usually requires relaxing incisions or mesh for closure. It is important to measure UBP during all attempts at closure so as not to re-create an AACS (Saggi et al, 1998).

COMPLICATIONS OF AN AACS

Additional complications include loss of fascia, organ system failure, sepsis, and death. A reperfusion syndrome often follows abdominal decompression, with profound and sometimes irreversible hypotension. This is secondary to a rapid increase in venous capacitance in the abdominal and pelvic vessels and a washout of potassium, acids, and other products of anaerobic metabolism that markedly compromise cardiac contractility. One study reports a 12% incidence of asystole due to the toxic effects of these metabolites on the heart. Management of the reperfusion syndrome is two-fold: first, avoidance by early recognition and decompression of an AACS; second, volume loading prior to decompression and inotropic support as needed. Finally, when the patient is decompressed, the abrupt increase in tidal volume delivered to the patients may cause a respiratory alkalosis.

OUTCOMES

Based on a review of the surgical literature, surgical decompression is 93% effective in reversing organ dysfunction, with an overall survival of 59%. The majority of deaths are due to MSOF or sepsis.

SELECTED READINGS

Doty JM, Saggi BH, Sugerman HJ, et al: Effect of increased renal parenchymal pressure on renal function. Under review.

Doty JM, Saggi BH, Sugerman HJ, et al: Effect of increased renal venous pressure on renal function. J Trauma 1999;47:1000.

Eddy V, Nunn C, Morris JA: Abdominal compartment syndrome, the Nashville experience. Surg Clin North Am 1997;77:801.

Ivatury RR, Diebel L, Porter JM, Simon RJ: Intra-abdominal hypertension and the abdominal compartment syndrome. Surg Clin North Am 1997;77:783.

Ivatury RR, Porter JM, Simon RJ, et al: Intra-abdominal hypertension after life-threatening penetrating abdominal trauma: Prophylaxis, incidence and clinical relevance to gastric mucosal pH and abdominal compartment syndrome. J Trauma 1998;44:1016.

Mayberry JC, Goldman RK, Mullins RJ, et al: Surveyed opinion of American trauma surgeons on the prevention of the abdominal compartment syndrome. J Trauma 1999;47:509.

Meldrum DR, Moore FA, Moore EE, et al: Prospective characterization and selective management of the abdominal compartment syndrome. Am J Surg 1997;174:667.

Moore EE, Burch JM, Franciose RJ, et al: Staged physiologic restoration and damage control surgery. World J Surg 1998;22:1184.

Morris JA, Eddy VA, Blinman TA, et al: The staged celiotomy for trauma. Ann Surg 1993;217:576.

Pickhardt PJ, Shimony JS, Heiken JP, et al: The abdominal compartment syndrome: CT findings. AJR Sept. 1999;575–579.

Saggi BH, Sugerman HJ, Ivatury RR, Bloomfield GL: Abdominal compartment syndrome. J Trauma 1998;45:597.

CRITICAL CARE

Chapter 16
Acute Renal Failure
Paul Bankey

Acute renal failure (ARF) is an important contributing factor in perioperative and post-traumatic morbidity and mortality. As an isolated organ system failure, ARF has an associated mortality of 8%; however, ARF in association with septic shock and multiple organ dysfunction syndrome has a mortality that has remained significantly higher (70% to 80%) despite aggressive critical care, newer treatment modalities, and increased understanding of the pathophysiology. Renal replacement therapy and the intensive care required for general surgery patients who develop ARF place a large burden on health care resources. The most cost-effective intervention in ARF is its *prevention*, by effectively ensuring adequate circulating intravascular volume and treating surgically reversible contributing causes. The outcome of ARF is most often linked to the resolution of the patient's underlying problems; however, the consequences can also be minimized by the preoperative identification of high-risk surgical patients, prompt recognition, and intervention while the condition is still in reversible stages. Ongoing investigation is determining the role for specific mediator antagonists and renal protective agents as additional therapies for ARF.

It is rare for the general surgery patient to require direct operation on the kidney, renal vasculature, or urinary tract for treatment of ARF; however, deteriorating renal function is often a harbinger of a perioperative complication requiring management by the general surgeon. In most patients, ARF is reversible if recognized and treated early.

CLINICAL PRESENTATION

Acute renal failure is traditionally defined as the abrupt decline in previously stable or normal glomerular and tubular function, clinically characterized by the retention of nitrogenous (azotemia) and other metabolic waste products. The incidence of ARF is relatively common (as many as 5% of hospitalized patients); medical intervention is often a contributing cause. The three most common causes of ARF are as follows: (1) volume depletion or hypotension; (2) aminoglycoside antibiotics; and (3) radiocontrast exposure frequently associated with care provided by general surgeons in the course of major surgery.

In ARF, the loss of function occurs over a period of hours to days and results in a decreasing glomerular filtration rate (GFR). Glomerular filtration rate is the most direct indicator of renal function; however, it is difficult to measure directly in clinical practice. Serum concentrations of blood urea nitrogen (BUN) and creatinine (Cr) are more commonly used to assess renal function. In most instances, the serum creatinine level is an excellent barometer of renal function because a steady-state relationship exists between serum creatinine and GFR; however, the relationship is not linear, and initial large decreases in clearance or GFR produce only small changes in serum creatinine. The clinical significance of this is that an increase in a patient's Cr from 1 to 2 mg/dL signifies a 50% reduction in GFR, and an increase from 1 to 4 mg/dL a 75% reduction. The correlation between Cr and GFR depends on the assumption that it is delivered to the serum from tissue at a constant rate. Patients with hypercatabolic states, such as trauma and sepsis, and patients with diminished muscle mass have conditions that alter the rate of Cr production, reducing the correlation of the serum concentration with renal function. Nomograms are available that accurately correlate age, ideal body weight, and Cr with GFR.

Patients with ARF may be classified on the basis of their urine output. Patients that produce less than 50 mL/day are considered anuric. *Oliguria* is defined as a urine output less than 400 mL/day. This volume represents the minimum amount of urine in which a normal daily solute load of 500 mOsm can be excreted if the kidney is maximally concentrating urine to 1200 mOsm/kg of water. *Nonoliguric ARF* is defined as a lack of homeostasis (electrolyte imbalance or azotemia) despite a production of urine exceeding 400 mL/day. *High-output ARF* is defined as renal insufficiency with urine outputs greater than 1000 mL/day and frequently as much as several liters per day. The clinical relevance of this classification is that nonoliguric renal failure patients have a better prognosis than that of those with oliguric or anuric failure; therefore, management should be directed toward preventing progression of nonoliguric renal failure to oliguric or anuric ARF. Fluids and electrolytes are easier to manage in patients with nonoliguric ARF, and these patients have a significantly lower number of days on dialysis, overall mortality, and higher incidence of recovery avoiding either permanent dialysis or renal transplantation. In one study of 35 patients with post-traumatic ARF, the complications of hyperkalemia and pulmonary edema were halved and overall mortality decreased from 70% to 38%.

Acute renal failure is often clinically divided into three categories, based principally on the pathophysiology of the disease (Table 16–1). *Prerenal ARF* is defined as a rapidly reversible rise in serum Cr caused by renal hypoperfusion. In prerenal ARF, there is no apparent renal parenchymal damage and the reduction in GFR merely reflects a drop in glomerular perfusion. Restoration of renal perfusion rapidly restores GFR and normal serum Cr levels. Other diagnoses—that is, intrarenal or post-renal ARF—should be pursued if renal function does not respond promptly to restoration of renal perfusion.

Renal perfusion and GFR can be maintained at moderate levels of hypovolemia largely through the actions of sympathetic stimulation and activation of the renin-angio-

Table 16–1	Major Causes of Acute Renal Failure		
	PRERENAL	**INTRARENAL**	**POSTRENAL**
	Intravascular volume depletion	Ischemic ATN	Neoplasm
	Hemorrhage	Shock	Prostate
	Vomiting	Septic	Cervix
	Third-spacing	Cardiogenic	Colorectal
	Burns	Hypovolemic	
	Fever		
	Diarrhea		
	Decreased cardiac output	Nephrotoxic ATN	Dysfunctional bladder
	Congestive failure	Aminoglycosides	Anticholinergic drugs
	Pulmonary hypertension	Radiocontrast agents	Catheter obstruction
	Myocardial ischemia	Myoglobinuria	Prostatic enlargement
		Hemoglobinuria	
		Chemotherapeutic agents	
		Amphotericin B	
	Decreased renal perfusion with normal or high cardiac output	Glomerulonephritis	Nephrolithiasis
	Sepsis	Immune complex–mediated	
	Cirrhosis	Postinfectious	
	Drugs	Vasculitis	
	Nonsteroidal anti-inflammatory agents	Tubulointerstitial disease	Papillary necrosis
	Angiotensin-converting enzyme inhibitors	Allergic interstitial nephritis	
		Other vascular	Abdominal compartment syndrome
		Thrombotic microangiopathy	
		Vascular trauma	
		Cholesterol embolization	

tensin system (autoregulation). Angiotensin II activity results in constriction of the glomerular *efferent* arteriole, producing increased *efferent* arteriolar resistance. This increases hydrostatic pressure in the glomerular capillary. The *afferent* arterioles are less susceptible to constriction, possibly owing to increased nitric oxide activity. Efferent arteriolar constriction maintains intraglomerular hydrostatic filtration pressure (GFR) and increases the filtration fraction (GFR/renal blood flow [RBF]). Compensated hypovolemia also results in the stimulation of intrarenal vasodilating prostaglandins. Further hypovolemia results in profound sympathetic stimulation and renin-angiotensin activation that constricts the *afferent* arteriole. Mesangial cells also constrict, reducing glomerular surface area, so that the GFR and the filtration fraction declines. Eventually, hypoperfusion overwhelms these compensatory mechanisms, resulting in progression to renal ischemia and acute tubular necrosis (ATN). The use of nonsteroidal anti-inflammatory drugs (NSAIDs), which block synthesis of prostaglandins and are frequently used in the perioperative management of pain, are particularly hazardous in the setting of prerenal hypovolemia. Another class of drugs to avoid in the setting of prerenal hypovolemia is the angiotensin-converting enzyme (ACE) inhibitors, which block production of angiotensin II. Both of these groups of agents interfere with glomerular autoregulatory mechanisms and may precipitate severe renal hypoperfusion and ATN.

Intrinsic or *intrarenal ARF* reflects direct injury to the renal parenchyma. Acute tubular necrosis is the most common form of intrarenal ARF and may be caused by a variety of insults, such as ischemia and nephrotoxins, that lead to necrosis of the tubular epithelia (see Table 16–1).

In the surgical setting, ATN is frequently encountered

following episodes of hypotension, commonly following resuscitation for septic or hemorrhagic shock. Acute tubular necrosis may also occur postoperatively; however, many factors contribute to postoperative ATN in addition to hypotension, as evidenced by the observation that in 50% of cases no hypotension is documented. In severe renal hypoperfusion, renal tubular epithelial cells develop hypoxia and necrose, especially in areas where the metabolic rate is high. The renal tubule has two areas that have extremely active metabolic function: the proximal tubule and the medullary thick ascending loop of Henle as part of the countercurrent mechanism. The tubular epithelium is rich in the energy-requiring sodium-potassium (Na^+,K^+-ATPase) pumps, which are susceptible to ischemia. Despite a large fraction of cardiac output going to the kidney (20%), a delicate balance exists between oxygen delivery and oxygen consumption within regions of the cortex and medulla. Even in the presence of relatively adequate RBF, severe hypoxia of tubular epithelium can develop. Ischemic epithelia slough into and obstruct the tubular lumen, producing clinically diagnostic granular casts and increased tubular backpressure. Backleak of tubular fluid exacerbates renal ischemia by further intensifying intrarenal vasoconstriction and decreasing GFR. In experimental models, the use of individual renal protective agents, such as volume loading with saline, osmotic diuresis with mannitol, vasodilatation with dopamine, furosemide, or prostaglandin E_1, can lessen the tubular ischemia and backleak, resulting in less oliguria and a more rapid recovery.

Ischemic ATN secondary to renal artery occlusion is a rare cause of ARF that the general surgeon encounters primarily in the setting of blunt or penetrating trauma. The diagnosis is suggested by nonvisualization of the kidney on computed tomography (CT) evaluation or intravenous pyelogram. Irreversible renal injury develops rapidly in the setting of warm ischemia; thus, revascularization within 6 hours is the treatment goal. Controversy exists regarding the role of revascularization when the diagnosis of renal artery thrombosis is made beyond 4 to 6 hours and overall renal salvage is low (<10%); however, case reports indicate salvage in kidneys revascularized up to 12 hours after injury. Furthermore, in situations in which a patient's solitary kidney is at risk, harvesting, cooling, and autotransplantation has been successfully performed.

A number of agents frequently used or encountered in the care of general surgery patients can result in nephrotoxic ATN (see Table 16–1). Antimicrobial agents commonly used in surgical patients reported to cause ATN include aminoglycosides and amphotericin B. Aminoglycoside nephrotoxicity occurs in a startling 5% to 15% of patients treated with these drugs. In the setting of renal insufficiency, aminoglycosides also cause ototoxicity. Recognition of injury is delayed from its onset, since creatinine does not begin to increase until 7 to 10 days later. Aminoglycoside ARF is dose-dependent and nephrotoxicity is related to the serum concentration, particularly trough levels. Clinical guidelines have been developed for the drug concentration monitoring and dosing of aminoglycosides, including both peak and trough levels, typically for gentamicin. Improved understanding of the pharmacodynamics and toxicity of aminoglycoside antibiotics has resulted in the study of once-daily dosing regimens. Although studies have suggested a therapeutic advantage and possibly a decrease in toxicity with once-daily administration, these effects have been modest. However, the cost savings and simplicity with once-daily dosing makes this approach appealing.

Aminoglycosides are filtered into the proximal tubule, bind to anionic brush-border membrane phospholipids, and become absorbed into intracellular lysosomes where, when released, they damage membranes and inhibit oxidative phosphorylation, resulting in ATN. Aminoglycoside nephrotoxicity is enhanced by the interaction of NSAIDs, endotoxin, cyclosporin A, and amphotericin B and electrolyte disorders, such as hypercalcemia, hypomagnesemia, hypokalemia, and metabolic acidosis. Increased nephrotoxicity is also reported in patients receiving concurrent antimicrobial therapy with cephalosporins. In the setting of concurrent risk factors, it is recommended to utilize equally effective non-nephrotoxic antibiotics, such as extended-spectrum penicillins, cephalosporins, carbapenems, and monobactams.

Amphotericin B used for systemic fungal infections causes nephrotoxicity in most patients. It is strongly bound to cellular membranes and alters permeability. This effect on the renal tubular epithelium leads to failure of hydrogen ion excretion and urinary loss of potassium, resulting in the development of a distal type of renal tubular acidosis with hypokalemia. The loss of renal function is proportional to the dose of amphotericin, and irreversible renal failure occurs at high doses (>2 g). Saline loading at the time of administration may reduce toxicity. Encapsulation of amphotericin B in liposomes or complexing of the compound with other lipid carriers

brings about a major reduction in toxicity, and these formulations are being utilized with increasing frequency. In patients with evidence of baseline or acquired renal insufficiency, transition to these formulations should be considered.

Another drug-related form of intrarenal ARF is interstitial nephritis, which has been classically reported following methicillin use; however, it has also been observed with other antibiotics and medications (sulfamethoxazole, rifampin). Drug-induced interstitial nephritis is considered to be of allergic origin and is often associated with a skin rash and eosinophilia. Radiocontrast-associated ARF is relatively common because of its ubiquitous use in the diagnostic and interventional treatment of general surgery patients. Contrast-induced ARF usually presents within 48 hours of exposure, with the serum Cr peaking at 3 to 5 days. Frequently, these patients have underappreciated pre-existing intrinsic renal insufficiency concurrently with other risk factors, such as advanced age, diabetes mellitus, volume depletion, and a large dye load. The risk of contrast-associated ARF can be reduced by the administration of intravenous saline to ensure a replete intravascular volume prior to exposure. Osmotic or loop diuretics have been used in addition to saline but have not consistently improved renal preservation over intravenous fluid alone.

Myoglobinuria is a frequent cause of nephrotoxic ARF in the surgical population. Patients with crush injuries, electrical burns, necrotizing soft-tissue infections, or ischemia-reperfusion syndromes, such as after revascularization, or who develop compartment syndromes are at high risk for rhabdomyolysis and myoglobinuria. Myoglobin is filtered and precipitates in the renal tubules, obstructing fluid flow, while the heme molecule causes direct toxicity to the tubular epithelium. Patients with myoglobinuria present with dark port-wine or tea-colored urine, which may be confused with gross hematuria initially. Serum levels of creatine phosphokinase (CPK) characteristically are sky-high, greater than 10,000 U/mL, in patients with the full-blown disease.

Postrenal ARF results from obstruction of the urinary collection system at one of several levels. Obstruction must usually be prolonged and bilateral to result in ARF, and the prognosis for recovery is dependent on the duration of obstruction. A palpable bladder on examination indicates more than 500 mL of retained urine, consistent with obstruction. In the perioperative or postinjury patient, it is important to demonstrate that indwelling bladder catheters are patent and are not obstructed, and thus are not the cause of ARF.

The acute development of abdominal compartment syndrome is increasingly being recognized as a cause of ARF, requiring intervention by the general surgeon. Surgical patients can develop this syndrome following large volume resuscitation, placement of intra-abdominal packing for control of hemorrhage, prolonged operation with "tight" abdominal fascial closure, and diffuse peritonitis. The diagnosis is made clinically in a patient with high peak inspiratory pressures and carbon dioxide retention on the ventilator, progressive oliguria, and abdominal rigidity. Bladder pressures are measured in complex cases to confirm the clinical diagnosis, with more than 20 to

30 mm Hg considered significant to warrant abdominal decompression, although no absolute level of intra-abdominal hypertension is considered to be an indication for decompression. In the setting of acute abdominal compartment syndrome, ARF can be caused by decreased venous return from the vena cava, resulting in reduced cardiac output; increased pressure on the renal parenchyma, causing reduced renal blood flow; and increased renal venous pressure. Recent laboratory work suggests that increased renal venous pressure is the major contributing mechanism. In experimental models, decreasing renal venous pressure while holding constant both renal parenchymal pressure and cardiac output can reverse oliguria completely.

DIAGNOSTIC EVALUATION

The evaluation of the patient with ARF has two major goals: to determine the cause and potential therapy; and to assess the extent of complications and need for supportive care. The history and physical examination may provide evidence suggesting the cause; however, they are even more important in assessing the severity of the sequelae of ARF.

Evaluation of volume status is critical in the setting of low urine output and rising BUN and Cr. Body weight, daily input and output, neck vein distention, peripheral edema, ascites, fever, gastrointestinal losses, diuretic use, and maintenance intravenous fluids all take on increased importance in determining whether the patient has a prerenal component to ARF. Direct measurement of central venous pressure or pulmonary capillary occlusion pressure is recommended as an aid in the determination of intravascular volume status and in optimizing renal perfusion in the perioperative or postinjury patient.

Serum and urine chemistries can assist the clinician in the diagnosis and management of the patient with oliguria (Table 16–2). The fractional excretion of sodium (FENa) and urine sodium are useful measurements of how actively the kidney is resorbing sodium and reflect renal perfusion and intravascular volume status. In prerenal ARF, the kidney is hypoperfused; therefore, it actively resorbs Na, and both the urine Na and FENa are *low*. In contrast, renal parenchymal damage results in the loss of resorption of Na, and the urine Na and FENa are *high*.

Table 16–2	Indices That Distinguish Prerenal ARF From ATN	
MEASUREMENT	**PRERENAL ARF**	**ATN**
Specific gravity	>1.020	< or ≃1.010
FENa	<0.1 to 1%	>1% preferably >3%
Urine osmolality	>500	<350 or ≃300
Urine sodium	<20	>40
Serum BUN/Cr	>20	<15 or 10–15
Microscopic sediment	Hyaline casts	Brown granular casts

FENa = Fractional excretion of sodium(%) = 100 × (urine Na × serum Cr)/(urine Cr × serum Na).

BUN/Cr = blood urea nitrogen–to–creatinine ratio.

CrCl = creatinine clearance = urine Cr × [timed urine volume (mL/min)]/serum Cr.

The use of diuretics, particularly loop diuretics, can confound these measurements. Thus, measurements are best taken prior to their administration. Creatinine clearance, which measures GFR, can be estimated from a 2-hour timed urine collection (see Table 16–2). The urine sediment is also useful in establishing a diagnosis. Muddy-brown coarse granular casts in the urine sediment are the classic finding in ATN, while white cell casts with eosinophiluria are seen in interstitial nephritis. Urine that dips positive for blood in the absence of red blood cells (RBCs/HPF) on microscopic examination suggests that hemoglobinuria or myoglobinuria is present. This combination suggests rhabdomyolysis or hemolysis as the cause of ARF.

Renal ultrasound imaging should be considered early, to exclude obstruction in ARF. It documents that both kidneys are present and may identify other pathology, while duplex scanning can demonstrate RBF. Renal ultrasound also allows determination of kidney size; for example, small kidneys indicate a chronic condition with superimposed acute deterioration; a thin renal cortex indicates a diminished chance for recovery of function.

THERAPY

Therapeutic options (Fig. 16–1) for ARF depend on its cause. Prerenal ARF is diagnosed and treated by restoration of renal perfusion. Postrenal ARF frequently requires mechanical intervention, which may be as simple as the placement of a Foley catheter or the more complicated placement of nephrostomy tubes or a laparotomy. *There is no known therapy for modifying the course of ATN once it has become established.* The clinician must strive to remove the cause of the disease and provide supportive care until the return of adequate renal function.

RESTORATION OF INTRAVASCULAR VOLUME. The initial goal in the management of the perioperative or postinjury patient with ARF is the optimization of the patient's hemodynamic status and, by inference, renal perfusion. Even in patients clinically suspected of having ATN, intravascular volume should be normalized, as assessed by clinical findings and the monitoring of arterial blood pressure and cardiac filling pressures (preload) utilizing either central venous pressure or pulmonary capillary occlusion pressure. If the patient does not respond appropriately to volume loading with increased central venous pressure and increased urine output, a pulmonary artery catheter should be utilized to measure cardiac output and oxygen delivery. Sepsis indicates decreased ventricular compliance and the need for higher-than-normal filling pressures to generate the same cardiac output. Despite concerns of fluid overload resulting from falling urine output, surgical patients frequently require generous amounts of intravenous fluid or blood to optimize preload. Even if hemodynamic parameters appear adequate, a trial of fluid is recommended early in the course of oliguric ARF.

DIURETICS. If renal function does not improve significantly after optimization of intravascular volume, a trial of furosemide (40 to 320 mg IV in increasing doses) or mannitol (12.5 to 25 g IV) is recommended. These agents

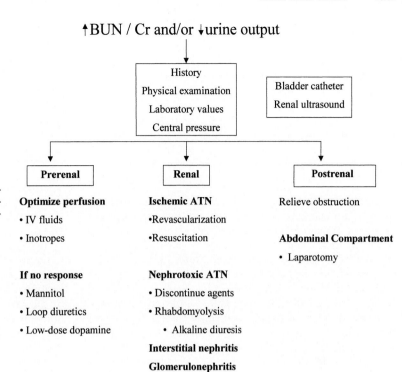

↑BUN / Cr and/or ↓urine output

History
Physical examination
Laboratory values
Central pressure

Bladder catheter
Renal ultrasound

Prerenal

Renal

Postrenal

Optimize perfusion
• IV fluids
• Inotropes

Ischemic ATN
•Revascularization
•Resuscitation

Relieve obstruction

Abdominal Compartment
• Laparotomy

If no response
• Mannitol
• Loop diuretics
• Low-dose dopamine

Nephrotoxic ATN
• Discontinue agents
• Rhabdomyolysis
  • Alkaline diuresis

Interstitial nephritis

Glomerulonephritis

Figure 16–1. Simplified therapeutic approach to oliguric renal failure indicating three major classifications—prerenal, renal, and postrenal—and indicated therapies.

dilate renal arterioles, increase solute clearance, and help to relieve tubular obstruction. Furthermore, these agents help convert oliguric ARF to nonoliguric ARF. If the urine output does not respond to the initial dose of mannitol, it should be stopped. Intravascular osmotic load exacerbates fluid overload and can cause pulmonary or cerebral edema. Furosemide, if ineffective alone, can be combined with metolazone (5 to 10 mg orally) or chlorothiazide (500 mg IV) to improve urine output. It is important to exercise care in patients with anuria. Repeated doses of furosemide can lead to complications, such as deafness and allergic interstitial nephritis. In patients who respond to diuretics, an individual agent or a combination furosemide-mannitol drip can be used and titrated to response (a common recipe is 250 mL of 5% dextrose in water (D_5W), 200 mg of furosemide, and 12.5 g of mannitol).

DOPAMINE. Low-dose dopamine (1 to 3 μg/kg per minute), administered alone or with diuretics, has been used to increase RBF in patients with sepsis or liver failure. Many clinicians believe that low-dose dopamine confers renal protection even though no controlled, prospective data support it. The lack of data on the efficacy of renal dose dopamine in preventing the need for dialysis and improving patient mortality has done little to dampen its use for patients with sepsis and oliguria. Low-dose dopamine activates renal dopaminergic receptors, thus producing increased RBF, GFR, and urine sodium excretion. It benefits renal perfusion without affecting systemic cardiac output. Experimental data do suggest a role for dopamine in the management of oliguric ARF. In subjects receiving a norepinephrine infusion between 0.2 and 1.6 μg/kg per minute, the addition of dopamine increased RBF by 40% to 50%. Thus, the administration of low-dose dopamine seems rational, especially when the clini-

cal situation requires the concomitant infusion of other inotropic or vasopressor agents, such as norepinephrine or dobutamine.

In patients with septic shock, profound hypotension, and oliguria, vasopressor therapy with norepinephrine may actually *improve* renal function by enhancing renal perfusion pressure to a greater extent than its vasoconstriction effects would normally allow. This enhancement may be applicable as well to patients with chronic hypertension who normally have higher mean arterial pressures (MAP) and require perfusion pressures at these levels to maintain RBF. In a study of 25 patients with septic shock and profoundly low systemic vascular resistance (MAP consistently <50 mm Hg), it was found that renal function was refractory to intravascular volume loading and low-dose dopamine infusion. When an infusion of norepinephrine was added at 0.5 to 1.5 μg/kg per minute and dopamine was maintained at a "renal" dose (2 to 3 μg/kg per minute), the cardiac index did not change, but MAP increased significantly and urine flow and creatinine clearance also increased significantly. This and other studies demonstrating increased urine output with the addition of dopamine to diuretic and vasopressor therapy strongly suggest that renal autoregulation is impaired in sepsis and the maintenance of adequate renal perfusion pressure is critical to renal protection and optimal recovery.

ATRIAL NATRIURETIC PEPTIDE. Although no new therapies have been identified that modify the clinical course of ATN, several promising agents are under investigation. Investigators have compared the effect of hemorrhage and myocardial ischemia on renal function following a 50% reduction in cardiac output and aortic pressure. After hemorrhage, RBF decreased 90% with cortical ischemia and oliguria, while during cardiogenic shock RBF decreased only 25% with preservation of urine flow. The difference is that in cardiogenic shock, left atrial pressure is maintained at normal or elevated levels. This suggests that an important renal protective effect of atrial distention is attributable to the release of atrial natriuretic peptide (ANP). Subsequent investigation has identified ANP as an endogenous hormone that has improved renal function in animal models of ARF due to ATN. In a recent multicenter, randomized, double-blinded, placebo-controlled study, 504 subjects with all types of ATN received a synthetic form of ANP; however, no beneficial effect on dialysis requirements or mortality was observed.

SPECIFIC THERAPIES. Patients with myoglobinuria require additional specific therapy in addition to the optimization of renal perfusion and diuresis to minimize the extent of ARF. First, it is necessary to push urine output much higher than is necessary for fluid and electrolyte balance. Urine output should be maintained at more than 150 mL/hr through the initial phases of treatment in order to dilute and clear precipitated and free myoglobin from the tubules. In the normovolemic patient with ongoing intravenous fluid resuscitation, mannitol (1 g/kg initially) is added to further induce an osmotic diuresis. Second, urine pH should be increased above 7, since myoglobin precipitation is lower at alkaline pHs. This is accomplished by adding sodium bicarbonate to the intravenous fluids, monitoring urine pH at frequent intervals, and utilizing diuretics that promote an alkaline urine such as the carbonic anhydrase inhibitor acetazolamide rather than furosemide, which tends to create an acidic urine. The overall goal is to produce a high-output alkaline diuresis.

In patients with acute abdominal compartment syndrome, laparotomy relieves intra-abdominal hypertension. The response to abdominal decompression is usually dramatic and lifesaving, although standard treatments for ARF involving volume loading and inotropes are not effective here.

Several approaches to wound closure have been recommended, which include leaving the fascia open and closing the skin; however, bridging the fascial defect with prosthetic mesh is recommended, preferably with absorb-able material to reduce the risk of fistulization and to leave the skin open. The remaining wound is covered with an impermeable plastic drape to reduce fluid losses through the mesh. Reoperation to perform fascial closure within 3 to 5 days is not uncommon if the underlying process is successfully controlled and the patient starts to "auto-diurese."

COMPLICATIONS

The mainstay of therapy for intrarenal ARF is controlling the complications of volume, osmotic, and mineral balance until the return of adequate renal function (Table 16–3).

In oliguric patients, fluid intake must be rigorously monitored. Medications should be given in the smallest volume acceptable. Parenteral nutrition should be concentrated. A reasonable goal is for input to equal output, or the volume of maintenance fluids to equal measured fluid losses (urine, gastrointestinal fluid, surgical drains) plus insensible losses, which can be estimated at 600 mL/day (or higher if the patient is febrile). Nutritional support in the setting of ARF should have the same goals of caloric and nitrogen equilibrium as in the surgical patient without ARF. Protein support should not be withheld for fear of causing uremic complications, as this exacerbates the wasting of lean body mass and vital organs (liver, heart, gut, diaphragm) and leads to deficits in wound healing, immune response, and the patient's ability to wean from the ventilator. Nutritional support should take priority, and the development of uremic symptoms or other complications should be treated with renal replacement therapy, not a reduction in nutrition.

Potassium should almost never be administered to an oliguric patient. A particularly deceptive and dangerous situation is the patient with high-output ATN in which potentially large volumes of urine are produced but potassium is not excreted. Hyperkalemia can develop rapidly in this situation if normal urine losses are assumed and electrolyte replacement is performed empirically. Potassium replacement should be governed by direct measure-

Table 16–3	**Complications of Acute Renal Failure**		
COMPLICATION	**CLINICAL CONSEQUENCE**		**THERAPY**
Volume overload	Pulmonary edema		Fluid and sodium restriction
	Respiratory failure		Diuretics
Hyperkalemia	Arrhythmia		Potassium restriction
	Ventricular tachycardia		Calcium gluconate (10%)
	Heart block		Glucose (D_{50}) and insulin
			Sodium bicarbonate (7.5%)
			Cation-exchange resin
Metabolic acidosis	Hyperventilation		Sodium bicarbonate for <15 mEq/L
Hyponatremia	Water imbalance		Fluid restriction
Hypocalcemia	Carpopedal spasm		Phosphate-binding antacids
Hyperphosphatemia	Arrhythmia		Avoid magnesium antacids
Hypermagnesemia			Supplemental calcium
Uremic syndrome	Nausea and vomiting		Renal replacement therapy
	Pericarditis or pleuritis		Hemodialysis
	Mental status changes		Hemofiltration
	Anemia		
	Platelet dysfunction		

ment of urine electrolytes at frequent intervals if the urine output is high (>500 mL/hr). Another worrisome situation for rapid development of hyperkalemia is clinical rhabdomyolysis. Here, the muscle necrosis releases large amounts of potassium and phosphorus, frequently resulting in the need for aggressive therapy and, not infrequently, early dialysis. The first and immediate treatment of symptomatic hyperkalemia (K^+ >6.5, or significant electrocardiographic findings of peaked T waves, widening of the QRS complex) is 10% calcium gluconate (5 to 10 mL IV over 2 minutes), which antagonizes the cardiac and neuromuscular effects. Glucose (50 mL of D_{50}), insulin (5 to 10 units regular IV over 5 minutes), and sodium bicarbonate (50 mL IV over 5 minutes) have an onset of 30 to 60 minutes and work primarily by shifting potassium into cells. Binding resins (15 to 30 g of resin in 50 to 100 mL of 20% sorbitol PO, or by enema every 4 hours) have an onset of several hours and exchange potassium for sodium.

RENAL REPLACEMENT. Several approaches to renal replacement therapy are available for the surgical patient in ARF. Intermittent hemodialysis has the greatest experience and established efficacy; however, over the last decade, the availability of highly permeable membranes has allowed development of continuous renal replacement therapy (CRRT), which gradually removes fluids and solutes, resulting in better hemodynamic stability and fluid and solute control (Table 16–4). Dialysis therapy is indicated when the level of waste products in the blood is toxic or when fluid balance cannot be maintained with the use of medication or restriction. There is no evidence that dialysis shortens the course of ARF, and because of potential complications of this therapy it should be reserved for well-documented complications of ARF. These are listed in Table 16–3 and include volume overload, acidosis, hyperkalemia, coma or seizure, uremic bleeding, and pericarditis. Absolute levels of BUN or Cr are not as important a factor in the decision to start dialysis as is the patient's overall condition.

Dialysis alters the solute composition of blood by exposing it to a dialysate through a semipermeable membrane. Solute removal is affected by several factors, including (1) the molecular size of the solute; (2) its concentration gradient between blood and the dialysate solution;

(3) the rate of blood flow through the dialyzer; (4) the area of the membrane and its ultrafiltration capacity; (5) the transmembrane pressure; and (6) time. Regular dialysis, done three times per week for 4 hours at a blood flow rate of 200 mL/min gives the patient the equivalent of an average weekly GFR of 10 to 15 mL/min. Unfortunately, intermittent hemodialysis in the intensive care unit setting is frequently associated with hypotension, hypoxemia, and cardiac arrhythmias, which limit the actual time for solute and fluid removal. Extensive evidence indicates that hemodialysis also activates circulating leukocytes, which exacerbate renal injury and may prolong or prevent recovery.

Patients who do not tolerate intermittent hemodialysis can be provided renal replacement through the use of a variety of continuous, low-flow techniques that differ in the access utilized and in the principal method of solute clearance. The simplest is slow continuous ultrafiltration (SCUF), which uses MAP as the driving force. A dialysate solution can be added to the hemofiltration to assist solute removal. This is termed *continuous arteriovenous hemodialysis* (CAVHD). If MAP is inadequate (<70 to 80), the use of a pump within a venovenous circuit can be an alternative. This is termed *continuous venovenous hemofiltration* or *hemodialysis* (CVVH or CVVHD). The advantage of continuous techniques, compared with intermittent dialysis, is that they are well tolerated in hypotension and allow a greater volume of fluid removal, facilitating nutritional support. The disadvantages of this approach are the need for anticoagulation and the high volume of replacement fluid that must be closely monitored. The use of CRRTs associated with the clearance of inflammatory mediators from the circulation suggests that these methods may also have an impact on the course of renal failure, multiple organ dysfunction, and ultimately mortality in patients with sepsis or systemic inflammation. Experimental evidence in models of sepsis suggests that hemofiltration has a beneficial impact in severe sepsis; however, because human evidence of mediator-derived benefits of hemofiltration is anecdotal, the primary indications for continuous renal replacement for ARF patients are refractory volume overload, the need for large amounts of blood products, and intolerance to intermittent hemodialysis due to hypotension or arrhythmias.

Table 16–4	Comparison of Continuous Renal Replacement Therapy Techniques (CRRT)				
	SCUF	**CAVH**	**CVVH**	**CAVHD**	**CVVHD**
Access	A-V	A-V	V-V	A-V	V-V
Pump	No	No	Yes	No	Yes
Filtrate (mL/hr)	100	600	1000	300	300
Filtrate (L/day)	2.4	14.4	24	7.2	7.2
Dialysate flow (L/hr)	0	0	0	1.0	1.0
Replacement fluid (L/day)	0	12	21.6	4.8	4.8
Urea clearance (mL/min)	1.7	10	16.7	21.7	21.7
Simplicity	1	2	3	2	3

Simplicity ranked 1–4; 1 = most simple; 4 = most difficult.
SCUF, slow continuous ultrafiltration; CAVH, continuous arteriovenous hemofiltration; CVVH, continuous venovenous hemofiltration; CAVHD, continuous arteriovenous hemodialysis; CVVHD, continuous venovenous hemodialysis.
Modified from Mehta RL: Continuous renal replacement therapies in the acute renal failure setting: Current concepts. Adv Ren Replace Ther 4(2 suppl 1):81–92.

Pearls and Pitfalls

PEARLS

- The initial goal in the management of the perioperative or postinjury patient with ARF is the optimization of the patient's hemodynamic status. Even if hemodynamic parameters appear adequate, a trial of fluid is recommended early in the course of oliguric ARF.
- An anastomotic leak or intra-abdominal abscess can cause renal failure with or without signs of systemic infection.
- Prerenal ARF results from the loss of effective circulating volume without direct parenchymal damage to the kidney unless the hypoperfusion is unrecognized or undertreated, resulting in progression to ATN.
- Low-dose dopamine (1 to 3 μg/kg per minute), administered alone or in combination with vasopressors such as norepinephrine, has been used to increase RBF in disease processes associated with renal vasoconstriction, such as sepsis or liver failure.
- Patients with myoglobinuria require additional specific therapy in addition to the optimization of renal perfusion and diuresis to minimize the extent of ARF. Urine output should be maintained at more than 150 mL/hr through the initial phases of treatment so as to dilute and clear precipitated and free myoglobin from the tubules. Second, urine pH should be increased above 7, since myoglobin precipitation is lower at alkaline pHs. The overall goal is to produce a high-output *alkaline diuresis.*

- Nutritional support in the setting of ARF should have the same goals of caloric and nitrogen equilibrium as the surgical patient without ARF.
- The primary indications for CRRT for ARF patients are refractory volume overload, the need for large amounts of blood products, and intolerance to intermittent hemodialysis due to hypotension or arrhythmias.
- In patients who are still producing urine, a loop diuretic, such as furosemide, administered in combination with a thiazide (cortical collecting tubule) diuretic, such as hydrochlorothiazide or metolazone, may improve urine output.

PITFALLS

- The decision to use once-daily dosing of aminoglycoside agents in perioperative or postinjury patients must also take into account the altered and shifting drug volume of distribution and clearance in these patients. Nephrotoxicity occurs in a startling 5% to 15% of patients treated with these drugs.
- In the setting of concurrent risk factors, it is recommended to utilize equally effective non-nephrotoxic antibiotics, such as extended-spectrum penicillins, cephalosporins, carbapenems, and monobactams.
- Nutritional support should take priority, and the development of uremic symptoms should be treated with renal replacement therapy, not a reduction in nutrition.

PROGNOSIS

The prognosis of the patient with ARF is highly dependent on resolution of the underlying disease. No patient should die of uremia or its metabolic consequences. In the oliguric patient with ARF whose underlying disease process resolves, renal function returns, on average, in 10 to 21 days. Statistically, about 10% of patients demonstrate no recovery of function and about 30% show only partial recovery; therefore, surviving patients have a high likelihood of becoming dialysis independent.

SELECTED READINGS

Corwin H, Lisbon A: Renal dose dopamine: Long on conjecture, short on fact. Crit Care Med 2000;28:1657.

Doty J, Saggi B, Blocher C, et al: Effects of increased renal parenchymal pressure on renal function. J Trauma 2000;48:874.

Fisman D, Kaye K: Once-daily dosing of aminoglycoside antibiotics. Infect Dis Clin North Am 2000;14:475.

Hesselvik J, Brodin B: Low-dose norepinephrine in patients with septic shock and oliguria: Effects on afterload, urine flow, and oxygen transport. Crit Care Med 1989;17:179.

Johnson J, Rokaw M: Sepsis or ischemia in experimental acute renal failure: What have we learned? New Horizons 1995;3:608.

Lewis J, Salem M, Chertow G, Weisburg L, McGrew F, Marbury T, Allegren R, and Anaritide Acute Renal Failure Study Group: Atrial natriuretic factor in oliguric acute renal failure. Am J Kidney Dis 2000;36:767.

Mindell J, Chertow G: A practical approach to acute renal failure. Med Clin North Am 1997;81:731.

Rogiers P: Hemofiltration treatment for sepsis: Is it time for controlled trials? Kidney Int 1999;56(suppl 72):S99.

Rosenberg M: Acute renal failure. In Abrams J, Cerra F (eds): Essentials of Surgical Critical Care. St. Louis, Quality Medical Publishing, 1993.

Solomon R, Werner C, Mann D, et al: Effects of saline, mannitol, and furosemide to prevent decreases in renal function induced by radiocontrast agents. N Engl J Med 1994;331:1416.

Thadani R, Pascual M, Bonventre JV: Acute renal failure. N Engl J Med 1996;334:1448.

Chapter 17

Adrenal Insufficiency
David T. Efron, Gershon Efron, and Adrian Barbul

The adrenal glands are formed by the fusion of two embryologically distinct entities. At about the fourth week of gestation, the cortex develops from the mesoderm adjacent to the urogenital ridge, whereas the medulla is derived from neuroectoderm after the sixth week of development.

The cortex itself is highly structured and comprises three different histologic and hormone-secreting layers. The outer layer, designated the zona glomerulosa, is the source of mineralocorticoid secretion. The intermediate layer, the zona fasciculata, secretes primarily glucocorticoids and, to a lesser degree, androgens. The inner layer, the zona reticularis, secretes primarily androgens, but it is also a source of some glucocorticoid production.

The adrenal medulla, which produces catecholamines (epinephrine and norepinephrine), is regulated principally by neuronal stimulation. The production of catecholamines and the physiologic response to their release depend on adequate levels of glucocorticoids.

NORMAL ADRENAL PHYSIOLOGY

The accurate diagnosis and successful treatment of patients with potentially lethal adrenal insufficiency necessitate an understanding of the normal physiology of the adrenal gland. Although all three types of adrenocortical hormones exert important biologic effects, disruption of glucocorticoid and mineralocorticoid activity is life-threatening. The secretion of each of these hormones is controlled by discrete physiologic autoregulatory systems. Disturbances of androgen physiology have a profound effect on sexual development and physical characteristics, but they are not life-threatening, and have a minor role in the treatment of adrenal insufficiency.

Glucocorticoids play an essential role in maintaining physiologic homeostasis and the regulation of both the inflammatory and metabolic responses exhibited during major stress, such as occurs with trauma, hemorrhage, surgery, and sepsis. These responses include regulation of blood pressure, immune reactivity, and modulation of energy production from glucose, proteins, and lipids. Normally, cortisol secretion is stimulated directly by adrenocorticotropin (ACTH) released from the anterior pituitary. ACTH release, itself, is stimulated by corticotropin-releasing hormone (CRH), which is produced in the hypothalamus. Production of both ACTH and CRH are inhibited by cortisol in a feedback loop. In times of stress and injury, glucocorticoid production is increased in response to heightened metabolic demand.

Although ACTH can stimulate aldosterone secretion, mineralocorticoid physiology is regulated primarily by the renin-angiotensin pathway. Disruption of aldosterone activity results in an inappropriately low serum sodium (hyponatremia) and high serum potassium (hyperkalemia) concentrations. Both the hypothalamo-pituitary-adrenal axis and the renin-angiotensin-aldosterone axis are detailed in Figure 17–1.

Glucocorticoids and mineralocorticoids have distinct regulatory pathways; thus, identifying whether the renin-aldosterone pathway is intact is helpful in discerning whether the existing adrenal insufficiency is primary or secondary in origin. The distinction is important, as the treatment of primary adrenal insufficiency necessitates mineralocorticoid replacement in addition to glucocorticoid therapy. It should be remembered that glucocorticoids have some mineralocorticoid activity and that mineralocorticoid replacement may not be required until glucocortiocoid replacement is tapered below a daily dose of 50 mg of hydrocortisone equivalent.

DEFINITION AND DIAGNOSIS OF ADRENAL INSUFFICIENCY

Adrenal insufficiency, which is defined as the inability of the adrenal gland to secrete corticosteroids, is classified as being primary or secondary. The onset may be acute or chronic. Primary adrenal insufficiency results from the destruction of the adrenals themselves, which thereby deletes the source of the hormones. Secondary adrenal insufficiency is due to impaired adrenal gland stimulation either from hypothalamic or pituitary dysfunction, but it occurs more commonly as the result of protracted glucocorticoid therapy. Intake of exogenous glucocorticoids suppresses the hypothalamo-pituitary-adrenal axis. As with other forms of secondary adrenal insufficiency, impaired ACTH stimulation results in adrenocortical atrophy and the subsequent inability of the adrenal gland to produce appropriate levels of glucocorticoids. A comprehensive list of the causes of adrenal insufficiency is given in Figure 17–2. Since destruction of the cortex affects all the resident cell types, with the rare exception of isolated glucocorticoid deficiency, reduced glucocorticoid secretion noted in primary adrenal insufficiency is always accompanied by decreased or absent mineralocorticoid secretion.

The signs and symptoms of adrenal insufficiency are nonspecific (see Fig. 17–2). However, a number of findings that result from the underlying cause of adrenal insufficiency may aid in diagnosis. It is important to note that several causes of secondary adrenal insufficiency are associated with endocrinopathies that result from disruption of other pituitary-dependent endocrine glandular axes.

Addison's disease is due to chronic primary adrenal insufficiency secondary to the destruction of the cortex, leading to a deficiency of both glucocorticoids and miner-

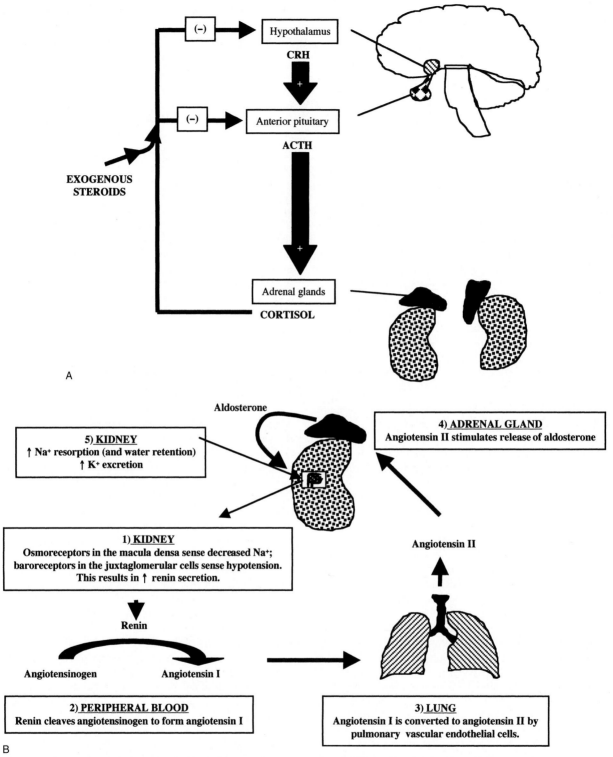

Figure 17–1. *A,* The hypothalamo-pituitary-adrenal axis. CRH, and arginine-vasopressin, produced in the hypothalamus stimulate ACTH secretion in the anterior pituitary. ACTH, in turn, stimulates cortisol secretion in the adrenal glands. Cortisol secretion occurs in a diurnal pattern, with maximal secretion in the early morning. Cortisol inhibits both CRH and ACTH secretion in a negative-feedback loop. *B,* The renin-angiotensin-aldosterone axis. Sodium sensors in the macula densa and baroreceptors in the juxtaglomerular cells of the kidney respond to a change in electrolyte balance and to decreased arterial pressure, respectively, leading to increased renin production and release. Renin, in turn, cleaves the plasma protein angiotensinogen to form angiotensin I. Angiotensin I is subsequently converted to angiotensin II by the vascular endothelial cells of the lung. In addition to being a potent vasoconstrictor, angiotensin II stimulates aldosterone secretion, which in turn acts at the distal renal tubules to increase Na^+ resorption from the urine, thereby retaining intravascular volume.

Primary Adrenal Insufficiency

Inflammatory
  Autoimmune adrenalitis
Infectious
  Tuberculosis
  Fungus
  Opportunistic (HIV/AIDS)
Neoplastic
  Primary (carcinoma)
  Metastases (lung, breast, kidney)
Resection
  Bilateral adrenalectomy
  s/p Unilateral adrenalectomy for
    secreting adrenocortical tumor
Hemorrhage/Necrosis
  Coagulopathy
  Hypotension
Functional adrenal suppression
  Sepsis

Secondary Adrenal Insufficiency

Suppression
  Protracted glucocorticoid Rx
Erosion/Destruction/Necrosis
  Sellar tumor (primary or brain mets)
  Craniopharyngioma
  Hypothalamic tumor
  Sarcoidosis
  Histiocytosis
  Sheehan's syndrome (hemorrhage)
Resection/Trauma
  Hypophysectomy (surgical/XRT)
  Head trauma (blunt/penetrating)
Congenital
  Empty sella syndrome

SIGNS ASSOCIATED WITH PRIMARY INSUFFICIENCY

Hyperpigmentation
Vitiligo
Associated autoimmune thyroid disease

SYMPTOMS OF ADRENAL INSUFFICIENCY

Acute

Fever
Nausea/Vomiting
Abdominal pain/distention
Hypotension (often refractory)
Hyponatremia/hyperkalemia
Obtundation/depressed mental status

Chronic

Fatigue
Orthostatic hypotension
Weight loss/anorexia
Nausea/vomiting
Diarrhea
Dizziness
Hypoglycemia
Anemia

SIGNS ASSOCIATED WITH SECONDARY INSUFFICIENCY

Headache, optical disturbances, diabetes insipidus
Paucity of axillary and pubic hair
Amenorrhea
Small testicles
Decreased libido/potency
Prepubertal growth deficit, delayed puberty
Secondary hypothyroidism

Figure 17–2. The causes of adrenal insufficiency with associated signs and symptoms. (Adapted from Oelkers W: Adrenal insufficiency. N Engl J Med 1996;335:1206–1211.)

alocorticoids. In the absence of negative-feedback inhibition by cortisol, excess CRH is produced. Excessive amounts of melanocortin (which is formed in concert with the secretion of CRH) are responsible for the hyperpigmentation characteristic of this disease.

Acute adrenal insufficiency, commonly referred to as addisonian crisis, is a medical emergency. The signs and symptoms include fever, nausea or vomiting, abdominal pain, and hypotension often refractory to fluids and pressors, abdominal distention, hyponatremia, hyperkalemia, and depressed mental status. Immediate treatment includes fluid resuscitation with normal saline (2 to 3 L) and rapid glucocorticoid replacement. In suspected cases of acute adrenal insufficiency, blood should be drawn to assess basal cortisol and ACTH levels and diagnostic tests for adrenal insufficiency should be initiated. Treatment should commence promptly and should not await the availability of laboratory results.

The diagnosis of adrenal insufficiency is accomplished first by demonstrating decreased plasma cortisol levels, and then by assessing the responsiveness of the adrenals to stimulation. The various tests are outlined in Table 17–1.

SURGICAL IMPLICATIONS OF ADRENAL INSUFFICIENCY

Adrenal insufficiency impacts surgeons in a number of ways:

I. The management of patients who are rendered adrenally insufficient as the result of surgery
  A. Bilateral adrenalectomy is rarely performed at the present time. Historically, this operation was performed as an adjunct in the treatment of androgen-sensitive malignancies as well as for bilateral adrenal hyperplasia (a misdiagnosed cause of Cushing's disease). Following bilateral adrenalectomy, lifelong maintenance glucocorticoid and mineralocorticoid therapy is required. In addition, supplemental doses of steroids must be administered to replicate the normal stress response that is seen even during routine illness. These are frequently given as a "stress-dose" regimen (see later). If maintenance therapy composed of glucocorticoids is tapered below 50 mg/day (hydrocortisone equivalent), mineralocorticoids must

Table 17–1	Tests for the Diagnosis of Adrenal Insufficiency

REASON FOR TEST	HORMONE TEST	NORMAL RANGE	INTERPRETATION RESULTS
Rule out adrenal insufficiency	Measurement of basal plasma cortisol between 8 and 9 AM	Plasma cortisol, 6–24 μg/dL	If plasma cortisol ≤ 3 μg/dL, adrenal insufficiency confirmed; if ≥19 μg/dL, adrenal insufficiency ruled out
	Conventional corticotropin test	Basal or post-corticotropin plasma cortisol, ≥20 μg/dL	Insufficient increase in plasma cortisol in most cases of adrenal insufficiency
	Low-dose corticotropin test	Basal or post-corticotropin plasma cortisol, ≥18 μg/dL	Probably insufficient increase in plasma cortisol in all cases of adrenal insufficiency
Primary adrenal insufficiency	Conventional corticotropin test	Basal or post-corticotropin plasma cortisol, ≥20 μg/dL	No increase in plasma cortisol in primary adrenal insufficiency
	Measurement of basal plasma cortisol and corticotropin	Plasma cortisol, 6–24 μg/dL; plasma corticotropin, 5–45 pg/mL	Plasma cortisol low or in the low-normal range, but plasma corticotropin always > 100 pg/mL in primary adrenal insufficiency
Secondary adrenal insufficiency suspected	Insulin-induced hypoglycemia	Plasma glucose, <40 mg/dL; plasma cortisol, ≥20 μg/dL	Little or no increase in plasma cortisol in secondary adrenal insufficiency
	Short metyrapone test	Plasma 11-deoxycortisol at 8 hr, ≥7 μg/dL; plasma corticotropin, >150 pg/mL	Insufficient increase in plasma corticotropin (very sensitive) and 11-deoxycortisol in secondary adrenal insufficiency
	Corticotropin-releasing hormone test	Depends on dose, time of administration, and species of origin (human, ovine) of corticotropin-releasing hormone	Insufficient increase in plasma corticotropin and cortisol in secondary adrenal insufficiency
	Low-dose corticotropin test	Basal or post-corticotropin plasma cortisol, ≥18 μg/dL	Probably insufficient stimulation in all cases of secondary adrenal insufficiency
Secondary adrenal insufficiency due to hypothalamic disease suspected	Insulin-induced hypoglycemia	Plasma glucose, <40 mg/dL; plasma cortisol, ≥20 μg/dL	Little or no increase in plasma cortisol in secondary adrenal insufficiency due to hypothalamic disease
	Corticotropin-releasing hormone test on different day	Transient increase in plasma corticotropin and cortisol	Prolonged, exaggerated plasma corticotropin response; weak plasma cortisol response in hypothalamic disease

From Oelkers W: Adrenal insufficiency. N Engl J Med 1996;335:1206–1211. Copyright 1996 Massachusetts Medical Society. All rights reserved.

be added (usually fludrocortisone at a dose of 0.1 to 0.2 mg/day).

B. *Unilateral adrenal resection for a glucocorticoid-secreting tumor* may result in postoperative adrenal insufficiency because of suppression of the hypothalamo-pituitary-adrenal axis, the consequence of excessive steroid production by the tumor. The contralateral (nonpathologic) adrenal gland may be atrophied and initially unable to produce enough cortisol to maintain homeostasis after the surgery. Postoperative glucocorticoid therapy with subsequent tapered dosing is indicated as the opposite adrenal gland recovers function.

C. *Pituitary resection (or other base-of-skull surgery)* may disrupt the hypothalamo-pituitary-adrenal axis and accordingly requires cortisol replacement. The hypothalamo-pituitary-thyroid axis is also disrupted; thus, thyroid hormone needs to be administered.

D. *Hypoaldosteronism, which occurs rarely after adrenalectomy* for an aldosteronoma, presents with significant hyperkalemia and hypotension and can last for days to months after the surgery. Treatment with 0.1 to 0.2 mg/day of fludrocortisone corrects the electrolyte imbalance.

II. Patients with known adrenal insufficiency presenting with a surgical problem
   A. *Steroid replacement therapy is essential in the absence of adrenal function.* In addition to the normal daily cortisol requirement, the increased steroid requirement during the stress of surgery and critical illness needs to be covered by supplemental doses of steroid.
   B. *Iatrogenic hypoadrenalism secondary to glucocorticoid therapy* is the most common cause of adrenal insufficiency in the surgical population. As the result of suppression of the hypothalamo-pituitary-adrenal axis, patients may not respond to surgical stress with appropriate glucocorticoid secretion. In all patients rendered adrenal insufficient, adequate steroid coverage is a necessity.

   Traditionally, patients receiving routine steroid therapy who are scheduled for surgery have been treated automatically with "stress-dose" steroids. The standard regimen consists of the administration of 100 mg of hydrocortisone just prior to surgery followed by 50 to 100 mg every 6 hours for 24 to 48 hours thereafter. Subsequently, the dose is tapered to preoperative levels. The rationale of the regimen is to mimic, and perhaps supersede, the body's normal endogenous adrenocortical response to stress.

   The validity of this uniform treatment in all patients receiving steroid therapy has been questioned. The adrenal glands normally produce about 30 mg of cortisol per day, which is equivalent to 7.5 mg of prednisone per day. Many patients who are receiving an equivalent daily dose of steroids do not demonstrate suppression of hypothalamo-pituitary-adrenal axis and therefore are being overtreated by the standard stress-dose regimen. In a comprehensive evidence-based review, Salem and colleagues outlined consensus recommendations for perioperative

steroid replacement that are stratified for the degree of operative stress and designed to mimic the expected endogenous adrenal production of cortisol. The guidelines are summarized in Table 17–2.

   Glucocorticoid replacement should be tailored to the individual patient. It is important that all physicians caring for these patients be vigilant for signs of addisonian crisis, which must be recognized early and treated promptly. Although overtreatment with corticosteroids carries the potential morbidity from impaired healing and immunosuppression, undertreatment is immediately life-threatening.
   C. *Adrenogenital syndrome* is due to a congenital deficiency of the enzyme 21-hydroxylase and results in the failure to produce cortisone from steroid precursors in the adrenal cortex (Fig. 17–3). The excessive accumulation of androgen precursors is exacerbated by the absence of ACTH suppression by cortisol feedback. Additionally, 30% of these patients demonstrate a severe disruption of 21-hydroxylase activity and have salt wasting because of mineralocorticoid deficiency. Patients with adrenogenital syndrome are treated with glucocorticoid therapy to suppress ACTH secretion and the subsequent bilateral adrenal hyperplasia. Awareness of both the degree of the patient's enzyme deficiency and the steroid replacement requirement is essential before one contemplates surgery in these patients and will avoid a potentially disastrous outcome.

III. New-onset adrenal insufficiency in the setting of critical illness
   A. The clinical syndrome of acute adrenal insufficiency is often masked and difficult to diagnose in the setting of the complex pathophysiology associated with critical illness. Adrenal insufficiency can occur in a critically ill patient as the result of either infarction of the adrenals due to protracted hypotension or hemorrhage into the adrenals secondary to coagulopathy. Any patient with hypotension unresponsive to fluid resuscita-

Table 17–2	Perioperative Glucocorticoid Replacement		
	MINOR STRESS	**MODERATE STRESS**	**MAJOR STRESS**
Example of operative stress	Inguinal hernia	Open CCY R hemicolectomy TAH Total joint replacement	Whipple Esophagogastrectomy Total proctocolectomy
Steroid replacement* (duration) Dosing	25 mg (day of) Normal oral steroid dose given immediately preoperatively	50–75 mg (1–2 days) Normal oral steroid dose given immediately preoperatively plus 25–50† mg hydrocortisone IV q8h thereafter	100–150 mg (2–3 days) Normal oral steroid dose given immediately preoperatively plus 25–50† mg hydrocortisone IV q8h thereafter

CCY, cholecystectomy; R, right; TAH, total abdominal hysterectomy.
*Doses given represent daily requirements given in hydrocortisone equivalents.
†Actual dose is dependent on the preoperative steroid dose. If the patient is maintained on 5 mg/day prednisone, 25 mg of hydrocortisone q8h may be appropriate, whereas patients normally receiving 40 mg prednisone/day will probably require 50 mg hydrocortisone q8h.

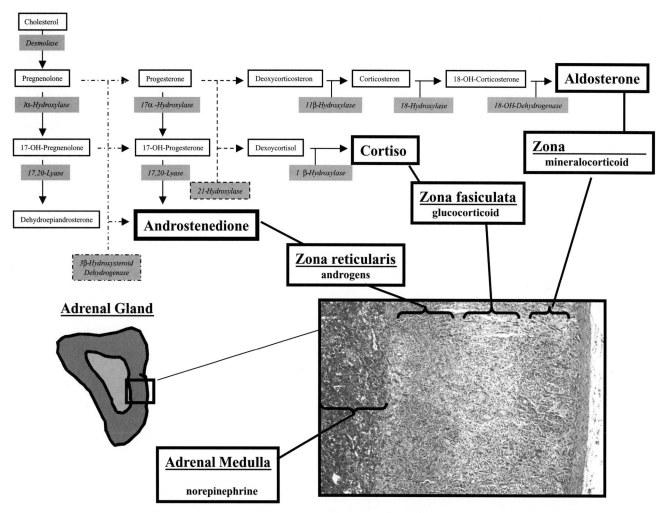

Figure 17–3. Histologic section of the adrenal gland showing all layers and the hormones primarily produced by each. The corticosteroid-forming metabolic pathways are outlined. 21-Hydroxylase deficiency is the most common congenital enzyme deficiency resulting in bilateral adrenal hyperplasia pathologically and female pseudohermaphroditism clinically (low-power hematoxylin and eosin stain of normal human adrenal tissue). (Courtesy of Deepa Dutta, MD, Department of Pathology, Sinai Hospital of Baltimore.)

Pearls and Pitfalls

PEARLS

- Differentiation between primary and secondary causes of adrenal insufficiency is key to appropriate treatment.
- Autoimmune adrenalitis is currently the most common cause of primary adrenal insufficiency (Addison's disease); glucocorticoid therapy is the most common cause of secondary adrenal insufficiency.
- Hyperpigmentation is a feature of primary adrenal insufficiency.
- Petechiae in the patient with acute adrenal insufficiency suggests hemorrhagic infarction of the adrenal glands secondary to meningococcemia (Waterhouse-Friderichsen syndrome).
- Prophylactic perioperative steroid replacement should be individualized to the operative stress that is anticipated.

- The management of adrenogenital syndrome with cortisol requires evaluation for salt wasting, which, if present, needs to be corrected prior to surgery.
- Perioperative steroid support is recommended in patients with Cushing's syndrome who undergo adrenalectomy for a secreting tumor.
- *Acute adrenal insufficiency is life-threatening and needs immediate steroid replacement prior to the return of diagnostic test results.*
- *Shock that does not respond to intravenous fluid boluses and pressor support in the setting of hyponatremia and hyperkalemia is suggestive of adrenal insufficiency.*
- In the critically ill patient, normal values of steroid production and function may be misleading and should prompt further evaluation of the patient.

tion and pressor support in the setting of unexplained hyponatremia and hyperkalemia should be assessed and simultaneously treated for new-onset adrenal insufficiency.

B. Frequently, critically ill patients are noted to have cortisol levels (both basal and poststimulated) in the normal range for normal individuals. Such levels in critically ill patients may be inappropriately low, presenting a picture of *relative adrenal insufficiency*. It has been estimated that plasma cortisol levels should exceed 15 to 20 μg/dL during critical illness, whereas healthy subjects have a normal range of 5 to 24 μg/dL. Adrenal activity is defined by both the ability to maintain a basal daily production of cortisol and the ability to respond appropriately to metabolic and physiologic stress by increased output. The response to ACTH stimulation testing in these patients is difficult to interpret, as "no increase" may denote adrenals that are maximally active and have no additional reserve, or adrenals that are unable to respond appropriately; either interpretation implies a relative inability to respond to stress.

Routine use of glucocorticoid therapy in pa-

tients in septic shock has been shown to decrease the requirement for pressor support and generally to improve the immediate clinical picture. Notwithstanding, the use of glucocorticoid therapy in the treatment of septic states remains controversial.

SELECTED READINGS

Barquist E, Kirton O: Adrenal insufficiency in the surgical intensive care unit patient. J Trauma 1997;42:27.

Briegel J, Forst H, Haller M, et al: Stress doses of hydrocortisone reverse hyperdynamic septic shock: A prospective, randomized, double-blind, single-center study. Crit Care Med 1999;27:723.

Glowniak JV, Loriaux DL: A double-blind study of perioperative steroid requirements in secondary adrenal insufficiency. Surgery 1997;121:123.

Lamberts SWJ, Bruining HA, de Jong FH: Corticosteroid therapy in severe illness. N Engl J Med 1997;337:1285.

Oelkers W: Adrenal insufficiency. N Engl J Med 1996;335:1206.

Orth DN, Kovacs WJ: The adrenal cortex. In Wilson JD, Foster DW, Kronenberg HM, Larsen PR (eds): Williams Textbook of Endocrinology, 9th ed. Philadelphia, WB Saunders, 1998, pp 517–664.

Richards ML, Caplan RH, Wickus GG, et al: The rapid low-dose (1 μg) cosyntropin test in the immediate postoperative period: Results in elderly subjects after major abdominal surgery. Surgery 1999;125:431.

Salem M, Tainish RE, Bromberg J, et al: Perioperative glucocorticoid coverage: A reassessment 42 years after emergence of a problem. Ann Surg 1994;219:416.

Chapter 18

Monitoring Respiratory Function and Weaning from the Ventilator

Soumitra R. Eachempati and Philip S. Barie

Advances in the management of the mechanically ventilated patient represent some of the most notable changes in critical care in the last decade. These advances are especially important because improved resuscitation and operative care mean that many critically ill and injured patients who previously might not have survived their acute insults are now requiring long-term supportive care, including prolonged mechanical ventilation. To assist in the management of these chronically ventilated patients, monitoring techniques have become increasingly sophisticated. Additionally, it has been reported that more sophisticated strategies have enhanced and predicted successful ventilator weaning.

VENTILATOR SUPPORT

Indications for Ventilator Support

Most patients require intubation and mechanical ventilation for a short period to facilitate the performance of a procedure or operation. Prolonged ventilator support is required in a minority of patients for one of several indications. Severe metabolic derangements, such as shock, sepsis, and acidosis, represent some of the most common reasons for ventilatory support. The inability to perform adequate gas exchange as the result of an acute pathophysiologic insult to the lungs, such as pneumonia, pulmonary contusion, or pulmonary embolism, may require mechanical ventilation. Severe systemic processes, such as sepsis, pancreatitis, burns, multiple injuries, and coagulopathies, can affect pulmonary function indirectly by creating a massive systemic inflammatory response, which in turn can promote increased pulmonary microvascular permeability, pulmonary edema, and local cellular infiltration. The common indications for the maintenance of an artificial airway with or without ventilatory support include patients with altered mental status, oropharyngeal edema, or other upper airway obstruction, or maxillofacial trauma in which airway protection is required. The inability to control and mobilize secretions poses another reason for long-term ventilatory support.

Assist-Controlled Ventilation

After the establishment of an adequate endotracheal or transtracheal airway, any of several standard ventilator modes may be used. In assist-controlled ventilation, the machine exerts some control over every breath, depending on the precise settings. The magnitude of the breaths may be volume limited, flow limited, or pressure limited, and the ventilator also allows for patient-triggered machine breaths. Traditionally, a volume-limited, patient-triggered, time-cycled mode of ventilation has been the most common method of ventilation. With this mode, the patient receives a fixed number of machine breaths with a set tidal volume (V_T), but the patient's spontaneous breaths are also able to trigger the machine to deliver a breath with this same V_T.

In patients with acute lung injury and loss of lung compliance, volume-limited ventilation can contribute to alveolar injury from the force of the delivered breath itself. To decrease this iatrogenic "volutrauma," or lung injury, some clinicians employ the ventilator modality, referred to as "pressure-controlled ventilation" (PCV). This term is actually a misnomer, when one considers that the mode actually utilizes a pressure-limited basis, not a pressure-controlled basis of ventilation, because the delivered breaths are limited from exceeding a designated set pressure. This technique is usually a machine-triggered, time-cycled mode of ventilation. In both volume-limited and pressure-limited ventilation, the machine can be patient triggered and will deliver a desired V_T after the initiation of a spontaneous patient breath. Consequently, these techniques are best avoided in spontaneously breathing patients, because they can lead to ventilator dysynchrony, air trapping, hypoxemia, hypocapnia, and patient discomfort.

Intermittent Mandatory Ventilation and Pressure-Support Ventilation

Two commonly practiced modes of ventilation in more alert patients include synchronous intermittent mandatory ventilation (SIMV) and pressure-support ventilation (PSV). In SIMV, the machine delivers a set minimal number of breaths per minute with a set V_T, but patient effort is sensed so as not to deliver a breath from the machine during any patient breath. Therefore, IMV should be more comfortable for the spontaneously breathing patient. In PSV, the patient's spontaneous breaths are augmented by inspiratory gas flow to a predetermined inspiratory airway pressure, thereby increasing inspiratory gas flow. Hence, the patient can be relieved completely from the work of breathing (WOB), or it can be shared by the machine and the patient, depending on the amount of pressure set by the clinician, because the inspiratory pressure can be adjusted to regulate V_T. Pressure-support ventilation may be used with a set IMV rate or without a set rate—that is, only continuous positive airway pressure (CPAP) between patient-initiated breaths—but must not be used in apneic patients because the mode does not provide a backup ventilatory rate.

Complications of Ventilator Support

The complications of prolonged ventilator support frequently relate to the underlying process that has created the pulmonary decompensation. Complications arising purely from the force of the ventilation include volutrauma, muscular overdistensibility, and patient discomfort. Volutrauma is due to the forced overdistention of the remaining healthy alveolar units by the ventilator breaths. This effect may be difficult to predict or identify, but it is most likely to occur in the patient with acute lung injury, alveolar collapse, and decreased pulmonary compliance. Increased afterload and the decreased venous return generated by pulmonary hyperinflation and increased transpulmonary pressure can also result in hypotension or a low cardiac output state.

Other complications of ventilator support relate to the patient's need for ventilation. Prolonged mechanical ventilation can lead to muscle atrophy and systemic weakness. Most importantly, prolonged ventilation can produce a significant, life-threatening risk of nosocomial infection related to the duration of the ventilation. Ventilator-associated pneumonia has a complex pathogenesis. The bacterial pathogens typically are endogenous flora and may be resistant to multiple drugs if the process of care has been a prolonged one. The inability to clear secretions, as well as recurrent microaspirations, may allow bacteria from the oropharynx and alimentary tract to enter the lower airway. Several methods of prophylaxis may be beneficial in decreasing this pneumonia risk, including keeping the head of the bed elevated, intragastric feedings performed according to strict protocol to minimize the risk of aspiration, and the use of new endotracheal tubes that permit the removal of subglottic secretions. Some practitioners believe that the application of topical and oral antibiotics or "selective digestive decontamination" may also be of some use.

MONITORING TECHNIQUES

Capnography

A vital monitoring advance, from the gas-exchange standpoint, has been the increased use of capnography, or the monitoring of carbon dioxide in end-tidal expired gas ($ETCO_2$). Capnography relies on either mass spectroscopy or infrared light absorption to detect the presence of carbon dioxide during different phases of the ventilatory cycle. Capnography is useful in the assessment of tracheostomy or endotracheal tube placement, weaning, and ongoing monitoring. With the ability of capnography to detect hypercapnia during ventilator weaning of intubated patients, its use has diminished the need for the measurement of blood gases. With the use of capnography in conjunction with pulse oximetry, many patients can be entirely weaned from mechanical ventilation without the meaurement of arterial blood gases.

Other information is acquired from the $ETCO_2$ as well.

Prognostically, an $ETCO_2$-$PaCO_2$ gradient above 13 mm Hg after resuscitation has been associated with an increased mortality rate in trauma patients. Additionally, a sudden perturbation of the $ETCO_2$ can be correlated with some undetected pathology, such as dislodgment or occlusion of the airway, a state of low cardiac output, and pulmonary embolism. Finally, the characteristics of the waveform can indicate information regarding whether the patient harbors obstructive or reactive airway disease.

Measuring Auto-PEEP

In certain critically ill patients, hyperinflation at end-expiration occurs when the lung develops limitations in gas outflow and begins to develop air trapping. This hyperinflation results from dynamic airway collapse or a ventilatory cycle that does not allow time for complete pulmonary exhalation. This scenario can occur in any situation in which expiratory air flow resistance is increased, such as acute lung injury or acute respiratory distress syndrome (ARDS), but is most pronounced in chronic obstructive pulmonary disease (COPD), in which a high tidal volume or a high respiratory rate preclude adequate exhalation. Normally, the recoil pressure of the lung at end-exhalation generally approximates zero because the lung volume at this time equals the relaxation volume. Elevated recoil pressure at end-expiration during conditions of pulmonary hyperinflation is termed *auto-PEEP* (positive end-expiratory pressure) or *intrinsic PEEP*. Mechanical ventilator settings that are unsuited for the patient's pathophysiology, notably inverse-ratio ventilation used for management of severe, refractory ARDS, can cause iatrogenic auto-PEEP.

The presence of auto-PEEP has multiple deleterious effects. The air trapping increases pulmonary airway and vascular pressures and can decrease left ventricular preload as well as increase right ventricular afterload. Additionally, intrinsic PEEP predisposes the lungs to alveolar injury through volutrauma and substantially increases the work of breathing. The management of auto-PEEP, once detected, involves decreasing the respiratory rate and the applied VT.

Measuring auto-PEEP is possible in several ways. The most common method in use is the "end-expiratory occlusion technique." This method is employed to determine the level of auto-PEEP in patients who are sedated and paralyzed. Here, the expiratory port of the ventilator is occluded, and the steady state pressure is measured. Another method for measuring auto-PEEP in a patient with no spontaneous breaths uses continuous flow and pressure readings. In this technique, the pressure that must be applied by the ventilator to initiate inspiratory flow is approximately the auto-PEEP. A method of performing measurements of auto-PEEP in the patient who is breathing spontaneously uses an esophageal balloon catheter system and determines the change in esophageal pressure from the start of inspiratory effort to the onset of inspiratory flow.

Effective Static Compliance

Pulmonary compliance refers to the distensibility of the lung in response to a given amount of inspiratory pressure. In actuality, it is a combination of lung and chest wall compliance that is of clinical significance. In patients with severe acute lung injury as well as many chronic interstitial or fibroproliferative lung diseases, pulmonary compliance decreases. In states of poor compliance, ventilation-perfusion mismatch causes impaired gas exchange, leading to hypercapnia and hypoxemia. To restore balanced gas exchange, the clinician may be forced to increase applied distending volumes or pressures. The effect on compliance is unpredictable; therefore, the use of compliance as an indicator of the response to changes in the mechanical ventilation strategy may be unreliable. However, the absolute value of static lung compliance (C_s) has prognostic implications.

If the patient is completely sedated and is not initiating any spontaneous respiration, "effective C_s" can be calculated as the total volume delivered by the ventilator until zero gas flow occurs at end-inhalation divided by the distending transthoracic pressure, a value approximated by the pressure difference at the airway opening and the atmospheric pressure. The total volume delivered to the patient is the delivered V_T minus the compression volume in the ventilator tubing (C_{tub}). To achieve conditions of zero gas flow and allow the calculation of C_s, a maneuver called an "inspiratory hold" must be performed. In this maneuver, the expiratory port needs to be occluded long enough (usually 2 seconds) for the airway pressure to reach a constant value called a "plateau pressure" (P_{plat}). The total distending pressure for the system will be the P_{plat} minus the total PEEP (external and auto-PEEP). Therefore,

$$C_s = \frac{V_T}{(P_{plat} - PEEP)} - C_{tub}$$

where C_{tub} is 0.3 mL/cm H_2O for high-compliance tubing and 4.5 mL/cm H_2O for low-compliance tubing. Calculations should be based on three breaths. A normal range of C_s for a healthy adult would 0.06 to 0.10 L/cm H_2O and 0.02 to 0.03 L/cm H_2O or less for patients with ARDS.

Effective Dynamic Compliance

The "effective dynamic compliance" (C_d) is a more easily measured approximation of compliance for the ventilated patient. This variable is calculated by dividing the ventilator-delivered tidal volume by the peak airway pressure (P_{aw}) minus the PEEP, or

$$C_d = \frac{V_T}{(P_{aw} - PEEP)}$$

In some centers, this method of approximating compliance is popular for determining the optimal amount of PEEP to be applied, but to do so is problematic because the response is not always predictable. Static compliance is more reliable and reproducible than is C_d for determining optimal PEEP support, but this method has not proved superior to others in determining the best level of PEEP for ventilated patients.

Pressure-Volume Curves

Another technique for the measurement of pulmonary compliance involves the construction of a pressure-volume curve. To create this curve, the ventilated patient should be sedated and paralyzed in order to minimize the effects of any patient-initiated breaths. As described originally, the patient is disconnected from the ventilator and a 1.5- to 2.0-L syringe is connected to the endotracheal tube. This syringe is equipped with a pneumotachygraph and a pressure transducer. The chest is then inflated stepwise in 50- to 100-mL increments with a 2- or 3-second pause between steps until a volume of 1.7 L or an airway pressure of 40 to 50 cm H_2O has been reached. The chest is then deflated in a similar stepwise manner, and the deflation values are recorded.

After the procedure has been repeated three times, the results are averaged and plotted. Theoretically, these results produce a sigmoid-shaped curve with three distinct slopes. The initial slope produces the "starting compliance," whereas the slope after about 250 mL of air has been instilled is called the "inflation compliance." In the plot, the clinician can approximate an area between the two lower slopes, called the "lower inflection point" (Fig. 18–1), which is assumed to represent the alveolar closing volume or the volume at which alveoli and airways reopen during inspiration. Some authors have suggested that this inflection point corresponds to the optimal end-expiratory pressure or applied PEEP needed by patients with acute lung injury or ARDS in order to optimize alveolar recruitment.

Other information can also be derived from pressure-volume curves. The difference between the inflation and the deflation curves may represent "hysteresis," or the amount of trapped air in the airways. The higher portion of the upper inflection point may represent the boundary of total lung capacity above which volume any inflation may contribute to lung injury.

Although the construction of pressure-volume curves appears attractive and informative, many patients with severe lung injury and high oxygen and PEEP requirements may not tolerate being taken off the ventilator, even for short periods of time, to allow the study. Currently, some ventilators allow the instillation of air without removal of the patient from the circuit. Nonetheless, the construction of these curves, in general, remains difficult and cumbersome for routine use in most ventilated patients.

Work of Breathing

For certain patients in whom weaning poses difficulties owing to chronic weakness and fatigability, a commercially available WOB monitor (CP-100, Bicore, Riverside, Calif.) is available. This device is an easily placed esophageal balloon catheter (for estimation of intrapleural pressure) with pressure and flow transducers placed in the ventilator circuit for calculation of the WOB. The physiologic WOB is normally about 0.5 to 0.6 J/L and successful extubation is more probable when physiologic WOB is less than 0.8 J/L. The clinician can regulate the ventilator

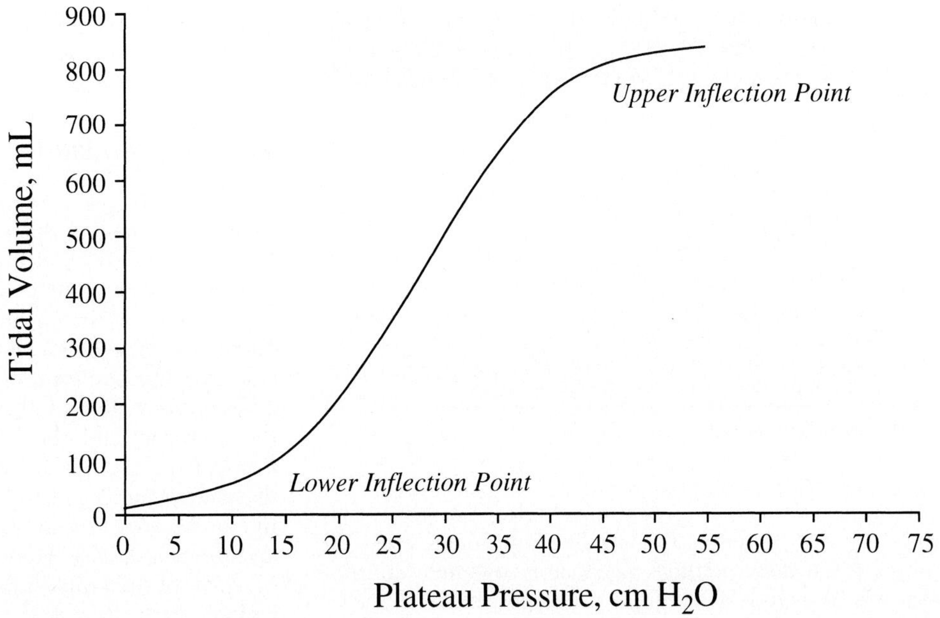

Figure 18–1. A pressure-volume curve. The initial flat portion at the lower plateau pressures reflects small volumes due to unopened alveoli. The lower inflection point represents the pressures where the alveoli are opened. After the lower inflection point, the volumes increase proportionately to the pressures. At the higher inflection point, the lungs are maximally inflated and the volumes can no longer increase despite increased plateau pressures.

and adjust the level of the machine and patient support using any of the conventional weaning modalities so that patients are using no more than this level of energy for their respirations. In this manner, the inability to wean does not become a function of preventable patient fatigability. Although this device and other similar devices have gained sporadic popularity, no large-scale consensus trials have shown that WOB measurements decrease number of days on the ventilator or patient mortality.

WEANING TECHNIQUES

Candidates for Weaning

When the ventilated patient is no longer perceived as needing ventilatory support, he or she may be taken off the ventilator. Occasionally, health care providers misjudge the patient's ability to perform spontaneous respirations, and the patient subsequently requires the reinstitution of ventilator support. For patients with a tracheostomy, this maneuver simply entails reattaching the ventilator circuit to the patient's tracheostomy. For patients who previously were supported via an oral or endotracheal airway, failure of machine-independent breathing requires reintubation. Failed extubation is clearly a morbid event in terms of increased mortality and surrogate end-points, such as prolonged length of stay. In addition to complications relating to aspiration, hypoxia, and cardiac ischemia, many patients also become functionally more fatigued after a failed extubation and are unable to be successfully weaned for some time. As described earlier, infectious and noninfectious complications associated with prolonged intubation may be substantial. Consequently, the decision to extubate a patient may be a critical decision for that patient's welfare.

Criteria for Extubation

For successful extubation to occur, the pathophysiology that required the ventilatory support must have become

sufficiently controlled and the patient should be free from major reversible metabolic derangements. The most important derangement that clinicians sometimes underestimate is metabolic acidosis. If a patient with metabolic acidosis is extubated prematurely, the patient may have a drive to breathe rapidly, become fatigued quickly, and possibly require reintubation. Less critical but more common as a reason for extubation failure is metabolic alkalosis, which in surgical patients develops when patients mobilize their perioperative "third-space" fluid sequestration and become hypokalemic, often with the assistance of loop diuretics.

Other criteria for extubation are equally important. The patient must be able to oxygenate and ventilate capably without the respirator and have the fortitude to do so indefinitely. Also, the patient must be able to protect his or her own airway. Generally, this last requirement means that the patient must have a functional gag reflex, an adequate ability to cough, and an alert sensorium. Adequate pulmonary hygiene is crucial to successful weaning. Many patients with copious secretions fail ventilatory weaning because they are unable to clear these secretions. The clinician must be alert to the possibility of glottic dysfunction even after relatively brief periods of intubation, both from the perspective of weaning and the restitution of oral feedings.

Weaning Parameters

Researchers have described many parameters that aid the clinician in determining whether the patient is a candidate for extubation (Table 18–1). These parameters have been studied to different degrees and enjoy variable popularity. The simplest weaning parameters represent the patient's ability to oxygenate and ventilate, and to follow commands that require physical strength. An arterial blood gas can be drawn while the patient is on minimal ventilator settings, such as CPAP or a T-piece with an F_{IO_2} less

Table 18–1	Commonly Used Weaning Parameters and Criteria*

PaO_2 >60 mm Hg on FIO_2 ≤0.4
$PaCO_2$ 35–45 mm Hg
Arterial pH 7.35–7.45
Spontaneous respiratory rate >30 breaths per minute
Spontaneous V_E <10 L/min
Spontaneous V_T >5 mL/kg
f/V_T <105 breaths per minute per liter
Vital capacity >10 mL/kg
Increase or decrease in heart rate >20 beats per minute during weaning
Increase or decrease in systolic blood pressure >20 mm Hg
Negative inspiratory force less than −25 cm H_2O

*See text for abbreviations.

than 0.5. Blood gases are usually determined after 30 minutes. On these settings, satisfactory weaning parameters would include PaO_2 greater than 60 mm Hg, $PaCO_2$ between 35 and 45 mm Hg, pH of 7.35 to 7.45, respiratory rate less than 30 breaths per minute, and mean V_T greater than 5 mL/kg. Some clinicians believe that other physiologic criteria, including a heart rate increase of more than 20 beats per minute from baseline or a mean blood pressure increase of more than 15 mm Hg, demonstrate that spontaneous WOB is excessive and some ventilatory support must be continued.

The intensity of the respiratory excursion achieved by the ventilated patient is believed to correlate with successful ventilator weaning, but an awake and cooperative patient is crucial in obtaining interpretable data. Narcotics and sedatives should be minimized insofar as possible, and their effects allowed to subside. Importantly, the interior diameter of the endotracheal tube should be at least 8 mm for best accuracy. Several different parameters may be obtained. The first, the "maximal inspiratory force" or "negative inspiratory force" (NIF), represents the maximal pressure generated by a voluntary effort from functional residual capacity. In studies, an NIF of less than −25 cm H_2O has been correlated weakly with the ability to be weaned. Another parameter, the single-breath vital capacity, when greater than 10 mL/kg, has also been advocated as a predictor of adequate respiratory function, but the correlation is similarly weak.

Several calculated values may be indicative of the patient's ability to breathe spontaneously. Minute ventilation (V_E) measured after several minutes of spontaneous breathing has been predictive of successful extubation when it is less than 10 L/min. Patients whose "maximal voluntary ventilation," or V_E, generated when breathing maximally over 12 to 15 seconds was twice spontaneous V_E also fare better after extubation.

The measure of successful weaning that is simplest and has been demonstrated to be most predictive of successful weaning is the "rapid shallow breathing index" (RVR or f/V_T). The RVR measures the respiratory rate–to–V_T ratio during a 1-minute trial of spontaneous breathing by the ventilated patient. When the RVR is less than 105 breaths per minute per liter, multiple studies have shown that the patient is highly likely to wean success-

fully. Even more predictive is the RVR obtained after 30 minutes of spontaneous breathing.

Weaning Modalities

Researchers have proposed different techniques for optimizing the chances of a successful extubation of chronically ventilated patients. In addition to weaning parameters, it has been purported that the ventilatory mode affects the expediency of weaning. Although no definitive studies favor one type of weaning strategy over another, several different strategies are widely used, depending on the preference of the clinician and the institution. Recently, many institutions have demonstrated that protocol-directed weaning reduces the duration of mechanical ventilation, increases the chances of successful extubation, and decreases cost. However, successful implementation of protocol-driven weaning requires clinicians to be comfortable with the withdrawal of ventilator support whenever preset criteria are met, even in the middle of the night. Moreover, most interactions according to the protocol are performed by nursing or respiratory therapy personnel, which may cause some discomfiture.

There are no data that suggest that the gradual withdrawal of ventilator support increases the chances of a successful extubation or decreases the number of days that the patient is on the ventilator. Consequently, some clinicians favor weaning by a single 2-hour T-piece or CPAP trial in the presence of less than 8 cm H_2O of PSV. If the patient does not tolerate the entire 2-hour trial, the patient is placed back on the ventilator and the trial is repeated the next day. The rationale behind this strategy implies that if a patient can breathe efficiently through an endotracheal tube and ventilator circuit for 2 hours, the patient has the muscle strength to withstand extubation.

In the opinion of the authors, patients who are breathing spontaneously are best weaned while the ventilator is on settings of IMV with PSV. Weaning by IMV and PSV can be done independently or concurrently. Some clinicians keep the PSV at 5 cm H_2O and wean the IMV set rate by 1 to 4 breaths per minute per day as the patient's physiology allows. Intolerance to IMV weaning is shown by tachypnea, tachycardia, and the use of accessory muscles and is usually due to an increased respiratory muscle load (Table 18–2). To perform this type of IMV weaning, the IMV rate can be held constant or can be increased while the PSV is increased up to 20 cm H_2O to diminish the WOB performed by the patient. Other clinicians prefer to wean the IMV rate to 0 (essentially, CPAP mode), while weaning the PSV from 20 cm H_2O to 5 to 8 cm H_2O at a rate of 1 to 4 cm H_2O per increment. Both of these methods require the patient to be breathing spontaneously and oxygenating adequately without a need for FIO_2 greater than 0.5. If these conditions are not met, the patient is at risk for having potentially dangerous hypoxic episodes during the weaning process, and may require reinstitution of full mechanical ventilation.

Table 18–2	Factors Associated with Increased Respiratory Muscle Load

Increased carbon dioxide production (catabolism, inappropriate fuel mix)
Increased dead space ventilation (ARDS, pulmonary embolus)
Central hyperventilation
Drug or alcohol withdrawal
Airway obstruction (tracheal stenosis, tracheomalacia)
Pulmonary edema
Anemia
Atrophy of respiratory musculature
Decreased chest wall compliance (circumferential chest wall bandages or burns)
Malnutrition
Electrolyte abnormalities (hypokalemia, hypophosphatemia, hypomagnesemia, hypocalcemia)

Noninvasive Ventilation

Noninvasive ventilation is a possible alternative for gas exchange in critically ill patients who require ventilatory support or who are failing extubation. This type of ventilation is usually administered as noninvasive positive-pressure ventilation (NIPPV) via a face mask or nasal mask. The attached mask with auxiliary pressure can be used for up to several days. Different types of support can be applied to the mask to augment respiratory excursion. The most popular pressure mode with NIPPV has been CPAP or intermittent positive pressure (IPP), but recently, the use of bilevel positive airway pressure (BiPAP) has become more popular. BiPAP operates as a noninvasive mode of ventilation applied by mask. Unlike CPAP, BiPAP also includes an exhalation valve that permits maintenance of expiratory positive pressure as well. This aspect of the modality improves the exhalation of carbon dioxide.

In selected patients with respiratory compromise who need only short-term support, NIPPV or BiPAP may be able to avert the need for endotracheal intubation or reintubation after extubation. Patients who may benefit from NIPPV include those with difficult airway access and those with reversible pathologic processes of moderate severity, such as exacerbations of COPD, cardiogenic pulmonary edema, certain neurologic disorders, and even ARDS. The disadvantages of this technique include the lack of a secure airway, failure of the mask to achieve a proper seal, the inability of the clinician to suction the airway or perform bronchoscopy without disrupting the seal of the face mask, and patient noncompliance with wearing the uncomfortable mask.

Pearls and Pitfalls

Weaning and Extubation

PITFALLS

- Extubation of the patient unable to protect his or her airway
- Extubation of the patient with untreated metabolic acidosis or alkalosis
- Inadequate diuresis for pulmonary congestion
- Excessive or prolonged narcotic or benzodiazepine use
- Prolonging ventilation unnecessarily

SELECTED READINGS

Butler R, Keenan SP, Inman KJ, et al: Is there a preferred technique for weaning the difficult-to-wean patient? A systematic review of the literature. Crit Care Med 1999;27:2331.
Chao DC, Scheinhorn DJ: Weaning from mechanical ventilation. Surg Clin North Am 1998;14:799.
Dries DJ: Weaning from mechanical ventilation. J Trauma 1997;43:372.
Eachempati SR, Barie PS: Minimally invasive and noninvasive diagnosis and therapy in critically ill and injured patients. Arch Surg 1999;134:1189.
Ely EW, Baker AM, Dunagan DP, et al: Effect of the duration of mechanical ventilation on identifying patients capable of breathing spontaneously. N Engl J Med 1996;335:1864.
Horst MH, Mouro D, Hall-Jenssens RA, Pamukov N: Decrease in ventilation time with a standardized weaning process. Arch Surg 1998;133:483.
Johanningman JA, Davis K Jr, Campbell RS, et al: Use of the rapid shallow breathing index as an indicator of patient work of breathing during pressure support ventilation. Surgery 1997;122:737.
Jubran A: Monitoring patient mechanics during mechanical ventilation. Surg Clin North Am 1998;14:629.
Kollef MH, Shapiro SD, Silver P, et al: A randomized-controlled trial of protocol-driven versus physician-directed weaning from mechanical ventilation. Crit Care Med 1997;25:567.
MacIntyre NR: Issues in ventilator weaning. Chest 1999;115:1215.
Manthous CA, Schmidt GA, Hall JB: Liberation from mechanical ventilation: A decade of progress. Chest 1998;114:886.
Nava S, Ambrosin N, Clini E, et al: Noninvasive mechanical ventilation in the weaning of patients with respiratory failure due to chronic obstructive pulmonary disease: A randomized controlled trial. Ann Intern Med 1998;128:721.
Tobin MJ, Van de Graaff WB: Monitoring of lung mechanics and work of breathing. In Tobin MJ (ed): Principles and Practice of Mechanical Ventilation. New York, McGraw-Hill, 1994, pp 967–1003.

Chapter 19
Coma

Mark A. Mittler, Gordon Anderson, and Curtis Doberstein

Coma and Altered Mental Status in the Surgical Critical Care Setting

Mark A. Mittler

The evaluation and management of patients with altered mental status can vary dramatically in the vast array of situations encountered in surgical critical care environments. Typically, the cause of diminished level of consciousness can be broadly categorized into the following: traumatic, metabolic, and pharmacologic. While this chapter addresses each of these categories individually later, there are some common themes that are applicable to all patients.

The evaluation of level of consciousness is easy. Clearly, the hardest part is remembering to do it. In an acute setting, such as a trauma room, the patient is generally receiving enough stimuli that a few seconds of simple "hands-off" observation provides crucial information. Are the patient's eyes open? Is he or she speaking? Are all extremities moving? In fact, the answers to these three questions provide enough information to calculate a patient's Glasgow Coma Score (GCS) (Teasdale, 1974).

Caring for patients with altered mental status, however, does not end with the initial assessment in the case of trauma. All patients in a critical care setting, regardless of diagnosis, should be assessed from a neurologic standpoint throughout their stay. This is an ongoing process that is relatively easy to overlook. All too often, neurologic compromise is noted at terminal stages despite otherwise excellent care. While there are many reasons for this, generally one common theme prevails—inadequate communication among care providers.

LEVEL OF CONSCIOUSNESS: PATIENT COMMUNICATION AND PHYSICIAN EVALUATION

The neurologic assessment of the patient with a significantly compromised level of consciousness generally consists of calculation of the GCS, examination of pupillary responses to light, asymmetry of motor responses, corneal reflexes, gag reflex, oculocephalic-oculovestibular reflexes, and respiratory effort. Obviously, patients who are awake and alert can be more thoroughly assessed as needed (Valadka, 2000, p. 383).

Since the introduction of the GCS (Table 19–1), it has clearly become the most commonly used objective measure of neurologic status in trauma settings. The distinct advantage of GCS utilization is the extremely low interobserver and intraobserver variability within the scoring system. The score is a value from 3 to 15 based on best motor response, best verbal response, and eye opening.

Although there are clear limitations to applying the GCS to all patients—such as endotracheal intubation precluding verbal scoring, or orbital trauma affecting eye opening—the system is quite valuable in providing a means of following the patient's mental status over time in the context of multiple care providers.

RADIOGRAPHIC EVALUATION FOR DIMINISHED LEVEL OF CONSCIOUSNESS

During the past three decades, advances in cranial imaging have been dramatic. The role of brain imaging in dealing with alterations of patient consciousness is quite simple. To rule out acute reversible structural causes of deteriorating mental status, nonenhanced computed tomography (CT) is clearly the test of choice, given availability, rapidity of procedure, and ease of interpretation. Extra-axial or intra-axial hematomas can be identified.

Table 19–1	Glasgow Coma Scale	
Eye Opening	4	Spontaneously
	3	To speech
	2	To pain
	1	Never
Verbal Response	5	Oriented
	4	Confused
	3	Inappropriate words
	2	Incomprehensible sounds
	1	Silent
Motor Response	6	Obeys commands
	5	Localizes pain
	4	Withdrawal
	3	Abnormal flexion
	2	Extends to pain
	1	No response
Total (E + V + M) 3–15		

Hypoxic-ischemic injury can be detected, and some toxic etiologies, such as methanol-induced lucencies in the basal ganglia, can also be noted.

ELEVATED INTRACRANIAL PRESSURE

The most commonly encountered scenario for neurologic compromise in a surgical critical care setting is head trauma. It is well established that the vast majority of patients with life-threatening traumatic injuries have some component of head injury. While we are unable to reverse initial brain injury, the treatment goal for head-injured patients is to prevent secondary injury. The control of elevated intracranial pressure (ICP) is a well-established means of preventing secondary brain injury.

There are some basic principles that provide a foundation for understanding intracranial pressure. Elevated intracranial pressure can be due to hematomas between the skull and the dura (epidural), between the dura and the brain (subdural), or within the brain (e.g., cerebral contusion). Elevation of ICP is also encountered with obstruction of cerebrospinal fluid (CSF) outflow and with cerebral edema. Since the brain is encased in a rigid container, an increase in volume within that container results in an increase in pressure. The effect of raised ICP on brain function or level of consciousness is related to the impairment of cerebral perfusion. The cerebral perfusion pressure (CPP) is a measure of the mean arterial pressure (MAP) minus the ICP. In general, a CPP of 70 mm Hg or greater is adequate to provide perfusion to the central nervous system.

In addition to a declining level of consciousness, the patient with elevated ICP may develop signs of "Cushing's triad"—hypertension, bradycardia, and/or alterations of respiratory rate and rhythm.

From a practical standpoint, there are three "compartments" or "volumes" within the calvarium—brain tissue volume, vascular volume, and CSF volume. In order for ICP, and therefore CPP, to remain stable, an increase in volume of one compartment must be compensated for by a decrease in volume of another compartment. Therapy for raised ICP is based on this basic principle. Surgical removal of mass lesions (e.g., hematomas) allows the three compartments to exist without compromise. Ventriculostomy placement not only allows for accurate measurement of ICP but also provides a means of decreasing the CSF compartment volume. Hyperventilation, although rarely indicated, causes hypocapnia, leading to alkalosis-induced cerebral vasoconstriction, thereby decreasing the intracranial vascular volume. The diuretic mannitol creates an osmotic gradient between the blood and the brain parenchyma, resulting in the movement of water out of the cranium, decreasing brain volume (Lee and Hoff, 1996, p. 511). Although it is beyond the scope of this text to detail the intensive care unit management of elevated ICP, readers can consult *Guidelines for the Management of Severe Head Injury* for evidence-based treatment strategies.

BRAINSTEM AND DIFFUSE CORTICAL INJURIES

In addition to intracranial hypertension, other causes of coma exist in the head-injured patient. Brainstem or bilateral cortical dysfunction from trauma can account for profoundly decreased levels of consciousness. The reticular activating system (RAS) is a diffuse network that receives input from and is stimulated by every major somatic and special sensory pathway (Plum and Posner, 1982, p.13). Brainstem trauma involving the RAS by direct injury or transmitted shearing forces causes impairment of consciousness, often without any localizing signs. Bilateral cortical dysfunction may be seen in cases of both open and closed head injuries. The most common scenario of head injury causing prolonged coma is that of diffuse axonal injury (DAI). Sudden acceleration or deceleration causes a shear injury to axons throughout the brain. Although a spectrum of severity exists in cases of DAI, in its classic form small punctate hemorrhages and intraventricular blood are seen on CT in the absence of large hematomas or elevations of ICP (Liau et al, 1996, p. 1562).

Unilateral cortical injuries, for the most part, do not cause prolonged alterations of consciousness unless there is secondary elevation of ICP or some other metabolic derangement.

There are hundreds of causes of coma and altered level of consciousness, the vast majority of which are diffuse, multifocal, or metabolic. Table 19–2 provides an organizational scheme for many of these causes. Further discussion of these causes is limited to those that are most frequently encountered in the surgical critical care setting.

OXYGEN DEPRIVATION

Disturbances in the supply of oxygen to the brain can be divided into three categories—anoxic anoxia, anemic anoxia, and ischemic anoxia, representing problems with oxygen supply, oxygen-carrying capacity of blood, and blood supply, respectively (Plum and Posner, 1982, p. 208). While each of these categories has a variety of causes, the common denominator is insufficient oxygen to meet the metabolic demands of the brain. Under otherwise normal physiologic circumstances, a total lack of oxygen delivery will result in brain cell death beginning at about 4 minutes. In cases in which the metabolic demand has been lowered, such as hypothermia or barbiturate "protection," this time period may be extended.

In a surgical critical care setting, oxygen delivery tends to be closely monitored and is rarely the source of idiopathic coma. Arterial blood gas determination and pulse oximetry readily alert caregivers to poor oxygenation of blood. Alteration may indicate processes such as pulmonary embolus, pulmonary edema, and airway obstruction. Hemoglobin quantitation identifies most instances of anemia, and blood pressure monitoring can help ensure adequate perfusion of the central nervous system. While embolic or thrombotic stroke may evade the aforemen-

Table 19–2	Some Diffuse, Multifocal, or Metabolic Causes of Delirium, Stupor, and Coma

A. Deprivation of oxygen, substrate, or metabolic cofactors
  1. Hypoxia (interference with oxygen supply to the brain—cerebral flow (CBF) normal).
    a. Decreased blood PO_2 and O_2 content
      Pulmonary disease
      Alveolar hypoventilation
      Decreased atmospheric oxygen tension
    b. Decreased blood O_2 content, PO_2 normal—"anemic anoxia"
      Anemia
      Carbon monoxide poisoning
      Methemoglobinemia
  2. Ischemia (diffuse or widespread multifocal interference with blood supply to brain)
    a. Decreased CBF, resulting from decreased cardiac output
      Stokes-Adams; cardiac arrest; cardiac arrhythmias
      Myocardial infarction
      Congestive heart failure
      Aortic stenosis
      Pulmonary infarction
    b. Decreased CBF resulting from decreased peripheral resistance to systemic circulation
      Syncope
      Carotid sinus hypersensitivity
      Low blood volume
    c. Decreased CBF associated with generalized or multifocal increased vascular resistance
      Hyperventilation syndrome
      Hyperviscosity (polycythemia, cryoglobulinemia or macroglobulinemia, sickle cell anemia)
      Subarachnoid hemorrhage
      Bacterial meningitis
      Hypertensive encephalopathy
    d. Decreased CBF owing to widespread small-vessel occlusions
      Disseminated intravascular coagulation
      Systemic lupus erythematosus
      Subacute bacterial endocarditis
      Fat embolism
      Cerebral malaria
      Cardiopulmonary bypass
  3. Hypoglycemia
    a. Resulting from exogenous insulin
    b. Spontaneous (endogenous insulin, liver disease, etc.)
  4. Cofactor deficiency
    a. Thiamine (Wernicke's encephalopathy)
    b. Niacin
    c. Pyridoxine
    d. Cyanocobalamin
    e. Folic acid
B. Diseases of organs other than brain
  1. Diseases of nonendocrine organs
    a. Liver (hepatic coma)
    b. Kidney (uremic coma)
    c. Lung (CO_2 narcosis)
    d. Pancreas (exocrine pancreatic encephalopathy)
  2. Hyper and/or hypofunction of endocrine organs
    a. Pituitary
    b. Thyroid (myxedema-thyrotoxicosis)
    c. Parathyroid (hypo- and hyperparathyroidism)
    d. Adrenal (Addison's disease, Cushing's disease, pheochromocytoma)
    e. Pancreas (diabetes, hypoglycemia)
  3. Other systemic diseases
    a. Diabetes
    b. Cancer
    c. Porphyria
    d. Sepsis

C. Exogenous poisons
  1. Sedative drugs
    a. Barbiturates and nonbarbiturate hypnotics
    b. Tranquilizers
    c. Bromides
    d. Ethanol
    e. Opiates
  2. Acid poisons or poison with acidic breakdown products
    a. Paraldehyde
    b. Methyl alcohol
    c. Ethylene glycol
    d. Ammonium chloride
  3. Psychotropic drugs
    a. Tricyclic antidepressants and anticholinergic drugs
    b. Amphetamines
    c. Lithium
    d. Phencyclidine
    e. Phenothiazines
    f. LSD, mescaline
    g. Monoamine oxidase inhibitors
  4. Others
    a. Penicillin
    b. Anticonvulsants
    c. Steroids
    d. Cardiac glycosides
    e. Cimetidine
    f. Heavy metals
    g. Organic phosphates
    h. Cyanide
    i. Salicylate
D. Abnormalities of ionic or acid-base environment of CNS
  1. Water and sodium (hyper- and hyponatremia)
  2. Acidosis (metabolic and respiratory)
  3. Alkalosis (metabolic and respiratory)
  4. Magnesium (hyper- and hypomagnesemia)
  5. Calcium (hyper- and hypocalcemia)
  6. Phosphorus (hypophosphatemia)
E. Disordered temperature regulation
  1. Hypothermia
  2. Heat stroke, fever
F. Infections or inflammation of CNS
  1. Leptomeningitis
  2. Encephalitis
  3. Acute "toxic" encephalopathy
  4. Parainfectious encephalomyelitis
  5. Cerebral vasculitis
  6. Subarachnoid hemorrhage
G. Primary neuronal or glial disorders
  1. Creutzfeldt-Jakob disease
  2. Marchiafava-Bignami disease
  3. Adrenoleukodystrophy
  4. Gliomatosis cerebri
  5. Progressive multifocal leukoencephalopathy
H. Miscellaneous disorders of unknown cause
  1. Seizures and postictal states
  2. Concussion
  3. Acute delirious states
    a. Sedative drug withdrawal
    b. "Postoperative" delirium
    c. Intensive care unit delirium
    d. Drug intoxications

From Plum F, Posner J: The Diagnosis of Stupor and Coma, 3rd ed. Philadelphia, FA Davis, 1982, p 178.

tioned monitoring, these events would probably present with focal neurologic deficit, rather than coma.

Syncopal episodes, despite multiple potential etiologies, can also be discussed in this context. Most often, in a hospital setting, syncopal events are due to circulatory embarrassment with postural changes, and generally do not occur while patients are lying in bed.

DISORDERS OF GLUCOSE REGULATION

Hypoglycemic coma in the critical care setting is generally iatrogenic in origin, with excessive administration of insulin or acute withdrawal of hyperalimentation after the induction of endogenous hyperinsulinism. Initial delirium may progress to transient mania or directly to lethargy and coma. Rapid intravenous infusion of 50 mL of 50% dextrose in suspected hypoglycemic states should be performed even before formal laboratory values return. Hypoglycemic states may also be encountered in severe pancreatic insufficiency, acute fulminant hepatic failure, acute adrenal insufficiency, and insulinoma (Schwartz et al, 1989, p. 481). Primary hypoglycemia is extremely rare although frequently suspected, owing to the similarity of prodromal symptoms to those of syncopal episodes—such as pallor, sweating, and yawning.

Other disturbances of glucose regulation can cause an altered level of consciousness. Although only 10% of patients who present to acute care with diabetic ketoacidosis (DKA) will arrive in coma, 80% will have diminished levels of consciousness (Plum and Posner, 1982). DKA generally develops in patients with severe diabetes who either neglect the control of their disease or develop an acute infection. Thirst, polyuria, anorexia, dehydration, tachycardia, and hypotension are among the signs and symptoms. Nausea, vomiting, and acute abdominal pain may initially obscure the diagnosis, but laboratory confirmation of metabolic acidosis in the appropriate setting generally leads to this relatively common diagnosis. Hyperosmolar nonketotic states can also present with profound depression of mental status. Although poorly understood, the predominant metabolic features of this condition are hyperglycemia, hypernatremia, and a considerable increase in serum osmolarity.

Once a patient loses consciousness from a disorder of glucose regulation—regardless of etiology—there is a significant risk of subsequent seizure activity (Patten, 1996, p. 396). Therefore, as with any loss of consciousness, airway management is of paramount importance in preventing secondary brain injury.

PHARMACOLOGIC ETIOLOGIES OF COMA

Ethanol intoxication is a common finding in emergency rooms and trauma centers throughout this country. "Alcoholic stupor" can present with classic vasodilatory effect, such as a flushed face, rapid pulse, low blood pressure, and hypothermia, with serum ethanol levels of 250 to 300 mg/dL. As the serum concentration increases over 300 mg/dL, patients become pale and quiet, with sluggishly reactive pupils. As the patient's level of consciousness

falls, respiratory depression ensues and cardiovascular collapse may follow (Plum and Posner, 1982, p. 244). When intoxication is associated with the simultaneous use of other substances, the clinical picture can be less clear. Careful history taking and toxicology studies are essential in the formation of a treatment strategy, but airway, respiratory, and circulatory support remain the most crucial elements in maximizing outcome.

Barbiturates, opiates, benzodiazepines, and antipsychotics such as haloperidol are among the most commonly utilized drug classes in the critical care setting. Evaluation of an altered level of consciousness in the hospital absolutely requires an evaluation of the patient's medication profile. Reversal agents such as naloxone for opiate overdose, or flumazenil for benzodiazepine overdose, have dramatic effects when appropriately administered. These agents, however, often have half-lives shorter than those of the drugs they reverse, so multiple administrations and continuous observation may be necessary.

METABOLIC DISORDERS ASSOCIATED WITH ALTERED LEVELS OF CONSCIOUSNESS

Disorders of thyroid or adrenal function can lead to depression of mental status. Acute thyrotoxicosis (e.g., thyroid storm) can present with tremor, choreiform movements, fever, delirium, seizures, and coma (Patten, 1996, p. 426). Control of these peripheral effects can be rapidly obtained with the use of beta-blockade. The initial clinical picture of myxedema, on the other hand, is most commonly seen as mental apathy, physical inertia, and hypothermia. The onset of myxedema coma is generally acutely precipitated by infection, heart failure, trauma, or anesthetic drug administration in an untreated hypothyroid patient (Patten, 1996, p. 426; Plum and Posner, 1982, p. 238).

Hepatic encephalopathy and coma have been related to hyperammonemia. Exogenous and endogenous sources of ammonia may contribute to this entity. Breakdown of dietary protein via gastrointestinal flora as well as gastric ammonia production from urea, combined with hepatic dysfunction and the inability of ammonia to appropriately enter the Krebs cycle, accounts for this elevation in serum ammonia level. Early in the hepatic failure, there is confusion and exaggerated reflexes ("hepatic flap"). This is followed by generalized muscular hypertonicity, rigidity, and eventually flaccidity and coma. Serum ammonia levels at this stage are often over 125 µg/dL (Schwartz et al, 1989, p. 1362).

Although adrenocortical insufficiency is rare in the surgical patient, it can be seen in patients after adrenalectomy, those with metastatic cancer, or those treated with chronic steroids. The most common cause of acute adrenal insufficiency is the inadvertent withdrawal of chronic steroid therapy. Weakness, nausea, vomiting, abdominal or flank pain, fever, lethargy, and confusion are among the signs and symptoms of this often-missed diagnosis. Suspicion of acute adrenocortical insufficiency should be followed immediately by treatment with a water-soluble

Pearls and Pitfalls

PITFALLS

- The absence of a documented neurologic baseline prevents the identification of subsequent changes in the patient's mental status.
- A delay in the assessment of altered neurologic status in the patient may have a significant negative effect on outcome.
- Abrupt cessation of exogenous steroids to patients on long-term steroid therapy can be fatal.

PEARLS

- The meticulous documentation of initial and interval neurologic status, including GCS, allows caregivers to identify problems.
- After the rapid assessment of physiologic parameters, such as blood pressure and oxygenation, as well as a review of administered medications, non–contrast-enhanced brain CT may identify reversible causes of coma.
- A careful medication history must always be obtained on every patient. Chronic steroid administration should not be terminated abruptly.

corticosteroid. This can be a lifesaving treatment if the condition is identified (Schwartz et al, 1989, p. 1575).

ADDITIONAL CENTRAL NERVOUS SYSTEM CAUSES OF ALTERATION OF CONSCIOUSNESS

Although there is little difficulty in recognizing the generalized tonic-clonic seizure, nonconvulsive seizure or even subclinical status epilepticus can account for an acutely diminished level of consciousness. Additionally, generalized seizure activity is often associated with a postictal period of time during which consciousness is altered. Even in the surgical intensive care unit, brief generalized tonic-clonic episodes may, in fact, be missed despite frequent neurologic assessments. Often, a dramatic change in mental status may represent a postictal state after a

seizure, or may be due to complex partial seizure activity. Electroencephalography (EEG) may help distinguish these episodes from other causes and may lead to treatment with antiepileptic drugs (AEDs).

Acute bacterial meningitis, if unrecognized, can be rapidly life-threatening. In a premorbid state, there is often a period of lethargy or coma. Rapid treatment is essential, and any significant suspicion on the part of the physician should be followed by immediate antibiotic therapy, even before cranial imaging or CSF collection.

There are two additional causes of coma that, although rarely observed, deserve some mention. Acute hydrocephalus may be due to otherwise asymptomatic intraventricular hemorrhage, late-onset aqueductal stenosis, or cerebellar infarction or hemorrhage. Loss of consciousness is due to elevated ICP, and treatment, once recognized, can be rapidly instituted by way of ventriculostomy placement in any acute care setting. The other infrequently encountered cause of coma is cerebral venous sinus thrombosis. Although most commonly seen in dehydrated infants, this can occur in any setting of significant dehydration. The diagnosis is easily missed unless the physician keeps the diagnostic suspicion in mind. CT findings are quite subtle and may require magnetic resonance venography (MRV) or conventional cerebral angiography with late-phase venous assessment. Treatment ranges from simple hydration to anticoagulation to direct angiographic thrombolysis.

SELECTED READINGS

American Association of Neurological Surgeons/Congress of Neurological Surgeons: Guidelines for the Management of Severe Head Injury: Joint Section on Neurotrauma and Critical Care, 1995.

Lee K, Hoff J: Intracranial pressure. In Youmans JR (ed): Neurological Surgery, 4th ed. Philadelphia, WB Saunders, 1996, p 511.

Liau L, Mergsneider M, Becker D: Pathology and physiology of head injury. In Youmans JR (ed): Neurological Surgery, 4th ed. Philadelphia, WB Saunders, 1996, p 1562.

Patten J: Neurological Differential Diagnosis, 2nd ed. London, Springer-Verlag London Ltd, 1996.

Plum F, Posner J: The Diagnosis of Stupor and Coma, 3rd ed. Philadelphia, FA Davis, 1982.

Schwartz S, Shires G, Spencer F: Principles of Surgery, 5th ed. New York, McGraw-Hill, 1989.

Teasdale G, Jennet B: Assessment of coma and impaired consciousness: A practical scale. Lancet 1974;2:81.

Valadka A: Injury to the cranium. In Mattox K, Feliciano D, Moore E (eds): Trauma, 4th ed. New York, McGraw-Hill, 2000, p 383.

Diagnosis of Brain Death

Gordon Anderson and Curtis Doberstein

As the ability of medical science to prolong organ function has increased, new concepts for clarifying and expanding the definition of brain death have evolved. The concept that the irreversible loss of cerebral function constitutes death has been generally accepted by the public at large

and has been enacted into law in most states. The need for a precise definition of brain death stems from the fact that vegetative functions, such as cardiac activity, can be maintained for prolonged periods of time even in the total absence of cerebral function. In addition, the increased demand for organs needed for transplantation procedures has pushed the need for the prompt declaration of brain death in appropriate donor patients. It is also ethically and practically important to convey the definition of brain death to families who might otherwise be given a false sense of hope by the persistence of a loved one's heartbeat even though there is no chance of recovery from the neurologic insult. It should be emphasized that there have been no reports of patient survival with the use of a strict criteria of brain death. The modern criteria used to document brain death in adults derive from the *President's Commission for the Study of Ethical Problems in Medical, Biomedical, and Behavioral Research* (1981), which advocates that laws define brain death as irreversible cessation of all functions of the entire brain. The determination of brain death in children younger than the age of 5 years is not reviewed in this chapter given the plasticity of the developing brain and the fact that the brain death examination in this age group should be completed by pediatric specialists. The purpose of this chapter is to review the criteria for completing the clinical brain death examination in adults, and to discuss the potential role of confirmatory diagnostic tests.

CLINICAL BRAIN DEATH EXAMINATION

Most criteria suggest that the diagnosis of brain death be agreed on by two licensed physicians with a period of observation of 12 to 24 hours prior to the final declaration. The use of confirmatory tests (described later) may shorten the period of observation. Typically, the diagnosis is made by neurosurgeons, neurologists, or specialists staffing intensive care units or emergency departments. Brain death can occur after a variety of insults, such as blunt and penetrating trauma, space-occupying intracranial lesions including cerebral hematomas and stroke, or cerebral ischemia-hypoxia. It is crucial to differentiate brain death from reversible coma secondary to metabolic causes, such as uremia, hepatic failure, and hypothermia. In addition, pharmacologic coma from agents such as opioids, barbiturates, alcohol, or neuromuscular blockade can mimic brain death and must be ruled out. Identifying the underlying cause of brain death is essential, and neuroimaging studies such as computed tomography, magnetic resonance imaging, and angiography can prove helpful in this regard. Diagnostic studies also increase the certainty with which the underlying brain injury can be said to be irreversible.

The basic requirement for the declaration of brain death is to document the irreversible loss of brainstem and cerebral cortical activity. The clinical examination is relatively simple to perform and can be reliably and reproducibly performed at the bedside in a short period of time (Table 19–3). Before performing the examination, it is important to document that the patient is not hypothermic (core temperature above 90°F[32°C]) and not hypotensive (systolic blood pressure >90 mm Hg). Brain-dead patients are uniformly intubated and unresponsive. These patients have no motor response to deep central pain, such as sternal rubbing or firm pressure applied to the orbital rim. Spinal cord–mediated reflex movements

Table 19–3	**Summary of the Clinical Brain Death Examination**

Absence of reversible causes
   Hypothermia
   Shock
   Drug intoxication or metabolic disorders
Stable vital signs
   Core temperature above 32.2°C
   Systolic blood pressure greater than 90 mm Hg
Loss of brainstem function
   Fixed and dilated pupils
   Absent gag, corneal, and oculovestibular reflexes
   No spontaneous respiration
No response to deep, central pain

can be seen, including the flexor plantar reflexes of the legs, abdominal or cremasteric reflexes, and complex movements such as the Lazarus sign (sitting up in bed). If complex movements do occur and it is difficult to determine whether they are reflexive in nature, confirmatory tests (described later) may prove useful. Brainstem reflexes are then assessed. The pupillary examination should be completed in a semidark room. The pupils should be midposition. A flashlight is shone sequentially into each eye, and the direct and consensual responses are assessed. Brain death is excluded if any response is seen. The corneal reflex, which tests for function at the level of the midbrain, is tested by applying a piece of cotton on the cornea, with the practitioner taking care not to touch the conjunctiva. No eyelid movement should be seen. The oculocephalic (doll's eye) reflex is tested by turning the patient's head from side to side while holding the eyes open. The eyes should remain in midposition. Any reflex movement of the eyes away from the direction of head turning excludes brain death. This test also evaluates cerebral function at the level of the midbrain. The vestibulocephalic stimulation test (cold water caloric) is done with the head of the bed elevated 30 degrees so as to orient the horizontal semicircular canal in a true horizontal position. Approximately 50 mL of ice water is then irrigated into each ear canal, after establishing that there is no tympanic membrane perforation or cerumen impaction. The eyes are held open and observed for 60 seconds after irrigating each side. No eye movement should be seen. The gag test is performed by moving the endotracheal tube while checking for retching or movement of the uvula. Cough assessment is done by passing a cannula down the endotracheal tube and observing for reaction.

The apnea challenge is generally performed as the last test in the brain death evaluation because of the potential for causing hypotension or raised ICP. The patient must first be documented to have an arterial partial pressure of carbon dioxide (PCO_2) reflective of normocapnia. Preoxygenation with 100% fraction of inspired oxygen (FIO_2) is then done via the endotracheal tube for 10 to 15 minutes. The patient is subsequently disconnected from the ventilator and observed for any signs of respiratory effort over a period of 10 minutes. The test is aborted if any signs of breathing activity are noted or of hemodynamic instability, such as hypotension or cardiac arrhythmia, are noted. Arterial blood gases are obtained at the end of the trial. If no respiratory efforts are noted and the arterial P_{CO_2} is greater than or equal to 60 mm Hg, the patient is documented as apneic. If the P_{CO_2} does not meet or exceed 60 mm Hg, the test must be repeated. If hemodynamic changes preclude the completion of the apnea challenge, the completion of confirmatory diagnostic testing is required.

After completion of the brain death examination, a signed note should be written in the patient's chart describing the findings on examination as well as the date and time of declaration of brain death. Completed confirmatory tests should also be described. The family should then be made aware as to the findings on examination, the implications of the diagnosis of brain death (i.e., irreversible with no chance of recovery), and potential options, such as withdrawal of life support or enrollment in an organ donation program.

Observation Interval

The clinical brain death examination needs to be repeated after an appropriate interval to confirm the diagnosis of brain death. The interval between serial examinations varies, depending on the cause of the patient's loss of neurologic function and on whether any confirmatory tests have been performed. In cases in which an irreversible condition has been documented and no confirmatory tests are obtained, the typical period of observation between clinical examinations is 12 hours. This can be reduced to 6 hours if a confirmatory test is obtained. In cases in which massive cerebral damage is documented (e.g., gunshot wounds or large cerebral hematomas), some experts recommend that only a single clinical examination be performed if a confirmatory test will also be completed.

Confirmatory Diagnostic Tests

Several confirmatory diagnostic tests are available to aid in diagnosing brain death. These tests can also prove beneficial by shortening the observation time required between clinical examinations. These tests either give measures of cerebral blood flow (CBF) or provide information about the integrity of cerebral and brainstem functions. Since the brain suffers irreversible damage after only minutes of CBF cessation, a test that demonstrates absent CBF helps confirm brain death. Cerebral angiography is considered the gold standard for documenting absent CBF and confirming brain death. However, the invasive nature, cost, requirement for patient transport, and potential renal damage from contrast load in potential organ donors have caused angiography to be used less frequently, particularly in light of the availability of other less invasive tests.

Radionuclide angiography estimates CBF and has the advantages of being noninvasive, less costly, rapidly performed, and free from contrast medium requirements. The test is performed by intravenously injecting a radioisotope such as technetium and obtaining serial cranial images at 2-second intervals for 60 seconds. A confirmatory brain death study documents cessation of blood flow

with absent radiotracer uptake in the anterior and middle cerebral artery distributions. Delayed flow in the dural venous sinuses, which can arise from the external carotid circulation, does not exclude the diagnosis of brain death. This test can be confounded by technical factors such as the lack of a good bolus injection and poor sensitivity for detecting low values of posterior fossa CBF.

Another useful CBF confirmatory test is transcranial Doppler ultrasonography (TCD). Transcranial Doppler imaging can be used to evaluate the velocity and direction of blood flow in the internal carotid, middle cerebral, anterior cerebral, and basilar arteries. Oscillating TCD flow (i.e., blood traveling in both forward and backward directions) or the observation of characteristic systolic peaks can prove to be reliable ancillary TCD indicators of brain death. Doppler ultrasound has the advantage of being portable, noninvasive, and readily repeatable. However, technician experience is required in cases of brain death confirmation.

Electroencephalography (EEG) and brainstem auditory evoked responses (BAER) are functional tests that can provide important information regarding cerebral function. Electroencephalograms yield information about cortical function only, but share with Doppler ultrasound the advantage of being fast, inexpensive, and portable. An EEG that documents electrocerebral silence (i.e., "flatline") can be helpful in confirming the diagnosis of brain death, although EEG alone is not sufficient to distinguish brain death from reversible coma. Brainstem auditory evoked responses provide information about the integrity of sensory function in the pons and lower brainstem. Electrodes placed in the scalp and ear ipsilateral to a click stimulus can measure five distinct waves. The waves are seen within 10 milliseconds of the stimulus. Wave I is thought to derive from cranial nerve 8, while waves II through V arise from different areas of the medulla, pons, and midbrain. The BAER is useful in brain death because it is relatively unaffected by the presence of drugs or altered metabolic states (e.g., uremia). Wave I should be elicited on at least one side in order to establish the validity of the test. This will establish that signals are propagated through the nerve to the brainstem so that the lack of waves II through V may be interpreted as indicating the lack of function in the lower brainstem.

DIFFICULTIES IN DIAGNOSING BRAIN DEATH

In performing the clinical brain death examination, the physician may encounter confounding factors that make the assessment difficult to complete. The presence of facial trauma, for example, can render the execution of any or all of the brainstem tests difficult or impossible. The persistence of spinal reflexes, such as the triple flexion response that can be seen in the lower extremities as a response to pain, is not mediated by cortical or brainstem functions. Their presence, therefore, does not exclude brain death as a diagnosis but may be confusing to family members who observe motor activity. The presence of preexisting chronic obstructive pulmonary disease (COPD) may call into question the validity of the apnea test, owing to altered responses in these patients to hypercapnia. There may also be instances in which a clear history of stroke, hypoxia, or trauma cannot be obtained, and the etiology of the coma remains unclear despite obtaining appropriate neuroimaging and metabolic studies. It is in instances such as these that a confirmatory test can prove helpful. Confirmatory tests may be used to corroborate the clinical examination and to reduce the interval needed between serial examinations before brain death can be declared. This last point becomes especially important in the unstable patient who is being maintained for organ transplantation. The various technical pitfalls and limitations of each of the confirmatory tests must also be kept in mind, so that false-positive or false-negative results are not overlooked, which can be a source of not only confusion and angst for the family, but also needless prolongation of the declaration process. Also of use in difficult cases or cases in which the etiology is not clear is the consultation of a physician experienced in declaring brain death, typically a neurologist or neurosurgeon. Families who are distraught at the diagnosis of brain death may also be put more at ease by the corroborating opinion of a specialist.

Errors can also arise during brain death evaluation if the diagnosis is taken for granted and steps are omitted from the examination. Not only can this lead to the erroneous confirmation of brain death, but also it can damage the ability of the physician to form a rapport with a family that could potentially have agreed to participate in an organ donation program.

ORGAN DONATION

If consent is obtained for organ donation from the patient's legal guardian, a transplant coordinator should be contacted as soon as possible. The transplant coordinator is an excellent resource for obtaining the appropriate investigations (e.g., electrocardiogram, serology, and microbiology tests) as well as aid in managing the patient's current medical problems (see later) and providing support and information for the family. In addition, the state medical examiner may need to be contacted, particularly in homicide or accident cases.

Complete cardiorespiratory failure typically occurs 3 to 5 days following brain death; however, prior to this, multiple physiologic alterations can occur that potentially harm viable organs. Every effort should be made to maintain adequate vital signs and electrolyte homeostasis. Hypotension should be controlled through volume expansion. Crystalloid solutions (D_5 1/4 NS + 20 mEq KCl) are typically used in the initial setting and are administered at 100 mL/hr, in addition to replacing urine losses milliliter for milliliter. If hypotension occurs despite adequate crystalloid infusion, colloid (e.g., albumin) administration is indicated. Vasopressors (e.g., dopamine) can be used if volume expansion fails to maintain blood pressure; however, at high doses these agents may damage organs by limiting perfusion. Therefore, start with a low dose and slowly titrate upward as needed.

Endocrine dysfunction is common among brain-dead patients and requires appropriate treatment. Diabetes insipidus often will ensue following necrosis of hypophyseal tissue, with resulting impairment of antidiuretic hormone release. Urinary output is usually greater than 300 mL/hr; however, it may soar into the range of 800 mL/hr. Serum sodium can quickly rise into the range of 170 mm/dL, which can be damaging to potential donor organs. Antidiuretic hormone analogues may be used to replace antidiuretic hormone, either in boluses or as a continuous drip. Aqueous vasopressin (Pitressin) is preferred over DDAVP to avoid renal compromise. Euvolemia and electrolyte homeostasis must be maintained. Early anticipation and treatment of diabetes insipidus can help maintain electrolyte and volume balance in patients being considered for organ donation.

Pearls and Pitfalls

PEARLS

- The diagnosis of brain death can be made by the use of standardized criteria and appropriate ancillary tests, prerequisites for which include the following:

  Knowledge of the underlying cause of the loss of function, supported by neuroimaging studies.
  Establishment of normothermia and hypotension.
  Absence of drugs or medical conditions that can confound the examination.
  Absence of brainstem reflexes and cortical activity on clinical examination.
  Waiting for a sufficient observation period.
  Ancillary tests, such as angiography, TCD, radionuclide scintigraphy, EEG, and BAER, can corroborate the clinical diagnosis and shorten the waiting period between serial examinations.
  The ability to declare brain death, as distinct from cardiorespiratory death, allows families a sense of closure in the setting of devastating neurologic injury and opens the opportunity to save other lives through organ transplantation.

PITFALLS

- Serious consequences may result from the misdiagnosis of brain death. Errors in diagnosis can arise if the following occur:

  Brain death is taken for granted, and steps are omitted from the examination process.
  Spinal reflexes are confused with brainstem or cortical motor activity.
  Potential errors of ancillary tests are not taken into account.

SELECTED READINGS

Beresford HR: Medical-legal issues facing neurologists: Brain death. Neurol Clin 1992;17:295.

Black PM: Conceptual and practical issues in the decision of death by brain criteria. Neurosurg Clin North Am 1991;2:493.

Kaufman JJ, Brick J, Frick M: Brain death. In Youmans JR (ed): Neurological Surgery, 3rd ed. Philadelphia, WB Saunders, 1991, pp 439-451.

Plum F, Posner JB (eds): Brain death. In The Diagnosis of Stupor and Coma 3rd ed. Philadelphia, FA Davis, 1982, p 319.

President's Commission for the Study of Ethical Problems in Medical, Biomedical and Behavioral Research: Defining Death: Medical, Legal and Ethical Issues in the Determination of Death. Washington, DC, U.S. Government Printing Office, 1981.

Surgeon General's Workshop on Increasing Organ Donation. Proceedings. Washington, DC: U.S. Department of Health and Human Services, 1991.

Task Force for the Determination of Brain Death in Children: Guidelines for the Determination of Brain Death in Children. Pediatrics 1987;80:298.

Chapter 20

Acute Systemic Hypertension

Neil A. Davis and Lunzy D. Britt

Acute elevations of blood pressure are potentially life-threatening events that require expeditious but careful evaluation and treatment to avoid injury to the central nervous system, heart, and kidneys. Acute hypertension in the surgical patient is complicated by the increased potential for bleeding. The surgeon must evaluate potential etiologies of acute hypertension, which may include preexisting hypertension, anxiety, pain, fluid imbalances, and electrolyte abnormalities. Although blood pressure variations are common in patients undergoing surgery, a recognized association exists between operative mortality rate and inadequately controlled hypertension. It is imperative that the surgeon has a comprehensive understanding of the pharmacologic management of acute hypertension and the associated etiologies. Choice of agent varies by indication and requires careful consideration of concomitant disease states and potential contraindications (see Table 20–1).

CLINICAL PRESENTATION

Acute elevations in blood pressure are categorized as *hypertensive urgencies* (elevated blood pressure without evidence of end-organ damage) or *hypertensive emergencies* (severe elevations in blood pressure associated with end-organ damage). The absolute blood pressure values are less important than the presence or absence of end-organ damage. Treatment of hypertensive emergencies requires immediate blood pressure reductions, whereas blood pressure reduction in treatment of hypertensive urgencies may be accomplished over a period of 24 to 48 hours. An understanding of cerebral autoregulation is important for the treatment of acute hypertension. Cerebral vascular autoregulation maintains constant cerebral perfusion pressure over a mean arterial pressure (MAP) range of approximately 50 to 150 mm Hg. As the MAP decreases, cerebral vasodilation occurs; as MAP increases, cerebral vasoconstriction occurs, maintaining a relatively constant cerebral perfusion pressure. If MAP goes below the lower limit of cerebral autoregulation, symptoms of cerebral ischemia may occur. Chronic hypertension impairs cerebral autoregulation such that a loss of autoregulation and cerebral hypoperfusion may occur at a higher blood pressure than normal. Therefore, reduction of MAP by no more than 20% to 25% within the first 2 hours has been advocated to reduce the risk of iatrogenic injury by exceeding the lower limit of autoregulation. Further reduction may be accomplished slowly over 2 to 6 hours, carefully avoiding excessive declines.

PREOPERATIVE MANAGEMENT

Patients with diastolic blood pressures greater than 110 mm Hg before induction have a greater incidence of perioperative complications, such as arrhythmias and myocardial ischemia. Patients taking chronic antihypertensive medications should take the morning dose of medication before surgery to minimize intraoperative hypertensive episodes.

INTRAOPERATIVE MANAGEMENT

Most intraoperative hypertension results from activation of the sympathetic nervous system, especially in patients with chronic hypertension. The clinician must exclude pain, inadequate sedation, and anxiety as potential causes of hypertension.

POSTOPERATIVE MANAGEMENT

Often occurring in the first 10 to 20 minutes after surgery, postoperative hypertension may result in adverse sequelae, such as bleeding, cerebrovascular accidents, and myocardial ischemia. Systolic blood pressures greater than 180 mm Hg have been associated with increased bleeding from wound sites or chest tubes.

DRUG THERAPY

Nitroglycerin

Nitroglycerin is a direct vasodilator of peripheral capacitance and resistance vessels. The dominant effect of nitroglycerin is venodilation, reducing venous return. It is a weak arterial vasodilator with a greater effect on large arteries than on smaller arteries and arterioles. Low doses produce venodilation and large vessel arterial dilation with much higher doses producing systemic arteriolar dilation. Nitroglycerin decreases preload, left ventricular diastolic pressure, volume, and myocardial oxygen demand. It dilates ischemic coronary arteries and increases oxygen delivery to ischemic myocardium. Nitroglycerin tends to induce cerebral venodilation, which may increase cerebral blood volume and exacerbate intracranial hypertension. Nitroglycerin has a rapid onset of action and an elimination half-life of minutes, allowing for return of baseline blood pressure within 10 minutes after infusion discontinuation. Nitroglycerin is the preferred agent for treatment of ischemic heart disease and is also effective for acute left ventricular failure. However, its predominant effect on venous vasculature may limit its effectiveness as an antihypertensive (Table 20–1).

Sodium Nitroprusside

Sodium nitroprusside is a potent vascular smooth muscle relaxant that produces balanced vasodilation of resistance

Table 20–1	Drug Therapy for Hypertension	
INDICATION	**AGENT OF CHOICE**	**CONTRAINDICATIONS**
Hypertensive encephalopathy	Nitroprusside, labetalol	Clonidine
Cerebral vascular events	Nitroprusside, labetalol	Diazoxide, hydralazine
Left ventricular failure	Nitroprusside, enalaprilat, nitroglycerin	Labetalol, β-blockers
Myocardial ischemia	Nitroglycerin	Diazoxide, hydralazine, fenoldopam
Dissecting aortic aneurysm	β-Blockers ± nitroprusside	Diazoxide, hydralazine
Catecholamine crisis	β-Blockers + nitroprusside, labetalol, phentolamine	β-Blockers alone
Renal insufficiency	Nitroprusside, labetalol	Enalaprilat
Eclampsia	Hydralazine, methyldopa, labetalol	Nitroprusside

and capacitance vessels. It reduces preload and afterload, allowing improvement in left ventricular function and pulmonary edema in congestive failure. Nitroprusside induces cerebral vasodilation and may increase cerebral blood volume and intracranial pressure. It should not be used as monotherapy with aortic dissection because reflex increases in sympathetic tone may increase shear forces on the aorta. A β-blocker may be used in conjunction with nitroprusside to inhibit reflex increases in heart rate and myocardial contractility. Nitroprusside is nonenzymatically degraded to cyanide, which is then metabolized via the liver to thiocyanate. Thiocyanate is excreted renally. Caution should be given to nitroprusside use in severe hepatic or renal dysfunction, because cyanide toxicity may occur in hepatic failure and thiocyanate accumulation may occur in renal failure. Sodium nitroprusside can be used relatively safely in the setting of renal failure if the dose and duration are limited. It has a very rapid onset and its effects dissipate within 1 to 2 minutes after stopping the infusion. With very few exceptions, nitroprusside is effective first-line therapy for most acute hypertensive crises.

Esmolol

Esmolol is a short-acting β₁-selective β-blocker. It competitively blocks adrenergic stimulation of β-adrenergic receptors within the myocardium and vascular smooth muscle. β-blockers reduce blood pressure by blocking peripheral (especially cardiac) adrenergic receptors (decreasing cardiac output), decreasing sympathetic outflow from the central nervous system, diminishing peripheral sympathetic tone, and suppressing renal renin release. Esmolol produces negative chronotropic and inotropic effects and generally leads to a decrease in myocardial oxygen consumption. Patients with high plasma renin levels have the greatest hypotensive response to esmolol.

Even though it is β₁-selective, the agent should be used with caution in reactive airway disease. Abrupt withdrawal of β-blocking agents may precipitate hyperadrenergic withdrawal syndrome, potentially producing ischemia and arrhythmias. β-adrenergic receptor antagonists do not appear to adversely affect intracranial hypertension in traumatic brain injury patients. Esmolol has a short onset of action and a terminal half-life of only 9 minutes. Its main utility lies in its extremely short duration of action.

Labetalol

Labetalol is an α-blocker and a nonselective β-blocker. It shares similar pharmacologic activity to other β-blocking agents. The β-adrenergic blocking activity of labetalol is approximately three or seven times more potent than its α-adrenergic effects following oral or intravenous administration, respectively. Onset after intravenous administration occurs within 5 minutes. Labetalol has an elimination half-life of 6 to 8 hours. Although it has a relatively long half-life, labetalol reduces blood pressure in a steady and controlled fashion. Labetalol may be given via intermittent bolus or continuous infusion. Intravenous administration does not significantly affect cerebral blood flow and can effectively be used to treat hypertension in traumatic brain injury patients. It may also be given to patients with coronary artery disease. Labetalol may be used to treat catecholamine crises, but concomitant therapy with an α-blocking agent may be required as a result of the predominance of β-adrenergic activity.

Enalaprilat

Enalaprilat is an angiotensin-converting enzyme (ACE) inhibitor that inhibits conversion of angiotensin I to angiotensin II. It reduces blood pressure by decreasing systemic vascular resistance via its vasodilatory properties on arteries and arterioles. Enalaprilat is most effective in patients with increased renin levels. It decreases renal vascular resistance and improves renal blood flow. Enalaprilat decreases left ventricular filling pressure and improves left ventricular function in patients with congestive heart failure. Increases in serum creatinine or oliguric renal failure may be seen in states of low cardiac output or intravascular depletion. Enalaprilat is contraindicated in patients with bilateral renal artery stenosis. Effects of ACE inhibitors on intracranial pressure have not been widely studied, but they appear to have the potential to exacerbate intracranial hypertension. After intravenous enalaprilat administration, hypotensive effects are apparent within 5 to 15 minutes with maximum effect occurring within 1 to 4 hours. Duration of action in most patients is approximately 6 hours. All ACE inhibitors impair the breakdown of bradykinin, which may result in life-threatening angioedema. Potassium levels should be monitored during therapy because ACE inhibitors may precipitate hyperkalemia. Enalaprilat may cause precipitous decreases in blood pressure in patients dependent on high systemic vascular resistance for maintenance of blood pressure. Enalaprilat may offer unique benefit in high renin states of hypertension or acute left ventricular failure.

Nicardipine

Nicardipine is a dihydropyridine calcium channel antagonist. The principal physiologic action is to inhibit the transmembrane influx of extracellular calcium ions across the membranes of myocardial and vascular smooth muscle cells. Specificity for vascular smooth muscle predominates with minimal negative inotropic effects appreciated. Nicardipine is a potent vasodilator that causes selective dilation of arterial resistance vessels. It appears to augment coronary blood flow and improve perfusion to ischemic coronary vessels. It is a cerebral vasodilator and may exacerbate intracranial hypertension. Intravenous nicardipine has an onset of action of 5 to 10 minutes and duration of 1 to 4 hours. Flushing, headache, and peripheral edema appear to be the most common side effects. It is extensively metabolized in the liver and dosages should be reduced in patients with hepatic impairment or decreased liver blood flow. The calcium channel blocking properties of nicardipine position it as an effective alternative to first-line antihypertensive agents.

Fenoldopam

Fenoldopam is a peripheral dopamine-1 (DA_1) agonist. Postsynaptic DA_1 receptors mediate arterial vasodilation. Fenoldopam also dilates the renal vasculature, leading to increased renal perfusion, natriuresis, and diuresis. Its DA_1 receptor agonist properties are six to nine times more potent than those of dopamine. Fenoldopam, therefore, may be useful for treatment of hypertensive patients in the setting of renal dysfunction. It may elicit reflex tachycardia and therefore should be used with caution in patients with ischemic heart disease. Fenoldopam has an onset of action of approximately 5 minutes with peak activity occurring in 15 minutes, allowing for rapid titration of the drug. The hypotensive effects dissipate within 5 minutes after discontinuation of the infusion. The renal vasodilatory properties of fenoldopam may provide advantages over other agents in the setting of renal dysfunction, but further research is necessary to elucidate its place in therapy.

Hydralazine

Hydralazine is a direct arteriolar vasodilator that acts on precapillary arterioles. Diastolic blood pressure is usually affected more than systolic pressure. The hypotensive effects are often accompanied by reflex increases in heart rate, cardiac output, and stroke volume. Increased cardiac output partially offsets the hypotensive effect of arteriolar dilation and may limit the antihypertensive effectiveness. Sodium and water retention may lead to increases in plasma volume. Concomitant use of a diuretic may inhibit sodium and water retention during therapy. Hydralazine is extensively metabolized by the liver. Onset of action after intravenous administration is approximately 5 min-

utes with duration of 3 to 4 hours. Patients with severe brain injury demonstrate increased intracranial pressure and defective cerebral autoregulation after hydralazine administration. Because of the cardiac adverse effects and the unpredictable activity in comparison with other agents, hydralazine is usually second line therapy.

Diazoxide

Diazoxide reduces peripheral vascular resistance and blood pressure by direct vasodilatory effects on smooth muscle in peripheral arterioles. Resistance to the hypotensive effects of diazoxide occur in patients receiving multiple doses secondary to sodium retention and extracellular volume expansion. Concomitant use of a diuretic has been advocated to inhibit sodium and water retention during therapy. The hypotensive effects of diazoxide are accompanied by reflex increases in heart rate, cardiac output, and left ventricular ejection rate. Coronary and cerebral perfusion are maintained and there is no change in myocardial oxygen consumption. Diazoxide should be avoided in the treatment of aortic dissection or coarctation of the aorta because increases in cardiac output and heart rate may be deleterious. Diazoxide has an onset of action of 3 to 5 minutes after intravenous administration and, although the duration is somewhat variable among patients, it is usually less than 12 hours. The half-life of diazoxide may be prolonged in patients with renal dysfunction. Routine diazoxide use has been replaced by newer agents with fewer adverse effects and easier use.

COMPLICATIONS

Most complications related to intravenous antihypertensive therapy involve extensions of pharmacologic action. A preventable pitfall lies in reducing blood pressure too rapidly or too low for a chronic hypertensive. Excessive reductions in blood pressure may create secondary insults that worsen end-organ damage. A thorough knowledge of pharmacologic options to treat acute hypertension enables

---

Pearls and Pitfalls

PEARLS

- Excessive reductions in blood pressure may create secondary insults that worsen end-organ damage. A preventable pitfall lies in reducing blood pressure too rapidly or too low for a chronic hypertensive patient.
- Reduction of MAP by no more than 20% to 25% within the first 2 hours reduces the risk of iatrogenic injury by exceeding the lower limit of cerebral autoregulation.
- Patients with diastolic blood pressures greater than 110 mm Hg before induction have a greater incidence of perioperative complications, such as arrhythmias or myocardial ischemia.
- Postoperative hypertension most often occurs in the first 10 to 20 minutes after surgery.
- With very few exceptions, nitroprusside is effective first-line therapy for most acute hypertensive crises.

the clinician to weigh efficacy, adverse effects, and phar-macodynamic profile when choosing an agent.

OUTCOMES

Circumventing an unfavorable outcome, defined as end-organ damage or loss of life, is the paramount goal in the management of acute systemic management. Specific treatment paradigms have been previously described. However, patient variations are key factors in the overall outcome of an individual. Even though some patients appear to tolerate a significantly high blood pressure, other patients suffer catastrophic end-organ damage and possible death with lower blood pressure.

SELECTED READINGS

Calhoun DA, Oparil S: Treatment of hypertensive crisis. N Engl J Med 1990;323:1177.
Chernow B, eds: The Pharmacologic Approach to the Critically Ill Patient, 3rd ed. Baltimore, Williams & Wilkins, 1994.
Erstad BL, Barletta JF: Treatment of hypertension in the perioperative patient. Ann Pharmacother 2000;34:66.
Gifford RW: Management of hypertensive crisis. JAMA 1991;266:829.
Tietjen CS, Hurn PD, Ulatowski JA, et al: Treatment modalities for hypertensive patients with intracranial pathology: Options and risks. Crit Care Med 1996;24:311.

Chapter 21

Do Not Resuscitate, Do Not Treat

Dan W. Brock

Resuscitation as used here is the life-giving restoration of heartbeat or respiration in a patient who has suffered cardiac or respiratory arrest. Do Not Resuscitate (DNR) orders state that no resuscitation attempt should be made for a particular patient. Do Not Treat or Comfort Measures Only (CMO) orders state that treatment interventions, including interventions that might extend life, should be undertaken only if they will improve the comfort of the patient. This chapter addresses some of the main ethical issues in practice and policy regarding DNR and CMO orders in the hospital setting.

RESUSCITATION

The ability sometimes to bring a patient back from the brink of death by resuscitation is surely one of the great successes of modern medicine. While originally developed for otherwise healthy patients who had suffered loss of heartbeat and respiration following surgery or near drowning, resuscitation techniques were increasingly improved and more widely applied during the 1960s and 1970s. Because a resuscitation attempt must begin within minutes of cessation of heartbeat (if it is to have any hope of success in restoring cardiac and respiratory function without debilitating neurologic consequences for the patient from prolonged loss of oxygen to the brain), it became common to attempt it in all hospital patients who suffered cardiac arrest. At the same time, it was increasingly recognized that resuscitation would not benefit some patients, and so some hospitals developed policies in the mid-1970s for orders not to attempt resuscitation. At the present time, virtually all hospitals have a policy that, in the absence of an order not to resuscitate, resuscitation will be attempted on any patient who suffers cardiac or respiratory arrest. The reasons for such policies are obvious and sound. Taking the time to decide whether a patient will be resuscitated is incompatible with the need to begin resuscitation or a code immediately. This means that every hospitalized surgical patient, in effect, has a standing order to resuscitate unless a DNR order is written. Ensuring that a patient's code status is addressed in a timely and appropriate manner is of great importance for both patients and physicians: for patients, attempts to resuscitate would then take place only when wanted and warranted; for physicians, few interventions can be more disturbing than having to run a "code" when it only brutalizes the patient for no benefit at the end of the patient's life.

Several questions need to be addressed. How should resuscitation decisions be made? Who should be involved in the decision making? What ethical values should guide the decisions? When should decision making take place? How should conflicts be resolved?

CODE STATUS DECISIONS WITH COMPETENT PATIENTS

Even though code status should be decided well in advance of a need for resuscitation, the decision-making process in most respects should be like that for other medical interventions. Medicine has a long tradition in which the physician–patient relationship was understood in paternalist terms with decision-making authority resting with the physician. That tradition has probably been stronger and more persistent in surgery than in other aspects of the medical field. The patient was not seen to have a substantial role in deciding treatment, although it was recognized that the patient's consent to treatment was needed and that the patient usually needed a sufficient understanding of what would be done to comply effectively with treatment. This view of the physician–patient relationship and of treatment decision making has been largely rejected in favor of a process of shared decision making in which the physician and patient each have important and necessary roles. Roughly (and oversimplifying), physicians use their training, experience, and expertise to provide information about diagnosis and prognosis without treatment and about treatments that might provide an improved prognosis together with their risks and benefits. Patients bring their own aims and values that enable them to select, together with their physicians, the alternative intervention that is best for them.

This is the process of obtaining *informed consent* for treatment generally and for surgery in particular. Two values form the fundamental ethical basis for shared decision making—patient well-being and self-determination. Serving the patient's well-being is the fundamental aim of medicine. I use the concept of "well-being" instead of "health and extending life" to signal that which intervention will be best for a particular patient depends, in part, on that patient's particular values and plan of life, which cannot be determined by medical science alone. Self-determination is simply the interest of ordinary persons in making important decisions about their lives for themselves and according to their own values and aims, not according to what someone else might consider best for them. Physicians' task then is to use their training and skills to promote their patient's well-being, consistent with respecting patients' self-determination by securing an informed consent for treatment.

CODE STATUS DECISIONS WITH INCOMPETENT PATIENTS

Sometimes shared decision making with patients is not possible because the patient is incompetent and unable

163

to participate. In that case, a surrogate must be identified to act for the patient. The surrogate should be whomever the patient has designated, or would want, to act for him, typically a close family member. The surrogate's decisions should be guided by any pertinent advance directive, if one exists. In the absence of an advance directive, the surrogate's decision should be guided by what the patient would have wanted in the circumstances if competent; in the absence of knowledge of the patient's wishes, the decision should be guided by an assessment of what will best serve the patient's interests. An important responsibility of surgeons in shared decision making with surrogates is to help surrogates understand that their job is to decide together with the surgeon what the patient would have wanted, not to decide what they want for the patient. If surrogates understand that their principal role is to provide evidence of the patient's wishes, not to take the full burden of responsibility for the decision, then the responsibility for the choice is left with the patient as much as possible given the patient's incompetence. The emotional and psychological burdens of the decision about code status then become easier to bear for surrogates.

Sometimes, especially with incompetent patients, decisions about treatment must be made in emergency circumstances in which there is no time to involve the patient or to locate and involve a surrogate in decision making. Emergency conditions in which the patient would likely suffer serious harm or death if time were taken to secure the patient's or a surrogate's consent to treatment constitute a long-standing exception to the requirement that treatment not be rendered without consent, recognized in both the law and medical ethics. In this situation, it is the surgeon's responsibility to follow the patient's advance directive if such exist; if there is no advance directive, then the surgeon must follow what the patient would have wanted, or if that is not known, what most reasonable people would want in the circumstances.

SURGEONS' RESPONSIBILITIES

Whether decision making about code status is with a competent patient or an incompetent patient's surrogate, the surgeon has an important responsibility to enable patients or surrogates to make an informed choice. That includes ensuring that they understand the patient's prognosis with whatever treatments will be pursued, together with whatever uncertainties attend the prognosis. Most important is the surgeon's responsibility to ensure that patients or surrogates are well informed about resuscitation itself, because they are often either uninformed or misinformed. In particular, they must be given an estimate, based on relevant data, about the likely benefits of resuscitation, especially the likelihood of the resuscitation attempt being successful in restoring cardiac and respiratory function, as well as in achieving other end points important to the patient such as surviving to leave the hospital or recovering or retaining some level of functional status or quality of life. In some cases, data can be provided about resuscitation outcomes specific to the patient's condition, for example, for patients with meta-

static cancer or multiorgan system failure. Many patients and families overestimate the likelihood of benefit from a resuscitation attempt without clear and specific information from their surgeon. Equally important is information about the burdens and risks of resuscitation. This includes a frank description of what the process of resuscitation is like, the risks such as permanent respirator dependence or broken ribs from the process, as well as the likelihood of a worsened quality of life after a successful resuscitation.

The discussion about code status can be difficult and uncomfortable for a patient or surrogate, as well as for the surgeon. It is important to provide a full and accurate description of the process, burdens, and risks of resuscitation. Even though a sanitized description may make the discussion psychologically and emotionally easier, it can lead to uninformed or misinformed decisions that are harmful to the patient and not what the patient would have wanted with a sound understanding of the nature of the choice. Finally, it is important that patients or surrogates understand that a DNR order applies only to resuscitation in the case of cardiac or respiratory arrest; it does not result in any other treatment or care being withheld. Sometimes the reasons for deciding on a DNR order may support decisions to forego other treatments as well, but those other decisions must remain distinct from the DNR decision. Patients or their families should not have to be reluctant to have a DNR order for fear that other desired care will be withheld or less aggressive because of a DNR order. And surgeons must ensure, as well, that all members of the care team understand that the DNR order applies only to resuscitation, not to any other aspect of the patient's care.

THE TIMING OF DECISIONS ABOUT CODE STATUS

When should the issue of code status be raised with patients or their surrogates? First, it is the surgeon's responsibility to raise the question with the patient or surrogate, not to wait until they raise the question. A few commentators have argued that code status should be raised with all hospital patients, because any patient could suffer a cardiac or respiratory arrest. Even if the question is not posed to all patients, it is important for the surgeon to address code status promptly with patients who have a higher likelihood of suffering cardiac or respiratory arrest. Moreover, physicians should be aware of their limited ability to predict when a patient is likely to code. One study of more than 200 consecutive codes run in a teaching hospital found that approximately 70% of the patients' physicians, both house staff and attending physicians, did not expect the patient to suffer an imminent cardiac arrest. The implication is that, if the patient's code status is to be addressed and settled appropriately when the patient suffers a cardiac or respiratory arrest, then it is necessary for physicians to address the issue with patients before they believe it is necessary to do so. Erring on the side of raising the issue early rather than late is important as well because a significant amount of time and discussion is often needed before the patient's code status can be resolved. Furthermore, if a surgeon has any significant reason to believe that the patient would not want to be resuscitated or that the patient's wishes about resuscitation may have changed, then the question of code status should be raised promptly with the patient. Finally, depending on the nature of the surgery, there is often a significant enough, even if low, risk of cardiac arrest following the surgery to require raising the question of code status with the patient.

Sometimes patients who are to undergo surgery already have a DNR order before surgery; a DNR order need not be inconsistent with pursuing surgery for a number of reasons, such as when the surgery would increase the comfort or quality of life of a terminally ill patient. When the hospital's or individual surgeon's policy is that the DNR order must be suspended during surgery, patients must always be informed of that fact as part of the informed consent for the surgery, including the time parameters during which the DNR order will be suspended. While the issue remains highly controversial, some hospitals, surgeons, and anesthesiologists in unusual circumstances will permit a patient to undergo surgery without suspending a DNR order that was in place before the surgery.

RESOLVING CONFLICTS

Sometimes conflict arises between the surgeon and the patient or surrogate regarding the patient's code status. Such conflict can take several forms. If a competent patient wants a DNR order but the surgeon believes that it would not be in the patient's interests, it is the surgeon's responsibility to ensure that the patient understands all information relevant to the choice and to advocate the course of action he or she believes to be in the patient's best interests. However, the law, public policy, and professional codes of ethics are clear that a competent patient's refusal of treatment must be respected, even if the patient's physician or others believe the patient has made a bad choice. If the surrogate for an incompetent patient insists on a DNR order for the patient that the surgeon believes the patient would not have wanted or is not in the patient's interests, the same steps of ensuring the surrogate's understanding and advocating for what the surgeon believes is in the patient's interests are appropriate. However, further steps may also be required when a surrogate is acting for an incompetent patient. If the surgeon believes that the surrogate is acting from a conflict of interest with the patient or that there is clear evidence that the patient did or would not have wanted a DNR order, it is the surgeon's responsibility to take further steps to protect the patient's interests. These can include seeking the participation of other family members, consulting with an ethics committee, or, if all else fails, going to court to clarify the surrogate's authority.

FUTILITY

The more difficult cases occur when a patient, or more commonly the surrogate for an incompetent patient, insists on the patient being a "full code" when the surgeon believes that an attempt to resuscitate the patient would be futile. The proper response to demands for futile care is controversial and unsettled in the law, medical practice, and medical ethics. Some institutions, commentators, and professional organizations have proposed specific policies concerning patients' or surrogates' demands for futile care, although there is no consensus about what these policies should be. One difficulty is how futility should be understood. The strongest ethical basis for physicians refusing demands for futile care is when it is known with virtual certainty that the resuscitation attempt would not succeed in restoring cardiac or respiratory function; however, there are few cases in which data support that a resuscitation attempt would be virtually certain to fail. More common is when a patient is near death and the physician believes that resuscitation even if successful would only delay death for a very short time and that doing so would not benefit the patient because of the patient's suffering and extremely poor quality of life. Here, the fundamental ethical issue is whose judgment should prevail in deciding whether resuscitation would provide the patient any benefit or benefit sufficient to justify its burdens. The American Medical Association's Ethical and Judicial Council has developed a reasonable proposal for these cases that requires a further discussion among the involved parties, referral to an ethics committee, and, if the ethics committee supports the patient or surrogate, transfer of the patient's care within the institution to a physician willing to carry out those wishes. Whereas, if the ethics committee supports the physician, the care need not be provided and the patient would be transferred to another institution. This approach to conflicts about futile care ensures a fair procedure in which all parties can air their views. The patient's or surrogate's decision is respected if it is supported by the process, and physicians are not required to act contrary to their own deeply held moral or professional values.

TIMING OF CMO DECISIONS

Do Not Treat, or more commonly Comfort Measures Only (CMO), orders are herein understood as orders not to continue or initiate any further diagnostic, monitoring, or therapeutic interventions whose purpose is to extend the patient's life. Interventions are to be undertaken only when they have a reasonable prospect of maintaining or improving the comfort of a dying patient. These orders raise many of the same issues as those discussed concerning resuscitation. The ethical framework sketched earlier regarding who should be involved in decision making, what their different roles should be, and the ethical values that should guide the decision-making process apply equally here.

Unlike the decision regarding resuscitation and DNR orders, which has to be made in advance of the need for resuscitation, the time needed for the decision to make the patient's status CMO can typically be taken without seriously harming the patient. The question of changing the patient's status to CMO can appropriately be raised by the surgeon or by the patient or surrogate. Surgeons should raise the issue with a patient or surrogate when they believe that further attempts to extend the patient's life would no longer provide any benefit to the patient or when they believe that further life-extending interventions would not be wanted by the patient. Alternatively, patients may raise the issue with their surgeon when they no longer wish to have further life-extending interventions, and surrogates should raise the issue with the surgeon when they believe the patient would no longer want those interventions. The decision to shift to CMO status can often be difficult for patients, and especially for some family members acting as surrogates; surgeons have a responsibility to take the time necessary to help them work through their emotional and psychological conflicts in order to resolve the issue.

CONFLICTS

The same sorts of conflicts that arise when deciding code status also arise when deciding CMO status. However, because a CMO order amounts to a refusal of care aimed at extending life, the patient's or surrogate's authority to insist on the order is clearer than it is to demand cardiopulmonary resuscitation judged by the surgeon to be futile. There is often ambiguity about the precise meaning and implications of a CMO order for a particular patient. Differences can arise among members of the treatment team, or with patients or families about

whether a particular intervention is likely to contribute to the patient's comfort. Special difficulties can arise when an intervention has a reasonable prospect of contributing to the patient's comfort, but is likely to extend life further. In these cases of a conflict in treatment goals, the surgeon, together with the patient or family, must decide the relative importance of the conflicting goals for the specific circumstances and intervention. Because of the unavoidable ambiguity of CMO orders, it is important to make them as specific as possible. Surgeons should attempt to anticipate diagnostic, monitoring, or therapeutic questions likely to arise in the patient's care and to be attentive to inevitable ambiguities and uncertainties in the interpretation of a CMO order as they arise.

Finally, just as with DNR orders, it is important that patients and families be assured that a CMO order will not result in abandonment of the patient. All measures to optimize the patient's comfort must be vigilantly pursued, especially necessary palliative care, and all measures that maintain the patient's dignity must always be provided. With dying patients, a referral to hospice care should be considered and offered to the patient and family when appropriate. When aggressive surgical interventions have failed to improve the patient's condition and prognosis and when a decision is made to make the patient CMO, disappointment, sadness, and even anger are natural. However, surgeons must not allow difficulty in coming to terms with the patient's impending death to result in physical or psychological withdrawal from the patient at the time when support may be most needed and important.

SELECTED READINGS

Brock DW: Death and dying. In Life and Death: Philosophical Essays in Biomedical Ethics. Cambridge, Cambridge University Press, 1993.

Brody H, Campbell ML, Faber-Langendoen K, Ogle KS: Withdrawing intensive life-sustaining treatment: Recommendations for compassionate clinical management. N Engl J Med 1997;336:652.

Council on Ethical and Judicial Affairs, American Medical Association: Guidelines for the appropriate use of do-not-resuscitate orders. JAMA 1991;265:1868.

Council on Ethical and Judicial Affairs, American Medical Association: Medical futility in end-of-life care. JAMA 1999;281:937.

Fitzgerald JD, et al: Functional status among survivors of in-hospital cardiopulmonary resuscitation. Arch Intern Med 1997;157:72.

Gazelle G: The slow code—should anyone rush to its defense? N Engl J Med 1998;338:467.

McCann RB, Hall WJ, Groth-Juncker A: Comfort care for terminally ill patients: The appropriate use of nutrition and hydration. JAMA 1994;272:1263.

President's Commission for the Study of Ethical Problems in Medicine and Biomedical and Behavioral Research: Deciding to Forego Life-Sustaining Treatment, A Report on the Ethical, Medical, and Legal Issues in Treatment Decisions. Washington, DC, US Government Printing Office, 1983.

Task Force on Ethics of The Society of Critical Care Medicine: Consensus report on the ethics of foregoing life-sustaining treatments in the critically ill. Crit Care Med 1990;18:1435.

Tomlinson T, Brody H: Futility and the ethics of resuscitation. JAMA 1990;264:1276.

Tomlinson T, Brody H: Ethics and communication in do-not-resuscitate orders. N Engl J Med 1988;318:43.

Chapter 22

Multisystem Organ Dysfunction and Failure: The Systemic Response to Critical Surgical Illness

Kenneth Burchard

In 1973, Tilney, Bailey, and Morgan described "sequential systems failure" in patients who initially survived surgery for abdominal aortic aneurysm rupture, a concept of progressive organ malfunction reemphasized and amplified by Arthur Baue in 1975. Since then, surgeons and critical care specialists have become increasingly cognizant of the many surgical patients who survive an initial critical surgical illness to only be threatened again from organ dysfunction or failure that may or may not have been evident at the time of the original insult. This later threat is not inconsequential, with reports of mortality rates exceeding 50%.

Dr. Baue recognized that severe inflammatory illness (one type of "hit" to cellular function) was as likely to be associated with multisystem organ dysfunction syndrome (MODS)/multisystem organ failure syndrome (MOFS) as the severe hypoperfusion-ischemic illness (another "hit") described by Tinley and colleagues. Twenty-five years of investigation have provided evidence of an increasingly complex linkage between these insults (the multiple "hit" hypothesis) that cause cellular and organ damage. This chapter outlines the pathophysiological and clinical manifestations of this linkage between hypoperfusion-ischemia and severe systemic inflammation. The management principles presented emphasize prevention of MODS/MOFS as well as several emerging strategies that attempt to ameliorate the severity or duration of MODS/MOFS.

DEFINITIONS

The definitions most germane to the concept of MODS/MOFS regard (1) organ dysfunction or failure, (2) shock, (3) hypoperfusion-ischemia, and (4) systemic inflammation.

Organ Dysfunction or Failure

Measurement tools that quantify severity of illness or organ malfunction have assisted both bedside clinical assessment and clinical research. For instance, the APACHE score quantifies overall severity of illness, whereas individual organ alterations can be measured with the Multiple Organ Dysfunction Score (ODS) described by Marshall (Table 22–1). The association of increased mortality risk with MODS/MOFS is well characterized by such a scoring system, with mortality rates less than 5% for scores of 0 to 4 and reaching 100% for

scores of 21 to 24. More important than a single time measurement of the ODS is an increase in ODS over time (termed the delta ODS) as a predictor of mortality. Therefore, the definition of organ dysfunction or failure becomes numerical; in this chapter, MODS/MOFS is present when the ODS is greater than 9.

Shock

Traditional descriptions of shock often use systolic hypotension (<90 mm Hg) as the defining variable for the presence or absence of shock. Using this criterion, classification schemas that use categories such as hypovolemic, septic, cardiogenic, and neurogenic shock are common. However, certain causes of hypotension (e.g., neurogenic vasodilation after spinal cord injury) do not necessarily result in threatening cellular or organ injury. In addition, cellular and organ injury may develop without hypotension reaching the 90 mm Hg requirement. Therefore, definitions of shock based on systolic blood pressure are potentially misleading and narrow in scope.

In 1872, S. D. Gross described shock as "a rude unhinging of the machinery of life." Using a similar, broader concept, shock can be defined as *a condition in which total body cellular metabolism is dysfunctional and sometimes lethal to cells, organs, and the individual.*

In the past 2 decades, experimental and clinical studies have accrued data that demonstrate two mechanisms of cellular injury (hypoperfusion and inflammation) that are neither competitive nor exclusive, but are most often additive during shock states. Simply stated, *hypoperfusion-ischemia begets inflammation and inflammation begets hypoperfusion-ischemia.* Therefore, most patients in whom MODS/MOFS has developed have suffered shock wherein cells suffer from both the effects of too little oxygen and too many inflammatory toxins (multiple "hits").

Hypoperfusion-Ischemia

The provision of adequate oxygen supply to cells depends on the variables listed in Table 22–2. Ischemia is present when cellular oxygen demand is greater than the oxygen supply. Ischemia can result from marked reductions in hemoglobin concentration (<7 g/dL) and from low arterial oxygen saturation (<90%). Therapeutic intervention for these deficiencies (i.e., transfusion of red blood cells,

Table 22–1	**Multiple-Organ Dysfunction Score**					
			SCORE			
ORGAN SYSTEM	0	1	2	3	4
Respiratory° (Po_2/Fio_2 ratio)	>300	226–300	51–225	76–150	75
Renal† (serum creatinine)	**100**	101–200	201–350	351–500	>500
Hepatic‡ (serum bilirubin)	**20**	21–60	61–120	121–240	>240
Cardiovascular§ (PAR)	**10.0**	10.1–15.0	15.1–20.0	20.1–30.0	>30.0
Hematologic‖ (platelet count)	>120	81–120	51–80	21–50	**20**
Neurologic¶ (Glasgow Coma Score)	15	13–14	10–12	7–9	**6**

°The Po_2/Fio_2 ratio is calculated without reference to the use or mode of mechanical ventilation, and without reference to the use or level of positive end-expiratory pressure.

†The serum creatinine concentration is measured in μmol/L, without reference to the use of dialysis.

‡The serum bilirubin concentration is measured in μmol/L.

§The pressure-adjusted heart rate (PAR) is calculated as the product of the heart rate (HR) multiplied by the ratio of the right atrial (central venous) pressure (RAP) to the mean arterial pressure (MAP): PAR = HR × RAP/mean BP.

‖The platelet count is measured in 10^{-3} platelets/mL.

¶The Glasgow Coma Score is preferably calculated by the patient's nurse and is scored conservatively (for the patient receiving sedation or muscle relaxants, normal function is assumed, unless there is evidence of intrinsically altered mentation).

From Marshall JC, Cook DJ, Christou NV, et al: Multiple organ dysfunction score: A reliable descriptor of a complex clinical outcome. Crit Care Med 1995; 23:1638–1652.

mechanical ventilation) can usually rapidly improve these oxygen supply variables. Continuing deficits in arterial blood flow (i.e., hypoperfusion) are a more common cause of prolonged oxygen supply deficits.

Hypoperfusion is present when one or more regions of blood supply are inadequate to supply cellular oxygen demands. When sufficiently prolonged, severe global hypoperfusion by itself is a recognized etiology of shock and MODS/MOFS.

Systemic Inflammation

Inflammation is a normal response to tissue injury and infection and is necessary for tissue repair, wound healing, and host defenses. However, whereas a localized inflammatory response to an insult is usually beneficial, severe tissue damage from a variety of causes (Table 22–3) can result in inflammation distant from the original disease (systemic inflammation) that may then cause cellular malfunction and death in remote organs. This generalized inflammatory state is similar to, but not limited to, the reaction to life-threatening infection that has been called *sepsis*. The concept of the "systemic inflammatory response syndrome," or SIRS, developed by The American Society of Chest Physicians/Critical Care Society Consensus Conference has been advanced as recognition that systemic inflammation has multiple etiologies.

To meet the definition of SIRS, a patient must manifest two or more of the following conditions: (1) temperature greater than 38.5°C or less than 36°C, (2) heart rate greater than 90 beats per minute, (3) respiratory rate greater than 20 breaths per minute or $Paco_2$ less than 32 torr, and (4) total leukocyte count greater than 12,000 cells/mm³, less than 4000 cells/mm³, or greater than 10% immature forms. Many patients with inflammation but without evidence of significant cellular and organ malfunction (i.e., not in shock, no development of MODS/MOFS) may meet the definition of SIRS. The SIRS variables of hypothermia (<36°C) and leukopenia (<4000 cells/mm³) are associated with more severe inflammation, as are systolic hypotension and evidence of organ malfunction (e.g., elevated blood urea nitrogen and creatinine, oliguria, altered mental status, decreased arterial oxygenation, increased bilirubin, decreased platelets). When sufficiently prolonged, severe systemic inflammation by itself is a recognized cause of shock and MODS/MOFS.

MECHANISMS OF CELLULAR INJURY

Hypoperfusion-Ischemia as a Cause of MODS/MOFS

The primary etiologies of decreased cardiac output are decreased venous return and diminished function of the

Table 22–2	**Cellular Oxygen Supply Variables**

Oxygen content of arterial blood
Hemoglobin concentration
Oxygen saturation
Dissolved oxygen
Cardiac output (flow of arterial blood to capillaries)
Diffusion from capillaries to cells
Oxygen demand of the cells

Table 22–3	**Partial List of Etiologies of Systemic Inflammation**

Infection (systemic inflammation from infection is called sepsis)
Trauma
Burns
Ischemia-reperfusion
Pancreatitis
Drug reactions
Hemolytic transfusion reactions

cardiac ventricles. Certainly, the primary mechanism for cell and organ injury secondary to decreased cardiac output is a deficit in oxygen supply. Information germane to cardiovascular physiology and the diagnosis and management of circulatory disorders is presented elsewhere in this text.

Mechanisms that link hypoperfusion-ischemia with inflammation are listed in Table 22–4. Polymorphonuclear cell (PMN) activation and cytokine release have been documented during hemorrhagic hypoperfusion, presumably because hypoxia alone can stimulate inflammatory cell activation. Resuscitation of the circulation after severe or prolonged ischemia (ischemia-reperfusion) is a well-recognized mechanism of inflammation stimulation, especially via PMN activation. Localized ischemia-reperfusion can result in systemic inflammation via such mechanisms as activation of Kupffer cells (gastrointestinal tract ischemia-reperfusion) and pulmonary endothelial cells and macrophages (extremity ischemia-reperfusion). Ischemia sufficient to produce tissue death (infarction) results in a local inflammatory response that may become systemic with sufficient tissue injury. Severe hypoperfusion can result in a decrease of gastrointestinal tract mucosal barrier function that inhibits the migration of intestinal microorganisms or their breakdown products from the lumen to extraluminal sites (lymphatics, bloodstream, peritoneal cavity). This "translocation" can happen without frank ischemic necrosis of the bowel. Migration of these intraluminal materials to extraluminal sites can serve as a stimulus for systemic inflammation.

Inflammation as a Cause of MODS/MOFS

The mechanism whereby severe inflammation results in cell malfunction and death is not as well understood as the effects of inadequate oxygen supply. In fact, many investigators consider inadequate oxygen supply to be a primary mechanism (see later text), but several recent investigations have demonstrated inflammation-induced injury to cell function despite excellent quantities of oxygen. The injured cell still behaves as if an energy deficit is present, a condition termed *cytopathic hypoxia,* which is more in keeping with the concept that a toxin is inhibiting cellular energy production from oxygen. Similar to the effects of a deficit in oxygen supply, cell membrane function worsens, lactate levels increase, and calcium accumulates in the cells. Once again, these toxic effects on cell function are difficult to separate from the hypoperfu-

Table 22–4	Hypoperfusion-Ischemia Begets Inflammation

Activation of inflammatory cells during hemorrhage
Ischemia-reperfusion
Regional
Gastrointestinal (GI) tract
Extremity
Total body
Infarction
Translocation of organisms or inflammatory stimulants across the GI tract

Table 22–5	Inflammation Begets Hypoperfusion-Ischemia

Decreased venous return
Vasodilation
Loss of plasma volume
Increased capillary permeability (local and systemic)
Intracellular fluid accumulation
Lumen of GI tract
Deficits in the microcirculation
Depressed myocardial function
Metabolic
Anatomic
Increased pulmonary vascular resistance

sion-ischemic insults associated with inflammation (Table 22–5).

The most common etiology of inadequate cardiac output during inflammation is decreased venous return, which results from vasodilation as well as a loss of intravascular volume. Vasodilation of systemic veins and arterioles is characteristic of severe inflammation, and several inflammatory mediators have been implicated as causative (e.g., histamine, kinins, prostacyclin, nitric oxide). Increasing the capacitance of veins can result in decreased venous return.

Collectively the exudation of plasma volume into inflammatory foci, the accumulation of fluid in the gastrointestinal tract, and the migration of fluid into the interstitium and cells is termed the *third space* to distinguish it from normal plasma and interstitial fluid spaces. The magnitude of the third space effect is roughly proportional to the magnitude of the tissue injury or infection that has stimulated the inflammatory response. The primary effect of third space fluid accumulation is to deplete plasma (and thereby intravascular volume) and impair venous return.

Once intravascular volume and venous return is restored, systemic inflammation is frequently associated with an increase in cardiac output and oxygen delivery, commonly referred to as a *hyperdynamic* circulation. Despite this increase in total body blood flow, regions of the circulation, especially regions of the microcirculation (arterioles, capillaries, venules), may exhibit deficits in flow sufficient to result in inadequate oxygen delivery to the cells in that region. Therefore, systemic inflammation can cause cell injury because of insufficient oxygen supply even when overall blood flow and oxygen delivery appear to be enhanced.

Restoration of intravascular volume sometimes does not result in a hyperdynamic circulation, but rather a hemodynamic state more consistent with depressed ventricular function. This is most often recognized in patients who have underlying cardiac disease, but, on occasion, systemic inflammation is sufficiently severe to impair the function of previously normal heart muscle. As might be expected from the previous description of mechanisms of cell injury during inflammation, two mechanisms have been proposed as a cause of these alterations: (1) a metabolic disturbance in cardiac myocyte function (e.g., cytopathic hypoxia) and (2) an anatomic injury to cardiac myocytes from microcirculatory deficits in oxygen delivery. The former mechanism is supported by studies that demonstrate that isolated heart muscle works less well when bathed with plasma from inflamed individuals, the latter from studies that demonstrate elevated blood troponin levels in individuals with severe inflammation.

Therefore, cardiac output may be impaired in a fashion that results in a physiology consistent with an *excess* of intravascular volume rather than a deficit. Recognition of such cardiogenic states of hypoperfusion during inflammation is important for proper therapeutic intervention.

In addition, severe inflammation is associated with increased pulmonary vascular resistance. This increase in right ventricular afterload may result in dilation of the right ventricle, decreased right ventricular ejection, and impaired filling of the left ventricle. Right atrial pressure may then increase and impair venous return.

CLINICAL DIAGNOSIS OF MODS/MOFS

The Patient at Risk

As listed in Table 22–6, the patient at risk for MODS/MOFS frequently is suffering a disease or injury that results in both inadequate oxygen supply and the stimulation of an inflammatory response. For instance, the patient with rib fractures, a pulmonary contusion, and massive hemorrhage from a ruptured spleen has both "hits" in place at the time of initial medical evaluation and management.

Recognition of the Patient in "Severe" Shock

The bedside recognition of the patient in severe shock is usually not a diagnostic challenge. Most often, hypotension (systolic pressure <90 mm Hg), tachycardia, tachypnea, peripheral vasoconstriction, oliguria, mental status alterations, and so on alert the clinician to the severity of organ malfunction. However, sometimes physical exami-

Table 22–6	Diseases Associated with MODS/MOFS

Severe hypovolemic hypoperfusion
  Hemorrhage
  Trauma
  Burns
  Pancreatitis
  Infection
  Bowel obstruction
  Peritonitis
Severe cardiogenic hypoperfusion–cardiogenic shock
Severe inflammation
  Infection
  Trauma
  Burns
  Pancreatitis
  Peritonitis
  Bowel obstruction
  Ischemia/reperfusion
  Allergic reaction
  Other drug toxicity

Table 22–7	Markers of Severe Cellular Insults from Shock

Sustained elevation in arterial lactate (>5 mmol/L)
Hypothermia (<36°C)
Markedly decreased ionized calcium (<3.8 mg/dL)
Hypoglycemia (<60 mg/dL)
Decreased oxygen consumption (<130 mL/min/m²)

nation and simple measures of organ function (e.g., urine output) are not sufficiently sensitive to recognize the patient in severe shock. Under these circumstances, other indicators of the "rude unhinging" of cellular function can alert the clinician to this magnitude of illness (Tables 22–7 and 22–8).

Metabolic acidosis with high arterial lactate levels at admission to the hospital and acidosis that continues for 24 hours or longer has been associated with MODS/MOFS and death. An elevated arterial lactate can develop as a consequence of ischemia as well as the cytotoxic hypoxia and increased pyruvate production associated with severe inflammation. Therefore, increased arterial lactate concentration and metabolic acidosis can be present despite the augmented oxygen delivery commonly measured during severe inflammation. Even though an elevated arterial lactate measurement does not prove that ischemia is present, a level greater than 5 mmol/L is still evidence of *severe* cellular malfunction.

Hypothermia can accompany severe hypoperfusion as well as severe inflammation and has been associated with poor outcome in each circumstance. The etiology of hypothermia in these patients is difficult to discern, but alterations in hypothalamic function as well as energy production deficits have been implicated. A deficit in energy production is most in keeping with the abnormalities in acid-base, ionized calcium, and oxygen consumption that are characteristic of the most critically ill patients with MODS/MOFS.

A decrease in serum ionized calcium, despite a metabolic acidosis, is a characteristic of severe hypoperfusion and inflammation and is not peculiar to such entities as pancreatitis or massive transfusion. The magnitude and duration of decreased ionized calcium at the time of intensive care unit admission has been associated with death days later. Increased intracellular calcium (e.g.,

Table 22–8	More Sensitive Markers of Cellular Insults from Shock

Indicators of hypoperfusion/ischemia
  Moderate elevations in arterial lactate (>2.4, <5.0 mmol/L)
  Moderate decrease in ionized calcium (>3.8, <5.0 mg/dL)
  Decreased mixed venous oxygen saturation (<65%)
  Decreased gastric intramucosal pH (pHi <7.32)
Indicators of inflammation
  Moderate elevations in arterial lactate (>2.4, <5 mmol/L)
  Moderate decrease in ionized calcium (>3.8 <5.0 mg/dL)
  Decreased gastric intramucosal pH (pHi <7.32)
  Decreased platelets, elevated d-dimer

leukocytes, red cells, liver cells, and muscle cells) has been measured in experimental animals and humans following hypoperfusion and inflammatory insults. Active cell membrane and organelle function is necessary to maintain normal cytosolic calcium concentrations, and increased cytosolic calcium is in keeping with the concept of cellular energy deficits. High concentrations of free intracellular calcium have been implicated as an etiology of further cell injury and death. This, along with recognition that exogenous calcium administration can increase mortality risk in inflamed animals, makes the benefits of exogenous calcium administration during shock and MODS/MOFS speculative at best.

The metabolic response to hypoperfusion and inflammation includes an increase in blood epinephrine, glucagon, and cortisol concentrations that stimulate an increase in blood glucose levels. Hypoglycemia during critical illness implies sufficient deficits in cellular (especially hepatic) metabolism to disrupt this gluconeogenic physiology and results in the reduction of a primary energy source. Severe metabolic acidosis (pH <7.0), high lactic acid levels, and hypoglycemia portend a grave prognosis.

One of the most consistent markers for a poor prognosis during critical illness is evidence that total body oxygen consumption is not increasing despite aggressive efforts to improve oxygen delivery. This deficit in total body oxygen utilization and the associated high mortality rate (30% to 50%) are consistent with the concept of "cytopathic hypoxia" as an etiology of cell malfunction during MODS/MOFS.

Defining the Patient with MODS/MOFS

Once the diagnosis of shock is made, then the ODS can be calculated and followed over ensuing days. As stated earlier, for this discussion, MODS/MOFS is present when the ODS is greater than 9. An increase in ODS of 5 points or greater, despite an initial value of less than 9, is especially indicative of a poor outcome.

THE CLINICAL MANAGEMENT OF THE PATIENT WITH MODS/MOFS

Prevention and treatment of MODS/MOFS depends on recognizing the patient at risk and rapid reversal of shock, whether it is moderate or severe. The guiding principles for reversal of shock are (1) attainment of excellent total body oxygen delivery and (2) interruption of moderate and severe systemic inflammation. The primary methods of achieving these principles are listed in Table 22–9.

The primary challenge for attainment of excellent total body oxygen delivery is improvement in cardiac index, with the best outcomes realized when the circulation becomes hyperdynamic as measured by a cardiac index of at least 4.5 L/min per m². Attainment of this hyperdynamic state commonly requires an accurate hemodynamic diagnosis using such adjuvants as the pulmonary artery catheter and echocardiograms. Patients who achieve a hyperdynamic state with fluid infusion alone are the most

Table 22–9	**Principles for Prevention of MODS/ MOFS Management of Shock**

Excellent oxygen delivery
　Red cells for hemoglobin <7.0 g/dL
　Supplemental oxygen and ventilator therapy to attain an arterial
　　oxygen saturation >90%
　Achievement, if possible, of a hyperdynamic circulation (cardiac
　　index ≥4.5 L/min/m²)
　　　Accurate hemodynamic diagnosis
　　　Therapy based on fluid loading and improving venous return
　　　? If adding inotropes/pressors improves outcome
　Interruption of inflammation
Interruption of inflammation
　Rapid achievement of an excellent circulation
　Locate/treat inflammatory focus (foci)
　Early diagnosis of infection
　Early gastrointestinal tract feeding
　Supplemental anti-inflammatory strategies
　　Physiologic hydrocortisone
　　Continuous venovenous hemofiltration
　　Antioxidants
　　Type of fluid for resuscitation

likely to avoid MODS/MOFS and survive. The use of inotropes and pressors in addition to or instead of fluid to reach a specified cardiac index and oxygen delivery has not been proven beneficial. Because inflammation begets hypoperfusion, the management of the circulation includes efforts to limit inflammation.

As complex as aggressive attention to the circulation may be, strategies to interrupt or lessen inflammation are even more multifaceted. This is especially true because the inflammatory response is usually an early component of any critical surgical illness. Because hypoperfusion begets inflammation, attention to the first principle stated earlier is integral to the inhibition of systemic inflammation. At first review, a patient may not exhibit overt evidence of an inflammatory site (i.e., lower extremity compartment syndrome, traumatic pancreatitis), and clinical or laboratory evidence of moderate or severe inflammation should prompt a search for an occult inflammatory focus. Patients at risk for MODS/MOFS are at increased risk for invasive infection. Anticipating this risk (e.g., removing central venous access placed in haste, obtaining surveillance cultures, conducting early imaging and sampling of fluid collections) may prevent or allow early detection of infection as the next inflammatory challenge.

Pearls and Pitfalls

PEARLS

- MODS/MOFS is caused by shock.
- Surgical shock is secondary to hypoperfusion-ischemia or inflammation.
- Hypoperfusion-ischemia begets inflammation.
- Inflammation begets hypoperfusion-ischemia.
- Recognition of the patient in shock and rapid shock reversal are the primary methods of avoiding and treating MODS/MOFS.

As mentioned earlier, the gastrointestinal tract may be the focus for inflammatory stimuli even when the bowel wall is not anatomically compromised. Early feeding of the jejunum appears to enhance gastrointestinal mucosal barrier function and inhibit the migration of microorganisms and inflammatory mediators across the lumen to extraluminal sites. Besides improving the local host defense of the gastrointestinal tract mucosa, enteral feedings improve distant host defenses (especially in the lung) and particular dietary formulations may inhibit systemic inflammation as well as reduce the risk of invasive infection.

SUMMARY AND CONCLUSIONS

The systemic response to surgical critical illness, multisystem organ dysfunction and failure, is a manifestation of the cellular injury that accrues from hypoperfusion/ischemia and systemic inflammation, the two "hits" of the multiple hit hypothesis for MODS/MOFS. Successful prevention or amelioration of MODS/MOFS is based on the principles of rapidly reversing or diminishing the effects of these cellular damaging processes, using commonly available techniques of beside and laboratory evaluation as well as prudent and timely medical and surgical therapy.

SELECTED READINGS

American College of Chest Physicians/Society of Critical Care Medicine Consensus Conference: Definitions for sepsis and multiple organ failure, and guidelines for the use of innovative therapies in sepsis. Crit Care Med 1992;20:864.

Baue AE: MOF/MODS, Sirs: An update. Shock 1996;6:S1.

Deitch AE: Multiple organ failure: Pathophysiology and potential future therapy. Ann Surg 1992;216:117.

Eastridge BJ, Darlington DN, Evans JA, Gann DS: A circulating shock protein depolarizes cells in hemorrhage and sepsis. Ann Surg 1994;219:298.

Garrison RN, Spain DA, Wilson MA, et al: Microvascular changes explain the "two-hit" theory of multiple organ failure. Ann Surg 1998;227:851.

Hayes MA, Timmins AC, Yau EHS, et al: Oxygen transport patterns in patients with sepsis syndrome or septic shock: Influence of treatment and relationship to outcome. Crit Care Med 1997;25:926.

Hoffmann JN, Werdan K, Hartl WH, et al: Hemofiltrate from patients with severe sepsis and depressed left ventricular contractility contains cardiotoxic compounds. Shock 1999;12:174.

Jacobs S, Zuleika M, Mphansa T: The multiple organ dysfunction score as a descriptor of patient outcome in septic shock compared with two other scoring systems. Crit Care Med 1999;27:741.

Kudsk KA, Minard G, Croce MA, et al: A randomized trial of isonitrogenous enteral diets after severe trauma: An immune-enhancing diet reduces septic complications. Ann Surg 1996;224:531.

Marshall JC, Cook DJ, Christou NV, et al: Multiple organ dysfunction score: A reliable descriptor of a complex clinical outcome. Crit Care Med 1995;23:1638–1652.

Peng RY, Bongard FS: Hypothermia in trauma patients. J Am Coll Surg 1999;188:685.

Schwartz DR, Malhotra A, Fink MP: Cytopathic hypoxia in sepsis: An overview. Sepsis 1999;2:279.

Tilney NL, Bailey GL, Morgan AP: Sequential system failure after rupture of abdominal aortic aneurysms: An unsolved problem in postoperative care. Ann Surg 1973;178:117.

Trump BF, Berezesky IK: Calcium-mediated cell injury and cell death. New Horizons 1996;4:139.

Welbourn CR, Goldman G, Paterson IS, et al: Pathophysiology of ischaemia reperfusion injury: Central role of the neutrophil. Br J Surg 1991;78:651.

Chapter 23

Basic and Advanced Mechanical Ventilation

Stephen A. Rowe and William G. Cheadle

Successful management of the mechanically ventilated surgical patient necessitates that the surgeon has knowledge of the respiratory physiology, the pitfalls and complications of positive pressure ventilation, the available methods of ventilation, and the criteria for terminating support.

There are multiple indications for intubation and positive pressure ventilation. Even though there are some objective, published criteria for intubation (Table 23–1), clinical experience and common sense often provide the best guidelines. Intubation under controlled elective conditions is safer for the patient than the emergent intubation that follows unnecessary delay in controlling the airway.

Normal respirations rely on negative pressure, and positive pressure ventilation has important physiologic consequences. An understanding of these is essential for appropriate ventilator management. Mechanical ventilation has potentially deleterious effects on cardiac performance. The increase in intrathoracic pressure leads to a decrease in both afterload and preload. The decrease in preload results in poor ventricular filling and can decrease cardiac output. The decreased afterload improves systolic ventricular emptying and can potentially improve cardiac output in a similar fashion to chest compressions given in cardiopulmonary resuscitation. The net result to cardiac output is dependent on whether diastolic filling of the heart is compromised; therefore, hypovolemia in a mechanically ventilated patient tends to decrease cardiac output.

Mechanical ventilation also carries the risk of increasing parenchymal lung injury. An FIO_2 greater than 60% is directly toxic to normal lungs, and an FIO_2 of 50% is potentially toxic to injured lungs. This injury is mediated through the development of reactive radicals. Additionally, there is the risk of volutrauma and barotrauma, particularly with large inflation volumes. Volutrauma de-

velops in 4% to 15% of mechanically ventilated patients, especially those with adult respiratory distress syndrome (ARDS) and aspiration pneumonia. Poor compliance of the diseased alveoli leads to overexpansion of normal alveoli, resulting in excessive pressures locally and the development of shear forces. The recognition of ventilator-induced pulmonary injury has led to the use of lower volumes and pressures in an effort to protect the lung (Table 23–2).

The use of positive end-expiratory pressure (PEEP) deserves special consideration. The advent of PEEP has allowed the use of lower tidal volumes by stenting open alveoli and preventing their collapse at the end of expiration. The resultant recruitment of unused alveoli increases the functional residual capacity (FRC) and improves both compliance and oxygenation. Thus, FIO_2 can be reduced to less than toxic levels. However, PEEP can also lower cardiac output and consequently lower oxygen delivery. The delivery of oxygen is dependent on both cardiac output and arterial oxygen content ($\dot{D}O_2 = CO \times CaO_2$). If cardiac performance is compromised, the improvement in arterial oxygenation does not translate to improved oxygen delivery to the tissues. Therefore, many authors recommend that cardiac performance should be monitored if high PEEP (>5 to 10 mm Hg) is used. This can be accomplished by monitoring $S\dot{V}O_2$ or by use of a Swan-Ganz catheter. PEEP can also develop from hyperinflation that occurs during rapid ventilation. This is known as intrinsic or auto-PEEP. The effects of PEEP are summarized in Table 23–3.

MODES OF VENTILATION

Assist-control ventilation (ACV) provides complete respiratory support (Table 23–4). The patient can initiate a breath that is then carried to a preset tidal volume and flow rate. If the patient initiates no breaths, the ventilator provides breaths at a preset rate. Because ACV provides

Table 23–1	Indications for Intubation
	Relieve airway obstruction
	Decreased mental status
	Inability to clear secretions
	Respiratory acidosis
	Respiratory failure:
	$PaO_2 < 60$ while $FIO_2 > 0.50$
	Intrapulmonary shunt > 15%
	A-a gradient >300 mm Hg
	Respiratory rate > 30
	$PaCO_2 > 60$

Table 23–2	Lung Protective Ventilation		
PARAMETER	TRADITIONAL	LUNG PROTECTIVE	
Volume	12–15 mL/kg	6–10 mL/kg	
Sigh	20–30 mL/kg 8–12/hr	None	
Peak pressure	50 cm H_2O	<35 cm H_2O	
Positive end-expiratory pressure	Rarely	Usually 5–15 cm H_2O	

Table 23–3	**Physiologic Effects of Positive End-Expiratory Pressure**
BENEFICIAL	**ADVERSE**
Increased functional residual capacity	Decreased cardiac output
Increased alveolar recruitment	Increased dead space ventilation
Improved ventilation-perfusion matching	Increased barotrauma
Redistribution of lung water	

total ventilatory support, there is little work of breathing done by the patient. Some authors believe that this can lead to atrophy of respiratory musculature and subsequent difficulty in weaning. Other disadvantages of ACV occur in the awake tachypneic patient. Because each breath is carried to full tidal volume, tachypnea can lead to hyperventilation and respiratory alkalosis. Guidelines for initial setting in ACV are tidal volume of 8 to 10 mL/kg, flow rate of 60 to 80 L/min, and a backup rate of 8 breaths per minute.

Intermittent mandatory ventilation (IMV) provides a preset respiratory rate. The patient is able to breathe spontaneously over the ventilator. In synchronized intermittent mandatory ventilation (SIMV) the machine breaths are triggered when the patient initiates an inhalation. This mode provides improved patient comfort. The advantages of this mode include reduced occurrence of hyperventilation and the ability to use IMV for weaning. Because work of breathing is high in this mode, it may not be appropriate in patients with respiratory muscle weakness. Recommended initial settings for SIMV are tidal volume of 10 to 12 mL/kg, respiratory rate of 8 to 10 per minute, and inspiratory time of 1.5 to 2 seconds. ACV and SIMV are the two most common modes of ventilation in the postsurgical patient, and numerous studies have failed to demonstrate improved outcome with either mode.

Pressure controlled ventilation provides a similar breathing pattern to IMV. The rate is set, but instead of a volume, a peak pressure is set for each breath. This mode is useful in neonates and in clinical situations in which the avoidance of high pressures is essential (ARDS). The major disadvantage of pressure controlled ventilation is the inconsistency of tidal volume. As lung compliance decreases and airway resistance increases, the tidal volumes decrease for a given pressure. PCV can be used with prolonged inspiratory times to prevent alveolar collapse. This is known as inverse ratio ventilation. The

resultant theoretical advantage of improved oxygenation has not been realized in controlled, double-blinded studies. Improved ventilation was noted, but at a cost of decreased cardiac output. Inspiration to expiration ratio is normally 1:2, allowing adequate time for exhalation and a return to the FRC. With the reversal of this normal ratio and inadequate exhalation time, auto-PEEP can develop and lead to decreased cardiac output. Additionally, tidal volume can suffer, with subsequent hypoventilation and hypercapnia.

A newer mode of ventilation, pressure regulated volume control (PRVC), allows ventilation in patients with high airway pressures while limiting barotrauma. The pattern of breathing is identical to that for ACV, but the ventilator controls the flow rate to minimize peak pressures. The advantages of this mode are the theoretical prevention of barotrauma and improved patient comfort. There are no major disadvantages except the limited availability of ventilators that provide this mode (i.e., Servo 300).

STRATEGIES FOR THE DIFFICULT TO VENTILATE PATIENT

Occasionally, conventional methods fail to provide adequate ventilation or oxygenation. Recently, there has been interest in nonconventional modes of ventilation to support these patients.

High-frequency ventilation (HFV) uses very high rates (greater than 100 breaths per minute in an adult and greater than 300 breaths per minute in a neonatal or pediatric patient) and small tidal volumes. HFV provides two major advantages. The minute volume is greater than that in conventional ventilation despite small tidal volumes. This allows improved alveolar recruitment without risk of alveolar overdistention and injury. The high flow rates also improve gas mixing and possibly ventilation–perfusion matching. Several pilot studies have demonstrated efficacy of HFV in ARDS in adults, but controlled studies remain to be done. Outcome studies in the pediatric population, however, have established a clear role for HFV.

Liquid ventilation (LV) has shown benefits in recent human and animal studies. LV relies on perfluorocarbons, which can accommodate high contents of oxygen. Several advantages are realized by LV: there is improved recruitment of alveoli, improved lung compliance, and apparent protection against lung injury. Although LV shows promise as a mode of supporting the ARDS patient, further

Table 23–4	**Modes of Ventilation**		
MODES OF VENTILATION	**ADVANTAGES**	**DISADVANTAGES**
SIMV—Set volume at a set rate times breaths with patient efforts	Allows weaning Works with patient	High work of breathing
ACV—Breaths are initiated by patient and carried to preset volume	Low work of breathing Patient comfort	Cannot wean in this mode May hyperventilate
PCV—Similar pattern to IMV, but carries breath to preset pressure	Less barotrauma	No guaranteed tidal volume
PRVC—Similar to SIMV but regulates flow to control pressure	Less barotrauma Improved comfort	Only available on certain ventilators

Table 23–5	Extubation Parameters	
Tidal volume	5 mL/kg
Respiratory rate	<35/min
Vital capacity	<10 mL/kg
Minute ventilation	<10 L/min
Negative inspiratory pressure	−25 cm H_2O
Rapid shallow breathing index	<80

randomized trials need to be performed. Additionally, the long-term effects of LV and perfluorocarbon absorption are unknown.

Surgeons are occasionally faced with patients who are essentially impossible to support on ventilators. Extracorporeal life support (ECLS) is an alternative mode of support. A cardiopulmonary bypass pump supports the patient, allowing the lungs to "rest." Changing the flow rate of the circuit or the FIO_2 to the membrane oxygenator controls oxygenation. Altering the gas flow across the membrane controls ventilation. The advantages of ECLS are the ability to support a patient despite poor pulmonary or cardiac performance, and the prevention of ventilator-induced lung injury. However, ECLS requires specialized equipment and trained personnel to manage the bypass circuit. In addition, the patient is at risk for complications such as stroke from circuit emboli and bleeding from systemic heparinization.

WEANING

Many criteria and methods have been proposed for discontinuing mechanical ventilation. The decision to begin weaning initially depends on the resolution of the process that led to artificial respiration and on signs of improving pulmonary function. After a prolonged period of mechanical ventilation, a period of gradually decreasing support precedes extubation. This paradigm has recently been challenged; a recent study concluded that no weaning period is necessary before extubation. Conventionally, however, IMV or T-piece weaning has been used. In IMV weaning, the respiratory rate is gradually decreased until the patient is essentially supporting his own respirations. T-piece weaning involves gradually increasing periods during which the patient supports his own respirations. Usually pressure support is added to overcome the innate resistance of the endotracheal tube. Once it seems the patient is able to breathe without the support of the ventilator, respiratory parameters are taken. These are listed in Table 23–5. Of those listed, negative inspiratory pressure and rapid shallow breathing index (RSBI) provide the best predictive value. Multiple studies have yielded varying results, but a recent outcomes-based trial found that an RSBI less than 80 predicted an excellent chance of successful extubation, whereas an RSBI greater than 100 predicted a very high likelihood of failure. Tachy-

Pearls and Pitfalls

PEARLS

- Intubate electively rather than emergently when possible.
- Oxygen delivery is dependent on arterial O_2 content *and* cardiac output; do not sacrifice cardiac output to improve oxygen content.
- Increase ventilation to lower CO_2; increase PEEP or FIO_2 to improve oxygenation.
- If a patient is tachypneic, check blood gas and tidal volumes. Sedate patient if tidal volumes are low and patient is hypocapnic.
- Beware of PEEP: If cardiac output is decreasing or if the patient is getting inadequate tidal volumes, consider lowering PEEP.
- Tachypnea in ACV mode may lead to hyperventilation.
- Tracheostomy not only provides a safe airway but also lowers airway resistance and work of breathing.
- RSBI is the single most predictive index for success or failure of extubation.

pnea alone does not necessarily correlate with failed extubation. If tidal volumes are normal, and the patient is hypocapnic, the tachypnea is likely the result of anxiety. In this situation, the patient should be sedated. Difficulties in weaning may arise from several situations. First, it is essential to ensure that whatever process led to the need for mechanical ventilation has improved. Malnutrition can be a contributing factor in poor weaning. Paradoxically, overfeeding can also lead to difficulties in weaning by increasing CO_2 production. Electrolytes should be checked and corrected if necessary. Magnesium and phosphorous are particularly important for respiratory muscle strength. The liberal use of tracheostomy in such patients often facilitates weaning by reducing the work of breathing and is also a safer option than outright extubation.

SUGGESTED READINGS

Chao DC, Scheinhorn DJ: Weaning from mechanical ventilation. Crit Care Clin 1998;14:799.

Leonard RC: Liquid ventilation. Anaesth Intens Care 1998;26:11.

MacIntyre NR: High-frequency ventilation. Crit Care Med 1998;26:1995.

McKibben AW, Ravenscraft SA: Pressure controlled and volume cycled mechanical ventilation. Clin Chest Med 1996;17:395.

Michaels AJ, Schriener RJ, Kolla S, et al: Extracorporeal life support in pulmonary failure after trauma. J Trauma 1999;46:638.

Pierce JD, Gilliland E: Effects of volume control, pressure control, and pressure regulated volume control on cardiopulmonary parameters in a normal rat lung. Mil Med 1998;163:625.

Price JA, Rizk NW: Postoperative ventilatory management. Chest 1999; 5s:130s.

Sandur S, Stoller JK: Pulmonary complications of mechanical ventilation. Clin Chest Med 1999;20:223.

Yanos J, Watling SM, Verhey J: The physiologic effects of inverse ratio ventilation. Chest 1998;114:834.

Chapter 24
Hepatic Failure

Patrick K. Kim and Clifford S. Deutschman

The liver plays a central role in the host response to injury, in that it is a key organ in protein synthesis, metabolic substrate utilization, drug and toxin metabolism, and host defense (Fig. 24–1). In surgical patients, chronic liver disease is the most common risk factor for the development of perioperative hepatic dysfunction and the most important factor influencing outcome. In patients without chronic liver disease, acute hepatic dysfunction has a variety of etiologies, including sepsis, the systemic inflammatory response syndrome (SIRS), trauma, and hemorrhage. Regardless of etiology, hepatic dysfunction is associated with increased risk of perioperative morbidity and mortality. Complications of hepatic failure include coagulopathy, gastrointestinal and variceal bleeding, encephalopathy, cerebral edema, respiratory failure, and renal failure. Several classification systems attempt to provide prognostic information based on the degree of hepatic dysfunction. Therapy of hepatic dysfunction is supportive and includes close monitoring of fluid and electrolyte status, nutritional support, repletion of coagulation factors, and support of respiratory and renal function. Most cases of acute hepatic dysfunction are transient and resolution is uneventful. In some cases, hepatic dysfunction may progress to frank hepatic failure. Death is usually a consequence of refractory coagulopathy or encephalopathy. In patients with decompensated liver failure, liver transplantation is the only curative therapy. In the future, bioartificial liver support systems may routinely bridge patients to transplantation or even become a viable option to liver allografting.

DIAGNOSIS

The presence of hepatic disease greatly impacts perioperative morbidity and mortality. Thus it is important to

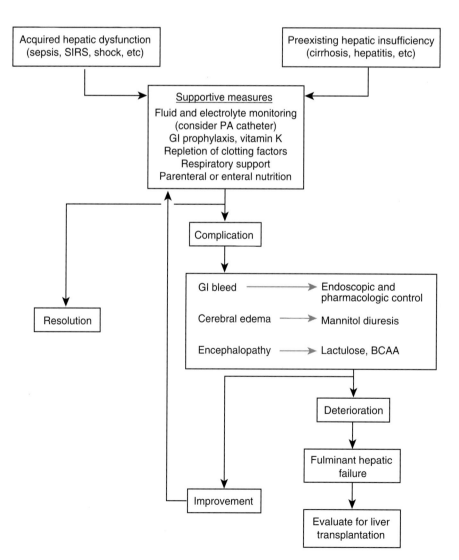

Figure 24–1. Suggested algorithm for the management of perioperative hepatic dysfunction.

identify hepatic disease before elective surgery. In preoperative patients, liver disease may be suspected based on history and physical examination, in which case liver function tests and hepatitis panels should be obtained. In surgical patients, the most common etiology of hepatic dysfunction is preexisting chronic hepatic disease, most often reflecting long-term alcohol consumption. Findings of chronic hepatic insufficiency include jaundice, icterus, ascites, asterixis, and encephalopathy. Laboratory studies may demonstrate hyponatremia, hypoproteinemia, hyperbilirubinemia, elevated prothrombin (PT) and partial thromboplastin time (PTT), and hyperammonemia. In patients with chronic hepatic insufficiency, the diagnosis is usually known or suspected and the primary challenge is perioperative management.

In patients without a history of liver disease, the differential diagnosis of acquired hepatic dysfunction includes sepsis, SIRS, trauma, major surgery, hypovolemic or cardiogenic shock, massive hemorrhage, prolonged hypotension, ischemia-reperfusion injury, hepatotoxic drugs, extrahepatic bile duct obstruction, and calculous or acalculous cholecystitis. The classic findings are jaundice and hyperbilirubinemia, although hyperbilirubinuria often precedes either finding. Laboratory studies may demonstrate hyperglycemia and elevations of serum transaminases, alkaline phosphatase, lactate dehydrogenase, PT, and PTT. Extrahepatic disease is ruled out by ultrasonography, computed tomography, or, if necessary, traditional cholangiography or endoscopic retrograde cholangiopancreatography. In sepsis- or SIRS-related hepatic dysfunction, hyperbilirubinemia results from excess of both conjugated and unconjugated forms of bilirubin, suggesting defective bilirubin handling. Elevations of transaminases, alkaline phosphatase, and lactate dehydrogenase are common but not sensitive indicators of hepatic dysfunction. Elevated PT and PTT measurements are due to impaired protein synthesis, indicative of marginal hepatic function.

CLINICAL COURSE

The course of acquired hepatic dysfunction varies widely but roughly parallels the patient's biphasic stress response to injury. The hypodynamic "ebb" phase of the stress response begins with injury and immediate release of catecholamines and cytokines, an adaptive response designed to restore overall homeostasis. However, the injury and the initial host response may have detrimental effects on the liver by altering portal venous or hepatic arterial flow or impairing hepatic microcirculation, resulting in hepatic necrosis and its clinical correlate, "shock liver." Timely, adequate resuscitation after injury minimizes the duration of the ebb phase in the liver and other organ systems and promotes the transition to the hyperdynamic "flow" phase. This phase peaks from 1 to 10 days after injury and correlates temporally with clinical and laboratory manifestations of hepatic dysfunction, as well as with cytokine activity, hepatic leukocyte activation, and alterations in hepatic gene expression. Acquired hepatic dysfunction typically occurs after respiratory insufficiency but before or synchronous with dysfunction of other organ systems. Among patients with multiple organ dysfunction syndrome (MODS), only respiratory dysfunction occurs more frequently than hepatic dysfunction. In general, with adequate support measures, acute hepatic dysfunction resolves uneventfully. Full recovery may require weeks, depending on the magnitude of insult and the functional reserve of the liver. However, in patients with preexisting hepatic insufficiency, uncomplicated recovery is less likely.

PREDICTION OF PERIOPERATIVE MORBIDITY AND MORTALITY

Several classification systems attempt to predict perioperative mortality in patients with chronic hepatic insufficiency. Liver-specific scoring systems include the original Child score, the modified Child-Pugh classification, and the Mayo Risk Score. The Child-Pugh classification stratifies hepatic dysfunction based on serum bilirubin and albumin, PT, and degree of encephalopathy and ascites (Table 24–1). In a retrospective study, preoperative Child-Pugh class correlated with mortality after abdominal surgery, and serum albumin and PT independently predicted perioperative mortality. Another retrospective study identified additional risk factors for perioperative mortality. These include male sex, elevated serum creatinine, presence of chronic obstructive pulmonary disease, active infection, preoperative upper gastrointestinal bleeding, high American Society of Anesthesiologists (ASA) score, major surgery, pulmonary surgery, and intraoperative hypotension.

Refined versions of the Acute Physiology and Chronic Health Evaluation (APACHE) are the most widely used comprehensive classification systems. APACHE II and APACHE III classifications assess variables from major organ systems as well as age and overall health and have been validated in predicting perioperative morbidity and mortality and length of intensive care unit stay.

COAGULOPATHY AND RELATED COMPLICATIONS

Coagulation is intimately related to liver function in several ways. Hepatic protein synthesis is impaired in severe

Table 24–1	Modified Child-Pugh Classification of Hepatic Dysfunction		

| CRITERION | POINTS | | |
	1	2	3
Serum bilirubin, mg/dL	<2.0	2.0–3.0	>3.0
Serum albumin, g/dL	>3.5	2.8–3.5	<2.8
Prothrombin time, sec prolonged	<1.7	1.7–2.3	>2.3
Ascites	None	Slight	Moderate
Encephalopathy	None	Minimal	Advanced
For primary biliary cirrhosis:			
Serum bilirubin, g/dL	<4.0	4.0–10.0	>10.0

Total points	Class
5–6	A
7–9	B
10–15	C

From Pugh RNH, Murray-Lyon IM, Dawson JL, et al: Transection of the oesophagus for bleeding oesophageal varices. Br J Surg 1973;60:646–649.

liver disease. This has profound effects on blood coagulation, because the liver synthesizes virtually all coagulation factors (and fibrinolytic proteins) except von Willebrand factor and tissue-type plasminogen activator (t-PA) and urinary plasminogen activator (u-PA). Malnutrition may lead to vitamin K deficiency, contributing to coagulation factor deficiency. Fibrinolysis is potentiated as a result of decreased hepatic breakdown of plasminogen activator and plasmin. Furthermore, splenomegaly, a common finding in portal hypertension, leads to splenic sequestration of platelets, resulting in thrombocytopenia.

Coagulopathy in the presence of altered PT/PTT is treated by administration of fresh-frozen plasma, which repletes coagulation factors. Cryoprecipitate may be considered instead of fresh-frozen plasma if excessive intravascular volume is a concern. A caveat is that cryoprecipitate does not contain vitamin K–dependent factors. Vitamin K should be administered intramuscularly preoperatively if deficiency is suspected. In acute situations, vitamin K may be given intravenously, although anaphylaxis can occur. Platelets are administered only if severe thrombocytopenia and life-threatening bleeding are present. Active gastrointestinal bleeding, which reflects both coagulopathy and impaired gastric mucosal substrate delivery, is treated with combined intravenous H_2 receptor antagonist (or proton pump inhibitor) and endoscopy to localize the bleeding source and stop hemorrhage.

Variceal Bleeding

In cirrhotic patients, the presence of portal hypertension contributes to risk of bleeding from esophageal or gastric varices. Reduction of portal pressure by β-blockade has been shown to be effective in prophylaxis of variceal bleeding. The goal is a hepatic venous pressure gradient of 12 mm Hg or reduction to 80% of baseline. Active bleeding is managed by a combined endoscopic and pharmacologic approach. Both endoscopic sclerotherapy and band ligation have been shown to be effective, but endoscopic banding is technically simple and safe, making it popular among endoscopic treatments. Pharmacologic options in the management of acute variceal bleeding include somatostatin, octreotide, vasopressin, and terlipressin. Both somatostatin and terlipressin are considered effective first-line drugs, with somatostatin having a better side-effect profile. The use of vasopressin has waned in popularity because of questionable efficacy and because of the incidence of adverse cardiac effects. Transjugular intrahepatic portosystemic shunt (TIPSS) is effective in controlling refractory variceal bleeding. Its complications include hepatic encephalopathy and shunt malfunction, particularly stent thrombosis or stenosis. In this high-risk group of patients, the advent of TIPSS has decreased the need for surgical shunting. TIPSS placement is rapidly gaining favor as a bridge to liver transplantation in patients with portal hypertension caused by end-stage liver disease.

Hepatic Encephalopathy

Hepatic encephalopathy probably results from impaired hepatic detoxification of blood ammonia, and abnormal transport and metabolism of amino acids and amines in the brain. However, the blood ammonia level correlates poorly with clinical encephalopathy and is therefore probably not useful for determining response to therapy. The treatment is oral or rectal administration of lactulose, which decreases the absorption of ammonia by colonocytes. In the past, restriction of protein intake was practiced with the intention of decreasing the substrate for ammonia production. However, protein restriction has not been demonstrated to be beneficial. The critically ill patient with hepatic dysfunction is hypercatabolic and requires an excess of protein intake to remain in nitrogen balance. Solutions enriched in branched chain amino acids (leucine, isoleucine, and valine) are effective for nutritional support of patients with hepatic failure and have been shown to relieve the symptoms of hepatic encephalopathy.

FLUID AND ELECTROLYTE DISORDERS

Chronic liver disease is associated with a state of total body sodium excess and paradoxical hyponatremia. It is thought that hepatic insufficiency causes decreased clearance of vasodilators (e.g., nitric oxide, prostacyclin, glucagon, adenosine, lipopolysaccharide), resulting in peripheral and splanchnic vasodilation, which is sensed as a decrease in effective circulating volume. This stimulates tubular sodium retention and reduces renal blood flow via stimulation of the sympathetic nervous system and by the renin-angiotensin-aldosterone axis. It is prudent to practice sodium restriction in these patients.

Hepatorenal syndrome is a condition of unexplained acute renal failure with absence of clinical, laboratory, or anatomic evidence of renal disease in the setting of primary liver disease (e.g., cirrhosis). Hepatorenal failure may occur as the result of simultaneous involvement of the kidney and liver by the same primary process, or by a primary process in the kidney with secondary liver involvement or vice versa. It is necessary to rule out prerenal sources, intrinsic renal sources (glomerulonephritis, including glomerulosclerosis, IgA nephropathy, cryoglobulinemia resulting from hepatitis C liver disease, acute tubular necrosis, toxins, drugs, hypoxia, interstitial nephritis), and postrenal obstruction. Although the cause of hepatorenal syndrome is unknown, the behavior of renal dysfunction is similar to that of prerenal oliguria. Thus, management is directed toward achieving and ensuring adequate circulating volume and kidney perfusion. A pulmonary artery catheter may be necessary to guide fluid administration.

CEREBRAL EDEMA

Intracranial hypertension resulting from cerebral edema is the leading cause of death and the most immediately life-threatening consequence of fulminant hepatic failure. Treatment of cerebral edema is directed toward decreasing intracranial pressure or improving cerebral perfusion pressure. To minimize psychomotor agitation, the patient should be sedated. Mechanical ventilation may be necessary. Fluid status requires constant monitoring, and a pulmonary artery catheter should be considered. Adjuvant treatment includes osmolar therapy with mannitol. Hyperventilation, once a mainstay of treatment, is now thought to be contraindicated because it reduces cerebral blood flow.

CARDIOVASCULAR AND RESPIRATORY DYSFUNCTION

Patients with chronic liver disease have decreased systemic vascular resistance and increased cardiac output. Although hepatic blood flow in these patients is equal to or greater than that in normal subjects, it is likely that the liver is sensitive to decreases in hepatic blood flow, and thus hypotension is poorly tolerated by the liver. Factors responsible for acute hepatic dysfunction may also cause cardiovascular dysfunction, impairing hepatic perfusion and worsening hepatic function. In general, adequate preload should be assured, and a pulmonary artery catheter should be considered if perfusion does not respond appropriately. Inotropic support may be necessary to maximize cardiac function and organ perfusion.

Hepatopulmonary syndrome is a condition of chronic liver disease and concomitant unexplained pulmonary insufficiency. Hypoxemia is thought to be due to intrapulmonary arteriovenous shunting. Patients may also have pulmonary hypertension, ventilation-perfusion mismatch, and evidence of interstitial or restrictive disease. Treatment is supportive, with supplemental oxygen being the mainstay of therapy. Mechanical ventilation may be necessary.

LIVER TRANSPLANTATION

Rarely, acute hepatic dysfunction fails to resolve despite maximal supportive measures, progressing to fulminant hepatic failure. Currently, the only cure for fulminant hepatic failure is liver transplantation.

THE BIOARTIFICIAL LIVER

No liver support system has achieved wide clinical use. Hemodialysis and hemoperfusion using charcoal or resin have been shown in some studies to improve encephalopathy. Ex vivo perfusion with porcine liver has been attempted, but hyperacute rejection limits clinical use. One promising modality is the bioartificial liver system (BAL), which uses intact porcine hepatocytes attached to microcarrier beads and contained in a hollow-fiber bioreactor. Blood is removed from the venous system and separated into cells and plasma. The plasma is filtered through an activated charcoal column and perfused through the hepatocyte bioreactor. It then is recombined with blood cells and returned to the body. The BAL is conceptually appealing because xenogenic hepatocytes should provide metabolic and synthetic as well as detoxification capabilities. Another promising modality is the molecular adsorbent recycling system (MARS), which dialyzes water-soluble and albumin-bound molecules, but not albumin or other proteins. Albumin-related binding sites on the dial-

---

Pearls and Pitfalls

PEARLS

- Chronic liver disease is the most common risk factor for the development of perioperative hepatic dysfunction.
- Most cases of acquired perioperative hepatic dysfunction resolve uneventfully with adequate supportive measures.
- The most lethal complications of fulminant hepatic failure are refractory coagulopathy and cerebral edema.
- Abnormalities of PT, PTT, and albumin suggest deficient protein synthetic capacity by the liver and correlate with risk of hepatic dysfunction.

PITFALLS

- *Patients with hepatic encephalopathy do not require protein restriction.* Adequate protein administration is crucial to maintaining nitrogen balance in patients with hepatic failure.
- *Hyperventilation is not the mainstay of treatment of cerebral edema related to liver failure.* Hyperventilation decreases cerebral blood flow, worsening cerebral perfusion pressure.
- *Renal failure in hepatorenal syndrome is responsive to fluid administration.* Although the pathophysiology of hepatorenal syndrome is not understood, renal dysfunction should be considered prerenal and treatment directed accordingly.

---

ysis membrane compete for toxins bound to plasma albumin, whereas low molecular weight substances diffuse through the membrane by size exclusion. MARS performs detoxification but has no intrinsic metabolic or synthetic capabilities. However, MARS has the advantage of avoiding the use of xenobiological tissue. In a small series of patients with acute decompensation of chronic liver insufficiency, MARS therapy was associated with improvements in Child score, hepatic encephalopathy, and biochemical markers of liver function.

Summary

Hepatic dysfunction increases the risk of perioperative morbidity and mortality. Patients with chronic liver disease may have abnormalities in fluid and electrolyte status, coagulation, and nutrition, which increase the risk of surgery. In patients with normal hepatic function, acquired hepatic dysfunction may occur in the setting of sepsis or SIRS, hypotension, or major surgery. Therapy of hepatic dysfunction is primarily supportive, and in the absence of chronic liver disease, recovery is typically uneventful. Fulminant hepatic failure carries a high mortality risk, and if it is refractory to intensive medical management, transplantation is indicated.

SELECTED READINGS

Andrejko KM, Deutschman CS: Altered hepatic gene expression in fecal peritonitis: Changes in transcription of gluconeogenic, β-oxidative, and ureagenic genes. Shock 1997;7:164.

Arkadopoulos N, Detry O, Rozga J, Demetriou AA: Liver assist systems: State of the art. Int J Artif Organs 1998;21:781.

Barie PS, Hydo LJ, Fischer E: Utility of illness severity scoring for prediction of prolonged surgical critical care. J Trauma-Injury Infect Crit Care 1996;40:513.

Beal AL, Cerra FB: Multiple organ failure syndrome in the 1990s. Systemic inflammatory response and organ dysfunction. JAMA 1994;271:226.

Blom HJ, Ferenci P, Grimm G, et al: The role of methanethiol in the pathogenesis of hepatic encephalopathy. Hepatology 1991;13:44.

Davison AM: Hepatorenal failure. Nephrol Dial Transplant 1996;(11 Suppl 8):24.

Garrison RN, Cryer HM, Howard DA, et al: Clarification of risk factors for abdominal operations in patients with hepatic cirrhosis. Ann Surg 1984;199:648.

Jalen R, Hayes PC: Hepatic encephalopathy and ascites. Lancet 1997; 350:1309.

Kim PK, Deutschman CS: Inflammatory responses and mediators. Surg Clin North Am 2000;80:885.

Lochs H, Plauth M: Liver cirrhosis: Rationale and modalities for nutritional support—The European Society of Parenteral and Enteral Nutrition consensus and beyond. Curr Opin Clin Nutr Metab Care 1999;2:345.

Mizock BA: Nutritional support in hepatic encephalopathy. Nutrition 1999;15:220.

Mammen EF: Acquired coagulation protein defects. In Bick RL (ed): Hematology: Clinical and Laboratory Practice. St. Louis, Mosby–Year Book, 1993:1449.

Stange J, Mitzner SR, Risler T, et al: Molecular adsorbent recycling system (MARS): Clinical results of a new membrane-based blood purification system for bioartificial liver support. Artif Organs 1999;23:319.

Zimmerman JE, Wagner DP, Seneff MG, et al: Intensive care unit admissions with cirrhosis: Risk-stratifying patient groups and predicting individual survival. Hepatology 1996;23:1393.

Ziser A, Plevak DJ, Wiesner RH, et al: Morbidity and mortality in cirrhotic patients undergoing anesthesia and surgery. Anesthesiology 1999; 90:42.

Chapter 25

Status Epilepticus

Michelle Aizenberg and Curtis Doberstein

Status epilepticus is an emergent condition that can result in significant morbidity and mortality if not treated appropriately. It is essential that this condition be promptly identified and treated emergently. Approximately 45,000 to 250,000 people develop status epilepticus each year and as many as one third of these patients have no previous history of epilepsy (Gastaut, 1983; Rowland, 1995; Gumnit et al; Payne and Bleck, 1997; Runge and Allen, 1996). This demonstrates that status epilepticus is not a rare event and that it cannot be excluded based on a patient's benign past medical history. In critically ill patients, as many as 4% will develop new-onset seizures. Even though more than half of the cases of status epilepticus occur in children, it has been suggested that patients older than 60 years of age are also more susceptible to developing this disorder (Hauser, 1990). The surgeon will most often encounter this condition in the trauma or critical care setting, although stable in-patients may also develop status epilepticus, particularly from withdrawal of their antiepileptic drugs (AEDs) or from metabolic derangements. The morbidity and mortality resulting from status epilepticus is strongly correlated to the duration of seizure activity, the etiology, and related medical conditions. In children, the overall mortality rate associated with status epilepticus is estimated to be less than 8%. In adults, it is estimated to be less than 30% (Bone, 1993).

DEFINITION AND CLASSIFICATION OF SEIZURE TYPE

Status epilepticus is defined as ongoing seizure activity lasting 30 minutes or multiple seizures without the return of consciousness between episodes. However, most often, continuous seizure activity is treated promptly so as to halt the activity and prevent the sequelae of continued neuronal stimulation. It would be inappropriate to allow seizure activity to propagate for 30 minutes before one establishes a definitive diagnosis of status epilepticus and initiates appropriate interventions. There are many detrimental effects of prolonged seizure activity that can affect the nervous, respiratory, cardiac, metabolic, renal, and musculoskeletal systems. Therefore, the strict definition of one-half hour should not be used as a criterion for intervention; and when seizure activity is obvious, treatment should be instituted immediately. However, it may be more difficult to diagnose epileptic activity in a patient who is in subtle convulsive or nonconvulsive status epilepticus.

The general classification of types of status epilepticus is outlined in Table 25–1. Convulsive status epilepticus is manifested by generalized seizure activity characterized by tonic-clonic movements. If a tonic, clonic, or my-

oclonic seizure occurs with sufficient frequency, it may also develop into status epilepticus. Convulsive seizure activity may initially begin as a generalized seizure or as a partial or focal seizure with subsequent secondary generalization. If seizures are secondarily generalized, the patient may initially present with lateralized movements (simple partial seizure) or changes in consciousness (complex partial seizure). Subtle convulsive status epilepticus presents with mild motor activity in a comatose patient that may not initially be picked up by the examiner.

Nonconvulsive status epilepticus may be characterized by slowness in mentation, stupor, confusion, or coma. Young and colleagues (1996) described various presentations of nonconvulsive status epilepticus (Table 25–2). The diagnosis can be difficult to make clinically because of the variation and subtlety in presentation. If nonconvulsive status epilepticus is suspected, an electroencephalogram (EEG) should be promptly obtained. A delay in diagnosing nonconvulsive status epilepticus often occurs and is associated with the greater mortality rate reported in this patient group (Young et al, 1996). From their assessment of nonconvulsive seizure, Young and co-workers have concluded that seizure activity should be suspected in patients with the following: prolonged postictal states; prolonged recovery of alertness from operative procedures or neurologic insults; acute onset of impaired consciousness or fluctuating mentation; impaired mentation with the presence of myoclonic or nystagmoid movements, episodic blank staring, aphasia, automatisms, or perseverative activity; or acutely altered behavior without obvious etiology. As many as 25% of patients admitted to a neurologic ICU can present with nonconvulsive status epilepticus (Jordan, 1992). Nonconvulsive status epilepticus can also result from partially treated generalized convulsive status epilepticus. Epilepsia partialis continua is a focal motor epilepsy that can be thought of as a restricted focal motor status epilepticus and is characterized by clonic movements of one muscle group. The face, arms, or legs are most often affected. In the face, the eyelids or mouth manifest symptoms. The distal muscles of the upper and lower extremities are affected more frequently than the proximal ones (Adams and Victor, 1993). Most patients with epilepsia partialis continua show

Table 25–1	Status Epilepticus Classification	
GENERALIZED		**PARTIAL**
Convulsive (tonic-clonic or clonic)		Simple (epilepsy partialis continuans)
Absence		
Secondarily generalized (most common)		Complex
Myoclonic		Secondarily generalized
Atonic (drop attack)		

Table 25–2	**Presentations of Nonconvulsive Status Epilepticus**

Unresponsiveness	Facial twitching
Marked diminution in alertness	Limb myoclonus
Obtundation	Aphasia
Altered behavior	Hallucinations
Acute confusion	Epileptic nystagmus

focal EEG abnormalities; however, the cause in these cases can be difficult to determine and it generally is unresponsive to AED therapy.

ETIOLOGY

The precipitants of status epilepticus are many, and the condition can be associated with acute or remote neurologic insults or may be idiopathic. Table 25–3 outlines the various causes of status epilepticus. In one half to two thirds of cases, an acute precipitant is the cause (Rowland, 1995; Bone, 1993). Acute metabolic derangements that may precipitate status epilepticus include hyponatremia, hypocalcemia, hypoglycemia, hypomagnesemia, and hyperosmolar states. Conditions such as hepatic, uremic, or anoxic encephalopathy can also lead to status epilepticus. Acid-base disturbances such as acidosis, respiratory alkalosis, and hypercapnia are known to decrease seizure threshold. Intoxication with various drugs, such as tricyclic antidepressants, cocaine, phencyclidine (PCP), theophylline, isoniazid, imipenem, lidocaine, steroids, and immunosuppressives, as well as withdrawal from narcotics, alcohol, or AEDs can be the cause of status. Infectious causes include sepsis, meningitis, and encephalitis. Sepsis enhances capillary permeability, altering the blood-brain barrier, which may allow for toxins to cross into the brain parenchyma more easily. Fever is a common cause of seizures in children and results in status epilepticus in approximately 35% of cases (Rowland, 1995). In addition, acute or remote head injuries are a frequent cause. Prior insults are found to be the culprit in cases of status epilepticus in approximately 3% to 23% of cases (Bone, 1993). Finally, structural lesions such as intracranial tumors or arteriovenous malformations provide an irritable focus that can lead to generalized seizure or status epilepticus.

In general, status epilepticus in adults usually results from withdrawal of AEDs or alcohol or from stroke or anoxia. In contrast, in children the most frequent etiologies include infections, metabolic disorders, or congenital malformations (DeLorenzo et al, 1992).

PATHOPHYSIOLOGY

As mentioned previously, a number of derangements occur within multiple-organ systems as the result of ongoing seizure activity. During the first half hour of seizure activity, the body has adequate reserves for compensating for the resulting pathophysiologic alterations. However, as seizure activity continues, these compensatory mechanisms fail and permanent damage to the central nervous system can ensue. Initially, systolic blood pressure is elevated as the result of circulating catecholamines. Cerebral blood flow increases as the result of increased cardiac output and increased mean arterial pressure. The mean cerebral arterial-venous oxygen difference decreases. Central nervous system venous pressure increases as the result of sustained muscle contractions. Circulating epinephrine and cortisol result in hyperglycemia. After 20 to 30 minutes of seizure activity, metabolic demand becomes greater than supply, and tissue damage can occur. At this point, blood pressure decreases, as does cardiac output and cerebral blood flow. The arterial-venous oxygen difference increases, resulting in decreased brain parenchymal oxygenation. Patients may return to normoglycemia or become hypoglycemic if gluconeogenesis fails.

Central nervous system disturbances resulting from prolonged seizure activity include cerebral edema and cerebral vasodilatation secondary to increased lactate production in the brain, resulting in increased intracranial pressure. Prolonged exposure to excitatory amino acid neurotransmitters, such as glutamate, leads to excessive excitation, with toxic levels of calcium building up in the cytosol of the neuron. A consequence of this is activation of autolytic enzymes and production of oxygen free radicals and nitric oxide, which are toxic to neurons. Furthermore, the phosphorylation of receptors and enzymes increases the likelihood of continued seizure activity. Membrane pump failure leads to increased cellular osmolality, which results in cytotoxic edema. These are the mechanisms by which neuronal death can occur. Autoregulation of cerebral blood flow ceases, and cerebral blood flow becomes dependent on the mean arterial pressure. As blood pressure falls, so does cerebral perfusion. This, in turn, may further propagate lactate production. The autonomic nervous system malfunctions, and this results in hyperpyrexia and excessive sweating. There is also impairment of the inhibitory system by way of GABA, which promotes further seizure activity (Payne and Bleck, 1997).

Pulmonary complications consist of respiratory acidosis, increased secretions in the tracheobronchial tree, and hypoxia. Carbon dioxide exchange and ventilation are impaired as the result of poor diaphragm function secondary to sustained muscular contractions. Subsequent elevations in carbon dioxide levels are one of the most potent cerebrovascular dilators. In addition, hypoxia also causes cerebrovascular dilatation, becoming quite significant around PO₂ levels of 50 mm Hg. Both of these alterations can contribute to cerebral edema. Neurogenic pulmonary

Table 25–3	**Precipitants of Status Epilepticus**	
	ACUTE	**CHRONIC AND REMOTE**
	Metabolic	Tumor
	Drug intoxication	Cerebrovascular accident
	Drug withdrawal	Anoxia
	Infection	Trauma
	Trauma	
	Fever	

edema can also occur. The exact mechanism is not clear, although it may be related to increased sympathetic nervous system activity, peripheral vasoconstriction, elevated blood pressure, and shifts of blood away from the periphery. These factors may lead to decreased left ventricular compliance, which results in increased atrial pressures that may be sufficient to initiate pulmonary edema.

Some of the cardiovascular effects of seizure activity have already been mentioned. Tachycardia occurs from increased levels of catecholamines, whereas increased vagal tone may induce bradycardia. Fatal arrhythmias may result from hyperkalemia or hypercalcemia secondary to acidosis or muscle necrosis. Peripheral vasoconstriction from the increased catecholamines produces decreased skin circulation. This makes it more difficult for the patient to dissipate the heat generated from sustained muscle contractions and contributes to the observed hyperpyrexia.

Metabolic changes include hyperglycemia initially and normoglycemia or hypoglycemia with prolonged seizure activity. Metabolic acidosis occurs from lactate production. The hypercalcemia that results can induce arrhythmias or further potentiate seizure activity. Patients also become dehydrated and hyponatremic. Endocrinologic changes include increased levels of growth hormone, prolactin, glucagon, adrenocorticotropic hormone (ACTH), cortisol, and epinephrine and norepinephrine. Hematologically, a leukocytosis is observed.

In convulsive status epilepticus, sustained muscle contractions contribute to heat production and a lack of ventilation. If the contractions are sustained for a long enough period of time, muscle necrosis and rhabdomyolysis can occur, with all of the resulting associated complications, including acute renal failure. If contractions are strong enough, compression fractures, joint dislocations, and tendon avulsions can occur.

TREATMENT

Once the diagnosis of status epilepticus has been established by witnessed continuous overt seizure activity and/or EEG monitoring, treatment should be initiated expeditiously. Status epilepticus becomes more difficult to effectively control as the duration of seizure activity increases and eventually may become refractory. A thorough but quick assessment as to the cause of status epilepticus should be made so that this may be corrected, if possible (Table 25–4). First and foremost, the ABCs of resuscitation must be addressed. Oxygen should be administered and the patient's head turned to the side to prevent aspiration. If motor activity terminates, an oral airway can then be introduced. Intubation is usually not necessary unless there is evidence of respiratory depression, cyanosis, or hypoxia, or if seizures last more than 30 minutes. If intubation is required, a short-acting neuromuscular blocking agent should be used so that paralysis will not mask ongoing seizure activity. It may be necessary to perform continuous EEG monitoring if paralytic agents are utilized or if the patient is in nonconvulsive status epilepticus. Cardiac and hemodynamic monitoring are essential, as arrhythmias and hypotension may occur as

Table 25–4	Timetable for Treatment of Status Epilepticus

0–10 Minutes

Assess patient. ABCs, oxygen, obtain IV access, administer normal saline infusion, send blood for CBC, chemistry, liver function, calcium, magnesium, AED levels, arterial blood gas, and toxicology if appropriate. Cardiac monitoring. Thiamine 100 mg + glucose 50%, 50 mL, if hypoglycemia is known or suspected (glucose 25%, 2 mL/kg in children).

10–40 Minutes

Administer lorazepam, 0.1 mg/kg IVP at 2 mg/min. If diazepam is used, 0.2 mg/kg IVP at 5 mg/min. Administer phenytoin, 15–20 mg/kg IV at 50 mg/min max (in children, 1 mg/kg/min), or fosphenytoin, 15–20 mg PE/kg at 150 mg PE/min.

40–60 Minutes

Additional doses of phenytoin or the equivalent of fosphenytoin can be administered to a maximum of 30 mg/kg if seizures persist. Call for neurology/EEG monitoring. Utilization of vasopressors and securing of the airway are almost always indicated at this point. Administer phenobarbital, 20 mg/kg IVP at 100 mg/min (in children, 15–20 mg/kg). Alternatively, phenobarbital, 10 mg/kg × 2, can be given. Arterial line and pulmonary catheterization are usually indicated for most patients at this point as well.

>60 Minutes

If seizures persist, they are considered refractory after administration of three AEDs. Continuous EEG monitoring is essential now. Pentobarbital, at a dose of 10–15 mg/kg, should be loaded at 50 mg/min. A continuous infusion of 2–3 mg/kg/hr should then be administered for maintenance. Burst suppression or cessation of seizure activity are titration endpoints. Every 12–24 hr, the drip should be discontinued to check for cessation of seizure activity (via EEG monitoring). If seizures still persist, consider other agents: thiopental, propofol, isoflurane, or etomidate. Arterial line and pulmonary artery catheterization are required by most patients at this stage. In addition, at this stage, midazolam should be started with a 0.2 mg/kg bolus and followed by a maintenance drip of 1–2 mg/kg/hr. Midazolam is short-acting, and a drip is required. Tachyphylaxis occurs that necessitates dose variation. It is important that the other AEDs that have been previously started (e.g., phenytoin) be continued so that when a patient is weaned from midazolam or general anesthetics, they have therapeutic levels of long-term AEDs.

IVP, intravenous push; PEs, phenytoin equivalents.

the result of seizure activity or drug administration. If hypotension does develop, vasopressors should be utilized to maintain normal or higher blood pressures so as to ensure adequate cerebral perfusion, particularly if cerebral autoregulation fails. A large-bore intravenous line should be placed if access has not been obtained already, and blood should be sent for analysis of electrolytes, including Mg^{2+}, and Ca^{2+}, glucose, anticonvulsant drug levels, complete blood count (CBC), liver and renal function tests, and toxicology if appropriate. Arterial blood gases should also be analyzed. An infusion of normal saline should be started, as solutions containing glucose cause some AEDs, especially phenytoin, to precipitate. If hypoglycemia is known or suspected, 100 mg of thiamine followed by 50 mL of 50% glucose solution should be administered. In children, 2 mL/kg of 25% glucose solution should be used. Thiamine must be administered in adult patients to prevent precipitation of Wernicke's encephalopathy, particularly when a history of alcohol abuse is known or suspected. Naloxone should also be administered to reverse the effect of any potential narcotic overdosage. Hyperpyrexia may necessitate the use of a cooling blanket. Rectal temperature monitoring is recommended, and the core temperature should not be allowed to climb, as this may exacerbate neuronal damage. The acidosis that results from ongoing seizure activity does not usually need to be treated, as the pH will correct with cessation of seizure activity.

Pharmacologic intervention should be started if seizure activity continues after approximately 10 minutes. Administration of medications should always be by the intravenous route. Other routes of administration do not provide reliable absorption or dosing of AEDs. They are also not as rapid in onset of action. Diazepam is available in a rectal gel formulation that can be effective in the treatment of repetitive seizures but should not be utilized by outpatients with seizure disorder unless it becomes impossible to obtain intravenous access in a timely fashion. Diazepam used to be the initial agent of choice, but its duration of action is short-lived. In addition, it rapidly redistributes into the body fat stores, reducing brain and blood levels, which leaves the patient susceptible to recurrence of seizure activity. This will occur within 20 to 30 minutes after initial administration of diazepam (Treiman, 1997). If diazepam is used, the patient should also be loaded with phenytoin or fosphenytoin. The dose of diazepam for the treatment of status epilepticus is 0.2 mg/kg administered at a rate of 5 mg/min. The dose may be repeated if seizure activity continues after 5 minutes. Respiratory depression may occur, and intubation may be necessary. It is important to note that if intubation is performed and neuromuscular blocking agents are utilized, AEDs must still be administered. The paralytics will mask any motor activity of the seizure while ongoing brain electrical activity will cause irreversible neuronal injury. EEG monitoring is essential at this point.

Lorazepam is the preferred initial agent, as it has a prolonged duration of action in comparison with diazepam, as well as a smaller volume of distribution, because it is less lipid soluble (Payne and Bleck, 1997). Lorazepam is also not as highly protein bound as diazepam, which results in more free drug being available for target tissues. Lorazepam has an effective duration of action of 12 to 24 hours, whereas diazepam has one of only 15 to 30 minutes (Bone, 1993). The dose of lorazepam is 0.2 mg/kg administered at a rate of 2 mg/min. Both lorazepam and diazepam may cause respiratory depression or hypotension, and patients receiving these medications should be monitored closely.

Phenytoin or fosphenytoin should be administered in conjunction with initial benzodiazepine treatment. Even if lorazepam or diazepam has been efficacious in halting seizure activity, a long-acting agent should be administered for the prevention of later recurrence. Phenytoin is a very effective anticonvulsant with a duration of action of about 24 hours. Phenytoin is administered by the intravenous route only. The dose is 15 to 20 mg/kg administered at a maximal rate of 50 mg/min in adults and 1 mg/kg per minute in children. The therapeutic serum level of phenytoin is 10 to 20 mg/L. After a dose of 18 mg/kg, most patients will achieve a serum level of 25 to 30 mg/L (Gumnit et al). Phenytoin is highly lipid soluble,

but redistribution is slower than with diazepam. Peak brain levels are reached in 6 to 10 minutes and stay elevated for several hours (Payne and Bleck, 1997; Runge and Allen, 1996). Several problems can arise with administration of phenytoin, such as hypotension or cardiac arrhythmias. If hypotension occurs, the rate of infusion should be lowered. If arrhythmias or widening of the QT interval occurs, the rate of infusion should also be slowed and ultimately stopped if it does not resolve with a slower rate of infusion. Phenytoin is highly insoluble, will precipitate out in dextrose-containing solutions, and is toxic to veins because of the drug vehicle. There is a risk of thrombophlebitis and frank tissue necrosis at the injection site. Fosphenytoin is a prodrug with an active metabolite of phenytoin. It is rapidly converted in the body by phosphatases to phenytoin. The benefit of fosphenytoin is that it can be infused at a faster rate and is not as toxic to veins. The dose of fosphenytoin is given in phenytoin equivalents (PEs). One vial of fosphenytoin contains 75 mg/mL of fosphenytoin, which is equivalent to 50 mg/mL of phenytoin. The dose of fosphenytoin for status epilepticus is 15 to 20 mg PE/kg to be administered no faster than 150 mg PE/min. Therapeutic concentrations are achieved in less than 10 minutes (Payne and Bleck, 1997).

If the aforementioned treatments have not succeeded in eliminating seizure activity, it becomes necessary to administer further medications. The third-line agent is phenobarbital and has been used for many years. It causes significant respiratory depression and suppression of consciousness. An intubation kit should be nearby prior to administration. Often, patients may be intubated prior to administration, as it is assumed they will need ventilatory support after administration of both benzodiazepines and phenobarbital. At this point, EEG monitoring should be initiated if it has not been done so up to this point. After phenobarbital is given, patients will have depressed consciousness and it will be difficult to assess their recovery from prolonged seizure activity. This can last for several days in some cases. The dose of phenobarbital is 20 mg/kg administered at a maximal rate of 100 mg/min. Dosing is sometimes given as 10 mg/kg for two doses. The dose in children is 15 to 20 mg/kg. The maximal single dose of phenobarbital to be given should not exceed 400 mg. Side effects of phenobarbital include respiratory depression, suppression of consciousness, and hypotension. If a patient becomes hypotensive, the rate of infusion should be slowed.

If status epilepticus persists after all of the aforementioned treatments, the patient is said to be in refractory status epilepticus, which is defined as failure of three or more AEDs. The patient should be intubated at this time, and general anesthetic agents are initiated. The best first-line general anesthetic is pentobarbital, which is given as a loading dose of 15 mg/kg at a rate of 50 mg/min. Maintenance doses (typically 2.5 mg/kg per hour) are then given to maintain the EEG in burst suppression.

The effectiveness of different AEDs has been studied by Trieman and colleagues (1998) for both overt and subtle generalized convulsive status epilepticus. In the randomized, double-blind study, they compared lorazepam and diazepam followed by phenytoin, phenobarbi-

Pearls and Pitfalls

PEARLS

- Status epilepticus is defined as ongoing seizure activity lasting more than 30 minutes or multiple seizures without return of consciousness between episodes.
- Precipitants of status epilepticus include the following: acute—metabolic alterations, drug intoxication, drug withdrawal, infection, trauma, and fever; chronic and remote—structural lesions such as tumor or cerebrovascular, anoxia, and trauma.
- The longer the duration of seizures, the more difficult the condition is to treat.
- Treatment consists first of the basics of resuscitation, followed by pharmacologic intervention (by the intravenous route) with concurrent cardiac and hemodynamic monitoring, performance of EEG, and additional measures as required.

PITFALLS

- Morbidity and mortality in status epilepticus strongly correlate to duration of seizure, etiology, and related medical conditions.
- There are many detrimental effects of prolonged seizure activity to all bodily systems; status epilepticus is a medical emergency.
- Careful attention to the treatment timetable and to specific related conditions is necessary.

tal, and phenytoin. Their analysis revealed a statistically significant difference ($P = 0.008$) in the frequency of success of the different treatments. Lorazepam was successful in eliminating seizure activity as the initial treatment in 52.2%, phenobarbital in 49.2%, diazepam followed by phenytoin in 43.1%, and phenytoin alone in 36.8%. Lorazepam was significantly better than phenytoin in a pairwise comparison ($P = 0.002$). In patients with subtle convulsive status, there were no significant differences in the success of the various treatments. There were no significant differences in the rates of recurrence in either the overt or the subtle convulsive status groups over a 12-hour period. The researchers concluded that lorazepam should be the initial treatment because even though it is not more efficacious, it is easier to use than phenobarbital or diazepam followed by phenytoin. It is more effective than phenytoin alone.

SELECTED READINGS

Adams RD, Victor M: Epilepsy and other seizure disorders. In Lamsback WJ, Navrozov M (eds): Principles of Neurology, 5th ed. New York, McGraw-Hill, 1993.

Bone RC (ed): Epilepsy Foundation of America: Treatment of Convulsive Status Epilepticus. Recommendations of the Epilepsy Foundation of America's Working Group on Status Epilepticus. JAMA 1993;270:854.

DeLorenzo RJ, Towne AR, Pellock JM, et al: Status epilepticus in children, adults, and the elderly. Epilepsia 1992;33(suppl 4):S15.

Gastaut, H: Classification of status epilepticus. In Delgado-Escueta AV, Wasterlain CG, Treiman DM, Porter RJ (eds): Advances in Neurology, vol 34: Status Epilepticus. New York, Raven Press, 1983, p 15.

Gumnit RJ, Risinger M, Leppik B, et al (eds): Clinical Neurology: The Epilepsies and Convulsive Disorders, vol 3, Chapter 31. Philadelphia, Lippincott–Williams & Wilkins.

Hauser WA: Status epilepticus: Epidemiologic considerations, sequelae. Neurology 1990;40(suppl 2):9.

Jordan KG: Nonconvulsive status epilepticus in the neuro ICU detected by continuous EEG monitoring. Neurology 1992;42(suppl 1):194.

Payne TA, Bleck TP: Update on neurologic critical care: Status epilepticus. Crit Care Clin 1997;13:17.

Rowland LP (ed): Paroxysmal disorders. In Merritt's Textbook of Neurology, 9th ed. Philadelphia, Williams & Wilkins, 1995, pp 837–884.

Runge JW, Allen FH: Emergency treatment of status epilepticus. Neurology 1996;46:20.

Treiman DM: Treatment of status epilepticus. In Engel J Jr, Pedley TA (eds): Epilepsy: A Comprehensive Textbook. Philadelphia: Lippincott-Raven, 1997, pp 1317–1323.

Treiman DM, Patti DM, Walton NY, et al: A comparison of four treatments for generalized convulsive status epilepticus. N Engl J Med 1998;339:792.

Willmore LJ: Epilepsy emergencies: The first seizure and status epilepticus. Neurology 1998;51:34.

Young GB, Jordan KG, Doig GS: An assessment of nonconvulsive seizures in the intensive care unit using continuous EEG monitoring: An investigation of variables associated with mortality. Neurology 1996;47:83.

Chapter 26

General Principles of Sepsis

Mitchell P. Fink

Although the term *sepsis* has been defined as the systemic response to infection, this definition is not entirely satisfactory for several reasons. First, the systemic manifestations of infection are inconstant. For example, most infected patients are febrile, but some are hypothermic; a few have neither fever nor hypothermia. Although most patients with "sepsis" have an elevated blood leukocyte count, profound leukopenia also can occur. Second, other conditions, such as acute pancreatitis and multiple trauma, are associated with the systemic release of proinflammatory mediators that can trigger the development of clinical findings virtually identical to those characteristic of severe infection. Indeed, many systemic hemodynamic, hematologic, and hormonal responses to infection can be reproduced by infusing volunteers or patients with certain proinflammatory cytokines, including tumor necrosis factor (TNF), interleukin-1 (IL-1), or interleukin-2 (IL-2). Thus, sepsis probably does not reflect the systemic response to infection per se; rather it reflects the effects of the proinflammatory mediators that are released during infections as well as other conditions. Accordingly, a new term, the *systemic inflammatory response syndrome*, or *SIRS*, has been adopted to describe the clinical syndrome associated with the release of proinflammatory mediators, regardless of the underlying cause. Third, considered one by one, most of the systemic signs of infection are nonspecific. Thus, tachycardia, which has been considered to be one of the cardinal features of both sepsis and SIRS, also can be a manifestation of pain, anemia, hypovolemia, or many other conditions that are not necessarily related to the presence of infection (or even inflammation).

Even so, in general medical usage, the term *sepsis* denotes the continuum of acute and subacute responses by the host to the invasion of normally sterile tissues by microbes. The term *septic shock* denotes circulatory collapse (i.e., systemic arterial hypotension) that results from overwhelming infection. *Bacteremia* implies the presence of bacteria in the blood as defined by positive blood cultures. *Fungemia* is the equivalent term used for bloodstream invasion by mycotic organisms. The term *endotoxicosis* denotes the syndrome induced in animals or human volunteers by the injection of lipopolysaccharide (LPS), a component of the outer cell wall of gram-negative bacteria. *Endotoxemia* is defined by the detection of LPS in blood or plasma samples.

EPIDEMIOLOGY

The criteria for establishing the diagnosis of sepsis are neither universally accepted nor uniformly applied in practice; thus, truly reliable data regarding the incidence of this syndrome are hard to obtain. The best current estimates, some of which are as yet unpublished, suggest that the annual incidence of sepsis in the United States is approximately 3 cases per 1000 persons, or roughly 750,000 total cases per year. Based on broad epidemiologic studies as well as a review of outcomes for patients given placebo in clinical trials of new agents for the adjuvant treatment of sepsis, the mortality rate for this condition is approximately 30% to 40%. The risk of death is higher still for patients whose presenting symptom is hypotension (i.e., septic shock) or dysfunction of multiple organ systems. Thus, sepsis represents an extremely serious public health problem.

CLINICAL PRESENTATION

Some older studies suggested that the clinical presentation of sepsis caused by gram-positive bacteria was different from the presentation associated with serious gram-negative infection; most recent reports, however, suggest that it is probably impossible to reliably distinguish gram-positive from gram-negative bacterial infection or even fungal infection on the basis of clinical findings alone. Common signs and symptoms of sepsis include fever (or, less commonly, hypothermia), chills, tachypnea, and altered mental status. In the "typical" case of well-compensated sepsis, the patient is tachycardic (i.e., heart rate > 90 beats per minute. Cardiac output indexed to body surface area (Q_t) is usually supranormal (i.e., >3.5 L/min per m^2), whereas calculated systemic vascular resistance index (SVRI) is usually subnormal (i.e., <2000 dyne-sec/ cm^5 per m^2). In well-compensated sepsis, mean arterial blood pressure is normal; however, by definition, in septic shock, mean arterial blood pressure is low (or there is a requirement for the infusion of vasoactive drugs to preserve normal mean arterial blood pressure). In the typical case of septic shock, Q_t is normal or elevated and SVRI is very low.

In addition to these hemodynamic findings, patients with sepsis often manifest signs or symptoms that are indicative of organ dysfunction. The most common finding is evidence of pulmonary dysfunction, which is called *acute lung injury*, when the quotient of arterial oxygen tension (PaO_2) divided by fractional inspired oxygen concentration (FIO_2) is 200 to 300 and *acute respiratory distress syndrome* when the PaO_2/FIO_2 ratio is less than 200. Other features of both acute lung injury and acute respiratory distress syndrome include pulmonary edema (secondary to increased alveolar capillary permeability and decreased alveolar epithelial fluid clearance), pulmonary arterial hypertension, and decreased pulmonary compliance ("stiff lungs").

Another common manifestation of sepsis, as well as the closely related *multiple organ dysfunction syndrome*, is the development of renal dysfunction, as manifested by azotemia with or without oliguria. Hepatic dysfunction also is probably very common but is difficult to quantify. The most common indicator of hepatic dysfunction is the development of cholestatic jaundice, characterized by roughly proportional increases in the circulating concentrations of both conjugated and unconjugated bilirubin. Thrombocytopenia is common in patients with sepsis and, when present, is associated with an increased risk of mortality. Frank *disseminated intravascular coagulation* is relatively uncommon, but biochemical evidence of coagulopathic abnormalities, such as mild prolongation of the prothrombin time (or the *International Normalized Ratio*), are common.

PATHOPHYSIOLOGY

A major breakthrough in current understanding of the pathophysiology of sepsis and septic shock occurred during the 1980s with the publication of a series of landmark papers by investigators from the Department of Surgery at Cornell University Medical School and the Rockefeller University in New York. These papers showed that injecting rodents with a protein called "cachectin" by the investigators, but which has come to be called TNF, induces clinical features and pathologic findings that are indistinguishable from those elicited by injecting experimental animals with purified LPS from gram-negative bacteria. Furthermore, these investigators showed that circulating TNF levels increase in endotoxemic animals and that passive immunization of animals with antibodies against TNF prevents death following the injection of either LPS or a large number of viable *Escherichia coli* bacteria. Thus, a modern version of Koch's postulates were satisfied and TNF (cachectin) was identified as a pivotal mediator of endotoxic and bacteremic shock in animals. These studies clearly indicated that the manifestations of sepsis were not primarily caused by the infecting microorganisms (or their products) per se, but rather by a mediator or, as was later recognized, a network of mediators, produced by the host in response to the infection. This recognition prompted an explosive growth in modern understanding of the inflammatory response, in general, and of the pathophysiology of sepsis and septic shock, in particular.

TNF is a pluripotent mediator capable of triggering a wide range of biologic responses. When human beings are injected with recombinant TNF, many of the responses observed are remarkably similar to those observed in patients with sepsis. Some of these responses are summarized in Table 26–1. It has become apparent, however, that TNF is far from being the only, or even the most important, mediator responsible for organ dysfunction or for mortality in sepsis. The proinflammatory mediators implicated in the pathogenesis of sepsis include a diverse array of secreted proteins, cell surface proteins, lipids, and small molecules ("autocoids"). The secreted proteins are called *cytokines*, and include TNF, IL-1, other interleukins (e.g., IL-6 and IL-18), interferon-γ (IFN-γ), and another recently described molecule, called high mo-

Table 26–1	**Some Biologic Responses Elicited When Humans Are Infused with Recombinant Tumor Necrosis Factor**

Fever
Headache
Anorexia
Hypercortisolemia
Systemic arterial hypotension
Transient neutropenia followed by neutrophilia
Increased plasma acute phase protein levels
Hypoferremia
Hypozincemia
Activation of coagulation cascades
Pulmonary edema

bility group (HMG)-1. Among the cytokines are a specialized group of proteins, called *chemokines*, that function to attract polymorphonuclear leukocytes and macrophages to the sites of infection and inflammation. One important chemokine is IL-8. Important cell surface proteins involved in the inflammatory response, and hence the pathogenesis of sepsis, include the receptors for various microbial products, such as LPS, and the receptors for endogenous mediators, such as the two receptors for TNF, called TNF-R1 and TNF-R2. Other important cell surface molecules are involved in the adherence of neutrophils to endothelial surfaces at sites of infection and in the lung and other organs as a consequence of SIRS. Important lipid mediators include platelet-activating factor, an ether-linked derivative of glycerol, and derivatives of the essential polyunsaturated fatty acid, arachidonic acid, which are collectively referred to as *eicosanoids*. The enzyme that produces a major subgroup of eicosanoids, the prostaglandins, is called cyclooxygenase and exists in two isoforms. One of the cyclooxygenase isoforms, COX-2, is induced when inflammatory cells, such as monocytes and macrophages, are exposed to certain bacterial products, notably LPS, or proinflammatory cytokines (e.g., TNF or IFN-γ).

One of the most important small molecules involved in pathogenesis of sepsis and septic shock is nitric oxide (NO•). One of the simplest stable molecules in nature, NO• is produced by many different types of cells and serves as both a signaling and effector molecule in mammalian biology. NO• is synthesized in a complex oxidation-reduction reaction that requires molecular oxygen and the amino acid L-arginine as substrates, and a family of enzymes called nitric oxide synthases (NOS) as catalysts. Whereas NOS-1 (also called neuronal NOS or nNOS) and NOS-3 (also called endothelial or eNOS) tend to be expressed constitutively in various cell types, iNOS (also called inducible NOS or NOS-2) is expressed for the most part only following stimulation of cells by proinflammatory cytokines (particularly, IFN-γ, TNF, and IL-1) or LPS. NOS-1 and NOS-2 produce small "puffs" of NO• in response to transient changes in intracellular ionized calcium concentration. In contrast, iNOS, once induced, produces large quantities of NO• for a prolonged period of time.

Many of the biologic actions of NO•, including vasodilation, induction of vascular hyperpermeability, and inhibition of platelet aggregation, are mediated through activation of the enzyme, soluble guanylyl cyclase. Binding of NO• to the heme moiety of soluble guanylyl cyclase activates the enzyme, enabling it to catalyze the conversion of guanosine triphosphate to cyclic guanosine monophosphate. Excessive production of NO• as a result of iNOS induction in vascular smooth muscle cells is thought to be a major factor contributing to the loss of vasomotor tone and the loss of responsiveness to vasopressor agents ("vasoplegia") in patients with septic shock.

Another group of small molecules that are thought to be important in the pathogenesis of septic shock are various partially reduced forms of molecular oxygen that are commonly referred to collectively as *reactive oxygen species*. Key reactive oxygen species include the free radicals superoxide anion (O_2^-) and hydroxyl (OH•) as well as the potent oxidizing agent hydrogen peroxide (H_2O_2). Reactive oxygen species can injure tissues and hence impair organ function by promoting lipid peroxidation in cytosolic and organellar membranes, damaging nuclear DNA, altering mitochondrial membrane permeability, and oxidizing key sulfhydryl groups on cellular proteins. A particularly toxic moiety, peroxynitrite ($ONOO^-$), can be formed during inflammation when NO• reacts rapidly with O_2^-. $ONOO^-$ has been implicated as being particularly crucial in the pathogenesis of vasoplegia and organ dysfunction in sepsis and septic shock.

Excessive activation of the coagulation cascade also seems to be important in the pathophysiology of sepsis. In experimental animals, treatment with anticoagulant proteins, such as recombinant activated protein C or recombinant tissue factor pathway inhibitor, improves survival, even when the therapy is started well after the onset of the septic process. A recent multicentric phase III clinical trial of recombinant human activated protein C documented that adjunctive treatment with this agent improves survival in patients with severe sepsis. A similar trial of recombinant human tissue factor pathway inhibitor currently is in progress.

Although excessive and diffuse inflammation is a critical component of the pathogenesis of sepsis, it has become apparent that an excessive counterregulatory component that leads to immunosuppression and decreased host resistance to infection is equally important. The counterregulatory anti-inflammatory component of the septic response is mediated by several cytokines and other factors. One of the most important of these counterregulatory factors is the cytokine IL-10, a protein that is produced primarily by a subset of helper lymphocytes, called Th2 cells. IL-10 inhibits production of numerous proinflammatory cytokines, including IL-1, TNF, IL-6, IL-8, IL-12, and granulocyte-macrophage colony-stimulating factor, by monocytes and macrophages; conversely, IL-10 increases synthesis of another counterregulatory cytokine, IL-1 receptor antagonist (IL-1RA), by activated monocytes. Other key counterregulatory factors that are released during sepsis include the soluble forms of the extracellular domains of the TNF receptors, called sTNF-R1 and sTNF-R2, and IL-1RA.

MANAGEMENT

The treatment of patients with septic shock has two major components: (1) specific treatment directed against the source of infection ("source control"), and (2) interventions designed to maintain adequate perfusion of vital tissues or substitute for the functions of dysfunctional or failing organs ("supportive care"). A third component of care, namely specific treatment directed at the inflammatory mediators responsible for the septic process, may be available soon in the form of recombinant human activated protein C (see earlier).

Source control consists of treatment with appropriate antimicrobial chemotherapeutic agents as well as timely and appropriate surgical or radiologic intervention to drain purulent collections, resect or débride devitalized tissues, and prevent ongoing contamination of the peritoneal or pleural spaces. The initial selection of antimicrobial agents for patients with sepsis should be empirical, guided by patient's underlying condition and a reasonable guess regarding the most probable pathogens involved. When more definitive microbiologic data are available, the initial regimen, which is typically designed to cover a very broad spectrum of organisms, can be tailored to treat the specific pathogens involved. Some reasonable empirical regimens are summarized in Table 26–2.

The importance of timely and appropriate surgical therapy cannot be underestimated. Although patients with septic shock are hemodynamically unstable by definition and, thus, are likely to tolerate general anesthesia and blood loss poorly, it is imperative to drain infected fluid collections and prevent ongoing contamination of the peritoneal or pleural cavities. In some instances, drainage can be achieved using minimally invasive radiographic approaches. However, operative intervention is often necessary. In these cases, intravascular volume deficits should be rapidly corrected and appropriate surgical resection, débridement, drainage, or diversion achieved without undue delay.

Despite intensive investigation, the appropriate endpoints (i.e., therapeutic goals) for the resuscitation of patients with sepsis or septic shock have not been established with certainty. Some experts have advocated titrating therapy to achieve "supranormal" values for cardiac output, systemic oxygen delivery (Do_2), and systemic oxygen utilization (Vo_2). However, the value of this approach is not supported by well-controlled clinical trials, and the aggressive volume loading that is necessitated by this approach can exacerbate pulmonary edema, prolong the necessity for mechanical ventilation, and possibly worsen the survival rate. Moreover, infusing inotropic agents, such as dobutamine or dopamine, may increase tachycardia and myocardial oxygen demand, risking myocardial infarction in patients with fixed occlusive lesions in the coronary circulation. Accordingly, a more moderate approach to hemodynamic resuscitation is probably more appropriate. In critically ill patients with sepsis or septic shock, invasive monitoring using a Swan-Ganz pulmonary artery catheter is probably helpful, although conclusive evidence in support of this view is lacking. Hemodynamically unstable patients with sepsis should be infused with

Table 26–2	Initial (Empirical) Antimicrobial Chemotherapeutic Regimens for Patients with Sepsis or Septic Shock

SOURCE OF INFECTION	ANTIMICROBIAL REGIMEN
Community-acquired peritonitis	Fluoroquinolone[1] + metronidazole[2] ± ampicillin[3]; aminoglycoside[4] + metronidazole[2] ± ampicillin[3]; third-generation cephalosporin[5] + metronidazole[2]; ticarcillin/clavulanic acid; piperacillin/tazobactam; carbipenem[6]; aztreonam + metronidazole[2] ± ampicillin[3]
Hospital-acquired peritonitis[8]	Fluoroquinolone[1] + metronidazole[2] ± APBL[7]; aminoglycoside[4] + metronidazole[2] ± APBL[7]; carbipenem[6] ± fluoroquinolone[1]; carbipenem[6] ± aminoglycoside[4]
Urinary tract infection	Fluoroquinolone[1]; third-generation cephalosporin[5]; aztreonam; aminoglycoside[4]
Community-acquired lower respiratory tract infection	Levofloxacin; third-generation cephalosporin[5] ± erythromycin[9]; ticarcillin/clavulanic acid ± erythromycin[9]; piperacillin/tazobactam ± erythromycin[9]
Hospital-acquired lower respiratory tract infection	Levofloxacin ± APBL[7] ± vancomycin[11]; ASP[10] + aminoglycoside[4] ± APBL[7] ± erythromycin[9]; piperacillin/tazobactam ± levofloxacin ± vancomycin[11]; carbipenem[6] ± aminoglycoside[4] ± erythromycin[9]
Hospital-acquired infection in neutropenic or profoundly immunosuppressed patients	Levofloxacin + APBL[7] + vancomycin; piperacillin/tazobactam + levofloxacin + vancomycin; carbipenem[6] + levofloxacin + vancomycin; carbipenem + aminoglycoside[4] + vancomycin
Necrotizing soft-tissue infection	Fluoroquinolone[1] + metronidazole[2]; aminoglycoside[4] + metronidazole[2]; third-generation cephalosporin[5] + metronidazole[2]; piperacillin/tazobactam; carbipenem[6]; aztreonam + metronidazole[2]

[1]Ciprofloxacin or ofloxacin or levofloxacin.

[2]Clindamycin can be substituted for metronidazole to provide coverage against obligate anaerobic species.

[3]Ampicillin can be added to regimen to provide coverage against *Enterococcus* spp, although many experts believe such coverage is unnecessary. Vancomycin can be substituted for ampicillin in penicillin-allergic patients.

[4]Gentamicin or tobramycin or amikacin.

[5]Cefotaxime or ceftizoxime or ceftriaxone.

[6]Imipenem/cilastatin or meropenem.

[7]APBL stands for antipseudomonal beta-lactam and includes piperacillin or azlocillin or mezlocillin or ceftazidime or cefepime; piperacillin has good activity against enterococci.

[8]Some experts recommend including two-drug antipseudomonal coverage for cases of sepsis caused by hospital-acquired peritonitis.

[9]Added to provide coverage against *Legionella* spp.

[10]ASP stands for antistaphylococcal penicillin and includes nafcillin or oxacillin; vancomycin can be substituted in penicillin-allergic patients or in hospitals with a high incidence of infections caused by methicillin-resistant *Staphylococcus* spp.

[11]Vancomycin should be added in hospitals with a high incidence of infections caused by methicillin-resistant *Staphylococcus* spp.

a colloid or crystalloid solution to increase intravascular volume sufficiently to maintain the pulmonary artery wedge pressure in the 12- to 15-mm Hg range. If cardiac output is very low (i.e., <2.0 to 2.5 L/min per m²), dobutamine should be infused to provide inotropic support. If cardiac output is greater than 2.5 L/min per m², vasopressor should be infused as necessary to maintain mean arterial blood pressure greater than 70 mm Hg. Most clinicians use norepinephrine as a first-line agent for this purpose. Rarely, a patient fails to respond adequately to infusion of norepinephrine. In such a case, an adequate increase in SVRI and mean arterial pressure often can be achieved by infusing relatively low doses of arginine vasopressin. Many clinicians use so-called "renal" doses of dopamine (approximately 1 to 4 μg/kg per minute) to support perfusion to the kidneys. Data supporting this approach are lacking, and this practice is no longer advocated.

For patients with acute lung injury or acute respiratory distress syndrome, mechanical ventilation is virtually mandatory. It is increasingly apparent that using the proper ventilatory management strategy can have a large impact on outcome. Specifically, it is important to avoid high plateau airway pressures while attempting to maximize alveolar recruitment with application of appropriate levels of positive end-expiratory pressure. In general, patients should be ventilated with a tidal volume of 6 mL/kg of ideal body weight. If plateau pressure exceeds 30 cm H_2O, then tidal volume should be decreased (or the patient should be switched to a pressure-controlled mode

of ventilation). Positive end-expiratory pressure and F_{IO_2} should be adjusted as necessary to maintain arterial oxygen saturation between 88% and 95%. Ventilator rate should be adjusted as necessary to maintain arterial pH between 7.30 and 7.45, recognizing that arterial carbon dioxide tension (Pa_{CO_2}) may be greater than the normal range with this strategy.

Beyond supportive care, there remains a need for

Pearls and Pitfalls

PEARLS

- Common signs and symptoms of sepsis include fever (less commonly, hypothermia), chills, tachypnea, and altered mental status.
- Sepsis is commonly associated with pulmonary dysfunction, renal dysfunction, and coagulopathy.
- Excessive production of nitric oxide is thought to be a major factor contributing to loss of vasomotor tone in patients with septic shock.
- Reactive oxygen species, including superoxide anion (O_2^-), hydroxyl radical (OH•), and hydrogen peroxide (H_2O_2), are also important in pathogenesis of organ injury caused by sepsis or septic shock.
- Current treatment of sepsis or septic shock focuses on *source control* (i.e., specific interventions directed at the source of infection) and *supportive care* (i.e., interventions for maintaining tissue perfusion or support or replace organ function).

therapeutic approaches that are directed against the underlying pathophysiologic mechanisms responsible for the development of sepsis and septic shock. During the past 15 years or so, more than 20 large-scale clinical trials have been carried out involving immunotherapeutic adjuvants for the management of sepsis. Agents that have been investigated include the following: glucocorticoids such as methylprednisolone administered in very high doses, monoclonal antibodies directed against core-region epitopes on LPS, monoclonal antibodies against TNF, recombinant human IL-1RA, fusion proteins that combine the extracellular domains of TNF-R1 or TNF-R2 with the immunoglobulin heavy chain molecules, and various platelet-activating factor receptor antagonists. None of these agents have been shown to improve survival rates, at least in a convincing way, and none have been approved by the U.S. Food and Drug Administration (FDA) for the adjuvant treatment of sepsis or septic shock. Recombinant human activated protein C is currently undergoing review by the FDA. If approved, this agent will be the first therapeutic directed specifically at a mediator cascade implicated in the pathogenesis of sepsis.

SELECTED READINGS

The Acute Respiratory Distress Syndrome Network: Ventilation with lower tidal volumes as compared with traditional tidal volumes for acute lung injury and the acute respiratory distress syndrome. N Engl J Med 2000;342:1301.

Beutler B, Milsark IW, Cerami AC: Passive immunization against cachectin/tumor necrosis factor protects mice from lethal effect of endotoxin. Science 1985;229:869.

Landry DW, Levin HR, Gallant EM, et al: Vasopressin deficiency contributes to the vasodilation of septic shock. Circulation 1997;95:1122.

Natanson C, Esposito CJ, Banks SM: The sirens' songs of confirmatory sepsis trials: Selection bias and sampling error. Crit Care Med 1998;26:1927.

Wang H, Bloom O, Zhang M, et al: HMG-1 as a late mediator of endotoxin lethality in mice. 1999;285:248.

Chapter 27

Neurologic Physiology: The Brain and Its Response to Injury

Gordon K. Nakata and Gerhard M. Friehs

BRAIN INJURY CLASSIFICATIONS

Primary brain injury may be either penetrating or blunt. *Penetrating injuries* are stab or missile injuries. Stab wounds lack the concussive zone of injury accompanying missile injuries. Thus, the location and depth of penetration dictate the severity of stab injuries. Unless there is vascular injury, there is usually blood along the track of penetration only. Especially thin areas of the cranium are the squamous temporal bone and the anterior cranial base. Stab wounds in these locations can involve the brainstem and circle of Willis, respectively. A missile's mass, velocity, and fragmentation pattern mainly dictate the extent of injury induced. The shock waves initiated by the missile cause tissue cavitation centimeters beyond the primary bullet track, accounting for the large amount of primary brain injury. Military missiles, in particular, achieve a higher velocity and produce a higher morbidity than those from civilian weapons. Additionally, high-velocity missiles carry force sufficient to cause skull fractures and extra-axial hematomas even with tangential impact.

Blunt injuries most frequently lead to skull fractures, subdural hematomas, epidural hematomas, contusions, and shear injuries. Subarachnoid hemorrhage is also a common sequela of head trauma. Trauma is the most common cause of subarachnoid hemorrhage. It occurs most frequently at the convexities—in contrast to aneurysmal subarachnoid hemorrhage, which is usually primarily in the basilar or sylvian cisterns. Vasospasm can occur as the result of traumatic subarachnoid hemorrhage, although less often than with aneurysms.

Subdural hematomas occur as the result of rupture of bridging veins usually from acceleration-deceleration injuries. They are most commonly located frontally and temporally. The bleeding with subdural hematomas is relatively low pressure (as opposed to epidural hematomas); thus, they may have a slow clinical course, often presenting as chronic subdural hematomas. The forces involved in creating subdural hematomas are often significant enough to cause accompanying contusions, traumatic subarachnoid hemorrhage, or shear injuries.

Epidural hematomas form from arterial bleeding. They are usually accompanied by skull fractures. The squamous portion of the temporal bone is particularly prone to fractures. The underlying middle meningeal artery is the most frequently lacerated, accounting for the high frequency of temporal epidural hematomas. A total of 70% to 80% of epidural hematomas occur in the temporal region. The clinical course with this disease is typically more rapid than with subdural hematomas. Only 20% to 50% of cases display the classic lucid interval during which the patient recovers after the initial blow, only to lose consciousness again as the epidural hematoma increases in size.

Cerebral contusions can underlie the primary site of contact *(coup)* or occur opposite the site of impact *(contrecoup)*. These are areas of bruised, hemorrhagic, and necrotic brain resulting from the translational force of the brain within the cranial vault. Contusions often develop over the course of 48 to 72 hours and cause late neurologic deterioration. They occur commonly at sites where the brain abuts bony protuberances; that is, temporal and frontal poles.

Intraventricular hemorrhage is not commonly seen as the only evidence of injury. It is often associated with other injuries and is an indication of a poor prognosis. Intraventricular hemorrhage may result from either rupture of subependymal veins or extension from subarachnoid hemorrhage.

PHYSIOLOGIC MONITORING OF THE CNS

In addition to general systemic parameters with obvious influence on the central nervous system (CNS), there are specific needs regarding measuring output parameters from the CNS. Probably the most commonly performed procedure is ICP monitoring. The different devices that allow us to obtain ICP values are shown graphically in Figure 27–1. The epidural, subdural, intraparenchymal, and intraventricular pressure sensors have achieved general acceptance, requiring a small burr hole to be introduced into their respective locations. However, only the intraventricular probe allows measurement of ICP and access to the cerebrospinal fluid (CSF) for diagnostic purposes or therapeutic drainage in case of pathologically increased CSF. Measuring oxygen saturation within the brain can be achieved by direct insertion of a probe into the brain parenchyma or by sampling the venous oxygen content through the jugular bulb. Another parameter often discussed is cerebral blood flow. A Xenon computed tomography (CT) measurement allows for generalized and regional readings. Percutaneously applied infrared sensors that estimate regional blood flow through the unopened skull perform another method of blood flow measurement. Several monitoring techniques utilize repetitive stimuli through various input organs to evoke a specific neural response that aids in the diagnosis of specific disease processes. Brainstem auditory evoked potentials (BAEPs) have shown usefulness for certain surgi-

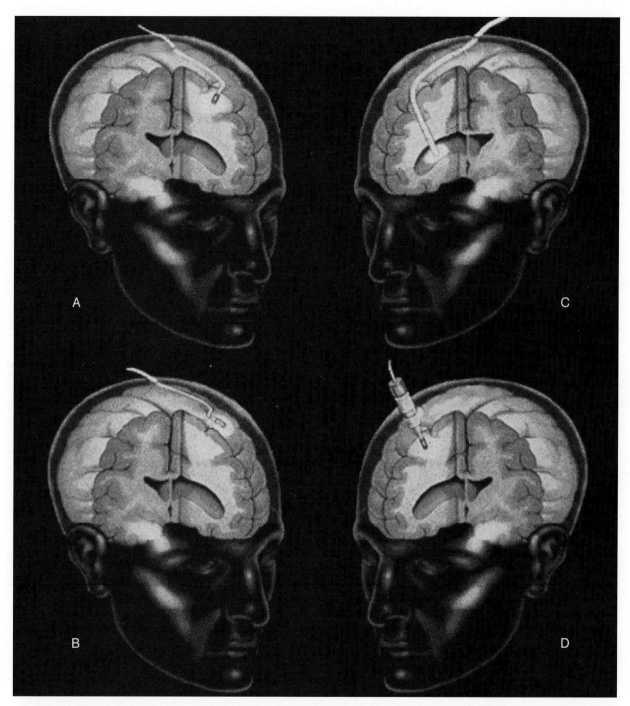

Figure 27–1. Different methods of measuring intracranial pressure: *A,* Free intraparenchymal pressure sensor. *B,* Epidural pressure sensor. *C,* Intraventricular catheter. *D,* Intraparenchymal sensor with skull fixation (ICP bolt).

cal procedures and in the prediction of brain death. Similarly, SEPs (sensory evoked potentials) and VEPs (visual evoked potentials) are useful in the diagnosis of conditions such as multiple sclerosis and spinal tumors.

Despite its relatively small weight of 1400 g, which translates into about 2% of adult total body weight, the brain receives 20% of the cardiac output and utilizes 20% of all glucose and oxygen. CNS cellular architecture has larger intercapillary distances than other organs. Accordingly, the diffusion distances from capillaries to brain tissue are longer, which accounts for the high susceptibil-

ity of the CNS to hypoxic conditions. An adapted mechanism of blood—and subsequently oxyhemoglobin—delivery is necessary for the provision of adequate tissue oxygenation. As the result of this requirement, the CNS has developed a blood-flow regulatory system that is controlled through a carbon dioxide (CO_2)–dependent positive-feedback loop. If the CO_2 partial pressure increases (hypoventilation-induced hypercapnia), the regional or general blood flow through the CNS increases within physiologic limits. In the setting of hypocapnia (e.g., hyperventilation-induced), the blood flow decreases, again within a certain range. This mechanism of blood flow autoregulation allows for sufficient cerebral perfusion, even in situations of significant variability in systemic mean arterial pressure (MAP). Another variable affecting cerebral perfusion is intracranial pressure (ICP). In contrast with the peripheral nervous system (PNS), which is located inside soft tissue, the CNS is encased within bone. This is a good protector against potential injury, but it limits the amount of space allocated to the CNS in the setting of increased demands. ICP is the resistance provided by the brain parenchyma and CSF spaces against cerebral perfusion pressure (CPP). The three variables ICP, CPP, and MAP are in linear relationship to each other in the following way:

$$CPP = MAP - ICP$$

ANATOMIC OVERVIEW

The CNS is composed of the brain and spinal cord. It is made up of three compartments, which stay in balanced relationship to each other: the CNS proper, the vascular compartment (blood vessels, venous sinuses), and the cerebrospinal fluid compartment (intraventricular and subarachnoid spaces). The CNS contains several different subsystems. It is surrounded by three layers of tissue: the dura mater, which separates the intracranial space into a left and right compartment, and a superior and inferior compartment known as the supratentorial and infratentorial spaces, respectively. The dura also gives rise to the large venous drainage system (venous sinuses), which drains deoxygenated blood from the brain surface through bridging veins into extracranial venous structures. The second layer, the arachnoid, defines a space filled with CSF, and through its spider web-like space all major blood vessels of the brain and spinal cord find their target structures. A balance is maintained between CSF production by convoluted capillaries in the choroid plexus and CSF absorption in specialized arachnoid structures (Pacchioni's granulations) on the brain. The control mechanisms of CSF dynamics are poorly understood. The third layer, the pia mater, which is attached to the CNS, increases surface tension of the otherwise gel-like CNS substance. Only penetration of these three meningeal layers allows access to the CNS.

PHYSIOLOGIC FUNCTION AND CONTROL

Shear injury, also known as *diffuse axonal injury (DAI),* is the result of disrupted nerve fibers. It usually occurs in the setting of motor vehicle accidents or other high-speed injuries, such as falls. Radiographically, one sees small hemorrhages, most typically in the brainstem and corpus callosum. On histology, retraction balls of Cajal can be seen at the cortical gray-white interface. These are swellings at both cut ends of the axon. This injury is less frequently associated with increased ICPs than with focal mass lesions.

Secondary brain injury has many possible causes, including increased intracranial pressure and subsequent

drop in CPP, brain shift and herniation, seizures, vascular injury, hypoxia, hypotension, hyperthermia, hypo- or hyperglycemia, anemia, or sepsis. Most of the emphasis in brain injury treatment is on the prevention of secondary injury. With the advent of neural transplantation and neural prosthetics, our impact on primary brain injury will hopefully improve.

TREATMENT OF BRAIN INJURY

In 1996, the Brain Trauma Foundation, in conjunction with the American Association of Neurological Surgeons, formed guidelines for head injury management. The Severe Head Injury Guidelines are briefly summarized as follows:

- Systemic hypotension of less than 90 mm Hg increases morbidity and mortality.
- Indications for ICP monitor: Severe head injury (Glasgow Coma Score [GCS] of 8 or less) with an abnormal CT scan. In the presence of a normal CT, monitoring is recommended for age greater than 40 years, unilateral or bilateral motor posturing, and systolic blood pressure less than 90. In the mildly or moderately head-injured patient, ICP monitoring may be indicated if he or she has a traumatic mass, such as a hematoma.
- Treatment threshold of increased ICPs is 20 to 25 mm Hg. The ICPs should be corroborated by examinations and CPP measurement.
- There are insufficient data regarding the relationship between CPP and outcome. Recommendations are to keep the CPP above 70 mm Hg.
- Use of hyperventilation, defined as less than or equal to 35 mm Hg. The standard of care is that $PaCO_2 \leq 25$ mm Hg should be avoided after severe traumatic brain injury. Prophylactic hyperventilation should be avoided during the first 24 hours. It may be used for brief periods of neurologic decline or for longer periods if ICPs are refractory to other methods (sedation, paralysis, CSF drainage, osmotic diuretics). A randomized prospective trial has shown worse outcomes for traumatic brain injury patients when treated with chronic prophylactic hyperventilation. Cerebral blood flow less than 15 to 20 mL/100 g per minute causes ischemic injury to the brain, confirmed by positron emission tomography.
- When one uses mannitol, intermittent boluses are more effective than is continuous infusion in lowering ICP. Indications for the placement of an ICP monitor include signs of transtentorial herniation and neurologic deterioration not attributable to systemic pathology. Serum osmolality should be kept less than 320 mOsmol/kg. Maintenance of euvolemia and the placement of a Foley catheter are important. More recently, 3% saline has been advocated as a safe and effective means of lowering ICP while maintaining a euvolemic state.
- Barbiturates can be used for medically and surgically refractory ICPs. The patient must be hemodynamically stable.
- Glucocorticoids are not indicated in head trauma patients.
- Nutritional support is standard in surgical patients. Nu-

trition should be instituted by the end of the first postoperative week.
- Antiseizure prophylaxis is not indicated beyond 1 week post surgery and has not been shown to prevent development of late post-traumatic seizures.

In recent years, the outcome of severe head injury has improved with implementation of early detection and response systems, advanced ICU care, particularly ICP management. The ICP monitor was first introduced in the 1960s. Since the observation that secondary injury plays a major role in the progression of brain damage, there has been much advance in ICU care as well as prehospital systems. There has also been much interest in measuring brain oxygenation. Microdialysis and jugular bulb monitoring are two such techniques in use. One of the difficulties with these methods is whether focal measurements accurately reflect overall brain perfusion. Jugular bulb monitoring takes global measurements and yields varying results. Brain temperature has been another area of interest. So far, hypothermia has not been conclusively shown to improve outcomes. Hyperthermia, however, is generally thought to be deleterious to an injured brain. A number of neurochemical processes are thought to contribute to ongoing brain injury. Many of these are undergoing current investigation:

- Excitatory amino acids: glutamate influx, leading to calcium influx and subsequent apoptosis
- Work with NMDA (N-methyl-D-aspartate) antagonists: selfotel, a receptor antagonist; Cerestat, a noncompetitive antagonist that blocks the Mg^{2+} channel
- Antioxidants: tirilizad, free radical scavenger; desferrioxamine, iron chelator; pegorgotein, free radical scavenger
- Cytokines: recent work indicates that interleukin-10 (IL-10) may reduce inflammation. Tumor necrosis factor (TNF) and IL-1 may worsen brain injury
- Apoptosis
- Glutamate or voltage gated influx of calcium is a factor in irreversible neuronal injury
- Axonal stretch: among other things, induces calcium influx and activation of calpain, leading to apoptosis and activation of excitatory amino acids

Regarding regeneration and transplantation, research is ongoing. Tissue transplants in movement disorders give hope of applications in head injury. Nerve growth factors in animal models have suggested improvements in both morphologic and functional recovery. A large amount of research is going on in the field of neuroprosthetics as well. Cochlear implants have shown preliminary success in humans. Visual and even motor implants are also rapidly approaching human trials. Both peripheral and central nervous system implants have great implications for focal nervous system disease.

Pearls and Pitfalls

PEARLS

- Neurosurgery has been in existence only for about a century.
- Our understanding of brain function is still primitive, our ability to treat injury to the brain limited. The brain has to rely on unimpaired massive blood flow to allow for continuous transport of nutrients, such as glucose and oxygen, since even short-term impairment of such delivery may cause irreversible damage.
- In an effort to streamline different approaches to the treatment of brain injury, the Brain Injury Association has funded the development of evidence-based guidelines, which were introduced in 1996 and have since become widely accepted.
- Treatment of brain injury is, strictly speaking, still limited to the prevention of secondary damage to the brain, rather than repair of primary damage, which is still not possible.
- Contrary to what is widely believed, brain cells are now thought to have the potential to regenerate after injury, even in the adult central nervous system.
- Although a treatment for human brain regeneration does not yet exist, intensive research is being conducted worldwide to make possible what was previously thought impossible.

SELECTED READINGS

Becker DP, Doberstein CE, Hovda DA: Craniocerebral trauma: Mechanisms, management, and the cellular response to injury. In Current Concepts. Kalamazoo, Mich, Upjohn Company, 1994, pp 4–47.

Brain Trauma Foundation, American Association of Neurological Surgeons, Joint Section on Neurotrauma and Critical Care: Guidelines for the management of severe head injury. J Neurotrauma 1996; 13:641.

Janny P, Joan JP, Janny L: A statistical approach to long-term monitoring of intracranial pressure. In Brock M, Dietz H (eds): Intracranial Pressure. Berlin, Springer-Verlag, 1972, pp 59–64.

Liau LM, Bergsneider M, Becker DP: Pathology and pathophysiology of head injury. In Youmans JR (ed): Neurological Surgery, 4th ed. Philadelphia, WB Saunders, 1996, pp 1549–1594.

Luerssen TG, Hults K, Klauber M, Marshall LF, and the TCDB Group: Improved outcome as a result of recognition of absent and compressed cisterns on initial CT scans. In Hoff JT, Betz AL (eds): Intracranial Pressure VII. New York, Springer-Verlag, 1989, pp 598–602.

Marshall LF: Head injury: Recent past, present, and future. Neurosurgery 2000; 47:546.

Miller JD, Sweet RC, Narayan R, Becker DP: Early insults to the injured brain. JAMA 1978; 240:439.

Popp AJ, Feustel PJ, Kimelberg HK: Pathophysiology of Traumatic Brain Injury. In Wilkins RH, Rengachary SS (eds): Neurosurgery, 2nd ed. New York, McGraw-Hill, 1996, pp 2623–2638.

Tuszynski MH, U HS, Amaral DG, Gage FH: Nerve growth factor infusion in the primate brain reduces lesion-induced cholinergic neuronal degeneration. J Neurosci 1990; 10:3604.

Tuszynski MH, Gabriel K, Gage FH, et al: Nerve growth factor delivery by gene transfer induces differential outgrowth of sensory, motor, and noradrenergic neurites after adult spinal cord injury. Exp Neurol 1996; 137:157.

Chapter 28

Thyroid Abnormalities Encountered in Surgical Critical Care

Glenn W. Geelhoed

Thyroid abnormalities may be severe enough to warrant admission to surgical critical care units, or they may be encountered as unanticipated problems complicating some other primary medical or surgical disorder causing the patient's hospitalization. Whether a cause of primary or secondary morbidity in critical care, the thyroid gland and its abnormal functioning must be managed with a high degree of medical and surgical skill. The possible abnormalities in form are less variable than the functional aberrations; the former are considered first.

CLINICAL PRESENTATION OF THYROID MASSES

Thyroid masses may be diffuse (goiter) or focal (nodule). Goiters are further differentiated into diffuse (such as the hyperplastic goiter of Graves' disease) or multinodular (such as the nontoxic multinodular goiter of endemic hypothyroidism). Particularly with multinodular goiters of massive size or strategic positioning in the submanubrial thoracic inlet, the thyroid mass itself becomes an imperative surgical indication when it causes upper airway obstruction or interferes with food or fluid swallowing, particularly in certain positions of neck flexion or turning. Such disturbances of vital function pose the danger of a life-threatening airway compromise, but it is a rare problem associated with thyroid mass lesions. The majority of masses that come to clinical differentiation are for the concern that a neoplasm may be present.

Thyroid Nodules

Thyroid nodules may be differentiated by a number of clinical means (see Table 28–3). The most significant findings are the size of the nodule, the age and gender of the patient, and clinical features of its mobility or fixation to tissues around it. With a few exceptions, most often suspected by family history or exposure to radiation, there are almost no significant thyroid abnormalities that are not palpable. The incidence of thyroid cancer in male and female patients is nearly equal, but there is a very large predominance of benign thyroid abnormalities in female patients; therefore, the very presence of a dominant mass in the thyroid of a male patient is a more significant finding. Description of palpable masses may be aided by scintiscanning, which reveals blood flow (technetium) or functional isotope concentration (iodine). Ultrasound may further assist the clinical impression as to whether the lesion is solid or cystic. Various contrast studies may help describe the extent of impingement on cervical or mediastinal structures, but few of these studies are as valuable as the chest radiograph.

After the clinical confirmation of a thyroid nodule's presence and gross characteristics given the circumstances of the patient, the next question becomes—what is the nature of this mass and the cells of which it is composed? Fine-needle aspiration (FNA) cytology gives this critical additional information only if it is positive. FNA cytology that shows the psammoma bodies, or the "Orphan Annie nuclei" of invaginated cytoplasm into the nuclei of the cells is pathognomonic of papillary cancer, which can also be said of the foamy pink cytoplasm of medullary thyroid cancer or the lymphocytes of thyroiditis. Much more difficult to interpret are follicular cells that have no such convenient cytologic markers of malignancy, because the hallmark of follicular carcinoma is microvascular invasion, a histologic feature. The description "follicular neoplasm" begs the question as to whether the neoplasm is benign or malignant. A negative cytologic study can be wrongly used to reassure patients; the determination "inadequate cytologic smear" does not necessarily rule out cancer. FNA is a "one-way test" that yields information if it is positive, and, if negative, it is "noninformation" because such a result can as easily be based in a sampling error. With such noninformation dismissed, the clinician returns to the clinical base of information previously obtained, and, on the basis of his or her suspicions (e.g., young male with a large, hard solitary mass versus a female with a smaller, softer, less defined mass) may recommend operation for the former. A period of a few months' observation, with or without thyroid hormone administration for thyroid-stimulating hormone (TSH) suppression, and reexamination and possibly repeat FNA to determine whether the nodule is bigger, may be recommended for the latter.

Preoperative Management: Thyroid Masses

A mass lesion from which a positive FNA is reported needs little further workup, except those studies needed for the safety of the patient in the operating room. A scan at this point would not dissuade operation and surgical exploration is the most definitive diagnostic study after the FNA report. Clinical information can usually rule out hyperfunction, such as results from a toxic adenoma, and there are few patients who are unable to tolerate an operation such as thyroid exploration unless there is evidence of hyperthyroidism or an associated pheochromocytoma if the patient has been found to have a medullary thyroid cancer, particularly with a positive family history.

As seen in the case of Lugol's iodine pretreatment of the goiter of Graves' disease, such pretreatment remarkably reduces the size and blood flow through the iodoprival multinodular goiter and should generally be used preoperatively for such diffuse goiters. Thyroid hormone may be given preoperatively at the same time as the cold iodine to the patient with hypothyroidism to restore cardiac responsiveness in preparation for operation. For the euthyroid patient (and most particularly, the hyperthyroid patient), thyroid hormone is contraindicated, because the half-life of the thyroid hormone in circulation is several weeks and no acute hypothyroidism should be expected in the perioperative thyroidectomy period.

Thyroid Inflammation

Thyroiditis may mimic some forms of thyroid masses and have the additional consideration that they may be linked with hyperfunction or hypofunction. In many cases, inflammatory conditions of the thyroid, like the mass lesion, raise the concern that the airway may be compromised, either through direct impingement or interruption in the normal neuromotor control of the larynx. This is particularly true for the intrathoracic gland, which may be affected by massive hypertrophy or inflammation and effect compromise of the subglottic airway in the submanubrial mediastinum. These problems demand careful observation of the larynx and its function during intubation, particularly in patients who require ventilatory support. A concern for the airway does not automatically translate to the removal of the thyroid impinging on the airway without a consideration of the status of the tracheolaryngeal integrity in the absence of the thyroid. In some cases of long-standing compressive goiter, particularly when some element of thyroiditis is involved, tracheomalacia rarely may be a residual problem following thyroidectomy.

In nearly all instances of operation on the thyroid, endotracheal intubation for the security of the airway is mandatory. Particular care must be taken in changing the position of the patient after cervical hyperextension, so that the ventilating tube is not advanced down beyond the carina into the mainstem bronchus. This may sometimes take the form of nasotracheal intubation, most often accomplished over a fiberoptic endoscope, in those cases in which the goiter is obstructive to more normal transoral intubation laryngoscopic technique.

CLINICAL PRESENTATION: FUNCTIONAL ABNORMALITIES

First considered is the group of functional thyroid abnormalities that may be most controversial with respect to surgery, because of competing claims from other treatments. Hypothyroidism is disposed of quickly, because treatment is by replacement with daily synthetic thyroid hormone oral administration and TSH guided by the patient's clinical response until stable. Hypothyroidism may be accompanied by goiter, and such mass lesions are considered separately with their different indications for surgical intervention.

Thyroid hyperfunction is of several types, with characteristic patient patterns seen in each that help determine

Table 28–1	Differential Diagnosis of the Clinical Causes of Hyperthyroidism

Diffuse toxic goiter (Graves' disease)
Toxic multinodular goiter (Plummer's disease)
Toxic adenoma ("hot nodule")
Toxic thyroiditis (Hashimoto's struma, or "Hashi-tox")
Ectopic toxic thyroid tissue (struma ovarii)
Overdosing exogenous thyroid hormone (iatrogenic or factitial thyrotoxicosis)
Iodine treatment complication in endemic goiter (Jod-Basedow disease)
Paraneoplastic hyperthyroidism (excess TSH-like paraendocrine tumor)

treatment (Table 28–1). Diffuse toxic goiter (Graves' disease) is most frequently seen in young women in their early reproductive years and is the type of hyperthyroidism most frequently encountered. Its etiology is multifactorial from familial, behavioral, and environmental causes, but it is expressed through an immunologic stimulation of the thyroid gland by a group of incomplete thyroid antibodies called thyroid-stimulating immunoglobulins (TSI). The TSI cause an increase in thyroxin synthesis and release, which suppresses pituitary TSH. The TSI also, rather independently, cause an infiltrative dermatomyopathy, accounting for the atrophy of some facial and cervical muscles, changes in texture of hair and skin, pretibial myxedema, and, most notably, the eye signs classically associated with Graves' disease. These findings, absent in the other four types of hyperthyroidism, as well as the factitial overfeeding of thyroid hormone, do not come from the hyperthyroidism itself, but from its cause—the TSI—which are unique to Graves' disease.

The other features of thyrotoxicosis, such as the cardiovascular, central nervous system, and gastrointestinal responses, are related to the hypermetabolism from excess thyroid hormone, and are also common symptoms with the other kinds of hyperthyroidism. These clinical symptoms can be confidently predicted to be controllable by reducing thyroid hormone output or blocking its effect, particularly by ablating the overactive thyroid. But, because exophthalmos, lid lag, and a dozen other eye signs, as well as the dermatomyopathy, are related to TSI rather than products of the thyroid gland secretion, resolution of these clinical features of Graves' disease may be more variable than those directly interdicted from hyperthyroidism.

Toxic multinodular goiter (Plummer's disease) occurs in older women, typically beyond reproductive years, and is associated with an antecedent multinodular goiter that has become hyperfunctioning. The toxicity manifested is typically that of cardiac and central nervous system disorders, with congestive failure prominent among them, and "T_3 (triiodothyronine) toxicity" is implicated.

Toxic adenoma may be seen with equal frequency in male and female patients, usually occurring within the third decade of life. This more rare form of hyperthyroidism is most frequently managed as treatment of the thyroid nodule, because a hyperfunctioning nodule that suppresses TSH and causes hypofunction of the adjacent thyroid gland is most often benign, but its functioning status does not exonerate the possibility of a thyroid malignancy.

Toxic thyroiditis (Hashimoto's struma) is an inflammatory disease of the thyroid with lymphocytic infiltration that results in both a symptomatic thyroiditis and stimulation to hyperthyroidism. As is the case with the resolution of almost all inflammation, which heals by scarring, the end stage of this form of thyroiditis is often a "burned out" thyroid gland, however it is treated.

Ectopic toxic thyroid tissue (struma ovarii) behaves as an ectopic source of excessive thyroid hormone, as would be seen in an overdosing of synthetic thyroid, and treatment is directed at the source of the hyperthyroidism, which lies outside the thyroid.

Preoperative Management

Medical management of hyperthyroidism (Table 28–2) may be instituted as preoperative treatment, or, in some cases, as definitive therapy, depending on the patient and the type of hyperthyroidism. When the patient is a candidate for operative therapy, he or she undergoes medical treatment in order to come to the operating room in as nearly euthyroid condition as possible. A nearly normal metabolic status may help to prevent the serious complication of operative induction of thyrotoxicosis, which in severe cases has been called thyroid storm.

Of the three types of drug therapy, the administration of Lugol's iodine solution for a preoperative preparation diminishes both the size of the gland and the blood flow through it; it makes the operation safer by decreasing thyroid hormone release. Thyroid hormone synthesis blockade is useful for protracting the process preoperatively, if tolerated by the patient (many of whom may experience skin rashes or blood dyscrasias on either PTU [propylthiouracil] or MTZ [methimazole]), and has been used for long-term control of some patients with hyperthyroidism. If hyperthyroidism recurs after cessation of the synthesis blockade for up to a year, or if it breaks through on increasing or ill-tolerated doses, surgical therapy moves up to first or second place as a treatment option, depending on the circumstances—age, sex of the patient, and type of hyperthyroidism. β-Blocker therapy diminishes the catecholamine-mediated response to the hyperthyroidism and is particularly useful in accelerated preoperative or intraoperative management.

Radioiodine ablation of the thyroid gland may be considered for selected patients, depending on the patient's age and the size of the goiter. Carcinogenesis following an ablative dose of radioiodine is a moot point with respect to the thyroid in an older patient, but it becomes an important consideration for illnesses such as leukemia or lymphoma, because higher doses are repeated in the treatment of younger patients. Teratogenesis is a serious concern, contraindicating radioiodine treatment in patients who are or plan soon to become pregnant. Hypothyroidism is the single most predictable problem following radioiodine treatment of hyperthyroidism that does not persist or recur. It is typically late in onset after radioiodine therapy, often following some time after the original treatment. Occult hypothyroidism can manifest as a surprise as congestive heart failure.

For these reasons, drug therapy should be used in all hyperthyroid patients to control the hypermetabolism, with additional measures being taken, such as administering Lugol's iodine, which has additional local advantages in reducing the size and blood flow through the thyroid. Radioiodine might be a good choice for older patients with smaller hyperfunctioning goiter, such as some patients with Plummer's disease. For younger female patients in active reproducing years, for patients who have large hyperfunctioning goiters, or for those who have failed earlier medical or radioisotope treatment, operation is considered a treatment of choice.

SURGICAL CRITICAL CARE

Patients in surgical critical care for nonthyroid indications often seem to have metabolic problems that are either regulated by the thyroid or mimic them. More important for diagnostic determinations is that tests of thyroid function become confusing or unreliable for patients who have critical illness or injury (Table 28–3).

Silent Hypothyroidism and Myxedema Coma

Myxedema coma can be a complication of therapy for the overactive thyroid or an end stage in inflammatory thyroid burnout for those who have had a significant degree of thyroiditis; however, it can be treated. The "hidden diagnosis" of hypothyroidism in the industrialized world has recently been estimated at about 10% of the random population. This estimate is only a fraction of the much higher incidence among the larger population of the developing world where iodine deficiency disorders are more prevalent. For patients with a global lethargy, hypotonia, hyporeflexia, or, particularly, cardiac abnormalities compounding other presenting complaints, a rapid TSH determination can unmask the hypothyroidism component. Many other patients in critical care may appear to be hypermetabolic with generally low or confusing determinations of thyroid hormones.

Thyroid Hormone Abnormalities in Critical Illness

Very sick patients may have metabolic failure with normal thyroxine (T_4) levels—a syndrome described as the "sick-euthyroid syndrome." As previously discussed, T_4 is not the active species of thyroid hormone in circulation, how-

Table 28–2	**Medical Therapy for Hyperthyroidism**

Decrease Thyroid Hormone *Release*
  Iodide (Lugol's iodine solution)
  Lithium
Decrease Thyroid Hormone *Production*
  Thiocyanates, perchlorates
  Thionamides (PTU)
  Methimazole (MTZ)
Decrease Thyroid Hormone *Response* by Adrenergic Interference
  Catecholamine depletion (reserpine, guanethidine)
  Beta-adrenergic blockade (propanolol)

Table 28–3	Changes in Thyroid Function and Tests Thereof in Settings of Surgical Critical Care					
CRITICAL CONDITIONS	T_4	**FREE T_4**	T_3	rT_3	**TSH**	**TRH-TEST**
Neonates	−	N	−	+	N	O
Aging	N/−	N	−	N	N/+	N/−
Starvation	N	N/+	−	+	−	−
Sepsis	−	+	−	+	N/−	N
Operation	N/−	N/−	−	+	N/−	−/N/+
Diabetes, controlled	N	N	N/+	N/+	N	N
Diabetic ketoacidosis	−	N/+	−	+	N	−
Cardiac failure	N	N	−	+	N	−
Liver failure	N/−	+	−	+	+/N	N
Renal failure	N/−	N/−	−	N	N/+	−

−, decreased; N, normal; +, increased; O, not done; TSH, thyroid-stimulating hormone; TRH, thyroid-releasing hormone.
Modified from Zaloga GP, Chernow B: Thyroid function in acute illness. In Geelhoed GW, Chernow B (eds): Endocrine Aspects of Acute Illness, (Clinics in Critical Care Medicine). New York, Churchill Livingstone, 1985.

ever, where it is peripherally metabolized to the active T_3. Many of these patients are under stress with elevated endogenous catecholamine, and they may even be getting infusions of pharmacologic doses of catechols. The 5'-deiodinase that activates T_4 to the functioning T_3 is catecholamine sensitive, so that the true T_3 levels are defi-

cient, and the T_4 degradation is to another inactive form of the reverse 5'-iodine position, or rT3. Furthermore, some patients may have an antecedent deficit in thyroid binding (e.g., liver disease, renal failure, sepsis, starvation, fluid shifts with major operation) as well as the faulty deiodination that limits peripheral conversion to active T_3. Because T_4 is normal, the anterior pituitary "reads" the thyroid status as normal and no TSH elevation follows—hence "sick euthyroid."

Later in serious illness, the T_4 as well as true T_3 may decrease in patients who may be moribund. This measured decrease in thyroid hormone species may be a marker of severe illness rather than its determinant, because in some of these conditions, such as late in sepsis, the pituitary does not seem to respond with an elevation of TSH. That the pituitary itself has not failed may be reflected in a positive TSH response to thyrotropin-releasing hormone (TRH) infusion.

In other conditions, there may be variable results in testing thyroid function because of changes in thyroid binding. These changes may result because of changes in the thyroid-binding protein or inhibitors that compete for the binding sites, the T_4 to T_3 conversion, or a genuine decrease in pituitary TSH output, which may reflect a process of adaptation to severe illness. This may be a shared inhibitory response on the pituitary by elevated corticosteroids and opioid peptides. No clinical benefit has yet been demonstrated by administering rapid-acting thyroid supplementation in such patients, and, in the normal response to critical illness, the crisis is usually definitively settled within the 100-day body store of thyroid hormone that most patients carry into the critical care unit.

Pearls and Pitfalls

PEARLS

- The single biggest advantage to surgical treatment of young patients with Graves' disease is immediate control of hyperthyroidism and a return to drug-free pituitary-thyroid autoregulatory balance.
- The risks of the operation include anesthesia and injury to the parathyroids and laryngeal nerves.
- For multinodular goiter, airway management is the key factor, with preoperative cold iodine and thyroid hormone pretreatment making subtotal thyroidectomy safer for the patient and relatively easier for the surgeon in operating on these large goiters.
- The greatest additional yield of critical information about a thyroid mass following clinical findings is FNA cytology. "Shadow-producing procedures" are often expensive, inefficient, and only marginally helpful and rarely definitive.
- Thyroid function may appear abnormal in patients under surgical critical care for nonthyroid indications.
- Myxedema coma is underdiagnosed (and quickly confirmed by TSH testing), and the "sick-euthyroid syndrome" (normal T_4 and TSH, but elevated to rT3 and lower T_3) results from changes in thyroid hormone binding and T_4 conversion.
- Decreased thyroid response in those not proven to be hypothyroid may even be adaptive to serious illness, and no benefit has been demonstrated through thyroid hormone supplementation for sick-euthyroid patients in critical care.
- A surgeon becomes experienced in total thyroidectomy by approaching each meticulous thyroid dissection as a preservation procedure of parathyroids and laryngeal nerves and their blood supplies. Halsted (1918) put it thus: "The extirpation of the thyroid gland for goiter typifies, perhaps better than any other operation, the supreme triumph of the surgeon's art."

SELECTED READINGS

Geelhoed GW: Problem Management in Endocrine Surgery. Chicago, Yearbook Medical Publishing, 1983.
Geelhoed GW: Tracheomalacia from compressing goiter: Management following thyroidectomy. Surgery 1988;104:1100.
Geelhoed GW: Metabolic maladaptation: Individual and social consequences of medical intervention in correcting endemic hypothyroidism. Nutrition 1999;15:908.
Geelhoed GW: Surgical Endocrinology: Tests of Clinical Judgment. Alexandria, Va, J and S Publishing, 2000.
Zaloga GP, Chernow B: Thyroid function in acute illness. In Geelhoed GW, Chernow B (eds): Endocrine Aspects of Acute Illness (Clinics in Critical Care Medicine). New York, Churchill Livingstone, 1985.

Chapter 29
Pulmonary Embolism
Lorrie A. Langdale

Despite heightened awareness and advances in technology, the nonspecific clinical presentation of pulmonary embolism continues to pose a diagnostic and management challenge. In autopsy studies by Legere and co-workers, pulmonary emboli (PE) were detected in more than 25% of deaths, but in 70% of these emboli were not clinically apparent prior to the patient's demise. Although most emboli do not result in death, early diagnosis and intervention are essential if fatalities, which most often occur within hours of the initial event, are to be prevented. In addition to the well-recognized risk factors of previous pulmonary embolism, age, obesity, trauma, malignancy, and inherited hypercoagulable states, stimulation of coagulation in response to injury and perioperative immobilization predispose patients to developing deep venous thrombosis (DVT) and secondary thromboembolism. Thromboses involving the deep venous system of the lower extremities proximal to the popliteal fossa present the highest risk of PE, although more distal clots are associated with emboli in as many as 13% of patients. In addition, approximately 10% of upper extremity thrombi embolize to the pulmonary vasculature, an incidence that is further increased when thrombi are associated with central venous catheters. Overall, PE complicated the course in approximately 10% of patients with DVT, but it should be noted that as many as 50% of patients with pulmonary emboli have no leg symptoms or identifiable source of clot.

Physiologically, PE is defined primarily as a ventilation-perfusion (V̇/Q̇) abnormality in which areas of ventilated lung are not perfused. Rarely is this purely a perfusion defect. Incomplete redistribution of regional blood flow without changes in ventilation, right-to-left shunting of deoxygenated blood, resistance-induced decreases in regional capillary transit time, increased oxygen extraction (secondary to decreased cardiac output), and release of vasoactive mediators from platelets within thrombi and damaged endothelium contribute to the varying degrees of shunt and V̇/Q̇ mismatch that underlie the broad spectrum of clinical presentation. Thus, small emboli that pass through the pulmonary vasculature and then lodge in the periphery of the lung are often asymptomatic. However, when emboli are associated with pulmonary infarction, the more classic symptoms of pleuritic chest pain, hemoptysis, and dyspnea are observed. Moderate-sized emboli, trapped in proximal segmental pulmonary vasculature, are associated with more severe dyspnea and hypoxemia, while larger emboli obstructing the pulmonary outflow tract are responsible for hemodynamic instability and sudden death (Stein and Henry, 1997).

Although hypoxemia, respiratory alkalosis, and tachycardia are common features and often trigger the clinical suspicion of pulmonary embolism, these characteristics are neither universal nor specific. Infectious diseases, cardiogenic and noncardiogenic pulmonary edema, traumatic lung injuries, and other forms of respiratory distress are often associated with a similar constellation of symptoms. On the other hand, while the degree of hypoxemia does correlate with the severity of the clinical PE syndrome, it should also be noted that a normal A-a gradient and a normal $PaCO_2$ when the patient is breathing room air are insufficient evidence to *rule out* the diagnosis. As many as 10% of patients with documented PE may have normal findings on measurement of blood gases. In a study of patients with suspected PE, the Prospective Investigation of Pulmonary Embolism Diagnosis (PIOPED) group determined that a low probability of PE, based on clinical assessment (0 to 19% probability of PE), correlated with exclusion of the diagnosis in 91% of cases, but high clinical probability predictions were associated with only 68% accuracy. Hence, while the degree of clinical suspicion remains the driving force for further investigation, the spectrum of clinical presentation emphasizes the need for sensitive and specific means of distinguishing pulmonary embolism from other etiologies of respiratory distress.

STRATEGIES FOR THE DIAGNOSIS AND MANAGEMENT OF PULMONARY EMBOLISM

DIAGNOSTIC TOOLS. (Tai et al, 1999.) A cost-effective diagnostic strategy is essential to rapid diagnosis and management. While an integral part of the assessment of respiratory distress, chest radiography is usually of little value in confirming the presence of PE. Increased lucency of a lung field (due to occlusion of the central pulmonary artery), atelectasis, small pleural effusions, or pleural-based wedge defects secondary to pulmonary infarctions are considered to be classic radiographic abnormalities, but they are absent in the majority of patients. As many as 40% of patients with PE have a normal study. The primary value of chest radiography is to rule out other etiologies of pulmonary dysfunction and to provide correlation for matching defects identified on V̇/Q̇ scan.

Pulmonary angiography remains the reference standard for the diagnosis of PE, but it is not without complication and may not be readily available in many communities. Ventilation-perfusion scanning (Fig. 29–1) circumvents these limitations and therefore has been generally accepted as the initial procedure of choice. Areas of mismatch characterized by an absence of perfusion in the presence of normal ventilation suggest PE, whereas areas of matching ventilation and perfusion deficits are more consistent with intrinsic lung disease. The sensitivity and specificity of V̇/Q̇ scanning are such that a high-probability scan, coupled with moderate to strong clinical

201

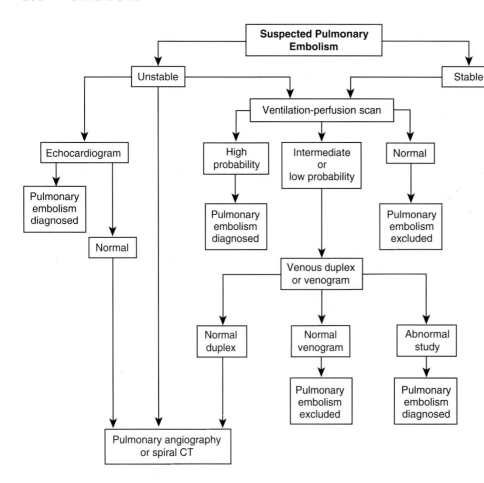

Figure 29–1. Suspected pulmonary embolism. Algorithm for the diagnosis of a suspected pulmonary embolism, based on the patient's clinical status.

indicators, yields a true positive diagnosis in 85% to 96% of cases. Fewer than 5% of patients for whom there is a low clinical suspicion of PE and a low-probability scan are ultimately determined to have a thromboembolism. Thus, patients for whom there is a relatively high clinical suspicion of PE and a high-probability scan may be reliably diagnosed and treated on the basis of V̇/Q̇ scan without further testing. The patients who are unlikely to have a PE and who also have a low-probability scan may be safely managed without anticoagulation. The large percentage of patients with suspected PE and intermediate- or mixed-probability groups (e.g., low clinical suspicion, high-probability scan), however, remain problematic and require further work-up before therapy can be started (Legere et al, 1999; Miettinen et al, 1998).

Spiral computed tomography (CT) and magnetic resonance imaging (MRI) are under investigation as adjuncts to V̇/Q̇ scanning (Tai et al, 1999; Stein et al, 1999). Both of these noninvasive techniques yield multiplanar images of pulmonary vasculature and parenchyma. Although spiral CT has a sensitivity of 94% and a specificity of 96%, when compared with pulmonary angiography the accuracy of this study is lower than that of angiography in evaluating peripheral lesions and is highly dependent on the interpretation and experience of the radiologist. MR angiography with gadolinium enhancement offers visualization of both pulmonary and lower extremity vasculature without the use of ionizing radiation. Consensus has not been reached among radiologists as to the most appropriate MRI modality (spin and gradient echo versus pulse contrast sequences versus MR angiography). With further refinements, these techniques may become especially useful adjuncts in the diagnosis of patients with indeterminate V̇/Q̇ scans.

When noninvasive studies are inconclusive, pulmonary angiography is advocated to provide definitive diagnosis. Despite angiography's potential for complications, its relative risks and cost outweigh those of missed PE or inappropriate anticoagulation. The incidence of complications, while low at 1% to 2%, may be further reduced if angiography is reserved for patients with hemodynamic compromise or inconclusive noninvasive studies, and avoided in patients with renal failure, congestive heart failure, or underlying pulmonary hypertension. Intravenous digital subtraction angiography has been advocated as a means of avoiding pulmonary catheterization, but satisfactory images are less sensitive and specific than are traditional angiography techniques. Enhancement of digital images by delivering contrast medium via the distal port of a Swan-Ganz catheter remains controversial among invasive radiologists.

DIAGNOSTIC STRATEGIES. (Perrier et al, 1996.) Several decision-analysis strategies combining noninvasive studies have been proposed for maximizing diagnostic acumen while minimizing the need for confirmation with pulmonary angiography. One approach is to look for evidence of a potential source of thromboembolism when the clinical presentation, chest radiography, and V̇/Q̇ scanning suggest an intermediate probability of PE. The most common imaging modality for suspected DVT is compression ultrasonography, enhanced when available by color Doppler imaging. Although the sensitivity of color Doppler ultrasonography in symptomatic patients has been reported to be as high as 98%, diagnosis of asymptomatic venous thrombosis, even in high-risk patients, has shown a disappointingly high degree of variability, ranging from 38% to 83%. In addition, since 56% to 67% of patients with angiographic evidence of PE also have negative lower-extremity Doppler ultrasonographic examinations, the absence of ultrasonic evidence of DVT does not eliminate the possibility that PE has already occurred. Ascending contrast-enhanced venography, while more accurate, is invasive and is generally reserved for patients with a technically inadequate Doppler examination. Kruit and co-workers have demonstrated that patients with intermediate-probability V̇/Q̇ scans and negative lower-extremity venography carry the same risk of subsequent thromboembolism as that of patients with a negative V̇/Q̇ scan. Impedance plethysmography and radioisotope techniques have not been widely adopted in clinical practice owing to limitations in sensitivity and specificity.

Another decision-analysis strategy, which has been tested in critically ill, ventilated patients at risk for a variety of respiratory complications, incorporates additional physiologic alterations associated with PE into the overall assessment of clinical probability (Anderson et al, 1999). Physiologic dead space is typically increased with significant thromboembolism and may be calculated by measuring end-tidal carbon dioxide. D-dimer, a highly sensitive but nonspecific laboratory assay (enzyme-linked immunosorbent assay [ELISA]), may be used to assess the presence or absence of venous thrombosis. Neither test is specific to the diagnosis of PE, but their combination does provide some predictive value. When a change in dead space of less than 10% and an absolute dead space of less than 45% are combined with D-dimer levels of less than 1000 ng/mL, PE may be safely eliminated from the clinical differential for patients with indeterminate V̇/Q̇ scans. The positive impact of these tests, however, is less certain, and further development of noninvasive decision strategies is necessary in order to minimize the need for confirmation with spiral CT, MRI, or pulmonary angiography.

TREATMENT STRATEGIES. (Hyers et al, 1998; Bick and Haas, 1998.) For the majority of patients, anticoagulation with heparin remains the therapeutic mainstay for PE (Table 29–1). In addition to minimizing the recurrence of PE, anticoagulation limits the long-term sequelae of lower extremity venous stasis associated with an underlying thrombotic obstruction. The immediate goal is to prevent further clot formation. Clot dissolution proceeds through endogenous fibrinolysis and is largely unaffected by heparin. Therapeutic anticoagulation, as measured by an activated partial thromboplastin time (PTT) of 1.5 to 2.5 times control values, should be achieved as rapidly as possible, since mortality increases in direct proportion to delays in treatment. Patients with excessive levels of plasma heparin-binding proteins will require more than

Table 29–1	**Guidelines for Use of Unfractionated and Low-Molecular-Weight Heparin in the Management of Suspected and Confirmed Pulmonary Embolism**

GUIDELINES FOR ANTICOAGULATION: UNFRACTIONATED HEPARIN

Suspected PE/DVT—no contraindication for treatment
  Obtain baseline APTT, PT, CBC
  Unfractionated heparin, 5000 U IV
  Begin imaging sequence to confirm
Confirmed PE/DVT
  Administer bolus again with heparin 80 IU kg IV and begin maintenance infusion at 18 U/kg
  Check APTT at 6 hr to keep APTT in therapeutic range
  Check daily platelet count
  Start warfarin therapy on day 1 at 5 mg and adjust to daily INR
  Stop heparin therapy after at least 4 to 5 days of combined therapy (INR >2.0 for 2 consecutive days)
  Anticoagulate with warfarin for at least 3 months at an INR of 2.0 to 3.0

GUIDELINES FOR ANTICOAGULATION: LOW-MOLECULAR-WEIGHT (LMW) HEPARIN

Suspected PE/DVT—no contraindication for treatment
  Obtain baseline APTT, PT, CBC
  Unfractionated heparin 5000 U IV
  Begin imaging sequence to confirm
Confirmed PE/DVT
  Begin LMW heparin (enoxaparin) 1 mg/kg SC q12h
  Start warfarin therapy on day 1 at 5 mg and adjust the subsequent dose according to INR
  Check platelet count day 3
  Stop LMW heparin therapy after at least 4 to 5 days of combined therapy (INR >2.0 for 2 consecutive days)
  Anticoagulate with warfarin for at least 3 months at an INR of 2.0 to 3.0

APTT, activated partial thromboplastin time; CBC, complete blood count; INR, international normalized ratio; PT, prothrombin time.

the typical loading dose of 100 to 200 U/kg, followed by continuous 30,000 U per 24-hour infusion of unfractionated heparin to achieve effective anticoagulation. The side effects of heparin include bleeding, hyperkalemia, and thrombocytopenia. Heparin-induced thrombocytopenia and the associated thrombosis syndrome occur in approximately 3% of patient treated with unfractionated heparin and are the result of antibodies to heparin–platelet factor 4 complexes.

In light of these potential complications and following successful trials demonstrating efficacy in DVT prophylaxis, low-molecular-weight heparins (LMWHs) have been proposed as therapeutic alternatives to unfractionated heparin for the treatment of PE (Hull et al, 2000). To date, investigations comparing LMWH to intravenous heparin have shown similar PE recurrence rates and mortality and bleeding complications, but no significant therapeutic advantage to LMWH. These drugs have longer half-lives; thus, LMWHs do offer the benefit of single-dose, subcutaneous administration without the need for vigilant monitoring of clotting times. However, LMWHs are more difficult to reliably reverse than is unfractionated heparin, posing a potentially significant problem should bleeding complications occur, especially in a post-surgical or post-trauma patient. Conversion to oral warfarin should be started within 3 days of beginning heparin.

A transient hypercoagulable state is paradoxically associated with the initiation of warfarin; thus, treatment should overlap intravenous therapy until the international normalized ratio (INR) stabilizes in the therapeutic range (2.0 to 3.0) for at least 48 hours.

The choice of initial treatment depends on the severity of physiologic compromise. For patients with hemodynamic instability, right-heart failure secondary to massive thromboembolism in the pulmonary outflow tract is usually fatal unless aggressive interventions to relieve the acute obstruction can be employed. In patients for whom there is a high suspicion of PE and no contraindication to therapy, one should initiate anticoagulation before imaging studies confirming the diagnosis are obtained. In addition to supplemental oxygen, mechanical ventilation, invasive hemodynamic monitoring, and inotropic support all have a place in management. Thrombolysis with streptokinase, urokinase, or recombinant tissue-type plasminogen activator (rt-PA) has been advocated as a means of relieving acute pulmonary hypertension and right-heart failure. Although results vary with the regimen tested, most studies have shown a trend toward improved mortality with thrombolysis (5% vs. 11%), especially for those with massive PE and hemodynamic instability, and a reduced rate of recurrent PE (8% vs. 19%) (Arcasoy and Kriet, 1999). Unlike heparin, thrombolytics are also effective for the dissolution of established thrombi and thus may also be useful in the management of patients who present late in their clinical course (up to 14 days after PE). Debate remains as to the most effective thrombolytic agent. Confounding variables include allergic reactions to streptokinase and urokinase, local versus systemic administration, and the relative balance of clot resolution with the frequency of bleeding complications.

While directed thrombolysis offers an effective means for improving pulmonary outflow, the unavoidable systemic effects of clot dissolution pose a significant relative contraindication to its use in the post-trauma or post-surgical patient with coincident massive PE. Surgical embolectomy (Trendelenburg procedure) and catheter embolectomy are safe alternatives in these hemodynamically unstable patients for whom thrombolytic therapy presents an equally life-threatening, potential risk of bleeding (Tai et al, 1999). Surgical pulmonary embolectomy may be life-saving, although it is not readily available in most centers. Transvenous catheter pulmonary embolectomy, on the other hand, can be performed at the time of pulmonary arteriography, avoiding median sternotomy and the potential need for cardiopulmonary bypass. Massive thrombi may be disrupted or extracted (aspirated) in as many as 76% of cases, with significant reductions in pulmonary artery pressure and improvement in cardiac function. Treatment should be followed by anticoagulation with standard heparin or warfarin therapy. To date, no formal clinical trials comparing directed thrombolysis with embolectomy have been conducted. However, nonrandomized trials comparing rt-PA and heparin to surgical embolectomy and vena cava clipping show similar survival rates.

The use of inferior vena cava filters as primary prophylaxis in patients at risk from PE is controversial (Tai et al, 1999; Hyers et al, 1998; Langan et al, 1999). The placement of a filter is clearly indicated in patients with an absolute contradiction to anticoagulant therapy (e.g., head trauma), complications requiring cessation of anticoagulation, or recurrent embolism in the setting of appropriate therapy. The indications for filter placement when continued anticoagulation is planned remain open to debate, but a filter should be considered in patients undergoing thrombolysis or if free-floating thrombus is identified on venography or duplex ultrasonography. Trials comparing the use of vena cava filters plus anticoagulation with anticoagulation therapy alone have documented early protection against recurrent PE in the filter group, although long-term follow-up suggests that the period of anticoagulation should be extended beyond 3 months to decrease the incidence of recurrent DVT and postphlebitic syndrome.

OUTCOMES

Resolution of DVT and respiratory compromise associated with primary and recurrent PE depends on the clinical treatment strategy. Whereas recanalization occurs in 99% of leg vein segments after anticoagulation therapy, a single episode of DVT increases the risk of developing chronic lower extremity valvular incompetence by a factor of 10. The postphlebitic syndrome, characterized by status ulcerations and limitations to ambulation, carries the added personal and economic costs of poor wound healing of stasis ulcers and limitations to activity with secondary work restrictions.

The duration of warfarin anticoagulation after DVT complicated by PE is the subject of ongoing debate (Bick and Haas, 1998; Clagett et al, 1998; Kearon et al, 1999). For nonsurgical patients, treatment for a minimum of 3 months results in significantly fewer recurrent pulmonary emboli and failures of disease resolution than does therapy for shorter periods. For patients with postoperative DVT and PE, however, treatment failures and recurrent PE are equivalent at 4 weeks or 3 months of therapy, suggesting that a shorter course of therapy may be adequate. Recommendations for patient with underlying coagulation disorders have not been established with clinical trials. However, patients with an associated malignancy; factor V Leiden defect; deficiencies of plasminogen, plasminogen activator, anti–thrombin III, or protein C or S; myeloproliferative disorders, including polycythemia vera; systemic lupus erythematosus; and homocystinuria should probably remain on anticoagulants indefinitely after a single episode of venous thrombosis.

A small percentage of patients develop chronic thromboembolic pulmonary hypertension after PE despite appropriate anticoagulation therapy. This frequently underdiagnosed syndrome is surgically correctable but must be distinguished from primary pulmonary hypertension complicated by right-sided heart failure. These patients present with gradual onset of worsening exertional dyspnea, hypoxemia, and right-sided heart failure after an asymptomatic period. The early clues to the diagnosis include disproportionately severe symptoms that are unexplained by spirometric measurements and the presence of flow murmurs over the lung field. Pulmonary and hemodynamic signs and symptoms progress without evidence of new perfusion defects on serial V̇/Q̇ scans, suggesting the involvement of smaller, peripheral pulmonary vessels in the presence of a partially recanalized proximal pulmonary vasculature. A modest degree of resting pulmonary hypertension, which may be demonstrated with echocardiography, is markedly worsened by exercise. Right-sided heart catheterization is essential to the quantitating the degree of pulmonary hypertension, to ruling out competing diagnoses, and to defining the surgical accessibility of the obstructing thrombotic lesions. This procedure should be delayed, however, for several months after an acute embolic event to allow for maximal resolution and organization of the embolus and to avoid an interruption of anticoagulant therapy.

Surgical treatment of chronic pulmonary thromboembolism is currently confined to three centers across the United States and requires a multidisciplinary approach to diagnosis and management (Archibald et al, 1999). Careful selection, especially with respect to comorbidities is mandatory because of the procedural morbidity and mortality. The majority of patients who have undergone surgery have a pulmonary vascular resistance in excess of 300 dynes-sec/cm^5 at rest or with exercise. Vena cava filters are routinely employed to decrease recurrent embolization. With the patient cooled and on full cardiopulmonary bypass, pulmonary artery embolectomies are performed through a median sternotomy, with the surgeon taking care to extract an intact thrombus out into the subsegmental vessels. Prostacyclin analogues are used in the perioperative period.

PREVENTION

Clearly, if improved clinical outcomes are to be realized and the complications of PE avoided, practitioners should focus on prevention (Bick and Haas, 1998; Clagett et al, 1998). The high incidence and potentially devastating consequences of venous thromboembolism mandate the use of DVT prophylaxis in patients at risk. Well-controlled clinical trials have documented the positive impact of prophylactic pharmacologic regimens and intermittent pneumatic compression devices in patients with two or more significant risk factors. Despite wide acceptance of these data, however, preventive measures are often omitted from routine medical practice.

Assessment of clinical risk is crucial to appropriate prevention strategies. The majority of controlled trials delineating the risk of thromboembolism have focused on surgical patients. Available data, however, suggest that relative risk reductions in the incidence of DVT are comparable between medical and surgical patients. Although numerous factors that increase the risk of developing DVT have been identified, special attention should be paid to patients older than 40 years of age and those with a previous history of thrombosis, hypercoagulable states (including postmenopausal hormone therapy), morbid obesity, cancer, stroke, trauma, or acute spinal cord injury. In addition, patients undergoing specific procedures (laparoscopic and pelvic surgeries, hip fractures, and hip and knee replacement) or those for whom a prolonged

period of immobilization is anticipated should receive DVT prophylaxis. The assessment of thromboembolism risk in an individual patient should reflect both the type of surgery and an accumulation of predisposing factors.

For patients considered to be at low risk for thromboembolism (minor surgery, age under 40 years, no other risk factors), prophylactic measures beyond the use of graduated compression stockings, coupled with early ambulation and maintenance of an adequate volume, do not appear to be warranted. Subcutaneous low-dose heparin (5000 U every 12 hours) or LMWH (drug-specific dosage) is recommended for moderate-risk patients (major surgery, age over 40 years, no additional risk factors). Alternatively, intermittent pneumatic compression devices and graduated elastic compression stockings may be substituted in this group if bleeding complications are of significant concern. For high-risk patients (major surgery, age over 60 years, additional risk factors), the heparin or LMWH anticoagulation regimen should be combined with compression devices. Although more expensive, sub-

---

Pearls and Pittfalls

Diagnosis

PITFALLS

- Clinical presentation is variable.
- Hypoxemia, respiratory alkalosis, and tachypnea are common but are not diagnostic.
- Normal A-a gradient does not exclude a pulmonary embolism (PE).

Use of the V̇/Q̇ Scan

PEARLS

- Low clinical suspicion + low probability scan = no further work-up or treatment of PE.
- High clinical suspicion + high probability scan = anticoagulation on vena cava filter.
- All other combinations require further investigation (see Fig. 29–1).

Treatment Strategies (see Table 29–1)

PEARLS

- After confirmation of the diagnosis, initial treatment depends on the degree of physiologic compromise:
  1. If the patient is unstable, consider thrombolysis; consider surgical or radiologic embolectomy if thrombolysis is contraindicated or unavailable
  2. If the patient is stable, use unfractionated heparin or low-molecular-weight heparin
  3. Anticoagulate with warfarin early
  4. If anticoagulation is contraindicated, consider inferior vena cava filter

Prevention

PEARLS

- Prevention is underutilized.
- Assessment of clinical risk is crucial to prophylaxis strategies.

cutaneous LMWH (5000 U every 8 hours) has been shown to be as safe and, in some series, more effective than standard heparin therapy as prophylaxis in patients at high risk. Sustained anticoagulation with warfarin may be warranted in patients with coagulation disorders.

SELECTED READINGS

Anderson J, Owings J, Goodnight J: Bedside noninvasive detection of acute pulmonary embolism in critically ill surgical patients. Arch Surg 1999;134:869.

Archibald C, Auger W, Fedullo P: Outcome after pulmonary thromboendarterectomy. Semin Thorac Cardiovasc Surg 1999;11:164.

Arcasoy S, Kriet J: Thrombolytic therapy of pulmonary embolism: A comprehensive review of current evidence. Chest 1999;115:1695.

Bick R, Haas S: International consensus recommendations: Summary statement and additional suggested guidelines. Med Clin North Am 1998; 82:613.

Clagett G, Anderson F, Geerts W, et al: Prevention of venous thromboembolism. Chest 1998;114:531S.

Hull R, Raskob R, Brant R, et al: Low-molecular-weight heparin vs. heparin in the treatment of patients with pulmonary embolism. Arch Intern Med 2000;160:229.

Hyers T, Agnelli G, Hull R, et al: Antithrombotic therapy for venous thromboembolic disease. Chest 1998;114:561S.

Kearon C, Gent M, Hirsch J, et al: A comparison of three months of anticoagulation with extended anticoagulation for a first episode of idiopathic venous thromboembolism. N Engl J Med 1999;340:901.

Kruit W, de Boer A, Sing A, van Roon F: The significance of venography in the management of patients with clinically suspected pulmonary embolism. J Intern Med 1991;230:333.

Langan E, Miller R, Casey W, et al: Prophylactic inferior vena cava filters in trauma patients at high risk: Follow-up examination and risk/benefit assessment. J Vasc Surg 1999;30:484.

Legere B, Dweik R, Arroliga A: Venous thromboembolism in the intensive care unit. Clin Chest Med 1999;20:2.

Miettinen O, Henschke C, Yankelevitz D: Evaluation of diagnostic imaging tests: Diagnostic probability estimation. J Clin Epidemiol 1998;51:1293.

Perrier A, Bounameaux H, Morabia A, et al: Diagnosis of pulmonary embolism by a decision analysis–based strategy including clinical probability, D-dimer levels, and ultrasonography: A management study. Arch Intern Med 1996;156:531.

PIOPED Investigators: Value of the ventilation/perfusion scan in acute pulmonary embolism: Results of the prospective investigation of pulmonary embolism diagnosis (PIOPED). JAMA 1990;263:2753.

Stein P, Henry J: Clinical characteristics of patients with acute pulmonary embolism stratified according to their presenting syndromes. Chest 1997;112:974.

Stein P, Hull R, Pineo G: The role of newer diagnostic techniques in the diagnosis of pulmonary embolism. Curr Opin Pulmon Med 1999;5:212.

Tai N, Atwal A, Hamilton G: Modern management of pulmonary embolism. Br J Surg 1999;86:853.

Chapter 30
Right Ventricular Failure and Cardiogenic Shock

Pankaj H. Patel and David H. Livingston

Shock is a clinical syndrome resulting from inadequate tissue perfusion and oxygen delivery required for the maintenance of normal cellular metabolism. The clinical manifestations of shock are end-organ dysfunction and sympathetic and neuroendocrine effects caused by hypoperfusion. Cardiogenic shock is caused by impaired cardiac function, resulting in low cardiac output and inadequate tissue perfusion.

CLINICAL PRESENTATION

The etiology of cardiogenic shock may be the result of myocardial, structural, or electrical abnormalities of the heart intrinsically, or the result of extrinsic factors that either compress the heart and impair ventricular filling or severely obstruct ventricular inflow or outflow (Table 30–1). Cardiogenic shock resulting from an acute left ventricular myocardial infarction, the most common cause, occurs when more than 40% of the left ventricle is involved and may occur in 5% to 15% of all infarcts. The most common cause of right ventricular (RV) failure is failure of the left ventricle. RV infarction occurs in up to one third of all inferior wall myocardial infarctions, and only occasionally is extensive enough to cause cardiogenic shock. Other causes of RV failure are secondary to RV afterload (e.g., pulmonary embolus, pulmonary hypertension, or mitral stenosis) or secondary to decreased RV filling (e.g., tension pneumothorax or cardiac tamponade).

Clinical manifestations develop as a consequence of the inability of the heart to accommodate venous return from the lungs or from the systemic circulation, and the associated adrenergic response with resultant failure of peripheral perfusion. Clinical findings of cardiogenic shock may thus be similar to those of hypovolemic shock because both involve induction of the adrenosympathetic response. In left ventricular failure, accumulation of blood in pulmonary vasculature results in pulmonary edema, whereas in RV failure, accumulation of blood in systemic veins results in peripheral edema and hepatomegaly without pulmonary edema.

Patient history may reveal ischemic pain or history of coronary artery disease, valvular disease, or heart failure. Physical examination may find tachycardia, hypotension, tachypnea, change in mental status (agitation deteriorating to obtundation), S_3 gallop or mitral regurgitation (MR) murmur, signs of peripheral vasoconstriction (cool, clammy, pale, mottled, decreased capillary refill), and oliguria. In left-sided cardiogenic shock, there may be rales and evidence of hypoxia resulting from pulmonary edema. Jugular venous distention, Kussmaul's sign (prom-

inent cervical venous pulse or distention during inspiration), hepatomegaly, and peripheral edema with clear lungs may be seen in right-sided failure.

Cardiac isoenzymes (creatine kinase [CK], lactate dehydrogenase [LDH], troponin I) may help diagnosis myocardial infarction, but tests for these isoenzymes are often negative in the first 4 to 6 hours. An electrocardiogram often has nonspecific findings, but it may provide evi-

Table 30–1	Causes of Cardiogenic Shock

Myocardial

Infarction
    Reduced left ventricular (LV) function (>40% LV infarcted or with ischemic dysfunction)
    Extensive right ventricular infarct
    Acute mitral regurgitation (ischemic or ruptured papillary muscle)
    Ventricular septal rupture
    Ventricular wall rupture with cardiac tamponade
Cardiac contusion
Dilated cardiomyopathies
Myocarditis (viral, autoimmune, parasitic)
Pharmacologic/toxic depression (beta-blockers, Ca-channel blockers, tricyclic antidepressants, anthracycline)
Intrinsic depression (SIRS-related, i.e., "depressants," acidosis, hypoxia)
Postcardiopulmonary bypass

Structural

Valvular stenosis (mitral, aortic)
Valvular regurgitation (mitral, aortic)
Ventricular septal defects
Ventricular wall defects and aneurysms
Severe hypertrophic cardiomyopathy

Electrical

Supraventricular arrhythmias
Ventricular arrhythmias
AV blocks/complete heart block

Extracardiac Obstructive and Compressive

Tension pneumothorax
Pericardial tamponade (trauma, myocardial rupture, Dressler's syndrome, inflammatory, autoimmune, infectious, malignancy, uremia, anticoagulation)
Pericarditis (constrictive)
Mediastinal hematoma (s/p cardiac surgery)
Herniation or abdominal viscera through a diaphragmatic hernia
Positive-pressure ventilation with high positive end-expiratory pressure
Pulmonary embolus (>50%–60% pulmonary vascular bed)
Air embolus
Acute pulmonary hypertension
Aortic dissection (tamponade, aortic insufficiency)
Aortic coarctation
Myxoma
Miscellaneous (hyperviscosity syndrome, sickle cell crisis, polycythemia vera)

SIRS, systemic inflammatory response syndrome; s/p, status post.

207

dence of an old or acute infarct (ST segment elevations in right-sided precordial leads V_{3R} and V_{4R} for RV infarction), ischemia, pericarditis, or pulmonary embolism. A chest radiograph may show pulmonary edema, cardiomegaly (in the case of preexisting congestive heart failure or cardiomyopathy), pleural effusions, or other findings specific to the etiology of the cardiogenic shock. An echocardiogram can be extremely helpful in identifying the cause of heart failure, especially if structural abnormalities exist. Echocardiography reveals wall motion abnormalities; provides estimation of left ventricular (LV) (and to some extent RV) ejection fraction, thereby differentiating between left and right ventricular failure; and reveals pericardial effusion, in which concomitant RV diastolic collapse would be consistent with tamponade. An arterial blood gas measurement confirms the presence of hypoxia, assesses the adequacy of ventilation, and determines acid-base status. Other studies, such as a ventilation-perfusion scan or a pulmonary arteriogram, may be necessary as the clinical situation warrants.

Invasive hemodynamic monitoring often establishes the specific nature of shock and allows the appropriate treatment to be delivered effectively and expediently. The hemodynamic patterns found in different types of shock are listed in Table 30–2. Left-sided cardiogenic shock is usually associated with hypotension, a left ventricular ejection fraction (LVEF) less than 30%, a cardiac index less than 2.2 L/min per m², increased peripheral resistance, a pulmonary capillary wedge pressure (PCWP) greater than 18, a normal or somewhat increased central venous pressure (CVP), a decreased mixed venous oxygen saturation, and an increased arteriovenous difference.

MANAGEMENT

Initial management of any form of shock is prompt restoration of perfusion. If the cause is not immediately apparent, one must initiate empirical therapy to include volume resuscitation to prevent progression to an irreversible state. Optimization of cardiovascular dynamics and institution of supportive care must be in progress while performing diagnostic maneuvers. Early recognition of heart

failure can allow for intervention before progression to shock. The earliest sign of LV dysfunction is an increase in PCWP, with maintained stroke volume (SV) and cardiac output (CO). More severe dysfunction results in decreased SV with a compensatory tachycardia, so CO is still maintained. Therefore, there is a value to monitoring SV as an earlier marker of heart failure, rather than measuring CO (therefore interpretation of CO should be in relation to the heart rate to detect early changes in SV). Finally, when tachycardia cannot compensate for worsening SV, CO declines, and early compensated heart failure progresses to cardiac decompensation. As a compensatory mechanism to maintain blood pressure, systemic vascular resistance increases, further compromising perfusion and reducing CO further.

As in other forms of shock, restoration of peripheral perfusion is accomplished through optimizing cardiovascular and respiratory mechanics. The goals in management of cardiogenic shock are to maintain systemic oxygenation and perfusion and, in the setting of myocardial ischemia, to improve myocardial oxygen delivery while minimizing myocardial oxygen consumption.

Initial therapy while determining the exact etiology of cardiogenic shock should include supplemental oxygen, with the consideration of early mechanical ventilation to decrease the work of breathing, especially in the obtunded, hypoxic patient with an acid-base disturbance or decreased pulmonary compliance from pulmonary edema. Although the optimal hemoglobin concentration remains controversial, we recommend maintaining the hemoglobin concentration around 10 g/dL to ensure adequate tissue and myocardial oxygen delivery. Whereas sinus tachycardia is a compensatory mechanism for decreased SV, other tachyarrhythmias are hemodynamically compromising and should be immediately electrically cardioverted in the presence of shock. Furthermore, excessive tachycardia results in an increased myocardial oxygen demand and should be controlled. Bradyarrhythmias should be treated with atropine, and if recurrent or persistent, managed with sequential atrioventricular (AV) pacing.

Central venous access and insertion of a pulmonary artery catheter should be performed for invasive hemody-

Table 30–2	**Hemodynamic Patterns in Shock**				
	CO	SVR	PCWP	CVP	SVo₂
Hypovolemic	↓	↑	↓	↓	↓
Cardiogenic					
Left ventricular (LV) failure	↓	↑	↑	nl- ↑	↓
Right ventricular (RV) failure	↓	↑	nl- ↓ °	↑ °	↓
Extracardiac obstructive					
Pericardial tamponade	↓	↑	↑ †	↑ †	↓
Massive pulmonary embolism	↓	↑	nl- ↓ ‡	↑	↓
Distributive					
Early	↓ -nl- ↑	↓ -nl- ↑	nl	nl- ↑	nl- ↓
Early after IV fluids	↑	↓	nl- ↑	nl- ↑	↓ -nl- ↑
Late	↓	↑	nl	nl ↓ (rare ↑)	↓ (rare ↑)

°Equalization of pressures in RV myocardial infarction may suggest pericardial tamponade.
†Equalization (± 3 mm Hg) of pressures is characteristic, including pulmonary artery diastolic (PAD) and right ventricular end-diastolic pressure (RVEDP).
‡May be clinically unobtainable or uninterpretable.

namic monitoring, allowing for optimization of cardiac function through manipulation of preload, afterload, and inotropy. Even before cardiac parameters are obtained, judicious administration of intravenous fluid to increase preload is usually warranted. Once hypovolemia has been corrected, inotropic support is the mainstay of therapy. Adequacy of resuscitation can be monitored with additional laboratory data, such as serum lactate and base deficit measurements.

Pharmacologic measures are often required to optimize preload, afterload, and contractility. The goal is improvement of cardiac output and perfusion while maintaining mean arterial blood pressure. Commonly used inotropic agents in cardiogenic shock are the catecholamines dopamine and dobutamine, and phosphodiesterase inhibitors such as amrinone and milrinone. Digitalis glycosides have limited utility as an inotropic agent in cardiogenic shock, partly because they cause renal, coronary, and mesenteric vasoconstriction, but they remain most useful in the treatment of supraventricular tachycardias, including atrial fibrillation and flutter. Dopamine in moderate doses (5 to 8 μ/kg per minute) can increase cardiac output through its inotropic and chronotropic effects while maintaining blood pressure. However, it does this at the expense of increasing myocardial oxygen consumption. A pure β-adrenergic agonist such as dobutamine does not significantly increase myocardial oxygen consumption and is the therapy of choice for low cardiac output without hypotension. But, it is less valuable in cardiogenic shock because it often does not elevate blood pressure; the increase in CO is offset by the decrease in systemic vascular resistance. Dobutamine may be added to dopamine once blood pressure has improved (systolic blood pressure greater than 80 mm Hg). Amrinone and milrinone are potent inotropes as well as venous and arterial vasodilators, resulting in increased contractility and decreased preload and afterload without increasing myocardial oxygen consumption. Phosphodiesterase inhibitors amplify the effects of dobutamine.

Preload can be manipulated with intravenous fluids, diuretics, nitrates, and opiates. Volume is preferred to hemodynamic drugs for improving blood flow, and volume expansion to a PCWP of 15 to 20 (or higher in a poorly compliant left ventricle) should be instituted before administration of vasoactive agents. The venodilatory effects of the aforementioned medications can improve pulmonary congestion, and nitroglycerin has the added benefit of coronary vasodilatation. However, they can exacerbate hypotension and should be used judiciously, sometimes in conjunction with vasopressor agents.

Afterload reduction can prompt increases in CO through a decrease in systemic vascular resistance, but require blood pressure stability and close hemodynamic monitoring. In addition to the aforementioned nitroglycerin, dobutamine, and amrinone, nitroprusside is an ideal afterload reducer. It is a potent venous and arterial vasodilator that has no effect on myocardial contractility or regional distribution of blood flow. Vasopressors that increase afterload are dopamine in higher concentrations and norepinephrine with some inotropic activity.

Left Ventricular Failure

The management of cardiogenic shock resulting from LV failure can be based initially on ventricular filling pressures (Fig. 30–1). If the PCWP is low, volume should be administered to an optimal PCWP (i.e., the highest pressure that will augment cardiac output without producing pulmonary edema), as high as 18 to 24 mm Hg. Once optimal PCWP has been reached, treatment is based on blood pressure. If the blood pressure is low, dopamine may be used, followed by dobutamine. In the presence of normal blood pressure, treatment is with dobutamine or amrinone (combination therapy is more effective in patients with severe heart failure). With high blood pressure, nitroprusside is preferred for afterload reduction. For patients with coronary artery disease, nitroglycerin has the advantage improving myocardial oxygen supply and demand. If the cardiogenic shock is the result of aortic dissection, β-blockers will decrease the ratio of the change in pressure to the change in time (dP/dT). Finally, if the PCWP is elevated (pulmonary edema), management is based on the cardiac output; if the CO is diminished, dobutamine or amrinone are used. Dopamine should be avoided because it increases PCWP, possibly

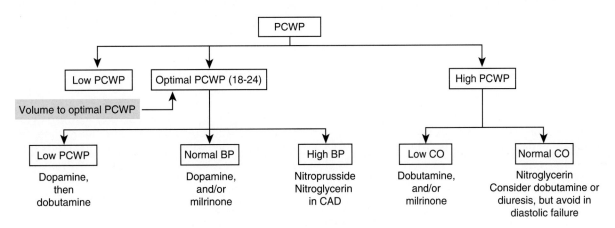

Figure 30–1. Management of left ventricular failure.

by constricting pulmonary veins. Vasodilators may increase the shunt fraction and worsen hypoxemia in patients with pulmonary edema. If the CO is normal, nitroglycerin will reduce PCWP while also reducing arterial resistance to maintain CO. A normal CO with pulmonary edema suggests diastolic failure; high filling pressures are helping to maintain CO, so aggressive diuresis is not recommended as first-line therapy. If nitroglycerin is unsuccessful, low-dose dobutamine may help, but increased heart rate suggests inadequate filling (i.e., diastolic failure) and dobutamine should be discontinued.

When cardiogenic shock is secondary to myocardial infarction, protection of the peri-infarct zone of ischemic myocardium is important to recovery. β-Blockers, nitroglycerin, and morphine can improve the myocardial oxygen supply and demand ration, but have a limited role in the presence of hypotension secondary to cardiogenic shock. Early reestablishment of coronary perfusion with thrombolytics, coronary angioplasty, or surgery can improve survival.

Right Ventricular Failure

RV dysfunction has been increasingly recognized as a significant contributor to low cardiac output and cardiogenic shock. RV failure can be due to the direct myocardial injury from an inferior wall myocardial infarction (one third of all inferior wall infarcts, with cardiogenic shock occurring in only 10% to 20% of patients with RV infract), but it is also commonly seen without infarction and in conjunction with respiratory failure, trauma, and sepsis. The RV is twice as sensitive to afterload as is the LV, so RV function is significantly impaired by pathologic processes that increase RV afterload, such as LV myocardial infarction, mitral stenosis, pulmonary embolus, hypoxic pulmonary vasoconstriction, essential pulmonary hypertension, fluid overload, and increased pulmonary airway pressures. Increased RV afterload increases RV myocardial oxygen consumption, possibly resulting in ischemia, which worsens RV failure. The contribution of the RV also becomes an important factor of cardiac function when there is decreased RV preload, secondary to hypovolemia, pericardial tamponade, tension pneumothorax, or increased positive end-expiratory pressure. Changes in the function of one ventricle can result in corresponding functional changes in the other.

Classically, CVP increases, PCWP may be normal or decreased, and CVP increases relatively more than PCWP with volume administration. Sometimes equalization of CVP and PCWP may mimic pericardial tamponade. RV failure can also impact on LV function through the interventricular septum—significant RV enlargement can push the septum to the left and compromise LV function by decreasing LV end-diastolic volume (EDV). Echocardiography can be helpful in differentiating right versus left ventricular failure. In RV failure, there is an increase in RV chamber size (if the patient has been adequately volume resuscitated), in RV wall motion abnormalities, and in paradoxical motion of the interventricular septum.

The right ventricle is a thin-walled, low-pressure chamber whose compliance can change significantly in critical illness. RV EDV can increase with minimal increases in end-diastolic pressure (estimated by CVP). In addition, CVP and PCWP are affected by positive end-expiratory pressure and by increased intra-abdominal pressures. Therefore, in critically ill patients, CVP correlates poorly with RV EDV. Right ventricular end-diastolic volume, which correlates with cardiac output through the Frank-Starling curve, can be calculated by measuring ejection fraction (EF) with echocardiography (when heart size is normal), radionuclide studies, or ventriculography. Stroke volume is calculated from heart rate and measured cardiac output, and then EDV is calculated (EDV = SV/EF).

Calculation of RV EDV can also be performed repetitively at the bedside with RV EF thermodilution catheters, which are Swan-Ganz catheters that are modified to measure RV EF using fast-response thermistors linked to the cardiac cycle with two intracardiac electrocardiogram electrodes. This method of EDV calculation correlates well with the aforementioned methods unless the ventricular rate is greater than 150 bpm or the cardiac rhythm is irregular (as in atrial fibrillation or frequent ectopy). Normal RV EF is 0.4 to 0.6, and normal RV EDV index (RVEDVI) is 60 to 100 mL/m². An RVEDVI of less than 140 predicts a preload recruitable increase in cardiac index. The assessment of preload status using RVEDVI eliminates the variables of RV compliance and airway pressures, and has been shown to be a better predictor than CVP or PCWP as to which patients will respond to a fluid challenge. Other studies have had contradictory results and suggest that response to an empirical fluid challenge may be superior in assessing adequacy of preload.

Treatment of RV failure is with fluid administration to improve preload (up to an RVEDVI of 140 mL/m², an increased CVP, or based on response to empirical fluid administration), which can partially restore CO that has been diminished by increased pulmonary vascular resistance. Aggressive volume infusion beyond an RVEDVI of 140 mL/m² may reduce CO as a result of compression of the LV by the interventricular septum (thereby decreasing LV filling). Once RV preload has been optimized, inotropic support and afterload reduction with dobutamine can further improve cardiac output; such support has proven efficacy in RV failure from acute myocardial infarction and pulmonary embolus. Cardiac contractility may be depressed in patients with sepsis and may benefit from the early institution of inotropic support. Additionally, afterload reduction can be effected by addressing the causes of increased pulmonary vascular resistance, for example, positive-pressure ventilation and increased mean airway pressures, pulmonary embolus, and mitral stenosis. Vasodilators that reduce venous return to the RV are not recommended. Ischemia to the AV node is common in patients with RV infarction because the AV node is often supplied by the right coronary artery. There is a risk for complete heart block, which requires sequential AV pacing.

Systolic Versus Diastolic Failure

Cardiac failure can result from systolic or diastolic dysfunction, or a combination of both. Diastolic failure is the

Pearls and Pitfalls

PEARLS

- Stabilization and partial or complete reversal of shock state must be effected before evaluation for the exact diagnosis. However, a precise diagnosis is necessary to guide appropriate therapy.
- Cardiac output may not be reduced in the early stages of heart failure because the ventricle is still responsive to preload and an increase in heart rate can compensate for the decrease in stroke volume.
- If hypotension does not improve with volume or if signs of congestive heart failure are evident, hemodynamic monitoring with a pulmonary artery catheter should be initiated early. Even though the utility of these measures is debatable, when the information is used properly under these circumstances, such measures are helpful in defining the prognosis associated with severe pulmonary edema and in guiding fluid, inotropic, and vasopressor therapies.
- Failure to recognize RV failure or surgically correctable causes of cardiogenic shock may result in failure of appropriate management; that is, vigorous volume expansion or surgery, respectively.
- Patients with cardiogenic ischemic events should be expeditiously screened for thrombolysis if the blood pressure improves, or they should be prepared for emergent cardiac catheterization. Similarly, suspicion of a massive pulmonary embolus requires rapid evaluation for possible embolectomy or thrombolysis. Early coronary reperfusion after myocardial infarction can limit the incidence of cardiogenic shock. Once in shock, there is still a 70% mortality rate after reperfusion with thrombolysis. Coronary angioplasty can significantly improve survival statistics in patients with cardiogenic shock.
- Liberal use of morphine, nitroglycerin, or diuretics (as with pulmonary edema from other causes) may produce untoward hemodynamic effects by lowering preload. These medications should be used cautiously while monitoring left heart pressures and cardiac output.

PITFALL

- Failure of prompt recognition of cardiogenic shock is the most significant error. Delays in treatment result in irreversible deterioration in cardiac function.

cause of 30% to 40% of acute heart failure. In systolic failure, there is a failure of contractility and a depression of the Starling curve downward. In diastolic dysfunction, ventricular compliance is decreased without a significant change in contractility at any given end-diastolic *volume*. Whereas increases in end-diastolic pressure (as measured by CVP or PCWP) result in a concomitant increase in EDV in the setting of systolic failure, in diastolic failure there is a minimal increase in EDV. In the management of diastolic failure, volume administration to increase EDV is the mainstay of treatment, but increased CVP and PCWP will result in peripheral and pulmonary edema. Medications to improve diastolic compliance, such as calcium-channel blockers, may be helpful. Inotropes should be avoided.

If preload and afterload manipulation, in addition to pharmacologic inotropic support, fail to improve perfusion adequately, *temporary* circulatory support can be provided with intra-aortic balloon counterpulsation or ventricular assist devices until the myocardium has recovered or while preparations are made for some other intervention. Other measures that may be indicated in severe cardiogenic shock are urgent myocardial revascularization, correction of other anatomic cardiac defects, and, in some instances, cardiac transplantation.

OUTCOMES

In-hospital mortality rate among patients with cardiogenic shock following myocardial infarction exceeds 70% unless a surgically correctable lesion, such as a ventricular aneurysm or valvular dysfunction, is found. Of the few hospital survivors, the 5-year survival rate is only 40%. Patients with RV infarction and preserved LV function have a 1-month survival rate of 75% and a 1-year survival rate of 60%.

SELECTED READINGS

Alpert JS, Becker RC: Mechanisms and management of cardiogenic shock. Crit Care Clin 1993;9:205.
Creamer JE, Edwards JD, Nightingale P: Mechanism of shock associated with right ventricular infarction. Br Heart J 1991;65:63.
Farmer JA: Cardiogenic shock. In Civetta JM, Taylor RW, Kirby RR (eds): Critical Care. Philadelphia, Lippincott-Raven, 1997.
Hochman JS, Boland J, Sleeper LA, et al: Current spectrum of cardiogenic shock and effect of early revascularization on mortality: Results of an International Registry. SHOCK Registry Investigators. Circulation 1995;91:873.
McGhie AI, Goldstein RA: Pathogenesis and management of acute heart failure and cardiogenic shock: Role of inotropic therapy. Chest 1992;102(5 Suppl 2):626S.
Nelson LD: The new pulmonary arterial catheters: Right ventricular ejection fraction and continuous cardiac output. Crit Care Clin 1996;12:795.
Serrano CV Jr, Ramires JA, Cesar LA, et al: Prognostic significance of right ventricular dysfunction in patients with acute inferior myocardial infarction and right ventricular involvement. Clin Cardiol 1995;18:199.

Chapter 31

Nosocomial Pneumonia
Mark A. Malangoni

Pneumonia is the third most common nosocomial infection. More patients die of pneumonia than of any other hospital-acquired infection. Whereas much has been written about this disease in seriously ill patients, it only recently has been recognized that nosocomial pneumonia is an important cause of morbidity and death in surgical patients.

In the past, nosocomial pneumonia developed in many patients following an emergent or elective operation; often, these patients had not received prolonged ventilatory support. With advances in critical care, more patients are surviving after serious illness and injury and, as a result, nosocomial pneumonia develops in patients while on mechanical ventilation. Thus, ventilator-associated pneumonia now comprises approximately 90% of cases of nosocomial pneumonia. Understanding the risk factors for the development of pneumonia, its clinical presentation, and the principles of management are essential to optimize outcome in patients in whom this infection develops.

CLINICAL PRESENTATION

Risk Factors

The traditional risk factors for the development of pneumonia include age greater than 60 years, the presence of an ultimately or rapidly fatal underlying disease, a recent upper abdominal or thoracic operation, altered consciousness, long preoperative hospital stay, a history of smoking, preexisting chronic obstructive pulmonary disease, a high American Society of Anesthesiologists status score, and malnutrition, usually indicated by a low serum albumin. These risk factors define patients at greater risk for development of pneumonia following an elective operation. Risk factors for the development of ventilator-associated pneumonia include the duration of intubation, the duration of mechanical ventilation, altered consciousness, emergency intubation, poor infection control practices, and preexisting pulmonary disease. For injured patients, there is a direct correlation between the likelihood of nosocomial pneumonia development and the Injury Severity Score. Other indices of disease severity such as the Acute Physiology and Chronic Health Evaluation (APACHE) II Score correlate with the development of nosocomial pneumonia and other nosocomial infections. Many of the parameters used to calculate these scores cannot be controlled (e.g., age, preexisting disease), yet these factors do serve an important purpose by identifying patients who are at higher risk for this infection. It is this high-risk group in whom interventions can best be tested for their preventive effects.

When patients are hospitalized, there is an early and dramatic change in the bacterial flora of the oropharynx as well as of the rest of the gastrointestinal tract. There is a shift from gram-positive cocci as the predominant bacteria colonizing the oropharynx in healthy persons to a predominance of gram-negative bacilli within 2 to 3 days of hospitalization. These new organisms often are resistant to multiple antibiotics. Nonpathologic aspiration, which can occur in 25% or more normal patients, allows the upper airways to become colonized with pathogenic bacteria. Endotracheal intubation bypasses the normal glottic barrier and exposes the proximal airways to large numbers of microorganisms. Aspiration of pooled oropharyngeal secretions is common and provides an additional pathway for bacteria to colonize the tracheobronchial tree. Bacterial colonization of the normally sterile upper airways generally precedes the development of ventilator-associated pneumonia.

Diagnosis

The traditional features of community-acquired pneumonia (i.e., fever, elevated white blood cell count, a new infiltrate on chest radiograph, and the presence of productive sputum) are not always present in patients with nosocomial pneumonia. The Centers for Disease Control and Prevention have defined the criteria necessary to establish the diagnosis of nosocomial pneumonia (Table 31–1). Although these criteria are sensitive for the occurrence of nosocomial pneumonia, they lack the specificity necessary to be highly accurate.

A recent International Consensus Conference (ICC) has developed more thorough definitions for the presence of ventilator-associated pneumonia (Table 31–2). These criteria are predicted on the use of more invasive diagnos-

Table 31–1	**Centers for Disease Control and Prevention Criteria for Diagnosis of Nosocomial Pneumonia**

1. Rales or dullness to percussion on chest examination and any of the following:
   a. New onset of purulent sputum or change in sputum character
   b. Organism isolated from blood culture
   c. Pathogen isolated from transtracheal aspirate, bronchial brushing, or biopsy
2. New or progressive infiltrate, consolidation, cavitation, or pleural effusion on chest radiograph and any of the following:
   a. a, b, or c, as above
   b. Isolation of virus or detection of viral antigen in respiratory secretions
   c. Diagnostic antibody titers
   d. Histopathologic evidence of pneumonia

Adapted from Garner JS, Jarvis WR, Emori TG, et al: CDC definitions for nosocomial infections, 1988. Am J Infect Control 1988;16:128–140.

Table 31–2	**Definitions of Ventilator-Associated Pneumonia**

Definite Pneumonia

New, progressive, or persistent infiltrate, purulent tracheal secretions, and one of the following:
1. Radiographic evidence of pulmonary abscess and positive aspirate
2. Histologic proof on open lung biopsy or at autopsy (abscess formation or consolidation with PMN accumulation) plus culture of >10⁴ microorganisms/g of lung tissue

Probable Pneumonia

New, progressive, or persistent infiltrate, purulent tracheal secretions, and one of the following:
1. Quantitative culture of lower respiratory tract secretions obtained by bronchoalveolar lavage or protected specimen brush
2. Positive blood culture of an organism found within 48 hr of isolation of the same organism in lower respiratory tract secretions
3. Positive pleural fluid culture of an organism identical to the organism found in lower respiratory tract secretions
4. Histologic proof on open lung biopsy or at autopsy (abscess formation, or consolidation with PMN accumulation) plus culture of <10⁴ microorganisms/g of lung tissue

PMN, polymorphonuclear lymphocytes.
Adapted from Cook DJ, Brun Buisson C, Guyatt GH, Sibbald WJ: Evaluation of new diagnostic technologies: Bronchoalveolar lavage and the diagnosis of ventilator-associated pneumonia. Crit Care Med 1994;22:1314–1322.

tic techniques in order to improve the overall accuracy of diagnosis. Many of the common clinical situations that are consistent with the diagnosis of pneumonia according to the Centers for Disease Control and Prevention criteria are not addressed by the ICC recommendations.

Fever, abnormal pulmonary findings on physical examination, the presence of purulent tracheobronchial secretions, and the development of new infiltrate on the chest radiograph define the presence of pneumonia with a high degree of accuracy in previously healthy patients. However, surgical patients may have fever and leukocytosis from other causes (Table 31–3), which also can result in an abnormal pulmonary examination. The development of a new or progressive infiltrate on chest radiograph of a patient who is receiving mechanical ventilation is not always due to pneumonia (see Table 31–3). The chest radiograph is particularly difficult to interpret when patients have preexisting disease or when the adult respiratory distress syndrome or bilateral pulmonary infiltrates are present.

A Gram stain of the sputum is a sensitive but nonspecific test to diagnose nosocomial pneumonia. The negative predictive value of a sputum Gram stain is excellent. This test is most useful to confirm the adequacy of a sputum specimen. When at least 25 white blood cells per low

Table 31–3	**Noninfectious Causes of Pulmonary Infiltrates**

Adult respiratory distress syndrome	Neoplasm
Aspiration	Pleural effusion
Atelectasis	Pulmonary contusion
Congestive heart failure	Pulmonary edema (noncardiogenic)
Hemorrhage	Pulmonary emboli

power field and 10 or fewer epithelial cells per low power field are seen, the likelihood that the specimen is from the distal tracheobronchial tree is high. The finding of a large number of organisms with similar morphologic characteristics on Gram stain also has a strong correlation with the presence of bacterial pneumonia.

It is important to obtain a representative culture of the tracheobronchial secretions to establish the diagnosis of pneumonia as well to determine the antimicrobial susceptibility of the pathogens. Cultures obtained from expectorated sputum or by endotracheal suction can be contaminated by oropharyngeal secretions, which lowers the sensitivity of the sputum culture. Approximately 30% to 40% of patients in whom ventilator-associated pneumonia develops will have disease caused by multiple pathogens that can confound the diagnosis, because the presence of multiple organisms on culture also can indicate that the specimen is contaminated by oropharyngeal secretions. Quantitative cultures of an uncontaminated sputum specimen have been demonstrated to improve the overall accuracy of the sputum culture. A threshold of 10⁵ bacteria colony-forming units (CFU)/mL is used to indicate the presence of pneumonia. The positive predictive value of quantitative cultures is 50% to 60%, whereas the negative predictive value is approximately 90%. The accuracy of quantitative sputum cultures decreases when recent or concomitant antibiotics have been administered.

Limitations in the accuracy of sputum cultures has led to a greater reliance on more invasive techniques in order to improve the accuracy of sputum sampling. Both protected specimen brush (PSB) sampling and bronchoalveolar lavage (BAL) are useful to improve the accuracy of diagnosis. PSB sampling is usually done through the flexible bronchoscope. Care should be taken to minimize contamination of the bronchoscope by secretions during insertion. The bronchoscope should be placed into a subsegmental bronchus in the area of an infiltrate and the PSB catheter is advanced out of the side channel and a protective inert plug is extruded. The PSB catheter is manipulated to sample any secretions. The brush is then retracted, removed, and the tip of the brush is placed in a sterile specimen cup. One milliliter of 0.9% normal saline solution is added to the specimen container to prevent desiccation of the specimen. A quantitative culture of the specimen should be plated within 30 minutes. Growth of more than 10³ CFU/mL is considered a positive culture. The overall sensitivity rate of PSB pneumonia is approximately 88% and the specificity is approximately 95%. Recent or concomitant antibiotic use reduces the accuracy of PSB and it has been suggested that the threshold for diagnosis should be decreased to 10² CFU/mL in this situation. There are some limitations to the use of PSB. Contamination with oropharyngeal secretions can result in a false-positive test and results are generally not available for up to 48 hours. Hemorrhage is an uncommon but important complication of PSB sampling.

BAL is another method of sampling lower airway secretions. After the flexible bronchoscope is advanced and wedged into an affected bronchial subsegment, five or six 50-mL aliquots of sterile 0.9% normal saline are infused and aspirated through the bronchoscope. The aspirate is sent for quantitative culture. BAL is simpler and less expensive to perform than PSB and it provides a more sensitive test with the lower incidence of complications. The sample volume of BAL is approximately 1000 times greater than PSB, which may account for its greater sensitivity. A threshold of 10^4 or 10^5 CFU/mL is used to define pneumonia. The lower value is generally selected for patients who have been receiving antibiotics. The sensitivity and specificity of BAL are approximately 93% and 100%, respectively. Temporary hypoxemia can be associated with the use of BAL. Therefore, it is important to maintain the patient on 100% oxygen for approximately 10 minutes before performance of BAL and for 30 minutes after this study. Even with these precautions, temporary hypoxemia can still occur, which limits the use of BAL in patients maintained on a fractional inspired oxygen concentration (FIO_2) of at least 80%.

Patients with pneumonia should have an arterial blood gas study done. A high alveolar-arterial oxygen gradient ($PAO_2 - PaO_2$, or $AaDO_2$) at the time of diagnosis is predictive of successful treatment (Fig. 31–1). The $AaDO_2$ also is useful for monitoring the progress of patients with nosocomial pneumonia.

Prevention

A number of interventions have been demonstrated to decrease the incidence of ventilator-associated pneumonia. These include elevation of the patient's head, the use of aseptic technique during patient care including suctioning, application of a chlorhexidine solution to the oropharynx as part of a daily care program, and continuous aspiration of subglottic secretions. These measures are meant to reduce the aspiration of secretions and to decrease the number of bacteria in these secretions. Infection control practices also help reduce the degree of

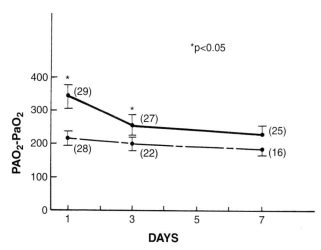

Figure 31–1. Relationship of $PAO_2 - PaO_2$ for successfully *(dashed line)* and unsuccessfully *(solid lines)* treated patients. Numbers in parentheses reflect the number of patients in whom these observations were made. (From Malangoni MA, Crafton R, Mocek FW: Pneumonia in the surgical intensive care unit: Factors determining successful outcome. Am J Surg 1994;167:250–255. With permission from Excerpta Medica Inc.)

bacterial contamination during tracheobronchial suctioning.

Management

Antimicrobial therapy is an essential component of the management of nosocomial pneumonia. The goal of antimicrobial treatment is to effectively eradicate pathogens causing the infection. Additional treatments include appropriate pulmonary toilet to assist with the clearance of secretions and to prevent the development of atelectasis, aerosol treatments as needed for associated diseases, and adherence to the general principles that guide overall patient management.

Antibiotic treatment can either be empirical or directed. The initial selection of antimicrobials is an empirical decision. Once the pathogens are identified, antibiotic use should be modified. The Gram stain generally is useful to guide empirical therapy, particularly when a dominant organism is found.

Empirical treatment can be initiated with either a single drug or a combination of antibiotics. The indications for the use of single-drug therapy include the following: a single organism on Gram stain, particularly when multiply antibiotic-resistant bacteria are not suspected; multiple organisms susceptible to a single antimicrobial agent; and the presence of pneumonia resulting from *Staphylococcus aureus*. Most gram-negative pneumonias in this category are due to pathogens that are susceptible to either a second- or third-generation cephalosporin, a beta-lactam antibiotic combined with a beta-lactamase inhibitor, or aztreonam. A fluoroquinolone should be used for patients who are allergic to penicillins. Patients who have staphylococcal pneumonias should be given either nafcillin for oxacillin-sensitive *S. aureus* or vancomycin for oxacillin-resistant *S. aureus*.

Ventilator-associated pneumonia, which develops within the first 5 days of hospitalization, is usually due to either *Haemophilus influenzae*, *Streptococcus pneumoniae*, methicillin-sensitive *S. aureus*, or *Enterobacter*. These organisms can be effectively treated with a single drug and have a relatively low incidence of antibiotic resistance as long as a second- or third-generation cephalosporin is not used to treat *Enterobacter* pneumonia. This situation has resulted in development of antibiotic resistance resulting from derepression of beta-lactamases.

The presence of multiple pathogens often requires selection of a combination of antibiotics. This situation is common when both gram-positive and gram-negative organisms are identified on the Gram stain. Additionally, some gram-negative bacteria that are multiply antibiotic-resistant should also be treated with combination therapy. These bacteria include *Pseudomonas aeruginosa*, *Serratia*, *Acinetobacter*, and some *Enterobacter* infections. Many *Enterobacter* species develop antibiotic resistance, particularly if a second- or third-generation cephalosporin is used as empirical single-agent treatment; therefore, combination antibiotic therapy may be needed by the time directed treatment is begun. When combination therapy is used, antibiotics that have different mechanisms of bacterial killing should be selected to minimize the devel-

Table 31–4	**Empirical Choices for Combination Antimicrobial Therapy of Ventilator-Associated Pneumonia**

Aminoglycoside or ciprofloxacin plus any of the following:
  Beta-lactam/beta-lactamase inhibitor
  Antipseudomonal penicillin
  Carbapenem
  Aztreonam
  Antipseudomonal third-generation cephalosporin (e.g., ceftazidime or cefoperazone)
  Fourth-generation cephalosporin (e.g., cefepime)

opment of resistance while on treatment. Acceptable choices for empirical combination antibiotic treatment are listed in Table 31–4.

After the culture results are available, the antibiotic choice should be reevaluated to select a single agent or combination of agents that are effective against the pathogens isolated. Preference should be given to agents that have a low incidence of adverse effects in order to minimize pharmacy expenses and to reduce pressures for the development of antimicrobial resistance in the hospital environment. Although combination therapy is often needed for the empirical treatment of ventilator-associated pneumonia resulting from gram-negative bacteria or mixed gram-positive and gram-negative organisms, treatment with a single drug may be appropriate once the pathogens have been identified. Combination therapy is necessary when multiple organisms are isolated on culture or when ventilator-associated pneumonia is due to "high-risk organisms," such as *P. aeruginosa*. It may not be possible to identify a single drug that is effective against multiple pathogens, particularly if methicillin-resistant *S. aureus* is isolated. Varying patterns of antibiotic resistance among both gram-positive and gram-negative bacteria, as well as other factors such as allergies, can influence the selection of antibiotic therapy.

Once treatment has begun, oxygen saturation, arterial blood gases, the white blood cell count, temperature, and the chest radiograph should be monitored. Patients with ventilator-associated pneumonia should have continuous noninvasive monitoring of oxygen saturation and need intermittent arterial blood gas determinations. An improvement in $AaDo_2$ generally indicates an improvement in the pneumonic process. Likewise, a decrease in leukocytosis and remission of fever are other indicators of response to treatment. The chest radiograph findings usually lag behind the clinical findings. Therefore, patients may be markedly improved and ready to stop therapy even though the infiltrates seen on chest radiograph may not be completely resolved.

Outcome

The outcome of ventilator-associated pneumonia is influenced by a variety of parameters. A number of reports have shown that the initial selection of appropriate empirical antimicrobial therapy for nosocomial pneumonia is associated with a lower mortality rate. This suggests that

the initial drug selection should be effective against the pathogens suspected based on the sputum Gram stain. It is important to treat all pathogens identified on sputum culture. The mortality rate of patients with nosocomial pneumonia has been reported to be between 20% and 40%. The attributable mortality rate of nosocomial pneumonia is less than that, generally 12% to 30%. This paradox occurs because many patients who have nosocomial pneumonia die of other illnesses and the pneumonia may be an incidental infection that does not contribute to death. In other situations, pneumonia can occur in terminally ill patients as the final event before death. The attributable mortality rate of nosocomial pneumonia caused by multiple antibiotic-resistant organisms such as *P. aeruginosa* and *Enterobacter* is greater than for other bacteria.

We have previously demonstrated that a high $AaDo_2$ on the day of diagnosis, as well as a shorter duration of mechanical ventilation, is associated with a greater likelihood of successful treatment of pneumonia (Table 31–5). Because nosocomial pneumonia represents a pathophysiologic spectrum of disease, it is possible that these parameters reflect the magnitude of the physiologic derangement or an increased severity of preexisting pulmonary disease, both of which intrinsically predict a worse outcome for treatment.

Patients who have nosocomial pneumonia with an associated bacteremia are at higher risk for death. The presence of bacteremia often indicates that normal host defense mechanisms have been overwhelmed by the bacterial inoculum or that host defenses are due to preexisting conditions. Other parameters associated with poor outcome with this illness are an increased APACHE II score and the development of multiple organ failure, in particular, respiratory failure. The presence of pneumonia in patients with adult respiratory distress syndrome also is associated with a higher mortality rate.

Approximately 30% to 40% of patients with nosocomial pneumonia fail initial therapy. Treatment failure can be due to either persistent or recurrent disease. *Pseudomonas aeruginosa* and *S. aureus* are the most common organisms isolated from sputum culture in patients with treatment failure. Our previous study indicates that treatment failure resulting from the development of antibiotic resistance while the patient is receiving antibiotic therapy is twice as common as pneumonia resulting from a new bacterial species. Recurrent pneumonia after successful treatment is often due to gram-negative bacteria, and multiply antibiotic-resistant organisms are common.

Table 31–5	**Variables Predictive of Successful Treatment**

	ODDS RATIO (95% CONFIDENCE INTERVALS)
Duration of intubation (days)	7.81 (2.32–26.38, $P = 0.0004$)
Duration of ventilation (days)	6.43 (1.90–21.68, $P = 0.0015$)
$AaDo_2$, day 1 (mm Hg)	3.97 (1.40–11.26, $P = 0.0082$)

Adapted from Malangoni MA, Crafton R, Mocek FW: Pneumonia in the surgical intensive care unit: Factors determining successful outcome. Am J Surg 1994;167:250–255. With permission from Excerpta Medica Inc.

Pearls and Pitfalls

PEARLS

- Early pneumonia has predictable pathogens.
- There is no agreement on a "gold standard" for diagnosis.
- BAL and PSB sampling are highly specific for the diagnosis.
- Endotracheal cultures have a high false-positive rate.
- The initial assessment of physiologic dysfunction ($AaDo_2$) helps predict the outcome of therapy.
- Diagnosis is more difficult for patients with adult respiratory distress syndrome.
- Pneumonias resulting from infection with *P. aeruginosa*, *Enterobacter*, *Acinetobacter*, and *S. aureus* have a high rate of treatment failure.
- Criteria for diagnosis often overlap with the systemic inflammatory response syndrome.
- Computed tomography of the chest is helpful to identify complications.

PITFALLS

- No agreement on a gold standard for diagnosis.
- Endotracheal cultures have a high false-positive rate.
- Diagnosis is more difficult for patients with ARDS.
- Criteria for diagnosis often overlap with the systemic inflammatory response syndrome (SIRS).

There are a variety of reasons for treatment failure. The selection of an antibiotic that is not effective against the isolated pathogens allows the pneumonic process to progress even though the patient may be receiving pharmacotherapy. In some patients, an unrecognized complication such as a lung abscess or empyema can develop, which requires a longer duration of treatment. In addition, these localized infections may need to be drained. Computed tomography of the chest is a useful aid for the diagnosis of these infections. Extrapulmonary infections also may occur, leading to confusion when assessing the effectiveness of antimicrobial therapy for nosocomial pneumonia.

Persistent infection caused by antibiotic-resistant organisms usually results in a rapid deterioration in patient condition. In contrast, the development of a recurrent pneumonia usually occurs after a period of initial improvement. These patients suffer a relapse that is often heralded by an increasing oxygen requirement. Patients who have recovered enough to be extubated may require reintubation for recurrent pneumonia.

SELECTED READINGS

American Thoracic Society: Hospital-acquired pneumonia in adults: Diagnosis, assessment of severity, initial antimicrobial therapy, and preventative strategies. Am J Respir Crit Care Med 1995;153:1711.

Croce MA, Fabian TC, Shaw B, et al: Analysis of charges associated with diagnosis of nosocomial pneumonia: Can routine bronchoscopy be justified? J Trauma 1994;37:721.

Garibaldi RA, Britt MR, Coleman ML, et al: Risk factors for postoperative pneumonia. Am J Med 1981;70:677.

Malangoni MA: Single vs. combination antimicrobial therapy for ventilator-associated pneumonia. Am J Surg 2000;179:585.

Malangoni MA, Crafton R, Mocek FC: Pneumonia in the surgical intensive care unit: Factors determining successful outcome. Am J Surg 1994;167:250.

Meduri GU, Mauldin GL, Wunderink RG, et al: Causes of fever and pulmonary densities in patients with clinical manifestations of ventilator-associated pneumonia. Chest 1994;106:221.

Polk HC, Heinzelmann MH, Mercer-Jones MA, et al: Pneumonia in the surgical patient. Curr Probl Surg 1997;34:117.

Polk HC Jr, Livingston DH, Fry DE, et al: Treatment of pneumonia in mechanically ventilated trauma patients: Results of a prospective trial. Arch Surg 1997;132:1086.

Yaffe MB, Fink MP: Hospital-acquired pneumonia in the postoperative setting. Semin Respir Crit Care Med 1997;18:121.

Chapter 32

Basic Pharmacokinetics, Pharmacodynamics, and Important Drug Interactions

David S. McKindley and Virginia Glen

Critically ill patients, particularly high-risk surgical patients, require the use of many more drugs than other patient populations. This is not only due to the acute nature of the illness but also due to the frequent comorbid disease states present. Therefore, it is essential that the surgeon be familiar with primary pharmacology issues that include general pharmacokinetic principles, how the pharmacokinetics of certain drugs differ in this patient population, and clinically significant drug interactions that are likely to be encountered. A growing number of studies in the field of critical care pharmacology have been directed at investigating pharmacokinetic differences between critically ill and non–critically ill patients; less is known about the differences in the pharmacodynamics between these two general populations of patients. For this reason, this chapter emphasizes pharmacokinetics with general pharmacodynamic concepts also reviewed.

PHARMACOKINETIC PRINCIPLES

The study of pharmacokinetics involves investigation of the concentration-versus-time drug profiles with particular interest in the absorption, distribution, metabolism, and elimination of these compounds. Each of these points is discussed separately; however, perturbations in one parameter may cause changes in other parameters. For example, altered protein binding that produces changes in distribution characteristics of a drug may also lead to changes in metabolism and elimination of the drug.

Absorption

Extent and rate of drug absorption are important considerations when discussing the amount of drug that reaches systemic circulation following extravascular drug administration. Extent of absorption, known as bioavailability (F), is the percentage of the administered dose that reaches circulation. *Bioavailability* alone does not provide information concerning the rate of drug absorption, which is equally important. An example where knowledge of both factors is critically important would be a drug that is highly bioavailable (>95%) but has an extremely slow rate of absorption. This could lead to maximum concentrations below a desired therapeutic concentration and would, therefore, not produce the desired effect.

There are many factors that can influence drug absorption. Some of these factors include the dosage form of the drug (e.g., enteric tablet coating, liquid-filled capsule, elixir), stability of the drug compound at the site of absorption (e.g., stomach, duodenum, nasal pharynx, subcutaneous), and the chemical form of the drug. In addition, the extent of liver metabolism of a drug will affect the amount of drug that reaches the systemic circulation. Orally administered drugs that are significantly metabolized by the liver before they reach the systemic circulation are designated as having a high "first-pass metabolism." Examples of drugs that have an extensive first-pass metabolism include lidocaine, morphine, and metoprolol. The first-pass metabolism is the highest with lidocaine, which reduces its oral bioavailability to the point where serum concentrations are undetectable. In the case of morphine and metoprolol, oral doses are much higher than intravenous doses in order to overcome the significant amount of drug lost to the first-pass metabolism.

Distribution

The distribution characteristics of a drug in the body depend upon the degree of plasma and tissue protein binding, solubility, and ionization of the drug compound. The pharmacokinetic parameter that describes drug distribution is volume of distribution (V_d). This parameter simply relates total amount of drug in the body to concentration of drug in plasma using the formula:

$$V_d = X_o \div Cp \qquad [1]$$

where Cp is the plasma concentration of the drug and X_o is the total bolus dose administered. Estimated V_d of a drug is not a physiologic volume and, therefore, is frequently referred to as an "apparent V_d." In many situations, the V_d of a drug far exceeds the volume of total body water (i.e., 42 L per 70 kg), which indicates significant distribution into tissues. Furthermore, perturbations in plasma and tissue binding characteristics can greatly affect the V_d of a drug.

V_d is a clinically useful pharmacokinetic parameter because it can be used to determine the loading dose required to achieve a desired drug concentration. For example, a loading dose of phenytoin ($V_d = 0.7$ L/kg) can be determined by rearrangement of Equation 1 to solve for X_o. If the desired therapeutic Cp following the loading dose is 20 mg/L and the Cp before the dose is zero, then the dose can be determined as follows:

217

X_o = 49 L × 20 mg/L. The calculated dose would be 980 mg assuming an average 70-kg patient. This is an approximate calculation because the dose would need to be infused at a rate of less than 50 mg/min to prevent complications. Therefore, the actual Cp would be less than 20 mg/L because a portion of drug will distribute out of the plasma compartment and be available for metabolism by the end of infusion.

Metabolism

Various organs in the body can metabolize drugs, such as the lungs, gastrointestinal tract, and the kidney. However, the liver is the site for most drug metabolism. Two major types of reactions are responsible for drug metabolism. Phase I reactions (including the cytochrome P-450 system [CYP450]), which add or expose functional groups, involve oxidation, reduction, and hydrolysis and are located in the smooth endoplasmic reticulum of hepatocytes. Phase II reactions are biosynthetic in nature and involve conjugation reactions with small endogenous substrates such as glucuronic acid, sulfate, or glycine. Biotransformation of lipophilic drugs to more polar compounds is essential for urinary excretion.

Elimination

A drug or its metabolites can be eliminated from the body by several mechanisms and depends on the solubility, ionization, and protein binding of the compound. The primary routes of elimination include hepatic, biliary, pulmonary, and renal, which is the predominant mechanism. Hydrophilic compounds are excreted, while lipophilic drugs tend to be reabsorbed by the kidney for further metabolism to a more hydrophilic compound. Renal routes of drug elimination involve filtration and active secretion mechanisms, while drug reabsorption in the nephron also affects the degree of drug elimination. Only unbound drug in the plasma is filtered by the glomerulus while bound drug can be eliminated by renal secretion using active transport systems. Clearance is the pharmacokinetic term that describes the rate of drug elimination. The definition of clearance is the volume of fluid (usually plasma) from which drug is removed per unit of time. The clearance of a drug can be divided into renal and nonrenal clearances. The sum of these clearances makes up total drug clearance (CL).

The degree of protein binding can significantly affect the CL of a drug. Therefore, conditions that alter the concentration of plasma protein or displace drug from the protein binding site can lead to significant changes in CL. Alterations in blood flow to the eliminating organ can also alter the CL of some drugs, particularly drugs that are highly extracted by the organ because the CL of these drugs is primarily dependent on the rate at which the drug is delivered to the organ (i.e., bloodflow). Alterations in the enzymatic activity of systems, particularly the hepatic enzymes responsible for drug elimination, can also lead to changes in the CL of drugs.

PHARMACOKINETIC ANALYSIS

Pharmacokinetic Parameters

The V_d and CL are considered to be independent pharmacokinetic parameters. That is, when there are changes in one parameter, the other parameter is not directly affected by that change. In contrast, the frequently referenced pharmacokinetic parameter, half-life ($t\frac{1}{2}$), is a dependent parameter. By definition, the $t\frac{1}{2}$ of a drug is the time required for Cp to decrease by half. The equation that describes $t\frac{1}{2}$ is as follows:

$$t^{1}\!/_{2} = \frac{0.693 \times V_d}{CL} \qquad [2]$$

where 0.693 is the natural logarithm of 2 because the Cp is reduced by half. One misconception of $t\frac{1}{2}$ is that it is completely dependent on CL; however, as described in Equation 2, V_d can also produce alterations in $t\frac{1}{2}$ without a change in CL. Another dependent pharmacokinetic parameter is the elimination rate constant (k_e). As with $t\frac{1}{2}$, the k_e is also dependent on V_d and CL as represented by the equation:

$$k_e = CL \div V_d \qquad [3]$$

Therefore, $t\frac{1}{2}$ and k_e are directly correlated by the relationship

$$t^{1}\!/_{2} = 0.693 \div k_e \qquad [4]$$

The k_e is estimated by taking the negative slope of the concentration versus time profile; therefore, the units of measure for k_e are inverse time.

Compartmental Pharmacokinetic Models

The plasma concentration-versus-time profile of a drug can be described using a compartmental model approach. These models represent either a single compartment, which usually represents the intravascular compartment, or multiple compartments, which can represent skeletal muscle, adipose tissue, lung tissue, or cerebral spinal fluid, for example. Figure 32–1 illustrates a one- and two-compartment model of two hypothetical drugs as they would appear on a normal and log Cp axis. The two drugs have vastly different pharmacokinetic properties with exception of the $t\frac{1}{2}$ (terminal $t\frac{1}{2}$ for the two-compartment drug), which is identical and represented by the same slope. Use of compartmental models allows for estimation of pharmacokinetic parameters such as V_d, CL, and $t\frac{1}{2}$. Drugs that exhibit relatively small V_d (i.e., hydrophilic drugs and low tissue-binding characteristics) can often be described using a single-compartment model. However, even these drugs may display an initial central compartment or distribution phase followed by a postdistribution compartment if early blood sampling for drug concentrations were conducted. One example of a drug that follows a single-compartment model is gentamicin because plasma concentrations are not drawn until 30 to 60 min-

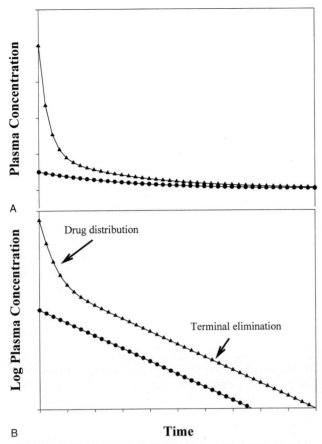

A

B   **Time**

Figure 32–1. Plasma concentration versus time profile of two hypothetical drugs represented on a normal y-axis *(A)* and on a log y-axis *(B)*. The line with triangles (▲) illustrates a drug that is best represented by a two-compartment model, while the line with circles (●) illustrates a drug that follows a one-compartment model. The drug that follows two-compartment characteristics in *B* clearly shows the prolonged distribution phase required for the drug to reach equilibrium between the plasma and the tissue compartments, followed by the linear terminal elimination phase.

utes after the dose is infused. When blood samples are collected earlier than 30 minutes following the dose, a two-compartment model better describes the concentration-versus-time profile. A three-compartment model has been used to describe the concentration-versus-time profile of some highly lipophilic drugs such as anesthetics and antiarrhythmics. When more than one compartment is used to describe the concentration-versus-time profile, the slope of each compartment (i.e., on log scale) has a different elimination rate constant. For example, a two-compartment model would have an α (distribution) and a β (terminal) rate constant; therefore, each of these slopes would also have an associated t½, hence the terms *distribution t½* and *terminal t½*.

LINEAR VERSUS NONLINEAR PHARMACOKINETICS. All discussion up to this point has focused on linear, or first-order, pharmacokinetics. Linear pharmacokinetics is present when CL remains the same irrespective of Cp. Therefore, t½ and k_e do not change when Cp changes. Nonlinear elimination pharmacokinetics, on the other hand, occurs when CL changes as a function of Cp. In other words, Cp changes disproportionally with dose and

is due to the changes in CL. This type of pharmacokinetics is also called Michaelis-Menten, dose- or concentration-dependent, or saturable elimination. Most drugs that are eliminated by an active process (e.g., hepatic enzymes) can display Michaelis-Menten pharmacokinetics as long as the dose is high enough to saturate the eliminating mechanism. In clinical practice, however, the concentration required to produce Michaelis-Menten pharmacokinetics for many of these drugs is not achieved and, therefore, can be described using linear pharmacokinetics. Drugs that do exhibit Michaelis-Menten pharmacokinetics within the therapeutic range of Cp (e.g., phenytoin), however, need to have the dosage adjusted in a conservative manner because of the disproportionate increase in Cp that can occur as the dosage is increased, as illustrated in Figure 32–2. The equation that describes Michaelis-Menten pharmacokinetics is as follows:

$$\text{Velocity} = \frac{V_{max} \times Cp}{K_m + Cp} \qquad [5]$$

where V_{max} is the maximum velocity reached by the system and K_m is the concentration at which half V_{max} is achieved.

PHARMACOKINETIC DIFFERENCES IN THE CRITICALLY ILL PATIENT

The purpose of this section is not to review each individual pharmacokinetic alteration described in the critically ill but rather provide a description of the general types of alterations that can lead to clinically significant pharmacokinetic changes. In many cases, the clinician can predict pharmacokinetic alterations depending on patient characteristics (e.g., physiologic changes, renal function, capillary leak syndrome) and pharmacokinetic characteristics of the drug (e.g., hydrophilic, highly protein bound, primary rate of elimination).

Critically ill patients frequently receive drugs that are

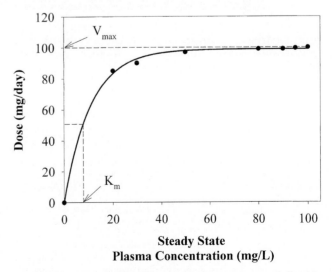

Figure 32–2. The fitted line represents the nonlinear relationship between steady-state plasma concentration and dose of a drug that has a V_{max} of 100 mg/day and a K_m of 7.5 mg/L.

monitored using serum concentrations such as anticonvulsants, antiarrhythmics, and antibiotics. Drugs in these categories have at least one of the following four characteristics that necessitate serum concentration determination: (1) serum concentrations that correlate better with clinical response than does the drug dosage, (2) a narrow therapeutic range, (3) significant interpatient variability in serum concentrations that results from identical dosage regimens, and (4) intrapatient variability as a function of time. Many drugs administered to this population are not monitored in the clinical laboratory because there are no rapid drug assays available. An increasing number of drugs have been found to have significant differences in pharmacokinetics when compared with the same drugs in the non–critically ill patient. Unfortunately, standard drug dosage ranges are determined from pharmacokinetic studies in non–critically ill patients and may not be appropriate for the critically ill patient. In many instances when "approved" dosage regimens are administered to critically ill patients, the serum concentrations produced are not optimal for either safety or efficacy of the drug. This can lead to inappropriate drug dosing, which oftentimes goes unrecognized, particularly for drugs that are not pharmacokinetically monitored. Evidence is mounting (e.g., antibiotics, sedatives, and analgesics) for the need to develop appropriate dosing guidelines for drugs that display significantly different pharmacokinetics in critically ill versus non–critically ill patients.

Each of the four general pharmacokinetic processes (i.e., absorption, distribution, metabolism, and elimination) can be significantly altered in critically ill patients compared with non–critically ill patients. In most instances, critically ill patients demonstrate highly variable pharmacokinetic parameters, which strongly support the need to individualize drug therapy and frequently reassess pharmacokinetics throughout the intensive care unit admission. Pharmacokinetic alterations in critically ill patient populations are summarized in Table 32–1.

Absorption

The rate and extent of drug absorption from any extravascular site of drug administration can be significantly altered due to cardiovascular instability, which may lead to variable perfusion of the site of absorption. Gastrointestinal drug absorption can be significantly affected by the binding of drugs to other orally administered drugs or enteral feeds. One example of highly variable oral bioavailability has been shown with ciprofloxacin in patients who were cardiovascularly stable. Oral bioavailability of this antibiotic ranged from 31% to 83% in stable critically ill patients who received the drug via nasogastric tube. Although absorption of some drugs has been shown to be unaffected by critical illness, many other drugs are unpredictable. For these reasons, we recommend that the more expensive, intravenous route be used whenever possible in the critically ill patient to avoid poor and highly variable bioavailability.

Distribution

The V_d of drugs used in the critically ill patient is one of the most well described pharmacokinetic alterations in this population (see Table 32–1). These changes often occur as a result of variations in drug protein binding and fluid shifts. Critically ill patients frequently display significant reductions in serum albumin concentrations, either as the result of acute illness or comorbid disease states. Albumin is the primary serum protein that binds acidic drugs like phenytoin. The serum α_1-acid glycoprotein concentration is markedly increased in the critically ill patient because it is an acute phase protein. α_1-Acid glycoprotein is the primary serum protein that binds basic drugs like lidocaine. Decreases in albumin and increases in α_1-acid glycoprotein serum concentrations can lead to major changes in fraction unbound of highly protein

Table 32–1	**Representative Pharmacokinetic Alterations in the Critically Ill Patient**			
POPULATION	**DRUG**	**DRUG CHARACTERISTICS**	**PHARMACOKINETIC ALTERATION**	**COMMENTS**
SICU	Aminoglycosides	Renal elimination Low protein binding	↑V_d	Wide variability Mean V_d greater than in non–critically ill patients
ICU	Midazolam	Hepatic metabolism High protein binding (albumin)	↑V_d, ↓k_e, ↓ plasma protein binding	Compared with non–critically ill patients
Neurotrauma	Phenytoin	Hepatic metabolism High protein binding (albumin)	↑V_{max} and ↓ plasma protein binding over time that correlated with albumin concentrations	Time-variant model compared with time-invariant model
Trauma	Sulfamethoxazole	Renal and hepatic elimination Moderate protein binding	↑V_d, ↑CL	Compared to nontrauma patients
Renal failure	Digoxin	High tissue binding (Na$^+$,K$^+$-ATPase) Renal elimination	↓V_d, ↓CL	Unknown mechanism for altered V_d. Likely due to ↓ tissue binding
ICU	Aztreonam	Moderate protein binding (albumin) Renal elimination	↑V_d, ↑CL, ~$t_{1/2}$, ↓ plasma protein binding	Compared with noninfected subjects
Severe burns	Ticarcillin	Moderate protein binding (albumin) Renal elimination	↑V_d, ↑CL, ↑CL_R	Compared with healthy volunteers

V_d, volume of distribution; k_e, elimination rate constant; CL, total drug clearance; CL_R, renal clearance; $t_{1/2}$, half-life.

bound drugs (i.e., >70%). For example, the V_d of midazolam (i.e., highly bound to albumin) was significantly increased in critically ill patients compared to volunteers. It is unclear as to the etiology of this altered V_d, but it is likely due to marked hypoalbuminemia. Lidocaine binding to α_1-acid glycoprotein has been described as having a linear relationship between the degree of binding and the α_1-acid glycoprotein concentrations in trauma patients. The α_1-acid glycoprotein concentrations were fourfold higher than controls in some patients, resulting in marked reductions in the free lidocaine concentration, while the total lidocaine concentrations reported by the laboratory were normal. This scenario occurs when there are protein binding alterations that occur with a high hepatic extraction ratio (E_H) drug (e.g., lidocaine). The E_H is the percentage of drug that is removed in a single pass through the liver. A high E_H indicates that a significant fraction of drug (i.e., >70%) is removed in this manner. In the case where α_1-acid glycoprotein concentrations increase, the lidocaine dose would need to be increased even though the total concentration was reported normal because less unbound drug is available to interact at the receptor.

Alterations in the V_d also result from expanded extracellular fluid compartments secondary to fluid shifts. Fluid shifts primarily affect drugs that are hydrophilic and have a low un-ionized fraction at physiologic pH. The V_d may be affected by changes in tissue binding properties of drugs that are highly bound to tissue. Plasma protein binding of a drug is an important factor in predicting the magnitude at which fluid shifts will alter the V_d. Examples of altered drug V_d resulting from fluid shifts or tissue binding include aminoglycosides and digoxin, respectively.

METABOLISM. Multiple physiologic changes in the critically ill can lead to altered hepatic drug metabolism, which can lead to changes in the clearance of hepatically eliminated drugs (CL_H). These changes and review of the primary literature regarding drug metabolism in the critically ill patient are discussed in detail elsewhere. In general, alterations in hepatic blood flow (Q_H), hepatic enzyme activity, and drug protein binding can affect CL_H. Knowledge of the E_H of a drug can greatly enhance the ability of a clinician to predict how changes in liver blood flow, hepatic enzyme activity, or drug protein binding will affect CL_H. Predicting how these factors would affect CL_H can be simplified by investigating the extremes of E_H. Drugs with a high E_H (i.e., > 0.7), which include fentanyl, furosemide, lidocaine, and metoprolol, will have a CL_H that approaches Q_H. The CL_H of these drugs would be highly dependent on Q_H and minimally affected by changes in protein binding and hepatic enzyme activity. These effects would be clinically important for these drugs in conditions where reduced Q_H is present, such as septic shock, administration of vasopressors, or high positive end-expiratory pressure. These conditions significantly reduce CL_H secondary to decreased drug delivery to the liver. On the other hand, hyperdynamic patients who display elevated cardiac outputs and subsequently increased Q_H would observe increases in CL_H. In contrast, a drug with a low E_H (i.e., <0.3), such as clindamycin,

lorazepam, and metronidazole, would have a CL_H that would be minimally affected by changes in Q_H, but rather by changes in hepatic enzyme activity and protein binding. The CL_H for a low E_H drug that has a low degree of protein binding is considered to be *binding insensitive*. That is, the CL_H is dependent primarily on hepatic enzyme activity and varies minimally with changes in protein binding characteristics. However, low E_H drugs that are highly protein bound are considered to be *binding sensitive* agents. Therefore, the CL_H is dependent on both enzyme activity and degree of protein binding.

Alterations in the protein binding of drugs frequently occur in the critically ill patient and can ultimately affect hepatic drug metabolism because only unbound drug is available for metabolism. High protein bound drugs (i.e., >70% bound) are particularly vulnerable to clinically significant changes in metabolism, since only a small fraction (i.e., <30%) of the total drug present in the blood is pharmacologically active. Therefore, small changes in protein binding may occur secondary to changes in plasma protein concentration leading to pronounced changes in the unbound concentration.

Although drugs with intermediate E_H (i.e., midazolam, haloperidol, meperidine) have been eliminated from this discussion, it is important to understand that the CL_H of these agents is dependent on both Q_H and hepatic enzyme activity. The degree at which Q_H, hepatic enzyme activity, and protein binding would affect the CL_H would depend on where the E_H falls between 0.3 and 0.7.

Elimination

Given the multiple factors (e.g., organ blood flow, protein binding) that affect elimination of drugs, it is reasonable to suspect that significant changes in pharmacokinetic parameters are likely to occur in the critically ill. Elimination of drugs excreted primarily by the kidney has been studied in various subpopulations of critically ill patients. Patients with greater than 20% total body burns had a significantly greater CL_R of ticarcillin compared with controls. The CL of sulfamethoxazole, which is eliminated primarily by the kidney, was significantly greater in trauma patients compared with historical controls. The increased drug clearance is likely secondary to the elevated cardiac output observed in hyperdynamic patients, which leads to increased kidney blood flow. Aminoglycoside CL in critically ill patients has been reported to be highly variable, with only 53% of the CL explained by creatinine clearance. Histamine-2 receptor antagonists (e.g., cimetidine) are another class of renally eliminated drugs that have been shown to have significantly higher CL estimates in the critically ill compared with controls.

As one would expect, many physiologic alterations that could affect drug CL occur in the critically ill patient, which frequently results in non–steady-state conditions. As the patient's kidney blood flow fluctuates as the result of hemodynamic changes, the clinician needs to be able to identify potential effects on drug CL. Drug dosage adjustments for renal insufficiency are frequently conducted; however, increased drug CL resulting from hyperdynamic physiology is not fully appreciated and is likely to be overlooked. Failure to recognize these alterations could lead to ineffective drug therapy and may explain some therapeutic failures observed in critically ill patients.

PHARMACODYNAMIC PRINCIPLES

Knowledge of drug pharmacokinetic parameters aids the clinician in predicting which drugs may be affected by critical illness; however, the pharmacokinetics of a drug can be similar in two patients but the therapeutic effect observed in these patients can be significantly different. For this reason, study of pharmacodynamics is important in describing these differences in response. By definition, pharmacodynamics is the study of drug effects and the mechanisms of action. Most drugs interact with a receptor, which results in a cascade of biochemical and physiologic events and ultimately produces the drug effect. Investigation into the relationship between drug concentration and effect can permit determination of the dose-response curve. This curve is useful in identifying the therapeutic range of a drug and will allow for evaluation of drug toxicity as the concentration increases throughout the dosage range. Unfortunately, pharmacodynamics in the critically ill has been less emphasized than pharmacokinetics. Clearly, a better understanding of pharmacodynamic alterations in this population is critical and requires significant consideration.

Drug Interactions

The hepatic drug interactions discussed in this section will focus on those involved with the CYP450 enzyme system. Hundreds of clinically significant drug interactions have been described in the literature and many more newly discovered drug interactions are being reported monthly; therefore, it is likely that numerous interactions go unrecognized, particularly with drugs that have been recently introduced to the market. There are numerous published tables of hepatic drug interactions that the reader should review if a drug interaction is suspected. Additional information concerning specific drug interactions can be obtained from a clinical pharmacist or drug information service.

To determine the clinical significance of drug interactions, it is important to distinguish between drugs that are substrates, inhibitors, and inducers of CYP450. Examples of these drugs, as well as some clinically significant interactions involving drugs commonly used in the critically ill, are illustrated in Table 32–2. The primary isozymes involved in drug metabolism are CYP1A2, CYP2C, CYP2D6, and CYP3A4. Any drug metabolized by these isozymes is called a substrate.

ENZYME INHIBITION. The most common mechanism for an enzyme inhibition interaction occurs as the result of reversible inhibition at the CYP450 active site, which can be classified as competitive or noncompetitive. Competitive inhibition occurs when an inhibitor drug prevents binding of the substrate to the active site on the enzyme and can be overcome with increasing concentrations of

Table 32–2	Hepatic Extraction Ratio (E_H) for Drugs Induced by CYP 450 Isozymes		
	LOW E_H (<0.3)	**INTERMEDIATE E_H (0.3–0.7)**	**HIGH E_H (>0.7)**
	Chlordiazepoxide	Alfentanil	Fentanyl
	Clindamycin	Diphenhydramine	Flumazenil
	Diazepam	Droperidol	Furosemide
	Erythromycin	Haloperidol	Ketamine
	Lorazepam	Meperidine	Lidocaine
	Methadone	Midazolam	Metoprolol
	Metronidazole		Morphine
	Pentobarbital		Naloxone
	Phenytoin		Propofol
			Sufentanil
			Verapamil

the substrate. Noncompetitive inhibition occurs when the inhibitor drug binds to another site on the enzyme to form an inactive complex regardless of normal substrate binding. This type of inhibition is overcome after new isozymes are produced.

Numerous drugs inhibit metabolism of a substrate. The clinical relevance depends on several factors, with one of the most important being the therapeutic index of the altered drug. Drugs with narrow therapeutic indexes (e.g., phenytoin) are more likely to be clinically relevant when involved in a drug interaction. Drug toxicities associated with inhibition may occur insidiously (e.g., nystagmus with inhibition of phenytoin metabolism) or produce serious adverse effects (e.g., hemorrhage due to warfarin inhibition by amiodarone). Competitive inhibition can also lead to decreased efficacy of a drug whose pharmacologic action resides in its metabolites. In general, inhibition of a drug can occur after the first dose. The time needed for maximal inhibition depends on the time to reach a new steady-state concentration.

ENZYME INDUCTION. Enzyme induction is an adaptive response that protects cells by increasing the detoxification activity of the liver. The major isozymes induced by drugs include CYP3A4, CYP1A2, and CYP2C. Several clinical problems can arise in the management of critically ill patients due to induction of drug metabolism, including exacerbation of the disease due to diminished drug efficacy or increased drug toxicity after removal of the inducer. Induction of CYP450 enzymes may occur as early as 24 hours after initial drug administration. Induction is overcome only by discontinuation of the inducer. The time required to reach a noninduced state after drug discontinuation is similar to the induction time-course.

PHARMACODYNAMIC DRUG INTERACTIONS. Pharmacodynamic drug interactions occur when two or more drugs have either a synergistic or an antagonistic effect. These interactions can occur at the same or different cellular receptor sites where the pharmacokinetics of the drugs do not have to be affected in order to produce the interaction. An example of a synergistic interaction would occur when diazepam and phenobarbital are administered together.

The response can be pronounced depression of the

Pearls and Pitfalls

PEARLS

- V_d and CL are independent parameters; therefore, alterations in one parameter do not necessarily lead to alterations in the other parameter; whereas $t\frac{1}{2}$ and k_e are parameters dependent on *both* V_d and CL.
- Conservative dosage adjustments need to be conducted with drugs that follow Michaelis-Menten pharmacokinetics because of the unpredictable disproportionate changes that occur between dosage and Cp.
- Numerous clinically significant pharmacokinetic alterations can occur in critically ill patients that may lead to poor therapeutic drug effect or toxicity. These changes can occur in the drug's bioavailability, distribution, metabolism, and elimination.
- The V_d of drugs in the critically ill patient is one of the most well-described pharmacokinetic alterations. This parameter has a high interpatient and intrapatient variability and is generally increased with most drugs during the acute phase of illness. Therefore, larger doses may need to be administered in order patients to achieve therapeutic concentrations.
- Drug protein binding, hepatic enzyme activity, and hepatic blood flow are important considerations in determining the effect of critical illness on hepatic drug clearance.
- Many hepatic drug interactions can occur in the critically ill patient as a result of the multiple drugs administered. Becoming familiar with those drugs that produce CYP 450 inhibition or induction aids the clinician in identifying drug combinations that have a high likelihood of a clinically significant drug interaction.

central nervous system due to the combined effect of both drugs on the chloride channels. Two examples of antagonistic interactions employed in the intensive care unit include flumazenil and naloxone, which antagonize the effects of the benzodiazepines and opioids, respectively. Both of these antagonists compete at the receptor site.

Although it is difficult to predict every drug interaction, there are strategies that aid in anticipation of potential interactions and minimize the adverse effects. These strategies include (1) ascertaining information on the mechanism of potential drug interactions with multiple medications, (2) determining the expected therapeutic and adverse effects of the medications, (3) increasing therapeutic drug monitoring during the expected onset

or offset of medications with a narrow therapeutic index, and (4) adding medications only when necessary and using the lowest effective dose.

SELECTED READINGS

Adam D, Zellner PR, Koeppe P, Wesch R: Pharmacokinetics of ticarcillin/clavulanate in severely burned patients. J Antimicrob Chemother 1989;24:121.

Boccazzi A, Langer M, Mandelli M, et al: The pharmacokinetics of aztreonam and penetration into the bronchial secretions of critically ill patients. J Antimicrob Chemother 1989;23:401.

Brouwer KLR, Dukes GE, Powell JR: Influence of liver function on drug disposition. In Evans WE, Schentag JJ, Jusko WJ (eds): Applied Pharmacokinetics: Principles of Therapeutic Drug Monitoring, 3rd ed. Vancouver, Canada, Applied Therapeutics, 1992;6:1–59.

Dasta JF, Armstrong DK: Variability in aminoglycoside pharmacokinetics in critically ill surgical patients. Crit Care Med 1988;16:327.

Edwards DJ, Lalka D, Cerra F, Slaughter RL: Alpha$_1$-acid glycoprotein concentration and protein binding in trauma. Clin Pharmacol Ther 1982;31:62.

Flockhart DA: Drug interactions and the cytochrome P450 system. The role of cytochrome P450 2C19. Clin Pharmacokinet 1995;29:45.

Forrest A, Nix DE, Ballow CH, et al: Pharmacodynamics of intravenous ciprofloxacin in seriously ill patients. Antimicrob Agents Chemother 1993;37:1073.

Hess MM, Boucher BA, Laizure SC, et al: Trimethoprim-sulfamethoxazole pharmacokinetics in trauma patients. Pharmacotherapy 1993;13:602.

Hyatt JM, McKinnon PS, Zimmer GS, Schentag JJ: The importance of pharmacokinetic/pharmacodynamic surrogate markers to outcome. Focus on antibacterial agents. Clin Pharmacokinet 1995;28:143.

Koup JR, Jusko WJ, Elwood CM, Kohli RK: Digoxin pharmacokinetics: Role of renal failure in dosage regimen design. Clin Pharmacol Ther 1975;18:9.

Lin JH, Lu AY: Inhibition and induction of cytochrome P450 and the clinical implications. Clin Pharmacokinet 1998;35:361.

McKindley DS, Boucher BA, Hess MM, et al: Effects of the acute phase response on phenytoin metabolism in neurotrauma patients. J Clin Pharmacol 1997;37:129.

McKindley DS, Hanes S, Boucher BA: Hepatic drug metabolism in critical illness. Pharmacotherapy 1998;18:759.

Mimoz O, Binter V, Jacolot A, et al: Pharmacokinetics and absolute bioavailability of ciprofloxacin administered through a nasogastric tube with continuous enteral feeding to critically ill patients. Intensive Care Med 1998;24:1047.

Morgan DJ, Smallwood RA: Clinical significance of pharmacokinetic models of hepatic elimination. Clin Pharmacokinet 1990;18:61.

Romac DR, Albertson TE: Drug interactions in the intensive care unit. Clin Chest Med 1999;20:385.

Schentag JJ, Smith IL, Swanson DJ, et al: Role for dual individualization with cefmenoxime. Am J Med 1984;77:43.

Schwinn DA, Watkins WD, Leslie JB: Basic principles of pharmacology related to anesthesia. In Miller RD, ed: Anesthesia. New York, Churchill Livingstone, 1994, pp 4–43.

Tholl DA, Shikuma LR, Miller TQ, et al: Physiologic response of stress and aminoglycoside clearance in critically ill patients. Crit Care Med 1993;21:248.

Vree TB, Shimoda M, Driessen JJ, et al: Decreased plasma albumin concentration results in increased volume of distribution and decreased elimination of midazolam in intensive care patients. Clin Pharmacol Ther 1989;46:537.

Wagner BK, O'Hara DA: Pharmacokinetics and pharmacodynamics of sedatives and analgesics in the treatment of agitated critically ill patients. Clin Pharmacokinet 1997;33:426.

Chapter 33

Pericardial Tamponade

Heitham T. Hassoun and Frederick A. Moore

Pericardial tamponade is a potentially lethal condition that requires accurate diagnosis and prompt intervention. The practicing surgeon encounters this condition most commonly after penetrating thoracic trauma and occasionally after blunt torso trauma. A bleeding heart wound fills the pericardial cavity, which is constricted by the inelastic pericardium, often leading to the physical findings of acute cardiac compression including pulsus paradoxus and Beck's triad (hypotension, increased jugular venous pressure, and quiet heart sounds). Pericardial tamponade can also occur in a number of other medical conditions with a more insidious onset (Table 33–1). These patients usually have preserved systemic blood pressures with a steady elevation in intrapericardial pressures. Regardless of the etiology, occult tamponade can decompensate rapidly with life-threatening consequences.

PATHOPHYSIOLOGY

Pericardial tamponade is defined as a hemodynamically significant compression of the heart by accumulating pericardial contents including effusions of blood, pus, or gas, singly or in combinations. The pericardial space usually contains 15 to 35 mL of fluid. With increasing pericardial fluid accumulation, the intrapericardial pressure increases based on three factors: (1) the volume of fluid, (2) the rate of accumulation, and (3) compliance of the pericardium. Rapid accumulation of as little as 150 mL of intrapericardial fluid causes a marked increase in intrapericardial pressure and subsequent critical reduction in cardiac output. On the other hand, with slowly accumulating fluid collections, the normal pericardium can stretch, allowing the pericardial space to tolerate more than 1 L of fluid without an increase intrapericardial pressure. The spectrum between a pericardial effusion and tamponade is a continuum. It is important to recognize that the relationship between intrapericardial fluid volume and pressure is not linear (Fig. 33–1). Initially, fluid accumulation in the pericardial cavity has little effect on the intrapericardial pressure (flat portion of the curve). The steep portion of the curve represents clinical tamponade, when small increments in volume cause rapid and significant increases in intrapericardial pressure. Slowly developing fluid collections allow for pericardial "stretch" and subsequent increased intrapericardial volume before onset of clinical tamponade. This is represented by the longer flat portion of the pressure-volume curve.

The heart and the pericardial contents continuously compete for the relatively fixed intrapericardial volume. As the intrapericardial pressure increases, the atria and ventricles are compressed, leading to a progressive reduction in cardiac filling and subsequent stroke volume. Compensatory mechanisms (e.g., adrenergic stimulation) increase heart rate, mean arterial pressure, and ventricular diastolic pressure in order to support cardiac output. Tachycardia leads to decreased diastolic filling time, which decreases myocardial perfusion and can cause subendocardial ischemia and lethal arrhythmia. Tamponade occurs when the intrapericardial pressure exceeds intracardiac pressures. In critical tamponade, cardiac output has usually decreased by 30% and transmural pressures are zero (normally 15 to 30 mm Hg). At this point, there is a marked shift of the ventricular septum into the left ventricle as inspiration fills the right heart, causing a decrease in left ventricular end-diastolic volume and subsequent stroke volume. This phenomenon is known as *pulsus paradoxus* and is defined as 10 mm Hg or greater decrease in arterial pressure during inspiration.

DIAGNOSIS

The diagnosis of pericardial tamponade relies heavily on clinical suspicion. The classic features of Beck's triad and pulsus paradoxus are not consistently present. The clinical manifestations vary based on how rapidly the tamponade develops as well as the individual's cardiac function and volume status. Rapid accumulation of fluid in the pericardial space can quickly lead to a decompensated pericardial tamponade. In this case, the patient appears critically ill, demonstrating restlessness and marked jugular venous pressure. However, post-traumatic patients are often hypovolemic and *low pressure tamponade* may occur at much lower central venous pressures. These patients are often asymptomatic until volume loading precipitates a decompensated tamponade. On the other hand, a patient with a slowly developing pericardial tamponade displays subtle initial signs and symptoms such as fatigue, shortness of breath, dizziness, chest pain, tachycardia, and atrial arrhythmias. Pericardial tamponade can also occur days to weeks after an injury or cardiac operation if pericarditis with significant effusion develops.

There are several diagnostic techniques for the evaluation of patients with equivocal clinical findings of pericardial tamponade. Noninvasive studies include transthoracic two-dimensional echocardiography, computed tomography (CT), magnetic resonance imaging, chest radiograph,

Table 33–1	Nontrauma Causes of Pericardial Tamponade	
Malignancy	Postpericardiotomy	
Uremia	Connective tissue diseases	
Radiation	Idiopathic	
Infection		

RELATIONSHIP BETWEEN INTRAPERICARDIAL VOLUME AND PRESSURE IN PERICARDIAL TAMPONADE

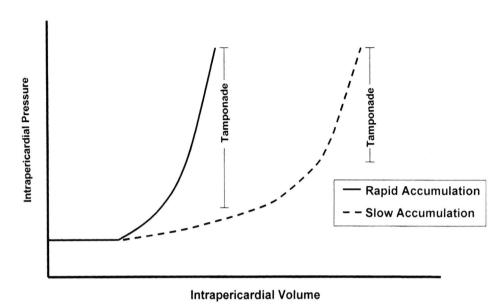

Figure 33–1. Schematic showing nonlinear relationship between intrapericardial volume and pressure in pericardial tamponade. The solid line represents rapid accumulation of intraperitoneal fluid. Under these conditions, the inelastic pericardium cannot stretch, causing a rapid increase in intrapericardial pressure once the pericardial reserve volume has been reached. The dashed line represents slow accumulation of intraperitoneal fluid. In this case, the pericardium can stretch, allowing a large volume increase with minimal change in pressure and no hemodynamic consequences until the limit of pericardial dilation is reached.

and electrocardiogram. Two-dimensional echocardiography is the method of choice for diagnosing and following up cases of suspected pericardial tamponade in patients who are hemodynamically stable. Echocardiographic features of tamponade include right atrial compression during diastole, right ventricular collapse during diastole, and a dilated inferior vena cava with lack of inspiratory collapse. CT imaging, especially helical CT, has been increasingly beneficial in screening stable patients with suspected blunt thoracic aortic injuries. In these cases, CT can also demonstrate abnormal pericardial contents including fluid, blood, and air, as well as direct cardiac injuries. Whereas a chest radiograph can show an enlarged cardiac silhouette if a significant pericardial effusion is present, it is rarely helpful in the setting of acute tamponade. Electrocardiogram findings in pericardial tamponade include electrical alternans (alternating positive-negative P wave) and decreased QRS voltage. Invasive hemodynamic monitoring can also be used to diagnose pericardial tamponade. A central venous pressure greater than 20 mm Hg suggests tamponade, especially if there is a trend of increasing central venous pressure with decreasing systolic blood pressure. A pulmonary artery catheter demonstrating elevated and equal diastolic pressures in the right atrium, right ventricle, and pulmonary artery is pathognomonic for pericardial tamponade.

Until recently, the use of echocardiography in trauma patients was reserved for the evaluation of blunt cardiac injury. Most patients with penetrating cardiac injuries are in overt shock upon arrival to the emergency center (EC). These patients should undergo emergent thoracotomy, decompression of the pericardium, and repair of the cardiac injuries. In patients who are more hemodynamically stable, diagnostic choices in the past included pericardiocentesis, subxyphoid pericardial window, or transthoracic echocardiography by a cardiologist. Diagnostic pericardiocentesis is not an ideal study because of its invasiveness

and high rate of both false-positive and false-negative results. Whereas subxyphoid pericardial window is very sensitive and specific, it is an even more invasive procedure, requiring general anesthesia with a high rate of negative explorations. Over the past 10 years, a number of studies have shown that ultrasonography performed in the EC is the diagnostic test of choice for traumatic cardiac injuries. A recent prospective, multicenter study found that pericardial ultrasound examination performed in the trauma resuscitation room is a rapid and accurate modality for the diagnosis of hemopericardium. A positive examination is based on three findings: (1) separation of the pericardial layers with an anechoic area, (2) a decrease in the motion of the parietal pericardium, and (3) identification of a swinging motion of the heart within the pericardial sac. An example of pericardial tamponade diagnosed by EC ultrasound is depicted in Figure 33–2.

MANAGEMENT

The definitive treatment of pericardial tamponade is prompt evacuation of the pericardial cavity. Several methods are available for the drainage of pericardial contents

Table 33–2	Options for Pericardial Drainage

Percutaneous
    Blind needle pericardiocentesis
    Echo-guided pericardiocentesis
    Pericardiocentesis with catheter drainage
    Balloon pericardiotomy
Surgical
    Subxyphoid pericardial tube drainage
    Subxyphoid pericardial window
    Video-assisted thoracoscopy
    Thoracotomy

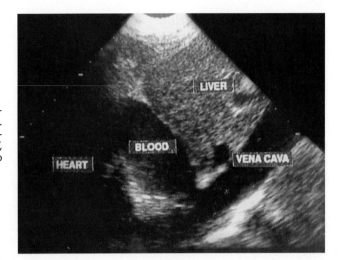

Figure 33–2. Pericardial tamponade diagnosed by surgeon-performed ultrasound in the emergency center using a 3.5-MHz probe. (From Mirvis SE, Hastings G, Scalea TM: Diagnostic imaging, angiography, and interventional radiology. In Mattox KL, Feliciano DV, Moore EE [eds]: Trauma, 4th ed. New York, McGraw-Hill, 2000, p 269, with permission.)

(Table 33–2). The choice of procedure depends on urgency as well as the etiology of the tamponade. An algorithm for the management of patients with suspected pericardial tamponade is depicted in Figure 33–3. For moribund patients who have sustained penetrating thoracic injuries with loss of vital signs in the EC, an emergent left anterolateral thoracotomy with opening of the pericardium is indicated. The patient should then be taken to the operating room for definitive cardiac wound repair and chest wall closure. For unstable patients with a palpable blood pressure, intravenous fluids should be rapidly administered as the diagnosis is confirmed by EC ultrasound or blind pericardiocentesis if ultrasound is not available. Patients with a positive examination should be transported to the operating room expeditiously. A catheter can be placed in the pericardium as a temporizing measure until definitive treatment can be given in the

operating room. Stable trauma patients with evidence of pericardial tamponade by EC ultrasound should undergo treatment in the operating room by subxyphoid pericardial window or sternotomy, or both, depending on etiology and associated injuries. Pericardial effusions are occasionally identified by chest CT after blunt trauma. These patients should undergo transthoracic echocardiography for confirmation and to evaluate for evidence of tamponade physiology.

Echocardiography-guided percutaneous pericardiocentesis is the initial treatment of choice in hemodynamically stable patients with non–trauma-related tamponade. It is simple, safe, and effective in removing pericardial fluid, improving hemodynamics, and relieving symptoms. However, a high incidence of recurrence, especially within the first 48 hours, is associated with echocardiography-guided drainage alone. The use of a pericardial drainage catheter

PERICARDIAL TAMPONADE

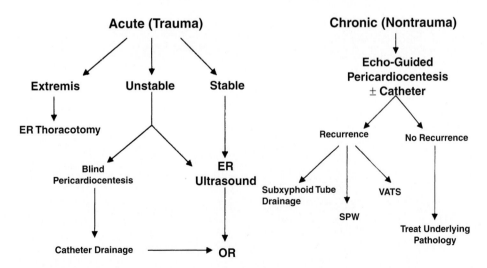

Figure 33–3. Algorithm for the management of suspected pericardial tamponade in both acute and chronic conditions. SPW, subxyphoid pericardial window; VATS, video-assisted thoracoscopic surgery.

Pearls and Pitfalls

PEARLS

- Rapid EC decompression can be lifesaving.
- The relationship between intrapericardial fluid volume and pressure is not linear (see Fig. 33–1).
- Pericardiocentesis can be used for diagnosis.
- Emergency center ultrasonography is the diagnostic test of choice if available.
- Placement of an intrapericardial catheter during initial drainage can reduce the incidence of recurrence.

PITFALLS

- Clinicians may fail to consider diagnosis in postinjury shock.
- Chronic pericardial fluid collections can rapidly progress to acute tamponade.
- The classic features of Beck's triad, which is used for diagnosis, are not consistently present.
- Chronic effusions frequently reaccumulate after echocardiography-guided pericardiocentesis.

---

can significantly reduce the incidence of recurrence and subsequent need for surgical drainage.

SELECTED READINGS

Ball JB, Morrison WL: Cardiac tamponade. Postgrad Med J 1997;73:141.

Beck CS: Two cardiac compression triads. JAMA 1935;104:714.

Chan D: Echocardiography in thoracic trauma. Emerg Med Clin North Am 1998;16:191.

Feliciano DV, Rozycki GS: Advances in the diagnosis and treatment of thoracic trauma. Surg Clin North Am 1999;79:1417.

Harken AH, Hammond GL, Edmunds LH: Pericardial diseases. In Edmunds I H (ed): Cardiac Surgery in the Adult. New York, McGraw Hill, 1997, pp 1303–1317.

Knoop T, Willenberg K: Cardiac tamponade. Semin Oncol Nursing 1999;15:168.

Mullins RJ: Management of shock. In Mattox KL, Feliciano DV, Moore EE (eds): Trauma, 4th ed. New York, McGraw-Hill, 2000.

Reddy PS, Curtiss EI, Uretsky BF: Spectrum of hemodynamic changes in cardiac tamponade. Am J Cardiol 1990;66:1487.

Rozycki GS, Feliciano DV, Ochsner MG, et al: The role of ultrasound in patients with possible penetrating cardiac wounds: A prospective multicenter study. J Trauma 1999;46:543.

Spodick DH: The Pericardium: A Comprehensive Textbook. New York, Marcel Dekker, 1997.

Spodick DH: Pathophysiology of cardiac tamponade. Chest 1998;113:1372.

Tsang TSM, Oh HK, Seward JB: Diagnosis and management of cardiac tamponade in the era of echocardiography. Clin Cardiol 1999;22:446.

Chapter 34
Gastrointestinal Failure
Thomas Genuit and Lena M. Napolitano

The gastrointestinal (GI) tract is a complex organ system. Its functions include mechanical and enzymatic digestion of food, absorption of nutrients, minerals and water, excretion of processed toxins and waste products, and barrier functions associated with both humoral and cellular immune elements. This chapter focuses mainly on problems related to the loss of intestinal mucosal integrity and barrier function that are encountered in the practice of general surgery, especially when caring for critically ill patients.

To properly understand the functions of the gut mucosal barrier, as well as the pathogenesis and implications of its failure, it is important to have a comprehensive knowledge of the intestinal anatomy and physiology. This chapter concentrates on certain key aspects of gut anatomy. The *gut mucosal barrier* is composed of a surface epithelial layer and a subepithelial immune cellular component (Fig. 34–1). Immature enterocytes proliferate in the mucosal crypts and mature while migrating to the villous tips, where apoptosis and cellular sloughing take place. The enterocytes are joined by tight cellular junctions that prevent free diffusion and passage of macromolecules.

In certain areas of the gut (i.e., duodenum), specialized cells in the depth of the crypts secrete bactericidal components (i.e., lysozyme) into the lumen, and, throughout the intestine, epithelial goblet cells secrete surface-protecting mucus. Interspersed within the lamina propria and submucosa are numerous immune competent cells

(e.g., lymphocytes, monocyte-macrophages, neutrophils), which may form organized aggregates (Peyer's patches) in certain areas of the gut and constitute approximately 25% of the total intestinal cell mass. Overall, the intestinal immunocytes form the largest aggregation of cellular immune components in the body. These cells secrete immunoglobulins (IgA) and other mediators into the gut lumen, combat local violation of mucosal integrity (bacterial translocation), process antigen, and release mediators to modulate the systemic immune response.

The integrity of this intestinal mucosa–submucosal complex is critically dependent on several essential factors, most importantly adequate perfusion. The intestine features a segmental *arterial blood supply* with limited intersegmental collateral flow (arcades, marginal artery). The innermost (mucosal) layer with its factor 10^3 to 10^4 surface enlargement is the most metabolically active part of the intestinal wall and receives approximately 80% of the total intestinal flow (approximately 20% of the cardiac output at rest). It is important to understand that the mucosa is positioned at the capillary end of the blood supply, beyond extraintestinal and intraintestinal arteriolar resistance vessels, regulating flow (see Fig. 34–1).

In terms of total body homeostasis, the intestine is an "organ of secondary importance"; adequate perfusion may be compromised at the systemic, as well as the local level. Any state of systemic hypoperfusion (e.g., cardiac insufficiency, hypovolemia) elicits counterregulatory mechanisms aimed at maintaining perfusion to "vital or-

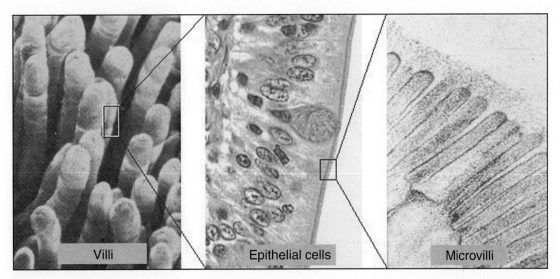

Figure 34–1. Histologic structure of the intestinal mucosal surface. The panels depict the intestinal mucosal surface, showing villi, epithelial cells that cover the villi, and the microvilli of the epithelial cells. In the middle panel (light micrograph), the microvilli are visible and look something like a brush. For this reason, the microvillus border of intestinal epithelial cells is referred to as the "brush border." In the panel showing villi, the mucosa forms multitudes of projections that protrude into the lumen and are covered with epithelial cells. In the panel showing microvilli, the luminal plasma membrane of absorptive epithelial cells is studded with densely packed microvilli.

229

gans" (brain, kidney, heart), at the cost of intestinal blood flow. In addition, the intestinal blood supply (celiac, superior mesenteric, and inferior mesenteric arteries) is derived from an anatomic area commonly involved in arteriosclerotic and aneurysmal disease (abdominal aorta). It is second only to the carotid artery and lower extremity territories as a target for cardiovascular thromboemboli. Less commonly, it also constitutes the target of certain arterial inflammatory conditions (e.g., panarteritis nodosa, Wegener's granulomatosis, giant cell arteritis).

Apart from problems related to arterial perfusion, the unique anatomic arrangement of the intestinal *venous drainage* (via the mesenteric and the portal veins to the liver) makes it vulnerable to disturbance. Liver disease may cause portal venous hypertension with gut edema and systemic shunting; tumors and intra-abdominal inflammation may lead to mesenteric venous thrombosis, as can systemic hypoperfusion and hypercoagulable states. Finally, conditions that elevate the gut intraluminal pressure (i.e., intestinal obstruction) or intra-abdominal pressures (abdominal compartment syndrome) may also compromise the critical mucosal blood supply both on the arterial and venous side.

Intestinal *lymphatics* (beginning as capillaries in the villus, draining through submucosal plexus and subserosal lacteals to mesenteric and paravascular lymph nodes, and from there going into the cisterna chyli and thoracic duct) form a pathway for systemic shunting of bacteria and inflammatory mediators that may play an important role in GI failure.

The *intestinal luminal contents* also are intimately related to the function of the mucosa-submucosal complex. Proximal mucosal injury may result from gastric acid, pancreatic enzymes, and bile contents. Distally, the amount of bacterial colonization increases (stomach and proximal intestine are essentially free of bacteria, but the bacterial count increases to 10^9 in the terminal ileum and 10^{11}/g feces in the colon), and injury may result from toxic waste products and bacterial endotoxins and exotoxins. The balance between different enteric bacterial species that prevent overgrowth of a particular pathogen and invasive infection may be disturbed by the use of (enteral or parenteral) antibiotics, intraluminal stasis (obstruction, blind loop), gut ischemia, and global immunosuppression (human immunodeficiency virus, steroids, diabetes, malnutrition). These complex anatomic and physiologic relationships between aggressive and defensive factors may explain why GI failure is commonly associated with critical illness.

CLINICAL PRESENTATION

To evaluate a patient with GI failure, one must always first obtain a detailed history and physical examination, paying particular attention to the sequence, duration, and quality of signs and symptoms related to the GI tract. The clinician must inquire about previous GI related problems, abdominal operations, and the patient's family history. It is equally important to search for evidence of extraintestinal disease and drugs that might cause secondary GI failure. Finally, systemic complications of GI fail-

ure (volume loss, electrolyte abnormalities, anemia, infection, malnutrition) must be recognized early and treatment often begun before completion of the sometimes time-consuming diagnostic workup of a specific problem.

The *signs and symptoms of GI failure* depend, to a certain degree, on the underlying disease process but ultimately reflect the disturbed transport, digestive, absorptive, mucosal barrier, and immune surveillance functions of the intestine. Disturbance of one function may cause alteration of the others, and systemic illness and GI failure are intimately related. Therefore, in most circumstances, GI failure results in a mixed clinical picture.

Disturbance of the transport function may result from drugs, or from intrinsic GI or extraintestinal disease. It may lead to increased transit times (ileus, obstruction) with accumulation of luminal contents, resulting in intestinal dilatation, increased luminal pressure (decreased mucosal perfusion), and bacterial overgrowth. Presenting signs and symptoms of this type of dysfunction include nausea, vomiting, obstipation, alteration of bowel sounds, abdominal distention, and pain. Altered transport may also lead to a more rapid transit with increased frequency and volume of stools (diarrhea), as well as altered consistency and composition (fat, mucus, blood). *Disturbance of the digestive and absorptive process* may result from these transport abnormalities, or from primary enterocyte dysfunction or abnormalities related to the gut-associated glandular organs (hepatobiliary and pancreatic disease). GI failure, however, is most commonly due to the disruption of gut mucosal integrity by inflammation and ischemia. This dysfunction results in an increased distal luminal solute load, which, in conjunction with bacterial fermentation, may lead to further mucosal irritation, increased secretion of mucus, and alteration of bowel motility with flatulence, foul-smelling stools, and diarrhea.

Any process that interferes with mucosal perfusion and integrity may lead to *erosion* (peptic, inflammatory, ischemic) of the mucosal surface. This may lead to pain, ulceration, bleeding (acute and chronic, occult or overt), and perforation (with intra-abdominal contamination, peritonitis, or abscess). Finally, loss of mucosal integrity and barrier function by any of the aforementioned mechanisms may lead to *translocation* of bacteria and toxins with activation of both local and systemic immune mechanisms (Fig. 34–2). Some degree of translocation occurs in otherwise healthy individuals with normal gut flora after elective GI (and other) surgeries, trauma, and thermal injuries. The increase in gut mucosal permeability seems to be correlated with the magnitude of mucosal insult and overall systemic performance. A more severe initial injury or superimposed secondary insult (e.g., hypotension, sepsis, abdominal compartment syndrome), as well as the addition of intestinal luminal factors (dilatation, bacterial overgrowth, lack of intestinal nutrition), leads to more extensive translocation. Resulting local infections (peritonitis, peritoneal abscess, fistula formation), sepsis, and systemic inflammatory response may lead to multiple organ dysfunction and a high mortality rate.

Almost universally with GI failure there is significant *loss of intravascular volume* (vomiting, diarrhea, and intraluminal, intraperitoneal, or systemic third-space

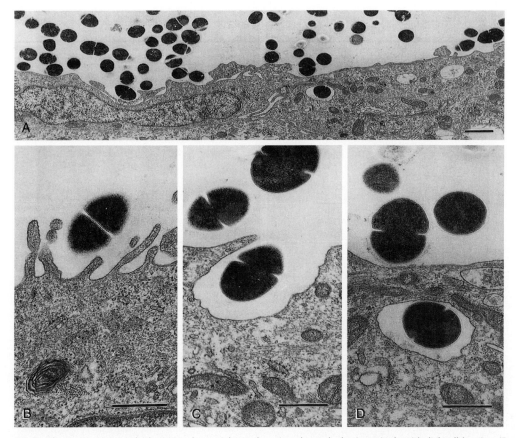

Figure 34–2. Electron micrograph depicting bacterial translocation through the intestinal epithelial cell barrier. (From Olmsted SB, Dunny GM, Erlandsen SL, Wells CL: A plasmid-encoded surface protein on *Enterococcus faecalis* augments its internalization by cultured intestinal epithelial cells. J Infect Dis 1994;170:1549–1556, with permission of the University of Chicago Press.)

losses), electrolyte and acid-base abnormalities, vitamin and trace element deficiencies, and calorie-protein malnutrition with associated anemia, coagulopathy, and susceptibility to infection. Fever and leukocytosis may relate to dehydration, inflammation, infection, or significant tissue ischemia. The severity of these disturbances and their systemic effects are related to host factors (e.g., age, comorbid conditions, immune status) and the duration and severity of the underlying GI process or systemic illness causing secondary GI failure.

All patients with GI failure require basic *laboratory studies,* including serum electrolytes, blood urea nitrogen, creatinine, complete blood count, and coagulation studies. Arterial blood gas analysis and serum lactate should be obtained in more severely ill patients and those who manifest any degree of metabolic acidosis on serum chemistries. The *radiologic workup* (including plain abdominal films, computed tomography, ultrasound, magnetic resonance imaging, angiography) and other specialized studies should be directed by the suspected underlying disease process and potential complications of GI failure.

Endoscopy can be an excellent means of diagnosing problems from the esophagus to the duodenum (esophagogastroduodenoscopy) and from the anus to the terminal ileum (colonoscopy, sigmoidoscopy). It is well suited for the diagnosis of mucosal inflammation and ischemia, as well as intestinal bleeding and obstruction. In the latter two cases, it may serve as a tool for initial or definitive therapy. Endoscopy can also be used to aid a planned operation (localization of lesions by intramural dye injection or intraoperative endoscopy). Great caution should be exerted when using endoscopy in severely inflamed and ischemic bowel, as well as with significant dilatation, because the risk of iatrogenic injury and perforation can be significant.

Gastrointestinal tonometry, a monitoring method that measures indirectly the pH of gastric mucosal cells (intramucosal pH, pHi), has also been used as a diagnostic tool for GI failure. Early studies have documented an intimate relationship between gut mucosal perfusion and overall volume status and cardiovascular performance. Gut mucosal acidosis reflects intestinal hypoperfusion and, in states of volume loss or cardiovascular dysfunction, the need for further resuscitation. There have been no convincing studies, however, that document an improvement in patient outcome when pHi is normalized. More recent studies have determined that pHi is simply a marker of disease (GI failure) and concluded that the routine use of gastric tonometry cannot be supported at the present time. The future development of newer probes and sites of measurement at easy to reach locations (sublingual, rectal) may make tonometry a more universally useful tool.

PREOPERATIVE MANAGEMENT

All patients with GI failure require aggressive *supportive therapy* to correct the significant volume losses, electrolyte and acid-base disturbances, anemia, and coagulopathy that are commonly present. In fact, restoration of intravascular volume and adequate cardiac flow (tissue oxygen delivery) is one of the single most important factors required throughout the therapy of GI failure. Longerstanding or more severe GI failure, especially in the elderly patient with significant comorbid conditions, should lead to transfer to an *intensive care environment.* Invasive cardiovascular monitoring with arterial, central venous, or pulmonary artery catheters may guide volume resuscitation and the need for inotropic support, especially in patients with significant cardiopulmonary disease or sepsis.

More recently, noninvasive methods of measuring preload and cardiac output (transesophageal hemodynamic monitor) are available for real-time comprehensive hemodynamic monitoring. This noninvasive method uses a transesophageal probe that houses an ultrasound transducer that measures the cross-sectional diameter and velocity of the descending aorta, and provides estimates of cardiac output, total systemic vascular resistance, aortic stroke volume, and peak velocity of aortic blood flow.

Critically ill patients are particularly susceptible to mesenteric ischemia related to multiple risk factors, which are common (Table 34–1). The evaluation of abdominal pain in intensive care patients should include a careful assessment of the patient's risk for mesenteric ischemia syndromes, and diagnostic evaluation (colonoscopy, angiography) should be initiated early in these patients (Fig. 34–3). Early appropriate intervention (including anticoagulation, fibrinolytic or vasodilator therapy, embolectomy, and methods to improve cardiac output) may result in salvage of bowel that is at risk for ischemia

| Table 34–1 | **Risk Factors for Mesenteric Ischemia** |

Visceral Arterial Thrombosis

Risk factors or overt manifestations of coronary artery, peripheral vascular, or cerebrovascular disease (e.g., age, male gender, smoking, hypertension, diabetes, hypercholesteremia)

Visceral Arterial Embolism

Atrial fibrillation, s/p myocardial infarction
Cardiac thrombus (e.g., ventricular aneurysm, mural thrombus)
Paradox embolism with deep venous thrombosis
Aortic aneurysmal and ulcerating arteriosclerotic disease
Hypercoaguable state (e.g., history of recent venous thorombosis, previous arterial embolization, known antithrombin III, protein C or S deficiency, dysfibrinogenemia)

Mesenteric Venous Thrombosis

Hypercoaguable states
Abdominal inflammation or sepsis, abdominal malignancy

Nonocclusive Mesenteric Ischemia

Cardiogenic or septic shock, hypovolemia, use of inotropes
Cardiopulmonary bypass
Abdominal compartment syndrome (e.g., trauma, laparotomy, massive resuscitation, hepatic ascites)

s/p, status post.

and prevent the need for massive enterectomy and resultant short gut syndrome in these patients.

Endotracheal intubation and mechanical ventilation are commonly required in patients with GI failure, to protect patients with altered mental status, protracted vomiting, respiratory failure, or shock. Furthermore, blood loss must be replaced and coagulation deficits quickly corrected in patients with acute GI hemorrhage.

With evidence of systemic infection, empirical *parenteral broad-spectrum antibiotic coverage* should begin immediately after cultures (blood, urine, sputum, and stool as indicated) have been obtained. The antibiotic regimen should cover the most common aerobic and anaerobic enteric pathogens. Consideration should also be given to antibiotic coverage of more resistant nosocomial pathogens if the patient had been hospitalized for more than a few days. Once a specific focus of infection has been identified, the antibiotic therapy should be tailored to the culture results.

Patients with GI failure should initially be kept NPO (given nothing by mouth). *Intestinal decompression* via a nasogastric tube may be necessary with recurrent emesis or significant intestinal dilation. Although gastric decompression is effective for the proximal intestine, it may be incomplete with intestinal ileus and distal intestinal obstruction. The use of prolonged preoperative decompression or long enteral tubes in this setting is controversial.

Most critically ill patients require *stress ulcer prophylaxis* as part of the supportive regimen. Patients with respiratory failure and coagulopathy are at highest risk for clinically important GI bleeding. There is significant controversy as to whether H_2-antagonists, proton-pump inhibitors, or antacids should be used to raise the intragastric pH to levels greater than 4.5 to 5, because this has been documented to cause increased proximal GI bacterial colonization and nosocomial pneumonia rates. Gastric mucosal protective therapy with sucralfate can be administered as an alternative, but it is associated with a significantly higher rate of clinically important GI bleeding in critically ill patients. Proton-pump inhibitors are currently available only in oral formulation and may not be adequately absorbed in patients with GI failure. An intravenous formulation of a proton-pump inhibitor is currently undergoing clinical trial and in the future may be the optimal stress ulcer prophylaxis therapy in critically ill patients with GI failure.

Finally, once a specific diagnosis has been established, *nonoperative treatment modalities* directed at the underlying process may be available to manage the patient (e.g., endoscopic decompression of sigmoid volvulus or hemostasis of GI bleeding, percutaneous drainage of infected intra-abdominal fluid collections, thrombolysis of vascular thromboembolism). If patients with GI failure require surgical intervention, consideration should be given to performance of a gentle preoperative *bowel preparation* (mechanical or antibiotic) in an attempt to decrease the risk of postoperative surgical site infections.

INTRAOPERATIVE MANAGEMENT

The decision to operate must be individualized for each patient. The components of GI failure most frequently

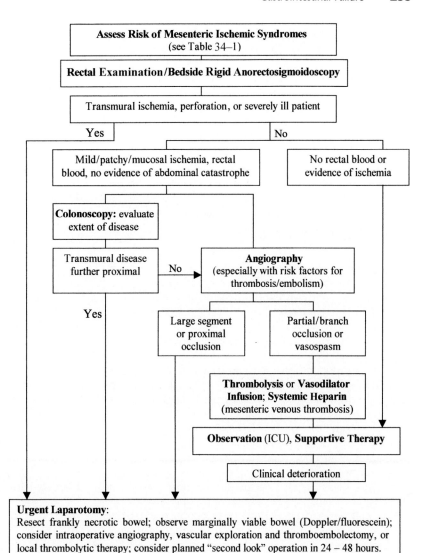

Figure 34–3. Algorithm for diagnostic evaluation of mesenteric ischemia.

requiring surgical intervention are intestinal obstruction, GI bleeding, severe inflammation, intestinal ischemia or gangrene, and perforation. In the operating room, it is essential that communication be established between the surgeon and anesthesiologist, operative nurses, and ancillary staff (e.g., radiology technician) about the planned procedure.

The choice of incision depends on the underlying problem and planned procedure. In most operations for GI failure there is some degree of intra-abdominal inflammation, adhesions, and friable bowel. It is *important to proceed carefully* to avoid unnecessary loss of intestine or injury of other abdominal structures. Extensive adhesiolysis should be avoided to relieve a defined obstruction because it increases the risk for iatrogenic injury and recurrent obstruction. In certain *inflammatory conditions* (e.g., Crohn's disease), obstructions might be relieved by stricturoplasty rather than resection. In some cases (e.g., severe diverticulitis), proximal diverting intestinal decompression (enterostomy–mucous fistula) allows bowel rest, and antibiotic or anti-inflammatory therapy resolves extensive inflammation and reduces the extent of necessary resection. With *bowel ischemia,* careful intraoperative

evaluation (inspection, palpation, Doppler, fluorescein, and Wood's lamp) and preservation of all viable bowel is essential.

When questions about the viability of intestinal segments arise, it may be best to limit the initial operation to controlling overt bleeding, mending perforation, and removing frankly necrotic tissue. The patient is then stabilized in the intensive care unit and returned to the operating room in 24 to 72 hours for a planned "second look," to reevaluate intestinal viability and complete the operation. This concept of *"damage control"* may be applied to all operations for GI failure and severely ill patients. The underlying principle is to quickly define and treat the cause or complication of GI failure that is fueling the patient's critical illness, while avoiding additional extensive operative insults and any unnecessary loss of intestine. Similarly, deciding between primary anastomosis and diversion after resections for GI failure, the bowel to be anastomosed must be well perfused, free from gross disease, and allow tension-free anastomosis. In case of marginal viability of the intestinal segment, severe patient illness (hypotension, hypothermia, coagulopathy), significant intraperitoneal contamination, unprepared bowel, and significant caliber difference, consideration should be given to a primary diverting procedure with delayed anastomosis.

A growing body of literature is demonstrating the negative effects of increased abdominal compartment pressures on intestinal perfusion and multiple organ dysfunction. Consideration should be given to delaying fascial abdominal closure (open packing, Ioban composite dressing, or temporary mesh closure) when there is a chance of significant intra-abdominal swelling (e.g., massive resuscitation, significant gut ischemia or inflammation, coagulopathy) or a need for a second-look operation.

POSTOPERATIVE MANAGEMENT

Postoperative management focuses primarily on supportive therapy with volume resuscitation, cardiovascular and respiratory support, antibiotic therapy, and correction of anemia and coagulopathy. Stress ulcer prophylaxis should be maintained. Whenever possible *enteral nutrition should be instituted as early as possible.* Intestinal mucosal epithelial cells (enterocytes) require enteral luminal nutrients for maturation and replication. There is substantial evidence that early enteral nutrition decreases gut mucosal atrophy, improves barrier function, and reduces bacterial translocation. Enteral nutrition, by contributing to maintaining the proper luminal milieu of nutrients and bacteria, GI hormone release, and gut-hepatic axis function, has also been shown to reduce septic complications and multiple organ dysfunction in surgical patients.

On the other hand, total parenteral nutrition should be considered early with evidence of preoperative malnutrition and anticipated periods of intolerance to enteral nutrition of greater than 14 days. Absolute indications for total parenteral nutrition include short gut syndrome, high-output enterocutaneous fistula, complete bowel obstruction, and severe malabsorption. Even in these cases, however, consideration should be given to the supplementation of small amounts of (iso-osmolar, elemental) enteral nutrition to support the intestinal epithelium whenever possible.

There is a growing body of literature that suggests that immunonutrition (enteral nutrition supplemented with certain nutrients, such as arginine, glutamine, omega-3 fatty acids, and nucleotides) may play an important role in enhancing intestinal integrity and supporting overall immune function and wound healing. Numerous studies have documented that the use of immunonutrition in trauma and critically ill patients results in improved outcomes, decreased length of stay, and significant reductions in infectious complications.

Patients with GI failure, systemic inflammatory response, and multiple organ dysfunctions often are first seen in a hypermetabolic or catabolic state and their ability to process nutrients may be severely altered by sepsis or renal or hepatic dysfunction. Careful monitoring of nutritional adequacy (wound healing, weight gain, serial serum prealbumin or transferring concentrations, nitrogen balance) in these patients is important. Accurate determination of caloric requirements by indirect calorimetry is recommended in critically ill patients to provide

adequate nutritional support, adjust for proper nutrient composition, and prevent underfeeding or overfeeding.

OUTCOMES

The short-term outcomes in the surgery for GI failure are dependent on several factors. The severity, extent, and nature of the GI disease, host factors (e.g., age, comorbid conditions, nutritional, and immune status), and the timeliness of supportive care all influence the incidence of secondary complication, systemic inflammatory response, and multiple organ dysfunctions. Comprehensive modern intensive care with cardiovascular and protective pulmonary support, prevention and aggressive therapy of infections, and nutritional support has decreased short-term mortality rates in these critically ill patients.

One potential complication of massive enterectomy in patients with ischemic bowel, necrotizing enterocolitis, or midgut volvulus is short gut syndrome. These patients generally require long-term parenteral nutritional support and cannot tolerate enteral nutrition secondarily to loss of intestinal absorptive area. The common complications of short gut syndrome include infection, malnutrition, and hepatic dysfunction. Recent advances, using a regimen of high-dose glutamine and growth hormone, have resulted

---

Pearls and Pitfalls

PEARLS

- Comprehensive knowledge of intestinal anatomy and physiology is needed in order to understand the functions of the gut mucosal barrier.

Symptoms of GI Failure

- Disturbance of transport function
- Disturbance of digestive/absorptive process
- Erosion of mucosal surface (pain, ulceration, bleeding, perforation)
- Translocation of bacteria and toxins, resulting in infection
- Loss of intravascular volume as a result of diarrhea, emesis, fistulas

Diagnosis and Treatment May Require

- Laboratory studies
- Radiologic studies
- Endoscopy
- Surgery

PITFALLS

- Neglect of supportive therapy to correct significant hypovolemia, electrolyte and acid-base disturbance, and coagulopathy
- Improper assessment of intensive care unit patients manifesting abdominal pain, a sign of risk of mesenteric ischemia
- Failure to tailor treatment to individual case and to take careful consideration of nonoperative and operative treatment modalities for specific etiology of GI failure

in successful conversion to partial or complete enteral nutritional support in patients with short gut syndrome.

Patients with significant GI failure may not return to their previous functional state and may require prolonged rehabilitation. Recent studies have shown that SIP (Sickness Impact Profile) scores as a measure of functional performance may not return to baseline for as long as a year after critical illness. Long-term results are mainly dependent on the amount of functional GI tract left, residual organ dysfunction (renal, hepatic, pulmonary), and the patient's age and preexisting comorbid conditions.

SELECTED READINGS

Beale RJ, Bryg DJ, Bihari DJ: Immunonutrition in the critically ill: A systematic review of clinical outcome. Crit Care Med 1999;27:2799.

Bower RH, Cerra FB, Bershadsky B, et al: Early enteral administration of a formula (Impact) supplemented with arginine, nucleotides, and fish oil in intensive care unit patients: Results of a multicenter, prospective, randomized, clinical trial. Crit Care Med 1995;23:436.

Cook D, Guyatt G, Marshall J, et al: A comparison of sucralfate and ranitidine for the prevention of upper gastrointestinal bleeding in patients requiring mechanical ventilation. N Engl J Med 1998;338:791.

Galban C, Montejo JC, Mesejo A, et al: An immune-enhancing diet reduces mortality rate and episodes of bacteremia in septic intensive care unit patients. Crit Care Med 2000;29:643.

Gomersall CD, Joynt GM, Freebairn RC: Resuscitation of critically ill patients based on the results of gastric tonometry: A prospective, randomized, controlled trial. Crit Care Med 2000;28:607.

Kirton OC, Civetta JM: Splanchnic flow and resuscitation. In Civetta JM, Taylor K, Kirby R (eds): Critical Care, 3rd ed. Philadelphia, Lippincott-Raven, 1996, pp 443–455.

Lemaire LC, van Lanschot JJ, Stoutenbeek CP, et al: Bacterial translocation in multiple organ failure: Cause or epiphenomenon still unproven. Br J Surg 1997;84:1340.

Liebermann MD, Shou J, Torres AS, et al: Effects of nutrient substrates on immune function. Nutrition 1990;6:88.

Napolitano LM, Bochicchio G: Enteral feeding of the critically ill. Curr Opin Crit Care 2000;6:136.

O'Boyle CJ, MacFie J, Mitchell CJ, et al: Microbiology of bacterial translocation in humans. Gut 1998;42:29.

Rowlands BJ, Gardiner KR: Nutritional modulation of gut inflammation. Proc Nutr Soc 1998;57:395.

Saggi BH, Sugerman HJ, Ivatury RR, Bloomfield GL: Abdominal compartment syndrome [review]. J Trauma 1998;45:597.

Sanchez-Garcia M, Prieto A, Trjedor A, et al: Characteristics of thoracic duct lymph in multiple organ dysfunction syndrome. Arch Surg 1997;132:13.

Swank GM, Deitch EA: Role of the gut in multiple organ failure: Bacterial translocation and permeability changes. World J Surg 1996;20:411.

Upperman JS, Deitch EA, Guo W, et al: Post-hemorrhagic shock mesenteric lymph is cytotoxic to endothelial cells and activates neutrophils. Shock 1998;10:407.

Wells CL, VandeWesterlo EM, Jechorek RP, et al: Effect of hypoxia on enterocyte endocytosis of enteric bacteria. Crit Care Med 1996;24:985.

Wells CL, Jechorek RP, Gillingham KJ: Relative contributions of host and microbial factors in bacterial translocation. Arch Surg 1991;126:247.

Wilmore DW, Byrne TA, Persinger RL: Short bowel syndrome: New therapeutic approaches. Curr Probl Surg 1997;34:398.

Zelenock GB: Visceral occlusive disease. In Greenfield L, Mulholland M, Oldham K, et al (eds): Surgery: Scientific Principles and Practice, 2nd ed. Philadelphia, Lippincott-Raven, 1996, pp 1764–1780.

Chapter 35

Diabetes Mellitus and Diabetes Insipidus

Timothy L. Pruett

Polyuria can be perplexing in the critical care unit. Effective patient management requires accuracy of diagnosis and effective intervention. Surgical and trauma patients commonly have endocrinologic disorders at the root of their polyuria, in particular relative or absolute deficiencies of insulin or vasopressin. To prevent serious deterioration, prompt recognition and initiation of therapy is needed.

CLINICAL PRESENTATION

The surgical patient is often a fluid and perfusion challenge. In the surgical setting, the root cause of polyuria can sometimes be obscure and multifactorial. An essential early evaluation is to determine the likely cause of the excessive urine formation, either an osmotic induced diuresis or a failure of renal concentration of urine.

Diabetes Mellitus

In the surgical setting, the classic signs of polydipsia, polyuria with subsequent identification of glycosuria, can be obscured by the traumatic or surgical events that are more pressing. Knowledge that the patient is dependent on insulin (or an oral agent) to maintain metabolic control clearly triggers suspicion that polyuria is related to a relative or absolute insulin deficiency. Failure to recognize abnormalities in glucose homeostasis leads to serious physiologic consequences. The significant elevation of blood glucose induces an osmotic diuresis, leading to hyperosmolality, hypoperfusion, hemoconcentration, and urinary loss of sodium, potassium, magnesium, and phosphorus. In some elderly patients, hyperosmolar coma can be the consequence. In surgical patients, hyperglycemia is often confounded by other events, such as hyperosmolar feedings, drugs (steroids), or volume replacement fluids.

In addition to problems associated with reduced intravascular volume, the consequences of impaired glucose metabolism can lead to a significant metabolic acidosis (with compensation through abnormally deep, rapid pattern of *Kussmaul's respirations*), electrolyte abnormalities (with impaired cardiac rate and function), and increased osmolality (with changes in mental status). In surgical patients, ventilatory control and anesthesia may mask these classic clinical patterns.

Diabetes Insipidus

Failure of the kidney to concentrate urine can come from either central nervous system interruption of vasopressin release (central diabetes insipidus) or failure of the kidney to respond to vasopressin (nephrogenic diabetes insipidus). The most common form confronting the surgeon is either post-traumatic or postoperative central diabetes insipidus. In the setting of the head-injured patient, prodigious amounts of dilute urine can be made. It is not uncommon for the urine output to exceed 1000 mL/hr. Depending on the amounts and types of replacement fluids, changes in osmolality follow. The classic clinical picture of hypotonic polyuria with excessive thirst is predicated on an ability of the patient to consume free water to compensate for the fluid and electrolyte loss. In the surgical setting, this typically does not occur. The clinical setting of a patient with a head injury or surgery, in whom polyuria subsequently develops, leads one to suspect central diabetes insipidus.

PATHOGENESIS

Diabetes Mellitus

Blood glucose homeostasis is the product of a plethora of hormonal, activity, environmental, and dietary interactions. In the surgical setting, glucose-containing intravenous fluids are commonly used. The effect of surgical or traumatic stress renders a relative resistance to the effect of insulin. In the acutely injured patient, the stress of the event may be sufficient to trigger the relative insulin resistance. In a hospitalized patient, the development of significant increases in the insulin requirement is often the consequence of a process such as nosocomial infection or pancreatitis. Treatment of the insulin resistance is difficult without simultaneously addressing the underlying event.

The mechanisms of this relative insulin resistance include impairment of insulin stimulation of glucose transport across cellular membranes and changes of gluconeogenesis related to catecholamines and corticosteroids. Hyperglycemia requiring modest amounts of insulin therapy is common in the perioperative patient. This transient requirement for exogenous insulin does not predict a subsequent dependency on exogenous insulin. However, severe hyperglycemia can easily develop in the patient with baseline relative or absolute insulin deficiency after surgical stress. An obligate diuresis occurs when the transport threshold for glucose of the renal tubule is exceeded. If not recognized and corrected, significant hyperosmolality and intravascular volume loss can occur, resulting in hypoperfusion and mental status changes.

In a minority of cases, the deficit of insulin is associated with a relative or absolute increase in glucagon concentration and results in diabetic ketoacidosis. This clinical syndrome is the combination of (1) severe hyperglycemia and volume contraction as noted earlier and (2) the activation of the ketogenic state with the attendant overproduction of ketones by the liver. Ketosis occurs when free fatty acids are released from peripheral stores and are *not* significantly re-esterified within the liver and stored or sent back into the circulation as very low density lipoproteins, but rather are oxidized within the liver. Glucagon is the primary agent controlling the accelerated hepatic oxidation of fatty acids through at least two mechanisms. It appears to have a direct action on the carnitine palmitoyltransferase enzyme system. This enzyme system facilitates the entry of fatty acids into the hepatic mitochondria where β-oxidation occurs and ketone bodies are produced. The second mechanism for inducing ketosis is through a reduction of malonyl-coenzyme A, with a subsequent increase of carnitine within the liver. This results in the activation of carnitine acyltransferase and increased ketogenesis.

The clinical consequences of the hyperglycemia and ketogenesis are significant. Volume contraction varies depending on the duration of the diuresis and the attentiveness to volume replacement. In the typical medical patient with diabetic ketoacidosis, a fluid deficit in excess of 3 to 5 L is usually assumed. The diuresis is associated with significant loss of body electrolytes, particularly sodium, potassium, phosphates, and magnesium. Hypertonicity is virtually always the consequence of increased plasma glucose concentrations. Because of the associated hyperlipidemia, calculated serum osmolality can be misleading, making a measured osmolality more reliable. Metabolic acidosis follows the accelerated ketogenesis and the accumulation of acetoacetate and β-hydroxybutyrate within the blood. Acidosis can be profound with pH less than 7.0. The consequence of the acidosis can result in significant elevations in the serum potassium, despite a total body deficit of several hundred milliequivalents.

Diabetes Insipidus

Vasopressin facilitates the concentration of urine through the V_2 receptor of the principal cell of the renal conducting duct. Flow of water from the lumen of the duct into the medulla is enhanced. In addition, through an effect on the thick limb of the ascending loop of Henle, increased sodium absorption and urea permeability is affected.

Vasopressin is synthesized in the anterior hypothalamus as a preprohormone, converted to a prohormone that is stored within secretory granules, and transported along axonal pathways to the posterior pituitary. There, under varying control, the prohormone is cleaved and vasopressin is released into the circulation. The control upon vasopressin release is multiple. The primary stimulus for vasopressin release is a change in plasma osmolality. These receptors reside within the hypothalamus. In addition, stretch receptors in the left atrium respond to blood volume changes and baroreceptors within the ca-

rotid and aorta effect vasopressin release in response to hypotension. Under more normal conditions, osmolality is the dominant stimulus. However, in the case of severe hypotension, the baroreceptor response may counterbalance the osmolality effect and stimulate vasopressin release and override a simultaneous inhibitory stimulus. A variety of drugs alter vasopressin release, but typically not to the extent to cause serious clinical problems.

Diabetes insipidus can be classified as central (four types) or nephrogenic. Unless a patient is admitted with a known abnormality of hyporesponsiveness to vasopressin, the majority of cases confronting the surgeon will be the consequence of traumatic or surgical disruption of central vasopressin release. For the surgical patient without the ability to drink, unrecognized diabetes insipidus can lead to severe dehydration, tachycardia, weakness, mental status changes, fever, vascular collapse, and death. Electrolyte abnormalities are proportional to the mismatch of fluid replacement to urinary losses. If there is no stimulus to drink and no fluids are replaced, such as occurs with a hypothalamic injury, severe hypernatremia results. Even in observed patients with head injury, mismatch of amounts and concentrations of sodium replacement can result in serious hypernatremia. It is not uncommon to find serum sodium concentrations in excess of 170 mEq/L in patients with diabetes insipidus, who eventually become organ donors. In the typical patient who is cared for by a surgeon, the kidney responds to the effects of therapeutically administered vasopressin (analogues).

DIAGNOSIS

The clinical finding of polyuria (defined as urine output greater than 30 mL/kg per 24 hours) requires some investigation. Within the acute care setting, clinical assessment of injury and underlying disease conditions in combination with easily available laboratory tests (serum electrolytes, glucose, arterial pH, urinalysis) will quickly guide to therapy.

Diabetes Mellitus

Hyperglycemia, usually in excess of 500 mg/dL, is associated with significant glycosuria. The urine contains significant concentration of glucose with a significant specific gravity. This can lead to the significant volume contraction and prerenal azotemia. This can further lead to hypoperfusion and a modest amount of lactic acidosis, but the major cause of the anion gap acidosis in diabetic ketoacidosis is the high concentration of serum acetoacetate and β-hydroxybutyrate. Because the routine serum ketone strip assays are not quantitative, it is necessary to perform serial dilutions to estimate the severity of the ketosis and to monitor therapy.

Starvation can induce a ketotic state, but it does not cause an anion gap and the serum ketone strip assay typically turns negative with one dilution. The only other significant disease process, which a surgeon should seriously entertain within the differential diagnosis, is alcoholic ketoacidosis. The condition occurs in chronic alcoholic patients (typically after a binge, but may be delayed for more than a day from the last drink) after a period of starvation. The frequent association with abdominal pain, vomiting, and pancreatitis may bring the surgeon into consultation. There may be a severe ketotic anion gap acidosis associated with high levels of serum lipids. It is rare that the serum glucose concentration exceeds 250 to 300 mg/dL and, in most patients, blood glucose measurements are less than 150 mg/dL. This is the only serious discriminatory finding with diabetic ketoacidosis (other than history) allowing for differentiation. The treatment of alcoholic ketoacidosis is glucose and volume replacement, without the need for exogenous insulin.

Diabetes Insipidus

The clinical diagnosis of diabetes insipidus is the most suggestive in the setting of hypotonic (low specific gravity, less than 1.010, and osmolality less than 250 mOsm) polyuria in combination with head trauma. In this setting, one must differentiate iatrogenic water intoxication from the true diabetes insipidus condition of lack of vasopressin regulation of urinary solute concentration. Assessment of urine and serum osmolality will suggest whether hypotonic diuresis is appropriate. Maintenance of vascular volume and physiologic concentrations of serum sodium is important. Monitoring of central vascular pressures and cardiac output helps facilitate assessment of vascular volume. In true posttraumatic diabetes insipidus, administration of 5 U of vasopressin produces a significant reduction of urine output with increased osmolality. If the vascular volume is adequate and water intoxication is entertained, then slowly decreasing volume replacement in combination with normal saline infusion allows for normalization of serum electrolytes. With significant hyponatremia (<120 mEq/L) or rapid decreases in serum sodium concentrations, replacement with hypertonic saline may be necessary to prevent or treat the neurologic, muscular, or cardiac sequelae. Other causes of hypotonic polyuria, such as psychogenic polydipsia and drug-induced diabetes insipidus, are not commonly seen by the surgeon. Differentiation of solute-induced polyuria is necessary, but typically a high urine specific gravity (>1.020) suggests an osmotic diuresis.

TREATMENT

The goals of therapy for the surgical patient are reconstitution and maintenance of intravascular volume and tissue perfusion and correction of abnormalities of the physiologic state. The methods of therapy are significantly different in these two diseases.

Diabetes Mellitus

Plasma Volume

The volume status in the surgical patient can be variable. Depending on the vigilance of the observation and replacement of urinary losses, the intravascular volume may be depleted minimally or by several liters. Isotonic expansion of a contracted plasma volume should be expeditiously performed. The need to stop the obligate solute diuresis requires more or less insulin depending on the extent of ketogenesis. Patients with hyperosmolar coma without ketosis need rapid isotonic volume expansion and small amounts of insulin to control blood glucose after the plasma volume has been reconstituted. In diabetic patients with ketosis, therapeutic amounts of insulin are required in addition to plasma expansion. However, in this setting, the ultimate goal of insulin therapy is not the normalization of blood glucose, but stopping ketogenesis. In fact, normalization of blood glucose levels commonly occurs *before* ketosis is cleared. After plasma volume has been reconstituted, it is important to give the patient free water to allow the reconstitution of the normal osmotic condition.

Insulin Therapy

Insulin therapy is given to counteract the effects of glucagon and to stop ketogenesis. Insulin should be administered intravenously until the episode of ketoacidosis is eradicated. Although there is no universal dose, an initial bolus of 20 to 50 U of insulin, followed by a continuous insulin infusion of 10 to 20 U/hr is reasonable. If acidosis persists or worsens early in therapy, additional boluses of insulin should be used to achieve the therapeutic goals. It is crucial to monitor the effect of therapy by following pH and anion gap and by assessing serum ketones by dilution positivity. The latter can stabilize or "worsen" in the face of improving anion gap, because the ketone strips measure only acetoacetate efficiently. Although the total ketone concentration may decrease, the dilution measurement can appear to remain stable or increase as β-hydroxybutyrate is converted to acetoacetate. As the ketosis is cleared, the serum ketone dilutions and the pH and anion gap become more congruent. One should continue intravenous insulin infusion until the anion gap is normal, the pH is normal, and the serum is negative for ketones. As noted earlier, blood glucose levels may normalize before the correction of ketoacidosis, necessitating the administration of glucose-containing intravenous fluids. As a general principle, the surgical patient should be given glucose-containing fluids when the serum glucose has decreased to 300 to 350 mg/dL. Fluid replacement should match volume losses after euvolia is achieved and with an electrolyte composition to maintain or obtain physiologic blood concentrations.

Acidosis

There has been considerable debate regarding the utility of sodium bicarbonate administration for patients with severe acidosis (pH <7.10). There does not appear to be any specific benefit for patients with a pH between 6.9 and 7.1. Concerns of cardiac dysfunction and arrhythmias with pH less than 6.9 may warrant bicarbonate therapy. The concern about administering bicarbonate to this type of patient is the development of metabolic alkalosis with the conversion of the ketones into bicarbonate.

Electrolytes

Potassium replacement is always required in the treatment of diabetic ketoacidosis. The timing of its administration is the only issue. With severe metabolic acidosis, a significant hyperkalemia can be present despite a severe total body deficit. With insulin therapy, potassium is transported intracellularly with glucose. In combination with the correction of the acidosis, the serum potassium also decreases. If neglected, severe hypokalemia can result, with the attendant cardiac and muscular disturbances. Once it is clear that the acidosis is correcting and the serum potassium is stable and decreasing, addition of potassium salts to replacement fluids is necessary. If severe hypokalemia results (K^+ <2.0 mEq/24 hr), insulin therapy should be stopped while administering 40 mEq of potassium. The type of potassium salt should be chosen as either potassium chloride or potassium phosphate. It is common for this patient population to have a significant total body deficit in *phosphate* as well as potassium and severe hypophosphatemia can occur. Monitoring of serum phosphate concentration facilitates the choice of potassium salt replacement. Serum *magnesium* often decreases as vascular stabilization and ketosis corrects, necessitating the administration of magnesium sulfate.

Osmolality

In young patients, rapid reduction in serum osmolality can result in cerebral edema. This does not appear to be such a significant problem for the adult population, but the prospect of cerebral edema associated with rapid osmolality changes should be recognized.

Diabetes Insipidus

Volume Maintenance

Accurate assessment of volume status is crucial. A combination of physical examination and monitoring devices is useful in this setting. The treatment of water intoxication is gradual depletion of intravascular volume, allowing the correction of serum sodium. In diabetes insipidus, volume loss can be prodigious, making volume replacement challenging. The hypotonic urine and a rapid replacement of intravascular volume can result in significant changes in the serum electrolyte composition. Assessment of urine osmolality and electrolyte composition compared with the serum osmolality and composition helps guide intravenous volume replacement. It is necessary to obtain serial measurements (every 1 to 6 hours) depending on the volume loss and rate of fluid replacement and to adjust fluid replacement accordingly. Change can occur quickly and assumptions of appropriateness of volume replacement strategy may be erroneous.

Vasopressin Replacement

After volume resuscitation has been started, a subcutaneous injection of 5 U of arginine vasopressin confirms the responsiveness of the kidney to the hormone. This is typically manifest by a doubling of the urinary osmolality (UOsm) within several hours. The duration of action of arginine vasopressin is relatively short, being cleared within 3 to 6 hours. If there is a question of early recovery of neurohypophysis or difficulty with hyponatremia and fluid balance, the use of the short-acting agent is desirable. If the diagnosis is clear or the patient is experiencing arrhythmias or hypertension, desmopressin (DDAVP) has a duration of action of 10 to 14 hours in most patients. It can be given either subcutaneously or intravenously (1 to 4 μg). This agent has very few pressor and cardiac rhythm effects (unlike vasopressin), which allows for its intravenous use. Although it can be given through intranasal (5 to 20 μg) application, in the surgical patient with multiple tubes and potential trauma, it is often not practical. In the acute setting, care must be taken to carefully follow the composition of serum electrolytes. With rapid diuresis and volume resuscitation, water intoxication or serious hypernatremia can become problematic without careful monitoring and adjustments. In addition, with rapid volume correction, reductions of serum potassium, phosphate, and magnesium are common.

Hypothalamic-Pituitary Dysfunction

Essential to long-term management is comprehensive understanding of the extent of hypothalamic-pituitary dysfunction. After the patient has been stabilized, thorough radiographic and endocrinologic evaluation is required.

Prompt diagnosis and therapy minimize the risk for the patient with significant diabetes mellitus or diabetes insipidus. Both of these conditions can clinically abate after the surgical stress has resolved, without the need for chronic therapy; however, a long-term condition can ensue. Optimal care involves the integration of medical teams to ensure effective education and management of a potentially chronic problem.

Pearls and Pitfalls

Out-of-Control Diabetes Mellitus

PITFALLS

- Stopping insulin therapy when the blood sugar has normalized and ketosis is ongoing
- Failure to give exogenous glucose to allow the safe administration of insulin
- Failure to recognize the severity of potassium and phosphate deficiency
- Inducing a late metabolic alkalosis by giving bicarbonate to correct the early acidosis

Diabetes Insipidus

PITFALLS

- Inducing severe serum electrolyte abnormalities through rapid volume replacement
- Arrhythmias, hypertension, abdominal pain with the use of aqueous vasopressin

SELECTED READINGS

Atkinson MA, MacLaren NK: The pathogenesis of insulin-dependent diabetes mellitus. N Engl J Med 1994;331:1428.

Bendz H, Aurell M: Drug-induced diabetes insipidus: Incidence, prevention and management. Drug Saf 1999;21:449.

Chen JM, Cullinane S, Spanier TB, et al: Vasopressin deficiency and pressor hypersensitivity in hemodynamically unstable organ donors. Circulation 1999;100(19 suppl):II244.

Cunnah D, Ross G, Besser GM: Management of cranial diabetes insipidus with oral desmopressin (DDAVP). Clin Endocrinol 1986;24:253.

Foster DW: Diabetes mellitus. In Fauci AS, Braunwald E, et al (eds): Harrison's Principles of Internal Medicine, 14th ed. New York, McGraw-Hill, 1998, p 2060.

Foster DW, McGarry JD: The metabolic derangements and treatment of diabetic ketoacidosis. N Engl J Med 1983;309:159.

Hensen J, Henig A, Fahlbush R, et al: Prevalence, predictors and patterns of postoperative polyuria and hyponatremia in the immediate course after transsphenoidal surgery for pituitary adenomas. Clin Endocrinol 1999;59:431.

King LS, Yasui M, Agre P: Aquaporins in health and disease. Mol Med Today 2000;6:60.

Kitabchi AE, Wall BM: Management of diabetic ketoacidosis. Am Fam Physician 1999;60:455.

Laffel L: Ketone bodies: A review of physiology, pathophysiology and application of monitoring to diabetes. Diabetes Metab Res Rev 1999;15:412.

Mahoney CP, Vicek BW, DelAguila M: Risk factors for developing brain herniation during diabetic ketoacidosis. Pediatr Neurol 1999;214:721.

Moses AM: Osmotic thresholds for AVP release using plasma and urine AVP and free water clearance. Am J Physiol 1989;256:R892.

Moses AM, Streeten DHP: Disorders of the neurohypophysis. In Fauci AS, Braunwald E, et al (eds): Harrison's Principles of Internal Medicine, 14th ed. New York, McGraw-Hill, 1998, p 2003.

Robinson AG: dDAVP in treatment of central diabetes insipidus. N Engl J Med 1976;294:507.

Siperstein MD: Diabetic ketoacidosis and hyperosmolar coma. Endocrinol Metab Clin North Am 1992;21:915.

Viallon A, Zeni F, Lafond P, et al: Does bicarbonate therapy improve the management of severe diabetic ketoacidosis? Crit Care Med 1999;27:2690.

Yan SH, Sheu WH, Song YM, Tseng LN: The occurrence of diabetic ketoacidosis in adults. Intern Med 2000;39:10.

Yoshioka T, Sugimoto H, Uenishi M, et al: Prolonged hemodynamic maintenance by the combined administration of vasopressin and epinephrine in brain death: A clinical study. Neurosurgery 1986;8:565.

Chapter 36
Aspiration Pneumonitis

Byron E. Wright and Michael A. West

Since the time of the ancient Greeks, the aspiration of fluids, particulate matter, or both, has been recognized as a dangerous and life-threatening event. Perhaps Anacreon's death after inhaling a seed marked the beginning of the journey to understand, treat, and ultimately prevent this phenomenon. More than 2000 years later, despite all that is known about the etiology and consequences of this condition, death remains a frequent outcome.

The classic description by Mendelson in 1946 of 66 consecutive cases of aspiration in obstetric anesthesia patients was the first to document the association between surgery, anesthesia, decreased levels of consciousness, and this syndrome. In 1975, Bartlett and Gorbach proposed dysphagia, interruption of the gastroesophageal junction, and altered mental status as the "triple threat" of aspiration. Although aspiration was initially recognized as an anesthesia and perioperative complication, it is currently known to occur in a wide variety of clinical settings. This potentially devastating event is a particular concern in the ICU where an ever-increasing number of critically ill patients require long-term enteral and ventilatory support.

ETIOLOGY

Multiple predisposing factors and clinical conditions increase the risk of aspiration. These factors can be placed into one of three categories: (1) conditions of altered mental status, (2) neurogenic alteration of the normally coordinated acts of swallowing and secretion clearance, and (3) structural or functional aerodigestive abnormalities. These factors are summarized in Table 36–1. Aspiration is not an uncommon event. There is a documented incidence of aspiration of gastroesophageal contents in 10% of elective anesthesia cases and the incidence is up to 25% for emergent cases. These aspiration events are clinically significant less than 5% of the time. Aspiration has also been estimated to occur in 30% to 70% of critically ill patients and represents a leading cause of death in this population. Most aspiration events remain clinically silent. In an otherwise healthy individual, these episodes may be of no consequence because the normal defenses of the tracheobronchial tree clear and minimize the aspirate.

Clinical consequences of aspiration include pneumonitis, pneumonia, obstruction, and abscess formation (Table 36–2). Whether an aspiration event produces clinical complications depends on the amount, the pH, the character, and the source of the aspirate. A large number of studies have suggested that the two most important factors are volume and pH. Aspiration rarely produces pneumonitis or acute lung injury unless the aspirate volume exceeds 25 mL and the pH is less than 2.5. Low volume aspirates with a pH greater than 2.5 are not clinically significant. However, another significant factor is the presence of particulate in an aspirate. Knight and colleagues demonstrated a synergistic acute lung injury when both low pH (<2.5) and particulate matter are present in aspirate given in a rat model. Additionally, acute lung injury and pneumonitis was documented by Schwartz and his group when particulate material was present in the aspirate, even at a pH greater than 5.

PATHOPHYSIOLOGY

The precise mechanism of postaspiration lung injury has remained the subject of debate. As noted earlier, the single most important component of injury is parenchymal exposure to acid. Multiple animal studies have confirmed that the lower the pH, the more severe the injury. In the absence of other variables, such as particulate debris, no injury is seen if the pH is greater than 2.5. Although clinical manifestations may become apparent immediately, Knight and colleagues described a biphasic pattern of acute injury. The initial insult is thought to arise as a result of the chemical or acidic exposure. Acid exposure results in local tissue damage with increased basement membrane permeability and associated fluid

Table 36–1	Risk Factors for Aspiration	
ALTERED MENTAL STATUS	**NEUROMUSCULAR ABNORMALITIES**	**AERODIGESTIVE DISEASE**
Anesthesia	Multiple sclerosis	Achalasia
Sedation	Muscular dystrophy	Esophageal dysmotility
Ethanol intoxication	Parkinson's disease	Tracheoesophageal fistula
Head injury	Head injury	Esophageal stricture
Drug overdose	CVA	Esophageal neoplasm
Seizure	Cerebral palsy	Gastroesophageal reflux
Cerebrovascular accident (CVA)		Tumors of the larynx
		Tumors of the oropharynx

Adapted from Shifrin RY, Choplin RH: Aspiration in patients in critical care units. Radiol Clin North Am 1996;34:83–96.

Table 36–2	Pulmonary Complications of Aspiration
	Pneumonitis
	Pneumonia
	Airway obstruction
	Abscess formation
	Empyema
	Adult respiratory distress syndrome

and protein leak. These acute alterations peak approximately 1 hour after exposure to acid.

The second phase of injury is seen 2 to 3 hours after acid exposure and is associated with a neutrophil-mediated acute inflammatory response. This response is maximized at 4 hours. Aspiration injury can be defined and quantitated by measuring an increase in membrane protein permeability. A permeability index (pi) is measured based on leakage of radioactive-labeled albumin across the pulmonary vasculature. The importance of neutrophil-mediated injury in this process was confirmed by following the pi values in animals made neutropenic before acid exposure. The postinjury pi levels in this group of animals were identical to the pi levels seen after the initial phase of injury in animals with normal neutrophil levels. This suggests that the second phase of injury does not occur in the absence of the neutrophil response. Neutrophils induce tissue damage through the release of reactive oxygen species and tissue proteases. Further evidence of oxidative injury by neutrophils came from the demonstration of marked elevation in serine protease activity in lavage samples from acid-induced lung injury in rats. Other studies have established a protective role of protease inhibitors in lung injury models. In contrast, the role of reactive oxygen species in aspiration pneumonitis remains somewhat unclear. Deferoxamine and catalase, both known antioxidants, failed to demonstrate beneficial effects in an acid injury animal model. Subsequent studies using the same antioxidants did demonstrate protection when injured lung was exposed to higher levels of inspired oxygen.

Exposure to acid is highly injurious to the tracheal and bronchial mucosa. A nonparticulate spread of acidic fluid produces a diffuse pattern of injury, whereas aspiration with particulate matter produces a more localized, patchy pattern of disease. Histologically, contact with acid results in absent or damaged type II pneumocytes, increased proliferation of type I pneumocytes, and intense bronchorrhea. The resultant increased capillary permeability also results in interstitial edema and alveolar flooding. Extensive atelectasis develops as a result of obstruction of small airways and increased surface tension from the alveolar flooding. Surfactant loss from damage to type II pneumocytes also contributes to atelectasis. A severe tracheobronchitis is usually seen, with the distribution of inflammation depending on the nature of the aspirate (liquid or particulate). Mucosal damage results in areas of peribronchial hemorrhage and necrosis. A granulocytic infiltrate predominates 2 to 3 hours after the initial injury as neutrophils migrate into the injured area.

Alveolar collapse leads to localized release of vasoconstrictors with a resultant increase in vascular resistance and significant pulmonary shunting. Lung compliance decreases dramatically and severe bronchospasm may result. The presence of particulate matter in the aspirate can produce additional alveolar hypoventilation through obstruction of smaller airways. In addition, if food particles are present in the aspirate, they can induce a foreign body reaction with subsequent monocytic infiltration and eventual granuloma formation. This may set the stage for a chronic inflammatory process in affected areas of the lung.

CLINICAL MANIFESTATIONS

Aspiration of fluids from the stomach, small bowel, or the oropharyngeal pool is a relatively frequent event in a variety of clinical situations. As previously stated, the majority of the episodes are of minimal consequence and do not cause significant symptoms. When the volume, pH, and amount of particulate material in the fluid are sufficient to overwhelm the clearance mechanisms and induce injury, a predictable syndrome results.

The typical clinical picture of aspiration pneumonitis develops quickly. The first signs and symptoms of severe aspiration injury become noticeable within 1 to 2 hours. These include dyspnea, tachypnea, and tachycardia. Some degree of cyanosis along with cough and an audible wheeze may be present as well. Chest auscultation at this time reveals rales, rhonchi, and wheezing. As the pathophysiology of the injury proceeds along the biphasic pattern discussed earlier, clinical manifestations progress accordingly. Respiratory impairment may become severe and even life threatening, necessitating positive pressure ventilation and full ventilatory support. The threat of ongoing aspiration or a lack of airway protection may mandate endotracheal intubation to prevent further exposure and injury.

As progressive pulmonary edema develops, a relative intravascular fluid deficit may exist, resulting in profound hypotension and vasomotor collapse. Ongoing resuscitation is frequently required. Less frequently, a massive aspiration of gastric contents presents with acute bronchospasm, airway obstruction, and acute respiratory failure. Cardiopulmonary collapse and death may rapidly ensue.

Infectious complications related to an aspiration event develop in a significant number of patients. Some type of pleuropulmonary infection develops in approximately 25% to 50% of patients who aspirate gastric contents. Although an acidic gastric aspirate contains very low levels of bacteria, or may even be sterile, the acute injury makes the affected area of lung highly susceptible to secondary bacterial infection. The increased susceptibility to pulmonary infection arises because of fluid stasis, compromised tracheociliary clearance, and overall impaired local tissue immunity.

A large number of critically ill patients receive acid suppression therapy or are on antimicrobials for unrelated issues. These patients frequently have bacterial overgrowth and gastroesophageal colonization. In these patients, aspiration may be heavily contaminated with bacteria, with a resultant primary infection arising much more often as a consequence of the initial event. More frequently, the source of bacterial infection results from the high bacteria counts present in aspirated oropharyngeal, rather than gastric, secretions. For example, quantitative cultures of saliva yield bacteria counts of 10^8 colony-forming units. Under normal, nonhospitalized circumstances, anaerobic bacteria predominate in the oropharynx. Again, patients who are hospitalized, on antimicrobials, or have oropharyngeal or esophageal pathology or other underlying illness are much more likely to have a mixed aerobic and anaerobic oropharyngeal flora. When these patients have an aspiration event, they are more likely to sustain a polymicrobial infection. Infectious complications of aspiration may present as a "simple" pneumonia in this clinical setting but may also progress to parenchymal abscess with necrosis, complicated parapneumonic effusion, or empyema.

Leukocytosis, fever, and radiographic infiltrates are frequently present in patients who are at risk for a significant aspiration event. Thus, these indicators of infection are not reliable. In many instances the clinical course of the patient over the 36- to 48-hour interval after a presumed aspiration is more helpful to make the diagnosis. An increase in the degree of leukocytosis with bandemia, increasing temperatures, and worsening infiltrates are strongly suggestive of infection. Appropriately collected (bronchoalveolar lavage, bronchial brushings) positive tracheobronchial cultures are reliable indicators of an infectious process. In contrast, simple sputum cultures are often misleading in this setting. The primary benefit of a sputum culture may be to help identify an unanticipated pathogen.

Radiographic abnormalities in aspiration pneumonitis are seen frequently. The findings are not specific for the syndrome, nor do they correlate with the severity of the injury. The pattern of lung injury, as well as the radiographic representation of that injury, is dependent on where the aspirate goes. Because aspirate is primarily in liquid form, it tends to settle in the most gravitationally dependent portions of the tracheobronchial tree. Hospitalized patients, in general, and critical care patients, in particular, tend to be in a supine or semisupine position at the time of aspiration. This typically focuses the severity of the injury in the posterior portions of the lung. The superior segment of both lower lobes (B6 segment) is the most dependent portion for supine patients. Because of the less acute angle of the right mainstem bronchus to the trachea compared with the left, the right lung is more frequently involved than the left. Nonetheless, bilateral lung involvement is the rule rather than the exception. In Mendelson's original series, 23% of the 66 cases described had bilateral lung involvement and Landay and colleagues, in 1978, described bilateral infiltrates in 41 of 60 patients. The lower lung fields are much more commonly involved. Most authors agree that infiltrate severity on the initial radiograph bears no correlation to outcome or severity of disease. A worsening pattern of infiltrate 2 to 3 days after the initial event may be indicative of either an evolving pneumonia or the development of adult respiratory distress syndrome.

TREATMENT OPTIONS

Initial management after aspiration should be directed toward optimizing oxygenation and ventilation, preventing further aspiration with appropriate patient positioning, and removing any airway obstruction caused by aspiration of a high amount of particulate matter. If an aspiration event is witnessed, some authors have advocated positioning the patient head down and tilted toward their right side in an attempt to localize the aspirate to a single lobe. However, given the fact that severity of injury seems to correlate well with volume of aspirate, in addition to pH,

it might be more reasonable to minimize this volume with aggressive suctioning and other airway protection maneuvers. As discussed earlier, an occasional patient will aspirate either such a large volume of gastric contents or have such a high amount of particulate matter in the aspirate that severe bronchospasm and airway obstruction result. In this setting, immediate positive pressure ventilation, with or without mechanical ventilation, and bronchoscopy to relieve solid particle airway obstruction are required.

After stabilizing measures have been undertaken, care is largely supportive. Prevention of ongoing aspiration and adequate airway protection are key to avoiding further injury. Daily radiographs early in the hospital course are necessary to monitor for the development of pneumonia, effusions, and adult respiratory distress syndrome. As the pulmonary edema and alveolar flooding of early injury develop, relative intravascular volume deficits may require judicious resuscitation. Some patients, particularly those with underlying cardiac disease, require invasive central venous and pulmonary artery pressure monitoring to appropriately manage the volume status issues that arise.

A long-standing issue in the management of aspiration is the use of corticosteroids. Given the inflammatory nature of the biphasic injury it seems reasonable to suppose that steroids might be of some benefit, but multiple studies have been unable to confirm this. Some authors have even demonstrated a detrimental effect on outcome. Given this lack of data, along with their immunosuppressive effects on an already highly susceptible patient population, there is little current support for their use.

Indicators of infection merit initiation of empirical antimicrobial therapy. Pneumonia occurring as a result of out-of-hospital aspiration events typically involves anaerobic organisms. The most common bacterial isolates in this setting are *Peptostreptococci, Fusobacterium,* and *Bacteroides.* Hospitalized patients have a differing bacteriology. Pleuropulmonary infections related to aspiration in this group are much more likely to involve aerobic, nosocomial pathogens such as *Pseudomonas, Klebsiella,* or *Escherichia coli.* Empirical antibiotics for hospitalized patients should be broad spectrum with good anaerobic and gram-negative aerobic coverage. Second- or third-generation cephalosporins are commonly used in this setting. If primarily anaerobic organisms are suspected, then penicillin or clindamycin are excellent therapy choices. The use of prophylactic antibiotics has failed to result in fewer infectious complications, has not lowered mortality rate, and has not improved outcome.

Optimizing oxygenation is the mainstay of the supportive care. This inevitably involves the use of high levels of supplemental oxygen. The human lung is able to tolerate markedly increased levels of inspired oxygen for up to 24 hours. However, several authors have postulated that in the setting of acute lung injury, the protective mechanisms for clearing radical oxygen species might be significantly compromised, resulting in greater injury over a much shorter period of time from supplemental oxygen. Proper pulmonary toilet, recognition and treatment of infection, drainage of large effusions, use of adequate positive end-expiratory pressure in ventilated patients, and acceptance of reasonably low levels of arterial oxygen tension are key to minimizing the level of supplemental oxygen. Treatment options are summarized in Table 36–3.

OUTCOME

Overall mortality rate after aspiration of gastric contents remains high. Fatality rate estimates range from 20% to 40% and have been as high as 60% in some series. Acute aspiration episodes account for 20% of all anesthesia related deaths and are the leading cause of death in obstetric anesthesia. The majority of patients suffering a significant aspiration event require a period of supportive care, typically 48 to 72 hours, followed by clinical and radiographic resolution of their pneumonitis. A small percentage of patients suffer such a severe initial injury that their course consists of a rapid and progressive decline in pulmonary function, or even death. A final group of patients whose condition is stabilized from the initial injury suffer a secondary complication, such as pneumonia or adult respiratory distress syndrome.

Adverse clinical consequences of aspiration injury tend to be relatively acute and self-limited. Most patients recover without long-term pulmonary impairment. An exception to this is patients who suffer repetitive "silent" aspiration episodes. Recurrent aspiration can induce cumulative chronic inflammatory changes and produce long-term impairment in pulmonary function. In addition, solid particle aspirate can induce chronic inflammatory, granulomatous type changes that can lead to long-term lung impairment.

PREVENTION

Because lung injury occurs and progresses so quickly after an aspiration event, and because risk factors for aspiration in a variety of clinical situations are readily identified, prevention of this complication should be a strong focus of patient care. Critically ill patients possess multiple risk factors for ongoing aspiration. Recumbent positioning, altered mental status, feeding or decompressive tubes across the lower esophageal sphincter, and mechanical vent support via either a tracheostomy or endotracheal tube all heavily predispose such patients to episodes of aspiration. Complicating matters further, the underlying pathology of these patients worsens their outcome if a significant aspiration takes place.

The most effective therapy for aspiration is prevention. Preventive measures include use of protective intubation

Table 36–3	**Management Summary for Aspiration Injury**

USE	AVOID
Preventive measures	Corticosteroids
Pulmonary toilet	Prophylactic antibiotics
Positive pressure ventilation	High level supplemental O_2
Fluid resuscitation	Ongoing aspiration
Bronchoscopy (consider)	
Empirical antibiotics	

Pearls and Pitfalls

PEARLS

- Altered mental status, alteration of coordinated swallowing and secretion clearance, and structural aerodigestive abnormalities increase the risk of aspiration.
- Aspiration occurs in 30% to 70% of all critically ill patients and accounts for significant morbidity and mortality in this population.
- The *primary* determinants of lung injury (pneumonitis) are the volume (>25 mL) and pH (<2.5) of the aspirate.
- Tissue damage results from *both* the initial acid exposure and subsequent neutrophil-based inflammatory response.
- Patients *should* be managed by optimizing oxygenation and ventilation, protecting the airway to prevent further aspiration, fluid resuscitation, and initiating appropriate *empirical* antibiotics.

PITFALLS

- There is *no* beneficial role for managing patients with *prophylactic* antibiotics, corticosteroids, *routine* bronchoscopy, or unnecessarily high levels of supplemental oxygen.

with high volume–low pressure cuffs, feeding through gastrostomy or jejunostomy tubes whenever possible, selective gastric decompression, and appropriate suctioning of oropharyngeal secretions. Alkalinization of gastric contents is also of potential importance. Because the single most important factor in the pathogenesis of acute lung injury after aspiration is the pH of the fluid, there is a sound rationale for the use of antacid therapy to maintain pH at greater than 4.5 in high-risk patients. H_2 blockers are the most widely used agents and are unquestionably effective, when properly dosed, at maintaining desired pH. Other available agents include orally administered antacid suspensions or proton-pump inhibitors. Reasonable questions have been raised concerning increased risk of not only infectious pulmonary complications but also overall infectious complications from gastroesophageal bacterial overgrowth in this patient population as a result of acid suppression therapy.

CONCLUSION

Aspiration and subsequent aspiration pneumonitis are frequent complications in surgery and surgical critical care units. The logical approach to this problem begins with recognition of high-risk situations and preemptive initiation of preventive steps. Understanding the mechanism and sequence of injury and the components of supportive care, and having a heightened awareness of the possible infectious and inflammatory complications will help to optimize the outcome for management of these patients.

SELECTED READINGS

Bartlett JG, Gorbach SL: The triple threat of aspiration pneumonia. Chest 1975;68:560.

Chastre J, Fagon JV, Trouillet JL: Diagnosis and treatment of nosocomial pneumonia in patients in intensive care units. Clin Infect Dis 1995;21(suppl 3):s226.

Kennedy TP, Johnson KJ, Kunkel RG, et al: Acute acid aspiration lung injury in the rat: Biphasic pathogenesis. Anesth Analg 1989;69:87.

Kirsch CM, Sanders A: Aspiration pneumonia. Otolaryngol Clin North Am 1988;21:677.

Knight PR, Druskovich G, Tait AR, et al: The role of neutrophils, oxidants, and proteases in the pathogenesis of acid pulmonary injury. Anesthesiology 1992;77:772.

Knight PR, Rutter T, Tait AR, et al: Pathogenesis of gastric particulate lung injury: A comparison and interaction with acidic pneumonitis. Anesth Analg 1993;77:754.

Landay MJ, Christensen EE, Bynum LJ: Pulmonary manifestations of acute aspiration of gastric contents. AJR Am J Roentgenol 1978;131:587.

LoCicero J III: Bronchopulmonary aspiration. Surg Clin North Am 1989;69:71.

Mendelson CL: The aspiration of stomach contents into the lungs during obstetric anesthesia. Am J Obstet Gynecol 1946;52:191.

Nader-Djalal N, Knight PR, Davidson BA, et al: Hyperoxia exacerbates microvascular lung injury following acid aspiration. Chest 1997;112:1607.

Roberts RB, Shirley MA: Reducing the risk of acid aspiration during cesarean section. Anesth Analg 1974;53:859.

Schwartz DJ, Wynne JW, Gibbs CP, et al: The pulmonary consequences of aspiration of gastric contents at pH values greater than 2.5. Am J Respir Crit Care Med 1980;121:119.

Shifrin RY, Choplin RH: Aspiration in patients in critical care units. Radiol Clin North Am 1996;34:83.

Teabeaut JR II: Aspiration of gastric contents: An experimental study. Am J Pathol 1952;28:51.

HEAD AND NECK

Chapter 37

Incidence, Etiology, Diagnosis, and Staging of Head and Neck Cancer

Richard J. Wong and Jatin P. Shah

The majority of head and neck cancers are malignancies of the upper aerodigestive tract. Malignancies of the skin, the paranasal sinuses, the salivary glands, the thyroid gland, and the parathyroid glands are also included in this category, as well as less common tumors originating from soft tissue, bone, and neurovascular structures within the head and neck. This discussion of head and neck cancer focuses primarily on squamous cell carcinoma of the upper aerodigestive tract and summarizes the incidence, the demographics, the major risk factors, and the basic etiologic theories of head and neck cancer. An overview of the diagnosis of these malignancies from history, physical examination, imaging studies, and biopsy methods is reviewed, with an emphasis on the concerns that should be addressed for each specific head and neck site. Finally, the American Joint Committee on Cancer staging system (1997) for head and neck cancer is outlined.

INCIDENCE AND DEMOGRAPHICS

The incidence of oral cavity and pharyngeal cancer in the United States was estimated to be approximately 29,800 new cases in 1999, representing 2.4% of all new cancers. In this same period, there were about 10,600 new cases of laryngeal cancer (0.9%) and 18,100 new cases of thyroid cancer (1.5%). Taken together, these malignancies constituted 4.8% of all new cancer cases in the United States. Approximately 8100 deaths from oral cavity and pharyngeal cancer, 4200 deaths from laryngeal cancer, and 1200 deaths from thyroid malignancies were expected during this period, together representing 2.3% of all cancer deaths in the United States. Worldwide, the relative incidence of head and neck malignancies is higher than in the United States. The combined worldwide incidence of oral cavity, pharyngeal, laryngeal, and thyroid cancer was approximately 586,000 new cases in 1999, or 7.2% of all new cancer cases. The worldwide mortality from these malignancies was estimated to be 291,000, representing 5.6% of all cancer deaths. It should be noted that other sites of head and neck cancer (e.g., cutaneous, paranasal sinus, and salivary gland malignancies) are not included in these figures.

The patterns of head and neck cancer development are influenced by a variety of demographic factors, including geographic location, gender, and age. Melanesia, a group of islands in the Pacific, holds the highest worldwide incidence of oral cavity and pharyngeal cancer in males at 39.0 cases per 100,000 people. The next two highest incidences of these cancers are seen in Western Europe and south central Asia, at 21.8 and 20.5 cases per 100,000,

respectively. In India and Southeast Asia, oral cavity cancer represents about 35% of all malignant tumors (Shah and Lydiatt, 1995). This high incidence is related to the practices of tobacco and betel consumption, which significantly increase the risk of developing oral cancer. Nasopharyngeal carcinoma has the highest prevalence in southeastern China, where the consumption of dry salted fish is a well-established risk factor.

There are gender differences in the occurrence of head and neck cancer, with a significantly higher prevalence in men than in women. Oral and pharyngeal cancer is about 2.5 times more common in men than in women, and has the seventh highest incidence (3%) of all malignancies in males in the United States. Laryngeal cancer is approximately seven times more common in men than in women, the highest gender ratio of any cancer site. In recent years, however, a trend toward an increased occurrence of head and neck cancer in women may be related to an increase in tobacco and alcohol use. Thyroid cancer is three times more common in females than in males and is responsible for 2% of all cancers in women in the United States, making it the ninth most common malignancy in this group. Other demographic factors related to an increased incidence of head and neck cancer include increasing age and low socioeconomic status.

ETIOLOGY

The majority of patients with head and neck cancer have a history of tobacco and alcohol consumption. Both substances have long been implicated as independent risk factors for developing oral and pharyngeal cancer. Nonsmoking males who consume more than four alcoholic drinks per day have a sixfold increase in the risk of developing oral and pharyngeal cancer, and nondrinking males who smoke more than two packs of cigarettes per day have greater than a sevenfold increase in risk. In males who consume more than four drinks and two packs of cigarettes per day, the risk increases more than 37-fold, reflecting a multiplicative rather than an additive effect of the two factors combined (Blot, 1988). Other studies have also found a synergistic effect between tobacco and alcohol in the pathogenesis of oral and pharyngeal cancer (Rothman and Keller, 1972). It is estimated that approximately 75% of all oral and pharyngeal cancers in the United States are caused by smoking and drinking, with the majority of these influenced by the synergism between these two factors.

The deleterious effects of smoking may be related to the nitrosamines and the polycyclic aromatic hydrocarbons in tobacco, which can act as both initiators and promoters of carcinogenesis. Drinkers carry an increased risk of developing head and neck cancer at sites that come in direct contact with the alcohol (e.g., oral cavity and oropharynx) compared with other sites not in direct contact with the alcohol. This suggests that the carcinogenic effects of alcohol act through topical exposure. An association between the use of mouthwash, which contains ethanol, and head and neck cancer also supports this idea. The risk of development of oral and pharyngeal cancer in chronic mouthwash users is 40% greater in males and 60% greater in females after adjusting for alcohol and tobacco consumption; this risk increases in proportion to the duration and the frequency of mouthwash use. Ethanol has not been shown to be carcinogenic in laboratory animals, and the exact mechanism by which alcohol induces cancer remains unknown. Theories suggest that alcoholic drinks may (1) contain other carcinogenic compounds, (2) act as a solvent that enhances the penetration of tobacco or other carcinogens into tissues, (3) generate metabolites that are carcinogenic, (4) enhance nutritional deficiencies, and (5) catalyze the activation of other compounds into carcinogens (Blot 1992).

Slaughter and coworkers proposed that the entire epithelial lining of the upper aerodigestive tract undergoes widespread cytologic changes on prolonged exposure to carcinogens that make it prone to the development of multifocal cancers. This "field cancerization" theory is supported by the association of alcohol and tobacco exposure with the development of multiple primary squamous cell carcinomas within the field of mucosa at risk. Patients with oral or pharyngeal cancer develop second primary tumors at a rate of approximately 4% annually. Both tobacco smoking and alcohol consumption contribute to the risk of developing second primary cancers, with the effects of smoking more pronounced than those of alcohol. Active smokers experience a fourfold increased risk of developing second primaries compared with nonsmokers and former smokers. This increased risk is reduced by more than half 5 years after cessation of smoking and is nearly completely resolved by 10 years (Day and Blot, 1992, 1994).

Other methods of tobacco consumption related to the culture and the customs of various geographic areas may increase the carcinogenic potential of the tobacco and may increase the incidence of head and neck cancers. In Southeast Asia, for example, chewing betel nut and betel leaf, smoking bidi (a tobacco preparation rolled in betel leaf), and reverse smoking (in which the lighted end of the cigarette is held within the mouth) are common practices. These customs promote carcinogenesis and contribute to the high incidence of oral cavity cancer in this region. Snuff dipping—placing finely ground or powdered tobacco between the gum and the cheek—is another practice that has been associated with an increase in oral cancer. In women living in the southern United States who use snuff, a fourfold increase in the risk of oral cancer was detected. Among chronic snuff users, this risk approached 50-fold for cancers of the gum and the buccal mucosa.

Diet and nutrition have also been shown to affect the incidence of head and neck cancer. Consumption of dry salted fish has been implicated as an important environmental factor in the development of nasopharyngeal carcinoma in southeastern China, a region where this malignancy has a particularly high incidence. Dimethylnitrosamine is a volatile carcinogen found in salted fish that may be responsible for this association. The deficiencies of iron, riboflavin, and other vitamins seen in Plummer-Vinson syndrome are associated with an increased incidence of postcricoid hypopharyngeal squamous cell carcinoma. Within normal dietary ranges, the risk of oral and pharyngeal cancer in women has been shown to decrease as the consumption of fresh fruit, vegetables, breads, and cereals increases.

Viral infection is also correlated with the development of head and neck cancer. The Epstein-Barr virus has long been implicated in the development of nasopharyngeal carcinoma. The nonkeratinizing and undifferentiated types of nasopharyngeal carcinoma (World Health Organization types 2 and 3) have been shown to be highly associated with Epstein-Barr virus by means of polymerase chain reaction studies in biopsy samples. The human papillomavirus is a well-established cause of benign recurrent respiratory, oral, and nasal papillomas. Two types of head and neck cancer, verrucous carcinoma and tonsillar carcinoma, are strongly correlated with human papillomavirus infection based on molecular epidemiologic data. Carcinomas of the tongue, the nasal cavity, and the nasopharynx are less well correlated with human papillomavirus, which may be a factor in only a subset of these tumors.

Certain types of occupational exposure have well-established effects on the incidence of head and neck malignancies. There is a strong association between sinonasal squamous cell carcinoma and nickel exposure. Workers at a nickel refinery in Norway developed squamous cell carcinoma at 250 times the expected rate, with a latent period of 18 to 36 years. There is a similar relationship between exposure to wood dust particles and sinonasal adenocarcinoma. In woodworkers in the furniture industry in southern England, there was estimated to be an approximately 875-fold increase in the incidence of sinonasal adenocarcinoma in comparison to the rate in the normal population. Nickel and asbestos exposure have been correlated with an increased risk of developing laryngeal carcinoma.

Cutaneous malignancies of the head and neck, which are largely basal and squamous cell carcinomas, are strongly correlated with exposure to ultraviolet B radiation in sunlight. The incidence of cutaneous carcinoma is related to outdoor occupations, leisure time spent in sunlight, ozone layer depletion, and geographic habitation, with people living at lower latitudes at higher risk. Exposure to ionizing radiation is a well-established risk factor for the development of thyroid cancer. Low-dose irradiation has also been implicated in the development of benign and malignant salivary gland neoplasms. Poor dentition and poor oral hygiene have been correlated with lower socioeconomic status and higher incidences of oral cavity cancer.

MOLECULAR BASIS OF CARCINOGENESIS

The behavioral and the environmental factors that cause increased development of head and neck cancer ultimately result in DNA changes by a variety of mechanisms. Many smoking-related mutations are alterations of GC base pairs, with 75% being G→T substitutions. Such alterations may result in the activation of a proto-oncogene or the inactivation of a tumor suppressor gene (TSG) and may lead to a malignant phenotype. Cyclin D1 is a proto-oncogene required for cell cycle progression that may become amplified and contribute to uncontrolled proliferation. TSGs, on the other hand, encode proteins that normally exert a regulatory control on cell growth. One of the most commonly inactivated TSGs in head and neck carcinoma is p53, a gene normally involved in arresting cell growth at the G_1-S cell cycle checkpoint to permit DNA repair. The genetic alteration and the inactivation of the p53 TSG may therefore lead to both an accumulation of DNA damage and a loss of growth control. The frequency of p53 mutations in head and neck cancer has been found to be significantly higher in patients exposed to tobacco and alcohol (58%) than in those not exposed (17%). This finding forms an important link between well-established head and neck cancer epidemiologic data and our molecular understanding of carcinogenesis.

Genetic alterations gradually accumulate with continued exposure of the upper aerodigestive tract to carcinogens. With an increasing number of genetic alterations, mucosa may progress along a spectrum from normal histologic structure to hyperplasia, atypia, dysplasia, and carcinoma in situ before finally displaying the frankly malignant behavior of invasive carcinoma. This genetic progression model correlates well with the predisposition of head and neck squamous cell carcinoma to arise from previously existing, precancerous epithelial lesions that appear clinically as leukoplakia or erythroplakia. The progression model also supports Slaughter's field cancerization theory: A field of upper aerodigestive tract mucosa chronically exposed to carcinogens is at increasing risk of multifocal carcinogenesis through the continued accumulation of genetic alterations.

HISTORY

A thorough history and physical examination are essential in directing the examiner toward the site of disease and lending insight into the extent of disease. Details of the patient's presenting symptoms are elicited, including specific characteristics, duration, and rapidity of changes. The growth pattern of any mass lesions is established. Symptoms such as pain, numbness, odynophagia, dysphagia, trismus, change in voice or articulation, respiratory difficulty, nasal obstruction, epistaxis, change in vision, otalgia, hearing loss, vertigo, tinnitus, headache, malaise, weight loss, and other constitutional symptoms are elicited. Particular attention should be directed to the anatomic site involved. Questions should address symptoms that might be expected if anatomic structures adjacent to the primary site are invaded by tumor, with the goal of ascertaining the limits of extension.

A social history establishes risk factors for head and neck cancer. Tobacco use may be quantified by multiplying the number of years that the patient has smoked by the number of packs per day that he or she consumes; the product is expressed as the number of "pack years." Alcohol consumption is also quantified by assessing the number and the type of drinks consumed by the patient as well as any history of alcohol dependence. It should be kept in mind that patients will often underestimate the quantity of alcohol that they consume. Inquiries into other risk factors should be made, including previous radiation exposure, occupational exposure, sun exposure, dentition problems, oral hygiene, and preexisting chronic lesions. A family history of malignancy as well as potentially inheritable coexisting medical conditions should be determined. Certain head and neck tumors (e.g., medullary thyroid carcinoma) may have a familial pattern of transmission and may warrant a particularly detailed family history.

PHYSICAL EXAMINATION

General

The overall appearance of the patient is assessed initially, with an immediate overview of functional status, obvious deformities, level of comfort, respiratory status, voice and articulation, and nourishment. All facial, scalp, and cervical skin lesions are inspected.

Face, Ears, and Eyes

Any facial weakness or asymmetry is noted, and the function of both the facial and the trigeminal nerve is tested. The pinna and the external auditory canal are examined. Postauricular and preauricular (parotid gland) regions are palpated. The tympanic membrane is visualized by means of otoscopy to assess the middle ear space. Obstruction of the eustachian tube due to nasopharyngeal or paranasal sinus tumors may manifest as serous otitis media. The eyes are examined for visual acuity, pupil reactivity, extraocular motility, and globe position. Diplopia may coincide with restriction in motility or a displaced globe secondary to mass compression from a paranasal sinus tumor.

Nasal Cavity, Paranasal Sinuses, and Nasopharynx

The external nose and the cheek are assessed for any swelling due to an underlying mass (Fig. 37–1). Endoscopic examination of the nasal cavity and the nasopharynx is routinely performed. Inspection of the entire nasal mucosal lining is directed toward identifying mass lesions or mucosal irregularities. Within the nasopharynx, attention should be paid to Rosenmüller's fossa, a recess posterior to the eustachian tube orifice that is a common originating site for nasopharyngeal carcinoma. Inspection of the dentition, the hard palate, and the alveolar ridge in the oral cavity may reveal signs of an inferior maxillary sinus mass. Cheek numbness indicates involvement of the infraorbital nerve. Trismus may indicate extension of a tumor into the pterygoid musculature. Orbital extension

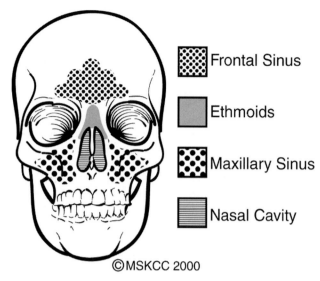

Figure 37–1. Anatomy of the paranasal sinuses.

can result in globe displacement, restriction of extraocular movement, and loss of vision.

Oral Cavity and Oropharynx

Examination of the oral cavity includes a careful inspection of the teeth, the tongue, the floor of the mouth, the alveolar ridge, the buccal mucosa, and the palate for any visible lesions or masses. The tonsillar fossa, the tongue base, the retromolar trigone, the soft palate, and the posterior pharyngeal wall are examined in the oropharynx (Fig. 37–2). The surface characteristics of the mucosa are studied for any irregularities. Palpation is essential to determine a lesion's full extent in three dimensions. Bimanual palpation is particularly helpful in the assessment of masses of the floor of the mouth as well as submental, submandibular, and buccal masses.

The relationship between an oral cavity or oropharyngeal mass and the mandible is of significance with respect to both staging and treatment planning. The most common route of mandibular invasion into the cancellous bone is through a tooth socket or the occlusal surface of an edentulous mandible. Tongue deviation on protrusion indicates hypoglossal weakness, and restriction of tongue motion suggests deep invasion with infiltration of the intrinsic and the extrinsic tongue musculature. Impaired sensation of the tongue, the lower alveolus, or the lower lip occurs with involvement of the mandibular division of the trigeminal nerve. If trismus is present, the pterygoid musculature, the masseter muscle, or the temporomandibular joint may be invaded by tumor.

Larynx and Hypopharynx

The examiner first assesses the patient's voice quality. Fiberoptic visualization of the larynx and the hypopharynx is an essential part of routine head and neck examination in the office. The identification of any mass lesion, ulceration, or mucosal irregularity specifies the subsites in-

volved within the supraglottis, the glottis, or the hypopharynx (Fig. 37–3). Vocal cord mobility (fully intact, decreased, or fixed) is noted. Sensation of the supraglottis indicates superior laryngeal nerve function. The piriform sinuses and the postcricoid space are not well visualized on office examination, and rigid endoscopy under anesthesia is required for full evaluation. External palpation of the anterior neck should assess the thyroid and the cricoid cartilages, the thyrohyoid and the cricothyroid membranes, the cervical lymph nodes, the thyroid gland, and laryngeal mobility over the prevertebral fascia.

Neck

The neck is palpated with particular attention to the regions at highest risk of regional nodal metastases (Fig. 37–4). Bimanual examination of the submandibular region is performed. Palpable masses or lymph nodes should be assessed for size, texture, mobility or fixation, involvement of overlying skin, and proximity to other structures. The thyroid and the cricoid cartilages and the thyroid gland are palpated. Shoulder movement is assessed to document the function of the spinal accessory nerve.

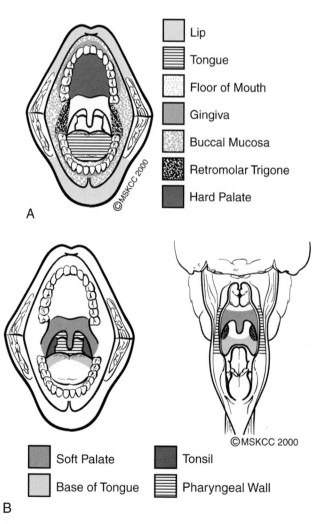

Figure 37–2. Anatomy of the oral cavity (A) and the oropharynx (B).

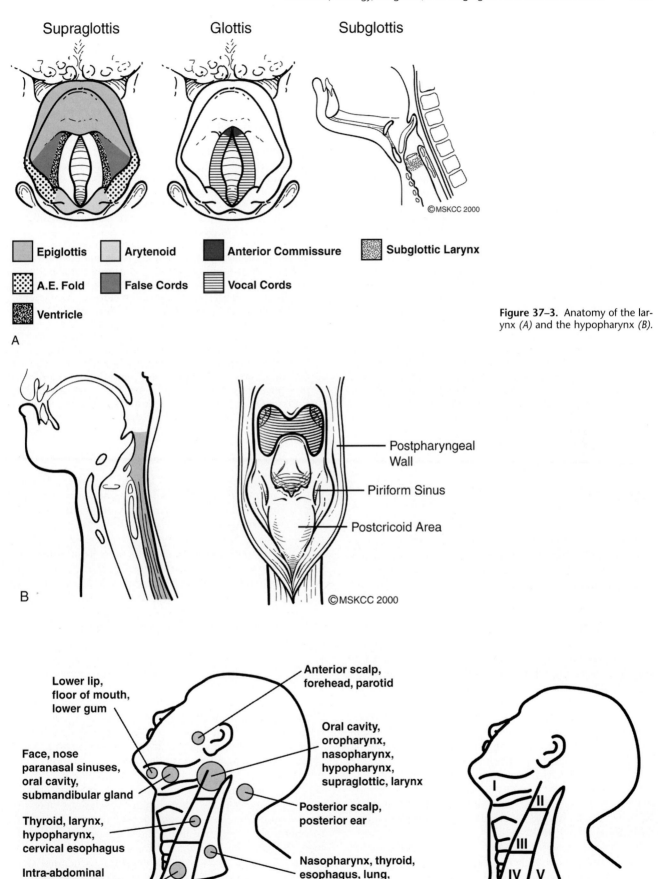

Supraglottis   Glottis   Subglottis

©MSKCC 2000

- Epiglottis
- A.E. Fold
- Ventricle
- Arytenoid
- False Cords
- Anterior Commissure
- Vocal Cords
- Subglottic Larynx

Figure 37–3. Anatomy of the larynx *(A)* and the hypopharynx *(B).*

A

Postpharyngeal Wall

Piriform Sinus

Postcricoid Area

B   ©MSKCC 2000

Lower lip, floor of mouth, lower gum

Anterior scalp, forehead, parotid

Oral cavity, oropharynx, nasopharynx, hypopharynx, supraglottic, larynx

Face, nose paranasal sinuses, oral cavity, submandibular gland

Posterior scalp, posterior ear

Thyroid, larynx, hypopharynx, cervical esophagus

Nasopharynx, thyroid, esophagus, lung, breast

Intra-abdominal organs: breast, lung, esophagus, thyroid

©MSKCC 2000

I
II
III
IV V

Figure 37–4. Regions of the cervical lymph nodes.

Pearls and Pitfalls

PEARLS

- The combined incidence of oral cavity, pharyngeal, laryngeal, and thyroid cancer was 4.8% of all new cancer cases in the United States in 1999; worldwide, this figure was 7.2%.
- Head and neck squamous cell carcinoma is more common in men than in women. Oral and pharyngeal cancer is 2.5 times more common in men, and laryngeal cancer is seven times more common in men. In contrast, thyroid cancer is three times more common in women.
- The major risk factors for head and neck squamous cell carcinoma are tobacco use and alcohol consumption, which have a synergistic effect. Approximately 75% of all oral and pharyngeal cancers in the United States are caused by smoking and drinking, with the majority influenced by the synergism between these two factors.
- The high incidence of head and neck squamous cell carcinoma in southeastern Asia is related to the customs of chewing betel nut and betel leaf, smoking bidi, and reverse smoking, all of which promote carcinogenesis. Nasopharyngeal carcinoma in southeastern China is related to the consumption of dry salted fish and the Epstein-Barr virus. Sinonasal squamous cell carcinoma and adenocarcinoma have been linked with occupational exposure to nickel and wood dust, respectively.
- A field of upper aerodigestive tract mucosa chronically exposed to carcinogens is at increased risk of development of multifocal cancers through the accumulation of genetic alterations. With an increasing number of these alterations, the mucosa may progress along a spectrum from normal histologic structure to hyperplasia, atypia, dysplasia, and carcinoma in situ before displaying the malignant behavior of invasive carcinoma.
- In eliciting a patient's history, questions should address symptoms that might be expected if anatomic structures adjacent to the primary cancer site are invaded by tumor. A complete head and neck examination is performed, with attention to determining the local extent of disease at the primary tumor site and possible cervical lymph node metastases.
- Further work-up may include imaging studies and fine needle aspiration biopsy. An examination with the patient under anesthesia permits (1) a more detailed inspection of the primary site with the patient relaxed, (2) the surveillance of the rest of the aerodigestive tract for detection of second primary cancers, and (3) the performance of tumor biopsies for histologic diagnosis.
- Cancer staging is an essential method of categorizing patients for the rapid communication of disease extent, the planning of treatment strategies, the comparison of results after treatment, and the provision of prognostic information to patients. The American Joint Commission of Cancer's staging system is based on the TNM system, in which T describes the primary tumor, N the regional lymph nodes, and M distant metastases.

IMAGING

Many patients with a head and neck tumor will require radiologic imaging to assess fully its relationship to adjacent anatomic structures. These images may provide important information about the tumor's proximity to the carotid artery, the cranial nerves, the laryngeal or the tracheal cartilage, the dura, the bone, the prevertebral fascia, and the orbit. The invasion or the close proximity of such structures will have a direct impact on staging, treatment planning, and prognosis. For example, tumors involving the suprastructure of the maxillary sinus are in close proximity to the orbit and the skull base and have a worse prognosis than tumors confined to the infrastructure of the maxillary sinus. The pattern of tumor extension into anatomic spaces or tissue planes is another factor that should be examined. Malignancies may track along tissue planes or neurovascular structures or into potential spaces of less resistance. The invasion of the paraglottic space and the pre-epiglottic space by laryngeal carcinoma, for example, carries prognostic and treatment implications. Cervical metastatic nodal involvement that may not be palpable on physical examination may also be detected on imaging of the neck.

Computed tomography and magnetic resonance imaging are the predominant imaging modalities used in the head and neck. Computed tomography has several advantages over magnetic resonance imaging, including superior bone detail, lower cost, and better availability. Magnetic resonance imaging offers a better differentiation of tumor from adjacent soft tissue and may be superior to computed tomography in assessing tumor invasion of cranial nerves, dura, brain, and muscle. Magnetic resonance imaging is often preferred for nasopharyngeal tumors and deep tumors of the tongue base. Tumor invasion of major vessels may be further investigated by angiography or magnetic resonance angiography to assess patency, collateral circulation, and vessel contour. Ultrasonography is useful for evaluating, following, and guiding fine needle aspiration biopsy of thyroid masses, indeterminate lymph nodes, and cystic lesions.

BIOPSY

Once the tumor has been evaluated by means of physical examination and imaging studies, a tissue specimen is required to establish a pathologic diagnosis. Palpable cervical lymph nodes or masses, thyroid nodules, and parotid gland masses may all require fine needle aspiration. Fine needle aspiration is a highly sensitive procedure, carries very few associated risks, and may be conveniently performed in an office setting. Cutaneous lesions may require a punch or an excisional biopsy. Shave biopsies fail to obtain an adequate full-thickness specimen for histologic diagnosis and should be universally condemned. A general principle is to plan the biopsy in a manner that minimally violates the integrity of normal surrounding tissue planes and structures. This approach avoids tumor contamination of uninvolved tissues and facilitates later surgical removal.

Table 37–1	Staging of Head and Neck Cancer*

LIP AND ORAL CAVITY

Primary Tumor (T)

TX	Primary tumor cannot be assessed
T0	No evidence of primary tumor
Tis	Carcinoma in situ
T1	Tumor 2 cm or less in greatest dimension
T2	Tumor more than 2 cm but not more than 4 cm in greatest dimension
T3	Tumor more than 4 cm in greatest dimension
T4 (lip)	Tumor invades adjacent structures (e.g., through cortical bone, inferior alveolar nerve, floor of mouth, skin of face)
T4 (oral cavity)	Tumor invades adjacent structures (e.g., through cortical bone or into deep [extrinsic] muscle of tongue, maxillary sinus, or skin. Superficial erosion alone of bone/tooth socket by gingival primary is not sufficient to classify as T4)

NASOPHARYNX

T1	Tumor confined to the nasopharynx
T2	Tumor extends to the soft tissues of oropharynx and/or nasal fossa
	T2a Without parapharyngeal extension
	T2b With parapharyngeal extension
T3	Tumor invades bony structures and/or paranasal sinuses
T4	Tumor with intracranial extension and/or involvement of cranial nerves, infratemporal fossa, hypopharynx, or orbit

OROPHARYNX

T1	Tumor 2 cm or less in greatest dimension
T2	Tumor more than 2 cm but not more than 4 cm in greatest dimension
T3	Tumor more than 4 cm in greatest dimension
T4	Tumor invades adjacent structures (pterygoid muscles, mandible, hard palate, deep muscle of tongue, larynx)

MAXILLARY SINUS

TX	Primary tumor cannot be assessed
T0	No evidence of primary tumor
Tis	Carcinoma in situ
T1	Tumor limited to the antral mucosa with no erosion or destruction of bone
T2	Tumor causing bone erosion or destruction, except for the posterior antral wall, including extension into the hard palate and/or the middle nasal meatus
T3	Tumor invades any of the following: bone of the posterior wall of the maxillary sinus, subcutaneous tissues, skin of cheek, floor or medial wall of orbit, infratemporal fossa, pterygoid plates, ethmoid sinuses
T4	Tumor invades orbital contents beyond the floor or medial wall, including any of the following: orbital apex, cribriform plate, base of skull, nasopharynx, sphenoid, frontal sinuses

ETHMOID SINUS

T1	Tumor confined to the ethmoid with or without bone erosion
T2	Tumor extends into the nasal cavity
T3	Tumor extends to the anterior orbit and/or maxillary sinus
T4	Tumor with intracranial extension or orbital extension including apex or involving sphenoid, frontal sinus, and/or skin of external nose

STAGE GROUPING

All Except Nasopharynx

I	T1	N0	M0
II	T2	N0	M0
III	T3	N0	M0
	T1	N1	M0
	T2	N1	M0
	T3	N1	M0
IVA	T4	N0	M0
	T4	N1	M0
	Any T	N2	M0
IVB	Any T	N3	M0
IVC	Any T	Any N	M1

Nasopharynx

I	T1	N0	M0
IIA	T2a	N0	M0
IIB	T1	N1	M0
	T2	N1	M0
	T2a	N1	M0
	T2b	N0	M0
	T2b	N1	M0
IIIT1	N2	M0	
	T2a	N2	M0
	T2b	N2	M0
	T3	N0	M0
	T3	N1	M0
	T3	N2	M0
IVA	T4	N0	M0
	T4	N1	M0
	T4	N2	M0
IVB	Any T	N3	M0
IVC	Any T	Any N	M1

*See Chapter 39 for staging of cancer of the hypopharynx, the supraglottis, the glottis and the regional lymph nodes as well as distant metastases.
Used by permission of the American Joint Committee on Cancer (AJCC®), Chicago, Illinois. AJCC Cancer Staging Manual, 5th ed. Philadelphia, Lippincott-Raven, 1997.

A complete endoscopic examination of the upper aero-digestive tract with the patient under anesthesia serves several purposes: (1) It permits the most detailed inspection of the site and the extent of the primary tumor with the patient relaxed under anesthesia; (2) it permits surveillance of the rest of the upper aerodigestive tract for detection of second primary tumors; and (3) it allows for the performance of tissue biopsies for histologic diagnosis. During the examination under anesthesia, palpation of the oral cavity and the oropharynx should be performed. Lesions of the tongue base may be best detected through bimanual palpation with one finger in the mouth and the other hand on the neck. A systematic examination of the oropharynx, the hypopharynx, and the larynx is performed during direct laryngoscopy. Lesions extending into the subglottis may be visualized with angled rigid endoscopes. Esophagoscopy and bronchoscopy should be performed when clinically indicated by the patient's symptoms and when the risk of multiple primary tumors is high. The routine performance of these procedures in all patients with head and neck cancer, however, is of low yield and remains controversial. Intraoperative frozen section analysis allows multiple biopsies to be taken in the event that an initial negative sample is not representative of the tumor. Highly suspicious lesions warrant the performance of multiple biopsies with frozen section analysis until the diagnosis can be more clearly established.

STAGING

The purpose of a staging system is to provide a universal measurement of the extent of cancer. Staging is an essential method of categorizing patients for (1) the rapid communication of disease extent to others, (2) the planning of treatment strategies, (3) comparing results after treatment, and (4) the provision of prognostic information. An optimal staging system employs criteria that may be assessed accurately, easily, and objectively with low cost.

The American Joint Commission of Cancer has published the most widely accepted staging system (Table 37–1). It is based on the TNM staging system, in which T describes the primary tumor, N describes regional cervical lymph node involvement, and M indicates the number of distant metastases. Other factors (e.g., functional status, comorbidity, and molecular prognostic factors) have not been incorporated into a staging system but may eventually assist in providing more accurate predictions of outcome in the future.

SELECTED READINGS

Acheson ED: Nasal cancer in the furniture and boot and shoe manufacturing industries. Prev Med 1976;5:295–315.
American Joint Committee on Cancer: AJCC Cancer Staging Manual. New York, Lippincott-Raven, 1997.
Blot WJ: Alcohol and cancer. Cancer Res 1992;52(Suppl 7):2119s–2123s.
Blot WJ, McLaughlin JK, Winn DM, et al: Smoking and drinking in relation to oral and pharyngeal cancer. Cancer Res 1988;48:3282–3287.
Brennan JA, Boyle JO, Koch WM, et al: Association between cigarette smoking and mutation of the p53 gene in squamous-cell carcinoma of the head and neck. N Engl J Med 1995;332:712–717.
Day GL, Blot WJ: Second primary tumors in patients with oral cancer. Cancer 1992;70:14–19.
Day GL, Blot WJ, Shore RE, et al: Second cancers following oral and pharyngeal cancers: Role of tobacco and alcohol. J Natl Cancer Inst 1994;86:131–137.
Landis SH, Murray T, Bolden S, Wingo PA: Cancer statistics, 1999. CA Cancer J Clin 1999;49:8–63.
Pedersen E, Hogetveit AC, Anderson A: Cancer of the respiratory organs among workers at a nickel refinery in Norway. Int J Cancer 1973;12:32–41.
Rothman K, Keller A: The effect of joint exposure to alcohol and tobacco on risk of cancer of the mouth and pharynx. J Chronic Dis 1972;25:711–716.
Shah JP, Lydiatt W: Treatment of cancer of the head and neck. CA Cancer J Clin 1995;45:352–368.
Slaughter DP, Southwick HW, Smejkal W: "Field cancerization" in oral stratified squamous epithelium: Clinical implications of multicentric origin. Cancer (Phila) 1953;6:963–968.
Winn DM, Blot WJ, McLaughlin JK, et al: Mouthwash use and oral conditions in the risk of oral and pharyngeal cancer. Cancer Res 1991;51:3044–3047.
Winn DM, Blot WJ, Shy CM, et al: Snuff dipping and oral cancer among women in the southern United States. N Engl J Med 1981;304:745–749.
Winn DM, Ziegler RG, Pickle LW, et al: Diet in the etiology of oral and pharyngeal cancer among women from the southern United States. Cancer Res 1984;44:1216–1222.

Chapter 38
Cancer of the Oral Cavity and Oropharynx

Jay O. Boyle

Carcinomas of the oral cavity and oropharynx are a significant cause of morbidity and mortality worldwide. The incidence of oral cancer is highest in India and Southeast Asia; the incidence of oropharyngeal cancer is highest in France and Eastern Europe. In the United States in the year 2000, there were an estimated 30,200 oral and oropharyngeal cancer cases, causing 7800 deaths (Landis et al, 1999). Clinically, these tumors are classified and staged as two separate sites, and they demonstrate some differences in biology and treatment. The oral cavity extends from the lips to the circumvallate papilla of the tongue (Fig. 38–1); the oropharynx includes the tonsils, base of the tongue, soft palate, and posterior pharyngeal wall (Fig. 38–2).

Head and neck squamous cell carcinoma is strongly linked to exposure to carcinogens in tobacco smoke and to the promoter effects of alcohol. Patients who smoke 2 packs of cigarettes daily and consume 30 alcoholic drinks per week have a nearly 40-fold increased risk of oropharyngeal cancer (Blot et al, 1988). Squamous cell carcinoma constitutes 90% of oral and oropharyngeal cancer; the remainder is composed predominantly of lymphomas and minor salivary gland tumors. Chronic carcinogen exposure leads to "field carcinogenesis" of the upper respiratory tract. Therefore, patients form second primary carcinomas of the upper respiratory tract at a rate of 3% to 4% per year to 25% at 10 years (Day and Blot, 1992).

The most common sites of primary carcinoma are head and neck, lung, esophagus, and bladder. The clinical and histopathologic progression of head and neck cancers is well defined. Carcinogen exposure causes genetically abnormal clonal populations that may form precancerous leukoplakias. Histologically, there is a progression from hyperplasia, to dysplasia, to invasive cancer. Once invasive, tumors spread first regionally and later to distant organs.

Surgery is the mainstay of treatment for oral and oropharyngeal cancer. Improved locoregional control and survival in advanced oral cancer have been achieved with the addition of postoperative radiation therapy. The morbidity of oropharyngeal cancer treatment with regard to speech and swallowing has been improved in recent years by the use of primary radiation therapy, concomitant radiation and chemotherapy, or brachytherapy at the primary site for selected cases. Chemotherapy alone is palliative treatment for recurrent or unresectable disease.

ANATOMY

The functions of oral and oropharyngeal tissues include articulation of speech, facial expression, respiration, mastication, deglutition, and taste. The oral cavity is bounded anteriorly by the skin and vermilion border of the upper and lower lips. The oral cavity extends posteriorly to the circumvallate papillae of the tongue, the junction of the hard and soft palates, and the anterior tonsillar arch. Laterally, the oral cavity is bounded by the buccal mucosa. The oral cavity is divided into the following subsites: the lip, anterior two thirds of the tongue, floor of the mouth, gingiva, retromolar trigone, buccal mucosa, and hard palate (see Fig. 38–1). The oropharyngeal subsites are the tonsils, soft palate, and posterior third of the tongue and posterior pharyngeal wall (see Fig. 38–2).

The oral cavity and oropharynx are lined with squamous epithelium. The submucosa contains copious minor salivary glands and lymphatics. These lead to regional metastases in the local lymph nodes in the neck, which are divided into five levels (Fig. 38–3). The blood supply is from the branches of the external carotid artery, and the venous return is via the common facial vein and the pharyngeal plexus of veins to the internal jugular vein. Sensation in the mouth is provided by the branches of the lower two divisions of the trigeminal nerve and by the glossopharyngeal nerve in the oropharynx. These nerves are the afferent loop for the swallowing reflex. The pharyngeal constrictors and soft palate are innervated by the vagus nerve (cranial nerve X), and the tongue muscles are innervated by the hypoglossal nerve (cranial nerve XII).

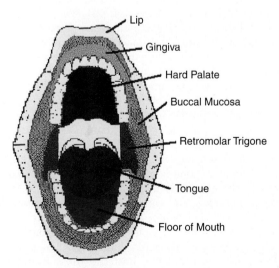

Figure 38–1. Diagram of oral cavity subsites. (Modified from Shah JP: Head and Neck Surgery 2. St. Louis, Mosby–Year Book, 1997.)

Labels: Lip, Gingiva, Hard Palate, Buccal Mucosa, Retromolar Trigone, Tongue, Floor of Mouth

257

Anterior View

Posterior View

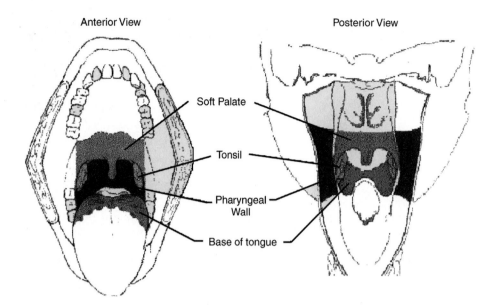

Soft Palate

Tonsil

Pharyngeal Wall

Base of tongue

Figure 38–2. Diagram of oropharynx subsites. (Modified from Shah JP: Head and Neck Surgery 2. St. Louis, Mosby–Year Book, 1997.)

The tonsil is made up of lymphoid tissue covered by stratified squamous mucosa, with prominent folds and crypts. The bed of the tonsil is formed by the superior constrictor muscle, lateral to which is the parapharyngeal space and the carotid sheath. The soft palate comprises the tissue superior to the tonsil laterally and from the uvula inferiorly to the junction of the hard palate anteriorly. The nasal surface of the soft palate is also included in the oropharyngeal anatomy. The soft palate consists of muscle fibers of the tensor veli palatini and the levator veli palatini.

The mandible consists of the bilateral ascending rami with condylar and coronoid processes, the body, and the anterior arch. It contains the inferior alveolar canal, artery, and nerve. The teeth reside in the alveolar process, which resorbs in the edentulous patient.

ASSESSMENT

Assessment of patients with oral and oropharyngeal cancer involves a detailed history and physical examination, supplemented by imaging studies, pathologic biopsy, staging, and then treatment planning. The history begins with a detailed history of the present illness, focusing on the duration and severity of symptoms. The most common symptoms are pain, bleeding, presence of a mass, nonhealing ulcer, weight loss, voice change, velopalatine insufficiency, and dysphagia. Patients commonly have been treated by their primary care physician for pharyngitis with one or more courses of antibiotics, without significant improvement in the symptoms. Most patients with oral and oropharyngeal carcinoma are in their 6th and 7th decades, and the majority have had heavy exposure to tobacco and alcohol. This leads to significant comorbidities identified in the past medical history. Cardiovascular disease, chronic obstructive pulmonary disease and emphysema, liver dysfunction, and peripheral vascular disease are common. The family history provides information regarding the familial predisposition to cancer, and the social history provides important information regarding the patient's occupation, family support and home environment, and exposure to carcinogens.

The most important aspect of the assessment of oral and oropharyngeal cancer patients is the physical examination, which provides the major part of staging information. A detailed complete head and neck examination, including the tympanic membranes, a complete cranial nerve examination, and careful palpation of the neck are first performed. The tumor is then examined through the open mouth and measured, if possible, with calipers. The measurement is recorded in centimeters. The epicenter of the tumor is identified and the mass is palpated through the open mouth, if possible. The boundaries of

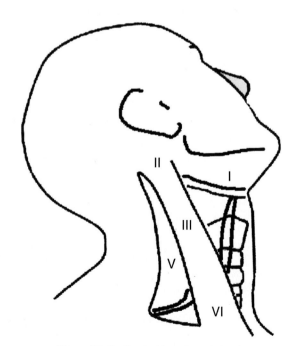

Figure 38–3. Cervical lymph node levels.

the tumor are determined in all directions, including depth, by palpation and proximity to the mandibular or maxillary bone. The inferior extent of most oropharyngeal tumors and the function of the larynx and hypopharynx must be visualized with fiberoptic nasopharyngoscopy. Often, it is possible to biopsy oral and oropharyngeal lesions through the open mouth with a straight or curved cup forceps. Some tumors require biopsy under anesthesia, which is especially appropriate if the extent is not certain on the office examination and the patient needs a staging examination under anesthesia. Some oropharyngeal tumors can be adequately examined in all dimensions with visualization and palpation.

If the third dimension of the tumor is not apparent or if documentation of the tumor size and location is necessary, tomographic imaging is appropriate. Computed tomography (CT) scanning with contrast enhancement demonstrates oral and oropharyngeal tumors well. Magnetic resonance imaging (MRI) is also excellent for imaging the soft tissues of the oropharynx. The advantages of MRI over CT include improved tissue resolution, routine sagittal and coronal imaging, and lack of radiation exposure. The disadvantages of MRI compared with CT scanning are poor discrimination of the cortical bone of the maxilla, mandible and skull base; greater expense; and the inability of some patients to tolerate the noisy, closed space of the MRI unit. Tumors obviously invading the carotid artery, brain, or cervical spine are generally considered inoperable for cure.

Some patients benefit from examination under anesthesia for biopsy and staging purposes. General anesthesia for biopsy may be necessary if the tumor is not visible, the gag reflex is severe, or there is a concern for the control of hemorrhage, for control of the airway, or for trismus. It is sometimes difficult to adequately localize a tumor in the base of the tongue or the lateral pharyngeal wall, where irregular mucosa normally exists. Mapping biopsies may be helpful. Tumors that obviously extend into the larynx and hypopharynx should be evaluated with the patient under general anesthesia with direct laryngoscopy and a consideration of esophagoscopy or flexible bronchoscopy. This should also be done if symptoms are referable to the esophagus or bronchi.

The appropriate metastatic workup consists of posteroanterior and lateral chest x-radiographs, liver function tests, and further imaging based on symptoms. Routine CT scanning of the chest, abdomen, and pelvis is not cost effective. CT-guided needle biopsy can be helpful in documenting distant metastases.

When all the assessment data are available, the patient's tumor is staged by the American Joint Committee on Cancer (AJCC) staging system (Table 38–1). The T stage of the primary tumor is based on tumor size. The N stage is based on the size and anatomic distribution of metastasis to regional lymph nodes. Tumors that are T3 or that demonstrate cervical lymph node metastases are stage III, and those that are T4 or N2 or M1 disease are stage IV. Treatment planning should be undertaken in a multidisciplinary tumor board setting, including surgeons, chemotherapists, and radiation therapists. The participation of dentists, social workers, speech and language pathologists, and nurses is helpful.

| Table 38–1 | UICC/AJCC Tumor Staging |

PRIMARY TUMOR (T)

TX	Primary tumor cannot be assessed
T0	No evidence of primary tumor
Tis	Carcinoma in situ
T1	Tumor 2 cm or less in greatest dimension
T2	Tumor more than 2 cm but not more than 4 cm in greatest dimension
T3	Tumor more than 4 cm in greatest dimension
T4	*(lip):* Tumor invades adjacent structures (e.g., through cortical bone, tongue, skin of neck). *(oral cavity):* Tumor invades adjacent structures (e.g., through cortical bone, into deep [extrinsic] muscle of the tongue, maxillary sinus, skin). *(oropharynx):* Tumor invades mandible, palate, larynx.

REGIONAL LYMPH NODES (N)

NX	Regional lymph nodes cannot be assessed
N0	No regional lymph node metastasis
N1	Metastasis in a single ipsilateral lymph node, 3 cm or less in greatest dimension
N2	Metastasis in a single ipsilateral lymph node, more than 3 cm but not more than 6 cm in greatest dimension; or in multiple ipsilateral lymph nodes, none more than 6 cm in greatest dimension; or in bilateral or contralateral lymph nodes, none more than 6 cm in greatest dimension
N2a	Metastasis in single ipsilateral lymph node more than 3 cm but not more than 6 cm in greatest dimension
N2b	Metastasis in multiple ipsilateral lymph nodes, none more than 6 cm in greatest dimension
N2c	Metastasis in bilateral or contralateral lymph nodes, none more than 6 cm in greatest dimension
N3	Metastasis in a lymph node more than 6 cm in greatest dimension

DISTANT METASTASIS (M)

MX	Presence of distant metastasis cannot be assessed
M0	No distant metastasis
M1	Distant metastasis

STAGE GROUPING

Stage 0	Tis	N0	M0
Stage I	T1	N0	M0
Stage II	T2	N0	M0
Stage III	T3	N0	M0
	T1	N1	M0
	T2	N1	M0
	T3	N1	M0
Stage IV	T4	N0	M0
	T4	N1	M0
	Any T	N2	M0
	Any T	N3	M0
	Any T	Any N	M1

UICC, Union Internationale Centre Cancer; AJCC, American Joint Committee on Cancer.

Used with the permission of the American Joint Committee on Cancer (AJCC®), Chicago, Il. From AJCC Cancer Staging Manual, 5th ed. Philadelphia, Lippincott-Raven, 1997.

CHOICE OF TREATMENT MODALITY

The surgeon's goal is complete removal of the primary tumor and any cancer cells in regional lymph nodes, while preserving the uninvolved structures. The radiotherapist's goal is to damage the cancer cells irreparably while sparing normal tissue. Either modality is effective in controlling early oral and oropharyngeal carcinomas, but the use of both modalities or a combination of chemotherapy and radiation is necessary to control locally advanced disease. The role of chemotherapy alone in localized disease is palliative. Currently, distantly metastatic disease is incurable but can often be effectively palliated with chemotherapy or radiation or both.

Treatment choices are best made after considering tumor factors, patient factors, and resource factors. Tumor factors include site and subsite, T stage, N stage, histologic characteristics, endophytic versus exophytic morphology, and the proximity of tumor to bone. Patient factors include the patient's age, comorbidities, convenience, rehabilitation potential, and the patient's wishes. Resource factors include the availability of a well-trained surgeon or radiotherapists with a dedicated interest in head and neck cancer, the availability of advanced hardware for the planning and delivery of radiation, and the availability of funds to pay for the treatment.

The best treatment of early T1 and T2 oral cancer is usually surgery. Radiation therapy alone is effective for some early superficial lesions of the tongue or floor of the mouth, but the resulting xerostomia, the risk of mandible necrosis, and the long duration and expense of treatment make radiation a poor choice. Bone involvement by oral cancer often limits the effectiveness of external beam radiation, so lesions of the gingiva and hard palate are best treated with surgery owing to the close proximity of bone and the high incidence of bone invasion. Advantages of surgery for T1 and T2 oral cancer, compared with radiation, include decreased cost, decreased time of treatment, generation of a surgical specimen for examination of potential prognostic features, and, in some instances, an opportunity to sample the regional clinically negative nodes for occult disease. Advantages of radiation therapy for early lesions are avoidance of surgery and no general anesthetic.

Advanced T3 and T4 lesions of the oral cavity are best treated with surgery followed by adjuvant radiation therapy. Improvement in locoregional control of advanced oral and oropharyngeal cancer is attributable to the addition of postoperative radiation (Vikram et al, 1984a and b). Brachytherapy utilizing afterloading catheters can sometimes be employed for oral cancers, especially tumors of the tongue. However, resection of small lesions is usually simpler and less morbid, and surgery followed by radiation is more appropriate for treating the large tumor bed. The proximity of the tumor to the mandible, the complex surface anatomy, and the uncertainty of the tumor margins also limit brachytherapy approaches to oral cavity cancers. In contrast to tumors of the oropharynx, tumors of the oral cavity are poorly responsive to traditional organ-sparing approaches combining either sequential or concomitant chemotherapy and radiation therapy. The control rates for oral cavity cancers using these regimens are the lowest of all head and neck sites (Wolf et al, 1999).

In the treatment of oropharyngeal cancer, radiation alone, combined chemotherapy and radiation, and brachytherapy all play a significant role. Surgery is effective for early T1 and T2 lesions of the soft palate, tonsil, and base of the tongue and remains the treatment of choice when functional results are anticipated to be good. However, lesions with expected poor function after surgery may be well treated by nonsurgical means, reserving surgical salvage for nonresponders. For example, large T2

lesions of the base of the tongue respond well to a combination of external beam radiation and brachytherapy (Harrison et al, 1998). Tumors of the tonsil are particularly responsive to external-beam radiation therapy.

Advanced oropharyngeal cancer has traditionally been treated with combination surgery and postoperative radiation therapy. This surgery often requires specialized microvascular free flap reconstruction and intensive rehabilitation. Data are accumulating to support an organ preservation chemotherapy-radiation approach for advanced tumors of the oropharynx (Pfister et al, 1995). This approach is derived from the experience with larynx preservation, and surgical salvage is employed for nonresponders. Occasionally, the swallowing function is severely impaired after chemoradiotherapy. Invasion of the mandible indicates the need for surgical treatment.

Chemotherapy alone for oral and oropharyngeal cancers is palliative. Although some complete clinical responses can be obtained, they are not durable. Preoperative chemotherapy does not reduce the extent of surgical resection or the morbidity of oral cancer surgery.

SURGERY FOR ORAL AND OROPHARYNGEAL CANCER

Preoperative considerations are critical in treating patients with these tumors. Comorbidities are high in this patient population, and preoperative medical, cardiac, or anesthesia clearances are often indicated. Airway management is critical, and many oral and nearly all pharyngeal resections require tracheotomy.

The lip is the most common site of oral cancer, and it behaves like skin with cancer. T1 and T2 lesions are usually cured by wedge resection of the lip with primary closure, although primary radiation therapy is also effective. As many as 50% of the lower lip can be resected and closed primarily in three layers. Larger resections require an Abbe or Estlander lip switch reconstruction or Karapandzic advancement flaps. Large T3 or T4 lesions require resection of involved tissues, bilateral upper neck dissections, complex reconstruction, and postoperative radiation therapy.

The anterior two thirds of the tongue is the most common site of oral cancers. Oral tongue lesions tend to present in earlier stages because of early symptoms.

Tongue cancer may spread by deep invasion between muscle fascicles, which offer little resistance to tumor spread, so at least a 1-cm margin of normal tongue muscle should be taken around the tumor. Peroral partial glossectomy of T1 and T2 lesions of the oral tongue is easily performed using electrocautery. Intraoperative margin specimens for frozen section are taken with a scalpel. When feasible, the resection is planned in a transverse wedge fashion, and the defect of a partial glossectomy is closed horizontally. The resulting tongue function is excellent.

Tumors of the posterior portion of the tongue, floor of the mouth, or oropharynx are best approached through a mandibulotomy (Spiro et al, 1985). This provides the exposure required to perform an oncologically sound resection, and the morbidity is low. These patients benefit

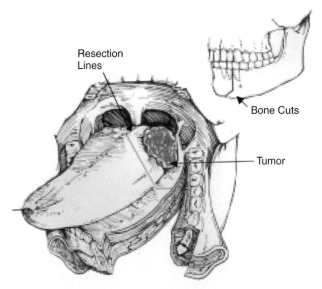

Figure 38–4. Mandibulotomy. (Adapted from Booth W: Maxillofacial Surgery. New York, Churchill Livingstone, 1999.)

from staging elective supraomohyoid neck dissection or therapeutic modified radical neck dissection, which provides the neck exposure needed for the mandibulotomy approach (Fig. 38–4). The neck dissection is performed, the lower lip is split, and the mandible and floor of the mouth mucosa and muscles are divided to allow the mandible to be retracted laterally. The mandible is plated after the resection, restoring form and function. Reconstruction of large or total tongue defects is best with pedicled pectoralis myocutaneous flaps or with free tissue transfer from the forearm or rectus muscle of the abdomen.

Early tongue cancers demonstrate occult spread to the cervical lymph nodes in 20% to 30% of cases. Except for oral cancers less than 2 mm thick, all early staged oral cancer patients should receive elective supraomohyoid neck dissection (Spiro et al, 1986). On the other hand, elective radiotherapy to the neck should be employed if radiation therapy is the treatment selected for the primary tumor. Clinically positive disease in the neck is treated with modified radical neck dissection and postoperative radiation.

The floor of the mouth is the second most common oral subsite, accounting for 20% of oral cancers. Because of the frequent involvement of the mandible by floor of the mouth tumors, management of the mandible is an important aspect of planning resections of the floor of the mouth. Resection of the full thickness of the mandible requires complex reconstruction or it can leave severe anterior defects. Reconstruction with the fibula free-flap has revolutionized the postoperative form and function of patients after anterior arch resection, and this reconstruction is preferred for all segmental mandibular defects. However, lateral defects can be adequately restored with reconstruction bars if they are well covered with soft tissue, or small lateral defects can be left unreconstructed in elderly edentulous patients.

In an effort to preserve continuity of the mandible,

the upper half of the mandible can be resected with the tumor (marginal mandibulectomy; Fig. 38–5) as a margin or if there is only minimal cortical involvement (Shaha, 1992). If there is gross bone invasion, a segmental resection and reconstruction are indicated.

An alternative surgical approach to T3 and T4 floor of the mouth lesions that do not require segmental mandibular resection is the transcervical pull-through procedure. After bilateral upper neck dissections, the primary tumor specimen is delivered into the neck, with or without marginal mandibular resection, by dividing the floor of the mouth muscles. Total glossectomy can also be performed by this approach in some cases.

Tumors of the gingiva and hard palate are often identified early but usually require bone resection owing to the early bone involvement. Small T1 lower gingival lesions are removed with marginal mandibulectomy and primary closure. Upper lesions require alveolectomy or partial or total maxillectomy, depending on the stage. Total maxillectomy may indicate the need for a Weber-Ferguson facial incision (Fig. 38–6) and upper cheek flap to ensure adequate visualization for the upper bone cuts. Rehabilitation and reconstruction of even large maxillary defects are excellent with a dental obturator. A temporary obturator should be prepared before surgery and placed for 5 days at the time of surgery as an immediate repair. Split-thickness skin grafting of the maxillectomy defect shortens healing time.

Tumors of the retromolar trigone occur with a disproportionately high frequency (15% of oral cancers), considering the small surface area. Tumors of this site are difficult to assess and treat because of their posterior location, mucosal irregularity, and trismus. Surgical access to this region is challenging. Bone resection is nearly always indicated, and recurrence is difficult to diagnose. A lip-splitting incision and a lower cheek flap allow access.

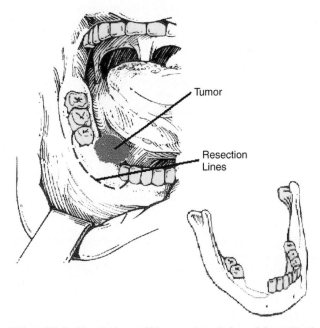

Figure 38–5. Marginal mandible resection. (Adapted from Booth W: Maxillofacial Surgery. New York, Churchill Livingstone, 1999.)

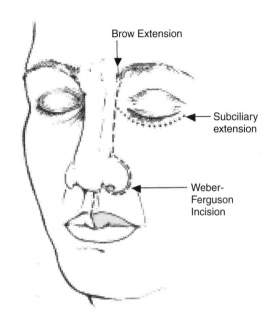

Brow Extension

Subciliary extension

Weber-Ferguson Incision

Figure 38–6. Weber-Ferguson skin incisions. (Adapted from Booth W: Maxillofacial Surgery. New York, Churchill Livingstone, 1999.)

Most T1 and T2 tumors of the soft palate can be resected perorally. Electrocautery or handheld CO_2 laser can be used to efficiently excise these tumors in a bloodless field. A through-and-through resection of the soft palate is nearly always indicated. The resulting defect can be left to granulate, or it can be closed primarily. T3 and T4 tumors of the soft palate may extend into the nasopharynx, hard palate, tonsil, parapharyngeal space, base of the tongue, or lateral pharyngeal wall. Peroral resection is sometimes possible. Nasal endoscopy can be helpful to perform necessary cuts on the nasal septum or lateral wall of the nasopharynx. Significant posterior and inferior extension to the lateral pharyngeal wall or the parapharyngeal space suggests the need for a mandibulotomy approach to ensure excellent access and visualization of the deepest portions of the tumor. Trismus is an ominous sign of pterygoid muscle involvement and is a poor prognostic factor.

Large defects of the soft palate are best reconstructed with an obturator with a nasopharyngeal bulb. This will allow swallowing without nasal regurgitation of food into the nasal cavity. Free-flap reconstruction of the soft palate does not provide a functional, mobile soft palate and should be avoided. Defects of the tonsil and the lateral pharyngeal wall are well reconstructed with the radial forearm free-flap.

T1 and T2 tumors of the base of the tongue are amenable to surgical resection with primary closure. The principal concern in all operations on the base of the tongue is the postoperative swallowing function; therefore, the planning of base of the tongue surgery must include saving the lingual and hypoglossal nerves when-

ever possible and preserving the structure and function of the supraglottic larynx to help prevent aspiration. In my experience, very few, if any, squamous cell carcinomas of the base of the tongue are amenable to an endoscopic resection. The base of the tongue is difficult to visualize with the laryngoscope, and the depth of invasion and the third dimension assessment of the tumor during the resection cannot be easily palpated, leading to uncertainty in the resection margins. The fascicles of the tongue musculature provide no resistance to the spread of a tumor; therefore, an aggressive, deep resection of the tongue musculature is indicated. Similarly, very few, if any, base of the tongue cancers can be adequately excised perorally.

Base of the tongue cancers are approached by mandibulotomy, transhyoid pharyngotomy, or lateral pharyngotomy. The transhyoid pharyngotomy avoids the mandibulotomy, but the visualization of the tongue base tumor is not as good. After neck dissection, the suprahyoid musculature is divided off the hyoid and the contralateral vallecula is entered. The tumor is palpated, and the base of the tongue exposed. The tumor is resected under vision and palpation. Small defects can be closed primarily. The lateral pharyngotomy can also expose small base of the tongue and pharyngeal tumors. After neck dissection, the pharynx is entered laterally, and the tumor is resected under direct vision. The pharyngotomy can be closed primarily or with complex flap reconstruction. Injury to the superior laryngeal nerve will increase the chance of postoperative aspiration because of poor sensation. Flap reconstruction of the base of the tongue will lead to aspiration if there is not enough sensate and mobile tissue immediately above the larynx. Every effort should be made to close the base of the tongue primarily near the larynx and interpose flaps more laterally if possible.

Small tumors of the posterior pharyngeal wall sometimes can be resected endoscopically or through a lateral pharyngotomy or midline mandibulotomy. If possible, healing by second intention will allow better swallowing function than does flap reconstruction in this location.

Surgery for tonsil cancers is effective, but surgery is often reserved for more advanced tonsil lesions because they are highly radioresponsive, and radical resection of the tonsil leads to functional deficits. Rarely, if ever, is simple tonsillectomy adequate treatment for even T1 tonsil cancer. Rarely can one be confident that the superior constrictor, the bed of the tonsil, is free from tumor involvement. A resection of the constrictor muscle with the tonsil is usually indicated. For advanced tumors that involve the mandible or those that have failed radiation, a radical resection through a mandibulotomy approach or with a segmental resection of the ascending ramus of the mandible is indicated. Free-flap reconstruction of soft tissue or bone is state of the art.

REHABILITATION

Head and neck cancer treatment can lead to significant impairment of function. The rehabilitation of speech and swallowing function after oral and oropharyngeal surgery is critical. This process requires the head and neck surgeon, plastic surgeon, speech and language therapist, nurses, dentists, prosthodontists, and oral and maxillofacial surgeons.

The first important element of rehabilitation is optimizing the patient's resection and reconstruction at the time of surgery. Preserving vital structures when appropriate and restoring form and function with state-of-the-art reconstruction maximizes the chances that a motivated patient will succeed in rehabilitation. After surgery, oral prostheses, modified barium swallow evaluations, and swallowing therapy help patients regain swallowing capacity. Still, some patients remain PEG-tube dependent for enteral nutrition, but this need not impair normal daily activities. Speech therapists can help patients maximize phonation, articulation, and alternative communication methods as needed.

Because head and neck cancer is caused by exposure to tobacco and alcohol, many patients are in need of active programs to assist in tobacco and alcohol cessation. Continued exposure increases the risks of subsequent cancer formation and decreases the efficacy of rehabilitation.

COMPLICATIONS

Surgical complications can be minimized by appropriate patient selection and preoperative evaluation, including medical, cardiology, and anesthesia clearance. Patients in negative nitrogen balance should be considered for a nasogastric feeding tube placement and several weeks of nutritional therapy prior to surgery. Properly selected patients should have a low incidence of major complications (Sessions and Hudkins, 1993).

The most common complications after oral and oropharyngeal cancer surgery are wound related. Minor wound breakdown, epidermolysis, and minor wound infections are common. The excellent blood supply to the head and neck helps ensure good healing of soft tissues. Careful surgical technique will minimize complications. It is important to handle tissues atraumatically, observe careful hemostasis, obliterate dead spaces, and minimize bacteria by antiseptic skin preparation and copious irrigation before closure. Twenty-four hours of IV antibiotics, initiated at least 1 hour prior to surgery, helps reduce the rate of wound infection.

The majority of wound complications will heal with aggressive cleansing and infection control. Management of comorbidities such as diabetes mellitus, malnutrition, and hypothyroidism in order to maximize wound healing is critical. Persistent nonhealing or a persistent orocutaneous fistula may result from the presence of a foreign body, such as hardware, nonabsorbable suture, or sequestered bone. Persistent tumor must be ruled out by biopsy in any nonhealing wound after oral cancer surgery. The frequency, complexity, and duration of wound complications are greater in the irradiated patient.

Major cardiovascular, pulmonary, and systemic complications are few. Major head and neck resections, which do not violate the chest or abdominal cavity, allow for early ambulation and enteric feeding and normalization

of physiology. Carotid artery exposure to fistula saliva and subsequent dehiscence remains a feared and fatal complication, which is now uncommon following improvement in flap reconstruction.

OUTCOMES

Outcomes in oral and oropharyngeal cancer surgery can be divided into survival and functional outcomes. Five-year survival rates for early T1 and T2 cancers are reported in the 70% to 90% range. In all head and neck sites, the presence of metastatic nodes to the neck decreases the survival by 50%. Five-year survival for patients with stage IV disease, especially with bulky or bilateral lower neck metastases, is less then 20%.

In resectable stage III and stage IV tumors with N0 or N1 disease, 5-year survival has been increased to the 50% to 60% range by the aggressive addition of postoperative radiation therapy (Vikram et al, 1984a and b). With improved local control rates in recent years, a higher percentage of deaths is due to distant disease and second primary carcinomas, rather than from uncontrolled locoregional disease.

Factors that predict survival of head and neck cancer patients are low T-stage, low N-stage, low overall stage, and the absence of significant comorbidities. Even though the study of the molecular genetics of squamous cancer is rapidly evolving, currently no molecular markers have been shown to predict survival in head and neck cancer patients in a large prospectively gathered series. Functional outcomes of surgery for early oral and oropharyngeal cancers are excellent. It is rare for patients to suffer significant loss of speech and swallowing function after surgical resection of T1 or T2 lesions.

Functional outcomes diminish with increasing volumes of resected tissue. Tissues impacting most on function

---

Pearls and Pitfalls

PEARLS

- Ninety percent of head and neck cancers are squamous cell carcinomas caused by tobacco and alcohol.
- Patients with oral and oropharyngeal cancer have a high incidence of comorbidities and of second cancers of the upper aerodigestive tract.
- Early T1 and T2 oral cancers are best treated surgically.
- Advanced T3 and T4 oral cancers are best treated with surgery and postoperative radiation.
- Radiation or surgery is used for early oropharyngeal cancer.
- Surgery and radiation, or brachytherapy, or chemotherapy and radiation are used for advanced oropharyngeal disease.
- Improved reconstruction has dramatically improved functional outcome.
- Rehabilitation of speech and swallowing is critical for quality of life.
- Early local disease is cured in 90% of cases. Advanced regional metastases indicate a less than 20% 5-year survival rate.

include base of tongue, hypoglossal nerve, lingual nerve, anterior mandibular arch, and soft palate. When extensive or multiple resections of these structures are undertaken for advanced disease, patient function may be poor even with the most advanced reconstructive and rehabilitative techniques.

SELECTED READINGS

Blot WJ, McLaughlin JK, Winn DM, et al: Smoking and drinking in relation to oral and pharyngeal cancer. Cancer Res 1988;48:3282.

Day GL, Blot WJ: Second primary tumors in patients with oral cancer. Cancer 1992;70:14.

Harrison LB, Lee HJ, Pfister DG, et al: Long-term results of primary radiotherapy with/without neck dissection for squamous cell cancer of the base of tongue. Head Neck 1998;20:668.

Landis SH, Murray T, Bolden S, Wingo PA: Cancer statistics, 1999. CA Cancer J Clin 1999;49:8.

Pfister DG, Harrison LB, Strong EW, et al: Organ function preservation in advanced oropharynx cancer: Results with induction chemotherapy and radiation. J Clin Oncol 1995;13:671.

Sessions RB, Hudkins C: Complications of surgery of the oral cavity. In Eisele DW (ed): Complications in Head and Neck Surgery. Baltimore, Mosby, 1993, pp 218–222.

Shaha AR: Marginal mandibulectomy for carcinoma of the floor of the mouth. J Surg Oncol 1992;49:116.

Spiro RH, Gerold FP, Shah JP, et al: Mandibulotomy approach to oropharyngeal tumors. Am J Surg 1985;150:466.

Spiro RH, Huvos AG, Wong GY, et al: Predictive value of tumor thickness in squamous carcinoma confined to the tongue and floor of the mouth. Am J Surg 1986;152:345.

Vikram B, Strong EW, Shah JP, Spiro R: Failure at the primary site following multimodality treatment in advanced head and neck cancer. Head Neck Surg 1984a;6:720.

Vikram B, Strong EW, Shah JP, Spiro R: Failure in the neck following multimodality treatment for advanced head and neck cancer. Head Neck Surg 1984b;6:724.

Wolf GT, Forastiere A, Ang K, et al: Workshop report: Organ preservation strategies in advanced head and neck cancer—current status and future directions. Head Neck 1999;21:689.

Chapter 39

Larynx and Hypopharynx

John F. Carew

Cancers of the head and neck are relatively uncommon, representing fewer than 5% of all cancers in the United States and accounting for 21,500 cancer deaths in 1998. Head and neck cancers, however, rank as the sixth most common cancer worldwide, a major health care problem. More than 90% of these tumors are squamous cell carcinomas (SCCs) arising from the mucosa of the upper aerodigestive tract. The risk factors most strongly associated with the development of head and neck cancers are tobacco and alcohol use. Alcohol potentiates tobacco-related carcinogenesis and is also an independent risk factor. A strong epidemiologic association also exists between smokeless tobacco and oral carcinogenesis.

Of the 295,000 cases of cancer of the head and neck accrued by the National Cancer Data Base over a 10-year period, the larynx was the most common site affected, accounting for more than 20% of all head and neck cancers (Hoffman et al, 1998). The larynx performs several unique and vital functions related to speaking, breathing, and swallowing, and the treatment of patients with neoplasms of the larynx or hypopharynx requires consideration of these critical functions. Specifically, the impact of therapeutic options on both the quantity and the quality of life needs to be taken into consideration. This chapter addresses the treatment of cancers of the head and neck, and specifically of the larynx and hypopharynx. These two sites are intimately related, and so they are discussed together. Any differences in the presentation, treatment, or outcome are contrasted in the discussion of these two subsites of the upper aerodigestive tract.

CLINICAL PRESENTATION

The most common presenting symptom in patients with cancer of the larynx is hoarseness. Any patient who complains of hoarseness lasting longer than 2 weeks requires examination of the larynx with adequate visualization of the vocal cords in order to determine whether a cancer is the etiology of the hoarseness. Specifically, in patients with risk factors such as significant tobacco or alcohol exposure, the index of suspicion should be high and any duration of hoarseness should lead one to obtain an adequate examination of the larynx. In contrast, patients who have cancers of the hypopharynx often have more subtle clinical presentations. Often, they complain of progressive odynophagia dysphagia that is more pronounced with solids than with liquids, and hoarseness. In general, patients with cancers of the vocal cords are seen in the early stage of disease because these tumors become symptomatic early in the course of the disease. Patients who have tumors of the supraglottic larynx or hypopharynx have more subtle symptoms and hence are first seen with more advanced primary tumors. Additionally, the hypopharynx can be difficult to visualize on examination in the office, especially the apex of the piriform sinus. This also contributes to the higher incidence of advanced-age disease seen in patients with cancers of the hypopharynx. As tumors become more advanced, other symptoms that may be noticed include the presence of a neck mass, representing regional metastasis, otalgia, weight loss, hemoptysis, and finally stridor and difficulty in breathing.

Once a tumor of either the larynx or the hypopharynx is suspected by the clinical history, a thorough head and neck examination with good visualization of the larynx and hypopharynx is critical. A laryngeal mirror provides an excellent view of both the larynx and the upper hypopharynx in the cooperative patient. Occasionally, because of body habitus or a prominent gag reflex, the mirror examination may be inadequate and further examination with the use of a fiberoptic or rigid telescope gives more information regarding the larynx and hypopharynx. The fiberoptic and the rigid telescope offer a detailed view of the larynx and hypopharynx and provide an opportunity to obtain photographic documentation, which may be useful in treatment planning and follow-up. The critical aspects of the tumor that can be ascertained from inspection include locating the epicenter of the tumor, discerning mucosal involvement, and assessing vocal fold mobility on film. It may be difficult, however, to determine the third dimension, or depth, of the tumor on physical examination, even with the aid of these fiberoptic and rigid telescopes. For this reason, high-resolution computed tomography (CT) scans are invaluable in assessing primary tumors at both the laryngeal and the hypopharyngeal positions. Specifically, CT scanning aids in determining the depth of the tumor and any pre-epiglottic or paraglottic space involvement in these tumors. Along with examination of the primary, these patients must also have adequate assessment of the regional lymph nodes that are at risk from primaries of the larynx and hypopharynx. Levels II, III, and IV are the regional lymph nodes at greatest risk for primaries of the larynx and hypopharynx. Even though clinical examination often reveals any regional lymph node metastasis, again CT scans give complementary information on early regional metastasis.

The staging of tumors of the larynx and hypopharynx, including the neck, is listed in Table 39–1. A chest x-ray examination and serum liver function tests provide adequate metastatic evaluation in the absence of any systemic complaints. In patients at high risk for distant metastases, such as advanced bilateral neck metastases or bulky metastases low in the neck, consideration may be given to chest CT to assess early metastatic disease, which would profoundly affect treatment planning.

PREOPERATIVE MANAGEMENT

The most critical aspect of the preoperative evaluation of patients with cancer of the larynx or hypopharynx involves

Table 39–1	AJCC Staging of Carcinoma of the Larynx and Hypopharynx

Larynx: Supraglottis
T1: Tumor limited to one subsite of the supraglottis with normal vocal cord mobility
T2: Tumor invades mucosa of more than one adjacent subsite of the supraglottis or glottis or region outside the supraglottis (e.g., mucosa of the base of tongue, valleculae, medial wall of piriform sinus) without fixation of the larynx
T3: Tumor limited to the larynx with vocal cord fixation and/or invades any of the following: postcricoid area, pre-epiglottic tissues
T4: Tumor invades through the thyroid cartilage, and/or extends into the soft tissues of the neck, thyroid and/or esophagus
Larynx: Glottis
T1: Tumor limited to the vocal cords (may involve anterior or posterior commissure) with normal vocal cord mobility
   T1A: Tumor limited to one vocal cord
   T1B: Tumor involves both vocal cords
T2: Tumor extends to the supraglottis and/or subglottis, and/or with impaired vocal cord mobility
T3: Tumor limited to the larynx with vocal cord fixation
T4: Tumor invades through the thyroid cartilage and/or extends to other tissues beyond the larynx (e.g., trachea, soft tissues of the neck, including thyroid, pharynx)
Larynx: Subglottis
T1: Tumor limited to the subglottis
T2: Tumor extends to the vocal cords with normal or impaired mobility
T3: Tumor limited to the larynx with vocal cord fixation
T4: Tumor invades through the cricoid or thyroid cartilage and/or extends to other tissues beyond the larynx (e.g., trachea, soft tissues of the neck, including thyroid, esophagus)
Hypopharynx
T1: Tumor limited to one subsite of the hypopharynx and 2 cm or less in greatest dimension
T2: Tumor involves more than one subsite of the hypopharynx or an adjacent site, or measures more than 2 but not more than 4 cm in greatest diameter without fixation of the hemilarynx
T3: Tumor measures more than 4 cm in greatest dimension or with fixation of the hemilarynx
T4: Tumor invades adjacent structures (e.g., thyroid/cricoid cartilage, carotid artery, soft tissues of the neck, prevertebral fascia/muscles, thyroid and/or esophagus)
Neck
N0: No regional lymph node metastasis
N1: Ipsilateral lymph node metastasis ≤3 cm
N2: Lymph node metastasis in a single ipsilateral lymph node >3 cm and ≤6 cm, or in multiple lymph nodes none more than 6 cm (including bilateral nodal metastasis)
N2A: Lymph node metastasis, a single ipsilateral lymph node >3 cm and ≤6 cm
N2B: Lymph node metastasis, multiple ipsilateral lymph nodes, all ≤6 cm
N2C: Lymph node metastasis, a bilateral or contralateral lymph node, all ≤6 cm
N3: Lymph node metastasis >6 cm

adequate endoscopic assessment of the primary tumor. This is done by direct laryngoscopy and esophagoscopy with the patient under general anesthesia. The extent of the primary tumor is assessed and rigid telescopes with 0-, 30-, 70-, and 120-degree lenses are extremely helpful in assessing the primary tumor. Specifically, they aid in determining subglottic extension and in mapping out the exact extent of the tumor. This information is critical in treatment planning in that partial laryngectomies can be designed for various tumors, depending on their location. In patients whose primary tumors arise in the hypopharynx, adequate endoscopic assessment is critical to treatment planning. The practitioner needs to determine the resectability of the tumors, the potential need for sacrificing the larynx at the time of surgery, and the amount of pharynx that will need to be sacrificed and thus reconstructed. Additionally, the lower extent of the tumor must be assessed in relationship to the cricopharyngeus and upper esophagus. It is critical to understand that the hypopharynx is a funnel-shaped structure and that the more distal the location of the lesion, the greater the likelihood of circumferential sacrifice of the pharyngeal wall. With this in mind, surgical resection of bulky hypopharyngeal tumors that approach the cricopharyngeus and upper esophagus often necessitates circumferential sacrifice in the form of a total laryngopharyngectomy and thus requires reconstruction of the resected segment. Such

reconstruction is most often performed with the use of a free jejunal transfer.

Once the tumor has been adequately assessed, a treatment plan must be designed that will give the patient the highest chance of survival along with the least functional morbidity. The optimal treatment for each patient requires consideration of both tumor as well as patient factors. The single most important tumor factor is the extent of the tumor, as seen on detailed endoscopic evaluation. Mapping out the tumor during this preoperative evaluation allows one to consider whether the tumor would be amenable to a partial laryngectomy or would require a total laryngectomy or total laryngopharyngectomy. Other characteristics of the tumor are also important and include whether the tumor is endophytic or exophytic. Exophytic tumors tend to be more radioresponsive and thus may yield higher control rates in a radiation therapy–based treatment paradigm.

The other factors involved in the treatment decision-making process include the occupation, general medical status, and mental status of the patient. Specifically, patients who are candidates for partial laryngectomy must have adequate pulmonary reserve to tolerate a small amount of aspiration. Additionally, the importance of the voice to the patient's livelihood and lifestyle is also critical in deciding on treatment. Finally, the length of time the patient is willing to be out of work to undergo treatment may influence the decision, in that a patient with an early cancer treated with surgical resection may be able to return to work earlier than one whose cancer is treated with radiation therapy.

Even though the optimal treatment must be determined for each individual patient, several broad statements may be made regarding treatment options for laryngeal and hypopharyngeal cancers. In general, most patients with early-stage disease (stage I or II) can experience higher rates of local control with a single mode of treatment. The two treatments that can be considered for early-stage disease include either surgical resection or external-beam radiation therapy. For early-stage glottic cancers, good local control can be achieved with either external-beam radiation therapy or surgical resection. A superior quality of voice, however, is usually seen in patients who undergo external-beam radiation therapy. In selected patients, however, endoscopic resection of early tumors with microlaryngoscopic techniques may yield a good result with regard to vocal quality. In patients with more bulky primary tumors, surgical resection may be considered if a conservation procedure that spares the voice can be performed. In patients with advanced-stage disease, multimodality therapy is usually required. In the past, this usually included surgical resection followed by adjuvant radiation therapy (see Selected Readings, including Harwood et al [1983] and Myers and Alvi [1996]). In the past 20 years, however, treatment paradigms combining chemotherapy with radiation therapy have evolved and have yielded equivalent survival rates when evaluated in a randomized prospective fashion (Lefebvre et al [1996] and Department of Veterans Affairs Laryngeal Cancer Study Group [1991]). Given this, patients who wish to use a treatment paradigm that may preserve their larynx and hypopharynx, such as chemotherapy and radiation therapy, should be offered this nonsurgical option. However, patients considering chemotherapy and radiation therapy as a treatment option must be reliable and must enroll a multidisciplinary team experienced in treating advanced cancers of the larynx and hypopharynx. Finally, tumors of the larynx and hypopharynx that show extension outside of the larynx or hypopharynx and that have soft-tissue involvement, are endophytic, or impair the airway to such an extent that tracheostomy is required often demonstrate aggressive clinical behavior and have poor responses to treatment. In these patients with aggressive primary tumors, early surgical intervention may improve the chances for local control and thus improve quality of life, which otherwise would deteriorate with persistent or recurrent disease. A surgical treatment plan in these cases may not improve survival, but it may improve the quality of life in these patients who can suffer from airway obstruction and intractable pain as their tumors progress.

In patients in whom a surgical treatment approach is considered, there is a vast array of potential surgical procedures that are as diverse as the tumors themselves. Although there are general classifications of the surgical procedures, each one is designed specifically to encompass, in an oncologic fashion, each patient's individual tumor as assessed on endoscopic examination. These various broad classifications of surgical procedures are presented in the next section on intraoperative management.

INTRAOPERATIVE MANAGEMENT

The surgical procedures that can be used in carefully selected patients with cancer of the larynx or hypopharynx are presented in broad categories. As previously mentioned, operations are designed on the basis of the endoscopic evaluation of each individual patient's tumor to afford the optimal oncologic resection while minimizing functional morbidity. For early tumors of the larynx or hypopharynx, endoscopic resection of the primary lesion in the properly selected patient can yield high local control rates. Endoscopic resections are more commonly performed in patients with laryngeal primaries, because hypopharyngeal primaries more often present with advanced-stage disease. For early T1 lesions, simple endoscopic resection with negative surgical margins often is curative. For more advanced lesions, an endoscopic approach using the laser to assist in resection of tumors has been reported by Steiner as well as Zeitels. These approaches attempt to limit surgical morbidity while achieving good oncologic results.

For more advanced lesions of the larynx and hypopharynx, partial laryngectomy or partial laryngopharyngectomy can be considered, based on the endoscopic assessment of the tumor. Tumors that arise on the true vocal cord, with limited involvement of the arytenoid or anterior commissure, can be resected with a vertical partial laryngectomy. In this procedure, a horizontal incision is made over the thyroid cartilage, which is widely exposed. The majority of the thyroid cartilage on the side of the lesion and the true vocal cord and portions of the subglottic mucosa and false vocal cord are resected, as dictated by the extent of the tumor. The strap muscles are then closed over the defect, helping to reconstruct the larynx. A tracheostomy is placed and left in place for approximately 4 to 7 days until the patient is able to tolerate its being capped and until endoscopic evidence of an adequate airway is present. If anterior commissure involvement is seen, the vertical partial laryngectomy can be extended to include the anterior commissure. This operation is called a frontal lateral partial laryngectomy. When a vertical partial laryngectomy is performed, voice quality is quite good, but when a significant amount of the anterior commissure is sacrificed, voice results are less predictable. This procedure, however, should not be contemplated if there is significant posterior commissure involvement, subglottic extension, or inadequate pulmonary reserve.

For tumors involving the supraglottic larynx, supraglottic laryngectomy can be performed. It is critical to assess the pulmonary reserve in these patients, however, because at least a small amount of aspiration is almost uniformly present temporarily postoperatively. Patients are selected for this surgery based on assessment of the tumor as mapped out on preoperative endoscopic evaluation. Detailed examination with the rigid telescope is critical when one selects patients who are appropriate for this operation. Specifically, assessing the proximity of the lower border of the tumor to the anterior commissure and true vocal cords is crucial. A horizontal incision is made in the neck, and the supraglottic larynx is exposed and resected. The resection usually includes the upper half of the thyroid cartilage, the thyrohyoid membrane, the hyoid and the epiglottis, and the aryepiglottic folds and false vocal cords. The surgeon performs closure by suturing the base of the tongue to the remaining thyroid cartilage with interrupted sutures. A tracheostomy is required temporarily following supraglottic laryngectomy. Relative contraindications to supraglottic laryngectomy include involvement of the posterior or anterior commissure, preepiglottic space involvement, fixation of the vocal cord, extension into the piriform sinus, or inadequate pulmonary reserve.

For more advanced lesions, extended partial laryngectomies have been designed, as described by Pearson, with the near-total laryngectomy, and Laccourreye, with the supracricoid laryngectomy. These extended partial laryngectomies are designed for oncologic resections of bulky primary tumors while preserving as much normal mucosa as possible. The resection is designed to afford an oncologic resection of the tumor while minimizing functional morbidity. A horizontal incision is made for wide exposure of the laryngeal framework. The appropriate oncologic resection is performed, and the cricoid and at least one arytenoid are preserved. Closure is achieved by approximating the cricoid to either the hyoid or the epiglottis, depending on the extent of resection. These patients invariably require a temporary tracheostomy, and their functional outcome is less predictable with regard to decannulation and swallowing. In most properly selected patients, decannulation and adequate peroral intake are achieved.

As mentioned earlier, nonsurgical treatment paradigms exist for advanced cancers of the larynx and hypopharynx. In patients who would require a total laryngectomy or total laryngopharyngectomy, a nonsurgical treatment option should be considered. In those who either fail nonsurgical treatment or whose tumors are aggressive, total laryngectomy or total laryngopharyngectomy may be necessary. These procedures are done through a horizontal incision with wide exposure the larynx. In a total laryngectomy, the larynx is resected from above the hyoid to the trachea. Closure can usually be achieved primarily so long as a significant amount of the hypopharynx did not require sacrifice. If a tension-free closure cannot be done primarily, a flap may be used to reconstruct the anterior wall and facilitate a tension-free closure, thus minimizing the risk of fistula. When a tumor involves the hypopharynx, occasionally a partial laryngopharyngectomy can be performed, which preserves the contralateral vocal cord. In properly selected patients, this yields an adequate airway and a reasonable voice, and preserves the ability of the patient to swallow. These are done in a fashion similar to that for partial laryngectomies, with wide exposure of the laryngeal framework through a horizontal incision. The components of the larynx and hypopharynx that are involved with tumor are resected. In the case of partial laryngopharyngectomy, caution must be used because hypopharyngeal tumors often have a significant amount of submucosal extension, which may be greater than clinically apparent. For this reason, this procedure must be

done in carefully selected patients. In these procedures, a tracheostomy is again necessary to maintain an adequate airway. For more advanced lesions of the hypopharynx, however, a total laryngopharyngectomy is often necessary. In this procedure, a horizontal incision is also used to widely expose the larynx and the hypopharynx. In most cases, a circumferential resection of the larynx and hypopharynx is necessary. In these cases, reconstruction is usually performed with a jejunal free tissue transfer. Alternatively, a gastric pull-up may be used to reconstruct the circumferential defect. In carefully selected patients, in whom part of the hypopharyngeal wall on the contralateral side is preserved, a flap may be used to reconstruct the defect and thus preclude the necessity of a circumferential reconstruction technique.

Appropriate management of the neck is critical to maximizing survival in patients with advanced cancer of the larynx. The treatment of the neck depends, in part, on the treatment of the primary. If the primary is to be treated by surgical means, an elective dissection of the lymph nodes at risk should be planned in the clinically negative neck in patients at significant risk for occult regional lymph node metastases. For a lesion of the vocal cord or hypopharynx, the ipsilateral levels II to IV should be cleared, whereas for a supraglottic lesion bilateral levels II to IV are at risk and should be dissected. The incidence of occult metastasis for glottic primaries is much lower than that for supraglottic or hypopharyngeal primaries. In this context, elective neck dissection is rarely done for early glottic tumors, compared with supraglottic or piriform sinus tumors. If there is clinically apparent lymph node metastasis in the neck and the primary is to be treated with surgery, a comprehensive neck dissection (levels I to V) should be performed.

Alternatively, if a patient with clinically negative sides of the neck is to undergo chemotherapy and radiation therapy for the primary lesion, the side or sides of the neck at risk should also be treated electively with radiation therapy. A somewhat more controversial situation exists if there is a clinically positive neck and the primary is to be treated by chemotherapy and radiation therapy. In this case, the options include performing a comprehensive neck dissection before chemotherapy or radiation therapy, performing a planned comprehensive or selective neck dissection after chemotherapy or radiation therapy, or assessing the response following chemotherapy or radiation therapy and performing appropriate neck dissection based on this response. At this time, data for substantiating an advantage to any of these approaches are lacking, and all are acceptable.

POSTOPERATIVE MANAGEMENT

As expected, the postoperative management of the aforementioned surgical procedures varies, depending on the extent of resection. For patients with early-stage lesions who undergo endoscopic resection, the postoperative airway is usually adequate, and therefore tracheostomy is not needed. Additionally, the patients are often able to swallow within 24 to 48 hours following the procedure, and thus a feeding tube is not necessary. In patients undergoing more extensive endoscopic resection for bulky tumors, the return of swallowing and the adequacy of airway must be assessed at the completion of resection and decisions must be made regarding stabilization of the airway and the necessity for a feeding tube. For partial laryngectomies, such as a vertical partial laryngectomy or a supraglottic laryngectomy, a tracheostomy is often necessary to maintain the airway for the first several days postoperatively, during the time of maximal edema. Often, these tracheostomies can be downsized 5 to 7 days postoperatively and decannulated once the patient tolerates having the tracheostomy capped. However, patients who undergo supraglottic laryngectomy often have difficulty in swallowing postoperatively. Removal of the tracheostomy facilitates laryngeal elevation and enhances swallowing. At times, however, prolonged tracheostomies are necessary to ensure an adequate pulmonary toilet if significant aspiration occurs. For this reason, the decision to decannulate must take into consideration the degree of aspiration the patient has, the patient's pulmonary reserve, and the patient's general medical condition. A feeding tube is usually placed for patients undergoing both vertical partial laryngectomies as well as supraglottic laryngectomies to ensure adequate nutrition in the immediate postoperative period. In patients undergoing vertical partial laryngectomies, often adequate peroral intake can be seen at 5 to 7 days, and at that time the feeding tube can be removed. In patients who undergo supraglottic laryngectomy, however, swallowing may be slightly delayed, and the overall clinical picture must be taken into account when one decides when to remove the feeding tube and allow the patient to begin swallowing. Likewise in patients who undergo partial pharyngolaryngectomies, a feeding tube is left in place for a week, after which swallowing is assessed. Additionally, the tracheostomy is removed once the patient is able to tolerate its being capped.

Patients undergoing total laryngectomy or total laryngopharyngectomy have a stoma and thus do not require a tracheostomy tube. Occasionally, a temporary soft Silastic stent is placed in the stoma to decrease crusting and allow healing. In a correctly designed stoma, there should not be a need for long-term stenting with a soft Silastic tube. In patients undergoing total laryngectomy and laryngopharyngectomy, a feeding tube is placed and the patient is maintained on tube feeds for a week to 10 days following surgery. If the patient remains afebrile and the neck looks good, the patient is given a trial of peroral feeds at 7 to 10 days postoperatively. If the patient has received prior chemotherapy and radiation therapy, often the trial of peroral intake is delayed for a slightly longer period. Finally, in patients who undergo free jejunal reconstruction, often a Gastrografin swallow is obtained to exclude a leak before peroral intake is allowed. A fistula should be suspected in any patient who remains febrile without another source of fever or whose neck incision shows significant edema, erythema, or fluctuance. If a fistula is identified, the wound should be opened widely and local wound care begun.

COMPLICATIONS

The complications associated with laryngectomy or laryngopharyngectomy can be divided into acute and chronic categories. The acute complications include those related to surgery and general anesthesia. These include bleeding, infection, pneumonia, and fistula. The most troublesome of these is the pharyngocutaneous fistula. The fistula rate following total laryngectomy remains relatively high, ranging from 8% to 22%. Appropriate treatment of a pharyngocutaneous fistula requires early recognition and then wide opening of the wound with appropriate wound care. The patient should stop all oral intake, and an alternative route of alimentation should be established. If significant carotid exposure is seen, consideration should be given to coverage with a regional flap to afford carotid protection, especially in the setting of previous radiation therapy. Often, the fistula closes spontaneously with aggressive wound care. In the cases that do not close, however, local, regional, and even free flaps may be used to obtain closure.

The most common complications of partial laryngectomy are related to inadequacy of the airway and swallowing, resulting in delayed decannulation and peroral feeding. Pharyngocutaneous fistulas are much less common in patients undergoing partial laryngectomies but are managed in a similar fashion, as described earlier.

The most common chronic complication of total laryngectomy and laryngopharyngectomy is stricture formation with dysphagia. It is crucial to exclude recurrent tumor whenever new dysphagia or worsening dysphagia develops. This is usually best evaluated by endoscopy with direct visualization of the mucosa of the neopharynx. Preoperative esophagograms are often helpful in defining the location and extent of stricture. If a stricture is seen, these can usually be dilated, although repeated treatments are often required. Ultimately, if a stricture is unresponsive to these conservative measures, consideration can be given to free tissue transfer to reconstruct an adequate neopharynx.

The early sequelae of radiation therapy relate primarily to the acute tissue reactions with characteristic skin changes and mucositis. These are managed symptomatically with oral hygiene and topical medications. The late sequelae of radiation therapy include skin changes, xerostomia, and very rarely, chondroradionecrosis of the laryngeal skeleton. Xerostomia is treated symptomatically with oral hygiene and humidification. In severe cases of chondroradionecrosis, which profoundly impairs swallowing and breathing, a total laryngectomy may be needed to restore the patient's ability to swallow.

Treatment protocols that use chemotherapy and radiation therapy to preserve organ function have successfully demonstrated their ability to anatomically preserve the larynx without compromising patient survival. One aspect of these protocols that is often underappreciated, however, is the functional capacity of the retained organs. Few investigators have clearly documented the functional sequelae of chemotherapy and radiation therapy. Lazarus retrospectively studied patients treated with chemotherapy and radiation therapy and found that 40% had swallowing difficulties. Certainly, patients who successfully undergo chemotherapy and radiation therapy to preserve their larynx have a much improved quality of life compared with patients who have undergone total laryngectomy. Nevertheless, anatomic preservation does not translate into functional preservation. Very rarely, total

Table 39–2 | Results of Conventional Treatment of Advanced Carcinoma of the Larynx

AUTHORS	N	Rx	STAGE III/IV	5-yr SURVIVAL*
Kirchner	308	S/RT	100%	54%–56%
Harwood	353	RT	54%	70%
Harwood	410	RT	66%	57%
Yuen	192	S	100%	77%
	50	S/RT	100%	91%
Mendenhall	100	RT	100%	74%
	65	S ± RT	100%	63%
Nguyen	116	S/RT	100%	68%
Myers	65	S ± RT	100%	62%†

*Survival refers to disease-free survival when available; otherwise reference is to overall survival.
†2-yr survival.
S, surgery; RT, radiation therapy.

laryngectomy is performed to restore the ability to swallow when a larynx is incompetent and nonfunctional but clinically free from cancer following these nonsurgical treatment paradigms.

OUTCOMES

Historically, surgery in the form of total laryngectomy followed by adjuvant postoperative radiation therapy has been the standard treatment for most patients with advanced-stage cancer of the larynx (Kirchner and Owen, 1977; Mendenhall et al, 1992; Yuen et al, 1984; Nguyen et al, 1996; Myers and Alvi, 1996). Additionally, selected patients with advanced-stage larynx cancer have undergone definitive radiation therapy alone (Harwood et al, 1979, 1983; Mendenhall et al, 1992). The results of these treatments are summarized in Table 39–2 with 5-year survival rates ranging from 54% to 91%.

More recently, chemotherapy and radiation therapy have evolved into an effective treatment for advanced-stage cancer of the larynx. A summary of results from the various studies evaluating chemotherapy and radiation therapy in the treatment of patients with advanced-stage laryngeal cancer, with the goal of larynx preservation, are listed in chronologic order in Table 39–3. In all but one study, more than 90% of patients evaluated had stage III

or IV disease. Most studies included only those patients who would have required a total laryngectomy if treated by conventional means with surgery and postoperative radiotherapy. Treatment results for patients given chemotherapy and radiation therapy in these studies are fairly consistent, with 2-year survival rates ranging from 50% to 77%, larynx preservation rates ranging from 64% to 79%, local-regional failure rates ranging from 20% to 33%, and distant failure rates ranging from 8% to 21%. However, only one of these studies was limited only to patients with laryngeal primaries (Department of Veterans Affairs Laryngeal Study Group, 1991); the remainder of the studies included patients with oropharynx, oral cavity, and even paranasal sinuses as sites of primary tumors. The majority of the studies that included nonlaryngeal sites did so because surgical treatment of the primary would have required total laryngectomy. The data presented in Table 39–3 refer to the subset of patients with laryngeal primaries whenever possible, although this information was not always available. Analogous results for the treatment of patients with cancer of the hypopharynx are presented in Table 39–4. As can be seen, chemotherapy and radiation therapy yield results similar to those with conventional treatment. The overall results for hypopharyngeal tumors, however, are much worse than those seen with laryngeal tumors.

In several of the aforementioned studies, single-mo-

Table 39–3 | Results of Treatment of Advanced Carcinoma of the Larynx Using Chemotherapy and Radiation Therapy

AUTHORS	N	Rx	STAGE III/IV	2-yr SURVIVAL*
Jacobs	30	C/RT	100%	52%†
Demard	50	C/RT	64%	74%†
				(Response rate)
Veterans Affairs Larynx Group	166	C/RT	100%	68%
	166	S/RT	100%	68%†
Pfister	13	C/RT	98%	77%†
Karp	14	C/RT	92%	50%†
Urba	8	C/RT	93%	75%†
Clayman (includes data from Shirinian)	26	C/RT	96%	68%†
	52	S/RT	96%	81%†

*Survival refers to disease-free survival when available; otherwise reference is to overall survival.
†Study included both laryngeal and nonlaryngeal sites
C, chemotherapy; S, surgery; RT, radiation therapy.

| Table 39–4 | Results of Treatment of Advanced Carcinoma of the Hypopharynx |||||

AUTHORS	N	Rx	STAGE III/IV (%)	2-yr SURVIVAL (%)*
Kraus	25	C/RT	96	32
Lefebvre	100	C/RT	93	43
	94	S/RT	93	32
Zelefsky	26	C/RT	92	30†
	30	S/RT	100	42†
Beauvillain	45	C/RT	—	19†
	47	C/S/RT	—	37†
Kraus	132	S/RT	78	41†

*Survival refers to disease-free survival when available; otherwise reference is to overall survival.
†5-yr survival.
C, chemotherapy; S, surgery; RT, radiation therapy.

dality therapy in the form of definitive radiotherapy was used and yielded disease-specific survival rates similar to those seen with the combination of induction chemotherapy and radiation therapy. Although the selected cohort of patients who received radiation therapy alone had fewer stage IV and node-positive patients, the contribution of chemotherapy to these larynx preservation protocols remains undetermined. Whereas previous randomized prospective trials have not included a radiation therapy–only arm, an ongoing prospective randomized trial has included a radiation therapy–only arm to address this question. This phase III trial has three treatment arms, including (1) radiotherapy alone, (2) sequential chemotherapy and radiotherapy, and (3) concomitant chemotherapy and radiotherapy. Data from this study will help to further define the optimal treatment for patients with advanced larynx cancer.

Finally, researchers continue to develop novel treatment strategies to further improve the survival and functional outcomes in patients with advanced cancers of the larynx. One such unique strategy uses high-dose, intra-arterial cisplatin with a systemic neutralizing agent along with conventional radiotherapy (Robbins et al, 1996). In this study, in which the majority of patients had stage IV disease (86%) and clinically involved regional lymph nodes (79%), a major response rate was seen in 95% of patients. Nine of 10 patients retained their larynx, and the 2-year disease-specific survival rate was 76%. A total of 3 of the 42 patients experienced central nervous system complications as the result of catheretization of the carotid system. Nevertheless, this option remains a promising and novel approach in the treatment of advanced-stage laryngeal cancer.

SELECTED READINGS

Beauvillain C, Mahe M, Bourdin S, et al: Final results of a randomized trial comparing chemotherapy plus radiotherapy with chemotherapy plus surgery plus radiotherapy in locally advanced resectable hypopharyngeal carcinomas. Laryngoscope 1997;107:648.

Clayman GL, Weber RS, Guillamondegui O, et al: Laryngeal preservation for advanced laryngeal and hypopharyngeal cancers. Arch Otolaryngol Head Neck Surg 1995;121:219.

Demard F, Chauvel P, Santini J, et al: Response to chemotherapy as justification for modification of the therapeutic strategy for pharyngolaryngeal carcinomas. Head Neck 1990;12:225.

Department of Veterans Affairs Laryngeal Cancer Study Group: Induction chemotherapy plus radiation compared with surgery plus radiation in patients with advanced laryngeal cancer [see comments]. N Engl J Med 1991;324:1685.

Harwood AR, Beale FA, Cummings BJ, et al: Supraglottic laryngeal carcinoma: An analysis of dose-time-volume factors in 410 patients. Int J Radiat Oncol Biol Phys 1983;9:311.

Harwood AR, Hawkins NV, Beale FA, et al: Management of advanced glottic cancer: A 10-year review of the Toronto experience. Int J Radiat Oncol Biol Phys 1979;5:899.

Hoffman HT, Karnell LH, Funk GF, et al: The National Cancer Data Base report on cancer of the head and neck. Arch Otolaryngol Head Neck Surg 1998;124:951.

Jacobs C, Goffinet DR, Goffinet L, et al: Chemotherapy as a substitute for surgery in the treatment advanced resectable head and neck cancer: A report from the Northern California Oncology Group. Cancer 1987;60:1178.

Karp DD, Vaughan CW, Carter R, et al: Larynx preservation using induction chemotherapy plus radiation therapy as an alternative to laryngectomy in advanced head and neck cancer: A long-term follow-up report. Am J Clin Oncol 1991;14:273.

Kirchner JA, Owen JR: Five hundred cancers of the larynx and pyriform sinus: Results of treatment by radiation and surgery. Laryngoscope 1977;87:1288.

Kraus DH, Pfister DG, Harrison LB, et al: Larynx preservation with combined chemotherapy and radiation therapy in advanced hypopharynx cancer. Otolaryngol Head Neck Surg 1994;111:31.

Kraus DH, Zelefsky MJ, Brock HA, et al: Combined surgery and radiation therapy for squamous cell carcinoma of the hypopharynx. Otolaryngol Head Neck Surg 1997;116:637.

Laccourreye H, Laccourreye O, Weinstein G, et al: Supracricoid laryngectomy with cricohyoidopexy: A partial laryngeal procedure for selected supraglottic and transglottic carcinomas. Laryngoscope 1990;100:735.

Lazarus CL, Logemann JA, Pauloski BR, et al: Swallowing disorders in head and neck cancer patients treated with radiotherapy and adjuvant chemotherapy. Laryngoscope 1996;106:1157.

Lefebvre JL, Chevalier D, Luboinski B, et al: Larynx preservation in pyriform

Pearls and Pitfalls

PITFALLS

- **Admonitions.** Do not contemplate surgical resection of a laryngeal or hypopharyngeal tumor until adequate endoscopic assessment has been performed.
- **Common errors of practice.** The most common error of practice is underestimating the clinical extent of disease.
- **Anatomic considerations.** The most critical anatomic consideration is using the endoscopic assessment in planning an oncologically sound resection.
- **Pathology change.** Squamous cell carcinomas account for more than 90% of tumors of the larynx and hypopharynx. Occasionally, the practitioner may encounter other histologies, such as lymphoma, spindle cell carcinoma, neuroendocrine carcinoma, minor salivary gland carcinomas, mucosal melanomas, and various sarcomas.

sinus cancer: Preliminary results of a European Organization for Research and Treatment of Cancer phase III trial. EORTC Head and Neck Cancer Cooperative Group [see comments]. J Natl Cancer Inst 1996;88:890.

Mendenhall WM, Parsons JT, Stringer SP, et al: Stage T3 squamous cell carcinoma of the glottic larynx: A comparison of laryngectomy and irradiation. Int J Radiat Oncol Biol Phys 1992;23:725.

Myers EN, Alvi A: Management of carcinoma of the supraglottic larynx: Evolution, current concepts, and future trends. Laryngoscope 1996;106:559.

Nguyen TD, Malissard L, Theobald S, et al: Advanced carcinoma of the larynx: Results of surgery and radiotherapy without induction chemotherapy (1980–1985). A multivariate analysis. Int J Radiat Oncol Biol Phys 1996;36:1013.

Pearson BW: Subtotal laryngectomy. Laryngoscope 1981;91:1904.

Pfister DG, Strong E, Harrison L, et al: Larynx preservation with combined chemotherapy and radiation therapy in advanced but resectable head and neck cancer. J Clin Oncol 1991;9:850.

Robbins KT, Fontanesi J, Wong FS, et al: A novel organ preservation protocol for advanced carcinoma of the larynx and pharynx. Arch Otolaryngol Head Neck Surg 1996;122:853.

Shirinian MH, Weber RS, Lippman SM, et al: Laryngeal preservation by induction chemotherapy plus radiotherapy in locally advanced head and neck cancer: The M.D. Anderson Cancer Center experience. Head Neck 1994;16:39.

Steiner W: Results of curative laser microsurgery of laryngeal carcinomas. Am J Otolaryngol 1993;14:116.

Urba SG, Forastierre AA, Wolf GT, et al: Intensive induction chemotherapy and radiation therapy for organ preservation in patients with advanced resectable head and neck carcinoma. J Clin Oncol 1994;12:946.

Yuen A, Medina JE, Goepfert H, Fletcher G: Management of stage T3 and T4 glottic carcinomas. Am J Surg 1984;148:467.

Zeitels SM, Vaughan CW, Domanowski GF: Endoscopic management of early supraglottic cancer. Ann Otol Rhinol Laryngol 1990;99:951.

Zelefsky MJ, Kraus DH, Pfister DG, et al: Combined chemotherapy and radiotherapy versus surgery and postoperative radiotherapy for advanced hypopharyngeal cancer. Head Neck 1996;18:405.

Chapter 40

Sinuses and Skull Base

Paul A. Kedeshian

The paranasal sinuses (ethmoid, maxillary, sphenoid, frontal) and skull base are the sites of numerous non-neoplastic and neoplastic entities. The overwhelming majority of pathologies seen in this region are infectious/inflammatory and include nasal polyposis and bacterial and fungal sinusitis. These disorders are typically treated with medical therapy (antibiotics, antihistamines, topical steroids, allergic avoidance); however, endoscopic surgical drainage is employed in cases when medical therapies have failed.

In contrast to the relatively common occurrence of infectious and inflammatory sinus disease, neoplasms of the sinuses, whether or not they extend to the anterior skull base, are exceedingly rare (<5% of all head and neck neoplasms). Moreover, the treatment of these neoplasms can be quite challenging secondary to their proximity to the brain, eyes, and other critical neurovascular structures. Consequently, the management of skull base and paranasal sinus tumors depends upon the cooperative efforts of a multidisciplinary management team that includes head and neck surgeons, maxillofacial surgeons, neurosurgeons, plastic or reconstructive surgeons, medical oncologists, and radiation oncologists.

CLINICAL PRESENTATION

Malignancies of the paranasal sinuses may initially give rise to symptoms of unilateral sinus or facial pressure, nasal obstruction, or epistaxis. However, these symptoms are often absent or quite nonspecific and therefore, these tumors may go unrecognized until they have extended beyond the bony confines of the sinuses. Anterior extension may cause cheek/malar swelling or hypoesthesia (secondary to invasion of the infraorbital nerve) while inferior extension may cause palatal or gingival swelling. Extension into the orbit may cause proptosis, visual changes, or alterations in extraocular muscle movement, whereas posterior extension may compromise pterygoid muscle function, resulting in trismus. When paranasal sinus tumors extend superiorly, they can cause anosmia, headache, cerebrospinal fluid rhinorrhea, and a variety of neurologic symptoms.

A comprehensive head and neck physical examination that includes anterior rhinoscopy and nasal endoscopy may demonstrate a lesion arising in the sinonasal cavity or anterior skull base (Table 40–1). A careful assessment of facial contour, specifically in the area of the maxilla and malar area, should be performed. Intraoral inspection and palpation of the palate, gingiva, and buccogingival sulcus, as well as noting any trismus, is crucial. A complete evaluation must also include a detailed eye examination, testing both extraocular movement and visual acuity. Neurologic examination specifically testing the function of cranial nerves I through VI to detect any sensory or

motor deficits must also be performed, with particular attention to minor sensory deficits in the skin overlying the maxilla.

Radiographic imaging is critically important in the accurate assessment of neoplasms of the paranasal sinuses and anterior skull base. Computed tomography (CT) in both the axial and coronal planes yields unparalleled information regarding the integrity of the bony sinus walls and can demonstrate whether the tumor has eroded the lamina papyracea adjacent to the eye or cribriform plate at the skull base. Magnetic resonance imaging (MRI) permits a more precise definition of the soft tissue extent of the tumor as well as an assessment of its vascularity. This can be of tremendous assistance in assessing involvement of either the dura of the anterior cranial fossa or the soft tissue contents of the orbital cone. Consequently, depending upon the clinical presentation and observed physical findings, CT and MRI examinations may serve as complementary studies.

The tissue diagnosis of neoplasms of the paranasal sinuses and skull base can usually be obtained via endoscopic visualization and biopsy of the tumor mass directly through the nasal cavity. Such a biopsy can often be performed under local anesthesia following adequate topical decongestion of the mucosa. However, prudence must be exercised when performing a biopsy if a lesion appears vascular or if it is located in the superior nasal vault and its potential connection with the anterior cranial fossa could precipitate a cerebrospinal fluid leak. This

Table 40–1	Lesions of the Sinuses and Skull Base

Physical Examination—Signs and Symptoms
Bilateral/longstanding: usually infectious or inflammatory
Unilateral: more often malignant; search for visual, neurologic, intraoral, or facial soft tissue findings

Imaging
Perform *prior to* biopsy
CT for bony definition
MRI for soft tissue
Consider additional studies (angiogram/embolization) as warranted

Biopsy
Perform in a way that does not compromise subsequent surgical resection

Treatment—Surgical
Proposed surgical approach should accommodate unexpected intraoperative findings
Anticipate all reconstructive and functional needs preoperatively and obtain necessary consultations
Assume the need for postoperative adjuvant therapy

Treatment—Nonsurgical
Precisely define the rationale for proceeding with nonsurgical treatment and whether salvage surgery is a potential future consideration

endoscopic biopsy approach, in contrast to an open biopsy through the anterior maxillary wall (Caldwell-Luc), avoids potential tumor contamination of normal tissues of the cheek and preserves the anatomic integrity of the surrounding structures, as well as their relation to the tumor mass.

The differential diagnosis of neoplasms that involve the paranasal sinuses and anterior skull base includes a range of both benign and malignant histologies. The most commonly seen benign tumors are inverting papillomas (schneiderian papilloma) and juvenile nasopharyngeal angiofibromas (JNA). However, the majority of tumors in this region are malignant and include squamous carcinomas arising from either the sinonasal cavity or the nasopharynx, adenocarcinomas and adenoid cystic carcinomas arising from the minor salivary glands of the sinonasal tract, chondrosarcomas or osteogenic sarcomas arising from the various bony and cartilaginous elements of the sinonasal cavity, soft tissue sarcomas, mucosal melanomas, esthesioneuroblastomas, and extensive skin cancers of the midface with deep penetration and skull base extension. In addition to these neoplasms, lymphomas (particularly in patients with HIV) and small cell neuroendocrine carcinomas (plasmocytomas) may also involve the paranasal sinuses and anterior skull base, although their treatment is generally nonsurgical. Although there are significant differences in the biologic behavior and overall prognoses of the various malignant histologies, the details of their surgical treatment do not differ significantly and they will therefore be discussed as a group.

PREOPERATIVE MANAGEMENT

Due to the varied histologies of the tumors in this region, objective comparisons of treatments (surgical resection versus nonsurgical therapies) are impossible. However, a multidisciplinary management team approach to the treatment of these tumors has resulted in dramatic improvements in surgical morbidity and improvements in safety. Consequently, most malignant paranasal sinus and anterior skull base lesions are best treated with surgical resection followed by external beam radiotherapy. When surgery is contraindicated, nonsurgical treatment protocols have been employed (discussed later) that may offer an equivalent likelihood of benefit with less morbidity.

Although absolute contraindications to surgery for malignant tumors in this region do not exist, a tumor's histology and biologic behavior are exceedingly important (particularly in the case of esthesioneuroblastoma). Important considerations include (1) whether gross total tumor resection can be accomplished—particularly when extensive dural and/or brain parenchymal invasion is present, and (2) whether surgical resection would cause unacceptable morbidity—such as tumors involving an only-seeing eye, tumors involving the optic chiasm, or tumors encasing the internal carotid artery.

External beam radiotherapy has been employed, with good reported success, for the treatment of JNAs (Cummings et al, 1984; Kasper et al, 1993). Rather than cause cell necrosis or death in these benign vascular tumors,

radiotherapy is thought to act by causing vascular fibrosis, thus preventing any continued tumor growth or enlargement. However, secondary to the effectiveness of surgical resection and the potential effects of radiation on the growth of the facial skeleton in adolescents, most radiotherapy use for primary JNA treatment has been limited to the setting of very extensive tumors whose surgical resection might entail significant morbidity. External beam radiotherapy has also been employed as the primary treatment modality for tumors of the paranasal sinuses with extension to the anterior skull base. These treatments combine a combination of both anterior and lateral portals, with every effort made to minimize the dose delivered to the eye, optic nerve or chiasm, spinal cord, and lacrimal ducts (Parsons et al, 1994).

Nonsurgical treatment of malignant paranasal sinus or anterior skull base tumors has also been used by our group at the Memorial Hospital over the past decade. We have employed a regimen of concomitant chemotherapy and/or radiotherapy for patients with tumors of the head and neck deemed to be surgically unresectable (Harrison et al, 1998). Within this larger cohort of "unresectable" patients, a subset presented with tumors of the paranasal sinuses, many of which involved the anterior skull base. They were treated with a protocol that consists of an initial 4-week course of conventionally delivered external beam radiotherapy (1.8 Gy/d) to the sites of both gross and potential microscopic disease, during which concomitant cisplatin (100 mg/m^2) is delivered on days 1 and 22. During the subsequent 2 weeks, hyperfractionated radiotherapy (1.8 Gy every morning and 1.6 Gy every evening), is delivered, with the evening dose directed exclusively to the site(s) of gross disease. The total radiotherapy dose therefore approximates 70 Gy.

In addition to these experiences with the use of radiotherapy either with or without chemotherapy for tumors of the anterior skull base, the use of chemotherapy specifically for esthesioneuroblastomas is well described. Although chemotherapy is still employed as part of a combined treatment protocol in selected centers, (Levine et al, 1994), we have found esthesioneuroblastomas to have the most favorable prognosis of all malignant anterior skull base histologies (Shah et al, 1997). Consequently, although esthesioneuroblastomas are chemotherapy-sensitive tumors, we consider systemic chemotherapy only for those esthesioneuroblastomas that have locally unresectable disease or distant metastases.

Finally, selective centers have employed combination chemotherapy (delivered intravenously, intra-arterially, or topically), external beam radiotherapy, and routine tumor débridement for the treatment of malignant maxillary sinus neoplasms (Knegt et al, 1984; Sakai et al, 1983; Sakata et al, 1993). Although these centers report some success with these regimens, en bloc surgical resection followed by external beam radiotherapy still offers the greatest likelihood of total disease eradication and control of tumors in this region.

Once a surgical resection is planned for a tumor of the paranasal sinuses or anterior skull base, the extent of the anticipated surgical defect must be considered. For patients with malignant tumors whose removal will likely require resection of the hard palate, preoperative evaluation by a maxillofacial prosthedontist should be arranged. At this evaluation, dental impressions are made and a palatal obturator can be fabricated that will be applied to the surgical defect at the time of resection. For more extensive tumors whose resection might require resection of the soft palate, orbital floor, orbital contents, or anterior fossa dura, preoperative plastic surgical evaluation is imperative. More extensive soft tissue defects that result from these resections are most effectively reconstructed, from both a cosmetic and a functional standpoint, with free tissue transfers.

INTRAOPERATIVE MANAGEMENT

For benign tumors of the paranasal sinuses (JNA, inverting papilloma), or malignant tumors without extension to the anterior skull base, a maxillectomy provides adequate en bloc resection. Spiro and associates (1997) recently proposed a classification of these procedures as limited, subtotal, or total, in order to simplify their description. Limited maxillectomies encompass a single wall of the maxilla, with a medial maxillectomy being the typical example. Subtotal maxillectomy involves removal of at least two walls of the maxillary sinus (including the palate), and a total maxillectomy removes the entire maxilla. The soft tissue approach chosen for each of these bony resections also needs to be specified and usually is either a midfacial degloving–open-mouth approach for limited maxillectomies, or a lateral rhinotomy (that can be extended superiorly, inferiorly, or laterally as needed) for both the subtotal and total maxillectomy.

As previously noted, based upon a combination of clinical examination and radiographic imaging, the soft tissue approach and type of maxillectomy are chosen in an effort to achieve adequate en bloc tumor resection. The surgical defect thus created will range in scope from a medial maxillectomy in which only the lateral nasal wall, a portion of the lamina papyracea, and anterior ethmoid air cells are removed, to a total maxillectomy (with or without orbital exenteration) in which the entire maxilla is resected, including the ipsilateral hard palate, orbital floor, and pterygoid plates. Particularly in the case of more extensive maxillectomies, split-thickness skin grafts are employed as a means of relining the raw mucosal surfaces. These grafts are secured in place and then additionally bolstered by the intraoperative placement of the palatal obturator.

Prior to the resection of anterior skull base tumors, all patients receive intravenous steroids and antibiotics whose spectrum includes broad coverage for skin flora and upper aerodigestive tract flora, and a cephalosporin with good cerebrospinal fluid (CSF) penetration. Following the introduction of general endotracheal anesthesia, a lumbar spinal drain is placed, and, depending on the posterosuperior tumor extent, controlled CSF drainage, hyperventilation, or mannitol diuresis is used to minimize the need for frontal lobe retraction (Shah et al, 1997; Shah et al, 1992).

The surgical procedure commences with a bifrontal craniotomy. The bicoronal skin incision in the scalp is deepened to a level just superficial to the pericranium, which is then incised 5 cm posterior to the scalp incision. The galea and pericranium are elevated to the level of the supraorbital rims and the nasofrontal suture line, preserving the neurovascular (supraorbital) pedicle as it emerges from the supraorbital notch. Then, a frontal craniotomy is performed utilizing a single burr hole on either side of the saggital sinus and a side-cutting craniotome (Midas-Rex) for the bone flap. This frontal bone flap is later cranialized by removing the posterior bony sinus wall and stripping the mucosa from the anterior sinus wall to prevent the formation of a frontal sinus mucocele. The dura overlying the frontal lobe is then carefully explored, and the decision whether to proceed by an extradural or intradural route is made; based on the tumor's extent on dissection of the anterior cranial fossa floor, the olfactory bulbs are sharply divided, and their dural sleeves are oversewn to prevent a CSF leak. Frontal lobe relaxation by controlled CSF drainage then permits visualization of the bony anterior fossa floor. The superior bone cuts can then be made at the anterior skull base.

After the tumor has been adequately encompassed superiorly and all the bone cuts at the anterior cranial base have been performed, facial exposure of the tumor is obtained. Depending on the extent of the tumor, this is accomplished via either an isolated lateral rhinotomy or a Weber-Ferguson approach. If significant lateral extension of the tumor is present, the Weber-Ferguson approach can be modified through a Dieffenbach extension, which we prefer to carry out through a transconjunctival incision into the ipsilateral fornix of the conjunctiva, rather than through a subciliary incision. With this exposure, the tumor can be successfully mobilized, encompassing complete anatomic units (maxilla, orbit, sinus) en bloc with the bony skull base.

Following complete tumor resection, reconstruction of the anterior skull base defect can proceed. When orbital exenteration or total maxillectomy is performed and a significant soft tissue defect is present, free tissue transfer offers the best option for satisfactory reconstruction. However, if a significant soft tissue defect has not been created, the reconstruction will focus mainly on establishing a watertight seal around the intracranial contents and isolating the sinonasal tract. To achieve this, the scalp flap that includes both galea and pericranium is now dissected in a plane superficial to the galea, leaving galea on each side of the incision to allow for closure. This well-vascularized galeal-pericranial flap is then sutured to the basal dura and the perimeter of the bony defect (Kraus et al, 1994; Shah et al, 1992; Snyderman et al, 1990).

When tumors of the anterior skull base closely approach (if not directly invade) the orbital periosteum and orbital soft tissues, resection of the majority of the bony and fascial support of orbit may be required. Such a resection results in the loss of support for an otherwise normal eye and can decrease the likelihood of subsequent eye function, especially when postoperative radiotherapy is employed. A potential solution to improve eye function and cosmesis following the loss of the orbit's physical support was recently described by Cordeiro and colleagues (1998) who reconstructed the bony orbital floor using a combination of a bone graft (either split calvarium or rib) and a vascularized flap (either pedicled or free).

POSTOPERATIVE MANAGEMENT

For patients who undergo resection of neoplasms of the paranasal sinuses, the palatal obturator that secures the split-thickness skin graft in place and closes the palatal defect also permits these patients to resume an oral diet immediately postoperatively. The obturator is typically removed after 1 week, and the take of the skin graft to the surgical bed is assessed. A critical component of these patients' subsequent management is performing frequent nasal saline irrigation of the nose and sinus cavity to facilitate adequate healing and prevent the development of crusting and infection within the surgical cavity.

In those patients who undergo anterior skull base resection, the lumbar drain is allowed to remain in place for 5 postoperative days, and a controlled drainage of 10 mL/hour is usually maintained during this time. These patients require careful ophthalmologic and neurologic monitoring during the initial perioperative period and are fed via a nasogastric feeding tube for 5 to 7 days before any attempts at oral feeding are made. When free tissue transfer is employed for soft tissue reconstruction, these patients also will require careful monitoring of the flap's color, capillary return, and vascular status. In our experience, the average length of hospital stay for patients who undergo resection of the anterior skull base is 10 to 14 days.

COMPLICATIONS

Although decreases in the morbidity and mortality associated with anterior skull base resection have occurred since their initial description, the reported complication rate for malignant tumors is still close to 40% (Kraus et al, 1994). The incidence of complications can be difficult to compare among different centers secondary to differences in reporting and the definition of major and minor complications. Complications include a variety of infectious complications (abscesses, meningitis, bone and scalp flap infections), cerebrospinal fluid leaks, pneumocephalus, diabetes insipidus, retrobulbar hematoma, blindness, transient impairment in neurologic function, coma, stroke, and death. Therefore, although anterior skull base resection is unavoidably associated with a variable degree of operative morbidity, if careful patient selection, adequate perioperative preparation, and meticulous surgical technique are employed, the complication rate and morbidity of craniofacial resection can be maintained at an acceptable rate.

OUTCOMES

For all malignant histologies of the anterior skull base, the combined 5-year survival for patients who undergo anterior craniofacial resection is approximately 50% to

Pearls and Pitfalls

PEARLS

- Select a surgical approach that allows the tumor to be fully encompassed in all its dimensions, especially if superior extension to the base of the skull is seen.
- Tailor the aggressiveness of the treatment to the inherent biologic behavior of the tumor type and its natural history in the patient.
- Always plan on encountering a larger and more extensive tumor than either clinical examination or radiographs might suggest, and communicate this to the patient.
- Actively involve all members of the multidisciplinary treatment team at initial patient evaluation to achieve a consensus about the treatment plan.
- There is no substitute for a meticulously performed operation.

60% (Shah et al, 1997). However, within our own series of 115 consecutive anterior skull base resections treated at the Memorial Hospital, the 5-year disease-specific survival for patients with esthesioneuroblastomas is 100%, compared with 67% for patients with squamous carcinoma arising from the skin, 50% to 60% for sinonasal carcinomas/sarcomas/minor salivary tumors, and only 33% for patients with mucosal melanomas. More specifically, local tumor control was obtained in 65% of patients, and the disease-specific survival was 58% at 5 years and 48% at 10 years. These results emphasize the critical importance of tumor histology and biology in the prognosis of anterior skull base lesions and serve to reiterate the vital importance of preoperative tumor assessment and tumor biology when formulating a treatment plan and to confirm the role of postoperative radiotherapy.

Compared with these results with surgery, the reported 5-year survival for patients with extensive tumors that involve the anterior skull base treated with primary radiotherapy is 10% to 15% (Parsons et al, 1994). In contrast, when the results of concurrent chemotherapy and radiotherapy (unresectable treatment protocol) in the subgroup of patients with paranasal sinus tumors is examined, there was a 42% overall survival at 3 years' follow-up (Harrison et al, 1998). Local control was successfully achieved in 78% of patients whereas regional control was obtained in 57%. All these patients did not have a tumor that involved the anterior skull base, but these very-advanced-staged lesions were all judged to be surgically unresectable by a multidisciplinary disease management team, and, therefore, this nonsurgical treatment protocol merits consideration in patients with advanced tumors of the anterior skull base.

SELECTED READINGS

Cordeiro PG, Santamaria E, Kraus DH, et al: Reconstruction of total maxillectomy defects with preservation of the orbital contents. Plastic Reconstruct Surg 1998;102:1874.
Cummings BJ, Blend R, Keane T, et al: Primary radiation therapy for juvenile nasopharyngeal angiofibroma. Laryngoscope 1984;94:1599.

Dandy WE: Orbital Tumors: Results Following the Transcranial Operative Attack. New York, Oskar Priest, 1941.

Harrison LB, Raben A, Pfister DG, et al: A prospective phase II trial of concomitant chemotherapy and radiotherapy, with delayed accelerated fractionation in unresectable tumors of the head and neck. Head Neck 1998;20:497.

Kasper ME, Parsons JT, Mancuso AA, et al: Radiation therapy for juvenile angiofibroma: Evaluation by CT and MRI, analysis of tumor regression and selection of patients. Int J Radiat Oncal Biol Phys 1993;25:689.

Knegt PP, de Jong PC, van Andel JG, et al: Carcinoma of the paranasal sinuses: Results of a prospective pilot study. Cancer 1984;56:57.

Kraus DH, Shah JP, Arbit E, et al: Complications of craniofacial resection for tumors involving the anterior skull base. Head Neck 1994;16:307.

Levine PA, Debo RF, Meredith SD, et al: Craniofacial resection at the University of Virginia (1976–1992): Survival analysis. Head Neck 1994;16:574.

Parsons JT, Stringer SP, Mancuso AA, Million RR: Nasal vestibule, nasal cavity, and paranasal sinus. In Million RR, Cassisi NJ (eds): Management of head and neck cancer—A multidisciplinary approach. Philadelphia, JB Lipincott, 1994.

Sakai S, Hohki A, Fuchihata H, Tanaka Y: Multidisciplinary treatment of maxillary sinus carcinoma. Cancer 1983;52:1360.

Sakata K, Aoki Y, Karasawa K, et al: Analysis of the results of combined therapy for maxillary carcinoma. Cancer 1993;71:2715.

Shah JP, Kraus DH, Arbit E, et al: Craniofacial resection for tumors involving the anterior skull base. Oto-Head Neck Surg 1992;106:387.

Shah JP, Kraus DH, Bilsky MH, et al: Craniofacial resection for malignant tumors involving the anterior skull base. Arch Oto-Head Neck Surg 1997;123:1312.

Snyderman CH, Janecka IP, Sekhar LN, et al: Anterior cranial base reconstruction: Role of galeal and pericranial flaps. Laryngoscope 1990;100:607.

Spiro RH, Strong EW, Shah JP: Maxillectomy and its classification. Head Neck 1997;19:309.

Smith RR, Klopp CT, Williams JM: Surgical treatment of cancer of the frontal sinus and adjacent areas. Cancer 1994;7:991.

Chapter 41

Neck Metastasis and Unknown Primary Tumor

Bhuvanesh Singh

The presence of metastasis to the cervical lymphatics at presentation is the single most important factor determining the outcome of patients with head and neck squamous cell carcinoma (HNSCC) (Shah et al, 1993). Nodal metastasis can occur in one of three settings in patients with HNSCC: clinically detectable metastasis from a known primary site, metastasis from an unknown primary tumor, or clinically occult metastasis. The overriding issues are similar with respect to management in each of these clinical scenarios; namely, control of disease above the clavicles. In this chapter, each clinical scenario is considered individually.

HEAD AND NECK LYMPHATIC ANATOMY

Regional lymphatic metastasis from head and neck neoplasms occurs in a predictable, sequential fashion to specific regional lymph node groups. Accordingly, designated regional lymph node groups should be appropriately addressed in treatment planning for a given primary site. Conversely, specific primary sites should be investigated in cases of lymph node metastasis from an unknown primary tumor. Moreover, all regional lymph node groups are usually not initially at risk of nodal metastases from a given primary site. In the absence of grossly palpable metastatic lymph nodes, understanding the patterns of neck metastasis can facilitate selection of neck dissection.

Lymphatic nodal group anatomy in the head and neck is as follows:

Preauricular, Periparotid, and Intraparotid Lymph Nodes. These are the first-echelon lymph nodes for the anterior half of the scalp, the skin of the forehead, and the upper part of the face.

Postauricular and Suboccipital Group of Lymph Nodes. They provide initial drainage to the posterior half of the scalp and the posterior aspect of the external ear.

Parapharyngeal and Retropharyngeal Lymph Nodes. These are mainly at risk for metastatic dissemination from tumors of the pharynx.

Cervical Lymph Nodes in the Lateral Aspect of the Neck. These drain primarily the mucosa of the upper aerodigestive tract. These include submental, perivascular facial, and the submandibular group of lymph nodes located in the submental and submandibular triangles of the neck. Deep jugular lymph nodes include the jugulodigastric, jugulo-omohyoid, and supraclavicular group of lymph nodes adjacent to the internal jugular vein. Lymph nodes in the posterior triangle of the neck include the accessory chain of lymph nodes located along the spinal accessory nerve and the trans-

verse cervical chain of lymph nodes in the floor of the posterior triangle of the neck. The lymph nodes in the lateral neck are grouped as follows:

Level I. Submental Triangle. The nodal tissue located between the anterior bellies of the digastric muscles and cephalad to the hyoid bone.

Submandibular Triangle. Nodal tissue in the triangular area bounded by the anterior and posterior bellies of the digastric muscle and the inferior border of the body of the mandible. The lymph nodes adjacent to the submandibular salivary gland and along the facial artery are included in this group.

Level II. Upper Jugular Group. Nodal tissue around the upper portion of the internal jugular vein and the upper part of the spinal accessory nerve, extending from the base of the skull up to the bifurcation of the carotid artery or the hyoid bone. The posterior limit for this level is the posterior border of the sternocleidomastoid muscle, and the anterior border is the lateral limit of the sternohyoid muscle.

Level III. Midjugular Group. Nodal tissue around the middle third of the internal jugular vein from the inferior border of level II up to the omohyoid muscle or the cricothyroid membrane. The anterior and posterior borders are the same as those for level II.

Level IV. Lower Jugular Group. Nodal tissue around the lower third of the internal jugular vein from the inferior border of level III up to the clavicle. The anterior and posterior borders are the same as those for levels II and III.

Level V. Posterior Triangle Group. Nodal tissue around the lower portion of the spinal accessory nerve and along the transverse cervical vessels. It is bounded by the triangle formed by the clavicle, posterior border of the sternocleidomastoid muscle, and the anterior border of the trapezius muscle.

Central Compartment of the Neck. This includes the delphian lymph node overlying the thyroid cartilage in the midline draining the larynx and perithyroid lymph nodes adjacent to the thyroid gland. Lymph nodes in the tracheoesophageal groove provide primary drainage to the thyroid gland as well as the hypopharynx, subglottic larynx, and cervical esophagus.

Anterior Superior Mediastinal Lymph Nodes. These provide drainage to the thyroid gland and the cervical esophagus, and serve as a secondary lymphatic basin for anatomic structures in the central compartment of the neck.

RISK OF METASTASIS

The risk of regional lymphatic metastasis by primary squamous cell carcinomas of the upper aerodigestive tract can

279

be assessed according to anatomic location of the primary tumor, size, tumor (T) stage, and histomorphologic characteristics. In general, the risk of nodal metastasis increases from the anterior to the posterior aspect of the upper aerodigestive tract; that is, the lips (less than 5%), oral cavity (19% to 50%), oropharynx (22% to 66%), and hypopharynx (38%) (Fig. 41–1) (Shah et al, 1993; Lindberg, 1972). For tumors of the larynx and pharynx, the risk of nodal metastasis increases from the center of the laryngopharyngeal compartment to the periphery (Shah et al, 1993; Lindberg, 1972). The risk of regional lymph node metastasis from carcinoma of the true vocal cord is exceedingly small and increases as one progresses from the true vocal cords to the false vocal cords, aryepiglottic fold (16% to 26%), piriform sinus (38%), and pharyngeal wall (66%) (Shah et al, 1993). Within the oral cavity, a significantly higher risk of occult nodal metastases occurs in floor-of-the-mouth (40% to 50%), gingival (19%), and oral tongue cancers (25% to 54%), than in those originating from the hard palate (less than 5%) (Shah et al, 1993).

The risk of nodal metastases increases with increasing primary tumor burden at any site, as reflected by the T-stage. The risk of nodal metastasis increases from less than 14% for T1 lesions to 30% for T2, 45% for T3, and 55% to 75% for T4 lesions. Occult involvement increases from 19% for T1 and T2 lesions to 26% to 32% for T3 and T4 (Shah et al, 1993). Tumors showing endophytic growth, which reflects a higher potential for invasion, have a higher propensity for metastasis than do exophytic tumors. The risk of nodal metastases is also related to the depth of invasion for tongue and floor-of-the-mouth cancers. Fukano and colleagues found that clinically negative necks were pathologically positive in 30% of cases with a depth of invasion of less than 5 mm, compared with 43% when the tumor depth exceeded 5 mm (Fukano et al, 1997). Spiro and colleagues showed that the tumor thickness was an important and independent prognostic factor, with a 7.5% prevalence of neck failure for tumors less than 2 mm thick compared with 34% for 2 to 8 mm and 47% for those over 8 mm in thickness (Spiro et al, 1986). In addition, pathologic features such as differentia-

tion and the host-to-tumor interface have also been suggested as predictors of the risk of nodal metastasis.

LOCATION OF METASTASIS

For primary tumors in the oral cavity, the regional lymph nodes at highest risk for early dissemination by metastatic cancer are limited to levels I, II, and III (Fig. 41–2) (Shah et al, 1993, p. 274; Lindberg, 1972). Anatomically this translates into regional lymph node groups contained within the supraomohyoid triangle of the neck, including the submental, submandibular, perivascular facial, jugulodigastric, upper deep jugular, superior spinal accessory chain of lymph nodes, and midjugular lymph nodes. Skip metastases to level IV and level V, in the absence of metastatic disease at level I, II, or III, occur in fewer than 5% of cases at the time of the initial presentation (Shah et al, 1993; Lindberg, 1972). Therefore, for clinically negative necks, level IV and level V lymph nodes are generally not at risk for metastases from primary squamous carcinomas of the oral cavity. However, Byers and colleagues (1997) suggested that there is a relatively high presence of subsequent failure at level IV after supraomohyoid neck dissection. This pattern of metastasis can be effectively encompassed in a supraomohyoid neck dissection. Finally, given the increased risk of skip metastasis, consideration should be given to the inclusion of level IV lymphatics as part of the routine supraomohyoid neck dissection.

The first-echelon lymph nodes at highest risk for harboring metastases for tumors on the lateral aspect of the oropharynx and hypopharynx, in the clinically negative neck, are the ipsilateral deep jugular lymph nodes at levels II, III, and IV (Shah et al, 1993; Lindberg, 1972). Contiguous lymph nodes lateral to the internal jugular vein overlying the cutaneous roots of the cervical plexus are usually considered a component of levels II, III, and IV. In patients with primary carcinomas of the oropharynx, the risk of micrometastases to levels I and V is exceedingly small, and skip metastases to levels I and V in the absence of disease at levels II, III, or IV are

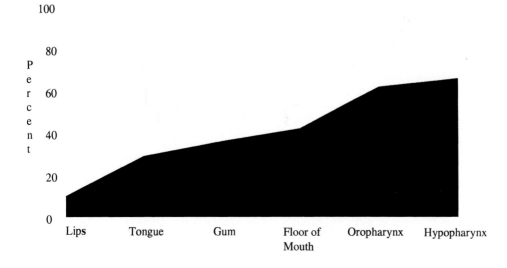

Figure 41–1. Incidence of nodal metastases at presentation in relation to primary site.

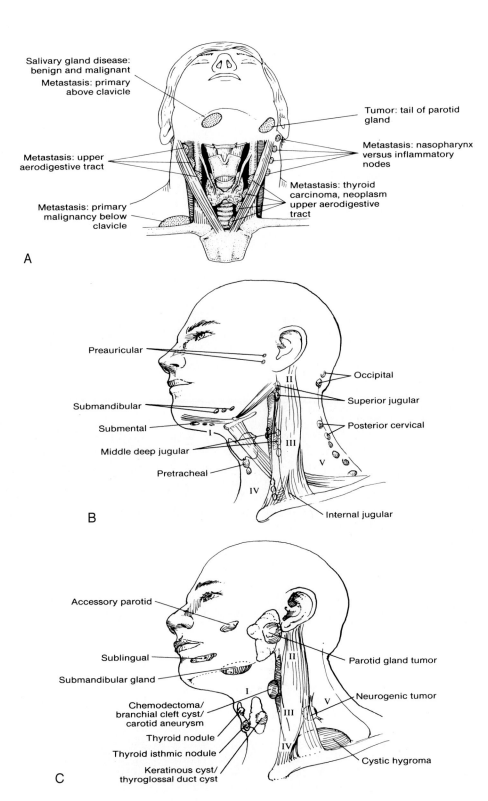

Figure 41–2. Potential sites of metastasis based on the location of the primary tumors. (From Bland KI: Neck masses. In Polk HC Jr, Gardner B, Stone HH [eds]: Basic Surgery, 5th ed. St Louis: Quality Medical Publishing, 1995, pp 342–343.)

unusual. Primary tumors, which involve both sides of the midline, have a potential for microscopic dissemination of metastatic disease to jugular lymph nodes on both sides of the neck. A jugular or lateral neck dissection, which encompasses the removal of all lymph nodes in levels II, III, and IV in the neck, is ideally suited for tumors in these anatomic locations.

OCCULT NODAL METASTASIS

Several studies report diminished survival in patients found to have occult lymphatic metastasis to the cervical lymphatics. Tulenko and co-workers showed that the 5-year cure rate decreased from 79% in patients without any evidence of metastasis, to 29% in those with occult disease detected on pathologic examination, to 11% in those with clinically evident disease (Tulenko et al, 1966). Similarly, Alvi and Johnson showed that disease control rates decreased from 82% for patients without metastasis to 47% for those with occult metastasis and 31% when extracapsular spread was present in lymph nodes containing occult metastasis (Alvi and Johnson, 1996). Accordingly, identification and treatment of patients with occult metastasis appears warranted.

Since there is no statistical difference in regional control rates or survival between patients undergoing elective neck dissection for micrometastasis and those undergoing therapeutic neck dissection for N1 disease at presentation, extrapolation suggests that patients with N0 necks can be followed until metastasis becomes clinically evident (Shah et al, 1993). Unfortunately, not all patients at risk for micrometastasis to the cervical lymphatics progress in a consistent, predictable manner. A report by Andersen and colleagues showed that the majority of patients initially observed with N0 neck, clinically have greater than N1 nodal involvement at the time of definitive treatment, even with close follow-up (Andersen et al, 1996). In fact, the majority of patients (77%) had metastatic disease greater than N1 or associated extracapsular spread on pathologic analysis. In addition, the rate of distant metastasis in patients with N0 necks is higher in patients who develop subsequent nodal recurrence (11%) than in patients who remain disease free (3%). This suggests early intervention is warranted in patients at high risk for occult nodal involvement.

Theoretically, identification and treatment of patients with metastatic squamous carcinoma to regional cervical lymph nodes would be expected to have a favorable impact on overall survival. However, prospective studies have failed to confirm this association. Conversely, improved disease-free survival has been observed in both prospective and retrospective analyses. Kligerman found that the disease-free survival increased from 49% to 72% with the addition of elective supraomohyoid neck dissection (Kligerman et al, 1994). Similarly, Fakih also reported increased disease-free survival with the addition of elective neck treatment (67% versus 47%) (Fakih et al, 1989). Accordingly, it can be summarized that elective neck dissection aids in prognostication, identifies cases requiring adjuvant treatment, and improves initial disease control rates.

No established clinical parameters reliably identify patients with clinically occult lymphatic metastasis. Accordingly, most authors have adapted an arbitrary cutoff of 10% to 15% incidence of occult nodal involvement in selecting patients requiring elective intervention (Andersen et al, 1996; Kligerman et al, 1994; Fakih et al, 1989). Decision analysis, based on statistical analysis of data from the available medical literature, suggests that a 20% risk should be the accepted threshold for providing treatment.

Augmentation of clinical examination with various radiologic studies, including computed tomography (66%), magnetic resonance imaging (MRI) (75%), and ultrasound examination (68%), enhance the accuracy of the identification of patients who have nodal metastasis (van den Brekel and Castelijns, 2000). The 92% accuracy rate for the identification of cervical metastasis reported with the use of positron emission tomography (PET) scanning is tainted by sample size constraints. Molecular and sentinel node biopsy assessments of occult metastasis are variable and need to be investigated. Both mathematical models and molecular studies have also met with variable results. Overall, no reliable methods have been identified for reproducibly predicting the presence of nodal metastasis in individual patients with clinically detectable disease.

At present, elective treatment of lymphatics at high risk for metastases from upper aerodigestive tract cancers is warranted. Effective treatment can be provided with the use of either radiation therapy or surgery. The use of selective neck dissections is sufficient for identifying patients with occult metastasis. Adjuvant treatment is warranted in cases in which metastasis is identified. The lack of improvement in survival in the patient population with occult nodal metastasis can be attributed to several factors, including false-negative pathologic examinations and inadequate adjuvant treatment. The presence of metastasis, which is missed on routine pathologic examination, is confirmed in studies that use supplemental subserial sectioning, immunohistochemistry, or molecular analysis. Most strikingly, using p53 mutation analysis, Brennan and colleagues identified a 21% rate for missed lymphatic metastases (Brennan et al, 1995). The inadequacy of currently available adjuvant treatment is shown in the lack of benefit of adjuvant chemotherapy in patients with extracapsular spread associated with lymphatic metastasis except in one series (Johnson et al, 1985).

CLINICALLY DETECTABLE METASTASIS

Primary Site Identified

The presence of a clinically palpable, unilateral, firm enlarged cervical lymph node in an adult should be considered metastatic until proved otherwise, and it should initiate a systematic search for the primary site. The search for a primary tumor should precede any therapeutic intervention. The important features of cervical lymph nodes are the location, size, consistency, number, and signs of extracapsular spread, such as invasion of the overlying skin, fixation to deeper soft tissues, or paralysis of cranial nerves (Shah et al, 1993). Histologic diagnosis of metastatic carcinoma is usually established by a needle aspiration biopsy and cytologic examination of the smears. Open biopsy is rarely indicated. If an open biopsy is planned, incisions should be made in congruence with neck dissection incisions and the possibility for a comprehensive neck dissection entertained.

Radiographic evaluation for palpable cervical lymph nodes is not required in the majority of cases. In the case of massive metastatic disease, radiographic evaluation by CT scan with intravenous contrast enhancement or MRI with gadolinium contrast enhancement is desirable for assessing the extent of the nodal disease. Particular attention is directed to the relationship of the mass to the carotid artery, skull base, and parapharyngeal space on the ipsilateral side. In addition, lymph node groups that are not accessible for clinical examination are best assessed by a CT scan or MRI scan, such as those in the parapharyngeal, retropharyngeal, and superior mediastinal regions. The radiographic features suggestive of metastatic involvement are size, rim enhancement, central necrosis, and extranodal invasion.

As indicated earlier, the single most important factor in the prognosis for squamous cell carcinoma of the head and neck is the presence or absence of cervical lymph node metastasis. Cure rates for patients with cervical lymph node metastasis are nearly one half of those achieved in patients who present with tumors localized to the primary site (Shah et al, 1993). The extent of nodal metastasis in the neck and several characteristics of the regional lymph nodes directly influence prognosis. These include the size and number of involved nodes, and their anatomic location. The presence of extranodal spread of metastatic disease with invasion of the soft tissues clearly has an impact on prognosis. Patients with multiple-level involvement develop recurrence in the dissected neck twice as often as those with single-level involvement. Lower cervical lymph node (level IV) and lower posterior-triangle lymph node (level V) involvement by metastatic cancer usually implies an ominous prognosis. Perivascular and perineural infiltration by tumor and the presence of tumor emboli in regional lymphatics also have an adverse impact on prognosis. Therefore, these factors must be considered in developing a treatment strategy for patients in whom regional lymph nodes are involved by metastatic disease, particularly for planning adjuvant therapy and for the assessment of prognosis. Adjuvant postoperative radiation therapy significantly enhances regional control in the dissected neck. This improvement in regional control is seen in patients with limited neck disease (N1), as well as in patients with extensive nodal disease (N2B).

Unknown Primary Tumor

Unknown primary cancer is defined as the histologic evidence of malignancy in the cervical lymph nodes with no apparent primary site for the origin of the metastatic tumor. This descriptor is misleading, for primary cancers are eventually identified in more than 90% of the 8% to 13% of patients presenting with a neck mass as their only complaint. Accordingly, the proper nomenclature for this entity should be unidentified primary cancers. A con-

founding factor with regard to an unidentified primary is its differentiation from branchial-cleft cyst carcinoma. Skepticism has surrounded the existence of branchial-cleft carcinoma since the entity was first described in 1882 (Singh et al, 1998). The landmark work of Hays Martin established four criteria for the diagnosis of branchial-cleft carcinoma, the most important criterion being histologic proof of carcinoma arising from epithelium of a normal cyst. Of the 43 cases found in an extensive review of the literature, only 9 cases satisfied all four of the criteria, making this entity more of an academic point of discussion than a conundrum for therapeutic decision making (Singh et al, 1998).

Overall, in the United States, 850 cases, or 2% of all head and neck cancers, annually are designated as unknown primaries. However, many of these cases represent cases in which the primary disease went undiagnosed. The reasons for missed diagnosis include insufficient examination, inaccessible sites, and inaccessible or microscopic primaries. Clearly, the most important aspect of the assessment of patients with metastatic cancer in the neck in absence of an obvious primary is a detailed examination, both in the office and with the patient under general anesthesia. Improvements in examining techniques, specifically the advent of fiberoptic telescopes, are reflected in the changing location of subsequently detected primary tumors from 31% in a series from Memorial Hospital from 1950 to 1964, to 15% from 1965 to 1976 and 12% from 1977 to 1990 (Fig. 41–3) (Barrie and Strong, 1970; Davidson et al, 1994; Spiro et al, 1983). Similarly, the sites of subsequent primary tumors have changed from the nasopharyngeal majority in the series from 1950 to 1964, to the hypopharynx and base of the tongue in sequential series covering patients from 1965 to 1990 (Fig. 41–4). Our service does not advocate the use of "random biopsies," but rather directed biopsies from clinically suspicious regions. An exception may be the addition of ipsilateral tonsillectomy, given the accumulating evidence in support of its efficacy.

The vast majority of unidentified primaries tend to be epidermoid carcinomas (60%), followed by adenocarcinomas (22%), anaplastic tumors (10%), and melanomas (8%), which can be effectively analyzed with the use of

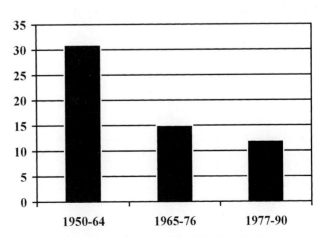

Figure 41–3. Rate of subsequent identification of primary tumor: The MSKCC experience.

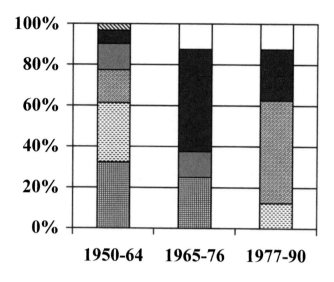

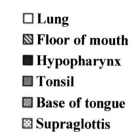

Figure 41–4. Location of subsequent primary tumor after treatment of unidentified primary tumor: The MSKCC experience.

fine-needle aspiration (Spiro et al, 1983). Open biopsy should be considered in very limited circumstances, with preparedness to perform neck dissection if needed. Studies suggest that inappropriately planned neck biopsies lead to higher rates of wound necrosis, neck recurrence, and distant metastasis. Recent evidence has disputed these findings, suggesting that an excisional biopsy followed by radiation treatment results in no deleterious effects.

The outcome of patients with unknown primaries can be associated with several clinical and pathologic parameters. The most important determinant of outcome is the extent of nodal involvement at presentation (Spiro et al, 1983). The 5-year survival decreases precipitously from N1 to N2 to N3 nodal disease. The management of unknown primaries has changed with time. At our institution, surgery alone was the treatment of choice from 1950 to 1964 and 1965 to 1976 (Barrie and Strong, 1970; Spiro et al, 1983). Since then, adjuvant radiation therapy has been utilized in the majority of cases. This has resulted in improved locoregional control and diminished subsequent identification of primary tumors (Fig. 41–5) (Barrie and Strong, 1970; Davidson et al, 1994; Spiro et al, 1983).

MANAGEMENT OF CLINICALLY DETECTABLE METASTASIS

Clearly, the goal of treatment of cervical lymph node metastasis is regional control of the disease. Micrometastases and minimal gross metastases may be controlled with radiotherapy alone. However, surgery remains the mainstay of treatment of cervical metastases, since it provides comprehensive clearance of all grossly enlarged lymph nodes and offers accurate histologic information on the lymph nodes at risk for micrometastasis in the clinically negative neck.

The classic radical neck dissection, originally described by Crile, has traditionally been the "gold standard" for the management of the neck in patients with head and neck cancer. Although oncologically sound, the classic approach was associated with significant cosmetic and functional debility. Chronic pain from the shoulder was common, a result of accessory nerve sacrifice. Better understanding of head and neck cancer metastases has led to the use of modified radical neck dissection to reduce morbidity without compromising regional control rates or survival.

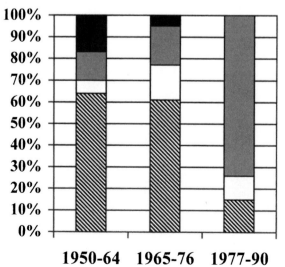

Figure 41–5. Patterns of treatment of unidentified tumors at MSKCC.

Modified radical neck dissection type I (MRND-I) achieves that goal without an adverse impact on prognosis. Five-year survival rates, regional failure rates in the dissected neck, and the location of recurrence are comparable in patients with palpable metastatic disease undergoing classic radical neck dissection and modified radical neck dissection that preserves the spinal accessory nerve (Shah et al, 1993). Regional recurrence rates in the dissected neck following classic radical neck dissection and MRND-I are comparable (Shah et al, 1993). Similarly, regional failure rates in patients undergoing classic radical neck dissection and MRND-I for N1 and N2 disease are also comparable. The presence of extranodal spread by metastatic disease does not seem to influence regional recurrence rates following classic radical neck dissection or MRND-I so long as the accessory nerve is not directly involved by cancer. At present, it is inadvisable to perform MRND-I for N3 disease.

Our current management philosophy is to perform a comprehensive MRND-I preserving the spinal accessory nerve in patients with grossly enlarged lymph nodes. Classic radical neck dissection is still warranted in patients with N3 disease, matted metastases involving multiple levels, recurrent metastatic disease in a previously irradiated neck, grossly apparent extranodal spread with invasion of the spinal accessory nerve and/or internal jugular vein at the base of the skull, and the presence of skin involvement. Given the improved control rates, postoperative radiation therapy is recommended in all patients with multiple metastatic lymph nodes, extranodal spread of tumor, or other ominous histopathologic features.

MANAGEMENT OF OCCULT METASTASIS

Although the indications for comprehensive surgical clearance of regional lymph nodes in the neck with clinically palpable metastatic lymph nodes are obvious, the indications for elective treatment of the N0 neck are less clear. No statistical differences in regional control rates or survival rates are seen between patients undergoing elective neck dissection for micrometastases and those undergoing therapeutic neck dissection for N1 disease at presentation. Not all patients at risk for micrometastases present for subsequent therapeutic neck dissection with N1 disease. The prognosis of a patient with metastatic squamous carcinoma of regional cervical lymph nodes depends on the extent of nodal disease in the neck. When there is a significant risk of micrometastases to regional lymph nodes, based on the characteristics of the primary tumor, an elective dissection of regional lymph nodes should be considered.

Lymphatic basins at risk for metastasis can be managed effectively with either surgery or radiation therapy (Shah et al, 1993). Accordingly, the selection of the appropriate modality should be based on the assessment of other tumor parameters. In patients with locally advanced lesions, where adjunctive treatment is required, the neck can be effectively managed with radiation therapy alone. Studies have shown a greater than 90% control rate with the use of elective irradiation. However, several questions remain regarding the use of radiation in this setting.

Critics of the use of radiation therapy note that the reported failure rate of 10%, in the setting of elective treatment for occult metastasis, indicates a 33% failure rate, since only about 30% of cases treated in this manner actually contain metastases. Proponents of elective radiation therapy counter with the finding that the control rate with radiation in patients without recurrence at the primary site is 96% to 99%, extrapolating that radiation is highly effective in the setting of N0 necks.

In patients with surgically treated primary lesions not requiring adjuvant radiation therapy, surgical management of the neck should be performed, guided by the location of the primary lesion. Given the significant functional and aesthetic morbidity following classic radical neck dissection, modification of the operation to reduce morbidity without compromise of regional control rates or survival is indicated. With elective treatment of the neck, it is seldom necessary to do a comprehensive neck dissection to excise all five levels of lymph nodes. Since cervical lymph node metastases to the first-echelon lymph nodes occur in a predictable and sequential fashion, elective neck dissection can be limited to addressing only the lymph node groups at highest risk for a given primary site. The limitation of dissection of lymph nodes levels is considered a "staging procedure," although authors argue whether selective neck dissections are therapeutic in certain settings. Nonetheless, the histologic information derived from the study of the excised lymph nodes facilitates selection of adjuvant therapy in patients who are at increased risk for neck failure and spares the need for a morbid operation or adjuvant radiotherapy in others who are at reduced risk.

CLASSIFICATION OF NECK DISSECTION

The understanding of the biologic progression of metastatic disease from primary sites in the head and neck region to cervical lymph nodes has allowed the development of several modifications of the classic radical neck dissection to reduce morbidity and maintain therapeutic efficacy. In order to standardize the terminology of various types of neck dissections, the following classification scheme is recommended:

COMPREHENSIVE NECK DISSECTION. The term *comprehensive neck dissection* is applied to all surgical procedures on the lateral neck, which comprehensively remove cervical lymph nodes from level I through level V. Under this broad category are included the following operative procedures:

Classical Radical Neck Dissection. Resection of levels I to V in continuity with the sternocleidomastoid muscle, internal jugular vein, and the accessory nerve.
Extended Radical Neck Dissection. Resection of additional regional lymph nodes or sacrifice of other structures, such as cranial nerves, muscles, and skin.
Modified Radical Neck Dissection Type I (MRND-I). This procedure selectively preserves the accessory nerve.
Modified Radical Neck Dissection Type II (MRND-II). This procedure preserves the accessory nerve and the sternocleidomastoid muscle but sacrifices the internal jugular vein.

Modified Radical Neck Dissection Type III (MRND-III). This procedure requires preservation of the spinal accessory nerve, internal jugular vein, and sternocleidomastoid muscle.

Selective Neck Dissection. These operations selectively remove lymph node groups at designated levels only and do not comprehensively dissect all five levels of lymph nodes. Selective neck dissections are usually employed as staging procedures for the clinically negative neck where the lymph nodes are at risk for micrometastases. These operations include the following:

Supraomohyoid Neck Dissection. This procedure encompasses dissection of lymph nodes at levels I, II, and III and is recommended as an elective procedure for primary tumors of the oral cavity. Some authors have scrutinized the extent of nodal excision required in the supraomohyoid neck dissection. One study questioned the benefit from the dissection of the supraspinal accessory lymphatic as a part of the procedure, reporting only a single case in which metastasis was identified in this region, which also contained coexistent metastasis in the level II region of the neck (Kraus et al, 1996). Dissection and retraction along the accessory nerve can be minimized if the supraspinal doses do not require excision, but this limitation in dissection requires further corroboration. A study by Byers and colleagues, reporting a failure rate of 15% outside the traditional confines of the supraomohyoid neck dissection, advocated the extension of the neck dissection to include level IV of the neck (Byers et al, 1997). The efficacy of this extension in limiting neck nodal recurrence needs to be confirmed.

Jugular Neck Dissection (Anterolateral Neck Dissection). This procedure encompasses dissection of lymph nodes at levels II, III, and IV.

Central Compartment Neck Dissection. This procedure encompasses clearance of lymph nodes in the central compartment of the neck adjacent to the thyroid gland and in the tracheoesophageal groove.

Posterolateral Neck Dissection. This operation encompasses lymph nodes in the occipital triangle, posterior triangle of the neck, and the deep jugular chain of lymph nodes at levels II, III, and IV. This operation is recommended for melanomas and squamous carcinomas of the posterior scalp.

OTHER CONSIDERATIONS

Regional recurrence of metastatic disease in the dissected neck is dependent on the volume of neck metastasis at the time of neck dissection; for multiple metastatic lymph nodes, it is prohibitively high. Therefore, to enhance the regional control rate, postoperative radiation therapy is recommended. The need for adjuvant postoperative radiation therapy, however, depends on the extent of disease in the neck and the presence or absence of extracapsular spread. Regional control of metastatic disease in the neck is significantly enhanced with postoperative radiotherapy. The indications for postoperative radiotherapy include the presence of gross residual disease, multiple positive

---

Pearls and Pitfalls

PEARLS

- The presence of a clinically palpable, unilateral, firm enlarged cervical lymph node in an adult should be considered metastatic until proven otherwise, and should initiate a systematic search for the primary site.
- A detailed patient history and physical examination and fine-needle aspiration biopsy are the cornerstones of the evaluation of enlarged cervical nodes.
- Branchial-cleft carcinoma is more of an academic point of discussion than a conundrum for therapeutic decision making and should be entertained only as a diagnosis by exclusion.
- Regional lymphatic metastases from head and neck neoplasms occur in a predictable and sequential fashion to specific regional lymph node groups.
- Metastases to the cervical lymphatics at presentation constitute the single most important factor that determines the outcome of patients with head and neck squamous cell carcinoma.
- The presence of a 10% to 15% risk of occult nodal involvement in a clinically negative neck in a patient with head and neck cancer should lead to the consideration of elective intervention.
- Outcomes are comparable in patients with palpable metastatic disease who have undergone classic radical neck dissection and modified radical neck dissection that preserves the spinal accessory nerve.
- Radical neck dissection is usually required for N3 disease.
- Postoperative radiotherapy should be considered in the setting of the presence of gross residual disease, multiple positive lymph nodes in the neck, extracapsular extension by metastatic disease, perivascular or perineural invasion by tumor, and other ominous findings, such as tumor emboli in lymphatics, cranial nerve invasion, or extension of disease to the base of the skull.

---

lymph nodes in the neck, extracapsular extension by metastatic disease, perivascular or perineural invasion by tumor, and other ominous findings, such as tumor emboli in lymphatics, cranial nerve invasion, or extension of disease to the base of the skull.

SELECTED READINGS

Alvi A, Johnson JT: Extracapsular spread in the clinically negative neck (N0): Implications and outcome. Otolaryngol Head Neck Surg 1996;114:65.

Andersen PE, Cambronero E, Shaha AR, Shah JP: The extent of neck disease after regional failure during observation of the N0 neck. Am J Surg 1996;172:689.

Barrie J, Strong E: Cervical nodal metastasis of unknown origin. Am J Surg 1970;120:466.

Brazilian Head and Neck Cancer Study Group: Results of a prospective trial on elective modified radical classical versus supraomohyoid neck dissection in the management of oral squamous carcinoma. Am J Surg 1998;176:422.

Brennan JA, Mao L, Hruban RH, et al: Molecular assessment of histopathological staging in squamous-cell carcinoma of the head and neck. N Engl J Med 1995;332:429.

Byers RM, Weber RS, Andrews T, et al: Frequency and therapeutic implications of "skip metastases" in the neck from squamous carcinoma of the oral tongue. Head Neck 1997;19:14.

Davidson BJ, Spiro RH, Patel S, et al: Cervical metastases of occult origin: The impact of combined modality therapy. Am J Surg 1994;168:395.

Fakih AR, Rao RS, Borges AM, Patel AR: Elective versus therapeutic neck dissection in early carcinoma of the oral tongue. Am J Surg 1989;158:309.

Fukano H, Matsuura H, Hasegawa Y, Nakamura S: Depth of invasion as a predictive factor for cervical lymph node metastasis in tongue carcinoma. Head Neck 1997;19:205.

Johnson JT, Myers EN, Srodes CH, et al: Maintenance chemotherapy for high-risk patients: A preliminary report. Arch Otolaryngol 1985;111:727.

Kligerman J, Lima RA, Soares JR, et al: Supraomohyoid neck dissection in the treatment of T1/T2 squamous cell carcinoma of oral cavity. Am J Surg 1994;168:391.

Kraus DH, Rosenberg DB, Davidson BJ, et al: Supraspinal accessory lymph node metastases in supraomohyoid neck dissection. Am J Surg 1996;172:646.

Lindberg R: Distribution of cervical lymph node metastases from squamous cell carcinoma of the upper respiratory and digestive tracts. Cancer 1972;29:1446.

Shah JP, Medina JE, Shaha AR, et al: Cervical lymph node metastasis. Curr Probl Surg 1993;30:1.

Singh B, Balwally AN, Sundaram K, et al: Branchial cleft cyst carcinoma: Myth or reality? Ann Otol Rhinol Laryngol 1998;107:519.

Spiro RH, Huvos AG, Wong GY, et al: Predictive value of tumor thickness in squamous carcinoma confined to the tongue and floor of the mouth. Am J Surg 1986;152:345.

Spiro RH, DeRose G, Strong EW: Cervical node metastasis of occult origin. Am J Surg 1983;146:441.

Tulenko J, Priore RL, Hoffmeister FS: Cancer of the tongue: Comments on surgical treatment. Am J Surg 1966;112:562.

van den Brekel MW, Castelijns JA: Imaging of lymph nodes in the neck. Semin Roentgenol 2000;35:42.

Chapter 42
Salivary Glands
Joseph Califano and Jatin P. Shah

Salivary gland disease often requires surgical management under the direction of a head and neck surgeon. Proper surgical evaluation of salivary gland pathology, however, requires knowledge of both the medical and the surgical aspects of the many different systemic and local pathologic processes that affect the salivary glands.

ANATOMY AND PHYSIOLOGY

The salivary glands consist of paired, major salivary glands, including the parotid, submandibular, and sublingual glands. In addition, approximately 600 to 1000 small, minor salivary glands are distributed thoughout the upper aerodigestive tract.

The parotid gland (Fig. 42–1) is the largest salivary gland, located beneath the preauricular skin and subcutaneous tissues. Composed almost entirely of serous glands, it accounts for the majority of salivary flow in an active state but provides approximately 25% of the total volume of saliva. It is bounded posteriorly by the external auditory canal, inferiorly by the styloid process and the styloid musculature, and superiorly by the zygoma. Portions of the gland extend anteriorly to the masseter muscle, and posteriorly in a plane superficial to the sternocleidomastoid muscle, and can extend through the stylomandibular

membrane into the parapharyngeal space. The facial nerve exits from the stylomastoid foramen, turns anterolaterally to enter the parotid gland, and branches at the pes anserinus, dividing into the frontal, zygomatic, buccal, marginal mandibular, and cervical branches that innervate the mimetic facial musculature. Although the facial nerve serves to divide the gland into a superficial and deep lobe, no true anatomic division exists to divide these two portions of the gland. The parotid gland is drained by Stensen's duct, which exists from the anterior border of the gland, 1.5 cm below the zygoma. The duct courses anteriorly and superficial to the masseter muscle, turning medially to enter through the buccinator muscle and open intraorally in the buccal mucosa opposite the second maxillary molar.

The submandibular gland, composed of both mucous and serous secretory cells, is the second largest salivary gland, supplying approximately 70% of the total volume of saliva. It is located in the submandibular triangle, bounded inferiorly by the anterior and posterior bellies of the digastric muscle, superiorly by the body of the mandible and the floor of the mouth, and superficially by the facial vein and marginal mandibular branch of the facial nerve. It extends anteriorly, with portions that extend superficial and deep to the mylohyoid muscle. Whar-

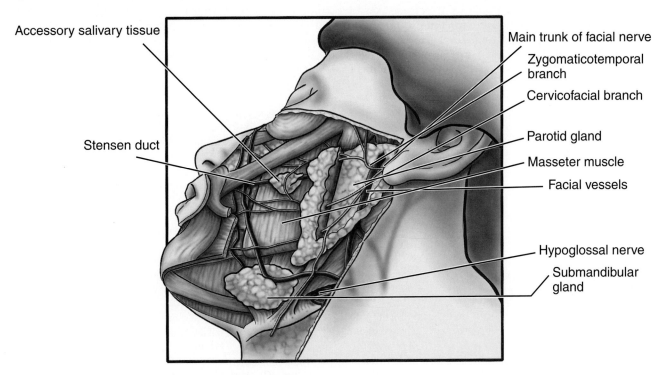

Figure 42–1. Anatomic relationships of the parotid and submandibular salivary glands. (From Shah JP: Salivary gland tumors. Curr Probl Surg 27[12]:782, 1990.)

ton's duct drains the gland, exiting medially before traveling anteriorly between the mylohyoid and the hyoglossus muscles onto the genioglossus muscle and deep to the sublingual gland, eventually opening a few millimeters lateral to the midline lingual frenulum in the anterior floor of the mouth.

The sublingual gland is the smallest of the major salivary glands, produces predominantly mucous secretions, and lies just beneath the mucosa of the anterior floor of the mouth. Approximately 10 small ducts exit the superior aspect of the gland directly into the oral cavity. The gland is bordered laterally by the mandible and genioglossus, and inferiorly by the mylohyoid muscle, with the lingual nerve and Wharton's duct traveling between the genioglossus and the sublingual gland.

The minor salivary glands, approximately 600 to 1000 in number, are simple, submucosal glands that empty directly into the upper aerodigestive tract. They are ubiquitously located at the mucosal surface of the oral cavity, as well as in the nasopharynx, oropharynx, larynx, and other upper aerodigestive mucosal surfaces. They account for a small percentage of total saliva production.

CLINICAL PRESENTATION AND EVALUATION

The diagnosis and evaluation of salivary gland disease relies on a comprehensive history and physical examination, appropriately supplemented by laboratory and imaging studies. A complete examination of the head and neck, including otoscopy, rhinoscopy, indirect laryngoscopy, examination of all mucosal surfaces, and bimanual palpation of head and neck structures as well as a complete cranial nerve examination, is the cornerstone of initial evaluation. Pain, fever, salivary hypersecretion or hyposecretion, nerve dysfunction, purulent discharge, aberrant taste sensation, swallowing and voice dysfunction, gland enlargement, trismus, and evidence of masses in extrasalivary head and neck sites are important findings. Any evidence of concurrent systemic disease must be actively sought, including infectious (human immunodeficiency virus [HIV]), autoimmune, or lymphatic disease (lymphoma, Sjögren's syndrome).

All major salivary glands should be palpated bimanually, with one hand in the oral cavity to precisely define suspected masses, and define involvement of tumors with adjacent normal structures. Palpation of stones in Wharton's or Stensen's duct may yield a diagnosis of sialolithiasis in the context of recurrent sialadenitis. Secretions may be milked from parotid and submandibular glands, cultured, and their character noted (cloudy, purulent, or bloody). Careful evaluation of all cranial nerves, in particular the facial, lingual, and hypoglossal nerves, is performed, owing to the anatomic proximity of these structures to the major salivary glands.

Serologic studies and cultures may be performed to evaluate patients for systemic diseases with salivary gland manifestations, including immunologic (Sjögren's syndrome) and infectious (tuberculosis, cat-scratch disease, HIV).

Computed tomography (CT) of the neck with intrave-

nous contrast enhancement is perhaps the most common imaging modality currently used to evaluate salivary gland pathology. CT is used to define the location of salivary gland masses, define masses as cystic or solid, look for evidence of invasion of adjacent structures, and define significant cervical lymphadenopathy associated with infectious and neoplastic processes. Magnetic resonance imaging (MRI) may also be used for many of the same reasons, but it also has the advantage of providing a multiplanar imaging capability and may be advantageous in delineating extension of the pathology into the skull base. CT remains superior in defining the nature and extent of bony erosion secondary to an infectious or neoplastic pathology.

Fine-needle aspiration (FNA) may be used to evaluate suspected neoplasms or abscesses, either in the office setting or with CT guidance. Plain radiography is a time-honored modality used for confirming the diagnosis of salivary calculi. Sialography, once the mainstay of salivary gland imaging, is now only rarely used.

COMMON DISEASE ENTITIES

Bacterial Sialadenitis

Historically, bacterial sialadenitis has occurred frequently with patients in whom dehydration and salivary stasis occur owing to prolonged anorexia and uncompensated fluid losses in the postoperative period. Subsequent retrograde migration of intraoral bacteria results in acute sialadenitis, resulting in the term *surgical parotitis*. Hence, bacterial infections of the major salivary glands are typically the result of mechanical blockage of salivary ducts or are due to stasis of salivary secretions. Sialolithiasis, the formation of calculi in the ductal system of salivary glands, may also result in blockage of salivary flow. Patients with salivary calculi, therefore, are at risk for episodes of acute and chronic sialadenitis.

Signs and symptoms of acute bacterial sialadenitis include pain, tenderness, swelling, and induration of the involved gland, with erythema of the overlying skin or oral mucosa. The involved gland or glands may be milked to yield purulent discharge from the duct orifice, which may be cultured. It must be kept in mind that if a stone completely obstructs the duct, no fluid will be milked from the gland, and a stone in the duct of the involved gland may or may not be palpable. Fever or leukocytosis are often present, but are occasionally absent. Plain radiography may be able to confirm the presence of a salivary stone. Etiologic bacterial species include *Staphylococcus aureus*, *Streptococcus*, *Haemophilus*, and anaerobic species. Many of these isolates produce β-lactamase.

Management includes administration of appropriate parenteral or oral antibiotics, adequate hydration, sialagogues, oral hygeine, warm compresses, and bimanual massage to milk purulent drainage from the gland. Stones located close to a distal duct orifice may be expressed manually or removed after enlarging the duct orifice with a small incision over a lacrimal probe used to cannulate the duct. Stenting or marsupialization of the duct may be required if it is explored.

Failure to respond to conservative therapy may indicate abscess formation and requires surgical drainage. This diagnosis may be confirmed by CT, by ultrasonography, or by aspiration of pus from the abscess cavity. Drainage of the parotid gland is accomplished by elevation of a standard anteriorly based flap over the superficial parotid fascia, incision of the parotid fascia parallel to the branches of the facial nerve, blunt dissection in the gland parenchyma parallel to the direction of the facial nerve branches to drain any loculated abscess, and placement of an external drain.

Chronic sialadenitis is characterized by repeated episodes of salivary gland pain and inflammation, with or without overt, acute bacterial infection. Obstructions of salivary flow from ductal stricture, mucus plugging, or calculi are common etiologies of this entity. A vicious cycle of obstruction, followed by inflammation, followed by worsening obstruction is characteristic of the clinical course. To date, the only reliable method of treatment for chronic or recurrent sialadenitis is surgical removal of the gland.

Viral Salivary Gland Disease

Paramyxovirus causes mumps, the most common cause of acute viral sialadenitis. Mumps is characterized by tender, bilateral, parotid gland swelling, low-grade fever, arthralgia, malaise, and headache. It occurs predominantly in children and is usually treated supportively. Diagnosis can be made with the use of hemagglutination inhibition and complement fixation tests, but is usually made on clinical grounds.

Infection with HIV is associated with salivary gland lymphoproliferative disorders and with cystic enlargement of the major salivary glands. These lesions evolve as gradual, painless enlargement of one or more salivary glands that usually represent epithelium-lined simple cysts, but they may represent HIV-associated lymphoma. Diagnosis is made by FNA and characteristic cystic appearance on CT or MRI in the appropriate clinical context. These lesions are usually managed conservatively by clinical observation. Suspicion of lymphoma or other solid neoplasm indicates standard surgical excision for diagnostic and therapeutic purposes.

Granulomatous Disease

Previously uncommon tuberculous mycobacterial infection of the salivary glands has been increasing owing to the contribution of tuberculosis associated with HIV infection. Infection of the salivary glands by *Mycobacterium tuberculosis* may occur via the lymphatic network intrinsic to the parenchyma of the parotid gland and the lymphatics adjacent to all of the major salivary glands, either as a primary infection or as a secondary infection related to a primary pulmonary focus. This infection presents in the parotid gland as diffuse enlargement, or as a solid, slowly growing, painless mass. Attempts at diagnosis with FNA are difficult, so that most cases of parotid tuberculosis are diagnosed after a superficial parotidectomy to remove a suspicious mass.

Atypical (nontuberculous) mycobacterial infections present as a rapidly increasing mass in the neck or parotid gland in children 1 to 3 years of age. Systemic signs and symptoms are few, and the natural history of these lesions involves spontaneous rupture into the skin. Treatment consists of excision and/or curettage of involved tissue after a clinical diagnosis has been made, with simultaneous culture of purulent cyst contents to confirm diagnosis. Curettage is the recommended treatment when this lesion involves the parotid gland, to minimize any injury to facial nerve branches.

Actinomyces includes many species of gram-positive anaerobic bacteria that also present as painless, indurated, infected cervical or parotid lymph nodes that may necrose and spontaneously drain. Diagnosis is confirmed by FNA or swab showing sulfur granules and filamentous gram-negative rods. Penicillin is the mainstay of treatment.

Cat-scratch disease is a granulomatous lymphadenitis resulting from inoculation via skin trauma from a domestic cat, accompanied by systemic signs and symptoms ranging from absent to severe. A clinical diagnosis is made by the history and clinical presentation in the context of a sterile abscess culture or a characteristic histologic appearance of excised lymph nodes. Treatment is essentially supportive.

Toxoplasmosis presents as both a disseminated form of disease and a form resulting in localized lymphadenopathy, transmitted by a parasite found in raw meat or cat feces. Diagnosis is confirmed by antibody titers. *Franciscella tularensis* is a gram-negative organism transmitted by insect bite, subsequently followed by local lymphadenopathy and constitutional symptoms (i.e., tularemia). Aggressive, early drainage of involved lymph nodes in the acute stages of infection is contraindicated, as it may result in systemic dissemination of disease. After diagnosis by antibody titers and antibiotic therapy, remaining cysts may be excised or drained.

Systemic Disease

Sialadenosis is a syndrome of bilateral, nontender parotid swelling attributable to innumerable underlying disease states, including cirrhosis, diabetes, alcoholism, malnutrition, bulimia, ovarian insufficiency, hypothyroidism, pancreatic insufficiency, and pharmacologic site effects. Symptoms and signs of primary Sjögren's syndrome include bilateral parotid gland swelling associated with xerophthalmia and xerostomia. Association with another connective tissue disorder gives a diagnosis of secondary Sjögren's syndrome. Mucosal lip biopsy is used to confirm the diagnosis by characteristic lymphocytic infiltration of the minor salivary glands. Of note, these patients are at risk for neoplastic disease, as approximately 5% of patients eventually develop a lymphoproliferative neoplasm.

Trauma

Management of trauma to the salivary glands includes treatment of important anatomic structures related to the salivary glands as well as treatment of the injured glandular structures. A comprehensive physical examination, as outlined previously, must be performed. Injuries to the facial nerve medial to an imaginary line drawn between the lateral canthus and the mental foremen are not usually treated by reanastomosis owing to their propensity to recover spontaneously. Nerve injuries lateral to this line are candidates for exploration and tension-free reanastomosis or grafting of severed or damaged nerve fibers. It is noted that 36 hours post injury it is unlikely that distal, severed nerve endings may be reliably located with the use of electrical stimulation. Salivary duct injuries may be evaluated with sialography, and repaired with microvascular anastomosis over Silastic stents to prevent subsequent stricture. The failure to repair major ductal injuries may result in post-traumatic sialocutaneous fistula or sialocele formation. The management of sialocele consists of repeated aspiration of saliva and placement of compression bandages. Surgical exploration or pharmacologic therapy is reserved for cases that fail conservative management.

Acquired and Congenital Cysts

Congenital cysts of the first branchial cleft present as preauricular or parotid masses and are essentially duplications of the membranous (type I) or membranous and cartilaginous (type II) external auditory canal. These developmental anomalies are often intimately associated with the facial nerve. Appropriate treatment of these cysts mandates careful identification and dissection of the facial nerve, usually resulting in the performance of a superficial parotidectomy.

Ranulae are acquired cysts of the sublingual glands and present as translucent, cystic masses in the floor of the mouth. When they enlarge and extend inferiorly, resulting in a cystic neck mass, they are called plunging ranulae. Excision of the entire cyst, as well as the sublingual gland from which the cyst usually arises, prevents recurrence.

Salivary Gland Neoplasms

General Considerations

Approximately 80% of salivary gland neoplasms originate in the parotid gland, 15% develop in the submandibular gland, and the remaining tumors arise in the sublingual and minor salivary glands. A total of 70% to 80% of parotid neoplasms are benign, 50% of submandibular neoplasms are benign, and fewer than 40% of sublingual and minor salivary gland tumors are benign. Most salivary gland neoplasms (95%) occur in adults. The most common benign pediatric salivary gland tumor is the hemangioma, followed by the pleomorphic adenoma. The most common malignant salivary gland tumor in children is mucoepidermoid carcinoma.

Most major salivary gland neoplasms present as asymptomatic masses. Pain in and of itself is not an indicator of malignancy, but it is associated with a poorer prognosis when found in association with malignancy. Minor salivary gland tumors may present as painless masses almost anywhere in the upper aerodigestive tract, although usually they are found in the hard palate, sinonasal tract, and other sites.

A thorough head and neck examination, as outlined previously, should be performed. Special attention is paid to cranial nerve function, tumor fixation to local structures, and associated cervical adenopathy. For example, facial nerve paralysis in patients with parotid gland carcinoma is an indicator of an extremely poor prognosis, with 5-year survival rates varying between 0 and 15% in patients with parotid malignancy who present with paralysis. Fine-needle aspiration biopsy may be used to aid in diagnosis with essentially no risk of seeding the biopsy needle track. CT and MRI scans do not differentiate benign from malignant tumors, and rarely do they alter the therapeutic approach to major salivary gland neoplasms. However, CT and MRI are used to evaluate malignant or recurrent neoplasms, large tumors, parapharyngeal space involvement, suspected carotid artery involvement, and involvement of structures that suggest inoperability. Minor salivary gland malignancies involving the nose or paranasal sinuses are commonly imaged with MRI to evaluate orbital, dural, neural, or cranial involvement.

Benign Neoplasms

Pleomorphic adenoma makes up 65% of all salivary gland neoplasms and is the most common tumor of the parotid gland. Grossly, this tumor has a well-defined capsule, but microscopically it demonstrates incomplete encapsulation and transcapsular growth with pseudopodial extensions. This is thought to account for the high rate of recurrence after attempts at simple enucleation of these tumors. Therefore, pleomorphic adenomas must be excised with an adequate cuff of normal parotid tissue, usually via a superficial parotidectomy.

Warthin's tumor is the second most common benign neoplasm of the parotid gland and accounts for 6% to 10% of all parotid tumors, but it is rarely found in other salivary gland sites. Warthin's tumors are often cystic, can occur multicentrically, and occur bilaterally approximately 10% of the time. Most tumors are found in older men, and an increased risk of occurrence in smokers is noted.

Oncocytomas occur almost exclusively in the parotid gland, constitute fewer than 1% of all salivary gland neoplasms, and commonly occur in patients who are in the sixth decade of life. These tumors are solid, and are removed by superficial parotidectomy with facial nerve preservation.

Monomorphic adenomas describe a group of rare salivary gland neoplasms, including basal cell adenoma, clear cell adenoma, glycogen-rich adenoma, and other rare tumors. The monomorphic adenomas are considered benign, nonaggressive neoplasms and are treated by resection with a margin of normal tissue, including superficial parotidectomy in the parotid gland.

Malignant Neoplasms

Mucoepidermoid carcinoma is the most common malignant tumor involving the parotid gland and the second most common malignant tumor of the submandibular gland, after adenoid cystic carcinoma. These tumors are divided into high, intermediate, and low-grade types. Low-grade tumors behave more like benign neoplasms but may invade locally and metastasize. High-grade mucoepidermoid carcinoma resembles squamous cell carcinomas, and diagnosis is confirmed by mucin staining to differentiate them from squamous cell carcinoma. These neoplasms are aggressive, with a high propensity for metastasis.

Adenoid cystic carcinoma accounts for 6% of all salivary gland neoplasms, and it is the most common malignancy of the submandibular gland and minor salivary glands. Perineural invasion is a nearly omnipresent feature of this tumor, accounting for the difficulty in eradicating this tumor despite wide surgical excision, and the tendency for late recurrence, sometimes after a decade or more of disease-free status. Adjuvant radiation therapy is recommended for this tumor type.

Acinic cell carcinoma represents 1% of all salivary gland neoplasms and 2% to 4% of parotid gland neoplasms. Almost all acinic cell carcinomas (95%) are found in the parotid gland, and are rarely found in the submandibular gland. Patients are usually women in the fifth decade of life. Acinic cell carcinoma exhibits a benign course early after treatment, but 20-year follow-up studies have shown a 50% survival rate. Bilateral involvement of the parotid gland is noted approximately 3% of the time.

Adenocarcinoma occurs most commonly in the minor salivary glands, followed by the parotid gland, and represents 15% of malignant parotid neoplasms. These are aggressive tumors that are likely to recur and metastasize.

Polymorphous low-grade adenocarcinoma is the second most common malignancy of the minor salivary glands, presenting as a firm, painless mass on the palate, buccal mucosa, or upper lip during the sixth decade of life. These tumors also exhibit perineural spread, and are treated with wide local excision.

Carcinoma expleomorphic adenoma describes a malignant tumor that has arisen from a preexisting pleomorphic adenoma, and representing 2% to 5% of salivary gland tumors. A typical history describes a mass present for 10 to 15 years that suddenly increases in size. This tumor has a very poor prognosis, and surgical excision followed by postoperative radiation is recommended.

Squamous cell carcinoma is a rare malignancy of the salivary glands that constitutes fewer than 2% of salivary gland tumors, and occurs most commonly in the submandibular gland. The diagnosis of a true, primary squamous cell carcinoma of the salivary glands requires exclusion of contiguous spread of an adjacent squamous cell carcinoma into the gland, distant metastases to the gland from a cutaneous malignancy, and high-grade mucoepidermoid carcinoma. These tumors present in the seventh decade of life, and more commonly in males. They are associated with a high rate of regional and distant metastases, and surgical excision followed by radiation therapy is recommended.

Sarcomas of the salivary glands are rare. Diagnosis requires exclusion of metastatic spread of a sarcoma from another primary site and invasion of the gland from an adjacent soft tissue sarcoma. Behavior of these tumors is analogous to that of sarcomas found in other anatomic sites, depending on size, tumor type, and grade.

Primary lymphoma of the salivary glands is rare. This diagnosis requires proof of no known extrasalivary lymphoma, proof that the lymphoma arose from salivary gland parenchyma, and standard pathologic confirmation of the diagnosis. Surgical intervention is usually reserved for diagnosis.

Therapy

Surgical biopsy, tumor enucleation, and excisional biopsy of parotid neoplasms are mentioned here only to recommend avoidance of these techniques. All of these are associated with a high rate of recurrence, especially for a pleomorphic adenoma. The proper approach to most parotid neoplasms is to perform a superficial parotidectomy, with preservation of the facial nerve and its branches, so that the tumor is removed with an adequate cuff of normal tissue (see Fig. 42–1). Superficial parotidectomy is curative for most benign parotid neoplasms and superficial, low-grade malignant neoplasms. Total parotidectomy, in which both superficial and deep lobes are excised, is recommended for high-grade malignancies that involve both lobes of the parotid gland, and for benign tumors of the deep lobe of the parotid. The facial nerve is preserved during excision of the malignancy unless grossly involved with tumor. If resected, the facial nerve is usually immediately grafted intraoperatively. Neck dissection is indicated for clinically positive cervical metastases or if suspicious nodes found during the primary resection are positive. There is no proven benefit of elective neck dissection for a clinically negative neck; however, an elective neck dissection is acceptable for high-grade neoplasms with a high risk of lymph node metastasis (e.g., squamous cell carcinoma and high-grade mucoepidermoid carcinoma). Parapharyngeal space tumors may be removed via a transcervical approach, reflecting the submandibular gland anteriorly after identification of the facial nerve to allow access to the anterior compartment of the parapharyngeal space. Neoplasms involving the submandibular gland are usually limited to the gland itself, and surgical resection is usually confined to the submandibular triangle. All nerves are preserved unless involved by tumor.

Radiation therapy in combination with surgery has improved locoregional control and survival in patients with carcinoma of the major salivary glands, and it benefits patients with minor salivary gland malignancies who are at high risk for local failure. Indications for adjuvant radiation therapy include high tumor stage, high grade, or concerns regarding adequacy of resection. The salivary glands are sensitive to radiation, and most patients treated with therapeutic radiation that involves the salivary glands experience significant xerostomia and alterations in taste sensation and are at risk for dental caries.

Chemotherapy has been shown to be of little benefit in the treatment of salivary gland malignancy, and it is usually reserved for attempts at palliation in unresectable, previously irradiated tumors.

Surgical Technique

A brief description of the techniques of superficial parotidectomy is presented here. For approaches to the resection of submandibular gland tumors, deep lobe parotid tumors, salivary tumors of the sinuses, parapharyngeal space, and other minor salivary gland sites, the reader is referred to the selected readings that follow.

The patient is placed under general anesthesia, in a supine position with head extended and rotated in a direction contralateral to the side with the parotid tumor in preparation for a superficial parotidectomy. A standard parotidectomy incision extends from the preauricular skin crease, curves around the earlobe, extends posteroinferiorly before extending along a cervical skin crease approximately 3 cm below the angle of the mandible. An anteriorly based skin flap raised superficial to the parotid fascia is raised to the anterior border of the parotid gland. The posterior skin flap is raised for a short distance in order to expose the sternocleidomastoid muscle and the pretragal cartilage. As the tail of the parotid gland is raised anteriorly from the anterior border of the sternocleidomastoid muscle, the greater auricular nerve may need to be divided. Occasionally, a posterior branch of the greater auricular nerve may be preserved by retracting this branch posteriorly. The parotid gland is divided off the deep attachments to the sternocleidomastoid muscle, exposing the posterior belly of the digastric muscle. At this point, meticulous hemostasis is imperative, so that early identification of the facial nerve may be accomplished and inadvertent injury to the nerve may be avoided. The use of bipolar cautery and fine suture is encouraged, as unipolar cautery may result in electrical injury to neural tissue.

The substance of the parotid gland is meticulously dissected from the cartilaginous external auditory canal and the soft tissue of the tympanomastoid sulcus with the use of a fine hemostat. Using gradual step-by-step dissection, the main trunk of the facial nerve is identified as it emerges from the stylomastoid suture line. Dissection then proceeds in a plane superficial to the nerve anteriorly toward the periphery of the gland. A curved hemostat is used to spread the parotid tissue over the nerve and its branches. The overlying tissue between the two tines of the hemostat is divided, while the underlying nerve branch is constantly visualized and preserved. Tissue between adjacent nerve branches is carefully divided, ensuring that an adequate cuff of tissue is maintained around the tumor. Nerve branches directly adjacent to the tumor may be carefully dissected off the tumor, taking care to preserve the adjacent tumor capsule. Sequential dissection of all nerve branches essentially lifts the superficial portion of the parotid gland of the facial nerve, with the tumor encompassed in the superficial portion of the gland. Once hemostasis has been ensured, a Penrose drain is placed through the portion of the wound directly behind the earlobe, the incision is closed in two layers, and a light pressure dressing is placed.

Complications

Complications of surgery for salivary gland disorders obviously depend on the nature of the pathology; that is, infectious, traumatic, neoplastic, the site of the operative

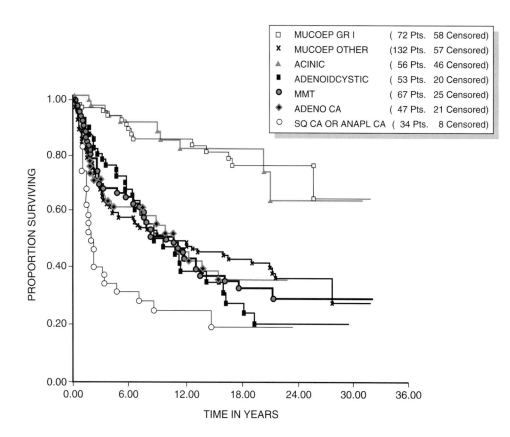

Figure 42–2. Kaplan-Meier survival curves for salivary gland malignancies by histologic diagnosis. Low-grade mucoepidermoid carcinoma (MUCOEP GR 1) and acinic cell carcinoma (ACINIC) have favorable survival. Adenoid cystic (ADENOIDCYSTIC), medium- and high-grade mucoepidermoid carcinoma (MUCOEP OTHER), malignant mixed tumor (MMT), and adenocarcinoma (ADENO CA) have an intermediate survival. Anaplastic and squamous cell carcinomas (SQ CA OR ANAPL CA) have poor survival outcomes. (From Spiro RH: Management of malignant tumors of the salivary glands. Oncology 1998; 12:671–683.)

procedure, and extent of procedure. Most documented complications related to salivary gland surgery are those related to superficial parotidectomy, as this is the most common procedure associated with salivary gland pathology.

Temporary facial nerve paralysis occurring in one or two facial nerve branches has been reported in 10% to 30% of parotidectomies, with rates of permanent paralysis in fewer than 3% of patients. The most commonly injured branch of the facial nerve is the marginal mandibular branch.

Hemorrhage and hematoma are uncommon, and are treated by exploration and ligation of any bleeding vessels. Infection is rare and is treated with adequate drainage with or without antibiotics. Occasionally, necrosis may be noted in the distal tip of the postauricular skin flap, which is avoided by designing a widely based posterior skin flap.

Postoperative development of a sialocele occasionally occurs. Treatment consists of repeated aspiration with or without placement of compression dressings. The treatment of salivary fistulas consists of placement of pressure dressings.

Lack of sensation in the distribution of the greater auricular nerve is almost an expected sequela of superficial parotidectomy. Occasionally, the development of a painful neuroma occurs at the severed end of the nerve, requiring subsequent excision.

Frey's syndrome, or gustatory sweating, is caused by aberrant innervation of cutaneous sweat glands by severed postganglionic parasympathetic nerve endings. When examined for this complication carefully, the majority of patients are found to have developed this complication, although only about 10% find the symptoms bothersome. Treatment includes topical glycopyrrolate and the placement of an interposition graft between the residual gland and the skin, as well as other methods.

Submandibular gland complications are related to the adjacent anatomic structures.

Outcomes

The essential predictors of outcome in salivary gland malignancy include tumor histology, stage, grade, and adequacy of surgical resection. Kaplan-Meier survival curves for the major types of salivary gland malignancy are depicted in Figure 42–2. Studies show that low-grade mucoepidermoid carcinoma and acinic cell carcinoma have a more favorable prognosis, and squamous cell carcinoma, salivary duct carcinoma, and anaplastic carcinoma have relatively poor survivals, with other types falling into an intermediate group. Recurrence may occur more than 10 years following treatment for some salivary gland tumors (see Fig. 42–2). In patients with adenoid cystic carcinoma in particular, disease-related deaths can occur after more than 20 years of follow-up. Therefore, disease-free survival may differ significantly from cumulative survival.

Clinical stage is, by far, the best predictor of survival and is determined by tumor size and the presence or absence of cervical nodal and distant metastasis (Fig. 42–3). T stage increases, regardless of size, when there is extension of tumor into the skin, adjacent soft tissues, or bone, or when the facial nerve is involved.

Tumor grade also appears to have an influence on survival (see Fig. 42–3). Bony involvement is an indicator of poor prognosis in univariate analysis. Of note, stage for stage, however, there are no significant survival differences between patients treated for malignant major salivary gland tumors and those treated for malignant minor salivary gland tumors.

The adequacy of surgical resection is another important prognostic factor. The presence of microscopic tumor at the border of resection portends poorer local control in multiple studies. Adjunctive external-beam radiation therapy is indicated when microscopic residual

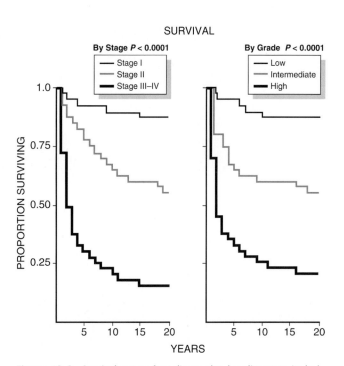

Figure 42–3. Survival curves for salivary gland malignancy, including adenocarcinoma, mucoepidermoid carcinoma, and squamous cell carcinoma, by stage and grade. (From Spiro RH: Management of malignant tumors of the salivary glands. Oncology 1998; 12:671–683.)

disease is suspected, especially when one deals with a high-grade neoplasm.

SELECTED READINGS

American Joint Committee for Cancer: AJCC Cancer Staging Manual. Philadelphia, Lippincott-Raven, 1998.

Batsakis JG: Tumors of the major salivary glands. In Batsakis JG ed: Tumors of the Head and Neck: Clinical and Pathological Considerations. Baltimore, Williams & Wilkins, 1979, p 1.

Batsakis JG: Neoplasms of the minor and "lesser" major salivary glands. In Batsakis JG (ed): Tumors of the Head and Neck: Clinical and Pathological Considerations. Baltimore, Williams & Wilkins, 1979, p 65.

Eisele DW, Johns ME: Salivary gland neoplasms. In Bailey BJ (ed): Head and Neck Surgery–Otolaryngology, 2nd ed. Philadelphia, Lippincott-Raven, 1998, p 1485.

Gayner SM, Kane WJ, McCaffrey TV: Infections of the salivary glands. In Cummings CW (ed): Otolaryngology–Head and Neck Surgery, 3rd ed. St. Louis, Mosby–Year Book, 1998, p 1234.

Haller JR: Trauma. In Cummings CW ed: Otolaryngology–Head and Neck Surgery, 3rd (ed): St. Louis, Mosby–Year Book, 1998, p 1247.

Shah JP: Color Atlas of Head and Neck Surgery: Mouth, Pharynx, Larynx, Thyroid, Parotid, Soft Tissues, and Reconstructive Surgery. London, Mosby-Wolfe, 1990.

Spiro RH: Salivary neoplasms: Overview of a 35-year experience with 2,807 patients. Head Neck Surg 1986;8:177.

Spiro RH: Management of malignant tumors of the salivary glands. Oncology 1998;12:671.

Spiro RH, Armstrong J, Harrison L, et al: Carcinoma of major salivary glands: Recent trends. Arch Otolaryngol Head Neck Surg 1989;115:316.

Chapter 43

Neurovascular and Soft Tissue Tumors of the Head and Neck

Snehal G. Patel and Jatin P. Shah

Neurovascular and soft tissue tumors of the head and neck constitute a group of diverse neoplasms, the vast majority of which are benign. Although most benign neurovascular and soft tissue tumors are relatively innocuous, the potential for local destruction does exist, whereas malignant tumors can metastasize in addition to causing local pathology. Malignant tumors of mesenchymal origin or soft tissue sarcomas of the head and neck also comprise a wide variety of biologically diverse neoplasms that constitute only about 10% of all sarcomas. Surgical excision, which is the most effective form of treatment in most instances, may result in unacceptable cosmetic and functional deformity, and this must be taken into account when one plans the treatment approach.

CLINICAL PRESENTATION

Tumors of the neck in children are most commonly congenital or inflammatory and may be associated with minimal signs and symptoms. Benign soft tissue masses of the neck in adults may also be otherwise asymptomatic, but pressure effects on adjoining structures such as the aerodigestive tract may result in difficulty in swallowing or breathing, hoarseness of the voice, and cranial nerve deficits or altered sensation from compression of cranial nerves. Tumors of the nasal cavity may cause nasal obstruction or epistaxis, but the majority of paranasal sinus tumors remain asymptomatic and are detected at a relatively advanced stage. Although local tissue destruction and invasiveness are hallmarks of malignant tumors, some benign tumors located in restricted anatomic spaces, such as the skull base, can also present with signs and symptoms such as cranial nerve deficits that are usually associated with malignant tumors. Symptoms from metastases to regional lymph nodes and/or distant sites develop during the course of the progression of the disease, but they may infrequently be the only presenting symptoms. Certain tumors, such as neurofibromas, develop in the background of more widespread systemic disease, often as a component of familial syndromes. The specific clinical features of each of the individual types of lesions are described later, along with their other salient features.

Differential Diagnosis

A complete description of all benign as well as malignant soft tissue and neurovascular lesions of the head and neck is clearly beyond the scope of this book. Table 43–1 presents a list of some of the more common lesions that may be encountered in clinical practice.

HEMANGIOMAS. Hemangiomas are most common in the neonate or infant and most frequently present at cutaneous sites, such as the scalp, face, and neck. They may also arise within the mucosa of the aerodigestive tract or the deep soft tissue of the neck. The clinical appearance is characteristic, and most lesions present at or soon after birth as raised, erythematous cutaneous masses. Deep-seated lesions, on the other hand, may be discovered incidentally (Fig. 43–1) or may present as an ill-defined neck mass with normal overlying skin. Hemangiomas of the upper aerodigestive tract may present with intermittent stridor or hemoptysis, and about half will have an obvious cutaneous lesion at the same time. As most lesions involute spontaneously before puberty, hemangiomas in children are managed expectantly, but lesions in critical locations such as the periocular region or the airway may require early intervention to prevent functional compromise. Nonsurgical treatment modalities include the use of lasers, intralesional steroid injection, and treatment with agents such as interferon α-2a and TNP-470.

CYSTIC HYGROMAS. Cystic hygromas are malforma-

Table 43–1

Differential Diagnosis of Neurovascular and Soft Tissue Tumors of the Head and Neck

I. **Vascular Tumors**
   A. Benign
      1. Hemangiomas
      2. Lymphangiomas
      3. Juvenile nasopharyngeal angiofibromas
      4. Paragangliomas
   B. Malignant
      1. Hemangiopericytomas
II. **Neurogenic Tumors**
   A. Benign
      1. Neurilemmomas
      2. Neurofibromas
   B. Malignant
      1. Malignant peripheral nerve sheath tumors
      2. Esthesioneuroblastomas
III. **Soft Tissue Tumors**
   A. Benign
      1. Lipomas
      2. Fibromatoses
   B. Malignant (soft tissue sarcomas)
      1. Malignant fibrous histiocytomas
      2. Fibrosarcomas
      3. Dermatofibrosarcoma protuberans
      4. Angiosarcomas
      5. Liposarcomas
      6. Rhabdomyosarcomas

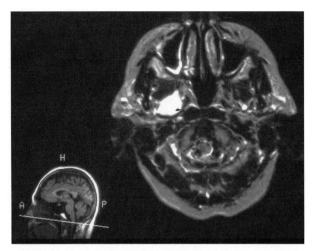

Figure 43–1. An MRI scan of the brain done for investigation of cerebrovascular stroke in this 69-year-old woman revealed a contrast-enhancing lesion in the right parapharyngeal space. The lesion was excised via a transcervical approach, and pathologic examination of the specimen confirmed the diagnosis of cavernous hemangioma.

tions of the lymphatic system that also present during infancy, but unlike hemangiomas they rarely involve spontaneously and therefore almost always require treatment. The majority of lesions are seen before the child is 2 years old, and present as soft, easily compressible, ill-defined lateral neck masses. Histologically, the lesion demonstrates multiple superficial and deep extensions that burrow into the surrounding tissue. This makes complete excision difficult and predisposes to the commonly cited complications, such as cranial nerve injury, lymphatic fistula, and local recurrence.

JUVENILE NASOPHARYNGEAL ANGIOFIBROMAS (JNAs).
JNA is a benign vascular neoplasm that arises from the fibrovascular stroma of the nasopharynx in the area of the sphenopalatine foramen. The common clinical presentation is with nasal obstruction and intermittent epistaxis in an adolescent male. Endoscopy reveals a vascular mass in the nasal cavity or nasopharynx that shows contrast enhancement on computed tomography (CT) or magnetic resonance imaging (MRI). Biopsy is fraught with danger and can result in life-threatening epistaxis owing to the extremely vascular nature of the mass. These tumors are generally supplied by the internal maxillary and ascending pharyngeal branches of the external carotid artery, but vessels from the internal carotid or vertebral basilar systems may also contribute. With the recognition that the lesion can be locally invasive, several staging systems have been developed based on the extent of spread outside the nasopharynx. Surgical excision is the mainstay of treatment of extracranial tumors and those with minimal intracranial extension. Preoperative carotid and vertebral angiography can determine the contribution of the intracranial circulation to the vascular supply, and embolization of the tumor has been reported as a means of reducing intraoperative blood loss. The traditional contraindications to surgery have included intracranial extension and/or vascular supply from the internal carotid artery, but these lesions can now be treated with the use

of craniofacial and skull base approaches. Tumors with extensive intracranial extension are treated nonsurgically with the use of radiation, chemotherapy, or antiandrogen treatment.

PARAGANGLIOMAS. Paragangliomas arise from extraadrenal neural crest–derived rests that migrate in association with cranial nerves and the aorta and its branches during embryonic development. The paraganglia are composed of sustentacular cells that are modified Schwann cells, and chief cells that are capable of producing catecholamines and other neurotransmitters. Paragangliomas are classified according to the neurovascular structures with which they are associated; the carotid body tumor, the glomus jugulare, and the glomus intravagale are the most common within the head and neck. Approximately 10% of tumors are familial and are associated with an autosomal dominant pattern of inheritance of a gene located on the long arm of chromosome 11. Compared with the more common sporadic type, these familial tumors are more often multicentric and bilateral and are more prone to secreting neurotransmitters or demonstrating malignant behavior. Functioning tumors produce symptoms such as tachycardia, palpitations, headache, and flushing, and patients with these symptoms should be screened preoperatively for plasma and urinary levels of catecholamines and their metabolites. The carotid body is a chemoreceptor located in the adventitia of the posteromedial aspect of the carotid bifurcation, and it regulates ventilation in response to fluctuations in arterial oxygen, carbon dioxide, and pH. Chronic hypoxia, as in individuals who live at high altitudes, predisposes to the development of sporadic carotid body tumors. The usual clinical presentation is that of a painless, pulsatile neck mass near the angle of the mandible, classically described as having limited mobility in the craniocaudad direction. Radiologic imaging with CT or MRI demonstrates the characteristic splaying of the internal and external carotid arteries with intense contrast enhancement, which on MRI appears as a "salt-and-pepper" pattern owing to the presence of flow voids within the tumor.

Carotid body tumors have been classified as group I tumors, which are small and easily dissected from the vessels; group II, which partially surround the vessels and are more adherent; and group III, which are large and intimately adherent to the entire circumference of the carotid bifurcation. These tumors have been estimated to grow about 5 mm a year, and surgical excision is the treatment of choice. Paragangliomas of the jugulotympanic region are classified as either (1) glomus tympanicum, arising from the posterior auricular branch of the vagus (Arnold's nerve) or the tympanic branch of the glossopharyngeal nerve (Jacobson's nerve), or, most commonly, (2) glomus jugulare, arising from the jugular bulb itself. These lesions generally remain silent until expansile growth causes dysfunction of cranial nerves IX to XII, which are in close proximity. The clinical features may include hoarseness of the voice, hearing loss and tinnitus, diminished gag reflex, and deviation of the tongue. A vascular mass may be visualized medial to an intact tympanic membrane. The radiologic imaging is optimally achieved with the use of CT for details of bony erosion at the skull base, and with MRI for delineating the relationship to adjacent neurovascular structures. Surgical resection of these tumors can result in severe morbidity owing to dysfunction of the facial and lower cranial nerves. Older patients, who may not be able to compensate for these deficits, may be treated with nonsurgical options, such as external-beam radiation therapy. Glomus intravagale are rare tumors that arise from the paraganglionic tissue located in the perineurium of the vagus nerve. The usual site of these tumors is at the level of the inferior vagal ganglion, but they have been reported to arise as far down as the carotid bifurcation or as far superiorly as the jugular foramen. The patient typically presents with a neck mass associated with hoarseness of the voice from a paralysis of the ipsilateral vocal cord. More advanced lesions may present with multiple cranial neuropathies or Horner's syndrome. These tumors can be radiologically differentiated from other masses in the region by the fact that they displace the contents of the carotid sheath anteriorly. In contrast with other paragangliomas, glomus intravagale tumors metastasize in almost 20% of patients and the lungs are the site most commonly affected. Complete surgical excision of these tumors results in considerable laryngeal dysfunction, as the vagus nerve needs to be sacrificed in the vicinity of the base of the skull.

HEMANGIOPERICYTOMAS. Hemangiopericytomas are malignant tumors that arise from the capillary pericytes of Zimmermann located in the outer wall of the capillaries. Within the head and neck, the sinonasal tract is the most commonly involved site, followed by the neck and the orbit. Tumors of the neck present as painless, slow-growing vascular masses, while nasal obstruction and epistaxis are common presenting symptoms of sinonasal hemangiopericytomas. An erythematous mass may be evident on endoscopy, and radiologic imaging may demonstrate a contrast-enhancing mass associated with bony erosion or destruction. En bloc surgical resection of sinonasal hemangiopericytomas may require an anterior craniofacial approach. The role of radiation therapy as primary treatment or adjuvant therapy remains unproven, and chemotherapeutic agents have not been reported to produce any significant clinical benefit. Local recurrence of the tumor has been reported in as many as 50% of patients, but in general the prognosis is better than that for hemangiopericytomas at other sites in the body.

SCHWANNOMAS. Schwannomas, or neurilemmomas, arise from the Schwann cells of the sheaths of peripheral nerves. As many as 50% of these benign tumors occur within the head and neck as solitary, well-encapsulated lesions. The most commonly affected nerves are the eighth (acoustic neuroma), the tenth, and the sympathetic chain, but other nerves, including smaller peripheral branches (Fig. 43–2A to C), can be affected. Radiologic imaging, especially MRI, demonstrates a moderately enhancing mass in close proximity to a nerve. A preoperative histologic diagnosis is usually not available, as diagnostic interpretation of cytology specimens is difficult. Surgical excision is the most effective form of treatment; and as these tumors grow in an expansile fashion within the substance of the nerve generally without actual infiltra-

tion, it may be possible for the tumor to be dissected and separated from the nerve, thus preserving the nerve's integrity. The sequelae of neural deficit following surgical excision, however, must always be factored in when one selects the type of treatment. The rate of growth of these tumors is generally slow; thus, close observation of lesions that are at significant risk for postoperative morbidity may be justified, especially in the elderly and the infirm. Alternative modalities, such as external-beam radiation therapy, have been used and reported to be effective in arresting the progression of these lesions. A very small proportion of schwannomas behave like malignant tumors, demonstrating high mitotic activity and local aggressiveness with higher local and distant failure rates. In addition to the size of the primary tumor, the ability to achieve complete surgical excision of the tumor is a major factor that determines outcome.

NEUROFIBROMAS. In contrast with schwannomas, neurofibromas are unencapsulated tumors that cause a fusiform dilatation of the peripheral nerve of their origin. They commonly occur as multiple, discrete nodules in one of two types of presentation. Neurofibromatosis type 1, or von Recklinghausen's disease, is an autosomal dominant disorder characterized by multiple café au lait spots with central nervous system, bony, and ocular lesions. Malignant transformation has been reported in as many as 30% of individuals with von Recklinghausen's disease. Neurofibromatosis type 2 is also inherited as an autosomal dominant disorder but is considerably rarer than type 1, and only rarely do these lesions undergo malignant transformation. Bilateral acoustic neuromas and meningiomas are the most commonly associated tumors. A neurofibroma can also present as a solitary mass without any suspicious family history. Surgical excision is the treatment of choice for these solitary lesions, and the nerve of origin almost always has to be sacrificed because of the diffuse, fusiform nature of the pathologic involvement.

MALIGNANT PERIPHERAL NERVE SHEATH TUMORS (MPNSTs). MPNSTs, or malignant schwannomas, can present as a solitary mass or may arise as the result of malignant degeneration of a von Recklinghausen lesion in 5% to 15% of patients and are heralded by nerve dysfunction or pain. Tumors arising from a given nerve involve it in a fusiform or nodular pattern, and gadolinium-enhanced MRI may demonstrate perineural extension of the tumor. Adverse prognostic factors include existing neurofibromatosis, previous radiation, size larger than 5 cm, and glandular or rhabdomyomatous differentiation. Complete surgical resection with negative margins is desirable, and adjuvant radiation therapy may be used to enhance the chances of local control.

ESTHESIONEUROBLASTOMAS. These are malignant tumors of the olfactory neuroepithelium that have a characteristic bimodal age distribution involving patients in their second and sixth decades of life. Presenting signs and symptoms are generally vague and can include nasal obstruction, epistaxis, and headache, but invasion into surrounding structures can result in proptosis, diplopia, and increased intracranial pressure. Nasal endoscopic examination may reveal a polypoid superior nasal mass that

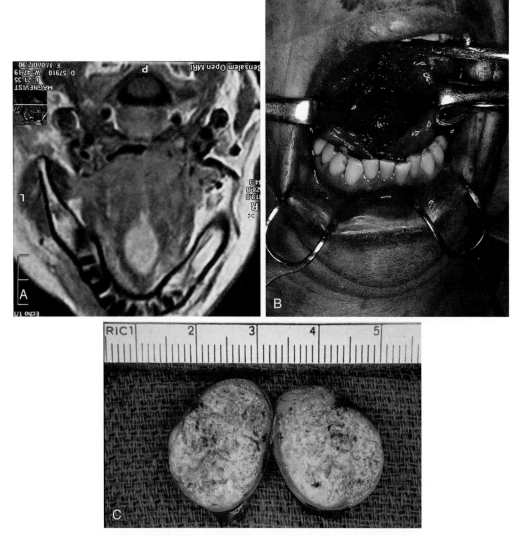

Figure 43–2. *A,* A contrast-enhancing lesion was incidentally discovered on MRI within the substance of the tongue of a 52-year-old woman. *B,* The tumor was approached in the midline of the ventral aspect of the tongue after cannulating and protecting the openings of the submandibular salivary ducts. *C,* Cut section revealed a well-encapsulated, fleshy tumor that on microscopic examination proved to be a typical schwannoma.

enhances with contrast medium and is locally destructive on radiologic imaging. Lymph node or distant metastases can occur in as many as 20% of cases. Although esthesioneuroblastomas form neural rosettes and stain for neuron-specific enolase on immunohistochemistry, these tumors may be difficult to differentiate from other small round cell tumors such as melanoma, lymphoma, and sinonasal undifferentiated carcinoma (SNUC). Surgical resection with the use of an anterior craniofacial approach is the treatment of choice. Radiation therapy should be reserved for treatment of microscopically involved surgical margins or surgically unresectable recurrent disease. Chemotherapy has been reported to produce transient objective responses, but it should generally be used for the treatment of unresectable disease or distant metastases.

FIBROMATOSES. The fibromatoses are locally aggressive lesions of fibroblastic or myofibroblastic origin that tend to recur locally after resection. They constitute a spectrum of diseases that are broadly categorized into infantile

fibromatosis (e.g., fibromatosis colli, diffuse infantile fibromatosis, hereditary gingival fibromatosis, juvenile nasopharyngeal fibroma) and adult fibromatosis (e.g., plantar and palmar fibromatosis, Peyronie's disease, and desmoid fibromatoses). These fibromatoses can be difficult to distinguish histologically from a fibrosarcoma. The head and neck region is involved in as many as one third of all extra-abdominal desmoids, most commonly affecting the neck, followed by the face, scalp, and oral cavity and other sites. They present as an indolent, firm to hard mass that may recently have increased in size, causing pain. Desmoids have been reported to arise in surgical scars and previously irradiated tissue. Grossly, the lesion arises from fascia or aponeurosis or from within a muscle, and resembles scar tissue. The microscopic extent of disease is generally more extensive than is apparent at operation, and conservative surgical resection is likely to result in positive margins. Radical surgical excision, on the other hand, can be mutilating, and adequate treatment must encompass the lesion with as wide a margin as possible within the constraints of the local anatomy. External-beam radiation may be used in the postoperative adjuvant setting when indicated, but there have been reports of partial and even complete responses to primary radiation therapy. Other nonsurgical modes of therapy have included tamoxifen, progesterone, and nonsteroidal anti-inflammatory agents.

MALIGNANT FIBROUS HISTIOCYTOMAS (MFHs). MFH is a pleomorphic sarcoma that is thought to arise from fibroblasts and is now recognized as the most common soft tissue sarcoma in adults. The sinonasal tract is involved in as many as one third of patients, and the rest are evenly distributed among the neck, larynx, craniofacial skeleton, salivary glands, and oral cavity. Wide local excision with adequate margins is the treatment of choice, but radiation and doxorubicin (Adriamycin)-based chemotherapy have also been used. Advanced age, male gender, tumor size greater than 6 cm, and bony origin are adverse prognostic factors, and overall 5-year survival rates have been reported at around 50%.

FIBROSARCOMAS. These lesions are currently thought to constitute only 5% to 10% of all sarcomas and, within the head and neck, most frequently involve the face, neck, scalp, and paranasal sinuses. They commonly present as a painless, slow-growing mass that, on biopsy, may be difficult to differentiate from MFH, the fibromatoses, and malignant peripheral nerve sheath tumors. Accurate classification of these histologically similar lesions has been facilitated by the advent of immunohistochemistry and molecular markers. Fibrosarcomas are generally radioresistant, and the treatment of choice is aggressive surgical resection.

DERMATOFIBROSARCOMA PROTUBERANS. This is a locally aggressive, nodular cutaneous tumor of uncertain origin. The usual clinical presentation is that of an elevated, firm, slowly growing mass in the scalp or neck. Although the tumor may appear to be well encapsulated, microscopic extension into the adjacent tissue may be present to a distance of around 3 cm and the deep fascia may be involved. Wide local excision, therefore, must ensure margins of at least 3 cm, along with the underlying deep fascia. Postoperative radiation therapy may be used, as appropriate, to improve the chances of local control.

ANGIOSARCOMAS. These are rare but aggressive neoplasms that commonly involve the scalp or the face. The typical patient is a white male who presents with an ulcerating, nodular, or diffuse lesion. Most of these tumors are high-grade lesions, and their size is an important determinant of outcome. Complete surgical excision is desirable but is often impossible owing to their propensity to spread laterally within the dermis. Adverse prognostic factors include multicentricity, deep extension, and positive surgical margins, and postoperative radiation therapy may enhance local control.

LIPOSARCOMAS. Liposarcomas account for only about 1% of head and neck sarcomas and most commonly affect elderly males. They have a predilection for the neck, but the larynx and pharynx may also be affected. Histologic grade is a significant predictor of outcome, and approxi-

mately two thirds of patients survive 5 years after treatment.

Investigation

Attempts at tissue diagnosis must generally be made only after adequate noninvasive imaging of the area, as surgical manipulation can distort anatomic planes, and potentially serious bleeding can be avoided if a vascular mass is identified on radiologic imaging. Although CT scans are widely used as the first-line imaging modality, the additional multiplanar capabilities and soft tissue resolution of MRI may be used to advantage in the appropriate situations. Invasive carotid angiography has been replaced largely by the use of MR angiography, but it retains its value in determining the adequacy of cerebral perfusion (balloon occlusion testing) in patients in whom carotid ligation or resection is anticipated. Ultrasonography has been used to guide accurate placement of a needle for aspiration of masses that are clinically inaccessible. Other modalities, such as bone scans and [18]fluorodeoxyglucose positron emission tomography (FDG-PET) scans, may be used under the appropriate circumstances to assess the extent of disease. After the extent and spatial anatomic relationships of the lesion have been accurately and satisfactorily delineated, attempts must be made to obtain a histologic diagnosis. There are exceptions to this rule, however, and vascular lesions such as hemangiomas, paragangliomas, and juvenile nasopharyngeal angiomas should not be biopsied, for obvious reasons. Fine-needle aspiration (FNA) cytology is a well-established biopsy technique, and its accuracy may be enhanced by using special immunocytochemical stains. Open biopsy is attempted only if FNA is inconclusive and there is a clinical suspicion of a tumor, such as lymphoma, that requires no surgical treatment. In any event, the biopsy incision must be planned so as not to compromise surgical access, if required, and to allow for its en bloc excision with the definitive surgical specimen. Malignant tumors require metastatic evaluation, and patients with paragangliomas must be screened for abdominal disease if they have a family history or if the lesions are associated with signs and symptoms of catecholamine overactivity. Functional paragangliomas also require evaluation for estimation of levels of plasma and urinary catecholamines and their metabolites, such as metanephrine and vanillylmandelic acid. Appropriate measures, including the perioperative use of α- and β-adrenergic blockers, must be undertaken to ensure the safe induction of anesthesia in these patients. Lesions that arise from or are in close proximity to the upper aerodigestive tract must be carefully evaluated with the patient under general anesthesia to evaluate their exact extent.

PREOPERATIVE MANAGEMENT

Patients scheduled for surgical management not only must be adequately evaluated, as described earlier, but also should be in optimal physiologic condition to minimize intraoperative and postoperative complications. Apart from routine preoperative evaluation to assess nutritional and cardiopulmonary status, patients with head and neck tumors require specialized investigations, depending on the diagnosis and surgical plan. Balloon occlusion testing of the carotid artery is indicated if surgical excision of the tumor carries the risk of resecting, or necessitates resection of, the carotid.

Debilitated patients, especially the elderly, may not be acceptable candidates for surgery, and alternatives, including radiation therapy, may be considered even for benign lesions such as paragangliomas. In the treatment of malignant lesions, if the need for postoperative radiation therapy is anticipated, multidisciplinary planning not only allows continuity in care but also facilitates utilization of options such as brachytherapy. Preoperative consultations with members of other surgical teams, such as the neurosurgeon, plastic surgeon, vascular surgeon, and maxillofacial prosthetist, and other specialists, such as speech, swallowing, and physical therapists, must also be obtained when relevant.

INTRAOPERATIVE MANAGEMENT

Patients who undergo surgery for tumors of the head and neck require special attention to intraoperative airway management in order to maximize exposure and to facilitate the conduct of the surgical procedure. Routine orotracheal intubation is adequate for most patients, but a nasotracheal tube is more appropriate for operations on the oral cavity and oropharynx. The extra space afforded by the ability to close the jaw completely following nasotracheal intubation may also be valuable during operations on the parapharyngeal space. Patients who need major resection and reconstruction of the oropharynx or mandible should undergo an intraoperative tracheostomy that may be decannulated during the early postoperative period as the edema subsides.

Most neck masses can be approached satisfactorily with the use of standard neck incisions (Fig. 43–3), depending on the extent of exposure required. Benign tumors of the nasal cavity and paranasal sinuses may be treated endoscopically, but more extensive resections are required for malignant lesions. Limited lesions of the lateral nasal wall can be adequately excised with a medial maxillectomy via a lateral rhinotomy. Advanced lesions of the region may require a total maxillectomy to encompass the posterolateral extent or an anterior craniofacial approach to encompass the superior extent. Appropriate soft tissue and/or bony reconstruction facilitates optimal rehabilitation, but a detailed description of these complex procedures is outside the scope of this discussion.

Parapharyngeal space tumors are approached with the use of one of three approaches: the cervical approach, the transparotid approach, or the combination of either of these with a mandibulotomy. The space may be entered through the neck inferiorly by either excising or mobilizing the submandibular salivary gland anteriorly for resection of small extraparotid lesions. For lesions in relation to the parotid gland, a superficial parotidectomy is undertaken, and the facial nerve and its branches are carefully preserved. Access to the parapharyngeal space may be enhanced by dividing the stylomandibular ligament and,

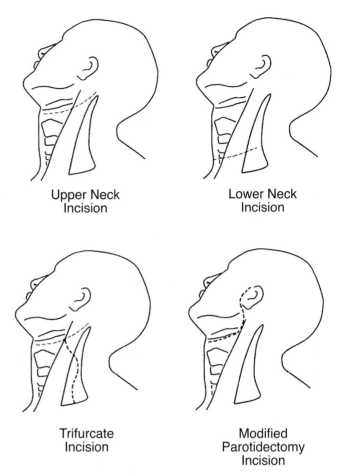

Figure 43–3. Diagrammatic representation of some commonly used incisions that may be used to access tumors of the neck.

even, the styloid process if necessary. Invasive, malignant tumors require wider exposure, and the transparotid or transcervical approach may be combined with a paramedian mandibulotomy. An elective tracheostomy is prudent in all patients whose mandibular continuity has been disrupted. Tumors abutting or involving the skull base can be adequately resected with the use of complex craniofacial procedures.

Carotid body tumors are approached through a standard transverse skin crease incision, and proximal and distal control of the common external and internal carotid arteries is obtained. Group I and small group II lesions can be easily excised by careful dissection in the subadventitial plane, ligating the vessels that feed the tumor on the posterior aspect of the carotid bifurcation. For more advanced lesions, ligation of the external carotid artery reduces the blood flow to the tumor and provides extra maneuverability. Partial or circumferential carotid resection is only rarely necessary, and this eventuality should be anticipated with adequate preparations as described earlier.

The majority of patients who have had surgery for tumors of the neck can resume an oral diet postoperatively as soon as they have recovered from the general anesthetic, but a fine-bore nasogastric feeding tube must be temporarily used to provide nutrition when oral intake is not practical or safe. Rarely, patients with advanced malignant lesions in whom adjuvant postoperative radiation therapy is anticipated may benefit from the intraoperative placement of a percutaneous endoscopic gastrostomy.

With appropriate preoperative evaluation, there should be very little scope for unexpected findings during the operative procedure. However, certain issues, such as minimal bony erosion, invasion of the prevertebral fascia, and adventitial invasion of the carotid, can be resolved only during surgery, and the surgeon should be adequately prepared to modify the operative approach as necessary.

POSTOPERATIVE MANAGEMENT

The immediate postoperative management consists of maintaining a secure airway and a stable cardiopulmonary status. Patients who have had a tracheostomy need extra nursing care to suction secretions and to provide humidification and nebulizers. The patient is generally nursed with the head end of the bed elevated to 30 degrees, and, once the effects of general anesthesia have passed, ambulation should be encouraged. Patients undergoing combined craniofacial surgery are optimally managed in a neurosurgical observation unit, and those who have complex flap reconstruction also need intensive nursing and observation. Acute postoperative pain following major resections is managed by opioid analgesics administered intravenously either as patient-controlled analgesia or at regular fixed intervals. The regimen is then changed to oral or enteral analgesics as postoperative recovery continues, and the majority of patients can subsequently be maintained on nonopioid analgesics. If the upper digestive tract has not been violated, oral intake is allowed when the patient has recovered from anesthesia. For all other patients, nutrition is maintained by enteral feeds via a nasogastric feeding tube or a percutaneous endoscopic gastrostomy. Commencement of oral intake in these patients generally requires a period of 7 to 10 days to allow healing, but it may take longer if there is associated aspiration. The input of a swallowing therapist and a dietitian can be invaluable in the rehabilitation of these patients. Postoperative nursing care also includes maintenance of suction or Penrose drains and meticulous wound care. Patients undergoing major resections continue to use inflation stockings while confined to bed, but early ambulation is encouraged if there are no medical contraindications, and this helps reduce the risks of deep vein thrombosis, pulmonary embolism, or respiratory complications.

COMPLICATIONS

Surgical treatment of tumors of the neck carries a risk of injury to major neurovascular structures, and the sequelae of these complications can be devastating (Table 43–2). The use of a combined craniofacial approach places the cranial cavity at risk for contamination from the upper aerodigestive tract, with all its attendant sequelae. Systemic complications, such as deep vein thrombosis, pulmonary embolism, and myocardial infarction, are not as

Table 43–2	Complications of Surgery for Neurovascular and Soft Tissue Tumors	
COMPLICATION	**SEQUELAE**	
Injury to nerves		
Marginal mandibular nerve	Deformity of angle of the mouth	
Hypoglossal nerve	Difficulty in moving the tongue	
Vagus nerve	Hoarseness, aspiration	
Sympathetic chain	Horner's syndrome	
Phrenic nerve	Paralysis of ipsilateral diaphragm	
Brachial plexus	Weakness or paralysis of limb muscles	
Facial nerve	Facial paralysis, exposure keratitis	
Injury to thoracic or major lymphatic duct	Chyle leak	
Injury to pharynx or esophagus	Salivary fistula	
Stimulation of carotid bulb	Bradycardia	
Injury to internal carotid artery	Hemorrhage, cerebrovascular stroke	
Major venous injury	Air embolism, hypotension, mortality	
Complications of craniofacial surgery		
Major wound infection	Meningitis	
CSF leak, pneumoencephalus	Headache, meningitis	
Lack of orbital support	Diplopia	
Other complications	Oroantral fistula, epiphora due to nasolacrimal duct stenosis, ectropion	
Intermediate and late complications		
Reactionary or secondary hemorrhage	Hematoma, airway compromise	
Carotid artery exposure and rupture	Mortality or cerebrovascular stroke	
Mandibular nonunion or osteonecrosis	Pain, persistent sinus or recurrent infections	

common as following other major surgery, primarily because most patients can be ambulated relatively early in their postoperative course. However, patients with an antecedent history of cardiopulmonary disease must be carefully monitored.

OUTCOMES

Approximately 50% of hemangiomas involute spontaneously by the age of 5 years, and almost 90% regress by the onset of puberty. Cavernous lymphangiomas almost always recur after partial excision, but as many as 20% have been reported to recur even after complete excision because of their infiltrative nature. Surgery for juvenile nasopharyngeal angiofibromas results in local recurrence rates of less than 10% in small lesions, but more extensive tumors may fail in as many as 40% of instances. Overall complication rates for carotid body tumor surgery have been reported at around 40%, with mortality ranging up to 13%, cerebrovascular stroke in 8% to 20%, and cranial nerve deficits from 30% to 45%. Meticulous surgical technique is therefore paramount to safe conduct of these operations. A 10-year survival rate of approximately 65% has been reported following surgical excision of esthesioneuroblastoma. Five-year survival rates of 50% to 75% have been reported in patients with solitary malignant peripheral nerve sheath tumors, but only a third of those with co-existing neurofibromatosis survive 5 years. Local recurrence rates for desmoid tumors range from 19% to 40% following adequate wide local excision. Multiple recurrences are common, and as many as 90% of tumors will recur if they are treated with marginal or lesional excision. Five-year survival rates for malignant fibrous histiocytomas have been reported at around 50% and those for liposarcoma at around 67%. Although local recurrences after surgery for dermatofibrosarcoma protruberans are not uncommon, an overall 5-year survival rate of around 95% has been reported. At the other end of the spectrum, the clinical course of angiosarcomas is often relentless in spite of aggressive management, and only about a third of patients survive 5 years.

Summary

Open biopsy of a neck mass before one obtains imaging and/or FNA should be avoided, as anatomic planes are compromised and this limits the usefulness of the imaging. In addition, if the vascular nature of a mass is apparent on imaging, potential hemorrhage from an open biopsy can be avoided. If open biopsy of a lesion is deemed necessary, the skin incision must be placed carefully so as not to compromise subsequent exposure should definitive surgery become necessary. As discussed earlier, transoral biopsy of a parapharyngeal mass should also be avoided. Surgery for tumors around the great vessels of the neck and the skull base is complicated by the need to preserve these vessels and the cranial nerves in their vicinity. Meticulous dissection technique and a thorough knowledge of the regional anatomy are essential to a successful outcome.

A considerable degree of interobserver variability exists, even among experienced pathologists, in histologic typing and grading of soft tissue sarcomas, with diagnostic discrepancies reported in as many as 25% to 40% of lesions. The routine use of immunohistochemistry has facilitated classification, but a great deal of experience is still required for the interpretation of these results. Therefore, it is imperative to seek an expert opinion in case of doubt.

Surgical excision is generally the most effective form of treatment for most neurovascular and soft tissue tumors of the head and neck, but adequate excision of

malignant tumors may result in unacceptable cosmetic and functional deformity. It is therefore important for the treating surgeon to be able to judge when alternative, nonsurgical treatment may be offered to advantage in a particular patient.

Pearls and Pitfalls
Common Errors of Practice
- Open biopsy before relevant imaging is obtained
- Inappropriately sited incision for open biopsy of a neck mass
- Transoral biopsy of a parapharyngeal mass

Anatomic Danger Points
- Facial nerve in the vicinity of the styloid process
- Marginal mandibular nerve in the upper neck
- Lower cranial nerves at the skull base
- Hypoglossal nerve where it crosses the carotid artery
- Vagus nerve in the carotid sheath
- Sympathetic chain and ganglia
- Major lymphatic ducts in the lower neck
- Brachial plexus and phrenic nerve

SELECTED READINGS

Conley J, Healey WV, Stout AP: Fibromatosis of the head and neck. Am J Surg 1966;112:609.

Farr HW, Carandang CM, Huvos AG: Malignant vascular tumors of the head and neck. Am J Surg 1970;120:501.

Farr HW: Carotid body tumors: A 40-year study. CA Cancer J Clin 1980;30:260.

Grabb WC, Dingman RO, Oneal RM, Dempsey PD: Facial hamartomas in childhood: Neurofibroma, lymphangioma, and hemangioma. Plast Reconst Surg 1980;66:509.

Hodge KM, Byers RM, Peters LJ: Paragangliomas of the head and neck. Arch Otolaryngol Head Neck Surg 1988;114:872.

Kraus DH, Dubner S, Harrison LB, et al: Prognostic factors for recurrence and survival in head and neck soft tissue sarcomas. Cancer 1994;74:697.

Lack EE, Cubilla AL, Woodruff JM, et al: Paragangliomas of the head and neck region: A clinical study of 69 patients. Cancer 1977;39:397.

Shah JP: Soft tissue sarcomas. Probl Gen Surg 1988;5:58.

Shah JP: Head and Neck Surgery: Diagnostic Approaches, Therapeutic Decisions, Surgical Techniques and Results of Treatment. 2nd ed. Barcelona, Mosby-Wolfe, 1996.

Som PM, Biller HF, Lawson W: Tumors of the parapharyngeal space: Preoperative evaluation, diagnosis and surgical approaches. Ann Otol Rhinol Laryngol 1981;90(suppl 80):3.

Wanebo HJ, Koness RJ, MacFarlane JK, et al: Head and neck sarcoma: Report of the Head and Neck Sarcoma Registry. Society of Head and Neck Surgeons Committee on Research. Head Neck 1992;14:1.

GASTROINTESTINAL

Esophagus and Paraesophageal Region: Benign

Chapter 44

Gastroesophageal Reflux Disease

C. Daniel Smith

Gastroesophageal reflux disease (GERD) is defined as the failure of the antireflux barrier, allowing abnormal reflux of gastric contents into the esophagus. GERD is a mechanical disorder most commonly caused by a defective lower esophageal sphincter (LES). This abnormality results in a spectrum of disease, ranging from the symptom "heartburn," to acute or chronic esophageal tissue damage with subsequent complications of stricture, bleeding, or metaplastic mucosal changes (Barrett's esophagus). GERD is an extremely common condition, accounting for nearly 75% of all esophageal pathology. Nearly 44% of Americans experience monthly heartburn, and 18% of these individuals use nonprescription medication directed against GERD.

Considerable debate abounds regarding optimal treatment of GERD. Because up to 10% of Americans experience daily heartburn and because of the impact of this condition on an individual's quality of life, it is no surprise that there is a tremendous amount of interest and effort going into understanding this condition and establishing effective treatment algorithms (Fig. 44–1). Medical therapy is the first line of management for GERD. Esophagitis heals in approximately 90% of patients with intensive medical therapy; however, medical management does not address the condition's mechanical etiology; thus, symptoms recur in more than 80% of patients within 1 year of drug withdrawal. Additionally, while medical therapy may effectively treat the acid-induced symptoms of GERD, esophageal mucosal injury may continue as a result of

ongoing alkaline reflux. Finally, medical therapy may be required for the rest of one's life. The expense and psychological burden of a lifetime of medication dependence, undesirable lifestyle changes, uncertainty as to the long-term effects of some newer medications, and the potential for persistent mucosal changes despite symptomatic control all make surgical treatment of GERD an attractive option, especially with the use of a minimally invasive approach.

Historically, antireflux surgery was recommended only for patients with refractory or complicated gastroesophageal reflux. Through the early 1990s, several major developments changed modern thinking regarding the long-term management of patients with GERD. First, the introduction of proton pump inhibitors provided a truly effective medical therapy for GERD. Therefore, very few patients have "refractory" GERD. Second, laparoscopic surgery became available, thereby significantly changing the morbidity and recovery after an antireflux procedure. Third, the widespread availability and use of ambulatory pH monitoring and esophageal motility testing dramatically improved the ability to recognize true GERD and select patients for long-term therapy. Fourth, it has become known that patients with GERD have a greatly impaired quality of life, which normalizes with successful treatment.

With this, the management goals of GERD have changed. Rather than focusing therapy only on *controlling* symptoms, modern treatment of GERD aims to *eliminate*

307

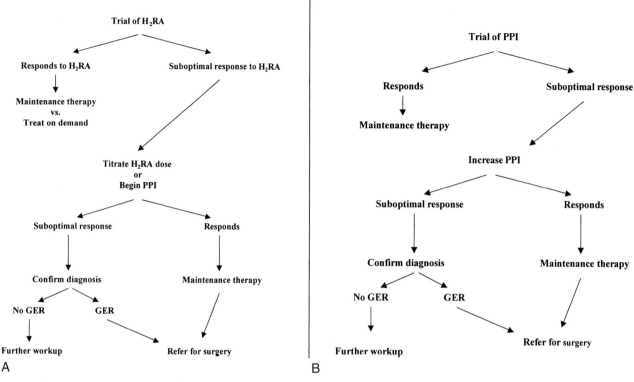

Figure 44–1. Management algorithm for the treatment of uncomplicated *(A)* and complicated *(B)* gastroesophageal reflux, based on endoscopic findings. GER, gastroesophageal reflux; H₂RA, H₂ receptor antagonist; PPI, proton pump inhibitor.

symptoms, improve quality of life, and institute a lifelong plan for management.

CLINICAL PRESENTATION

Gastroesophageal reflux leads to symptoms related to the reflux of gastric content into the esophagus, lungs, or oropharynx, or to damage to the esophageal mucosa and respiratory epithelium with subsequent changes related to repair, fibrosis, and reinjury. Manifestations of GERD are typically classified as esophageal and extraesophageal. Esophageal manifestations of GERD include heartburn, chest pain, water brash, or dysphagia (Table 44–1). Dysphagia often suggests a complication of GERD such as esophageal ulcer, stricture, or Barrett's metaplastic changes in the mucosa. Extraesophageal manifestations are generally pulmonary, resulting from pulmonary aspiration of refluxate or a vagally mediated reflex inducing bronchospasm when refluxate stimulates the distal esophagus. In fact, up to 80% of patients with asthma have endoscopic evidence of GERD, and 50% of patients in whom a cardiac cause of chest pain has been excluded have acid reflux as a cause of their pain. Other extraesophageal manifestations include chronic cough, laryngitis, dental damage, and chronic sinusitis. Before assuming that extraesophageal symptoms or the *atypical* symptom of chest pain is caused by GERD, primary cardiac or pulmonary etiologies for these symptoms must be excluded. Dysphagia requires special attention because esophageal malignancy most commonly presents with dys-

phagia. Esophagogastroduodenoscopy (EGD) is critical in the workup of all patients with dysphagia to rule out malignancy.

The clinical diagnosis of GERD is fairly straightforward if the patient reports the classic symptom of heartburn that is readily relieved after ingesting antacids. Many patients have undergone treatment with their primary care physician with an empirical trial of H₂ blockers or proton pump inhibitors, and resolution of symptoms with such treatment may be diagnostically helpful.

A careful history should confirm both typical and atypical symptoms of GERD and any response to medical therapy. Atypical symptoms, no response to high doses of proton pump inhibitors, or patients with dysphagia, odynophagia, gastrointestinal bleeding, or weight loss suggests complications of GERD or another disease process entirely, and should prompt a more thorough, symptom-directed workup looking for another explanation for symptoms.

Even though a barium swallow is often the first test obtained, an EGD is necessary in all GERD patients and frequently confirms the diagnosis. An esophageal mucosal biopsy should be obtained to confirm esophagitis, and esophageal length and the presence of a hiatal hernia or stricture can be assessed and may eliminate the need for a confirmatory barium swallow. With these findings, no other tests beyond EGD are necessary. However, in many patients, the EGD results are normal because of the empirical treatment of symptoms attempted by primary care physicians. In this setting, 24-hour pH testing is necessary to objectively establish the diagnosis of GERD.

Table 44–1	**Patient Symptoms and Likely Etiologies**	
SYMPTOM	**DEFINITION**	**LIKELY ETIOLOGY**
Heartburn	Burning discomfort behind breast bone Bitter acidic fluid in mouth Sudden filling of mouth with clear/salty fluid	Gastroesophageal reflux disease (GERD)
Dysphagia	Sensation of food being hindered in passage from mouth to stomach	Motor disorders Inflammatory process Diverticula Tumors
Odynophagia	Pain with swallowing	Severe inflammatory process
Globus sensation	Lump in throat unrelated to swallowing	Psychiatric or neurologic problems
Chest pain	Mimics angina pectoris	GERD Motor disorders Tumors
Respiratory symptoms	Asthma/wheezing, bronchitis, hemoptysis, stridor	GERD Diverticula Tumors
Ear, nose, throat symptoms	Chronic sore throat, laryngitis, halitosis, chronic cough	GERD Diverticula
Rumination	Regurgitation of recently ingested food into mouth	Achalasia Inflammatory process Diverticula Tumors

Ambulatory 24-hour pH monitoring is the gold standard in diagnosing GERD and is of unquestionable benefit in patients in whom the diagnosis is unclear or in those with nonerosive esophagitis. However, this test is lengthy, cumbersome, and uncomfortable, particularly in patients with severe GERD who must stop antisecretory medication for 5 to 10 days before the test. Ambulatory pH monitoring is *not* mandatory in patients with typical reflux symptoms and erosive esophagitis on EGD. However, it *is* mandatory when an objective diagnosis of GERD is lacking. Barium swallow is the test of choice in evaluating the patient with dysphagia, suspected stricture, paraesophageal hernia, or shortened esophagus. Other studies may be helpful, including tests of gastric emptying or acid secretion studies in patients with significant bloating, nausea, or vomiting, or with no response to proton pump inhibitors. One should seriously question the diagnosis of GERD in any patient who has no symptomatic improvement with proton pump inhibitors.

PREOPERATIVE MANAGEMENT

The preoperative evaluation should both justify the need for surgery and direct the operative technique to optimize outcome. At a minimum, all patients being considered for surgery should undergo a thorough history and physical examination, have objective evidence of GERD based on the finding of esophagitis on EGD or a positive 24-hour pH study, and undergo esophageal manometry.

Esophageal manometry allows evaluation of the LES and is diagnostic in differentiating GERD from achalasia. Equally important is its use in assessing pressures generated in the body of the esophagus and in identifying individuals with impaired esophageal clearance who may not do well with a 360-degree fundoplication (Nissen procedure). Reliable esophageal clearance occurs with distal esophageal contractions of 30 to 40 mm Hg. In patients with impaired peristalsis as evidenced by mean distal esophageal pressures less than or equal to 30 mm Hg or esophageal peristalsis in 60% or less of wet swallows, many advocate modifying the surgical approach by performing a partial fundoplication (270-degree Toupet fundoplication). Finally, results of esophageal manometry may be completely normal, including no evidence of LES weakness, in patients with GERD, but one should consider further testing when these normal findings are present.

The most critical aspect of preoperative management is confirming the diagnosis and identifying those patients with conditions associated with GERD that may require special consideration. Specifically, patients with associated esophageal motor disorders identified during esophageal motility testing or those with a shortened esophagus may require a tailored approach to GERD. Esophageal body dysfunction (body pressure less than 30 mm Hg or less than 60% peristalsis with wet swallows) may require a partial fundoplication, and a shortened esophagus should undergo esophageal lengthening (Collis gastroplasty). Failure to recognize these associated problems, and surgeon-derived anecdotal "modifications" to proven techniques have led to increasing numbers of patients "failing" laparoscopic antireflux surgery.

INTRAOPERATIVE MANAGEMENT

The goal of antireflux surgery is to establish an effective LES pressure. To realize this goal, most surgeons believe it is necessary to position the LES within the abdomen where the sphincter is under positive (intra-abdominal) pressure and to close any associated hiatal defect. To accomplish this, several surgical techniques have been developed. Recently, advancements in laparoscopic technology and technique have nearly eliminated open antireflux surgery. The laparoscopic techniques reproduce their open counterparts while eliminating the morbidity of an upper midline laparotomy incision. Open antireflux operations remain indicated when the laparoscopic technique is not available or is contraindicated. Contraindications to laparoscopic antireflux surgery include uncorrectable coagulopathy, severe chronic obstructive pulmonary disease, and pregnancy. Previous upper abdominal operation, particularly prior open antireflux surgery, is a relative contraindication to a laparoscopic approach and should only be undertaken by very experienced laparoscopic surgeons.

The laparoscopic Nissen fundoplication is the most widely applied antireflux operation (Fig. 44–2). In many centers, it is the antireflux procedure of choice in patients with normal esophageal body peristalsis. Key elements of the procedure include the complete dissection of the esophageal hiatus and both crura, mobilization of the

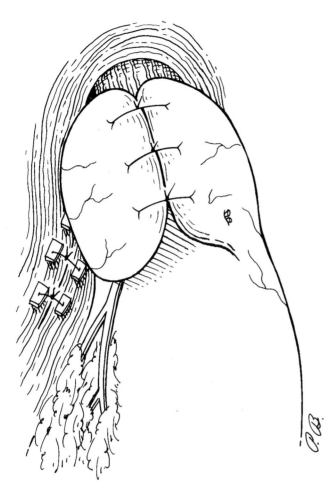

Figure 44–2. Depiction of Nissen 360-degree fundoplication.

gastric fundus by dividing the short gastric vessels, closure of the associated hiatal defect, creation of a tension-free 360-degree gastric wrap at the distal esophagus around a 50- to 60-French intraesophageal dilator, limiting the length of the wrap to 1.5 to 2.0 cm, and stabilizing the wrap to the esophagus by partial thickness bites of the esophagus during creation of the wrap.

The Toupet fundoplication (Fig. 44–3) is identical to the Nissen except that the fundoplication is a 270-degree wrap rather than a 360-degree wrap. The gastric fundus is brought posterior to the esophagus and sutured to either side of the esophagus, leaving the anterior surface bare. This 270-degree fundoplication has the theoretical advantage of limiting postoperative bloating and dysphagia, especially in those with impaired esophageal body peristalsis. Some clinicians have advocated that the routine use of the Toupet fundoplication on all GERD patients could eliminate the need for preoperative esophageal manometry in many patients. However, a partial fundoplication is not as durable as a total fundoplication, and its use in the most severe cases (grade IV esophagitis, Barrett's esophagus, stricture) is questioned.

Figure 44–4 depicts the operating room setup and patient positioning for laparoscopic foregut procedures. An orogastric tube and Foley catheter are used to decompress the stomach and bladder. If operative time is expected to be less than 90 minutes and the patient voids

preoperatively, the Foley can be avoided. Pneumoperitoneum is induced via an infraumbilical incision and then cannulas are placed (see Fig. 44–4, *inset*). The esophageal dissection is really a crural dissection in that once the crura have been completely dissected, the distal esophagus has thereby been safely encircled. The esophagus is mobilized out of the mediastinum until at least 3 cm of distal esophagus is comfortably below the diaphragm, and the vagus nerves are left against the esophagus. Any hiatal defect is sutured closed until the crura efface the nondilated esophagus. The gastric fundus is then mobilized by dividing all the short gastric vessels and freeing any attachments between the back wall of the stomach and the anterior surface of the pancreas. The mobilized gastric fundus is brought through the retroesophageal window and plicated around the distal esophagus. A 56- to 60-French intraesophageal dilator is in place to ensure creation of a "floppy" fundoplication. Plication sutures incorporate the anterior esophageal wall to prevent migration of the wrap.

POSTOPERATIVE MANAGEMENT

Patients are allowed to drink liquids immediately postoperatively. Carbonated beverages are specifically avoided because of the resulting gastric distention. Because of edema at the fundoplication, patients are maintained on a liquid diet for 5 to 7 days and then a soft diet for the next 2 weeks. Hospital dismissal is usually on the first postoperative day, with follow-up in 3 weeks. In difficult cases (extensive paraesophageal dissection, redo surgery, or paraesophageal hernia repair), a contrast swallow on the first postoperative day is recommended to rule out a small leak or other anatomic problem. Patients are released from the hospital with prescriptions for a liquid

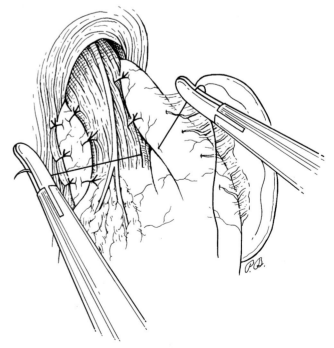

Figure 44–3. Depiction of Toupet 270-degree fundoplication.

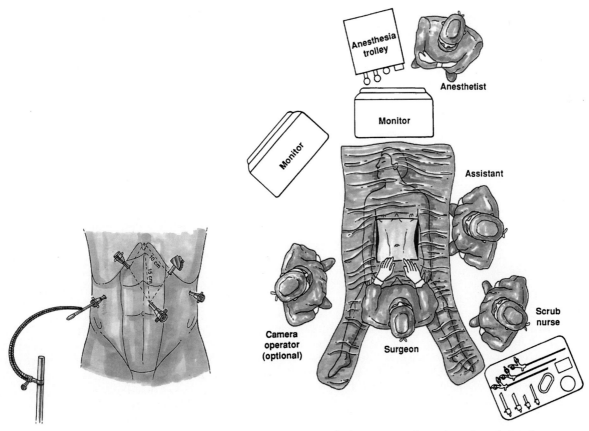

Figure 44–4. Depiction of operating room setup for laparoscopic foregut procedures. *Inset,* Cannula locations.

pain medicine, liquid stool softener, and an antiemetic, which can be administered rectally if nausea occurs. A dietitian sees the patients before discharge to instruct them on the soft diet, emphasizing the avoidance of carbonated beverages, breads, and other dry foods that tend to lodge at the fundoplication. There are no limitations on physical activity unless a paraesophageal hernia was repaired, in which case avoidance of heavy lifting is suggested for approximately 4 to 6 weeks. Preoperative antisecretory or prokinetic medications are stopped.

Postoperative nausea and vomiting or retching remains the most significant and controllable postoperative event associated with significant complications. Most patients receive preemptive antinausea medication, and staff caring for patients postoperatively are instructed to respond immediately with medication to any patient complaint of nausea. If any early postoperative retching occurs, a contrast swallow is immediately obtained in case wrap disruption or herniation has occurred. If this occurs and is detected with the first 24 to 48 hours, immediate reoperation can be undertaken to correct the problem. If these anatomic problems are not found until outpatient follow-up 1 to 2 weeks later, a 6- to 12-week delay is necessary before undertaking reoperation because of the adhesions that will have formed by this time.

COMPLICATIONS

The laparoscopic approaches to the operative management of GERD have significantly altered the pattern and frequency of early postoperative complications seen during the era of open fundoplication. After open antireflux surgery, pneumonia, wound infection, incisional hernia, cardiac events, or deep venous thrombosis occurred in as many as 25% of patients. With laparoscopic approaches, these complications are unlikely and occur in less than 1% of patients. It remains unclear how much of this change is due to the laparoscopic approach itself or to the modernization of the management of GERD (offering surgery early in the disease process before advanced age or comorbidity is present) and more aggressive early postoperative ambulation and hospital dismissal. The most vexing postoperative complication is nausea and retching. During episodes of retching, breakdown of the fundoplication or herniation of the wrap through the diaphragm can occur. Therefore, postoperative nausea should be treated aggressively. Antinausea medication and counseling from a dietitian regarding the liquid diet prescribed early postoperatively helps patients avoid dietary indiscretions that may prompt retching or induce dysphagia.

OUTCOMES

Thousands of patients undergoing laparoscopic Nissen fundoplication have been reported in the world literature, with 93% of patients being symptom-free at 1 year postoperatively. Only 3% have required some medical therapy to control their symptoms. Overall, 97% of these patients are satisfied with their results. Transient dysphagia occurs in nearly 50% of patients and resolves within 3 weeks

Table 44–2	**Medical versus Surgical Treatment of Barrett's Esophagus**					

	NO. PATIENTS		SYMPTOM CONTROL		STRICTURE/ ESOPHAGITIS	
AUTHOR	**Medical**	**Surgical**	**Medical**	**Surgical**	**Medical**	**Surgical**
Attwood, 1992* (p)	26	19	22%	81%	38%	21%
Ortiz, 1996 (pr)	27	32	85%	89%	53%/45%	5%/15%
Sampliner, 1994 (p)	27	—	70%	—	50%	—
Csendes, 1998 (pr)	—	152	—	46%	—	64%

*Before availability of proton pump inhibitors
pr, prospective randomized; p, prospective.

of surgery. Late complications of wrap migration and paraesophageal herniation may also be related to postoperative retching but are more likely due to either failure to close the esophageal hiatus or a shortened esophagus. Long-term dysphagia is emerging in 10% to 15% of patients, but is frequently well accepted by them in the context of the excellent control of GERD symptoms they experience. In 3% to 4% of patients, unremitting dysphagia or recurrent reflux require reoperation for correction. When redo fundoplication is undertaken, 93% of patients experience good to excellent results. Troubling long-term side effects such as gas bloat have been virtually eliminated by the floppy nature of the fundoplication.

Barrett's Esophagus

Barrett's esophagus is the condition in which the tubular esophagus normally lined by squamous epithelium becomes lined with metaplastic columnar epithelium that may transform into adenocarcinoma. Most recently, it has been recognized that the specialized intestinal metaplasia (not gastric type columnar changes) constitutes true Barrett's changes with the risk of progression to dysplasia and adenocarcinoma.

Barrett's esophagus develops in 7% to 10% of people with GERD, and many believe this represents the end stage of the natural history of GERD. Clearly, Barrett's esophagus is associated with a more profound mechanical deficiency of the LES, severe impairment of esophageal body function, and marked esophageal acid exposure. In contrast, some patients are asymptomatic and have only short segments of columnar lined epithelium in the distal esophagus (<3 cm), which does not have this same strong association with GERD. Additionally, there seems to be a lower incidence of metaplastic epithelium in these "short segments" of Barrett's, and therefore a lower malignancy potential. Considerable debate remains regarding the significance of short-segment Barrett's esophagus.

Endoscopically obvious Barrett's esophagus with intestinal metaplasia is a major risk factor for adenocarcinoma of the esophagus, with the annual incidence of adenocarcinoma in this condition estimated at approximately 0.8%, which is 40 times higher than in the general population. Once high-grade dysplasia is identified in more than one biopsy from columnar lined esophagus, nearly 50% of patients already harbor a foci of invasive cancer. This finding is the basis for recommending careful endoscopic surveillance in patients with Barrett's esophagus with intestinal metaplasia and in recommending esophagectomy when high-grade dysplasia is identified.

Treatment goals for patients with Barrett's esophagus are similar to those for patients with GERD, that is, relief of symptoms and arrest of ongoing reflux-mediated epithelial damage. Additionally, those with Barrett's esophagus regardless of type of treatment (surgical or medical) require long-term endoscopic surveillance with biopsy of columnar segments looking for progressive metaplastic changes or progression to dysplasia. Patients with Barrett's esophagus typically have the most severe GERD and likely require long-term therapy. Several studies have compared medical and surgical therapy in patients with Barrett's esophagus (Table 44–2). These data support the notion that Barrett's esophagus is associated with more severe and refractory GERD, and antireflux surgery is effective at alleviating these symptoms in 75% to 92% of patients.

Table 44–3	**Antireflux Surgery and Regression of Barrett's Esophagus**				

AUTHOR	**NO. PATIENTS**	**FOLLOW-UP (yr)**	**DECREASED LENGTH BARRETT'S**	**NO BARRETT'S**	**CANCER**
Skinner, 1983	10	4	1	1	0
Williamson, 1990	37	4.2	4	0	—
Martinez, 1992	16	6.6	0	0	3
Sagar, 1995	56	5.5	24	5	0
Ortiz, 1996	32	5	8	0	1
TOTAL	151		37	6	4

Table 44–4	Antireflux Surgery and Progression of Barrett's to Dysplasia or Adenocarcinoma			
	NO. PATIENTS		**DEVELOPMENT OF DYSPLASIA**	
AUTHOR	**Medical**	**Surgical**	**Medical (%)**	**Surgical (%)**
McCallum, 1990	152	29	19	3.4
Ortiz, 1996	27	32	22	3.1
McDonald, 1996	—	118	—	2.5

Pearls and Pitfalls

PEARLS

- Antireflux surgery is indicated in patients with GERD refractory to medical management or in those whose symptoms return when medicine is withdrawn.
- In patients with classic symptoms, EGD and esophageal manometry may be all the preoperative evaluation necessary.
- Laparoscopic Nissen fundoplication is safe and effective in long-term management of GERD.
- Toupet fundoplication may be used in patients with impaired peristalsis in the esophagus.
- Barrett's esophagus is a premalignant metaplasia of the esophageal mucosa resulting from severe chronic reflux.
- Severe dysplasia in Barrett's esophagus justifies esophagectomy.
- The potential of antireflux surgery to lessen the risk of malignant transformation of Barrett's esophagus has been suggested but is as yet unproven.

Even though effective therapy controls GERD symptoms in patients with Barrett's esophagus, it appears that appropriate treatment of GERD does not induce regression of the Barrett's epithelium. Results in a combined series of 151 patients over 4 to 6 years found rare occurrences of regression of Barrett's epithelium (Table 44–3). However, there is growing evidence to suggest that antireflux surgery may prevent progression of Barrett's changes and thereby protect against dysplasia and malignancy (Table 44–4). In the series reported from the Mayo Clinic,

three cancers occurred over an 18-year follow-up period. The clustering of these three patients within the first 3 years of follow-up after operation suggests that these patients may have already progressed to dysplasia at the time of operation. Clearly, GERD associated with Barrett's changes remains poorly understood and a significant concern.

SELECTED READINGS

Anvari M, Allen C, Borm A: Laparoscopic Nissen fundoplication is a satisfactory alternative to long-term omeprazole therapy. Br J Surg 1995;82:938.

Heitmiller RF, Redmond M, Hamilton SR: Barrett's esophagus with high-grade dysplasia. An indication for prophylactic esophagectomy. Ann Surg 1996;224:66.

Hunter JG, Smith CD, Branum GD, et al: Laparoscopic fundoplication failures: Patterns of failure and response to fundoplication revision. Ann Surg 1999;230:595–604; discussion 604–606.

McDonald ML, Trastek VF, Allen MS, et al: Barrett's esophagus: Does an antireflux procedure reduce the need for endoscopic surveillance? J Thoracic Cardiovasc Surg 1996;111:1135–1138; discussion 1139–1140.

Patti MG, Bresadola V: Gastroesophageal reflux disease: Basic considerations. Probl General Surg 1996;13:1.

Peters JH: The surgical management of Barrett's esophagus. Gastroenterol Clin North Am 1997;26:647.

Sampliner RE: Practice guidelines on the diagnosis, surveillance, and therapy of Barrett's esophagus. The Practice Parameters Committee of the American College of Gastroenterology. Am J Gastroenterol 1998;93:1028.

Smith CD, Fink AS, Applegren K: Guidelines for surgical treatment of gastroesophageal reflux disease (GERD). Society of American Gastrointestinal Endoscopic Surgeons (SAGES). Surg Endosc 1998;12:186.

Spechler SJ: Epidemiology and natural history of gastro-oesophageal reflux disease. Digestion 1992;51:240.

Spivak H, Smith CD, Phichith A, et al: Asthma and gastroesophageal reflux: Fundoplication decreases need for systemic corticosteroids. J Gastrointest Surg 1999;3:477.

Waring JP, Hunter JG, Oddsdottir M, et al: The preoperative evaluation of patients considered for laparoscopic antireflux surgery. Am J Gastroenterol 1995;90:35.

Chapter 45
Barrett's Esophagus
Jeffrey H. Peters

Norman Barrett described the condition that bears his name in 1950. He incorrectly believed that he was observing a congenitally short esophagus and an intrathoracic stomach. Phillip Allison, in 1953, carefully examined seven esophagectomy specimens of patients with the changes that Barrett had described and conclusively showed that it was indeed the tubular esophagus lined with columnar epithelium. Barrett's esophagus is now known to be an acquired abnormality, occurring in 10% to 15% of patients with gastroesophageal reflux disease (GERD). Although historically the definition of Barrett's esophagus was confined to the presence of columnar mucosa extending 3 cm or more into the esophagus, it is currently considered to be present given any length of endoscopically visible tissue that is intestinal metaplasia on histology. Recent data indicate that specialized intestinal-type epithelium, the hallmark of which is the presence of goblet cells, is the only tissue predisposed to malignant degeneration, and a similar risk of malignancy exists in segments of intestinal metaplasia less than 3 cm long ("short-segment Barrett's").

CLINICAL PRESENTATION

Before World War II, the finding of columnar epithelia in the tubular esophagus was uncommon in clinical practice. Its prevalence has increased from approximately 1 in 1000 endoscopies in the early 1980s, 10 in 1000 in the late 1980s, to 55 to 60 per 1000 in the late 1990s. At present, long-segment Barrett's esophagus is found in 4% to 6% of patients with reflux symptoms, 1% of all upper endoscopies, and 0.3% of the U.S. population. Short-segment Barrett's esophagus (<3 cm) is probably equally prevalent, effectively doubling the incidence.

Reflux symptoms develop in patients with Barrett's esophagus at an earlier age, and these patients have more severe symptoms than age- and gender-matched patients with GERD. Complications of reflux, including esophagitis, stricture, and ulceration, also occur more frequently in patients with Barrett's esophagus. Physiologic studies reveal markedly abnormal esophageal acid exposure, an incompetent lower esophageal sphincter, and poor esophageal body clearance of acid in more than 90% of these patients. Both the frequency and the duration of reflux episodes are increased in comparison with patients with no columnar metaplasia. Contractility of the esophageal body is often impaired in patients with Barrett's esophagus and may be profoundly reduced, resulting in prolonged contact of refluxed acid with esophageal mucosa. The clinical and physiologic severity in patients with short-segment Barrett's esophagus is generally intermediate between those with long-segment Barrett's and erosive esophagitis. Thus, regardless of any concern for the development of dysplasia and cancer, the presence of Barrett's esophagus is an indication of severe gastroesophageal reflux and, as such, an indication to consider surgical treatment.

PREOPERATIVE MANAGEMENT

Nondysplastic Barrett's Esophagus

The long-term relief of symptoms remains the primary force driving antireflux surgery in patients with nondysplastic Barrett's esophagus; the prevention of disease progression is an important secondary goal. Patients with Barrett's esophagus are not different from the broader population of patients with GERD and should be considered for antireflux surgery when factors suggest severe disease or predict the need for long-term medical management, both of which are almost always true in patients with Barrett's esophagus.

Endoscopic Ablation

The conceptual need to ablate Barrett's epithelium stems from its potential to degenerate into adenocarcinoma. This fact is important, because the foundation upon which ablation rests (in nondysplastic Barrett's) disappears if antireflux surgery is shown to prevent the development of cancer. The best use of ablative technology may be to eliminate Barrett's epithelium before antireflux surgery. Ablative methods currently in use include electrosurgery, laser and argon-directed light waves, photodynamic therapy, and endoscopic mucosal resections. To date, the risk–benefit of the techniques used has not been adequately evaluated, particularly in the absence of dysplasia. Furthermore, once the epithelium has been ablated, gastroesophageal reflux must be controlled.

Ablation of high-grade dysplasia or early adenocarcinoma has greater merit. The critical issues yet to be resolved are (1) whether the absence of a cancer can be accurately predicted and (2) if present, whether the depth of the tumor (intramucosal versus submucosal) and the presence or absence of regional nodal metastases can be correctly predicted before surgery. The accuracy of endoscopic ultrasonography in determining the depth of tumors confined to the esophageal wall is not sufficient to predictably differentiate the fine detail of tumor infiltration when the tumor is limited to the esophageal wall.

Antireflux Surgery

Antireflux surgery is an excellent treatment option in most patients with Barrett's esophagus. However, Barrett's esophagus implies severe GERD, with its attendant sequelae such as large hiatal hernia, stricture, shortened esophagus, and poor motility. These anatomic and physiologic features make successful antireflux surgery a particular challenge. Indeed, antireflux surgery in patients with Barrett's esophagus may not be as successful in the long term as in those without Barrett's (see later discussion). The most important features to identify before surgery are the presence of esophageal shortening, poor esophageal body function, and dysplasia; each has significant bearing on the decision for surgical treatment as well as the approach and type of antireflux procedure selected.

Large hiatal hernias are often associated with shortening of the esophagus, which can compromise the ability to perform an adequate tension-free antireflux repair. This fact may account for the emerging observation of an increased failure rate in patients with Barrett's esophagus after laparoscopic fundoplication. Before surgery, esophageal length should be assessed using a video barium study in concert with endoscopic findings. The possibility of a short esophagus should be considered in patients with strictures or those with hiatal hernias greater than 5 cm. These cases, which are common in the setting of long-segment Barrett's esophagus, are likely best approached transthoracically. The transthoracic approach allows esophageal lengthening via complete mobilization from the diaphragmatic hiatus to the aortic arch.

Traditionally, a partial fundoplication has been the procedure of choice in the presence of poor esophageal body function characterized by contraction amplitudes of 20 to 30 mm Hg or less in the distal esophageal segments or greater than 40% simultaneous waves on manometry. In the presence of poor esophageal body function, there is a risk of dysphagia secondary to a complete 360-degree Nissen fundoplication. The magnitude of this risk is not well documented, however. The decision is complicated by recent reports that have shown an unacceptably high prevalence of recurrent reflux following partial fundoplications (see later discussion). The clinician and the patient may be left with selecting the "lesser of two evils" in such a circumstance, recurrent reflux versus postoperative dysphagia.

Dysplastic Barrett's Esophagus

The presence of dysplasia is based on histologic changes currently classified as (1) no dysplasia, (2) indefinite for dysplasia, (3) low-grade dysplasia, and (4) high-grade dysplasia. Some degree of dysplasia is present in 15% to 25% of patients at presentation and develops in 5% to 10% of patients per year. Barrett's esophagus complicated by dysplasia should be treated aggressively. Patients who are indefinite for dysplasia should be given 60 to 80 mg of proton pump inhibitor therapy for 3 months and then have another set of biopsies. The presence of severe inflammation makes the microscopic interpretation of dysplasia difficult. If it remains indefinite, treatment should be as if low-grade dysplasia were present, with continued medical therapy or antireflux surgery and biopsy every 6 months. Patients with low-grade dysplasia are perhaps the most difficult group to manage because

of the potential difficulty in surveillance after antireflux surgery. Biopsies within the wrap may be difficult for the inexperienced. Either aggressive medical treatment by an experienced endoscopist or antireflux surgery is appropriate. High-grade dysplasia should be confirmed by two pathologists knowledgeable in gastrointestinal pathology and is generally treated by esophagectomy. On average, 45% to 50% of these patients harbor invasive cancer when the specimen is removed. It is not possible with present technology to differentiate which patients harbor a cancer. Five-year survival rate, however, approaches 90% in this setting.

INTRAOPERATIVE MANAGEMENT

Antireflux Surgery

Partial Versus Complete Fundoplication

Partial fundoplications may be constructed around the esophagus anteriorly (Watson/Dor) or posteriorly (Toupet) as well as through the abdomen or chest (Belsey). Because of concern over recurrent reflux, partial fundoplications are rarely used routinely, generally being reserved for patients with abnormal esophageal motility. Even in this circumstance, their use is being challenged, largely because the population of patients with GERD-induced motility abnormalities have the most severe reflux, and thus are most likely to have recurrence after a partial fundoplication. Recent reports have questioned the durability of partial fundoplications, with 24-hour pH studies showing reflux in up to 50% of patients 2 to 3 years after this operation. Risk factors for failure included the presence of a defective lower esophageal sphincter, an aperistaltic distal esophagus, and the presence of erosive esophagitis. Although current dogma holds that a partial fundoplication is the procedure of choice in patients with poor esophageal body motility, many surgeons employ a complete fundoplication, particularly in patients with Barrett's esophagus in whom the control of acid secretion may play an important role in the propensity for dysplastic degeneration. As stated before, the clinician and the patient may be left with selecting the "lesser of two evils" in such a circumstance, recurrent reflux versus postoperative dysphagia.

Technique of Fundoplication

Although the technique of Nissen fundoplication is slowly becoming more standardized, several features remain controversial. Debate continues regarding the importance of crural closure, fundic and esophageal mobilization, and anchoring of the fundoplication to the diaphragm. No randomized studies have evaluated the role of routine crural closure, but compelling evidence indicates that closure should be standard. Several studies have shown a higher incidence of recurrent herniation in patients in whom the crura were not closed. One group identified postoperative paraesophageal herniation in 3% of 253 patients who had and 11% who had not undergone crural repair. Perhaps most compelling is the fact that recurrent hernia has emerged as the leading cause of failure after laparoscopic fundoplication, even with routine crural closure. Most researchers would now agree that routine crural closure should be an integral part of the operation.

Postoperative dysphagia may be secondary to undue tension on the fundoplication resulting from incomplete fundic mobilization in the absence of division of the short gastric vessels. Although the fundus relaxes in concert with the sphincter, a phenomenon termed *receptive relaxation*, the gastric body does not. If the fundus of the stomach is not completely mobilized, the body of the stomach can be wrapped around the sphincter, often too tightly and under too much tension, both of which can interfere with relaxation and compliance of the sphincter to a bolus. In a prospective study, ligation of the short gastric vessels was associated with significantly less dysphagia than in the group without short gastric vessel ligation. Others have found a higher incidence of dysphagia when laparoscopic Nissen with and without short gastric division were retrospectively compared. Taken together, these and other data support the contention that complete fundic mobilization is important to allow construction of a tension-free fundoplication.

Operative Management of High-Grade Dysplasia

Because of the high risk of present and future adenocarcinoma, high-grade dysplasia is best treated by a total esophagectomy removing all Barrett's tissue. Options for resection include transhiatal or transthoracic esophagectomy or, more recently, vagal-sparing esophagectomy. The vagal-sparing approach is suitable only when clinicians are confident that there is no regional nodal disease. Reconstruction is accomplished with either the stomach (transhiatal) or colon (vagal-sparing) with the anastomosis in the neck.

Recent data from the author's experience suggest that, in the absence of an endoscopically visible lesion, any cancer in the esophagus is predominantly intramucosal and nodal metastases are rare. Whether this fact will suffice to select the extent of surgical resection awaits further study. In the presence of an endoscopically visible lesion, the possibility of a submucosal tumor is high. Because tumors that invade into the submucosa have a 60% or more incidence of lymph node metastasis, it seems prudent to perform an en bloc esophagectomy for treatment of visible lesions, regardless of the histologic findings on biopsy (e.g., high-grade dysplasia or intramucosal carcinoma). Recent studies indicate that, in early adenocarcinoma in Barrett's esophagus, metastases do not appear to involve the splenic artery nodes and the spleen. Splenic artery dissection consequently is not part of the en bloc resection for this condition, nor is an extended gastric resection. Gastrointestinal continuity is reestablished by pulling the stomach up into the neck and performing an esophagogastrostomy. This approach, however, is not universally accepted.

POSTOPERATIVE MANAGEMENT
Perioperative Management

After laparoscopic hiatus herniorrhaphy, a nasogastric tube is not necessary. Pain is managed with parenteral narcotics or ketorolac for the first 24 hours and oral hydrocodone thereafter as necessary. A Foley catheter is placed after induction of anesthesia and left in until the morning after surgery. Oral liquids are allowed the morning after surgery. Soft solids are begun on the second postoperative day and continued for 2 weeks. The patient should be instructed to eat slowly, chew carefully, and avoid untoasted bread and meats for 2 weeks.

The perioperative care of esophagectomy patients has steadily improved over the past several decades. The postoperative stay after transhiatal esophagectomy averages 7 to 10 days in high-volume centers. Many patients can be managed without the need for transfusion or ventilator support, and patients are eating soft solid diets at the time of discharge.

Long-Term Follow-Up

Temporary dysphagia is common after surgery (perhaps even desirable because it signifies a functionally effective wrap) and generally resolves within 3 months. Dysphagia before surgery usually improves after laparoscopic fundoplication. Dysphagia persisting beyond 3 months has been reported in up to 10% of patients. In the author's experience, occasional difficulty swallowing solids is present in 7% of patients at 3 months, 5% at 6 months, 2% at 12 months, and rarely 24 months after surgery. The dysphagia induced by laparoscopic fundoplication is usually mild, need not require dilatation, and is temporary. Other side effects common to antireflux surgery include the inability to vomit and increased flatulence. Most patients cannot vomit through an intact wrap, although it is rarely clinically relevant. Flatulence is a common and noticeable problem likely related to increased air swallowing present in most patients with GERD.

Patients with Barrett's esophagus should remain in an endoscopic surveillance program after antireflux surgery because there is no reliable evidence to indicate that the Barrett's mucosa will regress. Current recommendations call for surveillance endoscopy every 1 to 3 years. The cost effectiveness of surveillance has been shown to be equal or superior to mammographic screening of breast lesions. Little data exist to guide the clinician regarding the need for, and benefit of, continued assessment of reflux postoperatively, although recurrence is likely in 5% to 10% of patients. As data emerge regarding the importance of lifelong elimination of pathologic reflux in patients with Barrett's esophagus, postoperative pH monitoring at selected intervals (3 to 5 years) may become commonplace.

Long-term functional results of esophagectomy in the setting of high-grade dysplasia are "good." Most patients (60% to 70%) enjoy an unrestricted diet and report their alimentary ability as excellent to good. Occasional regurgitation and diarrhea are reported in 30% to 40%. Although studies assessing quality of life after esophagectomy are only beginning to be reported, those that are available suggest surprisingly little variation from normal.

COMPLICATIONS
Morbidity and Mortality Rates of Antireflux Surgery

Elective antireflux surgery is a safe procedure, with a mortality rate similar to that of cholecystectomy (0.2%).

Many large series have been reported with no perioperative deaths. Complications occur in 8% to 10% of patients after laparoscopic antireflux surgery. Approximately 2% of these procedures require conversion to an open operation. Three fourths of conversions are related to technical problems, and one fourth are for intraoperative complications such as bleeding arising from the short gastric vessels or spleen, retractor trauma to the liver, injury to the left inferior phrenic vein, or an aberrant left hepatic artery. Pneumothorax and pneumomediastinum can occur related to breach of either pleural membrane, usually the left, during the hiatal dissection but do not require chest tube insertion because accumulated carbon dioxide is rapidly absorbed after release of pneumoperitoneum.

Intraoperative injury to the esophagus or stomach occurs rarely (0.5% to 0.8%) but can lead to serious morbidity if unrecognized. Gastric and esophageal perforation during laparoscopic fundoplication has been shown to occur early during the course of a surgeon's experience (first 10 patients) and is related to technical errors, including improper dissection behind the gastroesophageal junction, passage of a bougie, and suture disruption caused by excessive tension on the wrap. Patients whose injury is recognized and repaired at the time of surgery do well.

Morbidity and Mortality Rate of Esophagectomy

Transhiatal or transthoracic simple esophagectomy presently carries a mortality rate of 2% to 5% in expert centers, and the rate continues to decrease. Anastomotic leak occurs in 10% to 15% of patients but is generally well tolerated because of the cervical anastomosis. Other complications include reoperation for bleeding (1% to 2%), recurrent laryngeal nerve paresis (1% to 4%), pneumonia (2% to 3%), and chylothorax (<1%). The most prevalent postoperative problem is anastomotic stricture, which occurs in 25% to 30% of patients after esophagectomy and gastric interposition. Orringer has reported that up to 70% of patients received at least one postoperative dilatation.

OUTCOMES

Outcome of Antireflux Surgery in Barrett's Esophagus

Surprisingly few studies have focused on the symptomatic outcome after antireflux surgery in patients with Barrett's esophagus. Those that are available document excellent to good results in 72% to 95% of patients 5 years after surgery. Several have compared medical and surgical therapy. In a prospective but nonrandomized study, 45 patients underwent either medical or surgical treatment of Barrett's esophagus. Heartburn or dysphagia recurred in 88% of patients who underwent medical treatment and in 21% after antireflux surgery. Reflux complications, primarily esophageal stricture, occurred in 38% of medically treated and 16% of surgically treated patients ($P < 0.05$).

Esophageal adenocarcinoma developed in one patient in each group. Antireflux surgery was superior to acid suppression for both control of symptoms and prevention of complications in patients with Barrett's esophagus. Other nonrandomized comparisons have reported similar results.

Ortiz et al. (1996) reported a prospective randomized comparison of medical and surgical therapy in 59 patients with Barrett's esophagus. Medical therapy consisted of either H_2 blockade or proton pump inhibitors. Symptomatic improvement occurred in 85% receiving medical therapy and 89% after antireflux surgery. In contrast, in the group receiving medical therapy, 53% and 45% of patients had persistent esophagitis or stricture, respectively, compared with 5% and 15% of patients having antireflux surgery. These studies document the ability of antireflux surgery to provide long-term symptomatic relief in patients with Barrett's esophagus.

The outcome of laparoscopic Nissen fundoplication in patients with Barrett's esophagus has been assessed at 1 to 3 years after surgery. Farrell and colleagues (1999) reported that mean scores for heartburn, regurgitation, and dysphagia improved dramatically after Nissen fundoplication in 50 patients with both long- and short-segment Barrett's esophagus. Importantly, there was no decrement in symptom scores when 1-year results were compared with those at 2 to 5 years postoperatively. They did, however, find a higher prevalence of "anatomic" failures requiring reoperation in patients with Barrett's esophagus when compared with non-Barrett's patients with GERD. A comparison of 42 patients with symptomatic Barrett's esophagus with 101 patients with typical symptoms of GERD without Barrett's after laparoscopic fundoplication revealed no difference in outcome. An excellent to good outcome was achieved in 90% of the Barrett's patients and 92% of the non-Barrett's group, even though patients with Barrett's esophagus had higher esophageal acid exposure, more commonly had impaired esophageal clearance, and had later stage of disease as indicated by lower mean esophageal contraction amplitudes and higher number of reflux episodes with long duration. Esophageal acid exposure was restored to normal in all 10 patients with Barrett's esophagus who volunteered for pH monitoring after antireflux surgery.

The Fate of Barrett's Esophagus After Antireflux Surgery

Neither medical nor surgical therapy reliably results in complete regression of Barrett's epithelium once it is firmly established. After antireflux surgery, loss of intestinal metaplasia in patients with visible Barrett's esophagus was rare but occurred in 73% of patients with intestinal metaplasia of the cardia, suggesting that the metaplastic process may be reversible if reflux is eliminated early in its process. Antireflux surgery was associated with regression of dysplasia in 70% of patients with low-grade dysplasia. The possibility of reversal of short-segment Barrett's has recently been confirmed. Fourteen patients with short-segment Barrett's esophagus were evaluated a mean of 25 months after antireflux surgery. Two of 14 patients

(14%) had no evidence of intestinal metaplasia on repeated postoperative biopsies, and four regressed from low-grade dysplasia to nondysplastic Barrett's. If further studies confirm the ability of antireflux surgery to promote regression of even a small portion of patients with short-segment Barrett's esophagus, the clinical implications would be significant.

Evidence suggests, although by no means is it proven, that fundoplication may protect against dysplasia and invasive malignancy. Four recent studies suggest that effective antireflux surgery may impact the natural history of Barrett's esophagus. One hundred and nineteen patients with nondysplastic Barrett's received medical treatment, and 42 underwent antireflux surgery. Dysplasia developed in 10 of 119 patients in the medically treated group (20%) and in 2 of 42 (3%) in the surgical group. Another retrospective review of 118 patients with Barrett's esophagus undergoing antireflux surgery revealed three cancers occurring over an 18.5-year follow-up, all within the first 3 postoperative years. Development of adenocarcinoma clustered in the early years after antireflux surgery and not randomly dispersed throughout the follow-up strongly suggests that antireflux surgery altered the natural history of the Barrett's esophagus, particularly given the fact that once dysplasia has developed, prospective studies show that carcinoma ensues in an average of 3 years.

The Veterans Administration outcomes group retrospectively reviewed 102 patients undergoing annual surveillance for a total of 563 patient-years of follow-up. New-onset low-grade dysplasia developed in 19 patients, high-grade dysplasia developed in four, and adenocarcinoma developed in three. Antireflux surgery was associated with a decreased risk of development of dysplasia; indeed, dysplasia did not appear in any of the patients after antireflux surgery. Finally, dysplasia developed in 6 of 27 (22%) patients on medical treatment and in only 1 of 32 (2%) patients at a median of 5 years after antireflux surgery.

Outcome of Esophagectomy in High-Grade Dysplasia

Most of these tumors are limited to the wall of the esophagus, and few spread to regional lymph nodes. Esophageal adenocarcinoma associated with high-grade

Pearls and Pitfalls

PEARLS

- Barrett's esophagus is an epithelial metaplasia of the distal esophagus resulting from severe gastroesophageal reflux.
- The prevalence of Barrett's esophagus is increasing in incidence, and it is clearly linked to esophageal adenocarcinoma, a highly lethal cancer.
- Identification of the risk factors predisposing to Barrett's esophagus may allow early and aggressive antireflux treatment to prevent the development of metaplastic epithelium.
- When Barrett's esophagus is established, treatment priorities are focused on elimination of reflux to alter the natural history of the disease, techniques of successful epithelial ablation, and molecular and epidemiologic prediction of patients at high risk for deterioration to adenocarcinoma.

dysplasia on surveillance biopsies, identified with surveillance endoscopy, is highly curable. Five-year survival rate approaches 90% in this setting.

SELECTED READINGS

Chandrasoma P: Norman Barrett: So close, yet 50 years away from the truth. J Gastrointest Surg 1999;3:7.

Csendes A, Braghetto I, Burdiles P, et al: Long-term results of classic antireflux surgery in 152 patients with Barrett's esophagus: Clinical radiologic, manometric and acid reflux tests before and late after operation. Surgery 1998;123:645.

Falk GW, Catalano MF, Sivak MV, et al: Endosonography in the evaluation of patients with Barrett's esophagus and high-grade dysplasia. Gastrointest Endosc 1994;40:207.

Farrell TM, Smith CD, Metreveli RE, et al: Fundoplication provides effective and durable symptom relief in patients with Barrett's esophagus. Am J Surg 1999;178:18.

Orringer MB, Marshall B, Iannettoni MD: Transhiatal esophagectomy: Clinical experience and refinements. Ann Surg 1999;230:392.

Ortiz A, Martinez de Haro LF, Parrilla P, et al: Conservative treatment versus antireflux surgery in Barrett's oesophagus: Long-term results of a prospective study. Br J Surg 1996;83:274.

Pera M, Trastek VF, Carpenter HA, et al: Barrett's esophagus with high-grade dysplasia: An indication for esophagectomy. Ann Thorac Surg 1992;54:199.

Peters JH, Clark GWB, Ireland AP, et al: Outcome of adenocarcinoma arising in Barrett's esophagus in endoscopically surveyed and non-surveyed patients. J Thorac Cardiovasc Surg 1994;108:813.

Sampliner RE: Practice guidelines on the diagnosis, surveillance and therapy of Barrett's esophagus. Am J Gastroenterol 1998;93:1028.

Chapter 46
Achalasia
Amjad Ali and Carlos A. Pellegrini

The word *achalasia* means "lack of relaxation" in Greek. Idiopathic achalasia, the most common primary esophageal motility disorder, has an incidence of about 1% per 100,000 and a prevalence of 8 per 100,000. It affects men and women with equal frequency, and most patients are first seen between the third and fifth decades of life. Since its first description by Thomas Willis in 1674, the etiology of the idiopathic form still remains elusive. Treatment has evolved from use of the cork-tipped whalebone used by Thomas Willis to the application of the latest laparoscopic and thoracoscopic techniques of esophageal myotomy popularized since 1991.

The disease is characterized by a triad of

- Incomplete or absent relaxation in the lower esophageal sphincter (LES)
- Progressive loss of peristalsis in the body of the esophagus
- Resultant esophageal dilatation

The primary defect is the neuronal degeneration in the myenteric plexus of the esophageal wall, which results from an inflammatory process leading to ganglion and nerve cell damage. Loss of activity of the inhibitory neurons results in an incomplete relaxation of the LES. Myotomy specimens from patients with achalasia show a hypersensitivity to cholinergic drugs consistent with denervation sensitivity. Additionally, investigations have shown decreased levels in the LES of nitric oxide (NO) synthetase, the enzyme that makes NO, a potent smooth muscle relaxant. This decrease, proposed as a contributing factor to the tonic contraction of the LES, received further support by a recent finding that sildenafil (Viagra), known to augment the smooth muscle relaxant effects of NO, reduces LES pressure in patients with achalasia. On the other hand, substance P, another neurotransmitter that stimulates LES contraction, is not affected in achalasia, which suggests that the cholinergic system is intact in these patients. The use of botulinum toxin for the treatment of achalasia is based on this information, because botulinum is a potent inhibitor of acetylcholine release from presynaptic nerve terminals. The etiology of neuronal damage is not known. The striking similarity between idiopathic achalasia and the esophageal motor dysfunction seen in patients with Chagas' disease caused by the protozoan *Trypanosoma cruzi* in Central America points to an infectious etiology. Some evidence suggests that previous infection with varicella zoster virus or measles virus may be responsible for the disease. Also, there is some similarity in the pathologic changes of achalasia and neuronal damage seen with Parkinson's disease and hereditary cerebellar ataxia. A syndrome similar to idiopathic achalasia can be reproduced in animals by damage to the dorsal motor nucleus or the nucleus ambiguus, which are both associated with the vagus nerve.

Obstruction at the gastroesophageal junction from a tumor of the cardia (pseudoachalasia), a tight Nissen fundoplication, or an Angelchik prosthesis can produce a condition with radiologic and manometric features similar to achalasia. Removal of the distal obstruction in many cases results in a return of peristalsis, suggesting distal obstruction as a primary defect leading to a loss of peristalsis in the body of the esophagus.

CLINICAL PRESENTATION

All patients with achalasia have a history of *dysphagia*. Many patients describe exacerbation of dysphagia with ingestion of cold liquids and emotional stress. The patients accumulate food in the esophagus until the hydrostatic pressure at the bottom of the column overcomes the resistance of the LES and pushes some food into the stomach. The sensation of dysphagia disappears over time in some patients as the esophagus becomes distended and food collects in the distended esophagus instead of passing into the stomach. At that stage, patients may feel heartburn as a result of bacterial fermentation of retained food in the esophagus. Regurgitation and aspiration pneumonia may then develop. Two thirds of patients with achalasia experience *regurgitation*. Distinguishing regurgitation from vomiting may be difficult. Regurgitation generally occurs during or at the end of a meal, and the regurgitated material tastes bland rather than sour or bitter. These patients are usually slow eaters, and they frequently have to leave the table to regurgitate. Regurgitation during sleep may cause coughing, in some instances staining of the pillows, and often leads to aspiration. One third to one half of patients suffer from *chest pain*. Chest pain is a prominent complaint in patients with a variant of the disease called *vigorous achalasia*. Symptoms usually are present for several years before the diagnosis is made. In some patients, a distal esophageal diverticulum develops as a result of chronic distal obstruction, and these patients are at a higher risk of esophageal perforation with pneumatic dilatation.

Diagnostic Workup

Radiologic Studies

Radiologic findings depend on the stage of the disease. Nonspecific findings on chest radiograph include mediastinal widening, presence of an air-fluid level in the esophagus, absence of a gastric air bubble, and abnormal pulmonary markings caused by chronic aspiration. The

319

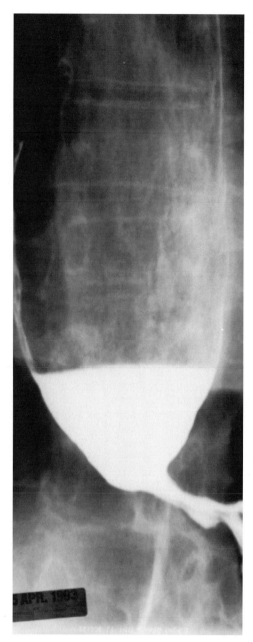

Figure 46–1. Barium esophagogram in a patient with advanced achalasia. The x-ray study shows a dilated sigmoid esophagus with tapering bird's beak appearance of the distal esophagus.

barium upper gastrointestinal study is normal in the early stages of the disease but later in the disease shows a dilated, tortuous esophagus with an air-fluid level. When the cardia is well visualized on the barium study, it shows a tapering bird's beak appearance (Fig. 46–1). It should be noted, however, that the "typical" bird-beak configuration may also be seen in patients with pseudoachalasia caused by a neoplasm in this area. The inability to push swallowed air into the stomach leads to the absence of a gastric air bubble. Barium studies also pick up epiphrenic diverticula when present. Many patients are referred to surgeons with a diagnosis of achalasia based on a barium swallow. However, it is important to fully evaluate the

patient with an upper endoscopy and an esophageal manometry before proceeding with treatment.

Upper Endoscopy

Endoscopy reveals a dilated tortuous esophagus with residual liquid or food in the lumen. Esophagitis is usually the result of fermentation of esophageal contents in untreated patients and a result of gastroesophageal reflux in patients who have previously undergone treatment for achalasia. The LES appears puckered and does not open with air insufflation, but unlike a stricture, it easily permits passage of the endoscope with a characteristic popping sensation. Endoscopy helps rule out the possibility of pseudoachalasia, but careful examination of the gastroesophageal junction with the scope retroflexed is required to avoid missing a small cancer in that area. However, endoscopy cannot rule out pseudoachalasia caused by a mural or extramural tumor. When this is suspected on the basis of the patient's history (rapid weight loss, weight loss of more than 20 lb, or symptoms with duration of less than 6 months), endoscopic ultrasonography is recommended. Endoscopy also picks up yeast esophagitis, which can obliterate the submucosal plane as a result of inflammation and scarring, and contaminate the mediastinum in case of a procedural perforation of the esophagus during therapy. Therefore, yeast esophagitis should be aggressively treated with oral antifungal agents before treating achalasia. Endoscopy also identifies the presence of a hiatal hernia or an epiphrenic diverticulum, which places patients at a higher risk for esophageal perforation with balloon dilatation.

Manometry

Manometry is the gold standard for diagnosing achalasia. The classic features of achalasia on manometry are

- Incomplete LES relaxation
- Absence of esophageal body peristalsis
- Elevated LES pressure
- Positive intraesophageal body pressure

Incomplete relaxation of LES is the most characteristic finding, occurring in 80% of patients. Normal LES relaxation is more than 90% versus 35% in achalasia (Fig. 46–2A and B). However, interpretation of LES relaxation may be misleading if the tip of the manometry catheter is placed in the lower part of the LES. Under these conditions upward movement of the LES during swallowing brings the tip of the catheter into the stomach briefly and gives a false impression of relaxation. It is important to place the transducer in the proximal part of the LES to evaluate relaxation.

Lack of peristalsis in the distal (smooth muscle) segment of the esophagus is another hallmark of achalasia. Typical peristaltic waves are of very low amplitude (see Fig. 46–2C and D), and peristalsis is absent with a massively distended esophagus. Normal intraesophageal pressure is subatmospheric, but it is positive in patients with achalasia as a result of outflow obstruction and retention

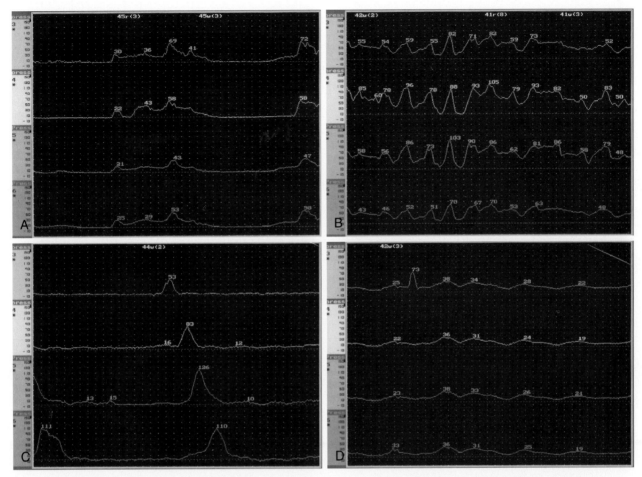

Figure 46–2. *A,* Normal lower esophageal sphincter (LES) relaxation after a wet swallow. *B,* Absence of LES relaxation after a wet swallow in a patient with achalasia. *C,* Normal peristalsis in the body of the esophagus after a wet swallow. *D,* Low-amplitude simultaneous contractions in the body of the esophagus of a patient with achalasia.

of food and secretions. All four findings are *not* always present. LES pressure may be normal, but it is usually not subnormal in untreated achalasia. In patients with a massively distended esophagus, it may be impossible to pass the manometry catheter through the LES even under fluoroscopy. In these patients, an esophageal body study demonstrating lack of peristalsis is sufficient documentation to proceed with treatment.

Presence of characteristic findings on barium swallow and normal manometry should raise the suspicion for pseudoachalasia. These patients should be evaluated for the presence of a tumor that may be local and directly compressing the esophagus (e.g., an aortic aneurysm, a hepatic tumor, or a tumor of the diaphragm) or a remote tumor (causing a paraneoplastic syndrome).

Patients with vigorous achalasia may have high amplitude, simultaneous esophageal contractions. These patients are usually younger and have chest pain as a prominent symptom. Most investigators believe vigorous achalasia to be an early form of the disease. The cutoff pressure for esophageal contractions used by most gastroenterologists is 40 mm Hg. Patients with nonperistaltic pressure waves exceeding 40 mm Hg are classified as having vigorous achalasia, whereas those with esopha-

geal body pressure waves less than 40 mm Hg are said to have classic achalasia.

24-Hour pH Study

Gastroesophageal reflux is usually not present in patients with untreated achalasia. However, patients may complain of heartburn as a result of fermentation of retained esophageal contents with production of lactic acid, which may lead to a falsely positive 24-hour pH study. However, the pH tracing does not have the deflections seen with gastroesophageal reflux. The other reason for this kind of tracing is the migration of the sensor into the stomach. In some achalasia patients, abnormal esophageal acid exposure despite high LES pressure is a result of reflux and not fermentation. A careful review of the 24-hour pH study is required to differentiate these patients from the ones with intraesophageal fermentation.

Esophageal Emptying Studies

Radiolabeled semisolid meal has been used to assess esophageal emptying and peristalsis in patients who cannot tolerate manometry. Although less specific than manometry, this test is noninvasive and can be used to assess treatment. A timed barium swallow is a simple and reproducible alternative technique to evaluate esophageal emptying. The patient ingests 100 to 200 mL of low-density barium over 30 to 45 seconds. Three-on-one spot x-ray films are obtained at 1, 2, and 5 minutes after ingestion. The degree of emptying is estimated qualitatively by comparing the 1- and 5-minute films. The degree of emptying may also be estimated quantitatively by measuring the height and width of the barium column for both films, calculating the area for both and determining the percentage of change in the area. Both qualitative and quantitative assessments were shown to be accurate methods of estimating esophageal emptying.

TREATMENT

Achalasia is an irreversible condition; thus, treatment aimed at alleviating symptoms is broadly divided into four strategies:

- Medical
- Mechanical
- Botulinum toxin injection
- Surgical

An algorithm for managing patients with achalasia is shown in Figure 46–3.

Medical Treatment

Smooth muscle relaxants including long-acting nitrates and calcium-channel blockers that act by reducing the LES tone are the mainstay of medical treatment. A number of nonplacebo controlled trials based on small patient populations have shown satisfactory response to long-acting nitrates and calcium-channel blockers. However, these results have not been reproduced by other investigators. Therefore, their use is limited to very mild cases or for patients unsuitable for mechanical or surgical therapies. Recently, sildenafil (Viagra) has been shown to reduce LES pressure in achalasia by augmenting the smooth muscle relaxation caused by NO. The role of this new modality in treatment of achalasia remains to be defined.

Mechanical Esophageal Dilatation

Dilatation of the LES is widely employed for the treatment of achalasia. The type of dilators and the techniques of dilatation have improved considerably. A comparison of pneumatic dilatation with the mercury bougie and other studies have established pneumatic dilatation as the standard form of esophageal dilatation for treating achalasia. Dilatation to a diameter of at least 3 cm (>90 French) is recommended to achieve long-term results. Low compliance balloon dilators such as Rigiflex and Witzel balloon systems are preferred over high-compli-

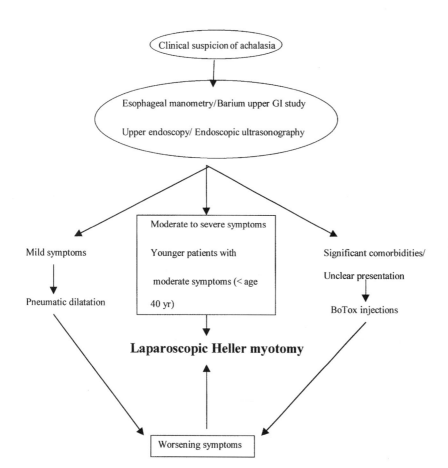

Figure 46–3. Algorithm for management of achalasia.

ance balloons to minimize risk of esophageal rupture. Low-compliance balloon dilators have a maximal designated diameter and further inflation results in an increase in the pressure within the balloon lumen only. High-compliance balloon dilators adapt to the surrounding esophagus, which results in an increase in esophageal wall tension in the more dilated esophagus proximal to the obstruction, increasing the risk of perforation. However, a recent trial comparing low-compliance with high-compliance balloon dilators did not show a significant difference in complication rate or clinical outcome. The Rigiflex pneumatic dilatation is performed under fluoroscopic guidance, and the Witzel balloon dilator allows endoscopic positioning of the balloon without fluoroscopy.

Immediate complications of mechanical dilatation include intramural hematoma, gastrointestinal bleeding, and esophageal perforation. Most complications manifest within 6 hours after the procedure, so patients should be closely observed for that time period. The most feared complication is esophageal perforation, the incidence of which ranges from 1% to 13%. Factors that increase the risk of esophageal perforation include massively dilated esophagus, a large hiatal hernia, an epiphrenic diverticulum, the aggressiveness with which dilatation is performed, and the size of the balloon. Patients with suspected esophageal perforation should undergo a Gastrografin swallow followed by a barium swallow if no leak is identified. Some patients with localized perforation may be managed conservatively with bowel rest and broad-spectrum antibiotics, but most patients need an emergency thoracotomy.

The reported success of resolution of dysphagia is between 60% and 80%, and relief is immediate for most patients. However, long-term results show that only 60% of patients remain in remission at 1 year, and recurrence of symptoms develops in more than half of patients by 5 years. A second dilatation is equally effective in patients who respond to the first dilatation, but there is a less than 20% chance of success in patients who did not respond to the first dilatation. The success rate of esophageal myotomy is not different in patients with prior pneumatic dilatation, but dissection and myotomy are more challenging in these patients. Patients younger than 40 years of age have a lower success rate with esophageal dilatation. Postprocedure gastroesophageal reflux has been reported in 2% to 30% of patients, but it responds well to medical therapy.

Botulinum Toxin

Injection of botulinum toxin (BoTox) into the LES is a newer modality and is an adaptation of successful use of this toxin in treatment of skeletal muscle disorders. BoTox is a potent inhibitor of acetylcholine release from presynaptic nerve terminals. The proposed mechanism of action is reduction in cholinergic excitation. Early results were encouraging, with an immediate clinical response in 90% of patients. However, results have not been nearly as good on follow-up; in 39%, recurrence developed within 3 months. Treatment failure was observed in 14 patients as a result of lack of initial response or rapid relapse.

Only 3 of the 11 nonresponders had a positive effect from a second injection. Sustained remission at 6 months persisted in 65%. Among patients who responded to the treatment, the probability of remaining in remission at 1 year was 68%, and the average duration of sustained response was 1.3 years. Patients who were older and had symptoms of vigorous achalasia responded better. Others have reported similar results.

BoTox therapy is an option for debilitated patients unable to tolerate balloon dilatation or surgical myotomy. BoTox has also been used in the diagnosis and management of patients with unclear presentation. These patients can be divided into three groups. The first group includes patients with symptoms consistent with achalasia but insufficient manometric criteria to make the diagnosis. The second group of patients has factors in addition to achalasia contributing to their symptoms, and the third group includes patients with advanced achalasia in whom it is not clear whether sphincter-directed therapy would be of benefit before esophagectomy. The short duration of action of BoTox can be used to the advantage of these patients because little harm is done if BoTox injection does not help relieve symptoms. Because of its ease of administration, intrasphincteric injection of BoTox can be used safely to decide whether sphincter-directed therapy would benefit a particular patient with unclear presentation before more invasive and permanent treatment modalities are recommended.

One disadvantage of the use of BoTox is the increased technical difficulties that result if an esophagomyotomy is required subsequently. In a recent review of laparoscopic Heller myotomy after BoTox treatment at our institution, we noted considerable technical difficulties in 8 of 15 patients with previous BoTox injections compared with 3 of 42 patients with no previous BoTox injections. Previous treatment with dilatation did not seem to confer a worse effect because dilatation causes a disruption of the muscularis in one area; thus, healing and scarring are limited to that part of the esophageal wall. BoTox is injected at multiple sites, and injections are frequently repeated. This repeated injury causes the muscularis and the mucosa to seal the area and eliminate the plane that needs to be developed by the surgeon to accomplish a satisfactory esophageal myotomy.

Surgical Therapy

Surgical treatment of achalasia consists of a longitudinal myotomy of the distal esophagus and gastroesophageal junction. The original technique of esophageal myotomy described by Heller in 1914 involved an anterior and posterior myotomy of the esophagus. The technique has been modified to a single anterior myotomy. A minimally invasive approach was first applied for the treatment of achalasia in 1991. Before the advent of laparoscopy, most myotomies in the United States were carried out through the chest. A transabdominal laparoscopic approach has been gaining wider acceptance, although some surgeons still prefer a thoracoscopic approach. Our experience involves laparoscopic myotomy with partial fundoplication in 133 patients and left thoracoscopic myotomy in 35 patients. We found better relief of dysphagia (93% versus 85%), less postoperative reflux (17% versus 60%), and shorter hospital stay (48 hours versus 72 hours) in the laparoscopic group.

Both laparoscopic and thoracoscopic approaches for myotomy are well established and offer the benefits of minimally invasive surgery to the patients. However, the thoracoscopic approach requires a double-lumen endotracheal intubation with collapse of the left lung. Although thoracoscopy obviates the need for gas insufflation, it does not offer an axial alignment of the operating instruments with the esophagus as in the laparoscopic approach, and makes dissection and suturing more difficult. The most distal part of the dissection is technically more difficult and less clearly visualized during a thoracoscopic myotomy. Finally, many surgeons believe that conversion to an open procedure is associated with more morbidity in the chest than in the abdomen.

Surgical Technique

For the average patient, we prefer an abdominal (laparoscopic) approach done in a semilithotomy position. Five trocars are placed in the upper abdomen in an arrangement similar to that for laparoscopic antireflux operations. The hiatus is identified, and the peritoneum over the hiatus and the left crus of the diaphragm are divided. The phrenogastric ligament and short gastric vessels are divided and ligated with an ultrasonic coagulating instrument to mobilize the stomach. The phrenoesophageal membrane is divided circumferentially, and dissection is continued into the mediastinum. The anterior vagus nerve is dissected free from the esophagus. A 52-French lighted bougie is inserted into the esophagus both to help in the identification of the esophagus and to provide a hard surface over which the myotomy can be performed. After the fat pad at the cardioesophageal junction is resected to precisely identify the gastroesophageal junction, a plane is developed anterior to the stomach and the esophagus. A very long myotomy of 8 to 10 cm in length carried down to the level of the mucosa is performed with a 2- to 3-cm extension on the stomach. A partial antireflux wrap without closure of the crura is performed at the end, and the bougie is removed.

Addition of an antireflux procedure at the time of the myotomy is controversial. Myotomy destroys the lower esophageal sphincter. A transthoracic myotomy that does not disrupt the hiatus and extends only 1 cm onto the stomach does not require a wrap. However, long-term follow-up has shown a disturbingly high incidence of reflux after this surgery for achalasia of between 25% and 48%. It is virtually impossible to perform a long enough myotomy to relieve the obstruction and not cause reflux. With the addition of an antireflux wrap, the incidence decreases to 5% to 10%, most of which cases are of mild to moderate reflux and can be managed medically.

The type of antireflux wrap is also controversial. There is a general consensus that a complete 360-degree wrap may cause significant obstruction at the distal end of the esophagus and lead to worsening of esophageal function in these patients who already have impaired peristalsis.

However, there is less agreement on the most suitable partial wrap. A Belsey Mark IV is popular among surgeons performing the myotomy through the chest. Partial posterior wrap (Toupet) and anterior wrap (Dor) are equally popular among surgeons performing a laparoscopic transabdominal myotomy. One multi-institutional study has shown a higher incidence of postoperative reflux after anterior partial fundoplication than after posterior partial fundoplication. Proponents of Toupet fundoplication also believe it keeps the myotomy edges separated and prevents the recurrence of obstruction. Believers in the Dor fundoplication propose that it provides an excellent patch in case there is a tiny perforation of the esophageal mucosa not identified during the operation.

Many retrospective studies have compared the outcome of surgical myotomy with balloon dilatation. Only one controlled, randomized study compares the two modalities (see Csendes and colleagues, 1989). Most have shown superior long-term results with surgery. Repeat pneumatic dilatations increase the effectiveness of dilatation from 66% to 80%, but they also increase the risk of esophageal perforation by twofold to threefold. Younger patients (younger than 40 years) should probably undergo treatment primarily with a myotomy, because pneumatic dilatation is less than 50% effective in these patients.

Complications

The most feared early complication of all invasive treatments of achalasia is unrecognized esophageal perforation. It should be suspected and aggressively sought in all patients with persistent fever or left-sided pleural effu-

---

Pearls and Pitfalls

PEARLS

- Achalasia is characterized by dysphagia, incomplete relaxation of the LES, progressive loss of esophageal peristalsis, and esophageal dilatation.
- Every patient with suspicion of achalasia should undergo esophageal manometry, barium upper GI study, and upper endoscopy.
- Patients with suspected achalasia with shorter duration of symptoms and a history of substantial weight loss should also undergo endoscopic ultrasonography to rule out the possibility of pseudoachalasia.
- Pneumatic dilatation may be offered once or twice to patients with mild to moderate disease.
- BoTox therapy should be reserved for patients who are unable to tolerate surgery because of significant comorbidities or whose clinical presentation is complicated and the diagnosis of achalasia is in doubt.
- Laparoscopic Heller myotomy should be offered as early as possible to young patients (younger than 40 years) with achalasia because they have a higher incidence of failure with dilatation and BoTox injections.
- Long-term results of surgical myotomy are superior to repeated esophageal dilatation.
- Patients with achalasia are at risk for development of squamous cell cancer of the esophagus.

sion. Early postoperative dysphagia is usually a result of an incomplete myotomy. Late dysphagia results from a reflux-induced peptic stricture or from healing of the myotomy with subsequent reobstruction of the gastroesophageal junction. Early postoperative dysphagia is usually a technical complication of the procedure and responds to extension of the myotomy or takedown of the wrap. Patients with late dysphagia are more difficult to treat, especially when the LES pressure is less than 10 mm Hg. The cause of dysphagia in these patients is extremely poor esophageal body function or a peptic stricture. Further division of the LES may be of benefit in this group of patients; pneumatic dilatation or even BoTox injection may also be tried and found to be effective. A second myotomy is less likely to be successful, and these patients often need esophageal resection.

ASSOCIATION WITH ESOPHAGEAL CARCINOMA

Achalasia is a premalignant condition. One study found that squamous cell cancer of the esophagus developed in 5% of patients with achalasia within 20 years after the diagnosis of achalasia. These tumors develop at an age 10 years younger than in the general population and carry a worse prognosis because of late diagnosis. Surveillance endoscopy is recommended every 2 years for screening of cancer in these patients. A change in the esophageal mucosa to a "tree bark" appearance should increase the suspicion of cancer. The effect of treatments on the incidence of cancer is not known.

SELECTED READINGS

Csendes A, Braghetto I, Henriquez A, Cortes C: Late results of a prospective randomised study comparing forceful dilatation and oesophagomyotomy in patients with achalasia [see comments]. Gut 1989;30:299.

Meijssen M, Tilanus HW, Van Blakenstein M, et al: Achalasia complicated by esophageal squamous cell carcinoma: A prospective study in 195 patients. Gut 1992;33:155.

Moonka R, Patti MG, Feo CV, et al: Clinical presentation and evaluation of malignant pseudoachalasia. J Gastrointest Surg 1999;3:456.

Patti MG, Arcerito M, Tong J, et al: Importance of preoperative and postoperative pH monitoring in patients with esophageal achalasia. J Gastrointest Surg 1997;1:505.

Patti MG, Pellegrini CA, Horgan S, et al: Minimally invasive surgery for achalasia: An 8-year experience with 168 patients. Ann Surg 1999;230:587; discussion 593.

Pellegrini C, Wetter LA, Patti M, et al: Thoracoscopic esophagomyotomy: Initial experience with a new approach for the treatment of achalasia. Ann Surg 1992;216:291–296; discussion 296.

Raiser F, Perdikis G, Hinder RA, et al: Heller myotomy via minimal-access surgery. Arch Surg 1996;131:593.

Spiess AE, Kahrilas PJ: Treating achalasia: From whalebone to laparoscope. JAMA 1998;280:638.

Vaezi MF, Baker ME, Richter JE: Assessment of esophageal emptying post-pneumatic dilation: Use of the timed barium esophagram. Am J Gastroenterol 1999;94:1802.

Vaezi MF, Richter JE, Wilcox CM, et al: Botulinum toxin versus pneumatic dilatation in the treatment of achalasia: A randomised trial [see comments]. Gut 1999;44:231.

Chapter 47
Esophageal Perforation
Daniel L. Miller

The management of esophageal perforation continues to be a surgical challenge. Although uncommon, the condition is frequently fatal if not recognized early. Esophageal perforation involves traumatic injury to the esophagus, occurring iatrogenically or spontaneously or associated with trauma. The increase in diagnostic and therapeutic endoscopy has made instrumentation the most common cause of esophageal perforation. Iatrogenic injuries are usually treated successfully because of earlier detection and prompt attention. Spontaneous perforations, however, usually have a fatal outcome because of diagnostic delays. Overall improvement in the care of these patients has decreased mortality because of a high degree of clinical suspicion combined with timely intervention. Management of esophageal perforation requires a mastery of multiple operative procedures. A thorough understanding of treatment options is required to successfully manage patients with such a potentially devastating injury.

IATROGENIC INJURIES OF THE ESOPHAGUS

Iatrogenic injuries account for more than half of all esophageal perforations. The instrumentation intervention that most frequently causes perforation includes esophagoscopy, pneumatic dilatation, bougienage, and sclerotherapy. Esophageal perforation has also been described with placement of nasogastric tubes, endotracheal tubes, endoesophageal prostheses, Sengstaken-Blakemore tubes, and transesophageal echocardiography.

The actual risk of perforation during instrumentation of the esophagus is extremely low. A review of more than 210,000 flexible esophagoscopies revealed a perforation rate of 0.03%. The rate of perforation for mercury bougienages is 0.09%, and that of pneumatic dilatation varies from 1.1% to 4.0%. Perforation associated with transesophageal echocardiography is on the rise with the increased use of this procedure in emergency situations.

Areas at risk for instrumental perforation are weak regions or narrowed areas of the esophagus. The cervical and intrathoracic portions of the esophagus are the areas most frequently perforated. The most common area of weakness is Lanier's triangle, which is the region within the neck where a Zenker's diverticulum originates. Anatomic areas of narrowing more susceptible to perforation include the physiologic sphincters, but also the esophagus adjacent to the aortic arch and the left mainstem bronchus. Perforation can also occur after dilatation of esophageal strictures, which can occur at any site within the esophagus.

Presentation

The symptoms of esophageal perforation depend on the cause, location, and duration since perforation. The pre-

sentation of a patient with esophageal perforation secondary to instrumentation varies with the site of injury. The classic triad is pain, fever, and subcutaneous or mediastinal air. Pain is the most frequent symptom, occurring in almost all patients. The pain from cervical perforation is usually low in the neck, overlying the sternocleidomastoid muscle. In patients with thoracic perforations, the pain is usually experienced in the substernal or upper abdominal areas. Fever usually develops *after* the pain in the majority of patients.

Emphysematous crepitus in the neck is very common after cervical perforation and can be detected by palpation in 60% of patients and radiographically in more than 95% of patients (Fig. 47–1). In contrast, mediastinal emphysema after thoracic perforation is appreciated by palpation in only 30% of patients and radiographically in 40%. Mediastinal emphysema may also be detected by the presence of a crackle on auscultation in cadence with normal cardiac sounds, so-called Hamman's sign or mediastinal "crunch," in 20% of patients.

Dyspnea may also be present because of the development of pleural effusions associated with pleural suppuration. Effusions occur in 50% of patients with thoracic

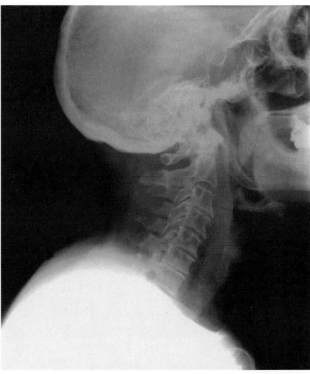

Figure 47–1. Lateral cervical radiograph demonstrating emphysema within the paraesophageal space; perforation related to endoscopy for reflux symptoms.

perforations, compared with only 10% in patients with cervical perforations. The clinical presentations resulting from iatrogenic injuries may be quite variable, and the findings may be very subtle. Therefore, a high index of clinical suspicion is crucial to avoiding a potentially fatal delay in the diagnosis of an esophageal perforation.

Diagnosis

Radiologic studies are often essential in establishing the diagnosis of esophageal perforation. Chest and upright abdominal radiographs should be performed in all patients suspected of having an esophageal perforation. Abnormalities are found on plain radiography in 90% of patients (Fig. 47–2). Significant changes can be absent if radiographs are performed within the first several hours after perforation (Fig. 47–3). Cervical radiographs should also be included if clinical suspicion is high for a cervical esophageal injury.

Contrast-enhanced studies may be performed to confirm the diagnosis and identify the site of perforation. A water-soluble contrast agent such as diatrizoate (Gastrografin) is used initially because barium can cause an acute inflammatory response in the mediastinum. Dilute barium should be used if any Gastrografin study is negative because its excellent coating properties make it more sensitive in the detection of smaller perforations.

Computed tomography (CT) of the chest can be extremely helpful in patients for whom there is a high

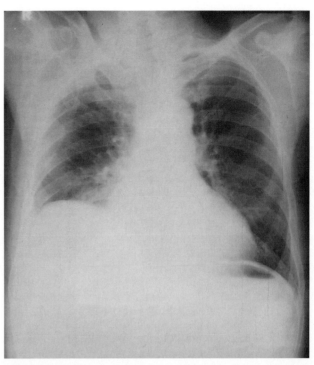

Figure 47–3. Anteroposterior chest radiograph demonstrating an elevated right hemidiaphragm 3 hours after the patient experienced substernal pain associated with vomiting.

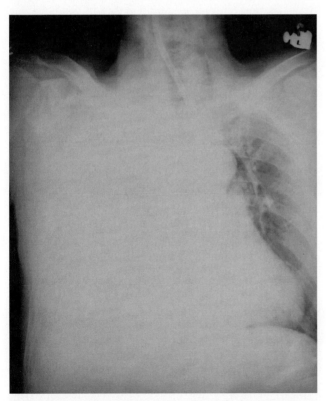

Figure 47–2. Anteroposterior chest radiograph demonstrating an opacified right side of the chest secondary to pleural effusion 24 hours after the patient experienced substernal pain associated with vomiting.

suspicion of perforation and in whom standard contrast-enhanced radiography fails to confirm the diagnosis of esophageal perforation. CT findings include pneumomediastinum, periesophageal abscesses, or communication between the esophagus and a mediastinal air-fluid collection or the pleural cavity.

Early after instrumentation-induced perforation, laboratory tests are normal. Serial testing shows leukocytosis and possible acidosis secondary to evolving sepsis from a delay in the diagnosis of an esophageal perforation. Oliguria and hypotension may rapidly become established owing to the sepsis that develops from the anaerobic organisms in the extravasated saliva.

Management

The optimal management of iatrogenic esophageal perforations is controversial. Most series in the literature deal with a small number of patients and multiple causes of the perforation. Also, there are no prospective randomized studies comparing operative versus nonoperative management of iatrogenic esophageal perforations. Therefore, the therapy chosen should be individualized to the clinical setting of the patient. Regardless of the type of therapy chosen, delays in the diagnosis and treatment are associated with increased morbidity and mortality.

NONOPERATIVE THERAPY. The role of nonoperative treatment in healthy patients who are a low risk for surgical intervention is controversial. The main reason for considering nonoperative management is the considerable morbidity and mortality associated with emergency esophagectomy if the clinical situation determines its necessity. Several studies have attempted to identify selection criteria for nonoperative management after iatrogenic instrumentation perforations. In general, patients with minimal symptoms and fever, without signs of shock and sepsis, and with a nontransmural or "contained" leak may be considered for nonoperative management. Patients with cervical perforations tend to have better results with nonoperative therapy than those of patients with thoracic perforations. This difference in outcome is due to the fact that the majority of cervical perforations are confined within the neck and do not result in such extensive mediastinal contamination as a thoracic perforation.

Nonoperative management consists of appropriate fluid resuscitation, broad-spectrum antibiotics, parenteral alimentation, and diversion of oropharyngeal secretions away from the site of perforation. The decision to proceed to surgical intervention is made whenever the patient's status deteriorates or does not show improvement. Antibiotics are continued until extramural extravasation is no longer present, and clinical improvement is evident (10 to 14 days). A clear liquid diet can be started as soon as no extravasation is seen on a follow-up contrast study. If an extraesophageal extravasation persists that drains freely back into the esophagus and there is good clinical improvement, the patient can be started on clear liquids, but the diet should be advanced cautiously with the practitioner observing for signs of contamination.

OPERATIVE THERAPY. Operative intervention is the treatment of choice in patients with either large, noncontained esophageal perforations or clinical signs of sepsis or shock. The surgical techniques used in the management of esophageal perforations are drainage alone, drainage and primary repair, and drainage and esophageal diversion or esophagectomy.

Cervical perforation may be managed, with excellent results, by simple drainage of the paracervical space, although some authorities still recommend primary closure of the defect. Thoracic perforations, because of their poor prognosis and increased risk of sepsis, generally require primary repair with reinforcement or esophagectomy, depending on the underlying pathology. If gross contamination is present, with evidence of extensive esophageal necrosis, primary repair is not possible. In this situation, exclusion and diversion are performed. This management strategy necessitates a second operation to restore esophageal continuity. Management of a transmural perforation after pneumatic dilatation for achalasia usually consists of primary closure of the perforation, with contralateral myotomy and possible antireflux procedure.

BAROGENIC INJURY OF THE ESOPHAGUS

Barogenic, or spontaneous, perforation of the esophagus refers to perforation of the esophagus in the absence of instrumentation or external force. In 1724, Herman Boerhaave described the clinical course and subsequent autopsy of a barogenic esophageal rupture in Baron van Wessenaer, the High Admiral of the Dutch Navy, who feasted then induced vomiting for prevention of an exacerbation of gout. Thus, barogenic esophageal rupture is referred to as Boerhaave's syndrome.

The mechanism of spontaneous perforation is thought to involve a sudden increase in esophageal intraluminal pressure incurred by rapid distention of the distal esophagus through vomiting or retching. The tear usually develops in the distal left lateral wall of the esophagus, 3 to 5 cm above the gastroesophageal junction. The esophageal tear is usually a full-thickness injury and communicates with the left pleural cavity in 80% of patients. However, the perforation may also communicate with the right chest cavity or peritoneum, depending on its exact location. Some cases have resulted from other causes of increased intraluminal pressure within the esophagus, such as blunt trauma, straining, weight lifting, severe coughing, childbirth, and vomiting induced by medication.

Presentation

The classic triad of symptoms associated with spontaneous perforation of the esophagus was first described by Mackler in 1952. Mackler's triad is vomiting or retching, thoracic pain, and subcutaneous emphysema. Initially thought to be present in one third of patients, the literature suggests that the triad may be even more uncommon, on the order of fewer than 10% of patients with barogenic rupture of the esophagus.

The signs and symptoms of barogenic perforation are usually nonspecific but may mimic those of instrumentation perforations. Chest pain, abdominal pain, dyspnea, dysphagia, and fever all are found in various combinations or altogether. Pain is the most common presenting symptom in the majority of patients. Because of the nonspecific nature of symptoms, the diagnosis is often confused with other life-threatening illnesses, such as pancreatitis, pneumonia, myocardial infarction, spontaneous pneumothorax, acute aortic dissection, and perforated peptic ulcer.

The physical findings depend on the location and duration of perforation. Fever and tachypnea are found in the majority of patients regardless of location. Crepitus is less common in thoracic perforations. Rales, tubular breath sounds, dullness to percussion, and egophony are manifestations of pleural effusion found with thoracic and abdominal perforations. Perforation of the esophagus at the gastroesophageal junction can present as an acute abdomen. If a delay in diagnosis has occurred, some patients manifest signs and symptoms of hypoperfusion, such as hypotension, tachycardia, and cyanosis, which can be the presenting symptom in 25% of patients.

Diagnosis

The workup of suspected barogenic esophageal perforation is similar to that for instrumentation perforations. A plain chest radiograph suggests esophageal perforation in 90% of the patients with barogenic rupture, whereas the history and physical examination are diagnostic in only approximately 15% of patients. Pleural effusion, pneumothorax, pneumomediastinum, atelectasis, and subcutaneous emphysema are the most common findings. Chest radiographs may be normal in approximately 10% of the patients.

Contrast studies continue to be the standard for the diagnosis and determination of the site of barogenic esophageal perforation (Fig. 47–4). Controversy continues about the use of water-soluble contrast material versus barium sulfate. The superior mucosal detail of barium and its ability to stain the tissues, thereby demonstrating not only the primary leak but also unusual additional esophageal mucosal abnormalities, make the use of dilute barium sulfate the often-recommended contrast agent for diagnosing and localizing spontaneous esophageal perforations. One should keep in mind that contrast studies continue to have a false-negative diagnosis rate of 10%.

Esophagogastroduodenoscopy and CT are adjunct radiologic modalities that can improve the diagnosis of esophageal perforation. The primary goals of these procedures are the diagnosis of chronic perforation when other studies have been nondiagnostic and the exclusion of associated esophageal pathology. CT findings suggestive of esophageal perforation include pneumomediastinum, air-fluid levels within the contaminated chest cavity, pleural effusions, and free flow of contrast material into a chest tube or a pleural cavity (Fig. 47–5).

Management

The goal of management of barogenic esophageal perforations is to prevent further contamination, eliminate gross infection, restore gastrointestinal continuity, and initiate nutritional support. The principles of the treatment of spontaneous esophageal perforation are débridement of infected and necrotic tissue, elimination of distal esophageal obstruction, primary closure of the perforation, wide drainage, establishment of enteral access, and initiation of antibiotic therapy. Factors that affect outcome include

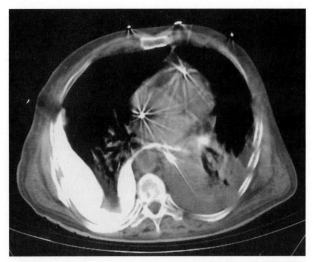

Figure 47–5. Computed tomography of the chest, demonstrating the free flow of contrast material from an esophageal perforation into the right chest cavity. A left pleural effusion is also shown, but contrast material was not evident within the left side of the chest.

the patient's age, the clinical response to the injury, underlying esophageal disease, the cause and size of the perforation, and the period of time from perforation to initiation of treatment. Treatment options are nonoperative or operative.

NONOPERATIVE THERAPY. Nonoperative management of spontaneous esophageal perforations is rarely successful. The only patients that are potential candidates for nonoperative treatment are those who present late after the event and experience minimal symptoms. The patient should first be resuscitated to eliminate hypoperfusion. Broad-spectrum antibiotics are started immediately. The pleural cavity contaminated by the perforation is then drained with multiple chest tubes to ensure evacuation of all infected material. A nasogastric tube is placed to divert secretions from the site of perforation. Finally, nutritional support is administered. Only a very select group of patients can be treated successfully by this approach.

OPERATIVE THERAPY. Absolute indications for operation are sepsis, shock, respiratory failure, pneumothorax, pneumoperitoneum, extensive mediastinal emphysema, or nonoperative therapy eventuating in abscess or empyema. Operative options include primary closure with or without external esophageal reinforcement, resection, exclusion and diversion, periesophageal drainage alone, T-tube drainage, and continuous irrigation and drainage of perforation. The operative approach depends on accurate identification of the perforation.

Cervical esophageal perforations are usually approached through the left neck anterior to the sternocleidomastoid muscle, medial to the carotid sheath, but lateral to the thyroid and trachea. The upper two thirds of the thoracic esophagus is approached through a right thoracotomy via the fourth or fifth intercostal space. The lower third of the thoracic esophagus is exposed via a left thoracotomy through the seventh intercostal space. The abdominal esophagus is reached through an upper midline laparotomy or thoracoabdominal incision if necessary.

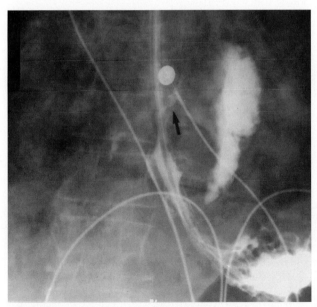

Figure 47–4. Radiograph of a water-soluble contrast swallow study showing the free flow of contrast material into the left chest cavity. The *arrow* identifies the site of perforation in the distal esophagus.

Primary repair of an esophageal perforation was first performed successfully over 50 years ago. The components of primary repair include débridement of necrotic tissue, myotomy to expose the full extent of mucosal disruption, mucosal closure, and widespread drainage of the area to minimize contamination. Characteristically, the tear in the muscle of the esophagus is smaller than the rent in the mucosa; therefore, the muscle must be opened to expose the full extent of the mucosal tear. Failure to do this leads to persistent leaks and disruption of the repair.

External reinforcement of a primary repair is always necessary. Reinforcement of the repair provides an extra layer of protection to reduce the risk of leak and contain a small leak if it occurs. This maneuver is especially warranted in primary repairs performed after 24 hours. Cervical perforations are best reinforced with strap muscles. In the chest, the intercostal muscle is preferred because of its bulk, vascular supply, and large arc of rotation. Omentum, which has a rich blood supply, may also be used. The success of reinforced primary repair depends on the ability of the esophageal tissue to hold the suture of the reinforcing tissue; therefore, tissue necrosis and infection cannot be too extensive. Reinforced primary repair is doomed to failure or leads to death if performed on an organ with distal obstruction.

Distal esophageal obstruction requires treatment. Perforated carcinoma necessitates resection or placement of an intraluminal stent if the tumor is nonresectable. If achalasia is present and has not been relieved by performing the procedure that led to perforation, treatment should consist of a myotomy 180 degrees opposite the perforation repair site. If gastroesophageal reflux is present, an antireflux procedure should accompany the esophageal repair. A Belsey repair is preferred for thoracic perforation and a Nissen for abdominal perforation. The stomach wrap is then used as the tissue for external reinforcement.

Drainage alone is reserved for small cervical perforations. Drainage alone is usually unacceptable in thoracic perforation, because continued contamination is not prevented. Irrigation and drainage of a perforation diagnosed late after primary closure can also be performed. Precise chest tube placement at the site of perforation is established at operation after débridement. The perforation can be irrigated with saline solution either continuously through a nasogastric tube or by frequent oral saline intake. As the chest tube output diminishes, the chest tubes are advanced and eventually removed. The late diagnosis of a thoracic perforation can also lead to the development of an obvious fistula to the pleural cavity. The use of T-tube drainage can be performed, which would create a controlled esophagocutaneous fistula that should eventually heal if no distal obstruction is present.

Resection is reserved for massive necrosis or malignant obstruction. Resection eliminates the perforation as a source of sepsis, as well as removing the underlying esophageal disease and provides alimentary continuity; however, resection requires some form of anastomosis in a contaminated field. Transhiatal esophagectomy has been recommended as the method of resection after perforation. Transhiatal esophagectomy has the advantage of achieving anastomosis in the neck, far removed from the area of contamination, thus avoiding necrotic tissue and a perianastomotic infection. On rare occasions with severe contamination, resection without reanastomosis with cervical end-esophagostomy and closure of the distal gastroesophageal junction may be necessary to completely defunctionalize the area; this is a very radical procedure that subjects the patient to a long, difficult postoperative course and thus is used very selectively.

Multiple techniques have been described for repair of an esophageal perforation. The treatment principles are the same regardless of the technique chosen. These principles include primary closure of the perforation (even if it has existed for more than 24 hours), wide drainage of the proximal and distal esophagus to prevent further contamination, reinforcement of the repair, and placement of access for enteral nutrition.

OUTCOME

The cause and location of the perforation, delay in diagnosis and treatment, the method of treatment, and the underlying esophageal disease all affect the outcome of patients with esophageal perforation. Iatrogenic and instrumental injuries are associated with a mortality of 10% to 20%, whereas spontaneous perforation carries a mortality rate of 30% to 40%. Traumatic perforations of the esophagus have a somewhat lower mortality (less than 10%), probably related to the decreased time interval between perforation and treatment in the acute setting of multiple injuries. The overall mortality of a cervical perforation is 6% compared with 29% and 34% for abdominal and thoracic perforations, respectively. The mortality of cervical perforation is less because of the well-contained fascial compartments within the neck, which

---

Pearls and Pitfalls

- Early recognition and treatment of esophageal perforation require a high index of suspicion.
- Successful outcome depends on early diagnosis and early aggressive treatment.
- Signs and symptoms of esophageal perforation are pain, fever, and mediastinal or subcutaneous air.
- Spontaneous esophageal perforation (Boerhaave's syndrome) should be suspected when chest or esophageal pain, fever, and a left pleural effusion follow an episode of vomiting or retching.
- Repair of esophageal perforation depends on site of perforation, delay to time of treatment, local conditions, and the presence or absence of an underlying esophageal disorder.
- Cervical perforations are usually best treated with simple drainage.
- Intrathoracic perforations may be repaired primarily, with the suture line reinforced externally by autogenous tissue flaps.
- When an obstructing lesion, cancer, or achalasia is present, either esophageal resection or relief of the distal obstruction (e.g., stent or myotomy) is required.

prevent infectious spread; also, the absence of reflux of gastric content into the cervical esophagus reduces contamination.

Timely recognition and initiation of treatment have long been recognized as essential to a favorable outcome. Delay in treatment of esophageal perforation more than 24 hours leads to a marked increase in complications and the risk of death. If treatment is initiated within the first 24 hours after perforation, the mortality is 15%, whereas treatment started more than 24 hours after injury bears a 33% mortality. Basing a treatment plan on the interval between perforation and presentation has also been associated with reduction in mortality. Clearly, a gravely ill patient with overwhelming sepsis fares worse no matter what treatment is given. However, the influence of treatment delay continues to decrease because of improvements in critical care, antibiotic therapy, and nutritional support.

Primary repair, which is usually performed on patients in the best of conditions, has the best overall results. Patients who undergo drainage alone, esophagectomy, or exclusion and diversion have higher mortality rates. Nonoperative treatment has a mortality of approximately 20%. This mortality is higher than that of primary repair.

CONCLUSION

A high index of suspicion that leads to early diagnosis and intervention produces the best results in treatment of esophageal perforation. Operative treatment should include primary repair, reinforcement, and elimination of distal obstruction. Nonoperative therapy is usually reserved for patients who experience iatrogenic instrument perforation and consists of broad-spectrum antibiotics and nutritional support. Surgeons who treat esophageal perforation must be knowledgeable about all therapeutic options. No single approach is always correct in dealing with this devastating injury.

SELECTED READINGS

Bladergroen MR, Lowe JE, Postlethwait RW: Diagnosis and recommended management of esophageal perforation and rupture. Ann Thoracic Surg 1986;42:235.

Buecker A, Wein BB, Neurerburg JM, Guenther RW: Esophageal perforation: Comparison of use of aqueous and barium-containing contrast media. Radiology 1997;202:683.

Gouge TH, Depan HJ, Spencer FC: Experience with the Grillo pleural wrap flap in 18 patients with perforation of the thoracic esophagus. Ann Surg 1989;209:612.

Jones WG, Ginsberg RJ: Esophageal perforation: A continuing challenge. Ann Thorac Surg 1992;53:534.

Michel L, Grillo HC, Malt RA: Operative and non-operative management of esophageal perforation. Ann Surg 1981;194:57.

Sarr MD, Pemberton JH, Payne WS: Management of instrumental perforations of the esophagus. J Thorac Cardiovasc Surg 1982;84:211.

Walker WS, Cameron EW, Walbaum PR: Diagnosis and management of spontaneous transmural rupture of the oesophagus (Boerhaave's syndrome). Br J Surg 1985;72:204.

Chapter 48

Esophageal Diverticula

Douglas E. Wood

An esophageal diverticulum is an outpouching of the esophageal wall beyond the true lumen. Food and secretions collect in these diverticula, which can lead to regurgitation and aspiration as well as dysphagia due to compression of the true lumen or due to the underlying esophageal motility disorder. Esophageal diverticula are rare, accounting for only 2% to 3% of patients presenting with dysphagia and are discovered in fewer than 1% of esophagograms.

Esophageal diverticula have been classified by etiology, anatomic structure, time of formation, and anatomic location. Although congenital diverticula have been identified in infants and children, the majority of diverticula are acquired and occur in adults older than 50 years of age. Acquired esophageal diverticula can be classified as traction or pulsion diverticula, based on the pathogenesis. Traction diverticula result from granulomatous inflammation of mediastinal lymph nodes that subsequently involve the adjacent esophageal wall. As acute inflammation resolves, contracting scar may then form a full-thickness outpouching of the esophageal wall. Traction diverticula are commonly found at the tracheal bifurcation and mainstem bronchi. They rarely cause symptoms, and so they require no therapy and can simply be considered a sign of healed mediastinal granulomatous infection. The only exception is when ongoing infection results in fistula to a bronchus, great vessel, or pericardium.

Pulsion diverticula involve outpouchings of mucosa and submucosa that arise from conditions associated with increases in intraluminal pressure. These typically occur proximal to an area of functional obstruction, most commonly just proximal to the location of the upper or lower esophageal sphincter. Peristalsis proximal to an unrelaxing sphincter produces high intraesophageal pressure, expanding the esophageal mucosa proximal to the area of functional obstruction and usually in areas of muscular weakness or blood vessels perforating the musculature, as with colonic diverticulitis.

Diverticula are sometimes classified as false or true diverticula, based on the presence or absence of the muscular layer. Pulsion diverticula are typically false diverticula, consisting of only mucosa and submucosa without the muscular layers. In contrast, traction diverticula are typically full-thickness outpouchings, or true diverticula. However, even "false" diverticula usually do have some component of the muscular layer intact, although usually thinned and splayed out as the diverticulum progresses. This classification has little real clinical utility and is of academic interest only.

The classification of esophageal diverticula by anatomic location is the most common and most clinically useful because etiology, evaluation, surgical treatment, and outcomes are similar within each anatomic category. The esophageal diverticula are generally divided into four groups and include the pharyngoesophageal (Zenker's) diverticula, midesophageal diverticula, epiphrenic diverticula, and intramural pseudodiverticulosis.

PHARYNGOESOPHAGEAL (ZENKER'S) DIVERTICULA

Pharyngoesophageal, or Zenker's, diverticula occur when the hypopharyngeal mucosa protrudes between the oblique fibers of the inferior pharyngeal constrictor and the transverse fibers of the cricopharyngeus muscles. Various theories about the pathogenesis of Zenker's diverticulum have mostly emphasized the lack of coordination between pharyngeal contraction and relaxation of the upper esophageal sphincter (UES). Functional obstruction occurs owing to UES spasm, failure of UES relaxation, or delayed UES relaxation. Each of these motor abnormalities results in pressure being exerted by the pharyngeal bolus, where the esophageal wall is weakest, i.e. between the inferior pharyngeal constrictors and the transverse fibers of the cricopharyngeus muscle. Although several studies have provided cineradiographic and manometric evidence of UES dysfunction, other studies in patients with Zenker's diverticulum have been unable to demonstrate evidence of dysfunction. Although the pathophysiology is unproven, there is general agreement that such a functional disturbance of the UES is the most likely etiology in the formation of pharyngoesophageal diverticula.

Clinical Presentation

Many patients with Zenker's diverticula are asymptomatic, and the abnormality is noted incidentally during an esophagogram. Signs and symptoms of Zenker's diverticula are frequently subtle but progressive. In early stages, patients may complain of a vague sensation or "sticking" in their throat. Patients may also have excessive salivation, intermittent dysphagia, or a paroxysmal cough. As the diverticular sac enlarges, spontaneous regurgitation of retained food can occur—a highly specific symptom of Zenker's diverticulum. Other signs and symptoms can be halitosis, gurgling sounds during swallowing, voice change, a sense of a neck mass, low cervical or retrosternal pain, dysphagia, or airway obstruction from progressive enlargement of the diverticulum. Patients with dysphagia may develop elaborate maneuvers for facilitating both swallowing and emptying of the diverticulum, including clearing the throat, placing pressure on the neck, or coughing. The most serious complication of Zenker's diverticulum is aspiration, usually manifested by coughing, choking, or wheezing. This complication frequently occurs with the patient in the recumbent position and may cause the patient to awaken at night with respiratory distress. At this stage, patients may present with aspiration pneumonitis or lung abscess.

The vague findings of an early Zenker's diverticulum are nonspecific, allowing the consideration of a wide variety of head and neck and upper esophageal pathologies. However, the classic signs and symptoms of dysphagia and regurgitation are unique for an esophageal diverticulum. Other potential diagnoses include midesophageal or epiphrenic diverticula, achalasia, esophageal carcinoma, and gastroesophageal reflux disease. However, these potential diagnoses can be readily differentiated with a contrast-enhanced esophagogram.

In most patients, a barium esophagogram is the only study necessary in confirming the presence of Zenker's diverticulum, eliminating other diagnoses, and providing anatomic and functional information necessary prior to consideration of surgery. Very early Zenker's diverticula are small and transient and may be captured only on cinepharyngoesophagogram. Most symptomatic diverticula are readily identified on a standard barium-enhanced esophagogram. The origin of these diverticula are posterior and require lateral projections for identifying the neck of the diverticula. Although the diverticular neck commonly lies at the C6–7 level, a large sac may develop inferiorly and laterally, so anteroposterior views of the esophagogram are necessary in confirming the size and extent of the diverticular sac. The esophagogram performed in the evaluation of Zenker's diverticulum should also confirm the presence of a persistent cricopharyngeal bar, which represents the incompletely relaxed or hypertrophied cricopharyngeal muscle. The cinepharyngoesophagogram is helpful in excluding concomitant oropharyngeal dysfunction. The esophagogram should also evaluate the remainder of the esophagus for signs of other esophageal pathology. Other causes of dysphagia, such as esophageal carcinoma or esophageal dysmotility, should be excluded.

Preoperative Management

With a diagnosis of Zenker's diverticulum established by esophagogram, further evaluation is not usually required. Computed tomography and magnetic resonance imaging are generally not indicated. Endoscopic examination is unnecessary except in patients with suspected malignancy, as it does not refine the diagnosis, improve the anatomic detail, or improve information crucial for planning for surgery. In fact, endoscopic examination may be hazardous owing to the risk of perforation. If endoscopy is necessary for examination of other upper gastrointestinal pathology, the esophagus should be intubated with the use of direct visualization with avoidance of forceful manipulation of the endoscope. Sometimes, endoscopy may require fluoroscopy to ensure passage of the endoscope into the true lumen. Similarly, manometric testing is of little value in the management of patients with Zenker's diverticula. Manometry may be difficult to perform, since the catheter may tend to coil in the diverticulum. Careful study of the UES may provide confirmatory data on the

pathogenesis of Zenker's diverticulum, but since it does not change the clinical management it should be predominantly for clinical research. The assessment of other suspected disorders, such as gastroesophageal reflux disease (GERD), with manometry, 24-hour pH studies, and esophagoscopy, is usually reserved until after surgical correction of Zenker's diverticulum.

Surgical correction of Zenker's diverticulum is a cervical or endoscopic procedure. The physiologic consequences of surgery are relatively minor and do not require extensive preoperative preparation or cardiopulmonary evaluation. Some patients that have had progressive dysphagia may have an associated weight loss. In most patients, it is preferable to proceed to surgical correction to restore the dysphagia and normal oral nutrition, rather than delaying surgery. The rare nutritionally debilitated patient can have his or her condition optimized for surgery with enteral alimentation. Patients with the aspiration complications of pneumonia or lung abscess should not be operated on urgently but, instead, should be treated with appropriate antibiotics until their pulmonary infection is controlled, allowing for safer elective surgical correction of the diverticulum.

Operative Management

There are five methods of surgical correction of Zenker's diverticulum: (1) diverticulectomy, (2) cricopharyngeal myotomy, (3) diverticulectomy with cricopharyngeal myotomy, (4) suspension of the diverticulum (diverticulopexy) with cricopharyngeal myotomy, and (5) endoscopic diverticulotomy.

Diverticulectomy has been the most commonly employed surgical procedure. A large surgical series from the Mayo Clinic had a 1% mortality, 5% morbidity, and a 93% effective control of signs and symptoms with diverticulectomy alone. Other authors have shown a high radiologic and symptomatic recurrence in patients treated with diverticulectomy alone. Although unproven, functional obstruction due to dysmotility or uncoordinated relaxation of the upper esophageal sphincter appears as the most probable etiology of Zenker's diverticulum, creating increased pressure in the hypopharynx during passage of a food bolus. This assumption has led most investigators to agree that UES myotomy is essential in the treatment of Zenker's diverticulum. The surgical principles of the other four techniques in use today for the treatment of Zenker's diverticulum are (1) relief of functional obstruction at the UES by cricopharyngeal myotomy and (2) prevention of food retention in a dependent diverticulum.

A cricopharyngeal myotomy may be chosen as the only therapy for the very small but symptomatic Zenker's diverticulum. Myotomy of the UES treats the underlying etiology and decreases the resistance to food passage from the pharynx into the esophagus. A myotomy alone has the advantages of avoiding a mucosal suture line, allowing rapid restoration of feeding and a shorter hospital stay. However, this is only useful for a small (less than 1 cm) diverticulum, where myotomy prevents continued growth of the diverticulum. The diverticulum must be broad-based and must not lead to persistent difficulties in food retention. Cricopharyngeal myotomy should be accompanied by a procedure to resect or suspend the diverticulum in patients with larger diverticula.

Diverticulectomy removes the redundant mucosal pouch that results in food retention and persistent signs and symptoms even after cricopharyngeal myotomy. Diverticulectomy has the advantages of restoration of the normal anatomic contours of the hypopharynx and proximal esophagus. However, this is at the cost of a suture line with its attendant risk of suture-line leak and fistula formation.

Some authors have recommended suspension of the diverticulum, or diverticulopexy, as an alternative to diverticulectomy. Diverticulopexy consists of suspending and fixing the sac to the prevertebral fascia so that the diverticulum is no longer dependent. Cricopharyngeal myotomy is always performed in association with diverticulopexy. The advantages of diverticulopexy relate to the theoretical decreased morbidity due to the avoidance of a mucosal suture line and the attendant suture line complications. Proponents of diverticulopexy believe that one can resume oral feeding sooner with a decreased hospital stay compared with patients undergoing diverticulectomy. However, comparison of myotomy and diverticulectomy versus myotomy and diverticulopexy have shown equally good clinical outcomes and a similar incidence of complications; fistula formation still occurs in 2% of patients undergoing either procedure. Most authors would only consider diverticulopexy for the small (1 to 4 cm) diverticulum and prefer diverticulectomy for large (more than 4 cm) Zenker's diverticulum.

Diverticulectomy, diverticulopexy, and cricopharyngeal myotomy all are performed through the same surgical field, most commonly with the patient under general anesthesia. The patient is placed in a supine position with the head hyperextended and turned to the right for the standard left cervical approach. An 8- to 10-cm incision is made along the anterior border of the left sternocleidomastoid muscle, centered at the level of the cricoid cartilage. The omohyoid muscle is divided, and the dissection carried medial to the carotid sheath and deepened to the level of the prevertebral fascia. The larynx is retracted medially and rotated to expose the posterior aspect of the hypopharynx. Care is taken during the dissection to prevent injury to the recurrent laryngeal nerve lying within the tracheoesophageal groove. The diverticulum will often be seen as a bulge at or below the level of the cricoid cartilage and should be grasped and dissected free from the overlying cricopharyngeal muscle and soft tissues to expose the diverticular neck. After mobilization of the diverticulum, a 40- to 45-French bougie should be placed carefully—the surgeon guiding it into the distal esophagus—which will prevent narrowing of the lumen during diverticulectomy and also provide some structural rigidity and muscular tension to aid in the performance of the myotomy. The myotomy is typically carried out posteriorly, with the cephalad extent beginning at the inferior margin of the diverticular neck. The myotomy is extended distally through approximately 2 cm of hypopharyngeal muscle and through the cricopharyngeus at the UES, ending in the cervical esophagus approximately

2 cm below the cricoid cartilage, and should measure approximately 6 cm in length. The myotomy should allow visualization of the underlying mucosa from the diverticular neck to the proximal esophagus. Other authors prefer a lateral myotomy that allows a posterior muscular closure after the diverticulectomy. The extent of lateral myotomy should be identical to the more common posterior myotomy.

For small (1 to 4 cm) diverticula, a diverticulopexy may be considered. This procedure requires full mobilization of the diverticular sac, with the tip of the diverticulum suspended to the posterior pharyngeal wall or prevertebral fascia. Placement of suspending sutures should not be full thickness, so that fistula formation can be avoided. If a diverticulectomy is preferred, the neck of the diverticulum is either stapled with a linear stapler or transected and oversewn with inverting interrupted sutures. The indwelling bougie helps prevent narrowing of the lumen during closure. If a lateral myotomy has been performed, the posterior pharyngeal muscle can be closed over the mucosal suture line as reinforcement. However, in the more common scenario of a posterior myotomy, the posterior pharyngeal muscle should not be closed as it may re-create the functional obstruction corrected by cricopharyngeal myotomy. Some authors test the mucosal integrity of their closure with 50 mL of air injected through a nasoesophageal tube positioned at the level of the diverticulectomy. Although suction drainage may be employed, this has not been shown to have a clear benefit over closure in the absence of external drainage.

In the 1950s, Dohlman described an endoscopic technique for management of Zenker's diverticulum that involved cautery division of the wall between the diverticulum and the esophagus. This approach created both an extensive diverticulotomy in which the dependent portion of the diverticulum was continuous with the body of the esophagus and a concomitant cricopharyngeal myotomy, thereby accomplishing the two surgical principles required in the management of Zenker's diverticulum. Development of the endoscopic surgical staplers has improved this technique, producing an esophagodiverticulostomy with stapled edges that reduces the risks of cervical or mediastinal contamination.

The endoscopic diverticulotomy procedure is performed with the patient under general anesthesia with endotracheal intubation. The patient is positioned supine with the neck hyperextended and the surgeon sitting behind the patient's head. The Weerda distending diverticuloscope (Karl Storz, Tuttlingen, Germany) is introduced with the upper blade of the double-lipped diverticuloscope in the esophageal lumen and the lower blade in the diverticulum. A laryngoscope holder is utilized to hold the diverticuloscope in place, and a zero-degree telescope provides a magnified vision of the operative field on a video monitor. Retained food and secretions are evacuated, the mucosa examined, and the depth of the diverticulum measured with a graduated rod. An endoscopic linear stapler is placed along the midline and positioned across the septum between the diverticulum and the esophageal lumen. The diverticulum must be completely opened to avoid any dependent portions, which may require multiple applications of the endoscopic stapler. A modification of the stapler providing a shorter anvil allows tissue stapling and division to the end of the staple line. Alternatively, endoscopic scissors may be used to complete the division to the end of the staple line in order to prevent a small redundant pocket for food retention in this location. The advantages of this procedure are obvious: it is a minimally invasive approach that allows for an early return to oral feeding, short operative time, and shorter hospital stay. Although results have been encouraging, experience with this technique is limited, in terms of both the number of surgeons experienced with this technique and publications defining its efficacy and long-term outcomes.

Postoperative Management

Patients are treated with parenteral or oral analgesics as needed. A nasogastric tube and surgical drain are not needed. Oral liquids can be resumed on the first postoperative day and the patient discharged on the second or third postoperative day with a pureed or soft mechanical diet. Patients can then resume a regular diet after 7 to 10 days with no special dietary restrictions. No routine postoperative radiographs or laboratory studies are needed, although some surgeons prefer an early follow-up esophagogram to either confirm the adequacy of the surgical correction or to exclude early fistula formation. Certainly, an esophagogram is necessary in the presence of localized or systemic signs of infection. Likewise, follow-up manometry or esophagoscopy is not needed, except as part of the clinical research protocol or to evaluate other suspected pathology.

Complications

Complications of Zenker's diverticulum roughly fall in three categories: preoperative complications, early operative morbidity, and late postoperative morbidity. Preoperative complications consist primarily of the sequelae of food retention with regurgitation and aspiration. Aspiration can produce recurrent pulmonary infections and lung abscess. Dysphagia from the mass effect of the diverticulum may result in weight loss and malnutrition. Perforation may occur as a complication of the diverticulum, most commonly during iatrogenic manipulation, particularly when the presence of the diverticulum is unknown. Ulceration, bleeding, and carcinoma can also occur as complications of Zenker's diverticulum.

The complications of the open techniques for correction of Zenker's diverticulum consist of vocal cord paralysis (3%), wound infection (3%), and fistula (2%); operative mortality is 1%. Both morbidity and operative mortality are substantially increased after reoperative procedures for recurrent Zenker's diverticulum. Operative complications of the endoscopic treatment consist predominantly of an esophageal leak from the esophagodiverticulostomy.

Late complications result predominantly in incomplete correction or recurrence of Zenker's diverticulum and are discussed in the following section on outcomes.

Outcomes

A cricopharyngeal myotomy results in a satisfactory outcome in only 70% to 80% of patients and therefore should be reserved for the very small symptomatic diverticulum with no dependent portion remaining after myotomy. Cricopharyngeal myotomy combined with diverticulectomy or diverticulopexy result in 93% to 96% good to excellent results. Similar results are obtained with endoscopic esophagodiverticulotomy; approximately 5% of patients require reoperation, usually because of a small residual diverticular pouch. GERD is commonly associated with Zenker's diverticulum; cricopharyngeal myotomy of the UES may worsen the symptoms of GERD. In this instance, further medical or surgical management of the patient's reflux disease may be warranted.

MIDESOPHAGEAL DIVERTICULA

Midesophageal diverticula are found in the middle third of the esophagus, usually near the tracheal bifurcation. They are uncommon and frequently asymptomatic, and so the true prevalence is unclear. They account for approximately 10% of all esophageal diverticula. Most patients have abnormal peristaltic waves arising from a motility disorder, such as achalasia, diffuse esophageal spasm, or other nonspecific esophageal motility disorders. Functional obstruction with a high-pressure zone is considered as primary etiology in the formation of a midthoracic esophageal diverticulum. Symptomatic patients present with complaints of dysphagia, belching, regurgitation, retrosternal or epigastric pain, heartburn, or weight loss. These symptoms may be attributed to the diverticulum but may also be related to the underlying motility disorder. The complications are unusual and consist of ulceration with bleeding or perforation, aspiration, esophagorespiratory fistula, and carcinoma.

Clinical Presentation

Midesophageal diverticula are usually diagnosed incidentally during a contrast-enhanced esophagogram obtained for the evaluation of nonspecific symptoms. A contrast-enhanced esophagogram may also reveal the presence of an associated motility disorder. Esophageal manometry is useful in the evaluation of midesophageal diverticula to allow definition of the associated motility abnormality. However, manometry may be difficult, owing to an inability to pass the manometry catheter past the diverticulum. Esophagoscopy generally provides no useful information regarding the diverticulum but may be helpful in assessing associated esophageal abnormalities. Chest computed tomography is not indicated in the evaluation of these diverticula, but they may be important in assessing periesophageal and mediastinal abnormalities if a traction diverticula is suspected. Asymptomatic patients do not generally require surgical intervention, but the presence of signs and symptoms indicates operative repair.

Operative Management

The principles of surgical correction for esophageal diverticula are twofold: resection of the diverticulum and distal esophageal myotomy. A right thoracotomy is the preferred approach, providing wide access to the middle third of the esophagus without interference by the aortic arch. The majority of midesophageal diverticula lie posterior and displaced to the right, but a right-sided approach is optimal even for left-sided diverticula. After dissecting the diverticulum to the diverticular neck, a 40- to 45-French esophageal bougie is placed, and a diverticulectomy performed. The esophageal mucosa of the diverticular neck is closed with a linear stapler or sutured with either running or interrupted suture, and the muscular layer is reapproximated over the mucosal repair. This two-layer closure may be buttressed with pleura, pericardial fat, or intercostal muscle, but this maneuver is not necessary in the uncomplicated operation. The esophagus is rotated 180 degrees and a contralateral esophageal myotomy performed from the upper level of the diverticulum distally, generally extending to the gastroesophageal junction or as preoperative manometry indicates. This procedure can also be performed with video-assisted thoracoscopy (VATS). The same principles are applied in achieving a satisfactory surgical outcome. The thoracoscope approach should be performed by surgeons with experience in other minimally invasive esophageal procedures, such as thoracoscope-assisted esophagectomy, resection of esophageal leiomyoma, or Heller myotomy.

Postoperative Management

Patients are mobilized early after surgery with aggressive ambulation and pulmonary toilet, as in other post-thoracotomy patients. A nasogastric tube is optional, and the chest drain may be removed by postoperative day 2 or 3 and patients started on a liquid diet. The diet is advanced to a soft mechanical diet over 1 to 2 days, with the patient discharged 5 to 7 days postoperatively. Contrast-enhanced esophagogram is not necessary postoperatively, but it may be employed by some surgeons to exclude early occult suture line leak before progression of oral diet or patient discharge.

Complications

The rarity of midesophageal diverticula requiring surgical treatment means that few data exist regarding the incidence of postoperative complications. Complications consist of esophageal leak, with resulting mediastinitis, as well as post-thoracotomy pulmonary complications. Surgical mortality has been variably reported to range from 0 to 9%. In general, multiple reports have documented minimal morbidity and mortality with excellent short- and long-term outcomes.

EPIPHRENIC DIVERTICULUM

Epiphrenic diverticula are located in the distal 10 cm of the esophagus, typically 4 to 8 cm above the cardia. These make up the majority of diverticula below the UES. They usually project from the right posterior wall of the esophagus. As with other esophageal diverticula, esopha-

geal motility disorders are commonly associated, consisting of a hypertensive UES, diffuse esophageal spasm, achalasia, or nonspecific motility disorders. The pathogenesis is similar to that of the other esophageal diverticula in which functional obstruction leads to an area of increased intraluminal pressure through which outpouchings may occur and then develop into a diverticulum. Reflux esophagitis may also be associated and may be a factor in the pathogenesis of the condition, owing to the associated motor abnormalities.

Clinical Presentation

The most frequent symptoms in patients with an epiphrenic diverticulum are dysphagia, regurgitation, and chest pain. It is often difficult to determine whether signs and symptoms are related to the diverticulum itself or are due to the underlying esophageal motility disorder. Regurgitation is precipitated by a change in position, commonly occurring at night, and is frequently of large volume. As in other diverticula, pulmonary complications from aspiration can occur, but they are less frequent than in patients with Zenker's diverticulum. Local complications of ulceration with bleeding or perforation, distal esophageal obstruction, a diverticular phlegmon or bezoar, and carcinoma all are rare. The diagnosis of an epiphrenic diverticulum is typically established with the use of a contrast-enhanced esophagogram revealing the diverticulum in the distal esophagus. A large size of or low origin of the neck of the diverticulum may make it difficult to differentiate an epiphrenic diverticulum from an esophageal ulcer or gastric volvulus. However, careful examination of the contrast-enhanced esophagogram can usually distinguish between these diagnoses.

Preoperative Management

Esophageal manometry is necessary in establishing and defining the expected esophageal motility disorder. Esophagoscopy is not a requirement in the work-up except to evaluate other potential esophageal pathology. Computed tomography provides no useful information in a work-up of these patients in the absence of complications. Asymptomatic patients do not require surgical intervention, but diverticulectomy with esophageal myotomy should be performed in patients with signs or symptoms or complications of their diverticulum.

Operative Management

During anesthetic induction, careful attention must be paid to the avoidance of regurgitation of retained diverticular contents. A low left-lateral thoracotomy is the preferred approach for optimal exposure of the distal esophagus and esophagogastric junction. This approach also provides good exposure for a long esophageal myotomy up to the level of the aortic arch if indicated. Simple diverticulectomy has been associated with high recurrence as well as significant morbidity and mortality, and so the same principles of diverticulectomy combined with distal myotomy apply in the surgical correction of epiphrenic diverticula. With the diverticulum dissected to its neck, a 40- to 45-French bougie is placed in the esophageal lumen to aid in the myotomy and to prevent narrowing of the esophageal lumen. The diverticular sac is excised with the use of a linear surgical stapler or a handsewn technique of running or interrupted sutures, with closure of the neck of the diverticulum. The esophageal muscle is then reapproximated over the mucosal repair, and, if desired, the suture line can be buttressed with a pedicled flap or adjacent pleura. A myotomy should be performed from the level of the diverticular resection across the lower esophageal sphincter (LES) to the gastric muscularis. If there is a more proximal motor disorder, a long esophageal myotomy should be performed up to the level of the aortic arch. The myotomy is placed 180 degrees opposite the side of the diverticular suture line.

Myotomy of the LES may exacerbate pre-existing GERD or result in new reflux symptoms that did not previously exist. Because of this possibility, many authors recommend the routine addition of an antireflux procedure using a partial wrap, such as a Belsey Mark IV procedure. A circumferential antireflux procedure, such as a Nissen fundoplication, is contraindicated because of the associated esophageal motor disorder. Several other authors do not employ a routine antireflux procedure, preferring to medically manage reflux signs and symptoms and avoid any component of obstruction at the gastroesophageal junction. This is an area of significant controversy for which no compelling data exist to advise surgeons toward or away from an antireflux procedure after epiphrenic diverticulectomy and myotomy.

Video-assisted, minimally invasive treatment of an epiphrenic diverticulum may be approached from the thoracoscopic or the laparoscopic angle. The laparoscopic approach positions the ports as for a laparoscopic Nissen fundoplication, with circumferential dissection and downward traction of the intra-abdominal esophagus providing exposure to the distal esophagus in the mediastinum, including the epiphrenic diverticulum. A left thoracoscopic approach follows the same details of the open procedure. A laparoscopic or thoracoscopic antireflux procedure utilizes the same indications and reservations as those described for the open approach.

Postoperative Management

Postoperative management follows the same details as those described for the management of a midesophageal diverticulum with regard to the management of tubes as well as the resumption of oral feeding and avoidance of post-thoracotomy complications.

Complications and Outcomes

The complications and outcomes of epiphrenic repair are similar to those described previously for midesophageal diverticula. Although few results have been reported in the minimally invasive approaches, early reports are favorable, and it is anticipated that the outcomes should be similar to open procedures as long as the principles of surgical correction are followed.

ESOPHAGEAL INTRAMURAL PSEUDODIVERTICULOSIS

Diffuse intramural diverticulosis is a rare condition characterized by multiple minute, flask-shaped outpouchings of the esophagus. The pseudodiverticula are dilated excretory ducts of esophageal submucous glands. Multiple factors have been postulated regarding the etiology and pathogenesis of this disorder, but most authors believe that this is an acquired abnormality representing a chronic inflammatory process involving the ducts of the submucosal glands. The most common symptom is dysphagia, and as many as a quarter of these patients may have an episode of food impaction. Esophageal stricture and a variety of other esophageal conditions are associated with intramural diverticulosis. The diagnosis is established by contrast-enhanced esophagogram, which reveals multiple flask-shaped outpouchings that vary from 1 to 5 mm in depth. These lie perpendicular or oblique to the longitudinal axis of the esophagus. Approximately 50% of the patients have a segmental distribution, with the remaining others involving the esophagus diffusely. The major differential diagnostic consideration is esophageal candidiasis. Although endoscopy usually cannot identify the pseudodiverticula, it is frequently useful in evaluating associated strictures and excluding candidiasis or esophageal cancer. Esophageal manometry is not helpful in the diagnosis or management of intramural diverticulosis. Esophageal dilatation is employed for strictures associated with this condition, which in the majority of patients remains stable over a long period of time, with a third of the patients having reduction or disappearance of their pseudodiverticula.

Pearls and Pitfalls

- No symptoms—no surgery
- Frail, debilitated, and elderly patients with signs and symptoms need definitive surgical correction, not medical management
- Exercise extreme caution during esophagoscopy to avoid perforation
- Correct the cause, not just the symptoms—documented or occult motility disorders are the prevailing pathogenesis and require myotomy
- Principles of surgical correction: myotomy to correct functional obstruction; prevention of food retention by diverticulectomy, diverticulopexy, or diverticulotomy
- Avoid an iatrogenic stricture, close mucosa over an esophageal bougie
- Close suture line of diverticular neck with two layers, mucosa and muscle, with myotomy on the opposite side
- Without a myotomy, the complications of leak and recurrence are high
- Avoid the vagus
- No circumferential wrap when an antireflux procedure is performed

CONCLUSION

Most esophageal diverticula are acquired and occur in middle-aged and elderly adults. Diverticula are generally found at or above esophageal sphincters and have an underlying motility disorder as their primary cause. Signs and symptoms and complications increase as the diverticulum enlarges and may be difficult to distinguish from the signs and symptoms related to the underlying motility disorder. Contrast-enhanced esophagography provides the most definitive diagnosis, and esophageal manometry is used to define associated motility disorders. Esophagoscopy is not useful except as needed to exclude other esophageal pathology. The principles of surgical treatment are the same in any location: correction of distal functional obstruction by esophageal myotomy and correction of the dependent diverticulum, usually by diverticulectomy, although diverticular suspension is an acceptable alternative. Endoscopic approaches to Zenker's diverticulum and minimally invasive approaches to midesophageal

and epiphrenic diverticula show promise in obtaining outcomes similar to those that have been obtained by open procedures, with minimal morbidity and good long-term results in restoring the normal swallowing mechanism.

SELECTED READINGS

Brouillette D, Martel E, Chen LQ, et al: Pitfalls and complications of cricopharyngeal myotomy. Chest Surg Clin North Am 1997;7:457.
Eubanks TR, Pellegrini CA: Minimally invasive treatment of esophageal diverticula. Semin Thorac Cardiovasc Surg 1999;11:363.
Fulp SR: Esophageal diverticula. In Castell DO (ed): The Esophagus. Boston, Little, Brown, 1992, pp 351–366.
Narne S, Cutrone C, Chella B, et al: Endoscopic diverticulotomy for the treatment of Zenker's diverticulum: Results in 102 patients with staple-assisted endoscopy. Ann Otol Rhinol Laryngol 1999;108:810.
Payne WS, King RM: Pharyngoesophageal (Zenker's) diverticulum. Surg Clin North Am 1983;63:815.
Payne WS, Reynolds RR: Surgical treatment of pharyngoesophageal diverticulum (Zenker's) diverticulum. Surg Rounds 1982;5:18.
Rice TW, Baker ME: Midthoracic esophageal diverticula. Semin Thorac Cardiovasc Surg 1999;11:352.
Sideris L, Chen LQ, Ferraro P, Duranceau AC: The treatment of Zenker's diverticula: A review. Semin Thorac Cardiovasc Surg 1999;11:337.

Esophagus and Paraesophageal Region: Malignant

Chapter 49
Esophageal Cancer: Transhiatal Resection
Richard F. Heitmiller

Esophageal carcinoma is an uncommon neoplasm accounting for approximately 5% of all gastrointestinal malignancies. Although uncommon, these tumors are aggressive and have a profound adverse effect on both quality of life and survival. For patients with localized disease, surgery remains the gold standard of therapy. Historically, several operative strategies using different incisional approaches have been devised for esophagectomy with proponents for each one. Experience has shown that regardless of the incisional approach, the morbidity, mortality, and postsurgical stage-matched survival rates are the same. Nonetheless, each surgical approach has unique advantages and drawbacks, and esophageal surgeons should be aware of these.

The overall incidence of esophageal cancer has increased only gradually over time. However, in the United States, Canada, and Western Europe, there has been a dramatic change in the prevalence of esophageal tumors by cell type, with adenocarcinoma replacing squamous cell carcinoma as the most common tumor cell type diagnosed. Whereas the predominance of patients with adenocarcinoma has not changed the established diagnostic and treatment principles or posttreatment outcome, it has changed the specific techniques available to work up and manage these neoplasms. Specifically regarding management, the acceptance and widespread use of

transhiatal esophagectomy (THE) has been directly linked to the surge in new cases of esophageal adenocarcinoma. In this chapter, the diagnosis and staging of esophageal cancer, and the indications, contraindications, technique, and results of THE are discussed.

DIAGNOSIS

The typical patient with esophageal carcinoma presents with a history of progressive solid food dysphagia and weight loss. The amount of weight loss often seems greater than would be expected for the degree of dysphagia reported. Less commonly, a patient may be seen with anemia, Hemoccult-positive stools, or hematemesis. Midscapular or lower chest pain not associated with swallowing is an ominous finding suggestive of mediastinal invasion. Onset of new respiratory symptoms including cough, hemoptysis, excess sputum production, or hoarseness may signal airway invasion, tracheoesophageal fistula, or recurrent laryngeal nerve invasion. New onset headache or focal neurologic symptoms may indicate brain metastases. Likewise, new bone or joint pains should alert the clinician to the possibility of bone metastases.

Adenocarcinoma of the esophagus presents at a mean age of 62 years. Patients have a prominent history of

341

hiatal hernia and gastroesophageal reflux, have a history of smoking in 71%, and are almost invariably white males. In a review of patients with adenocarcinoma from our institution, 99% were white, 1% were African American, 87% were male, and 13% were female. Squamous cell cancers present at a mean age of 63 years, and most patients have a history of smoking (91%). Also in our review, 60% of patients were male and 40% were female. The distribution between whites and African Americans was 63% and 37%, respectively.

If esophageal carcinoma is suspected on clinical grounds, then a barium esophagogram is the best initial screening test. It is safe, readily available, and relatively inexpensive. Radiographically, symptomatic esophageal cancer classically appears as an "apple core" lesion. Other radiographic findings include a noncircumferential polypoid mass, a segment of mucosal irregularity, or focal mucosal ulceration. Contrast studies can also identify associated esophageal pathology and provide an "overview" of the esophagus and stomach, which helps with planning surgical therapy.

Even if a classic-appearing lesion is identified on contrast esophagogram, esophagoscopy with biopsy is necessary to pathologically confirm the diagnosis. Given the safety of flexible esophagoscopy, many cases proceed directly to endoscopy without prior barium swallow if clinical symptoms suggest esophageal cancer. The combination of endoscopic biopsies and brushings for cytologic screening has a diagnostic accuracy of greater than 90%. In addition to establishing the diagnosis of cancer, the endoscopist should also determine the location of the tumor, its length, the extent (if any) to which the stomach is involved, and whether there is any associated esophageal pathology such as Barrett's epithelium.

Bronchoscopy is indicated for patients with esophageal tumors adjacent to the mainstem bronchi or trachea, especially if symptoms suggestive of airway invasion or fistula are present. Bronchoscopy is more sensitive than esophagoscopy at identifying tracheoesophageal fistulas, especially smaller ones. Patients in whom new onset hoarseness develops should have indirect laryngoscopy to determine the presence, side, and extent of vocal cord dysfunction.

STAGING

The goal of pretreatment staging is to determine the TNM (tumor, node, metastasis) status of the patient's tumor. Staging techniques and treatment options are closely linked in clinical practice. The aggressiveness with which a patient is evaluated for staging depends on which treatments are being considered. Surgery remains the gold standard treatment for patients with localized esophageal cancer. In the past, as long as a patient was a candidate for esophagectomy from a medical standpoint, the only staging necessary was to rule out tumors that were unresectable because of local invasion (T4) or metastatic (M1) disease. Differentiating between earlier stages of disease preoperatively was unnecessary. Accurate tumor staging was established upon review of the resected pathologic specimen. The introduction of new treatment options for esophageal cancer and the accumulating data

suggesting improved survival rates for patients with stage II and III esophageal tumors with neoadjuvant chemoradiation therapy protocols have made pretreatment staging essential in order to triage patients to appropriate treatment options. Evaluation of the available staging modalities for patients with esophageal neoplasia is an area of active clinical evaluation.

The optimal staging test is computed tomography (CT) of the chest and abdomen. Not only is it widely available, quick, and well tolerated by patients, but CT also visualizes the tumor location, screens for mediastinal tumor invasion, detects lymph node enlargement, and identifies metastatic disease. Esophageal cancer tends to metastasize in a site-specific fashion to the lung, liver, and celiac lymph nodes. All these sites are imaged on chest and abdominal CT. Whereas CT is accurate at identifying mediastinal invasion (T4 tumors) and metastatic disease (M1 tumors), it is notably inaccurate at differentiating T1–3 tumors and N0 versus N1 disease. Therefore, chest and abdominal CT is an excellent initial screening test that can reliably detect advanced staged disease in which palliative (usually nonoperative) therapy is indicated. Magnetic resonance imaging for staging of esophageal tumors is equivalent to CT at detecting T4 tumors and M1 disease but is poor at differentiating between earlier staged tumors. It offers no specific advantage over standard CT.

The gold standard screening test to determine T status is endoscopic ultrasonography (EUS). EUS is recommended for patients in whom T4 and M1 disease has been ruled out by prior CT. Accuracy of EUS T staging ranges from approximately 60% for T1 tumors to 98% for T4 tumors. Overstaging and understaging occur in 6% and 5% of patients, respectively. EUS is also used to assess regional nodal status. Periesophageal nodal size, shape, and internal nodal echo patterns are the criteria used to determine the probability of nodal metastatic disease. Numerous studies have shown a direct correlation between depth of mural tumor invasion (T stage) and the probability of nodal metastasis. More recently, ultrasound-guided transesophageal biopsy techniques permit cytologic documentation of nodal metastatic disease in many patients. Limitations of EUS are that it requires expensive, specialized equipment not available in many medical centers, the accuracy of the results is dependent on the operator's experience, and, in approximately 25% of patients, the examination is incomplete or cannot be performed for technical reasons. Nonetheless, in experienced hands, the T and N stages can be determined with an accuracy of approximately 90% and 80%, respectively.

The introduction of laparoscopic staging is directly related to the increasing numbers of patients with esophageal adenocarcinoma. Adenocarcinoma originates in the distal esophagus in the region of the esophagogastric junction. Therefore, the tumor and the regional lymph nodes are accessible to visual inspection and biopsy using standard laparoscopic techniques. Laparoscopic staging of esophageal adenocarcinoma has been compared with mediastinoscopic staging of non–small cell lung tumors. Accurate pathologic determination of regional nodal status is obtained. When added to EUS and CT, laparoscopy improves staging accuracy. Laparoscopic findings change patient management in 10% to 15% of patients. These results, however, only refer to laparoscopic staging of distal esophageal cancers (generally adenocarcinoma) and not the more proximal, intrathoracic cancers that are more likely squamous in origin.

Bone metastases, more common in adenocarcinoma than squamous cell tumors, are important, albeit infrequent, sites of early metastatic disease in patients with esophageal cancers. Although routine screening with bone scans for all patients is not recommended, a bone scan is indicated for symptomatic patients or for patients with an increased serum alkaline phosphatase.

Positron emission tomography (PET) is a new staging modality whose role in the workup of patients with esophageal cancer is currently under investigation. Most studies demonstrate that PET and CT have equivalent accuracy at imaging the primary tumor site and in identifying regional lymph nodal metastases. PET seems more accurate at detecting distant metastatic disease. Therefore, PET and CT appear to be complementary staging techniques with a combined accuracy that exceeds the staging accuracy of either study alone.

TREATMENT: TRANSHIATAL ESOPHAGECTOMY

Patients with metastatic esophageal cancer, regardless of cell type, have limited survival expectations, and treatment goals are palliative and usually nonoperative. For patients with localized disease, surgery remains the gold standard therapy. Lymphatic drainage from the esophagus is arbitrarily organized into three fields: cervical, thoracic, and abdominal. The standard operation used to resect an esophageal cancer includes resecting the involved portion of esophagus, the proximal stomach, and the regional lymph nodes (cervical, thoracic, or abdominal). The operative resection is therefore termed a partial, near-total, subtotal, or, simply, esophagogastrectomy with regional or *one-field* lymphadenectomy. Historically, several incisional strategies have been devised for esophagogastrectomy, including transhiatal resection, Ivor-Lewis approach (midline abdominal and right thoracotomy), multi-incision (midline abdominal, thoracotomy, cervical), and left thoracoabdominal. Each has its own proponents. Regardless of the incisional approach, virtually the same operative procedure is performed—an esophagogastrectomy with regional lymphadenectomy. It is not surprising, therefore, that the accumulated data document equivalent surgical morbidity and mortality rates, regardless of the incisional approach used, as long as the operative procedure is performed by an experienced operator. Similarly, numerous large reviews have shown that postoperative survival is not a function of surgical approach, but rather tumor stage. If the principle objectives of surgical resection (listed earlier) are fulfilled, then any of the incisional techniques may be used. Experience in esophageal surgery using all of the available esophagectomy techniques has made the author an advocate for the THE approach for reasons outlined later. It should be noted, however, that no single incisional technique is applicable to all patients with esophageal cancer. Esophageal surgeons should be comfortable with several approaches.

The first description of THE is credited to Denk in 1913, but it was not until 1933 that Grey-Turner successfully performed a THE in a 58-year-old coal miner with esophageal cancer. The resection and subsequent esophageal reconstruction were performed in a staged manner. Grey-Turner commented on a dissection plane immediately adjacent to the esophagus, which he termed the "esophageal bursa." Subsequently, the development of open thoracotomy techniques overshadowed the THE approach until the technique was popularized by Orringer in 1978. The following developments led to the current widespread acceptance of the THE technique:

1. Anatomic studies detailed the description of esophageal blood supply, demonstrating the basis for Grey-Turner's bloodless esophageal bursa and confirming the clinical observation that transhiatal esophageal dissection can be performed safely with minimal blood loss.
2. The stomach can be mobilized, based solely on the right gastroepiploic artery, and pulled up to the neck for anastomosis without ischemic necrosis.
3. The predominance of adenocarcinoma has led to the widespread application of the THE technique. Adenocarcinoma invariably arises in the lower esophagus near the esophagogastric junction. Therefore, transabdominal exposure permits tumor mobilization under direct vision as well as regional lymphatic dissection, both of which are required to fulfill the surgical principles of standard esophagectomy.
4. Esophageal anastomotic complications, most notably leaks, are more simply and safely managed in the cervical versus the thoracic location.
5. Finally, the functional result of using the stomach to reconstruct the resected esophagus when it is pulled up to the neck is excellent and applicable for patients with both benign and neoplastic esophageal diseases.

The safety of the THE approach is optimized if two conditions are met. The first is that the portion of intrathoracic esophagus to be removed "bluntly" is extrinsically normal. If this is not the case, the operating surgeon cannot reliably remain in the appropriate plane adjacent to the esophageal wall. Dissection outside of this paraesophageal plane risks significant bleeding or injury to adjacent mediastinal structures, such as azygous veins, aorta, and membranous portion of trachea. Distal esophageal tumors, usually adenocarcinomas, meet this condition. By widening the esophageal hiatus, the esophageal tumor and regional lymph nodes can be mobilized under direct vision. The extrinsically normal proximal esophagus is then mobilized bluntly. The second condition for using the THE technique is the availability of options for long-segment esophageal reconstruction (most commonly stomach or colon) because the replacement conduit must reach to the neck for esophageal anastomosis.

Previous sternotomy for coronary artery revascularization or thoracotomy for lung resection is not necessarily a contraindication for using the THE approach. Similarly, preoperative open or endoscopic gastrostomy tube placement does not prevent THE with gastric pull-up to the neck, as long as the vascular arcades along the lesser and greater curvature of the stomach are intact. The gastrostomy tube is removed at surgery, and the gastrostomy site closed in two layers, protecting the right gastroepiploic vascular vessels.

Contraindications include dense paraesophageal adhesions from intrinsic esophageal disease, a history of caustic ingestion, previous posterior mediastinal adhesions, transmural middle third esophageal cancer, and patients without stomach or colon for long-segment esophageal replacement. Patients with previous neck surgery or cervical irradiation may not be eligible for the THE approach because of the difficulties with exposing and mobilizing the cervical esophagus. Patients who are extremely thin have such limited mediastinal space that it is often prudent to elect to mobilize the intrathoracic esophagus under direct vision via thoracotomy.

Preoperative evaluation of vocal cord function should be performed in patients who are hoarse or who are suspected of aspiration. It is essential to document preoperative ipsilateral vocal cord dysfunction and to rule out contralateral cord paralysis. This prevents the disastrous postoperative complication of bilateral vocal cord paralysis.

The technique of THE has recently been illustrated (see Heitmiller RF: Closed-chest esophageal resection, 1999). Briefly, under single lumen endotracheal general anesthesia, patients are positioned with the neck in slight extension. The operation is organized into three parts: gastric mobilization, esophageal mobilization, and esophagogastric anastomosis. The stomach is mobilized based on the right gastroepiploic vessels. The lesser curvature, lower paraesophageal, and celiac lymph nodes are included en bloc with the stomach. A Kocher maneuver and pyloromyotomy are added. The esophageal hiatus is widened. Transhiatal mobilization of the esophagus is performed to approximately the level of the aortic arch (Fig. 49–1). Much of the lower esophagus, including the tumor site, can be dissected out under direct vision. The left cervical incision is performed before completing the intrathoracic esophageal mobilization. A gastric tube is fashioned with a gastrointestinal anastomosis stapler (Fig. 49–2). The intrathoracic esophagus is removed, and the gastric tube is pulled up through the posterior mediastinum to the neck where a two-layered, hand-sewn end-to-side anastomosis is completed (Figs. 49–3 and 49–4). An adjuvant feeding jejunostomy tube is added.

The salient features of postoperative care include early postoperative monitoring in an intensive care unit, overnight endotracheal intubation, nasogastric tube drainage for 3 to 4 days, low-rate (10 to 30 mL per hour) enteral feedings via operatively placed jejunostomy tube beginning on day 3, videoesophagogram on day 5 before initiating oral feedings, and then the introduction of a postesophagectomy therapeutic diet, which regulates both the quantity and the consistency of feedings. Beginning in 1994, a clinical care pathway was initiated at our institution, standardizing the features listed above with the goal of reducing treatment costs without compromising outcomes.

The following results with THE are largely representative of the outcomes reported by others. Major respiratory complications, including the need for chest tube, bronchoscopy, thoracentesis, initiation of antibiotics, reintubation, or intensive care, occur in 10% of patients. Of note, pneumonia was observed in only 3% of patients. Although many clinicians believe that cervical esophageal anastomoses are more prone to anastomotic leakage, we have not found this to be the case. Our anastomotic leak rate is about 1% using a two-layered, hand-sewn technique. Approximately one fourth of patients require at least one anastomotic dilatation for anastomotic narrowing. Postoperative arrhythmias, most commonly atrial, occur in approximately 10% of patients. Hoarseness resulting from ipsilateral recurrent laryngeal nerve injury is seen in 10% to 15% of patients. Our surgical mortality rate in a large, unselected series was 3%. The goal of our critical care pathway projects patient discharge on the eighth postoperative day.

The advantages of the THE over other esophagectomy techniques are not measured by differences in morbidity and mortality. The THE approach uses a single operative patient positioning and surgical prep. Only the cervical esophagus is preserved. Because the THE approach is mostly used to resect distal esophageal tumors, this results in a generous proximal esophageal margin, ensuring complete removal of the tumor and any associated Barrett's epithelium without the need for intraoperative pathologic assessment of the proximal esophageal margin. Postoperative pain is less than with esophagectomy techniques that employ a thoracotomy. Anastomotic leaks are more simply and safely managed in the cervical versus the intrathoracic location. The same is true for management of anastomotic

---

Pearls and Pitfalls

PEARLS

- THE may be used for both benign and malignant esophageal disease.
- Location of esophageal pathology (i.e., upper, middle, or lower third) is important in selecting patients for the THE approach.
- "Standard" preoperative staging is used for patients with esophageal cancer.
- Operative technical tips: Use intraoperative nasogastric tube and upper hand retractor, widen the esophageal hiatus before transhiatal mobilization, and stay in the paraesophageal plane for safe esophageal mobilization.
- Use of adjunctive feeding jejunostomy is recommended.
- Use a postoperative plan that prevents aspiration.

PITFALLS

- Ipsilateral recurrent laryngeal nerve injury may occur in approximately 10% of patients. This may be associated with an increased risk of postoperative aspiration.
- Narrow anteroposterior diameter chest anatomy is a relative contraindication to THE. Blunt esophageal dissection may result in marked operative hypotension.
- Patients with reduced ejection fraction secondary to ischemic coronary artery disease or valvular dysfunction may not tolerate THE.
- Adhesions or transmural esophageal tumor involving the middle or upper esophagus does not permit blunt dissection in the paraesophageal plane and increases the probability of bleeding and airway injury.

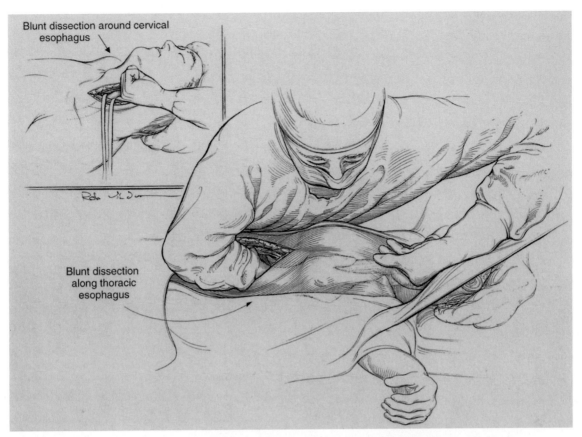

Figure 49–1. Technique of transhiatal esophageal mobilization. The *inset* shows that the distal cervical esophagus is encircled before completing the intrathoracic esophageal dissection. (From Heitmiller RF: Closed-chest esophageal resection. Operative Tech Thorac Cardiovasc Surg 1999;4:252.)

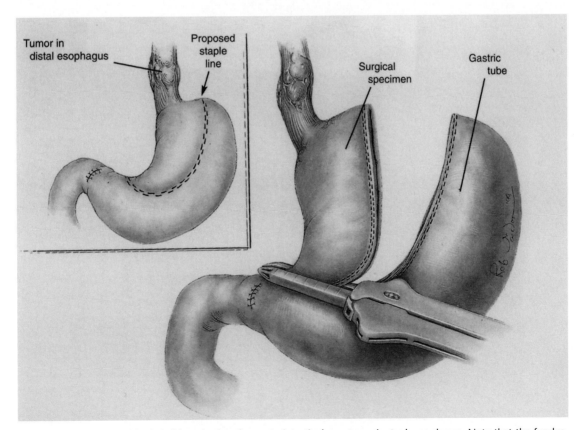

Figure 49–2. A gastric tube is fashioned using the gastrointestinal anastomosis stapler as shown. Note that the fundus, not the cardia, becomes the tip of this tube. (From Heitmiller RF: Closed-chest esophageal resection. Operative Tech Thorac Cardiovasc Surg 1999;4:252.)

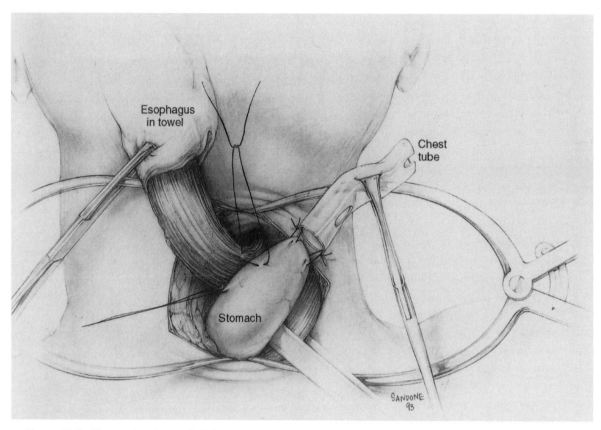

Figure 49–3. The gastric tube is pulled through the posterior mediastinum to the neck where it is positioned for an end-to-side esophagogastric anastomosis. (From Stone C, Heitmiller RF: Simplified, standardized cervical esophago-gastric anastomosis. Ann Thorac Surg 1994;58:259. Reprinted with permission from the Society of Thoracic Surgeons.)

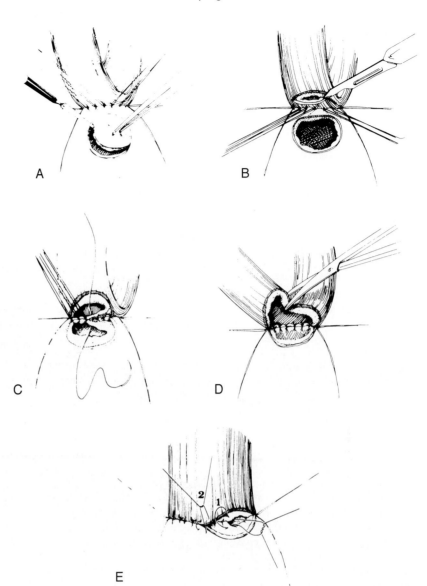

Figure 49–4. Anastomotic technique. *A,* A "back wall" of interrupted sutures is placed from esophageal muscle to seromuscular stomach before opening the stomach. *B,* The esophagus is opened anteriorly. *C,* An inner layer of sutures approximates the mucosal layers. *D,* The excess esophagus is removed after the back wall is completed. *E,* The anterior two layers are completed in an interrupted, inverting fashion. (From Heitmiller RF: Results of standard left thoracoabdominal esophagogastrectomy. Semin Thorac Cardiovasc Surg 1992;4:314.)

strictures. Finally, the quality of swallowing after THE with cervical esophagogastric anastomosis is excellent and therefore suitable for patients with benign as well as malignant esophageal disorders.

Summary

- Staging of esophageal cancer is as follows: T stage: EUS; N stage: chest and abdominal CT, EUS, laparoscopy; M stage: chest and abdominal CT, PET.
- Indications for THE: The portion of intrathoracic esophagus to be removed bluntly should be extrinsically normal, and there should be options for long-segment esophageal replacement. Previous sternotomy or thoracotomy *does not* prevent the use of the THE approach.
- Contraindications for THE: Paraesophageal adhesions, transmural tumor involving the intrathoracic esophagus, previous head and neck surgery, cervical radiation.
- Advantages of THE: Single operative positioning, wide

proximal esophageal margin, no thoracotomy pain, easier and safer management of anastomotic complications, excellent quality of swallowing.
- Results of THE are similar to those of a combined abdominal and thoracotomy approach.

SELECTED READINGS

Gillinov AM, Heitmiller RF: Strategies to reduce pulmonary complications after transhiatal esophagectomy. Dis Esophagus 1998;11:43.

Heitmiller RF: Closed-chest esophageal resection. Operative Tech Thorac Cardiovasc Surg 1999;4:252.

Heitmiller RF, Jones B: Transient diminished airway protection following transhiatal esophagectomy. Am J Surg 1991;162:442.

Heitmiller RF, Sharma R: Comparison of incidence and resection rates in patients with esophageal squamous cell and adenocarcinoma. J Thorac Cardiovasc Surg 1996;112:130.

Stone C, Heitmiller RF: Simplified, standardized cervical esophago-gastric anastomosis. Ann Thorac Surg 1994;58:259.

Zehr KJ, Dawson PB, Yang SC, Heitmiller RF: Implementation of standardized clinical care pathways for major general thoracic cases reduces hospital costs and length of stay. Ann Thorac Surg 1998;66:914.

Chapter 50

Esophageal Cancer: Transsthoracic Resection

Mark K. Ferguson

Carcinoma of the esophagus is relatively uncommon, comprising only about 2% of all adult malignancies. Squamous cell cancers of the esophagus, which are located primarily in the upper and middle thoracic esophagus, make up about half of all esophageal malignancies and are etiologically related to excessive tobacco and alcohol use. The majority of the remaining tumors are adenocarcinomas, which are located in the distal esophagus and at the esophagogastric junction. The etiology of these tumors is less well understood but appears to be related in part to gastroesophageal reflux disease and to dysplastic changes in Barrett's mucosa. The anatomic location of the esophagus, the debilitated condition of affected patients, and the relatively advanced stage of disease at the time of diagnosis all combine to create a challenging clinical problem for the surgeon.

CLINICAL PRESENTATION

Esophageal cancer develops most commonly in people in the sixth through eighth decades of life (Fig. 50–1). The most common presenting symptom is dysphagia, which is due to intraluminal growth of tumor and affects almost 80% of patients. This, in combination with general cancer cachexia, causes weight loss in about 50% of patients. Other symptoms may include odynophagia, regurgitation, and gastrointestinal bleeding manifested as melena or hematochezia. The initial evaluation of a patient suspected of having esophageal cancer includes upper gastrointestinal endoscopy and possibly a barium contrast–enhanced radiograph of the esophagus and stomach.

Once the diagnosis of esophageal cancer is established, a staging evaluation is performed to determine the TNM status of the tumor (Table 50–1). Computed tomography (CT) of the chest and abdomen should be the mainstay of staging. CT assesses the primary tumor and regional lymph nodes with an accuracy of only 60%, but it is fairly reliable in determining the presence of direct invasion of the airway or aorta, and it is highly accurate in identifying distant metastases in the lungs or liver. Endoscopic ultrasonography has been adopted routinely in some centers to provide a better assessment of T (tumor) and N (node) status, each of which is evaluated with about 80% accuracy. The inability to pass the ultrasound probe through the tumor, however, results in an incomplete examination in 30% of patients. Patients in whom the tumor abuts the trachea or mainstem bronchi should undergo bronchoscopy to rule out airway invasion if resection is contemplated. Bone scintigraphy is performed if symptoms suggest osseous metastases.

Positron emission tomography (PET) has recently been used for staging esophageal cancer and has the potential to identify asymptomatic distant metastases in up to 20% of patients. Minimally invasive staging techniques, including laparoscopy and thoracoscopy, are used routinely in some centers to improve the overall accuracy of TNM

Table 50–1	TNM Staging Criteria for Esophageal Cancer

Primary Tumor (T)

T0	No evidence of primary tumor
Tis	Carcinoma in situ
T1	Tumor invades lamina propria or submucosa
T2	Tumor invades muscularis propria
T3	Tumor invades adventitia
T4	Tumor invades adjacent structures

Regional Lymph Nodes (N)*

N0	No regional lymph node metastases
N1	Regional lymph node metastasis

Distant Metastasis (M)

M0	No distant metastasis	
M1	Distant metastasis	
	Tumors of the lower thoracic esophagus	
M1a		Metastasis in celiac lymph nodes
M1b		Other distant metastasis
	Tumors of the midthoracic esophagus	
M1a		Not applicable
M1b		Nonregional lymph nodes and/or other distant metastasis
	Tumors of the upper thoracic esophagus	
M1a		Metastasis in cervical nodes
M1b		Other distant metastasis

Stage Grouping

Stage 0	Tis	N0	M0
Stage I	T1	N0	M0
Stage IIA	T2	N0	M0
	T3	N0	M0
Stage IIB	T1	N1	M0
	T2	N1	M0
Stage III	T3	N1	M0
	T4	Any N	M0
Stage IV	Any T	Any N	M1
Stage IVA	Any T	Any N	M1a
Stage IVB	Any T	Any N	M1b

*Regional lymph nodes
Cervical esophageal tumor; scalene, internal jugular, upper cervical, periesophageal, supraclavicular, cervical not otherwise specified; intrathoracic esophageal tumor; tracheobronchial, superior mediastinal, peritracheal, carinal, hilar, periesophageal, perigastric, paracardial, mediastinal not otherwise specified.
From the American Joint Committee on Cancer: AJCC Cancer Staging Manual, 5th ed. Philadelphia, Lippincott-Raven, 1997.

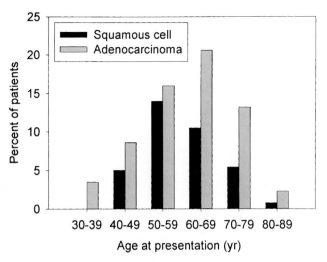

Figure 50–1. Age at presentation for adenocarcinomas and squamous cell cancers of the esophagus.

staging. Laparoscopy demonstrates unsuspected metastatic disease in up to 15% of patients and appears worthwhile for patients with tumors of the distal esophagus and cardia. Its role for squamous cell cancers remains to be determined. The role of thoracoscopic staging is uncertain at present considering the relatively high cost of the procedure and its associated morbidity.

Resection is the treatment of choice for patients in good general health with disease ranging from early stage I to regionally advanced stage III. Contraindications to resection include distant organ metastases; invasion by the primary tumor of the major airways, the vertebral bodies, or the aorta; and medical comorbidities that preclude major surgery. In the absence of resection, treatment should consist of cisplatin-based chemotherapy combined with radiation therapy, which offers improved tumor response and, most importantly, symptomatic palliation over chemotherapy or radiation therapy alone. Palliation of the dysphagia can be accomplished in selected patients with laser thermal coagulation, photodynamic therapy, or intraluminal stent placement.

PREOPERATIVE MANAGEMENT

Patients who are potential candidates for transthoracic resection should undergo a cardiopulmonary evaluation. Serious valvular or coronary artery disease that cannot be corrected is a contraindication to resection. Pulmonary function tests are indicated only for patients with chronic lung disease. Important respiratory impairment is a relative contraindication to thoracotomy, but other techniques for resection such as a so-called transhiatal esophagectomy may be considered. Evaluation of hepatic and renal function is performed routinely because impairment of either increases operative risk but is not a contraindication for surgery.

The role of neoadjuvant therapy before resection is controversial. Despite the growing interest in this modality, few randomized studies have been performed to evaluate its efficacy objectively. Combined chemoradiotherapy produces a better complete pathologic response rate than does chemotherapy alone. Radiotherapy as a preoperative adjuvant treatment offers no advantage over resection alone. Whether neoadjuvant chemoradiotherapy improves survival rate compared with surgery alone is not clear. At present, despite its enthusiasts, such treatment is considered investigational.

Smoking cessation is strongly encouraged because it substantially decreases the risk of postoperative pulmonary complications. Many surgeons suggest that a modified colon preparation be performed on an outpatient basis with a clear liquid diet for 2 days and cathartics and oral antibiotics on the day before operation. Patients are often admitted on the day of surgery. Prophylaxis for deep venous thrombosis with low-dose subcutaneous heparin or other suitable means is suggested. A thoracic epidural catheter is placed for postoperative analgesia. A urinary catheter is inserted. A radial artery catheter is useful in monitoring arterial pressures and oxygen concentrations but, under normal circumstances, central venous catheterization is not necessary unless cardiac dysfunction is evident preoperatively. Many esophageal surgeons prefer that the patient be intubated with a double lumen endotracheal tube to allow single lung ventilation.

INTRAOPERATIVE MANAGEMENT

Approaches to Resection

Appropriate positioning of the patient depends on the incisions to be used (Fig. 50–2). For some operations, the patient is placed in a true lateral position with the lowermost leg flexed and the uppermost leg extended. This positioning places some traction on the pelvis, which helps to widen the ipsilateral intercostal spaces. The lower arm is extended on an arm board and the upper arm is extended parallel to it on a suspended support device attached to the table to help displace the scapula off the chest wall. A modified lateral position is used when simultaneous access to the chest, abdomen, and neck is desired. The patient is placed supine and rolled into a semilateral position without turning the hips substantially. The head is turned slightly to the contralateral side, the contralateral arm is tucked at the side, while the ipsilateral arm is either positioned at the side to permit an anterolateral thoracotomy or is prepped circumferentially and left mobile to permit a standard lateral thoracotomy.

The most common approach involves a laparotomy and right thoracotomy through the fifth intercostal space (Ivor Lewis esophagectomy, or two-hole approach) possibly combined with a cervical incision (McKeown modification of the Ivor Lewis approach, or three-hole approach). Such an approach is appropriate for tumors in any location and of any cell type. This technique can be performed in the lateral or semilateral position, with the understanding that use of the full lateral position usually requires repositioning the patient to permit access to the abdomen and, when necessary, the neck. The operation is usually begun in the abdomen to permit an initial staging assessment

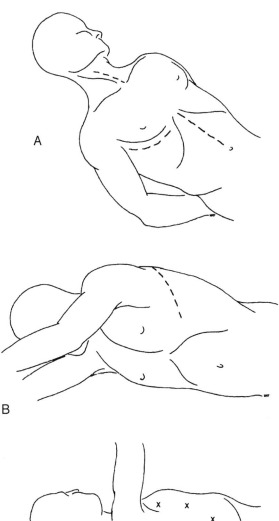

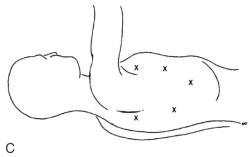

Figure 50–2. Positioning and incision options for transthoracic esophagectomy. *A,* Semilateral position for simultaneous laparotomy, right anterolateral thoracotomy, and cervical incision. *B,* Right lateral decubitus position for left thoracotomy. *C,* Left lateral decubitus position for right thoracoscopy (suggested port sites indicated) or right lateral thoracotomy.

before the thoracotomy is performed. If preoperative testing suggests the possibility of unresectable disease resulting from local invasion or intrathoracic metastases, exploratory thoracotomy is performed first.

An exclusive left thoracotomy or a left thoracotomy combined with a cervical incision is often appropriate for patients with tumors of the distal esophagus and esophagogastric junction. The patient is placed in a true lateral position or is possibly rolled slightly posterior to give access to the left upper quadrant of the abdomen. A lateral thoracotomy is performed through the left seventh or eighth intercostal space while access to the abdomen is provided using a peripheral incision in the diaphragm extending from near the sternum to the tip of the spleen. If necessary, the incision can be extended across the costal margin as a thoracoabdominal incision into the upper abdomen to provide additional exposure; however, this can be a very painful incision.

Minimal access techniques have recently been described which theoretically provide the means to perform a standard resection while minimizing postoperative morbidity and hospital length of stay. The thoracoscopic part of the operation is performed through the right chest with the patient in a true lateral position. The surgeon stands at the patient's back using two operating ports; an additional camera port and two retractor ports are usually necessary to provide adequate exposure. Thoracoscopy may also be combined with laparoscopic techniques for mobilization of the stomach and placement of the jejunostomy feeding tube.

Extent of Resection

A standard resection theoretically includes the portion of the esophagus containing the tumor with 5-cm margins proximal and distal to the gross extent of tumor. From a practical perspective, however, the entire esophagus distal to the cancer is usually resected (except in exceptional cases of a localized cervical esophageal cancer) and a margin of proximal stomach is also taken in continuity to permit adequate clearing of proximal perigastric lymph nodes. The proximal extent of resection is determined by the histologic subtype of tumor, the options available for reconstruction, and the desired site for the anastomosis. Squamous cell cancers are often multifocal, necessitating a near-total esophagectomy with either a high intrathoracic or a cervical anastomosis. Adenocarcinomas are rarely multifocal, but because they often extend submucosally for varying distances, documentation of a resection margin negative for malignancy is appropriate before concluding a resection. Also, many surgeons will try to remove all proximal esophagus involved with changes of Barrett's epithelium.

Controversy exists over whether the primary tumor should be resected with a small amount of adjacent surrounding tissue or whether a more extensive en bloc resection should be performed. A standard esophagectomy includes surrounding adventitial soft tissues and adjacent regional lymph nodes within 5 cm of gross tumor but does not typically include pericardium, contralateral pleura, azygos vein, or thoracic duct. A radical en bloc esophagectomy includes surrounding adventitial soft tissues within 10 cm of gross tumor as well as the azygos vein, thoracic duct, adjacent pericardium, contralateral pleura, and, in some instances, the spleen. No randomized studies have been performed comparing the two techniques, and no survival advantage has been demonstrated for the radical en bloc approach.

Extent of Nodal Dissection

A standard resection entails removal of the regional lymph nodes within 5 cm of gross tumor. Nodes in the celiac axis region (M1 lymph nodes) should also be dissected routinely. Recent studies suggest that 10% to 20% of patients with localized disease based on clinical staging have involvement of cervical or supraclavicular lymph nodes, indicating stage IV (M1) disease. The desire for improved accuracy in staging along with the benefit of a potential survival advantage has stimulated the use of more extensive nodal dissection in the mediastinum, upper abdomen, and neck. This extended, or three-field, lymphadenectomy typically includes proximal perigastric, hepatic artery, splenic artery, and celiac axis lymph nodes in the abdomen, all accessible mediastinal lymph nodes including subcarinal and bilateral recurrent laryngeal nerve chains in the thorax, and supraclavicular and superficial and deep cervical lymph nodes in the neck. The extended dissection is associated with a higher incidence of injury to the recurrent nerve. No randomized studies have yet been performed comparing the standard with the extended technique, and no convincing survival advantage for the latter technique has been demonstrated.

Options for Reconstruction

In most patients, the stomach is used for reconstruction. No clear advantage has been demonstrated for other reconstructive options with regard to long-term survival, nutritional indices, or quality of life. During the esopha-

gectomy, a proximal partial gastrectomy is performed to provide an adequate distal tumor-free margin and to permit removal of proximal perigastric lymph nodes. This resection preserves the gastric fundus, which is the site of the planned anastomosis. The stomach is usually fashioned into a tube by resection of the lesser curvature to the level of the fourth or fifth branch of the left gastric artery near the incisura. A generous Kocher maneuver permits this neoesophagus to reach easily into the neck and end-to-side anastomosis is performed along the greater curvature side to avoid vascular compromise to the lesser curvature line of gastric resection.

If the stomach is not appropriate for use in reconstruction because of prior disease or surgery, or because the extent of gastric resection does not permit it to reach to the remaining esophagus, alternative options include a colon interposition, jejunal interposition as a pedicled or free graft, or a composite reconstruction. A low or mid-intrathoracic anastomosis is easily achieved with a "short" segment of colon based on the ascending branch of the inferior mesenteric artery or with a segment of proximal jejunum. Long segment interpositions to the high thoracic or cervical esophagus are best accomplished with the transverse and descending colon. Bowel interpositions are passed posterior to the stomach and positioned in an isoperistaltic orientation. The distal anastomosis is made to the posterior wall of the stomach if it exists or directly to the duodenum, or to a loop of jejunum if the stomach cannot be used.

Other Considerations

Care must be taken during gastric mobilization to seek the presence of an aberrant left or common hepatic artery arising from the left gastric artery. Unintentional division of such a vessel may lead to acute hepatic ischemia. The thoracic duct is ligated just above the diaphragm during any transthoracic esophagectomy to minimize the chances of a postoperative chylothorax. A gastric emptying procedure is not performed routinely, although many surgeons perform at least a pyloromyotomy. A feeding jejunostomy is placed to provide early enteral alimentation. The reconstructive organ is drained with a nasoenteral tube, which is positioned during completion of the anastomosis. The esophageal hiatus is approximated to the reconstructive organ with several interrupted sutures to prevent intrathoracic herniation of abdominal contents. Drainage of the pleural space is accomplished with a single thoracostomy tube. Under most circumstances, it is appropriate to extubate the patient in the operating room.

POSTOPERATIVE MANAGEMENT

Initial management in an intensive care setting is appropriate in most institutions. Supplemental oxygen and fluid boluses are often necessary during the first 2 postoperative days. Antibiotics are continued for the first postoperative day. The head of the patient's bed is elevated 15 to 30 degrees to help prevent aspiration. Early physical mobilization with ambulation and frequent pulmonary toilet exercises such as coughing and use of an incentive

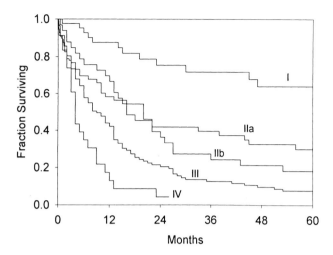

Figure 50–3. Survival by stage after esophagectomy for esophageal cancer.

spirometer helps avoid the development of pulmonary complications. Enteral feeding is begun within 24 hours of the operation. Daily chest radiographs are performed while the thoracostomy tube is in place.

The thoracostomy tube is removed when drainage is less than 200 to 300 mL daily. The nasogastric tube is removed when the output is minimal and after there is clinical evidence for resumption of bowel activity. In the absence of a clinical suspicion for an anastomotic leak, a contrast examination of the anastomosis adds little to the decision about beginning oral intake. If such an examination is performed, it is done either with a water-soluble contrast agent or with dilute barium. Most patients are advanced to a soft diet within 1 week of the operation. Patients are instructed to sleep with the head of the bed elevated. The jejunostomy tube is maintained for the first couple of weeks after hospital discharge, and tube feedings are provided at night until the patient is able to tolerate a relatively normal amount of oral intake. The typical duration of hospitalization in the absence of postoperative complications is 1 week.

COMPLICATIONS

The most frequent and troublesome complications after esophagectomy are pulmonary in nature, including pneumonia, aspiration pneumonia, and adult respiratory distress syndrome. Early institution of antibiotics and emphasis on pulmonary toilet are appropriate for patients in whom pneumonia is suspected to have developed. The antibiotics should cover gram-positive oral anaerobes as well as gram-negative aerobes.

Anastomotic leaks develop in 5% to 20% of patients. They are more common when a cervical anastomosis is performed but are more lethal when they develop in an intrathoracic anastomosis. The diagnosis of anastomotic leak should be entertained whenever a septic picture develops. Depending on the situation, appropriate evaluation may include endoscopy, contrast radiography, or CT. Management of cervical anastomotic leaks usually requires only opening the incision to provide adequate drainage, whereas intrathoracic leaks often need more aggressive intervention such as thoracostomy tube drain-

Pearls and Pitfalls

- Personally perform or view an endoscopic examination to assess the local and distal extent of disease.
- A visible esophageal mass on CT scan is usually indicative of T3 or T4 status.
- Use minimally invasive staging techniques to document suspected areas of metastatic disease.
- Insist that the patient cease use of tobacco and alcohol well in advance of the operation.
- Provide gastrostomy or jejunostomy tube feedings to patients undergoing neoadjuvant chemoradiotherapy before they begin to lose weight.
- The presence of a gastrostomy tube does not preclude use of the stomach as a reconstructive organ after esophagectomy.
- Allow a sufficient period of recovery after neoadjuvant therapy so that patients can regain their baseline performance status.
- Avoid thoracoabdominal incisions whenever possible

because transection of the costal margin often leads to chronic pain.
- Carefully palpate the celiac axis region before proceeding with transection of the left gastric artery to avoid inadvertent injury to an aberrant hepatic artery.
- Avoid performing a low or mid-intrathoracic esophagogastrostomy for patients with Barrett's adenocarcinoma; free reflux results in a high likelihood of recurrent Barrett's mucosa.
- Redundancy of an intrathoracic reconstructive organ delays emptying and promotes regurgitation and aspiration.
- In the presence of signs of sepsis, the cause is an anastomotic leak until proved otherwise.
- Have the patient practice swallowing sips of water for a day before performing an initial postoperative contrast-enhanced radiograph to improve coordination and reduce the likelihood of aspiration.

age and rarely reclosure and reinforcement of the anastomosis, takedown of the reconstruction, or salivary diversion.

Other common early complications include recurrent laryngeal nerve injury (5% to 20%), chylothorax (5%), and supraventricular arrhythmia (10%). Realistic operative mortality rate is 5% to 10%. Long-term complications include gastric emptying problems in 10%, dumping symptoms in 15%, mild weight loss in most patients, and anastomotic strictures that require dilation in 30%.

OUTCOMES

The quality of life is generally good for patients after they have recovered from the acute effects of surgery. Most are able to tolerate a general diet with few restrictions, although the quantity able to be ingested at a single sitting is somewhat reduced, and snacks between meals are encouraged. Long-term survival depends on the stage of disease at the time of diagnosis (Fig. 50–3). Recurrent disease is usually evident within 2 years of resection in patients who fail treatment. The likelihood of local recurrence after a technically satisfactory operation is 10%, and most recurrences develop distally.

SELECTED READINGS

Altorki N: The rationale for radical resection. Surg Oncol Clin North Am 1999;8:295.

American Joint Committee on Cancer: AJCC Cancer Staging Manual, 5th ed. Philadelphia, Lippincott Williams & Wilkins, 1997, pp 65–69.

Block MI, Patterson GA, Sundaresan RS, et al: Improvement in staging of esophageal cancer with the addition of positron emission tomography. Ann Thorac Surg 1997;64:770.

Bossett J-F, Gignoux M, Triboulet J-P, et al: Chemoradiotherapy followed by surgery compared with surgery alone in squamous cell cancer of the esophagus. N Engl J Med 1997;337:161.

Ferguson MK, Martin TR, Reeder LB, et al: Mortality after esophagectomy: Risk factor analysis. World J Surg 1997;21:599.

Krasna MJ, Flowers JL, Attar S, et al: Combined thoracoscopic/laparoscopic staging of esophageal cancer. J Thorac Cardiovasc Surg 1996;111:800.

Law S, Fok M, Chu KM, et al: Thoracoscopic esophagectomy for esophageal cancer. Surgery 1997;122:8.

Nishimaki T, Suzuki T, Suzuki S, et al: Outcomes of extended radical esophagectomy for thoracic esophageal cancer. J Am Coll Surg 1998;186:306.

O'Brien MG, Fitzgerald EF, Lee G, et al: A prospective comparison of laparoscopy and imaging in the staging of esophagogastric cancer before surgery. Am J Gastroenterol 1995;90:2191.

Walsh TN, Noonan N, Hollywood D, et al: A comparison of multimodal therapy and surgery for esophageal adenocarcinoma. N Engl J Med 1996;335:462.

Stomach: Benign and Malignant

Chapter 51
Peptic Ulcer Disease and *Helicobacter pylori*

Rhonda A. Cole and David Y. Graham

Peptic ulcer disease is described as a chronic, debilitating disease with lifelong implications and impairments. The epidemiology of peptic ulcer disease has changed. In Western countries in the 1960s and 1970s, the lifetime risk of developing a peptic ulcer was estimated to be 1 in 10, with approximately 25% of those with peptic ulcer experiencing a major complication such as bleeding. Fifteen thousand patients died each year as the result of ulcer-related complications. As late as 1990, although the burden of peptic ulcer disease in the United States was estimated at 4 million cases with 500,000 new cases annually, the prevalence of duodenal ulcer disease continues to decrease. Nevertheless, peptic ulcer remains a major cause of economic loss and health care expenditures as the direct result of the large number of days and dollars absorbed in lost productivity, restricted activity, physician visits, and hospitalizations. Recent expenditures in the United States alone for peptic ulcer disease have been in the range of $20 billion per year.

THE BACTERIUM

In the past 2 decades, the basic concepts of the pathogenesis of peptic ulcer, the medical and surgical treatments, and the outcome have undergone change. Peptic ulcer is no longer considered a medically incurable disease. The discovery that an infection with the bacterium *Helicobacter pylori* was the cause of the disease ultimately transformed peptic ulcer disease from a chronic condition ("once an ulcer, always an ulcer") into a treatable and curable infectious disease.

Helicobacter pylori is a gram-negative rod, curved or S-shaped, containing seven sheathed, unipolar flagella. The bacterium is highly mobile, propelling itself in a corkscrew motion through the viscous gel layer. One distinctive characteristic is its ability to produce highly active urease in large amounts. The hydrolysis of urea into carbon dioxide and ammonia allows *H. pylori* to use the nitrogen from the ammonia as well as create an alkaline microenvironment to buffer the harsh acidic environment of the stomach.

EPIDEMIOLOGY AND TRANSMISSION

The prevalence of *H. pylori* in a population is inversely related to the standard of living and hygiene. More than 80% of adults living in developing countries are infected. The primary host is the human, and transmission is primarily between humans (Table 51–1). Infection occurs when the bacterium gains access to the stomach in a sufficient concentration to cause an infection. The actual mode of transmission varies with the situation, with most infections originating by fecal-oral transmission. Oral-oral, water-borne, food-borne, and iatrogenic transmission from contaminated endoscopes and nasogastric tubes (gastric-oral) have also been reported.

Helicobacter pylori infection is typically acquired in childhood. The prevalence of infection in a cohort of adults is directly related to the risk they had of acquiring

Table 51–1	**Risk Factors for *Helicobacter pylori* Infection**

Native of a developing country
Low socioeconomic status during childhood
Exposure to gastric contents of infected individuals
Large families with infants
Crowded living conditions
Unsanitary living conditions
Unclean water or food
Lack of consistent hot water supply

it in childhood. In African-American and white Hispanic populations in the United States, the prevalence of *H. pylori* is high. This high prevalence is not a consequence of genetic predisposition to infection but rather to the fact that these two ethnic groups have only recently moved from the lower socioeconomic groups into the middle and upper socioeconomic groups. The prevalence for any such group is actually what one would expect based on the socioeconomic status of their families during their childhood.

Improved sanitation and standards of living break the pattern of transmission. In the middle class white population in the United States, the prevalence of *H. pylori* infection is typically less than 15%. This decreasing prevalence appears to account for the decline in the incidence of the various *H. pylori*–associated diseases. This rapid and natural loss of the infection in a population associated with improvement in standard of living confirms that *H. pylori* is not a commensal or beneficial bacterium that provides some important function, but rather it is consistent with the bacterium being a major pathogen.

DISEASE ASSOCIATIONS

Helicobacter pylori causes chronic destructive gastritis. The pattern of gastritis predicts the risk of different outcomes. For example, antral-predominant (or corpus-sparing) gastritis is associated with duodenal ulcer disease, and atrophic pangastritis is associated with gastric ulcer and gastric cancer. In most patients, the infection is latent, and the individual remains asymptomatic despite the presence of continuing gastric damage. The risk of a symptomatic outcome varies with the geographic region, which is, in turn, a reflection of the bacterium, host, and environmental interactions. In the United States, the risk of peptic ulcer among those with *H. pylori* infection is about one in six (17%) and the lifetime risk of gastric cancer is approximately 1% to 3%. In other countries, the risk of gastric cancer is higher. For example, in Korea, the risk of dying of gastric cancer for an adult male is greater than 7%. These different risks reflect different environments more than different genetics or different strains of *H. pylori*. This observation is clearly shown in the rapid change in disease presentation after migration or even within a single country over time. The major environmental changes responsible for the remarkable changes in prevalence of *H. pylori*–related disease appear to relate to diet and include the introduction of refrigerators, reduced use of salt as a preservative, and the year-round availability of fresh fruits and vegetables.

Helicobacter pylori has been etiologically associated with duodenal ulcer, gastric ulcer, gastric adenocarcinoma, and primary B-cell gastric lymphoma (gastric mucosa–associated lymphoid tissue [MALT] lymphoma). Cure of the infection results in healing of the gastritis, cure of peptic ulcer disease, remission of low-grade gastric MALT lymphomas, and prevention of gastric cancer. Gastric atrophy and intestinal metaplasia of the stomach either do not regress or regress minimally after appropriate treatment of the *H. pylori* infection.

HELICOBACTER PYLORI IN THE PATHOGENESIS OF DISEASE

Gastric Cancer

For half a century, it was recognized that both peptic ulcer and gastric cancer were tightly associated with gastritis. The association of gastric cancer with gastritis was responsible for a large number of epidemiologic studies designed to discover the cause of gastritis so that gastric cancer could be prevented. Even though the details of how *H. pylori* infection may produce cancer are still obscure, the general phenomenon of chronic inflammation, development of a metaplastic epithelium, followed by dysplasia and ultimately cancer is a common theme in epithelial cell cancer. One does not have to look farther than chronic viral hepatitis and hepatocellular carcinoma, smoking and lung cancer, acid reflux and adenocarcinoma in Barrett's esophagus, ulcerative colitis and colon cancer, or schistosomes and bladder cancer to find examples of this pattern. It appears likely that the environmental factors previously recognized to be associated with gastric cancer (e.g., high salt diet low in fresh fruits and vegetables) were actually descriptions of factors that allowed or promoted rapid progression of *H. pylori* gastritis to the stage of atrophic gastritis with intestinal metaplasia. Gastric cancer may simply be a reflection of the prevalence of this progression. Whether the bacterium plays a particular role is unclear.

Duodenal Ulcer

The association of duodenal ulcer with antral-predominant gastritis has been recognized for almost 100 years. The last half century saw a remarkable increase in modern understanding of the physiology and regulation of acid secretion. Recently, it has been possible to bring the large body of data regarding acid secretion together with what is known about *H. pylori* to produce unifying hypotheses regarding *H. pylori* and duodenal ulcer disease. One early question was "How can an infection in the antrum cause an ulcer in the duodenum?" *H. pylori* infection is restricted to gastric epithelium, and gastric epithelium in the form of gastric metaplasia is normally found in the duodenal bulb. The extent of gastric metaplasia in the duodenum is related to the gastric acid output or, better still, to the duodenal acid load. In addition, development of gastric metaplasia is part of the healing process after duodenal injury. Thus, the presence of a high duodenal acid load, which is characteristic of patients with duodenal ulcer disease, promotes the development of niches for colonization by *H. pylori*. The inflammatory response to *H. pylori* colonizing this gastric metaplasia promotes more gastric metaplasia, resulting in more *H. pylori* colonization.

Helicobacter pylori gastritis causes dysregulation of acid secretion (e.g., impaired shut-off of acid secretion when the antral pH declines to 3 or less) and the ability of the duodenal bulb to secrete bicarbonate in response to acid. Both of these dysregulations increase the functional duodenal acid load and promote *H. pylori* colonization in the duodenal bulb. The key to understanding why a duodenal ulcer could not be sustained when the acid secretion decreases to less than 12 mmol per hour and possibly why there is accelerated healing with antisecretory medical or surgical therapy is the fact that *H. pylori* growth is inhibited by bile. *Helicobacter pylori* should not be able to grow well in the duodenum. In fact, low pH precipitates glycine-conjugated bile acids and thus allows *H. pylori* to thrive in the duodenal bulb where its growth would normally be impaired or prevented. The duodenal acid load is typically unable to extend this low pH barrier much beyond the duodenal bulb, which may be why postbulbar ulcers are rare. Reducing the duodenal acid load impairs *H. pylori* growth and results in resolution of duodenal ulcer disease despite the continued presence of *H. pylori* in the stomach (e.g., after successful highly selective vagotomy). The actual ulcer is thought to form at the site of the *H. pylori* infected and inflamed gastric metaplasia. Not only is the gastric metaplasia inflamed, but the inflammation spills over into the normal duodenum at the junctions of the gastric metaplasia and the villus mucosa. This junctional epithelium appears to be particularly susceptible to damage and is where the ulceration begins.

Gastric Ulcer

The pathogenesis of gastric ulcer remains largely a mystery. Gastric ulcers tend to occur at another junctional epithelium (i.e., the line of advancing damage between the antral mucosal and the corpus mucosa). Why gastric ulcers are typically on the lesser curvature is unknown. Possibly, older speculations regarding blood flow and repair will be explanatory, but more studies are needed.

Dyspepsia

The most common symptom of peptic ulcer is dyspepsia. Nonulcer dyspepsia is a diagnosis made after a full evaluation, including endoscopy that excludes other diseases. Nonulcer dyspepsia responds poorly to therapy designed to eradicate *H. pylori*. Nevertheless, when a new patient is seen with dyspepsia, he or she should be evaluated for peptic ulcer, and a proportion will actually have peptic ulcer disease. The current approach is to evaluate these patients for *H. pylori* noninvasively and to treat those infections. This approach is based on the notion that this population is markedly increased in those with symptomatic *H. pylori* disease. Those with nonulcer dyspepsia will likely not respond symptomatically, but their potentially life-threatening *H. pylori* infection will be eliminated, sparing them the risk of subsequent development

of a serious *H. pylori* outcome. In addition, they will not be a risk to the community as a source of transmission. Endoscopy is performed in those patients with features that suggest an ulcer complication or a malignancy; otherwise, noninvasive testing is adequate. This approach is cost effective (Fig. 51–1).

APPROACH

The current approach has three components: test, treat, and confirm cure. No patient should receive *H. pylori* eradication therapy without having confirmation that *H. pylori* infection is actually present. Even the presence of a duodenal ulcer is not sufficient grounds to prescribe eradication therapy without prior testing because, in Western countries, an increasing proportion of ulcers are due to nonsteroidal anti-inflammatory drug use and are *H. pylori*–negative, especially in the elderly. The fact that the patient without the infection can only suffer harm from antibiotic therapy violates the principle of "do not harm." The diagnosis of latent *H. pylori* infection carries with it the obligation to treat just as the diagnosis of latent syphilis carries with it the obligation to cure the disease. Thus, treatment is typically offered to those with an increased risk of a serious symptomatic outcome (Table 51–2).

Diagnostic Tests

The methods of diagnosing *H. pylori* fall into two categories: noninvasive tests and those that require endoscopy.

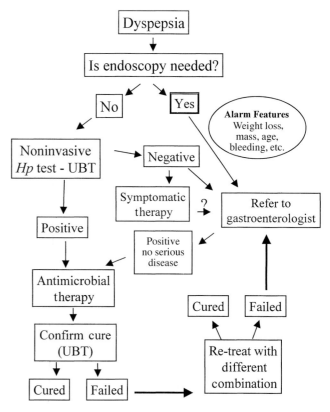

Figure 51–1. An approach to the patient presenting with dyspepsia is outlined. Most patients will not need referral for endoscopy, and can be treated based on the results of noninvasive *H. pylori* testing.

Table 51–2	**Indications for Diagnosis and Treatment of *Helicobacter pylori* Infection**

Current or past peptic ulcer
Unevaluated dyspepsia without alarm features
History of endoscopic or surgical resection of an early gastric cancer
First-degree relative with gastric cancer or peptic ulcer disease
Low-grade gastric mucosa-associated lymphoid tissue lymphoma
Patient requests diagnosis and, if positive, treatment

In most instances, noninvasive testing is all that is required. The most widely available are serologic tests that detect antibody to *H. pylori*. A number of such tests are available commercially, including rapid tests that can be done "in the office" or "near the patient." In addition, serum can be sent to the laboratory for more traditional enzyme-linked immunosorbent assays (ELISAs). Only tests that measure IgG antibody to *H. pylori* are FDA-approved. There are a number of companies offering anti–*H. pylori* IgA or IgM tests that are unreliable and should not be used or relied upon to make decisions. The rule of thumb is that physicians should demand that their laboratory use approved tests only. The approved tests have sensitivity and specificity consistently greater than 90%. A positive IgG antibody test to *H. pylori* in most patients denotes active infection. Antibody titers decrease very slowly after successful therapy and cannot be relied upon to provide an answer about the outcome of therapy, even if one measures the change in titer using paired serum samples.

The urea breath test (UBT) is the best noninvasive test in that it denotes active infection, whereas serology cannot distinguish between active and recent infection. The UBT will likely become the method of choice for determining *H. pylori* status, especially for follow-up to confirm cure. The breath test is based on the fact that *H. pylori* contains a high concentration of urease, which hydrolyzes ingested urea labeled with either ^{13}C or ^{14}C into ammonia and carbon dioxide. The carbon dioxide is captured in the expired breath and measured. An increase in enrichment of the stable isotope ^{13}C or appearance of the radioactive isotope ^{14}C confirms the presence of an active infection. The ^{13}C-UBT (Meretek Diagnostics, Nashville) is preferred because there is no radioactivity, and it is approved for both pretreatment and posttreatment testing.

The newest test is the stool antigen test in which a sample of stool is sent to the laboratory for an ELISA for *H. pylori* antigens. It has proven to be simple and reliable but has a slightly higher rate of false-positive results than the UBT for confirmation of cure. Both the UBT and the stool antigen test may yield false-negative results when the bacterial load is low, especially when the patient takes antibiotics, bismuth, or a proton pump inhibitor. H_2-receptor antagonists do not influence the ^{13}C-UBT but do adversely affect the ^{14}C-UBT. The effect on the stool antigen test is unknown. Thus, it is important to stop potentially interfering drugs before testing; proton pump inhibitors should be discontinued for 1 week and antibiotics or bismuth for approximately 4 weeks before testing.

Invasive methods require upper gastrointestinal endoscopy. During the endoscopy, gastric mucosal biopsies can be taken for culture, rapid urease tests, and/or histology. For accurate histologic assessment of *H. pylori* status, one should take a specimen from the antrum, corpus, and preferably from the gastric angle as well. These should not be handled but should be "shook off" into the formalin and then embedded "on edge." For accurate determination of *H. pylori* status, especially after therapy, a special stain must be used, such as hematoxylin and eosin plus a Diff Quik or single stains such as the Genta or El-Zimaity, which use triple stain methodology. Hematoxylin and eosin alone provide poor results.

Biopsy specimens can also be put into a rapid urease test. Several are available commercially. The principle is that the biopsy is put into a medium containing urea and a pH indicator. As *H. pylori* urease hydrolyzes the urea to produce ammonia, the increase in pH is seen as a color change. One specimen from the antrum and one from the corpus can be combined in a single test. Rapid urease tests are also very good (e.g., >90% accurate), but like histology and the noninvasive tests, they suffer when there is a low bacterial load. The use of a rapid urease test allows the clinician to diagnose an active *H. pylori* infection immediately and to start therapy that day before the patient leaves the office. Rapid urease testing also provides a check on the accuracy of the pathologist. If there are many discrepancies, it is likely that the pathologist is wrong and retraining or the use of other stains should be considered.

Culture of *H. pylori* is not commonly available but is increasingly needed because antibiotic resistance has become increasingly common among *H. pylori*.

THERAPY FOR *HELICOBACTER PYLORI* INFECTION

Sufficient data are available to devise therapeutic regimens effective for *H. pylori* eradication. Single antibiotics proved ineffective, and dual therapies consisting of a proton pump inhibitor or ranitidine bismuth citrate and one antibiotic proved poor choices because of less than desired cure rates and a high rate of development of resistant *H. pylori* when these therapies failed. Current therapies consist of an antisecretory drug, typically a proton pump inhibitor or ranitidine bismuth citrate, and two antibiotics (Table 51–3).

With other infectious diseases, few would be satisfied with cure rates less than 95%. Such cure rates have proven to be difficult to obtain consistently with *H. pylori*. There are few head-to-head comparisons of therapies or evaluations of the various components of any therapy such as dose, duration, dosing interval, and formulation. As such, there is no universally acceptable therapy. Treatment failure is typically due to poor compliance with the complex regimens or because of side effects of the treatment and antibiotic resistance. Therapy that is too short in duration may be another factor.

The antimicrobial drugs used for the eradication of *H. pylori* include bismuth salts, amoxicillin, metronidazole, tetracycline, clarithromycin, furazolidone, and the proton pump inhibitors. The initial successful therapy was a bismuth-based triple therapy (BMT) consisting of tetracycline 500 mg four times a day, metronidazole 250 mg

| Table 51–3 | **Antibiotic Regimens for Treating** *Helicobacter pylori* **Infection** |

Proton pump inhibitor (or ranitidine bismuth citrate) triple therapies for 14 days
    Proton pump inhibitor or ranitidine bismuth citrate bid
    Clarithromycin 500 mg bid
                  and
    Amoxicillin 1 g bid
                  or
    Metronidazole 500 mg bid
Traditional bismuth triple therapy for 14 days
    A bismuth (2 tablets) qid
    Tetracycline HCl 500 mg qid
    Metronidazole 250 mg tid or qid
    An H_2–receptor antagonist or proton pump inhibitor once daily
Bismuth quadruple therapy for 14 days
    A bismuth (2 tablets) qid
    Tetracycline HCl 500 mg qid
    Metronidazole 500 mg tid
    A proton pump inhibitor once or twice daily
Furazolidone salvage therapy for 14 days
    A bismuth (2 tablets) qid
    Tetracycline HCl 500 mg qid
    Furazolidone 100 mg tid
    A proton pump inhibitor once or twice daily

three times a day, and a bismuth such as bismuth subsalicylate or subcitrate, 2 tablets four times a day, all given for 14 days. An antisecretory drug was also given. The introduction of clarithromycin provided a substitute for metronidazole and became the basis of a number of new triple therapies containing a proton pump inhibitor (see Table 51–3). These new therapies had the potential advantage of twice-a-day dosing and were therefore more convenient. Both the initial BMT (Helidac) and one of the newer twice-a-day clarithromycin, amoxicillin, or proton pump inhibitor therapies (PREVPAC) are available in convenient dose packs that make prescription and compliance easy. However, this convenience is associated with increased cost compared with the components prescribed separately, and the regular price increases that have occurred are certainly not well justified for PREVPAC.

Clarithromycin resistance is increasing worldwide; in the United States, it is about 13%. Clarithromycin resistance effectively removes clarithromycin from the combination regimen such that the combination of a proton pump inhibitor, clarithromycin, and amoxicillin becomes, in essence, only the proton pump inhibitor and amoxicillin. Increasing the dose of clarithromycin does not increase the effectiveness with resistant *H. pylori*. In contrast, whereas metronidazole resistance is more common than clarithromycin resistance, it can be partially or completely overcome by increasing the dose and possibly the duration of metronidazole therapy. Metronidazole is a prodrug that must be reduced in the bacterial cell in order to become activated, and a number of enzymes in *H. pylori* can possibly serve as metronidazole nitroreductases. The amount of metronidazole available locally in the stomach is also large, and thus sufficient drug may become activated to kill the organism. The best and certainly the most complex current therapy is a bismuth quadruple therapy that consists of BMT with an increased

dose of metronidazole and a proton pump inhibitor. Salvage therapy should work when others have failed. The two current choices are bismuth quadruple therapy and furazolidone quadruple therapy, which consists of substitution of furazolidone (100 mg three times a day) for the metronidazole in bismuth quadruple therapy. Furazolidone is a monoamine oxidase inhibitor, and one should carefully research for side effects and interactions with foods and other drugs before prescribing it.

The optimum duration of therapy is unknown, but an overall longer duration has yielded better cure rates. Head-to-head comparisons show a rank order with 14 days being better than 10 days and 10 days being better than 7 days. We recommend no less than 10 days and preferably 14 days of therapy (see Table 51–3).

Side Effects of Therapy

Side effects of therapies for *H. pylori* are common but are typically mild and do not require stopping therapy. They are no different from when these antibiotics are used for other indications and include nausea (common), diarrhea (common), rash, dysgeusia (clarithromycin), black stools (bismuth), intolerance to alcohol (metronidazole), and monilial vaginitis (tetracycline). Pseudomembranous colitis is rare.

CONFIRMATION OF CURE

The widespread availability of the noninvasive tests for evaluating *H. pylori* status, (i.e., the ^{13}C-UBT and the

---

Pearls and Pitfalls

- *Helicobacter pylori* is a serious transmissible human pathogen that causes a chronic progressive destructive gastritis, peptic ulcer disease, and gastric cancer.
- Although duodenal ulcer occurs in the duodenum, the *H. pylori* infection is in the stomach and in gastric metaplasia in the duodenum.
- *Helicobacter pylori* infection is curable with antibiotic therapy, but reasonable cure rates require the combination of an antisecretory drug or bismuth and two antibiotics.
- Cure of *H. pylori* cures peptic ulcer disease. If there is no *H. pylori*, there is no ulcer; and if there is no ulcer, there are no ulcer complications, suggesting that surgery should be limited to persons with complications of the infection and should be as minimally destructive of normal function as possible.
- The current approach with peptic and gastric ulcer and with gastritis is to test, treat, and confirm cure.
- If infections persist after treatment, an aggressive approach at treatment is warranted.
- Currently there is no global or national effort to screen for latent *H. pylori* infection, but diagnosis of infection mandates treatment.
- Perforated or bleeding duodenal ulcer in patients younger than 50 years of age is probably *H. pylori* related. In contrast, in patients older than 70 years of age, especially those receiving nonsteroidal anti-inflammatory drugs, *H. pylori* is probably not involved.

stool antigen test) have made posttreatment confirmation of success the standard of care. Failure to cure the infection puts the patient at risk for recurrent ulcer disease with all its complications. The protocol is to test 4 to 6 weeks after therapy with at least 1 week abstinence from proton pump inhibitor therapy. Patients who have failed many treatments should have culture and susceptibility testing done to choose the best therapy. One may always choose to maintain the patient on acid-suppressing drugs (H_2-receptor antagonists or proton pump inhibitors) while awaiting the release of more effective therapeutic regimens.

TREATMENT FAILURES

Retreatment in the event of treatment failure should not involve the reuse of clarithromycin. If the original regimen used clarithromycin, metronidazole should be used and vice versa. If both were used, bismuth quadruple therapy is the treatment of choice. Furazolidone therapy should be reserved for multiple treatment failures.

SPECIAL CONSIDERATIONS REGARDING SURGERY AND *HELICOBACTER PYLORI* ULCER DISEASE

Helicobacter pylori is similar to tuberculosis in that, at one time, surgical therapy was commonly employed for treating the complications of pulmonary tuberculosis. This approach led to the widespread availability of excellent and experienced lung surgeons. The success of antibiotic therapy eliminated that need and that expertise has largely been lost. The same is now happening with surgery for the complications of peptic ulcer. There are few indications for major resections and reconstructions of the stomach to "cure" *H. pylori* peptic ulcers. Minimal surgery that targets the complication has become the rule, followed by eradication therapy later to cure the disease. There is actually no emergency to treat the *H. pylori* infection, and one can safely rely on the prior experience with antisecretory therapy while allowing the patient to heal. Our general approach is to use a proton pump inhibitor for several weeks and then start eradication therapy as an outpatient after the ulcer has healed (e.g., bleeding ulcer). It is important in complicated ulcer disease not to discontinue antisecretory therapy until one is confident that the infection has been cured.

The cure of *H. pylori* infection in patients with *H. pylori* peptic ulcers cures the disease and prevents complications. The dictum "no acid, no ulcer" has become "no *H. pylori*, no ulcer" and "no ulcer, no ulcer complications." Reinfection in adults is rare, and monitoring for reinfection is not needed.

SELECTED READINGS

El-Zimaity HM, Segura AM, Genta RM, Graham DY: Histologic assessment of *Helicobacter pylori* status after therapy: Comparison of Giemsa, Diff-Quik, and Genta stains. Mod Pathol 1998;11:288.
Graham DY: Therapy of *Helicobacter pylori*: Current status and issues. Gastroenterology 2000;118:s2.
Graham DY, Osato MS: *H. pylori* in the pathogenesis of duodenal ulcer: Interaction between duodenal acid load, bile, and *H. pylori*. Am J Gastroenterol 2000;95:87.
Howden CW, Hunt RH: Guidelines for the management of *Helicobacter pylori* infection. *Ad Hoc* Committee on Practice Parameters of the American College of Gastroenterology. Am J Gastroenterol 1998;93:2330.
Miehlke S, Graham DY: Antimicrobial therapy of peptic ulcer. Int J Antimicrob Agents 1997;8:171.
Ota H, Genta RM: Morphological characterization of the gastric mucosa during infection with *H. pylori*. In Ernst P, Michetti P, Smith PD (eds): The Immunobiology of *H. pylori* from Pathogenesis to Prevention. Philadelphia, Lippincott-Raven, 1997, pp 15–28.

Chapter 52

Massive Upper Gastrointestinal Hemorrhage

Carina G. Biggs and Philip E. Donahue

Upper gastrointestinal (UGI) hemorrhage occurs with regularity in many diverse clinical settings. Owing to the variation in severity of a single episode, clear guidelines outlining the most efficient approach for diagnosis and treatment are warranted. Endoscopic diagnosis and management continue to be the keystone of effective diagnosis and treatment because 90% of bleeding sites can be identified and more than 70% managed initially by this approach. The current reliance on endoscopic management is in marked contrast with the preinterventional treatment era (before 1990), when surgical intervention was frequently necessary for the treatment of bleeding lesions, most commonly for peptic ulcers.

As the result of rather remarkable endoscopic advances, operative intervention is now considered by many to be the last resort, a stance that, while attractive to many physicians and most patients, is clearly inappropriate in some situations. Experienced surgeons recognize that there are times when emergency surgical intervention is imperative, and the failure to undertake timely operative intervention risks missing the only opportunity to salvage a patient. This "last resort" mentality is illogical in the treatment of some lesions that not only cause recurrent bleeding but also may be lethal if not treated definitively. Surgeons who recognize the risks and benefits of the operations for controlling bleeding or other ulcer complications must continue to promote the role of elective and urgent surgical intervention for selected bleeding lesions.

Choice of Operation

The specific surgical approaches are decided on intraoperatively after the site of bleeding has been identified. An experienced surgeon makes a choice of operation based on individual factors, including his or her previous operative experience, personal preferences, and other possible factors. Although the tools and techniques for controlling bleeding have changed, the surgical principles that guide patient management remain constant and are herein restated in the perspective of current clinical practice.

INCIDENCE OF GASTROINTESTINAL BLEEDING

The incidence of UGI bleeding varies widely in different population subgroups. The National Hospital Discharge Survey and the National Ambulatory Medical Care Survey suggest that UGI bleeding is responsible for 500 of every 100,000 hospital admissions (0.5%); however, this figure may have unrecognized potential sources of error. Nevertheless, the number is useful for several purposes. First, it underscores the magnitude of UGI bleeding as a common

problem. Second, it serves as a convenient reference number for evaluating our statistics on UGI bleeding at Cook County Hospital because the incidence at our institution is somewhat higher for a variety of reasons.

Individual hospitals and communities have differing experiences with the various causes of bleeding. For example, differences in the incidence of peptic ulcer between Western and Asian population subgroups are tenfold. Inner-city hospitals, Veterans Administration medical centers, and community hospitals have a different experience with UGI bleeding as the result of their widely diverse populations that manifest a spectrum of etiologies of bleeding. At Cook County Hospital in Chicago during a recent 12-month period, the 1000 patients with UGI bleeding represented about 3% of admissions that year. It is interesting that a previous report from the West Side Veterans Administration Medical Center in Chicago found a 1.5% incidence of UGI bleeding in a largely elderly population of hospitalized veterans, 10% of whom required endoscopic therapy. These incidence rates are three times higher than the national rate and reflect the severity of disease as well as the intensity of service required in urban medical centers that serve aged and socioeconomically underprivileged populations.

A report from Europe found a yearly incidence of ulcer bleeding of 45 per 100,000 population, which is comparable to that in the United States. This report highlighted a high-risk group (median age of 71 years, 63% in shock on admission) of 951 patients who had an overall mortality of 14%. Most deaths occurred in elderly patients or in those with serious comorbid conditions, the same factors associated with death for the past 50 years. Some areas in Europe have higher rates of UGI bleeding, but this should not be surprising, since there are well-recognized differences in ulcer incidence in various populations. In Chicago in 1998, the rate of hospitalization of patients for gastric and duodenal ulcers was 60 per 100,000 population.

In all reports, mortality was higher in older patients and in the socioeconomically disadvantaged. The increased incidence of complications and mortality observed in higher-risk groups, such as those in Scotland, is similar to that observed in the highest-risk groups in the United States, where the death rate and the incidence of problems due to ulcer increase with each decade of life in the population at large.

THE SPECTRUM OF UPPER GASTROINTESTINAL BLEEDING SITES

Most sources of UGI bleeding are found in the stomach and duodenum, but the failure to consider sites in other portions of the aerodigestive tract can result in misdiagnosis or delay in treatment (Table 52–1). Other lesions, such as vascular malformations, pseudoaneurysms of the splanchnic vessels including late sequelae of chronic pancreatitis or pancreatic necrosis and infections of vascular prostheses, or coagulopathic states need to be at least considered and managed individually. Success in treating these lesions requires knowledge of the natural history of the lesion, the application of innovative diagnostic approaches, and the use of accepted, proven techniques. Other lesions that infrequently cause massive bleeding,

Table 52–1	**Differential Diagnosis of Upper Gastrointestinal Bleeding**	
	SPECIFIC LESIONS	**ENDOSCOPIC TREATMENT**
Mouth	Arteriovenous malformations	+
	Telangiectasia	+
	Traumatic tears or lacerations	No
Oropharynx	Telangiectasia	+
Nose	Hypertension	No
	Telangiectasia	+
	Trauma	No
Nasopharynx	Trauma	No
Esophagus	Esophagitis	+
	Esophageal varices	+
	Peptic ulceration	+
	Neoplasm	+, temporary
	Mallory-Weiss tear	+
Stomach	Acute gastric mucosal lesions	+
	Gastric ulcer	+
	Neoplasm	+, temporary
	Heterotopic tissue (pancreas)	+
	Gastric varices	+
	Dieulafoy's lesions	+
	Arteriovenous malformations	+
	Thrombocytopenia (any cause)	±
	Hereditary hemorrhagic telangiectasia	+
	Anastomotic bleeding	+
	Visible vessels ≤1.5 mm in diameter	+
	Visible vessels >1.5 mm in diameter	±
	Nasogastric tube–induced lesions	+
	Gastritis—acute gastric lesions	+
Duodenum and jejunum	Duodenal ulcer	+
	Duodenitis	+
	Neoplasm (adenoma, carcinoma)	+, temporary
	Duodenal varices	+
	Aortoenteric fistula (atherosclerotic or graft-related)	No
	Hemosuccus pancreaticus°	No
	Hemobilia°	No
	Telangiectasias	+
	Arteriovenous malformations	+
	Ulcerated diverticulum	±
	Visible vessels ≤1.5 cm in diameter	+
	Visible vessels >1.5 mm in diameter	±

°Consider therapeutic angiographic intervention.

such as submucosal tumors, are generally not life threatening, but the risk of future bleeding and malignancy justifies a role for operative intervention for those lesions that enlarge or change in character. The most common sites of UGI bleeding are in the stomach and duodenum.

Mallory-Weiss tears, a common cause of UGI bleeding, account for 10% of all UGI bleeding episodes. The shearing forces associated with abrupt changes in intragastric pressure cause the mobile portion of the gastric wall to be propelled toward the oropharynx. The relatively fixed posterior wall of the cardia and gastroesophageal junction acts as a fulcrum for this pressure, so that the gastric wall tears longitudinally. These tears disrupt small arterial branches of the gastric wall, which results in persistent bleeding. Vomiting either does not occur or is underreported in up to 50% of patients. Patients generally stop bleeding spontaneously, but when the bleeding persists, most Mallory-Weiss tears are quite amenable to control with one of several endoscopic techniques discussed later.

Ulcers of the stomach and duodenum often are heralded by the typical spectrum of dyspeptic complaints, but the absence of symptoms of ulcer disease is a well-established scenario. Elderly patients may be particularly insensitive to the local irritant effects of the ulcer, perhaps because of an age-associated decrease in nociceptive function. Other factors that may be involved in determining whether an ulcer causes symptoms are chronicity, location, and stage of healing. Endoscopic findings such as pulsatile bleeding or the presence of a clot, a visible vessel, or a pulsation in the ulcer base can predict the risk of ongoing or subsequent ulcer bleeding. When patients with these lesions are appropriately treated by interventional techniques (coagulation, injection of epinephrine or sclerosant, laser), the rate of rebleeding is 10% to 20%. Without therapy, rebleeding rates are between 50% and 75%. In contrast, there is renewed interest in the prognostic value of emergency department–based endoscopy in patients with UGI bleeding who have a clean ulcer base; such patients have been observed for a short period of time and discharged from the emergency department.

DIAGNOSIS AND TREATMENT

All data relating to causes of bleeding should be sought, including signs and symptoms of ulcer diathesis, alcohol abuse, cardiovascular disease, and bleeding tendency. A medication history is essential, since patients treated with long-term anticoagulant therapy or, more commonly, nonsteroidal anti-inflammatory drugs (NSAIDs) have a propensity to bleeding. Treatment of the bleeding may be incomplete unless the use of such drugs is taken into consideration. It is important to remember that the history as related by the patient or a relative is often misleading.

Physical examination is performed as soon as possible, with the patient supine. A rapid, systematic approach establishes the physiologic status of the patient. The pulse and its character, blood pressure, the presence or absence of neck vein distention, and the state of peripheral capillary perfusion are noted on the initial survey. This information about the effective blood volume should guide the pace of further maneuvers. When marked abnormalities (increased pulse, diaphoresis, and hypotension) are identified, intravenous lactated Ringer's solution or 0.9% sodium chloride are administered with an initial 1000-mL bolus.

The chest and heart deserve particular attention, because congestive failure or arrhythmia may force a revision of the usual sequence of examinations. The abdomen may reveal clues about an underlying disorder, such as ascites, spider nevi, hepatosplenomegaly, and masses. Although an epigastric bruit is not extremely unusual, especially in patients with a high-flow state, its presence may indicate an otherwise unsuspected aneurysm. The presence of melena or bright red blood per rectum (hematochezia) is noted. The most common cause of massive amounts of bright red blood per rectum is massive UGI bleeding. The color of the rectal blood helps reveal the source and duration of the bleeding as well. Melena indicates that acid-hematin is present following degradation of hemoglobin by gastric contents, whereas bright red blood may represent blood from an UGI source only minutes before.

As the physical examination is completed, enough blood for emergency studies and for cross-matching is collected. Two large-bore intravenous lines should be established. A Foley catheter and a nasogastric (NG) tube *must* be inserted. The type of NG tube depends on the situation, ranging from a simple sump tube in a patient suspected of having a low-grade episode of hemorrhage to an Ewald tube (32 French) in a patient suspected of having fresh clots within the stomach.

If the hypotensive patient has minimal or no increase in blood pressure in response to the first liter, a second liter of Ringer's lactate solution is administered over 10 to 15 minutes. If there is still no response in blood pressure, the presence of massive bleeding—or some other problem, such as cardiogenic shock or congestive heart failure—must be considered. Most patients will have an increase in blood pressure by the completion of the second liter of intravenous fluid.

As soon as the patient is identified as a candidate for endoscopic investigation, the endoscopy team should be notified. Timely warning allows preparation of monitoring equipment, such as a pulse oximeter, electrocardiographic monitor, and oxygen. Decisions about the timing or performance of endoscopic investigation are deferred until the response to resuscitation is determined. When the patient has been adequately assessed clinically and appropriate resuscitative fluid therapy begun, the clinician is ready to estimate the rate of hemorrhage based on the information at hand.

A small percentage of patients bleed so massively that immediate transfer to the operating room while continuing the resuscitation is indicated. The typical lesion causing this severity of hemorrhage is an arterial vessel more than 2 mm in diameter or an aortoenteric fistula. The urgency of the situation is reflected by ongoing hypotension and tachycardia, even after several liters of fluid resuscitation. In this situation, endoscopic examination is best deferred until the patient is intubated and partially anesthetized. The operating room is an ideal and maybe the *only* appropriate place for dealing with a patient who is bleeding to death.

The risks of hypotension and hypoxia during endoscopy are real, and the authors prefer to use minimal sedation during the procedure; pulse oximetry and appropriate monitoring of the patient's physical status, level of consciousness, and adequacy of perfusion must be measured and documented. Under the best of circumstances, the endoscopic examination should be performed with the help of an experienced assistant. The potential for complications is high during emergency procedures, and the endoscopist must take all steps necessary to minimize complications or deal with them if they occur. Whether the procedure is performed in the intensive care unit, the operating room, or the endoscopy suite, the equipment for cardiac resuscitation should be readily available.

ENDOSCOPIC EXAMINATION. The endoscope is inserted into the oropharynx while the examiner digitally explores for loose teeth or dentures that may become dislodged during the procedure. Positive findings within the esophagus include esophageal inflammation, ulcers, tumors, or tears of the gastroesophageal junction that extend into the esophagus. Alternatively, the absence of sources of bleeding within the esophagus helps determine the incision needed.

As the stomach is entered, there will usually still be large amounts of blood if massive bleeding has occurred. It is impossible to attempt to aspirate this material through the suction channel of the endoscope because the suction will become clogged. Therefore, it is advisable first to identify a path through the debris between the cardia and the pylorus and cautiously maneuver the scope toward the gastric outlet. The information to be gained is whether the visible mucosa appears normal or ulcerated and whether there is any information about the presence of mucosal pathology that can explain a massive hemorrhage. Sometimes, it is advantageous to rotate the patient from the left lateral decubitus position to either a supine or a right lateral position to ascertain the presence or absence of pathology.

Often the source of bleeding can be identified through the pylorus. Occasionally, peripyloric edema or inflammation is noted, which may suggest an actively bleeding ulcer nearby. If difficulty is encountered when the surgeon attempts to pass the endoscope through the pylorus, one must determine the presences of organic stenosis of the gastric outlet or spasm of the pyloric muscles. It may help maximize visualization to inject 1 ampule (1 mg) of glucagon intravenously to allow relaxation of the smooth muscle of the gut, which occurs within 30 to 60 seconds. Once the pylorus is traversed, the bulb and second and third portions of the duodenum can be examined sequentially.

ENDOSCOPIC INTERPRETATION. Certain lesions, such as a chronic peptic ulcer, are recognized by the presence of a mucosal defect, a whitish, fibrinous base, or a deformity in the gastric or duodenal contour. Clot is a constant challenge because active bleeding and clot formation can frustrate any examination; pre-examination lavage by a large-bore (≥32 French) orogastric tube is favored by most endoscopists.

The examiner should always look for "visible vessels" that have recently bled in the base of ulcers. When clot is attached to the base of an ulcer crater, irrigation or débridement to remove the clot may afford the endoscopist a clear view of the base of the lesion, but such an aggressive diagnostic approach should be taken *only* if the endoscopist has some capability to control the bleeding provoked by this approach.

ENDOSCOPIC TREATMENT OF A BLEEDING LESION. The easiest technique is use of a sclerosant injected into the four quadrants surrounding a bleeding point. Other techniques involve the use of a heater probe, which combines an irrigation system with a probe that coagulates the bleeding point. The bipolar coagulation device (BICAP) is equally effective. The choice of these approaches depends largely on the availability of the equipment and operator expertise. The advantages of all these techniques are that the treatment of the patient takes place at the bedside, with immediate evidence of treatment success or failure. Use of the various laser techniques is not recommended under emergency conditions.

Recurrent bleeding has been a major problem with all the endoscopic techniques. When a patient has a large visible vessel at the base of the ulcer (1.5 to 2.0 mm), the authors recommend consideration of operative intervention within 24 to 48 hours to avoid the risk of recurrent hemorrhage. This group of patients has a very high incidence of rebleeding between the second and the third days following initial coagulation. When the patient rebleeds, the authors strongly recommend operative intervention rather than another attempt at coagulation, unless the patient is not an operative candidate.

ROLE OF ANGIOGRAPHIC INTERVENTION

Angiography has never enjoyed a major role in either the diagnosis or the treatment of UGI bleeding. With the advent of direct endoscopic visualization, the need for angiographic demonstration of the site of bleeding has been limited to bleeding from the hepatobiliary tree (hemobilia) or from pancreatic pathology (pancreatic pseudocysts or hemosuccus pancreaticus). These sites rarely bleed massively but can be very difficult to diagnose because the site of bleeding is not visualized by the endoscopist. Clinical hints of their presence include either a history of recent biliary intubation, percutaneous transhepatic biopsy or cholangiography, or known acute or chronic inflammatory disease of the pancreas.

In these conditions, angiography may prove both diagnostic and therapeutic. Hemorrhage from post-traumatic intrahepatic pseudoaneurysms of the pancreas may be thrombosed via angiographic embolization and thereby treated definitively. The ability of therapeutic angiographic embolization to control bleeding from the more common causes of esophagogastroduodenal hemorrhage (e.g., ulcers, neoplasms) is limited for at least two reasons: first, the blood supply to these regions has multiple collateral input not amenable to embolization of a single vessel; and second, the sites of bleeding are usually not directly from a named vessel but involve secondary or tertiary

vessels that are difficult or impossible to cannulate directly for embolization (e.g., esophageal arteries, perigastric arcade, or branches off the gastroduodenal artery). Thus, angiography should not be considered as a part of the initial armamentarium in managing UGI hemorrhage.

PRINCIPLES IN OPERATIVE TREATMENT OF UPPER GASTROINTESTINAL BLEEDING

For the patient with life-threatening, severe hemorrhage, the surgeon is the best person to determine the relative risks of operative intervention in the context of the patient's clinical status and comorbidities. Basic overall principles are outlined here, followed by a more detailed description of operative choices for each entity (Tables 52–2 and 52–3).

ESOPHAGEAL BLEEDING. Hemorrhage from the esophagus rarely requires urgent operative intervention. If bleeding is from an esophageal ulcer or severe erosive esophagitis secondary to severe gastroesophageal reflux disease, a fundoplication should be considered, combined with simultaneous intraoperative coagulation of the worst bleeding points; severe acute hemorrhage from these lesions is quite rare. In general, esophagotomy or resection should be avoided unless the ulcer is malignant; in the latter situation, all attempts to avoid an emergency or semiurgent operation should be exhausted to allow adequate preoperative staging. Other more unusual, nonvariceal sources of hemorrhage (e.g., traumatic tears, esophagoaortic fistulas, infective esophagitis) require individualized management.

GASTRITIS. When severe hemorrhage complicates diffuse gastritis, an operative mortality of more than 50% complicates the management of these very rare but difficult patients. Once more than 6 units of blood have been given, an operation is usually indicated. Near-total gastrectomy is the procedure of choice, but gastric devascularization with ligation of the named vessels to the stomach has been described. For as yet unknown reasons, such severe gastritis is exceedingly uncommon today; it

Table 52–2	**Indications for Urgent or Emergency Surgical Treatment**

ABSOLUTE

1. Patients with unstable vital signs who do not respond to aggressive resuscitation
2. Significant rebleeding (hematemesis or hematochezia) within 72 hr after initial cessation of bleeding
3. Lesions that invariably rebleed (e.g., aortoenteric fistula)

RELATIVE

1. Previous hemorrhages from the same site
2. Large gastric or duodenal ulcers (≥2.0 cm)
3. Large, visible vessel
4. Shortage of blood

These recommendations are less detailed than those in previous chapters on bleeding. The rote application of guidelines, of course, is not desirable. All therapeutic interventions should be discussed thoroughly with the patient and relatives, since the risk of morbidity or mortality is high in most settings.

Table 52–3	**Endoscopic and Surgical Interventions in Gastroduodenal Hemorrhage**	
SITE OF BLEEDING	**ENDOSCOPIC TREATMENT**	**SURGICAL TREATMENT**
Esophageal ulcer, GERD	Coagulation, injection	Prevention of gastroesophageal reflux
Mallory-Weiss tear	Coagulation, injection	Oversew (rarely necessary)
Esophageal varices	Sclerosis, banding	Shunt, TIPS, liver transplantation
Chronic gastric ulcer (types I–IV require individual assessment)	Coagulation, injection (vessels <1.5 mm wide)	Resection (best), oversew (poor risk), vagotomy optional
		Highly selective vagotomy (not widely used)
Acute gastric ulcers	Coagulation, injection	Resection (subtotal gastrectomy)
Gastric cancer	Coagulation, injection	Appropriate operation
Gastric varices	Generally not done	Splenectomy (splenic vein thrombosis) or shunt (portal hypertension)
Anastomotic bleeding	Coagulation, injection	Oversew (rarely necessary)
Duodenal ulcer	Coagulation, injection (vessels <1.5 mm wide)	Individualized treatment by oversewing or excision of ulcer plus vagotomy (truncal or highly selective); antrectomy rarely indicated
Aortoenteric fistula	Not effective	Resection of infected graft, vascular bypass
Hemosuccus pancreaticus	Not effective	Ligation or resection of pancreatic vessels in addition to treatment of the primary pancreatic pathology
Duodenal diverticula	Coagulation, injection (if safe)	Oversew (occasionally necessary)

GERD, gastroesophageal reflux disease; TIPS, transjugular intrahepatic portosystemic shunt.

was more common 20 to 30 years ago prior to the advent of routine and comprehensive intensive care support.

GASTRIC ULCERS. Resection remains the best choice for these lesions. The amount of stomach varies, depending on the site of origin and the patient's history. High ulcers present a formidable challenge but can be approached by simple resection as well. The surgeon should consider whether the ulcer is malignant and act accordingly. A frozen section study often is warranted.

ANASTOMOTIC ULCERS. These ulcers result either from repeated acid hypersecretion, aspirin or NSAID use, or development of gastric cancer. With bleeding, the ulcerated anastomosis should be excised; further gastrectomy or vagotomy should be seriously considered and individualized.

DUODENAL ULCERS. Oversewing the bleeding ulcer, followed by pyloroplasty and vagotomy, is usually the approach of choice. If the patient is young, some thought should be given to duodenotomy with control of hemorrhage, and either parietal cell vagotomy, acid suppression, or both postoperatively, plus eradication of the likely etiology of *Helicobacter pylori*. As a general rule, resection is not necessary and has neither intrinsic nor essential benefit, since the overall morbidity of resection overshadows the benefit of a lower rate of ulcer recurrence.

INTRAOPERATIVE ENDOSCOPY

On rare occasions, the plan of management brings the patient with massive bleeding to the operating room to continue resuscitation with the thought that if there is no prompt improvement in the patient's condition, an emergency laparotomy will be performed. The timing of the endoscopy should be secondary to the overall management of the patient but not necessarily postponed until after the incision has been made. The primary goal of the endoscopic procedure is to determine whether or not there are esophageal varices or another esophageal source of bleeding.

If bleeding esophageal varices are present, there is no clear standard therapy since the mortality associated with variceal hemorrhage of this magnitude approaches 50%. The authors individualize their management. Given the unstable condition of the type of patient just mentioned, a Blakemore tube would probably be the more desirable, saving sclerotherapy for a more controlled interval, usually 24 to 48 hours later.

Even with the most severe hemorrhage, one can usually recognize a Mallory-Weiss tear with active bleeding at the gastroesophageal junction. Preoperative recognition of this site of bleeding is important because this area is hard to visualize intraoperatively. The use of an immediate intraoperative endoscopic examination is much more attractive than gastrotomy in defining the lesion. Moreover, with knowledge of the site of bleeding, the gastrotomy allowing access for oversewing can be made closer to the lesion high in the stomach.

DIEULAFOY'S LESION. These lesions represent focal aberrant large arterial vessels in the mucosa of the stomach or, rarely, the duodenum. They become ulcerated and can bleed quite massively. They tend to occur more frequently in alcoholic patients. Because these lesions are focal and not multicentric, and because the mucosal ulceration or erosion is only 1 to 2 mm, they can easily be missed at endoscopy. Many lesions stop spontaneously but will rebleed. When visualized endoscopically, they are readily amenable to definitive treatment with endoscopic techniques.

GASTRIC ULCER. There is little consensus among experienced surgeons about the "ideal" operation for gastric ulcer despite wide experience with diverse operations for the past 100 years. When treatment options are discussed, the "location-based" classification allows individualization of treatment, depending on the type of lesion. Type II and III ulcers are thought to be partially due to hypersecretion of acid. Therefore, optimal treatment of these lesions includes gastrectomy with or without vagotomy.

TYPE I GASTRIC ULCER (AT INCISURA ALONG THE LESSER CURVATURE). The most effective treatment for this lesion is surgical removal of the distal stomach, encompassing the ulcer in the gastric resection. This procedure usually involves a 50% resection. Since type I gastric ulcers are not associated with acid hypersecretion, a vagotomy is unnecessary unless there is evidence of previous duodenal ulcer. Although the authors prefer the Billroth I reconstruction, many surgeons use a Billroth II reconstruction. Little objective evidence supports the use of one over the other. The essential part of the procedure is that the resection should remove all the antral mucosa and the ulcer base. Simple oversewing of the bleeding base of the ulcer, combined with vagotomy and pyloroplasty, is not optimal but may be reserved for the unstable patient who may not tolerate a more physiologically demanding operation. Vagotomy and pyloroplasty, combined with excision of the ulcer base, are more attractive. However, vagotomy and pyloroplasty do not address the basic problem of diseased mucosal surfaces nearly as well as does gastric resection.

TYPE II AND TYPE III GASTRIC ULCER. For a type II ("combined") gastric ulcer or type III pyloric channel ulcer, vagotomy and pyloroplasty with oversewing of the bleeding ulcer is the minimal operative procedure indicated because hyperacidity is prominent in these patients. The potential for development of gastric atony and increased duodenogastric reflux makes a highly selective vagotomy preferable to some surgeons. The standard approach, however, for a stable patient with a type II or type III bleeding chronic gastric ulcer remains gastric resection.

TYPE IV GASTRIC ULCER. When surgeons operate for a bleeding type IV ulcer, the best approach involves a transmural resection of the ulcer with closure of the gastrotomy. No additional gastrectomy or vagotomy is necessary. Although recurrence rates may be somewhat higher (~5% to 10%), an extended gastrectomy is usually not indicated in an emergency situation. For a chronic type IV ulcer, if an antrectomy is planned it will be necessary to extend the tongue of the resected lesser curvature into the proximal stomach to include the ulcer. In such a case, the use of a Roux-en-Y jejunal limb offers the best reconstruction for restoration of gastrointestinal continuity. Total gastrectomy is the last choice of operation for this benign disease.

RECURRENT ULCERS

When a recurrent or anastomotic ulcer is discovered after previous gastric surgery, the approach includes three considerations: a new problem, unrelated to the previous operation; the primary ulcer diathesis, expressing itself despite the previous antiulcer operation; or a specific complication of the previous operation. This situation requires the insight of an experienced surgeon, because many of the possible problems may not be recognized by a practitioner not well versed in the complications of

surgical treatment. If a type I gastric ulcer recurs, the answer will usually be found in the extent of the gastric resection. When type II and type III ulcers recur, there is usually an incomplete vagotomy or need for an antrectomy or higher gastrectomy, and eradication of *H. pylori*. Other considerations should include the inordinate use of NSAIDs or development of a gastric remnant cancer. When a type IV ulcer recurs, the extent of the gastric

Pearls and Pitfalls

- Ulcers remain very common in the population at large, despite their relative disappearance from the list of routine operations performed in major medical centers.
- Endoscopic diagnosis and treatment of bleeding lesions, especially the pulsatile clot or the visible vessel in the base of an ulcer, are effective in 80% to 90% of bleeding ulcers.
- Bright red blood per rectum can occur in the setting of massive UGI bleeding.
- Although most UGI bleeding comes from gastric or duodenal lesions, one must consider sources from the nasopharynx, esophagus, hepatobiliary tree (hemobilia), or pancreas (hemosuccus pancreaticus).
- The initial evaluation and treatment are performed in the resuscitation phase, after the primary survey has been performed. Sufficient intravenous access, fluid infusion, and protection of vital processes are done prior to endoscopic investigation, which is the next step.
- Angiography has little role in UGI bleeding.
- Recognize the lesions that are very poor candidates for endoscopic treatment, such as "huge" (for an endoscopist, huge is greater than 1.5 to 2.0 mm) arterial bleeding sites, lesions that present a poor target (extremely irregular or undefined anatomy), or pseudoaneurysms.
- Absolute indications for operative treatment include the hemodynamically unstable patient, significant rebleeding within 72 hours of initial cessation of bleeding, and lesions that invariably rebleed (e.g., aortoenteric fistula).
- Operative techniques for bleeding ulcers involve oversewing of the site of bleeding combined with ulcer excision, a definite antiulcer operation, or gastrectomy dependent on type of ulcer and hemodynamic stability of patient.
- Repeated endoscopic treatment may be detrimental to the patient with medical comorbidities by delaying necessary definitive operative treatment.
- If endoscopic treatment cannot be performed in unstable patients who are "bleeding out," there is another opportunity after the induction of anesthesia: most surgeons prefer nonoperative treatment for acutely bleeding varices unless they are associated with splenic vein thrombosis.
- Choice of operation is individualized, depending on individual factors. For benign disease, "less is better" as a rule; extended highly selective vagotomy is the overall best choice for treatment in young patients because of the absence of side effects. Truncal vagotomy or antrectomy is the first choice for surgeons who want 99% certitude that the ulcer will not recur.

resection may have been insufficient, or a stagnant gastric remnant may have been created by the original operation.

SELECTED READINGS

Allison MC, Howatson AG, Torrance CJ, et al: Gastrointestinal damage associated with the use of nonsteroidal anti-inflammatory drugs. N Engl J Med 1992;327:749.

Bordley DR, Mushlin AJ, Dolan JG, et al: Early clinical signs identify low-risk patients with acute upper gastrointestinal hemorrhage. JAMA 1985;753:3282.

Donahue PE: Peptic ulcers in Cook County—1998: The modern face of a common problem. Chicago Med 1998;103:16.

Donahue PE, Nyhus LM: Massive upper gastrointestinal hemorrhage. In Nyhus LM, Wastell C, Donahue PE (eds): Surgery of the Esophagus, Stomach and Small Intestine, 5th ed. Boston, Little, Brown, 1995, pp 642–654.

Pollard TR, Schwesinger WH: Upper gastrointestinal bleeding following major surgical procedures: Prevlaence, etiology and outcome. J Surg Res 1996;64:75.

Wangensteen OH, Wangensteen SD, Dennis C: The history of gastric surgery. In Wastell C, Nyhus LM, Donahue PE (eds): Surgery of the Esophagus, Stomach and Small Intestine, 5th ed. Boston, Little, Brown, 1995, pp 354–385.

Chapter 53

Peptic Ulcer Disease: Perforation

Harry M. Richter, III

Duodenal ulcer (DU) is a disease in retreat. Even before the introduction of histamine (H_2) receptor blockers, the need for curative ulcer surgery was on the decline, at least in Western industrialized countries. Although potent antisecretory medicines, including H_2 blockers and proton pump inhibitors, greatly improve and facilitate medical treatment, they do not alter the underlying ulcerogenic diathesis that characterizes chronic DU. We currently recognize that most chronic DU disease depends on active gastric infection with the *Helicobacter pylori* organism. Eradication of this organism permanently cures the great majority of DUs. The diminishing prevalence of *Helicobacter* infection in modern, economically advantaged societies (the result of improved public hygiene) most likely explains the spontaneous amelioration of the DU problem.

NATURAL HISTORY OF ULCER PERFORATION

Surgeons have long recognized two distinct classes of perforated DU: perforated "acute" ulcers; and perforated "chronic" ulcers. Acute ulcers are those with no documented ulcer prior to perforation and dyspepsia for less than 3 months leading up to the perforation. The remainder are chronic ulcers that generally account for about 70% of DU perforations. The distinction between perforated acute and perforated chronic ulcer remains important. Simple surgical closure of a perforated acute ulcer is usually sufficient therapy; only a small fraction (usually the younger patients) will suffer further ulcer disease. Simple closure of a perforated chronic ulcer, on the other hand, merely overcomes the acute catastrophe. Many, possibly most, of these patients develop further ulcer complications or medical intractability. For this reason, many surgeons embraced the practice of immediate, definitive, antiulcer operation for perforated DU, provided the patient is stable. Several clinical trials have demonstrated that in selected patients, definitive surgery can be as safe as simple omental patch closure and will prevent further ulcer complications and distress.

The clinical picture of ulcer perforation has evolved since the 1980s. The marked male predominance is disappearing. Perforations now occur at a substantially older patient age, and patients tend to have more serious, chronic illnesses. Finally, a greater proportion of the DUs that perforate are deemed acute, rather than chronic, ulcers. Thus, a smaller proportion of patients is fit for definitive ulcer surgery, and it appears that a smaller proportion would benefit from an antiulcer operation.

What role does *H. pylori* play in DU perforation? Since nearly all patients with DU have evidence of *Helico-bacter* infection, patients with perforated chronic ulcer might be expected to be similarly infected. One early study disclosed that only about one half of patients with perforated DU were *Helicobacter* positive, a fraction not different from that of a suitably matched control group. The data suggest that *Helicobacter* is not necessarily directly related to the pathogenesis of perforated DU. It is interesting that among both the *Helicobacter*-positive and the *Helicobacter*-negative groups, only one quarter of the patients had a previous suspicion of ulcer disease, whereas the remainder appear to have had perforations of an acute DU. This impression was corroborated by the gross description of the ulcer at operation. The conclusions of this study therefore do not preclude a role for *Helicobacter* in chronic DUs that perforate. Subsequent reports demonstrate a much larger proportion of *Helicobacter*-positive patients presenting with DU perforation.

The importance of *H. pylori* infection was most emphatically demonstrated in a recent report from Hong Kong. Eighty percent of patients with perforated DU were found to be *Helicobacter* positive. The *Helicobacter*-positive patients were treated by patch closure of the perforation alone and were then randomized to receive either conventional antiulcer medication or a standard anti-*Helicobacter* antibiotic therapy. Those patients receiving only antisecretory therapy experienced a 38% ulcer recurrence within the first year, whereas the patients randomized to the anti-*Helicobacter* group had only a 5% recurrence of DU. In conclusion, patients whose chronic DU perforates very likely harbor *H. pylori* infection. Furthermore, eradication of the *Helicobacter* infection confers long-term protection against recurrent ulcer, no different from the experience with uncomplicated chronic DU. On the other hand, the role of *Helicobacter* in perforated acute DU remains uncertain.

PRESENTATION AND DIAGNOSIS OF PERFORATED DUODENAL ULCER

Perforated DU is the prototypical "acute abdomen," and most patients continue to present in this way. The non-hospitalized patient is usually well, albeit with a current or intermittent history of dyspepsia or ulcer disease, and suddenly he or she experiences the onset of severe epigastric pain, which rapidly spreads to involve the entire abdomen. The onset of pain is so abrupt that the patient is often able to note the exact minute at which it occurs. Most patients vomit early in the attack.

The intensity of the abdominal pain is usually sufficient to bring the patient to the hospital within several hours, although intoxication or simple stubbornness may delay arrival. The patient appears acutely ill and is often tachy-

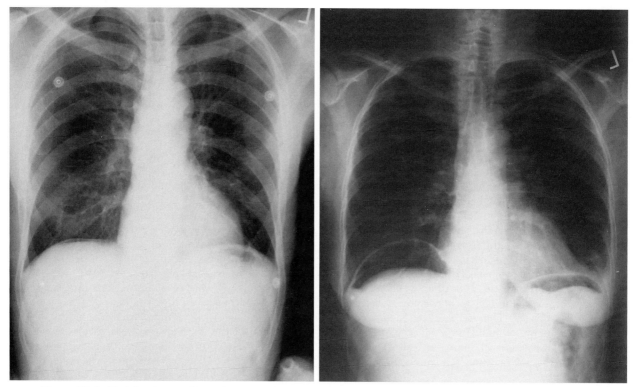

Figure 53–1. Upright chest radiographs demonstrating free intraperitoneal air. *Left Panel,* Subtle finding of a small amount beneath the right hemidiaphragm. *Right Panel,* Obvious free air beneath the right and left hemidiaphragms.

cardic. Hypotension is uncommon, as is fever. Usually the abdomen is silent, tender, and rigid in all quadrants. Digital rectal examination is uncomfortable and may disclose a trace of occult blood. The white blood cell count may be normal or slightly increased, and the serum amylase level is likewise normal or slightly increased, as amylase escaping the perforation is absorbed across the peritoneal surface. Although this picture is classic for perforated ulcer, the differential diagnosis must also include acute pancreatitis, closed-loop small intestinal obstruction, and leaking abdominal aortic aneurysm, among others.

An upright chest radiograph, seeking "free air" beneath the diaphragm, is the first diagnostic test (Fig. 53–1). If the patient can tolerate standing erect for several minutes before exposure of the radiograph, small volumes of free air may percolate upward, increasing the diagnostic yield. About three quarters of patients with perforated DU have demonstrable pneumoperitoneum on upright chest radiograph, the percentage being slightly lower as more time elapses after perforation. Patients who cannot tolerate standing upright may undergo a cross-table lateral x-ray exposure in the left decubitus position; the radiologist looks for free air outlining the right edge of the liver.

In the absence of demonstrable free air, the next diagnostic test is computed tomography (CT) of the abdomen after ingestion of oral contrast. CT may reveal minute amounts of intraperitoneal air, either around the liver or confined to the hepatoduodenal ligament. Should CT be unavailable, a diatrizoate (Gastrografin) upper gastrointestinal (GI) study is undertaken to establish the diagnosis

(Fig. 53–2). This study has the added advantage of identifying those patients whose perforated DU has spontaneously sealed.

A growing group of patients with other serious comorbidities develop perforated DU while hospitalized for

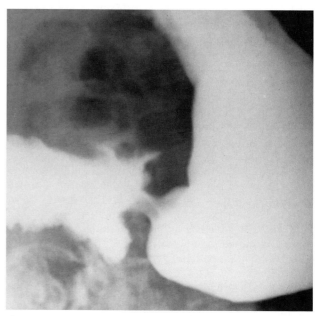

Figure 53–2. Gastrografin upper GI contrast study demonstrating leak of contrast material from a perforated duodenal ulcer. Note air bubble within the leaking contrast material.

another condition. In these patients, often already obtunded and perhaps even intubated, diagnostic delay is the greatest. The surgeon is called because the patient has "become distended" or "looks septic." Abdominal examination reveals distention and tympani, but involuntary guarding is less distinct than might be expected. Plain abdominal films, if negative, should be followed by CT when the patient can tolerate it. Otherwise, bedside paracentesis may reveal bile-stained fluid, confirming a GI catastrophe.

TREATMENT

Definitive antiulcer operation for perforated DU now has a vastly diminished role, for several reasons. First, long-term relief of ulcer disease is achieved by eradication of *H. pylori*, when present. Second, a greater percentage of patients have acute ulcers, which portend less risk of long-term ulcer disease. Third, patients are now more likely to be older and critically ill, as a result of comorbid diseases, and thus are not safe candidates for a prolonged operation. Finally, few surgeons trained within the past 2 decades are facile with the complexities of ulcer surgery.

Currently, the indications for definitive surgery in the setting of perforation include the following: (1) perforation with concomitant hemorrhage or gastric outlet obstruction; (2) a chronic ulcer history with documented negative *Helicobacter* status; (3) ulcer perforation too large to patch safely (greater than 1-cm diameter); and (4) leak following attempted patch closure. An as yet unanswered question is whether older patients who require and will continue to require aspirin or nonsteroidal anti-inflammatory agents should undergo a definitive antiulcer procedure. Patients with Zollinger-Ellison syndrome whose DUs perforate are not benefited by any of the standard antiulcer operations.

Initial treatment consists of aggressive intravenous fluid resuscitation, nasogastric suction, and a single-agent, broad-spectrum parenteral antibiotic. During resuscitation, monitoring of hemodynamic stability is important with a urinary catheter, central venous pressure catheter, and arterial line following standard indications, as does the provision of supplemental oxygen. Parenteral opioids for pain relief are appropriate once the diagnosis is made and whenever operation is to be delayed for more than 1 hour or if nonoperative therapy is elected. Likewise, prophylaxis against deep venous thrombosis is begun with a pneumatic calf compression device before or during operation and continued postoperatively; subcutaneous heparin is added postoperatively.

Nonoperative Treatment

This approach has often illogically been called "conservative" treatment. Many perforated DUs are found to be spontaneously sealed at the time of surgical exploration. If the goal of operation is simple closure of the perforation, then operation to achieve this goal is often, in fact, unnecessary. A deliberate program of nonoperative therapy can be successful if applied to carefully selected patients. The components of nonoperative treatment include intravenous hydration, nasogastric suction, parenteral antibiotics, gastric antisecretory medication, analgesia, and prophylaxis against deep vein thrombosis.

Appropriate candidates for a trial of nonoperative management are relatively young and healthy patients who, at the time of presentation, have localized as opposed to diffuse tenderness and rigidity. Some authorities require that a diatrizoate upper GI contrast study confirm spontaneous closure of the duodenal perforation.

Successful pursuit of nonoperative treatment avoids an operation but does not reduce hospital stay. Intraperitoneal infections requiring drainage are more common than postoperative closure with peritoneal lavage (Fig. 53–3). Moreover, endoscopy is mandatory after recovery to exclude the occasional perforated gastric carcinoma. The perforations of a substantial portion of patients initially treated nonoperatively will fail to seal and require operative closure. Unfortunately, those patients deemed to be at highest operative risk are exactly those most likely to fail a nonoperative approach. Nonoperative therapy for the seriously ill patient offers little hope of survival.

Techniques of Operative Management

Omental Patch

The abdomen is entered through a short upper midline incision centered about halfway between xiphoid and umbilicus, but protecting the falciform ligament in case it is needed as patch material. A perforated DU is found on the anterior aspect of the duodenal bulb by retracting the left lobe of the liver superiorly. The abdomen is irrigated thoroughly with warmed saline and aspirated dry. Almost always, a convenient tongue of omentum can be readily drawn over the duodenal bulb (Fig. 53–4).

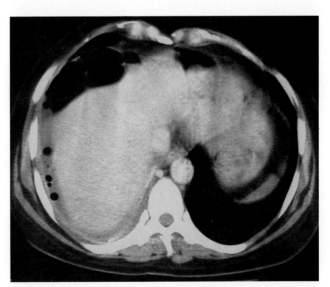

Figure 53–3. CT of the abdomen several days after unsuccessful nonoperative treatment of a perforated duodenal ulcer. Note residual free intraperitoneal air anterior to the liver and colon, and gas-containing fluid lateral to the right lobe of the liver.

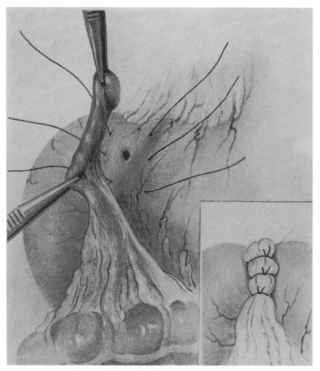

Figure 53–4. Omental patch closure ("Graham patch") of perforated duodenal ulcer. Note the placement of sutures, which are then tied over the omental tissue. (Reprinted from Maingot R: Abdominal Operations, 7th ed. New York, Appleton-Century-Crofts, 1980, with permission.)

Three or four interrupted sutures spanning the perforation are placed but are left untied. The sutures are taken as full-thickness bites of duodenum; accurate placement is facilitated by bringing the needle out through the perforation following the first bite, and then reintroducing the needle through the perforation to emerge through the opposite rim of the perforated ulcer. Substantial bites of the firm rim of the ulcer should be assured to avoid sutures tearing out; deep sutures do not risk narrowing the lumen. The previously identified tongue of omentum is then laid directly over the perforated ulcer, and the sutures are tied gently but snugly over the omental patch. For small ulcers, many surgeons will tie the sutures first to reapproximate the edges of the ulcer and then patch the closure with the omental patch, using the uncut ends of the previously tied sutures. Fascial closure is routine, and the skin is closed unless peritoneal contamination is purulent and extensive.

If the omentum is absent or atretic or cannot be mobilized, the falciform ligament provides suitable back-up tissue. The round ligament is divided between ties just above the umbilicus, and the falciform and round ligaments are then freed from the anterior abdominal wall, dissecting cephalad toward the liver. After sufficient mobilization, the pedicle thus developed will fit nicely in place as a viable, vascularized patch material. If necessary, it may be doubled upon itself to provide additional bulk and secured in place like an omental patch. Essentially the same omental or falciform patch procedure can be

accomplished laparoscopically, but no benefit has been confirmed to date.

Resection

Patch closure of perforations greater than 1 cm in diameter is best avoided, because the risk of leak is great. The most secure approach is to perform an antrectomy, closing the scarred and inflamed duodenal stump around an exteriorized catheter (mushroom or Malecot) and draining the stump with closed suction drains. A standard Billroth II gastrojejunostomy restores alimentary continuity. In stable patients, a truncal vagotomy is then undertaken. Because resumption of oral intake may be slow, a nasal-intestinal feeding tube is guided through the gastrojejunostomy and down the efferent jejunal loop.

Vagotomy

When the now-rare indications for definitive operation are met, the selection of an antiulcer procedure is a balance between optimal functional outcome on one hand and the surgeon's experience on the other. Those surgeons skilled in performing highly selective vagotomy (parietal cell vagotomy) advocate combining this procedure with omental patch closure of the perforation. If gastric outlet obstruction is suggested by history, a drainage procedure is added. Either the perforation is extended across the pylorus, and this opening closed transversely as a Heineke-Mikulicz pyloroplasty, or a gastrojejunostomy (posterior, retrocolic) is added. The surgeon inexperienced with highly selective vagotomy may opt for truncal vagotomy with pyloroplasty or gastrojejunostomy. In spite of its very low ulcer recurrence rate, vagotomy and antrectomy seem best reserved for managing the giant perforations, as described earlier.

POSTOPERATIVE CARE AND OUTCOME

Antibiotics are continued until culture of the peritoneal fluid is available. If the fluid is sterile, as is usually the

---

Pearls and Pitfalls

- The spectrum of perforated DU is changing from more chronic ulcers to more acute ulcers, probably as our population gets older.
- The hallmarks of a perforated ulcer are sudden onset of abdominal pain, peritonitis, and free air on upright abdominal or chest radiograph.
- Preoperative preparation requires aggressive fluid resuscitation and preoperative antibiotics.
- Surgical options include simple patch closure, vagotomy and pyloroplasty through the perforation, antrectomy/vagotomy, or patch closure with parietal cell vagotomy.
- Nonoperative treatment may be used selectively in hemodynamically stable patients with localized abdominal tenderness and a self-sealed ulcer.

case, the antibiotics are stopped. Otherwise, they are tailored as dictated by sensitivity. A pure culture of *Candida* species is not unusual and is merely a marker of upper GI tract perforation; antifungal agents are not necessary. Parenteral antiulcer medication is continued unless definitive operation has been performed. The nasogastric tube is removed as soon as the abdomen is soft, and oral intake may be resumed thereafter. The complications encountered include those routinely associated with major abdominal surgery, in particular myocardial infarction, pneumonia and/or respiratory failure, and pulmonary embolism. Septic complications, such as intraabdominal abscess or enteric leak, are uncommon. *Helicobacter* status is assessed several weeks after recovery and is treated if found.

Several studies document risk factors for death with DU perforation. Risk factors supported by several, if not all, studies, include preoperative hypotension, advanced age (greater than 70 years), serious comorbidity, and duration of perforation greater than 24 hours. Overall mortality rates range between 5% and 15% and are not improving.

SELECTED READINGS

Donovan AJ, Berne TV, Donovan JA: Perforated duodenal ulcer. Arch Surg 1998;133:1166.
Lau WY, Leung KL, Kwong KH, et al: A randomized study comparing laparoscopic versus open repair of perforated peptic ulcer using suture or sutureless technique. Ann Surg 1996;224:131.
Ng EKW, Lam YH, Sung, JJY, et al: Eradication of *Helicobacter pylori* prevents recurrence of ulcer after simple closure of duodenal ulcer perforation. Ann Surg 2000;231:153.
Reinbach DH, Cruickshank G, McColl KEL: Acute perforated duodenal ulcer is not associated with *Helicobacter pylori* infection. Gut 1993;34:1344.

Chapter 54

Peptic Ulcer Disease: Obstruction

Daniel T. Dempsey

Obstruction of the gastric outlet has represented the main indication for surgery in approximately 10% to 15% of patients operated upon for peptic ulcer disease. Although all population studies have shown that the incidence of elective operation for peptic ulcer has been declining dramatically for several decades, this decline started before introduction of antisecretory drugs and has persisted thereafter. Whereas some studies suggest a decline in the number of operations for obstructing peptic ulcer disease, others show that the small percentage of ulcer patients requiring operation for this complication has remained relatively constant. In virtually all large clinical series, surgery is more commonly performed for bleeding or perforation than for obstruction.

At least half of the patients admitted to hospital for obstructing peptic ulcer in the United States have *Helicobacter pylori* infection (see later discussion). Both gastric outlet obstruction as a complication of peptic ulcer disease and *H. pylori* infection are probably more common in developing countries, where both *H. pylori* infection and surgery for obstructing peptic ulcer are more prevalent. This may be an important issue for U.S. surgeons treating peptic ulcer disease in immigrant patients.

CLINICAL PRESENTATION

Patients with obstructing peptic ulcer disease have epigastric pain, bloating, and usually vomiting. Moreover, the patient notices early satiety with weight loss. The vomitus contains recognizable food fragments and is characteristically free of bile. Examination often shows a distended epigastrium, sometimes with visible peristalsis ("the stomach you can see"). Borborygmi are heard, and a succussion splash may be elicited ("the stomach you can hear"). The lower abdomen is typically scaphoid, but the distended stomach may be palpable in the upper abdomen ("the stomach you can feel"). The abdominal examination can change measurably with nasogastric decompression. Serology typically reveals a hypokalemic, hypochloremic metabolic alkalosis and hemoconcentration. Upright abdominal x-ray study usually shows a massively dilated stomach with a large air-fluid level.

Pathophysiology

Peptic ulcer disease is the most common cause of gastric outlet obstruction. In most patients, the disease is chronic and results in scarring and fibrosis of the prepyloric antrum, pylorus, or (most commonly) the first portion of the duodenum. Thus, both type II gastric ulcer (i.e., gastric ulcer with old or new duodenal ulcer) and type III gastric ulcer (i.e., prepyloric ulcer with or without

gastric or duodenal ulcer) may be associated with gastric outlet obstruction. But most patients with this problem from peptic ulcer disease have only duodenal ulcer. Acute peptic ulceration may create sufficient edema and motor dysfunction to block the gastric outlet, but more commonly this occurs in the setting of an already scarred pyloric channel. Endoscopic studies have shown that approximately 50% of patients admitted to hospital with benign gastric outlet obstruction have active ulceration, usually in addition to chronic cicatrix (Table 54–1). In addition to having aggressive medical therapy, approximately 75% of patients with obstructing peptic ulcer will require endoscopic ("balloon") dilation or surgery within 4 months of hospitalization. Although early and aggressive treatment of *H. pylori* may decrease the need for early intervention in the patient group not abusing nonsteroidal anti-inflammatory drugs (NSAIDs), definitive treatment should be considered during the initial hospitalization.

Diagnosis

The differential diagnosis of gastric outlet obstruction in the adult patient includes benign and malignant causes. Peptic ulcer disease, gastric cancer, and pancreatic cancer are the most common diagnoses. Other possibilities include duodenal webs, hypertrophic pyloric stenosis, submucosal tumors (e.g., Brunner's gland adenomas), polyps, and gastroparesis. Upper endoscopy is the most useful test. To perform this test safely and effectively, the stomach must first be decompressed with a large bore nasogastric or Ewald tube before endoscopic sedation. Biopsy samples should be obtained to rule out both malignancy and *H. pylori* infection. Other potentially useful tests in selected patients include computed tomography, upper gastrointestinal series, and gastric emptying scintiscan.

Obstructing Peptic Ulcer Disease in the *Helicobacter* Era

About half of the patients admitted to hospital with gastric outlet obstruction from peptic ulcer disease have *H. pylori* infection, and the prevalence is higher in developing countries. Two important questions regarding the management of these patients persist: (1) Does aggressive treatment of *Helicobacter* infection decrease the need for endoscopic or operative therapy? (2) Does aggressive treatment of *Helicobacter* infection after endoscopic or operative therapy decrease the incidence of recurrent ulceration or obstruction? If the answer to the second question is "yes," then it may be superfluous to do a bigger ulcer operation to lower the incidence of recurrence. If the answer to the first question is also affirma-

Table 54–1	Endoscopic Balloon Dilation for Obstructing Peptic Ulcer						
AUTHOR (YR)	PATIENTS	DILATIONS	PERF	SUCCESS[a]	OPERATION[b]	MEAN FOLLOW-UP (MONTHS)	ACTIVE ULCER[g]
DiSario (1994)	30	51	2	24	6	15	10 of 30
Kozarek (1990)[c]	23	?	1	16	5	31	12 of 23
Hewitt et al (1999)[d]	46	122	0	20	16	19	28 of 46
Griffin (1989)[e]	25	?	0	20	5	9	14 of 24
Lau et al (1996)[f]	54	73	4	20	25	39	20 of 54

[a]Success = acceptable symptoms and no operation.
[b]Includes patients operated on acutely for perforation.
[c]Twenty-eight patients were dilated, but 5 were lost to follow-up; 7 of 23 had anastomotic stricture.
[d]Forty-six patients attempted, but not feasible in 5.
[e]Twenty-five patients attempted but not feasible in 1.
[f]Fifty-four patients attempted but not feasible in 5; 4 with early restenosis had cancer.
[g]Active ulcer at initial endoscopy.

tive, then operating too soon may be equally misguided. Finally, it is essential for the surgeon to recognize that virtually all publications on operation for peptic ulcer predate modern understanding of *Helicobacter* as a causative factor in this disease. Most of these studies also predate the availability of proton pump inhibitors. The real answer to these questions depends on patient age, whether *II. pylori* infection is present, and whether the patient has been taking NSAIDs.

PREOPERATIVE MANAGEMENT

Most patients coming to hospital with obstructing peptic ulcer disease require either endoscopic or operative treatment within the next few months. Thus, the majority of hospitalized patients with *chronic* obstructing ulcer disease should undergo a trial of balloon dilation or be operated upon during the index hospitalization. Patients with *acute* disease or acute-on-chronic disease may respond to medical management alone, but many of these patients have recurrent obstruction within the first year of follow-up, necessitating more aggressive therapy.

Medical Treatment

Fluid resuscitation, nasogastric decompression, acid suppression, and nutritional support are the mainstays of medical therapy. Fluid and electrolyte deficits are replaced with normal saline. Potassium chloride may be added to the intravenous fluids once there is evidence of adequate renal function. Vital signs and urine output guide resuscitation. Invasive hemodynamic monitoring may on occasion be required for patients with severe cardiac or pulmonary compromise. Intravenous antisecretory agents are standard. Nasogastric suction should be continued until the drainage is less than 1 L per day, and a "clamping trial" may be useful before pulling the tube. If it is likely that endoscopic or operative therapy will be needed, nasogastric suction should be continued. If the patient improves with medical treatment alone, a diet may be tried. Once this is tolerated, antibiotics for *H. pylori* should be added if there is evidence of infection on endoscopic biopsy (histology or urease test) or if the

patient has positive serology and has never undergone treatment.

Endoscopic Treatment

Through-the-scope balloon dilation (see Table 54–1) of the strictured gastric outlet is initially successful in many patients with obstructing peptic ulcer disease, but recurrent future obstruction is common. Published series suggest that approximately one half to two thirds of patients can be helped for up to 3 years with this treatment as long as they have adequate treatment after dilation. The average diameter of the dilating balloon in most series is 15 mm, and perforation is unusual with this size balloon in the hands of an experienced endoscopist. Technical difficulties may preclude balloon dilation in up to 10% of patients with benign gastric outlet obstruction. Approximately 50% of patients in treatment remain relatively symptom-free for up to 3 years, but repeat dilation is often necessary to maintain this underwhelming result. One might expect the long-term success of balloon dilation to be further improved by routine eradication of *H. pylori* infection and aggressive antisecretory therapy. Lam (1997) suggests that balloon dilation for obstructing peptic ulcer is more durable in *H. pylori*–positive patients who receive treatment than in *H. pylori*–negative patients.

Considering the potency of current antisecretory drugs and the profound decrease in ulcer recurrence rates with successful *H. pylori* treatment, there is little rationale for the routine addition of laparoscopic highly selective vagotomy (HSV) to endoscopic balloon dilation for obstructing peptic ulcer disease. It should be noted that there are no randomized prospective studies comparing operative treatment with balloon dilation in this population, an important caveat because the indications for intervention may be different in published series of balloon dilation or surgery for obstructing peptic ulcer.

OPERATIVE MANAGEMENT

Over the past 2 decades, the emphasis in the literature on operation for obstructing peptic ulcer disease has been on the following procedures: HSV with pyloric dilation or duodenoplasty, HSV and drainage, truncal vagotomy and drainage, and vagotomy (either truncal or selective) and antrectomy (Table 54–2). Proponents of these antiulcer operations point out that most patients coming to operation have failed aggressive medical management and are therefore more likely to fail a minimalist operation, that is, big disease requires big surgery. Proponents of the lesser, more "physiologic" operations argue that patients who fail medical management are the very patients who are least likely to do well with a big operation, that is, often those elderly patients taking NSAIDs. They further argue that current understanding of *H. pylori* in ulcer pathophysiology (together with the development of proton pump inhibitors) greatly mitigates the worry about recurrent ulcer, heretofore a major reason for doing the bigger operations, at least in younger patients with *H. pylori* as the etiologic agent. Finally they point out that patients who fail the smaller procedures can safely undergo reoperation if necessary. The author is currently on the side of those who believe that "less is more."

Data from the era before both proton pump inhibitors and the discovery of *H. pylori* suggest that prepyloric and pyloric channel ulcers are notoriously liable to recur following HSV (25%). Thus, a formal antiulcer operation may still be appropriate for good-risk patients with gastric outlet obstruction and prepyloric ulcer disease, even though *H. pylori* treatment and proton pump inhibitor therapy may change this attitude.

Highly Selective Vagotomy and Dilation or Duodenoplasty

In most patients with gastric outlet obstruction from peptic ulcer disease, the stenosis is distal to the pylorus. Professor Johnston of Leeds therefore hypothesized that if the obstruction was relieved and ulcer recurrence prevented, the antropyloric mechanism should function normally and the patient would be rendered symptom-free. This hypothesis led to a trial of HSV to treat the ulcer

diathesis while leaving the antrum and pylorus innervated, combined with forceful operative dilation of the postpyloric stenosis in a series of patients with obstructing duodenal ulcer. The results were compared with a similar series of patients who underwent truncal vagotomy and drainage by another service in the same institution. Twenty-two of 23 (96%) patients who underwent HSV and dilation achieved a good to excellent clinical result (Visick I or II) at a mean follow-up of 24 months, compared with only 17 of 23 (74%) patients who underwent truncal vagotomy and drainage at a longer mean follow-up of 41 months. Subsequent studies have generally confirmed these results. Other researchers compared truncal vagotomy and pyloroplasty with truncal vagotomy and forceful dilation in a randomized prospective trial of 41 patients with obstructing chronic duodenal ulcer. Satisfactory results (Visick I and II) were achieved in 79% and 85%, respectively, at a mean follow-up of 34 months. In several series collected from the literature (including his own), Mentes (1990) identified 249 patients who underwent HSV and dilation and were followed up for up to 10 years (but most for less than 5 years). There was a 12% incidence of poor results, including a 7% restenosis rate.

It may be argued that there is little to commend HSV and operative dilation currently, because endoscopic balloon dilation and antisecretory drugs might accomplish the same goals in most patients. However, published studies of HSV and forceful operative dilation generally report better results than published studies of endoscopic dilation (see Table 54–1). Postpyloric peptic strictures not amenable to dilation can be treated effectively with HSV and duodenoplasty (success rate 90%—Visick I or II), thereby preserving antropyloric function.

It is generally agreed (even by advocates of these procedures) that HSV and dilation or duodenoplasty is a poor operation in patients with gastric outlet obstruction and type II or III gastric ulcer. Until better data are available, in this small group of patients, selective vagotomy and antrectomy may be the best treatment. Similarly, patients with isolated pyloric channel ulcers should not undergo HSV and dilation, but rather HSV and drainage (we prefer gastrojejunostomy).

Highly Selective Vagotomy and Drainage

Highly selective vagotomy and drainage is a safe and effective operation for obstructing peptic ulcer disease (see Table 54–2). A Jaboulay gastroduodenostomy is the "pyloroplasty" of choice, although the Finney technique can also be used. The extensiveness of the scarring or the length of the stricture frequently precludes the construction of a Heineke-Mikulicz pyloroplasty. Some authors favor gastrojejunostomy as a drainage procedure because it is easier to perform and easier to reverse or incorporate into a subsequent gastrectomy if necessary. It is hard to argue with that view. If a patient with a Jaboulay or Finney pyloroplasty requires a subsequent distal gastrectomy for persistent symptoms or ulcer recurrence, the closure of the duodenal stump can be formidable. The recurrent ulcer rate is no higher with gastrojejunostomy than it is with gastroduodenostomy. HSV is preferable to

| Table 54–2 | **Drainage or Resection for Obstructing Peptic Ulcer** |

Csendes et al, 1993 (Prospective, Randomized, Mean f/u = 98 mo)

	HSV + GJ	HSV + P	SV + A
N	30	30	30
Operative deaths	0	1	0
Visick I	24	19	21
Visick II/III	3	5	4
Visick IV	0	3	3
Lost to f/u	3	2	2

Gleysteen and Droege, 1988 (Retrospective Analysis of Perioperative Morbidity and Mortality)

	HSV + P	TV + P	TV + A
N	16	7	26
Operative deaths	0	1	2
Reop	1	1	3
Uneventful	94%	43%	46%
Delay GE	0%	33%	33%

A, antrectomy; f/u, follow-up; GJ, gastrojejunostomy; HSV, highly selective vagotomy; P, pyloroplasty; SV, selective vagotomy; TV, truncal vagotomy.

truncal vagotomy because it preserves antral motor function and avoids postvagotomy diarrhea.

HSV and gastrojejunostomy thus remains our choice of operation in patients who are not amenable to or who fail endoscopic dilation. We are not confident that HSV and operative dilation or duodenoplasty is sufficiently reliable in patients who have failed endoscopic balloon dilation and current medical treatment even if they are *H. pylori* positive. In the laparoscopic era, HSV and gastrojejunostomy is an especially attractive option. The Taylor operation (posterior truncal vagotomy and anterior HSV) may be substituted for the standard HSV. In this population with obstruction, special care must be taken to avoid denervating the antrum. Thus, it is prudent to denervate the anterior proximal stomach first so if the anterior nerve of Laterjet is damaged, the posterior branch can be preserved.

Vagotomy and Antrectomy

This irreversible operation remains the treatment of choice for obstructing peptic ulcer in some centers, but its popularity is waning. Although a seductively attractive surgical option for patients with gastric outlet obstruction because ulcer recurrence rate is so low (<2%), resection is often easier on the surgeon than it is on the patient. Most series that compare antrectomy with drainage in the treatment of obstructing peptic ulcer do not support the routine use of resection in this patient group (Table 54–3). It is the opinion of this author that vagotomy and antrectomy should be avoided as the initial operation for obstructing peptic ulcer disease unless the patient has a type II or III gastric ulcer (type I gastric ulcer does not cause obstruction). Resection is particularly appealing in these patients, because both the obstruction and the gastric ulcers are resected along with the "locus minoris resistentiae." If a difficult duodenal stump is anticipated, HSV and gastrojejunostomy with biopsy of gastric ulcers is a clearly acceptable alternative. Although vagotomy and antrectomy are excellent for patients who have failed vagotomy and drainage, these operations can sometimes be salvaged without resection (e.g., gastrojejunostomy for

failed pyloroplasty, thoracoscopic vagotomy and balloon dilation for failed HSV and duodenoplasty). Aggressive medical treatment should always be tried before elective reoperation.

The argument for vagotomy and antrectomy has been the enviably low ulcer recurrence rate (<2%). But this argument has been weakened by the elucidation of the role of *H. pylori* in peptic ulcer disease and by the recognition that successful eradication of *H. pylori* virtually eliminates ulcer recurrence. The operation should clearly be avoided if the duodenum is "difficult." It should also be avoided in asthenic individuals who can ill afford a Visick III or IV result. Some authors suggest a total gastric vagotomy (selective vagotomy) rather than a truncal vagotomy when doing an antrectomy for obstructing peptic ulcer disease, because this probably decreases the incidence of postvagotomy diarrhea.

POSTOPERATIVE MANAGEMENT

After operation, patients are maintained on nasogastric suction and intravenous fluids. A urinary catheter is helpful in the postoperative fluid management of many of these patients, because postoperative nasogastric drainage can be copious. Early ambulation, adequate analgesia, and incentive spirometry are used routinely. We also use antiemetics in the first 24 hours. Blood tests are ordered selectively as clinically indicated. If the patient has had a drainage procedure or dilation, the nasogastric tube is generally removed on the first or second postoperative day if the drainage is bilious and less than 600 mL per 24 hours. If the patient has had a gastric resection, the tube is generally removed on the third or fourth postoperative day. In this era of patient "fast-tracking," early postoperative water-soluble contrast studies are being used with increasing frequency in some centers by surgeons who believe that the documented absence of leak as well as gastric emptying warrant immediate feeding and possibly earlier discharge. Closed-suction peritoneal drains are occasionally used and remain for 5 days or until the patient is eating. Diet is advanced as tolerated after the nasogastric tube is removed. We avoid high-calorie liquids and high-fiber foods for the first 6 postoperative weeks.

COMPLICATIONS

Atelectasis and Pneumonia

It is absolutely crucial that the stomach be empty and the anesthesia personnel be aware of the preoperative diagnosis before administration of general anesthesia, lest potentially fatal aspiration pneumonia result. Atelectasis is minimized by early ambulation, adequate analgesia, and incentive spirometry. Postoperative vomiting and injudicious use or management of nasogastric suction may also predispose to pulmonary complications. A nonfunctioning nasogastric tube with a stomach full of secretions is worse than no tube; the tube serves as a wick by encouraging reflux and possible aspiration. Similarly, an unnecessary tube is unwise. Tubes should be checked frequently and

Table 54–3	Choice of Operation for Obstructing Peptic Ulcer Disease
ULCER TYPE	**TREATMENT OPTIONS**
Duodenal	Endoscopic balloon dilation
	HSV and forceful operative dilation
	HSV and duodenoplasty
	HSV and gastrojejunostomy
Pyloric	Endoscopic balloon dilation
	HSV and gastrojejunostomy
Prepyloric (i.e., some type III gastric ulcers)	Selective vagotomy and antrectomy
Duodenal and either pyloric or gastric ulcers (i.e., some type II and III gastric ulcers)	Selective vagotomy and antrectomy
	HSV and gastrojejunostomy and biopsy*

*If unsafe duodenal stump anticipated with resection.
HSV, highly selective vagotomy.

removed as soon as there is clinical evidence of adequate gastric emptying.

Delayed Gastric Emptying

Postoperative vomiting or copious nasogastric drainage is not uncommon in patients operated on for gastric outlet obstruction. Metoclopramide (if the antrum has not been removed) or erythromycin may improve gastric emptying in these patients. The operation should not be deemed a success or failure for at least 3 months, by which time the majority of patients are better.

Although many gastric operations can be done without the routine use of a nasogastric tube, we continue to use this apparatus in patients operated on for gastric outlet obstruction, hoping to prevent the occasional case of severe postoperative gastric distention or massive aspiration that can compromise anastomotic integrity and gastric motor function. Replacement of a nasogastric tube in the early postoperative period should be done carefully, because it is possible to perforate a gastric or duodenal suture line with a rigid plastic tube. If prolonged gastric intubation is anticipated, a gastrostomy tube should be seriously considered.

Wound Problems

Patients operated on for gastric outlet obstruction are at increased risk for wound infection for several reasons. Stasis and acid suppression increase bacterial loads in gastric contents that may contaminate the wound intraoperatively. These organisms may consist of resistant flora if the patient has been in hospital for several days before operation. In addition, these patients are often malnourished with altered host defenses. Wound infection can be minimized by avoidance of intraoperative contamination, the judicious use of prophylactic antibiotics, and possibly by intragastric lavage with antibiotic solution. Wound infection and malnutrition also increase the risk of dehiscence and hernia.

Dumping and Diarrhea

Severe dumping develops in at least 5% of patients in whom the pylorus has been destroyed or bypassed. Thus, if gastric outlet obstruction is due to a postpyloric stenosis, dilation or duodenoplasty should be the preferred procedure if technically possible. Postvagotomy diarrhea develops in 2% to 5% of patients who undergo truncal vagotomy, but severe postvagotomy diarrhea is less common (1%). Thus, selective or highly selective vagotomy is

---

Pearls and Pitfalls

- Gastric outlet obstruction is usually caused by peptic ulcer disease, but malignancy must be considered.
- Most patients with gastric outlet obstruction and chronic ulcer symptoms require some form of definitive endoscopic or operative therapy; others require balloon dilation or highly selective vagotomy and gastrojejunostomy or duodenoplasty.
- Although current literature suggests that long-term results are better with operation than with balloon dilation, there are no randomized prospective studies. Furthermore, almost all studies were done before the elucidation of the importance of *Helicobacter* and before the development of proton pump inhibitors.
- *Helicobacter pylori* infection is present in at least 50% of patients with peptic ulcer disease and gastric outlet obstruction. Successful treatment may improve long-term results after (but probably will not alter the need for) definitive therapy.
- In surgical patients requiring gastric drainage, highly selective vagotomy is preferable to truncal or selective vagotomy because it preserves antral motor function. In patients requiring antrectomy, selective vagotomy is preferable to truncal vagotomy because it avoids postvagotomy diarrhea.
- In the good-risk patient with type II or III gastric ulcer and outlet obstruction, antrectomy and selective vagotomy should be considered. If a difficult duodenal stump is anticipated, HSV and gastrojejunostomy with biopsy of gastric ulcers is acceptable.

---

preferable. The latter also preserves the antral pump, which may improve emptying in patients with peptic obstruction treated with a drainage procedure.

SELECTED READINGS

Bowden TA, Hooks VH, Rogers DA: Role of highly selective vagotomy and duodenoplasty in the treatment of postbulbar duodenal obstruction. Am J Surg 1990;159:235.

Csendes A, Maluenda F, Braghetto I, et al: Prospective randomized study comparing three surgical techniques for the treatment of gastric outlet obstruction secondary to duodenal ulcer. Am J Surg 1993;166:45.

Gleysteen JJ, Droege EA: Expedient surgical treatment of chronic ulcer stenosis. J Clin Gastroenterol 1988;10:619.

Hewitt PM, Krige JEJ, Funnell IC, et al: Endoscopic balloon dilation of peptic pyloroduodenal strictures. J Clin Gastroenterol 1999;28:33.

Lau JYW, Chung S, Sung JJY, et al: Through-the-scope balloon dilation for pylorostenosis: Long-term results. Gastrointest Endosc 1996;43:98.

Lam Y, Lau JY, Law KB, et al: Endoscopic balloon dilation and *H. pylori* eradication in treatment of gastric outlet obstruction. Gastrointest Endosc 1997;46:379.

Mentes AS: Parietal cell vagotomy and dilatation for peptic duodenal stricture. Ann Surg 1990;212:597.

Paimela H, Tuompo PK, Perakyla T, et al: Peptic ulcer surgery during the H2-receptor antagonist era: A population-based epidemiological study of ulcer surgery in Helsinki from 1972 to 1987. Br J Surg 1991;78:28.

Chapter 55

Gastric Ulcer

Diane M. Simeone and Kathleen Graziano

Approximately 4.5 million people suffer from peptic ulcer disease annually in the United States and, although the mortality rate improved in the 1960s, it has remained at approximately 5% over the past 30 years. Approximately 20% of these people suffer from gastric ulcers. Mortality rate for gastric ulcers is higher than that for duodenal ulcers, probably because of the increased age and frequent comorbid illnesses that occur in patients with gastric ulcer. Unlike patients with duodenal ulcers, most patients with gastric ulcers do not have increased basal or stimulated acid secretion. Indeed, gastric ulcers may develop in the presence of minimal amounts of acid. Although acid is an essential factor for gastric ulcer formation ("no acid, no ulcer"), it is generally accepted that gastric ulcers are most likely due to compromised mucosal defense rather than an excessive acid environment.

Ingestion of nonsteroidal anti-inflammatory drugs (NSAIDs) and colonization with *Helicobacter pylori* are the most important contributors to the pathogenesis of the majority of gastric ulcers. Occasionally, an idiopathic, nonmalignant gastric ulcer develops in the absence of an established cause, but this scenario accounts for less than 10% of occurrences. Recently, increasing use of therapeutic endoscopy, potent antisecretory drugs, and the identification of *H. pylori* as an etiologic agent in peptic ulcer disease have reduced the number of patients who require surgical intervention. Even so, it is critical that surgeons remain familiar with surgical therapy for gastric ulcers.

CLINICAL PRESENTATION

Patients classically describe a gnawing or burning epigastric pain, often most intense in the early morning hours, that is usually made worse by the ingestion of food and is not improved with eating, as occurs with duodenal ulcer disease. These symptoms are not specific to gastric ulcer disease, however, and other diseases need to be considered in the differential diagnosis. These disorders include pancreaticobiliary diseases (e.g., pancreatitis, cholecystitis), upper gastrointestinal tract neoplasms, gastroesophageal reflux, mesenteric ischemia, intestinal disorders, and coronary artery disease, which may also produce epigastric pain, thus mimicking ulcer pain. A number of patients are asymptomatic and have only a slow decline in hematocrit or a guaiac-positive stool. Approximately 10% to 20% of patients are first seen with a complication of a gastric ulcer such as hemorrhage, perforation, or obstruction without an antecedent history of abdominal pain.

Benign gastric ulcers have been divided into four types (Fig. 55–1). Type I ulcers are the most common (50%) and occur in the body of the stomach, usually along the lesser curvature, at the angularis incisura. Patients with type I ulcers have normal or low acid secretion. Type II ulcers (25%) also occur in the body of the stomach but are associated with either an active duodenal ulcer or a duodenal scar resulting from past ulceration. Type III ulcers (20%) are prepyloric in location. Both type II and type III ulcers are associated with acid hypersecretion. Type IV ulcers (<10%) occur high along the lesser curvature of the stomach, near the esophagogastric junction and are associated with low acid secretion.

MEDICAL MANAGEMENT

An argument has been made to treat otherwise healthy individuals with epigastric pain with antiulcer drugs without first evaluating their disease with endoscopy. This policy of "treat first" seems most appropriate for patients younger than 40 years of age with mild or intermittent epigastric symptoms with no evidence of systemic symptoms or ulcer complications. The treatment response must be monitored, and symptoms must not recur after therapy is discontinued. Early endoscopic evaluation should be performed in patients older than 50 years of age and in patients with clinical features of anorexia, weight loss, gastric outlet obstruction, a palpable abdominal mass, microscopic anemia, or guaiac-positive stool. Upper endoscopy allows the opportunity to confirm the diagnosis and to obtain biopsy specimens to rule out neoplasm and evaluate the presence of *H. pylori* infection. Obtaining at least seven biopsy samples of the ulcer is required to effectively exclude an underlying neoplasm.

Once malignancy has been excluded with the appropriate endoscopic evaluation, medical therapy is directed at decreasing basal and stimulated acid secretion by the use of H_2-receptor antagonists such as cimetidine or ranitidine or by proton pump inhibitors such as omeprazole (20 to 40 mg per day). Reduction of acid secretion with these agents promotes healing of the gastric ulcer. H_2-receptor antagonists have been shown to effectively heal more than 80% of gastric ulcers after 8 weeks of therapy, and proton pump inhibitors have performed similarly with greater than 90% healing after 8 weeks of continuous therapy.

The importance of recognizing and treating *H. pylori* infection cannot be underestimated. Failure to eradicate infection is a contributor to nonhealing. Assessment for *H. pylori* infection should be performed using one of the available diagnostic tests. Noninvasive methods to detect infection include serologic tests and a breath test for urea. These methods are less expensive than endoscopic biopsy and are nearly as sensitive and specific. If upper endoscopy is indicated, mucosal biopsy specimens can be obtained, and the presence of *H. pylori* can be determined by histologic examination or by the detection of bacterial

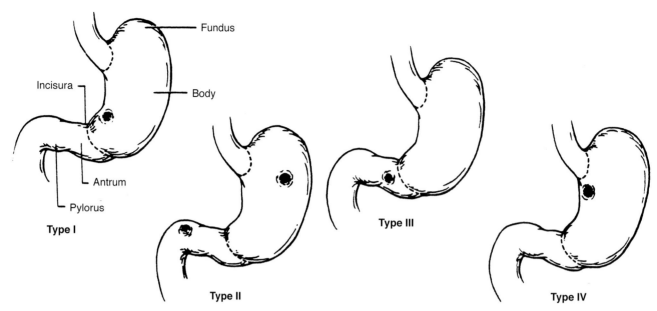

Figure 55–1. Types of gastric ulcers and their locations. (From Mulholland MW: Peptic ulcer disease. In Bell RH, Rikkers LF, Mulholland MW [eds]: Digestive Tract Surgery: Text and Atlas. Philadelphia, Lippincott-Raven, 1995, p 190.)

urease by specific dye tests. The mainstay of therapy is double or triple antibiotic therapy. The antimicrobial agents most commonly used for treatment of *H. pylori* infection are amoxicillin, bismuth, clarithromycin, metronidazole, and tetracycline. Antibiotic therapy may be taken alone or in combination with a proton pump inhibitor. Treatment for 14 days with triple therapy regimens has resulted in eradication rates of approximately 85%. Repeat endoscopy is indicated in all patients with gastric ulcers because even a malignant ulcer can demonstrate some evidence of healing. If any remaining ulcer or scar is present, it should be biopsied again.

OPERATIVE MANAGEMENT

The indications for elective surgery have decreased with the success of medical therapy, but situations still exist in which surgery should be considered. If an ulcer has failed to completely heal after 12 weeks of continuous medical therapy or if the patient has more than one recurrence, then the patient is considered to have intractable disease. There are several possible reasons that an ulcer may not heal and warrant further investigation. They include persistent *H. pylori* infection, Zollinger-Ellison syndrome, NSAID abuse, mesenteric ischemia, and microscopic malignancy. Very unusual causes of chronic ulceration include Crohn's disease, sarcoidosis, eosinophilic gastroenteritis, and infections such as tuberculosis and cytomegalovirus. In the presence of a nonhealed gastric ulcer, we recommend repeat upper endoscopy with multiple biopsies, testing for persistent *H. pylori* infection, and exclusion of Zollinger-Ellison syndrome by either a normal basal gastrin level or a secretin stimulation test. A careful history should be obtained to exclude NSAID use. After these measures have been taken, elective surgery may be undertaken.

The indications for elective operative treatment in patients with gastric ulcer are failure to heal following maximal medical therapy for 12 weeks and the inability to exclude an occult malignancy. Even though giant ($>$3 cm) ulcers have traditionally been considered an indication for elective surgery based on size alone, recent studies suggest that most patients with giant gastric ulcers may be managed successfully with aggressive medical treatment and that giant gastric ulcers may be approached like nongiant ulcers, with the same criteria for surgical intervention.

Type I ulcers are best treated by antrectomy to include the ulcer with reconstruction by a gastroduodenal (Billroth I) anastomosis. Gastrojejunostomy (Billroth II) is an acceptable alternative. Operative mortality rate after this procedure is 1% to 2%, and the 5-year ulcer recurrence rate is approximately 2%. A truncal vagotomy is not necessary in the treatment of type I ulcers because most of these patients do not hypersecrete acid. There is no scientific evidence that addition of truncal vagotomy improves ulcer cure rates in type I ulcers, and it may increase the occurrence of postvagotomy dumping, diarrhea, or gastroparesis. A secondary choice is transmural excision of the ulcer combined with a highly selective or parietal cell vagotomy. The recurrence rate after this procedure, however, is 4 to 6 times higher than after antrectomy.

For patients with type II ulcers, the operative procedure should be designed to decrease acid secretion as well as to remove the ulcer and the gastric mucosa at risk for ulceration. A truncal vagotomy and antrectomy with Billroth I reconstruction best accomplishes these goals with an operative mortality rate of 1% and a 5-year recurrence rate of less than 5%. If excessive scarring or inflammation is present in the duodenum, a gastrojejunostomy should be performed. Secondary options include ulcer excision combined with either highly selective vagotomy or truncal vagotomy and pyloroplasty; however, these procedures are associated with higher recurrence rates.

Patients with type III ulcers (prepyloric and pyloric) also tend to have higher rates of acid secretion. As with patients with type II ulcers, the operative procedure of choice is truncal vagotomy and antrectomy to include the ulcer. Highly selective vagotomy or truncal vagotomy with pyloroplasty are less acceptable surgical options for these patients, in that numerous reports have demonstrated a recurrence rate up to 40% for ulcers in this location.

Type IV ulcers require antrectomy with extension of the resection along the lesser curvature to include the ulcer (Pauchet maneuver). Because these patients do not have increased acid secretion, a vagotomy is not required. Operative mortality and recurrence rates are similar to those for the other ulcer types. If the ulcer is large or associated with considerable inflammation, a subtotal gastrectomy with Roux-en-Y jejunal reconstruction can be considered but introduces concomitant increases in morbidity and mortality risk.

Hemorrhage, perforation, and obstruction are the three most common complications of gastric ulcer, requiring surgical intervention. Hemorrhage occurs in approximately 15% of patients and perforation occurs in approximately 5% of patients. In patients with bleeding, fluid resuscitation, gastric lavage, and upper endoscopy are undertaken first. Interventional endoscopic therapy is effective in approximately 80% of patients in establishing hemostasis of an actively bleeding gastric ulcer or an ulcer with stigmata of recent hemorrhage (visible vessel, adherent clot). Angiographic embolization offers an additional means to control bleeding, but only in a patient with severe comorbid illness who may pose a prohibitive operative risk.

Emergency operations for the bleeding patient should address both the bleeding and the underlying disease. The operative procedure of choice is antrectomy with a Billroth I reconstruction with the addition of vagotomy in patients with type II and type III ulcers. With type IV ulcers, antrectomy with extension to include the ulcer is preferred. In unstable patients, simple vessel transfixion with oversewing of the ulcer may be performed. This, however, is not a definitive operative procedure and may result in a rebleeding rate of 25%.

In patients with a perforated gastric ulcer, an antrectomy to include the ulcer should be performed with an accompanying truncal vagotomy in type II and III ulcers. The mortality rate from perforation of a gastric ulcer is twice that seen with a perforated duodenal ulcer, probably because of increased patient age and frequent associated comorbid illnesses. In unstable patients with a gastric ulcer perforation, biopsy or excision only with closure of the ulcer with an omental patch is a viable option.

Gastric outlet obstruction is most typically seen with type III gastric ulcers but is also seen with type II ulcers. Obstruction may be due to the effects of acute edema or spasm or may be due to chronic scarring. The former tends to resolve with medical treatment, whereas the latter usually requires surgical intervention. Endoscopic balloon dilatation to relieve gastric outlet obstruction caused by a gastric ulcer has been used but has not been shown to maintain good long-term results. All patients should undergo preoperative gastric decompression, correction of fluid and electrolyte imbalances, and endo-

scopic evaluation with biopsies done before surgical intervention. For patients who fail initial conservative therapy, vagotomy with antrectomy is highly effective, but should be performed with caution if there is significant scarring of the duodenum, making duodenal stump closure difficult.

Laparoscopic surgery has been used under elective conditions to treat intractable disease and under emergent conditions to manage perforation. Proximal gastric vagotomy has been performed as an alternative to lifelong medical therapy with a recurrence rate of 8% and a complication rate of 2%. Laparoscopic repair of perforated ulcer with omental patch has successfully been performed using sutures as well as sutureless techniques that employ gelatin sponge and fibrin glue. Reported results appear comparable to those obtained using the open technique. Advantages include less postoperative pain and a shorter hospital stay. Laparoscopic truncal vagotomy and antrectomy have been performed in a number of centers, although the experience remains low and thus should be undertaken only by the experienced laparoscopic surgeon.

POSTOPERATIVE MANAGEMENT

Patients who undergo elective operative treatment for a gastric ulcer should have nasogastric suction continued for several days. Intravenous fluids should be maintained until there is evidence that the postoperative ileus is resolved and oral intake can be resumed. Antibiotics are required only in the immediate perioperative period. In patients who undergo emergent surgical intervention, complications may develop related to preexisting comorbid illnesses and the presence of preoperative shock, including cardiac ischemia or renal failure. Parenteral nutrition should be administered to malnourished patients or those suffering from advanced peritonitis. Patients with a prolonged gastric ileus may require supplemental enteric feeding through a feeding tube. Enteral feeding can be accomplished through placement of a nasojejunal tube at the time of the operative procedure; some surgeons may choose to create a jejunostomy at the time of the operative procedure if a prolonged ileus is anticipated.

COMPLICATIONS

The potential complications that may occur after gastric ulcer surgery are numerous. Early complications include infection, intraluminal and intra-abdominal bleeding, delayed gastric emptying, anastomotic leak, and duodenal stump leak. Late complications include recurrent ulcer formation and postgastrectomy sequelae. The incidence of recurrent ulcer depends on the pathophysiology of the underlying disease process and the type of operative procedure performed. In patients in whom recurrent ulcers develop, incomplete vagotomy, retained antrum, recurrent or persistent *H. pylori* infection, and Zollinger-Ellison syndrome must be considered.

Morbidity in the form of postgastrectomy sequelae may be experienced by as many as 25% of patients undergoing gastric surgery for ulcer disease. These sequelae include delayed gastric emptying, dumping syndrome, postvagotomy diarrhea, chronic gastroparesis, alkaline reflux gastritis, and afferent or efferent loop syndrome. The occurrence of severe postgastrectomy symptoms is low, involving only 2% of patients. One of the most common postgastrectomy sequelae is the dumping syndrome that results from ablation, resection, or bypass of the pyloric sphincter, usually in connection with a vagotomy. Dumping is characterized by postprandial vasomotor and gastrointestinal symptoms. The pathogenesis of dumping is not clearly understood but is thought to be related to rapid entry of ingested food into the proximal small intestine, resulting in fluid shifts and elaboration of vasoactive agents. Early dumping occurs immediately after a meal and is characterized by epigastric discomfort, nausea, diarrhea, dizziness, sweating, and palpitations. Late dumping is much more unusual and occurs 1 to 3 hours after eating; it manifests as reactive hypoglycemia and vasomotor symptoms and is relieved by ingestion of carbohydrates. In most patients with early dumping, simple dietary measures, including avoidance of carbohydrates and limited fluid intake at meals, are successful in all but 1% of patients. Octreotide, a somatostatin analogue, can be an effective agent in treating severe dumping symptoms not responsive to dietary manipulations, but it is very expensive.

OUTCOMES

Operative mortality rate for elective gastric ulcer surgery is approximately 2%. Patients who require emergency surgery for a complication of gastric ulcer, including perforation and bleeding, have operative mortality rates ranging from 10% to 40%. Risk factors that increase mortality rate in the emergent setting include a transfusion requirement of greater than 5 units, age greater than 60 years,

Pearls and Pitfalls

- Gastric ulcers constitute approximately 20% of all peptic ulcers.
- Types I and IV gastric ulcers are associated with low or normal acid secretion, whereas types II and III involve acid secretion.
- The wary surgeon maintains a high suspicion of underlying malignancy.
- Most gastric ulcers heal with antiacid therapy and treatment of *H. pylori* infection.
- Persistent gastric ulcers after 8 to 12 weeks of maximal therapy probably should be treated surgically.
- Choice of operative therapy depends on the type of gastric ulcer.
- Complications including bleeding, obstruction, or perforation complicate approximately 20% of cases of gastric ulcers.

preoperative shock, and significant comorbid illness. Delay exceeding 12 hours in operative treatment after gastric ulcer perforation has also been shown to result in significantly increased risk of death.

SELECTED READINGS

Graham DY: Therapy of *Helicobacter pylori*: Current status and issues. Gastroenterology 2000;118:52.
Laine L, Peterson WL: Bleeding peptic ulcer. N Engl J Med 1994;331:717.
Lau WY, Leung KL, Kwong KH, et al: A randomized study comparing laparoscopic versus open repair of perforated peptic ulcer using suture or sutureless technique. Ann Surg 1996;224:131.
Mulholland MW: Peptic ulcer disease. In Bell RH, Rikkers LF, Mulholland MW (eds): Digestive Tract Surgery: A Text and Atlas. Philadelphia, Lippincott-Raven, 1995, pp 167–199.
Simeone DM, Hassan A, Scheiman JM: Giant peptic ulcer: A surgical or medical disease? Surgery 1999;126:474.
Svanes C, Lie RT, Svanes K, et al: Adverse effects of delayed treatment for perforated peptic ulcer. Ann Surg 1994;220:168.

Chapter 56

Postgastrectomy and Postvagotomy Syndromes

Matthew M. Hutter and Sean J. Mulvihill

In the past, gastric surgery for ulcer was one of the mainstays of general surgical practice. Currently, gastric operations are primarily performed for neoplasm and morbid obesity. Recent advances in the medical management of peptic ulcer disease have remarkably decreased the frequency of ulcer operations, especially for intractability. Over the past 3 decades, the use of histamine H_2-receptor antagonists, proton pump inhibitors, endoscopic ulcer therapy, and antibiotic treatment of *Helicobacter pylori* have all led to a 10-fold decrease in the number of ulcer operations performed. Indeed, some chief residents in general surgery finish their training without having performed an elective gastric operation for ulcer; thus, the average surgeon's familiarity with postgastrectomy and postvagotomy syndromes is greatly reduced.

Overall, postoperative symptoms develop in approximately 25% of patients after gastric surgery, but in only 1% to 3% are the symptoms severe enough to require remedial surgery. The wise surgeon must understand these postgastrectomy syndromes in order to prevent them at the time of initial operation, to accurately diagnose the patterns of altered motility and function when postgastrectomy symptoms occur, to have the patience to allow an approach involving a "tincture of time" as well as dietary and medical therapies to work, and to perform the appropriate remedial operation only when necessary. This chapter examines the postgastrectomy and postvagotomy syndromes, as well as the management of these conditions.

DUMPING SYNDROME (RAPID GASTRIC EMPTYING)

The dumping syndrome refers to the rapid gastric emptying seen in patients with vasomotor and gastrointestinal complaints after gastrectomy with vagotomy. An increased rate of gastric emptying is caused by a combination of a reduction in the functional reservoir volume after gastrectomy, loss of receptive relaxation after vagotomy, loss of pyloric regulation of the release of hyperosmolar chyme into the duodenum and small bowel, and loss of duodenal feedback inhibition after gastrojejunostomy. Virtually all patients with dumping have had some form of a vagotomy, which, by abolishing receptive relaxation of the proximal stomach, induces a much more rapid gastric emptying of liquids. The severity of a patient's symptoms is largely proportional to the rate of gastric emptying. The incidence of the dumping syndrome depends on the type of gastric surgery performed, with highly selective vagotomy having the lowest incidence (1% to 3%). After gastrec-

tomy with vagotomy, 25% to 50% of patients have some symptom of dumping, although most symptoms improve with time, leaving only 1% to 2% of patients with persistent, disabling symptoms. Dumping symptoms include postprandial bloating, crampy abdominal pain, nausea, and explosive diarrhea. Vasomotor symptoms are composed of diaphoresis, weakness, dizziness, flushing, and an intense desire to lie down. The dumping syndrome has been classified into early and late forms, according to the timing of symptoms after a meal (Fig. 56–1).

Early dumping occurs within 10 to 30 minutes of a meal and results from the rapid emptying of hyperosmolar chyme into the small bowel. The "dumping" of this hyperosmolar chyme into the upper gut causes inappropriate release of vasoactive gut peptides; in addition, fluid shifts from the intravascular space into the small bowel. This fluid sequestration causes crampy abdominal pain and fullness, and leads to a relative hypovolemia and hypotension. Tachycardia and lightheadedness follow. Postprandial release of several gut hormones—including enteroglucagon, glucagon-like polypeptide, pancreatic polypeptide, vasoactive intestinal peptide, gastrin-releasing peptide, serotonin, bradykinin, motilin, and neurotensin—is exaggerated in patients during the dumping syndrome. The exact role these peptides play, however, in initiating the symptoms of dumping is unclear. Nevertheless, symptoms can occur within minutes of food ingestion and octreotide, a somatostatin analogue that inhibits or alters the release of the peptides, has been shown to be effective in treating symptoms, suggesting that these and other gut hormones are the major factors in the pathophysiology of this condition.

Late dumping occurs less frequently than early dumping. Symptoms develop 2 to 3 hours after eating and are mainly caused by hypoglycemia. The rapid emptying of high carbohydrate gastric contents into the proximal small bowel leads to an exaggerated peptide release, including enteroglucagon. These peptides sensitize the β-cell to stimulation by blood glucose levels, resulting in excessive insulin release. Once the absorbed carbohydrates are metabolized, the persistently increased insulin levels cause a late hypoglycemia. The symptoms of late dumping are similar to the vasomotor symptoms of hypoglycemia in a diabetic with an insulin reaction; interestingly, gastrointestinal symptoms are usually absent. Early dumping symptoms are exacerbated by eating carbohydrates, whereas the symptoms of late dumping are relieved with their ingestion.

Diagnosis

The diagnosis of dumping is usually suspected from the patient's clinical symptoms. Diagnostic studies may be

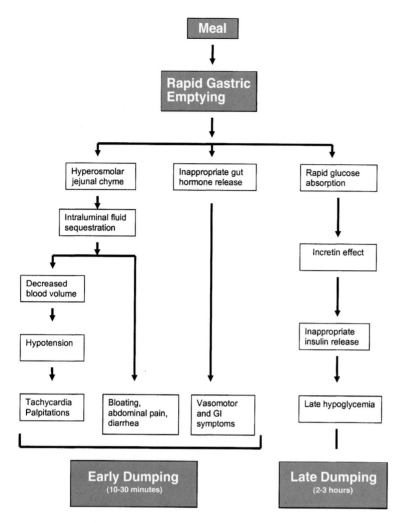

Figure 56–1. Patterns of dumping syndrome.

warranted to confirm the diagnosis and to differentiate it from other postgastrectomy syndromes. Radionuclide studies usually document an early rapid gastric emptying of a liquid meal and sometimes also the solid component. Endoscopy or barium studies can be helpful in defining the anatomy and excluding other postgastrectomy syndromes, such as bile reflux gastritis or afferent limb syndrome.

Medical Treatment

Most symptoms of dumping are mild and improve with time, dietary changes, and, occasionally, medications. Dietary changes are the mainstay of treatment and include taking small frequent meals, separating the ingestion of liquids and solids (i.e., drinking liquids 30 minutes after a "dry" meal), avoiding simple or concentrated carbohydrates, and adding fiber or complex carbohydrates to the diet. Lying supine after eating may slow gastric emptying and increase venous return, thereby minimizing symptoms. Adding gel-forming carbohydrates, such as pectin, to the diet or ingestion of amylase inhibitors delays glucose absorption and lengthens bowel transit time, although it may create the unwanted problem of malabsorption.

Octreotide, a somatostatin analogue, is effective in improving symptoms in most patients with severe dumping unresponsive to other medical therapy. Octreotide provides relief by slowing gastric emptying, inhibiting insulin release, and decreasing gut peptide secretion. An initial dose of 50 µg subcutaneously 30 minutes before each meal is usually effective. This dose can be increased to 100 or 150 µg per meal if necessary. The main side effect of octreotide is steatorrhea from inhibition of pancreatic enzyme secretion, although clinically significant steatorrhea is rare and generally responds to oral pancreatic enzyme replacement. Hyperglycemia from inhibition of insulin release can occur rarely, and fingerstick blood glucose levels should be measured at least for the first few days of treatment.

Surgical Treatment

Operative intervention is indicated only for the 1% of patients with persistently debilitating symptoms of dumping despite dietary modifications and octreotide treatment. A conservative approach is warranted because most patients with dumping improve with time and because remedial surgery is not uniformly successful. Many remedial procedures have been described, including surgical narrowing of the gastrojejunostomy stoma, conversion of a Billroth II to a Billroth I, jejunal interpositions, conversion to a Roux-en-Y gastrojejunostomy, and pyloric reconstruction. The choice of remedial operation depends on the initial operation (Table 56–1). For patients who initially had a pyloroplasty, the easiest and most logical remedial procedure is a pyloric reconstruction. The old, transverse pyloroplasty scar is opened, the pyloric muscular ring is reapproximated, and the incision is closed longitudinally. Gastric stasis is unusual after pyloric reconstruction. Approximately 80% of patients have relief from dumping symptoms.

Patients with prior Billroth I and Billroth II reconstructions are best served with the creation of a Roux-en-Y gastrojejunostomy. The anatomy of Roux drainage of the stomach slows gastric emptying. The Roux limb should be constructed at least 50 cm in length to prevent the reflux of bile into the stomach. This procedure is technically easier than jejunal interposition or the conversion of a Billroth II gastrojejunostomy to a Billroth I gastroduodenostomy and improves symptoms in 85% to 90% of patients. In patients with Billroth I anatomy, the prior anastomosis should be resected, with a retrocolic gastrojejunostomy erected in an end-to-side fashion with the Roux limb. In patients with Billroth II anatomy, if the gastric anastomosis is satisfactory, the afferent limb is divided proximal to the stomach and anastomosed to the jejunum downstream. The size of the gastric remnant is important because, if there is still an ulcer diathesis with high acid secretion, stomal ulceration becomes a very real concern in that the Roux anatomy brings an "unprotected jejunal mucosa" (the Roux limb is not bathed by the alkaline bile) in contact with the gastric lumen.

For patients with a previous Roux-en-Y gastrojejunostomy, constructing a 10-cm antiperistaltic jejunal segment within the Roux limb has been suggested. In this procedure, a site at the mid-aspect of the Roux limb is selected. The bowel is divided proximally and distally with linear cutting staplers. The mesentery is divided in parallel to vessels feeding the segment, preserving inflow. The segment is then rotated 180 degrees and reanastomosed in situ with the 10-cm segment now in an antiperistaltic direction. Care should be taken with these anastomoses to avoid narrowing the lumen. Rotated segments greater than 10 cm in length may cause stasis. Large series with this antiperistaltic approach do not exist, experience is anecdotal at best, and most surgeons who have performed this operation have failures.

Table 56–1	Remedial Operations for Dumping Syndrome	
PRIOR OPERATION		**REMEDIAL OPERATION**
Vagotomy and pyloroplasty		Pyloric reconstruction
Antrectomy and gastroduodenostomy		Roux-en-Y gastrojejunostomy
Antrectomy and gastrojejunostomy		Roux-en-Y gastrojejunostomy
Antrectomy and Roux-en-Y gastrojejunostomy		Antiperistaltic jejunal segment

POSTVAGOTOMY DIARRHEA

After truncal vagotomy, 20% of patients complain of postoperative diarrhea, and in 1% or less the diarrhea is debilitating. The incidence is lower after selective vagotomy, in which the celiac branch is preserved, and rare after highly selective vagotomy. Avoiding truncal vagotomy at the time of the initial operation prevents this syndrome. Diarrhea is usually episodic and in its severe form is characterized by frequent watery stools with occasional explosive delivery. Diarrhea often occurs immediately after eating.

The pathophysiology of this syndrome remains unclear, but total vagotomy is the precipitating factor that most likely interferes with central nervous system regulation of gut motility and secretion. Impaired gallbladder emptying and increased excretion of bile salts appear to play a role, and impaired pancreatic function, intestinal mucosal changes, and bacterial overgrowth have also been implicated as causes.

Diagnosis

Diarrhea after gastric surgery is common and usually is unrelated to vagotomy. Postvagotomy diarrhea is a diagnosis of exclusion after *all* other causes of diarrhea have been excluded. Other diagnoses to consider include bacterial overgrowth, *Clostridium difficile* colitis, partial obstruction, inflammatory bowel disease, parasites, gluten enteropathy, malabsorption, and laxative abuse. No specific tests are available to confirm that the diarrhea is, indeed, caused by vagotomy.

Medical Treatment

Dietary changes similar to those for the dumping syndrome may be effective for postvagotomy diarrhea, including giving small, frequent meals with liquids separated from "dry" solid meals. Increased fiber intake is helpful for some patients. Opiates are somewhat effective in decreasing bowel motility, as are other antidiarrheals such as diphenoxylate with atropine or loperamide. Cholestyramine binds bile salts and improves diarrhea in some patients. Octreotide is less effective in treating postvagotomy diarrhea than dumping syndrome. In some patients, diarrhea is worsened by inducing pancreatic insufficiency and steatorrhea. In refractory patients, no medical therapy works.

Surgical Treatment

Remedial surgery may be considered in patients with severe postvagotomy diarrhea unresponsive to medical therapy. The patient, referring physician, and surgeon should wait at least 1 year after the onset of postvagotomy diarrhea before considering remedial surgery so that medical therapies can be adequately assessed. Construction of one or two 10-cm antiperistaltic jejunal segments located 100 and 200 cm from the ligament of Treitz is the suggested approach. The best guess, however, is that only

60% of patients who undergo this operation have good results; many of these patients may not have had true postvagotomy diarrhea. Alternative approaches include a reversed ileal onlay graft with the reversed portion encompassing only one half of the diameter of the intestine. Experience with any of these procedures is limited. As with reversed jejunal segments for dumping, care should be taken to avoid technical anastomotic problems such as narrowing. Reversed segments longer than 10 cm may produce obstructive symptoms or bacterial overgrowth. Rarely, no therapy is effective. There are no series large enough to provide reliable data about the surgical treatment of this rare condition.

ALKALINE REFLUX GASTRITIS

Alkaline reflux gastritis is caused by the reflux of duodenal contents into the stomach through destruction, removal, or bypass of the pyloric sphincter. Although some bile reflux is seen in all patients after gastrectomy or pyloroplasty, severe symptoms of alkaline reflux gastritis develop in only 1% or less. Most patients have a Billroth II reconstruction, even though Billroth I anatomy and pyloroplasty are also associated with this syndrome. Another poorly understood form of bile reflux gastritis may occur rarely after simple cholecystectomy. It is not known why some patients are susceptible to pain and injury of the gastric mucosa by bile and pancreatic secretions and others are not.

Symptoms include a burning, constant epigastric pain, and nausea, which may be exacerbated with eating. Bilious emesis mixed with undigested food is common but often does not relieve the pain or nausea. This feature distinguishes this condition from afferent loop syndrome in which bilious emesis, without food, relieves the patient's discomfort.

Diagnosis

Endoscopy with gastric biopsy and radionuclide and barium studies should be done to confirm alkaline reflux gastritis and to rule out other postgastrectomy syndromes that can cause epigastric pain, nausea, and vomiting. Recurrent ulceration, afferent loop syndrome, gastroparesis, or anastomotic stricture can present with similar symptoms. At endoscopy, a beefy red gastritis is found with pooling of bile in the gastric remnant. Biopsy reveals gastritis (although gastritis can be seen in any patient after gastrojejunostomy). Gastric fluid analysis can diagnose persistent acid secretion caused by undiagnosed Zollinger-Ellison syndrome, retained antrum, or incomplete vagotomy. Quantitative biliary radionuclide scans may show biliary reflux and pooling within the stomach. Radionuclide gastric emptying studies can show delayed gastric emptying that may be amenable to prokinetic agents, and if medical therapy is not sufficient, then these functional studies can help identify patients at risk for gastroparesis if Roux conversion is chosen for a remedial procedure. Recently, use of a sensor probe for bile has documented bile reflux into the gastric lumen.

The wary clinician should be hesitant to arrive at a diagnosis of bile reflux gastritis in a large percentage of patients "at risk." Bile reflux gastritis is uncommon. In many patients with postvagotomy gastroparesis, bile reflux gastritis is diagnosed, conversion to a Roux anatomy is chosen, and the patient's symptoms worsen.

Medical Treatment

Medical treatment has disappointing efficacy for alkaline reflux gastritis. Prokinetic agents to improve gastric emptying and coating agents, such as sucralfate, to improve gastric mucosal defense have limited success in ameliorating symptoms. Dietary and behavior changes are not usually helpful. Cholestyramine, which binds bile salts, is only occasionally effective.

Surgical Treatment

The best surgical option is conversion to Roux-en-Y gastrojejunostomy. This procedure is effective in treating reflux symptoms in approximately 80% of patients with well-documented bile reflux gastritis (Fig. 56–2). The Roux limb must be of sufficient length, 50 cm, to prevent pancreaticobiliary secretions from refluxing into the gastric remnant. In some patients, however, conversion to Roux-en-Y gastrojejunostomy unmasks an underlying gastroparesis or the Roux stasis syndrome.

In patients with Billroth II anatomy, Braun enteroenterostomy, in which the afferent and efferent limbs are anastomosed to divert bile/pancreatic juice from the stomach, is an attractive option; however, this "diverting" anastomosis is not always effective in preventing bile from traversing the afferent loop. Patients must have sufficient length of the afferent limb to make this reconstruction feasible.

Another alternative, the duodenal switch procedure, has been described by DeMeester and colleagues (1987) as a remedy for alkaline reflux gastritis through an intact pylorus after, for instance, cholecystectomy. The duodenum is transected 5 to 7 cm distal to the pylorus, the distal end of the duodenum is oversewn, and the proximal end is anastomosed end-to-end to a Roux limb. Results in small numbers of patients are promising, and duodenal switch should be considered for patients with alkaline reflux gastritis who have not had previous surgery (primary alkaline reflux gastritis), or in the rare postsurgical patient whose previous surgery did not include a resection.

STASIS SYNDROMES: GASTROPARESIS AND THE ROUX SYNDROME—DELAYED GASTRIC EMPTYING

Postgastrectomy stasis syndromes include gastroparesis and the Roux syndrome. The exact cause of stasis is poorly understood, although preexisting gastric dysmotility, made worse by gastrectomy and vagotomy, are thought to play a major role. Vagotomy inhibits antral contractions and disrupts the gastric rhythm of pacemaker cells and migrating motor complexes, resulting in delayed gastric empty-

INITIAL OPERATION

Vagotomy and Pyloroplasty

Billroth I

Billroth II

REMEDIAL PROCEDURES

Roux-en-Y Gastrojejunostomy

Billroth II with Braun Enteroenterostomy

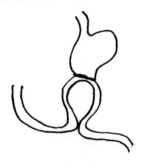

Figure 56–2. Remedial procedures for alkaline reflux gastritis.

ing. Preoperative gastric outlet obstruction is also a contributing factor, with a short-term postsurgical gastroparesis occurring in approximately 10% of patients. The overall incidence of postsurgical gastroparesis is 2% to 3%.

The Roux stasis syndrome describes stasis in the Roux limb often in combination with an element of gastroparesis in patients after a Roux-en-Y diversion. The pathophysiology is likely due to abnormal jejunal peristalsis with atonic or retrograde contractions in the Roux limb, coupled with gastroparesis. The incidence is as high as 25% to 30% after Roux-en-Y reconstruction, but is of a severity significant enough to affect nutritional intake in less than 5% of patients.

Symptoms of the stasis syndromes include epigastric fullness, early satiety, abdominal pain, nausea, and vomiting; severe gastroparesis, weight loss, and nutritional deficiencies result, leading to need for some form of nutritional supplementation or support. Bezoars develop in up to 12% of these patients.

Diagnosis

Diagnostic procedures are important to differentiate whether there is a mechanical or functional etiology to the delayed emptying. Barium studies and endoscopy can help visualize the flaccid gastric remnant seen in gastroparesis while ruling out mechanical obstruction or other causes of delayed gastric emptying such as stomal obstruction or alkaline reflux gastritis. Radionuclide gastric emptying studies with liquid and solid meals and radionuclide biliary scanning in Roux patients can provide

a functional assessment of motility and emptying. In some centers with a specialty interest in motility, upper gastrointestinal manometry studies can determine contractile patterns that may help differentiate the various potential etiologies.

Medical Treatment

Early acute gastroparesis responds best to conservative management. Once obstruction is excluded, nasogastric decompression, nutritional support, and patience are the mainstays of treatment. It is important to discontinue, if possible, medications that hinder gastric emptying, such as opiates, calcium channel blockers, β-agonists, and anticholinergics. Prokinetic agents, such as metoclopramide, bethanechol, and erythromycin may be helpful in the treatment of postoperative gastroparesis. Gastric bezoars can respond to proteolytic enzymes or to endoscopic fragmentation.

Surgical Treatment

Operative intervention should be considered for patients with mechanical obstruction and in those with gastroparesis who fail a suitable trial of medical therapy. As a rule, the intent of operative therapy is to remove all of the atonic stomach that functions as a nonmotile gastric reservoir with near total (>95%) gastric resection.

In patients who have undergone a previous vagotomy with pyloroplasty or gastrojejunostomy, distal gastrectomy with Billroth I or II reconstruction is often performed but is usually not successful; indeed, antrectomy leaves the body of the stomach in situ. This is the area of the stomach that normally functions as the reservoir of the stomach and, if nonmotile, gastric emptying is not accelerated. The most consistently successful remedial procedure is near total gastrectomy with Roux-en-Y cardiojejunostomy. This procedure is favored in patients with previous gastric resection and should be considered in patients with previous vagotomy and drainage procedures. This operation is successful in approximately 50% of patients. If alkaline reflux gastritis is thought to be playing a role, then the best treatment is near-total or total gastrectomy with Roux-en-Y drainage, or Billroth II gastrojejunostomy with Braun enterostomy. For patients with the Roux syndrome, there is no good remedial option.

AFFERENT AND EFFERENT LIMB SYNDROMES

Afferent and efferent limb syndromes are caused by mechanical obstruction. Afferent limb syndrome is a rare occurrence after Billroth II gastrojejunostomy caused by obstruction of the limb draining the biliary and pancreatic secretions. Obstruction is usually caused by kinking, volvulus, adhesions, internal herniation, or intussusception. At the gastrojejunostomy site, recurrent ulceration, stricture, and carcinoma may precipitate the afferent limb syndrome. The acute form of afferent limb syndrome is a closed loop obstruction of the duodenum and proximal jejunum. Afflicted patients have severe epigastric pain, nausea, nonbilious vomiting, tachycardia, and fever; it can also present as acute pancreatitis or jaundice caused by biliary obstruction. Acute afferent obstruction can be a surgical emergency, because unrelieved obstruction can lead to intestinal ischemia and perforation. The chronic form of afferent limb syndrome is more common and results from intermittent, partial obstruction of the afferent limb. Symptoms include postprandial epigastric pain and fullness as biliary and pancreatic secretions build up in the afferent limb after a meal. Explosive bilious vomiting devoid of foodstuff relieves symptoms.

Efferent limb syndrome is less common than afferent limb syndrome and is synonymous with postoperative small bowel obstruction. Symptoms include colicky abdominal pain, distention, diffuse tenderness, and frequent bilious vomiting. Because the obstruction is proximal, small bowel distention and air-fluid levels may not be appreciated on plain abdominal radiographs.

Diagnosis

In acute or chronic afferent limb syndrome, ultrasonography or computed tomography reveals a fluid-filled loop of bowel in the epigastrium or right upper quadrant. In efferent limb syndrome, barium studies or computed tomography with oral contrast can help diagnose the site of obstruction. Endoscopy should be performed to rule out alkaline gastritis, recurrent ulcer, anastomotic stricture, and carcinoma.

Surgical Treatment

Treatment of afferent and efferent limb syndromes is surgical. For afferent loop syndrome, the procedure of choice depends on the cause of the obstruction. If the obstruction is purely adhesive, then an enterolysis may suffice, although some surgeons advocate revision of the Billroth II anastomosis with Braun enteroenterostomy. If the obstruction is related to a stomal stenosis, the surgeon will need to exclude the presence of a carcinoma or a stomal ulcer. For the latter, a simple revision of the gastrojejunostomy does not treat the cause of the stomal ulcer (i.e., too much acid or use of aspirin or other nonsteroidal anti-inflammatory drugs). Unless a concomitant ulcer procedure is included (vagotomy or higher gastrectomy) or the offending nonsteroidal anti-inflammatory drug problem is addressed, the stomal ulcer will likely recur. In acute afferent limb syndrome, the limb must be inspected closely to assess viability. Afferent limb syndrome can be avoided at the initial surgery by performing a retrocolic gastrojejunostomy with a short (5 to 15 cm) afferent limb. All defects in the mesentery and mesocolon should be closed, and the gastrojejunostomy should lie in a horizontal plane without kinks.

Efferent limb syndrome is also best treated surgically, except for jejunogastric intussusception, which can be managed nonsurgically in two thirds of patients. If anastomotic stricture is the culprit, then balloon dilation or revision of the anastomosis is indicated, again noting and treating potential etiologies of a stomal ulcer. Lysing adhesions, closing internal hernias, or anchoring the efferent limb to the anterior abdominal wall or transverse mesocolon may prevent further herniation or kinking and twisting of the efferent limb.

ASSOCIATED POSTGASTRECTOMY CONDITIONS

Nutritional and Metabolic Changes

Although some degree of weight loss is common after gastric operations, improvement generally comes with time, and significant nutritional effects are rare. Fat malabsorption and steatorrhea are occasionally seen after gastric surgery. Bacterial overgrowth, stasis, or intestinal mucosal dysfunction can also cause malabsorption. Iron deficiency anemia occurs in 30% to 50% of patients and is likely due to failure to liberate and absorb the iron that is bound in organic molecules in food. Folate and vitamin B_{12} deficiencies are common and can lead to megaloblastic anemia. Osteomalacia resulting from impaired calcium and vitamin D absorption has been reported. These nutritional deficiencies are best treated with replacement therapy. Also, an as-yet poorly understood functional pancreatic exocrine insufficiency may occur after a Billroth II–like procedure or Roux-en-Y drainage; oral pancreatic enzyme supplements may help markedly.

Postvagotomy Dysphagia

Postvagotomy dysphagia results from either denervation of the distal esophagus, resulting in a failure of sphincter relaxation, or from postoperative esophageal hematoma or inflammation. If symptoms fail to resolve with frequent small soft meals, or liquid meals, then dilation with balloon or Maloney dilators is usually effective.

Small Gastric Remnant Syndrome

Small gastric remnant syndrome manifests as early satiety, postprandial fullness, and vomiting, and occurs most commonly in patients who have had 80% to 90% of their stomachs removed. Frequent, small dry meals can help prevent these symptoms, and antispasmodic and prokinetic agents can be helpful. This syndrome is similar to postgastrectomy gastroparesis (and may even be identical). If conservative treatments fail, then completion total gastrectomy and Roux-en-Y esophagojejunostomy often corrects the problem. Various pouches constructed from loops of jejunum have been described to help re-create a reservoir function for the absent stomach. However, when compared with objective parameters to esophagojejunostomy alone, pouches offer little benefit in most series.

Gastric Remnant Cancer

The risk for development of gastric remnant carcinoma increases twofold to sixfold in patients after antrectomy with Billroth II reconstruction compared with patients without prior partial gastrectomy. This is a late phenomenon, occurring 15 to 20 years after gastrectomy and has led some to screen at-risk patients with radiography or endoscopy. However, the routine use of endoscopic surveillance may not be warranted, because the overall rate of gastric remnant cancer is low. In addition, the natural history and time course of progression of gastric remnant dysplasia to carcinoma is unknown. The costs of such a program applied to all patients with a history of partial gastrectomy is high.

Pancreatic Cancer

Recent studies have suggested an increased risk for development of pancreatic cancer in patients after remote partial gastrectomy. After 20 or more years after gastric resection, the relative risk of pancreatic cancer varies from 1.6- to 5-fold. A higher level of suspicion in this patient population may lead to early detection.

Recurrent Ulcer

Recurrent ulcers can cause symptoms after prior gastric surgery. The incidence depends on the indication for operation as well as the type of surgery initially performed. Parietal cell vagotomy has the highest rate of recurrent ulceration, averaging 15% in most series. Main causes of recurrent ulceration include an inadequate initial operation, continued exposure to environmental ulcerogens (including *H. pylori*), and the Zollinger-Ellison syndrome. Incomplete vagotomy can be confirmed with a sham feeding test, and retained antrum and Zollinger-

Ellison syndrome can be diagnosed with gastrin measurements with or without secretin stimulation. Initial management with H_2-receptor blockers, proton pump inhibitors, and *H. pylori* treatment is appropriate. Operation is reserved for patients failing medical therapy, for those with gastrinoma, or for complications such as hemorrhage, perforation, or obstruction.

CONCLUSION

Postgastrectomy symptoms occur in up to 25% of patients after gastric surgery, so physicians involved in the care of these patients should be aware of the spectrum of postgastrectomy syndromes as well as their diagnosis and management. Future postgastrectomy problems may be minimized at the time of initial operation by fully understanding the potential pitfalls of gastric surgery. Highly selective vagotomy should be performed preferentially in the now rare patient undergoing elective ulcer surgery. Truncal vagotomy should be avoided when possible. Careful anastomotic technique and construction of Roux and Billroth II limbs can avoid mechanical difficulties such as kinking or obstruction. Billroth II gastrojejunostomy with the addition of Braun enteroenterostomy should be considered to avoid alkaline reflux gastritis, afferent limb syndrome, and gastroparesis.

When postgastrectomy symptoms develop, a focused evaluation using endoscopy, barium studies, and gastric emptying studies should identify the cause. Medical, dietary, and behavioral therapies should be tried for at least 1 year before consideration of remedial surgery. When

Pearls and Pitfalls

- Some form of postgastrectomy syndrome affects approximately 25% of patients after gastrectomy.
- Postgastrectomy syndromes involve rapid emptying (dumping), slow emptying (gastroparesis, stomal obstruction), bile reflux syndromes (bile reflux gastritis or esophagitis), or miscellaneous problems, such as gastric remnant carcinoma, postvagotomy diarrhea, afferent or efferent loop syndrome, and stomal ulcer.
- Dumping is usually a transient phenomenon; patience is required, as operative intervention is the last resort after trying octreotide.
- Postgastrectomy or postvagotomy gastroparesis is difficult to treat; operative intervention involves a near-total gastrectomy and is reserved for nutritional compromise.
- Bile reflux syndromes (especially gastritis) are rare; patients for operative intervention should be carefully screened to exclude gastroparesis.
- Postvagotomy diarrhea has no good proven treatment.
- Afferent or efferent loop syndromes involve some form of mechanical obstruction of the respective loop and require intervention.
- If the patient with gastric outlet obstruction has stomal stenosis—beware. Simple redoing of the anastomosis will not address the cause of the stenosis (acid, nonsteroidal anti-inflammatory drugs, cancer) and the stenosis will recur.

conservative therapy fails, a well-diagnosed remedial operation usually successfully controls most symptoms in the majority of patients.

SUGGESTED READINGS

Cheadle WG, Baker PR, Cuschieri A: Pyloric reconstruction for severe vasomotor dumping after vagotomy and pyloroplasty. Ann Surg 1985;202:568.

DeMeester T, Fuchs K, Ball C: Experimental and clinical results with proximal end-to-end duodenojejunostomy for pathologic duodenogastric reflux. Ann Surg 1987;206:414.

Forstner-Barthell AW, Murr MM, Nitecki S, et al: Near-total completion gastrectomy for severe postvagotomy gastric stasis: Analysis of early- and long-term results in 62 patients. J Gastrointest Surg 1999;3:15.

Glasgow RE, Mulvihill SJ: Postgastrectomy syndromes. Probl Gen Surg 1997;14:132.

Gray JL, Debas HT, Mulvihill SJ: Control of dumping symptoms by somatostatin analogue in patients after gastric surgery. Arch Surg 1991;126:1231.

Greene FP: Management of gastric remnant carcinoma based on the results of a 15-year endoscopic screening program. Ann Surg 1996;223:701.

Gustavsson S, Ilstrup D, Morrison P, Kelley K: Roux-Y stasis syndrome after gastrectomy. Am J Surg 1987;155:490.

Vogel SB, Drane WE, Woodward ER: Clinical and radionuclide evaluation of bile diversion by Braun enteroenterostomy: Prevention and treatment of alkaline reflux gastritis. An alternative to Roux-en-Y diversion. Ann Surg 1994;219:458.

Chapter 57

Bariatric Surgery

Rifat Latifi and Harvey J. Sugerman

Obesity is the second leading cause of preventable death in the United States and thus presents a major public health problem. An estimated 97 million adults in the United States are overweight or obese: 33% of the population are overweight, defined as a body mass index (BMI) of 25 to 29.9 kg/m², while 22% are obese, with a BMI of at least 30. Morbid obesity, on the other hand, has been arbitrarily defined as a weight 100 pounds above the ideal body weight, or a BMI of at least 35 kg/m². Severe obesity (more than 244 pounds for men or more than 225 pounds for women) is present in 5% (2.8 million) of men and 7% (4.5 million) of women in the United States. As the BMI increases, so does the mortality rate from all causes, especially from cardiovascular disease, which is 50% to 100% above that of persons with a normal BMI in the range 20 to 25 kg/m². Recent findings suggest that obesity is associated with a low-grade systemic inflammatory state, as manifested with elevated levels of proinflammatory cytokine interleukin-6 (IL-6) and C-reactive protein, thought to contribute to cardiovascular morbidity. Elevated C-reactive protein levels have been associated with an increased risk of myocardial infarction, stroke, peripheral arterial disease, and coronary heart disease.

Although the causes of severe obesity are probably multifactorial, surgical treatment of this condition (bariatric surgery) has gained much attention in recent years. To this end, surgical treatment of morbid obesity—that is, BMI greater than 40 kg/m² or BMI greater than 35 kg/m² with comorbid conditions—has gained acceptance among surgeons, physicians, and the public.

CLINICAL PRESENTATION

Severe obesity is associated with a large number of clinical syndromes (Table 57–1), some of which cause premature death in this growing population. Major comorbidities are cardiovascular-related problems, respiratory insufficiency due to obesity, hypoventilation and sleep apnea syndrome, diabetes mellitus, venous stasis, hypercoagulopathy, endocrine-related problems, intracranial and intra-abdominal hypertension and their consequences, and bone and joint disease. Other obesity-related conditions, such as urinary and sexual dysfunction, are prominent pathologic features of morbidly obese patients. The difficulties in diagnosing surgical conditions in obese patients, such as peritonitis, necrotizing panniculitis, necrotizing fasciitis, diverticulitis, necrotizing pancreatitis, and other intra-abdominal infections, are notable. Moreover, establishing a secure airway during or after surgery in morbidly obese patients is often very challenging.

INDICATIONS FOR SURGERY

Currently, bariatric surgery is indicated for patients with a BMI of 40 kg/m² or greater who do not have any comorbidity or with a BMI of 35 kg/m² or over who have associated comorbidity. Furthermore, there should be no evidence of an identified endocrine disorder that can cause massive obesity. Most insurance companies require that patients should have failed formally controlled nonsurgical attempts to reduce their weight. However, no nonoperative program has had long-term efficiency in maintaining weight loss.

PREOPERATIVE MANAGEMENT

Preoperative management of morbidly obese patients consists of detailed evaluation of the medical, dietary, and psychological histories. Moreover, it should involve a primary care physician, a surgeon, and a dietitian. Once the patient and his or her family have accrued sufficient information to consent to the operation, preadmission testing should be performed. This includes a chest radiograph, complete blood count (CBC), chemistry panel and electrocardiogram.

Patients with a history of peptic ulcer disease should undergo preoperative endoscopy. If an ulcer is present, it should be treated preoperatively and the operation should be postponed until there is no clinical or endoscopic evidence of an ulcer. The treatment should be combined with eradication of *Helicobacter pylori*, if present. Upper gastrointestinal (UGI) radiographic series are performed only in patients requiring revision of previous gastric procedures. Baseline arterial blood gases should be obtained in patients with a BMI greater than 50 or in those with a history of sleep apnea. Patients should be questioned for signs and symptoms of obstructive sleep apnea syndrome (multiple nocturnal awakenings, loud snoring, falling asleep while driving, morning and daytime somnolence). If these symptoms are present, patients should undergo sleep polysomnography. If sleep apnea is present, patients should be treated with nasal continuous-positive airway pressure (CPAP), and they will require postoperative monitoring in the intensive care unit. Preoperative insertion and optimization with a Swan-Ganz catheter is reserved for patients with heart failure and obesity hypoventilation (room air $PaO_2 \leq 55$ mm Hg, $PaCO_2 \geq 47$ mm Hg). Since intubation may be very difficult, particularly in severely obese patients with a difficult airway, an experienced anesthesia and surgical team should be present at the time of intubation and extubation.

Table 57–1	**Pathologic Conditions Associated with Morbid Obesity**

Cardiovascular Dysfunction
 Coronary artery disease
 Increased complications after coronary bypass operation
 Cardiomyopathy
 Left ventricular concentric hypertrophy: hypertension
 Left ventricular eccentric hypertrophy
 Right ventricular hypertrophy, pulmonary failure
 Prolonged QT interval with sudden death
 Heart failure
Respiratory Insufficiency of Obesity (Pickwickian Syndrome)
 Obesity hypoventilation syndrome
 Obesity sleep apnea syndrome
Metabolic Complications
 Type II diabetes mellitus
 Hypertension
 Elevated triglycerides
 Elevated cholesterol
 Nonalcoholic steatohepatitis (NASH)
 Cholelithiasis
 Cholecystitis
Increased Intra-abdominal Pressure
 Obesity hypoventilation syndrome
 Gastroesophageal reflux
 Stress overflow urinary incontinence
 Thrombophlebitis
 Venous stasis ulcers
 Pulmonary embolism
 Nephrotic syndrome
 Hernias (incisional, inguinal)
 Preeclampsia
 Pseudotumor cerebri
Sexual Hormone Dysfunction
 Amenorrhea, hypermenorrhea
 Stein-Leventhal syndrome: hirsutism, ovarian cysts
 Infertility
Cancer
 Endometrial carcinoma
 Breast carcinoma
 Colon cancer
 Renal cell carcinoma
 Prostate cancer
Degenerative Bone and Joint Disease
 Osteoarthritis of feet, ankles, knees, hips, back, and shoulders
 Chronic lower back pain
Psychosocial Impairment
 Decreased employability, work discrimination

CHOICE OF OPERATION, EVIDENCE-BASED

Bariatric surgical procedures have proved superior in inducing weight loss and correcting preoperative comorbid conditions of obese patients compared with all other modalities. Based on 14 randomized clinical trials that examined the effects of surgical procedures on weight loss, 8 of which were considered appropriate for evidence-based medicine, bariatric surgery is the treatment of choice for morbidly obese patients (evidence category B). Indeed, the National Institutes of Health (NIH) has sanctioned bariatric surgery as effective in the patient with morbid obesity. In these studies, all patients had a BMI of at least 40 kg/m² or had a BMI greater than 35 kg/m² with associated comorbid conditions. Both the weight loss and the improvement in the comorbid conditions in patients undergoing surgical interventions for morbid obesity were

significant. In these trials, gastric bypass induced weight loss from 50 kg to as much as 100 kg over a period of 6 months to 1 year, and it was superior to gastroplasty. On the other hand, when gastroplasty was combined with diet, it achieved better results than those of diet alone.

Over the last decade the safety and effectiveness of many surgical procedures have evolved. Although currently most bariatric surgical centers in North America and Europe perform Roux-en-Y gastric bypass (RYGBP), vertical banded gastroplasty (VBG), or adjustable gastric banding (AGB), several other procedures are briefly mentioned here.

Jejunoileal Bypass

Jejunoileal bypass (JIB) was the first popular surgical procedure for morbid obesity. During this procedure, a short length of proximal jejunum (8 to 14 inches) was connected to the distal ileum (4 to 12 inches) as an end-to-end or end-to-side anastomosis. Although this operation produced weight loss by obligatory malabsorption through bypass of a major portion of the absorptive surface of the small intestine, it was associated with a number of serious early and late complications.

The most serious postoperative complication of JIB was acute and chronic liver failure that on occasion required liver transplantation. Other serious late sequelae are an immune-complex arthritis, gallstones, hypocalcemia, oxalate kidney stones, osteoporosis, intractable malodorous diarrhea with associated potassium and magnesium abnormalities, metabolic acidosis, vitamin B_{12} deficiency, vitamin K deficiency, oxalate neuropathy with renal failure, pneumatosis intestinalis, and bypass enteritis associated with occult blood in the stools and iron-deficiency anemia. These complications have led some researchers to suggest that all JIB procedures should be reversed because cirrhosis can develop insidiously in the absence of abnormal liver function tests (LFTs). If the cirrhosis is Child's Class A, the patient should be converted from the JIB to a RYGBP, as simple takedown of the JIB has been associated with a regaining of all lost weight in about 90% of patients. Child's Class B cirrhosis, especially with esophageal varices, carries an excessive risk during conversion to RYGBP, and a simple "takedown" of the JIB should be performed. Standard JIB should no longer be performed because of these unacceptable complication rates. Also, randomized, prospective studies have shown that the GBP operation is associated with a comparable weight loss and a significantly lower complication rate than that with JIB.

Gastroplasty

The concept and the technique of gastroplasty was introduced and suggested as a safer and relatively easier method for restricting food intake. In gastroplasty, the upper stomach is stapled close to the gastroesophageal junction to create a small upper gastric pouch that communicates with the rest of the gastrointestinal (GI) tract through a small outlet. Gastroplasties are performed with either horizontal or vertical placement of the staples.

Horizontal gastroplasty, which usually requires ligation and division of the short gastric vessels between the stomach and the spleen, carries the risk of devascularization of the gastric pouch or splenic injury. Although theoretically attractive because there is no bypass of the gut, all gastroplasties have been associated with very high failure rates (>50%). The VBG is a current gastroplasty in which a "donut hole" opening is made in the stomach with an end-to-end anastomosis (EEA) stapling device 5 cm from the cardioesophageal junction (Fig. 57–1). A 90-mm stapling device is used to construct the pouch between this opening and the angle of His, and a 1.5 × 5 cm strip of polypropylene mesh is wrapped around the stoma on the lesser curvature and sutured to itself, but not to the stomach. VBG can be associated with severe gastroesophageal reflux, but it resolves after conversion to gastric bypass. VBG is more effective than horizontal gastroplasty, but is significantly less effective than RYGBP.

Gastric Bypass

In recent years, RYGBP (Fig. 57–2) is favored as the procedure of choice in morbidly obese patients because of superior long-term weight loss effects compared with VBG (71% vs. 53% loss of excess body weight). In four randomized, prospective trials and three retrospective studies, RYGBP was found to induce greater weight loss than VBG, especially for patients addicted to sweets. "Sweets eaters" do poorly after VBG with regard to their weight and do better after RYGBP because most develop signs and symptoms of dumping syndrome following the

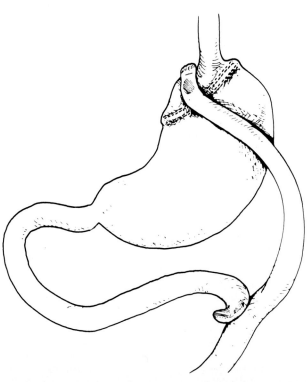

Figure 57–2. Roux-en-Y gastric bypass. (From Sugerman HJ, Starkey JV, Birkenhauer R: A randomized prospective trial of gastric bypass *versus* vertical banded gastroplasty for morbid obesity and their effects on sweets *versus* people who do not eat sweets. Ann Surg 1987;205:613–624, with permission.)

ingestion of foods rich in sugar early after RYGBP. Furthermore, many patients who have undergone VBG often fail to lose enough weight to correct their obesity-related comorbidity.

The high incidence of staple-line disruption has led some surgeons to recommend transecting the stomach for GBP patients, as it is done when this procedure is performed laparoscopically. However, with three to four superimposed applications of a 90-mm stapler, the incidence of staple-line disruption has been less than 2%. Currently, the authors' group performs gastric bypass by constructing a small gastric pouch (15 to 30 mL) with a 45-cm Roux-en-Y limb and stoma restricted to 1 cm. Superobese patients (BMI ≥50 kg/m²) achieve a better weight loss with a 150-cm Roux limb (long-limb gastric bypass). The small gastric pouch has a very small, almost nonexistent acid secretion and is associated with a low incidence of marginal ulcer. The RYGBP is associated with long-lasting weight loss in 70% of patients. The average weight loss at 2 years is 66% of excess weight, at 5 years it is 60%, and mid-50s at 10 years following surgery.

OPEN TECHNIQUE OF GASTRIC BYPASS

The abdomen is entered through a midline incision. On entering the peritoneal cavity, complete exploration is performed to exclude unanticipated pathology before the GBP is begun. If gallstones, sludge, or polyps are present on palpation or are found on intraoperative ultrasonogra-

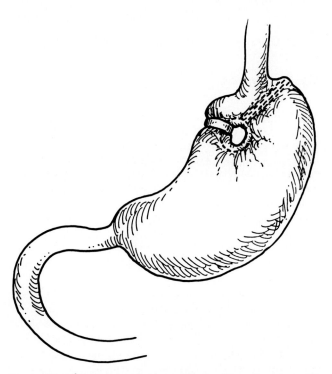

Figure 57–1. Vertical banded gastroplasty. (From Sugerman HJ, Starkey JV, Birkenhauer R: A randomized prospective trial of gastric bypass *versus* vertical banded gastroplasty for morbid obesity and their effects on sweets *versus* people who do not eat sweets. Ann Surg 1987;205:613–624, with permission.)

phy, cholecystectomy is performed. Some bariatric surgeons routinely remove the gallbladder.

The distal esophagus is mobilized and encircled with a soft rubber drain. The gastrohepatic omentum is entered overlying the caudate lobe. An aberrant left hepatic artery should be avoided. The phrenoesophageal ligament overlying the anterior and lateral distal esophagus is sharply incised. This incision facilitates blunt mobilization of the distal esophagus. Laterally, the dissection must be at the level of the esophagus. Low lateral dissection may lead to injury of the short gastric vessels or spleen. An opening is made in the mesentery alongside the stomach between the first and the second branches of the left gastric artery large enough to admit a right-angled clamp. Following blunt dissection of the avascular space on the posterior stomach wall, between the opening in the gastrohepatic omentum and the lateral angle of His, an encircling rubber tube is placed to serve as a guide for the introduction of the stapling device. Before staplers are applied, all intraluminal tubes (the nasogastric tube, the esophageal stethoscope) must be removed by the anesthesiologist.

The proximal jejunum is divided with a gastrointestinal anastomosis (GIA) stapling device and a Roux limb is created. A side-to-side jejunojenunostomy is created at 45 cm for standard bypass or at 150 cm for superobese patients. With blunt dissection, an opening is created in the transverse mesocolon and the Roux limb is brought through to reach the proximal stomach without tension. A 55-mm or 90-mm stapling device is placed across the stomach with the use of the rubber tube as a guide. Once the surgeon has ascertained that the staple line is across the stomach and that the stomach is not folded on itself, the stomach is stapled three times with superimposed staple applications.

A 1-cm gastrojejunal anastomosis is created between the proximal stomach and the Roux limb. This anastomosis is hand-sewn with the use of a two-layer technique. Once the posterior layer of the anastomosis is sewn, a No. 30 French dilator is placed per os by the anesthesia team and guided by the surgeon through the anastomosis to define the appropriate dimensions. After completing the anastomosis, methylene blue dye is injected through the nasogastric tube to assess for leak. Mesenteric defects at the jejunojenunostomy and in the mesocolon through which the Roux limb passes are closed to prevent an internal hernia. The abdominal fascia is closed with a running stitch, whereas the skin is approximated with skin staples.

LAPAROSCOPIC BARIATRIC SURGERY

Laparoscopic bariatric surgery is in its early phases of development. Although the long-term results of laparoscopic bariatric surgery are not known, the advantages should include a decreased length of hospital stay, less pain, and a lower risk of incision hernia, which is about 20% following open obesity surgery. In addition, as with other laparoscopic surgeries, it is hoped that there will be fewer and less severe adhesions, with the potential for fewer subsequent small bowel obstructions. The bariatric procedures currently performed laparoscopically include VBG, gastric banding (with adjustable bands), and RYGBP.

The success of laparoscopic bariatric surgery should be compared with the gold standard of open bariatric surgery. First, like other laparoscopic operations, this operation is performed according to the principles of open procedures. Second, it is hoped that a minimal-access approach, in addition to decreasing the recovery time, will reduce the perioperative complications of wound infections.

Adjustable Gastric Banding

The adjustable silicone gastric band was developed to be placed laparoscopically. The device contains a balloon that is adjusted by injecting saline into a subcutaneously implanted port. This procedure is very popular in Europe. However, no long-term studies validate its safety and efficacy. A United States Food and Drug Administration (FDA)–approved trial is currently in progress in the United States. There have been problems with band slippage leading to gastric obstruction with the subsequent need to revise the position of the band, esophageal dilatation, band erosion into the lumen of the stomach, port infections, and inadequate weight loss. Other complications include food intolerance, reflux esophagitis, pouch dilatation, and stoma occlusion. A number of patients with the laparoscopically placed gastric band have been converted to a GBP. In some patients, removal of the gastric band and conversion to RYGBP can be performed laparoscopically, however, these operations are technically challenging owing to adhesions from the previous operation.

Gastric Bypass

The initial experience with 75 patients who underwent laparoscopic RYGBP (LRYGBP) with a 21-mm EEA was reported to be comparable with that of those who underwent open gastric bypass. Furthermore, the follow-up from 3 to 60 months on 500 patients who underwent LRYGBP has been reported, with an incidence of major complications of 11% and an anastomotic leak rate of 5%, and no mortality. The stapled circular gastrojejunal anastomosis is created by pulling the anvil through the mouth and down the esophagus. This procedure has been associated with a higher frequency of wound infection, and incisional hernia.

As experience is gained with this laparoscopic operation, the complications related to the complex technical nature of the procedure will probably decrease. Most surgeons perform LRYGBP in patients with a BMI of 40 kg/m² or less, although a few groups have reported on successful LRYGBP procedures in patients with BMIs up to 70 kg/m². The results are relatively comparable to an open technique; however, the operations take longer. The mastering of this procedure is difficult, and the learning curve is very steep.

Partial Biliopancreatic Diversion and Duodenal Switch Operation

The partial biliopancreatic diversion was developed as both a gastric restrictive and a malabsorptive procedure that does not have a blind intestinal limb where bacterial overgrowth can occur. This operation involves a subtotal gastrectomy, leaving a 400-mL gastric pouch for the average obese patient and a 200-mL gastric pouch for the superobese patient. The distal small bowel is transected 250 cm proximal to the ileocecal valve, and the proximal bypassed bowel is anastomosed to the ileum 50 cm proximal to the ileocecal valve. This leaves a 200-cm "alimentary tract," a 300- to 400-cm "biliary tract" of bypassed intestine, and a 50-cm "common absorptive alimentary tract" where the ingested food mixes with bile and pancreatic juices for the digestion and absorption of all complex foodstuffs to occur. This operation has produced an excellent weight loss in patients and does not appear to be associated with the high incidence of bacterial overgrowth seen in the JIB, as bile and pancreatic juices wash out the bypassed small intestine. However, the biliopancreatic diversion may be associated with severe protein-calorie malnutrition, necessitating hospitalization and total parenteral nutrition. Frequent, foul-smelling steatorrheic stools lead to fat-soluble vitamin deficiencies and calcium loss secondary to chelation with fat, producing severe osteoporosis. A randomized, prospective trial using a much smaller stomach (50 mL) without gastric resection and a longer common absorptive intestinal tract (150 mL) in superobese patients, called a distal GBP, was associated with a much greater weight loss than that with a standard GBP but had a 25% incidence of severe malnutrition, necessitating conversion to the standard GBP. The authors currently reserve this distal GBP for superobese patients who fail a standard GBP and have severe obesity-related comorbidity (e.g., diabetes, obesity hypoventilation syndrome). These patients require fat-soluble vitamin supplementation and may develop severe malnutrition.

A modified malabsorptive procedure, known as the duodenal switch operation, has been developed with the hope that there will be less protein and fat-soluble vitamin malabsorption. This procedure involves wedge resection of the greater curvature of the stomach, division of the duodenum in the distal bulb, and division of the ileum 250 cm proximal to the ileocecal valve, with anastomosis of the proximal duodenal segment to the distal ileal segment; the distal end of the transected duodenum is oversewn as a duodenal stump. The segment that carries the biliary and pancreatic secretions is anastomosed to the ileum 100 cm proximal to the ileocecal valve. It is not yet clear whether this operation will prevent the protein malnutrition or the calcium and fat-soluble vitamin deficiencies associated with a malabsorptive procedure.

POSTOPERATIVE MANAGEMENT

Most of the patients who undergo bariatric surgery do not require special postoperative management. However, those who have sleep apnea, obesity hypoventilation, or a history of congestive heart failure may require mechanical ventilation in the intensive care unit until their arterial blood gases and weaning parameters confirm that it is safe to extubate them.

COMPLICATIONS OF GASTRIC SURGERY FOR MORBID OBESITY

The most feared early complication of gastric surgery for morbid obesity is a postoperative gastric leak, with development of peritonitis (Table 57–2). Perforation of the distal stomach, although rare, can occur because of marked dilatation of the excluded stomach secondary to afferent limb obstruction at the jejunojenunostomy. This complication is usually heralded by frequent hiccups and can be diagnosed by noting a large gastric bubble on a plain abdominal radiograph. Impending gastric perforation requires urgent decompression performed via a percutaneous technique or with operative decompression. In patients who undergo reoperation, such as conversion from JIB to GBP or in patients with extensive adhesions from previous abdominal surgery, a gastrostomy tube should be inserted prophylactically for decompression. The gastrostomy tube can also be used for feeding until the patient's oral intake permits weight stabilization or for

Table 57–2	Complications of Bariatric Surgery

Perioperative
Splenic or other organ injuries
Dilation of excluded stomach
Perforation of distal stomach (rare)
Afferent limb obstruction
Difficult to recognize abdominal catastrophe
Deep vein thrombosis and pulmonary embolus
Cardiac events
Wound infections
Wound dehiscence
Anastomotic leak
Abdominal sepsis
Multiple organ system failure
Gastrointestinal fistulas
Prolonged ventilatory dependency
Difficult tracheostomy
Death
Nutritional
Protein-calorie malnutrition
Malabsorption of micronutrients
Vitamin deficiencies (vitamins B_{12} and folate, and fat-soluble vitamins A, D, E, and K)
Acute thiamine deficiency
Iron deficiency anemia
Mineral deficiencies (Ca, Mg)
Dehydration
Failure to lose weight
Gastrointestinal
Food intolerance
Dumping syndrome
Nausea, vomiting
Marginal ulcers
Stomal stenosis
Diarrhea
Long-Term Surgical
Incisional hernia
Gallstones
Intra-abdominal (internal) hernia
Bowel obstruction

enteral nutritional support in patients who develop a leak from the proximal gastric pouch.

The inability to readily recognize an abdominal catastrophe is one of the most significant aspects of the surgical care of morbidly obese patients. The classic signs and symptoms of peritonitis are often absent in these patients. Thus, if the patient experiences worsening abdominal pain, back pain, or left shoulder pain, urinary frequency, or rectal tenesmus, one should suspect a leak. Tachycardia, tachypnea, fever, leukocytosis, or metabolic acidosis also should raise a strong suspicion of an abdominal catastrophe. A significant leak can often be confirmed with UGI series using water-soluble contrast medium. If a leak is observed or even if the study is negative but the suspicion is high, the patient's abdomen must be urgently explored. An attempt to repair the leak should be made, and a large sump drain placed nearby, because the repair frequently breaks down. This approach may lead to a controlled fistual, which requires therapy with total parenteral nutrition and a feeding gastrostomy or jejunostomy.

Other complications early after obesity surgery include deep vein thrombosis, pulmonary embolus, and superficial or deep wound infections. Although these complications are not unique to bariatric surgery, they are more common in this patient population. The incidence of lower leg venous thrombosis and pulmonary embolism can be reduced with the use of intermittent venous compression boots placed prior to the start of the operation and low-dose heparin (LDH) or low-molecular-weight heparin (LMWH) given 30 minutes prior to surgery. Although there are no data to support the use of LMWH in these patients, if LMWH is used, higher doses may be needed based on heparin anti–factor X levels. A vena cava filter may be placed in patients with either obesity hypoventilation or severe venous stasis disease prophylactically at the time of obesity surgery; however, there is no evidence to support the routine use of the vena cava filter in this population. Early ambulation is also important in patients who undergo bariatric surgery.

A marginal ulcer develops in about 10% of GBP patients. This usually responds to acid suppression therapy (H_2-receptor blocker or omeprazole). Other causes include the use of nonsteroidal anti-inflammatory drugs (NSAIDs). Stomal stenosis can develop in patients following RYGBP. Outpatient endoscopic balloon dilation of the stoma should be attempted. This is usually successful in GBP patients but is effective in fewer than half of the stenoses in VBG patients.

LATE COMPLICATIONS

GALLSTONES. Rapid weight loss after either VBG or GBP is associated with a high incidence (35%) of gallstone formation and with a 10% need for subsequent cholecystectomy for biliary complications within 3 to 5 years of obesity surgery. Although some surgeons perform prophylactic cholecystectomy at the time of bariatric surgery, others perform cholecystectomy only with sonographic evidence of gallstones. In a randomized, prospective clinical trial, prophylactic ursodeoxycholic acid, 300 mg orally twice daily, reduces the risk of gallstone forma-

tion from 32% to 2% when given for 6 months after bariatric surgery; moreover, there is a very low risk of subsequent gallstone formation for the 6 months after discontinuation of the medication.

NUTRITIONAL COMPLICATIONS. After bariatric surgery, nutritional complications, such as protein-calorie malnutrition, may develop. A rare syndrome of polyneu-

---

Pearls and Pitfalls

PEARLS

- Obesity is a national epidemic; morbid obesity (BMI >35 kg/m²) affects 5% of men and 7% of women.
- Bariatric surgery is the most effective weight reduction technique and has been sanctioned by the NIH.
- Roux-en-Y gastric bypass appears to be the most effective and safe bariatric procedure. Recently, it has been done laparoscopically.
- Roux-en-Y gastric bypass is successful in maintaining long-term weight loss in about 65% to 75% of patients.
- Weight loss reverses insulin-dependent diabetes mellitus, sleep apnea, and usually hypertension.
- Reoperative bariatric surgery can be effective, but it has a higher morbidity and mortality rate.

Preoperative Pearls

- Select patients carefully
- Have a frank conversation with the patient and his or her family

Intraoperative Pearls

- Achieve good surgical exposure
- Explore the entire abdomen
- Remove all tubes from the esophagus before stapling the stomach
- Close all intra-abdominal spaces for potential hernias
- Repair existing umbilical hernia
- Convert to open technique if needed, when the operation is attempted laparoscopically
- Perform a leak test or endoscopy at the end of the procedure
- Call for help if needed

Postoperative Pearls

- Recognize subtle signs and symptoms of peritonitis
- Beware of presence or absence of classic abdominal pain, guarding, tenderness, and rigidity
- Do not ignore the following:
  Shoulder pain
  Hiccups
  Chest pain
  Back pain
  Tenesmus
  Urinary frequency or emergency
  Anxiety
  Feeling of impending doom
  Tachycardia
  Tachypnea
  Respiratory failure
  Sudden hypotension
  Metabolic acidosis

ropathy has been reported after these operations. This syndrome usually occurs in association with intractable vomiting, severe protein-calorie malnutrition, and subsequent acute thiamine deficiency. The risk of vitamin B_{12} deficiency mandates long-term follow-up, with annual measurement of serum vitamin B_{12} concentrations. These patients should take 500 μg of oral vitamin B_{12} daily or 1 mg of vitamin B_{12} intramuscularly per month. Iron-deficiency anemia can occur in menstruating women and may be refractory to supplemental oral iron because iron absorption takes place primarily in the duodenum and upper jejunum. Occasionally, intravenous iron-dextran may be necessary. Menstruating women should take 2 iron sulfate tablets (325 mg/day) by mouth after GBP as long as they continue to menstruate. Magnesium deficiency may also occur and require supplementation. Patients with either a long-limb gastric or partial biliopancreatic bypass can develop calcium and fat-soluble vitamin deficiencies that need to be monitored and treated. Also, serum vitamin D concentrations should be followed yearly after the malabsorptive procedures.

OUTCOMES OF SURGERY FOR MORBID OBESITY

Gastric procedures for morbid obesity can yield dramatic and long-term weight reduction, with an average loss of two thirds of excess weight within 1 to 2 years. Weight usually stabilizes at this level in most patients as the reduced-caloric intake meets caloric expenditure. The patients must be followed carefully to ensure adequate protein, vitamin, and other micronutrient levels.

Weight loss corrects insulin-dependent (insulin-resistant) diabetes in almost all patients. No other therapy has produced more durable and complete control of diabetes mellitus. Hypertension is cured in two thirds of the patients; similar results occur with the headaches and associated cerebrospinal fluid pressure elevation in almost all patients with pseudotumor cerebri. The obstructive sleep apnea syndrome, which poses the greatest immediate risk to life of any of the morbid obesity complications, resolves with weight loss. The hypoxemia and hypercapnia seen in the obesity hypoventilation syndrome return toward normal with weight loss. Increased pulmonary artery and pulmonary capillary wedge pressures also improve after weight loss along with correction of abnormal arterial blood gases.

The loss of weight usually corrects abnormalities in the cyclic secretion of female sexual hormones, permits healing of chronic venous stasis ulcers associated with venous insufficiency, prevents reflux esophagitis, relieves stress-overflow urinary incontinence, and improves low back pain and joint pain. Furthermore, weight loss allows successful total artificial joint replacement. Surgically induced weight reduction is associated with significant improvement of left ventricular ejection fraction, decreased cardiac reserve, and improvements in cardiac chamber size and ventricular thickness. Improvement in the lipid profile of morbidly obese patients has been documented. The patient's self-image is often markedly improved after bariatric surgery.

Failed Gastric Surgery for Obesity

The inability to lose more than 40% of one's excess weight is considered a failure of bariatric surgery. About 10% to 15% of patients regain lost weight or fail to achieve an acceptable weight loss. Although some patients can overcome the GBP and regain weight by expanding either the stoma or the pouch, this finding is not common. The cause of this failure appears to be excessive, constant nibbling on foods with a high-caloric density.

Reoperation

Reoperation for failed bariatric surgery can be extremely challenging and heralds a significant risk of morbidity and possible mortality. Attempts to reverse or revise a failed gastroplasty are often unsuccessful because of recurrence of stomal dilation and problems with gastric emptying. Reoperation in these patients may be difficult because of adhesions to the liver and spleen. Results appear to be significantly better when these patients are converted to a RYGBP. Because of the technical difficulties, these patients must understand that the risks of serious complications are higher after a secondary procedure than after a primary one. It is probably inappropriate and dangerous to convert a failed GBP to a vertical banded gastroplasty. Furthermore, revision of a dilated gastrojejunal stoma has not been effective. Most patients who fail a GBP do so as a consequence of excessive fat ingestion. If the patient has significant obesity or comorbidity that has failed to resolve or has returned with weight regained, conversion to a malabsorptive distal GBP (modified partial biliopancreatic diversion) can be performed; however, this can be associated with protein-calorie malnutrition, steatorrhea, fat-soluble vitamin deficiencies, and osteoporosis and thus requires close surveillance.

SELECTED READINGS

Hess DS, Hess DW: Biliopancreatic diversion with a duodenal switch. Obes Surg 1996;6A:122.

Kellum JM, DeMaria EJ, Sugerman HJ: The surgical treatment of morbid obesity. Curr Probl Surg 1998;35:791.

NIH Technology Assessment Conference Panel, NIH Conference: Methods for voluntary weight loss and control. Ann Intern Med 1992;116:942.

Scopinaro N, Gianetta E, Civalleri D, et al: Two years of clinical experience with bilio-pancreatic bypass for obesity. Am J Clin Nutr 1980;33:506.

Sugerman HJ, Baron PL, Fairman RP, et al: Hemodynamic dysfunction in obesity hypoventilation syndrome and the effects of treatment with surgically induced weight loss. Ann Surg 1988;207:604.

Sugerman HJ, Starkey J, Birkenhauer R: A randomized prospective trial of gastric bypass versus vertical banded gastroplasty for morbid obesity and their effects on sweets versus nonsweets eaters. Ann Surg 1987;205:613.

Chapter 58
Gastric Adenocarcinoma

Martin R. Weiser and Kevin C. Conlon

Worldwide, approximately 800,000 new patients are diagnosed with stomach cancer and over 600,000 deaths are attributed to this disease annually. Gastric cancer is very common in Eastern Asia; age-standardized incidence rates are highest in Japan, where 78 per 100,000 population will develop the disease. In North America, the incidence of gastric cancer is considerably lower, at 8 per 100,000. Women are half as likely to develop gastric cancer. Gastric cancer patients have a 50% survival in Japan, a number that is significantly higher than the survival rate in North America. This difference is thought to be related to the earlier presentation of gastric cancer in Japan compared with Western countries, possibly because of nationwide screening programs.

EPIDEMIOLOGY

Many risk factors have been linked with gastric cancer, including low socioeconomic status, cigarette smoking, and alcohol abuse. Diets rich in salted or smoked foods and low in fruits and vegetables have been related to the development of gastric adenocarcinoma. Poorly preserved foods have increased levels of nitrates and nitrites, which can result in N-nitroso compounds known to be carcinogenic to gastric mucosa in multiple animal models. In support of this theory is the reduced incidence of gastric cancer in developed countries, where refrigeration and food preservation are common.

Gastric cancer is also associated with inflammatory precursor lesions such as chronic atrophic gastritis, pernicious anemia, and partial gastrectomy for benign disease. This association may in part explain the relationship between *Helicobacter pylori* infection and the incidence of adenocarcinoma. *Helicobacter pylori* infection leads to gastritis, gastric atrophy, metaplasia, and eventually dysplasia. Intestinal-type cancers located in the antrum and body of the stomach are more common in patients with *H. pylori* infection. Virulence is strain dependent, and bacteria possessing the *cag A* gene are more likely to produce atrophic gastritis and gastric cancer. These observations led the International Agency for Research on Cancer and the World Health Organization to designate *H. pylori* as a group I carcinogen in 1994. Treatment of asymptomatic carriers may be warranted, but no definitive data exist to substantiate this recommendation.

Screening for gastric cancer with endoscopy has been successful in countries with a high incidence of the disease. The dramatic increase in the number of curative resections in Japan, from 48% in the 1940s to 98% during the 1980s, has been attributed to early endoscopy. Western countries, with a significantly lower incidence of gastric cancer, have not adopted mass screening, since it is not considered to be cost-effective. In part the lack of mass screening may explain why two thirds of patients in the United States present with advanced gastric cancer (stage III or stage IV disease).

Recent data have suggested a shift in location of tumors within the stomach for patients in the United States. Adenocarcinoma of the gastroesophageal junction and cardia have increased, whereas distal stomach cancers have decreased. The etiology for this change is unknown, but its implications are important, since proximal cancer is more difficult to treat than are distal lesions.

PATHOLOGY

The majority of gastric malignancies are adenocarcinomas, followed by lymphoma, carcinoid, squamous cell carcinoma, and sarcoma. The histologic subtypes of gastric adenocarcinoma include papillary, tubular, mucinous, signet ring, adenosquamous, squamous, small cell, and undifferentiated carcinoma. A number of classification systems exist. The commonly utilized Lauren classification scheme divides adenocarcinoma of the stomach into two histologic groups: intestinal and diffuse. The intestinal type is frequently seen in countries with a high incidence of gastric cancer. These tumors are most commonly seen in the distal stomach of older men who have a history of gastritis. The diffuse type is equally distributed between men and women, is more often seen in the proximal stomach, and presents at a younger age (<40 years). Diffuse gastric cancer extends with indistinct margins, is difficult to diagnose, and often presents at an advanced stage.

A second classification scheme based on gross features has been described by Borrmann. Lesions are categorized as type 0 through IV. Type 0 lesions represent early gastric cancer and correlate with a low potential of metastatic disease. Type I lesions are polypoid, type II lesions are fungating, and type III lesions are excavated and ulcerated. Type IV lesions correspond to diffuse gastric wall thickening without a discrete mass. This classification has recently been employed in the treatment of early gastric cancer, since polypoid lesions (Borrmann type I) may be suitable for endoscopic resection.

CLINICAL MANIFESTATIONS

Early symptoms of gastric cancer are nonspecific and include abdominal pain and dyspepsia. These are often interpreted as ulcer related and are ignored. As the disease progresses, the symptoms become more pronounced and may cause anorexia, weight loss, nausea, and melena. Approximately one quarter of patients will have a history of gastric ulcer. In some patients, the symptoms may suggest the location of the primary tumor. Dysphagia is usually associated with tumors of the cardia or gastro-esophageal junction. Gastric outlet obstruction is associated with antral tumors, and early satiety can be seen with a diffusely infiltrating tumor.

The majority of patients have no physical findings until the disease is advanced or metastatic. The presence of an intra-abdominal mass, hepatomegaly, or ascites portends a poor outcome. Other physical findings consistent with metastatic disease include a palpable umbilical mass (Sister Mary Joseph's node), palpable supraclavicular lymph node (Virchow's node), peritoneal implants in the pelvis (Blumer's shelf), and an ovarian mass (Krukenberg's tumor).

DIAGNOSIS

Currently the most common mode of diagnosing gastric cancer is endoscopy. Barium meal is utilized in some centers, but endoscopy is usually required to confirm the diagnosis and to obtain histologic specimens. Endoscopy has become the standard as it allows visualization and immediate biopsy of both tumors and nonmalignant processes. This has become important in the aggressive treatment of *H. pylori* infection. The diagnostic accuracy of endoscopic biopsy is related to the number of biopsies taken per patient, the site of biopsy within the ulcer, and tumor type. In a series of more than 200 patients biopsied for esophageal and gastric cancer, a diagnosis was obtained in 70% of patients with one biopsy, 95% with four biopsies, and 98.9% with seven biopsies. Biopsy was most successful if taken from both the slough and the rim of an ulcerated lesion. Biopsy of diffusely infiltrating lesions compared with exophytic lesions was much less effective (50% versus 92%).

Mass screening is efficacious in regions with a high incidence of gastric cancer, such as Japan. In Western countries, early endoscopy in symptomatic patients in order to confirm benign disease and diagnose early malignant disease has been advocated. In a British prospective trial of 2659 patients, endoscopy found abnormalities in 75% of those older than 45 years of age suffering from dyspepsia; high-risk premalignant disease was diagnosed in 493 (19%), and malignancy in 115 (4%). Although not cost-effective, early endoscopy is advocated for diagnosing the rare malignancy and treating premalignant disease, such as *H. pylori*.

Although markers such as carcinoembryonic antigen (CEA), CA19-9, CA72.4, and alpha-fetoprotein can be abnormally increased in 15% to 60% of patients, these markers are not specific for gastric cancer and, therefore, are not used in the diagnostic algorithm for this disease. Some authorities advocate the measurement of serum markers preoperatively, since early recurrence may be detected by a postoperative rise in these markers.

STAGING

Gastric tumors are staged by depth of tumor invasion (T stage), extent of lymph node metastases (N stage), and presence of distant metastatic disease (M stage). There is

Table 58–1	TNM Staging for Gastric Cancer

Primary Tumor
T1 Invasion of lamina propria into submucosa
T2 Invasion of muscularis propria/subserosa
T3 Invasion of serosa
T4 Invasion of adjacent structures
Regional Lymph Nodes
N0 No regional lymph node metastasis
N1 Metastasis in 1 to 6 regional lymph nodes
N2 Metastasis in 7 to 15 regional lymph nodes
N3 Metastasis in more than 15 regional lymph nodes
Distant Metastasis
M0 No distant metastasis
M1 Distant metastasis

Used with permission of the American Joint Committee on Cancer (AJCC®), Chicago, Illinois. From the AJCC® Cancer Staging Manual, 5th ed. Philadelphia, Lippincott-Raven, 1997.

now international agreement among the American Joint Commission on Cancer (AJCC), the Union Internationale Contre le Cancer (UICC), and the Japanese Research Society for Gastric Cancer (JRSFC) to use the TNM staging system (Tables 58–1 and 58–2).

T1 tumors invade the mucosa or submucosa, T2 tumors penetrate through the muscularis propria or subserosa, T3 tumors penetrate the serosa, and T4 tumors invade other structures. The 1997 edition of the *AJCC Cancer Staging Manual* has adopted a new definition for N stage based on the number of positive lymph nodes: N1 disease is 1 to 6 positive nodes, N2 is 7 to 15 positive nodes, and N3 is more than 15 positive nodes. The older 1992 classification system was based on location of positive nodes and distance from the primary tumor. The N classification based on the number of positive nodes is superior in estimating prognosis to the old 1992 classification system. The new classification of N status, however, relies on a systematic and reproducible approach to resecting and analyzing perigastric lymph nodes; at least 15 negative nodes should be analyzed before the diagnosis of N0 is rendered, in order to improve the quality of staging.

Table 58–2	Gastric Cancer Staging		
Stage 0	Tis	N0	M0
Stage IA	T1	N0	M0
Stage IB	T1	N1	M0
	T2	N0	M0
Stage II	T1	N2	M0
	T2	N1	M0
	T3	N0	M0
Stage IIIA	T2	N2	M0
	T3	N1	M0
	T4	N0	M0
Stage IIIB	T3	N2	M0
Stage IV	T4	N1	M0
	T1–3	N3	M0
	T4	N2–3	M0
	T any	N any	M1

is, in situ.
Used with permission of the American Joint Committee on Cancer (AJCC®), Chicago, Illinois. From the AJCC® Cancer Staging Manual, 5th ed. Philadelphia, Lippincott-Raven, 1997.

Staging Modalities

Following diagnosis by endoscopy, patients may be assessed for extent of disease using endoscopic ultrasonography (EUS), computed tomography (CT), positron emission tomography (PET), and laparoscopy with laparoscopic ultrasonography. The use of peritoneal cytology and molecular staging are currently being investigated and may become a component of gastric staging in the future.

Endoscopic Ultrasonography

At the time of diagnosis, EUS can provide key staging information, especially in superficial tumors and those located at the gastroesophageal junction. EUS estimates depth of tumor invasion and the extent of perigastric adenopathy. The accuracy of EUS for depth of invasion ranges from 60% to 90% and depends on tumor morphology, stage of disease, and the endoscopist. Early polypoid cancers are more accurately staged by EUS than are advanced ulcerated lesions. The most common reason for misdiagnosis is the inability to differentiate inflammation and fibrosis from tumor. Tumor depth determined by EUS correlates with tumor behavior. Patients who are staged by EUS as T3 or T4 as opposed to T1 or T2 are at increased risk for recurrence after complete resection. EUS also has the ability to diagnose enlarged perigastric lymph nodes, but it is less accurate in detecting distant nodal disease.

Computed Tomography

Abdominal and pelvic CT is the most common staging tool for gastric cancer. CT accurately diagnoses locally advanced cancer in more than 95% of patients. Figure 58–1 is a CT from a patient with locally advanced disease along the lesser curve of the stomach and nodal metasta-

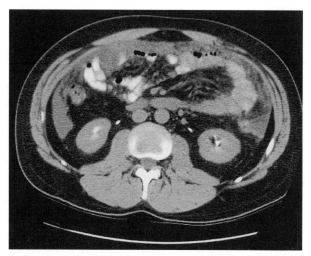

Figure 58–2. Computed tomography denoting carcinomatosis with omental caking.

ses in the lesser omentum. CT is similarly effective in detecting metastases and will accurately assess the liver in 85% of patients. Carcinomatosis with diffuse peritoneal seeding, malignant ascites, and adnexal and pelvic metastases are well depicted by CT (Fig. 58–2).

CT is less reliable in diagnosing lymph node metastases. Size has been the major criteria used to diagnose lymph node disease. CT detects only 45% of nodes less than 9 mm in size but over 70% of nodes larger than 9 mm. The chance of a lymph node that contains metastatic disease is related to size: 23% of nodes between 10 and 14 mm harbor metastases, whereas 80% of nodes greater than 14 mm contain disease.

The limitations of CT include not detecting small primary or metastatic tumors nor recognizing T4 disease. CT cannot differentiate inflammation from tumor invasion and therefore may not diagnose contiguous organ invasion. CT cannot detect small peritoneal metastasis and liver lesions less than 1 cm in diameter.

Positron Emission Tomography

PET is an investigational imaging tool with potential for detecting metastatic disease and measuring response of the primary tumor to chemotherapy. Malignant tissue consumes glucose more avidly than normal tissue. Intravenous ^{18}fluorodeoxyglucose (FDG) is taken up by tumor cells and emits positrons detected by a gamma camera. Early studies in esophageal cancer have demonstrated that PET can detect 20% of metastases missed by CT. There are few PET studies in gastric cancer, but early results indicate that gastric cancer is an avid consumer of FDG. At present, PET is used in the setting of investigational studies until its efficacy is proved.

Laparoscopy and Laparoscopic Ultrasonography

Laparoscopy has proved effective in staging gastric cancer patients. As many as 40% of clinically "resectable" pa-

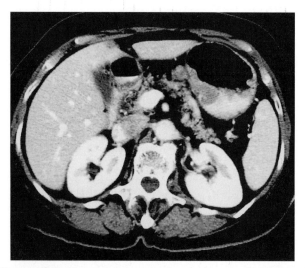

Figure 58–1. Computed tomography showing locally advanced gastric cancer, with disease along the lesser curve and nodal metastases in the lesser omentum.

tients will be diagnosed with M1 disease at laparoscopy. Laparoscopy is especially sensitive in detecting small peritoneal and hepatic metastases not detected by CT and EUS. Figure 58–3 shows peritoneal metastases noted on laparoscopy that would preclude a curative resection. This patient had no metastases evident on helical CT.

Laparoscopy diagnosed metastatic disease in 32 of 111 patients (29%) thought to be M0 by preoperative CT. The peritoneum and liver comprised 97% of metastatic disease noted by laparoscopy. Overall, laparoscopy accurately staged 94% of the patients for the presence or absence of metastatic disease. Patients noted to be M1 by laparoscopy did not undergo an open laparotomy and had an average hospital stay of 1 day compared with 7 days for patients who were subjected to laparotomy without resection. In contrast with previous surgical dogma, patients without bleeding or obstruction diagnosed with M1 disease by laparoscopy did not require reoperation for bleeding, perforation, or obstruction, and their survival was similar to that of historical control patients with M1 disease. These data indicate that prophylactic bypass or resection may not be necessary in the asymptomatic patient with M1 disease. Port site recurrences have not been problematic.

Currently, 10-mm probes are available to allow ultrasonography at the time of laparoscopy. Laparoscopic ultrasonography (LUS) has improved the staging of gastric cancer. Smith and associates (1993) studied 93 patients with resectable disease by routine preoperative imaging: 18 patients were found to have M1 disease by laparoscopy alone. An additional seven patients were noted to have incurable disease on LUS. In total, 25 of 93 patients avoided a laparotomy for incurable gastric cancer. LUS appears to improve the detection of nodal disease. Laparoscopy alone misses approximately 50% of lymph node metastases. LUS detects suspicious adenopathy and allows biopsy to diagnose metastatic disease.

Peritoneal Cytology

Growing evidence suggests that viable tumor cells in peritoneal fluid portend a poor outcome in gastric cancer

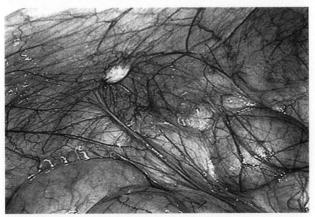

Figure 58–3. Laparoscopy identified small-volume peritoneal metastasis in a patient without evidence of distant disease on preoperative computed tomography.

patients. Peritoneal fluid sampling is easily performed at the time of laparoscopy. Positive peritoneal lavage is more likely to be found in patients with advanced disease. In a study of 127 patients in whom peritoneal cytology was analyzed, no T1 or T2, 10% of T3 and T4, and 59% of M1 patients had positive cytology. Even in the absence of M1 disease, positive cytology is associated with early recurrence and poor outcome. These patients behave more closely with stage IV patients, indicating that positive peritoneal lavage is an M1 equivalent.

The sensitivity of peritoneal fluid cytology can be dramatically increased by the use of immunohistochemistry and reverse transcriptase–polymerase chain reaction techniques. Using these methods, 46% to 64% of stage III and stage IV patients will have positive cytology. However, these methods also result in a 10% positive peritoneal cytology rate for stage I and stage II patients. The clinical relevance of such a sensitive method has yet to be determined.

Molecular Staging

Advances in molecular biology have provided new methods to predict outcome for patients with gastric cancer. The tumor suppressor gene $p53$ has been implicated in the gastric carcinogenesis sequence, and overexpression of $p53$ correlates with poor survival. Similarly, overexpression of adhesion molecules may have a role in tumor metastases, and tumor expression of the cell adhesion receptor sialyl-Le(x) is associated with venous invasion and poor outcome. The cell adhesion molecule CD44 is increased in patients with advanced gastric cancer and associated with an increased rate of metastases.

Abnormally high levels of tumor markers such as CEA, CA19-9, and CA72.4 are commonly noted. In general, elevated tumor markers are associated with advanced disease and poor outcome. Some series have also shown that a high serum level of some tumor markers is an independent predictor of poor outcome. For example, there is a 32% 5-year survival after resection for patients with an elevated preoperative CEA, compared with 77% for patients with a normal preoperative CEA. Similarly, high serum levels of CA72.4, a glycoprotein associated with gastric cancer, are associated with lymph node metastases, advanced disease, and poor outcome.

Staging Algorithm

The current staging algorithm at Memorial Sloan–Kettering Cancer Center is represented in Figure 58–4. The majority of our patients undergo endoscopy/EUS. CT is performed to detect obvious metastases that would preclude a curative resection. Metastatic disease is usually biopsied under CT guidance to avoid the general anesthesia required for laparoscopy. For patients without evidence of M1 disease, laparoscopy is performed to detect low-volume peritoneal and hepatic metastases. Patients with locally advanced disease (T3/T4 lesions with N1/N2 adenopathy) are at high risk for local recurrence and may be offered neoadjuvant chemotherapy followed by resection. Patients with T1 or T2 disease without detect-

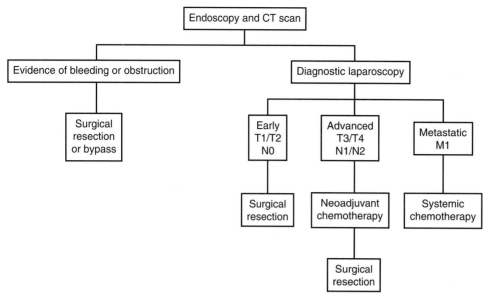

Figure 58–4. Work-up and treatment algorithm for patients with gastric adenocarcinoma.

able nodal disease undergo immediate resection at the time of the laparoscopy. Patients with M1 disease and no evidence of bleeding or obstruction are not resected and are candidates for chemotherapy. Peritoneal fluid sampling for cytology may be performed at the time of laparoscopy for research purposes.

TREATMENT

Surgery

Complete surgical resection is the most important prognostic factor for gastric cancer patients. The "R" staging classification represents the degree of resection and residual disease. An R0 resection denotes complete resection with no residual disease. An R1 resection indicates microscopic and an R2 resection implies gross residual disease. Current controversies in the treatment of gastric cancer involve the extent of gastric and lymph node resection and the use of adjuvant or neoadjuvant chemotherapy.

Gastric Resection

The effect of gastric resection on survival and morbidity for distal lesions has been investigated in randomized controlled trials. In a French prospective trial of 169 patients with antral cancers, 93 were randomized to total gastrectomy and 76 to subtotal gastrectomy. There was no difference in survival between the two groups. The Italian Gastrointestinal Study Group randomized 624 patients with distal stomach cancers to subtotal or total gastrectomy; no survival advantage was noted. For proximal lesions, no randomized trial exists. A retrospective study showed that total gastrectomy and proximal gastrectomy have the same survival and morbidity. Proponents of total gastrectomy and Roux-en-Y reconstruction note the morbidity of bile reflux in patients who undergo a subtotal resection. Proponents of subtotal resection report the benefit of preserving a gastric reservoir. No prospec-

tive trial has clearly addressed this issue. We favor subtotal gastrectomy for both proximal and distal lesions if complete resection can be performed.

Recently, the treatment options of early T1 gastric lesions have expanded to include endoscopic mucosal resection and gastrectomy without lymphadenopathy. Endoscopic resection involves submucosal injection of fluid to facilitate complete mucosal resection. This technique is suitable for well-differentiated, raised lesions (Borrmann types 0, I, and II) less than 3 cm in diameter. Tumors invading the submucosa are at risk for lymph node metastases and are not appropriate for endoscopic resection. Recurrences do occur, especially if tumors are removed in a piecemeal resection. In a series of 308 endoscopic resections for early cancer, 44 patients had residual or recurrent lesions. All recurrences were resected, and no patients died of gastric cancer. With increasing experience, fractional resections are becoming less common.

Resection without lymphadenectomy has also been advocated for patients with early T1 lesions because the risk of lymph node metastases is very low. One group showed that only 4% of patients with T1 lesions limited to the mucosa and less than 4.5 cm in diameter had lymph node metastases. In contrast, 56% of patients with T1 lesions invading the submucosa and greater than 4.5 cm in diameter had lymph node metastases. Thus, preoperative diagnosis is key in selecting patients for endoscopic mucosal resection or limited resection without lymphadenectomy.

Lymphadenectomy

The extent of lymph node dissection is an area of great controversy. A D1 resection indicates dissection of just the perigastric lymph nodes, whereas a D2 lymphadenectomy is more extensive and includes those nodes along the celiac, hepatic, and splenic vessels. The Japanese have long contended that extended lymphadenectomy improves accuracy of staging and overall survival. However, Western experts interpret the greater survival in

Japanese patients after extended lymphadenectomy as stage migration (i.e., upstaging of patients).

Large randomized prospective studies were initiated to answer these questions. The Dutch Gastric Cancer Group (Bonenkamp et al, 1999) updated their prospective randomized trial comparing D1 versus D2 lymphadenectomy. In this multicenter trial, 711 patients with gastric cancer were assigned to either D1 or D2 lymphadenectomy, and outcome was compared between the two groups. No difference in 5-year survival was observed, but an increased rate of complications and postoperative deaths was found in the D2 group. The increase in postoperative morbidity was predominantly associated with resection of the pancreas and spleen.

A British trial of 400 patients with gastric cancer randomized patients to either D1 or D2 dissection (Cushieri et al, 1999). As in the Dutch trial, there was no difference in survival between the two groups, and the D2 group had a higher morbidity related to the increased incidence of pancreatic and splenic resections with extended lymphadenectomy. These two prospective, randomized, multicenter trials found no survival benefit to extended lymphadenectomy.

Proponents of the D2 dissection note the 10-year results of the German Gastric Cancer Study, which revealed no difference in postsurgical morbidity and mortality rates among the 1654 patients assigned to either D1 or D2 lymph node dissection (Siewert et al, 1998). Further, this prospective observational trial described improved survival for patients with stage II tumors, independent of stage migration. Experienced centers report acceptable morbidity with splenic-sparing extended lymphadenectomy. At our institution, extended lymphadenectomy is routinely performed, as the authors believe it improves staging and may benefit patients with micrometastatic lymph node disease.

Adjuvant and Neoadjuvant Therapy

Adjuvant Chemotherapy

Many studies have investigated the use of postoperative chemotherapy, but lack of effective agents has resulted in few studies with beneficial reports. Two meta-analyses have been performed to assess the benefit of postoperative adjuvant chemotherapy. The Cancer Institute Hospital in Tokyo, Japan, examined six randomized studies involving 1177 patients given mitomycin-based chemotherapy. The combined odds ratio was 0.63 (95% confidence interval, 0.5 to 0.79), suggesting a benefit from adjuvant chemotherapy. Another larger meta-analysis reviewed 14 randomized trials involving 2096 patients, comparing surgery alone versus surgery and postoperative adjuvant chemotherapy. The combined odds ratio was 0.88 (95% CI, 0.78 to 1.08), suggesting that adjuvant chemotherapy did not increase survival over surgery alone. This meta-analysis was criticized because it included trials using methyl-CCNU, a drug that is now known to have limited activity in gastric cancer. An amended study that included two additional trials resulted in an odds ratio of 0.82 (95% CI, 0.68 to 0.98), indicating

an advantage to the use of postoperative chemotherapy. Many investigators remain skeptical of these meta-analyses, since many individual, well-planned studies have not shown benefit from adjuvant chemotherapy.

Neoadjuvant Chemotherapy

The majority of patients in North America will present with locally advanced disease (serosal invasion and perigastric adenopathy) and are at high risk for developing recurrent disease after resection. The limited efficacy of adjuvant chemotherapy has prompted the evaluation of neoadjuvant approaches. Preoperative chemotherapy has theoretical advantages, which include immediate treatment of micrometastatic disease, potential for down-staging of tumors to increase resectability, and monitoring response to chemotherapy, thereby identifying patients who may benefit from additional chemotherapy. Initial results with preoperative etoposide, doxorubicin, and cisplatin, or 5-fluorouracil, doxorubicin, and methotrexate, showed greater than 50% response rates. However, toxicity was significant. A recent study showed that response to neoadjuvant therapy was most predictive of overall survival.

Intraperitoneal Chemotherapy

Intraperitoneal (IP) chemotherapy has theoretic advantage in gastric cancer since the recurrence pattern is predominately intra-abdominal. Regional lymph nodes and peritoneum are usually affected before disease spreads to distant sites. In a prospective trial, 248 gastrectomy patients were randomized to either IP mitomycin C and 5-fluorouracil or no additional therapy. No difference in survival was seen. However, in a subgroup analysis, patients with stage III disease treated with IP chemotherapy had an improved 5-year survival. These results suggest that additional studies are needed to assess the utility of IP chemotherapy.

Combined Neoadjuvant and Intraperitoneal Chemotherapy

Preoperative chemotherapy with immediate postoperative IP chemotherapy has also been investigated. Intravenous chemotherapy, including 5-fluorouracil, doxorubicin, and methotrexate, was given to patients with advanced disease prior to gastrectomy. Patients received postoperative IP cisplatin and 5-fluorouracil. The median survival was 31 months in those patients undergoing a curative resection. These data indicate that neoadjuvant systemic and IP chemotherapy hold promise for patients with advanced disease.

Adjuvant Chemoradiotherapy

Postoperative radiotherapy is another approach to locally treat the peritoneum and remaining perigastric lymph nodes. In gastrectomy patients, adjuvant chemoradiotherapy was compared with surgery alone. Patients who received postoperative therapy had improved survival and decreased local recurrence. However, this study has been criticized because the 10 patients who refused adjuvant therapy had a longer survival than the remaining 29 patients randomized to treatment. A recently reported intergroup study randomized 603 resected M0 patients to follow-up or postoperative chemoradiation with 5-fluorouracil and leucovorin and 4500 cGy. With a median follow-up of 3.3 years, patients receiving postoperative chemoradiation had a 44% improvement in relapse-free survival and a 28% improvement in overall survival. These data are interesting but require verification.

Intraoperative radiation (IORT) is another method to deliver treatment to the site of resection. A randomized trial compared external beam radiotherapy (50 Gy) with IORT (20 Gy) in patients with stage III or stage IV gastric cancer. The IORT group had reduced complications and a trend toward improved survival and lower local recurrence.

CONCLUSION

Gastric cancer is a common disease worldwide. Eastern Asia has a high prevalence of this tumor, and mass endoscopic screening has resulted in early detection of resectable cancers and improved survival. This observation is in contrast to Western countries, where the majority of patients present with advanced gastric cancer. Recent advances in staging, including laparoscopy and endoscopic and laparoscopic ultrasonography, have improved our ability to find patients with locally advanced disease who may benefit from neoadjuvant therapy. Multicenter randomized trials in Western countries have not shown benefit for extended gastric resections, and we favor subtotal resections if all tumor can be removed with microscopic negative margins. Although large multicenter trials have not shown any benefit to extended lymphatic dissection, many major centers with extensive experience with gastric cancer believe these trials were flawed and routinely perform D2 resections to improve staging and potentially benefit patients with micrometastatic disease. Adjuvant chemotherapy is still controversial. The current treatment algorithm for locally advanced cancer at Memorial Sloan–Kettering Cancer Center includes neoadjuvant chemotherapy followed by surgical resection and postoperative IP chemotherapy.

Pearls and Pitfalls

- Gastric adenocarcinoma usually presents as locally advanced disease in Western countries. In Japan, gastric cancer is the most common malignancy, and mass screening programs exist.
- The incidence of proximal gastric cancer is increasing, while that of distal cancers is decreasing.
- *Helicobacter pylori* plays a role in the pathogenesis of some forms of gastric cancer.
- Diagnosis is based primarily on clinical suspicion and gastroscopy with biopsy. Symptoms may appear late.
- Staging involves CT and, when available, endoscopic ultrasonography and laparoscopy. PET is of potential benefit.
- Surgical treatment usually involves subtotal gastrectomy; the role of a *formal,* extended lymphadenectomy is still controversial.
- Although suggestive of benefit, the role of adjuvant or neoadjuvant chemoradiotherapy remains controversial.

SELECTED READINGS

Bonenkamp JJ, Hermans J, Sasako M, van de Velde CJ: Extended lymph-node dissection for gastric cancer. Dutch Gastric Cancer Group [see comments]. N Engl J Med 1999;340:908.

Brennan MF, Karpeh MS Jr: Surgery for gastric cancer: The American view. Semin Oncol 1996;23:352.

Burke EC, Karpeh MS Jr, Conlon KC, Brennan MF: Laparoscopy in the management of gastric adenocarcinoma. Ann Surg 1997;225:262.

Burke EC, Karpeh MS Jr, Conlon KC, Brennan MF: Peritoneal lavage cytology in gastric cancer: An independent predictor of outcome. Ann Surg Oncol 1998;5:411.

Conlon KC, Karpeh MS Jr: Laparoscopy and laparoscopic ultrasound in the staging of gastric cancer. Semin Oncol 1996;23:347.

Cuschieri A, Weeden S, Fielding J, et al: Patient survival after D1 and D2 resections for gastric cancer: Long-term results of the MRC randomized surgical trial. Surgical Co-operative Group. Br J Cancer 1999;79:1522.

Lawrence W Jr, Menck HR, Steele GD Jr, Winchester DP: The National Cancer Data Base report on gastric cancer. Cancer 1995;75:1734.

Niederhuber JE: Neoadjuvant therapy [editorial; comment]. Ann Surg 1999;229:309.

Siewert JR, Bottcher K, Stein HJ, Roder JD: Relevant prognostic factors in gastric cancer: Ten-year results of the German Gastric Cancer Study. Ann Surg 1998;228:449.

Smith JW, Brennan MF, Botet JF, et al: Preoperative endoscopic ultrasound can predict the risk of recurrence after operation for gastric carcinoma. J Clin Oncol 1993;11:2380.

Wanebo HJ, Kennedy BJ, Chmiel J, et al: Cancer of the stomach: A patient care study by the American College of Surgeons. Ann Surg 1993;218:583.

Chapter 59

Stromal Tumors of the Stomach and Small Bowel

Malcolm M. Bilimoria and Kelly K. Hunt

There are approximately 7000 new patients seen with sarcoma each year in the United States, but the vast majority of these arise in the extremities. Sarcomas can also originate in any of the visceral organs within the abdominal cavity, most commonly in the gastrointestinal (GI) tract. Three percent of all sarcomas, or 200 patients each year, are classified as GI sarcomas, with most of these developing in the stomach and small bowel. Most GI sarcomas are diagnosed during the fourth to sixth decades of life, with a median age at presentation of 55 years. There is a slight female to male predominance of 1.4:1; however, there appears to be no ethnic, geographic, or racial predisposition to this disease.

Because sarcomas of the GI tract involve a bizarre form of smooth muscle proliferation, the term *leiomyoblastoma* was introduced. Based on the examination of these tumors using standard light microscopy, pathologists initially believed that these tumors were of smooth muscle origin; hence the tumors were later referred to as *leiomyosarcomas*. More recently, the interstitial cell of Cajal, which lies in the stroma of the muscular layer of the gut and has elements of both smooth muscle and neural differentiation, has been proposed as a cell of origin for these tumors. The interstitial cell of Cajal functions as an intestinal pacemaker cell.

Improvements in pathology and clarification of the pathologic terms have led to a classification system that emphasizes the stromal description of the tumor. The classification is generally divided into two parts based on features of differentiation. Tumors with well-developed features of differentiation are referred to as leiomyomas, schwannomas, glomus tumors, neurofibromas, or ganglioneuromas. Some pathologists have further divided GI stromal tumors (GIST) into GI stromal sarcomas (GISS), representing those tumors with clear malignant features, and GIST, representing tumors with indeterminate malignant potential. GIST are classified into primitive or complete differentiation in myoid, neural, and autonomic nerve elements. A large part of the confusion regarding the nomenclature of these tumors stems from the relative rarity of the tumor, allowing only a few pathologists to have significant experience with these tumors. Recent reports largely use the term GIST to describe all stromal tumors with even the slightest dedifferentiation and, in essence, have combined GIST and GISS into a single classification referred to in the literature as GIST. As such, the term GIST is used in this chapter to describe gastric and small bowel stromal tumors with any evidence of malignant dedifferentiation.

CLINICAL PRESENTATION

Gastric sarcomas usually present with vague symptoms, including pain (40%), anorexia (40%), GI bleeding (45%),

and weight loss (30%). Approximately 10% of gastric sarcomas are found as a result of diagnostic evaluations for apparently unrelated conditions, the most common evaluation being esophagogastroduodenoscopy to rule out ulcer disease.

As might be expected, laboratory studies are nonspecific. A mild leukocytosis in conjunction with a microcytic anemia is often seen. The carcinoembryonic antigen (CEA) level is normal even with extensive disease. Upper GI barium studies usually reveal a smooth-walled lesion with central ulceration. Endoscopy is useful in visualizing the lesion, but biopsies are conclusive in only 40% of patients. Abdominal and pelvic computed tomography (CT) should be performed and is helpful in determining not only whether there is evidence of invasion of adjacent organs but also whether liver metastases are present.

At presentation, patients are generally placed into one of three groups: primary tumor (Fig. 59–1), local recurrence, or metastatic disease (Fig. 59–2). The percentage of patients with metastatic disease at presentation varies from 35% in a series by Ng and colleagues from The University of Texas M. D. Anderson Cancer Center to 47% in a series from Memorial Sloan-Kettering Cancer Center done by DeMatteo and coworkers. The most common sites of metastases include the liver (60%), peritoneal surfaces (30%), and lung (10%). Gastric sarcomas, like GI sarcomas, in general rarely metastasize to lymph nodes; the results of several large series have demonstrated the absence of a single positive lymph node.

Sarcomas constitute approximately 20% of all small bowel malignancies. The small bowel subdivisions are involved in proportion to their length, with one third of

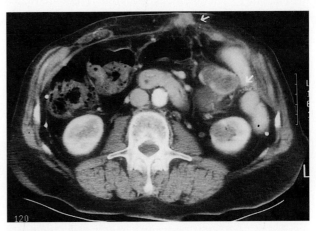

Figure 59–1. Preoperative computed tomography of a patient with a gastrointestinal stromal tumor originating in the small bowel. The patient has a lesion in the midline scar and on the left side of the abdomen (*arrows*).

405

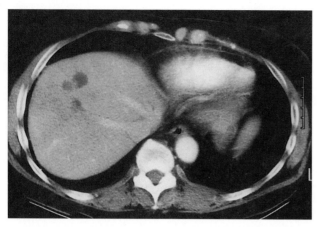

Figure 59–2. Abdominal computed tomography of a patient with a known gastrointestinal stromal tumor (GIST) of the small bowel found to have liver metastases on routine follow-up.

small bowel sarcomas originating in the duodenum, one third in the jejunum, and one third in the ileum. Adenocarcinoma of the small bowel is much more common than is sarcoma in all segments except for Meckel's diverticulum, where sarcomas comprise 44% of all the tumors. Sarcomas of the small bowel have been associated with metachronous malignancies at a rate of approximately 20%, but the nature of that association is not known.

Symptoms of small bowel sarcomas are also nonspecific, with pain and bleeding occurring in approximately 50% of patients and a palpable mass in only 20%. An upper GI series with small bowel follow-through identifies an intraluminal lesion in 50% of patients. Larger lesions can be detected by CT, whereas bleeding tumors can be detected by the tumor "blush" noted at angiography.

Finally, clinicians should be aware of a rare but well-documented paraneoplastic syndrome that can arise in patients with sarcomas at any site. Hypoglycemia can occur as a result of secretion of an insulin-like growth factor. More recently, Hoff and Sellin have advocated using a glucagon stimulation test to confirm the diagnosis. The best treatment for sarcoma-induced hypoglycemia is resection of the tumor; for patients with unresectable tumors, however, continuous glucagon infusion, usually through an implantable pump, can result in symptomatic relief of their hypoglycemia.

PREOPERATIVE MANAGEMENT

Initial evaluation of the patient with a stromal tumor of the stomach or small bowel should include a complete history and physical examination followed by abdominal and pelvic imaging with either CT or magnetic resonance imaging (MRI). Preoperative endoscopy should be considered, especially when a gastric or duodenal resection might be required. The histologic diagnosis should be confirmed, especially when imaging studies are not consistent with a GI stromal tumor.

A chest x-ray study is needed to rule out pulmonary chondromas or pulmonary metastases. Carney's syndrome—a triad of GI sarcomas, pulmonary chondromas, and extra-adrenal paragangliomas in young women—has

been well described and suggests that a genetic etiology may play a role in the development of these tumors. The GI sarcomas that develop as part of the syndrome are predominantly gastric and display a relatively indolent course when compared with GI sarcomas not associated with the syndrome. The pulmonary chondromas that arise after the development of the GI sarcomas have often been misinterpreted as pulmonary metastases from the GI sarcoma and are particularly troubling for the clinician.

Cases should be presented at a multidisciplinary conference with consideration for whether the tumor is potentially resectable. If the tumor is believed to be unresectable, thought should be given to the best form of palliation. Because radiation therapy and chemotherapy have not shown any benefit in the treatment of these tumors, there is no role for preoperative adjuvant therapy outside of a prospective clinical trial.

After proper preoperative staging, it is important to focus on the patient's overall health with specific attention to the patient's cardiac, pulmonary, and renal status. The goal of surgery is a margin-negative resection, which may require complex contiguous organ resection. Therefore, a thorough cardiac and pulmonary evaluation is needed to ensure that the patient is optimally prepared if a long, complex operation is needed.

Patients are generally given a full mechanical and antibiotic bowel preparation preoperatively in anticipation of intestinal resection and reanastomosis. Even when the tumor appears to be isolated to one segment of bowel, exploration may reveal that the tumor is adherent to the mesentery of another segment of intestine, requiring a more complex en bloc resection to achieve complete tumor resection with negative margins.

INTRAOPERATIVE MANAGEMENT

In the process of planning operative strategy, the surgeon must differentiate the patient whose treatment is for symptomatic relief in the face of unresectable disease versus the patient in whom cure is possible. Bulky gastric stromal tumors may best be approached through an upper abdominal (Chevron) incision, whereas a midline incision offers more versatility for small bowel stromal tumors, but this also varies with body habitus. Primary therapy involves surgical resection without the need for extensive lymphadenectomy. When evaluated, all series reported improved 5-year survival rates for patients undergoing complete resection versus those having an incomplete resection or debulking. The goal, therefore, is clearly centered on complete excision with negative margins. Care should be taken to avoid tumor rupture or spillage during the procedure, which is thought to be one mechanism for the high rate of peritoneal metastases from GI stromal tumors. Wedge resections or partial gastrectomies are viable options (as long as all margins are free of tumor); no survival advantage has been noted for more extensive resections.

The surgeon should prepare the patient for the possibility of an unresectable tumor when there is evidence of adjacent organ involvement on preoperative imaging.

Table 59-1	Five-Year Survival Rates in Patients with Gastrointestinal Stromal Tumors by Location and Tumor Grade		
AUTHOR, TUMOR GRADE	**NUMBER OF PATIENTS**	**TUMOR LOCATION**	**FIVE-YEAR SURVIVAL RATE, %**
Shui et al, 1983			
Grade not specified	41	Gastric	54
Lindsay et al, 1981			
Low grade	10	Gastric	55
High grade	25	Gastric	12
Shui et al, 1983			
Grade not specified	18	Small bowel	37
Evans, 1985			
Low grade	8	Small bowel	85
High grade	21	Small bowel	5
Ng et al, 1992			
Low grade	36	All gastrointestinal sites	40
High grade	45	All gastrointestinal sites	19

When the tumor is clearly unresectable, the extent of resection should be minimized because resection does not provide any survival advantage. Attention should be focused on addressing the patient's symptoms with respect to the tumor (i.e., GI obstruction, GI bleeding).

The liver should be evaluated at the time of exploratory laparotomy. There is no specific role for hepatic resection for metastatic disease except in patients in whom there is isolated small-volume disease that is easily resectable without adding significant morbidity to the patient's operation. Strong consideration should be given to enrolling patients with liver metastases into ongoing clinical trials. Some of the mechanisms under investigation for treating liver metastases include hepatic artery chemoembolization and radiofrequency ablation.

POSTOPERATIVE MANAGEMENT

Postoperative management is similar to that of any large intra-abdominal operation in that fluid management, pulmonary therapy, and early ambulation are important. Depending on the extent of the resection and the length of postoperative ileus, oral intake is initiated on postoperative day 3 to 5. For patients undergoing partial or subtotal gastric resection, Gastrografin swallow should be considered before initiating oral feeding. The average length of hospital stay is 7 days but is largely dependent on the extent of resection and any medical comorbidities in the individual patient.

There is no role for postoperative adjuvant chemotherapy or radiation therapy outside the context of a clinical trial.

COMPLICATIONS

Postoperative complications after resection of GI stromal tumors are similar to those seen with any complex intra-abdominal procedure requiring intestinal resection. The rate of wound complications remains 3% to 5% despite the use of prophylactic antibiotics during these clean/contaminated cases. Lower extremity sequential compression devices are used to prevent deep venous thrombosis, and systemic anticoagulation is considered for those patients with a history of deep venous thrombosis or with extensive pelvic disease. The incidence of cardiac complications is decreased by a thorough preoperative assessment that recognizes any limitations in cardiac function. The risk of pulmonary complications is reduced by aggressive pulmonary physiotherapy and early ambulation.

Complications of anastomotic leak or intra-abdominal bleeding are distinctly rare; these often require reopera-

---

Pearls and Pitfalls

PEARLS

- GI stromal tumors account for 3% of all gastric malignancies and 20% of all small bowel malignancies.
- Gastric and small bowel stromal tumors usually present with abdominal pain, GI bleeding, weight loss, or a combination of these.
- Patients with a gastric or small bowel stromal tumor and a history of syncope may be experiencing hypoglycemia resulting from tumor secretion of an insulin-like protein.
- During preoperative workup of a gastric or small bowel stromal tumor, one should not assume that a mass seen on chest x-ray film is a sign of metastatic disease. The patient may have Carney's syndrome, a triad of GI sarcomas, pulmonary chondromas, and adrenal paragangliomas.
- There is no evidence that more extensive gastric resection provides better results than does a simple wedge resection of a gastric stromal tumor as long as all margins are free of tumor.
- Adjuvant chemotherapy or radiation therapy are of little use in treating gastric or small bowel stromal tumors.
- Gastric and small bowel stromal tumors metastasize to the liver (60%), peritoneal surfaces (30%), and lung (10%). Metastases to lymph nodes are extremely rare.
- Survival in patients with gastric and small bowel stromal tumors depends on tumor grade, size, and resectability.

tion. Patients who have a prolonged postoperative ileus should be studied with abdominal and pelvic CT to rule out abdominal or pelvic abscess.

OUTCOMES

Follow-up of patients after resection for GI stromal tumors usually consists of a history and physical examination with abdominal and pelvic CT or MRI every 3 to 6 months for 5 years. Beyond 5 years, annual examinations are recommended. Endoscopy should be considered for gastric and duodenal primary cancers.

Survival expectations with gastric sarcomas are not different from those for sarcomas elsewhere in the GI tract, with a 5-year survival rate of approximately 30%. Patients with gastric sarcomas, like those with GI sarcomas in other sites, have a prognosis that depends on the grade and size of the sarcoma. Five-year survival rates in most series are similar to studies involving other GI sarcomas—50% to 85% with low-grade tumors and 5% to 15% with high-grade tumors (Table 59–1). Median survival rate depends on the presence of localized disease (46 months) or metastatic disease (19 months). DeMatteo and colleagues evaluated age, sex, tumor size, and surgical margins and found that only tumor size greater than 10 cm predicted poor survival outcome in patients with GI stromal tumors.

Most studies reveal that the actual GI location of the sarcoma has little bearing on the overall survival risk. As with gastric sarcomas, the most common sites of distant failure in patients with small bowel stromal tumors are the liver or peritoneal surfaces.

Finally, GI sarcomas have been associated with other primary tumors. Shiu and colleagues noted that 27% of GI sarcomas were associated with other malignancies, which usually develop years after the diagnosis of the GI sarcoma. More than 50% of the associated malignancies were adenocarcinomas of GI origin. This observation is important because it shows that clinicians must maintain a high index of suspicion for secondary malignancies and

a practice of close follow-up for their patients with GI sarcomas.

Close follow-up is important also because of the tendency of GI stromal tumors to recur despite removal of all gross disease. In 100 patients who died as a result of their GI sarcomas, 89% had peritoneal disease and 78% had liver metastases at the time of death. Extra-abdominal metastases were noted in only 28% of patients, with the metastases to the lungs accounting for the majority of this type of recurrence.

Interestingly, it appears that recurrent disease in the liver develops regardless of the prognostic factors associated with the primary tumor, whereas peritoneal recurrences are highly dependent on prognostic factors such as tumor grade and tumor size. Patients with isolated recurrent disease in the liver or on peritoneal surfaces may benefit from surgical resection if complete removal is possible. This is in contrast to patients with extra-abdominal metastases, who should be offered resection more judiciously; extra-abdominal metastases often indicate a biologically advanced disease state compared with intra-abdominal metastases. Consideration should always be given to enrolling patients with extra-abdominal metastases into existing clinical trials. Finally, a disease-free interval greater than 18 months has been associated with prolonged survival after metastasectomy compared with a shorter disease-free interval (median survival, 19 months versus 14 months).

SELECTED READINGS

DeMatteo RP, Lewis JJ, Leung D, et al: Two hundred gastrointestinal stromal tumors: Recurrence patterns and prognostic factors for survival. Ann Surg 2000;231:51.

Evans HL: Smooth muscle tumors of the gastrointestinal tract. Cancer 1985;56:2242.

Grant CS, Kim CH, Farrugia G, et al: Gastric leiomyosarcoma: Prognostic factors and surgical management. Arch Surg 1991;126:985.

Hoff AO, Sellin RV: The role of glucagon administration in the diagnosis and treatment of patients with tumor hypoglycemia. Cancer 1998;82:1585.

Lindsay PC, Ordonez N, Raaf JH: Gastric leiomyosarcoma: Clinical and pathological review of fifty patients. J Surg Oncol 1981;18:399.

Ng EH, Pollock RE, Romsdahl MM: Prognostic implications of patterns of failure for gastrointestinal leiomyosarcomas. Cancer 1992;69:1334.

Shui MH, Farr GH, Quan SHG, et al: Myosarcomas of the large and small bowel: A clinicopathologic study. J Surg Oncol 1983;24:67.

Chapter 60
Gastric Lymphoma
John H. Donohue

Despite the absence of nodal lymphoid tissue in the normal stomach, the stomach is the single most common site of extranodal lymphoma. *Helicobacter pylori* infection can be documented in more than 90% of patients with gastric lymphoma. Low-grade lymphomas of the stomach mimic mucosa-associated lymphoid tissue (MALT) and arise from the chronic inflammation caused by *H. pylori* infection. Eradication of *H. pylori* results in the complete histologic and molecular regression of most low-grade MALT lymphomas of the stomach; however, high-grade gastric MALT lymphomas and other gastric lymphomas, which histologically resemble nodal lymphomas, do not respond to therapy directed at eradication of *H. pylori*. These more aggressive neoplasms arise independently of *H. pylori* antigenic stimulation for their growth, and the adequate treatment of these lymphomas requires traditional cancer therapies. Because of the low incidence of gastric lymphoma (less than 10% of gastric malignancies), no conclusive controlled trials have been performed to determine the optimal method of management. Because nonoperative treatment approaches have shown comparable results to resection, gastric lymphomas are increasingly being managed with nonsurgical therapies.

CLINICAL PRESENTATION

Differential Diagnosis

The presentation of gastric lymphoma usually includes epigastric pain or dyspepsia indistinguishable from gastritis, peptic ulcer disease, or gastric adenocarcinoma. Upper gastrointestinal hemorrhage occurs in only a minority of patients and would be an unusual mode of presentation. More advanced stage gastric lymphomas more commonly produce B symptoms (weight loss, fatigue, fevers, and night sweats) and, infrequently, a palpable epigastric mass. Because gastric lymphomas generally remain localized to intra-abdominal lymph nodes, peripheral adenopathy is not present. The lack of specific symptoms or signs combined with the rarity of gastric lymphoma prevents making the diagnosis before tissue biopsy, although the diagnosis might be suspected when a very large gastric mass is present.

Diagnosis

Upper gastrointestinal endoscopy is the best method of obtaining an objective diagnosis of gastric lymphoma. Lymphomas of the stomach most commonly demonstrate a diffuse thickening of the mucosa, but ulcerated and polypoid lesions are not uncommon. Multiple deep endoscopic biopsies greatly improve the likelihood of de-

termining the correct diagnosis. Endoscopic ultrasonography provides useful information, especially in low-grade MALT lymphomas, by evaluating the depth of tumor invasion and the involvement of perigastric lymph nodes. Upper gastrointestinal radiographs provide no diagnostic data because there are no characteristic findings for gastric lymphoma. Computed tomography is often obtained for staging purposes (see later discussion); it adds little to diagnosis.

PREOPERATIVE MANAGEMENT

Staging

Determination of disease stage is important for therapeutic as well as prognostic reasons. The Musshoff modification of the Ann Arbor staging system is commonly used for gastric lymphomas (Table 60–1). Because most gastric lymphomas remain localized to the stomach and regional lymph nodes, abdominal computed tomography is a good method to stage the disease. Lymphangiograms are rarely done for gastric lymphoma. A head and neck examination (including endoscopy) should be performed to rule out secondary involvement of Waldeyer's ring MALT tissues. A routine chest x-ray study and bone marrow biopsy complete the staging workup. A serum lactic dehydrogenase measurement should be obtained because it correlates with the bulk of tumor, has prognostic implications, and can be used to monitor residual or recurrent disease after treatment.

TREATMENT

Neoadjuvant Therapy

The histologic type of gastric lymphoma determines the type of initial treatment. MALT lymphomas of the stomach are divided into two categories: (1) those of low-grade histology and (2) mixed or high-grade MALT lymphomas.

Table 60–1	Musshoff Staging System for Gastric Lymphomas	
STAGE	**DESCRIPTION**	
IE°	Tumor confined to the stomach	
IIEi	Tumor involvement of perigastric lymph nodes	
IIEii	Tumor with spread to para-aortic lymph nodes	
IIIE	Splenic involvement	
IV	Distant spread (i.e., bone marrow)	

°E denotes extranodal lymphoma.

409

Patients with predominantly low-grade MALT lymphoma and a small component of high-grade disease are usually treated as those with high-grade MALT lymphomas. Non-MALT lymphomas of the stomach are mostly intermediate-grade tumors according to the Working Formulation classification system.

Because *H. pylori* infection can be demonstrated in most patients with gastric lymphoma, eradication of this bacterium has been tested as a definitive treatment for this malignancy. In superficial, localized, low-grade MALT lymphomas of the stomach, effective treatment with antibiotics, bismuth compounds, and a proton pump inhibitor eliminates *H. pylori* and results in complete regression of the lymphoma in 60% to 90% of patients (Fig. 60–1). These clinical results are explained by recent experimental data. The B lymphocytes of MALT lymphomas proliferate only in the presence of both T lymphocytes isolated from the lymphoma and the specific strain of *H. pylori* for that patient. Whereas growth of early MALT lymphoma appears dependent on the continued stimulus of an *H. pylori* antigen, patients with more advanced disease (i.e., correlated to larger size, invasion into gastric musculature, nodal involvement, or a component of high-grade MALT lymphoma) are less likely to regress with eradication of *H. pylori*. These tumors have developed growth independent of the original antigenic stimulus.

Because of this unusual response to eradication of *H. pylori*, surgical treatment is not recommended for low-grade MALT lymphoma of the stomach. Treatment should first be with a combination of antibiotics and proton pump inhibitor for 2 weeks. Endoscopic reassessment with biopsies and ultrasonographic examination should be repeated every 3 months until complete histologic resolution of the MALT lymphoma occurs. This process generally requires several months (as long as 18 months). Even with no apparent residual microscopic disease, some patients retain a monoclonal population of B cells. With complete resolution of low-grade MALT lymphoma, endoscopic surveillance should be continued every 6 months. The total duration of follow-up necessary to ensure long-term freedom from disease relapse is unknown.

For the more unusual patient with low-grade MALT lymphoma unrelated to *H. pylori* infection (<10%) or

when the lymphoma does not disappear after eradication of *H. pylori*, surgical treatment is generally not necessary. Small clinical series with external beam radiation (30 Gy), single-dose chemotherapy (chlorambucil), and combination drug therapies have all shown excellent results for both disease-free and overall survival rates. Disease-specific survival rates of greater than 90% can be expected for low-grade MALT patients following all types of therapy.

For high-grade MALT and non-MALT lymphomas of the stomach, surgical resection may not necessarily be the treatment of choice (Fig. 60–2). Surgical resection was traditionally recommended before chemotherapy or radiation for patients with gastric lymphoma to avoid need for chemotherapy or radiation therapy and its treatment-related hemorrhage and perforation caused by tumor necrosis. In reality, the incidences of both these complications are minimal. In a review of nearly 250 patients with gastric lymphoma treated with primary chemotherapy (with or without radiation therapy), only seven (3%) experienced gastrointestinal hemorrhage. None required operative treatment or died of this complication. No treatment-related gastric perforations occurred in this collected review. For the unusual patient who requires emergency operation during chemotherapy, additional treatment for side effects of the therapy (i.e., thrombocytopenia) and higher complication rates resulting from immunosuppression and delayed wound healing need to be considered. Rarely, patients with gastric lymphoma are seen with life-threatening hemorrhage or perforation. Treatment is similar to that for any patient with an acute abdominal catastrophe. Adequate resuscitation and antibiotics are instituted, followed by surgical exploration as soon as possible.

Strategies in Patients Selected for Operative Treatment

Patients undergoing operation for gastric lymphoma are positioned supine. An upper midline or bilateral subcostal incision provides optimal exposure. Most early stage gastric lymphomas are amenable to total gross excision with a subtotal gastrectomy. Total gastrectomy is necessary

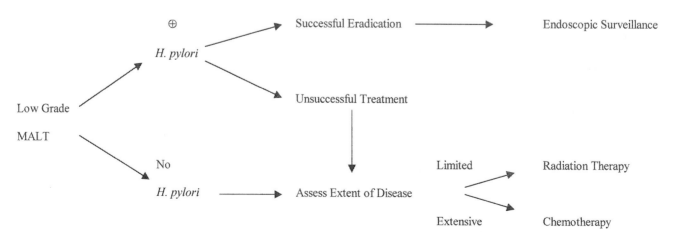

Figure 60–1. Management of low-grade gastric mucosa-associated lymphoid tissue (MALT) lymphomas.

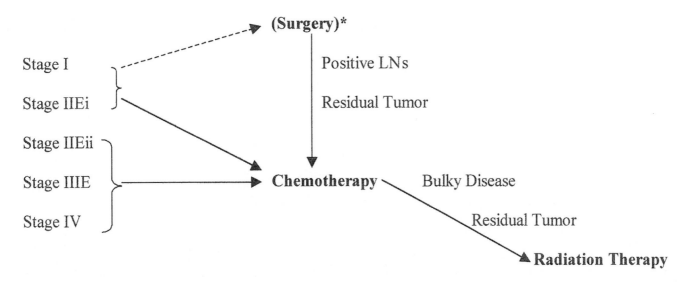

Figure 60–2. Management of high-grade mucosa-associated lymphoid tissue (MALT) and non-MALT lymphomas. LNs, lymph nodes.

only when diffuse infiltration of the stomach is present, and in this situation, primary chemotherapy may be preferred. Although all palpable tumor should be removed at the time of surgical exploration, negative microscopic margins are not of prognostic importance for patient outcome. The gastrectomy specimen should encompass enlarged perigastric lymph nodes. Para-aortic or other distant regional nodes should be sampled if they are worrisome for involvement. A radical lymphadenectomy has no role in the management of gastric lymphoma. Gastrointestinal continuity is most commonly reestablished with a loop gastrojejunostomy for subtotal gastrectomy and Roux-en-Y reconstruction for higher resections. Placement of a feeding jejunostomy tube should be considered in the malnourished patient.

Complex Presentations

With current preoperative imaging, extensive disease is rarely found unexpectedly at laparotomy. Direct involvement of adjacent organs may occur, usually with more advanced stage lymphomas. Extensive en bloc resections are not warranted, even if all gross tumor would be excised with such a procedure in deference to chemotherapy. Precise delineation of the tumor stage and a limited resection if preoperative bleeding or perforation is present constitute the best surgical treatment for locally advanced gastric lymphoma. Marking macroscopic residual tumor with radio-opaque clips helps direct postoperative radiation therapy.

Unexpected Findings

Many case reports of patients with concurrent gastric lymphoma and gastric adenocarcinoma have been reported, likely the result of the common etiologic factor *H.*

pylori. Wider surgical clearance of the adenocarcinoma (5 cm of proximal and distal stomach when feasible), sufficient resection of regional lymph nodes, and evaluation for intra-abdominal metastases of the carcinoma should all be completed intraoperatively as would be used for surgical treatment of a typical gastric cancer.

Postoperative Management

Because patients with gastric lymphoma are at increased risk for thromboembolic complications (risk factors include malignancy, older age), routine deep venous thrombosis prophylaxis should be initiated preoperatively and be continued until the patient is fully ambulatory. If postoperative chemotherapy or external beam radiation therapy is scheduled, these treatments can be initiated 4 weeks after the operation as long as the surgical incision is healing well and there is no evidence of postoperative infection.

Patients with stage IIE–IV disease should receive postoperative chemotherapy. An anthracycline-containing combination regimen, most commonly CHOP (cyclophosphamide, doxorubicin, vincristine, and prednisone), is used. Radiation therapy is unproven as a method to improve overall patient survival risk after a complete resection of gastric lymphoma; however, radiation therapy can provide benefit for local tumor control in patients with bulky disease. Patients with stage IE gastric lymphoma at higher risk for recurrence (i.e., high-grade disease, tumor larger than 10 cm, or transmural involvement) should receive adjuvant postoperative chemotherapy. Patients with low-grade stage IE MALT lymphoma of the stomach usually only require treatment to eradicate *H. pylori* if gastric resection removes all known disease.

Complications

Many previous surgical experiences for gastric lymphoma reported a postoperative mortality rate of 5% to 10%.

Recent experiences have more realistic mortality rates well below 5%. Significant or minor surgical complications occur in 25% of patients. In addition to intra-abdominal and wound infections, hemorrhage, and anastomotic complications, postoperative myocardial, pulmonary, cerebrovascular, and thromboembolic complications account for most patient morbidity.

OUTCOMES OF TREATMENT

Except for the surgical management of complications (bleeding, obstruction, perforation) or debulking of chemoresistant disease, the operative management of gastric lymphoma currently remains a controversial topic. Excellent long-term results have been accomplished with primary surgical resection of stage IE and stage IIE (when combined with adjuvant treatment) gastric lymphomas. The problems with surgical treatment include postoperative morbidity and mortality, the adverse impact on nutritional status, and occasional severe impairment of the patient's quality of life. The rationale for selecting gastrectomy as the treatment of choice has included (1) prevention of complications of primary chemotherapy, (2) exact pathologic staging, and (3) improved patient cure with complete tumor resection. Each of these indications has been challenged in the last decade because (1) spontaneous or treatment-induced complications are rare, (2) preoperative imaging provides highly accurate staging data, and (3) outcome of patients eligible for complete resection (mostly stage IE or IIEi) who have undergone treatment with primary chemotherapy has been comparable. Favorable results from patients with resectable early stage disease cannot be compared with the outcomes of patients with incompletely resected advanced stage gastric lymphoma. Many of the past surgical studies claiming better results for operative management have performed this type of analysis when comparing surgical and nonsurgical treatments.

Only two modest, randomized, prospective trials have evaluated different treatments for gastric lymphoma. One experience with 75 patients demonstrated an inferior 3-year survival rate for surgery alone (51%), compared with surgery plus chemotherapy (79%), which, in turn, was significantly less than the survival rate for patients who received radiation therapy followed by surgery and chemotherapy (100%). In a second study involving 52 patients, patients with gastric lymphoma were randomized to chemotherapy alone or debulking surgery plus chemotherapy. The incidence and severity of complications were greater in the surgical cohort, but the relapse-free and overall survival rates were identical. Although neither study conclusively proved an optimal form of therapy, the benefit and need for surgical management of gastric lymphoma patients, even those with stage IE disease, has been rightly questioned.

The results of all treatments for low-grade MALT lymphomas of the stomach are excellent. Because nearly all tumors are localized and will respond to conservative therapy, surgical resection should not be considered as primary treatment for low-grade gastric MALT lymphomas (see Fig. 60–1). Some patients are initially undertreated in this schema because higher grade lymphoma is not detected, but they will be recognized as such and treated appropriately thereafter.

At medical centers where high-grade MALT and non-MALT gastric lymphoma patients still undergo surgical resection, the clinical stage of disease determines the primary therapy (see Fig. 60–2). Patients with involvement of para-aortic lymph nodes (stage IIEii) or distant disease (stages IIIE and IV) require chemotherapy. Early stage patients have undergone treatment with a variety of therapies in recent years. Five-year survival rates for patients with stage IE gastric lymphomas treated primarily with surgery are 85% to 100%. Despite the potential for understaging, nonsurgical management for clinical stage IE gastric lymphoma patients also results in 5-year survival rates of 80% to 100%. Because surgery alone for gastric lymphomas with nodal involvement has a high failure rate (5-year survival rate of 35% to 45%), adjuvant chemotherapy, radiation therapy, or both, have been advocated. These combination treatments improve 5-year patient survival rates to 65% to 75%. Several authors have shown 5-year survival rates of 70% to 80% for stage IIE gastric lymphoma patients with chemotherapy alone or combined with radiation therapy. Because nonsurgical treatment results appear comparable to those for regimens including gastrectomy, many cancer centers have abandoned primary surgical treatment. Although a randomized, prospective trial of an appropriate sample size would be the best method of confirming the equivalency of nonoperative management, therapy without gastrectomy continues to gain in favor.

Treatment Failure

Low-grade gastric MALT lymphomas usually recur locally. This development may occur with pure low-grade MALT histology, but is more likely with a component of either overlooked high-grade MALT lymphoma or with a transformation. Non-MALT lymphomas of the stomach recur at local, regional, or distant sites. More advanced tumors have both higher incidences of incomplete tumor response and disease relapse. Undertreatment also results in higher failure rates. More intense therapy and combination therapies should be used for advanced stage disease, bulky tumors, and non-MALT gastric lymphomas. With early detection and adequate therapy, most patients with gastric lymphoma suffer limited toxicity, maintain an intact gastrointestinal tract, and remain disease free.

Pearls and Pitfalls

- Gastric lymphomas may be of the MALT variety (mucosa-associated lymphoid tissue) or non-MALT types.
- Approximately 80% of low-grade MALT lymphomas are treated successfully with eradication of *H. pylori*.
- In most patients, high-grade MALT and non-MALT lymphomas are probably best treated by primary chemotherapy (5-year survival rate, approximately 60%) and no longer by primary surgical resection.
- When surgical resection is indicated, a complete but conservative gastrectomy with perigastric (D1) lymphadenectomy of involved nodes is indicated. Residual disease is managed by adjuvant chemotherapy.

SELECTED READINGS

Aviles A, Diaz-Maqueo JC, de la Torre A, et al: Is surgery necessary in the treatment of primary gastric non-Hodgkin lymphoma? Leuk Lymphoma 1991;5:365.

Bartlett DL, Karpeh MS Jr, Filippa DA, Brennan MF: Long-term follow-up after curative surgery for early gastric lymphoma. Ann Surg 1996;223:53.

Bayerdorffer E, Neubauer A, Rudolph B, et al: Regression of primary gastric lymphoma of mucosa-associated lymphoid tissue type after cure of *Helicobacter pylori* infection. Lancet 1995;345:1591.

Bozzetti F, Audisio RA, Giardini R, Gennari L: Role of surgery in patients with primary non-Hodgkin's lymphoma of the stomach: An old problem revisited. Br J Surg 1993;80:1101.

De Jong D, Boot H, Van Heerde P, et al: Histological grading in gastric lymhoma: Pretreatment criteria and clinical relevance. Gastroenterology 1997;112:1466.

Ferreri AJ, Cordio S, Ponzoni M, Villa E: Non-surgical treatment with primary chemotherapy, with or without radiation therapy, of Stage I–II high-grade gastric lymphoma. Leuk Lymphoma 1999;33:531.

Isaacson PG, Spencer J: Gastric lymphoma and *Helicobacter pylori*. In De Vita VT, Hellman S, Rosenberg SA (eds): Important Advances in Clinical Oncology. Philadelphia, Lippincott-Raven 1996, pp 111–121.

Koch P, Grothaus-Pinke B, Hiddermann W, et al: Primary lymphoma of the stomach: Three-year results of a prospective multicenter study. Ann Oncol 1997;8(suppl 1):S85.

Maor MH, Velasquez WS, Fuller LM, Silvermintz KB: Stomach conservation in stages IE and IIE gastric non-Hodgkin's lymphoma. J Clin Oncol 1990;8:266.

Sackmann M, Morgner A, Rudolph B, et al: Regression of gastric MALT lymphoma after eradication of *Helicobacter pylori* is predicted by endosonographic staging. Gastroenterology 1997;113:1087.

Schechter NR, Portlock C, Yahalom J. Treatment of mucosa-associated lymphoid tissue lymphoma of the stomach with radiation alone. J Clin Oncol 1998;16:1916.

Shchepotin IB, Evans SRT, Shabahang M, et al: Primary non-Hodgkin's lymphoma of the stomach: Three radical modalities of treatment in 75 patients. Ann Surg Oncol 1996;3:277.

Steinbach G, Ford R, Glober G, et al: Antibiotic treatment of gastric lymphoma of mucosa-associated lymphoid tissue. Ann Intern Med 1999;131:88.

Thiede C, Alpen B, Morgner A, et al: Ongoing somatic mutations and clonal expansions after cure of *Helicobacter pylori* infection in gastric mucosa-associated lymphoid tissue B-cell lymphoma. J Clin Oncol 1998;16:3822.

Tondini C, Balzarotti M, Santoro A, et al: Initial chemotherapy for primary resectable large-cell lymphoma of the stomach. Ann Oncol 1997;8:497.

Small Bowel: Benign

Chapter 61
Small Bowel Obstruction
Robert E. Brolin

The topic of mechanical small bowel obstruction (SBO) continues to evoke controversy regarding proper management. In the 1920s, Wangensteen stressed the importance of early operative intervention in patients with strangulation obstruction and recognized the need to operate in patients with uncomplicated complete obstruction when nasointestinal tube decompression was unsuccessful. Better methods of tube decompression and a better understanding of the basic pathophysiology of intestinal obstruction led to gradual improvement in survival rates through the 1930s and 1940s. The past decade has witnessed two advances in the management of bowel obstruction. The diagnosis has been aided by more frequent use of computed tomography (CT). Treatment in some patients has been facilitated by use of minimally invasive techniques.

CLINICAL PRESENTATION

The diagnosis of mechanical bowel obstruction is based on historical, physical, and radiographic criteria. Acute mechanical SBO is characterized by nausea, vomiting, colicky abdominal pain, and obstipation. The vomiting is usually profuse and unrelenting. The cramping pains are frequently severe. On physical examination, the vital signs are usually normal unless the patient is severely dehydrated or has strangulation. Severely dehydrated patients appear ill with an ashen color, sinus tachycardia, and occasionally hypotension. The combination of fever, tachypnea, tachycardia, and hypotension suggests strangulation obstruction. Abdominal examination is typically characterized by distention and mild diffuse tenderness. Bowel sounds may range from the high-pitched, tinkling borborygmi, which are typically associated with early obstruction, to absent bowel sounds, which are usually associated with obstruction of several days' duration or occasionally with bowel infarction.

The clinical signs and symptoms of large bowel obstruction (LBO) are somewhat different from those of SBO (Table 61–1). LBO typically presents with significant bloating and abdominal pain, which is usually continuous rather than colicky in nature. Nausea and vomiting are not early or prominent symptoms. The most prominent sign is abdominal distention, which may be massive. Bowel sounds are variable, although rarely hyperactive. Tenderness is generally mild and diffuse. Guarding and rebound are usually absent except in cases with tense distention or obvious peritonitis. Dehydration is not a prominent finding in early LBO.

A specific battery of laboratory tests should be performed at the time of admission including a complete blood count (CBC), serum electrolytes, blood urea nitrogen (BUN), creatinine, and urinalysis. Although there are no laboratory tests that are diagnostic for SBO, there are several typical abnormalities. The CBC often shows hemoconcentration characterized by elevated Hgb levels. Approximately 25% of patients with SBO have abnormal serum electrolytes, most typically hypokalemic, hypochloremic metabolic alkalosis from loss of HCL in the vomitus. The BUN to creatinine ratio is likewise increased as a result of dehydration.

Other laboratory tests that are occasionally useful in the diagnostic evaluation of SBO are serum amylase, lipase, and arterial blood gases. Amylase and lipase should be performed when acute pancreatitis is possible in the differential diagnosis. Marked increase in lipase is suggestive of pancreatitis rather than SBO. Conversely, serum amylase may be slightly or moderately increased in some patients with SBO. Arterial blood gases are normal or show metabolic alkalosis. Metabolic acidosis is a late and ominous sign, typically associated with shock or necrotic bowel.

The battery of laboratory tests typically ordered in patients with LBO is similar to tests indicated in patients

Table 61–1	**Small Versus Large Bowel Obstruction**	
SIGNS AND SYMPTOMS	**SMALL BOWEL OBSTRUCTION**	**LARGE BOWEL OBSTRUCTION**
Abdominal pain	Colicky, severe	Variable in quality, intensity
Nausea, vomiting	Prominent	Variable, from none to prominent
Abdominal distention	Variable, none to obvious	Obvious, even massive
Abdominal tenderness	Variable, indiscrete	Vague, indiscreet
Bowel sounds	Variable, high pitched to absent	Usually hypoactive

with SBO. However, the probability of abnormal serum electrolytes and renal function tests is considerably lower (Table 61–2). An elevated white blood cell count may suggest ischemia or perforation, although leukocytosis is a nonspecific finding. Amylase and arterial blood gases are rarely of diagnostic usefulness in LBO, except when acute pancreatitis is considered in the differential diagnosis.

Plain abdominal radiographs should be obtained, including flat and erect views of the abdomen and an erect posteroanterior chest radiograph. The erect chest radiograph is obtained to rule out subdiaphragmatic air (free air), which is better visualized in this view than in abdominal radiographs. The signs of SBO are dilated loops of small bowel with air-fluid levels visible on the erect view (Fig. 61–1). In partial SBO, the clinical and radiographic features are similar to those of complete SBO except that obstipation is not a prominent clinical feature and radiographically, in addition to dilated loops of small bowel, there is gas in the colon above the peritoneal reflection. In most patients, the abdominal radiographs establish the diagnosis.

Until recently, plain supine and upright abdominal roentgenograms were considered essential in the diagnostic evaluation of bowel obstruction. However, an upper gastrointestinal contrast study or CT can be helpful in recognizing SBO when the clinical presentation and plain films are equivocal or nondiagnostic. Other indications include (1) to differentiate mechanical SBO from adynamic ileus, (2) to avoid delayed operative intervention in patients who have not responded to tube decompression, (3) to evaluate specific types of SBO including Crohn's disease and advanced abdominal carcinomatosis, and in patients during the early postoperative period.

Upper gastrointestinal studies can be performed using either barium or water-soluble agents; most authorities favor barium because it has no stimulant effect on the bowel, it is not easily diluted by enteric fluid, and mucosal detail is better. Air or water may be given with barium via a jejunal tube to perform small bowel enteroclysis.

This technique has been touted as superior to conventional upper gastrointestinal contrast studies in identifying both the level and etiology of obstruction. In our experience, the accuracy of conventional upper gastrointestinal contrast studies in differentiating patients with SBO who required operation from those who did not approach 100%. Patients who required operative intervention had either a discrete focus of obstruction or failure of the barium to enter the colon after 24 hours. Patients who did not require operation showed transit of barium throughout the full length of the small bowel, usually within 3 to 6 hours.

In LBO, plain abdominal radiographs show tremendous dilatation of the colon proximal to blockage. Volvulus of the colon may produce relatively specific gas patterns depending on the location of the torsion. When the diagnosis of LBO is suspected, determination of the site of blockage, best accomplished by a contrast enema, is the first order of business.

There are two contraindications for use of contrast enema in LBO. These studies should not be performed in suspected intestinal perforation or when the cecal diameter is greater than 10 cm; the risk of spontaneous cecal perforation becomes prominent when the diameter exceeds 9 cm. A barium enema performed in the setting of intestinal perforation can produce life-threatening barium peritonitis. There is virtually no indication for use of contrast enemas in patients with suspected SBO.

Use of CT is becoming increasingly popular in diagnosis of SBO. The role of CT is not universally established. Most authorities believe that CT should be reserved for patients whose initial treatment is with tube decompression but whose condition fails to improve after 24 hours. Hence, CT should not be done in patients who require operation shortly after hospital admission. In patients for whom a trial of tube decompression is chosen as initial treatment, CT has several advantages over other diagnostic techniques because CT (1) can identify a transition between dilated and collapsed bowel, (2) can identify mass lesions and hernias as the etiology of SBO, (3)

Table 61–2	**Small Versus Large Bowel Obstruction Laboratory and Radiographic Features**	
FEATURE	**SMALL BOWEL OBSTRUCTION**	**LARGE BOWEL OBSTRUCTION**
Complete blood count	Hemoconcentration, leukocytosis variable	No hemoconcentration, leukocytosis variable
Electrolytes, blood urea nitrogen	25% to 30% electrolyte abnormality; prerenal azotemia	Rarely abnormal
Amylase	Variable, may be elevated	Rarely abnormal
Plain radiographs	Dilated small bowel loops with fluid levels	Colonic distention prominent; occasional dilated small bowel loops

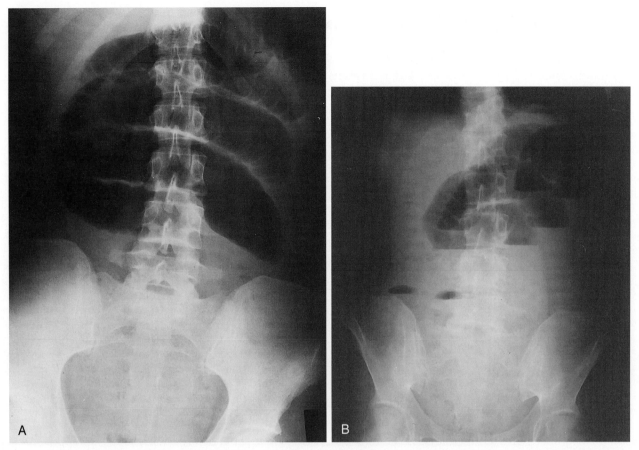

Figure 61–1. Flat *(A)* and erect *(B)* radiographs of a 36-year-old woman with complete SBO. There is obvious dilatation of the small bowel with fluid levels in the erect view and no gas in the colon.

can recognize features of strangulation, and (4) can aid resolution of ileus or partial obstruction by administration of Gastrografin. Although the sensitivity of CT in detecting strangulation is high, specificity is low with false-positive findings in the range of 20% to 30%.

No prospective studies show clear superiority of CT over other diagnostic modalities in management of SBO. CT is less reliable than barium contrast studies in determining which patients with partial SBO require operation. Conversely, CT is probably the best noninvasive method for detecting ischemic bowel. In early postoperative SBO, CT is highly reliable in distinguishing between ileus and mechanical obstruction. Use of CT in diagnosis of early postoperative SBO should obviate prolonged treatment by tube decompression in this group of patients.

PREOPERATIVE MANAGEMENT

Understanding the pathophysiology of mechanical SBO is essential to its appropriate management. When the small bowel becomes obstructed, the lumen proximal to the site of obstruction becomes progressively distended as it fills with air and enteric fluid. This produces nausea and vomiting, which will continue unabated until the bowel is decompressed. Vomiting leads to progressive dehydration,

which, if untreated, results in contraction of the plasma volume and ultimately hypovolemic shock. Frequently, shock at the tissue level produces patchy or segmental necrosis of the bowel, which is followed within hours by perforation and peritonitis. Renal shutdown and death are the end result. The end result of untreated LBO is perforation and peritonitis, which, without early operative intervention, is followed by septic shock and death.

Initial management in all patients with bowel obstruction should focus on decompression of the obstructed bowel and intravenous repletion of lost fluid. The bowel should be decompressed via a nasogastric or nasointestinal (long) tube. With SBO, fluid resuscitation should be aggressive and consist of a balanced electrolyte solution, usually normal saline. Intravenous lines should run "wide open" unless contraindicated by a history of heart failure. Supplemental potassium is necessary in the fluid to compensate for external losses, which occasionally may be severe. A Foley catheter should be placed to monitor the rehydration process. Operative intervention should not be carried out until the depleted plasma volume has been restored as indicated by normalization of the blood pressure and urine output. Perioperative broad-spectrum antibiotics are indicated because there is a potential for intestinal resection in obstructed bowel that has marked bacterial overgrowth in the lumen.

The timing of operative intervention is the most critical

decision during the initial evaluation of a patient with suspected SBO. In a review of 342 patients with SBO, we found that the plain abdominal radiographs obtained at the time of admission reliably predicted which patients required operation. In that review, 84% of patients with radiographic features of complete SBO required surgery compared with only 19% of patients with features of partial SBO. Most patients with radiographs consistent with complete SBO should undergo operation as soon as fluid losses are replenished, whereas patients with radiographic evidence of partial SBO should be given a nonoperative trial of tube decompression with the likelihood of avoiding operation. We also found that 95% of the patients whose obstruction was successfully treated by tube decompression showed either clinical or radiographic signs of improvement during the first 48 hours of treatment.

OPERATIVE MANAGEMENT

The timing of operation in patients with SBO frequently has a major impact on the degree of difficulty of the procedure and the subsequent postoperative course. Many operations for adhesive obstruction can be performed in less than an hour because they involve lysis of one or two adhesive bands. Conversely, operations performed late (after 4 to 5 days) in the course of this disease can be difficult because of the massively distended bowel, which presents several challenges for the surgeon. Long-standing distention results in thinning of the entire bowel wall, making handling of massively distended bowel extremely precarious. Full thickness injury may result from the most gentle manipulation. Enterotomy under these conditions can be disastrous, resulting in abrupt spillage of large volumes of infected enteric fluid. For the same reasons, resection of questionably viable bowel can be hazardous. Healing of enterotomy closures and anastomoses under these conditions is problematic. Decompression of massively distended bowel is also problematic because edema and atony prevent prompt reduction in luminal diameter after evacuation of intraluminal contents. Ineffective decompression may make incisional closure extremely difficult. These potential technical difficulties clearly favor earlier operation for acute mechanical SBO.

Other technical points may facilitate operations for SBO. The site of incision is occasionally important, particularly in patients who have had several major abdominal operations in the past. It is prudent if possible to avoid an incision directly overlying known adhesions involving the bowel. CT may facilitate the choice of incision by showing where the bowel is separated from the anterior abdominal wall.

Upon entering the abdomen, the first order of business is to identify decompressed bowel distal to the site of blockage. This facilitates location of the obstruction without eviscerating the distended proximal bowel, which is occasionally thin-walled and fragile. Avoidance of enterotomy is critical in minimizing the incidence of septic complications postoperatively.

Acute LBO, unlike SBO, is a surgical emergency in that the large bowel distends proximal to the site of a complete obstruction, and the risk of cecal perforation increases markedly if the ileocecal junction is competent. Thus, acute LBO is a surgical emergency. Primary resection *and* anastomosis are usually reserved for obstructing lesions of the ascending colon. Resection with proximal diversion is recommended for obstructing tumors or inflammatory diseases of the transverse and descending colon as long as that resection can be expeditiously accomplished. For fixed distal obstruction that cannot be relieved definitively (e.g., locally advanced or metastatic neoplasms, irradiated bowel), a proximal diversion is indicated.

Resection of questionably viable or necrotic bowel should be performed with great care. The surgeon must be careful to select the site of anastomosis using obviously viable bowel. Because there are no reliable objective methods available for determination of bowel viability, temporary intestinal ostomies, rather than primary anastomosis, should be considered when resection involves more than two thirds of the small bowel and viability of residual bowel is uncertain. A second-look type of approach is then mandatory. Bypass rather than resection is frequently an expeditious alternative in patients with SBO secondary to carcinomatosis because palliation, rapid recovery, and quality of life are the primary objectives.

During the past several years, successful treatment of SBO using minimally invasive techniques has been reported. Laparoscopic relief of SBO evolved from increasing experience with both enterolysis and bowel resection. One key technical point in a laparoscopic approach is finding safe ports of entry into the abdomen. CT may be useful toward that end. However, most minimally invasive surgeons recommend an open Hassan approach to creating the pneumoperitoneum. With massively distended bowel, safe entry is limited, and the ability to further expand the peritoneal cavity may be impossible. A minimally invasive approach to patients with SBO parallels the expertise and training of the general surgeons in this area.

POSTOPERATIVE MANAGEMENT AND OUTCOME

Postoperatively, patients remain on intravenous fluids and gastrointestinal tube decompression until return of bowel function. Return of bowel function is frequently anticipated by return of active bowel sounds rather than awaiting passage of stool or flatus. Fluids can be started orally soon after removal of the nasogastric tube. However, resumption of oral solid food may be met with resistance in patients with residual abdominal distention. A CBC and serum electrolytes test are indicated on the first postoperative day. Electrolytes are measured to assess the impact of fluid shifts resulting from resuscitation and aspiration of enteric fluid. Radiologic studies are not routinely indicated after uncomplicated operations for bowel obstruction. However, plain radiographs, contrast studies, and CT may be used in evaluation of postoperative patients with signs of recurrent SBO or intra-abdominal infection.

No convincing objective data demonstrate superiority of a long nasointestinal tube over a nasogastric tube in any clinical situation. In several published reviews, the use of a nasointestinal tube in an attempt to obviate operative intervention was no more successful than use of a nasogastric tube. Moreover, a number of negative features are associated with the use of nasointestinal decompression, including a greater number of postoperative complications, a longer duration of postoperative ileus, and a longer hospital stay for both the operative and nonoperative groups. Most importantly, there was a marked difference in the number of early operations—58% treated with nasogastric tubes versus 13% managed with nasointestinal tubes. Delayed operative intervention in patients initially managed preoperatively with nasointestinal tubes accounted for the greater number of complications, longer duration of ileus, and longer hospitalization. Time consumed in attempting to pass long tubes beyond the pylorus and in allowing the tube to progress through the bowel once it was passed likely contributed to the longer length of stay. In clear-cut cases of partial SBO, tube decompression is usually sufficient treatment. Our experience suggests that a nasogastric tube may be preferable to a nasointestinal tube for partial SBO.

There are several types of SBO in which immediate operative intervention is not usually indicated. Acute SBO caused by Crohn's ileitis usually resolves after 24 to 48 hours of treatment with parenteral steroids and antibiotics. However, repeated episodes of SBO resulting from Crohn's ileocolitis represent an indication for elective operative treatment. SBO in the early postoperative period frequently resolves after several days of tube decompression. With postoperative obstruction, many surgeons believe a nasointestinal tube to be superior to a short tube, having the theoretical advantage of internal enterolysis as it passes distally through the bowel. Conversely, the high mortality rate associated with early postoperative SBO has been attributed, in part, to unreasonable delay before re-exploration, suggesting that persistence with tube decompression for more than several days is unwise. In patients with suspected postoperative obstruction, both barium upper gastrointestinal contrast studies and CT can be helpful in distinguishing prolonged postoperative ileus from mechanical obstruction.

Obstruction related to abdominal malignancy has a high mortality rate, both because of the general debilitated state of these patients and because the bowel is often obstructed at multiple points by large tumor aggregates, precluding successful operative treatment. The reported mortality rate of malignant SBO is in excess of 50%. Occasionally these patients may elect not to undergo operative intervention and then go on to die without operation. Every possible nonoperative attempt at palliation of vomiting and other symptoms should be explored.

Perhaps the most difficult group of patients with SBO are those who have had multiple previous hospital admissions for adhesive SBO and several operations for lysis of adhesions. Generally, a conservative approach is taken at the outset with the hope of saving the patient another operation. Frequently, the presenting picture is that of partial SBO, which resolves after 24 to 48 hours of tube decompression. Conversely, withholding operation from

---

Pearls and Pitfalls

PEARLS

- SBO is not difficult to diagnose, but differentiating strangulation SBO from uncomplicated SBO is difficult.
- There is no good evidence that use of long (nasointestinal) tubes is better than using routine nasogastric tubes in resolving SBO.
- Complete SBO usually requires early operative intervention to prevent complications of overlooked strangulation SBO.
- Acute large bowel obstruction is a surgical emergency.
- Minimal access techniques (laparoscopic treatment) may have usefulness in selected patients with SBO.

---

patients with a clinical and radiographic picture of complete SBO may pose additional risk. CT may be useful in evaluating these patients.

POSTOPERATIVE COMPLICATIONS

Early postoperative complications are those typically associated with major abdominal operations including wound infection, dehiscence, deep vein thrombosis, atelectasis, anastomotic leak, and cardiac problems. Late complications include incisional hernia and recurrent SBO. Incisional hernias commonly occur in patients who have had wound infections. The incidence of early complications, particularly wound and pulmonary infections, is significantly higher in patients who have delayed operations, probably as a result of local problems with intestinal viability as well as marked bacterial overgrowth in the obstructed segment.

The use of antibiotics, balanced electrolyte solutions, and effective tube decompression, as well as improvements in operative technique have reduced the operative mortality rate of SBO to less than 5%. However, the mortality rate associated with strangulation obstruction remains 15% to 30%. Many studies have demonstrated the unreliability of clinical features such as fever, tachycardia, and leukocytosis in distinguishing uncomplicated SBO from strangulation SBO and have suggested that early operative intervention for complete SBO improves results. Conversely, in the absence of *all* clinical features of strangulation, "reasonable delay" in operative intervention may be warranted. What constitutes "reasonable delay" and what price is paid by patients in whom the nonoperative approach is taken is considerably less clear. This controversy has sparked the commonly quoted adage "the sun should never rise *and* set on a (complete) SBO," which still holds true.

SELECTED READINGS

Bizer LS, Leibling RW, Delany HM, Giliedman ML: Small bowel obstruction: The role of nonoperative treatment in simple intestinal obstruction and predictive criteria for strangulation obstruction. Surgery 1981;89:407.

Brolin RE: Partial small bowel obstruction. Surgery 1984;95:145.

Brolin RE, Krasna MJ, Mast BA: Use of tubes and radiographs in the management of small bowel obstruction. Ann Surg 1987;206:126.

Erickson AS, Brolin RE, Krasna MJ, et al: Use of GI contrast studies in small and large bowel obstruction. Dis Colon Rectum 1990;33:56.

Fleshner PR, Siegman MG, Brolin RE, et al: A prospective randomized trial of short vs. long tubes in adhesive small bowel obstruction. Am J Surg 1995;170:366.

Frager D, Baer JW, Medwid SW, et al: Detection of intestinal ischemia in patients with acute small bowel obstruction due to adhesions or hernia: Efficacy of CT. AJR Am J Roentgenol 1996;166:67.

Ha HK, Kim JS, Lee MS, et al: Differentiation of simple and strangulated small bowel obstructions: Usefulness of known CT criteria. Radiology 1997;204:507.

Sarr MG, Bulkley GB, Zuidema GD: Preoperative recognition of intestinal strangulation obstruction: Prospective evaluation of diagnostic capability. Am J Surg 1983;145:176.

Silen W, Hein MF, Goldman L: Strangulation obstruction of the small intestine. Arch Surg 1962;85:137.

Wolfson PJ, Bauer JJ, Gelernt IM, et al: Use of the long tube in the management of patients with small intestinal obstruction due to adhesions. Arch Surg 1985;120:1001.

Chapter 62

Small Intestinal Diverticular Disease

George A. Sarosi, Jr., and Richard H. Turnage

Diverticular disease may occur throughout the entire length of the small intestine. These lesions may be congenital in etiology such as the true ileal diverticulum (Meckel's diverticulum), or they may be acquired such as pseudodiverticula involving the duodenum, jejunum, and ileum. Although most patients with small intestinal diverticula are asymptomatic, a small number have complications related to hemorrhage, obstruction, inflammation, or perforation of the bowel. Because these lesions, whether symptomatic or asymptomatic, are often encountered unexpectedly, the clinician needs to be familiar with the clinical and pathologic spectrum of small bowel diverticular disease and its management. This chapter focuses on the clinical presentation, diagnostic tests and management of Meckel's diverticula, acquired jejunoileal diverticula, and acquired duodenal (peri-Vaterian) diverticula.

MECKEL'S DIVERTICULUM

Incidence and Pathology

The most familiar form of small bowel diverticular disease is Meckel's diverticulum. This is the most common congenital abnormality of the gastrointestinal tract, found in approximately 2% of individuals. There is no clear sex predominance. Unlike acquired jejunoileal or duodenal diverticula, which are pseudodiverticula, Meckel's diverticulum is a true diverticulum composed of all three layers of the bowel wall. It represents a failure of obliteration of the omphalomesenteric duct during embryonic development. The diverticulum, located on the antimesenteric border of the ileum within a meter of the ileocecal valve, is typically between 3 and 5 cm in length and may be attached to the anterior abdominal wall by a fibrous band. Ectopic gastric or pancreatic mucosal tissue is found in approximately one third of patients and is thought to increase the likelihood of symptoms.

Clinical Presentation and Diagnostic Studies

Meckel's diverticulum presents as an incidental finding at laparotomy or by development of complications, prompting urgent operative management. In adults, the incidental finding of an asymptomatic diverticulum is more common than a complicated diverticulum, whereas the converse is true in children. Although complicated, Meckel's diverticula seem to be found in patients before their fifth decade of life; a recent population-based epidemiologic study found a flat incidence of complications across age groups. The lifetime risk of a complication attributable to Meckel's diverticulum is between 4% and 6%.

The three most common complications attributable to Meckel's diverticula are hemorrhage, inflammation and perforation, and intestinal obstruction. The latter is the most common complication of Meckel's diverticula, representing approximately 40% percent of the complications. Obstruction may occur as a result of torsion around an omphalomesenteric band or by intussusception of the diverticulum. Small intestinal obstruction in a patient without a history of prior abdominal operation should at least raise the suspicion of the presence of Meckel's diverticulum.

The inflammatory complications of Meckel's diverticula include diverticulitis and perforation. Patients often have abdominal pain and physical findings of peritoneal irritation, a clinical scenario usually attributed preoperatively to acute appendicitis. In patients with signs and symptoms of peritonitis, preoperative radiographic studies such as enteroclysis or computed tomography will likely add little to successful management. In those patients undergoing laparotomy for presumed acute appendicitis in whom a normal appendix is found, the distal small intestine should be examined for Meckel's diverticulum. Although classically within 1 m of the ileocecal valve, they have been found up to 2 m proximally.

Almost all patients with bleeding from Meckel's diverticula are younger than 30 years old. The bleeding is due to ectopic gastric mucosa in the diverticulum causing peptic ulceration of normal mucosa adjacent to the diverticulum; the presence of hemorrhage has important implications in operative management. The patient may have a spectrum of bleeding ranging from the rare slow chronic blood loss to the much more common intermittent brisk lower intestinal hemorrhage manifested by the passage of maroon stools and clots. Preoperative localization of the site of hemorrhage may be facilitated by technetium[88m]-pertechnetate scintigraphy in which the isotope is sequestered by the ectopic gastric mucosa located within the diverticulum. The diagnostic accuracy of this study is much better in children than in adults (80% to 90% versus 46%, respectively). Enteroclysis is generally not useful in the evaluation of patients suspected of bleeding from Meckel's diverticulum because, although it may document the presence of the diverticulum, it does not provide information regarding the likelihood of hemorrhage. Furthermore, this study limits the ability to perform subsequent arteriography, a study that is more likely to localize the site of hemorrhage and hence guide subsequent therapy.

A common adage for Meckel's diverticulum is the rule of 2s: 2% of the population, 2 inches long, 2 feet from the ileocecal valve, 2 age peaks in presentation, 2 types of ectopic mucosa, 2 major types of complications, and the most important, 2 bad if you have one.

Operative and Perioperative Management

The preoperative preparation of patients with complications of Meckel's diverticula is similar to that of any patient who is to undergo an urgent abdominal procedure; specifically, the patient should undergo volume resuscitation and electrolyte repletion. Two large-bore intravenous lines should be placed for patients bleeding from Meckel's diverticulum and blood products typed and cross-matched. Broad-spectrum preoperative antibiotics appropriate for a procedure that enters the gastrointestinal tract should be administered.

In the operating room, patients should be positioned in the supine position. When the preoperative diagnosis is known, a periumbilical midline incision offers optimal access to the small intestine if a segmental bowel resection is required. Ultimately, the choice of operation performed depends on the mode of presentation of the diverticulum. For patients with intestinal obstruction or diverticulitis, a diverticulectomy is the procedure of choice unless the ileum is so inflamed that concerns exist regarding the integrity of the bowel wall closure. A diverticulectomy may be performed using a stapling device or by clamping the base of the diverticulum, excising it, and closing the bowel wall defect. Regardless of the technique chosen, it is important that the clamp or stapler be applied perpendicular to the long axis of the bowel to avoid narrowing the lumen of the intestine. If the bowel wall is severely inflamed, a segmental small bowel resection with primary anastomosis may be a more appropriate operation. Any bands between the diverticulum and the abdominal wall or the diverticulum, and the mesentery should be divided. Consideration might also be given to a laparoscopic minimal access technique.

When a patient is seen with hemorrhage associated with Meckel's diverticulum, the diverticulum and the adjacent small intestine should be resected en bloc to ensure inclusion of the bleeding site in the resected specimen because the site of bleeding is usually the ileal mucosa adjacent to or across from the diverticulum. Intestinal continuity may then be reestablished with an enteroenterostomy.

When Meckel's diverticulum is noted incidentally during an unrelated abdominal operation, the appropriate procedure depends on the age of the patient, the indications and scope of the original operative procedure, and the presence of fibrous bands between the diverticulum and abdominal wall or mesentery. Fibrous bands should always be cut when encountered. In patients younger than 40 years of age who are undergoing operative procedures in which excision of the diverticulum will not add significant incremental risk, the possibility of an incidental diverticulectomy should be entertained. However, there is little consensus (and even less data) regarding the most appropriate steps to take in this particular clinical setting unless an abnormality is palpated in the wall of the diverticulum.

The postoperative management of patients undergoing excision of Meckel's diverticulum depends on the indications for operation. Patients who undergo diverticulectomy for acute diverticulitis or perforation should be treated much the same as patients with acute appendicitis. An oral diet may be started upon resolution of ileus. Antibiotic therapy should be continued until the patient is afebrile with a normal white blood cell count and differential. For patients with uncomplicated intestinal obstruction or hemorrhage, postoperative antibiotics are unnecessary, and the patient may be advanced to a regular diet as tolerated.

Outcome

The outcome after resection of Meckel's diverticulum depends on the indications for the procedure. The complication rate for resection of an asymptomatic diverticulum ranges from 2% to 9% with most series reporting no deaths. In contrast, the postoperative complication rate for patients undergoing resection of a symptomatic Meckel's diverticulum is 7% to 15% with mortality rates of approximately 2%. Complications include wound infection, intestinal obstruction, anastomotic breakdown and intra-abdominal abscess. The incidence of future adhesive small bowel obstruction is 2% to 7%.

JEJUNOILEAL DIVERTICULOSIS

Incidence and Pathology

The incidence of jejunoileal diverticulosis is less than that of Meckel's diverticulum. The prevalence is approximately 2%. These lesions are usually found in the seventh decade of life with no apparent sex predilection. These lesions are acquired pseudodiverticula whose wall includes only the mucosal and submucosal layers of the bowel. They are found on the mesenteric side of the bowel wall and commonly lie within the mesentery. Eighty percent of patients have diverticula limited to the jejunum, 15% have lesions localized to the ileum, and 5% have diverticula throughout the small intestine. Most patients, particularly those with jejunal diverticula, have multiple lesions.

These acquired lesions are probably caused by a motility disturbance of the involved intestine, similar in principle to colonic diverticula. Poorly coordinated neuromuscular contractions allegedly lead to high intraluminal pressures and protrusion of mucosa through the muscular layers of the bowel wall at the point where the vessels enter the bowel wall. Concomitant pseudodiverticula are found in the colon and duodenum in 40% to 50% of patients with jejunoileal diverticulosis.

Clinical Presentation and Diagnostic Studies

Most patients (50% to 60%) are asymptomatic, with diverticula noted on radiologic study or found incidentally at laparotomy. These patients are likely to remain symptom-free; thus, there is no indication for resection. Twenty percent to 40% of patients are first seen with a nonspecific constellation of chronic abdominal complaints including pain, postprandial bloating, diarrhea, malabsorption, and vitamin B_{12} deficiencies; in only 10% to 15% of patients do acute complications requiring urgent operation occur.

Patients with chronic abdominal pain and malabsorption may constitute a preoperative diagnostic dilemma. Before the symptoms can be attributed to small bowel diverticulosis, other more common diagnoses should be considered. Upper gastrointestinal endoscopy, colonoscopy, biliary ultrasonography, and even computed tomography may be useful in detecting the presence of these more common diseases. Enteroclysis is the most sensitive study to detect jejunoileal diverticula, although the diverticula can usually be seen on a standard small bowel barium contrast study.

This symptom complex is thought to be due to bacterial overgrowth and poor intestinal motility. A regimen of a high-protein, low-residue diet coupled with vitamin B_{12} supplementation and intermittent courses of an oral broad-spectrum antibiotic results in improvement in 50% to 75% of patients. Only when this approach fails should surgery be contemplated for chronic symptoms.

The acute complications associated with jejunoileal diverticula are related to diverticulitis and hemorrhage. Patients with jejunoileal diverticulitis (with or without perforation) have acute abdominal pain, fever, abdominal tenderness (perhaps with evidence of peritonitis), and leukocytosis. Only rarely is the correct diagnosis suspected preoperatively. As with Meckel's diverticulitis, the severity of the patient's clinical presentation mandates laparotomy; hence, there is little utility in a lengthy and costly series of preoperative imaging studies that will not change the course of action.

Patients may have massive gastrointestinal hemorrhage from an ulceration of the mucosa and underlying artery at the neck of the diverticulum. The hemorrhage is painless and manifested by the passage of dark or maroon-colored stools. In contrast to colonic diverticular hemorrhage, bleeding from jejunoileal diverticula is rarely self-limiting, and misdiagnosis or delayed diagnosis is associated with an increased mortality risk. Because up to 50% of patients with bleeding jejunoileal diverticula also have colonic diverticula, preoperative localization of the bleeding source may be critical. Most authors believe that angiography, as opposed to radionuclide scanning, is the best study to localize active bleeding from small bowel diverticula. In patients whose bleeding is not brisk enough to be detected by angiography, scintigraphy may localize the bleeding to a particular segment of the small intestine (i.e., jejunum versus ileum). Colonoscopy and upper gastrointestinal endoscopy may be useful to rule out more common causes of hemorrhage such as peptic ulcer disease, colonic diverticula, or angiodysplasia.

Operative and Perioperative Management

The preoperative management of patients with complications of acquired jejunoileal diverticula is similar to that of patients with complicated Meckel's diverticula and includes volume resuscitation and broad-spectrum antibiotics. The most useful incision is a midline celiotomy. Because the diverticula are frequently multiple and may involve both the jejunum and ileum, the entire small bowel should be inspected before undertaking resection. Furthermore, the intramesenteric location of the diverticula may make their detection difficult. In patients with diverticulitis with or without perforation, the involved mesentery is thickened and inflamed. Resection of the involved intestine with a primary enteroenterostomy is the procedure of choice. In patients with hemorrhage, preoperative localization of the site of bleeding is crucial. Distending the bowel with air via the nasogastric tube or milking intestinal contents under pressure past the segment in question may facilitate the identification of the diverticula. Intraoperative enteroscopy may be useful in identifying the bleeding diverticulum in a patient with multiple diverticula involving the entire small intestine. The entire segment of involved bowel should be resected as long as an adequate length of intestine remains; diverticulectomy or inversion are associated with more complications such as fistula and intra-abdominal abscess.

The management of asymptomatic diverticula found incidentally at the time of laparotomy for another indication is controversial. Although no studies directly address this issue, most authors recommend leaving the diverticula in place, unless large diverticula are found in an isolated, dilated, and hypertrophied segment of bowel. With the latter findings, one should consider the original indications for laparotomy and the incremental addition of risk that a segmental small bowel resection would add to the operative procedure.

The postoperative care of patients after resection of acquired jejunoileal diverticula is as described earlier for Meckel's diverticula. The increased age and infirmity of these patients makes their recovery more complex, particularly in a patient requiring urgent laparotomy for bleeding or perforation.

Outcome

The reported morbidity rates for patients undergoing urgent laparotomy for complicated jejunoileal diverticular disease are in excess of 30% with mortality rates of 10% to 15%. The most common complications include wound infection, anastomotic leak, intra-abdominal abscess, and bowel obstruction.

DUODENAL DIVERTICULA

Incidence and Pathology

The duodenum is the portion of the small intestine most likely to harbor diverticula. The prevalence of duodenal diverticula is 2% to 27% in the general population. There is an increasing prevalence of these lesions with advancing age such that most patients with duodenal diverticula are in the sixth and seventh decades of life. Eighty percent of duodenal diverticula occur in the second portion of the duodenum, the majority of which are within 2 cm of the ampulla of Vater (peri-Vaterian). Unlike jejunoileal diverticula, the majority of these diverticula are solitary. Duodenal diverticula are pseudodiverticula at the mesenteric surface of the duodenum. They are postulated to be pulsion diverticula caused by a neuromuscular abnormality and resulting in duodenal dysmotility and high segmental pressures.

Clinical Presentation and Diagnostic Studies

The most common clinical presentation of a duodenal diverticulum is that of an asymptomatic diverticulum noted during the evaluation of abdominal symptoms. At least 90% of duodenal diverticula are asymptomatic. Vague symptoms of postprandial pain associated with bloating and nausea have been attributed to duodenal diverticula; however, careful evaluation usually reveals other causes for these symptoms. A clear association exists between periampullary duodenal diverticula, bacteriobilia, and primary and secondary choledocholithiasis. Less clear is an association between duodenal diverticula and cholecystolithiasis or pancreatitis.

Complications develop in approximately 10% of duodenal diverticula, most notably hemorrhage, diverticulitis, perforation, or obstructive jaundice. The most common complication is hemorrhage resulting from mucosal ulceration within the diverticulum. The resulting hematemesis and melena is indistinguishable from the bleeding of peptic ulcer disease. Upper gastrointestinal endoscopy enables the detection of peptic ulcerations, Mallory-Weiss tears, and gastroesophageal varices; however, visualization of bleeding from a duodenal diverticula may be difficult with standard forward-viewing endoscopy. A side-viewing endoscope may allow identification of the bleeding diverticulum. In those patients in whom endoscopy is unsuccessful, angiography may be diagnostic for those patients with rapid rates of bleeding. The hemorrhage is self-limiting in approximately 50% of patients; however, delays in surgical intervention are associated with higher mortality rates.

Patients may also have complications related to acute diverticulitis, most notably perforation. These patients are seen with abdominal pain, nausea, vomiting, leukocytosis, and right upper quadrant tenderness. Computed tomography may demonstrate the diverticulum with surrounding inflammation. Upper gastrointestinal barium studies are contraindicated given the likelihood of perforation, whereas contrast studies using a water-soluble contrast agent may show the diverticulum but will often fail to demonstrate the perforation.

The third mode of presentation for patients with complicated duodenal diverticula is that of biliary obstruction. These patients have the signs, symptoms, and laboratory findings of obstructive jaundice. Although biliary ultrasonography demonstrates intrahepatic and extrahepatic common bile duct dilation, endoscopic retrograde cholangiography (ERCP) is generally required to confirm the diagnosis and, most importantly, to rule out other more common causes of obstructive jaundice. Of note, the presence of a periampullary diverticulum has been shown

not only to markedly reduce the rate of successful ERCP from greater than 90% to 50% to 75%, but also to increase the rate of complications after endoscopic sphincterotomy for endoscopic interventions in the pancreaticobiliary systems.

Operative and Perioperative Management

The most frequent indication for operations in patients with duodenal diverticula is the management of acute perforation or hemorrhage. Because these patients are often elderly, preoperative optimization of their intravascular volume assumes particular importance. This may require central hemodynamic monitoring. Preoperative administration of a broad-spectrum antibiotic is also indicated.

An extended right subcostal or bilateral subcostal incision often provides excellent exposure of the second portion of the duodenum and, hence, management of most duodenal diverticula. For lesions near the ampulla of Vater, the operation of choice is a diverticulectomy with a two-layer closure of the duodenal defect. Because the diverticulum is usually located in the retroperitoneum posterior to the pancreatic head, an extensive Kocher maneuver with complete mobilization of the duodenum and pancreatic head is essential. Identification of the ampulla of Vater, common bile duct, and pancreatic duct is crucial for the safe management of most peri-Vaterian diverticula. This may be facilitated by the antegrade placement of a biliary catheter (via a choledochotomy or preferably the cystic duct) before beginning dissection. When the diverticulum is intrapancreatic or the ampulla is within the diverticulum, a duodenotomy may aid in performing the diverticulectomy from within the duodenal lumen. The presence of an abscess mandates the placement of closed suction drains.

The postoperative management may be aided by ad-

Pearls and Pitfalls

PEARLS

- Remember the rule of 2s for Meckel's diverticula.
- Most small bowel diverticular disease is asymptomatic and does not require surgical therapy.
- Operative therapy for vague gastrointestinal symptoms attributed to small bowel diverticular disease is rarely indicated.
- Complications related to small bowel diverticular disease usually require operative management.
- Consider the diagnosis of Meckel's diverticulum in negative explorations for appendicitis or rectal bleeding in younger patients.
- Diverticulectomy is usually adequate treatment for Meckel's and duodenal diverticula. Jejunoileal diverticula should be treated by segmental bowel resection.
- When one is operating on duodenal diverticula, the localization of the common bile duct and ampulla relative to the diverticulum is critical.

ministering octreotide to reduce the risk of pancreatic fistula in patients whose diverticula were contained within the substance of the pancreas.

Outcome

Operations for acute complications of duodenal diverticula are associated with an increased mortality rate and a 40% incidence of complications. The most frequently observed complications include duodenal leak, duodenal, pancreatic, or biliary fistula, intra-abdominal abscess, pancreatitis, injury to the pancreatic and common bile duct, and wound infection.

SELECTED READINGS

Akhrass R, Yaffe MB, Fischer C, et al: Small-bowel diverticulosis: Perceptions and reality. J Am Coll Surg 1997;184:383.

Chow DC, Babaian M, Taubin HL: Jejunoileal diverticula. Gastroenterologist 1997;5:78.

Cullen JJ, Kelly KA, Moir CR, et al: Surgical management of Meckel's diverticulum. An epidemiologic, population-based study. Ann Surg 1994;220:564.

Lobo DN, Balfour TW, Iftikhar SY, et al: Periampullary diverticula and pancreaticobiliary disease. Br J Surg 1999;86:588.

Longo WE, Vernava AM III: Clinical implications of jejunoileal diverticular disease. Dis Colon Rectum 1992;35:381.

Ludtke FE, Mende V, Kohler H, et al: Incidence and frequency or complications and management of Meckel's diverticulum. Surg Gynecol Obstet 1989;169:537.

Psathakis D, Utschakowski A, Muller G, et al: Clinical significance of duodenal diverticula. J Am Coll Surg 1994;178:257.

Tsiotos GG, Farnell MB, Ilstrup DM: Nonmeckelian jejunal or ileal diverticulosis: An analysis of 112 cases. Surgery 1994;116:726.

Chapter 63
Motility Disorders of the Small Bowel

Reginald V. N. Lord and Lelan F. Sillin

CLASSIFICATION OF SMALL BOWEL MOTILITY DISORDERS

The most prevalent type of small bowel motility disorder encountered by surgeons is the *adynamic* or *paralytic ileus* that occurs after intra-abdominal and other major operations. The two other principal types of small bowel motility disorder that may be seen are the postgastric surgery syndromes and the chronic small intestinal hypomotility, or pseudo-obstruction, syndromes. The postgastric surgery syndromes include postvagotomy, postgastrectomy, and postgastroenterostomy, including the Roux-en-Y, syndromes. Ileus, intestinal pseudo-obstruction, and the Roux syndrome are characterized by abnormally delayed transport of gastrointestinal contents, whereas the non-Roux postgastric surgery syndromes share features of abnormally rapid transit.

Paralytic Ileus

Paralytic ileus is an acute, reversible condition that results in a nonmechanical or "functional" intestinal obstruction. Ileus involves the entire gastrointestinal tract except the esophagus, although the ileus may resolve faster in some sections of the gut than others. Apart from its almost invariable development after intra-abdominal operations, paralytic ileus can occur after other major operations and after trauma, including isolated spinal or orthopedic injury. Ileus may also complicate intraperitoneal or generalized sepsis, myocardial infarction, pneumonia, and electrolyte disturbances, especially hypokalemia and hypophosphatemia. Clinical features of ileus appear to be less, and may be absent, after laparoscopic surgery compared with open abdominal surgery.

The pathogenesis of ileus is not well understood. Ileus is not simply a state of hypomotility, as evidenced by the fact that intestinal electrical and mechanical activity usually return rapidly after laparotomy, long before the clinical features of ileus disappear. Loss of the normal organization of the contractile activity appears to be more important than the loss of the contractile activity itself.

Intestinal Pseudo-obstruction

Intestinal pseudo-obstruction is a term applied to a group of syndromes that have in common permanent or recurrent hypomotility of either a part or the whole of the gastrointestinal tract. Although in sporadic cases the gut as a whole is abnormal, the most severely affected organ is usually the small intestine. Despite the name "pseudo-obstruction," patients with these conditions after previous abdominal surgery can also have true intestinal obstruction, sometimes requiring total parenteral nutrition (TPN). Although these syndromes are rare, an increased physician awareness of these disorders has resulted in an increase in their recognized prevalence. With the exception of acute colonic pseudo-obstruction (Ogilvie's syndrome), intestinal pseudo-obstruction syndromes are chronic diseases, with subacute and recurrent episodes in most patients that usually progress to chronic, nonresolving pseudo-obstruction.

The intestinal pseudo-obstruction syndromes are classified as either primary (idiopathic) or as secondary to a known disease. These syndromes are sometimes subclassified according to whether they have primarily a neuropathic or a myopathic etiology. Familial visceral myopathies and, less frequently, familial neuropathies have both been described, with a clear autosomal inheritance in many myopathic cases. Sporadic idiopathic forms have been termed chronic idiopathic intestinal pseudo-obstruction for the neuropathic patients and nonfamilial hollow visceral myopathy for the myopathic patients. A fibrotic myopathy is found in patients in whom the disease is secondary to connective tissue diseases, with scleroderma being the most common underlying disease. Individuals with myotonic dystrophy, progressive muscular dystrophy, and other muscle diseases have gut involvement but may have few alimentary tract symptoms. The more common neuropathic causes are diabetes mellitus, hypothyroidism, amyloidosis, and medication use (antidepressants, antipsychotics, anti-Parkinsonian drugs, narcotics, and some antihypertensive and chemotherapeutic agents). Abuse of laxatives, especially those containing anthraquinone, can cause a chronic pseudo-obstruction that predominantly affects the colon.

Postgastric Surgery Syndromes

The postgastric surgery syndromes include some symptom complexes that may also be classified as "postgastrectomy" syndromes. The postgastric surgery motility syndromes are the early and late postprandial dumping syndromes, postvagotomy diarrhea, and the Roux stasis syndrome. Other syndromes that, similar to these, produce postprandial symptoms in patients who have had a gastric operation are acute and chronic afferent loop obstruction, efferent loop obstruction, alkaline or bile reflux gastritis, and delayed gastric emptying.

Early Postprandial Dumping Syndrome

The early dumping syndrome consists of gastrointestinal and vasomotor symptoms that occur within the first 30 minutes after a meal in patients who have undergone gastric surgery. Up to 50% of patients may suffer early dumping symptoms after gastric surgery involving both a vagotomy and disruption of pyloric function (pyloroplasty or gastrojejunostomy). In contrast, early dumping syndrome is very uncommon after highly selective (parietal cell) vagotomy in which the pylorus is maintained intact or in patients after a distal gastrectomy in whom a vagotomy was not performed (e.g., gastric cancer or benign gastric ulcer).

Early dumping is thought to result from rapid emptying of hyperosmotic chyme from the stomach (or the residual stomach after distal gastrectomy) into the small intestine. The syndrome complicates partial gastrectomy because of loss of pyloric function in limiting the rate of gastric emptying. Dumping may also occur after vagotomy combined with a drainage procedure such as pyloroplasty or gastroenterostomy (because of a loss of the vagally mediated receptive relaxation in the proximal stomach, increasing the rate of liquid egress). The rapid delivery of hyperosmotic gastric contents into the small intestine is thought to cause a rapid shift of fluid from the intravascular space into the intestinal lumen, resulting in a minor decrease in the circulating plasma volume. This explanation is not entirely satisfactory, in that a good correlation between plasma volume and symptoms has not been found in all studies. More important in the pathogenesis is the release of vasoactive substances from the small bowel mucosa in response to the ingress of hyperosmolar intestinal contents.

Late Dumping Syndrome

The late dumping syndrome is much less common than early dumping. Symptoms occur 2 to 4 hours after meals, in contrast to the 15- to 30-minute interval between eating and symptoms for the early dumping syndrome. Rapid delivery of carbohydrates into the intestine is believed to produce an altered release of gastrointestinal hormones including insulin, neurotensin, and glucagon-like peptide-1 (GLP-1). GLP-1 and glicentin inhibit glucagon release, which, along with excessive insulin release, produces profound hypoglycemia, resulting in the clinical manifestations seen with the syndrome.

Postvagotomy Diarrhea

The reported frequency of change in bowel habit after vagotomy varies. However, 25% of patients experience some diarrhea, and between 2% and 5% will have troublesome diarrhea that persists for more than a few months after operation. Severe, incapacitating diarrhea that is essentially not treatable develops in 1% or less of patients after an abdominal (truncal) vagotomy (see later text). Postvagotomy diarrhea appears to be less frequent after highly selective vagotomy. Despite numerous studies, the pathophysiology of this condition remains unclear. One hypothesis is that unregulated delivery of bile salts by the denervated gallbladder is a causative factor, although one study reported that postvagotomy diarrhea was unchanged or even worse after cholecystectomy.

Roux Stasis Syndrome

Within the first month after construction of a Roux-en-Y gastroenterostomy, a syndrome known as post–Roux-en-Y gastroparesis, or Roux stasis syndrome, will develop in one fourth of those patients. The typical symptoms of this syndrome are nausea or vomiting, epigastric fullness, and abdominal pain. Slow emptying of the gastric remnant is the main abnormality present, and similar symptoms may occur in patients with postvagotomy gastric atony. Animal and human studies suggest that both impaired motor function of the gastric remnant and motility abnormalities of the small intestinal Roux limb contribute to the development of this clinical condition.

CLINICAL PRESENTATION AND DIAGNOSIS

Although it can be very difficult to distinguish either paralytic ileus or intestinal pseudo-obstruction from a mechanical small bowel obstruction resulting from adhesions, tumor, or other causes, there are important differences in the *typical* features of nonmechanical and mechanical bowel obstructions. These might alert a prudent surgeon and possibly avoid a nontherapeutic celiotomy in patients with pseudo-obstruction.

Paralytic Ileus

The diagnosis of ileus is suspected in the clinical situation in which it occurs. The diagnosis should be considered when signs of bowel obstruction develop in patients with known causes of ileus (such as myocardial infarction or spinal injury).

The clinical features of ileus are abdominal distention, obstipation, and either vomiting or a large quantity of nasogastric aspirate. Pain is usually absent, but, if present, it is noncolicky and is usually no more severe than would be expected with typical postoperative incisional pain and with the associated abdominal distention if the patient has not had a recent abdominal operation. Although the abdomen may be generally tender, it is usually not localized except at the wound. Whereas the abdomen is typically silent on auscultation without the groans and rushes of a mechanical obstruction, tinkles are common, and a succussion splash may result from the large volume of fluid contained within the distended stomach or bowel. Plain erect and supine films of the abdomen show both small and large bowel dilatation with scattered air-fluid levels.

Distinguishing paralytic ileus from mechanical obstruction in the postoperative period may be more difficult but is essential. Ileus is managed nonoperatively, whereas mechanical obstruction may require operation, including urgent surgery in some patients. Careful examination and investigation of patients with continuing signs of obstruction after operation are important in order to detect complications responsible for an ongoing ileus (such as an anastomotic leak) and to detect mechanical obstruction. Mechanical obstruction in the early postoperative period may be caused by fibrinous adhesions or by an internal hernia. Patients with persistent clinical features of bowel obstruction must be evaluated to rule out a mechanical obstruction. Passing of flatus or a bowel motion, followed by a return to absolute constipation, may be a sign that mechanical obstruction has occurred. Similarly, severe or colicky pain, localized tenderness, radiographic findings of one or more loops of dilated small intestine with a deflated colon, or the absence of gas in the colon is each a sign of mechanical obstruction and not ileus. A computed tomography scan with luminal contrast or a small bowel follow-through contrast examination may be needed to exclude mechanical obstruction.

Intestinal Pseudo-obstruction

Patients with intestinal pseudo-obstruction have a more gradual onset of progressively worsening intestinal obstruction or recurrent symptoms of subacute obstruction. Some patients come to attention only after complete cessation of bowel activity. Common symptoms include abdominal bloating, distention, and discomfort. Patients with colonic involvement may have severe constipation, although diarrhea may also occur as a result of bacterial overgrowth. Involvement of the foregut can cause nausea, vomiting, heartburn, dysphagia, and regurgitation. Children are frequently seen with failure to thrive and weight loss.

Except for those with a known causative disease such as scleroderma, the diagnosis of intestinal pseudo-obstruction is often not suspected or entertained. As a result, patients with these syndromes frequently undergo exploratory laparotomy to treat a presumed mechanical obstruction, and it is not uncommon for multiple laparotomies to have been performed without the correct diagnosis ever being reached. A careful history, including a detailed family and medication history, should prompt consideration of the diagnosis so that mechanical obstruction can be excluded by radiologic and endoscopic evaluation rather than by operation. The astute clinician may suspect intestinal pseudo-obstruction in the patient without a previous history of abdominal surgery (i.e., adhesions) in whom the clinical presentation is not characteristic of mechanical small bowel obstruction (e.g., slow onset, absence of crampy pain, history of less severe episodes). A slow-growing tumor may present with similar clinical features and needs to be excluded as does the diagnosis of sprue, which can mimic intestinal obstruction. Radiologic imaging often shows small bowel dilatation, although the diameter can be normal in early or mild cases. Foregut motility studies and gastrointestinal transit studies can be particularly helpful. If a full-thickness biopsy of the small bowel is needed to establish the diagnosis, a laparoscopic approach, in the appropriate setting, is preferred to reduce the risk of subsequent adhesions. The details of the tests used to establish the specific myopathic or neuropathic diagnosis in unclear cases are described in the review by Coulie and Camilleri (1999).

Postgastric Surgery Syndromes

Early Dumping Syndrome

Gastrointestinal symptoms of early dumping syndrome include nausea, epigastric fullness, abdominal pain, borborygmi, and diarrhea. Vasomotor features include diaphoresis, weakness, palpitations, tachycardia, dizziness, syncope, pallor followed by flushing, and blurred vision. Fear of food may result in weight loss.

Symptoms are worse after a high-carbohydrate, hyperosmolar meal with a large fluid volume, and they may be relieved when the patient reclines. In patients in whom the diagnosis is unclear, the clinical index proposed by Sigstad (1970) may help ascertain the diagnosis. Occasionally, patients are seen many years after gastric surgery, when details of previous gastric or "ulcer" operations may not be available. In these circumstances, a radiologic contrast study or an endoscopy is usually required to help clarify the anatomy and exclude other causes.

Special tests are usually not required to diagnose early dumping syndrome, but for patients with severe symptoms for whom remedial surgery is being considered, objective evidence of an increase in the rate of gastric emptying despite maximal medical therapy should be entertained. Rapid gastric emptying can be demonstrated with a radiographic contrast study, although it is not a particularly physiologic study. A scintigraphic study using a liquid radionuclide marker may be more useful. A provocative gastric infusion test, in which isotonic saline and 50 g glucose are given alternately in a blinded study, can be confirmative. Measurement of alterations in peripheral blood flow and plasma volume in response to a test meal may be needed for patients in whom the distinction between dumping and other postgastrectomy syndromes is unclear.

Late Dumping Syndrome

The clinical presentation of the late dumping syndrome differs from that of early dumping. Symptoms occur later, approximately 2 to 4 hours after meals, and patients typically experience marked vasomotor symptoms without gastrointestinal symptoms. Diaphoresis, tremulousness, lightheadedness, tachycardia, and even cognitive difficulty, confusion, and abnormal behavior are typical. The history may provide the diagnosis, but in uncertain cases the diagnosis can be confirmed by demonstrating hypoglycemia during symptomatic periods and by demonstrating that abnormally high peak glucose and insulin levels occur after a glucose challenge test.

Postvagotomy Diarrhea

Postvagotomy diarrhea is most common in the immediate postoperative period and is characterized by urgency and watery diarrhea. It usually resolves spontaneously. In rare patients, persistent bothersome diarrhea can have a continuation of this early symptom pattern. Alternatively, an episodic illness pattern in which diarrhea occurs for a few days with normal stools at other times can develop in patients with persistent diarrhea. The diarrhea episodes may be preceded by a nonspecific prodromal syndrome or they may occur without warning, resulting in soiling. The very rare patient may have unrelenting persistent diarrhea that is incapacitating. Microbiologic examination of the stool or a hydrogen breath test should be performed to exclude intestinal bacterial overgrowth.

Roux Stasis Syndrome

The diagnosis of the Roux stasis syndrome is made on the basis of the presence of the typical symptoms of nausea, intermittent and postprandial vomiting, epigastric fullness, and abdominal pain. The syndrome may be evident shortly after a Roux-en-Y reconstruction operation, but the later appearance of the Roux stasis syndrome with similar symptoms is more common. Patients with persistent late Roux stasis syndrome may have a significant disruption of lifestyle and severe nutritional difficulties. Both an upper gastrointestinal contrast study with small bowel follow-through and an upper gastrointestinal endoscopy should be performed. Although radiologic studies may suggest features of complete gastric outlet obstruction, the gastrojejunal anastomosis in patients with the Roux stasis syndrome is usually widely patent. Similarly, a portion of the Roux limb may be abnormally dilated without any evidence of distal obstruction. Abnormally delayed gastric emptying of solid food can be demonstrated on a radionuclide or barium study, and a bezoar may be present.

MANAGEMENT

Paralytic Ileus

The stomach should be decompressed with a nasogastric tube in patients with paralytic ileus to relieve vomiting and reduce the risk of aspiration. In patients with prolonged ileus, electrolytes should be checked regularly, and complications such as pneumonia or intra-abdominal sepsis should be excluded and aggressively treated when found. Ileus resolves spontaneously if the underlying cause or causes are identified and successfully treated. Nutritional support, including TPN, is not usually needed but may be helpful in patients who have both a prolonged ileus and antecedent malnutrition.

There is no convincing evidence that any pharmacologic treatments are beneficial. However, there are reports of occasional resolution of prolonged ileus after administration of either an adrenergic antagonist or a cholinergic agonist. Cisapride has been reported to have some benefit, but the use of this drug is associated with a risk of severe, life-threatening cardiac events. Although some investigators have attempted to pharmacologically shorten the duration of the ileus that normally follows

operations, the utility and wisdom of this approach has been questioned.

Intestinal Pseudo-obstruction

The treatment of known intestinal pseudo-obstruction syndromes is nonoperative. The goals of treatment are to provide nutritional support and to improve intestinal motility. High-calorie, high-protein soft or liquid diets may be indicated, along with vitamin and mineral supplementation. Antibiotic treatment is used for those patients with steatorrhea and diarrhea resulting from bacterial overgrowth. Promotility agents, including cisapride, erythromycin, and metoclopramide may be beneficial in some patients.

In those patients with the most severe myopathic disease and diffuse involvement of the gut, home TPN may be necessary. In patients with less severe disease, enteral feeding may be possible and is preferable to parenteral feeding. Oral feeding can be supplemented or replaced by enteral feeding via a feeding jejunostomy. Surgical resection or bypass is less effective for these syndromes than it is for isolated colonic hypomotility, but the rare patient with truly localized disease can benefit from resection. Studies of the regeneration of small intestinal motility in an animal model suggest that an end-to-end rather than an end-to-side anastomosis may be preferable for these patients.

Relief of distention and bloating by construction of a venting enterostomy has been reported to reduce the number of hospitalizations, nasogastric intubations, and laparotomies. This operation may even allow some patients to return to enteral feeding. In end-stage disease, small bowel transplantation is the future frontier and may be lifesaving.

Postgastric Surgery Syndromes

The natural history of postvagotomy diarrhea and dumping is that they eventually become less troublesome in most patients. Most patients experience spontaneous relief of symptoms within 6 months of surgery. At late follow-up, iron and vitamin B_{12} loss and abnormalities of bone and calcium metabolism are more likely to be problems than are any of the postgastrectomy syndromes.

Early Dumping Syndrome

The mainstay of treatment for dumping syndromes is dietary adjustment. Less severe symptoms are usually relieved by adoption of a diet pattern of frequent small, low-carbohydrate, high-protein, high-fat meals with minimal mealtime liquid consumption. Ingestion of the gel-forming carbohydrate pectin with meals may help delay gastric emptying. Those patients not adequately managed by dietary measures alone usually obtain sufficient relief of symptoms from the use of the synthetic somatostatin analogue octreotide. Octreotide significantly ablates the hormonal responses involved in the pathogenesis of dumping and improves the symptoms in many of these patients. Long-acting octreotide (octreotide-LAR) or the newer somatostatin analogue lanreotide-SR may be preferred to the conventional short-acting forms of these drugs. A recent report suggests that uncooked cornstarch, a complex carbohydrate that provides a slow and continuous glucose source and that may delay gastric emptying, is beneficial for children with severe dumping and may have some benefit in adults with this disorder.

Late Dumping Syndrome

Late dumping syndrome can usually be treated successfully by a reduction in the carbohydrate content of meals. In resistant patients, acarbose, an α-glucoside hydrolase inhibitor that decreases intraluminal digestion of starch and sucrose, can be combined with the gel pectin in an attempt to delay carbohydrate absorption. Octreotide is also reported to be helpful in patients with more severe symptoms.

The combination of spontaneous improvement, dietary modification, and medical treatments, including octreotide, has resulted in a reduced frequency of reoperations for both early and late dumping syndromes. Nonoperative therapies provide significant symptom improvement for most patients. For the patients who do not experience sufficient symptom relief, however, a variety of operations have been suggested. The reported success rate for treating dumping syndromes using an isoperistaltic jejunal segment interposed between the stomach and the duodenum (Henley loop operation) has been variable, and enthusiasm for this operation has waned. Interposition of separate double (Poth operation) or plicated triple limb jejunal pouch in the same position is controversial. The most commonly used operation is probably a Roux-en-Y diversion procedure, usually without but occasionally with a 10-cm reversed jejunal segment interposed between the gastric remnant and the Roux limb. Experience with any of these procedures is limited, and there are no good long-term studies addressing efficacy.

Postvagotomy Diarrhea

Postvagotomy diarrhea, like the other postgastric surgery syndromes discussed, is initially treated medically. Fluid restriction with meals and stool-firming agents such as kaolin-pectin, diphenoxylate, and loperamide may be beneficial. The most effective drug appears to be cholestyramine. Long-term low-dose use of this agent is usually required, thus exposing the patient to the potential complications of disordered coagulation and megaloblastic anemia. For the rare patient resistant to medical treatment, operative therapy can be considered. The most frequently used operation involves reversal of one (or two) 10- to 12-cm segment of jejunum at a level 90 to 100 cm below the ligament of Treitz. The jejunal segment should be divided along its mesentery, rotated 180 degrees in a counterclockwise direction, and reanastomosed in continuity using standard techniques. Postoperative abdominal pain and intermittent functional bowel obstruction can occur. There are no good long-term results available with this technique, and it should be used as a last resort.

Pearls and Pitfalls

- Although it may be difficult, a mechanical cause of intestinal obstruction should always be excluded before a functional one is diagnosed.
- Both a thorough history and clinical suspicion are important in recognizing and diagnosing small intestinal motility disorders.
- Whenever possible, enteral feeding is preferable to parenteral feeding.
- Postoperative ileus is normal, but prolonged ileus is not and needs to be investigated.
- The development of obstipation after apparent resolution of ileus, with passage of flatus or stool, is a sign of mechanical obstruction.
- Patients with intestinal pseudo-obstruction can have true, and even complete, nonmechanical bowel obstruction.
- Intestinal pseudo-obstruction may permanently involve either part or all of the gastrointestinal tract.
- If the diagnosis of chronic intestinal pseudo-obstruction is not considered, unnecessary laparotomy is often performed.
- Patients with suspected primary intestinal pseudo-obstruction require very specialized evaluations to precisely diagnose the type of myopathy or neuropathy present.
- Early dumping symptoms include (1) the gastrointestinal symptoms of nausea, vomiting, epigastric fullness, abdominal pain, borborygmi, and diarrhea, and (2) the vasomotor symptoms of diaphoresis, weakness, palpitations, tachycardia, dizziness, syncope, pallor followed by flushing, and blurred vision.
- Late dumping symptoms are predominantly vasomotor symptoms.
- As many as 50% of patients have dumping symptoms early after gastric surgery involving vagotomy and disruption of pyloric function.
- Patency of the gastrojejunostomy anastomosis should be confirmed by endoscopy in patients with suspected Roux stasis syndrome.
- Surgeons should not reoperate too early after gastric surgery. Most postgastric surgery syndromes improve significantly with nonoperative therapy.

Roux Stasis Syndrome

After excluding mechanical obstruction, the management of patients with this syndrome relies chiefly on supportive care and the use of prokinetic agents. Intermittent or continuous gastric decompression, usually via a nasogastric tube, may be needed. Enteral nutritional support is preferred if possible, but the enteral feeding tube should be positioned well beyond the gastroenterostomy. In severely symptomatic patients with nutritional compromise, permanent long-term TPN may be required. Drugs with reported benefit for treating this condition include cisapride and erythromycin, although cisapride must be used with great caution and not with concomitant use of erythromycin.

For patients with persistent symptoms despite these measures, total or near-total gastrectomy should be considered. In general, reported results have been encouraging in about half of the patients, suggesting that the gastric remnant plays a significant role in the genesis of this syndrome. However, the failure of these operations to achieve good symptom relief in a large number of patients (25% to 50%) suggests that abnormalities of small bowel motility also contribute. Also, because this syndrome can occur after a total gastrectomy without a functional gastric remnant, further support for incrimination of the Roux limb in the pathogenesis in selected patients is appropriate.

SELECTED READINGS

Coulie B, Camilleri M: Intestinal pseudo-obstruction. Annu Rev Med 1999;50:37.

Eckhauser FE, Conrad M, Knol JA, et al: Safety and long-term durability of completion gastrectomy in 81 patients with postsurgical gastroparesis syndrome. Am Surg 1998;64:711.

Forstner-Barthell AW, Murr MM, Nitecki S, et al: Near-total completion gastrectomy for severe postvagotomy gastric stasis: Analysis of early- and long-term results in 62 patients. J Gastrointest Surg 1999;3:15.

Miedema BW, Kelly KA: The Roux operation for postgastrectomy syndromes. Am J Surg 1991;161:256.

Murr MM, Sarr MG, Camilleri M: The surgeon's role in the treatment of chronic intestinal pseudoobstruction. Am J Gastroenterol 1995;90:2147.

Sarr MG: Appropriate use, complications and advantages demonstrated in 500 consecutive needle catheter jejunostomies. Br J Surg 1999;86:557.

Sigstad H: A clinical diagnostic index in the diagnosis of the dumping syndrome. Acta Med Scand 1970;188:479.

Sillin LF, Woodward A: The effects of vagotomy, gastrectomy, and the Roux-en-Y anastomosis on gastric motility and emptying. Probl Gen Surg 1993;10:290.

Vecht J, Masclee AA, Lamers CB: The dumping syndrome. Current insights into pathophysiology, diagnosis and treatment. Scand J Gastroenterol 1997;226(Suppl):21.

Chapter 64
Appendicitis

Michael S. Malian, Daniel C. Cullinane, and Michael P. Bannon

Acute appendicitis is the most common general surgical emergency. Reginald Fitz (1843–1913), who first realized that perforation of the appendix and subsequent peritonitis were frequently fatal, coined the term *appendicitis* for this disease process. Fitz began a crusade to convince physicians of the necessity to remove the appendix immediately if symptoms did not resolve. Richard Hall (1856–1897) heeded Fitz's advice and reported the first survival of a patient after removal of a perforated appendix. Thus, the successful surgical treatment of acute appendicitis began.

A detailed history and careful physical examination most frequently make the diagnosis. However, appendicitis may pose a significant diagnostic challenge. Despite advances, and interest, in imaging techniques, including high-resolution computed tomography (CT) and ultrasonography, the rate of pathologically negative appendectomy and perforated appendicitis remains high.

CLINICAL PRESENTATION AND DIAGNOSIS

Evaluation of the patient with suspected appendicitis requires a careful consideration of the history, duration, location, and quality of the pain as well as exacerbating and mitigating factors. Pain generally begins in the periumbilical region and is usually followed by anorexia, nausea, and sometimes vomiting. The pain subsequently migrates to the right iliac fossa, associated with localized tenderness. Fever and subsequent leukocytosis sometimes follows. Although the presence of a low-grade fever and mild leukocytosis (10,500 to 15,000 cells/mm^3) supports the diagnosis of an acute inflammatory condition, about 10% to 20% of patients have neither fever nor leukocytosis. This particular sequence of symptom progression represents the classic presentation of acute appendicitis.

Atypical presentations of acute appendicitis are not uncommon. Patients with a retrocecal or pelvic appendix may have relatively unimpressive tenderness in the right iliac fossa. Similarly, the very young (<4 years of age) or the elderly will present late in the course of the disease without the presence of symptomatology, or the ability to communicate the history of the progression of signs and symptoms. A large percentage of these patients will have perforated appendicitis by the time the diagnosis is made, and thus the clinician will need to maintain a high index of suspicion in this patient population. Indeed, so-called neglected appendicitis is a common presentation in the elderly population. These patients seek physician advice several days to several weeks after the onset of vague abdominal symptoms; they may have either a resolving phlegmonous process, an appendiceal abscess, or a distal small bowel obstruction.

Although abdominal pain is a constant feature of appendicitis, the diagnosis remains questionable in the absence of at least anorexia and tenderness. It is important that an exhaustive list of pathologic possibilities in the differential diagnosis be prepared and considered (Table 64–1). A careful history and physical examination remain the key to making the diagnosis of acute appendicitis. Pertinent laboratory studies should be obtained, including urinalysis to exclude a urinary tract infection and a beta-human chorionic gonadotropin (β-HCG) level to exclude pregnancy in women of child-bearing age. Flat and upright abdominal radiographs may be helpful in excluding other surgical and nonsurgical conditions; on occasion, the abdominal film shows an appendiceal calculus, which supports the diagnosis of appendicitis and also increases the likelihood of complicated appendicitis. As many as half of all patients admitted for observation for suspected appendicitis have this diagnosis excluded, and 15% to 30% of patients undergoing appendectomy have a normal appendix at the time of operation.

Improvements in techniques of CT over the last 10 years have resulted in a new tool in the evaluation and diagnosis of appendicitis. Several CT findings suggest acute appendicitis, including visualization of an abnormal appendix, stranding of the periappendiceal mesenteric fat, pericecal inflammation, and fluid in the right paracolic gutter. In particular, the combination of an abnormal-appearing appendix and pericecal inflammation together represent the most sensitive and specific signs. Proponents of the use of *routine* CT for the diagnosis of acute appendicitis cite a significant reduction in the number of negative appendectomies performed compared with historical controls at their institution. The accuracy of CT for the diagnosis of acute appendicitis ranges from 93% to 98%. Both false-negative and false-positive results occur, but clearly CT has a role in patients in whom the diagnosis is in question. High-risk patients, those with a nonclassic presentation, or selected patients (e.g., the very young or the elderly) may benefit most from the use of CT in the diagnostic approach. Several algorithms are

Table 64–1	Differential Diagnosis in the Patient with Suspected Acute Appendicitis
Influenza	Diaphragmatic pleurisy
Spinal disease	Gastroenteritis
Urinary tract infection	Renal colic
Acute cholecystitis	Acute diverticulitis (sigmoid or cecal)
Small bowel obstruction	Mesenteric adenitis
Meckel's diverticulitis	Terminal ileitis (Crohn's disease)
Ovarian torsion	Ruptured corpus luteum
Pelvic inflammatory disease	Ectopic pregnancy
Perforated peptic ulcer	

433

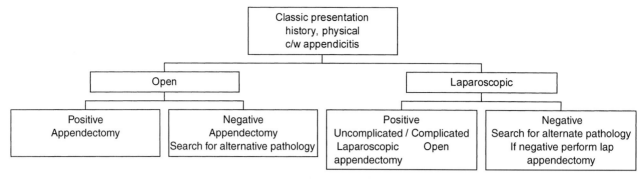

Figure 64–1. Treatment algorithm for the classic presentation of appendicitis, in which the history and physical examination results are consistent with the diagnosis.

offered for the evaluation and management of the patient with presumed appendicitis (Figs. 64–1 and 64–2).

PREOPERATIVE MANAGEMENT

During the evaluation of the patient for acute appendicitis, care should be dictated by clinical needs. Intravenous fluids and analgesics after the diagnosis has been established remain standard care. The need for a nasogastric tube and a urinary catheter is predicated on the severity of the illness and the patient's response to therapy.

When the diagnosis is established, an antibiotic should be administered preoperatively; the selection of an antibiotic is based on the level of expected contamination. *Escherichia coli, Pseudomonas,* and *Bacteroides* species are the most common organisms isolated. Second-generation cephalosporins are generally acceptable for the patient with a suspected nonperforated appendicitis. If perforation is suspected, broad-spectrum coverage of aerobes and anaerobes should include metronidazole or clindamycin and a cephalosporin, ampicillin with an aminoglycoside, or even a third-generation cephalosporin with anaerobic coverage.

OPERATIVE MANAGEMENT

Uncomplicated appendicitis may be managed with an open or laparoscopic technique. At this time, clinical studies are conflicting as to which approach is superior. The subgroups of patients who most clearly benefit from a laparoscopic approach are the very obese, in whom a large incision may be required, and young women, in whom the diagnosis is more often incorrect.

OPEN APPENDECTOMY. In the open technique, the abdomen should be palpated to ascertain the presence of a mass after induction of general anesthesia. If present, the mass is most often at McBurney's point (equidistant from the umbilicus and the anterior superior iliac spine). A transverse or slanting incision is made, measuring 5 to 10 cm as necessary, and is carried down to the abdominal wall musculature. Entry into the peritoneal cavity should be made lateral to the rectus sheath via a muscle-splitting incision.

The cecum is usually identified near the lateral peritoneal wall, grasped by its taeniae coli, and mobilized into the wound. If difficulty is encountered, the incision may be extended as necessary. In patients in whom the appen-

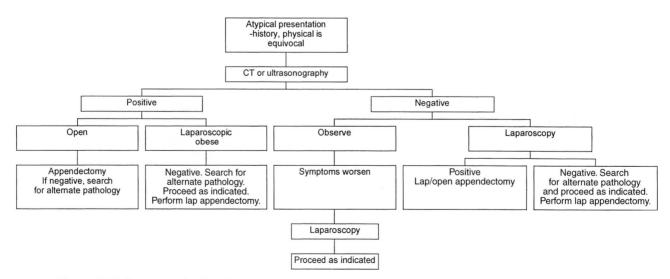

Figure 64–2. Treatment algorithm for the atypical presentation of appendicitis, in which the history and physical examination results are equivocal.

dix cannot be easily located, it is helpful to follow the colonic taeniae proximally to the point where they become confluent. The base of the appendix corresponds to the confluence of the taeniae coli.

Once the cecum has been delivered into the wound, the mesoappendix is divided between clamps. The base of the appendix is freed from peritoneal fat and is divided between clamps and doubly ligated (suture and free tie). The classic teaching of inverting the appendiceal stump has proved unnecessary, provided that the mucosa of the stump is cauterized to prevent a mucocele.

If the appendix intraoperatively is clearly normal, a vigorous search for alternative pathology is absolutely necessary. Inspection of the cecum and terminal ileum is imperative. Meckel's diverticulum, terminal ileitis, or cecal or sigmoid diverticulitis may present with classic features of appendicitis and may even appear similar on CT. In females, gynecologic pathology, such as ovarian torsion, ruptured corpus luteum cyst, or salpingitis, may be the source of the pathology. If the intraoperative investigation is nondiagnostic and significant pathology was suspected preoperatively, the surgeon must consider the need for further operative exploration by either extending the right lower quadrant incision or closing the appendectomy incision and making a midline incision. Ideally, the surgeon should have considered this possibility before making the appendiceal incision. Local factors suggesting significant distant pathology, which require further operative exploration, include bilious, purulent, or hemorrhagic peritoneal fluid. Usually when there is no peritoneal fluid and the omentum has not migrated to the right lower quadrant, other significant inflammatory pathology requiring operative therapy would be unusual.

In patients with complicated appendicitis (gangrene, perforation, abscess), consideration should be given to leaving the skin open and allowing the wound to heal by secondary intention or by delayed primary closure. Pediatric patients and very thin adults can often be managed with primary wound closure, even in the setting of complicated appendicitis with minimal morbidity.

LAPAROSCOPIC APPENDECTOMY. The laparoscopic technique affords the opportunity of a more complete evaluation of the abdominal cavity, particularly when alternative pathology is suspected or the diagnosis is in question. After general anesthesia, the bladder should be decompressed and an orogastric or nasogastric tube placed. A periumbilical incision is made, and pneumoperitoneum is achieved with a Veres needle or a trocar placed according to an open Hassan technique. After inspection of the peritoneal cavity, an additional 5- or 10-mm trocar is placed in the right upper abdomen well above McBurney's point. Through this trocar, an endoscopic Babcock clamp is used to grasp the cecum and elevate it anteriorly to expose the appendix. A 12-mm trocar may then be placed in the left lower quadrant or in the lower midline. This 12-mm port becomes the "operating port" through which the dissector, cautery, and endoscopic gastrointestinal stapler are introduced. The appendix is mobilized and the mesoappendix divided with bipolar cautery, ligaclips, or an endoscopic stapler with a vascular cartridge. The base of the appendix may be ligated with an endoscopic stapler or with an absorbable ligature. The appendix is

then deposited in a specimen retrieval bag for withdrawal without contamination through the 12-mm port. The fascia of the 10- or 12-mm trocar insertion sites are then closed with absorbable suture to prevent hernia formation.

POSTOPERATIVE MANAGEMENT

Patients may be discharged within 24 hours after uncomplicated appendectomy. Typically, they are given a regular diet within 12 hours of the operation. No further laboratory studies are usually obtained. No further antibiotics are given postoperatively to patients with uncomplicated appendicitis, other than the preoperative prophylactic antibiotic administered.

Gangrenous or perforated appendicitis usually requires 3 to 5 days of intravenous antibiotics and careful observation and attention to wound care. The authors' practice has been to continue antibiotics until the patient is afebrile and the leukocytosis has resolved. If after 3 to 5 days the patient continues to have fever and leukocytosis, a CT is generally obtained to search for an intra-abdominal abscess. Multiple studies have shown that intraoperative cultures obtained for perforated appendicitis rarely change the patient's therapy or outcome. Colonic flora are easily predicted, and appropriate antibiotic treatment with both gram-negative and anaerobic coverage should be initiated prior to operation or at the time of exploration when unsuspected perforated appendicitis is found.

Diet should be advanced as tolerated. If significant peritonitis is encountered, ileus is to be expected and may require nasogastric suction as well as delay in oral intake.

COMPLICATIONS

The most common complication after appendectomy is wound infection (approximately 5% to 25%). If wound infection is anticipated or of concern, the option of leaving the wound open for delayed primary closure should be considered. Children have the lowest incidence of superficial wound infection owing to their small amount of subcutaneous tissue.

If pain, fever, or leukocytosis continues after the operator has opened a wound infection, intra-abdominal or pelvic abscess must be considered. CT may achieve the diagnosis and guide percutaneous drainage. While most intra-abdominal abscesses can be successfully drained percutaneously, many pelvic abscesses require laparoscopy, laparotomy, or transrectal or transvaginal drainage. Abscesses of the pelvis have historically been drained through the anterior rectal wall or in the female through the posterior vaginal fornix. Postoperative small bowel obstruction and hernia formation are less common but may present as an early or late complication of adhesions and may require surgical intervention.

SPECIAL CIRCUMSTANCES

Appendicitis in the elderly often presents atypically and with a higher rate of perforation and intra-abdominal abscess. Exploration through a midline incision is sometimes advisable, as morbidity in general is higher with disseminated contamination, which requires extensive ir-

Pearls and Pitfalls

- Abdominal pain without tenderness generally excludes the diagnosis of appendicitis.
- Abdominal pain precedes the fever, nausea, and vomiting as primary complaints.
- CT of the abdomen is most useful in the setting of an atypical history and physical examination, but it should not overrule the clinical presentation.
- If widespread perforation or a markedly delayed presentation is highly suspected, a lower midline incision may improve exposure, facilitate extirpation, and control contamination.
- Diagnostic laparoscopy may be advantageous in females in particular, when the history, the physical examination, and imaging studies fail to confirm the diagnosis.
- Alternative pathology should be aggressively investigated in the event of negative appendectomy, especially with purulent, bloody, or bile-stained peritoneal fluid.
- Presentation of appendicitis in the young and elderly should prompt early exploration because of the high probability of perforation or delay.

rigation and drainage. The elderly also have a higher incidence of carcinoma of the cecum mimicking appendicitis. The delay in seeking medical attention (neglected appendicitis) and atypical presentations (often without leukocytosis) are the primary factors in this morbidity.

Appendicitis in pregnancy also poses a serious challenge. Appendicitis occurs in approximately 1 in 1500 pregnancies and is the most common acute surgical problem occurring in pregnant women. The incidence of acute appendicitis occurs with fairly even distribution throughout the trimesters of pregnancy. Ultrasonography in the left lateral decubitus position may be helpful in identifying acute appendicitis at any time during pregnancy. A high level of suspicion warrants exploration to avoid the morbidity of perforation. While the location of the appendix may vary with displacement due to the enlarged uterus, often the appendix will be in its usual right lower quadrant position. Diagnostic laparoscopy is not contraindicated, particularly in the first two trimesters of gestation, and may be helpful in identifying alternative pathology.

Crohn's disease with appendicitis also poses a dilemma. Under most circumstances, appendectomy can and should be performed as long as the disease does not involve the base of the appendix. However, if the base of appendix and cecum are inflamed, appendectomy alone is contraindicated because of a high rate of postoperative fistula formation, and consideration should be given to a distal ileocecectomy with either primary anastomosis or proximal stoma, depending on the local conditions.

Chronic and recurrent appendicitides are not entirely rare phenomena. Recurrent episodes of right lower quadrant pain for which there is no alternative explanation of symptoms or relief may warrant laparoscopic or open appendectomy if all other pathologic conditions are excluded. Approximately one third of patients with documented appendiceal inflammation by ultrasonography will develop recurrent right lower quadrant abdominal pain and chronic appendicitis. Most of these patients will develop recurrent appendicitis within 1 year of initial presentation. Interestingly, a few of these patients develop perforation or gangrene of the appendix.

SELECTED READINGS

Barber MD, McLaren J, Rainey JB: Recurrent appendicitis. Br J Surg 1997;84:110.

Bilik R, Burnweit C, Shandling B: Is abdominal cavity culture of any value in appendicitis? Am J Surg 1998;175:267.

Curtin KR, Fitzgerald SW, Nemcek AA Jr, et al: CT diagnosis of acute appendicitis: Imaging findings. AJR Am J Roentgenol 1995;164:1369.

Eldar S, Nash E, Sabo E, et al: Delay of surgery in acute appendicitis. Am J Surg 1997;173:194.

Franz M, Norman J, Fabri J: Increased morbidity of appendicitis with advanced age. Am Surg 1995;61:40.

Long KH, Bannon MP, Zietlow SP, et al: A prospective randomized comparison of laparoscopic appendectomy with open appendectomy. Surgery 2001;129:390.

McCall JL, Sharples K, Jadallah F: Systematic review of randomized controlled trials comparing laparoscopic with open appendectomy. Br J Surg 1997;84:1045.

Rao P, Rhea JT, Rattner DW, et al: Introduction of appendiceal CT: Impact on negative appendectomy and appendiceal perforation rates. Ann Surg 1999;229:344.

Silen W (ed): Appendicitis: The differential diagnosis of appendicitis. In Cope's Early Diagnosis or the Acute Abdomen, 19th ed. New York, Oxford University Press, 1996, pp 70–125.

Thompson JE Jr, Bennion RS, Schmit PJ, Hiyama DT: Cecectomy for complicated appendicitis. J Am Coll Surg 1994;179:135.

Wang Y, Reen DJ, Puri P: Is a histologically normal appendix following emergency appendectomy always normal? Lancet 1996;347:1076.

Weyant M, Eachempati SR, Maluccio MA, et al: Interpretation of computed tomography does not correlate with laboratory or pathologic findings in surgically confirmed acute appendicitis. Surgery 2000;128:145.

Chapter 65

Short Bowel Syndrome

Jon S. Thompson

Short bowel syndrome (SBS) is characterized by malabsorption and malnutrition, secondary to extensive intestinal resection. It generally occurs when less than 120 cm of functional intestine remains in adult patients. Several factors determine the severity and the spectrum of clinical features of the short bowel syndrome. These include the extent and site of the resection, underlying intestinal disease, the presence or absence of the ileocecal valve, the functional status of the remaining digestive organs, and potential for adaptation of the intestinal remnant. A number of pathophysiologic changes occur in SBS that may cause other specific metabolic problems of importance to the surgeon. The appropriate management of patients with SBS, beginning even in the preoperative period, should minimize the predictable complications that might occur and improve prospects for future survival (Table 65–1).

CLINICAL PRESENTATION

Mesenteric vascular disease and the treatment of cancer, including radiation therapy, are the intestinal conditions that most frequently lead to SBS (Table 65–2). Other tumors and benign conditions, such as Crohn's disease and intestinal obstruction, are also common underlying conditions.

The initial clinical presentation of these patients depends heavily on the underlying diagnosis. SBS results from a single massive intestinal resection in approximately three fourths of patients and from multiple lesser sequential resections in one fourth of patients. Patients undergoing massive resection are more likely to be elderly, present emergently, have mesenteric vascular disease, and have a worse nutritional and overall prognosis.

The most effective therapy for SBS is prevention. The surgeon should be aware of the need for timely intervention in patients with mesenteric ischemia, early operation for intestinal obstruction to avoid resection, and minimizing resection in patients with underlying chronic, persistent conditions, such as Crohn's disease, that might eventually lead to SBS.

PREOPERATIVE MANAGEMENT

When possible, discussion with the patient and family about the potential consequences of the SBS, including the need for prolonged parenteral nutrition (PN) support, should be undertaken before operative decision making. In the elderly patient with extensive comorbidity, it might be appropriate to consider not resecting diseased bowel that would result in SBS. Extensive resection could leave the patient as an intestinal "cripple" with numerous irre-

versible nutritional, financial, and quality-of-life issues; obviously, this can be a very difficult decision. For patients who have had previous resections and might predictably require further resection leading to the SBS, there should be greater discussion and consideration of management issues.

When considering further surgical procedures in patients who have had previous intestinal resection, the surgeon should try to gain as much information as possible about preexisting anatomy and intestinal disease. Contrast-enhanced studies of the intestinal tract are generally helpful in estimating the residual intestinal length and in assessing the presence of dilatation and potential points of obstruction and mucosal disease. Patients who have had previous resection are at increased risk for cholelithiasis, and preoperative ultrasonography should be obtained when appropriate. Nutritional status should be assessed so that appropriate nutritional support can be provided during the perioperative period.

In patients with acute intestinal conditions likely to require massive resection, management consists primarily of stabilizing the patient hemodynamically and correcting fluid and electrolyte deficits. Nasogastric decompression is usually appropriate. Preoperative antibiotics should cover colonic flora. If an ostomy is anticipated and time permits, consultation with a stomal therapist and picking the optimal site for the ostomy should be done preoperatively. These often become high-output stomas, and proper construction and positioning are important. Bowel preparation should always be considered when a colon remnant is present, if this is feasible.

INTRAOPERATIVE MANAGEMENT

An important intraoperative strategy is to avoid extensive resection when it is not clearly necessary. Decisions about

Table 65–1	Common Problems in the Management of SBS

Admonitions
  Prevention is the best treatment
  Avoid even limited resections when possible
  Consider prophylactic cholecystectomy
Common Errors in Practice
  Documenting only the intestine that has been removed, rather than that which remains
  Hasty decision to resect reversibly ischemic bowel
  Extensive resection for inflammatory disease
Anatomic Considerations
  Avoid blind loops
  Restore intestinal continuity when possible
Pathology Change
  Prevent irreversible hepatic disease

Table 65–2	**Underlying Disease in Adult Patients with Short Bowel Syndrome**

Mesenteric vascular disease	30
Cancer/radiation	30
Crohn's disease	9
Other benign conditions	26
Total	**95**

Data from Thompson JS: Comparison of massive vs. repeated resection leading to short bowel syndrome. J Gastrointest Surg 2000;4:101–104.

resection margins and management of intestinal lesions should not be carried out until the entire situation has been fully assessed. It may be prudent to consider the potential morbidity of additional anastomoses and thus to salvage even a few inches of small intestine in the setting of a severely shortened remnant. Strategies such as stricturoplasty, intestinal tapering, and serosal patching may be helpful in managing specific lesions that would otherwise require resection (Fig. 65–1).

Other important intraoperative issues relate primarily to the management of the intestinal disease. When one deals with intestinal ischemia, any constriction of the mesentery should be relieved, the bowel should be covered with warm, moist packs, and it should be observed for signs of viability. Palpation of pulses and the character of Doppler ultrasonic signals should be used to assess perfusion of the gut wall. Revascularization should be

performed when feasible. Viability is generally assessed by improved color, visible mesenteric pulsations, and peristalsis. Fluorescent staining and visualization with Wood's lamp to assess diffuse changes, and the use of a Doppler ultrasonic flow probe to evaluate blood flow at the margins of the bowel, continue to be the most useful modalities. Obviously, nonviable bowel requires resection. However, when viability is uncertain and recovery of viability is a possibility, a second-look procedure should be considered in retaining questionable bowel.

Intestinal obstruction should be excluded intraoperatively if this possibility has not been adequately assessed preoperatively. This procedure may require passing a balloon-tipped catheter (e.g., Baker's tube or Foley catheter) through the intestinal tract to identify possible stenoses. In patients who already have a short bowel, there may be opportunities to reconstruct the bowel to eliminate blind loops, which can lead to stasis and bacterial overgrowth.

Formation of ostomies may be advisable when the patient is unstable, intestinal viability is questionable, and the patient will be left with a very shortened intestinal remnant, for example less than 90 cm. Duodenal or high jejunal ostomies create difficult management problems. Occasionally, tube decompression is required rather than a stoma. However, in general, restoring intestinal continuity should be considered.

Since patients with SBS are at increased risk for development of cholelithiasis and acute biliary complications, a prophylactic cholecystectomy should be considered. This decision needs careful evaluation in the patient undergo-

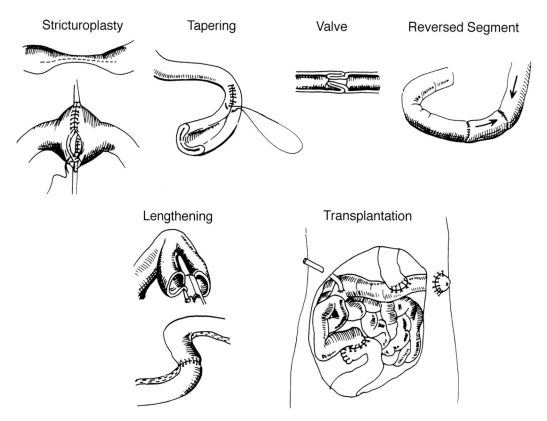

Figure 65–1. Surgical procedures for improvement of intestinal function in short bowel syndrome. (From Thompson JS, Langnas AN, Pinch LW, et al: Surgical approach to the short bowel syndrome. Ann Surg 1995;222:600–607, with permission.)

ing a massive resection in an emergent situation. Cholecystectomy would be more reasonably performed in patients who are undergoing elective procedures or who require subsequent reoperation.

POSTOPERATIVE MANAGEMENT

In the early postoperative period, the management of SBS is primarily the management of the critically ill surgical patient who has undergone an extensive resection. Control of sepsis, maintenance of fluid and electrolyte balance, and initiation of nutritional support are the key issues. As the patient recovers, the important priorities become maintaining adequate nutritional status, maximizing the absorptive capacity of the remaining intestine, and anticipating and preventing the development of complications related to the SBS and its management.

Nutritional support will be primarily in the form of PN during the early postoperative period. Fluid and electrolyte losses may be considerable. Most patients require approximately 35 kcal/kg per day and 1 to 1.5 g protein per kilogram per day with the appropriate electrolytes, minerals, trace elements, and vitamins. However, it is important to begin enteral nutritional support as early as possible once the ileus has resolved and then to gradually increase the proportion of enteral nutrients with time. Luminal nutrition maintains intestinal function, maximizes intestinal adaptation, and minimizes complications related to PN. In general, patients who have more than 180 cm of small intestine remaining will not require PN for an extensive period. The patients with approximately 90 cm of small intestine, and particularly those who have retained part or all of their colon, especially with an intact ileocecal valve, will require PN for less than 1 year. However, those who have less than 60 cm of small intestine are likely to require permanent PN.

The transition from parenteral to enteral support requires careful monitoring. The goals are to maintain a stable body weight and prevent large fluctuations in fluid status. Monitoring should be carried out to correct any metabolic abnormalities or nutrient deficiencies. PN should be gradually decreased as enteral intake increases. A marked increase in gastrointestinal fluid losses in response to enteral feeding usually signifies that increasing the feeding further will not be tolerated. As parenteral requirements diminish, this therapy can be used intermittently until weaning is achieved.

The optimal diet for a patient with the SBS is determined by the length and location of the intestinal remnant, the underlying intestinal disease, and the status of remaining digestive organs. For example, the presence of a stoma is important because diarrhea and perianal complications may markedly diminish oral intake. When the remnant is less than 90 cm, a program of more continuous feedings may be necessary to achieve satisfactory nutrient intake. Initially, a high-carbohydrate, high-protein diet appears to be appropriate to maximize absorption. Provision of simple nutrients will keep maldigestion from being a limiting factor during absorption. Fat requires more complex absorptive mechanisms, and stool fat will increase markedly when remnants are less

than 60 cm. The initial diet should be hypo-osmolar to minimize gastrointestinal fluid losses, but it may eventually be increased later.

The nature of the diet is also important for maximizing the adaptive response of the intestine to resection. The intestinal remnant will increase its surface area and absorptive capacity in the 6 to 12 months after resection. Provision of fat and dietary fiber may be particularly important in this process. The role of other specific nutrients is currently under investigation. Glutamine is a conditionally essential amino acid that is trophic to the gut. Growth factors, such as growth hormone, may also stimulate the adaptive response and improve fluid absorption. A great deal of experimental work is being directed at the provision of such growth factors to stimulate adaptation.

Medical treatment should be directed at minimizing gastrointestinal secretion and controlling diarrhea. Dietary fiber is useful in many patients. Narcotics such as codeine, Lomotil (diphenoxylate HCl and atropine sulfate), and loperamide may improve absorption via their antisecretory and antimotility effects. The somatostatin analogue, octreotide, will improve diarrhea, not only by reducing salt and water excretion but also by prolonging small bowel transit time and reducing gastric hypersecretion. Of potential side effects, octreotide probably should not be continued indefinitely but rather should be maintained over the time of adaptation (6 to 12 months). H_2 receptor antagonists and proton pump inhibitors are useful, particularly in the first few months after operation, to control the transient gastric hypersecretion and reduce fluid loss. Cholestyramine may be marginally beneficial for binding bile salts and ameliorating bile salt–induced colonic diarrhea when the colon is in continuity. This is most effective when the patient has had an ileal resection of less than 100 cm.

Patients who have had a stoma formed at the time of their resection should be given consideration at a future time for establishing intestinal continuity. There are both advantages and disadvantages to this. By restoring continuity, absorptive capacity may be increased and transit time prolonged. Energy from short-chain fatty acids reaching the colon may increase caloric intake. Obviously, there are psychologic advantages to eliminating the stoma. Furthermore, clinical evidence suggests that infective complications are reduced when the stoma is eliminated. However, colonic bile acids may induce diarrhea with associated perianal complications and dietary restrictions. One must weigh the potential of a functional "perianal ileostomy" with intestinal restoration versus a permanent stoma. Patients with colon incontinuity are at increased risk for nephrolithiasis. However, on balance, restoration of continuity is generally advisable when more than 90 cm of small intestine is present.

Repeat laparotomy is eventually required in approximately one half of patients who have SBS. This usually is required for intestinal complications. In these patients, careful planning should be carried out to avoid further resection. As mentioned previously, utilization of intestinal tapering to improve the function of dilated segments, employing stricturoplasty for strictures, and performing serosal patching for strictures and chronic perforations will help preserve the intestinal remnant. Other intestinal segments that might be recruited into continuity should be identified as well.

There has been long-standing interest in surgical treatment for SBS with several specific goals. One objective is to improve the function of existing intestine by using the strategies mentioned previously. Obstruction should be sought and remedied, ideally by a nonresectional approach. Dilated dysfunctional segments, which may aggravate malabsorption and lead to bacterial overgrowth, should be eliminated (e.g., by tapering enteroplasty). However, an intestine-lengthening procedure has been utilized in selected patients that permits using dilated segments of bowel to lengthen the intestinal remnant. These approaches are generally quite effective and appear to have durable long-term improvement. Another goal has been to slow intestinal transit and thus improve absorption. This approach has been done with the use of a variety of techniques, including artifical valves and sphincters, reversing intestinal segments, interposing colonic segments in the small intestine, and other innovative approaches. The outcome of these procedures is less predictable, and they should be applied cautiously in carefully selected patients. Finally, the intestinal remnant can be lengthened. With recent improvements in immunosuppression, the outcome of intestinal transplantation is improving. Intestinal transplantation has now become an acceptable clinical approach to this problem in selected patients.

The appropriate operation for the patient with SBS is determined by several factors. One of the most important factors is the type of nutritional support required. Patients who are able to sustain themselves with enteral nutrition alone should generally undergo surgery only if they demonstrate worsening malabsorption, are at risk for reacquiring PN, or have significant symptoms related to malabsorption. Patients who require PN but can tolerate a significant amount of enteral feeding may be candidates for surgical therapy with the goal being to discontinue PN. Patients who develop significant complications while receiving PN should clearly be considered for operative therapy. Many of these patients, especially when children, will require either combined liver–small bowel transplantation or isolated small bowel transplantation. While liver disease is an obvious indication for transplantation, difficult vascular access and persistent or recurrent sepsis are now acceptable reasons for considering such therapy. Obviously, other patient-related factors, such as age and underlying disease, should also be carefully considered. The choice of operation for patients can best be tailored in relation to the length of the intestinal remnant, the degree of intestinal function, and the caliber of the intestinal remnant (Table 65–3).

COMPLICATIONS

Metabolic complications are common in patients with SBS related to their tremendous fluid and electrolyte fluxes and the need for specialized nutritional support. These problems include metabolic alkalosis and acidosis, including d-lactic acidosis. Hypocalcemia is commonly related to both impaired absorption and binding by intra-

Table 65–3	**Surgical Management of Short Bowel Syndrome**
CLINICAL SITUATION	**SURGICAL APPROACH**
Patient receiving enteral nutrition with intestine of adequate length (>120 cm) and normal caliber	Recruit additional intestine if possible.
Patient with bacterial overgrowth and dilated bowel	Treat obstruction. Tapering enteroplasty if intestine of adequate length. Intestinal lengthening if short length.
Patient with intestine of marginal length (60–120 cm) of normal caliber and rapid transit, requires parenteral nutrition	Recruit additional intestine. Prolong transit (reversed segment, artificial valve, colon interposition).
Patient with intestine of short length (<60 cm) of normal caliber dependent on parenteral nutrition	Optimize intestinal function if no complications. Intestinal transplantation if complications. Combined liver-intestine transplantation if irreversible liver disease.

luminal fat. Both hyperglycemia and hypoglycemia occur in patients requiring PN. Patients with SBS need to be monitored closely to detect deficiencies of iron, other minerals, vitamins, and micronutrients.

Cholelithiasis occurs in approximately one third of patients with SBS related to malabsorption of bile acids with the formation of lithogenic bile, altered bilirubin metabolism, and biliary stasis. Thus, both pigment and cholesterol stones are frequently found. The natural history of cholelithiasis in this group of patients indicates that they tend to develop more biliary complications and require more complicated surgical treatment. Cholelithiasis should always be suspected in patients with abdominal pain and abnormal liver function tests and evaluated with ultrasonography. In patients dependent on PN, intermittent cholecystokinin injections may prevent stasis and reduce formation of sludge and gallstones. Early enteral nutrition should help reduce the risk of cholelithiasis. The risk of cholelithiasis significantly increases when there is less than 120 cm of small intestine, when PN is required, and when the terminal ileum has been resected. Prophylactic cholecystectomy should be considered in these patients, either at the time of initial resection or at subsequent laparotomy.

Patients with SBS develop gastric hypersecretion in the early postoperative period. This is usually a transient phenomenon and thus should be treated with medical therapy directed at the increased acid secretion. The need for operative treatment is infrequent, but if required, a procedure such as a highly selective vagotomy may be desirable to avoid gastric resection or small bowel denervation.

Nephrolithiasis occurs in one third of patients with SBS related to reduced intraluminal calcium and the resultant increased absorption of oxalate from the intestine. Since oxalate is absorbed from the colon, this complication occurs primarily in patients with a colon remnant in continuity. The management is to minimize oxalate in the diet, minimize intraluminal fat, provide calcium supplementation, and maintain a high urinary volume.

Bacterial overgrowth may be a problem but is difficult to diagnose and requires a high degree of suspicion. Bacterial overgrowth decreases the luminal concentration of conjugated bile acids, impairs fat absorption, leads to secretory diarrhea from malabsorbed fatty acids, increases formation of short-chain fatty acids, and results in an increased osmotic load and gas production. It also impairs vitamin B_{12} absorption. This is primarily a motor abnormality, which can be treated with intermittent antibiotic therapy. However, one should always consider a mechanical cause that may be relieved by operation.

Patients requiring long-term PN are at risk for catheter-related sepsis and catheter thrombosis, which can limit the clinician's ability to maintain nutritional support in the long term, when available access sites are exhausted. PN-induced liver disease occurs in approximately 15% of adult patients. This is a multifactorial problem related to the proportion of enteral calories, overfeeding, and recurrent sepsis. It can be prevented by increasing enteral calories, avoiding overfeeding, using mixed fuels (<30% fat), and eliminating nutrient deficiencies. Administration of ursodeoxycholic acid may also be beneficial. PN-related liver disease in children with SBS is more common than in adults and is poorly understood. Treatment is not very effective and may require strong consideration of liver–small bowel transplantation.

OUTCOMES

Patients with small intestinal remnants less than 90 cm, or less than 30 cm with an intact colon, are likely to have permanent intestinal failure. The requirement of PN for 2 years also indicates permanent intestinal failure and should lead to consideration of surgical treatment if severe symptoms or complications occur.

Survival in patients with SBS is approximately 85% at 2 years and 75% at 5 years. An end-jejunostomy, remnant length less than 50 cm, and mesenteric vascular disease have a negative impact on survival. Obviously, survival will also be influenced by patient age, other medical conditions, and underlying malignancy. PN-induced liver disease has an approximate survival of 1 year without transplantation.

Nontransplantation procedures for improving intestinal

Pearls and Pitfalls

PEARLS

- Short bowel syndrome (SBS) occurs after resection of enough small bowel to cause nutritional compromise.
- The best treatment is prevention by minimizing resection length and preserving viable small bowel.
- Postoperative management after extensive small bowel resection includes inhibition of hyperacidity, maintenance of fluid and electrolytes, and early enteral nutrition.
- Complications of SBS include metabolic acidosis, cholelithiasis, nephrolithiasis, bacterial overgrowth, and parenteral nutrition–induced hepatic failure.
- Surgical treatment of SBS may involve procedures for tapering, lengthening, or relieving obstruction.
- Severe SBS, especially with associated hepatic failure, may best be treated with small bowel transplantation.

---

function are successful in approximately 85% of patients. However, success is lowest (50%) in patients who undergo procedures for prolonging intestinal transit time. One-year patient survival after intestinal transplantation is approximately 85%, but it falls to 50% at 5 years. Isolated intestinal transplantation, in general, has a better prognosis than multiple-organ grafts.

SELECTED READINGS

Abu-Elmagd K, Reyes J, Todo S, et al: Clinical intestinal transplantation: New perspectives and immunologic considerations. J Am Coll Surg 1998;186:512.

Chan S, McCowen KC, Bistran BR, et al: Incidence, prognosis, and etiology of end-stage liver disease in patients receiving home total parenteral nutrition. Surgery 1999;126:28.

Messing B, Crenn P, Beau P, et al: Long-term survival and parenteral nutrition dependence in adult patients with the short bowel syndrome. Gastroenterology 1999;117:1043.

Thompson JS: The role of prophylactic cholecystectomy in the short bowel syndrome. Arch Surg 1996;131:556.

Thompson JS: Surgical approach to the short bowel syndrome: Procedures to slow intestinal transit. Eur J Pediatr Surg 1999;9:263.

Thompson JS, Langnas AN: Surgical approaches to improving intestinal function in the short bowel syndrome. Arch Surg 1999;134:706.

Thompson JS, Langnas AN, Pinch LW, et al: Surgical approach to the short bowel syndrome. Ann Surg 1995;222:600.

Vanderhoof JA, Langnas AN: Short bowel syndrome in children and adults. Gastroenterology 1997;113:1767.

Wilmore DW, Byrne IA, Persinger RL: Short bowel syndrome: New therapeutic approaches. Curr Probl Surg 1997;34:309.

Wilmore DW, Lacy JM, Soultanakis RP, et al: Factors predicting a successful outcome after pharmacologic bowel compensation. Ann Surg 1997;226:288.

Chapter 66
Radiation Enteropathy

Mary F. Otterson

Radiation is used for the treatment of approximately 50% of all malignancies, either as the sole therapy or as an adjunct. Depending on the dosing schedule, the site, and the volume of bowel exposed, radiation produces different effects on the gastrointestinal (GI) tract (Table 66–1). The early acute signs and symptoms of radiation injury include nausea, vomiting, abdominal cramping, and diarrhea. These are associated with changes in absorption and secretion as well as changes in specific contractile patterns of the small and large intestine and develop in the vast majority of patients receiving radiotherapy. Despite this, the early signs and symptoms associated with radiation are usually self-limited.

The late effects of radiation, while less common, are more difficult to manage (Table 66–2). Some disease states predispose the patient to the development of late complications. Preexisting diabetes increases the morbidity associated with irradiation, as do other vasculopathies. The morbidity of radiation enteropathy is also higher in the elderly. Interestingly, there does not seem to be increased radiation enteropathy in patients with inflammatory bowel disease, such as ulcerative colitis or Crohn's disease. Finally, postoperative radiotherapy appears to be associated with an increased risk of intestinal complications compared to preoperative irradiation.

The late effects of radiation are best avoided by shielding the bowel from exposure. If, however, radiation enteropathy develops, the signs and symptoms usually include diarrhea, obstructive symptoms, bleeding, and fistula formation. Management of these symptoms requires a variety of strategies.

CLINICAL PRESENTATION

Early Gastrointestinal Effects of Radiation
(Fig. 66–1)

Radiation injures rapidly dividing crypt cells in the small and large intestine, producing changes in epithelial electrolyte transport and nutrient absorption. This effect, combined with the continued migration of cells to the tips of the villi, results in epithelial cell loss. The magnitude of epithelial damage is dependent on the dose and frequency of radiation exposure. Some have suggested that elemental diets may assist in maintaining acceptable nutritional status. However, the vast majority of patients tolerate standard radiotherapy without supplemental feedings or fluids because of the limited volume of intestine irradiated.

Radiation increases the frequency of an ultrapropulsive contraction associated with vomiting called the retrograde giant contraction. These retrograde giant contractions begin midway in the small intestine and rapidly propel intestinal contents into the stomach immediately prior to vomiting. Antiemetic agents have varying degrees of effectiveness either as individual agents or in combination.

Giant migrating contractions (GMCs) are another type of GI contraction initiated by radiation. These contractions, which are of large amplitude and long duration and occur spontaneously in the distal small intestine, are associated with crampy abdominal pain and, when they propagate into the colon, defecation and diarrhea. The frequency of these contractions decreases abruptly after cessation of the radiation therapy.

CLINICAL PRESENTATION AND PREOPERATIVE MANAGEMENT

Late Gastrointestinal Effects of Radiation
(Fig. 66–2)

DIARRHEA. Because of the frequency of pelvic irradiation and proximity of the ileum to the radiation field, the ileum is the most common site of GI injury secondary to radiotherapy. The most common manifestation of ileal radiation enteropathy is diarrhea, especially if the ileocecal valve or a significant amount of bowel has been resected. Management of radiation-induced diarrhea is similar to that for ileal mucosal disease or resection. Abdominal cramping and diarrhea shortly after the patient eats suggests bile salt malabsorption. Antidiarrheals, such as loperamide and Lomotil, may not eliminate the abdominal cramping. As an initial strategy, bile salt–binding agents such as cholestyramine may be helpful. If this treatment is partially effective, the dose may be increased or divided throughout the day. If this approach is not effective, decreasing dietary fat may help. Fat intolerance suggests a larger volume of damaged small intestine and should raise the question of fat-soluble vitamin malabsorption. Limiting milk and dairy ingestion may decrease diarrhea owing to lactose intolerance. When the aforementioned strategies do not eliminate the entire problem, narcotics may be helpful, as may therapy designed to decrease gastric acid production.

Table 66–1	Early Gastrointestinal Effects of Radiation

Symptoms
  Nausea
  Vomiting
  Diarrhea
  Abdominal cramping
Caused by changes in intestinal secretion, absorption, and motility

The nutritional complications of radiotherapy due to bile, fat, or lactose intolerance should initiate a search for other nutrients that may not be effectively absorbed. Vitamin B_{12} malabsorption should be suspected because this vitamin is absorbed in the ileum; in addition to the hematologic and neurologic sequelae, another consequence of vitamin B_{12} malabsorption can be an elevated serum homocysteine, which is associated with accelerated cardiac and vascular disease. Treatment involves parenteral vitamin B_{12} replacement, folic acid supplementation, and consideration of the addition of pyridoxine. If this disorder results from long-standing radiation enteropathy, the damage is not likely to be reversed. The patient will redevelop the complication if therapy is stopped.

Electrolyte disturbances, when present, can be a difficult problem. Supplemental potassium and magnesium are often needed. Potassium supplements, in pill form, may lodge proximal to a radiation-induced stricture and further injure the bowel. Liquid supplements may be needed. Magnesium, because it generates additional diarrhea, may not be tolerated as an oral supplement.

A somatostatin analogue may help control radiation-induced chronic diarrhea. The need for parenteral administration, the cost of the drug, and the discomfort of injections result in somatostatin analogues being reserved for otherwise unmanageable diarrhea.

OBSTRUCTIVE SYMPTOMS. Strictures secondary to radiotherapy may be visible on a small bowel follow-through or enteroclysis because of proximal distention. Surgical intervention must be individualized to the patient's needs, since short bowel syndrome, fistula formation, or damage to adjacent structures may result from an attempt to resect bowel damaged by radiation. Intraperitoneal scar-

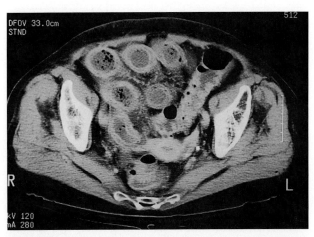

Figure 66–1. Acute effects of radiation on the bowel. This CT demonstrates the acute changes of intestinal irradiation. The bowel within the irradiated pelvic field is thickened and edematous. Although the patient was given oral contrast medium, because of the dysfunctional bowel within the pelvis, no intraluminal contrast medium is seen.

ring may be intense, particularly if the patient has had prior surgery. The patient may require a temporary or permanent ostomy. If a proximal small intestinal ostomy is necessary or a fistula occurs, volume supplementation or long-term total parental nutrition may be required. Surgical creation of the ostomy may be difficult if the mesentery is foreshortened. The discomfort of the patient who is left with a poorly functioning, proximal small intestinal ostomy that does not allow an appliance to be properly secured cannot be overestimated.

Patients with obstructive symptoms from radiation enteropathy often have malnutrition and thus face greater risk from their surgical procedure. Decreased serum albumin levels are directly correlated with an increased risk of surgical complication. In the patient who is partially obstructed and can tolerate only small volumes orally, a feeding tube with drip feedings administered at night can improve nutritional status. Occasionally, preoperative parenteral nutrition is required to prepare the patient for operation. Some authors suggest that long-term total parenteral nutrition with bowel rest may be appropriate treatment for radiation-damaged bowel.

If a previously asymptomatic patient with radiation-damaged bowel suddenly develops obstructive symptoms, causes other than irradiation, such as adhesive small bowel obstruction, recurrent malignancy, or a secondary malignancy should be considered. Although there is an increased risk of lymphoma and other tumors after radiation therapy, these new primary tumors are rare, and recurrent disease is far more likely. Computed tomography (CT) may be helpful. Surgical palliation by means of bypass or even gastrostomy tube decompression may improve the quality of life in the situation of carcinomatosis with unrelievable obstruction.

Some patients develop a form of intestinal pseudo-obstruction (lack of a true mechanical obstruction) as a consequence of radiotherapy. Pseudo-obstruction is extremely difficult to manage. The diagnosis is often made at laparotomy, when no source of the symptoms and

Table 66–2	Treatment of Late Gastrointestinal Effects of Radiation

Diarrhea
- Narcotics
- Bile salt–binding agents
- Low-fat diet
- Limit lactose
- Check for vitamin malabsorption
- Electrolyte disturbances
- Somatostatin

Obstruction
- Avoid surgery if possible
- Define the anatomy as much as possible
- Treat malnutrition aggressively
- Consider TPN
- Causes may include an adhesive obstruction, recurrent tumor, or secondary malignancy
- Pseudo-obstruction

Anal and Rectal Stricture
- Self-dilation
- Dilation with stent placement

Colonic Hemorrhage
- Formalin installation
- Electrocautery
- Laser ablation
- Hyperbaric oxygen

Enteric Fistula
- Somatostatin
- Surgery

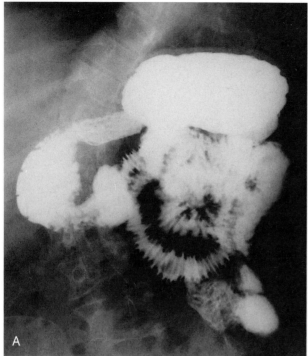

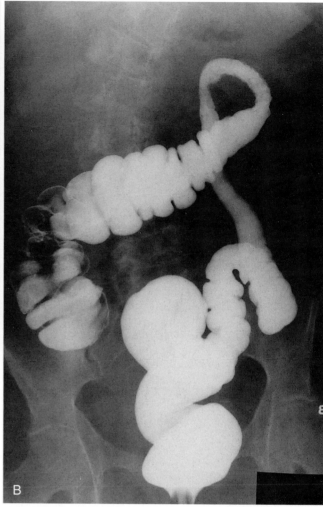

Figure 66–2. Chronic changes of the small and large intestine after irradiation. This patient received radiation therapy as a child for treatment of a Wilms' tumor. Thirty years after therapy, she developed crampy abdominal pain and guaiac-positive diarrhea. *A,* The small bowel barium study revealed thickened loops of small intestine within the left upper quadrant with sequential areas of stenosis. Note the patient's scoliosis, which is also a consequence of her previous radiation therapy. *B,* The barium enema demonstrates radiation-induced changes limited to the left upper quadrant. Note the lack of haustral markings, narrowing of the lumen, and mucosal changes.

radiographic findings can be found. If pseudo-obstruction is diagnosed, promotility agents such as erythromycin or cisapride may be helpful. If these agents are not successful, there is little to offer but prolonged total parenteral nutrition.

ANAL AND RECTAL STRICTURE. Patients who have received pelvic or perineal radiation may develop stricture of the anal canal or rectum. When the stricture is anal, simple dilation may be effective. The patient can be taught how to self-dilate. If the patient has concurrent diarrhea, anal dilation may result in partial incontinence. Rectal strictures can occasionally be managed with endoscopic dilation and stent placement. Repeated procedures may be required. Surgical diversion is reserved for patients who cannot otherwise be managed. Because of the distal obstruction, either a loop colostomy or end stoma with distal mucous fistula is required. The degree of concurrent scarring and morbidity determines the choice of surgical procedure.

COLONIC BLEEDING. Colonic hemorrhage from radiation proctitis is a rather late complication of irradiation. Bleeding from radiation proctitis represents a chronic problem in only 5% of patients receiving pelvic radiotherapy. On endoscopic examination, these patients have prominent mucosal telangiectasias. Local therapy includes installation of 4% formalin to decrease bleeding due to radiation proctitis; others have used the rectal instillation of sucralfate with minimal success. Endoscopic use of electrocautery or laser ablation is effective but demands persistent and repeated effort. Some authors suggest that hyperbaric oxygen may be helpful for patients with chronic radiation proctitis, but this approach mandates repeated administration and access to appropriate hyperbaric facilities.

Surgical resection of the involved rectum is the treatment of last resort. However, wound problems are common, and the perineum may not heal without adjunctive measures such as transfer of a muscle flap. Moreover, the patients are frequently elderly, with multiple health problems. Serious consideration of alternative therapy or referral to a center that handles a large number of these difficult patients is recommended.

ENTERIC FISTULA FORMATION. The development of a spontaneous or postoperative high-output fistula to the perineum, a second loop of bowel, vagina, bladder, or skin is a devastating complication for the patient with radiation enteropathy. These complications are frequently not amenable to conservative therapy. A trial of medical management including somatostatin may be advised. The best way of dealing with fistula formation is to avoid the initial fistula if possible. For example, if a patient who has received pelvic irradiation develops an unusual-appearing lesion at the end of the vaginal cuff, cytology determinations may prevent a full-thickness biopsy of the small intestinal wall.

SURGICAL MANAGEMENT TO PREVENT RADIATION ENTEROPATHY

Exposure of the small and large intestine is to be avoided if possible because of the risk of late consequences (Table 66–3). A variety of surgical, positioning, and radiation planning methods have been employed. These include, but are not limited to, the use of the omentum, tissue expanders, or Vicryl mesh to suspend the small bowel out of the radiation field, or radiation of tumor prior to surgery with resection of the most significantly irradiated bowel. Surgery may have occurred prior to the decision to employ radiotherapy, rendering these options not appropriate. During radiotherapy, radiation oncologists utilize techniques such as a full bladder to push the small bowel out of the pelvic field. Surgical therapy for irradiated bowel can be extremely difficult. Because of this, many practitioners recommend avoiding surgery. In addition, many signs and symptoms, particularly diarrhea, have no good surgical therapy. Each patient's treatment must be individualized according to signs and symptoms, anatomic findings, and the location and volume of bowel involved.

SURGICAL MANAGEMENT OF RADIATION-INJURED BOWEL

The surgeon must be extremely wary in treating all patients who have undergone previous radiotherapy. Even if such a patient is asymptomatic and is having surgery for other reasons, there is a serious risk of injury to the irradiated gut. When the patient presents with bowel obstruction, perforation, or massive hemorrhage, and surgery is required to preserve the patient's life, transfer to an outside facility or medical management may not be possible. In patients with perforation, peritonitis may be surprisingly localized despite the degree of scarring within the peritoneal cavity. Free air, likewise, may be absent. The surgeon may first realize the severity of the situation because a CT or contrast-enhanced study of the gut shows extravasation.

Prior to elective surgery, a modified bowel preparation

Table 66–3 | Surgical Methods for Preventing Radiation Enteropathy

Suspension of small bowel out of the pelvis
  Vicryl mesh
  Omentum
  Tissue expanders
  Radiation planning
Preoperative irradiation with removal of the most damaged tissue

Table 66–4 | Surgical Management of Irradiated Bowel

The morbidity and mortality rates of operating on irradiated bowel are very high; thus, be certain that you have maximally medically managed the patient.
Even incidental operations on irradiated bowel may become complicated.
Preoperative bowel preparation and nutritional therapy should be employed when possible.
Avoid excessive dissection.
If the bowel is injured, be certain there is no distal obstruction that will predispose to fistula formation or anastomotic breakdown.
Avoid situations that will lead to bacterial overgrowth in the remaining bowel, such as bypass.
Bowel that appears relatively normal may be damaged; remember that the pelvis has generally had the highest dose of radiation.
Avoid ostomy formation using irradiated bowel.
Resect fistulas whenever possible except in the case of the rectum. Removal of the rectum may require tissue flap transfer to close the perineal wound and has very high rates of morbidity and mortality. Diversion is safer.
Diversion to avoid a rectal or anal stricture may require a mucous fistula because of the distal obstruction.

may be helpful (Table 66–4). Oral and intravenous antibiotics that cover coliform bacteria are beneficial. Once the bowel has been opened, distal obstruction will guarantee failure of the surgical procedure, with resulting fistula or anastomotic leak. The surgeon may find a balloon catheter, such as a Foley, helpful when telescoped distally over the small bowel to ensure distal patency. This technique is not recommended if excessive surgical dissection is required.

Technically, surgery is often very difficult. The bowel may be matted without a discernible plane of dissection and is not as pliable as normal bowel. Even the mesentery is thickened and abnormal. Both the bowel and the mesentery may fracture when clamps are applied. Gentle surgical technique is essential. Unnecessary dissection of severely damaged bowel with excessive adhesiolysis is not indicated. While authors have claimed that stapled anastomoses are possible, a carefully fashioned anastomosis sewn by hand often is the best option.

If a stricture requires resection, the small intestine should be excised to a segment of normal-appearing bowel. Radiation damage may extend beyond the bowel that is obviously involved. The mucosa of radiation-strictured bowel does not generally contribute significantly to the absorptive capacity of the patient. Modification of a stricturoplasty technique has been suggested for patients with "isolated" strictures; however, use of this technique has not been widespread. In general, the length of involved bowel precludes a simple mucosal-preserving Heineke-Mikulicz stricturoplasty, and a longer stricturoplasty or bypassed loop may predispose to enteric stasis and bacterial overgrowth. Moreover, the stricturoplasty suture line is carried out in irradiated bowel with a resultant poor blood supply; that is why the stricture occurred.

It is preferable to resect, rather than to bypass, the involved segment of bowel. When the distal ileum is involved, resection and anastomosis to a segment of bowel out of the irradiated field (which is usually the pelvis) may decrease the rate of complication. This usually means also resecting part of the ascending colon to allow anastomosis to nonirradiated colon. Even in diseases such as ovarian cancer, in which the entire abdomen may have been irradiated, a pelvic boost of radiation has usually been administered. Bowel in the upper abdomen will have a reduced radiation exposure and thus should tolerate the anastomosis better.

Fistulas should be resected, rather than bypassed. In general, fistulas are not operated on under emergent conditions. Appropriate nutritional preparation of the patient, appropriate bowel preparation, and careful technique are essential. One possible exception in which resection of a fistula is often contraindicated is rectovaginal fistula. Resection of the irradiated rectum carries significant morbidity and mortality, and the patient may be better served by a proximal diversion. The distal sigmoid colon used for the ostomy may not heal as well as the more proximal colon because of its exposure to the radiation field. In general, it is better to avoid making a stoma from irradiated bowel.

OUTCOMES

Radiation enteropathy is a challenging clinical problem. Perioperative morbidity rates are between 30% and 50%, with mortality rates of 10% to 15%! Approximately half of all patients who require surgery for unrelenting problems have subsequent signs and symptoms of radiation enteropathy. Because of these discouraging results, a keen understanding of the medical therapies possible allows the surgeon to adequately care for this population. Care of these patients requires a clear understanding of the normal role of the small and large intestine as well as pharmacologic and surgical interventions for handling the pathophysiologic sequelae of radiation injury. The data that support therapeutic options for the patient with radiation enteropathy are limited and frequently anecdotal. There have been no large, randomized prospective studies on small intestinal, colonic, rectal, and pelvic floor function following irradiation. The region of bowel affected in each patient may vary widely; thus, it is unlikely that large studies will be possible. Therefore, the clinician

Pearls and Pitfalls

- Beware of unnecessary surgery in radiation enteropathy.
- Signs and symptoms of radiation-induced bowel damage include diarrhea, obstruction, perforation, and fistula.
- When surgical intervention is necessary, preoperative preparation of the patient should include optimization of nutritional state, perioperative antibiotics, and bowel preparation if possible.
- Operative outcomes are best when anastomoses involve nonirradiated segments of bowel; if possible and safe, avoid surgical bypasses.
- Radiation proctitis is treated with intrarectal formalin, endoscopic therapy, or proximal diversion.
- The best treatment of radiation enteropathy is to avoid gut radiation injury by preradiation planning of portals, preoperative radiation, and postoperative bowel exclusion.
- Confirmation of patent distal bowel is essential prior to resection/ostomy for obstructed bowel segment.

is left with anecdotal reports and personal experience to rely on in treating these challenging patients.

SELECTED READINGS

Chapuis P, Dent O, Bokey E, et al: The development of a treatment protocol for patients with chronic radiation-induced rectal bleeding. Aust N Z J Surg 1996;66:680.
Counter SF, Froese DP, Hart MJ: Prospective evaluation of formalin therapy for radiation proctitis. Am J Surg 1999;177:396.
de Almeida J: Extramucosal stricturoplasty: A new surgical technique for radiation enteritis. Dig Surg 1997;14:492.
Mann WJ: Surgical management of radiation enteropathy. Surg Clin North Am 1991;71:977.
Ooi BS, Tjandra JJ, Green MD: Morbidities of adjuvant chemotherapy and radiotherapy for resectable rectal cancer: An overview. Dis Colon Rectum 1999;42:403.
Otterson MF, Sarna SK, Moulder JE: Effects of fractionated doses of ionizing radiation on small intestinal motor activity. Gastroenterology 1988;95:1249.
Swan RW: Stagnant loop syndrome resulting from small-bowel irradiation injury and intestinal by-pass. Gynecol Oncol 1974;2:441.
Wang J, Zheng H, Sung CC, Hauer-Jensen M: The synthetic somatostatin analogue, octreotide, ameliorates acute and delayed intestinal radiation injury. Int J Radiat Oncol Biol Phys 1999;1:1289.

Chapter 67

Splanchnic Venous Thrombosis
Nicholas J. Zyromski and Michael G. Sarr

Venous thrombosis of the splanchnic circulation consists of four separate entities: mesenteric venous thrombosis (MVT), isolated splenic vein thrombosis, extrahepatic portal vein thrombosis, and hepatovenous occlusive disease (Budd-Chiari syndrome). All of these conditions share several potential pathogenic factors. This chapter examines the etiopathogenesis of splanchnic venous thrombosis, then considers each individual disease with primary emphasis on the most common splanchnic veno-occlusive disorder—MVT.

ETIOPATHOGENESIS

Most patients with splanchnic venous thrombosis have underlying pathology related to some combination of Virchow's triad of hypercoagulability, stasis, and endothelial injury (Table 67–1). Primary hypercoagulable states include protein C and protein S deficiency, activated protein C resistance caused by Factor V Leiden gene mutation, antithrombin III deficiency, and dysfibrinogenemia. Splanchnic venous thrombosis has also been reported in patients with secondary hypercoagulable states resulting from cancer, pregnancy, oral contraceptive use, polycythemia vera, paroxysmal nocturnal hemoglobinuria, myeloproliferative disorders, and splenectomy with subsequent thrombocytosis. In addition, conditions predisposing to a low flow state (such as congestive heart failure, portal hypertension, and cirrhosis), intra-abdominal inflamma-

tory diseases (such as pancreatitis, pelvic abscess, appendicitis, and diverticulitis), and blunt abdominal trauma have all been associated with splanchnic venous thrombosis.

MESENTERIC VENOUS THROMBOSIS

MVT, first reported by Elliot in 1895, accounts for 5% to 15% of all intestinal vascular occlusive disease with peak incidence occurring in the sixth and seventh decades of life. Although advances in imaging techniques and improved awareness have led to earlier diagnosis and treatment, MVT is still associated with a high degree of morbidity and mortality. Long-term prognosis of patients afflicted with this condition remains poor overall, because untreated acute MVT leads to intestinal necrosis and perforation. Rapid diagnosis and institution of therapy is essential for optimal outcome.

MVT has been defined as acute or chronic, depending on presentation, as well as primary or secondary, based on the absence or presence of an underlying disease process. Rhee and colleagues demonstrated that patients with minimal symptoms for greater than 4 weeks had significantly fewer complications from MVT than those with a more acute presentation, and they defined the cutoff point between acute and chronic MVT at 4 weeks. With increased availability and use of computed tomography (CT) in the diagnosis of abdominal disorders, a subgroup of asymptomatic patients with thrombus in the mesenteric venous system has been identified. In an autopsy series, bowel necrosis was present only in cases involving thrombosis of the venous arcades and vasa recta, suggesting that the bowel would remain viable if collateral vessels were free from occlusion. It is likely that patients with chronic MVT (asymptomatic or mild, chronic symptoms) have an adequate array of patent collateral vessels. Symptoms begin and progress as thrombus propagates to the small veins and intestinal ischemia develops.

CLINICAL PRESENTATION

Pain is the principal symptom of patients with MVT, ranging from intermittent generalized abdominal discomfort to severe, colicky, periumbilical pain. Symptoms often develop subtly, progressing in severity over the course of hours to days. The classic intestinal ischemic pain out of proportion to physical findings, as occurs frequently with arterial insufficiency to the gut, occurs in only approximately 20% of patients with MVT. Obstructive-like symptoms may also be present, with abdominal distention, nausea, vomiting, and constipation. Patients may mount a low-grade fever, and stool from rectal examination is often

Table 67–1	Etiology of Splanchnic Venous Thrombosis	
Inherited coagulopathy	Protein C deficiency
	Protein S deficiency
	Factor V Leiden deficiency
	Antithrombin III deficiency
	Dysfibrinogenemia
Secondary coagulopathy	Oral contraceptive*
	Malignancy
Hematologic coagulopathy	Polycythemia vera
	Paroxysmal nocturnal hemoglobinuria
	Hyperfibrinogenemia
	Myeloproliferative disorders
	Postsplenectomy thrombocytopenia
Splanchnic low-flow states	Congestive heart failure
	Cirrhosis with portal hypertension
Intra-abdominal pathology	Pancreatitis
	Inflammatory bowel disease
	Diverticulitis
	Appendicitis
	Perforated viscus
	Pelvic abscess
	Trauma

*In select patients

447

positive for occult blood. Grossly bloody diarrhea is a late sign; by this point, intestinal necrosis has almost invariably occurred. Findings of localized or generalized peritonitis also occur late in the course of the disease, usually related to transmural disease and thus dictating surgical intervention. A subset of patients with chronic MVT may be relatively asymptomatic or have mild complaints over a longer period of time. Early diagnosis is especially difficult in this group of patients.

DIAGNOSIS

A high degree of clinical suspicion is essential in making the preoperative diagnosis of MVT. This is key because the treatment of choice once the diagnosis is made involves immediate anticoagulation in an attempt to arrest progression of the thrombotic process. Thus, early diagnosis is crucial. A thorough history in patients with suspected MVT should include evaluation of factors predisposing to primary or secondary hypercoagulability, including a careful search for familial thrombotic disorders.

Laboratory evaluations are generally of little use in making the diagnosis of MVT. Leukocytosis, with a shift to the left, or bandemia is usually present, but serum enzyme levels of amylase, lactate, or lactate dehydrogenase are rarely elevated.

Plain abdominal radiography may be most useful in ruling out other intra-abdominal pathology, such as free air. The small bowel may have a thickened wall, many fluid-filled loops, and either a diffusely spaced gas pattern or even a nonspecific obstructive pattern. CT is currently the imaging modality of choice for diagnosis of MVT, offering greater than 90% sensitivity when the diagnosis is suspected. CT findings include visualization of clot in the superior mesenteric, portal, or splenic veins, thickening of the bowel wall with "thumbprinting" or pneumatosis intestinalis, and prominent inflammatory changes in the mesentery (Fig. 67–1). Air in the portal venous system is a late, grave finding consistent with intestinal necrosis. Improvements in magnetic resonance imaging of the gut vasculature are promising, with sensitivity being up to 100%; however, experience is limited, the test is expensive, and, overall, magnetic resonance imaging offers little advantage over CT. Ultrasonography may be helpful early in the course of the disease, but progressive inflammation and accumulation of intestinal air may hinder visualization of vascular structures. Mesenteric angiography with venous phase imaging is not routinely used in patients who are suspected to have MVT but it may be helpful. Thrombus extending into the superior mesenteric vein is the most common finding in this imaging modality.

In the past, some investigators have recommended diagnostic peritoneal lavage to rule out MVT. The presence of serosanguineous fluid is consistent with bowel ischemia, but this finding is not usually present until late in the course of the disease. Laparoscopy may be used to confirm the diagnosis of ischemic bowel but the utility of this approach is limited by the inability to evaluate the extent of vascular disease.

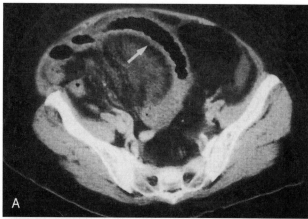

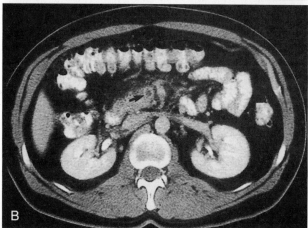

Figure 67–1. Computed tomography findings in mesenteric venous thrombosis. *A,* Thickened, distended small bowel with mesenteric streaking. *B,* Thrombus in superior mesenteric vein. (From Rhee RY, et al: Mesenteric venous thrombosis: Still a lethal disease in the 1990s. J Vasc Surg 1994;20:688–697, with permission.)

MANAGEMENT

As soon as the diagnosis of MVT is secured or highly suspected, intravenous anticoagulation with heparin should be instituted and maintained throughout the operation (if operation becomes necessary) and postoperative period. Anticoagulation reduces extension and recurrence of thrombosis and overall morbidity. Many authors also endorse early treatment with broad-spectrum antibiotics, and although there is no conclusive data to support this practice, it remains intuitively logical because of presumed bacterial translocation. Some patients with MVT may be successfully managed with resuscitation and anticoagulation alone. Rhee and colleagues reported a series of selected cases managed medically versus those requiring surgical intervention. Short- and long-term mortality rates were similar in both groups. Disease managed medically had a higher incidence of symptomatic recurrence than did disease treated surgically. Patients whose treatment consists of observation and anticoagulation should undergo frequent physical examination; prompt operative intervention is necessary if the patient's condition deteriorates or signs of peritonitis develop. Patients whose MVT is successfully managed medically must be maintained on lifelong anticoagulation with oral warfarin.

Scattered anecdotal reports of lytic therapy with urokinase, tissue plasminogen activator, and streptokinase have appeared in the literature, and in selected situations may offer a treatment alternative in high-risk patients. The possibility of hemorrhagic complications must be given serious consideration before this therapy is undertaken.

Operative intervention is indicated when signs of peritonitis develop or the patient's general condition deteriorates. At operation, the bowel is usually found to be cyanotic and edematous, with a thick, woody mesentery. Clot within the mesenteric veins is generally evident if resection is necessary. Intravenous fluorescein angiography and a Wood lamp have been used to determine bowel viability in attempts to minimize the length of bowel resected; however, margins of viable intestine may still be difficult to define. Strong consideration should be given to a planned second-look laparotomy 24 hours after initial operation. Occasionally, MVT involves necrosis of the entire jejunoileum, precluding treatment.

Although thrombectomy has been reported anecdotally in patients with MVT, clot may involve long segments of the venous system, making this procedure technically difficult or impossible. In addition, the venotomy itself may act as a nidus for new thrombus. Attempts at thrombectomy should be considered only in the acute situation when localized fresh clot is less than 3 days old.

Despite improvements in diagnosis and treatment, early and late mortality rates remain substantial (13% to 50%). Morbidity is also significant, often being related to the patient's underlying poor medical condition. Patients should be maintained on long-term oral anticoagulation to minimize the chance of recurrent MVT; even so, recurrence rates remain high, and long-term prognosis is generally poor. When an underlying primary hypercoagulable state is found to be the cause of MVT, immediate family members should be screened for this condition as well (Fig. 67–2).

SPLENIC VEIN THROMBOSIS

Isolated thrombosis of the splenic vein commonly arises as a result of pancreatic disease, such as severe acute or

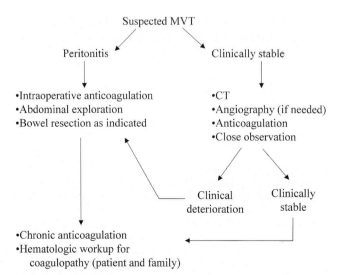

Figure 67–2. Algorithm for management of suspected mesenteric venous thrombosis.

chronic pancreatitis or malignancy. Presenting complaints are usually related to the underlying condition or involve upper gastrointestinal hemorrhage from gastric varices related to "left-sided" or "sinistral" hypertension. Diagnosis in asymptomatic patients is often secured serendipitously by CT. Treatment of splenic vein thrombosis is dependent on the underlying pathology and symptoms. The presence of splenic vein thrombosis in acute or chronic pancreatitis is not in itself an indication for surgical intervention; indeed, splenectomy in asymptomatic patients with splenic vein thrombosis (even in the presence of gastric varices) is unwarranted because complications do not develop in approximately 75% of these patients. Hemorrhage from gastric varices generally requires sclerotherapy or splenectomy. In the case of advanced pancreatic malignancy, treatment is precluded. Less aggressive tumors, such as islet cell tumors or cystic neoplasms, may be resectable regardless of splenic vein involvement.

HEPATOVENOUS OCCLUSIVE DISEASE (BUDD-CHIARI SYNDROME)

Budd-Chiari syndrome may result from several diverse etiologies, including primary or secondary hypercoagulable states (as discussed earlier), a poorly understood oblitierative veno-occlusive disease, and rarely from hepatic neoplasm or web in the suprahepatic inferior vena cava. The disease occasionally manifests acutely with right upper quadrant abdominal pain, tender hepatomegaly, ascites, and acute hepatic failure. More common, however, is the presentation of a subacute process evolving over days to weeks, with vague right upper quadrant abdominal pain, malaise, hepatomegaly, ascites, and signs of portal hypertension. The latter two findings in the absence of known liver disease should prompt consideration of this diagnosis. Diagnostic measures include evaluation of ascites, which reveals a very high protein content (>2.5 g/ 100 mL), a sharp contrast to the ascites of cirrhotic liver disease. Contrast-enhanced CT or liver–spleen nuclear isotope scan may show heterogeneous enhancement of the liver with an engorged caudate lobe. Retrograde hepatic venogram, if necessary, confirms hepatic venous occlusion and the presence of collateral vessels. Use of magnetic resonance imaging may be helpful in select patients.

Therapy proceeds based on underlying etiology and vascular or hemodynamic status, with acute presentations requiring emergent intervention to prevent fulminant hepatic failure (Fig. 67–3). The goal of therapy is to provide a low-pressure hepatic venous outflow. This may be accomplished with transjugular intrahepatic portosystemic shunt for emergent relief of variceal hemorrhage or ascites or with surgical portosystemic shunting in more elective situations. Both these options are generally well tolerated by the liver. In patients with retrohepatic caval occlusion, portocaval shunting is not possible because of high infrahepatic caval pressures; a mesoatrial shunt with ringed PTFE (polytetrafluoroethylene) may be used in this situation. Rarely, hepatic transplantation may be necessary in the case of permanent hepatic failure. In occa-

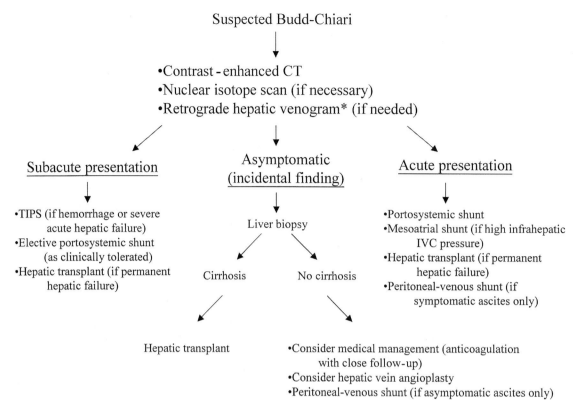

Suspected Budd-Chiari

• Contrast-enhanced CT
• Nuclear isotope scan (if necessary)
• Retrograde hepatic venogram* (if needed)

Subacute presentation

• TIPS (if hemorrhage or severe acute hepatic failure)
• Elective portosystemic shunt (as clinically tolerated)
• Hepatic transplant (if permanent hepatic failure)

Asymptomatic (incidental finding)

Liver biopsy

Cirrhosis   No cirrhosis

Acute presentation

• Portosystemic shunt
• Mesoatrial shunt (if high infrahepatic IVC pressure)
• Hepatic transplant (if permanent hepatic failure)
• Peritoneal-venous shunt (if symptomatic ascites only)

Hepatic transplant

• Consider medical management (anticoagulation with close follow-up)
• Consider hepatic vein angioplasty
• Peritoneal-venous shunt (if asymptomatic ascites only)

*include measurement of pressure gradient across retrohepatic vena cava

Figure 67–3. Algorithm for management of suspected Budd-Chiari syndrome.

sional patients with only symptomatic ascites, management has been by peritoneal-venous shunting. Optimal management of chronic or the recently described asymptomatic Budd-Chiari syndrome is less clear. If liver biopsy reveals cirrhosis, transplantation should be performed. Select asymptomatic cases have been managed with long-term anticoagulation, with or without hepatic vein angioplasty. Close follow-up of these patients is essential.

EXTRAHEPATIC PORTAL VEIN THROMBOSIS

Extrahepatic portal, mesenteric, or splenic vein thrombosis is a more chronic condition, usually recognized incidentally on CT or ultrasonography. Symptoms, when they occur, are usually sequelae of portal hypertension (gastric or esophageal hemorrhage) or from the underlying pathologic process—pancreatic inflammatory or neoplastic disease. As with MVT, many patients have an underlying hypercoagulable state, and aggressive workup for these conditions should be undertaken when the diagnosis of portal thrombosis is suspected or made. A unique subset of affected patients includes children with omphalitis or an omphalomesenteric catheter as a neonate.

As with MVT, systemic anticoagulation is the mainstay of therapy and should be maintained indefinitely in patients with documented hypercoagulable conditions. Anticoagulation has not been shown to increase the incidence or severity of gastrointestinal hemorrhage and paradoxically may be protective against hemorrhage. Surgical therapy is required only to correct complications of splanchnic

hypertension or the underlying etiologic process when aggressive, nonoperative management has failed. Select patients may benefit from portal-systemic decompressive procedures as long as the distal venous system is patent.

Pearls and Pitfalls

PEARLS

• Venous thrombosis of the gut may involve small veins of the mesentery (MVT), large extrahepatic splanchnic veins (superior mesenteric, portal, or splenic vein thrombosis), the isolated splenic vein (with or without "sinistral" or "left-sided" hypertension), or hepatic veins (Budd-Chiari syndrome).

• All patients with splanchnic venous thrombosis should be investigated for an underlying thrombotic disorder (acquired or familial).

• A high degree of clinical suspicion is essential for diagnosis; CT is the optimal imaging modality.

• Treatment of MVT and extrahepatic large splanchnic venous thrombosis is immediate and long-term anticoagulation.

• Treatment of sinistral portal hypertension is splenectomy if symptomatic (hemorrhage from gastric varices) or observation if asymptomatic.

• Treatment of Budd-Chiari syndrome ranges from observation to portosystemic shunt to hepatic transplantation, depending on acuity of presentation and severity of the disease.

Mesenteric/portal thrombectomy has been done in conjunction with shunting procedures but seems injudicial in light of the chronic nature of most portal thrombotic process.

SELECTED READINGS

Gehl H, Bohndorf K, Klose K, et al: Two-dimensional MR angiography in evaluation of abdominal vein with gradients refocused sequences. J Comput Assist Tomogr 1990;14:619.

Harward T, Green D, Bergan J, et al: Mesenteric venous thrombosis. J Vasc Surg 1989;9:328.

Hassan HA, Raufman J-P: Mesenteric venous thrombosis. South Med J 1999;92:558.

Loftus J, Nagorney D, Illstrup D, Kuuselman A: Sinistral portal hypertension. Ann Surg 1993;217:35.

Orloff MJ. Budd-Chiari syndrome: Shunt or transplant? HPB Surg 1998;11:136.

Poplausky M, Kaufman J, Geller S, et al: Mesenteric venous thrombosis treated with urokinase via the superior mesenteric artery. Gastroenterology 1996;110:1633.

Rhee RY, Gloviczki P, Mendonca CT, et al: Mesenteric venous thrombosis: Still a lethal disease in the 1990s. J Vasc Surg 1994;20:688.

Small Bowel: Malignant

Chapter 68
Adenocarcinoma of the Small Bowel

B. Mark Evers

INCIDENCE AND PATHOGENESIS

Small bowel cancers are exceedingly rare even though the small bowel constitutes approximately 80% of the total length of the gastrointestinal tract and makes up more than 90% of the mucosal surface area. Adenocarcinomas constitute approximately 50% of malignant tumors of the small bowel. In most reported series, the peak incidence occurs in the seventh decade of life and is slightly higher in men. Similar to colon cancer, the incidence tends to be higher in Western industrialized countries. The majority of adenocarcinomas are located in the duodenum and the proximal jejunum. In the duodenum, approximately 65% of adenocarcinomas occur adjacent to the ampulla of Vater but are entities separate from ampullary carcinomas.

Risk factors for adenocarcinoma of the small bowel include familial adenomatous polyposis syndromes (e.g., familial adenomatous polyposis, Gardner's syndrome, and Turcot's syndrome), hereditary nonpolyposis colorectal carcinoma, von Recklinghausen's disease, celiac disease, and Crohn's disease. It has been estimated that adenocarcinoma develops in 2% to 3% of patients with small intestinal Crohn's disease, with the majority of patients having had symptomatic disease for at least 5 years. Adenocarcinomas arising in association with Crohn's disease tend to occur in a younger age group, with a mean age of 46 years, as opposed to a mean age of about 60 years for sporadic small bowel adenocarcinomas. Other factors that have been suggested, but not proven, to contribute to small bowel cancer include a high fat intake, consumption of red meat or salt-cured or smoked food, cigarette smoking, and alcohol consumption. Although the molecular genetics of small bowel adenocarcinoma have not

been entirely characterized, similar to colorectal cancers, mutations of the *K-ras* gene are commonly noted.

CLINICAL MANIFESTATIONS

The clinical presentation of adenocarcinoma of the small bowel depends on the location of the tumor. Tumors of the periampullary region may present early with obstructive jaundice or bleeding. In the distal duodenum, the jejunum, and the ileum, symptoms are usually more nonspecific, with abdominal pain and weight loss due to progressive intestinal obstruction the presenting complaints in the majority of patients. Given the rarity of these cancers, a high index of suspicion is required.

In addition, patients may on rare occasion present with diarrhea, tenesmus, and passage of large amounts of mucus. Gastrointestinal bleeding, manifested by anemia and guaiac-positive stools or occasionally by melena or hematochezia, may occur. A palpable mass has been reported in approximately one fourth of patients with small bowel adenocarcinoma. Although patients may present with perforation and peritonitis, acute presentation indicative of an abdominal catastrophe is rare.

Adenocarcinomas of the small bowel may be flat and ulcerating, polypoid, or cicatricial (Fig. 68–1). The cancers typically infiltrate the intestinal wall, causing obstruction, and metastasize to regional lymph nodes; hematogenous spread is also common.

DIAGNOSIS

Barium contrast studies are the most useful diagnostic tests, with an abnormality noted in up to 90% of patients

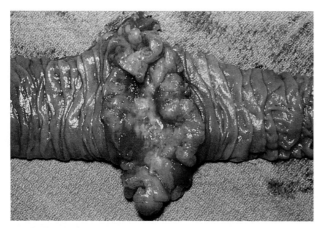

Figure 68–1. Polypoid adenocarcinoma of the jejunum. (Courtesy of Melvyn H. Schreiber, MD, The University of Texas Medical Branch, Galveston, Tex.)

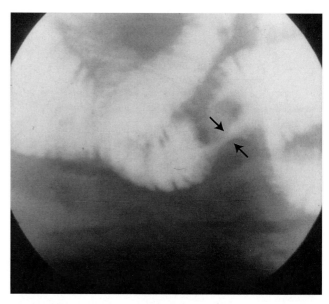

Figure 68–3. Barium radiograph demonstrating a typical apple-core lesion (*arrows*) caused by an adenocarcinoma of the jejunum. (Courtesy of Melvyn H. Schreiber, MD, The University of Texas Medical Branch, Galveston, Tex.)

with adenocarcinoma. Findings include filling defects and mucosal ulcerations (Fig. 68–2) or a typical apple-core constrictive lesion (Fig. 68–3). Upper endoscopy may be helpful in the diagnosis of duodenal lesions provided the lesion is in the proximal duodenum, but distal lesions (third and fourth portions of the duodenum) may not be evident with regular diagnostic endoscopy and often require an "extended" endoscopy. During colonoscopy, the colonoscope can on occasion be advanced into the

terminal ileum for visualization and biopsy of distal ileal neoplasms. Plain films may confirm the presence of an obstruction; however, for the most part, they are not helpful in establishing the diagnosis of small bowel cancer. Computed tomography of the abdomen may provide the most useful information regarding staging, the involvement of surrounding structures, and the distinction between primary and metastatic tumors (Fig. 68–4).

TREATMENT

The treatment of choice for adenocarcinoma arising in the periampullary duodenum is pancreaticoduodenectomy (Fig. 68–5). For tumors arising in the third or the

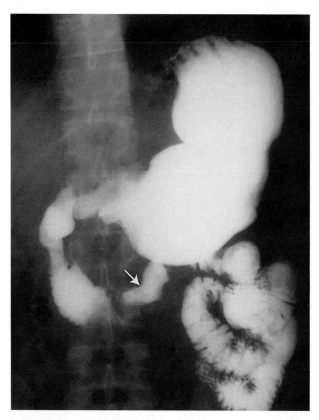

Figure 68–2. Adenocarcinoma of the third and fourth portions of the duodenum. A large filling defect is surmounted by an ulcer crater (*arrow*). (Courtesy of Melvyn H. Schreiber, MD, The University of Texas Medical Branch, Galveston, Tex.)

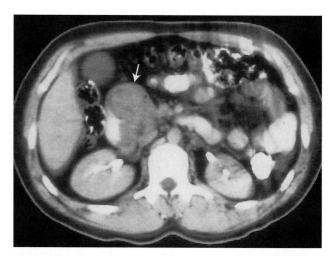

Figure 68–4. Computed tomography of the abdomen demonstrating duodenal adenocarcinoma (*arrow*). (Courtesy of Melvyn H. Schreiber, MD, The University of Texas Medical Branch, Galveston, Tex.)

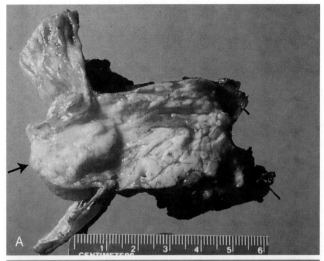

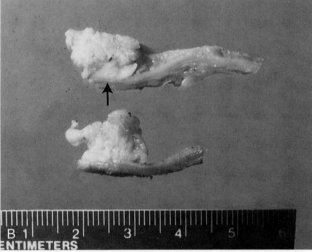

Figure 68–5. *A,* Pancreaticoduodenectomy performed for periampullary cancer (*arrow*). *B,* Cutting and fixation demonstrate that the cancer is arising from the ampulla (*arrow*). (Courtesy of Zoran Gatalica, MD, The University of Texas Medical Branch, Galveston, Tex.)

ble palliative results in poor-risk patients with unresectable disease. If bleeding is a significant symptom, endoscopic palliation using laser photocoagulation may be beneficial and would prevent the need for palliative resection.

For cancers arising in the jejunum or the ileum, wide en bloc resection of the primary tumor, including a wide wedge of mesentery with its regional lymph nodes, should be performed followed by primary end-to-end anastomosis (Fig. 68–6). In adenocarcinomas arising in the terminal ileum, right hemicolectomy and ileotransverse colostomy are best performed to maximize the lymphadenectomy. Even with the presence of metastatic disease, small bowel resection should be performed for palliation of jejunal or ileal cancers to prevent bleeding or subsequent obstruction.

The role of radiation and chemotherapy in the management of small bowel adenocarcinoma has not been entirely defined; however, these modalities do not currently appear to offer any significant benefit to overall survival. Based on the results with other gastrointestinal cancers, it appears that any beneficial role for radiation and chemotherapy in small bowel cancers may be limited to adjuvant treatment. Also, the use of newer chemotherapeutic agents, such as irinotecan (CPT-11), has yet to be evaluated for these cancers.

PROGNOSIS

The prognosis for resectable adenocarcinoma of the duodenum is relatively good, with a 5-year survival rate reported to be approximately 50% in most series. Most tumors of the distal duodenum, the jejunum, and the ileum present at a more advanced stage. The prognosis for these cancers is less favorable, with overall 5-year survival rates ranging from 5% to 30%. Less than 50% of patients with cancers of the distal duodenum, the jejunum, or the ileum will have tumors confined to the bowel wall; approximately 25% have distant metastases at the

fourth portion of the duodenum, segmental resection with duodenojejunostomy may be performed, because a classic pancreatoduodenectomy does not include the primary lymphatic drainage basin. Unlike cancers in the first and the second portions of the duodenum, neoplasms in this location tend to drain into the small bowel mesentery, and not through the head of the pancreas. Before extensive resection is performed, a thorough exploration should be carried out in an attempt to detect hepatic or serosal metastases. Metastasis to lymph nodes does not necessarily preclude resection, however. Although the survival rate for patients with negative lymph nodes is better, long-term survival can still be achieved after complete resection (R_0) with node-positive tumors, supporting an aggressive approach to treatment.

In patients with clearly unresectable duodenal carcinoma (e.g., with multiple hepatic metastases), gastrojejunostomy and biliary bypass can be performed for palliation. Alternative forms of palliative therapy involving endoscopically placed biliary stents can provide compara-

Pearls and Pitfalls

- Small bowel cancers are rare; adenocarcinomas constitute approximately 50% of malignant tumors of the small bowel.
- The majority are located in the duodenum and the proximal jejunum.
- Known risk factors include inherited polyposis syndromes and Crohn's disease.
- Presentation is dependent on location, with proximal duodenal tumors presenting as obstructive jaundice with bleeding and tumors of the jejunum and the ileum presenting with nonspecific abdominal pain and weight loss.
- Barium contrast studies are the most useful diagnostic tests.
- Treatment is resection; the role of radiation and chemotherapy has not been defined.
- Survival rates are 50% to 70% in the absence of nodal involvement but only 15% when positive nodes are found.

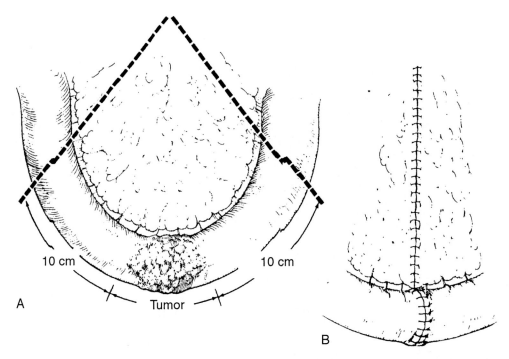

Figure 68–6. Surgical management of carcinoma of the small bowel. *A*, Malignant tumors should be resected with a wide margin of normal bowel and a wedge of mesentery to remove the immediate draining lymph nodes. *B*, End-to-end anastomosis of the small bowel and repair of the mesentery. (Adapted from Thompson JC: Atlas of Surgery of the Stomach, Duodenum and Small Bowel. St. Louis, Mosby-Year Book, 1992, p 299.)

time of diagnosis. In the absence of lymph node involvement, survival rates range from 50% to 70%. Survival rates drop to less than 15% when positive lymph nodes are identified.

SELECTED READINGS

Arber N, Neugut AI, Weinstein IB, Holt P: Molecular genetics of small bowel cancer. Cancer Epidemiol Biomarkers Prev 1997;6:745–748.

Ashley SW, Wells SA Jr: Tumors of the small intestine. Semin Oncol 1988;15:116–128.

Bakaeen FG, Murr MM, Sarr MG, et al: What prognostic factors are important in duodenal adenocarcinoma? Arch Surg 2000;135:635–641.

Buckley JA, Jones B, Fishman EK: Small bowel cancer. Imaging features and staging. Radiol Clin North Am 1997;35:381–402.

Cunningham JD, Aleali R, Aleali M, et al: Malignant small bowel neoplasms: Histopathologic determinants of recurrence and survival. Ann Surg 1997;225:300–306.

Evers BM: Small bowel. In Townsend CM Jr (ed): Sabiston Textbook of Surgery, 16th ed. Philadelphia, WB Saunders, 2001, pp 873–916.

Minardi AJ Jr, Zibari GB, Aultman DF, et al: Small-bowel tumors. J Am Coll Surg 1998;186:664–668.

Neugut AI, Jacobson JS, Suh S, et al: The epidemiology of cancer of the small bowel. Cancer Epidemiol Biomarkers Prev 1998;7:243–251.

O'Riordan BG, Vilor M, Herrera L: Small bowel tumors: An overview. Dig Dis 1996;14:245–257.

Rochlin DB, Longmire WP Jr: Primary tumors of the small intestine. Surgery 1961;50:586–592.

Rodriguez-Bigas MA, Vasen HFA, Lynch HT, et al: Characteristics of small bowel carcinoma in hereditary nonpolyposis colorectal carcinoma. Cancer 1998;83:240–244.

Sohn TA, Lillemoe KD, Cameron JL, et al: Adenocarcinoma of the duodenum: Factors influencing long-term survival. J Gastrointest Surg 1998;2:79–87.

Chapter 69

Lymphoma of the Small Bowel

Syed A. Ahmad, Jorge E. Romaguera, and Lee M. Ellis

Lymphomas are the third most common malignancy in the small bowel, with 1.6 cases diagnosed per 1,000,000 people each year; the gastrointestinal (GI) tract is the location of approximately 5% to 10% of all lymphomas and is the most common extranodal site of origin (24%). The stomach is the most common location of GI lymphoma, with small intestinal sites being second in frequency and contributing one quarter of the total number of GI lymphomas. In the West, small intestinal lymphomas account for about 2% of all malignancies of the alimentary canal.

The distinction between primary small bowel lymphoma and secondary involvement is critical. Primary small bowel lymphoma has previously been characterized as lymphoma that either presents with symptoms of GI involvement or has predominant small bowel involvement. A more stringent definition of primary small bowel lymphoma includes (1) absence of peripheral lymphadenopathy at clinical presentation; (2) absence of mediastinal adenopathy on chest radiography; (3) normal peripheral blood smear results; (4) involvement of the small bowel, the regional lymph nodes, or both at laparotomy; and (5) absence of liver and spleen involvement, except by direct spread from a contiguous focus. Primary lymphoma in the small bowel is rare, but secondary lymphomatous involvement of the GI tract in conjunction with disseminated disease is not uncommon.

Small bowel lymphoma occurs most often in the ileum (51%), followed by the jejunum (41%) and the duodenum (8%). The type and pattern of disease differ with respect to the extent of industrialization of the country. In developing countries, lymphoma, most often the alpha chain or the immunoproliferative small bowel type, is the most common small bowel cancer; it can arise anywhere in the small bowel, is most often found in young adults, and is associated with a poor survival rate. In industrialized countries, small bowel lymphoma is relatively rare, arises mainly in the ileum, is associated with relatively favorable survival (unless related to human immunodeficiency virus), and is most often of the diffuse, non-Hodgkin's B-cell type.

Numerous risk factors have been implicated in the development of small bowel lymphoma. Immunosuppression—whether from organ transplantation, acquired immunodeficiency syndrome, Wiskott-Aldrich syndrome, or other immunodeficiency syndromes—increases the risk of developing small bowel lymphoma. Small intestinal lymphoma has also been associated with small bowel enteropathies such as celiac disease and malabsorption syndromes. The Epstein-Barr virus has been implicated as a causative factor.

Supported by NIH T32 grant number CA09599 (Syed A. Ahmad).

CLINICAL PRESENTATION

The most common presenting symptom in 40% of patients is abdominal pain; also common are anorexia, weight loss, symptoms of small bowel obstruction, diarrhea, vomiting, and GI bleeding. Symptoms, particularly for those patients with existing enteropathy, may be present for 2 to 4 months before the patient seeks medical attention. Malnutrition may be apparent on physical examination, but fever, abdominal masses, peripheral lymphadenopathy, hepatosplenomegaly, and ascites do not appear until late in the course of the disease. Approximately 20% to 25% of patients will present with an abdominal catastrophe (e.g., perforation, obstruction, or bleeding). Symptoms vary with the type of lymphoma; for example, immunoproliferative B-cell lymphoma can present with digital clubbing, and enteropathy-associated T-cell lymphoma may present with exacerbation of preexisting celiac disease or dermatitis herpetiformis.

PREOPERATIVE MANAGEMENT

The nonspecific symptoms of small bowel lymphoma make early diagnosis difficult. Thus, the diagnosis of small bowel lymphoma should be considered when patients present with abdominal pain and obstructive symptoms. Contrast studies or enteroclysis is the diagnostic mode of choice for small bowel lymphoma because these tests can detect abnormalities in 90% of patients. Radiographic findings suggestive of small bowel tumors include intramural or intraluminal filling defects, mucosal abnormalities, intussusception, and complete obstruction (Fig. 69–1A). If a tumor is confirmed, abdominal computed tomography (CT) should be performed to identify extraintestinal extension, secondary mesenteric disease, or hepatic involvement. CT is also useful for staging the disease (Fig. 69–1B). Upper endoscopy may be useful for diagnosing lymphoma in the proximal small bowel. All patients should undergo either plain radiography or CT of the chest to rule out mediastinal and pulmonary involvement.

Biopsy is necessary to determine the histopathologic subtype of lymphoma. Biopsy samples can be obtained by means of esophagogastroduodenoscopy. Often, laparotomy or, more recently, laparoscopy is necessary to obtain adequate tissue. Blood tests for leukocytosis or serum tests for IgA heavy-chain or lactate dehydrogenase levels are unreliable for diagnosing small bowel lymphoma, although they may be useful as baseline measurements before beginning therapy.

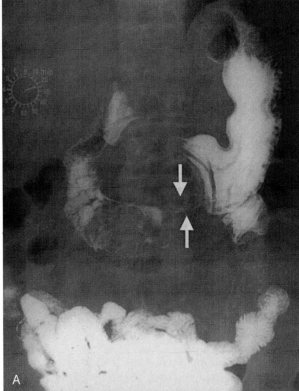

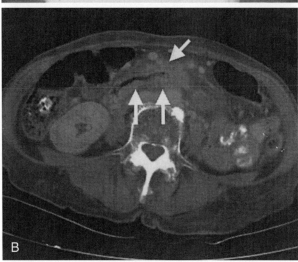

Figure 69–1. *A,* Upper gastrointestinal series/small bowel follow-through in a patient with lymphoma of the third portion of the duodenum. Note narrowing of the lumen. *B,* Computed tomographic scan of the abdomen demonstrating a mass surrounding the third portion of the duodenum.

CLASSIFICATION AND CLINICAL FEATURES

Most small bowel lymphomas are of non-Hodgkin's B-cell origin, and about 30% arise from T cells. Extranodal small bowel lymphoma has traditionally been staged according to a modified version of the Ann Arbor staging system (Table 69–1). Unfortunately, this classification fails to represent the unique histologic subtypes and clinical features associated with GI lymphomas. Because of this, the Re-

Table 69–1	Modified Ann Arbor Staging System for Extranodal Small Bowel Lymphoma

STAGE	DESCRIPTION
IE	Confined to primary organ
IIE	Involvement of adjacent lymph node
II2E	Involvement of regional, nonadjacent lymph node
III	Involvement of lymph nodes on both sides of the diaphragm, with or without involvement of extranodal sites (IIIE), spleen (IIIS), or both (IIIES)
IV	Diffuse or disseminated involvement of one or more extralymphatic sites (viscera or bone marrow?)

vised European American Classification of Lymphoid Neoplasms (REAL) was developed for pathologic classification and staging (Tables 69–2 and 69–3). Based on this, small bowel lymphomas can be further classified clinicopathologically as immunoproliferative small intestinal disease (IPSID), enteropathy-associated T-cell lymphoma (EATCL), or non-IPSID/EATCL lymphoma (Table 69–4).

Immunoproliferative Small Intestinal Disease

Originally known as Mediterranean lymphoma, the IPSID variant (also known as alpha chain disease) is classified as a low-grade B-cell lymphoma. In its early stages, IPSID is a diffuse mucosal infiltration of plasma cells and often terminates as large-cell immunoblastic lymphoma. Intestinal lesions appear grossly as thickened mucosal folds with small nodules, often with secondary involvement of mesenteric and abdominal lymph nodes. IPSID was originally found in the Mediterranean basin but is most prevalent among Arabs, non-European Jews, Iranians, and South African blacks. The disease appears most often between the ages of 15 and 35 years, and it is rare in the very young or the very old. Non-IPSID lymphomas, in contrast, usually present in patients older than 60 years. IPSID is the predominant form of GI lymphoma

Table 69–2	REAL Pathologic Classification of Lymphoma*

B-cell lymphoma
  Low-grade B-cell lymphoma of mucosa-associated lymphoid tissue (MALT)
  High-grade B-cell lymphoma of MALT
  Immunoproliferative small intestinal disease (IPSID), low-grade, mixed, or high-grade
  Mantle cell lymphoma
  Burkitt's-like lymphoma
  Other types of low- or high-grade lymphoma corresponding to peripheral node equivalent
T-cell lymphoma
  Enteropathy-associated T-cell lymphoma (EATCL)
  Other types not associated with enteropathy

*Revised European-American Classification of Lymphoid Neoplasms. From Harris NL, Jaffe ES, Stein H, et al: A revised European-American classification of lymphoid neoplasms. A proposal from the International Lymphoma Study Group. Blood 1994;84:1361–1392.

Table 69–3	Staging Classification for Primary Gastrointestinal Lymphoma

STAGE	DESCRIPTION
I	Tumor confined to GI tract Single primary site Multiple noncontiguous lesions

II	Tumor extending into abdomen from primary GI site
	Nodal involvement
	    Stage II$_1$: Local (i.e., paraintestinal lymphoma)
	    Stage II$_2$: Distant (i.e., mesenteric lymph node involvement)

IIE	Extension outside primary site to involve adjacent organs or tissues
	    Enumerate actual site of involvement (e.g., IIE [pancreas], IIE [posterior abdominal wall])
	    When there is both nodal involvement and penetration to involve adjacent organs, stage should be denoted using both a subscript and an E

IV	Disseminated extranodal involvement or a GI tract lesion with supradiaphragmatic nodal involvement

GI, gastrointestinal. From Rohatiner A, d'Amore F, Coiffier B, et al: Report on a workshop convened to discuss the pathological and staging classifications of gastrointestinal tract lymphoma. Ann Oncol 1994;5:397–400.

in lower socioeconomic strata and is the most-often-diagnosed form in people from nonindustrialized nations. Other non-Hodgkin's lymphomas occur in patients from all socioeconomic backgrounds.

The clinical presentation of IPSID is similar in most patients. Diarrhea is a common symptom and often leads to malabsorption and weight loss, although diarrhea may resolve spontaneously in the early stages of the disease. Also common are poorly localized abdominal pain, nausea, anorexia, digital clubbing, and peripheral edema. Abdominal catastrophes, such as perforation or formation of fistulas, are rare in IPSID, as are peripheral lymphadenopathy, fever, hepatosplenomegaly, and ascites.

Enteropathy-Associated T-Cell Lymphoma

Enteropathy-associated T-cell lymphoma is associated with poor clinical outcome. EATCL was originally described as malignant histiocytosis of the intestine, characterized by a pleomorphic infiltrate including multinucleated giant cells, histiocyte-like cells in the bases of ulcers, and dense infiltration of plasma cells. EATCL was later reclassified as a T-cell lymphoma. On pathologic examination, these lymphomas appear as ulcerated plaques or

strictures in the proximal small intestine, in contrast to B-cell lymphomas, which form annular or polypoid masses. Long-standing celiac disease or dermatitis herpetiformis (or both) is associated with a high risk of developing EATCL; people who have celiac disease have a 50 to 100 times higher risk of developing small bowel lymphoma. Most patients present with advanced disease that manifests as an exacerbation of the existing intestinal enteropathy; symptoms of malabsorption that do not respond to a gluten-free diet are common, and up to 25% of patients may present with intestinal perforation. Most patients are in their sixth or seventh decade of life. Surgery is reserved for patients who have resectable disease and for those who develop intra-abdominal catastrophes.

Non-IPSID, Non-EATCL Lymphoma

Primary small bowel lymphomas not associated with either IPSID or EATCL are usually of non-Hodgkin's B-cell origin and represent the overwhelming majority of small bowel lymphomas in western countries. All histologic subtypes in the REAL classification except for IPSID and EATCL fall into this category. Unlike IPSID and EATCL, these lymphomas tend to be localized, intermediate- or high-grade, and located in the ileum. Incidence peaks in the teen years or in the fifth decade of life (see Table 69–4). Patients usually present with abdominal pain, nausea, weight loss, and, occasionally, microcytic anemia or free perforation. B-cell symptoms such as fever and night sweats are uncommon. Most patients are treated with a multimodality approach. Localized lesions are typically treated with surgery; disease that is not confined to the abdomen or that is surgically unresectable should be treated with systemic chemotherapy.

TREATMENT AND OUTCOMES

Although several reports are available on the long-term outcome of patients treated for gastrointestinal non-Hodgkin's lymphoma, the rarity of the disease makes prospective studies impractical (Tables 69–5 and 69–6). Historically, most patients have been treated with surgery alone. The prognosis for patients with stage I or II disease (REAL classification) who have undergone complete surgical resection appears to be better than for those who have residual disease. Unfortunately, as many as 50% of patients with localized stage IE or IIE disease treated in

Table 69–4	Characteristics of Small Bowel Lymphoma Subtypes				

SUBTYPE	HISTOLOGIC FINDING	AGE AT ONSET	GEOGRAPHIC DISTRIBUTION	ANATOMIC LOCATION
IPSID	Low-grade B-cell	15–35 yr	Mediterranean, Middle East, South Africa	Duodenum, jejunum, ileum
EATCL	High-grade T-cell	>60 yr	Industrialized nations	Jejunum, ileum
Non-IPSID, non-EATCL	Intermediate- or high-grade B-cell	10–20 yr 40–50 yr	Industrialized nations	Ileum

EATCL, enteropathy-associated T-cell lymphoma; IPSID, immunoproliferative small bowel intestinal disease.

Table 69–5	Treatment Based on Clinicopathologic Staging			
		CHEMOTHERAPY	SURGERY	RADIATION
	Prelymphomatous IPSID	Tetracycline	—	—
	Advanced IPSID	Multiagent	+ + + °	±
	EATCL	Multiagent	+ + + °	±
	Non-IPSID, non-EATCL	Multiagent	+ + + °	±

°Not indicated in extensive small bowel involvement leading to short gut syndrome. EATCL, enteropathy-associated T-cell lymphoma; IPSID, immunoproliferative small bowel intestinal disease.

this way will experience a relapse. Although adjuvant abdominal radiation provides good local control, disease recurs at extra-abdominal sites in about half the patients so treated. These observations led many oncologists to suggest multimodal treatment, including surgery and adjuvant chemotherapy. The role of radiation given in combination with adjuvant chemotherapy has yet to be defined.

Immunoproliferative Small Intestinal Disease

Immunoproliferative small intestinal disease progresses in two distinct stages. The initial prelymphomatous stage eventually deteriorates into a lymphomatous stage characterized by synthesis of alpha chain proteins. Treatment for the prelymphomatous stage consists of antimicrobial therapy with tetracycline (2 g/day); lack of significant improvement over a 3- to 6-month period should prompt investigation whether the disease is more advanced. Treatment for the more aggressive lymphomatous stage should consist of surgery if the tumor is resectable. Unfortunately, the overwhelming majority of patients present with bulky, diffuse disease not amenable to resection. In this situation, treatment consists of chemotherapy, radiotherapy, or both. Combination chemotherapy regimens such as C-MOPP (cyclophosphamide, mechlorethamine, Oncovin, procarbazine, and prednisone), CHOP (cyclophosphamide, hydroxydaunomycin, Oncovin, and prednisone), or CVP (cyclophosphamide, vincristine, and prednisone) have been used as standard therapy for IPSID. No large prospective studies have been conducted to document the role of radiation in IPSID, although anecdotal evidence suggests that radiation in combination with

multiagent chemotherapy can improve survival. IPSID is a highly lethal disease with survival rates as low as 23% at 5 years. Patients with resectable stage I or II₁ disease have a 5-year survival rate of 40% to 47%, compared with 0% to 25% for unresectable or stage II₂ disease. More recently, using combination therapy based on doxorubicin, the survival rate for patients with all stages of IPSID was 67% at 3 years.

Enteropathy-Associated T-Cell Lymphoma

The management of EATCL is the same as for other histologic types of aggressive lymphoma. If the tumor is resectable, surgery should be undertaken, followed by chemotherapy. In advanced disease in which resection is not possible, treatment is usually anthracycline-based chemotherapy (i.e., C-MOPP, CHOP, or CVP). Some authors have also recommended whole abdominal radiation after chemotherapy. Unfortunately, because there are no randomized trials, the optimal treatment strategy is controversial. The prognosis for patients with EATCL is worse than for patients with B-cell lymphoma. Experience shows a 5-year survival rate of 75% for patients with B-cell lymphoma and only 25% for those with EATCL. Patients with EATCL have a higher perioperative complication rate, probably explained by the higher frequency of intestinal perforation at diagnosis.

Non-IPSID, Non-EATCL Lymphoma

The treatment of the different histologic subtypes in this category (mostly western B-cell lymphoma) incorporates a multimodality approach. In most patients, the tumor is

Table 69–6	Summary of Treatment Outcomes for Non-IPSID, Non-EATCL Small Bowel Lymphoma			
REFERENCE	NUMBER OF PATIENTS	SURGERY	CHEMOTHERAPY REGIMENS*	5-YEAR SURVIVAL RATES, %
Radaszkiewicz (1992)	63	Yes/No	Multiagent	24
Domizio (1993)	78	Yes/No	Single/multiagent	40 (high grade) 75 (low grade)
D'Amore (1994)	109	Yes	Multiagent	67
Liang (1995)	131	Yes	Multiagent	43

*Includes COPP (cyclophosphamide, Oncovin, procarbazine, prednisone), CHOP (cyclophosphamide, hydroxydaunomycin, Oncovin, prednisone), CVP (cyclophosphamide, vincristine, prednisone), MOPP (mechlorethamine, Oncovin, procarbazine, prednisone), or BACOP (bleomycin, Adriamycin, cyclophosphamide, Oncovin, prednisone).
EATCL, enteropathy-associated T-cell lymphoma; IPSID, immunoproliferative small bowel intestinal disease.

diagnosed at laparotomy, and surgical resection is standard. Chemotherapy should be used after surgery. In patients with unresectable tumor, chemotherapy followed by radiation therapy is recommended. Prognosis varies according to the grade and the stage of the tumor. The 5-year survival rate approaches 75% for low-grade B-cell tumors and 40% for high-grade histologic types. Treatment modalities vary; about 50% of patients have received either adjuvant chemotherapy or radiotherapy in addition to surgical resection. Patients who receive adjuvant therapy appear to fare better. The subset of patients who undergo complete surgical resection followed by adjuvant chemotherapy has a 5-year survival rate of 67%. Clinical stage, age greater than 59 years, and the presence of B-cell symptoms are factors with the strongest negative influence on survival.

Considerably worse survival has been reported by Radaszkiewicz and colleagues. In 63 patients with non-Hodgkin's lymphoma of the small bowel, the overall 5-year survival rate was 24%. Patients with Ann Arbor stage IE disease fared better (5-year survival rate of 45%) than patients with stage IIE disease (5-year survival rate of 17%). In addition, patients undergoing complete surgical resection fared better than those undergoing nonradical procedures (5-year survival rates of 46% and 0%, respectively).

Some oncologists advocate chemotherapy alone for treatment of gastrointestinal non-Hodgkin's lymphoma, but the literature supporting this practice is sparse. Whether radiation is useful in patients with small bowel lymphoma has yet to be determined. Administering radiation therapy with surgery has produced local control of disease, but extra-abdominal disease developed in as many as 50% of patients so treated. Given the lack to date of large, well-designed trials of radiation therapy used in conjunction with chemotherapy, the role of adjuvant radiation therapy remains to be elucidated.

In conclusion, it is difficult to establish absolute treatment recommendations for non-IPSID, non-EATCL small bowel lymphoma from the reports in the literature because of the lack of standardization of treatments and the retrospective nature of the reviews. It appears that complete surgical resection followed by chemotherapy, when feasible, offers the best survival advantage. The ability to achieve complete surgical resection is a prognostic factor for local and systemic relapse, as are stage and histologic grade. Five-year survival rates are reported to be 25% to 50% for high-grade or advanced disease and 60% to 80% for early-stage or low-grade histologic types. Small intestinal non-Hodgkin's lymphoma is potentially curable when both surgery and chemotherapy are undertaken; nevertheless, the optimal chemotherapeutic regimen and the role of radiotherapy in this disease remain to be identified through well-designed clinical trials.

Pearls and Pitfalls

- Gastrointestinal lymphoma is the third most common small bowel malignancy.
- The diagnosis of small bowel lymphoma should be considered when a patient presents with abdominal pain, GI bleeding, and obstructive symptoms.
- Enteroclysis and CT are the diagnostic modalities of choice.
- Small bowel lymphomas, differentiated as low-, intermediate-, or high-grade disease, can be classified into three categories based on clinicopathologic factors: IPSID, EATCL, and non-IPSID, non-EATCL lymphoma.
- All intermediate- and high-grade intestinal lymphomas that are **resectable** should be treated with surgery and Adriamycin (doxorubicin)-based chemotherapy.
- All intestinal lymphomas that are **unresectable** should be treated with multimodality doxorubicin-chemotherapy.
- Radiation therapy is useful for local control but does not prevent distant failure. Its role in treating small intestinal lymphoma remains to be determined.
- IPSID and EATCL are associated with a poor prognosis because patients present with advanced disease. Non-IPSID, non-EATCL lymphoma has a relatively better prognosis.

SELECTED READINGS

Al-Bahrani Z, Al-Mohindry H, Bakir F, et al: Clinical and pathologic subtypes of primary intestinal lymphoma: Experience with 132 patients over a 14-year period. Cancer 1983;52:1666–1671.

Bouvet M, JanJan NA, Jones DV Jr, Ellis LM: Small bowel tumors. In Torosian MH (ed): Integrated Cancer Management. New York, Marcel Dekker, 1999.

Cooper BT, Holmes GKT, Ferguson R, et al: Celiac disease and malignancy. Medicine 1980;59:249–261.

D'Amore F, Brincker H, Gronbaek K, et al: Non-Hodgkin's lymphoma of the gastrointestinal tract: A population-based analysis of incidence, geographic distribution, clinicopathologic presentation features, and prognosis. J Clin Oncol 1994;12:1673–1684.

Domizio P, Owen RA, Shepard NA, et al: Primary lymphoma of the small intestine: A clinicopathological study of 119 cases. Am J Surg Pathol 1993;17:429–442.

Fine KD, Stone MJ: Alpha-heavy chain disease, Mediterranean lymphoma, and immunoproliferative small intestinal disease: A review of clinicopathological features, pathogenesis, and differential diagnosis. Am J Gastroenterol 1999;94:1139–1152.

Harris NL, Jaffe ES, Stein H, et al: A revised European-American classification of lymphoid neoplasms: A proposal from the International Lymphoma Study Group. Blood 1994;84:1361–1392.

Iochim HL: Neoplasms associated with immune deficiencies. Pathol Annu 1987;22:177–222.

Liang R, Todd D, Chan TK, et al: Prognostic factors for primary gastrointestinal lymphoma. Hematol Oncol 1995;13:153–163.

Radaszkiewicz T, Dragosics B, Bauer P: Gastrointestinal malignant lymphomas of the mucosa-associated lymphoid tissue: Factors relevant to prognosis. Gastroenterology 1992;102:1628–1638.

Chapter 70
Carcinoid of the Small Bowel

Juan M. Sarmiento and David R. Farley

Small bowel carcinoid (SBC) tumors were first described in 1888 by Lubarsch, who found multiple small, unusual tumors in the distal ileum of two separate patients. In 1907, Oberndorfer coined the term *karzinoid* to indicate that this tumor resembled adenocarcinoma but had seemingly less aggressive behavior. Since then, carcinoid tumors have been reported throughout the entire gastrointestinal tract as well as in foregut structures, such as the thymus, the bronchi, and the lungs. In 1963, Williams and Sandler simplistically and importantly classified carcinoid tumors in the abdomen according to embryonic origin and blood supply, including foregut (celiac axis), midgut (superior mesenteric artery), and hindgut (inferior mesenteric artery) regions.

Carcinoid tumors arise from neuroendocrine cells and belong to the amine precursor uptake and decarboxylation system. Such totipotent cells produce a variety of substances that are metabolically active as hormones and biogenic amines (in the case of SBC, most commonly serotonin). Serotonin is synthesized from its precursor, 5-hydroxytryptophan, and is subsequently metabolized to 5-hydroxyindole acetic acid (5-HIAA), a measurable metabolite that is excreted in urine. Carcinoid tumors are also capable of secreting histamine, dopamine, substance P, prostaglandins, and other substances.

Although unique and seemingly unusual, carcinoid tumors are the second most common neoplasms of the small bowel, and a thorough understanding of these tumors is imperative for appropriate surgical and medical management.

CLINICAL PRESENTATION

Although appendiceal carcinoids represent 85% of all gastrointestinal carcinoid tumors, many or most appendiceal carcinoids are benign or incidental lesions noted during appendectomy. The vast majority are clinically irrelevant. Therefore, this discussion focuses on carcinoids residing within the small bowel. Typically occurring in the ileum (84%), SBCs are diagnosed in the sixth or seventh decade of life and usually present with nonspecific gastrointestinal symptoms, abdominal pain, or intestinal obstruction. An initial presentation of intestinal ischemia, abdominal mass, or hepatomegaly is rare. Given the slowly progressive nature of these carcinoids, patients may experience symptoms for years before the diagnosis is secured. In the 20-year experience with carcinoid tumors ($n = 58$) at the Massachusetts General Hospital, symptoms and signs of SBC were distributed as follows: pain (50%), vomiting (34%), weight loss (34%), diarrhea (22%), carcinoid syndrome (17%), flushing (12%), gastrointestinal blood loss (9%), asthma (9%), and tricuspid regurgitation (5%). Because SBC in most patients is undi-

agnosed before surgical exploration, the working preoperative diagnosis is typically small intestinal adenocarcinoma, Crohn's disease, adhesive obstruction, lymphoma, or colitis.

Small bowel carcinoid is frequently multicentric (in 30%), but, more important, patients with SBC typically (>90%) have metastases at the time of diagnosis, despite the size of the primary tumor. Although involvement of regional lymph nodes or hepatic metastases is the rule, only 6% of patients with SBC present with true carcinoid syndrome (sweating, tachycardia, hypotension, diarrhea, or flushing). In patients with carcinoid syndrome, the tumor burden is large, and the liver is unable to clear serotonin, substance P, and other biogenic amines from the bloodstream. Patients may present with the usual symptoms of flushing and diarrhea but also may have potentially severe bronchospasm. Carcinoid syndrome should tip off the astute physician to a *small bowel neoplasm,* because the syndrome is almost exclusive to such midgut neoplasms. Additionally, there is approximately a 17% rate of association with other nonendocrine malignancies. Colorectal adenomas and carcinomas are most frequently associated with SBC, but cancers of the stomach, lungs, and breast are also seen. Suspicion regarding the presence of concomitant neoplasms makes upper and lower gastrointestinal endoscopy, mammography, and chest radiography useful preoperatively.

Although suspicion regarding the possible presence of an SBC may be high, and numerous studies may help make the diagnosis, most carcinoids are in fact diagnosed definitively in the operating room. To make the diagnosis of SBC preoperatively requires a high index of suspicion, potential application of semiconfirmatory tests, and perhaps luck! The finding of elevated 5-HIAA levels in a 24-hour urine sample was heretofore the gold standard in detecting SBC, but normal levels are found in half of all patients with SBC. Plasma serotonin, substance P, neurotensin, neurokinin A, and neuropeptide K can be measured using immunofluorescent neuropeptide assays, but their sensitivity is similarly low, and most such substances are not increased in the majority of patients with SBC. Although chromogranin A levels are consistently high, this finding is not specific to carcinoid neoplasms.

Small bowel contrast studies, like serology tests, have been used to diagnose carcinoid tumors, although the accuracy is far from being satisfactory. Three typical imaging patterns have emerged: (1) solitary or multiple submucosal lesions; (2) mesenteric infiltration or retraction with or without associated intramural nodules; and (3) polypoid mass lesions with a mucosa-based appearance. The differential diagnosis includes benign tumors arising from the submucosa, a solitary metastasis, or aberrant gastric mucosa. If ulcerated, a "target" lesion is produced, and the differential diagnosis might include

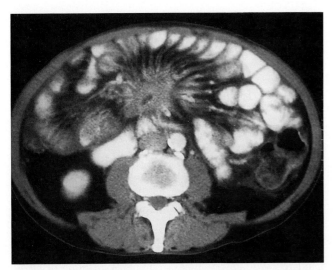

Figure 70–1. Abdominal computed tomography with enteric contrast material, depicting the desmoplastic reaction of the small bowel mesentery.

adenocarcinoma, lymphoma, melanoma, and Kaposi's sarcoma. In the presence of multiple nodules, either multicentricity or metastases need to be considered. Primary SBCs are typically small (<2 cm) and go undetected. Computed tomography, magnetic resonance imaging, ultrasonography, and angiography can be helpful in assessing the extent of carcinoid disease. Lymph node metastases are often bulky, and a desmoplastic reaction of the mesentery with swirling of the mesenteric tissue is common (Fig. 70–1). Although hepatic metastases are typically hypervascular, confirmatory liver function tests are invariably unreliable in this setting because the alkaline phosphatase level in the presence of multiple hepatic metastases is usually normal.

Somatostatin receptor scintigraphy (OctreoScan), based on the biologic activity of neuroendocrine tumors, visualizes carcinoid tumors (either primary or metastatic) in 80% to 95% of patients, a result that is clearly superior to that produced with the aforementioned serologic or imaging studies. This noninvasive technique has the potential to detect small tumors (≥1 cm) provided that they contain a high density of somatostatin receptors. Somatostatin receptor scintigraphy also has the capability of demonstrating extrahepatic metastases. The disadvantages include the inability to detect tumors less than 1 cm in diameter or those that are receptor negative outside the liver. The first-pass effect of the somatostatin analogue in the liver causes physiologic enhancement in the spleen and the genitourinary system, leading to high background activity in the left upper quadrant and the midabdomen. This may interfere with identification of tumors in these areas. Moreover, it is impossible to predict tumor size because the detection of the tumor is based on *density* of receptors and not on tumor *size*. Refinements currently in progress will allow eventual intraoperative use.

PREOPERATIVE MANAGEMENT

Although the primary goal is curative resection, careful preoperative preparation is mandatory to minimize mor-

bidity and potential mortality from this intervention (Fig. 70–2). The first crucial step is to detect symptoms characteristic of carcinoid syndrome (e.g., flushing, diarrhea). If the patient is asymptomatic, a surgical procedure may proceed with minimal preparation. In the presence of symptoms, patients are at risk of developing carcinoid crisis, which has a varying incidence (up to 50%) and is manifested as an attack of profound hypotension or bronchospasm during the induction of general anesthesia or during the operation. Ideally, every patient needs to be rendered symptom-free before the operation as a measure of reassurance that the carcinoid syndrome has been held in check. Symptomatic patients need to be given a somatostatin analogue to control symptoms. Most important, these patients need to receive a subcutaneous dose of a somatostatin analogue during induction of anesthesia to prevent carcinoid crisis intraoperatively.

Step two in preparation involves ruling out the presence of tricuspid insufficiency, which is present in about 5% of patients with SBC. A heart murmur or signs and symptoms of right-sided cardiac failure, if present, need to be evaluated appropriately. Transesophageal echocardiography should be used liberally.

If one is lucky or astute enough to make the diagnosis preoperatively, step three involves the use of somatostatin receptor scintigraphy to plan the operation and to maximize the chance that all tumor will be found and potentially resected to achieve a cure.

INTRAOPERATIVE MANAGEMENT

Small bowel carcinoids have more aggressive behavior and are associated with a greater risk of ultimate death than carcinoids in other locations. This information, coupled with a 30% rate of multicentricity and a greater than 90% rate of tumor spread, mandates meticulous surgical

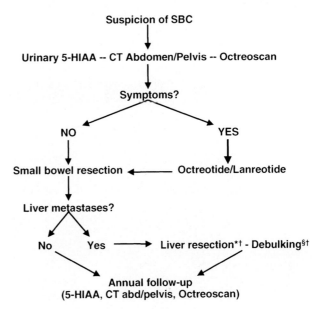

Figure 70–2. Flow chart of management of patients with small bowel carcinoids. *Wedge, segmentectomy, lobectomy in good-risk patients. †If symptomatic and suitable for resection of 90% or more of the macroscopic disease. §Consider chemotherapy.

treatment. There is no role for endoscopic treatments (as in rectal carcinoids) or limited resection (as in appendiceal carcinoids); a wide mesenteric resection, if possible, should involve the draining lymph nodes. A formal small bowel and mesenteric resection assesses nodal status and potentially reduces the risk of subsequent mesenteric desmoplastic reaction and bowel obstruction. Although knowing the size of the tumor is important in establishing the prognosis, the key to surgical treatment is rendering the patient disease free; in lieu of total extirpation, tumor debulking may be beneficial and warranted, depending on the clinical situation.

The patient is positioned supine with the arms tucked to the side. A midline incision is usually preferred. Whether identified by means of scintigraphic scans or the surgeon's fingers, all evident tissue involved by the tumor needs to be resected, if possible. Extensive dissection and resection in the face of unresectable disease must be tempered with mature surgical judgment individualized to the particular patient.

Small bowel carcinoids may be multicentric, and the surgeon should not spare any effort in localizing additional tumors, either multicentric carcinoids or associated malignancies. The limit of the intestinal resection needs to include the corresponding mesentery; careful palpation for nodal metastasis (wide en bloc resection) should be done (Fig. 70–3). Almost all patients can tolerate a primary anastomosis. For very distal ileal tumors—especially if larger than 2 cm—the surgeon should perform a right hemicolectomy.

Although bimanual palpation assists in the identification of liver metastases, intraoperative ultrasonography should be used routinely to confirm or rule out hepatic metastases. Treatment of liver metastases depends on tumor burden, symptoms, location, patient performance status, and underlying liver reserve. In most patients, nonanatomic liver resection is sufficient treatment for hepatic metastases from SBC. Resection of multiple hepatic lesions can be efficacious; a 5-year survival rate of 75% with fully resected neuroendocrine tumors metastatic to the liver can be expected. For patients with

metastatic carcinoid lesions that are not suitable for resection, recent experience with liver transplantation has achieved a 69% survival rate at 5 years with good control of symptoms. Such data speak to the indolent nature of metastatic carcinoid lesions and their favorable response to resective procedures.

POSTOPERATIVE MANAGEMENT

Care after intestinal resection for SBC is routine. Nasogastric decompression is useful temporarily. A liquid diet is initiated early and may progress promptly to a general diet. Dismissal occurs when the patient is ambulatory and is tolerating oral intake well.

There is no specific postoperative regimen for asymptomatic patients after surgical resection. These patients need to be followed; measurement of 24-hour urine 5-HIAA levels may be useful, especially in those patients with elevated preoperative levels. In patients with symptoms, somatostatin analogues are of paramount importance, especially in the presence of flushing and diarrhea. Octreotide, currently the most commonly used somatostatin analogue, lasts 6 to 8 hours but requires two or three daily subcutaneous injections. Octreotide binds to somatostatin receptors, which are expressed in more than 80% of carcinoid tumors, and inhibits both the secretion and the peripheral action of hormones and biogenic amines. Used in doses of 150 µg three times a day, symptoms improve in 88% of patients, and a decrease in urinary 5-HIAA excretion is seen in 72% of patients. Recently, a long-acting somatostatin analogue, lanreotide, which has similar efficacy and symptom control but minimal side effects, has shown promise; activity persists over 10 to 14 days after a 30-mg intramuscular injection. Because of this ease of administration, lanreotide might replace octreotide as first-line therapy in the management of patients with carcinoid syndrome. Regression of tumor has not been reported with the use of this or any other somatostatin analogue.

Other therapies for metastatic disease or carcinoid syndrome include α-interferon and a variety of chemotherapeutic agents. α-Interferon stimulates T lymphocyte function and controls secretion of tumor products. A 15% tumor regression rate has been documented with administration of this agent; α-interferon is particularly effective in patients unresponsive to somatostatin analogues alone. α-Interferon has many side effects (e.g., fever, anorexia, weight loss) that might interfere with the quality of life. Cytotoxic chemotherapy has similarly shown limited success in treating metastatic carcinoid tumors. The Eastern Cooperative Oncology Group, which used streptozocin plus cyclophosphamide or streptozocin plus 5-fluorouracil, reported response rates of 26% to 33%. Systemic chemotherapy with cisplatin and etoposide has similarly been ineffective.

Although beyond the scope of this chapter, therapy for hepatic metastases deserves mention. Complete resection is the management of choice, but when the patient is not a suitable candidate or resection is not possible owing to technical considerations, all is not lost. Hepatic artery embolization is often effective because metastases derive

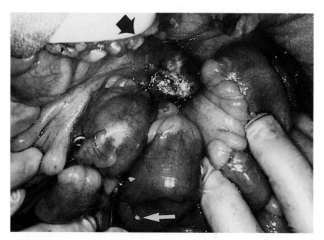

Figure 70–3. Intraoperative assessment reveals classic desmoplastic reaction of the small bowel mesentery (*black arrow*). Histologic confirmation of the 1.5-mm serosal lesion (*white arrow*) revealed a small bowel carcinoid.

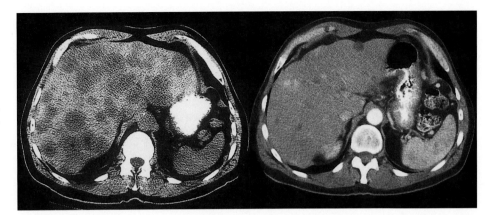

Figure 70–4. Computed tomography of a patient before and after hepatic artery embolization for metastatic small bowel carcinoid.

90% of their blood supply from the hepatic arterial flow (Fig. 70–4). Embolization can be performed with chemotherapeutic agents (doxorubicin). This approach results in effective palliation of symptoms, although it carries a significant morbidity rate, and the duration of effect may be short. As mentioned previously, liver transplantation is a potential option in an aggressive surgical armamentarium to treat metastatic SBC. Finally, even in the presence of widespread disease, tumor debulking is justified when 90% or more of the macroscopic disease is resectable in symptomatic patients.

COMPLICATIONS

Patients with resected SBC are at risk of development of anastomotic leak, intestinal obstruction, postoperative adhesions, fascial dehiscence, intra-abdominal hemorrhage or abscess, and infection of the surgical wound. In patients with SBC, especially those with manifestations of carcinoid syndrome, one must be alert to the development of bronchospasm; diarrhea and flushing, although not life-threatening, could be bothersome and could complicate a normal postoperative recovery. The best way of treating these "complications" is to prevent them by continuing the administration of somatostatin analogues

during the immediate postoperative period in previously symptomatic patients. In patients with tricuspid insufficiency, there is always the potential of right-sided cardiac failure. Judicious intravenous fluid administration is important, and in some patients, valve replacement needs to be considered.

OUTCOMES

Although 90% of patients with SBC present with lymphatic or hepatic metastases and 6% present with the carcinoid syndrome, the overall 5-year survival rate is better than 50%. Long-term survival correlates with the stage of the disease, with a 5-year survival rate of 65% in patients with localized or regional disease and a rate of 36% in patients with distant disease. In a patient with SBC with resectable nodal disease and no hepatic metastases, median survival is 15 years. Unresectable nodal disease (median survival = 5 years) or liver metastases (median survival = 3 years) confer diminished survival.

Not surprisingly, surgical patients with carcinoid tumor that is discovered incidentally (for whom there is only a 4% rate of lymph node involvement and hepatic metastases) and resected completely are invariably cured of the malignancy.

Summary

- Carcinoid tumors are the second most common primary neoplasm of the small bowel.
- Symptoms are often vague, chronic, and insidious and are usually precipitated by metastatic disease.
- Preoperative diagnosis is rare, and screening tests (5-HIAA, serum chromogranin A, computed tomography) are neither pathognomonic nor highly sensitive.
- Surgical treatment involves an aggressive approach: small bowel resection along with draining nodes and liver resection of hepatic metastases, if possible.
- Debulking for advanced symptomatic disease may be indicated.

SELECTED READINGS

Arnold R: Medical treatment of metastasizing carcinoid tumors. World J Surg 1996;20:203.
Kulke MH, Mayer RJ: Carcinoid tumors. N Engl J Med 1999;340:858.

Pearls and Pitfalls

PEARLS

- Primary SBC may be minute. Scrutinize and palpate the small bowel carefully.
- Look for concomitant malignancies (frequency of approximately 17%).
- Look for multiple SBCs (frequency of approximately 30%).
- Remember that metastatic disease is not synonymous with short survival.

PITFALLS

- Failure to suspect the diagnosis.
- Failure to take measures to prevent carcinoid crisis.
- Failure to perform a wide mesenteric resection.
- Failure to identify second carcinoids or cancers.

Modlin IM, Sandor A: An analysis of 8305 cases of carcinoid tumors. Cancer 1997;79:813.

Moertel CG, Sauer WG, Dockerty MB, Baggenstoss AH: Life history of the carcinoid tumor of the small intestine. Cancer 1961;14:901.

Morgan JC, Marks C, Hearn D: Carcinoid tumors of the gastrointestinal tract. Ann Surg 1974;180:720.

Que FG, Nagorney DM, Batts KP, et al: Hepatic resection for metastatic neuroendocrine carcinomas. Am J Surg 1995;169:36.

Shebani KO, Souba WW, Finkelstein DM, et al: Prognosis and survival in patients with gastrointestinal tract carcinoid tumors. Ann Surg 1999;229:815.

Strodel WE, Talpos G, Eckhauser FE, Thompson NW: Surgical therapy for small bowel carcinoid tumors. Arch Surg 1983;118:391.

Thompson GB, van Heerden JA, Martin JK Jr, et al: Carcinoid tumors of the gastrointestinal tract: Presentation, management and prognosis. Surgery 1985;98:1054.

Chapter 71

Stromal Tumors of the Small Bowel

Karen A. Yeh, Christina Kim, and Thomas R. Gadacz

Small intestinal tumors are relatively rare and may be quite difficult to diagnose. Gastrointestinal tumors of the small intestine (GISTs) are a heterogeneous group of intramural mesenchymal neoplasms composed of spindled or epithelioid stromal cells. These tumors are the most common nonepithelial neoplasm of both the stomach and the small bowel. For many years, these tumors were considered to arise exclusively from smooth muscle and were classified as either benign (leiomyoma) or malignant (leiomyosarcoma). Sophisticated pathologic examination has demonstrated that these tumors are diverse entities with different immunohistochemical and ultrastructural characteristics and varying clinical outcomes and prognoses. Currently, most connective tissue neoplasms of the GI tract that resemble smooth muscle neoplasms are categorized as "stromal" tumors. Although it is difficult to estimate the precise incidence of GISTs, this group of tumors is estimated to account for about 1% of all gastrointestinal malignancies and about 25% of all small bowel neoplasms. Controversy persists regarding the malignant potential of these tumors. Because of the difficulty in determining prognostic indicators, no standard staging system is yet available.

CLINICAL PRESENTATION

The clinical presentations of GISTs of the small bowel are as diverse as the pathologic characteristics. Although the tumors are more common in middle-aged and older patients, there are rare reports of these tumors occurring in the third decade of life. There is a slight male predominance but no apparent race predilection. Because of the rarity of these lesions, the incidence is difficult to estimate, but there seems to be a relatively equal distribution in the duodenum, the jejunum, and the ileum despite the shorter length of the duodenum. There are no identifiable etiologic agents or social risk factors.

It is not uncommon for GIST of the small bowel to be discovered incidentally during laparotomy performed for other indications, and up to one third of patients are reported to be asymptomatic at presentation. When present, symptoms are often vague and suggestive of nonspecific intra-abdominal disease. The most frequent presentation in the symptomatic patient is some form of gastrointestinal hemorrhage, which ranges from occult blood loss to melena or gross blood per rectum. Patients with ongoing gastrointestinal blood loss may present with the typical signs of anemia, including fatigue, shortness of breath, and tachycardia. Other symptoms may include vague abdominal pain or intermittent symptoms of partial obstruction. A palpable mass is a not-unusual presentation, suggesting an advanced and likely a locally invasive tumor. Laboratory studies may demonstrate normocytic

or microcytic anemia, but additional chemistry studies and liver function studies are not useful in diagnosis. At present, there are no identified tumor markers for GIST.

PREOPERATIVE EVALUATION AND MANAGEMENT

Diagnosis of a GIST may depend on a high index of clinical suspicion but may not be confirmed preoperatively. The picture is that of a patient with occult blood loss and nonspecific abdominal complaints or no real complaints. Frequently, patients will have undergone upper and lower gastrointestinal endoscopy with negative findings. Abdominal imaging may also have been performed, but this study is usually nondiagnostic. The exception may be the very large GIST that involves surrounding organs, but even positive imaging studies rarely lead to an accurate diagnosis.

The study most likely to lead to a correct preoperative diagnosis is esophagogastroduodenoscopy for duodenal GIST or "push" enteroscopy for proximal jejunal GIST. Visual inspection shows either endophytic or exophytic tumors or an intraluminal polypoid mass. Grossly, the tumors may have a smooth gray or whitish surface. Conversely, some tumors may erode the overlying mucosa and show areas of necrosis or hemorrhage (Fig. 71–1). Biopsy may be performed at the discretion of the endoscopist, but in the symptomatic patient, surgical resection is frequently warranted regardless of the histologic subtype of tumor. Rarely will tissue diagnosis alter the indication for surgical intervention.

Fluoroscopic studies of the small intestine may help localize the disease, and upper gastrointestinal series with small bowel follow-through or enteroclysis can demonstrate the site of intraluminal disease. These studies may also assist the surgeon in intraoperative location of smaller lesions.

For the patient with significant gastrointestinal hemorrhage, scintigraphic radionuclide-tagged red blood cell scanning (Fig. 71–2) or arteriography (Fig. 71–3) may help localize the source of the small intestinal lesion. These studies, however, are unlikely to lead the surgeon to the diagnosis of GIST. For those patients in whom a lesion is visualized on arteriography, leaving the arteriography catheter in place in the femoral artery with subselective catheterization of the appropriate small intestinal arterial branch may help the surgeon localize a small GIST in the operating room.

The majority of preoperative efforts at diagnosis are aimed at localizing the lesion. The preoperative preparation of the patient depends on the acuity of the presentation. For those who present with chronic and occult blood loss or intermittent partial bowel obstruction, attention

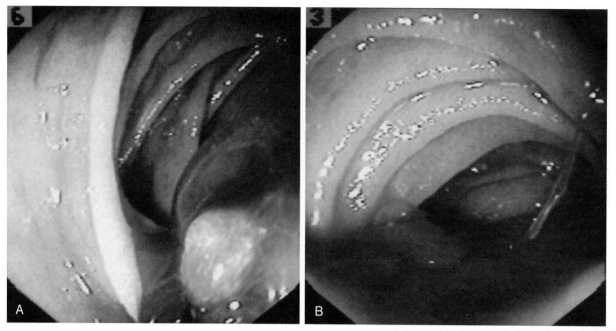

Figure 71–1. "Push enteroscopy" of a proximal jejunal gastrointestinal stromal tumor of the small intestine demonstrating ulcerated mucosa with hemorrhage.

should be given to the correction of anemia and electrolyte abnormalities and nutritional support. For those undergoing elective exploration, preoperative mechanical and antibiotic bowel preparation should be considered, because intraoperative findings frequently demonstrate invasion of surrounding organs. For those patients who present with massive gastrointestinal blood loss, rapid volume resuscitation and correction of anemia and possible coagulopathy should be performed, followed by emergent exploration if the lesion has been adequately localized.

SURGICAL MANAGEMENT

Because chemotherapy and radiation therapy are generally considered ineffective treatment modalities for GIST,

complete surgical resection remains the mainstay of therapy. Laparotomy is performed through a midline incision with the patient under general anesthesia. For jejunal or ileal tumors, there is controversy about the adequacy of resection margins, with recommendations ranging from 1 to 10 cm. Lymph node metastases are unusual (<10%) but are certainly documented. It is not yet determined how extensive lymphadenectomy should be, but regional nodes should be resected when feasible. During exploration, it is not uncommon to find direct invasion into adjacent organs, and involved organs should be resected en bloc whenever possible. For duodenal tumors of uncertain malignant potential, or when the size prevents the possibility of transduodenal resection, pancreaticoduodenectomy is warranted for medically fit patients. The tumor may be found to be unresectable for curative intent

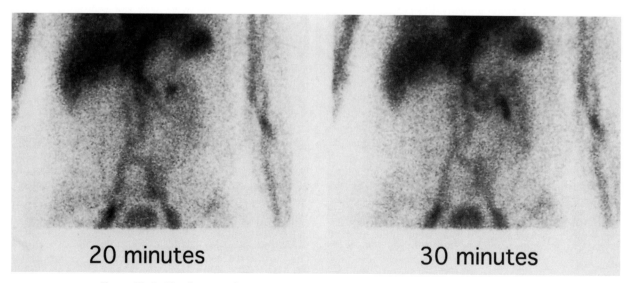

Figure 71–2. Bleeding scan demonstrating proximal small bowel hemorrhage on serial views.

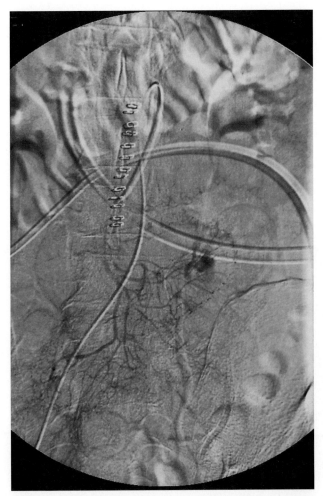

Figure 71–3. Arteriogram with selective catheterization of the ileal branch, showing the bleeding site.

owing to local invasion or distant disease. Nonetheless, resection of the small bowel should be performed when possible, with the intent of palliating bleeding or obstructive symptoms.

POSTOPERATIVE MANAGEMENT

After surgical resection, postoperative recovery is similar to that after any bowel resection. Foley and nasogastric catheters are removed in accordance with the surgeon's practice patterns. Drains are rarely required for limited small bowel resections. Serial determination of hemoglobin and electrolyte values should be performed. Early ambulation and antithrombotic prophylaxis are encouraged. The patient's diet should be advanced when there is evidence of return of bowel function.

During the postoperative evaluation, careful attention should be given to the surgical disease. GISTs of the small bowel are a heterogeneous group of tumors with diverse clinical outcomes. Although accurate pathologic evaluation does not typically change the management of GIST, it will allow the surgeon to counsel the patients and their families accurately about prognosis and expected outcome. A standard hematoxylin and eosin stain is shown

Table 71–1	Factors Affecting Metastatic Disease, Recurrence, and Prognosis		
GROSS FEATURES	**MICROSCOPIC AND IMMUNOHISTOCHEMICAL FEATURES**	**MOLECULAR MARKERS**
Size (>5 cm)	High cellularity	
Local invasion	>5 mitoses/10 hpf	p53 overexpression
Nodal metastases	Pleomorphism	High ki-67 index
Distant metastases	Nuclear atypia	

hpf, high-power field.

(Fig. 71–4), although a detailed description of the histopathologic characteristics of GIST is beyond the scope of this chapter. Over the years, a variety of classifications have been employed for these tumors, and adequate characterization may be difficult. Review by a pathologist with experience in GISTs is mandatory. A number of centers have performed multivariate and univariate analyses to determine which parameters correlate with metastatic disease, recurrence, and survival. Although diverse authors have found differing variables, most are in agreement that tumor size and mitotic counts are of significance. Other gross tumor characteristics and histologic findings that may be of importance are listed in Table 71–1. Guidelines for assessing malignant potential are described in Table 71–2.

Although adjuvant radiation therapy has been used with anecdotal success in patients with isolated pelvic stromal tumors, there is no evidence to suggest that adjuvant chemotherapy or radiation therapy is of benefit for those with GIST. The greatest experience with systemic therapy has been with doxorubicin- or ifosfamide-based regimens. Results have been disappointing, and response rates are low and have not translated into a survival advantage. These modalities may be employed for palliation of metastatic disease, but patients and families should be advised that limited data are available regarding the success of therapy. Because of the rarity of these tumors, phase 3 trials are not available.

FOLLOW-UP AND OUTCOME

Because of the relatively high frequency of recurrence, patients will require long-term follow-up. Researchers at Memorial Sloan-Kettering Cancer Center have recently

Table 71–2	Assessment of Malignant Potential, Risk of Metastatic Disease, or Recurrence	
MALIGNANT POTENTIAL	**TUMOR SIZE (cm)**	**MITOSES HPF**
Low	<5	<2
Intermediate	<5	>2
Intermediate	>5	<2
High	>5	>2

hpf, high-power field.

presented a review of 200 patients with GISTs of all sites, 80 of whom were treated at their facility (DeMatteo, 2000). Forty percent of patients developed recurrent disease. Approximately one third of patients developed local recurrence alone, 48% developed distant metastases, and 19% had both local and distant recurrence. Recurrence was primarily intra-abdominal. Their analysis found that tumor size greater than 10 cm was likely to predict recurrence, but other factors, including surgical margins, were not useful in this determination. Most patients who developed recurrent disease subsequently died.

Because of the high propensity of these patients to develop recurrence, regular follow-up examinations, including careful history taking, physical examination with fecal occult blood testing, and appropriate radiographic studies, should be performed. For duodenal lesions that have been excised without radical resection, esophagogastroduodenoscopy may be useful. For those individuals with a GIST with high malignant potential and a high probability of recurrence, imaging studies of the chest and the abdomen may be warranted. Despite careful and aggressive follow-up, early detection of recurrence may be difficult for the same reasons that detection of the initial tumor is difficult. Reoperation for local recurrence is warranted, as with other sarcomas.

The 5-year survival rate for GISTs of all sites ranges from 48% to 63%. Few data are available regarding large series of patients with GIST, but outcome generally ap-

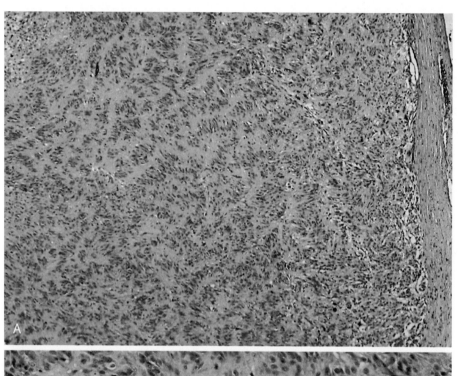

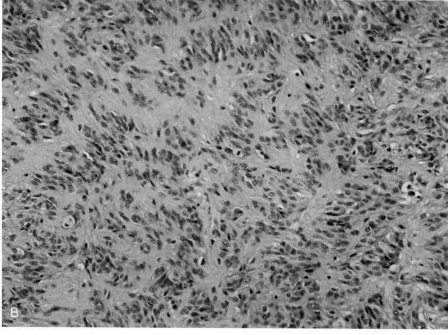

Figure 71–4. *A*, Photomicrograph of circumscribed spindle cell proliferation. *Arrow* marks pseudocapsule (magnification ×10). *B*, Photomicrograph demonstrating mitotically active spindle cells (*arrow*) with minimal atypia (magnification ×40).

Pearls and Pitfalls

- GISTs of the small bowel, previously termed *leiomyomas* or *sarcomas,* represent about 1% of all gastrointestinal neoplasms.
- When present, symptoms are nonspecific and usually involve gastrointestinal bleeding or obstruction.
- Diagnosis may be difficult; evaluation may show only a small bowel mass.
- Operative management involves a wide resection.
- Adjuvant chemotherapy or radiation therapy is of questionable value; thus, surgical resection is the mainstay of treatment.
- Prognosis is most affected by the size, grade, number of mitoses, and histopathologic stage as well as the ability to effect a curative resection.

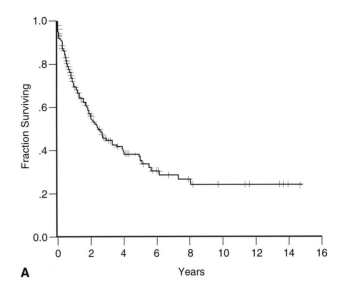

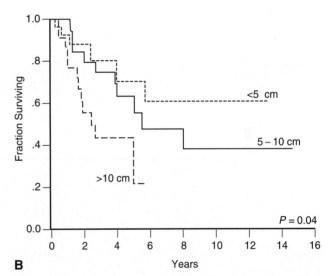

Figure 71–5. Survival in patients with gastrointestinal stromal tumors of the small intestine. *A,* Disease-specific survival (*n* = 200). *B,* Disease-specific survival by tumor size after complete resection (*n* = 80). (From DeMatteo RP, Lewis JJ, Leung D, et al: Two hundred gastrointestinal stromal tumors: Recurrence patterns and prognostic factors for survival. Ann Surg 2000;231:51–58.)

pears to parallel that of GIST of all sites. Survival data from the Memorial Sloan-Kettering Cancer Center are presented in Figure 71–5. These survival curves emphasize the importance of tumor size in predicting tumor recurrence and the importance of long-term follow-up, because failures may occur several years after diagnosis. Despite complete surgical resection with histologically negative margins, it can be anticipated that the disease will recur in many patients.

If recurrence is detected, surgical resection remains the only potentially curative therapy, and operative intervention should be planned if the recurrent disease appears resectable. The high rates of failure emphasize the need for effective adjuvant therapy. Current efforts appear to be directed at the development of intraperitoneal chemotherapy; a phase 1 trial is available through Memorial Sloan-Kettering Cancer Center.

CONCLUSIONS

Small bowel tumors are a rare entity, and GISTs (previously termed *leiomyoma* or *leiomyosarcoma*) are rarer still. Because of the changing terminology over the past several decades, interpretation of the literature may be confusing. Diagnosis is quite difficult and relies on a high index of clinical suspicion. Many radiographic and endoscopic studies may have been performed before surgical referral, and it is common for surgery to be undertaken without an accurate preoperative diagnosis. Most operations are performed for gastrointestinal hemorrhage. Small GISTs may be found incidentally at laparotomy for other indications. Surgical resection remains the only potentially curative therapy, and adjuvant chemotherapy or radiation therapy has not been shown to have an impact on survival. The extent of surgical resection remains controversial, but organs involved by direct extension should be resected when possible. Despite surgical resection to negative margins, many patients with large tumors or poor histologic indicators will develop recurrence and will ultimately die of this disease. The high rate of local and distant failure suggests that future re-

search efforts should be directed at the development of effective systemic therapy.

SELECTED READINGS

Chou FF, Eng HL, Sheen-Chen SM: Smooth muscle tumors of the gastrointestinal tract: Analysis of prognostic factors. Surgery 1996;119:171.

Coffman S, Deshmukh N: Gastrointestinal stromal tumors (GIST): Assessing their malignant potential. Contemporary Surg 1999;55:135.

DeMatteo RP, Lewis JJ, Leung D, et al: Two hundred gastrointestinal stromal tumors: Recurrence patterns and prognostic factors for survival. Ann Surg 2000;231:51.

Ludwig DJ, Traverso W: Gut stromal tumors and their clinical behavior. Am J Surg 1997;173:390.

Ng EH, Pollock RE, Munsell MF, et al: Prognostic factors influencing survival in gastrointestinal leiomyosarcomas: Implications for surgical management and staging. Ann Surg 1991;215:68.

Suster S: Gastrointestinal stromal tumors. Semin Diagn Pathol 1996;13:297.

Colon and Rectum: Benign

Chapter 72
Large Bowel Obstruction

Steven J. Hughes

Obstruction of the large intestine is a common diagnosis in Western cultures. Even with optimal management, the morbidity and the mortality associated with large bowel obstruction (LBO) are substantial. Complete LBO, in contrast to small bowel obstruction, is a surgical emergency because of the risk of colonic obstruction.

CLINICAL PRESENTATION

Etiology

The timing and the type of treatments for LBO are dependent on the cause of the obstruction and the presence or the absence of peritonitis. In the majority of patients, LBO is due to colon or rectal cancer. Carcinoma of the splenic flexure is associated with the highest risk of obstruction (approximately 50% of patients). Other much less common causes of LBO include diverticulitis, volvulus, hernia, fecal impaction, intussusception, ischemia, radiation injury, adhesions, endometriosis, and presence of a foreign body. These factors should be considered in the differential diagnosis of LBO.

Presenting Symptoms and Signs

Most patients with obstruction of the large intestine will present with acute complaints of abdominal distention and pain, failure to pass feces or flatus for a prolonged period (obstipation), anorexia, nausea, and, if the ileocecal valve is incompetent, emesis (often feculent). A history of abdominal distention and diarrhea is frequently obtained when a high-grade partial obstruction is present. Specific aspects of the antecedent history are helpful in determining the cause of the obstruction, including changes in bowel habits (e.g., reduced frequency or caliber of stools), presence of hematochezia or melena, changes in weight,

localized abdominal pain with fever, and duration of symptoms.

The physical examination should begin with an overall assessment of the relative condition of the patient, with scrutiny for signs of sepsis. Examination of the abdomen will determine the presence or absence of peritonitis, regional tenderness, a palpable mass, organomegaly, and ascites. Umbilical, incisional, inguinal, and femoral hernias should be either identified or specifically ruled out as the cause. Rectal cancer, carcinomatosis, inflammatory masses, fecal impaction, and foreign objects may be definitively diagnosed by means of digital examination of the rectum.

Laboratory and Radiographic Evaluation

Laboratory studies should include analysis of serum electrolytes and a complete blood count. Additional studies are obtained based on the patient's age and coexisting medical conditions, as recommended by the American Society of Anesthesiology. If malignancy is suspected as the likely cause, obtaining a preoperative serum carcinoembryonic antigen level should be considered.

An abdominal series, including an upright chest radiograph, usually provides most of the information needed to establish the diagnosis and the level of obstruction. The typical radiographic appearance of LBO is a dilated colon proximal to the obstruction with or without dilation of the small intestine (Fig. 72–1A). The presence of extraluminal air necessitates emergent celiotomy. The greatest diameter of the cecum should be determined. Perforation of the colon due to obstruction usually occurs in the cecum. A cecal diameter of greater than 15 cm usually results in perforation, whereas a cecal diameter of less than 11 cm is not generally associated with perforation. If indications for emergent surgical intervention

473

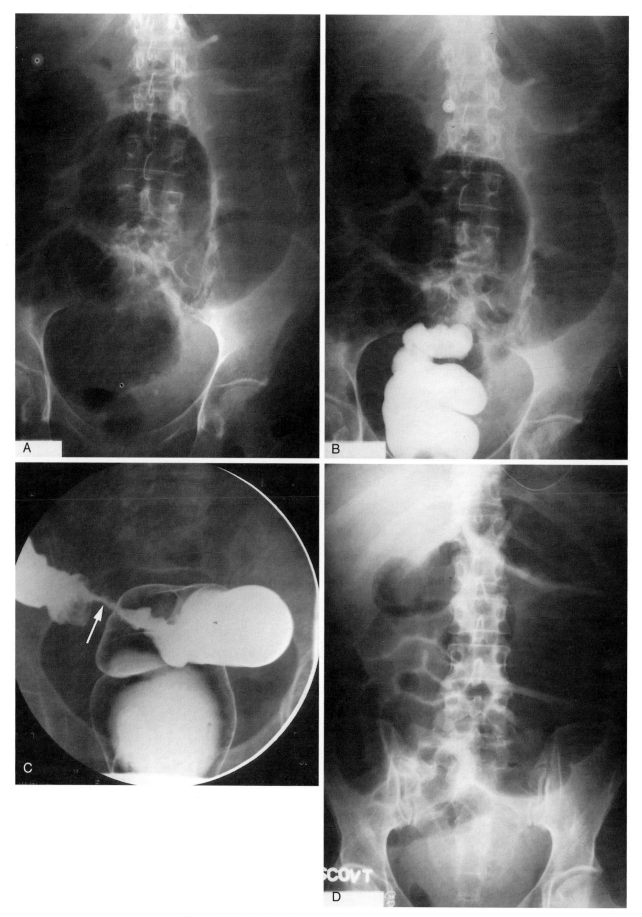

Figure 72–1. *See legend on opposite page.*

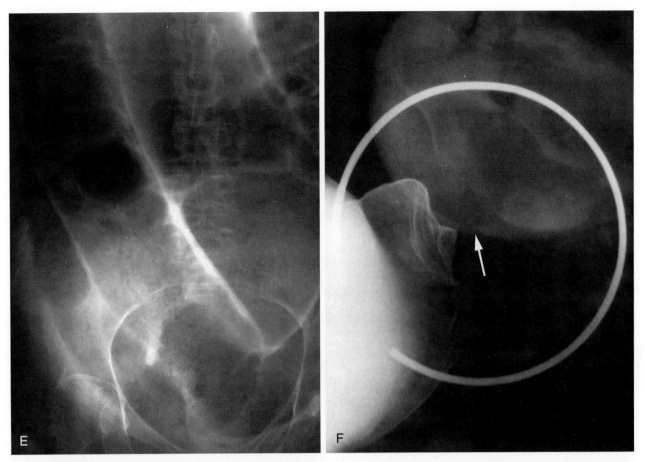

Figure 72–1. Radiographic findings in large bowel obstruction. *A,* Plain abdominal radiograph demonstrating dilated loops of large bowel consistent with mechanical obstruction in the rectum versus pseudo-obstruction. *B,* Water-soluble contrast enema from the same patient demonstrating obstructing rectal adenocarcinoma as the cause of obstruction. *C,* Water-soluble contrast enema of near-obstructing "apple core" lesion in the sigmoid colon. This lesion proved to be diverticular in origin. *D,* Cecal volvulus classically appears as dilated large intestine to the left of midline and dilated loops of small intestine. *E,* Abdominal radiograph of a sigmoid volvulus. *F,* Water-soluble contrast enema demonstrating characteristic bird's beak appearance (*arrow*). (Radiographs courtesy of Paul Sonda, MD, University of Michigan Department of Radiology, Ann Arbor, Mich.)

have been identified by means of physical examination or the acute abdominal series, further laboratory evaluation is usually not indicated.

A water-soluble contrast enema, which is useful in differentiating colonic pseudo-obstruction from mechanical obstruction, should usually be obtained if emergent operation is not deemed necessary (see Fig. 72–1*B*). The appearance of colon adenocarcinoma has classically been described as an apple-core lesion (see Fig. 72–1*C*), as compared with obstruction due to either extrinsic compression or ischemic or radiation-induced injury of the colon. The stricture associated with diverticular disease may be difficult to differentiate from malignancy on contrast enema study. If acute diverticulitis is suspected as the cause of the obstruction, computed tomography (CT) of the abdomen and the pelvis should be obtained rather than the contrast enema. Rectal contrast material is often necessary. CT accurately establishes the diagnosis of diverticulitis. If pericolic abscess or phlegmon without diffuse peritoneal contamination is identified, CT-guided percutaneous drainage of the inflammation may be performed. CT may also be helpful in the diagnosis and the

management of other causes of LBO; however, its routine use is controversial and probably not cost-effective.

SURGICAL MANAGEMENT

Preoperative Preparation

Before surgical exploration, resuscitation with intravenous fluids and correction of any electrolyte abnormalities are imperative. Pulmonary and radial artery catheterization and monitoring are often appropriate in the emergent situation or in patients with significant comorbid conditions. Nasogastric and Foley catheters should be placed. In carefully selected patients who have partial obstruction without evidence of proximal distention and impending perforation, mild mechanical bowel preparation may be attempted. The patient must be carefully monitored during this preparation for signs of distention. Oral antibiotics, including erythromycin base and neomycin, are also administered. Prophylaxis for peptic ulcer and deep venous thrombosis should be considered. Malnourished patients or those in whom the return of bowel function may be delayed for more than 4 to 7 days may benefit from initiation of total parenteral nutrition. Intravenous antibiotics with spectra that include skin and colonic flora should be administered before the incision is made. Ideally, the abdomen should be examined with the patient standing and sitting, and the optimal location for a stoma should be marked.

General Considerations

Exploration for LBO should be performed through a low midline incision with the patient in the supine position. The incision can be extended if necessary to mobilize the hepatic or the splenic flexure. The modified lithotomy position is appropriate if access to the anus for stapling or distal bowel irrigation is needed. The incision should be on the side of the umbilicus opposite the planned stoma site. A careful examination of the liver, the omentum, the retroperitoneal lymph nodes, and the peritoneum, particularly in the pelvis, should be performed for evidence of metastatic disease, and biopsy specimens of suspicious lesions should be obtained. Consideration should be given to the use of retention sutures in patients at risk of dehiscence or to open packing of the wound in patients at risk of wound infection.

Ascending and Transverse Colon Obstructions

It is now well accepted that LBO of the ascending or the transverse colon should be managed with right or extended right hemicolectomy, respectively, with primary ileocolic anastomosis. Creation of an ileostomy should be reserved for patients who are critically ill or who have diffuse contamination and peritonitis. Right hemicolectomy with primary anastomosis is also appropriate for cecal volvulus (see Fig. 72–1D).

Descending and Sigmoid Colon Obstructions

The surgical management of lesions in the descending or the sigmoid colon remains controversial. If the obstructing lesion is associated with a synchronous right-sided lesion, or if impending cecal perforation with serosal tears is present, subtotal colectomy with primary anastomosis is appropriate. Segmental resection of the left or the sigmoid colon with primary anastomosis may be performed with an acceptable leak rate of about 5% if on-table lavage of the proximal colon is done. On-table lavage requires a surgical team experienced in its use, and many surgeons prefer segmental resection with temporary proximal colonic diversion. Disagreement over which of these techniques is preferable remains. Delayed anastomosis is performed in only 70% of patients after colostomy formation and is associated with significant morbidity, but it minimizes the morbidity associated with the initial procedure. On-table lavage with primary anastomosis carries the risk of leak or the need for a second resection should

a nonpalpable synchronous lesion exist. In otherwise healthy patients, subtotal colectomy with primary anastomosis may be appropriate for left-sided lesions. It is associated with more frequent bowel movements than is segmental resection with on-table lavage and primary anastomosis, however, and is not well tolerated by elderly debilitated patients. Primary anastomosis should not be performed when peritonitis is present.

Rectal Obstructions

In contrast to the management of colon cancer, primary resection of obstructing rectal carcinomas is not indicated. Primary anastomosis below the peritoneal reflection is associated with an unacceptable risk of leak, and delayed reanastomosis is technically difficult. Diverting colostomy with mucous fistula formation should be undertaken for these lesions. There is some debate whether transverse or sigmoid colostomy is preferred. Following neoadjuvant therapy and evaluation of the colon for synchronous lesions, low anterior resection with primary anastomosis or abdominoperineal resection should be performed.

Colonic Pseudo-obstruction

The management of pseudo-obstruction (Ogilvie's syndrome) has traditionally involved nasogastric decompression, intravenous hydration, narcotic cessation, enemas, and decompressive colonoscopy when cecal distention reaches 11 to 12 cm. Recently, the use of intravenous neostigmine (1 to 2 mg) has significantly reduced the number of patients requiring colonoscopy. Cardiac monitoring should be implemented during this therapy. Surgical intervention is necessary only for perforation or failure of these modalities (see Chapter 75, Pseudo-Obstruction of the Colon).

Sigmoid Volvulus

Flexible sigmoidoscopy is successful in reducing 50% to 80% of sigmoid volvuli (see Fig. 72–1E and F). Recurrent volvulus may occur in as many as 90% of patients, and elective sigmoid colectomy with primary anastomosis should be recommended for most patients during the same hospitalization. In patients in whom reduction is not successful or gangrenous bowel is suspected, emergent exploration is indicated with resection and colostomy formation. Some surgeons have advocated mesosigmoidoplasty after detorsion if the colon is viable, thereby avoiding colostomy or primary anastomosis in an emergent setting. Recurrent volvulus is rare after this procedure. Operative detorsion alone is associated with an unacceptable recurrence rate. The extent of resection is controversial, but most surgeons prefer sigmoid colectomy over total abdominal colectomy.

Minimally Invasive Technique

The appropriate use of minimally invasive techniques in the treatment of LBO is in its infancy. Laparoscopically assisted colectomy, colostomy, and colocolostomy may be performed safely by experienced surgeons. Clinical trials comparing minimally invasive surgery of the large intestine with open procedures are lacking, and cost-effectiveness has also not been demonstrated. Nonetheless, some patients with LBO may be good candidates for minimally invasive techniques, including colectomy for benign causes of obstruction and diverting colostomy for rectal cancer. Further studies are necessary to delineate the role of minimally invasive surgery in LBO. Until further evidence-based data become available, the use of minimally invasive techniques for the management of LBO will remain controversial.

POSTOPERATIVE MANAGEMENT

In the absence of significant comorbid conditions or sepsis, patients typically require a 7- to 10-day hospitalization; however, longer stays are frequently necessary, and most retrospective reviews report mean stays of 18 to 21 days. Ambulation should be initiated on the first postoperative day. Catheter drainage of the bladder is continued until the patient has adequate mobility and frequent determinations of urine output are no longer necessary. Intravenous fluids and nasogastric decompression are required until the postoperative ileus resolves. Patients may then be started on a clear liquid diet and can be advanced to an appropriate diet as tolerated. After return of bowel function, conversion to oral medications for pain management is initiated. Prophylaxis for ulcer and deep venous thrombosis should be continued until discharge. Antibiotic therapy should be continued only for documented infections or ongoing sepsis.

COMPLICATIONS

Because urgent or emergent operation is often necessary for LBO, pulmonary, cardiac, renal, or infective complications may be expected in 15% to 30% of patients. Prophylaxis for peptic ulcer and deep venous thrombosis is strongly encouraged. By following the algorithms previously described, the rate of anastomotic leak should be 5% or less. Anastomotic leaks usually present 4 to 7 days postoperatively with fever and leukocytosis. In this setting, a water-soluble contrast enema should be obtained. Other potential complications are similar to those encountered during elective colon resection.

Pearls and Pitfalls

PEARLS

- Large bowel obstruction is most frequently due to malignancy. Other common causes include diverticulitis, volvulus, and pseudo-obstruction. Diagnosis is usually evident on plain radiography of the abdomen. Sepsis, the presence of free air, and impending perforation due to massive cecal dilation are indications for emergent operation.
- Large bowel obstruction, unlike small bowel obstruction, is a surgical emergency because of the risk of perforation. Obtain a contrast enema to rule out pseudo-obstruction. Mark a potential stoma site, get a preoperative carcinoembryonic antigen level, and place the patient in the lithotomy position if access to the anus may potentially be necessary.
- Minimally invasive techniques may have merit in selected individuals. Divert obstructing rectal cancers, and resect after neoadjuvant therapy.
- For ascending colon resection, consider primary anastomosis. Left-sided obstruction can be managed by means of limited resection with proximal colonic diversion or primary anastomosis (after on-the-table colonic lavage) or with subtotal colectomy with ileosigmoid anastomosis.

OUTCOMES

Large bowel obstruction requiring urgent or emergent surgical intervention is associated with a 10% to 20% mortality rate. The surgeon and the patient should recognize that obstructing large bowel adenocarcinomas are associated with a worse prognosis than are nonobstructing lesions of the same stage, and some consideration should be given to the use of adjuvant therapies.

SELECTED READINGS

Aldridge MC, Phillips RK, Hittinger R, et al: Influence of tumour site on presentation, management and subsequent outcome in large bowel cancer. Br J Surg 1986;73:663.

Lopez-Kostner F, Hool GR, Lavery IC: Management and causes of acute large-bowel obstruction. Surg Clin North Am 1997;77:1265.

Murray JJ, Schoetz DJ Jr, Coller JA, et al: Intraoperative colonic lavage and primary anastomosis in nonelective colon resection. Dis Colon Rectum 1991;34:527.

Ponec RJ, Saunders MD, Kimmey MB: Neostigmine for the treatment of acute colonic pseudo-obstruction. N Engl J Med 1999;341:137.

Single-stage treatment for malignant left-sided colonic obstruction: A prospective randomized clinical trial comparing subtotal colectomy with segmental resection following intraoperative irrigation. The SCOTIA Study Group. Subtotal Colectomy versus On-table Irrigation and Anastomosis. Br J Surg 1995;82:1622.

Chapter 73

Chronic Ulcerative Colitis

James M. Becker

Chronic ulcerative colitis is a diffuse inflammatory disease of the mucosal lining of the colon and rectum. Total removal of the colon and rectum provides a complete cure, and considerable progress has been made in the surgical management of inflammatory bowel disease. Newer surgical alternatives, developed over the last two decades, have eliminated the need for a permanent ileostomy following definitive resection of the involved colon and rectum.

EPIDEMIOLOGY

The incidence of ulcerative colitis varies greatly within particular geographic regions and within distinct populations. These differences within and between populations provide insights into the etiology and pathogenesis of ulcerative colitis. The annual incidence is about 6 to 12 per 100,000 in northern hemisphere countries, such as the United Kingdom, Norway, Sweden, and the United States, and about 2 to 8 per 100,000 in southern countries such as Australia, South Africa, and the countries of southern Europe. The incidences in Asia and South America are considerably lower. These trends suggest that the incidence of ulcerative colitis is highest in developed or urban regions and lowest in developing regions, although there are signs that the incidence rates of inflammatory bowel disease may be leveling off in developed countries and starting to increase in developing nations. Although still quite low, the incidence of ulcerative colitis is increasing in Japan, India, Thailand, and other countries in Asia. Epidemiologic studies support the earlier impression of a higher incidence of ulcerative colitis among Jews (two to four times the incidence in non-Jews) and in whites (four times the incidence in nonwhites).

Although the onset of ulcerative colitis typically occurs between ages 15 and 40 years, the age range extends from infancy to the elderly. In fact, 3% to 5% of new cases occur after age 60. Males and females are affected about equally. Genetic factors play a significant role in the pathogenesis of ulcerative colitis. A total of 10% to 25% of patients with ulcerative colitis have first-degree relatives with the disease. A number of families have been reported with as many as eight members affected over several generations. Both Crohn's disease and ulcerative colitis can occur within the same family, but there appears to be an 80% to 90% concordance for the same disease category within the family. Monozygotic twins have a higher concordance of inflammatory bowel disease than do dizygotic twins. In addition, the HLA phenotypes AW24 and BW35 are associated with ulcerative colitis, particularly in Israeli Jews of European origin. The frequency of the AW24 phenotype is increased in patients with early-onset chronic ulcerative colitis and moderate to severe disease. Geographic as well as racial differences can influence the occurrence of the disease, and there is no conclusive evidence regarding the genetic versus the environmental determination of familial patterns.

ETIOLOGY

The etiology of ulcerative colitis remains unknown (Fig. 73–1). While considerable scientific attention has been devoted to infectious and immunologic hypotheses, other avenues of investigation have included dietary, environmental, vascular, neuromotor, allergic, and psychogenic causes.

The investigation of bacterial and viral agents continues to be an active area, although there is considerable uncertainty as to the role that infectious agents play in the pathogenesis. Whether the infectious agents are more likely to trigger or perpetuate the disease is of great controversy. To be a trigger, an infectious agent would have to act by initiation or reactivation. Agents could initiate an autoimmune response by altering antigens, affecting molecular immunity, or increasing immune responsiveness. The microbial agent might also trigger the pathologic response by increasing mucosal permeability or by stimulating epithelial injury or localized ischemia. The microbial agent could reactivate the inflammatory process directly, by secondary infection, or by release of endotoxins.

Even though there is speculation regarding microbial initiation of inflammation, other investigators have suggested that infectious agents act primarily to perpetuate the disease. The full clinical expression of ulcerative colitis requires an intact mucosal immune system and also depends on normal intestinal flora and their products. Thus, alterations in the disease may result from subtle changes in intestinal flora.

Speculation that chronic ulcerative colitis is an autoimmune disease has considerable appeal. A number of immunologic studies have supported this concept, and there is a great deal of interest in the role of cytokines and immunoregulatory molecules in the control of the immune response in patients with inflammatory bowel disease.

Many investigators argue that the immunologic events observed in patients with ulcerative colitis are nonspecific epiphenomena and are not clinically useful disease markers. Little correlation exists between the systemic immunity and the clinical status of the patient. The changes are nonspecific, particularly those relating to heat-shock proteins and lymphocyte function. These changes in the systemic immune system may simply reflect inflammation, rather than being specific for the disease. In contrast,

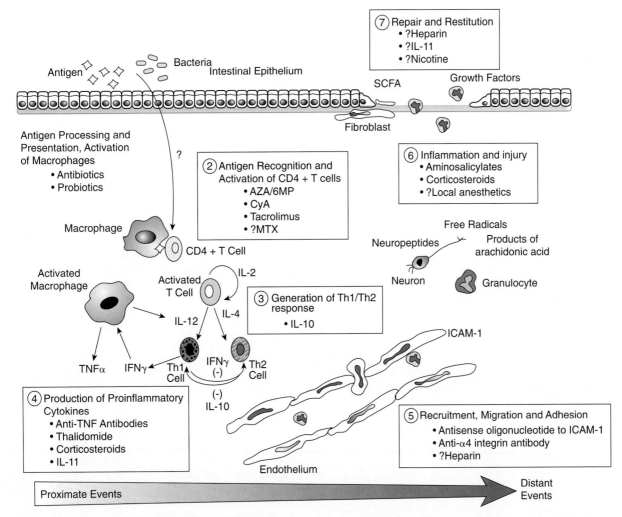

Figure 73–1. Pathogenesis of IBD as it relates to therapy. MTX, methotrexate; SCFA, short-chain fatty acids. (Adapted from Sands BE: Therapy of inflammatory bowel disease. Gastroenterology 2000;118[2 suppl 1]:S68–S82.)

many investigators believe that mucosal immunity plays a key role in mucosal defense and repair, and there is growing support for altered mucosal immunity in the pathogenesis of inflammatory bowel diseases.

Some have proposed that ulcerative colitis represents an energy-deficient state of the colonic epithelium, with decreased levels of free coenzyme A and a lower oxidation of butyrate to carbon dioxide in the colonic mucosal cells. Based on this theory, short-chain fatty acids might be therapeutically beneficial.

Despite the imperfections and differences, the accumulated evidence, especially the presence of chronic ulcerative colitis in three or more members of a family spanning several generations, the increased frequency among first-degree relatives, and the increased concordance rates of inflammatory bowel disease in monozygotic twins strongly suggest a genetic influence. The genetic mechanisms involved are poorly understood, although multiple gene alterations are likely. Genetic possibilities in ulcerative colitis include a polygenetic mode of inheritance, a specific form of somatic gene mutation in mesenchymal stem cells, the growth of a forbidden clone of cells whose mutant humoral products attack the colonic mucosa, and a rare additive major gene. During the past

decade, animal models of intestinal inflammation have substantially augmented our understanding of the pathogenesis of ulcerative colitis, particularly in the areas of inflammatory mediators and cytokine regulation, genetic susceptibility, and the influence of ubiquitous luminal bacterial constituents.

CLINICAL FEATURES

Ulcerative colitis usually manifests as bloody diarrhea, abdominal pain, and fever. Sixty percent of patients present with a relatively mild attack that occurs either as a segmental colitis involving the distal colon (80%) or as a pancolitis (20%). A total of 5% to 15% of patients with disease limited to the rectosigmoid area show eventual progression to involve most, if not all, of the length of the colon. Twenty-five percent of all patients present with a moderate attack in which bloody diarrhea is the major symptom. In 15% of patients, ulcerative colitis has an acute fulminating course, with relatively sudden onset of frequent bloody bowel movements, high fever, weight loss, and diffuse abdominal tenderness.

Extraintestinal manifestations of ulcerative colitis are

observed in a number of organ systems. Articular disorders, including peripheral joint disease, arthralgias, swelling, pain, and redness with migratory involvement, usually parallel the intensity of the colitis and respond to medical or surgical treatment. The joints of the lower extremities are most frequently involved. Overall, 20% of patients manifest endopathologic peripheral arthritis. Ankylosing spondylitis coexists in about 5% of patients, and sacroiliitis is observed in about 10% of patients. While lesions of the skin and oral cavity, including aphthous stomatitis and gingivitis and erythema nodosum, are observed less frequently in ulcerative colitis than in Crohn's disease, pyoderma gangrenosum is more frequent in ulcerative colitis (0.6%). Liver and biliary tract disorders occur commonly in patients with chronic ulcerative colitis, with 80% of patients demonstrating histologic evidence of pericholangitis on liver biopsy; hepatic involvement is more common in patients with pancolitis. About 70% of patients have fatty infiltration of the liver, 5% manifest chronic active hepatitis, about 1% develop biliary cirrhosis, and about 3% develop one of the most difficult complications, sclerosing cholangitis.

Patients with ulcerative colitis are at a slightly greater risk for thromboembolic disease and vasculitis. Rarely, they develop renal disease, clubbing, bronchial and pulmonary abnormalities, and amyloidosis in association with their inflammatory bowel disease.

DIAGNOSIS

The diagnosis is often one of exclusion. There are no pathognomonic laboratory, radiographic, or histologic features. In all patients presenting with diarrhea or bloody diarrhea, an infective cause must be excluded. Flexible sigmoidoscopy should be the first step in diagnosis because ulcerative colitis involves the distal colon and rectum in 90% to 95% of patients. Colonoscopy may be useful in determining the extent and activity of the disease, particularly in patients in whom the diagnosis is unclear, cancer is suspected, or there is a need to differentiate ulcerative colitis from Crohn's colitis. Barium enema examination of the colon may be of use in some patients, but it is potentially dangerous in those with toxic megacolon. A plain abdominal radiograph may be of help in recognizing and following toxic megacolon complicating ulcerative colitis.

MEDICAL MANAGEMENT

The principal categories of drug treatment of ulcerative colitis include symptomatic antidiarrheal and antispasmodic agents, sulfasalazine and its analogues, corticosteroids and adrenocorticotropic hormone (ACTH), immunosuppressive antimetabolites, and certain antibiotics (Table 73–1). Future treatments may also include such novel therapies as antigen-directed and immune mediator blockade, anti-inflammatory cytokines, neuroimmunodulators such as substance P antagonists, nitric oxide synthase inhibitors, oxygen radical scavengers, antisense blockade of gene expression, and potentially probiotic manipulation of luminal bacteria.

SURGICAL CONSIDERATIONS

Nearly half of patients with chronic ulcerative colitis will undergo colectomy within the first 10 years of their illness, primarily because of the chronic nature of the disease and the tendency for relapse. In addition, occasional fulminant complications occur, and there persists a significant risk of malignant degeneration. The indications for surgery vary widely, and these differing indications have different implications for the timing of surgery and the choice of operative procedure.

The indications for surgical intervention include (1) unrelenting hemorrhage, (2) toxic megacolon with impending or frank perforation, (3) fulminating acute ulcerative colitis unresponsive to steroid therapy, (4) obstruction from stricture, (5) suspicion or demonstration of colonic cancer, (6) systemic complications, (7) intractability, and, (8) in children, failure to mature at an acceptable rate (Table 73–2). For most patients with ulcerative colitis, a colectomy is performed when the disease enters an intractable, chronic phase and becomes a physical and social burden to the patient. With the available sphincter-sparing operations, it has become critically important to avoid standard proctectomy wherever possible and to distinguish diagnostically patients with ulcerative colitis from those with Crohn's disease.

SURGICAL EMERGENCIES

Approximately 10% of patients with ulcerative colitis present initially with an acute, catastrophic illness. Several well-identified complications of ulcerative colitis require urgent operation, including (1) unrelenting hemorrhage, (2) toxic megacolon with impending or frank perforation, (3) fulminating acute ulcerative colitis unresponsive to steroid therapy, (4) acute colonic obstruction from stricture, and (5) suspicion or demonstration of colon cancer.

Acute perforation occurs infrequently, with the incidence directly related to both the severity of the initial attack and the extent of disease. The overall incidence of perforation during a first attack is less than 4%, but if the attack is severe the incidence rises to about 10%, and if the pancolitis is associated with a clinically severe attack the perforation rate approaches 20%, with an associated mortality rate of 40% to 50%. Although free colon perforation occurs much more frequently in the presence of toxic megacolon, it is important to remember that toxic megacolon is not a prerequisite for development of perforation. In the presence of colonic perforation, the operation should be definitive without being overly aggressive. Abdominal colectomy with ileostomy and a Hartmann-type closure of the rectum is the procedure of choice.

Obstructions caused by benign stricture formation occur in 10% of patients, with one third of the strictures in the rectum. Strictures result from submucosal fibrosis and, occasionally, mucosal hyperplasia. Although they rarely cause acute obstruction, these lesions must be differentiated from carcinoma by biopsy or excision, and particular attention should be given to excluding Crohn's disease. In ulcerative colitis, strictures caused by carcinoma are less common than those caused by benign disease and are more prone to perforation.

| Table 73–1 | **Medications Commonly Used to Treat Ulcerative Colitis** |

| | ULCERATIVE COLITIS | | | |
| | Active Disease | | | |
CLASS/DRUG	Distal Colitis	Mild-Moderate	Moderate-Severe	Maintenance
5-ASA				
Enema	+	+[a]	−	+
Oral	+	+	−	+
Antibiotics (metronidazole, ciprofloxacin, others)	−	−	−	+[b]
Corticosteroids, classic and novel				
Enema, foam, suppository	+	+[a]	−	−
Oral	+	+	+	−
Intravenous	+[c]	−	+	−
Immunomodulators				
6-MP/AZA	+[c]	−	+[c]	+[c]
Methotrexate	−	−	−	−
Cyclosporine	+[c]	−	+[c]	−
Biologic response modifiers				
Infliximab	?	?	?	?

[a]For adjunctive therapy.
[b]Some data to support use; remains controversial.
[c]Selected patients.
5-ASA, 5-aminosalicylic acid; AZA, azathioprine; 6-MP, 6-mercaptopurine.
Adapted from Sands BE: Therapy of inflammatory bowel disease. Gastroenterology 2000;118(2 suppl 1):S68–S82.

Massive hemorrhage secondary to ulcerative colitis is rare, occurring in fewer than 1% of patients but accounting for about 10% of urgent colectomies performed for ulcerative colitis. Prompt surgical intervention is indicated after hemodynamic stabilization. Uncontrollable hemorrhage from the entire colorectal mucosa may be the one clear indication for emergency proctocolectomy. If possible, the rectum should be spared for later mucosal proctectomy and ileoanal anastomosis, but the surgeon and patient must realize that about 10% of patients will have continued hemorrhage from the retained rectal segment.

Acute toxic megacolon complicates ulcerative colitis in 6% to 13% of patients. Initial treatment of toxic megacolon includes intravenous fluid and electrolyte resuscitation, nasogastric suction, broad-spectrum antibiotics including both anaerobic and aerobic gram-negative coverage, and parenteral nutrition to improve nutritional status. Although the role of high-dose steroids in toxic megacolon is controversial, most patients with a severe attack of ulcerative colitis are already receiving steroid therapy and thus need stress doses of corticosteroids to prevent adrenal crisis. When toxic megacolon is treated promptly, immediate surgery is not inevitable. Even

among patients in whom prompt resolution has occurred, however, about half will require surgery within a year, and most will eventually require colectomy, but hopefully under elective conditions.

In the presence of acute toxic megacolon, surgery is associated with high operative morbidity and mortality. Postoperative complications, including sepsis, wound infection, abscess, fistula, or delayed wound healing, have been reported in as many as half of the patients. Postoperative mortality ranges between 11% and 16% and, for the subset of patients with perforation, 27% and 44%. The overall mortality rate after emergency surgery is 9%; the mortality rate is 6% for total abdominal colectomy and is as high as 15% for proctocolectomy, suggesting that conservative surgery may be most appropriate in the acute setting. With the popularity of anal sphincter–sparing procedures, the surgeon should always weigh the possibility that leaving the rectum intact allows its use for subsequent mucosal proctectomy and ileoanal anastomosis.

PROCTOCOLECTOMY AND ILEOSTOMY

Chronic ulcerative colitis is cured once the colon and rectum are removed; thus, single-stage total proctocolectomy and ileostomy has historically been the operation of choice for elective surgical treatment. Despite the fact that this operation eliminates all disease and risk of malignant transformation, it is poorly accepted by patients and their physicians, primarily because a permanent abdominal ileostomy is required after standard proctocolectomy. Patients receiving even the most carefully constructed ileostomies are incontinent with regard to gas and stool and must wear an external collecting bag both day and night.

Although 90% of patients with a Brooke ileostomy are

| Table 73–2 | **Ulcerative Colitis: Indications for Surgery** |

Severe or persistent hemorrhage
Toxicity and/or perforation
Suspected cancer
Significant dysplasia
Growth retardation
Systemic complications
Intractability

able to adequately adjust to the stoma, between 25% and 50% of patients with ileostomies complain of appliance-related problems. These complications include skin irritation or excoriation, discomfort, leakage, odor, the financial burden of caring for an ileostomy with modern disposable stomal devices, and the time and effort required. Perhaps more important than these problems are the significant psychologic and social implications of a permanent ileostomy, particularly for young and physically active patients. It is for this reason that surgeons have long sought other alternatives to total proctocolectomy and ileostomy.

SUBTOTAL COLECTOMY

Subtotal colectomy with either Brooke ileostomy and Hartmann closure of the rectum or ileorectal anastomosis (Fig. 73–2) has been employed in the surgical treatment of ulcerative colitis for decades. An abdominal stoma is eliminated if ileorectal anastomosis is performed, and the pelvic autonomic nerves are not disturbed, which means that impotence and bladder dysfunction should not be considerations. Subtotal colectomy with ileostomy is the procedure of choice in the emergency setting or if the diagnosis of ulcerative colitis, as opposed to Crohn's disease, cannot be clearly established. Although abdominal colectomy with ileorectal anastomosis is a lesser procedure that usually leaves the patient with full continence, it has not gained wide popularity because it is not a curative operation. The inflammatory process persists in the retained rectum, and there is an ongoing risk of malignancy that may be as high as 15% after 20 years.

CONTINENT ILEOSTOMY

In 1969, Kock described the continent ileostomy, constructed from terminal ileum and consisting of an intesti-

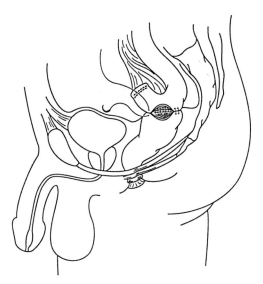

Figure 73–2. Ileorectal anastomosis after abdominal colectomy. This represents a nondefinitive operation for select patients with chronic ulcerative colitis. (From Becker JM: Surgery: Scientific Principles and Practice, 2nd ed. Philadelphia, Lippincott-Raven, 1997, pp 1100–1107, with permission.)

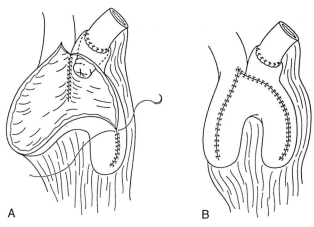

Figure 73–3. The continent ileostomy (Kock pouch) consists of an ileal reservoir and nipple valve constructed by intussuscepting the efferent limb and fixing it in place with sutures or staples (A). This provides a continent internal intestinal reservoir (B) that the patient can drain by intubating the pouch through the flush cutaneous stoma several times throughout the day. (From Becker JM: Surgery: Scientific Principles and Practice, 2nd ed. Philadelphia, Lippincott-Raven, 1997, pp 1100–1107, with permission.)

nal pouch that would serve as a reservoir for stool, with an ileal conduit connecting the pouch to a cutaneous stoma (Fig. 73–3). The operation was modified to include an intestinal nipple valve between the pouch and the stoma. Patients empty the pouch by passing a soft plastic tube through the valve via the stoma. The advantage of this operation is that it cures the disease and offers the patient a potentially new lifestyle by making the ileostomy continent and thereby avoiding an external appliance.

However, the continent ileostomy is associated with a high complication rate, usually related to displacement of the nipple valve, fecal incontinence, and difficulty in intubating and emptying the pouch. Valve failure has been reported in about 25% of patients. Although the Kock ileostomy has its advantages over the Brooke ileostomy, the high rate of mechanical, functional, and metabolic complications has limited its clinical usefulness. In centers that offer all surgical alternatives to patients with ulcerative colitis requiring colectomy, few Kock pouches are being constructed currently. The continent ileostomy, however, may be useful in selected patients who have already undergone total proctocolectomy and ileostomy and, after careful counseling, strongly desire an attempt at a continence-restoring procedure.

ILEOANAL ANASTOMOSIS

Rather then excising the entire rectum, anus, and anal sphincter, the surgeon can take advantage of the fact that ulcerative colitis is a mucosal disease. The rectal mucosa can be selectively dissected and removed down to the dentate line of the anus. This procedure preserves an intact muscular cuff of rectum and the anal sphincter complex. Continuity of the intestinal tract can be re-established by "pulling" the ileum down to the anus through the rectal cuff and circumferentially suturing it to the anus in an end-to-end fashion.

The potential advantages of this approach are that it eliminates all diseased tissue and is as definitive an operation as total proctocolectomy. The pelvic dissection is confined to the endorectal plane, and thus parasympathetic innervation to the bladder and genitalia are preserved, virtually eliminating problems with urinary dysfunction or impotence. Moreover, the often long-term draining perineal wound is eliminated. Although most surgeons use a temporary protecting loop ileostomy, a permanent abdominal stoma is unnecessary because of the ileoanal anastomosis. Finally, if performed carefully, the procedure maintains continence.

In the last two decades, there has been increasing interest in the ileoanal pull-through procedure. This interest was developed, in part, because other alternatives, such as the Kock pouch, were not as successful as had originally been hoped. In addition, important technical advances have been made. There was an inverse correlation between ileal compliance and capacity and stool frequencies in patients after the end-to-end ileoanal anastomosis. This process of ileal adaptation and dilatation could be hastened by surgical construction of an ileal pouch (reservoir) proximal to the ileoanal anastomosis (Fig. 73–4). Several types of ileal reservoirs were proposed, including the J-pouch, S-pouch, W-pouch, and lateral side-to-side isoperistaltic pouch (Fig. 73–5). Several studies have demonstrated a reduction in stool frequency in adult patients in whom an ileal pouch was constructed, particularly in the early postoperative period.

Another important technical addition to the operation is a temporary diverting loop ileostomy. This procedure allows fecal diversion during the early weeks of healing of the ileal pouch and ileoanal anastomosis, thereby re-

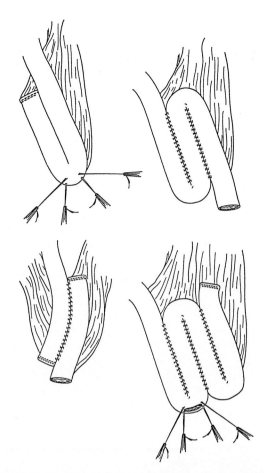

Figure 73–5. Creating the ileal pouch–anal anastomosis. The pouch is secured to the sphincter in each quadrant with a suture. The purse-string stitch closing the enterotomy is cut to allow the apex of the pouch to open. An anastomosis is then created between the apex of the pouch and the anoderm using interrupted absorbable sutures. (From Becker JM: Surgery: Scientic Principles and Practice, 2nd ed. Philadelphia, Lippincott-Raven, 1997, pp 1100–1107, with permission.)

ducing the incidence of pelvic sepsis and dehiscence of the ileal pouch and ileoanal anastomosis. Some surgeons have successfully eliminated the loop ileostomy in selected good-risk patients.

Although it was thought initially that only patients who were young and had relatively quiescent disease were candidates for ileoanal pull-throughs, the indications have liberalized during the past 10 years. Patients are not candidates if other medical problems or the severity of the colitis precludes a 4- to 6-hour operation. Whether younger patients have a superior result remains controversial. Many surgeons are comfortable in offering ileoanal anastomosis to patients in their sixth or seventh decade if they are in good health and have adequate anal sphincter function. Disease severity is not associated with a greater operative morbidity, nor with subsequent functional results. Crohn's disease is, however, an absolute contraindication to the operation. The most important criterion for performing an ileoanal pull-through is that the patient understands the physiology and technique of the operation and has realistic expectations about the outcome.

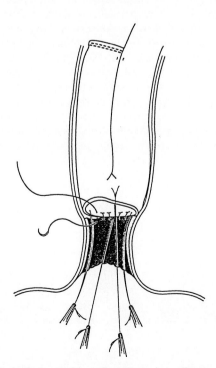

Figure 73–4. Ileal pouch configurations in patients undergoing ileal pouch–anal anastomosis. (From Becker JM: Surgery: Scientific Principles and Practice, 2nd ed. Philadelphia, Lippincott-Raven, 1997, pp 1100–1107, with permission.)

Postoperative morbidity and functional results in most large series after ileoanal pull-through have been encouraging (Fig. 73–6). In the author's series (1999) of more than 550 patients, 82% were operated on for ulcerative colitis and 18% for familial polyposis coli. The mean age was 35 years, with a range of 11 to 76 years. Sixty-two percent of the patients were male. The experience with ileoanal pull-through supports the absence of mortality and the low morbidity that can be achieved. No operative deaths occurred in the author's series, and the overall operative morbidity was about 10%.

The major operative morbidity after ileoanal pull-through is bowel obstruction, both early after the initial operation and later after closure of the loop ileostomy. The rate of bowel obstruction requiring reoperation is about 10%; however, this is no different from that after proctocolectomy and ileostomy. Pelvic and wound infections do occur in 10% to 20% of patients, although the overall infection rate was reduced to about 5% in several more recent large series. A 5% to 10% failure rate necessitating pelvic pouch resection and conversion to permanent ileostomy occurs and is, in part, related to patients with Crohn's disease in whom the original diagnosis prompting ileal pouch–anal anastomosis was incorrect.

Although the results with mucosal proctectomy and ileoanal pull-through have been excellent, differing views have arisen regarding the operative technique and its effect on anal physiology and the functional result. Some surgeons advocate an alternative approach that eliminates the need for distal mucosal proctectomy. Instead, the distal rectum is divided near the pelvic floor, about 2 cm proximal to the intact anal canal. The ileal pouch is then stapled to the top of the anal canal. The rationale for this approach is that by preserving the mucosa of the anal transition zone, the anatomic integrity of the anal canal would be preserved and the rate of fecal incontinence improved. While several studies suggest improved sensation and better functional results, these results have not been documented by any prospective, controlled study. The obvious concern is that by leaving disease-bearing mucosa in the anal canal, the patients are exposed to a lifelong risk of persistent or recurrent inflammatory disease, as well as the potential for malignant transformation. Among 50 patients treated with proctocolectomy for ul-

cerative colitis at the Mayo Clinic, 90% had disease present in the mucosa within 1 cm of the dentate line, where the specimens were examined histologically. This inflamed mucosa is left behind by this newer technique. In addition, dysplasia and adenocarcinoma have been described in the mucosa of the proximal anal canal in patients with ulcerative colitis. Until this technique is further evaluated, patients will require careful lifetime surveillance. Mucosectomy, although perhaps optimal in all patients, must be recommended in patients with rectal dysplasia, proximal rectal cancer, diffuse colonic dysplasia, and familial polyposis.

The most frequent late complication in patients undergoing ileoanal pull-through is pouch dysfunction or pouchitis, reported to occur in 10% to 50% of these patients. Pouchitis is an incompletely defined, poorly understood clinical syndrome consisting of increased stool frequency, watery stools, cramping, urgency, nocturnal leakage of stool, arthralgias, malaise, and fever. The syndrome is similar to that found in patients with the Kock continent ileostomy pouches. The etiology of this condition is unknown; speculation includes early Crohn's disease, bacterial overgrowth or bacterial dysbiosis, either primary or secondary malabsorption, stasis, ischemia, and nutritional or immune deficiencies. A small percentage of patients (<5%) with chronic pouchitis are eventually found to have Crohn's disease. A short course of metronidazole and ciprofloxacin is successful in treating two thirds of patients with pouchitis. The remaining patients have recurrent pouchitis that responds to cyclic metronidazole therapy or a chronic unresponsive form.

The functional results after ileoanal pull-through have been quite consistent across most large series. The number of bowel movements after ileoanal pull-through ranges from 4 to 9 daily, with an average of 6 per day. Nocturnal bowel movements occur one to two times nightly, with a mean of one. Nocturnal seepage of stool or staining is observed in 20% of patients in the early postoperative period, but by 1 year is observed infrequently. Patients have an extremely high level of satisfaction and performance, particularly compared with those who have undergone conventional Brooke ileostomy.

Eventually, a significant proportion of patients with ulcerative colitis require operation, with the realization

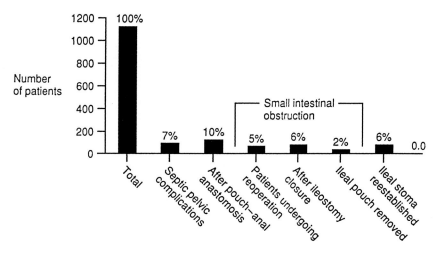

Figure 73–6. Operative morbidity after colectomy and ileoanal anastomosis in 12 clinical series. (From Becker JM: Surgery: Scientific Principles and Practice, 2nd ed. Philadelphia, Lippincott-Raven, 1997, pp 1100–1107, with permission.)

Pearls and Pitfalls

- The incidence of ulcerative colitis is highest in developed or urban regions of the world and lowest in developing regions.
- Current research suggests that infectious agents act primarily to perpetuate the disease.
- Many investigators believe that mucosal immunity plays a key role in mucosal defense and repair, and there is growing support for altered mucosal immunity in the pathogenesis of inflammatory bowel diseases.
- Ulcerative colitis usually presents with bloody diarrhea, abdominal pain, and fever.
- A small number of patients (15%) with ulcerative colitis have an acute and fulminating course.
- Extraintestinal manifestations of ulcerative colitis are observed in a number of organ systems, including articular disorders, lesions of the skin and oral cavity, liver and biliary tract disorders, thromboembolic disease, and vasculitis.
- The principal categories of drug treatment include symptomatic antidiarrheal and antispasmodic agents, sulfasalazine and its analogues, corticosteroids and adrenocorticotropic hormone (ACTH), immunosuppressive antimetabolites, and certain antibiotics.
- Indications for surgical intervention include unrelenting hemorrhage, toxic megacolon, fulminating acute ulcer

ative colitis unresponsive to steroid therapy, obstruction from stricture, suspicion of colonic cancer, systemic complications, intractability, and, in children, failure to mature.
- Subtotal colectomy with ileostomy is the procedure of choice in the emergency setting or if the diagnosis of ulcerative colitis, as opposed to Crohn's disease, cannot be clearly established.
- The continent "Kock" pouch ileostomy may be useful in selected patients who have already undergone total proctocolectomy and ileostomy and, after careful counseling, strongly desire an attempt at a continence-restoring procedure.
- Another important technical addition to the operation is a temporary diverting loop ileostomy in most patients.
- Ileoanal pull-through with mucosal proctectomy and abdominal colectomy should be the operation of choice.
- The major operative morbidity after ileoanal pull-through is bowel obstruction, both after the initial operation and after loop ileostomy closure.
- The most frequent late complication after ileoanal pull-through is ileal pouch dysfunction or pouchitis, in 10% to 50% of patients.

that colectomy should not reflect a therapeutic failure, but rather a permanent cure. Colectomy with mucosal proctectomy and ileoanal pull-through currently is the operation of choice for most patients requiring elective proctocolectomy for chronic ulcerative colitis. Total proctocolectomy with Brooke ileostomy should be reserved for patients who are not candidates for ileoanal pull-through or who, after careful counseling about the surgical alternatives, elect that alternative. Subtotal colectomy with ileostomy and a Hartmann-like closure of the rectum should be performed when emergency colectomy is indicated or if the diagnosis of ulcerative colitis versus Crohn's colitis is uncertain. The added morbidity of this staged approach means that attempts should be made to prepare the patient for a single-stage colectomy, mucosal proctectomy, and ileoanal pull-through. The continent ileostomy should be considered in a patient who is not a

candidate for ileoanal pull-through or in whom a total proctocolectomy and ileostomy has already been performed and when the patient wants some attempt at restoration of continence.

SELECTED READINGS

Becker JM: Surgical therapy for ulcerative colitis and Crohn's disease. Gastroenterol Clin North Am 1999;28:371.
Becker JM, Hillard AE, Mann FA, et al: Functional assessment after colectomy, mucosal proctectomy, and endorectal ileoanal pull-through. World J Surg 1985;9:589.
Heppell J, Kelly K: Pouchitis. Curr Opin Gastroenterol 1998;14:322.
Kirsner JB (ed): Inflammatory Bowel Disease, 5th ed. Philadelphia, WB Saunders, 2000.
Papadakis KA, Targan SR: Current theories on the causes of inflammatory bowel disease. Gastroenterol Clin North Am 1999;28:283.
Stein RB, Hanauer SB: Medical therapy for inflammatory bowel disease. Gastroenterol Clin North Am 1999;28:297.

Chapter 74

Crohn's Disease of the Small Bowel

Scott A. Strong, Bruce M. Belin, and Steven D. Wexner

Crohn's Disease of the Small Bowel

Scott A. Strong

Crohn's disease is a chronic inflammatory condition of uncertain etiology that affects the entirety of the alimentary tract and may involve extraintestinal sites as well. Whether it is related to an infectious etiology (unusual mycobacterium) or an autoimmune-type disease remains unknown, but the etiology is being actively investigated. Medical therapy remains the first-line treatment, with operative intervention reserved for patients who develop complications of the disease or fail repeated attempts at medical therapy. Surgeons must perform the appropriate operation or combination of procedures after considering a myriad of factors that involve disease distribution and clinical pattern. Although operative therapy generally improves the patient's quality of life, disease recurrence is common and to be expected, but it may be potentially impacted by several factors.

CLINICAL PRESENTATION

Crohn's disease should be considered when an individual presents with complaints of a chronic history of episodic abdominal cramping and diarrhea, especially when associated with constitutional symptoms such as fever, weight loss, and fatigue. Although the physical signs and laboratory features associated with Crohn's disease are generally nonspecific, the radiographic, endoscopic, and histologic characteristics usually discriminate Crohn's disease from other disorders. Conditions that may closely mimic the symptoms and findings of Crohn's disease include bacterial or fungal intestinal infections, amebiasis, sprue, lymphoma, tuberculosis, and, for those with inflammation limited to the large bowel, ulcerative colitis as well as other infectious colitides.

Despite current state-of-the-art medical suppressive therapy, the majority of patients with Crohn's disease will still require one or more operations during their lifetime. Disease distribution and clinical pattern influence the probability of operative intervention, but the overall incidence has persisted at 78% and 90% after 20 and 30 years, respectively, of disease symptoms. In general, the operative indications are categorized as acute and chronic complications of the disease or failed medical therapy with intractability (Table 74–1).

DISEASE COMPLICATIONS

Acute Disease Complications

Toxic colitis is a potentially fatal complication of Crohn's colitis. To minimize morbidity and potential mortality, this acute emergency warrants aggressive medical therapy and, at the least, early surgical consultation, even if an operation does not appear imminent. Because of the very real potential for operative intervention, the patient and family should be introduced to the surgeon very early after hospitalization, usually within the first 12 hours. Cooperation between gastroenterologist (or internist) and surgeon is crucial. Increasing colonic dilatation, free perforation, massive hemorrhage, peritonitis, and septic shock are indications for emergent operation after the patient has been adequately resuscitated. Otherwise, any worsening of the clinical course over the ensuing 24 to 72 hours of medical management should mandate urgent operative exploration. Furthermore, if the patient improves only minimally after 5 to 7 days of aggressive conventional therapy, the colitis should be considered refractory, and operative therapy is advised, as the probability of obtaining a remission is low.

Significant hemorrhage is a rare (~1%) complication, but it often represents a diagnostic as well as therapeutic challenge. A colonic ulcer is the usual source of bleeding

Table 74–1	Operative Indications for Patients with Crohn's Disease

Acute Disease Complications
  Toxic colitis or toxic megacolon
  Massive hemorrhage (rare)
  Perforation
Chronic Disease Complications
  Obstruction
  Malignancy
  Growth retardation
  Selected extraintestinal manifestations
Medical Failure
  Lack of a response with ongoing symptoms
  Failure to thrive, weight loss, malnutrition
  Incomplete response
  Intolerance of medication
  Noncompliance with medication

and can be identified as well as controlled during colonoscopy; operative treatment is necessary only 20% of the time. Overall, one third of patients will experience recurrent hemorrhage, typically within 3 years of their initial episode. Given the potential efficacy of endoscopic or medical treatment, a nonoperative approach should be aggressively pursued as first-line therapy in most patients.

Free *perforation* of the bowel is also infrequent (~2%) and typically occurs just proximal to a stricture or as a consequence of toxic colitis.

Chronic Disease Complications

Obstruction is the most common complication of Crohn's disease, particularly when the disease affects the small intestine. Acute obstruction is usually an incomplete obstruction due to inflammatory disease, and most often resolves with rehydration, pharmacologic medical therapy, bowel rest, and nasogastric decompression. Conversely, a chronic obstruction is typified by recurring episodes secondary to a fibrotic, fixed stricture or strictures that will not respond to long-term medical therapy and require elective operative treatment. In the latter scenario, contrast-enhanced radiographs often show a fixed narrowing evident both on multiple views and on repeated examinations with proximal dilatation. Colonic obstruction may herald a significant stricture that occasionally can be dilated endoscopically, provided that malignancy is excluded by biopsy and cytologic brushing.

The increased association between malignancies of the alimentary tract and Crohn's disease is well recognized. A variety of malignancies occur with greater frequency in Crohn's disease than in the general population. Small and large bowel adenocarcinoma complicating Crohn's disease is acknowledged and thoroughly described. Less reported associations, however, include gastric cancer, cholangiocarcinoma, carcinoid tumors, lymphoma, and malignant melanoma. This increased incidence of colorectal malignancy in Crohn's colitis has caused some clinicians to question whether an endoscopic surveillance program should be instituted. The now well-established colitis-dysplasia-carcinoma sequence of ulcerative colitis may not be as applicable in Crohn's disease; however, in support of this scenario, many researchers have suggested a strong correlation between remote as well as adjacent dysplasia and adenocarcinoma in Crohn's colitis. Given the difficult task of diagnosing colorectal cancer associated with long-standing Crohn's colitis and the relationship between dysplasia and carcinoma in this setting, the finding of dysplasia on colonoscopic biopsy or brushing, particularly in a worrisome area, warrants colonic resection.

Growth retardation occurs in one quarter of children affected by Crohn's disease. If retarded growth persists despite adequate medical and nutritional therapy, operative intervention is recommended early and before the onset of puberty. Otherwise, longitudinal growth will not occur because of epiphyseal closure.

Extraintestinal manifestations affect more than 25% of patients with Crohn's disease. Some of the manifestations are associated with the intestinal disease, while others are discordant. Typically, the cutaneous, ocular, and peripheral joint manifestations are linked to gut inflammation, while ankylosing spondylitis and primary sclerosing cholangitis behave independently. Resection of the grossly involved intestinal disease may have little, if any, impact on these extraintestinal manifestations.

Medical Failure (Intractability)

Medical therapy is initiated for most patients suffering from symptomatic Crohn's disease unless the presentation mandates emergent operative treatment. Huge advances have been made in the medical treatment of Crohn's disease over the last two decades, improving on the previous unimodel treatment with prednisone. Antibiotics, 5-aminosalicylate (5-ASA) compounds, steroids, immunosuppressive agents, and/or biologic modifiers are prescribed and delivered topically, enterally, or parenterally.

Patients started on medication for the treatment of their Crohn's disease should be counseled about potential side effects and adverse reactions. Additionally, the objectives of therapy should be detailed from the outset, clearly defining the goals for symptom control and duration of treatment. Treatment is not aimed at cure of the disease, but rather symptom suppression through anti-inflammatory medications. Lifelong medical follow-up will be necessary. If the treatment fails to adequately improve the specified symptoms within the dictated time interval, the medication should be supplanted or supplemented. If significant signs or symptoms persist after employing reasonable medical alternatives, operative intervention is warranted. Alternatively, some patients will become noncompliant with or will not tolerate the medications; in either instance, operative intervention should be considered.

OPERATIVE THERAPY

PREOPERATIVE MANAGEMENT. A variety of imaging and endoscopic modalities are used in the evaluation of a patient presenting for elective operative treatment of Crohn's disease. The particular strategy is individualized, depending on the symptoms and signs. In general, the small bowel and large bowel are examined with the use of contrast-enhanced radiographs and colonoscopy, respectively. Computed tomography is reserved for persons with complaints suggestive of intra-abdominal sepsis, while upper endoscopy is used for individuals with a history or symptoms suggesting gastroduodenal Crohn's disease. Nuclear medicine scans may be of use in discriminating whether chronic stenosing or acute inflammatory disease is the cause of obstructive symptoms.

Patients scheduled for operative treatment should be educated about their disease and the operative options because they commonly possess only rudimentary insight. Immunosuppressive medications should be discontinued 3 to 4 weeks prior to an *elective procedure* because they might interfere with the normal immune response and increase the likelihood of postoperative infection. Any physiologic, nutritional, or metabolic deficits should be corrected during the preoperative period, although malnutrition is usually difficult to reverse, even with the use of parenteral alimentation. Patients who might require temporary fecal diversion and those needing a permanent stoma should be appropriately counseled and marked preoperatively by either a stoma therapist or a nurse adequately trained in the vagaries of stomal management. This is crucial because the principal factor influencing satisfactory early rehabilitation of an ostomy patient is the correct location and construction of the stoma combined with adequate patient education about its care. Bowel preparation (nonobstructed patients), antibiotic prophylaxis, and stress-dosages of steroids (steroid usage within the past year) are used as indicated.

INTRAOPERATIVE MANAGEMENT. Several types of procedures are used in operative therapy for Crohn's disease. These may be classified as follows:

- intestinal resection with or without anastomosis
- bypass procedure: internal (e.g., gastroduodenostomy), external (e.g., ileostomy)
- stricturoplasty

Resection. Almost without exception, resection is the procedure of choice for Crohn's disease of the small bowel, when it is the patient's first operation. When the resection provides enough tissue for histologic examination, the procedure allows a certainty of diagnosis. Even with scattered proximal skip lesions that may be amenable to stricturoplasty, the distal ileal segment usually is the most inflamed site and typically warrants resection. The limits of resection should be to grossly uninvolved bowel; attempts to resect all "histologically involved" bowel are fraught with several complications. First, the length resected may be too extensive. Second, the histopathologic definition of "involvement" varies from center to center, and no universally accepted standards exist. Third, and most important, no studies have convincingly shown that complete "histologic" clearing of disease has any clinical benefit over clearance of just the grossly involved segment.

Resectional surgery is also the procedure of choice for Crohn's colitis. Despite high recurrence rates, segmental resection with colocolic or colorectal anastomosis provides many patients with Crohn's colitis with years of stoma-free life.

Bypass. Bypass operations are still considered desirable options, but only in specific circumstances. Exclusion bypass is a very reasonable option for a complicated ileocecal phlegmon with dense attachment to the iliac vessels or retroperitoneal structures (ureter), with plans for definitive resection in later months, especially if the patient has not received optimal attempts at medical therapy. Permanent treatment by bypass alone is not recommended because chronic complications can still occur in the bypassed segment, including the development of malignancy. In such patients, the proximal end of the excluded ileal segment should be exteriorized as a mucus fistula to vent the mucosal secretions that could cause ileal stump dehiscence. Continuity bypass (proximal-to-distal side-to-side bypass) is a preferred method of management of symptomatic gastroduodenal Crohn's disease that is refractory to medical treatment.

Ileostomy alone, proximal to complicated internal fistulous disease, is used infrequently in current times. Even for free perforation of the small bowel, resection of the perforated segment with exteriorization of the proximal bowel as an end-stoma is standard practice.

Stricturoplasty. The operative therapy for Crohn's disease has shifted increasing toward more conservative approaches over the past two decades. For patients with multiple strictures of the small bowel, intestinal conservation may be achieved by surgically widening the stricture via stricturoplasty. The technique was used initially for the successful treatment of tubercular strictures involving the small bowel and was then expanded to use in strictures secondary to Crohn's disease. Many centers have conducted comprehensive studies of patients undergoing stricturoplasty. Concerns about healing of the suture line and the occurrence of intra-abdominal abscesses or fistulas are minimized by appropriate patient selection (Table 74-2).

A Weinberg-type stricturoplasty technique is used for strictures less than 10 cm in length; a longer stricture is managed with a Finney-type stricturoplasty. Leakage and sepsis are more likely to occur with a long stricture, unless the bowel is supple enough to bend into a U-shape that still allows for a tension-free anastomosis. Alternatively, a side-to-side isoperistaltic stricturoplasty can be safely performed in this instance after resection of the strictured segment's middle third to facilitate the anastomosis. Increasingly more bold modifications of these functional, bowel-preserving "stricturoplasties" are being described, to treat longer segments of involvement (>15 cm). Their safety and utility has yet, however, to be determined. Thus, in general, strictures larger than 15 cm are probably best managed by resection.

PATTERNS OF DISEASE

SMALL INTESTINE DISEASE. "Isolated" small bowel Crohn's disease can present with varying degrees of intes-

Table 74–2	**Indications and Contraindications for Stricturoplasty in Crohn's Disease**

Indications for Stricturoplasty
Diffuse involvement of the small bowel with multiple strictures
Stricture or strictures in a patient who has undergone a previous major resection or resections of small bowel (>100 cm)
Rapid recurrence of Crohn's disease manifested as obstruction
Stricture in a patient with short bowel syndrome
Nonphlegmonous, fibrotic "burned-out" stricture
Contraindications to Stricturoplasty
Free or contained perforation of the small bowel
Phlegmonous inflammaton, internal fistula, or external fistula involving the affected site
Multiple strictures within a short segment easily amenable to resection (one suture line)
Stricture in close proximity to a site chosen for resection
Strictures generally longer than 10–15 cm
Colonic strictures*
Hypoalbuminemia (<2.0 g/dL)

*Many surgeons consider this controversial and conduct stricturoplasty in areas of limited colonic involvement.

tinal involvement. Among the variations seen is the scenario of "primary" distal disease separated from a more proximal "skip" lesion by a short segment that is normal appearing. When there is no concern about short bowel syndrome, as in most patients undergoing their first operation, the entire segment is resected, and a single anastomosis is performed.

Several stenotic segments separated from one another by noninvolved bowel typify another variation. These stenoses range in length from a few centimeters to more than 50 cm. Multiple stricturoplasties are preferred over resection or bypass for the symptomatic patient with diffuse jejunoileitis.

ILEOCOLIC DISEASE. The ileocecal region is the anatomic site most often involved with Crohn's disease, constituting approximately 40% of all patients undergoing operative therapy. In the majority of patients, resection with an ileal-ascending colon anastomosis is possible and desirable. The normal right colon is preserved to provide a larger surface area for water absorption and to avoid other potential sequelae (e.g., duodenal fistula) associated with recurrent disease at an ileal-transverse colon anastomosis.

Unilateral exclusion bypass may be a reasonable alternative for a fixed ileocecal mass, provided the associated sepsis is drained, and reoperation is planned for 6 months later after aggressive medical management. When the patient is explored after exclusion bypass, even in the remote past, it usually is possible to resect the terminal ileum and cecum, disconnect the ileal-transverse colon anastomosis, resect any disease proximal to the anastomosis, close the transverse colotomy, and create an ileal-ascending colon anastomosis. Consideration should be given to placing a ureteral stent immediately preoperatively in an attempt to avoid injury to the right ureter.

COLONIC DISEASE. The choice of operation for Crohn's disease affecting the large intestine depends on multiple variables, including patient age, disease distribution, extent of involvement, previous resections, rectal compliance, presence of perianal disease, and adequacy of fecal continence. Segmental resection with ileocolic or colocolic anastomosis and abdominal colectomy with ileoproctostomy are the procedures most commonly performed for Crohn's colitis.

Although the use of limited resection for Crohn's disease of the small intestine is widely accepted, the value of segmental resection in colonic Crohn's disease is more controversial. Among the large intestine's physiologic roles, the absorption of water and salt, particularly in the right colon, acts to protect against systemic dehydration and electrolyte imbalance. Therefore, although the large bowel is an "expendable" organ, attempts at its preservation are justified. Despite a high incidence of recurrence, the reoperative rate associated with segmental resection for Crohn's colitis should not relegate the patient with focal colonic disease to a total proctocolectomy with end-ileostomy. The use of stricturoplasty for limited disease remains controversial, although some groups claim good results.

A population of patients with symptomatic Crohn's colitis exists in whom a segmental resection is not feasible because of extensive colonic involvement. However, a subgroup of this population demonstrates relative rectal sparing, adequate fecal continence, and absence of active anoperineal sepsis; these individuals should be considered candidates for abdominal colectomy with ileoproctostomy. While some surgeons merely rely on subjective endoscopic evidence of rectal compliance, objective testing of anorectal physiology suggests that individuals who can adequately retain a 150 mL saline enema are suitable candidates for an ileoproctostomy.

In the rare patient with isolated Crohn's proctitis, resection of the rectum with end-colostomy is associated with an acceptable operative recurrence rate. However, the colostomy should be constructed as one does for an ileostomy with precise siting and spigot configuration, anticipating the high-volume, liquid effluent of Crohn's disease. Moreover, proctectomy alone should be avoided if the colon is segmentally involved, as pancolonic disease will most likely ensue. Therefore, unless significant small bowel has been resected or older age necessitates sparing of the absorbing surface of the large intestine, in these patients proctocolectomy with end-ileostomy is preferred over proctectomy and end-colostomy.

Total proctocolectomy with end-ileostomy is indicated in patients with Crohn's colitis whose proctitis, sphincter dysfunction, or anoperineal sepsis is too severe for rectal preservation and ileoproctostomy.

POSTOPERATIVE MANAGEMENT. Management of the patient in the postoperative period is individualized, depending on a myriad of considerations, including comorbid conditions, nutritional status, sepsis, operation performed, length of remaining bowel, duration of operation, blood loss, and the use of fecal diversion. In general, perioperative antibiotics are prescribed only on the day of operation, steroids are tapered to physiologic levels usually after 48 to 72 hours, ambulation is encouraged the night of operation or the next morning, and urethral catheters are continued for less than 3 days. Nasogastric tubes can be discontinued by the next morning, and a liquid diet is initiated. If the patient tolerates liquids without nausea, vomiting, or abdominal distention, the diet is advanced to solid foods without awaiting the passage of flatus or stool. Discharge is planned when the patient is afebrile, ambulating, tolerating a regular diet with return of bowel function, and comfortable with oral pain medication. This "modern" method of management, combined with realistic patient expectations, has reduced the length of patient hospitalization after an operation for Crohn's disease by several days without increasing the incidence of complications or re-admission.

If infected tissue is incompletely resected with the operation, long-term drainage is typically utilized in combination with prolonged outpatient oral antibiotic therapy. In this group, frequent follow-up is recommended. Otherwise, most patients are assessed approximately 6 weeks after discharge unless a stoma has been created. In the latter instance, follow-up at 4 weeks is recommended, because the aperture of the stoma appliance must be reduced as the peristomal edema subsides. For patients with a temporary stoma, a contrast-enhanced radiograph is obtained by the physician in 3 months, followed by elective stoma closure, assuming that all anastomoses are widely patent and without defect.

COMPLICATIONS

Operative therapy for Crohn's disease is associated with the complications typically encountered with intestinal resection, but patients with Crohn's disease are at particular risk for thromboembolic events linked to the disease, infection secondary to bacterial overgrowth in the affected small bowel, sepsis, malnutrition, or immunosuppression, and compromised healing because of chronic steroid therapy. Patients undergoing external fecal diversion alone are at the least risk for these complications, while multiple resections with anastomoses would seem to expose a patient to the greatest risk of postoperative complications. Contrary to this anticipated outcome, large series suggest that the morbidity associated with an operation that includes multiple stricturoplasties is comparable to that with a procedure in which a single resection with primary anastomosis is performed. Obviously, suitable patient selection, appropriate use of fecal diversion, and surgeon experience are critical to maintaining an acceptable operative morbidity in these patients with Crohn's disease, who are often difficult to manage.

OUTCOMES

Historically, morbidity, mortality, and recurrence rates were the sole measures of patient outcome after operative treatment of Crohn's disease. However, the recent introductions of new highly effective, yet costly treatments for Crohn's disease have forced physicians (internists and surgeons alike), patients, and society to make important choices regarding the allocation of resources. Cost-utility models relate the incremental cost of new treatments to improvements in health-related aspects of quality of life and should allow the decision-makers to arrive at sensible choices for patients and society.

Recurrence of Crohn's Disease

Patients with Crohn's disease are haunted by the likelihood of recurrence after resection of their disease. After all, Crohn's disease should be considered a chronic disease that virtually never goes away; symptoms and problems may abate, but if the disease is looked for histologically, evidence of it will be found. In an effort to better counsel patients about their relative risk of symptomatic recurrence, many centers have evaluated multiple factors thought to be harbingers of recurrence. Factors that may increase the recurrence rate include the following: young age at disease onset; gender; use of tobacco; ileocolonic pattern of disease; extraintestinal manifestations; long duration of preoperative symptoms; previous resections; operative indications, such as abscess and fistulization; blood transfusion; extent of resection; lack of fecal diversion; severely fistulizing features of resected bowel; and lack of suppressive chemotherapy after resection. Unfortunately, the role that these factors play in disease recurrence still remains poorly understood.

Some controversy exists regarding the best procedure for large bowel Crohn's disease because of concerns about disease recurrence weighed against the inconvenience of a permanent stoma for the patient. Total proctocolectomy and ileostomy offers a "low" operative recurrence rate—24% and 35% reoperative rates at 5 and 10 years, respectively. However, this procedure commits patients to a permanent ileostomy. In contrast, total colectomy or segmental resection can predispose patients to recurrence and further operation but may postpone or avoid surgery for a stoma in selected individuals. Crohn's colitis with relative rectal sparing can often be treated adequately with total colectomy with ileoproctostomy. After 10 years of follow-up, approximately 60% of patients will maintain intestinal continuity with a functioning ileoproctostomy. The success of this operation is independent of patient age and duration of symptoms, but is inversely linked, in part, to the presence of concomitant small bowel disease at the time of anastomosis. Segmental colonic disease treated with limited resection with colocolonic or colo-

Pearls and Pitfalls

- Crohn's disease is incurable. The long-term care of the patient should be considered, and procedures that jeopardize small bowel function or fecal continence should be avoided.
- Asymptomatic disease should be ignored. If a diseased segment is not a source of obstruction, hemorrhage, or malignancy, the surgeon should leave the bowel undisturbed, understanding that the principal goal of therapy is to minimize bowel resection.
- The operative options are influenced by multiple perioperative factors and intraoperative findings that influence the surgeon's decision making; the planned operative procedure must be often altered and, occasionally, aborted.
- Perforative disease can frequently affect nondiseased bowel segments as well as other intra-abdominal organs. In most instances, this target organ is bluntly teased from the diseased bowel, débrided, and closed primarily.
- Mesenteric division can be difficult because the mesentery is commonly thickened and friable; division requires overlapping placement of clamps and suture ligatures to maximize hemostasis and minimize the risk of dissecting hematoma.
- Resection margins should be conservative; macroscopically normal resection margins are associated with recurrence rates comparable to the more extensive resection margins.
- Septic foci require long-term drainage. Extensive, long-term drainage and omentum interposition will minimize the likelihood of recurrent sepsis and secondary involvement of a newly formed anastomosis.
- Bypass should be avoided whenever possible.
- Stricturoplasties will conserve bowel length and should be used appropriately.
- When possible, segmental resection of colonic Crohn's disease is preferable to colectomy and ileostomy.
- Overall, the therapy that minimizes symptomatic recurrence (operative or medical therapy) should be undertaken.

rectal anastomosis for Crohn's disease of the large bowel has been advocated by many institutions. While the majority of patients will experience symptomatic recurrence, about 75% will maintain intestinal continuity for more than a decade after the initial colonic resection with primary anastomosis.

Costs

Crohn's disease results in substantial morbidity as well as necessitating a high use of health services. Although patients spend nearly two thirds of their life after diagnosis in medical or surgical remission, the lifetime cost of suppressive treatment with aminosalicylates, corticosteroids, and immunosuppressive therapy is comparable to the lifetime cost of operative therapy. Operative therapy accounts for 50% to 60% of all hospitalizations and half of their total costs but is associated with the longest remissions. Therefore, treatment strategies that induce remission in mild disease, maintain remission with lower-cost maintenance therapy, and decrease the number of hospitalizations will have the largest effect on patient outcomes and costs.

Quality of Life

When patients with Crohn's disease express concerns about their disease, they emphasize worries about operation and fear of a permanent stoma. With the exception of patients who persist with chronic active disease, surgical intervention improves health-related quality-of-life scores to levels comparable to those of the general population. And the impact of operative therapy appears comparable to the effect of medication as long as the therapy results in disease remission. Therefore, to improve the quality of life of a patient with active Crohn's disease, the correct approach (i.e., medical versus surgical) is the one that leads to disease remission.

SELECTED READINGS

Casellas F, Lopez-Vivancos J, Badia X, et al: Impact of surgery for Crohn's disease on health-related quality of life. Am J Gastroenterol 2000;95:177.
Fazio VW, Aufses AH Jr: Evolution of surgery for Crohn's disease: A century of progress. Dis Colon Rectum 1999;42:979.
Fazio VW, Marchetti F, Church J, et al: Effect of resection margins on the recurrence of Crohn's disease in the small bowel: A randomized controlled trial. Ann Surg 1996;224:563.
Greenstein AJ, Lachman P, Sachar DB, et al: Perforating and nonperforating indications for repeated operations in Crohn's disease: Evidence for two clinical forms. Gut 1988;29:588.
Prabhakar LP, Laramee C, Nelson H, Dozois RR: Avoiding a stoma: Role for segmental or abdominal colectomy in Crohn's colitis. Dis Colon Rectum 1997;40:71.
Strong SA: Prognostic parameters of Crohn's disease recurrence. Baillieres Clin Gastroenterol 1988;12:167.

Crohn's Disease of the Colon

Bruce M. Belin and Steven D. Wexner

Crohn's disease is an inflammatory condition of the gastrointestinal tract that can occur anywhere from the mouth to the anus. A skip, or noncontinuous, distribution with transmural involvement and its sequelae of perforation and fistulization, fat wrapping or creeping, and mesenteric lymphadenopathy are characteristic of the disease. The disease most frequently involves the terminal ileum but may include the proximal ileum, jejunum, or even the duodenum. However, approximately half of patients with the condition exhibit perianal manifestations, such as fissures, fistulas, or abscesses, at least at some point during their disease course. A significant number of patients have involvement of the colon that varies in location, severity, and extent; the right side is more commonly involved than is the left, and the rectum is usually spared. While rectal sparing is characteristic of Crohn's disease, when the rectum is diseased the differentiation between Crohn's disease and other causes of proctitis can be difficult. The possibilities in the differential diagnosis may include mucosal ulcerative colitis, ischemic colitis, infectious colitis, diverticulitis, and malignancy; differentiation of Crohn's disease from mucosal ulcerative colitis may be particularly challenging in the setting of acute colitis.

PRESENTATION AND EVALUATION

Patients with Crohn's colitis usually present with diarrhea, abdominal pain, and weight loss. Since surgery is not curative, it is often recommended in North America only to treat complications of the disease. However, in Scandinavia, a more aggressive attitude has been adopted. This latter approach strives to decrease the morbidity of chronic immunosuppressive therapy and to limit the postoperative morbidity of surgery on a patient after septic complications have arisen. Although Crohn's disease most frequently presents in patients in their 30s, Crohn's colitis may also present in children and in the elderly. On presentation of a new patient, pertinent past radiographs, operative reports, discharge summaries, and pathology reports and slides should be obtained and reviewed. Special attention should be paid to nutritional evaluation, such as recent changes in the patient's diet, weight, and bowel function. Basic laboratory work should include at least a complete blood count as well as prothrombin time, partial thromboplastin time, and basic electrolyte panel. Problems encountered are leukocytosis from sepsis, anemia from insidious blood loss and malnutrition, coagulopathy from hepatic disease, and hypokalemia from diarrhea. Further evaluation, including measurement of albumin and prealbumin, as well as vitamin B_{12} and folate levels may be indicated. Both colonoscopy with biopsies, including examination of the terminal ileum and small bowel follow-through, or enteroclysis, are routinely performed to evaluate the distribution and severity of mucosal disease. If clinically indicated, a computed tomography is performed to delineate any extraluminal phlegmonous disease or retroperitoneal ureteric displacement or compression. Arrangements are made if resuscitation or preoperative nutrition is required—enteral nutritional support is preferred if small bowel function is adequate.

The clinical examination may reveal right iliac fossa fullness or distention secondary to chronic obstruction. It is important to identify patients with acute colitis suggested by abdominal pain, distention, pyrexia, dehydration, and leukocytosis; toxic dilation is more common in patients with new-onset disease. These patients require urgent resuscitation and surgical evaluation to avoid perforation and death. Other, more subtle extraintestinal manifestations of Crohn's disease include synovitis, ankylosing spondylitis, sclerosing cholangitis, erythema nodosum, pyoderma gangrenosum, and iritis. Significant rectal bleeding is not a common manifestation of Crohn's disease, compared with the aforementioned signs, symptoms, and findings.

Many patients with predominantly small intestinal or colonic Crohn's disease have a history of perianal disease or will have significant findings on examination, including eccentric and/or multiple anal fissures. These ulcers are frequently aggressive and may leave the underlying sphincter muscle exposed. Surprisingly, despite the severe appearance of the disease, patients experience deceptively little discomfort or pain. It is important to recognize these ulcers because in about 1% of patients they are the only manifestation of Crohn's disease. Since biopsy reveals granulomas in fewer than 40% of these ulcers, the diagnosis must often be made on the basis of clinical acumen, rather than histopathologic study. It is important to determine the patient's bowel function and continence, especially if surgery is planned. Many of the patients with perianal disease have concomitant rectal disease, while others will only later go on to develop intestinal involvement, further frustrating the diagnosis. Other anal problems may include abscesses and fistulas; these fistulas may be multiple and extensive or simple. Once again, an adequate knowledge of both the subjective continence and the objective sphincter function is an important prerequisite for fistula surgery. Endorectal ultrasonography, possibly with H_2O_2 instillation into the tract, helps delineate the course and nature of the fistula, while manometry quantitates resting and squeeze pressure as well as rectal capacity and compliance.

Ultimately, the diagnosis is usually confirmed by a combination of clinical examination, endoscopy, and radiographic studies. However, in the acute setting, these studies should be avoided. In the more elective setting, the findings may include discontinuous disease and linear *aphthous ulcers,* while biopsies may reveal granuloma. A contrast-enhanced enema can be useful when a complete colonoscopic examination is difficult or impossible owing to a stricture. In these cases, a double-contrast barium enema provides detail superior to a single-column study; however, if there is any possibility of perforation, a water-soluble agent is used. If a contrast-enhanced enema reveals any filling defects, endoscopic evaluation is necessary to exclude carcinoma. Strictures may also be seen in the setting of Crohn's disease and should be biopsied to exclude malignancy. If necessary, a pediatric colonoscope, a gastroscope, or even a pediatric gastroscope may be helpful in traversing a stricture. One must remember that even if multiple biopsies fail to reveal malignancy, carcinoma may still be present. Thus, surgery may be recommended as both a diagnostic and a therapeutic procedure in patients with colonic strictures.

MEDICAL TREATMENT

Similar to that for Crohn's disease of the small intestine, medical management is usually the first mode of treatment for Crohn's colitis. Medical therapy is continued either until the disease becomes quiescent and the therapeutic agents can be discontinued, they fail to alleviate symptoms, unacceptable side effects develop, or a complication of the disease arises that mandates surgery. Crohn's colitis frequently follows a prolonged course, and it is less likely to completely resolve with medical management than is ulcerative colitis. Figure 74–1 provides an overview for the medical and surgical management of Crohn's colitis.

Ninety percent of patients with Crohn's disease present with the symptoms and signs of chronic colitis: abdominal pain, diarrhea, and weight loss. The other 10% of patients present with acute colitis and therefore are at risk for toxic dilation, perforation, and even death unless urgent evaluation and intervention are initiated. Initial resuscitation includes intravenous hydration to achieve satisfactory urinary output with central venous pressure monitoring. Blood replacement and electrolyte supplementation are undertaken as needed. Antibiotics are often used empirically prior to evaluation and also as a therapeutic modality in the treatment of infective complications. Intravenous steroids, usually hydrocortisone 100 mg every 6 hours, are given if the patient has received steroids within the last 3 months. Bowel rest is initiated with parenteral nutritional support and, optionally, a nasogastric tube. If the abdomen is distended but soft, the patient may be monitored in an intensive care unit with hourly vital signs, frequent physical examinations, and evaluation of blood work, including arterial blood gas, complete blood count, and electrolytes at least every 12 hours. Abdominal girth and colonic diameter on plain abdominal radiographs are helpful parameters in following the disease course. Absolute indications for immediate surgery include a transverse colon diameter greater than 5.5 cm, or free air in the peritoneum or retroperitoneum. Patients who fail

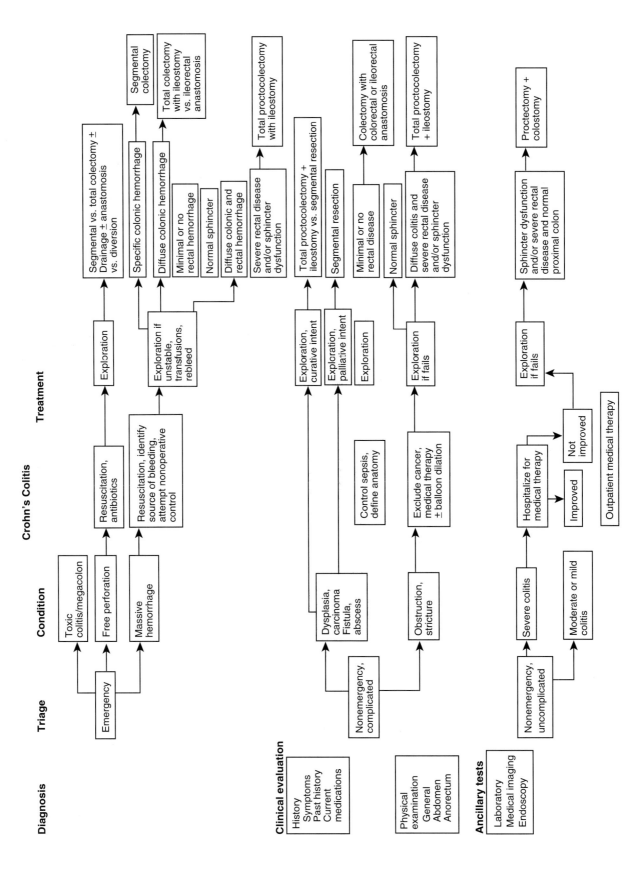

Figure 74–1. Algorithm for medical and surgical management of Crohn's colitis.

to improve or who deteriorate with this regimen should have surgery during the first 24 to 72 hours. Failure to expeditiously operate results in a significant increase in morbidity and mortality from perforation. Fortunately, the majority of patients present with chronic Crohn's colitis in the elective setting. They are usually treated with regimens that may include sulphasalazine, azathioprine, methotrexate, cyclosporine, and metronidazole, described in Table 74–3.

Sulphasalazine consists of 5-aminosalicylic acid (5-ASA) and sulfonamide. 5-ASA is an aspirin derivative that is the active component of the compound. The sulfonamide is a carrier that decreases absorption in the small bowel, ensuring delivery to the colon. Although the mechanism of action is unknown, 5-ASA is known to affect the lipoxygenase pathway and may function via the inhibition of free oxygen radicals. It has been proved to be of some efficacy in the treatment of acute Crohn's colitis. Side effects include nausea and vomiting, while hypersensitivity reactions and a dose-related hemolysis may rarely complicate therapy.

Corticosteroids decrease interleukin-2 production and block helper T-cell function. The side effects include hyperglycemia, hyperlipidemia, hypokalemia, fluid retention, hypertension, adrenal suppression, and fat redistribution. Recently, there has been interest in budesonide, a new steroid with allegedly fewer side effects.

Azathioprine and 6-mercaptopurine are purine antagonists that interfere with nucleic acid synthesis to achieve a nonspecific anti-inflammatory effect. Side effects include bone marrow suppression, nausea, fever, rash, and acute pancreatitis, all of which are reversible when the drug is stopped. Azathioprine has been shown to have a steroid-sparing effect that facilitates maintenance of remission.

Methotrexate is also an antimetabolite that inhibits dihydrofolate reductase to interfere with DNA synthesis, repair, and replication. Data suggest that it is beneficial in the treatment of active Crohn's disease, but its mechanism has not been described. Side effects include nausea, vomiting, stomatitis, and diarrhea; there is also a risk of leukopenia.

Cyclosporine suppresses antibody production by inhibiting helper T cells; it has been used cautiously, as its side effects include renal dysfunction, hypertension, paresthesias, hypertrichosis, and seizures. Some series have demonstrated a benefit in active Crohn's disease and anal fistula; however, the benefit does not appear to be sustained beyond 6 months.

Antibiotics, particularly metronidazole, have been used for Crohn's colitis and especially for perianal disease. The rationale for the use of metronidazole has been that the infective process of perianal disease is mostly due to anaerobes. The most common side effect is paresthesias, which usually limit its use as a chronic suppressive agent. Although metronidazole is not effective for ileocolic disease, benefit has been demonstrated in the setting of Crohn's colitis and perianal disease.

If the patient has Crohn's or indeterminate colitis and is managed with nonresective (medical) treatment for extended periods of time, surveillance for the development of colon cancer is imperative. While the risk is less than that of ulcerative colitis, increasing evidence suggests similar trends for the two diseases in the chronic setting. Thus, similar plans for screening should be employed, and resection, when performed, should always include the entire diseased segment.

Nonresectional medical therapy for anal and perianal disease is considered separately from medical therapy for the colon. Traditionally, anorectal surgery in the setting of acute perianal Crohn's disease was considered unwise, owing to fears of nonhealing wounds and fecal incontinence. As a result, both conservative medical therapy and procedures for establishing and maintaining adequate drainage were the mainstays of treatment. Abscesses may require drainage with the patient under general anesthesia; in fact, tenderness should prompt an examination with the patient under anesthesia if no etiology can be found. Recently, the long-held tenet of nonsurgical management was challenged in the setting of chronic anal and perianal Crohn's disease. Now, fistulotomies are more widely accepted for the treatment of intersphincteric and low transsphincteric fistulas. However, whenever uncertainty exists about the effects of the proposed fistulotomy

Table 74–3	Medical Agents for Crohn's Colitis and Crohn's Disease of the Perianal Region		
NAME	**DOSE**	**SIDE EFFECTS**
Anti-inflammatory Agents		
Sulphasalazine (Azulfidine)	Start 500 mg bid, increase by 1 g/day to 5–6 g/day	Nausea and vomiting; Hypersensitivity reactions; Dose-related hemolysis
Glucocorticoids (Hydrocortisone)	100 mg q 6 hours	Hyperglycemia, hyperlipidemia, hypokalemia, fluid retention, hypertension, adrenal suppression, fat redistribution
Immunomodulatory Agents		
Azathioprine	2–2.5 mg/kg/day	Bone marrow suppression, nausea, fever, rash, chronic pancreatitis
6-Mercaptopurine	1–1.5 mg/kg/day	Bone marrow suppression, nausea, fever, rash, chronic pancreatitis
Methotrexate	25 mg q week	Nausea, vomiting, stomatitis, diarrhea, leukopenia
Cyclosporine	4 mg/kg/day	Renal dysfunction, hypertension, paresthesias, hypertrichosis, and seizures
Antibiotic Agents		
Metronidazole	20 mg/kg/day in divided doses	Peripheral sensory neuropathy

on continence, draining setons and occasionally advancement flaps are good conservative alternatives.

Although there has been some short-term success with metronidazole and ciprofloxacin for perianal Crohn's disease, recent enthusiasm has clustered around immunosuppressive agents. Cyclosporine and 6-mercaptopurine reportedly achieve closure of fistula, but the response is not sustained. Infliximab (Remicade) for perianal disease in Crohn's disease was approved by the U.S. Food and Drug Administration (FDA) in May 1998. The early response of perianal disease in terms of closure of fistula tracts was followed by a lack of any demonstrable benefit, compared with placebo, after 18 weeks of therapy. There has also been concern about the risk of autoimmune antibodies and lymphoma. Further experience and prospective randomized trials are needed to elucidate the role of infliximab for perianal Crohn's disease.

PRINCIPLES OF SURGICAL MANAGEMENT

Goals of Surgery

The objectives of surgery are to treat the complications of the disease that led to surgery, to avoid the side effects of medical therapy, and to restore the patient's health. Approximately two thirds of patients with Crohn's colitis will ultimately require surgery, and half of the patients with Crohn's colitis eventually will have an ileostomy. Elective resection is safer and associated with a better outcome than is emergent resection. Sadly, it is often scheduled only after the patient has anemia, malnutrition, anorexia, and cachexia. In addition, by the time of referral to a surgeon, the patient has usually suffered many of the ill side effects of steroids. While insomnia, mood swings, psychosis, and water retention are reversible, aseptic necrosis of the femoral heads and disfiguring striae are not. Despite the misery secondary to the side effects of medical therapy, complications of the disease itself may also arise. All too often patients are told to avoid surgery because they may develop postoperative complications. Unfortunately, the immunosuppression compounded with the acute malnutrition and anemia often make operating on a septic sequela of Crohn's disease a self-fulfilling prophecy. Both physicians and patients must understand that although surgery is not curative, it can offer significant improvement in quality of life and can avoid many of the unpleasant side effects of medical management. It will also be accompanied by better results in the elective setting than in the emergent one.

Probability of Surgery and Recurrent Disease

The probability of requiring an initial operation for Crohn's colitis or surgery for recurrent disease is dependent on the location of disease and the length of intestine involved. About 90% of patients with right-sided disease will require at least one operation; right-sided disease is characteristically found in association with obstructing inflammatory disease of the terminal ileum. In comparison, only 50% to 60% of patients with left-sided disease require surgery. Left-sided disease may also require surgery for signs and symptoms of obstruction, but other indications frequently include abscess, fistula, and severe perianal disease. The chances of requiring surgery is less when the disease involves shorter and contiguous segments of intestine.

Recurrence or recrudescence occurs in 40% to 90% of patients after initial resection; the wide-ranging statistics probably result from differences in how recurrence is defined and variation in the length of follow-up. Factors influencing recurrence can be categorized into those introduced by the patient and those introduced by the surgeon. In general, younger patients with aggressive disease have an increased chance of recurrence. Smoking has also been repeatedly demonstrated to have a strong association with the need for further surgery. As in primary disease, right-sided disease and long-segment disease are more likely to require resection for recurrence.

Factors introduced by surgical management, such as length of surgical margins and anastomotic technique, have also been studied. While the extent of margins has been shown not to affect the recurrence rate in small bowel disease, the same is not true for colonic disease. It is generally agreed that the extent of resection and the type of operation has a major impact on recurrence and reoperation rates in Crohn's disease of the colon. The more colon that remains, the higher the chance for recurrent disease. For example, proctocolectomy has a 10-year recurrence rate of about 10% in comparison to the 50% recurrence rate observed after ileorectal anastomosis. Some evidence supports the use of postoperative immunomodulators and antibiotics for prophylaxis against recurrence. Anecdotal reports describe success with steroids, methotrexate, cyclosporine, and 6-mercaptopurine (6-MP). However, stronger evidence, based on prospective randomized trials, exists for metronidazole 20 mg/kg per day, and mesalamine (5-ASA) 3 mg/day.

Preparation for Surgery

Prior to surgery, patients are counseled about autologous blood donation and advised to avoid aspirin and nonsteroidal anti-inflammatories for 14 days prior to surgery. Even if the probability of a stoma is low, this contingency is always discussed; the patient consults with a stoma therapist for education and site selection. The possibility of intraoperative colonoscopy is discussed, and patient consent is obtained for both eventualities (stoma and colonoscopy). If significant iliac fossa or pelvic inflammation, such as a phlegmon, is suspected, intraoperative ureteric catheters are considered. They are especially useful in patients with iliac fossa phlegmon, or abscess, or if a fistula is identified. When unsuspected small bowel strictures are discovered, the patient should understand the principles of stricturoplasty. As always, informed consent is made available to patients to ensure that they and their family members are knowledgeable about the various risks, benefits, alternatives, and complications related to the operation.

On the day prior to surgery, the patient undergoes bowel preparation with 45 mL of sodium phosphate (Fleet Phospho-Soda, CB Fleet Co, Lynchburg, VA) at 4 PM and 8 PM, each administration followed by 4 to 5 separate 8-ounce glasses of water. One gram each of metronidazole and neomycin are given at 1, 2, and 10 PM to decrease the bacterial load of the colon. The patient is asked to eat a light lunch and kept NPO (nothing by mouth) after midnight the day prior to surgery, and is admitted the morning of surgery unless otherwise indicated. At that time, perioperative systemic antibiotics are given, including cefotetan 2 g "on call" to the operating room and for two postoperative doses, if the patient has normal renal function and no known medical allergies. Stress-dose steroids, such as hydrocortisone 100 mg, is given "on call" to the operating room and postoperatively tapered, if the patient has been on daily steroid medications during the last 3 months. Prior to induction of general endotracheal anesthesia, pneumatic compression stockings and subcutaneous low-molecular-weight heparin are utilized for prophylaxis against deep venous thrombosis.

Under general endotracheal anesthesia, the patient is placed in modified lithotomy position with the lower extremities in Allen stirrups (Allen Medical, Bedford Heights, OH). This position enables intraoperative colonoscopy. A bladder catheter and a nasogastric tube are inserted prior to the commencement of exploration. The abdominal wall is prepared and draped in the standard fashion, exposing the area from the xiphoid to the pubis and the width of the abdominal wall between the iliac spines. A thorough exploration of the small bowel and the entire length of the large intestine is mandatory. Despite small bowel series and enterolysis, unsuspected concomitant small bowel disease may be encountered.

SURGICAL OPTIONS

When surgery is required for acute fulminating colitis, the safest treatment is generally total abdominal colectomy and ileostomy. In the elective setting, treatment may involve segmental colectomy, total abdominal colectomy and ileostomy, abdominal colectomy and ileorectal anastomosis with or without "temporary" proximal diversion, and proctocolectomy and ileostomy. The merits of each procedure are considered in the following sections.

Abdominal Colectomy and Ileostomy

Abdominal total or subtotal colectomy and ileostomy is the treatment of choice for all emergent or urgent procedures for fulminant colitis that fails to respond to medical therapy. About one third to one half of patients presenting with fulminant colitis will have a diagnosis of Crohn's disease on follow-up, as opposed to ulcerative colitis or other proctocolitides. Uncertainty of diagnosis prevents consideration of ileoanal pouch surgery in the acute setting in order to minimize the need for further surgery and prevent ultimate resection of essential small bowel. Other advantages include avoiding the morbidity of a larger operation by leaving the defunctionalized rectum in

place and maintaining the ability to perform a subsequent ileoanal pouch procedure should further evaluation establish a firm diagnosis of ulcerative colitis. Abdominal colectomy removes the most diseased segment of intestine with an expeditious procedure that provides decompression of the gastrointestinal tract. If the rectal stump is severely inflamed, consideration should be given to a split mucous fistula or burying the distal stump underneath the skin superficial to the fascia so that a mucous fistula, instead of peritonitis, will result if the closure of the stump breaks down. The presacral space should not be entered, and the inferior mesenteric and superior rectal vessels should be left in situ. In the setting of an unknown diagnosis, mucous fistula allows access to the rectum for topical steroid therapy as well. Even with known proctitis, proctectomy should be avoided. Perianal disease in the emergent setting, but not proctitis, is predictive of the need for proctectomy. This procedure is not always inevitable, and, more importantly the morbidity and mortality associated with this procedure are prohibitive in the acute setting. Subsequent ileostomy closure with laparoscopic ileorectal anastomosis is possible and may offer significant benefit over laparotomy. However, if proctectomy becomes necessary, that operation is also well suited to the laparoscopic method.

Total Proctocolectomy (and Ileostomy)

Patients undergoing elective surgery with poor sphincter function and/or advanced rectal or perianal disease to the extent that restoration of gastrointestinal continuity is ill advised may be best served by a single stapled proctocolectomy and ileostomy. This procedure has the lowest recurrence rate of any operation for Crohn's disease, potentially because no anastomosis is created. Moreover, this operation removes the rectum, and so surveillance examinations are obviated. The most frequent complications of Crohn's disease after total proctocolectomy involve persistent infection, and delayed closure of the perineal wound or the ileostomy. Close rectal dissection limits the risk of impotence and retrograde ejaculation. Preoperative stoma marking and proper ileostomy construction should limit the occurrence of ileostomy complications.

Segmental Colectomy

Resection of 20 to 30 cm of colon with construction of a primary anastomosis is an attractive option in selected patients. This operation may be appropriate in that small subgroup of patients with only a segment of Crohn's colitis. This procedure is probably most frequently undertaken in the right colon in conjunction with disease of the terminal ileum. It may also be applicable in the sigmoid colon in cases of ileosigmoid fistulas, as in this latter group the ileum is the source of disease and the colon is actually normal. Although there is a higher recurrence rate with this more limited resection than with total abdominal colectomy or proctocolectomy, the operation does have a role.

Abdominal Colectomy and Ileorectal Anastomosis

Frequently, the rectum is spared or has mild disease. In these cases, when the patient has good preoperative sphincter function, an ileorectal anastomosis can be a good choice. Even in the setting of proctitis, it may offer a good choice because proctitis is not predictive of further perianal disease. Maintaining a functioning rectum prevents diversion proctitis that may result if a defunctionalized rectum is left in place and does not exclude a temporary proximal loop ileostomy. A proximal ileostomy should be considered in patients with a relatively normal rectum but significant symptomatic perianal disease, who refuse proctocolectomy. Although there is no clear evidence that proximal diversion expedites healing of perianal disease, proximal diversion certainly facilitates hygiene and improves quality of life if the patient has fecal incontinence. Although half of the patients treated with this procedure ultimately require proctectomy, the other half avoid it.

CONCLUSION

Despite the introduction of new immunomodulatory agents, such as infliximab, and advances in surgical techniques, such as laparoscopy, no panacea exists for the treatment or cure of Crohn's disease. On presentation, an attempt at medical treatment should be initiated unless emergency surgery is required. Embarking on such therapy usually allows for elective surgery after the patient has been thoroughly evaluated and physiologically optimized from an endocrinologic, hemodynamic, and nutritional standpoint. However, surgery must not be postponed in a patient who fails to respond to medical therapy. Such delay will result in profound morbidity.

When surgery is required for acute disease, the treatment of choice is usually total abdominal colectomy. In contrast, when surgery is performed for chronic disease, the operation of choice depends on many factors, including previous therapeutic interventions, certainty of pathologic diagnosis, anal sphincter function, and extent of perianal disease as well as the site, duration, and extent of colonic disease. Among the different procedures, total abdominal colectomy allows for the broadest array of subsequent options. After total abdominal colectomy, patients with ulcerative or indeterminate colitis may undergo ileal pouch anal anastomosis; patients with Crohn's disease may maintain their intestinal continuity and anal sphincter function. In carefully selected patients with Crohn's colitis, segmental resection may permit less intervention with superior function; however, surveillance for malignancy is obligatory whenever large intestine remains. While more limited procedures may increase the chance of recurrence and malignancy, patients with Crohn's disease are not doomed to eventual proctectomy. Even if the procedure is ultimately required, the interval between procedures may be very rewarding. If perianal healing or satisfactory fecal continence is unlikely, the patient may benefit most from proctectomy despite the potential for complications of the perineal wound.

SELECTED READINGS

Allan A, Andrews MB, Hilton CJ, et al: Segmental colonic resection is an appropriate operation for short skip lesions due to Crohn's disease in the colon. World J Surg 1989;13:611.

Corman ML: Crohn's disease and indeterminate colitis. In Colon and Rectal Surgery, 4th ed. Philadelphia, Lippincott-Raven, 1998.

Keighley MB, Williams NS: Crohn's disease. In Surgery of the Anus, Rectum, and Colon, 2nd ed. Philadelphia, WB Saunders, 1999.

Kelly DG, Fleming CR: Nutritional considerations in inflammatory bowel disease. Gastroenterol Clin North Am 1995;24:597.

Lewis JD, Deren JJ, Lichtenstein GR: Cancer risk in patients with inflammatory bowel disease. Gastroenterol Clin North Am 1999;28:459.

Lock MR, Fazio VW, Farmer RG, et al: Recurrence and reoperation for Crohn's disease: The role of disease location in prognosis. N Engl J Med 1981;304:1586.

Maunder RG, Cohen Z, McLeod RS, et al: Effect of intervention in inflammatory bowel disease on health-related quality of life: A critical review. Dis Colon Rectum 1995;38:1147.

Mavrantonis C, Wexner S: Crohn's disease. In Wexner SD (ed): Laparoscopic Colorectal Surgery. New York, John Wiley & Sons, 1999.

McKee RF, Keenan RA: Perianal Crohn's disease: Is it all bad news? Dis Colon Rectum 1996;39:136.

Michetti P, Peppercorn MA: Medical therapy of specific clinical presentations. Gastroenterol Clin North Am 1999;28:353.

Pastore RL, Wolff BG, Hodge D: Total abdominal colectomy and ileorectal anastomosis for inflammatory bowel disease. Dis Colon Rectum 1997;40:1455.

Prabhakar LP, Laramee C, Nelson H, Dozois RR: Avoiding a stoma: Role for segmental or abdominal colectomy in Crohn's colitis. Dis Colon Rectum 1997;40:71.

Present DH, Rutgeerts P, Targan S, et al: Infliximab for the treatment of fistulas in patients with Crohn's disease. N Engl J Med 1999;340:1398.

Sardinha TC, Wexner SD: Laparoscopy for inflammatory bowel disease: Pros and cons. World J Surg 1998;22:370.

Targan SR, Hanauser SR, van Deventer SJH, et al: A short-term study of chimeric monoclonal antibody cA2 to tumor necrosis factor α for Crohn's disease. N Engl J Med 1997;337:1029.

Wexner SD, Vernava AM: Crohn's colitis. In Clinical Decision Making in Colorectal Surgery. New York, Igaku-Shoin, 1995.

Yamada T, Alpers DH, Laine L, et al: Inflammatory bowel disease. In Textbook of Gastroenterology. Philadelphia, Lippincott–Williams & Wilkins, 1999.

Chapter 75

Pseudo-Obstruction of the Colon

W. Jay Suggs and Tonia M. Young-Fadok

INTRODUCTION

The entity known as Ogilvie's syndrome has evolved from Sir Heneage Ogilvie's original description in 1948. He described two patients with malignant infiltration of the celiac plexus that caused signs and symptoms of colon obstruction. Today, it refers to acute *pseudo*-obstruction of the colon from any cause; that is, dilatation of the proximal colon in the absence of mechanical obstruction. Differentiation from other causes of colonic dilatation is suspected by careful history taking and physical examination and is confirmed in combination with limited radiologic evaluation. Management is rarely surgical, but surgeons are frequently consulted because of the presenting abdominal distention. Moreover, general surgeons must be aware of the diagnosis, the risk of perforation, potential difficulties with colonoscopic decompression, and operative choices.

The pathogenesis of Ogilvie's syndrome is unknown. An imbalance between sympathetic and parasympathetic innervations to the colon has been postulated. Indeed, the success of the parasympathomimetic drug neostigmine is consistent with relative parasympathetic suppression.

CLINICAL PRESENTATION

Ogilvie's syndrome occurs infrequently. Of the more than 100,000 hospital admissions per year at Mayo Clinic, only 10 to 20 patients were identified annually.

Differential Diagnosis

Ogilvie's syndrome is a diagnosis of exclusion, so the history, physical examination, and investigations are directed toward excluding other causes of colonic distention, which require different treatment. First, the process is acute; chronic idiopathic pseudo-obstruction and chronic constipation are not causes of Ogilvie's syndrome. Second, no true mechanical obstruction of the colon is present; in contrast, fecal impaction, diverticular stricture, malignancy, and volvulus can cause a complete mechanical obstruction. Third, this process is limited to the colon, and usually to the right colon; radiographic and clinical findings are not usually mistaken for small bowel obstruction.

The History and Physical Examination

The typical patient is elderly, often with comorbidities. Rarely, the disease affects younger, healthier patients. In a series of 156 patients at the Mayo Clinic, the median age was 72 years, and there was a 5:2 male-to-female ratio. Two thirds had undergone an operation within the 30 days preceding the diagnosis. The median time from operation to diagnosis was 3 days. Renal and hepatic transplantation, and hip operations, had a high rate of association (Table 75–1). Other common comorbidities include trauma, alcoholism, dementia, treatment of mental illness with psychopharmacologic agents, bedrest, narcotics, cancer, and critically ill patients in the intensive care unit. A low threshold of suspicion is necessary, as many patients are incapable of complaining about symptoms.

The passage of flatus is variable but reduced. Constipation or diarrhea may be present. Vomiting and fever are not characteristic of pseudo-obstruction. Although some patients complain of abdominal cramping, pain is a surprisingly infrequent accompaniment of distention.

The most reliable physical finding is abdominal distention. Although there may be discomfort on palpation of the abdomen, peritoneal irritation is not present; peritoneal signs signify colonic perforation and are an indication for immediate laparotomy. Bowel sounds are nonspecific. Skin changes such as erythema or induration in the right lower quadrant are ominous signs of perforation and require immediate attention.

Investigations

Laboratory tests often show electrolyte abnormalities, the most common being hypokalemia. Leukocytosis should raise the suspicion of perforation or ischemic bowel.

The first imaging studies should be upright and supine abdominal radiographs. These will show a distended cecum and right colon with a variable amount of dilated transverse colon (Fig. 75–1). The cut-off is usually at the midtransverse colon or splenic flexure, where the colon

Table 75–1	Premorbid Operations in 156 Patients Later Developing Ogilvie's Syndrome, 1988–1997	
SURGERY TYPE	**NO. OF OPERATIONS**	**NO. OF PATIENTS (%)**
Cardiothoracic/vascular	112,631	25 (0.03)
Orthopedic: hip	9,563	22 (0.23)
Gynecologic/pelvic	36,429	17 (0.05)
Neurosurgery	26,962	10 (0.04)
Laparotomy	257,905	7 (0.003)
Kidney transplant	794	3 (0.38)
Obstetric	18,139	1 (0.04)
Liver transplant	734	1 (0.14)
Laparoscopy	11,451	1 (0.01)
Urology	45,480	0 (0)

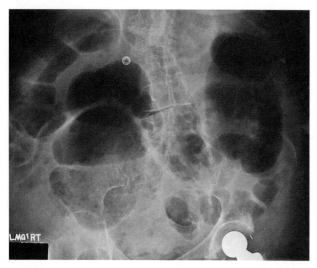

Figure 75–1. Plain abdominal radiograph demonstrating cecal and ascending and transverse colon dilatation, with relatively normal sigmoid gas pattern.

becomes innervated by the sacral plexus; however, there may be air in the rectum. Small bowel distention may occur with an incompetent ileocecal valve. The accepted maximal diameter of the normal cecum is 9 cm. A meta-analysis of 400 patients found that the risk of perforation increases with increase in cecal diameter: no risk if less than 12 cm, 7% if 12 to 14 cm, and 23% if more than 14 cm. In practice, the degree of discomfort associated with distention, at least in the fully competent patient, is a better clue to the urgency for decompression than is the absolute diameter. The greater the discomfort, the greater the rapidity of distention, and the more urgent the need for decompression.

Since colonic dilatation is also a feature of mechanical obstruction, it is essential to differentiate pseudo-obstruction from mechanical obstruction. Either water-soluble contrast-enhanced enema (with free flow of contrast medium from the rectum to the cecum) or colonoscopy will reliably differentiate the two.

PREOPERATIVE MANAGEMENT

The initial approach is to optimize the patient's medical condition. Oral intake should be discontinued, and a nasogastric tube inserted; however, it is unclear whether this helps in the patient with a competent ileocecal valve and no small bowel dilatation. It may, however, decrease the quantity of swallowed air passed into the colon. Intravenous fluids are started, and a urinary catheter is placed to monitor fluid balance carefully, as several liters of fluid may be sequestered in the dilated colon. Electrolyte imbalances are corrected, and, if possible, narcotics are withdrawn.

Treatment of Ogilvie's syndrome has evolved into four strategies: pharmacologic treatment with neostigmine, conservative medical management, colonoscopic decompression, and surgery. A water-soluble contrast-enhanced enema, performed to exclude mechanical obstruction, may be therapeutic in addition to being diagnostic. It

must be performed before any other intervention, unless the patient is proceeding directly to colonoscopy.

In the absence of contraindications to its use, the parasympathomimetic drug neostigmine has become first-line therapy. A randomized, prospective study showed that colonic decompression occurred within 30 minutes of administering 2 mg of intravenous neostigmine in more than 90% of patients; 75% required no further intervention. Neostigmine, however, must be administered in a monitored setting. If the first dose fails to decompress the colon, a second dose may be given. Bradycardia and increased tracheobronchial secretions are possible side effects. Atropine and an endotracheal intubation cart should be readily available. Relative contraindications to neostigmine use include recent myocardial infarction, arrhythmia, and airway lability. In no patients in this treatment group has a perforated colon developed.

Conservative medical management may be appropriate if there are contraindications to the use of neostigmine, if monitoring facilities are not available, and if the patient has only mild to moderate distention and minimal symptoms (the more symptomatic patient requires colonoscopy if neostigmine is not an option). Suppositories and ambulation may aid the passage of flatus. Although rectal tubes are frequently placed, there is little evidence of their efficacy other than as a rectal stimulant. They rarely reach the distal level of dilatation and so frequently become blocked as to be useless for decompression. Some have tried motility agents, such as metoclopramide, erythromycin, and cisapride, but no large randomized prospective trials confirm their efficacy. Surveillance by serial abdominal physical and radiographic examinations is crucial in avoiding perforation of a distended cecum. If there is deterioration, or no significant improvement in 24 hours, the next level of strategy should be implemented.

OPERATIVE MANAGEMENT

Colonoscopic Decompression

Colonoscopic decompression for Ogilvie's syndrome, first described in 1977, was the treatment of choice prior to the introduction of neostigmine. It would now be most appropriate in the patient with contraindications or failure to resolve with neostigmine. Colonoscopy is both diagnostic and therapeutic. It is technically more demanding than is elective colonoscopy because the colon is not prepared and may contain 1 to 5 liters of liquid stool, which hampers visualization. Patience is necessary to suction out the liquid as well as to use minimal air insufflation to avoid increasing the risk of perforation. Advancement to the hepatic flexure is usually adequate for decompression of the right colon, but the ascending colon must be visualized to confidently exclude obstruction if a Hypaque enema was not performed first. The use of a long colonic tube is controversial, but one may be placed at this time. The diameter of the cecum must decrease immediately or the examination was nontherapeutic. Serial examinations and abdominal radiographs are essential for follow-up.

Operative Management

If at any time there is evidence of ischemia or perforation, immediate laparotomy is mandatory. Surgical intervention is also indicated when less invasive measures fail. The patient is placed supine if it is clear that the level of dilatation is above the rectosigmoid junction and that per-anal stapling devices will not be used; otherwise, a modified lithotomy positioning is used. Placement of a cecostomy tube is the traditional and least invasive procedure for Ogilvie's syndrome. Be certain to use a large-diameter (>24 Fr) tube, since smaller tubes often become clogged with stool. These tubes need frequent irrigation to maintain patency and thus colonic decompression. It is appropriate when there is no evidence of bowel wall ischemia or compromise secondary to dilatation. The largest-diameter mushroom-tipped catheter or a balloon catheter may be used, secured by two pursestring sutures. It is helpful to bring the catheter through an interposing portion of the omentum before exiting it through the abdominal wall, to reduce the unpleasant leakage for which cecostomies are notorious. If ileocecectomy or right hemicolectomy is required, for example, for patchy ischemia, a primary anastomosis may be constructed even in the absence of a bowel preparation, as it is a right-sided anastomosis. The advisability of this must also be governed by standard factors, such as the absence of contamination, hemodynamic stability, lack of tension on the anastomosis, and adequate blood supply. Other techniques include laparoscopic cecostomy or percutaneous cecostomy tube placement.

POSTOPERATIVE MANAGEMENT

Postoperative management is determined primarily by two factors: the nature of the operation and any comorbid conditions. With perforation, the possibility of septic shock should be anticipated, and appropriate monitoring lines, fluid replacement, and antibiotic coverage instituted. Even in the absence of sepsis, many patients demonstrate electrolyte abnormalities that require aggressive correction. In the absence of small bowel dilatation, a nasogastric tube is probably unnecessary. When used, the nasogastric tube can be removed with resolution of postoperative ileus; e.g., passage of flatus and nondistended abdomen. These same considerations govern removal of a long colonic tube and introduction of clear liquids, with advancement to a regular diet as tolerated. A cecostomy should be irrigated frequently (every 2 hours) to maintain patency.

Some type of prophylaxis for deep venous thrombosis is usually considered mandatory, with elastic stockings, sequential compression devices, and/or subcutaneous heparin as indicated. Ambulation starts on the first postoperative day unless there are contraindications such as in the orthopedic patient. The patient who is to be discharged home with a cecostomy tube or stoma requires appropriate instructions regarding care. After resolution of colonic dilatation, a cecostomy tube may be pulled out after at least 4 to 6 weeks have passed to allow for maturation of the track. The resultant fistula should close spontaneously. The patient who has undergone creation of a stoma may be considered for stoma closure after 3 months.

COMPLICATIONS

The natural history of Ogilvie's is that without intervention, dilatation will either resolve or perforate. In accordance with the law of Laplace, the risk of perforation of the thin-walled cecum is much greater than that of the rest of the colon—about 3%. The authors' series noted two perforations in those undergoing colonoscopy (2%) and one in the surgical group (3%).

Postoperative morbidity is often the result of preoperative comorbidities rather than the operative intervention itself. The most common complications are sepsis (9% in the colonoscopy group and 24% in the surgical group), myocardial infarction (3% and 9%), and pulmonary embolus (1% and 6%).

OUTCOMES

Analysis of 156 patients managed at the Mayo Clinic over 10 years revealed that Ogilvie's syndrome resolved with medical management in 14 (9%), with colonoscopy in 108 (69%), and with operation in 34 (22%). Of those improving with colonoscopy, resolution occurred in 80% with one colonoscopy; over 90% resolved with two decompressions. The risk of operation did not rise with repeat colonoscopy.

Leaving long transanal tubes in the ascending colon during colonoscopy has been used in some centers. Although improved results have been demonstrated compared with colonoscopic decompression alone, the studies are small. Our analysis of 156 patients revealed that long tubes did not improve decompression rates ($P = .38$)

Pearls and Pitfalls

PEARLS

- Ogilvie's syndrome represents an acute pseudo-obstruction of the ascending colon.
- Predisposing factors include orthopedic, urologic, and transplant surgery, as well as trauma.
- Consider the diagnosis.
- Diagnosis is one of exclusion—exclude mechanical colonic obstruction.
- Water-soluble enema or colonoscopy can be both diagnostic and therapeutic.
- Treatment involves conservative management, intravenous neostigmine, colonoscopic decompression, or operative decompression.
- In the absence of contraindications, neostigmine is considered first-line therapy.
- Results depend in large part on the underlying comorbidities.
- Development of Ogilvie's syndrome is a marker of increased mortality.

and were associated with increased morbidity (35% versus 18%, $P = .043$).

The most striking outcome is the marked risk of mortality, at both 30 days and up to a year after operation. This risk is greatest in those who have required operative intervention, but it is still increased in patients responding to less invasive measures. Thirty-day mortality was 8% in the group managed medically, 9% in those undergoing colonoscopic decompression, and 22% in those requiring surgical intervention. The corresponding 1-year mortality rose to 15%, 25%, and 56%, respectively. It would seem that the development of pseudo-obstruction is a marker for increased risk of mortality related to associated comorbidities.

SELECTED READINGS

Geller A, Peterson BT, Gostout CJ: Endoscopic decompression for acute colonic pseudo-obstruction. Gastrointest Endosc 1996;44:144.

Hasler WL: Neostigmine for acute colonic pseudo-obstruction: New use for an old drug? Gastroenterology 2000;118:443.

Ogilvie H: Large-intestine colic due to sympathetic deprivation: A new clinical syndrome. BMJ 1948;2:671.

Ponec RJ, Saunders MD, Kimmey MB: Neostigmine for the treatment of acute colonic pseudo-obstruction. N Engl J Med 1999;341:137.

Schermer CR, Hanosh JJ, Davis M, Pitcher DE: Ogilvie's syndrome in the surgical patient: A new therapeutic modality. J Gastrointestinal Surg 1999;3:173.

Chapter 76

Diverticulitis

Christopher J. Sonnenday and Howard S. Kaufman

Diverticular disease of the colon is one of the most common and challenging clinical problems managed by general surgeons. Diverticulosis is common in Western countries and may occur in two thirds of adults by age 80. Although diverticula may be distributed throughout the entire colon, the majority of patients with symptomatic disease have involvement of the sigmoid colon. As many as 10% of individuals with diverticulosis will develop diverticulitis during their lifetime. Patients with symptomatic diverticulitis may present with acute or chronic symptoms, or both, and a spectrum of disease severity ranging from mild abdominal pain to fecal peritonitis. In addition, the clinical behavior of diverticulitis may mimic other diagnoses, such as adenocarcinoma of the colon, mesenteric ischemia, infective colitis, and inflammatory bowel disease.

For the purposes of management and discussion, diverticulitis is classified as uncomplicated or complicated. Most patients with acute uncomplicated diverticulitis respond to medical therapy and do not need surgical intervention. Alternatively, patients who fail to improve while receiving medical therapy or who develop associated complications, such as intestinal obstruction, abscess, fistula, or free perforation, will require operative management.

UNCOMPLICATED DIVERTICULITIS

Clinical Presentation

Uncomplicated diverticulitis is a clinical diagnosis and, many times, one of exclusion. Classically, patients present with left lower quadrant abdominal pain, constipation, and low-grade fever. Other associated symptoms may include nausea, vomiting, diarrhea, and dysuria. A history of similar attacks may be elicited. The physical examination should demonstrate left lower quadrant tenderness. Localized peritoneal signs may be present, but generalized peritoneal irritation suggests perforation and complicated disease. A left lower quadrant mass or fullness may be appreciated in some patients. Rectal examination often suggests fullness and tenderness, particularly toward the left pelvis. Fecal occult blood testing may be positive for trace heme, but frank blood is rare in diverticulitis and should lead to investigation for alternative diagnoses. Pelvic examination is essential in any female suspected of having diverticulitis in order to exclude gynecologic disease presenting with similar signs and symptoms.

In patients with a convincing clinical presentation for diverticulitis and a lack of signs and symptoms indicative of additional or alternative pathology, no further testing is necessary acutely. Extreme clinical acumen is necessary when the practitioner examines elderly patients or those patients receiving steroids, because findings of generalized peritonitis are often much less prominent (or absent) in these patient groups. A complete blood count, primarily to assess for leukocytosis, may be a helpful confirmatory test. The degree of leukocytosis may offer some prognostic value and aid in decision making regarding hospitalization versus outpatient management. Anemia suggests a different disease process and warrants further investigation. A urinalysis is useful in excluding urinary tract pathology; however, pyuria and hematuria may occur in uncomplicated diverticulitis.

The decision to pursue diagnostic imaging studies in uncomplicated diverticulitis depends on the severity of the patient's illness and the clinician's degree of confidence in the diagnosis. Supine and upright abdominal radiographs with an upright chest radiograph should be performed in patients with significant acute abdominal pain. Plain abdominal radiographs may demonstrate an obstructive pattern, extraluminal air, bowel wall thickening, or other findings that may favor alternative diagnoses, whereas the upright chest film should identify a pneumoperitoneum that would change the treatment plan.

Additional imaging may be obtained when the diagnosis is in question or if the patient is more severely ill and complicated diverticulitis is suspected. Water-soluble contrast enema and computed tomography (CT) are the most informative tests for confirming a diagnosis of diverticulitis. Although these tests have not been compared in a randomized prospective study, CT has gained widespread acceptance because it allows imaging of both intraluminal and extraluminal disease. The most common complications of diverticulitis, perforation and abscess, may be missed or underestimated by contrast enema. Recently, computed tomographic imaging with rectal contrast medium with or without oral and intravenous contrast medium has been used to improve the diagnostic accuracy of helical CT. Such techniques have been evaluated in a prospective fashion and have been shown to have 97% sensitivity, 100% specificity, and 99% overall accuracy. Moreover, CT suggested an alternative diagnosis in 60% of patients when diverticulitis was not present.

Endoscopy is usually avoided in the evaluation of patients with acute diverticulitis due to the risk of perforation. When necessary for confirming the diagnosis or excluding an obstructing cancer, limited flexible proctosigmoidoscopy may be carefully performed by an experienced endoscopist using minimal insufflation of air.

Management

In 1995, the American Society of Colon and Rectal Surgeons published practice guidelines for the management of uncomplicated diverticulitis. Standard therapy remains bowel rest and intravenous antibiotics. If marked clinical improvement does not occur within 48 to 72 hours, further evaluation to identify complications of diverticulitis, such as abscess, should be initiated. Localized infections in diverticulitis are polymicrobial, with gram-negative aerobic and anaerobic bacteria as the predominant pathogens. Broad-spectrum monotherapy and combination antibiotic therapy are equally effective in most patients.

Patients with uncomplicated diverticulitis and mild signs and symptoms have been managed increasingly as outpatients. Patients able to tolerate a liquid diet who have minimal systemic signs and symptoms and little tenderness may be treated safely without hospital admission. Oral antimicrobials should be selected on the basis of their broad spectrum and of patient tolerance. Close follow-up should be established to monitor the patient's response to therapy and to schedule appropriate evaluation of the colon after the inflammation has resolved. Most importantly, only reliable patients with sufficient social support should be treated as outpatients. Patients and their families require clear instructions to return for evaluation with any worsening of their signs and symptoms. There should be a low threshold for admission with any clinical decline in the patient's condition.

Although the majority of patients will recover uneventfully from a first attack of uncomplicated diverticulitis, 20% will progress and subsequently develop complications that require intervention. After the patient recovers from acute diverticulitis, a full evaluation of the colon should be performed to exclude additional or alternative pathology, particularly neoplasms. This evaluation may include either the combination of flexible sigmoidoscopy and barium enema or colonoscopy. Next, the decision to proceed with elective resection must be considered.

Two large retrospective studies have attempted to establish the natural history of diverticular disease in hopes of identifying a particular group of patients at high risk for recurrence who would most likely benefit from elective resection. Makela and co-workers (1998) recorded the clinical course of 366 Finnish patients over a 10-year period. Patients younger than the age of 40 years admitted for acute diverticulitis had a 40% incidence of recurrence over 10 years, whereas only 17% of patients older than 40 developed recurrent disease. Complicated diverticulitis developed in one third of patients after two admissions for uncomplicated diverticulitis and in one half of patients after more than two admissions. A similar study from New Zealand found a 30% incidence of recurrence in 418 patients over 5 years.

Based on the available literature, the current recommendations of the American College of Gastroenterology, the American Society of Colon and Rectal Surgeons, and the Society of Surgery of the Alimentary Tract are that patients undergo elective colon resection after two episodes of uncomplicated diverticulitis or after a single episode of complicated diverticulitis. Numerous series have clearly demonstrated that acute diverticulitis becomes less likely to respond to medical therapy, and patients are more likely to develop complications with each subsequent episode. In addition, any patient in whom the diagnosis of diverticulitis is in doubt and in whom colonoscopy and contrast enema cannot clearly exclude a colonic neoplasm should undergo elective resection.

Younger patients have been thought to have a more aggressive form of diverticulitis. For this reason, many believe that patients younger than age 40 should undergo elective resection after a single episode of diverticulitis. Immunocompromised patients are also at high risk for developing complicated diverticulitis. These patients should always be managed in hospital, as they may present indolently with what may become catastrophic disease. Immunocompromised patients are less likely to respond to medical therapy and have a higher rate of perforation. Therefore, resection should be considered early in the disease process.

Elective Colon Resection for Uncomplicated Diverticulitis

By definition, elective resection for recurrent uncomplicated diverticulitis should take place on a scheduled basis after the patient has undergone appropriate preoperative evaluation. An interval of at least 6 weeks for resolution of inflammation will allow for formal evaluation of the entire colon and a technically easier operation. Outpatient preoperative mechanical and oral antibiotic bowel preparation are used unless comorbid disease exists that would require a preoperative admission. A dose of intravenous antibiotics, typically a second-generation cephalosporin, is administered prior to the skin incision as prophylaxis.

Patients should be positioned carefully in the modified dorsal lithotomy position. Prophylaxis against deep venous thrombosis with antiembolism stockings and sequential pneumatic compression devices and subcutaneous heparin should be strongly considered in all patients. A Foley catheter and nasogastric tube should be placed. As the sigmoid colon is the most common area to be resected, the abdomen should be entered via an infraumbilical midline incision. Low transverse and Pfannistiel's incisions have also been described for use in colon resection for diverticular disease, but they limit the surgeon's ability to mobilize the splenic flexure if necessary and to deal with upper abdominal problems (e.g., gallstones, unrecognized malignancy), should they exist. There really is no good justification for a lower abdominal transverse incision.

The primary goal of elective surgery for uncomplicated diverticulitis is to resect the previously inflamed segment of bowel to prevent recurrence of disease. The distal margin of resection should be *below* (distal to) all diverticula and thus in the upper intraperitoneal rectum where the taeniae disappear. This should *not* routinely require entering the presacral space. The proximal margin of resection has not been demonstrated to have as significant an effect on the recurrence of disease. The involved segment, identified by serosal scarring, bowel wall thickening, and shortened mesentery, must be completely resected. If this segment extends into the descending colon, mobilization of the splenic flexure is usually needed to allow for a tension-free anastomosis to the rectum. No data demonstrate that all visible diverticula must be resected. The proximal margin of resection should be healthy-appearing bowel of normal caliber. If diverticula are left behind, they should not be included in the anastomosis. Depending on bowel wall thickness, the anastomosis may be performed in a hand-sewn or stapled fashion.

Since 1991, laparascopic techniques have been applied to colonic resection. The benefits of minimal access laparoscopic colorectal surgery include reduced postoperative narcotic requirements, early return of bowel and pulmonary function, shorter length of stay, and earlier return to work and other daily activities. Laparoscopic colorectal surgery requires complex dissection of the colon and rectum that involves a steep learning curve; this learning curve and level of technical difficulty initially discouraged many general surgeons from adopting these techniques. However, recent series have documented the safety and efficacy of laparoscopic surgery for diverticular disease.

For a minimal access (laparoscopic) approach, patients are prepared and positioned in a fashion similar to an open resection. Various combinations of port sites have been described, but most surgeons utilize four ports. The laparoscope is placed through an infraumbilical port. The main working ports are positioned in the right lower abdomen, and an additional port for retraction is placed into the left iliac fossa. Dissection is facilitated by the use of changes in the table position, with steep Trendelenburg and the patient's right side rotated down to keep the small bowel out of the pelvis while the surgeon dissects the sigmoid mesocolon. The patient therefore must be well secured to the operating table.

The goals of laparoscopic dissection should mirror those of the open technique: division of the lateral peritoneal reflection, identification of the left ureter, division of the mesenteric vessels, and mobilization of the proximal rectum. Mesenteric division may be performed prior to bowel mobilization according to surgeon preference and intraoperative findings. After distal mesenteric and bowel division, the sigmoid colon is exteriorized through an incision that extends the left lower quadrant port site. The involved segment of bowel is resected, and the anvil from a circular stapler is placed into the proximal colon. The circular stapler is advanced into the rectum by a transanal approach, and the anvil is engaged under laparoscopic vision. At this point, placement of the laparoscope into the right lower abdominal port site allows a better direct view of the engaged stapler. As with open resection, the donuts within the circular stapler should be intact, and a leak test should be negative. Fascial closure of the port sites greater than 5 mm is essential in decreasing the likelihood of postoperative hernia.

Numerous series have demonstrated that laparoscopic colon resection for diverticular disease can be performed safely, with morbidity comparable to the open procedure. Our group reported their initial experience with 397 laparoscopic colon resections. Morbidity varied from 5% to 9%, according to whether the operation was performed for acute or chronic disease. Patients with diverticular disease of any stage had slightly higher rates of conversion and intraoperative complications compared with patients with other pathologies. However, there was no difference in patient satisfaction or return to normal activity. The Laparoscopic Colorectal Surgery Study Group published a prospective multicenter study on the experience with 1118 patients, with 304 patients with diverticular disease.

The conversion rate among all patients with diverticulitis was 7% and 18% for complicated diverticulitis. Overall morbidity was 14%, with increasing morbidity clearly demonstrated in patients with more advanced disease (Hinchey's stages III and IV; see below). To date, no randomized clinical trials have been published that compare open laparotomy to laparoscopic resection for diverticular disease.

COMPLICATED DIVERTICULITIS

Complicated diverticulitis includes acute or chronic inflammatory disease with associated abscess, stricture, obstruction, fistula, or perforation. Although patients with chronic complications may present with well-described signs and symptoms, the diagnosis of diverticulitis as the underlying pathology may be made in the operating room during an emergent exploration for presumed intestinal obstruction or visceral perforation of unknown source. In these situations, intraoperative decisions must be made on the basis of the condition of the patient, the extent of disease, and an understanding of the appropriate options. When immediate exploration is not required, a focused clinical and radiologic evaluation can guide further intervention for abscess, stricture, or fistula. The presentation and the medical and surgical management of each complication are presented separately, as these clinical scenarios may be markedly different.

Diverticulitis Associated with Abscess or Phlegmon

In 1978, Hinchey and colleagues developed the classification system used to describe diverticulitis associated with perforation (Table 76–1). Patients with Hinchey stage I or II disease present in a manner similar to uncomplicated diverticulitis and may initially be thought to have a more benign course. However, persistence of fever, leukocytosis, abdominal pain and tenderness, or development of an abdominal mass should initiate diagnostic evaluation for an abscess. Helical CT with intravenous and enteric contrast medium (either colonic or oral) is the most accurate test for identifying a diverticular abscess (Fig. 76–1). Computed tomography also allows the opportunity to perform a guided percutaneous drainage when necessary.

Table 76–1	Hinchey Classification of Perforated Diverticulitis
Stage I	Microscopic perforation into the mesenteric border of the colon
	Pericolic or mesenteric abscess formation
Stage II	Perforation contained by adjacent structures
	Pelvic, intra-abdominal, or retroperitoneal abscess
Stage III	Perforation of stage I or II abscess into the peritoneal cavity
	No gross fecal spillage
	Generalized purulent peritonitis
Stage IV	Free perforation into the peritoneal cavity
	Generalized fecal peritonitis

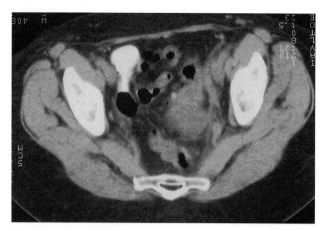

Figure 76–1. Diverticular abscess. Computed tomography performed with the administration of oral and intravenous contrast media demonstrates a 3-cm abscess adjacent to the sigmoid colon.

Small pericolic abscesses may be treated with bowel rest and intravenous antibiotics, with the majority of lesions expected to resolve without intervention. Antibiotic therapy should be selected to treat polymicrobial infection, including anaerobic coverage. Larger Hinchey stage II abscesses and stage I pericolic abscesses that do not respond to antibiotic therapy should be drained through either a percutaneous or, less commonly, an operative approach. Radiologically guided percutaneous drainage (Fig. 76–2) is the preferred choice for the treatment of diverticular abscess, with success rates of up to 90%. Successful percutaneous drainage allows for resolution of the septic focus and associated inflammatory process, thereby allowing a future semielective single-stage open or laparoscopic resection.

If percutaneous drainage is unsuccessful, the phlegmon worsens with ensuing obstruction, or the patient's clinical condition deteriorates, urgent operation becomes necessary. Initial intraoperative preparation and positioning of the patient undergoing exploration for complicated

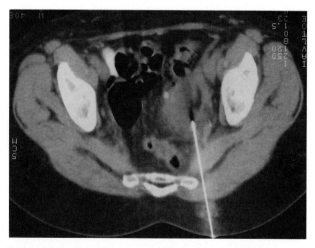

Figure 76–2. Computed tomography–guided drainage. The patient is in a prone position, and the abscess is accessed via a posterior approach through the left medial buttock. Follow-up CT in 4 days confirmed complete resolution of the pelvic abscess.

diverticulitis should be similar to that described earlier for uncomplicated diverticulitis. Placement of appropriate intravenous and arterial lines should be accomplished, depending on the patient's condition and need for invasive monitoring. An upper-body forced–hot air warming blanket may be used to maintain normothermia, especially because large-volume intravenous resuscitation and intraoperative irrigation or lavage may be necessary. Consideration should be given to cystoscopy with left-sided ureteral stenting to facilitate intraoperative identification of the ureter within the inflamed tissues of the retroperitoneum and sigmoid mesocolon. A lower midline incision is preferred with supraumbilical extension as necessary. The use of a disposable wound-protecting device should be considered in protecting the subcutaneous tissues from frank contamination.

Initial exploration focuses on careful entry into the peritoneal cavity, containment of any active fecal spillage, establishment of adequate exposure, and confirmation of the diagnosis. As many as 25% of patients explored for complicated diverticulitis will be found to have a perforated carcinoma. Identification of malignant disease may allow for adjustment of the extent of resection (another reason not to use a lower transverse incision). After the initial exploration, decisions relevant to the staging of the procedure should be made. Proximal diversion and drainage, the first step of the now archaic "three-stage" procedure, should be performed only in a patient who is so hemodynamically unstable that any prolongation of anesthesia would be fatal. Two large series have demonstrated that patients treated for perforated diverticulitis or abscess with proximal diversion, rather than resection, have a markedly increased mortality rate. A large review of the literature demonstrated a 25% mortality rate in patients treated without resection versus 11% in resected patients. Total hospital length of stay and the overall period of disability are also increased with a three-stage procedure.

The Hartmann procedure was applied to the management of patients with diverticulitis beginning in the 1940s. Recent mortality rates of 10% to 15% have been reported for patients with complicated diverticulitis treated with Hartmann's procedure. As many as 30% of patients will remain with a permanent colostomy, whereas those who undergo colostomy closure have a major complication rate of 4% to 10%. Although the Hartmann procedure has remained the standard procedure for complicated diverticulitis, *highly selected patients* with minimal fecal spillage, no hemodynamic instability, and healthy tissue at the proximal and distal margins of resection may be candidates for primary anastomosis with a proximal covering stoma. In addition, some authors advocate resection with primary anastomosis with an on-table bowel preparation by intraoperative colonic lavage. This technique involves irrigation of the colon via a catheter placed through the appendiceal stump or terminal ileum. Large-bore tubing (e.g., ventilator circuit tubing) is placed into the distal segment of colon to allow for extraperitoneal controlled drainage of stool and irrigant. The splenic flexure must be mobilized to facilitate manipulation of the colon and thorough irrigation. Seven published series utilizing on-table colonic lavage include 404 patients and report anastomotic leak and morbidity rates comparable to patients undergoing staged procedures. On average, an additional 20 to 50 minutes of operating room is required for performance of intraoperative lavage.

Regardless of the choice of operative procedure, the mobilization, dissection, and resection of the acutely inflamed sigmoid descending colon may be technically difficult. Dissection should be started proximal to the inflamed segment of bowel and may require complete mobilization of the splenic flexure. The more proximal portions of the left ureter and gonadal vessels are identified in an area relatively free from the surrounding inflammation. Attention may then be turned to the pelvis, where adhesions to the surrounding pelvic structures may be carefully divided. The surgeon's goal should be to initially avoid the most inflamed segment of colon, providing as much mobility as possible to facilitate the final dissection. It may be helpful to divide the colon at the proximal margin of resection and "peel" the proximal colon from the mesentery. The position of the left ureter should be frequently rechecked. Finger fracture techniques are often necessary for separation of the diseased colon from its inflammatory attachments to the left iliac fossa. The mesocolon should be divided carefully in small segments close to the colon. The indurated mesentery should be ligated and divided, rather than divided with cautery, owing to intense inflammation and hypervascularity. After the colon has been completely separated from the retroperitoneum, the ureter and gonadal vessels should be retraced distally to prove that they have not been injured during the dissection. As with an elective resection for diverticular disease, the distal margin of resection should be to the proximal rectum just distal to the taeniae coli. The colostomy or anastomosis is then performed.

Diverticulitis Associated with Perforation

Patients with Hinchey stage III and IV disease present in a manner similar to that of patients with a perforated viscus from any etiology, with peritoneal signs on physical examination and systemic signs of sepsis, potentially leading to eventual cardiovascular compromise and collapse. Preoperative work-up should be minimized, as peritonitis should be evident on physical examination. A complete blood count and electrolyte panel, electrocardiography, and chest radiograph should be obtained rapidly to identify comorbid conditions and guide the extent of resuscitation prior to operative intervention. Radiologic studies may reveal free air and fluid in the peritoneal cavity. After appropriate initial resuscitation with volume and, if indicated, vasopressors, surgical exploration of these patients should not be delayed. Broad-spectrum antibiotics should be administered.

In the operating room, invasive monitoring and volume lines are placed as indicated, and the patient is positioned supine or in the modified dorsal lithotomy position. An upper-body forced–hot air warmer should be used. A generous midline incision is wise. Intra-abdominal contamination should be cultured and washed out, and if the open colonic perforation is still leaking it should be

contained. Hartmann's procedure is the operation of choice and should be performed as described earlier. Similar to the procedure for a contained perforation, management with a three-stage procedure is currently outdated. Primary anastomosis should not be performed in the setting of gross purulent or fecal peritonitis. After closure of the fascia, consideration should be given to allowing the skin wound to heal by secondary intention or by performing a delayed primary closure. Mortality from perforated diverticulitis with fecal peritonitis can approach 35%, depending primarily on preoperative medical comorbidity.

Diverticulitis Associated with Fistula

Patients with fistula formation secondary to diverticular disease do not present with acute intra-abdominal sepsis but, rather, develop signs and symptoms following one or more episodes of diverticulitis. In some patients, a diverticular fistula develops without a clear history of diverticulitis. The subacute presentation of many of these patients provides some time for diagnostic work-up and elective management. The most common diverticular fistulae are colovesical, which account for 65% of patients. Pneumaturia, fecaluria, and/or recurrent urinary tract infections are the presenting signs. Computed tomography with enteric, but not intravenous, contrast medium is very sensitive in making the diagnosis of colovesical fistula with enteric contrast or, more commonly, an air-fluid level in the bladder. Colovaginal fistula is the second most common diverticular fistula, with the fistula extending nearly always to the vaginal cuff in women who are have undergone previous hysterectomy. Less common fistulas include coloenteric, colouterine, and colocutaneous.

The entire colon should be evaluated preoperatively either by colonoscopy or by contrast enema to eclude cancer and inflammatory bowel disease. Urosepsis should be controlled with appropriate antibiotics. A full-bowel preparation is given, and laparotomy or laparoscopy is performed to resect the involved segment of bowel, with primary anastomosis. The fistula tracts are usually short and cannot always be identified. If available, omentum or other healthy well-vascularized tissue should be placed between the anastomosis and previously contiguous organ. The bladder site of a colovesical fistula does not require any bladder resection, but only a simple oversewing.

Diverticulitis Associated with Obstruction

Diverticulitis-associated stricture or large bowel obstruction is often a diagnosis made intraoperatively, as patients may present with a large bowel obstruction without clear etiology. These patients should be handled in an emergent and efficient manner, as for any large bowel obstruction, because perforation may ensue from delayed recognition of a complete large bowel obstruction. Prompt hydration and nasogastric decompression should be performed with the intention of proceeding with the patient to the operating room shortly after admission. If partial obstruction exists, a gentle mechanical bowel preparation may be

Pearls and Pitfalls

Diagnosis

PITFALLS

- Beware of other diagnoses. Many diseases may resemble diverticulitis. Beware of missing diagnoses that require operative therapy, particularly mesenteric ischemia, appendicitis, and tubo-ovarian disease. Always admit patients, particularly the elderly and immunosuppressed, who do not have a secure diagnosis.
- *Diverticulitis does not bleed.* Hemorrhage may occur secondary to diverticular disease, but rarely in the setting of acute diverticulitis. Heme-positive stools in a patient suspected of having diverticulitis should lead to investigation of other diagnoses. Likewise, anemia in a patient with diverticulitis should not be attributed to diverticular disease without a complete work-up.
- *Is a urinalysis helpful?* Pyuria and microscopic hematuria may occur in acute diverticulitis. Clinical signs and symptoms should be carefully considered in excluding urinary tract disease from the differential diagnosis.
- *Endoscopy in patients with diverticulitis.* Lower endoscopy plays no role in the diagnosis of acute diverticulitis. All patients require evaluation of the colon after the acute attack has subsided.
- *Diverticulitis versus cancer.* As many as 25% of patients explored for diverticulitis have colorectal cancer. Careful exploration will help guide the necessary extent of resection. Furthermore, the failure to exclude malignancy in a patient investigated for diverticular disease is an indication for surgical resection.

Treatment

PITFALLS

- Use of antimicrobials. Intravenous and oral antibiotic regimens should cover both aerobic and anaerobic organisms. Common single-drug therapy regimens using metronidazole or a fluoroquinolone alone are not adequate.
- *Delay of surgical therapy.* Diverticulitis worsens with each subsequent attack. Resection is indicated for all patients with two attacks of uncomplicated diverticulitis, or after a single attack of complicated diverticulitis.
- *Extent of distal resection.* Resection for diverticular disease must include any previously inflamed bowel, with the distal margin extending onto the rectum. Failure to resect all distal sigmoid colon is associated with a high rate of recurrent disease.
- *Use of the "three-stage" procedure.* Surgical management of acute diverticulitis without resection, or proximal diversion and drainage, is associated with higher morbidity and mortality than those of the Hartmann procedure.
- *Beware the ureter.* The left ureter is frequently involved and distorted by the inflammation of diverticulitis. Preoperative cystoscopy and stenting, initial identification of the ureter proximal to the inflammation, and division of the mesentery close to the colon protect the ureter from injury.

---

attempted after resuscitation, but this procedure should be aborted immediately if recurrent symptoms develop. Hartmann's procedure with later colostomy closure is performed most often for obstruction secondary to diverticulitis. Selected patients without intraoperative instability may undergo on-table colonic lavage with primary anastomosis.

SELECTED READINGS

Elliot TB, Yego S, Irvin TT: Five-year audit of the acute complications of diverticular disease. Br J Surg 1997;84:535.

Kockerling F, Schneider C, Reymond MA, et al: Laparoscopic resection of sigmoid diverticulitis: Results of a multicenter study. Surg Endosc 1999;13:567.

Lee EC, Murray JJ, Coller JA, et al: Intraoperative colonic lavage in nonelective surgery for diverticular disease. Dis Colon Rectum 1997;40:669.

Makela J, Vuolio S, Kiviniemi H, Laitenen S: Natural history of diverticular disease: When to operate? Dis Colon Rectum 1998;41:1523.

Roberts P, Abel M, Rosen L, et al: Practice parameters for sigmoid diverticulitis: Supporting documentation; prepared by the Standards Task Force, American Society of Colon and Rectal Surgeons. Dis Colon Rectum 1995;38:126.

Rothenberger DA, Wiltz O: Surgery for complicated diverticulitis. Surg Clin North Am 1993;73:975.

Schoetz DJ: Diverticular disease of the colon: A century-old problem. Dis Colon Rectum 1999;42:703.

Stollman NH, Raskin JB: Diagnosis and management of diverticular disease of the colon in adults: Practice parameters of the American College of Gastroenterology. Am J Gastroenterol 1999;94:3110.

Chapter 77
Pilonidal Disease
David E. Beck

Pilonidal disease has been addressed since the 1800s, and the name is derived from the Latin *pilus,* meaning hair, and *nidus,* for nest. This term notes the association of trapped hair in this unusual form of natal cleft skin infection. Pilonidal disease is an acquired lesion that results from either a foreign-body reaction to hairs embedded in the skin or from inflammation or occlusion of hair follicles, which rupture into the subcutaneous fat. If the sinus cavity fails to heal promptly, epithelium migrates into the sinus from the edges of the follicle and forms an epithelium-lined tube.

CLINICAL PRESENTATION

Incidence

All forms of pilonidal disease are reported to be more common in men than in women with a relative frequency ratio of between 2.2 and 4 to 1. The greatest incidence of pilonidal disease occurs between puberty and age 40. Pilonidal disease was identified in 365 of 31,497 men (1.2%) and 24 of 21,367 women (0.11%) in a study of Minnesota college students. The same study noted an association between pilonidal disease and obesity.

Microbiology of Pilonidal Disease

A review of the predominant organisms cultured from infected pilonidal sinuses in 75 patients revealed anaerobic bacteria in 77% of aspirates, aerobic bacteria in 4%, and mixed aerobic and anaerobic bacteria in 19%. However, the presence of polymicrobial infection does not seem to require preoperative antibiotic therapy.

Classification and Physical Findings

There are three common presentations for pilonidal disease. Nearly all patients have an episode of acute abscess formation. When this abscess resolves, either spontaneously or with medical assistance, many patients develop a pilonidal sinus. Although most sinus tracts resolve, a minority of patients go on to have chronic or recurrent disease after initial treatment.

The physical examination usually demonstrates one or more small (1- to 2-mm) dermal pits at the base of the intergluteal cleft (Fig. 77–1). Tracking from these pits (usually in a cranial and lateral direction) will be an area of induration. With an associated abscess, the diseased area may have tenderness, erythremia, or draining pus. The greater the disease, the more prominent the findings. Treatment methods vary for each stage in pilonidal disease.

PREOPERATIVE MANAGEMENT

Preoperative preparation is similar to that for other anorectal procedures. Patients with abscesses and associated cellulitis should be administered therapeutic antibiotics in conjunction with drainage. Prophylactic antibiotics are not routinely administered unless wound closure is anticipated. Mechanical preparation of the bowel is not necessary, but some providers administer a small enema prior to surgery to minimize the possibility of a spontaneous bowel movement during anesthesia. Patients should be instructed on the chances of recurrence, the need for postoperative wound management, and the length of time that may be required for wound healing.

INTRAOPERATIVE MANAGEMENT

Abscess

The presence of an abscess mandates drainage. Simple incision and drainage of first-episode acute pilonidal abscesses results in an improvement in signs and symptoms in all patients and complete eradication of them in more than half of patients within 10 weeks. Between 20% and 40% of patients will develop recurrent disease after this form of treatment.

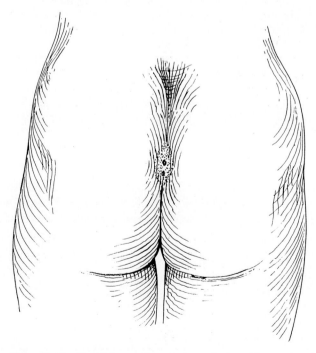

Figure 77–1. Pilonidal cyst disease. Dermal pits with associated sinus and abscess.

Incision and drainage of acute abscesses is readily performed in an office setting with the use of local anesthesia. In cases of simple abscess with minimal cellulitis, incision, drainage, and curettage of the wall of the cavity provide definitive treatment. The wound may be packed open with plain gauze initially to prevent premature closure of the skin over the cavity. The wound is kept clean by irrigating the area twice daily with warm tap water, with the use of either a shower attachment, sitz bath, or even Water-pik. It is important to keep the area dry to avoid maceration. The skin in the gluteal cleft is shaved prior to drainage and then during weekly office visits. Also during office visits, granulation tissue is cauterized and removed. Success in treatment results from diligent wound care by both the patient and the practitioner.

Sinus

As many as 40% of acute pilonidal abscesses treated with incision and drainage form a chronic sinus, which requires additional treatment. The majority of pilonidal sinuses resolve, regardless of treatment option, by age 40. It is theorized that changes in body habitus (altered and increased fat deposition alters the gluteal cleft) and softening of body hair account for this change with age.

Many treatments have been reported and then abandoned for nonhealing pilonidal sinuses. Table 77–1 presents a review of treatment methods used over the last 30 years grouped and analyzed by broad categories. *Closed techniques* (injection with phenol or coring out follicles and brushing the tracks) required shaving of the area but could be performed on an outpatient basis. Mean healing time was about 40 days, and recurrence rates were slightly higher than those for other forms of treatment. *Laying open,* or unroofing the tracks (Fig. 77–2A and B), with healing by granulation resulted in an average healing time of 43 days and required frequent outpatient dressing changes. The incidence of recurrent sinus formation was generally less than 20% with this technique. Local excision or the addition of cauterization of the cavity decreased the average healing time to 36 days and reduced the reported recurrence rates. *Wide and deep excision* of the sinus alone resulted in an average healing time of 73 days and recurrence rates similar to those for simple laying open of the sinus with wound granulation (see Fig. 77–2C and D). When partial closure of the wound

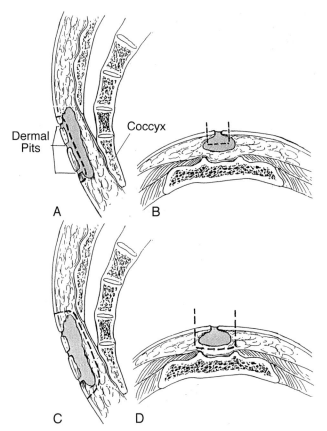

Figure 77–2. Laying-open technique (unroofing). Overlying tissue is excised. *A,* Sagittal view. *B,* Cross-sectional view. Wide and deep excision of sinus. *C,* Sagittal view. *D,* Cross-sectional view.

(marsupialization) is added to wide and deep excision of the sinus, healing time decreases to an average of 27 days. *Excision and primary closure* resulted in wound healing within 2 weeks in successful cases. However, as many as 30% of patients failed primary wound healing, and the average recurrence rate for patients treated by these experienced authors was 15%. The same time for wound healing was reported for excision and primary closure with the use of oblique or asymmetric incisions, but the recurrence rate was less than 10%.

Bascom reported fewer than 10% recurrence with *excision of follicles.* This procedure involved an incision lateral to the midline to scrub the chronic cavity free from hair

Table 77–1	Comparison of Techniques by Mean Time to Healing and Mean Recurrence Rate Based on Minimal Follow-Up in Several Review Articles		
PROCEDURE	**MEAN TIME TO HEALING (DAYS)**	**RECURRENCE RATE: <1 YEAR FOLLOW-UP (%)**	**RECURRENCE RATE: >1 YEAR FOLLOW-UP (%)**
Débride epithelial pit	42	10	18
Lay open sinus	43	4	13
Lay open sinus + cauterize base of sinus	36	4	13
Excision to fascia	73	14	13
Excision to fascia + marsupialization of edges	27	6	4

From Karulf RE, Perry WB: Pilonidal disease. In Beck DE, Wexner SD (eds): Fundamentals of Anorectal Surgery, 2nd ed. London, WB Saunders, 1998, pp 225–232. With permission.

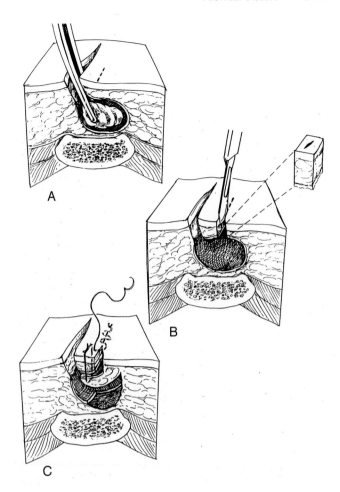

Figure 77–3. *A,* Lateral incision and débridement of cavity as described by Bascom. *B,* Removal of a midline pit with a small incision after lateral débridement. *C,* Closure of midline wounds without closure of the lateral incision. (From Karulf RE, Perry WB: Pilonidal disease. In Beck DE, Wexner SD [eds]: Fundamentals of Anorectal Surgery, 2nd ed. London, WB Saunders, 1998, pp 225–232, with permission.)

and granulation tissue (Fig. 77–3*A*). Removal of the small midline pits was carried out with small, 7-mm incisions (see Fig. 77–3*B*). When epithelial tubes were present, they were removed through the lateral incision. The lateral wound was then left open, but the midline incisions were closed with a removable 4-0 polypropylene subcuticular suture (see Fig. 77–3*C*).

CONSERVATIVE APPROACH TO PILONIDAL DISEASE

In an effort to preserve personal productivity, manage surgical problems on an outpatient basis, and reduce costs associated with health care, some authors perform lateral incision and drainage for acute abscess but avoid excisional treatment of pilonidal sinus in the majority of patients. Their protocol for conservative management consists of patient education about the nature of the condition and the need for perineal hygiene, meticulous hair control, and avoidance of exercises such as sit-ups and leg-lifts during periods of active disease. Hair control consists of a weekly 5-cm strip shave in the natal cleft from the anus to the presacrum until healing occurs. Another option for hair control, especially in patients living alone, is the use of a topical depilatory agent. The agent is applied to the natal skin while the patient is showering or bathing every 2 to 3 weeks.

POSTOPERATIVE MANAGEMENT

The general postoperative management of anorectal wounds involves efforts to keep the healing area clean and dry. If the wound is closed, the incision in washed once or twice daily (or after bowel movements) and dried with gauze, a towel, or a hair dryer on low setting. Open wounds are irrigated one to three times a day and loosely packed with gauze, as described earlier. It is important for the provider to inspect the healing wounds every 1 to 2 weeks to ensure adequate healing. Hypertrophic granulation tissue may require mechanical or chemical débridement. Failure of this débridement may prevent epidermal migration and closure.

COMPLICATIONS

Complex or Recurrent Disease

Even with proper treatment, a small subgroup of patients is left with persistent, nonhealing wounds. Repeated treatment of complex or recurrent disease with conventional measures rarely results in satisfactory healing. A number of more aggressive treatments have been described for treating complex or recurrent disease, including but not limited to wide excision and split-thickness skin grafting, cleft closure, excision and Z-plasty, modified

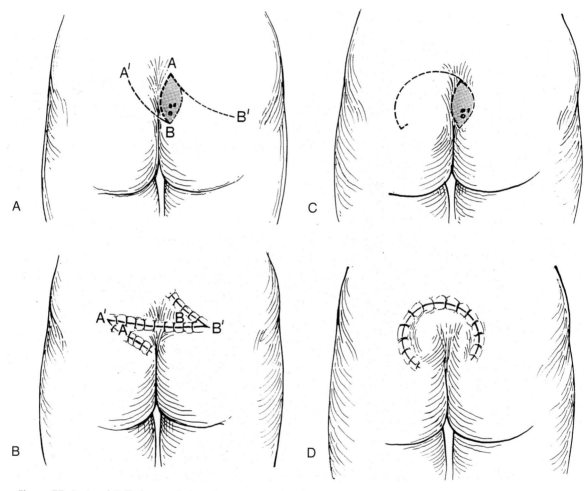

Figure 77–4. *A* and *B,* Z-plasty technique for recurrent pilonidal disease. *C* and *D,* Gluteus maximus myocutaneous rotational flap for recurrent disease. (From Karulf RE, Perry WB: Pilonidal disease. In Beck DE, Wexner SD [eds]: Fundamentals of Anorectal Surgery, 2nd ed. London, WB Saunders, 1998, pp 225–232, with permission.)

Table 77–2	Comparison of Techniques Using Primary Wound Closure by Failed Primary Healing and Mean Recurrence Rate Based on Minimal Follow-Up in Several Review Articles

PROCEDURE	FAILED PRIMARY HEALING (%)	RECURRENCE RATE: <1 YEAR FOLLOW-UP (%)	RECURRENCE RATE: >1 YEAR FOLLOW-UP (%)
Midline incision	8	8	15
Asymmetric or oblique incision	8	1	3
Skin-flap techniques	3	2	8

From Karulf RE, Perry WB: Pilonidal disease. In Beck DE, Wexner SD (eds): Fundamentals of Anorectal Surgery, 2nd ed. London, WB Saunders, 1998, pp 225–232, with permission.

Z-plasty, gluteus maximus myocutaneous flap, simple V-Y fasciocutaneous flaps, rhomboid fasciocutaneous flap, multiple flaps, and even reverse bandaging (Fig. 77–4). As a group, these techniques have resulted in primary healing in less than 14 days in 90% of patients. There are, however, disadvantages to these aggressive approaches (Table 77–2). Nearly all these techniques require hospitalization and general anesthesia. In addition, as many as 50% of the procedures that require skin flaps for wound coverage or closure develop loss of skin sensation or flap tip necrosis.

Another technique of "cleft closure" was described by Bascom. He removed skin from the more damaged side of the wound and covered the defect with a flap from the less damaged side (Fig. 77–5). While the wound was open, the base was scrubbed free from debris and granulation tissue. A drain was placed through a separate stab wound, and the incision was closed with a removable subcuticular polypropylene suture.

MALIGNANT DEGENERATION OF CHRONIC PILONIDAL DISEASE

An extremely rare complication of nonhealing pilonidal disease is squamous cell carcinoma arising from the sinus tract. Most of these tumors are slow growing but have a tendency to aggressive local invasion. Patients typically present after years of long-standing, untreated pilonidal disease. Patients with advanced disease, including inguinal metastasis, have a poor prognosis, and most die within 16 months. Long-term survivals have been reported in patients treated with aggressive surgical resection and adjuvant radiation therapy and chemotherapy to help reduce local recurrence.

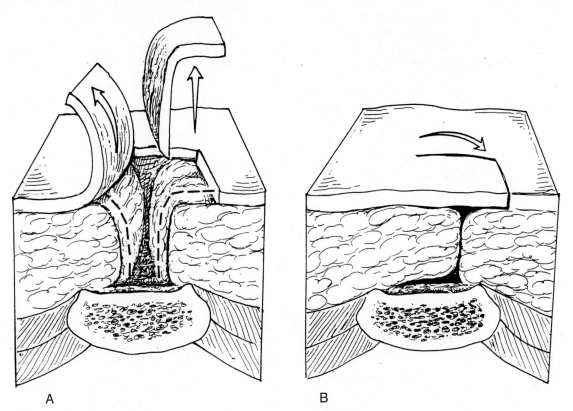

A   B

Figure 77–5. U-flap technique as described by Bascom for nonhealing midline wound. (From Karulf RE, Perry WB: Pilonidal disease. In Beck DE, Wexner SD [eds]: Fundamentals of Anorectal Surgery, 2nd ed. London, WB Saunders, 1998, pp 225–232, with permission.)

Pearls and Pitfalls

- Keep wounds as small as possible. The larger the wound, the longer it takes to heal.
- In getting wounds to heal, postoperative care is as important—if not more so—as intraoperative technique.
- Postoperative wounds need to be kept clean and free from hair and excess granulation tissue.
- During and after healing, the intragluteal region must be kept free from hair by shaving or the use of a depilatory agent to prevent recurrence. This should continue until the patient reaches the age of 30.
- If simpler methods have failed, consider excision with some type of flap closure.

OUTCOMES

Results of various operative methods are summarized in Tables 77–1 and 77–2. The numbers listed are average healing times from groups of experienced surgeons. Individual patient healing times will vary. Meticulous wound care helps, but in general the larger the wound, the longer the time required for healing.

Summary

Pilonidal disease has three basic presentations: acute abscess, simple sinus, and complex or recurrent disease. Simple incision and drainage of an acute abscess will result in relief of signs and symptoms in most patients. The treatment of a simple pilonidal sinus is eventually effective regardless of surgical techniques, so wound size should be minimized. Complex or recurrent disease often requires an aggressive approach, but consideration should

Table 77–3	**Author's Treatment Plan**

Acute Pilonidal Abscess
Lateral incision and drainage of abscess
Meticulous hair control by shaving natal cleft at presentation and weekly until healing occurs
Avoidance of trauma to the area during healing (avoiding exercises such as leg-lifts and sit-ups and prolonged periods of sitting)
Patient education about the need for improved perineal hygiene

Chronic Pilonidal Sinus
Conservative local care (hair removal and hygiene)
Minimal surgery (unroofing of sinus) for patients who fail conservative management
Healing by granulation

Complex or Recurrent Pilonidal Disease
Conservative excision of disease
Use of eccentrically placed incisions, rotation or U-flap for closure
Healing by granulation

be given to attempting conservative, nonoperative therapy in selected patients to minimize patient discomfort, time lost from work, and health care dollars spent on local wound care. The author's management plan for pilonidal disease is summarized in Table 77–3.

SELECTED READINGS

Allen-Mersh TG: Pilonidal sinus: Finding the right track for treatment. Br J Surg 1990;77:123.

Armstrong JH, Barcia PJ: Pilonidal disease: The conservative approach. Arch Surg 1994;129:914.

Bascom J: Pilonidal disease: Origin from follicles of hairs and results of follicle removal as treatment. Surgery 1980;87:567.

Karulf RE: Pilonidal disease. In Beck DE (ed): Handbook of Colorectal Surgery. St Louis, Quality Medical Publishing, 1997, pp 350–361.

Karulf RE, Perry WB: Pilonidal disease. In Beck DF, Wexner SD (eds): Fundamentals of Anorectal Surgery, 2nd ed. Philadelphia, WB Saunders, 1998, pp 225–232.

Patey DH, Scarff RW: Pathology of postanal pilonidal sinus: Its bearing on treatment. Lancet 1946;2:484.

Chapter 78
Anal Fissure and Fistula

Herand Abcarian

ANAL FISSURE

Anal fissure is a common painful anal disorder, which is often misdiagnosed as hemorrhoids. This may lead to inappropriate treatment, prolongation of symptoms, and even the wrong surgical procedure.

Clinical Presentation

Anal fissure presents as a small midline longitudinal ulcer or tear at the dentate line, causing pain after defecation that lasts from minutes to hours, the severity of which is disproportionate to the ulcer size. In patients with typical postcibal pain, digital rectal examination must be avoided (Table 78–1). Gentle eversion of the anal verge with lateral traction of the buttocks almost always demonstrates the small ulcer, which in 90% to 95% of patients is located in the posterior midline and in 5% to 10%, anteriorly. In acute fissures, the base of the ulcer is pink (corrugator ani muscle), but in chronic anal fissures, the internal anal sphincter with its typical white circular fibers is exposed.

Anal fissure is frequently associated with a tight or stenotic anus even when it is examined with the patient under anesthesia. The high resting pressure of the internal anal sphincter is postulated to impede the blood supply to the anoderm, and this relative ischemia (more in the midline due to the unequal distribution of vascular perfusion) worsens with increasing internal sphincter resting pressure. Straining on defecation causes trauma to the anoderm and produces the midline ulceration, which leads to indolence, failure to heal, and chronicity. In addition to the fissure, physical examination often reveals an external tag (sentinel pile) and a hypertrophic anal

papilla (hence, misdiagnosis as hemorrhoids). Infected fissures may extend through the intersphincteric plane to present as a small abscess or fistula. Fissures seen in nonmidline locations in the anal canal should raise suspicion for more serious illnesses, such as Crohn's disease, syphilitic chancre (which is painful in the anus), tuberculosis, and blood dyscrasias. Under these circumstances, an examination under anesthesia, with biopsy, dark field examination, and so on, may be indicated.

Preoperative Management

Most acute anal fissures respond to a high-fiber diet, increased water intake, and warm sitz baths. Anesthetic and steroid ointments are often ineffective. Conservative management results in an 80% to 90% healing of acute fissures, whereas 10% to 20% become chronic. Although currently the standard treatment for chronic anal fissure is lateral internal sphincterotomy, concern about anal incontinence has been the driving force for trials of alternative pharmacologic treatments.

NITROGLYCERIN. Nitric oxide receptors have been identified in the internal anal sphincter. Nitric oxide functions as an inhibitory neurotransmitter, thereby relaxing the internal anal sphincter. Topical application of nitric oxide donors such as nitroglycerin ointment to the anal verge causes reversible chemical relaxation of the internal sphincter. In uncontrolled trials, use of nitroglycerin ointment in 0.2% concentration for 8 weeks has shown a healing rate of 60% to 70% (compared with 30% for placebo) with no tolerance (tachyphylaxis). The major drawback of nitroglycerin is the frequent side effect of headaches in 35% to 75% of the patients, which causes

Table 78–1	Common Problems in the Treatment of Anal Fissure	
	PROBLEMS	**SOLUTIONS**
Diagnosis	Misdiagnosis of condition as hemorrhoids leads to prolonged ineffective medical care	Gentle eversion of the anus, looking for midline ulcer Avoid painful rectal examination
Pharmacologic treatment		
Nitroglycerin	Strong (>0.2%) concentration causes frequent headaches	Use only 0.2% strength to minimize headaches
	Application with patient in sitting or standing position increases the risk of headaches	Apply in Sims' position, and patient remains recumbent for 5 min
Botulinum toxin	Injection into external sphincter, higher doses cause incontinence	Inject only into internal sphincter, 0.4 mL only (0.2 mL both sides)
	Repeat injections, more than two times	Consider sphincterotomy
Intraoperative	Midline sphincterotomy causes keyhole deformity	Lateral sphincterotomy only to cephalad extent of fissure
	Fissure with abscess or fistula	Midline fistulotomy and sphincterotomy
Outcome	Inadequate sphincterotomy = recurrence	Judicious repeat sphincterotomy
	Excessive sphincterotomy = incontinence	Repair internal sphincter

515

10% of the patients to discontinue the treatment. Recurrence rate is high, and 30% to 50% of the patients will require subsequent sphincterotomy.

BOTULINUM TOXIN. Direct injection of botulinum toxin into the internal sphincter causes denervation by inhibiting the release of acetylcholine from presympathetic nerve terminals. No sedation or anesthesia is required. Injection of 0.2 mL of botulinum toxin on either side of the fissure, totalling 0.4 mL, with use of a 27-gauge needle, causes paralysis of the internal sphincter with pain relief within a few hours, which lasts for 3 to 4 months. In randomized trials, botulinum toxin injection resulted in 70% healing versus 13% in comparison with saline injection and was more effective in healing fissures in comparison with nitroglycerin ointment (96% versus 60% in 2 months). Tachyphylaxis occurred in 10%, but repeated injections are safe, albeit expensive.

CALCIUM CHANNEL BLOCKERS. These agents and anticholinergics reduce the internal sphincter pressure. Oral nifedipine (20 mg twice daily) resulted in a 36% reduction of the resting anal pressure and led to complete healing in 10 of 15 patients in 8 weeks. Topical nifedipine (2%) gel has the same results, with much fewer systemic side effects. Topical bethanecol 0.1% reduces internal sphincter pressure by 24% by blocking extrinsic cholinergic innervation and is just as effective as nifedipine in healing fissures. The two treatments may be additive.

Operative Management

By far the most effective treatment of chronic anal fissure is outpatient lateral internal sphincterotomy (LIS) (Fig. 78–1). With the patient in the prone jackknife position, this procedure can be done on either side of the anal canal with an open or closed technique with the patient under local anesthesia. Fibers of the internal sphincter should be divided only up to the cephalad extension of the fissure. Extensive or complete division of the internal sphincter causes anal leakage and fecal incontinence at rest, whereas inadequate sphincterotomy leads to recurrence. Midline sphincterotomy not only heals poorly but also is associated with a higher leakage rate due to anal "keyhole deformity." The anal fissure need not be excised; however, if it is surrounded by thick fibrotic scar tissue, this should be trimmed to allow rapid healing by secondary intention.

The only contraindication to LIS alone is the presence of an abscess/fistula at the base of the anal fissure. Under these circumstances, a midline intersphincteric fistulotomy, with unroofing of the abscess and trimming the fistula margins, results in reduction of the anal resting pressure and thereby obviates the need for a separate LIS.

Postoperative Management

Patients are encouraged to adhere to a high-fiber diet, increase their oral intake of water, and use non-narcotic oral analgesics. Although bowel movements may be uncomfortable or painful for a few days, relief from the severe long-lasting postcibal pain is appreciated immediately. Warm sitz baths (15 minutes three times daily) are followed by dry dressing to absorb wound drainage. Use

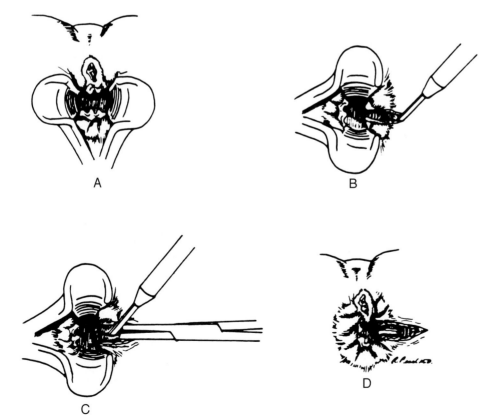

Figure 78–1. Lateral internal sphincterotomy. *A,* Posterior midline anal fissure. *B,* Anoderm is incised at the right lateral anal wall. *C,* Division of the distal internal sphincter. *D,* Completed sphincterotomy; an intact subcutaneous external sphincter is seen at the lateral end of the incision.

of topical anesthetic ointment increases perianal wetness and maceration.

Complications

LIS is associated with very few complications. Incontinence of flatus or leakage of loose stools in the days following surgery is common but subsides rapidly by the third postoperative week. Excessive bleeding is rare, and infection in the sphincterotomy incision, even if it is closed, is uncommon.

Outcome

The rate of healing of anal fissure after LIS exceeds 95%. Recurrence of fissure is almost always associated with persistent high anal resting pressure due to inadequate sphincterotomy, which can easily be documented by anal manometry. Judicious, conservative repeat sphincterotomy should result in permanent healing. Comparisons of LIS versus 0.2% nitroglycerin ointment showed healing rates of 90% and 92% in 6 weeks and 6 months, respectively, after LIS, in comparison with 29% and 25%, respectively, after nitroglycerin. Patient satisfaction was 100% versus 33%, and the operative rates after LIS were 2.6% versus 50% after nitroglycerin use. The incidence of long-term incontinence is variable because of the retrospective nature of the surveys, the lack of preoperative as well as postoperative assessments, and the variable length of follow-up.

ANAL FISTULA

Anal fistula, the chronic sequela of a cryptoglandular infection, is one of the most common anorectal disorders. If treated inappropriately, it can result in significant lifelong disability, such as fecal incontinence.

Clinical Presentation

Anal fistulas present as a draining perianal sinus. After spontaneous rupture or surgical drainage of an anorectal abscess, the wound may remain unhealed, with a bloody or purulent discharge. On occasion, the abscess heals,

only to recur later at the same location. Both clinical scenarios point toward the presence of a communication between the abscess and the anal canal—that is, a fistula resulting from infection in the anal glands, originally described as long ago as 1880.

Anal fistula is usually easy to diagnose and needs very little additional workup, except for anoscopy to identify the primary opening and for proctosigmoidoscopy to exclude inflammatory bowel disease. In patients with rectal bleeding, diarrhea, weight loss, or other systemic symptoms, a gastrointestinal workup is warranted to exclude Crohn's disease (Table 78–2). In some patients, the anorectal region is the only area affected by Crohn's disease, and in others involvement of the rectum, colon, or small bowel may follow after months or years of seemingly isolated anorectal disease. Multiple fistulous openings have to be differentiated from hidradenitis suppurativa.

Imaging studies are usually reserved for complex or recurrent fistulas. Computed tomography and magnetic resonance imaging have been utilized both with and without injection of contrast medium in the fistulous track. By far, the most useful information is obtained by direct fistulography, which may provide a "road map" for surgery. Endoanal ultrasonography with injection of hydrogen peroxide into the fistulous track may be helpful when the primary opening is hard to identify.

Preoperative Management

Anal fistulotomy (complete or staged), placement of setons, and injection of fibrin sealant into the fistula can be carried out without any bowel preparation. However, if the surgeon is planning to close a fistula with a dermal island flap anoplasty or an endorectal advancement flap, preoperative bowel preparation and perioperative intravenous antibiotics are indicated.

Intraoperative Management

ANESTHESIA. Simple fistulas can be treated with the patient under local infiltration anesthesia, using lidocaine with epinephrine, hyaluronidase, and sodium bicarbonate to minimize the burning sensation during injection. The supplemental use of intravenous sedation in longer procedures or in more nervous patients is helpful. However, in

Table 78–2	**Common Problems in the Treatment of Anal Fistula**	
Preoperative	Preoperative delays (antibiotics, repeated cauterizations) Extensive imaging and endoscopic studies	Expeditious examination with patient under anesthesia Selective endoscopy (suspecting Crohn's disease) Selective imaging (recurrent fistulas)
Intraoperative	Fistulectomy (causes incontinence) Aggressive unroofing of entire tract (causes incontinence) Forceful probing (causes false passage) Fistulotomy in all cases (increases incontinence rate) Unfamiliarity with anatomy	Fistulotomy (removal of entire tract unnecessary for healing) Careful probing, staging of fistula, and tailoring the operation Gentle probing, peroxide—methylene blue injection if needed Alternative procedures (flaps, setons, fibrin sealant) Refer if fistula persists or recurs
Postoperative	Persistence drainage treated with repeated cauterization and antibiotics	Examination with patient under anesthesia and alternative methods of treatment (recurrent fistula)
Outcome	Too conservative = persistence Too aggressive = incontinence	Refer to a more experienced surgeon

the more complex fistulas that require complete sphincter relaxation and longer operative time, it is best to utilize regional (spinal, caudal, epidural) or general anesthesia.

POSITIONS. Patients may be operated on in supine or lateral positions, but the prone flexed (jackknife) position with buttocks taped apart affords the best exposure for the surgeon and the assistants.

IDENTIFICATION OF TRACK. Gentle palpation of the perianal skin with the use of a water-soluble lubricant allows the surgeon to trace the fistula track from the secondary opening toward the anal canal. Superficial tracks can be palpated along their entire length, but transsphincteric fistulas dip under the sphincters short of the anal verge. The surgeon should then use a bivalve or moon-shaped (Ferguson) retractor to search for the primary opening of the fistula at the dentate line.

If the fistula has not been operated on before, Goodsall's rule is often very helpful in locating the primary opening (Fig. 78–2). Gentle insertion of a crypt hook into the primary opening and a fine blunt-tipped probe into the secondary opening may allow the probes to meet at the depth of the sphincters. Insertion of a probe into the secondary opening and progressive unroofing of the track must be avoided because it leads to complete division of the sphincter muscles. If the surgeon is unable to find the primary opening, hydrogen peroxide, colored lightly with 1 or 2 drops of methylene blue, may be gently injected into the secondary opening, while the operators look into the anal canal for telltale bluish bubbles. Forceful injection of hydrogen peroxide may cause dissection

of the surrounding tissue with typical crepitance. If too much methylene blue is used, the track may become deeply stained, thus interfering with identification of the beefy red granulation tissue.

Surgical Alternatives

Based on the intraoperative position of the primary and secondary openings and the depth of the track in relation to the sphincter mechanism, most anal fistulas can be easily categorized according to a classification proposed by Parks and associates in 1976 (Fig. 78–3). This is of paramount importance, because the more complex fistulas are associated with greater postoperative morbidity and incontinence after fistulotomy. At this time, the surgeon may choose to unroof the fistula tract by performing a fistulotomy (intersphincteric fistula) or placing a seton (braided suture) in the high (transsphincteric) fistula. Or the surgeon may simply abort the operation after a careful examination with the patient under anesthesia. Definitive surgery may be postponed for a later date, and the patient may even be referred to a more experienced surgeon.

If the fistula is a high transsphincteric or suprasphincteric fistula, it is better to avoid fistulotomy (sphincterotomy) and perform a dermal island flap anoplasty or endorectal advancement flap to close the primary opening. Alternatively, fibrin sealant (autologous or commercially available) may be used to close the fistula track, bearing in mind that this procedure is more effective in the long and narrow tracks than in the short, wide ones. Extrasphincteric fistulas are not amenable to fistulotomy

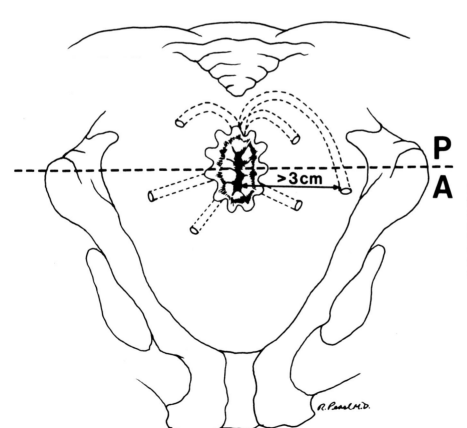

Figure 78–2. Goodsall's Rule (1900). All fistulas with secondary openings located anterior to a line bisecting the anus end radially into the anal canal. All fistulas located posteriorly or with a secondary opening over 3 cm from the anus converge to the posterior midline of the anal canal.

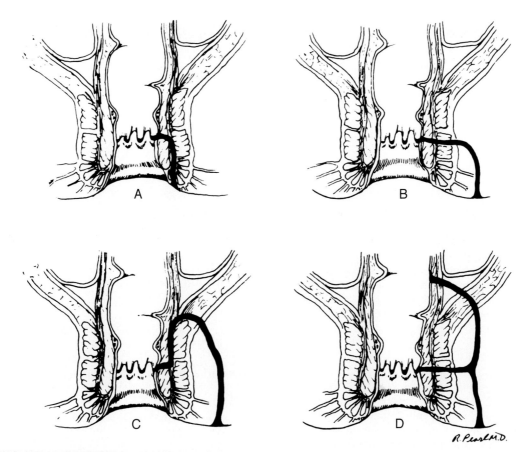

Figure 78–3. Classification of anal fistulas. (after Parks AG, Gordon PH, Hardcastle JD: A classification of fistula-in-ano. Br J Surg 1976;63:1.) *A,* Intersphincteric. *B,* Transsphincteric. *C,* Suprasphincteric. *D,* Extrasphincteric.

but can be temporized by insertion of braided suture or Silastic seton, which will keep the track draining and prevent recurrent abscesses. This technique is especially helpful in fistulas secondary to Crohn's disease, in traumatic or iatrogenic fistulas, and in fistulas of patients with acquired immunodeficiency syndrome (AIDS). A transsphincteric (York-Mason) approach for closing extrasphincteric fistulas may be attempted with or without diversion.

The most important intraoperative steps are (1) to come to the operating room well prepared; (2) be conservative, because recurrence is preferable to incontinence; (3) do fistulotomy, and not fistulectomy—removal of the fistula track is unnecessary and leads to gaping wounds and incontinence; (4) not hesitate to use a seton; and (5) consider referring the patient if the pathology is deemed too complex.

Postoperative Care

Most fistulas can be operated on an outpatient basis. Flap procedures require hospitalization for 1 to 2 days for pain control and for monitoring for urinary retention and flap viability. Patients are placed on nonconstipating analgesics whenever possible and on narcotics if pain is too severe. General diet, stool softeners, and increased water intake are encouraged. Sitz baths or showers (for flap procedures) three to four times daily are followed by careful drying of the wound, preferably with the use of a hair dryer on the cool setting. Plain gauze is placed on the wound and changed, as needed, to keep the area dry. The use of petroleum jelly, anesthetic, or steroid ointment is discouraged. The patient is seen every 2 weeks until the wound heals completely. Unhealed wounds after 8 weeks are suspicious for being persistent fistulas.

Pearls and Pitfalls

- Anal fissures are common painful disorders of the anal region.
- The goal of treatment is to reduce the increased tonic pressure of the internal anal sphincter.
- Topical nitroglycerin and injection of botulinum toxin are effective in some patients.
- The most definitive procedure is the lateral internal anal sphincterotomy.
- Anorectal fistulas arise from infection of anal glands at the dentate line.
- Anorectal fistulas are classified as intersphincteric, transsphincteric, suprasphincteric, and extrasphincteric.
- Treatment involves fistulotomy, placement of a seton, or complex flap closure.
- Multiple fistulas should raise the suspicion of Crohn's disease.

Table 78–3	Outcome of Fistulas by Type and Operation			
TYPE OF FISTULA	**OPERATION OF CHOICE**	**RESULTS**	**PERSISTENCE**	**INCONTINENCE**
Intersphincteric	Fistulotomy	Excellent	Rare	Rare
Transsphincteric	Fistulotomy vs. flaps	Good	Uncommon	Uncommon (5%)
Suprasphincteric	Flaps, fibrin sealant	Good	Common (20%)	20% after staged fistulotomy
Extrasphincteric	Seton, diversion	Poor	Frequent	Unknown

Complications

Fistulotomy is associated with very few early complications. Bleeding is a sign of poor interoperative hemostasis. When significant, it should be dealt with in the operating room and with the patient under anesthesia. Urinary retention secondary to pain and narcotic analgesics occurs in 1% to 2% of patients, mostly men, and is independent of the type of anesthesia. Flaps for closure of fistulas are more prone to infection and should be monitored more carefully.

Outcomes

The true incidence of recurrence or persistence of fistula is unknown but is related to the duration of the follow-up period. It is higher in more complex fistulas (Table 78–3). The success rate for intersphincteric fistula approaches 100%. Recurrence of transsphincteric and su-

prasphincteric fistulas could be as high as 5% to 10%. Recurrence of fistulas after flap procedures or fibrin glue injection is approximately 20%, but the procedures may be repeated because they do not entail sphincterotomy and therefore are not prone to resulting in fecal incontinence.

SELECTED READINGS

Brisinada G, Maria G, Bentivoglio AR, et al: A comparison of injections of botulinum toxin and topical nitroglycerin ointment for the treatment of chronic anal fissures. N Engl J Med 1999;342:65.
Cintron JR, Park JJ, Orsay CP, et al: Repair of fistula-in-ano using autologous fibrin tissue adhesive. Dis Colon Rectum 1999;42:607.
Del Pino A, Nelson RL, Pearl RK, Abcarian H: Island flap anoplasty for treatment of transsphincteric fistula-in-ano. Dis Colon Rectum 1996,29:224.
Parks AG, Gordon PH, Hardcastle JD: A classification of fistula-in-ano. Br J Surg 1976;63:1.
Pearl RK, Andrews JR, Orsay CP, et al: Role of the seton in the management of anorectal fistulas. Dis Colon Rectum 1993;36:573.
Ramanujam PS, Prasad ML, Abcarian H, Tan AB: Perianal abscess and fistulas: A study of 1023 patients. Dis Colon Rectum 1984;27:293.
Weisman RI, Orsay CP, Pearl RK, Abcarian H: The role of fistulography in fistula-in-ano. Dis Colon Rectum 1991;34:181.

Chapter 79

Polyposis Syndromes of the Colon

Eric J. Dozois and Roger R. Dozois

A polyp is an abnormal elevation of mucosa and submucosa from an epithelial surface. The numerous types of colorectal polyps include adenoma, hamartoma, and metaplastic lesions. Gastrointestinal polyposis syndromes share some similarities, such as a low incidence, autosomal dominant inheritance, and genetic predisposition to colorectal cancer and/or other extracolonic cancers. A clear understanding of the distinctions between these types of polyps is necessary for ensuring accurate recognition and proper management. This chapter briefly describes the clinical presentation, diagnosis, and management as they relate to the most common polyposis syndromes of the colon.

FAMILIAL ADENOMATOUS POLYPOSIS

Familial adenomatous polyposis (FAP) is a disorder inherited in a simple dominant fashion that affects both sexes equally and is characterized by the development of multiple adenomatous polyps (Fig. 79–1A and B) and an almost 100% risk of colorectal cancer. FAP is caused by a mutation of the *APC* gene located on chromosome 5q21–22 (Table 79–1). The number of adenomas can range from a few to a myriad, the often-cited number of 100 varying mostly according to the age of the patient.

Clinical Presentation

Symptoms and signs such as bleeding, change in bowel habit, and abdominal pain are most often due to large polyps and/or to cancer and are unusual before the age of 20 years. By the age of 40 years, cancer occurs frequently and is often unresectable in symptomatic patients. FAP may be associated with one or more extracolonic manifestations (ECM) such as osteomas, epidermoid cysts, dental abnormalities, desmoids (especially in the mesentery), and tumors of the central nervous system, thyroid, liver, adrenal cortex, biliary tract, and pancreas. The condition previously designated Gardner's syndrome is just a phenotypic variant of FAP. Congenital hypertrophy of the retinal pigment epithelium (CHRPE), which was used as a marker of the syndrome before the advent of genetic testing, is the most common extracolonic manifestation of FAP and is nearly 100% predictive of the syndrome if it has been demonstrated in the patient's kindred.

Three important extracolonic manifestations of FAP deserve lifelong surveillance. First, adenomas of the gastric antrum and of the small bowel, especially the duodenum and its periampullary region, may degenerate into cancer and serve as premalignant markers of this disease. Second, intra-abdominal desmoids (see Fig. 79–1C) may

occur in 10% of patients, and, despite their benign histology, they may possess a most aggressive behavior and lead to catastrophic and, even, fatal complications. Third, adenomas can develop within the ileal pouch (see Fig. 79–1D) several years after restorative proctocolectomy, but the long-term risk of cancer associated with them has yet to be determined.

An attenuated phenotype of FAP with fewer polyps (<100), later expression (third and fourth decade), and a more proximal colonic location may result from mutation in the *APC* gene and may be difficult to recognize if there is no family history. Genetic testing may be useful in helping decide whether proctocolectomy is advisable or not.

Diagnosis

The diagnosis of FAP is based on the history, physical examination, endoscopy, imaging, and genetic testing. FAP may be identified in symptomatic or asymptomatic patients at risk. Symptoms and signs such as bleeding, change in bowel habit, and abdominal pain are rare in patients younger than 20 years of age and are most often due to large polyps or to cancer or desmoid of the mesentery. Obstructive symptoms of the small bowel and/or ureters are usually associated with desmoid of the mesentery or retroperitoneum. Inquiries about a family history of colorectal cancer, duodenal cancer, or desmoid tumors are helpful.

The presence of multiple adenomatous polyps on flexible sigmoidoscopy, colonoscopy, or barium enema (see Fig. 79–1) helps establish the diagnosis. *Colonoscopy* may be preferable, especially if attenuated FAP is suspected. *Esophagogastroduodenoscopy* is recommended when the colorectal polyps are found initially. This test should be repeated at 1- to 3-year intervals after the age of 20 to 25 years if polyps are noted to be present in the stomach and/or duodenum. Computed tomography (CT) or magnetic resonance imaging (MRI) is most often reserved for patients known to have or suspected of having a desmoid.

GENETIC TESTING. Detection of the *APC* mutation can be achieved directly in blood (no other family members affected; sensitivity 80%; specificity 100%) or indirectly by linkage analysis (at least two other family members affected; sensitivity 95%; specificity 98% to 99%). Family members at risk and those with a positive *APC* mutation should undergo annual flexible sigmoidoscopy screening when they are 10 to 12 years old or at puberty. Several variations of APC mutations may affect the phenotype of FAP presentation.

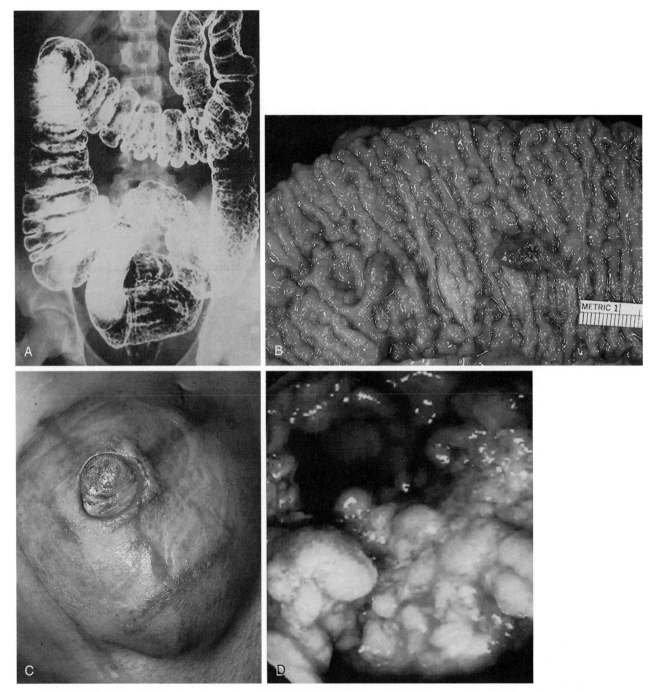

Figure 79–1. Familial adenomatous polyposis. Multiple filling defects on barium enema *(A);* numerous adenomas in re-sected colon specimen *(B);* desmoid of mesentery eroding into abdominal wall *(C);* and adenomatous polyps of ileum after ileal pouch–anal anastomosis *(D).*

Table 79–1	Polyposis Syndromes of the Colon			
GENETICS	**FAP**	**PJS**	**JP**	
Incidence	1:6,000–13,000	1:120,000	Rare	
Gene	*APC*	*STK11*	*DPC4/SMAD4*	
Chromosome	5q21–22	19p13.3	18g21.1	
Risk of cancer, %	100	Mildly increased	50	
Extracolonic cancer	Ampullary, duodenum, gastric (less common)	Pancreas, breast, endometrium, ovaries	—	
Surveillance				
Colonic	Yes	Yes	Yes	
Extracolonic	Stomach, duodenum	Breast, small intestine, pancreas, endometrium, and ovaries	—	

PJS, Peutz-Jeghers syndrome; JP, juvenile polyposis.

Management

Preoperatively, the surgeon should review with the patient and his or her family the role of prophylactic colectomy and the advantages and disadvantages of the various surgical options; namely, colectomy with either ileorectal anastomosis or restorative proctocolectomy with ileal pouch–anal anastomosis (IPAA). The patient should also meet the stoma therapist because of the possible need for a temporary or, rarely, permanent ileostomy. Most centers advocate IPAA because it theoretically eliminates the risk of colorectal cancer, is associated with functional results comparable with those of ileorectal anastomosis, and provides patients with a good quality of life (Tables 79–2 and 79–3). Abdominal colectomy with ileorectal anastomosis is reserved for the occasional patient with rectal sparing, patients with only scattered rectal polyps, and those with attenuated FAP. In the future, genetic testing may serve as a guide in tailoring the operation based on the type of *APC* mutation.

Inhibitors of cyclooxygenase—the so-called Cox-2 inhibitors—given orally as an adjunct to the usual care of FAP patients (i.e., surgery and endoscopy) appear to reduce the number of polyps in the duodenum and in the rectum. Whether the reduced medical polyp burden will alter the need for operation or reduce the risk of malignant transformation remains unknown.

PEUTZ-JEGHERS SYNDROME

Peutz-Jeghers syndrome is transmitted in an autosomal dominant manner and consists of mucocutaneous melanin pigmentation with coincidental intestinal polyposis and a family history. The polyps are hamartomas and are located in the following sites, in decreasing order of frequency: the small intestine; colon; rectum; and stomach. The gene responsible for Peutz-Jeghers syndrome is *STK11*, located on chromosome 19p13.3 (see Table 79–1).

Clinical Presentation

The characteristic pigmentation spots are seen on the lips, buccal mucosa, and dorsal aspect of the fingers and toes. Patients may be asymptomatic or present with abdominal cramping that can lead to small bowel obstruction due to intussusception caused by large polyps (Fig. 79–2). Chronic occult gastrointestinal bleeding may cause anemia. Colonic obstruction is rare. Hamartomas represent focal overgrowth in the proper proportion of tissues indigenous to that part of the body. The peculiar branching-tree arrangement of the smooth muscle, the presence of mitotic figures, and mucosal malformation within the intestinal wall (see Fig. 79–2) all have contributed to misinterpretation and "alleged" malignancy. Recent studies, however, would indicate that these patients do have an increased propensity, albeit mild, to the development of gastrointestinal and extraintestinal cancers. The cancer has a predilection for the colon and rectum, pancreas, breasts, ovaries, and endometrium (see Table 79–1).

Diagnosis

The diagnosis is based on the history, physical examination, endoscopy, and imaging. A family history of mucocutaneous pigmentation and bowel obstruction is pathognomonic of the syndrome. Careful examination of the lips, buccal mucosa, eyelids, dorsal aspects of the fingers, and toes should reveal the characteristic pigmentations (see Fig. 79–2). Enteroclysis may uncover a myriad of filling defects in not only the small intestine but also in the

Table 79–2	Outcome of Abdominal Colectomy with Ileorectal Anastomosis in Patients with FAP in the Literature						
					PERFECT CONTINENCE		
INSTITUTION	**N**	**MEAN AGE (YR)**	**POSTOPERATIVE COMPLICATIONS**	**MEAN NO. OF BM PER 24 HOURS**	**Day**	**Night**	**QUALITY OF LIFE (GOOD OR EXCELLENT)**
Cleveland Clinic	51	28	17	4	82	NA	93
Mayo Clinic	21	32	17	4	83	89	NA
St. Mark's	62	19°	21	3	72	NA	NA
Saint-Antoine	23	25.6	NA	3	98	96	NA
Toronto	60	31.5	23.3	<6 (75%)	90	87	80

BM, bowel movements; NA, not available.
Figures are percentages unless otherwise specified.
°Median.

						PERFECT CONTINENCE		
INSTITUTION	N	MEAN AGE (YR)	POSTOPERATIVE COMPLICATIONS	MEAN NO. OF BM PER 24 HOURS		Day	Night	QUALITY OF LIFE (GOOD OR EXCELLENT)
Cleveland Clinic	62	28.6	NA	5		75	74	95
Mayo Clinic	187	26	24	4		84	80	98
St. Mark's	37	31	60	5		60	NA	NA
Saint-Antoine	171	30	27	4		98	96	NA
Toronto	50	35.6	26	<6 (70%)		75	51	93

Table 79–3 Outcome of Proctocolectomy with Ileal Pouch–Anal Anastomosis in Patients with FAP in the Literature

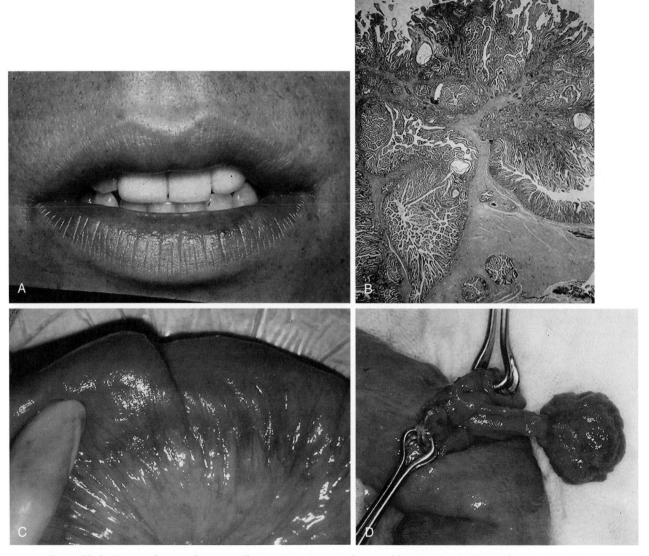

Figure 79–2. Peutz-Jeghers syndrome. *A,* Characteristic pigmented spots of lips. *B,* Jejunal polyp with mucosal malformation within the bowel wall misinterpreted as "malignant invasion." *C,* Large ileal polyp causing intussusception. *D,* Hamartomatous polyp after enterotomy before excision. (*A* and *B* from Dozois RR, Judd ES, Dahlin DC, Bartholomew LG: The Peutz-Jeghers syndrome: Is there a predisposition to the development of intestinal malignancy? Arch Surg 1969;98:509–517, with permission. *C* and *D* courtesy of E. J. Dozois.)

stomach and duodenum. Colonoscopy is ideal for assessing the colon and rectum and allows biopsies as well as removal of polyps. At times, patients with hamartomas may also harbor adenomas.

Management

Small bowel obstruction due to intussusception is relieved, at least temporarily, by operation with enterotomy and ablation of the offending large polyp or polyps (see Fig. 79–2). Occult bleeding resulting in anemia and the need for repeated transfusions requires clearing of polyps larger than 1 cm by endoscopy (stomach, duodenum, and colorectum) or at operation with or without intraoperative endoscopy for removal of small bowel polyps. Colon resection is reserved for colon cancer complicating Peutz-Jeghers syndrome, but prophylactic colectomy is not recommended.

JUVENILE POLYPOSIS

This polyposis syndrome is believed to be an autosomal dominant disorder. The polyps are hamartomatous, with a preponderance in the colon and the rectum, but they also occur in the stomach and small intestine. The gene responsible for the syndrome is *DPC4/SMAD4* and correlates with the *APC* gene.

Clinical Presentation

Patients with colonic involvement may be affected by numerous malformations of the skin (telangiectasias), heart (ventricular septal defect), and bones (polydactyly and macrocephaly). Juvenile polyposis is often diagnosed in adolescence and early adulthood, and in its rare, florid form it may be mistaken for FAP. Patients often complain of rectal outlet bleeding and, occasionally, of protrusion of polyp through the anus. The cumulative risk of colorectal cancer may be as high as 50%, and thus lifelong surveillance is necessary.

Diagnosis

The diagnosis is based on the clinical history, physical examination, and endoscopic evaluation.

Management

The increased risk of colorectal cancer that exists with polyps has resulted in some authors advocating prophylactic colectomy with either ileorectostomy or IPAA. If the number of colonic polyps is less than 20, endoscopic polypectomy is a reasonable alternative. If the number is more than 20, if dysplasia is present, and if the patient is symptomatic with rectal bleeding, colectomy is favored.

Other syndromes associated with hamartomatous polyps of the gastrointestinal tract have been described,

---

Pearls and Pitfalls

- The risk and primary sites of malignancy vary greatly with the form of polyposis syndrome.
- All polyposis syndromes appear to represent autosomal dominant transmissions; thus, if the patient has the genetic mutations, he or she will require lifelong surveillance.
- The risk of colorectal cancer in patients with FAP is virtually 100% by age 40; thus, all patients should undergo colectomy.
- Although Cox-2 inhibitors may decrease the number of polyps, the risk of malignancy may not decrease.
- Patients with FAP treated with abdominal colectomy with ileorectostomy are still at risk for developing rectal cancer.
- Peutz-Jeghers syndrome involves hamartomatous polyps throughout the gut, which are not premalignant. Nevertheless, these patients do have a slightly increased risk of gastrointestinal and extraintestinal cancer.
- Juvenile polyposis involves hamartomatous polyps primarily in the colon. Although the polyps do not appear to be premalignant, the risk of colon cancer is markedly increased, especially if there are more than 20 polyps in the colon.

---

but they are extremely rare. The conditions include the following:

1. Cronkhite-Canada syndrome, with hamartomas principally involving the stomach and colon and ectodermal changes such as hair loss, nail atrophy, and skin pigmentation
2. Cowden's syndrome, characterized by connective tissue polyps of the skin and gastrointestinal tract (most notably the rectosigmoid area), may be associated with an increased risk of breast and thyroid cancer
3. Ruvalcaba-Myhre-Smith syndrome, referring to hamartomas of the colon and ileum, pigmentation of the penis, and macrocephaly

Metaplastic polyposis is associated with 1- to 5-mm, hyperplastic lesions that have a pale, serrated appearance and no dysplasia. The lesions number 50 to 100 and can be visualized on radiograph or colonoscopy.

SELECTED READINGS

Berk T, Cohen Z: Hereditary gastrointestinal polyposis syndromes. In Nichols RJ, Dozois RR (eds): Surgery of the Colon and Rectum. New York, Churchill Livingstone, 1997, pp 390–410.

Boardman L, Thibodeau S, Schaid DJ, et al: Increased risk for cancer in patients with the Peutz-Jeghers syndrome. Ann Intern Med 1998;128:896.

Giardello FM: Gastrointestinal polyposis syndromes and hereditary non-polyposis colorectal cancer. In Rustgi AK (ed): Gastrointestinal Cancers: Biology, Diagnosis and Therapy. Philadelphia, Lippincott-Raven, 1995, pp 367–377.

King JE, Dozois RR, Lindor NM, Ahlquist DA: Care of patients and their families with familial adenomatous polyposis. Mayo Clin Proc 2000;75:57.

Nugent KP, Spigelman AD, Phillips RKS: Life expectancy after colectomy and ileorectal anastomosis for familial adenomatous polyposis. Dis Colon Rectum 1993;36:1059.

Nyam D, Brillant P, Dozois RR, et al: Ileal pouch–anal anastomosis for familial adenomatous polyposis. Ann Surg 1997;226:514.

Chapter 80
Fecal Incontinence

Giampaolo Ugolini and Fabio M. Potenti

Fecal incontinence is defined as the partial or total inability to control the passage of stools, liquid, or flatus. Fecal incontinence is a devastating problem that affects a small but select percentage of the population. The problem is often underestimated, with fewer than 50% of the patients reporting the symptoms to a physician. Although difficult to assess, the prevalence of fecal incontinence in the general population is probably somewhere around 2%, reaching a peak of 7% in independent adults older than the age of 65. The dimension of the problem increases exponentially in the nursing home population, of whom about 30% to 50% of the residents are incontinent. As many as 13% of women who have had their first vaginal delivery develop a degree of incontinence or urgency, with enormous psychosocial implications.

MECHANISM OF CONTINENCE

Maintenance of continence is a complicated mechanism that depends on a variety of factors: stool quality and volume, rectal reservoir and compliance, rectal sensory thresholds, and status of the anal sphincter complex. Undoubtedly, the functionality of the sphincters is one of the most important factors and depends not only on their morphologic integrity but also on preservation of sphincteric innervation. The internal anal sphincter (IAS), an involuntary muscle, is responsible for 50% to 85% of the resting tone, with the voluntary muscles making up the external anal sphincter (EAS) and the anal cushions responsible for the remainder. Although disruption of the IAS leads to passive incontinence (loss of stools without awareness), impairment of the EAS leads to urge incontinence (inability to postpone defecation).

ETIOLOGY

Multiple conditions can lead to fecal incontinence. A simple, but useful distinction is made between conditions associated with normal and abnormal pelvic floor function (Table 80–1).

CLINICAL PRESENTATION AND DIAGNOSTIC EVALUATION

Quantification of the severity of symptoms is very important. The use of an incontinence score serves as an objective and reproducible assessment of patient symptoms during the initial evaluation, and for comparison during follow-up visits after treatment. One of the most used and reliable is Wexner's incontinence score (Table 80–2). After a careful history and physical examination, tests of anorectal physiology provide the additional information required for planning treatment. These tests include endoanal ultrasonography, anorectal manometry, and pudendal nerve terminal motor latency.

ENDOANAL ULTRASOUND (EAUS). The introduction of EAUS in the late 1980s has radically changed the evaluation of patients with fecal incontinence. This modality of real-time imaging allows direct morphologic study of the anal sphincter complex with the ability to identify defects in the IAS and EAS at all levels of the anal canal (Fig. 80–1). This study is particularly important in patients with an obstetric history, previous anorectal surgery, and/or other direct injuries.

ANORECTAL MANOMETRY. This test allows a precise evaluation of important parameters, including resting and

Table 80–1	Etiology of Fecal Incontinence

Normal Pelvic Floor
  Diarrhea
  Proctitis (secondary to inflammatory bowel disease, infection, irradiation)
  Absent or small rectal reservoir (s/p proctectomy with low anastomosis)
  Neurologic disorders (multiple sclerosis, Alzheimer's disease, s/p brain or spinal injuries, cauda equina syndrome, tabes dorsalis)
  Encopresis
  Systemic disease affecting neuromotor coordination (diabetic neuropathy, collagen vascular diseases)
Abnormal Pelvic Floor
  Sphincter injuries (s/p obstetric tears of episiotomies, s/p anorectal surgery, s/p anal trauma)
  Pelvic floor denervation (pudendal neuropathy, perineal descent syndrome and rectal prolapse, neoplastic infiltration, irradiation, aging)
  Congenital disorders (spina bifida, imperforate anus, myelomeningocele)

s/p, status post.

Table 80–2	Incontinence Scoring System*				
TYPE OF INCONTINENCE	**FREQUENCY**				
	Never	**Rarely**	**Sometimes**	**Usually**	**Always**
Solid	0	1	2	3	4
Liquid	0	1	2	3	4
Gas	0	1	2	3	4
Wears pad	0	1	2	3	4
Lifestyle alteration	0	1	2	3	4

Never, 0 (never); rarely, <1/month; sometimes, >1/month, <1/week; usually, <1/day, >1/week; always, >1/day; 0 = perfect continence; 20 = complete incontinence.

After Jorge JMN, Wexner SD: Etiology and management of fecal incontinence. Dis Colon Rectum 1993;36:77–97.

squeeze pressures of the anal sphincteric complex, the rectoanal inhibitory reflex (RAIR) indicative of neuromotor coordination of the rectum and the anal sphincteric complex, and rectal sensory thresholds. The latter refers to the patient's first sensation of a step-wise inflated intrarectal balloon and the maximum tolerable volume of this balloon. A detailed mapping of the anal canal is provided, documenting the baseline level of sphincter function and rectal sensation prior to treatment.

PUDENDAL NERVE TERMINAL MOTOR LATENCY (PNTML). The advent of PNTML has allowed a simple evaluation of pudendal nerve function. The test is performed by recording activity in the sphincters in response to transrectal electrical stimulation of the motor nerve. Normal pudendal nerve latency is 2 ± 0.2 msec. A delay in nerve conduction is indicative of nerve injury.

Significant neuropathy can be present despite a normal examination, as the latency determination relies only on fast-conducting fibers.

TREATMENT OPTIONS

Several surgical and nonsurgical alternatives are available to clinicians. An overview of the most common and effective treatment options is shown in Table 80–3. These include the overlapping sphincteroplasty (Fig. 80–2), in which plication of the levator ani and the IAS is performed with overlapping of the EAS. Other procedures include attempts to re-create an anal sphincter either using an artificial valve (silicone balloon cuff; Fig. 80–3) or encircling the anorectum with a transposed gracilis muscle from the thigh. Proponents of these procedures

Table 80–3 | Treatment Options for Fecal Incontinence

SURGICAL TREATMENTS	INDICATIONS	TECHNIQUE	RESULTS
Overlapping sphincteroplasty	Focal anterior sphincter defect Normal PNTML has better outcome, but even patient with unilateral or bilateral pudendal neuropathy can have significant improvement	Identification of IAS, EAS, and levator ani muscles. Apposition of levator ani and plication of IAS are followed by overlapping repair of the EAS (see Fig. 80–2).	Success rate of this procedure is 70%–80%. Good results also in elderly patients. Wound infection is the most frequent complication (5%–10%).
Artificial bowel sphincter (ABS) (AMS Sphincter 800; American Medical Systems, Minnetonka, Minn.)	Multiple sphincter defects ± severe pudendal neuropathy Fecal incontinence secondary to neurologic or congenital disorders	The anus is encircled by a Silastic balloon cuff. The neosphincter is connected to a control pump in the scrotum (or in the labi major), and to a pressure-regulating balloon in the space of Retzius (see Fig. 80–3). The patient deflates the balloon, as needed, for the purpose of defecation.	Success rate of this procedure is about 75%. Infection and extrusion of the implant through the skin or the mucosa are the major complications.
Stimulated graciloplasty	Same as per ABS	The gracilis muscle is transposed from the leg around the anus and is sutured to the controlateral ischial tuberosity. Four to six weeks later, a nerve stimulator is implanted, with the battery inserted in a lower abdominal wall pocket.	Success rate of this procedure is about 70%. Unfortunately, complications are not uncommon and include technical problems with the muscle wrap and with muscle stimulation, perianal infection, infection of the stimulator and leads, and anorectal functional imbalance.

NONSURGICAL TREATMENTS	INDICATIONS	TECHNIQUE	RESULTS
Biofeedback	Partial neurogenic fecal incontinence (unilateral prolonged PNTML) Patients with mild sphincter injuries ineligible for or refusing surgery Patients who had undergone a previous anal sphincter reconstruction with residual incontinence	An anal plug with an EMG electrode is placed in the rectum. Exercise is performed with EMG tracings displayed on a computer monitor. Patients are also instructed to perform home Kegel exercises (10-sec relaxation and 10-sec contraction).	Biofeedback improves sphincter endurance and sphincter contraction, with a significant improvement of incontinence score in about 80% of patients. Bilateral and complete pudendal neuropathies are associated with poor outcome.
Procon Device (Ana-Tech LLC, Houston, TX)	Severe neurogenic fecal incontinence Patients with sphincter injuries ineligible for or refusing surgery Elderly or institutionalized patients	A catheter, with a motion-sensor electrode mounted at the distal tip, is placed in the rectum and held in place by a small balloon. A beeper is activated when stools reach the rectum, allowing the patient adequate time to reach the bathroom, deflate the ballon, and evacuate.	The device appears to be an effective and inexpensive method for improving quality of life in patients with fecal incontinence.

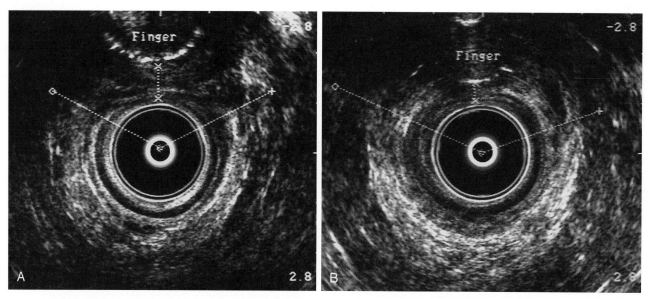

Figure 80–1. *A,* A 31-year-old female with fecal incontinence (Wexner's Incontinence Score of 12) status post fourth-degree obstetric tear. Endoanal ultrasonography (EAUS) shows an anterior defect of both external anal sphincter (EAS) and the internal (IAS). *B,* A 72-year-old female status post two episiotomies with fecal incontinence (Wexner's Incontinence Score of 15). EAUS shows anterior EAS and IAS defects.

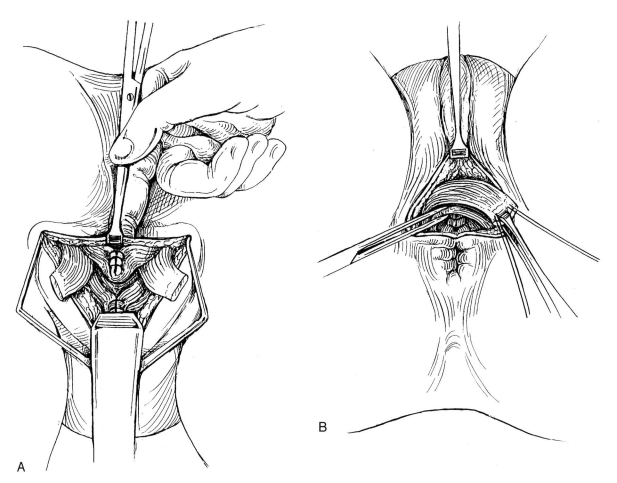

Figure 80–2. Overlapping sphincteroplasty. (From Anal incontinence. In Beck DE, Wexner SD [eds]: Fundamentals of Anorectal Surgery, 2nd ed. Philadelphia: WB Saunders, 1998, p 135.)

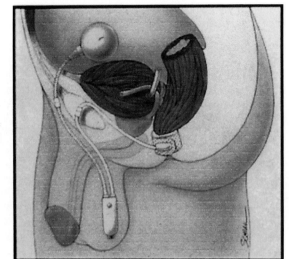

Figure 80–3. Artificial bowel sphincter. (Acticon Neosphincter. Courtesy of American Medical Systems, Inc. Minnetonka, Minn. Illustrations by Michael Schenk.)

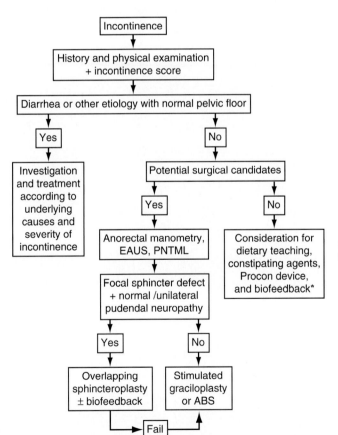

Figure 80–4. Decision-making algorithm for patients with fecal incontinence.

*Anorectal physiology tests are advisable before consideration of biofeedback.

Pearls and Pitfalls

- Fecal incontinence is more common than is reported because of psychosocial embarrassment.
- Fecal incontinence occurs from obstetric or postoperative injuries, mucosal diseases, neurologic disorders, and abnormal pelvic floor function.
- Fecal incontinence should be investigated by a combination of endorectal ultrasonography, anorectal manometry, and pudendal nerve terminal motor latency.
- Operative reconstruction or treatment includes sphincteroplasties or creation of a new anal sphincter mechanism.
- Nonoperative management includes attempts at biofeedback training or use of an intrarectal sensing device.

claim success rates of about 60%. A brief description of the technique, with its indications, is presented. Other treatments not described in the table include postanal repair, gluteal muscle transposition, sacral nerve stimulation, collagen injection, continence plugs, dietary teaching, and constipating agents. Nonsurgical methods include multiple approaches to biofeedback training in an attempt to "retrain" the sphincter to improve squeeze pressure and sphincter endurance. Another device has been developed that alerts the patient to the arrival of stool in the rectal vault, so that the patient can go to the bathroom for evacuation. An algorithm for decision making is also provided at the end of the chapter (Fig. 80–4).

SELECTED READINGS

Baeten CG, Geerdes BP, Adang EMM, et al: Anal dynamic graciloplasty in the treatment of intractable fecal incontinence. N Engl J Med 1995;332:1600.

Chen AS-H, Luchtefeld MA, Senagore AJ, et al: Pudendal nerve latency: Does it predict outcome of anal sphincter repair? Dis Colon Rectum 1998;41:1005.

Christiansen J, Hansen CR, Rasmussen O: Bilateral gluteus maximus transposition for anal incontinence. Br J Surg 1995;82:903.

Cook TA, Mortensen NJ: Management of faecal incontinence following obstetric injury. Br J Surg 1998;85:293.

Jameson JS, Speakman CT, Darzi A, et al: Audit of postanal repair in the treatment of fecal incontinence. Dis Colon Rectum 1994;37:369.

Johanson JJ, Lafferty J: Epidemiology of fecal incontinence: The silent affliction. Am J Gastroenterol 1996;91:33.

Jorge JMN, Wexner SD: Etiology and management of fecal incontinence. Dis Colon Rectum 1993;36:77.

Ko CY, Tong J, Lehman RE, et al: Biofeedback is effective therapy for fecal incontinence and constipation. Arch Surg 1997;132:829.

Kumar D, Benson M: GAX collagen injections: A novel treatment for faecal incontinence. Gut 1997;40(suppl 1):A52.

Law PJ, Bartram CI: Anal endosonography: Technique and normal anatomy. Gastrointest Radiol 1989;14:349.

Matzel KE, Stadelmaier U, Hohenfellner M, Gall FP: Electrical stimulation of sacral spinal nerves for treatment of faecal incontinence. Lancet 1995;346:1124.

Van Tets WF, Kuijpers JH, Bleijenberg G: Biofeedback treatment is ineffective in neurogenic fecal incontinence. Dis Colon Rectum 1996;39:992.

Wong WD, Jensen LL, Bartolo DCC, Rothenberger DA: Artificial anal sphincter. Dis Colon Rectum 1996;39:1345.

Chapter 81

Pruritus Ani

Santhat Nivatvongs

Pruritus ani is not a disease but a symptom of itching of the perianal skin. It is estimated to occur in approximately 1% to 5% of the population, with a male-to-female ratio of about 4:1. The onset of the condition is most commonly in the fifth and sixth decades of life. Most patients have only a mild form of the condition and respond quickly to proper treatment. To treat pruritus ani rationally, one must have a clear-cut concept of the etiologic factors involved in its production.

CLINICAL MANIFESTATION

Itching, usually combined with burning, is the prominent complaint. The itching may occur any time of the day or during sleep. Anything that keeps the anal skin moist causes itching. The itch-scratch cycle usually creates abrasion of the perianal skin, resulting in seepage of serum, which further irritates the perianal skin.

Careful history taking usually uncovers clues to the problem. Often, the patient has more problems at night or in hot, humid weather, although this is not always the case. The itching may also be exacerbated by friction from clothing, wool, and nylon. With time, the condition may progress to an unrelenting itching and burning with an insurmountable urge to scratch. Poor anal hygiene may be a major contributing factor. Questions regarding the patient's cleaning habits and how the perianal skin is cleansed are important to ask. Wiping with toilet paper only spreads and smears feces to the perianal skin. All cleaning wipes contain chemicals that also damage the sensitive perianal skin. Specific dietary ingredients and neurogenic, psychogenic, and idiosyncratic reactions with pruritus should be suspected whenever another factor is not readily identified. Because the diagnosis is made by exclusion, inquiries about diabetes mellitus, antibiotic use, and vaginal and anal discharge may establish the factors responsible for the symptoms. Stress and anxiety often exacerbate pruritus ani. Common complaints revolve around family, work, and finances.

PHYSICAL FINDINGS

In the early stage, examination of the perianal skin reveals minimal erythema and excoriation. As the symptoms progress, the perianal skin becomes friable, inflamed, and weeping from excoriation. Poor anal hygiene may be apparent with staining of stool or mucus, and a wet anal area. In the later stages, the typical findings of longstanding idiopathic pruritus ani include thickened, whitish, ulcerated, or abraded perianal skin from scratching, with deep furrows with radial ridges.

Flexible sigmoidoscopy or colonoscopy should be per-formed to rule out associated diseases, particularly in patients with chronic pruritus ani who are older than 50 years of age. Daniel and colleagues found associated colorectal disease in 35% of patients with chronic pruritus ani, including rectal cancer, 11%; proctitis, 5%; squamous cell carcinoma of anus, 5%; inflammatory bowel disease, 5%; adenomatous polyp, 4%; anal diseases, 2%; and colon cancer, 2%.

ETIOLOGIC FACTORS

Pruritus ani can be divided into a secondary type and an idiopathic type. With proper history, examination, and patch tests, the causes of the itching will eventually be discovered. The idiopathic type is diagnosed by means of exclusion.

SECONDARY PRURITUS ANI

From Within Anorectum

Prolapsed hemorrhoids (third and fourth degrees) cause mucous discharge, which, if not washed off, irritates the perianal skin. Treatment with rubber band ligation or hemorrhoidectomy is indicated. Anal fissures cause seepage of serum from the ulcer; anal fissures should be treated conservatively with bulk agents and warm sitz baths, nitroglycerine paste, or, if unresponsive to these measures, with lateral internal sphincterotomy. Discharge from anal fistulas is also caustic to the anal skin. Fistulotomy usually cures the problem. Other surgically correctable conditions include anal skin tags and prolapsed, hypertrophied anal papillae. Fecal incontinence, especially of liquid stool, can be a major problem. Radiation proctitis may cause leakage of mucus and liquid stool. Patients with pruritus ani have an abnormal rectal inhibitory reflex and abnormal transient internal sphincter relaxation. However, it is not known whether these abnormalities are the cause or the effect. Heavy coffee drinking is associated with relaxation of the internal sphincter, which may cause seepage of mucus and liquid stool. The main management of these problems is to eliminate the cause.

Anal hygiene is important in these situations. Patients should be discouraged from sitting in water to relieve itching because it causes maceration of the skin. Instead, washing with water by hand with or without glycerine soap is the best way to clean and relieve the irritation. In patients who have incomplete evacuation of stool, irrigation of the anal canal with a bulb syringe to wash out the anorectum after each bowel movement is helpful to prevent seepage of stool. Dietary measures to firm the stool should be instituted. For radiation proctitis, cortisone retention enemas may be helpful.

From Outside Anorectum

Sweating, particularly in overweight patients and in patients with a deep natal cleft, causes maceration of the skin with an eventual bacterial or fungal invasion. Wearing tight or nonporous underwear can also trap moisture. Proper washing with water by hand and wearing white, 100% cotton underwear helps improve the condition. Irritating vaginal discharge should also be ruled out.

From Perianal Skin Disease

In a study of patients with pruritus ani, Dasan and co-workers found 34 of 40 patients to have an underlying dermatosis that accounted for their symptoms, the most common form being psoriasis. Many of these patients also have a high incidence of sensitization to previously used topical preparations on patch testing. These patients should be referred to a dermatologist for proper tests and management. Anal condylomata acuminata can be easily diagnosed and should be treated with excision or electrocautery. Perianal Paget's disease and Bowen's disease can cause intense itching and mimic pruritus ani. Although they appear as a dermatitis, a biopsy confirms the diagnosis. Treatment consists of a wide local excision. Radiation to the perianal area, such as for carcinoma of prostate and cervix, damages the skin, causing erythema, ulceration, and seepage. The problem is usually temporary and improves with time. The area should be kept clean by hand washing. Cortisone cream usually helps as well.

Idiopathic Pruritus Ani

This category includes all patients with no known cause of the condition. Typically, the patients have a longstanding problem. The appearance of the perianal area varies from pale but otherwise normal looking, to ulcerated and seepy, to thickened with deep furrows. Many of these patients are excessively clean and have tried all kinds of topical preparations, including over-the-counter creams and steroid preparations. All of these agents should be stopped.

Proper washing of the area with water and glycerine soap (as long as the patient is not sensitive to it) instead of wiping with toilet paper should be strongly emphasized. Also, the psychological aspect of the condition should not be overlooked. In some patients, the anal itching may be the primary behavior, and this eventually perpetuates the itch-scratch cycle. Dietary measures are helpful for many patients with pruritus ani with the goal of achieving a nonwatery, bulky, formed stool. Fungal infection of the perianal skin is usually a secondary involvement from the moist and poor hygiene and is aggravated by antibiotic usage for this or other conditions.

The Last Resort

When all the etiologic factors have been excluded and other treatments have failed, one should consider injec-

---

Pearls and Pitfalls

PEARLS

- Diagnosis should be suspected when the perianal skin reveals erythema, excoriation, or ulcerated areas with deep furrows.
- Pruritus ani may be idiopathic or secondary to intra-anal disease (e.g., prolapsing hemorrhoids), extra-anal disease (e.g., excessive sweating), or perianal skin disease (e.g., dermatosis).
- Treatment involves improving perianal toilet and stopping all ointments.
- The rare patient with refractory disease may require treatment with subcutaneous methylene blue injection.

---

tion of the perianal skin with methylene blue as the last resort. The solution for injection is prepared as follows:

- 10 mL of 1% methylene blue
- 5 mL normal saline
- 7.5 mL 0.25 bupivacaine with 1:200,000 epinephrine
- 7.5 mL 0.5% lidocaine

The mixture is injected subdermally and subcutaneously in the anoderm and perianal skin. In their preliminary experience with 23 patients, Eusebio and colleagues found that cellulitis developed in three patients and full-thickness skin necrosis developed in three others when a 0.5% methylene blue solution alone was used; nevertheless, 21 of 23 patients had relief of their itching. In a subsequent experience, this same group, using the injection solution described earlier, noted no complications in 11 consecutive patients and good results in all.

Methylene blue causes death of nerve endings, and the injected area becomes numb for about 1 month. This temporary denervation breaks the itch-scratch cycle and allows the skin to heal and return to normal. Because the methylene blue solution alone can cause tissue necrosis, it should be diluted as described. The patient should be warned that his or her urine will turn blue for a few days. The skin in pruritus ani appears to have a low resistance to infection. The injected area should be cleansed with antiseptic before the injection. In some patients, prophylactic antibiotics should be considered as well.

SELECTED READINGS

Daniel GL, Longo WE, Vernava AM: Pruritus ani. Causes and concerns. Dis Colon Rectum 1994;37:670.

Dasan S, Neill SM, Donaldson DR, Scott HJ: Treatment of persistent pruritus ani in a combined colorectal and dermatological clinic. Br J Surg 1999;86:1337.

Eusebio EB, Graham J, Mody N: Treatment of intractable pruritus ani. Dis Colon Rectum 1990;33:770.

Eusebio EB: New treatment of intractable pruritus ani (Letter). Dis Colon Rectum 1991;34:289.

Farouk R, Duthie GS, Pryde A, Bartolo DCC: Abnormal transient internal sphincter relaxation in idiopathic pruritus ani: Physiological evidence from ambulatory monitoring. Br J Surg 1994;81:603.

Hanno R, Murphy P: Pruritus ani. Classification and management. Dermatol Clin 1987;5:811.

Mazier WP: Hemorrhoids, fissures, and pruritus ani. Surg Clin North Am 1994;74:1277.

Smith LE, Henrichs D, McCullah RD: Prospective studies on the etiology and treatment of pruritus ani. Dis Colon Rectum 1982;25:358.

Chapter 82

Rectovaginal Fistulas
Madhulika G. Varma and Ann C. Lowry

Rectovaginal fistulas are epithelium-lined tracks through the rectovaginal septum that give rise to embarrassing and debilitating problems for women and pose a therapeutic challenge to the surgeon. Fortunately, these fistulas are uncommon, constituting fewer than 5% of all anorectal fistulas. Rectovaginal fistulas can be congenital or, more likely, acquired. The most frequent cause of acquired rectovaginal fistulas is obstetric trauma (50% to 90%), but other disease processes and operations may result in these fistulas as well (Table 82–1).

CLINICAL PRESENTATION AND EVALUATION

Patients most frequently report passage of flatus or stool per vagina. Less common symptoms include vaginitis or persistent foul odor and discharge. Occasionally, these fistulas are asymptomatic or masked by more severe problems, such as associated fecal incontinence, undrained infection, or proctitis.

Appropriate evaluation of these patients includes a thorough history and physical examination. Detailed questioning helps to determine the etiology, any underlying disease processes, and associated symptoms, such as fecal incontinence. The importance of determining the functional status of the patient's anal sphincter muscle cannot be stressed enough, as it has a direct impact on the success of treatment. Most fistulas can be palpated on bimanual examination as an anterior midline crater. Digital rectal examination assesses evidence of abscess or induration, stricture, or sphincter defects. Further examination of the rectum by anoscopy or sigmoidoscopy will be adequate for most fistulas. If signs and symptoms suggest ulcerative colitis or Crohn's disease, other endoscopic or radiologic studies may be necessary. Patients with a history of radiation exposure should have a biopsy of the fistula to detect recurrent malignancy because as many as one third will have recurrent cancer on biopsy. Patients with an obstetric injury or symptoms of fecal incontinence should have endorectal ultrasonography to determine the presence of sphincter defects. One study found sphincter defects in 100% of women presenting with a rectovaginal fistula after delivery.

For the fistulas that are difficult to detect, a tampon can be inserted into the vagina and methylene blue or contrast medium instilled into the rectum. Evidence of dye, or contrast noted on radiography of the tampon, confirms the diagnosis. Saline can be instilled into patients placed in the lithotomy position, and the rectum insufflated with air to assess for the presence of bubbles. Radiographic studies are generally not useful in detecting these fistulas; indeed, endorectal ultrasonography was able to detect 100% of all sphincter defects but only 28% of associated fistulas.

CLASSIFICATION

Many classification systems exist to help the surgeon decide on an approach to surgical treatment. Our classification system (Table 82–2) defines fistulas as simple or complex based on size, location, and etiology. Low fistulas are those in which the rectal opening is in the transitional epithelium or distal to the dentate line, and the vaginal opening is near the vaginal fourchette. High fistulas open into the rectum in the upper half of the rectovaginal septum, with the vaginal opening behind or near the cervix. Simple fistulas tend to have healthy surrounding tissue and are more amenable to a local repair. Complex fistulas occur in diseased tissue, have often failed previous

Table 82–1	Etiology of Rectovaginal Fistulas

Obstetric Injury
- Fourth-degree tear—breakdown/infection of repair
- Forceps, episiotomy
- Septal necrosis

Trauma
- Operative—hysterectomy, low anterior resection, anorectal
- Sexual—instrumentation, coital injury
- Penetrating/Blunt Accidents—rectal/vaginal lacerations
- Fecal impaction

Inflammatory
- Inflammatory bowel disease—ulcerative colitis, Crohn's disease
- Endometriosis
- Drug reaction
- Chemical burns

Infection
- Cryptoglandular abscess, Bartholin's gland infection
- Diverticulitis
- Tuberculosis, amebiasis, schistosomiasis
- Lymphogranuloma venereum

Radiation
- Pelvic

Malignancy
- Rectum, anus, vagina, perineum, metastatic deposits, leukemia

Table 82–2	Classifications of Rectovaginal Fistulas		
	SIZE	LOCATION	ETIOLOGY
Simple	<2.5 cm	Low/mid	Trauma Infection
Complex	>2.5 cm	High	IBD Radiation Malignancy Previous repairs

IBD, inflammatory bowel disease.

repairs, and frequently require a more involved surgical strategy.

TREATMENT

The primary aims in treatment of rectovaginal fistulas are closure of the fistula and preservation of anal sphincter function (Table 82–3). Selection of the appropriate operative procedure, and its success, are dependent on the classification of the fistula, condition of the anorectal tissue, status of the anal sphincters, and any history of previous repairs. Surgical repair should be delayed until tissues are soft and pliable, without evidence of infection or inflammation. For women of childbearing age with significant symptoms, repair need not be delayed until childbearing is complete. Depending on the type of repair, subsequent children should be delivered by cesarean section.

For patients with simple fistulas and intact sphincters, the easiest local repair involves excision of the fistula track with a layered closure. This procedure can be performed from the rectum, perineum, or vagina and is dependent on the surgeon's preference and experience. Transanal and transperineal techniques are best approached via a prone jackknife position. An elliptical incision is made around the fistula and mucosal flaps are raised in a 2- to 3-cm circumference around the defect. The vaginal mucosa, rectovaginal septum, rectal muscle, and rectal mucosa are closed in successive order. Rates of successful fistula closure have ranged from 88% to 100%. Other transvaginal techniques include fistula inversion and vaginal mucosal advancement flaps.

The most common transanal approach is the rectal advancement flap (Fig. 82–1A to G). A trapezoidal flap of mucosa, submucosa, and some fibers of the internal anal sphincter muscle are mobilized at least 4 cm proximal to the fistula. The fistula track is then débrided and closed primarily by approximating the internal sphincter. The apex of the flap containing the fistula is resected, and the flap sutured to the distal mucosa. The vaginal side is left open for drainage. The success of this repair ranges from 40% to 100%. Factors that influence outcome include etiology of the fistula, presence of sphincter defects, and number of previous repairs. In one series,

more than one previous repair decreased the success rate from 85% to 55%.

Anocutaneous flaps have also been used to cover the defect by raising a flap of anoderm and perineal tissue and advancing this tissue into the anal canal. Fistulotomies are not recommended for rectovaginal fistulas, owing to the unacceptably high rate of postoperative fecal incontinence.

For patients with simple fistulas and associated sphincter defects, sphincteroplasty is the procedure of choice. The technique of sphincteroplasty is covered elsewhere in this text. The success of the repair and the functional outcome are directly dependent on repair of the sphincter defect. In one study, patients with advancement flaps had worse outcomes (40% versus 80% closure of fistula) than those of patients undergoing sphincteroplasty, and fewer patients reported satisfaction with the operation because of persistent incontinence. A recent study by Khanduja and co-workers (1999) combining advancement flap with sphincteroplasty reported a 100% success rate of fistula closure and 70% perfect anal incontinence; the remaining 30% had improved continence.

Another approach, perineoproctotomy, involves dividing the perineal tissues through the skin, sphincters, and rectovaginal septum to expose the fistula track. This creates a fourth-degree perineal laceration. The track is then débrided, and each layer is closed separately. While the technique is appropriate for patients with sphincter defects, the need to divide sphincter muscle makes it a less desirable choice for those with an intact sphincter. Success rates range from 88% to 100%, with little or no postoperative incontinence having been reported.

For patients with complex fistulas, the etiology and patient's medical condition usually determine the approach. More radical surgery is often required. In patients with high fistulas secondary to operative injury, temporary diversion is usually necessary to control sepsis and may, in itself, result in closure of the fistula. If not, subsequent colorectal resection may be required. In some patients, the fistula will heal with primary repair of the rectum and vagina and interposition of omentum or fascia. These techniques have also been reported laparoscopically. Therapy for rectovaginal fistulas secondary to malignancy is determined by the proper treatment of the underlying neoplasm.

Table 82–3	**Operative Approaches to Rectovaginal Fistulas**	
LOCAL	**ABDOMINAL**	**TISSUE TRANSPOSITION**
Vaginal	**Bowel Resection**	**Local**
Layered closure	Low anterior resection	Martius: bulbocavernosus
Fistula inversion	Coloanal anastomosis	Cadaveric dermal allograft
Mucosal advancement flap	Abdominoperineal resection	**Regional**
Transanal	**Layered Closure**	Gracilis
Layered closure	Open	Sartorius
Rectal advancement flap	Laparoscopic	Gluteus maximus
Cutaneous advancement flap	Tissue interposition (omentum)	Pudendal thigh
Perineal	**Diversion**	Rectus
Fistulotomy	Colostomy	**Other**
Perineoproctotomy	Ileostomy	Omentum
Sphincteroplasty	**Onlay Patch Anastomosis**	
	Bricker	

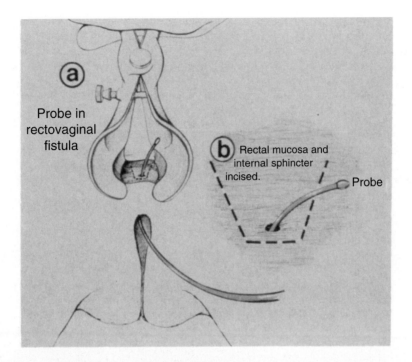

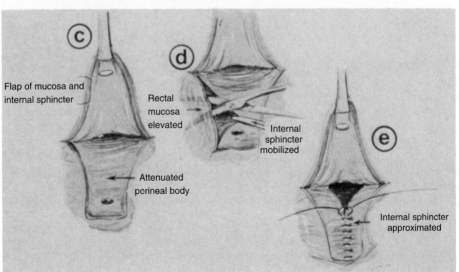

Figure 82–1. *A,* Probe in rectovaginal fistula with patient in prone jackknife position. *B,* Endorectal flap of mucosa, submucosa, and circular muscle is outlined. *C,* Width of flap is at least twice the base, and length sufficient to provide tension-free suture line. *D,* Internal sphincter muscle is mobilized laterally. *E,* Sphincter muscle may be approximated transversely as shown or longitudinally.

Illustration continued on following page

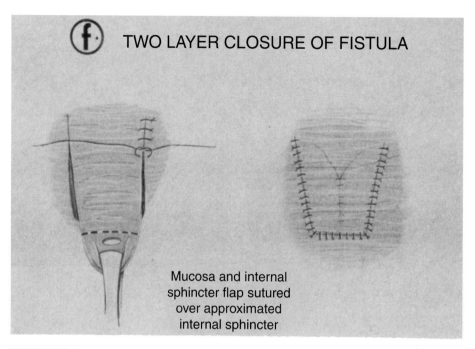

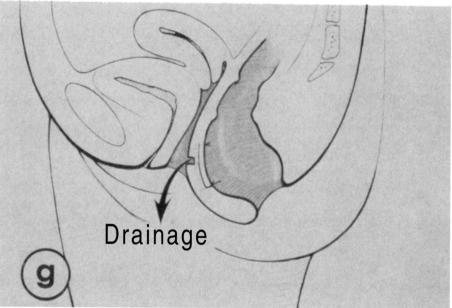

Figure 82–1 *Continued. F,* Excess flap containing the rectal fistula opening is excised, and flap sutured in place. End result is a two-layer closure. *G,* Vaginal mucosa is left open for drainage. (From Cameron JL [ed]: Current Surgical Therapy, 4th ed. Philadelphia, BC Decker, 1992, pp 246–247, with permission.)

Inflammatory bowel diseases pose a more difficult problem. Fistulas associated with ulcerative colitis are not amenable to local repairs and require proctocolectomy. Ileo-anal pull-through procedures have been performed successfully for these patients, but pouch-vaginal fistula is a potential postoperative complication of this procedure.

Patients with rectovaginal fistulas due to Crohn's disease may be treated with immunomodulators for their primary condition. Both cyclosporine and infliximab have been used with some success. However, most patients with inflammatory bowel disease require surgical intervention to treat these fistulas. Drainage of infection and abscesses with the use of setons helps to control local sepsis. The medical therapy may decrease inflammation to make the operation easier and subsequent wound healing better. A number of these patients ultimately require proctectomy, owing to active disease. If, however, there is no active proctitis and the patient is symptomatic, a local repair may be indicated. Endorectal advancement flaps, sleeve advancements, and vaginal repairs have been reported in this subset of patients. The use of diversion to improve outcome after surgical therapy is controversial.

Radiation-induced fistulas may be the most difficult to treat. Historically, local approaches had terrible results, owing to the ischemic damage of the tissue, and diversion was the only viable alternative. However, with prolonged diversion preoperatively to allow any surrounding inflammation to subside, a repair can be accomplished successfully. A low anterior resection or coloanal anastomosis may be a more reasonable choice for high or large fistulas. The use of a colonic J-pouch may improve the incontinence rate. The Bricker onlay patch anastomosis has also been used (Fig. 82–2).

Tissue interposition is an excellent way of introducing healthy, well-vascularized tissue in-between the rectal and vaginal defects. Grafts used for tissue transposition include the rectus abdominis, gluteus, gracilis, and sartorius muscles, which require a more extensive operation.

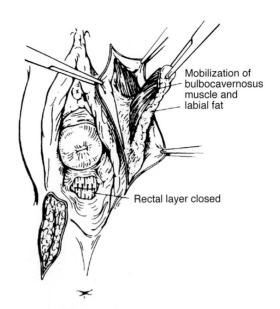

Figure 82–3. After the fistula has been exposed and the edges have been débrided, the rectal muscles are closed. The bulbocavernosus muscle and labial fat pad are mobilized. (From Goldberg SM, Nivatvongs S [eds]: Philadelphia, JB Lippincott, 1980.)

An elegant and simple tissue transposition technique is the Martius repair, which uses the bulbocavernosus muscle from the labia majora (Figs. 82–3 and 82–4). With the patient in lithotomy position, the fistula is identified through the perineal approach. The rectal defect is closed

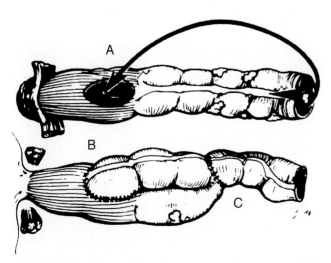

Figure 82–2. *A,* After the rectum is freed from the vagina and the fistula débrided, the sigmoid colon is divided. *B,* The sigmoid colon is rotated, and the end anastomosed over the fistula. *C,* After healing is complete, the proximal colon is anastomosed to the apex of the loop of sigmoid colon. (From Goldberg SM, Nivatvongs S [eds]: Philadelphia, JB Lippincott, 1980.)

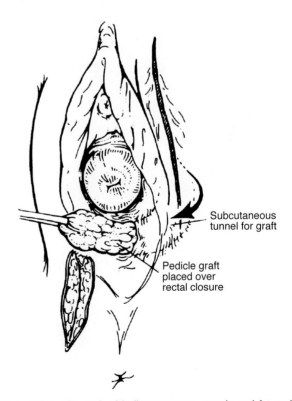

Figure 82–4. The graft of bulbocavernosus muscle and fat pad is passed through a subcutaneous tunnel to cover the rectal closure. (From Goldberg SM, Nivatvongs S [eds]: Philadelphia, JB Lippincott, 1980.)

after débridement of the track. A vertical incision is made on the labia majora, from the mons pubis to the posterior fourchette, and skin flaps are raised. The fat pad and bulbocavernosus muscle are mobilized and tunneled through the subcutaneous tissue and sutured over the rectal closure. The flap is based on the posteriorly located perineal branch of the pudendal artery. Success rates range from 75% to 85%.

NONOPERATIVE TREATMENT

For patients with significant medical risks, nonoperative therapies may be most appropriate. Fibrin glue has been used to occlude fistula tracks, but with quite variable success. The fistula track is curetted to remove granulation tissue, and then fibrin glue or tissue sealant is injected to create a coagulum. Reported success rates range from 60% to 80%, although experience is limited. The placement of an occlusive device was reported as an alternative to diversion for radiation-induced fistulas. A silicone-coated patch covering a nitinol frame was utilized with a success rate of 100%.

Rectovaginal fistulas remain a difficult problem. Many different therapies have been developed that usually attest to the poor success rate of most operative techniques. The preoperative evaluation is of utmost importance in determining which repair to use and its subsequent success. The etiology of the fistula, the anatomy of the sphincter complex, the condition of the rectovaginal tissues, and history of previous repairs all play an important role in determining the success of the repair chosen.

Pearls and Pitfalls

- Rectovaginal fistulas are most commonly related to obstetric injuries but may occur secondary to inflammatory bowel disease, radiation injury, or malignancy.
- Clinical symptoms include passage of flatus and/or stool via vagina.
- Rectovaginal fistulas are either low or high (with vagina) and either simple (involving healthy surrounding tissue) or complex (with diseased tissues).
- Primary aims in treatment include closure of the fistula and preservation of anal sphincter function.
- Repairs of simple fistulas have an 80% to 95% success rate.
- Repairs of complex fistulas involve advanced techniques and have a lower success rate.

SELECTED READINGS

Khanduja KS, Padmanabhan A, Kerner BA, et al: Reconstruction of rectovaginal fistula with sphincter disruption by combining rectal mucosal advancement flap and anal sphincteroplasty. Dis Colon Rectum 1999;42:1432.

Pinedo G, Phillips R: Labial fat pad grafts (modified Martius graft) in complex perianal fistulas. Ann R Coll Surg Engl 1998;80:410.

Radcliffe AG, Ritchie JK, Hawley PR, et al: Anovaginal and rectovaginal fistulas in Crohn's disease. Dis Colon Rectum 1988;31:94.

Shelton AA, Lowry AC: Management of rectovaginal fistulas. In Bailey HR (ed): Ambulatory Anorectal Surgery. New York, Springer-Verlag, 1999.

Tsang CBS, Rothenberger DA: Rectovaginal fistulas: Therapeutic options. Surg Clin North Am 1997;77:95.

Chapter 83

Pseudomembranous Enterocolitis
Michael Englesbee and Lisa Colletti

BACKGROUND

Diarrhea is a common side effect of antibiotic therapy. While it is usually more of a nuisance than a serious problem, fulminant forms of this disease can develop, with significant morbidity and mortality. The causes of most cases of antibiotic-associated diarrhea are unknown, but they are thought to be related to alterations in the colonic microflora. However, in 10% to 20% of patients, antibiotic-associated diarrhea is complicated by a bacterial toxin–induced colitis. The majority of these toxin-induced colitides and diarrhea are caused by *Clostridium difficile*. This diagnosis should be considered in the hospitalized patient with new-onset diarrhea because if it is left untreated, it may have potentially fatal complications. Other potential etiologic agents for toxin-induced colitis and diarrhea include *Staphylococcus aureus*, *Salmonella*, *Shigella*, *Yersinia*, and *Clostridium perfringens*. The human immunodeficiency virus (HIV) can also cause an inflammatory colitis that can be confused with *C. difficile* colitis. In the past decade, the prevalence of disease associated with *C. difficile* has markedly increased among hospitalized patients. This trend may be attributed to several factors, including increased awareness among hospital staff, widespread use of broad-spectrum antibiotics, greater numbers of elderly and immunocompromised patients, and the availability of faster and more accurate diagnostic tests.

Clostridium difficile is an anaerobic, spore-forming, gram-positive bacillus. The source of *C. difficile* may be the patient's native colonic flora, but nosocomial transmission has become recognized as being very common. Approximately 3% to 5% of healthy adults harbor *C. difficile* as part of their normal colonic flora. Current data suggest that *C. difficile* colitis is caused by a change in the normal colonic bacterial flora that allows overgrowth of toxin-producing strains of *C. difficile*. At least two toxins, toxin A and B, are enteropathogenic. *Clostridium difficile* can produce a wide spectrum of gastrointestinal disease, ranging from minor self-limiting diarrhea to life-threatening colonic perforation and sepsis. Pseudomembranous colitis is a particularly severe form of *C. difficile* colitis, manifested by diffuse colonic edema, multiple ulcerations, and the presence of an adherent pseudomembrane (Fig. 83–1). The pseudomembrane consists of dead leukocytes, mucosal epithelial cells, mucus, and fibrin adherent to the inflamed mucosa (Fig. 83–2).

Almost all antibiotics and some antineoplastic agents have been associated with predisposing the patient to *C. difficile* colitis. One series reported that 70% of cases were associated with cephalosporin administration, although this finding may be associated with the disproportionately greater use of cephalosporins among hospitalized surgical patients. Patients usually present within 5 to 10 days of initiation of antibiotic therapy, although some patients have presented as long as 10 weeks after discontinuation of antibiotics. The development of *C. difficile* colitis is not dependent on the duration of treatment or the total dose of antibiotic administered. Patients have developed *C. difficile* colitis after having received only one dose of preoperative antibiotic.

CLINICAL PRESENTATION AND DIAGNOSIS

Diarrhea is the most common symptom of *C. difficile* colitis and is found in 90% to 95% of affected patients. The amount of diarrhea varies widely, but 80% of patients have 4 to 10 bowel movements a day. Physical findings correlate with the severity of the disease, ranging from a normal examination to an acute abdomen and shock. Risk factors for *C. difficile* colitis include antibiotic therapy, elderly age, immunocompromised state, stay in an intensive care unit, burns, uremia, and possibly enteral feeding. In one study, after controlling for antibiotic use, patients receiving enteral feeding had a 20% chance of testing positive for *C. difficile*, while a control group tested positive only 8% of the time. Patients fed distal to the stomach were at increased risk compared with patients who were fed intragastrically.

Diarrhea may be absent in patients with a severe disease causing ileus or toxic megacolon. These patients may develop hypovolemic shock, cecal perforation, and/or toxic dilation of the colon, with secondary sepsis common in this group of severely ill patients. Abdominal films should be obtained to exclude free intraperitoneal air. The supine film in patients with toxic megacolon frequently demonstrates a dilated transverse colon, thickening of the bowel wall, loss of haustra, and occasionally pseudopolyps (Fig. 83–3). Evaluation with contrast-enhanced enema or endoscopy should not be pursued in patients when perforation or toxic megacolon is suspected. This clinical presentation is a surgical emergency associated with a 10% to 20% mortality rate. Occasionally, this clinical picture can develop in patients who are neutropenic secondary to treatment with antineoplastic agents, and can occur in the absence of antibiotic use; this is typically an ileocecitis or typhlitis (cecitis) caused by *C. difficile*. Another severe form of *C. difficile* colitis is occasionally seen in women undergoing cesarean section; altered colonic motility associated with pregnancy, in addition to the opiates given for postoperative pain management, as well as the preoperative prophylactic antibiotics contribute to development of *C. difficile* colitis. This form of *C. difficile* colitis is often associated with toxic megacolon and the

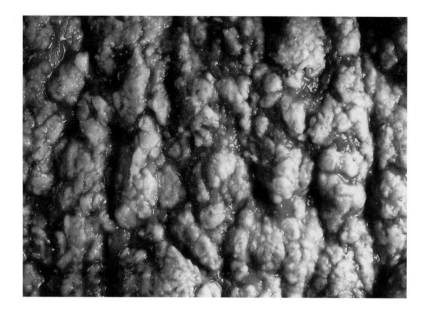

Figure 83–1. Gross pathology of florid pseudo-membranous colitis due to *Clostridium difficile*.

absence of diarrhea. Another situation in which *C. difficile* is a common etiologic agent is in the setting of enterocolitis associated with Hirschsprung's disease in infants and children.

Clostridium difficile generally does not produce an invasive infection. In contrast, the effects of the toxin on the colonic mucosa are responsible for the pathologic changes. Toxins produced within the colonic lumen bind to the colonic mucosa and attack the mucosal cell membranes and microfilaments. The resultant necrosis of epithelial cells induces inflammation, chemoattraction of neutrophils, increased capillary permeability, and loss of protein and fluid into the interstitium.

When the diagnosis of *C. difficile* colitis is suspected, a stool sample should be analyzed for both *C. difficile* toxins A and B. Two laboratory assays are currently available. The enzyme-linked immunosorbent assay (ELISA) is less expensive and much faster than tissue culture assays, with results obtained in 24 hours or less. In gen-

eral, it is not necessary to test for fecal leukocytes, as the results rarely alter management.

Limited endoscopy should be reserved for patients with a complicated differential diagnosis. This procedure, however, does allow direct visualization of the pseudomembranes, which are pathognomonic of *C. difficile* pseudomembranous colitis. These pseudomembranes appear as elevated, whitish plaques that range in size from a few millimeters to 2 cm (see Fig. 83–1). Although the presence of these lesions is diagnostic for pseudomembranous colitis, they may be absent in some severely ill patients. The mucosa adjacent to the pseudomembranes is often edematous and inflamed, but in patients with mild or moderate disease the mucosa is frequently normal or demonstrates nonspecific inflammation. In general, flexible sigmoidoscopy or rigid sigmoidoscopy is adequate for making the diagnosis. There is no apparent difference in the ability to detect pseudomembranes between rigid sigmoidoscopy (57%) and flexible sigmoidoscopy (50%).

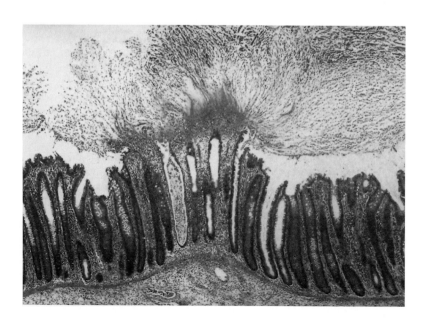

Figure 83–2. Microscopic section of severe pseudomembranous colitis due to *Clostridium difficile*. The pseudomembrane of dead leukocytes, mucosal epithelial cells, mucus, and adherent fibrin is obvious in the upper portion of photograph.

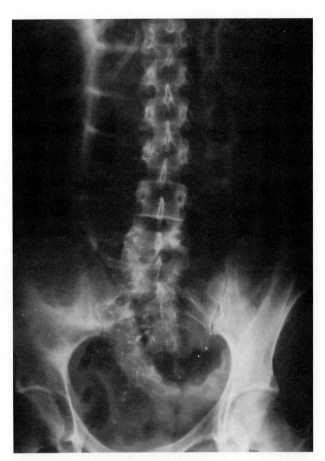

Figure 83–3. Plain abdominal radiograph of a patient with toxic megacolon due to severe *Clostridium difficile* enterocolitis; dilation involves primarily transverse colon.

Although surgical patients often have multiple risk factors for developing *C. difficile* colitis, determining the cause of hospital-acquired diarrhea is not always straightforward. Many patients fed enterally develop diarrhea, owing to the osmotic load delivered to the distal bowel. Also, it is frequently difficult to control the stool volume and number of bowel movements after a colectomy. Although the vast majority of patients with *C. difficile* disease manifest as colitis, *C. difficile* enteritis is an established entity that should not be overlooked in the postcolectomy patient. Several reports have documented fatal cases involving enteritis of both the ileum and the jejunum, although this entity is quite rare.

TREATMENT

Once the diagnosis of *C. difficile* colitis is made, treatment should include adequate fluid resuscitation and the discontinuation of the offending antibiotic. Recommended measures of infection control include patient isolation, the use of gowns and gloves for patient contact, strict hand washing, rigorous cleaning measures, and the restriction of staff and patient movement. Stopping the offending antibiotic is often sufficient to allow return of normal colonic flora and resolution of *C. difficile* enteritis in patients with mild disease. Antidiarrheal agents and

medications with slow transit times should be discontinued because they may inhibit clearance of the toxins.

For patients in whom the antibiotic therapy cannot be stopped or who have moderate to severe manifestations of colitis, treatment with oral metronidazole, 250 to 500 mg four times a day, is the treatment of choice. Metronidazole has nearly complete absorption and readily crosses the bowel wall. Successful treatment with metronidazole is well documented. Ten days of therapy is suggested for complete resolution of the infection, and symptomatic improvement should be noted within 48 hours of the initiation of therapy. Empirical therapy with metronidazole may be appropriate while one awaits the results of the stool toxin test, which should not take longer than 24 hours if the ELISA assay is used.

For many years, oral vancomycin was the standard treatment for *C. difficile* colitis. However, recently oral metronidazole has replaced vancomycin as the antibiotic of choice, as oral vancomycin is more expensive and has been implicated in the emergence of vancomycin-resistant enterococci. Multiple randomized prospective trials have demonstrated equal efficacy of oral metronidazole and oral vancomycin. In patients who do not tolerate oral metronidazole or who fail therapy with metronidazole, oral vancomycin should be started at a dose of 125 mg four times a day for a total of 10 days.

Surgical patients who cannot take oral medications or who have severe pseudomembranous colitis or toxic megacolon require intravenous metronidazole. In the critically ill patient, vancomycin enemas, 500 mg in 1 L of normal saline three times a day, may be added. Efficacy data for these regimens remain anecdotal, and treatment failures with intravenous metronidazole have also been documented.

Operative intervention may be necessary in the patient with perforation or toxic megacolon. Some patients with severe colitis may have an abdominal examination with rebound tenderness that raises concern, but if perforation is not present it may be appropriate to manage them with serial abdominal examinations and antimicrobials. In patients with fulminant disease, the procedure of choice is a total abdominal colectomy with ileostomy. The appearance of the proximal and distal extent of the colon may appear deceptively normal, but this should not preclude aggressive surgical resection. Multiple series have reported increased mortality if less than a total abdominal colectomy is performed. Lipsett and co-workers reported an overall mortality of 38%, with those undergoing a total abdominal colectomy having a 14% mortality, whereas those managed by a partial colectomy had a 100% mortality. This significant mortality rate may also reflect the underlying comorbidities in these patients.

Approximately 15% to 35% of patients treated with either oral metronidazole or vancomycin will relapse within 2 months. It is appropriate to repeat another 10-day course of the antibiotic initially used, for the recurrence rarely is associated with resistance. Ninety percent of patients will respond to this second course of therapy. For patients who repeatedly fail treatment with antibiotics, biotherapeutic techniques for changing the colonic bacterial flora have been described, with varying degrees of success.

Pearls and Pitfalls

- Antibiotic-associated diarrhea is common; fulminant forms of the disease may develop that can have significant morbidity and mortality.
- 10% to 20% of cases of antibiotic-associated diarrhea are complicated by a bacterial toxin–induced colitis.
- Etiologic agents of toxin-induced colitis include the following: *Staphylococcus aureus, Salmonella, Shigella, Yersinia, Clostridium perfringens,* and *C. difficile*.
- Most cases of diarrhea associated with a toxin-induced colitis are due to *C. difficile*.
- *Clostridium difficile* colitis should be considered in all hospitalized patients with new-onset diarrhea; failure to treat this disease can produce significant morbidity and mortality.
- *Clostridium difficile* colitis produces a range of signs and symptoms from minor self-limited diarrhea to colonic perforation and sepsis.
- All antibiotics and many antineoplastic agents can predispose to the development of *C. difficile* colitis.
- The development of *C. difficile* colitis is not associated with the duration or total dose of antibiotic treatment.
- Diarrhea is the presenting sign in *C. difficile* colitis in 90% to 95% of patients.
- Risk factors for *C. difficile* colitis include advanced age, antibiotic therapy, immunocompromised state, stay in the intensive care unit, burns, uremia, and, possibly, enteral feeding.
- Diarrhea may be absent in patients with severe *C. difficile* colitis causing ileus or toxic megacolon.

- Patients with toxic megacolon due to *C. difficile* colitis may develop hypovolemic shock, cecal perforation, and/or toxic dilation of the colon with secondary sepsis.
- Toxic megacolon due to *C. difficile* colitis is a surgical emergency with a 10% to 20% mortality rate.
- *Clostridium difficile* generally does not produce an invasive infection; the pathologic changes are due to the effects of the toxin on the colonic mucosa.
- The diagnosis of *C. difficile* colitis is made by testing a stool sample for toxins A and B.
- Endoscopy with the visualization of pseudomembranes is also diagnostic for *C. difficile* colitis.
- *Clostridium difficile* can rarely affect the ileum or jejunum in the postcolectomy patient.
- Treatment for *C. difficile* colitis includes fluid resuscitation, discontinuation of the offending antibiotic, and administration of the antibiotic metronidazole.
- Antidiarrheal agents should *NOT* be used in the treatment of *C. difficile* colitis, as they may inhibit the clearance of the toxins.
- Oral vancomycin is an alternative treatment for *C. difficile* colitis.
- Surgical intervention is necessary for the patient with toxic megacolon, owing to *C. difficile* colitis; the procedure of choice is total abdominal colectomy with ileostomy.

SELECTED READINGS

Bergstein JM, Kramer A, Wittman DH, et al: Pseudomembranous colitis: How useful is endoscopy? Surg Endosc 1990;4:217.

Bradbury AW, Barrett S: Surgical aspects of *Clostridium difficile* colitis. Br J Surg 1997;84:150.

Cheung A, Tank RE, Dellinger EP: Antibiotic-associated enterocolitis involving the small bowel. Surg Rounds 1991;14:821.

Fekety R: Guidelines for the diagnosis and management of *Clostridium difficile*–associated diarrhea and colitis. Am J Gastroenterol 1997;92:739.

Fekety R, McFarland LV, Surawicz CM, et al: Recurrent *Clostridium difficile* diarrhea: Characteristics of and risk factors for patients enrolled in a prospective, randomized, double-blinded trial. Clin Infect Dis 1997;24:324.

Gerding DN: Is there a relationship between vancomycin-resistant enterococcus infection and *Clostridium difficile* infection? Clin Infect Dis 1997;25(suppl 2):s206.

Gerding DDN, Johnson S, Peterson LR, et al: *Clostridium difficile*–associated diarrhea and colitis. Infect Control Hosp Epidemiol 1995;16:459.

Medich DS, Lee KKW, Simmons RL, et al: Laparotomy for fulminant pseudomembranous colitis. Arch Surg 1992;127:847.

Oliva SL, Guglielmo BJ, Jacobs R, et al: Failure of intravenous vancomycin and metronidazole to prevent or treat antibiotic-associated pseudomembranous colitis. J Infect Dis 1989;159:1154.

Wenisch C, Parschalk B, Hasenhundl M, et al: Comparison of vancomycin, teicoplanin, metronidazole, and fusidic acid for the treatment of *Clostridium difficile*–associated diarrhea. Clin Infect Dis 1996;22:813.

Chapter 84

Toxic Megacolon

Bruce A. Orkin and Sonya Krolik

Toxic megacolon may be described as a severe attack of inflammatory or infectious colitis resulting in total or segmental colonic dilatation to at least 6 cm associated with systemic toxicity. It is often a life-threatening illness and has traditionally been associated with high morbidity and mortality. Toxic megacolon is most commonly seen in patients with one of the inflammatory bowel diseases (IBD), such as ulcerative colitis and Crohn's disease. It may also be caused by severe infective colitis due to a variety of organisms including *Clostridium difficile, Salmonella, Shigella, Campylobacter, Yersinia, Entamoeba histolytica, Cryptosporidium,* and cytomegalovirus, and other viruses. It has been seen in patients undergoing antineoplastic therapy and in patients with human immunodeficiency virus (HIV) infection and acquired immunodeficiency syndrome (AIDS). Although many different pathologic entities may result in colonic dilatation, including ileus, Ogilvie's syndrome, Hirschsprung's disease, colorectal cancer with obstruction, and chronic constipation-dysmotility disorders, these entities are not typically associated with the systemic toxicity seen in toxic megacolon.

The incidence of toxic megacolon is difficult to define and is probably decreasing because of improved medical treatment of patients with IBD and with HIV infection. Also, patients with IBD are more likely to be referred for surgical resection earlier in their course because of the reconstructive procedures now available. About 6% of patients with IBD present with toxic megacolon, but this may be as high as 10% in patients with ulcerative colitis and as low as 2% in patients with Crohn's disease. About 15% of patients with fulminant or severe colitis will progress to toxic megacolon. Toxic megacolon is an uncommon complication of pseudomembranous or *Clostridium difficile*–associated colitis, occurring in about 2% of patients. When it does occur, it is an ominous sign, as mortality rates approach 75%. Acute colitis due to cytomegalovirus (CMV) occurs in immunocompromised patients. Affected HIV-positive patients are generally in more advanced stages of AIDS. When the process progresses to toxic megacolon, the prognosis is grave, with mortality rates greater than 80%. Overall, however, 90% of patients with toxic megacolon have inflammatory bowel disease as the underlying etiology.

The pathogenesis of toxic megacolon is related to the severity of the underlying colitis and to the depth of penetration of the process through the bowel wall. One explanation states that extension of the inflammatory process from the mucosa and submucosa into the smooth muscle layers leads to paralysis and consequent dilatation of the colon. In most patients with ulcerative colitis and infective colitis, the inflammation is histologically limited to the submucosa. In patients with toxic megacolon, this reaction is seen in the muscular layers and serosa. There may even be evidence of microscopic or frank perforation

in pathology specimens, lending support to this theory. On gross examination, there is thinning of the bowel wall and deep ulceration. Histologically, inflammation involves all layers of the colonic wall with invasion by polymorphonuclear leukocytes and lymphocytes, edema, myonecrosis, and abscess formation. Interestingly, destruction of the myenteric nerves (Auerbach's and Meissner's) is not a consistent finding, suggesting that toxic megacolon may not be neuropathically mediated. Recent studies suggest that nitric oxide may play a role in the development of this form of colonic dilatation. An additional mechanism is deep ulceration of the colonic mucosa, which disrupts the intestine's normal protective barrier and exposes the patient to luminal bacterial antigens and toxins, leading to local and systemic toxicity.

CLINICAL PRESENTATION

Typical patients with toxic megacolon have a history of IBD and a recent flare. They are often on steroids and other anti-inflammatory medications or even antidiarrheal agents. The copious diarrhea may be bloody and associated with nausea, pain, and abdominal distention. They "look toxic," with pallor, dehydration, fever, tachycardia, lethargy, and even shock. Yet, many patients do not present with this "typical" picture.

Toxic megacolon is a spectrum of severe inflammatory disease of the colon and is differentiated from toxic or fulminant colitis only by the radiographic finding of colonic dilatation. It may occur as the initial acute manifestation of inflammatory bowel disease or as a complication of the disease in a patient with a long history. It usually occurs in patients with pancolitis and is equally distributed among men and women and patients of all ages. Predisposing factors in patients with IBD include a recent flare of acute colitis, early discontinuation or rapid tapering of medications (especially steroids) and the use of antidiarrheal or anticholinergic agents, including antidepressants. Electrolyte abnormalities in potassium, calcium, and magnesium can contribute to the development of an ileus. Often, a patient has experienced an acute attack of colitis that has remained unresponsive to medical therapy for one or more weeks prior to the onset of toxic megacolon.

If there is no prior diagnosis of IBD in a patient with toxic megacolon, the underlying diagnosis may be difficult to discern. Inflammatory bowel disease should be suspected when there is a history of recurrent diarrhea, blood in the stool, recurrent abdominal pain with nausea, vomiting and dehydration, aphthous ulcers, perianal fistulas or abscesses, erythema nodosum, iritis, arthritis, or other extraintestinal manifestations of Crohn's or ulcerative colitis. An infective etiology should be strongly suspected in patients without a history of IBD. A detailed history of travel, dietary intake, contact with other ill individuals, HIV status, and recent antibiotic use should be obtained. Patients who are immunocompromised are at risk, and toxic megacolon may occur in the setting of antineoplastic therapy, immunosuppression in recipients of transplants, and HIV infection.

Clinically, toxic megacolon must be suspected in patients with a history of acute or chronic diarrhea who present with abdominal distention, abdominal pain, and signs of hemodynamic compromise. Clinical criteria used to define toxic megacolon were proposed by Jalan and colleagues in 1969 and include at least three of the following: fever greater than 38.0°C; white blood cell count greater than 10,500/mm³; heart rate greater than 120 bpm; or anemia. Associated findings include electrolyte disturbances (typically of magnesium and potassium), hypoalbuminemia, dehydration, more than nine episodes of diarrhea per day, changes in mental status, and hypotension or shock. Although patients defined by these criteria are clearly acutely ill, many other patients are just as ill but do not have all of these signs. Patients who are immunocompromised because of HIV infection, chemotherapy, or immunosuppression may not meet these criteria yet still may have toxic megacolon. Commonly, patients with known IBD present on high dosages of steroids and appear superficially to be much less ill; but physical examination, laboratory studies, and abdominal radiographs will alert the careful clinician to their condition. These patients are at a particularly high risk for perforation and delayed recognition because of their blunted symptomatic response, and thus a very high degree of suspicion must be maintained.

On physical examination, tachycardia, fever, malaise, pallor, and abdominal distention are usually present. The abdominal examination may vary from distention and tympani without significant pain on palpation to localized tenderness with rebound, suggesting impending perforation or peritonitis. Generalized pain, guarding, and rebound imply free perforation and a surgical abdomen. Analgesia, steroids, and decreased mental status all may affect the physical examination. Therefore, coupling the clinical picture with radiologic and laboratory findings is absolutely necessary.

Laboratory evaluation of the patient with suspected toxic megacolon should include a complete blood cell count with differential. Leukocytosis with a left shift and increased band forms is common. Anemia, often a prominent finding because of blood loss from the colon, may require transfusion. Full electrolyte, renal, and hepatic panels should be assessed. Patients often suffer from hypokalemia and hypomagnesemia because of the diarrhea. Alkalosis from volume depletion and electrolyte loss is associated with a poor prognosis. Acidosis may be prominent in the patient who is in shock. Serum protein measurements typically reveal low albumin from chronic disease and can be used to assess nutritional status. Erythrocyte sedimentation rate may be used to track the clinical course of disease. Initial management of all patients should always include stool cultures to help exclude infective causes of colitis.

Radiographic evaluation of the abdomen is imperative

for making the diagnosis of toxic megacolon. An abdominal series including flat and upright films and a chest radiograph is generally all that is needed to confirm the diagnosis. Computed tomography (CT) and ultrasonography are not typically necessary unless there is some question as to the etiology of the patient's problem. The presence of colonic dilatation of greater than 6 cm in the transverse colon with loss of haustral markings or evidence of edema (thumbprinting) is suggestive of toxic megacolon (Fig. 84–1). These findings, along with a clinical history of fever and leukocytosis, are diagnostic. Dilatation of the ascending and transverse colon is common, while that of the descending colon is less frequent, and that of the sigmoid and rectum is rare. Clinical suspicion and the trend of colonic dilatation, not the absolute size of the colon, are of greatest importance for diagnosis and monitoring of treatment. Other details that should be evaluated on the abdominal films include the presence of radiolucent linear ulcerations in the colon, suggesting deep ulceration, which may herald perforation. The presence of a continuous thin air column in the descending or transverse colon or increasing small bowel gas in a patient with clinical toxicity is a sign of progression to toxic megacolon. Serial examinations with abdominal films every 24 hours initially, and then less frequently, are extremely useful in monitoring progress and in evaluating for complications such as perforation.

When the patient carries the diagnosis of IBD, laboratory studies and plain films may be all that is needed prior to the initiation of medical therapy. If, however, this

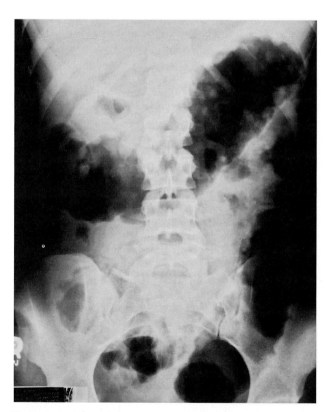

Figure 84–1. Plain abdominal radiograph of a patient with ulcerative colitis and toxic megacolon. Note massive dilatation of the transverse and descending colon with edema and thumbprinting and relative sparing of the ascending colon.

is the patient's first attack of colitis, a careful, limited sigmoidoscopy may be warranted to help make a diagnosis. Full colonoscopy is contraindicated in the setting of toxic megacolon because of the risk of colonic perforation. The endoscopic findings seen with many of the infective colitides, including *Shigella* and *Salmonella,* can be difficult to distinguish from Crohn's or ulcerative colitis. Biopsy evidence of colitis that does not distort crypt architecture may help separate infective colitis from inflammatory colitis. In pseudomembranous colitis due to *Clostridium difficile* infection, white or yellow plaques and ulcerations interspersed with normal mucosa may be visualized. In the HIV or AIDS patient, CMV colitis must be suspected, and biopsies should demonstrate CMV inclusion bodies.

MEDICAL MANAGEMENT

Optimal treatment of patients with toxic megacolon is provided by a multidisciplinary team, including both medical and surgical services. Early surgical consultation and frequent re-evaluation are critical. The initial therapy for all patients consists of admission to the intensive care unit, with aggressive rehydration and correction of electrolyte abnormalities. Patients who are anemic as the result of chronic colitis and acute bloody diarrhea (hemoglobin <8 to 9 g/dL) should be transfused. Coagulopathies should be corrected if abnormal and when there is active colonic bleeding. Broad-spectrum antibiotics, with coverage of both aerobic and anaerobic bowel flora, should be started promptly in most patients. Although antibiotics do not seem to influence the progression of toxic megacolon, they may reduce the consequences of bacterial invasion of the bowel wall and of perforation. The patient with toxic megacolon should be on bowel rest with nasogastric suction to minimize the addition of more gas to the gastrointestinal tract. Long tube decompression and rectal tubes probably add little to the evacuation of gas and carry additional risks. Use of all antimotility agents and anticholinergic agents should be discontinued immediately. Narcotics should be used judiciously, since they depress motility and may mask changes in the physical examination. All patients with toxic megacolon should probably have prophylaxis against peptic ulcer and deep venous thrombosis.

Frequent measurements of vital signs in association with serial physical examinations are imperative. Tachycardia is often the first sign of sepsis. Progression of the condition is associated with increasing abdominal distention, worsening pain, persistent or spiking fevers, and hemodynamic instability. The onset of peritoneal signs, such as rebound, guarding, and a rigid abdomen, herald colonic perforation, and the patient should be taken to the operating suite emergently. Free air on an abdominal film confirms the suspicion of perforation when the signs are not clear or are blunted, as in patients receiving steroids. At times, the only hint of perforation is a sudden and persisting tachycardia or a sudden increase in abdominal distention. Serial abdominal radiographs evaluate the extent of colonic distention and are central to the assessment of therapeutic response. Total parenteral nutrition

in the treatment of toxic megacolon is controversial because it has not been proved to reduce the need for surgery or the length of hospital stay. It is often used in the malnourished patient during recovery whether surgery has been necessary or not. Frequent changes in patient position (rolling and knee-to-chest) to redistribute colonic air and aid in elimination of flatus has been recommended, but whether it is really beneficial is unknown.

In the patient with toxic megacolon resulting from infective colitis, aggressive antibiotic therapy is paramount. Patients with *Clostridium difficile* colitis who develop toxic megacolon may have a rapidly progressive course despite treatment with intravenous metronidazole and oral vancomycin. If these patients fail to show clinical response or have continued clinical deterioration after 24 to 48 hours of treatment, operative therapy is indicated.

The mainstay of therapy in patients with IBD with toxic colitis has traditionally been high-dose intravenous steroids. Typical steroid dosages include 100 mg every 6 to 8 hours of hydrocortisone or the dose-equivalent of methylprednisolone or prednisone. Steroids should never be stopped acutely because of the risk of acute adrenal insufficiency and shock. As already mentioned, however, the astute clinician understands that steroid treatment may mask signs and symptoms of disease progression. Generally, improvement is seen within 1 to 2 days, and the patient may be transitioned to oral medications by 5 to 7 days with a tapering schedule. The majority of patients with a noncomplicated flare of IBD without toxic megacolon respond to steroid therapy and do not require operation. However, once megacolon develops, the success rate drops significantly. Steroid use should always be thought of as a short-term treatment option and should not be used for periods of more than several months, if at all possible, because of the complications that may ensue. Transition to anti-inflammatory medications or immunosuppressive agents may be considered, and, of course, operative resection is a reasonable alternative to continued steroid treatment, as indicated.

The anti-inflammatory medications, such as the 5-ASA compounds and sulfasalazine (Azulfidine), have no role in the treatment of toxic megacolon but may be added or resumed after resolution of the acute process. Most of the immunosuppressive medications (6-mercaptopurine, azathioprine) take weeks or months to have a significant effect and so are of no real use in the treatment of acute disease. Although cyclosporine has been promoted as an alternative to steroids for the treatment of toxic colitis, many groups have been unable to confirm the salutary experience of the Mount Sinai group in New York, and our own experience with this approach has been dismal, with several patients progressing to perforation within 24 hours of starting this medication. Therefore, we cannot recommend its use outside of controlled trials.

Indications that medical therapy has been successful include resolution of fever and leukocytosis, decreased fluid and blood product requirements, and decreased colonic distention by examination and radiographs. In most series, about 75% of patients required operative treatment during their hospital course. In one report, 60% did not respond to medical therapy and required surgery within a few days, 25% seemed to respond initially but then deteriorated, and only 15% were spared operation during that hospitalization. Even in the series successfully managed with cyclosporine, the majority went on to definitive surgical treatment within 6 months. Thus, development of toxic megacolon is thought by many to be a clear indication for colectomy. The only question becomes the timing. It is always preferable to operate electively on a well-nourished patient after a good preparation, since the lowest morbidity rate may be anticipated in this setting. Thus, medical management is still worthwhile in reducing the need for urgent surgery.

SURGICAL MANAGEMENT

The decision to proceed to operation is not a light one, but the indications should be well thought out and understood in advance so that, when necessary, there is no delay. It is important to discuss the possibility of operative intervention early in the hospitalization because when the decision is made to go to the operating room it is often necessary to do so rapidly. A patient and family who are prepared in advance will be less likely to hesitate and delay appropriate surgical intervention. The immediate indications for operation include evidence of perforation or peritonitis and major colonic hemorrhage. Operation may be recommended early in the patient's course when there is worsening dilatation, septicemia and shock, or persisting hemorrhage, or when the patient's general medical condition continues to deteriorate. Lack of a clinical response within 24 to 72 hours is a good general guideline. Some patients will have persistent toxicity and/or dilatation while receiving medical therapy, and a decision will be made to proceed with operation. Occasionally, a patient will show initial improvement but will worsen after starting a diet or tapering intravenous therapy while trying to transition to oral medications.

Colonic diameter is not a specific indication for surgery. There is no lower limit below which surgery is not needed. Many patients present with fulminant disease but without significant colonic dilatation and still require urgent operation. Most surgeons use a 5- to 6-cm dilatation of the transverse colon as a critical number, but this is an indication more of toxic dilatation in the ill patient than of the need for operation. More important is the trend on serial radiologic examination. Enlarging colonic diameter is an ominous factor (Fig. 84–2).

The operative procedure of choice depends on the clinical condition and disease process. The majority of these patients are critically ill, and complex restorative procedures are contraindicated. Surgical alternatives include loop ileostomy alone or with cecostomy, abdominal colectomy with end-ileostomy and rectal closure or mucous fistula, total proctocolectomy, and loop ileostomy with a colonic blowhole.

Loop ileostomy alone or with cecostomy is occasionally appropriate in selected patients with infective colitis, such as pseudomembranous colitis due to *C. difficile*. The goal is to decompress the colon and to irrigate the lumen with antibiotics via a cecostomy tube or a tube placed through the distal limb of the loop ileostomy into the cecum. This approach is not appropriate in patients with ulcerative colitis.

Abdominal colectomy with ileostomy and rectal stump closure is the operation of choice for most patients. This removes the majority of the diseased colon, diverts the fecal stream, and avoids an anastomosis that would be at inordinate risk for dehiscence. A more definitive procedure may be performed at a later date in a recovered, well-nourished and -prepared patient. The obvious disadvantages are the need for an ostomy, disease remaining in the residual rectal segment, and the need for a subsequent major operation. The ostomy site should be carefully marked preoperatively by an experienced surgeon or by the enterostomal therapy nurse. Broad-spectrum antibiotics are administered. The operation is performed through a generous midline incision. There is currently no role for laparoscopic approaches in this setting. Great care must be taken during this procedure, both when one enters the abdomen and during mobilization of the colon, because of the risk of iatrogenic perforation. The bowel may be massively dilated, filled with gas, fecal fluid, or blood, and tissue-paper thin. It is our practice to occlude the lumens of the terminal ileum and distal sigmoid with circumferential umbilical tapes. If the colon is very dilated, gas and some liquid may be evacuated with a 12- or 14-gauge needle or intravenous catheter and suction tubing. The field is first cordoned off with laparotomy pads and towels, and a purse-string suture is placed. The needle is passed through the middle of the purse-string suture, which will be tied down and covered with pads after partial evacuation of the bowel. The ileocolic vessels should be retained to facilitate future creation of a pelvic pouch. If there is no perforation or significant spillage, the incision may be closed primarily. The ileostomy is matured primarily at the time of surgery. Once the diseased colon is successfully removed, patients often recover quickly and regain a remarkable sense of well-being.

The rectal stump may be handled in several ways. Most surgeons will simply close the upper rectum with a linear stapler. Some bury this staple line by oversewing it with a row of inverting sutures. Rectal closure is usually performed at the rectosigmoid junction. In patients with extensive bleeding from the rectum, a lower transection may be performed, but this requires entering the presacral space, with its increased risks, and makes subsequent attempts at restoration more difficult. Our preferred approach is to leave just enough of the distal sigmoid colon to allow implantation of the closed end in the inferior fascial closure. The staple line lies in the subcutaneous tissue, so if it breaks down it will drain through the skin and not into the abdominal cavity; this results in a mucous fistula and avoids peritonitis. Other advantages of this approach include easy identification of the distal stump at a subsequent operation, a virgin pelvis for safer dissection, and easy access to the proximal end of the stump if disease persists. At the time of closure, the fascia is closed from the upper to the lower end. The closed end of the distal sigmoid is brought up through the lower end of the wound. The seromuscular layer of the stump is sewn to the anterior fascia, starting inferiorly on each side and running the two sutures superiorly to meet the lower end

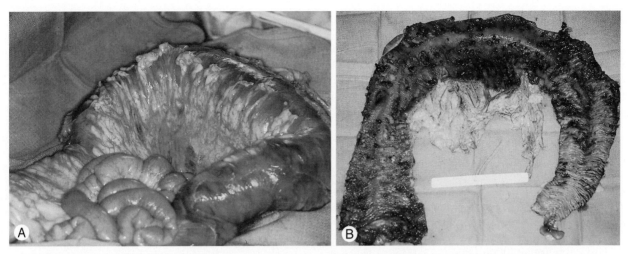

Figure 84–2. *A,* Intraoperative photograph of the patient from Figure 84–1. Note the marked dilatation, hyperemia, and thinning of the colon. *B,* The opened specimen. Extensive denuding of the mucosa with pseudopolyps and dilatation.

of the fascial closure, usually 4 to 5 cm above the lower end of the fascial defect. This row is placed 2 to 3 cm below the closed end of the stump so that the staple line lies comfortably in the subcutaneous plane with little tension on the stump. The skin is then closed over this. Alternatively, the stump may be primarily matured as a mucous fistula. The entire lumen does not need to be opened and everted. A corner of the staple line may be excised and sutured to 2 to 3 cm of the lower skin wound, closing the rest of the wound. If the colonic wall is so friable that it will not hold sutures, this stump should not be left in the peritoneal cavity. The Jones method of stump management is invaluable in this situation. The bowel is transected in the midsigmoid and brought through the lower end of the wound so that it protrudes 7 to 8 cm above the skin level. It is wrapped snugly in a damp gauze roll, and dressings are applied. About 7 days later, when adhesions have developed between the serosa and the wound, the end is trimmed and the edges matured secondarily at the bedside.

Total proctocolectomy is now rarely performed in patients with toxic colitis because of the increased morbidity of pelvic dissection and the advent of restorative procedures. It is generally better to leave the rectum in place at the time of an urgent resection.

Loop ileostomy with a colonic blowhole is a procedure that was devised by Rupert Turnbull and his colleagues at the Cleveland Clinic in the 1960s. It was designed for use in patients with severe toxic megacolon who were at high risk for intraoperative perforation because of marked thinning of the bowel wall or suspicion of walled-off microperforations. The location of the dilated transverse colon is noted on plain supine abdominal films just prior to operation, and the impression of the loop is marked on the patient's abdomen just prior to preparation. Additionally, the location of the transverse colon loop may be confirmed through the small incision made for the ileostomy or with intraoperative transcutaneous ultrasonography. An ileostomy incision is made in the right lower quadrant at the preoperatively marked ostomy site, and the anterior and posterior rectus fascias are divided vertically with the use of a muscle-splitting technique. The

terminal ileum is "fished out" while one retracts it with two small Richardson retractors. A spot 30 to 40 cm proximal to the ileocecal valve is selected to preserve the rest for later pouch construction. The transverse colon blowhole is created by making a 4-cm midline incision over the transverse colon in the epigastrium. The incision is carried down until the transverse colon is exposed. The incision may be slightly extended upward or downward, depending on the location of the colon. Two running absorbable sutures are placed from superior to inferior, one on each side, to secure the seromuscular layer to the posterior fascia and peritoneum, isolating the site from the peritoneal cavity. The loop is decompressed with a large-bore needle and suction, and is then incised vertically, leaving 0.5 to 1 cm at either end, and the cut edge

---

Pearls and Pitfalls

- The diagnosis of toxic megacolon is made on clinical grounds and plain abdominal films. Sigmoidoscopy may help when there is no prior diagnosis of IBD or to confirm an infective etiology. Colonoscopy and barium enema are generally to be avoided.
- Discuss the surgical alternatives with the patient and family early in the hospitalization to prepare them for this possibility.
- Perforation is the major risk factor. Operate early for failure of medical therapy to avoid this complication. Operative mortality is low in patients without perforation (~5%) and high in those with perforation (~50%).
- Operate immediately for suspected perforation.
- Operate urgently in patients who continue to deteriorate over the 1 to 2 days after admission.
- Do not delay operation in patients who do not respond to medical therapy in 2 to 4 days.
- Surgical options include
  - Abdominal colectomy with closure of the upper rectum—modified Hartmann's procedure.
  - Ileostomy and colonic venting-blowhole.
- Successful medical management in IBD patients is a precursor to elective colon resection.

is sutured to the skin. Patients generally do quite well after this procedure, with marked improvement in their clinical condition and resolution of the megacolon. A definitive resection is performed 3 to 6 months later. This operative approach is not appropriate when there is free perforation or marked hemorrhage. Although this procedure is rarely necessary now, it is a useful tool in selected patients.

OUTCOME

The mortality rate in patients with toxic megacolon due to IBD is about 15%. The major prognostic factor by far is the presence or absence of perforation prior to operation. Mortality rates are 5% without perforation, compared with 50% with perforation. Therefore, prompt surgical intervention should be undertaken when a patient shows signs of clinical deterioration or failure to respond to medical therapy to avoid this catastrophic complication. When toxic megacolon develops as a consequence of *C. difficile* or CMV infection, mortality rates approach 90%.

Most patients undergoing urgent operation for toxic megacolon will have an abdominal colectomy with end-ileostomy and closure of the upper rectum (modified Hartmann's procedure). The retained rectum is of concern in patients with IBD because of the likelihood of persistent disease in this segment. Most patients with ulcerative colitis will go on to have either an ileal pouch–anal anastomosis procedure or a completion proctectomy.

Patients with Crohn's disease and relative sparing of the anorectum may undergo closure of the ileostomy with ileorectal anastomosis. If the anorectum is diseased, attempts may be made to heal the process medically; however, the majority of patients will not have continuity re-established, and most will ultimately need a completion proctectomy. Even when the disease in the anorectum seems to resolve, recurrence is the rule, rather than the exception, once continuity is re-established.

Toxic megacolon is a potentially fatal complication of IBD or infective colitis. Although some patients will resolve their process with medical management, most will require surgical intervention. Proceeding with operation prior to colonic perforation results in less morbidity and mortality. The majority of patients who develop toxic megacolon will require operation at some point in their course, so early surgical consultation and discussions with the patient and family are critical.

SELECTED READINGS

Beaugerie L, Ngo Y, Goujard F, et al: Etiology and management of toxic megacolon in patients with human immunodeficiency virus infection. Gastroenterology 1994;107:858.

Heppell J, Farkouh E, Dubc S, et al: Toxic megacolon: An analysis of 70 cases. Dis Colon Rectum 1986;29:789.

Jalan KN, Sircus W, Card WI, et al: An experience of ulcerative colitis. I. Toxic dilation in 55 cases. Gastroenterology 1969;57:68.

Present DH: Toxic megacolon. Med Clin North Am 1993;77:1129.

Sheth SG, LaMont JT: Toxic megacolon. Lancet 1998;351:509.

Trudel JL, Deschenes M, Mayrand S, Barkun NI: Toxic megacolon complicating pseudomembranous enterocolitis. Dis Colon Rectum 1995;38:1033.

Colonic Volvulus
Stephen G. Pereira and Garth H. Ballantyne

Volvulus is defined as torsion or twisting of a segment of intestine along its mesentery that results in partial or complete luminal occlusion. When the occlusion is complete, a closed-loop obstruction arises, with the potential for compromised blood supply and increased intraluminal pressure. If the occlusion goes unalleviated, gangrene and perforation of the involved segment may ensue.

In Western societies, large bowel volvulus is responsible for about 5% of all colon obstructions. The sigmoid colon is by far the most common site of large intestine volvulus, accounting for 80% of patients with colonic volvulus, followed by the cecum in 15%; the transverse colon and the splenic flexure are very rare sites of volvulus. Sigmoid volvulus is more common in men (64%), with the highest incidence in the sixth decade. In addition, it appears to be more common in the black population. This condition is associated with laxative abuse, neurologic disease, and chronic constipation and is common among institutionalized and often debilitated patients.

Sigmoid volvulus is an acquired condition in the vast majority of patients. The process of sigmoid volvulus depends on three factors: (1) elongation of the sigmoid colon resulting in a redundant loop; (2) narrowing of the sigmoid mesentery with approximation of the points of fixation; and (3) a torque force that initiates the torsion process of the sigmoid colon.

In contrast with sigmoid volvulus, cecal volvulus is a congenital condition resulting from incomplete retroperitoneal fixation of the cecum or ascending colon. Cecal volvulus can occur by organoaxial torsion (true volvulus) or by mesenterioaxial torsion (cecal bascule). In contrast with sigmoid volvulus, which predominates in men, cecal volvulus more commonly affects women in the sixth decade of life.

Volvulus of the transverse colon is rare, constituting only 3% of all patients with colonic volvulus. It is more common in females (2:1) and seems to be more common in younger patients. Multiple physiologic, anatomic, and mechanical factors are involved in the development of transverse colon volvulus. Most common is the anatomic finding of an elongated, redundant transverse colon with close approximation of the points of mesenteric fixation. Chronic constipation and mechanical obstruction of the distal colon from carcinoma or inflammation have been associated with volvulus of the transverse colon.

Volvulus of the splenic flexure represents the rarest form of colonic volvulus, making up fewer than 2% of all patients with colonic volvulus. Splenic flexure volvulus has been reported more commonly in middle-aged women and appears to be caused either by a congenital insufficiency of fixation or by prior surgical procedures that increase the mobility of the splenic flexure. The latter has been implicated as the primary cause in as many as 70% of patients.

CLINICAL PRESENTATION

Sigmoid Volvulus

Patients with sigmoid volvulus typically present with signs and symptoms of colonic obstruction (Table 85–1). When a careful history is taken, as many as 60% of patients will report prior similar attacks that resolved spontaneously. Abdominal distention is the most common clinical sign. Patients also report obstipation and, less frequently, nausea, vomiting, and abdominal pain. Marked abdominal pain should suggest the possibility of compromised bowel and be taken seriously and evaluated aggressively. The onset of symptoms may be relatively rapid, developing over several hours, but, on the average, patients present with symptoms of 3 to 5 days' duration. The physical examination reveals a distended abdomen with marked tympany. Digital rectal examination usually demonstrates an empty rectal vault. Significant abdominal tenderness and signs of peritonitis suggest the presence of gangrenous bowel. Routine laboratory blood tests are usually unremarkable, although they may suggest mild dehydration. Severe dehydration, leukocytosis, and metabolic acidosis should also raise the suspicion of compromised bowel.

The differential diagnosis of colonic obstruction includes, in addition to sigmoid volvulus, neoplasia, diverticular disease, pseudo-obstruction (Ogilvie's syndrome), and volvulus of another segment of colon. The diagnosis of sigmoid volvulus can usually be made by plain abdominal radiographs. Upright abdominal radiographs demonstrate the characteristic "inverted loop" or "bent inner tube" sign, with the distended loop arising from the left pelvis and extending toward the right diaphragm (Fig. 85–1). In patients in whom the diagnosis remains uncertain, radiographs with a water-soluble contrast enema reveal the characteristic tapered narrowing of the bowel lumen, or "bird beak" sign. A contrast-enhanced enema study is clearly contraindicated in patients with signs and symptoms suggestive of gangrenous bowel, for fear of intraperitoneal spillage of contrast medium.

Cecal Volvulus

The presentation of patients with cecal volvulus is usually that of a large bowel obstruction, but the appearance may be that of a small bowel obstruction if the ileum is obstructed by the volvulus process. Most commonly, patients present with distention, crampy abdominal pain, nausea, and emesis. Physical examination typically reveals abdominal distention and tympany. The distention has been classically described as asymmetrical with an associated palpable mass, but this is present in only one third

Table 85–1	**Common Problems and Approaches**
Patient presents with signs and symptoms of bowel obstruction	*Sigmoid volvulus:* "Bent inner tube" sign with loop arising in left lower abdomen and extending to right upper abdomen
	Cecal volvulus: "Coffee bean" sign with "hilum" of bean directed downward to right lower abdomen
Abdominal radiographs nondiagnostic	Water-soluble contrast enema to confirm volvulus
Patient septic or hemodynamically unstable on presentation	Aggressive preoperative resuscitation in ICU setting; consider pulmonary artery catheter
Sigmoid volvulus diagnosed preoperatively	Attempt endoscopic detorsion and decompression of volvulized sigmoid colon to allow for bowel prep and semielective sigmoid resection with primary anastomosis during same hospital admission
Endoscopic decompression of sigmoid volvulus unsuccessful	Treat with Hartmann's procedure
Cecal volvulus (viable bowel)	Treat with right hemicolectomy and primary anastomosis (preferred) or cecopexy-cecostomy. Cecopexy alone is not recommended.
Transverse colon volvulus (viable bowel)	Treat with extended right hemicolectomy and primary anastomosis
Splenic flexure volvulus (viable bowel)	Treat with segmental resection or colopexy
Patient found to have a nonviable, or gangrenous, bowel at laparotomy	Resect all compromised bowel and construct ostomy. Avoid manual detorsion of volvulized segment until mesentery and bowel lumen have been clamped. Needle decompression of massively dilated bowel allows for easier handling of colon.

of patients. Abdominal tenderness and signs of peritonitis suggest gangrenous bowel. Laboratory data may demonstrate mild dehydration, but severe dehydration, leukocytosis, and metabolic acidosis should alert the surgeon to the possibility of compromised bowel.

The diagnosis of cecal volvulus is infrequently made clinically, and only 50% of radiographs show the characteristic features of cecal volvulus. The "coffee-bean" sign, with the "hilum" of the "bean" directed to the patient's right and downward toward the pelvis, is typical of true cecal volvulus (Fig. 85–2), while the "inverted teardrop" may be seen in the right lower abdomen with the more unusual cecal bascule, in which the cecum lops over onto the ascending colon anterorostrally (Fig. 85–3). Although a water-soluble contrast-enhanced study is controversial

owing to the risk of perforation and should probably be avoided, it is sometimes utilized when the diagnosis remains uncertain.

Transverse Colon Volvulus

The clinical presentation of transverse colon volvulus takes one of two forms—acute fulminating or subacute progressive. The acute form results from mesenteric vascular occlusion and is characterized by the sudden onset of severe pain, minimal abdominal distention, and rapid

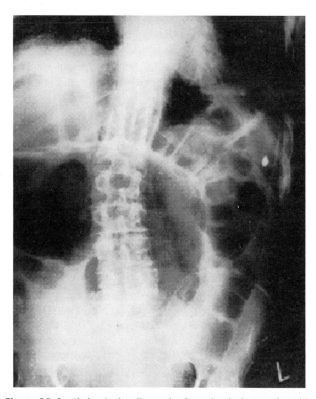

Figure 85–2. Abdominal radiograph of cecal volvulus produced by organoaxial torsion (true volvulus) of the cecum and ascending colon, demonstrating the "coffee bean" sign.

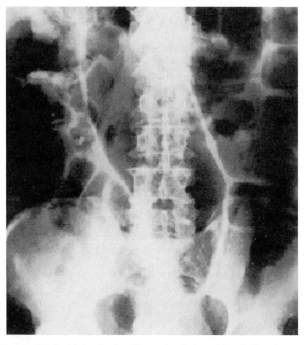

Figure 85–1. Abdominal radiograph of sigmoid volvulus demonstrating the "bent inner tube" sign.

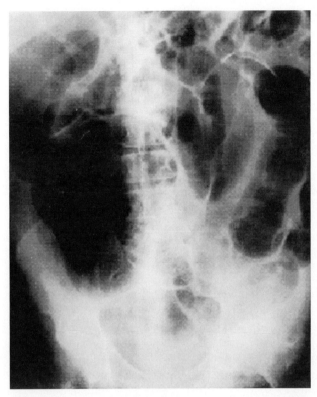

Figure 85–3. Abdominal radiograph of cecal volvulus produced by mesenterioaxial torsion (cecal bascule) of the cecum, demonstrating the "inverted teardrop" sign.

deterioration. In the subacute form, pain is gradual and less severe and there is usually marked abdominal distention. Laboratory studies are nonspecific, and plain radiographs demonstrate findings consistent with midcolonic obstruction. Radiographs with a water-soluble contrast-enhanced enema can provide the diagnosis.

Splenic Flexure Volvulus

The clinical presentation of volvulus of the splenic flexure is similar to that of any distal colon obstruction. Patients report crampy abdominal pain and have abdominal distention on examination. Vascular compromise in splenic flexure volvulus is rare. Preoperative diagnosis is difficult. As with other forms of colonic volvulus, the results of laboratory studies are nonspecific. Plain radiographs demonstrate findings consistent with a distal colonic obstruction. Radiographs with a water-soluble contrast-enhanced enema assist with the diagnosis.

PREOPERATIVE MANAGEMENT

The initial management of patients with colonic volvulus is identical to that of patients presenting with bowel obstruction. Patients without compromised bowel are usually only mildly dehydrated and require only 1 or 2 liters of intravenous volume resuscitation. Nasogastric tube decompression is helpful in patients presenting with nausea and emesis, particularly in patients with cecal

volvulus and small bowel obstruction. The subsequent preoperative management varies, depending on the type of volvulus present.

Sigmoid Volvulus

For patients in whom the diagnosis of sigmoid volvulus has been made on clinical and radiographic grounds and who do not have evidence of compromised bowel, an attempt at endoscopic decompression should be made. If detorsion of the volvulus is successful, the patient can then undergo a controlled bowel preparation with semielective surgery during the same hospitalization. Rigid sigmoidoscopy is the preferred technique. The large-caliber lumen of the rigid sigmoidoscope allows for better irrigation and aspiration of retained stool, and a rectal tube can be left in place. Alternatively, colonoscopic decompression can be utilized. Both techniques have an 85% to 90% success rate in detorsion of sigmoid volvulus. After successful derotation, a standard mechanical and antibiotic bowel preparation is performed and the patient is scheduled for elective colectomy during the same hospitalization. Endoscopic derotation alone, without subsequent surgical treatment, is associated with a 50% incidence of recurrent volvulus. If endoscopic decompression is unsuccessful, urgent laparotomy is performed.

For patients who present with gangrenous colon, emergency surgery should be planned. If the patient is toxic from sepsis or profound hypovolemia, they should be admitted to the intensive care unit for aggressive resuscitation followed by emergency laparotomy.

Cecal Volvulus

While successful endoscopic decompression of cecal volvulus has been reported, most patients should undergo emergency laparotomy, given the technical difficulty and lack of experience associated with endoscopy in the presence of cecal volvulus. Patients presenting with signs and symptoms of compromised bowel require aggressive resuscitation and emergency operation.

Transverse Colon and Splenic Flexure Volvulus

Successful endoscopic decompression has been reported and may play a role in its management. However, the majority of patients will require urgent operation. Patients with an acute fulminating course should be aggressively resuscitated and undergo emergency colectomy.

INTRAOPERATIVE MANAGEMENT

Sigmoid Volvulus

Patients who have undergone successful endoscopic decompression followed by a bowel preparation should be managed by a standard sigmoidectomy with primary anastomosis. More extensive resections are unnecessary. Nonresective procedures, such as colopexy, have recurrence rates as high as 50% and are not recommended. Laparoscopic sigmoidectomy may be considered in stable patients who have undergone successful preoperative endoscopic decompression.

The procedure is usually performed with the patient in the modified Lloyd-Davies position to allow for transrectal passage of a stapling device to perform an end-to-end anastomosis. A lower midline incision extending from umbilicus to pubis provides optimal exposure. If preoperative endoscopic detorsion has been unsuccessful, it should be expected that the sigmoid colon will be massively distended, and care must be taken not to inadvertently incise the sigmoid loop when one enters the abdomen. For patients who have undergone successful preoperative endoscopic decompression, the sigmoid colon is inspected for any evidence of ischemic changes or unsuspected perforation. If the sigmoid colon is viable and intact, a standard sigmoidectomy with primary anastomosis is performed. Takedown of the splenic flexure is rarely necessary. As mentioned previously, simple resection of the redundant sigmoid loop is all that is required for successful treatment.

For patients who present with compromised bowel or in whom endoscopic decompression has been unsuccessful, Hartmann's procedure is the treatment of choice. At laparotomy, needle decompression of the massively dilated sigmoid loop will make the bowel easier to handle. If possible, the colon should not be untwisted manually until the mesenteric vessels and bowel lumen have been clamped, particularly in the presence of compromised bowel. This maneuver will prevent toxins from the ischemic bowel from gaining access to the systemic circulation. The entire sigmoid colon is resected, along with any nonviable bowel. An end-colostomy is constructed in the usual fashion in the left lower abdomen. Takedown of the colostomy and reestablishment of colon continuity can be performed electively after a minimum of 6 weeks.

Cecal Volvulus

The majority of patients who present with cecal volvulus will undergo emergency surgical intervention. If the intestine is viable at laparotomy, two surgical options are available—resection or cecal fixation with cecostomy. Resection by right hemicolectomy is the authors' preferred management of cecal volvulus. In addition to preventing recurrence, this procedure relieves the obstruction and removes the bacteria- and endotoxin-filled dilated segment of colon, thereby reducing the potential for bacterial endotoxemia. A primary anastomosis is almost always possible. Contraindications to construction of a primary anastomosis include gangrenous bowel, perforation, peritonitis, sepsis, or any circumstances that make primary anastomosis hazardous. Laparoscopic right hemicolectomy is usually not advisable because of the usual marked dilatation and thin wall of the colon from obstruction.

Cecal fixation and decompression procedures, in the form of cecopexy and tube cecostomy, are acceptable alternatives to resection and are advocated by some sur-

geons. The advantages of cecopexy with cecostomy are that it is a relatively simple procedure, and the potential complications associated with an anastomosis are obviated. However, it has several potential disadvantages—the dilated segment of colon is left in situ, there is a risk of fecal contamination from the cecostomy and the cecopexy suture with abdominal wall sepsis, and there remains a potential for recurrence. Cecopexy alone is not recommended because decompression of the dilated colon is not achieved, and recurrence rates of 10% to 20% have been reported. The patient is placed in a supine position. The most versatile incision is a midline incision from midepigastrium to a point below the umbilicus. A standard right hemicolectomy with primary anastomosis is the treatment of choice. Contraindications to a primary anastomosis include gangrenous bowel or perforation with peritonitis, sepsis, or any circumstance that makes primary anastomosis hazardous. The surgeon must use good judgment; any situation that makes primary anastomosis hazardous should prompt the surgeon to perform a right hemicolectomy with ileostomy and mucous fistula.

CECAL FIXATION AND DECOMPRESSION. The volvulated colon is manually detorsed, and a colotomy is made through the anterior taeniae coli of the cecum. The cecum and ascending colon are decompressed with a large-bore suction catheter. Irrigation with saline is sometimes necessary to fragment solid fecal matter. Alternatively, the cecum can be decompressed and intubated via an appendectomy. For the cecostomy tube, two concentric purse-string sutures of 2-0 silk are placed around the colotomy. The cecum is then intubated with the largest available Malecot catheter (>30 French) and then secured in place with the purse-string sutures. Small-diameter cecostomy tubes easily become occluded. Thus, the largest tube available with frequent irrigation postoperatively usually maintains adequate cecal decompression.

A wide-based cecal fixation is then accomplished by suturing the antimesenteric border of the cecum and ascending colon to the lateral abdominal wall with multiple interrupted seromuscular sutures of 3-0 silk. A small stab wound is made in the right lower quadrant, and the end of the catheter is grasped with a clamp and pulled through the abdominal wall. Additional interrupted seromuscular sutures of 3-0 silk are placed around the catheter to fix the cecum to the anterior abdominal wall. The externalized catheter is then sutured to the abdominal wall skin with a heavy, nonabsorbable suture. After the abdominal incision is closed, a bulky dressing is placed around the catheter to prevent kinking of the catheter.

Transverse Colon Volvulus

Various resectional and colopexy procedures have been recommended for the treatment of volvulus of the transverse colon. The authors prefer resection, and, while a segmental resection has been advocated, an extended right hemicolectomy seems most prudent. A primary anastomosis can be accomplished if there are no signs of peritonitis or sepsis. The patient is placed in a supine position, and a midline incision is utilized. An extended right hemicolectomy with primary anastomosis is performed. In the presence of gangrenous bowel, peritonitis, or sepsis, resection with an ileostomy and mucous fistula should be performed.

Splenic Flexure Volvulus

The data on volvulus of the splenic flexure are too limited to draw any meaningful conclusions regarding the most appropriate surgical management. Segmental resection and splenic flexure colopexy have both been described as successful.

POSTOPERATIVE MANAGEMENT

Postoperative management is identical to that of patients undergoing bowel resection for other diseases. Patients are kept NPO and given maintenance intravenous fluids until passage of flatus. If a nasogastric tube had been placed, it can be removed on the first postoperative day. Routine postoperative laboratory tests are usually unnecessary. Deep vein thrombosis prophylaxis is maintained, and patients are encouraged to ambulate on the day after surgery. The urinary catheter is removed when the patient is ambulatory. After passage of flatus, patients are typically begun on a clear liquid diet and, if tolerated, advanced to a regular diet. Patients are usually ready for discharge 5 to 7 days postoperatively.

Patients with cecal volvulus who have undergone cecopexy and cecostomy require frequent attention to the cecostomy tube. It should be placed on continuous or intermittent suction and cautiously irrigated with water 3 or 4 times a day. Daily abdominal radiographs should be performed initially to confirm continued decompression of the cecum. The catheter is removed approximately 3 to 6 weeks postoperatively, and the resultant cecocutaneous fistula usually closes spontaneously. Patients who present with gangrenous bowel, perforation, or sepsis often require postoperative management in the intensive care unit with aggressive resuscitation and support. Many of these patients require large volumes of fluid resuscitation, with careful monitoring of fluid inputs and outputs.

COMPLICATIONS

Complications after surgery for volvulus of the colon are similar to that of other operations on the colon. The single most important determinant of morbidity and mortality is the condition of the colon at the time of surgery. If the involved segment of colon is found to be viable at surgery, mortalities of 6% to 20% have been reported (in large part related to underlying medical comorbidities), while in patients found to have strangulated, necrotic bowel,

Pearls and Pitfalls

- Colonic volvulus presents as a large bowel obstruction.
- Sigmoid volvulus is the most common form (~80%) and cecal volvulus is next most common (15%), whereas transverse colon or splenic flexure volvulus is rare.
- Diagnosis is often made by plain abdominal radiographs; contrast-enhanced enemas are usually not necessary.
- Sigmoid volvulus is best treated with endoscopic decompression, bowel preparation, and same admission elective sigmoid colectomy.
- Cecal volvulus is often not diagnosed preoperatively, presents as a small bowel obstruction, and is best treated with right hemicolectomy.
- Signs of peritonitis or vascular compromise in the patient with colonic volvulus requires aggressive resuscitation and emergent colectomy.

mortalities of 50% to 80% can be expected. The most common complications include infection, either intra-abdominal or at the wound. Resection with primary anastomosis also carries the risk of anastomotic leak. For cecal volvulus, cecopexy and cecostomy carry the risk of cecal necrosis, leakage, fistula (from the pexy sutures or at the site of cecostomy), and abdominal wall sepsis.

OUTCOMES

Recurrences of volvulus after sigmoidectomy are extremely rare, as expected, since the redundant segment of colon involved in the volvulus has been removed. Recurrence rates after surgery for cecal volvulus vary according to the technique employed. Recurrence does not occur after a right hemicolectomy and rarely with cecostomy. Recurrence rates following cecopexy alone are 5% to 10%.

SELECTED READINGS

Armstrong DN, Ballantyne GH: Colonic surgery for acute conditions: Volvulus of the colon. In Fielding LP, Goldberg SM (eds): Surgery of the Colon, Rectum and Anus. Oxford, Butterworth-Heinemann, 1993, pp 420–435.
Ballantyne GH: Review of sigmoid volvulus: History and results of treatment. Dis Colon Rectum 1982;25:494
Ballantyne GH, Brandner MD, Beart RW, Ilstrup DM: Volvulus of the colon: Incidence and mortality. Ann Surg 1985;202:83.
Eisenstat TE, Raneri AJ, Mason GR: Volvulus of the transverse colon. Am J Surg 1977;134:396.
O'Mara CS, Wilson TH, Stonesifer GL, Cameron JL: Cecal volvulus: Analysis of 50 patients with long-term follow-up. Ann Surg 1979;189:724.
Rabinovici R, Simansky DA, Kaplan O, et al: Cecal volvulus. Dis Colon Rectum 1990;33:765.
Welch GH, Anderson JR: Volvulus of the splenic flexure of the colon. Dis Colon Rectum 1985;28:592.

Chapter 86

Rectal Prolapse

Hannah Ngoc-Ha and Thomas E. Read

Although rectal prolapse has been recognized since biblical times, the optimal surgical procedure to correct rectal prolapse remains a subject of debate. There are a plethora of operations used to treat rectal prolapse, and the surgeon should select one that produces the best possible functional result for an individual patient with a low complication and recurrence rate. The choice of operation depends on many factors, including age, sex, associated constipation, degree of incontinence, history of prior repairs, comorbid conditions, and the expertise of the surgeon.

Part of the difficulty in treating patients with rectal prolapse results from our incomplete understanding of its pathophysiology. Rectal prolapse most likely results from a combination of the following factors: a sliding hernia through a defect in the pelvic fascia, an internal intussusception of the rectum as a result of repeated straining that eventually passes through the anus, a dysfunctional internal sphincter, and a lack of fascial fixation of the rectum to the sacrum. Internal intussusception (i.e., not protruding through the anus) probably represents an early form of rectal prolapse, although its significance in the absence of symptoms is uncertain in that many asymptomatic patients are found to have an internal rectal intussusception on defecography. Laxity of the pelvic floor is an important contributing factor in many patients with rectal prolapse, as evidenced by the finding that rectal prolapse is much more common in women who are more likely to have weakness of the pelvic floor and abnormal perineal descent.

CLINICAL PRESENTATION

Presenting signs include complete rectal prolapse (procidentia), occult prolapse (internal intussusception), or mucosal prolapse. Complete prolapse is a full-thickness, circumferential intussusception of the entire rectal wall through the anal canal presenting externally. Occult rectal prolapse is an internal intussusception of the mid or upper rectum that does not protrude through the anal orifice. Mucosal prolapse, not considered to be a true form of rectal prolapse, occurs when the connective tissue between the submucosa and the underlying muscle weakens and only the mucosa prolapses through the anal canal.

The degree of prolapse dictates the patient's symptoms. Patients with internal intussusception often complain of incomplete evacuation, with frequent and severe straining at defecation. Other symptoms include a bloody mucus discharge, perineal pain, and incontinence. Patients with complete rectal prolapse complain of a mass protruding from the anus, usually after bowel movements. If the prolapse is small, it is often mistaken for hemorrhoidal prolapse, both by patients and by physicians. If

the prolapse reduces spontaneously, the patient may only complain of passing mucus or blood per rectum, usually associated with some degree of anal incontinence. As the prolapsed segment lengthens, patients learn to manually reduce it after bowel movements. Occasionally, the prolapsed rectum becomes incarcerated, causing severe, acute discomfort.

Anal incontinence is frequently associated with rectal prolapse, which is not surprising given that the prolapsing rectum chronically dilates and stretches the sphincter musculature, causing traction injury to the pudendal nerves; this pathophysiology results in both mechanical and neurogenic incontinence. The pressure in the distal rectum caused by the presence of the intussuscepted segment may result in constant stimulation of the rectoanal inhibitory reflex, which reduces the tone of the internal anal sphincter.

Constipation is associated with rectal prolapse in about half of patients, although the cause of constipation and its relationship to rectal prolapse is controversial and poorly understood. In some patients, constipation may be primary, due to a delay in colonic transit, which causes chronic straining to evacuate hard stool, which in turn results in rectal prolapse. Alternatively, constipation may be secondary and result from obstruction of the colon at the pelvic outlet because of the prolapsing segment of rectosigmoid. The decision to perform colectomy at the time of repair of the rectal prolapse often hinges on the degree of constipation or colonic inertia present in an individual patient.

Rectal prolapse often presents in concert with other abnormalities of the pelvic floor such as rectocele, enterocele, cystocele, and uterine prolapse. Enterocele and rectocele may cause pelvic outlet obstruction and obstructed defecation, contributing to the chronic straining at stool. These entities should be sought out by the history and physical examination and, when suspected, confirmed by defecography, as patients may benefit from a combined pelvic floor repair.

PREOPERATIVE MANAGEMENT

The evaluation of a patient with suspected rectal prolapse begins with a directed history and physical examination. In addition to inquiring about continence status and constipation, other important factors in choosing the best surgical procedure include age, performance status, and comorbidity. A detailed obstetric history should be obtained from women, because a traumatic defect of the anal sphincter mechanism may contribute to incontinence and may be amenable to repair.

Anorectal examination begins by inspecting the prolapsed tissue for lesions that may serve as a lead point.

Table 86-1	Common Procedures for Repair of Rectal Prolapse				
PROCEDURE	APPROACH	RECURRENCE	ANESTHETIC RISK	RISK OF OTHER COMPLICATIONS
Sigmoid resection + rectopexy	Abdominal	Lowest	Moderate	Moderate
Rectopexy	Abdominal	Low	Moderate	Moderate-low
Perineal rectosigmoidectomy	Perineal	Low	Low	Low
Mucosal sleeve resection (DeLorme's procedure)	Perineal	Moderate	Low	Low
Anal encirclement	Perineal	High	Lowest	Moderate

Complete rectal prolapse appears as a mass protruding through the anus with concentric folds of mucosa lining the prolapsed segment. Hemorrhoidal prolapse can be differentiated by the deep radial folds separating the prolapsing tissue. Differentiation of true rectal prolapse from hemorrhoidal prolapse is critical because misdiagnosis leads to inappropriate treatment and creates significant morbidity. In patients in whom rectal prolapse is suspected but not visualized, the patient can be asked to strain while sitting on a commode to reproduce the prolapse.

Digital rectal and vaginal examinations may reveal a patulous anus, decreased sphincter tone, or a sphincteric defect. Uterine prolapse, rectocele, cystocele, or enterocele may also be present. Complete colonic evaluation with contrast enema or colonoscopy is warranted before considering repair, because a neoplasm may serve as the lead point of the intussusception. Endoscopic examination of the rectum may also reveal a solitary rectal ulcer on the anterior aspect of the rectum, which is thought to occur as a result of repetitive straining. This straining creates ischemia at the apex of the prolapsing rectum, ultimately leading to ulceration. Correction of rectal prolapse often heals a solitary rectal ulcer.

The role of anorectal physiologic testing in the evaluation of patients with rectal prolapse is controversial. Although studies of anal manometry and pudendal nerve terminal motor latency may help define the pathophysiology of anal incontinence in patients with rectal prolapse, these investigations are not accurate in predicting continence after surgical correction of the prolapse. If a combined pelvic floor disorder with multiple organ prolapse is suspected by physical examination, defecography is warranted. In addition, defecography is useful in patients with solitary rectal ulcer in the absence of overt rectal prolapse, because the study may reveal internal intussusception of the rectum. Defecography is not necessary for patients with isolated rectal prolapse. Colonic transit studies should be considered in constipated patients, because patients with colonic inertia should be considered for combined colonic resection and prolapse repair.

OPERATIVE MANAGEMENT

Although extremely high-risk patients with easily reducible rectal prolapse can be managed with laxatives and manual reduction of the prolapse, most patients benefit from surgical repair. The primary goals of surgery are to restore normal anatomy and improve symptoms of constipation and incontinence. Treatment options include

one or more of the following: narrow the anal orifice; obliterate the pouch of Douglas; restore the pelvic floor by plicating the levators; resect the prolapsing segment of rectosigmoid; and suspend or fix the prolapsing rectum to the sacrum.

Corrective procedures for rectal prolapse can be divided by approach: transabdominal or perineal (Table 86-1). Most transabdominal procedures have low recurrence rates; moreover, laparotomy allows the opportunity for colectomy in patients with severe constipation. In addition, pelvic floor disorders such as enterocele and rectocele may be corrected simultaneously. Most procedures performed using a perineal approach can be completed using local or regional anesthesia, thereby minimizing or avoiding anesthetic and cardiopulmonary risk. Although procedures using a perineal approach have higher recurrence rates than transabdominal procedures, they are excellent alternatives for the high-risk patient and for those patients who wish to avoid pelvic dissection, particularly so for male patients who will not accept the small risk of sexual dysfunction.

Regardless of the operative approach, all patients should undergo preoperative bowel preparation and should receive perioperative broad-spectrum antibiotic coverage and prophylaxis for deep venous thrombosis.

Abdominal Procedures

Good risk patients with rectal prolapse and constipation should be considered for *sigmoid resection and rectopexy.* The patient is placed in a dorsal lithotomy position. Through a midline laparotomy or low transverse incision, the left colon is mobilized from mid-descending colon to the sacral promontory. The presacral space is entered, and the rectum and mesorectum are mobilized posteriorly to the coccyx. The hypogastric nerves are preserved by sweeping them posteriorly. Anterior mobilization of the rectovaginal septum is usually unnecessary. The rectum is elevated and straightened, and several nonabsorbable sutures are placed between the lateral perirectal tissue and the presacral fascia just inferior to the sacral promontory. These sutures are tied after the redundant sigmoid colon is resected and end-to-end anastomosis is performed.

The advantages of resection-rectopexy are preservation of the native compliant rectum, removal of redundant sigmoid colon, alleviation of constipation, and low recurrence rate (less than 3%). Continence is improved in approximately half the patients. Disadvantages are related to the magnitude of the procedure. Most patients with rectal prolapse are older, debilitated, and tolerate laparotomy less well than younger, healthy patients. In addition, an anastomotic leak can be devastating. Anterior resection of the sigmoid and upper rectum without rectal fixation is not used commonly to treat rectal prolapse, because recurrence rates are much higher than after resection/rectopexy unless the rectum is fully mobilized and resected down to just above the levators—thus, in essence, performing a *low* anterior resection.

An alternative transabdominal procedure that avoids the complication of anastomotic leak is *sacral fixation* of the prolapsing rectum (rectopexy). The patient is placed in a dorsal lithotomy position and the rectum is mobilized to the pelvic floor as described earlier. The rectum is then straightened and suspended from the presacral fascia. The rectopexy can be performed using nonabsorbable sutures, as described, or, more effectively, by using a sling of prosthetic material. A variety of materials have been used to fashion the sling, although the most commonly used is prosthetic mesh (polypropylene or polytetrafluoroethylene, Fig. 86–1). The original sling technique, as described by Ripstein, created a circumferential wrap around the rectum. However, because obstructive symptoms or stool impaction proximal to the wrap developed in a substantial fraction of patients, most surgeons leave the anterior surface of the rectum free, using a partial wrap. A simple technique to avoid compression of the rectum by the wrap is to place a sterile proctoscope adjacent to the rectum when sizing the prosthetic material. There is no difference in the type of mesh used with regard to complication rate, recurrence rate, or functional outcome.

Rectopexy is an effective treatment, with recurrence rates of less than 5% in most series. However, constipation is not relieved by rectopexy and is sometimes worsened. Occasionally, a stricture can be demonstrated at the site of the wrap, but most constipation is probably secondary to preexisting colonic dysmotility. Preoperative colonic transit studies may help guide the selection of rectopexy alone versus resection/rectopexy for patients with rectal prolapse and constipation. Infection of the mesh and pelvic sepsis occur uncommonly (0 to 2% in most series).

Patients with rectal prolapse and enterocele or large rectocele may be considered for a *combined pelvic floor repair.* Most of these patients are women who have undergone hysterectomy and have laxity of the pelvic floor with perineal descent. Although the pursestring suture repair of the pouch of Douglas described by Moschcowitz has been associated with recurrence rates for rectal prolapse approaching 50%, a combined mesh rectopexy, pelvic floor repair, and elevation of the perineal body is more effective. The patient is placed in a dorsal lithotomy position, and a vaginal prep is performed. The redundant peritoneum overlying the vaginal cuff and anterior surface of the mesorectum is stripped. The rectovaginal septum is mobilized completely and the anterior surface of the levators exposed. A band of prosthetic mesh is sutured to the levators and the perineal body using sutures passed transabdominally. The mesh is secured to the presacral fascia just inferior to the sacral promontory, thus elevating the perineal body and pelvic floor. The rectum is elevated and sutured to the medial aspect of the mesh. The vaginal cuff is straightened and sutured to the anterior aspect of the mesh, thus obliterating the pouch of Douglas. If a cystocele is present, struts of mesh can be fashioned to prevent the bladder from prolapsing through the vaginal cuff.

The combined pelvic floor repair is effective in correcting prolapse but does not improve preexisting constipation. As with rectopexy alone, patients should be counseled that constipation will not be corrected by this procedure. Mesh erosion into the vagina or rectum occurs infrequently and rarely results in rectovaginal fistula.

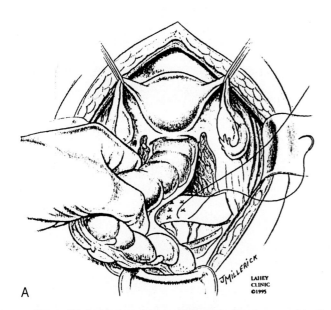
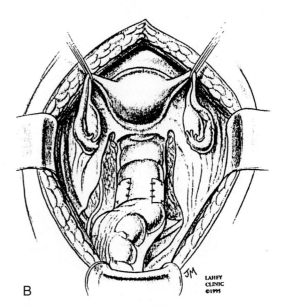

A   B

Figure 86–1. Mesh rectopexy. The mesh sling is secured to the periosteum of the sacrum *(A)* and then to either side of the rectum *(B),* leaving the anterior wall of the rectum free to distend and preventing formation of a stricture. (From Marcello P, Roberts P: Surgery for rectal prolapse. In Hicks T, Beck D, Opelka F, Timmcke A [eds]: Complications of Colon and Rectal Surgery. Baltimore, Williams & Wilkins, 1996:249, with permission.)

The *Ivalon sponge* procedure, described in 1959, uses a polyvinyl alcohol sponge to wrap the mobilized rectum in a posterior, noncircumferential fashion. Fixation occurs secondary to the vigorous inflammatory reaction induced by the sponge. Recurrence rates as great as 20% are thought to be a consequence of incomplete mobilization of the rectum or detachment of the sponge from the rectum before adhesion and fibrosis occur. When the fibrotic reaction from the sponge is overabundant, the rectum becomes stiff, and fecal impaction and stricture formation may occur, resulting in worsening constipation in 40% to 50% of patients. Pelvic abscess and sepsis, which occur in 0 to 3% of patients, require removal of the sponge either transabdominally or transrectally. The Ivalon sponge is not approved for use in the United States.

Laparoscopic Correction of Rectal Prolapse

Laparoscopic repair of rectal prolapse was first described in 1992; since then, numerous laparoscopic techniques have been reported, including sutureless rectopexy, suture rectopexy, proctosigmoidectomy, resection-rectopexy, and mesh rectopexy. The potential benefits of a minimal ac-

cess laparoscopic repair include early return of gastrointestinal function, less postoperative pain, better cosmesis, and shorter hospital stay. Short-term recurrence rates are similar to open transabdominal techniques. Postoperative incontinence and constipation are also comparable to open procedures, suggesting that the laparoscopic approach is an effective option in the treatment of rectal prolapse.

Perineal Procedures

Perineal rectosigmoidectomy has become our first choice for the vast majority of patients with rectal prolapse (Fig. 86–2). Regional anesthesia is adequate for most patients. The patient may be placed in the prone/jackknife or lithotomy position, although we find that the prone/jackknife position provides optimal exposure. The buttocks are taped apart, and the prolapse is re-created with gentle traction on the rectum. A full-thickness incision is made 1 cm proximal to the dentate line and the rectum is disconnected from the anal canal. A circumferential self-retaining retractor is placed to aid exposure. The rectum and sigmoid are mobilized circumferentially. The peritoneal cavity is entered, usually in the deep peritoneal cul-de-sac anteriorly, which can be encountered at a very

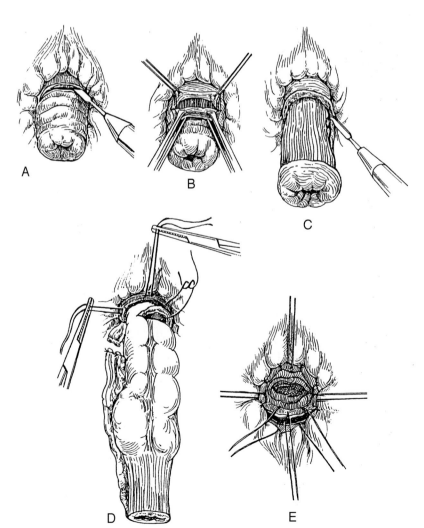

Figure 86–2. Perineal rectosigmoidectomy. A circumferential incision is made in the anal canal just above the dentate line *(A)*. The prolapsed rectum is separated and everted *(B and C)*. The peritoneal reflection is incised sharply, allowing the redundant bowel to be fully mobilized *(D)*. Once the mesentery is divided, the bowel is opened *(D)* and full-thickness interrupted sutures are placed between the divided colon and the anal canal *(E)*. (From Marcello P, Roberts P: Surgery for rectal prolapse. In Hicks T, Beck D, Opelka F, Timmcke A [eds]: Complications of Colon and Rectal Surgery. Baltimore, Williams & Wilkins, 1996:253, with permission.)

superficial level. The mesorectum is divided between clamps, staying close to the rectum, until the colon is straightened and there is resistance to further dissection. Care must be taken to ensure meticulous hemostasis in the mesentery, because vessels may bleed profusely when distal traction is released.

Levatorplasty is often combined with perineal rectosigmoidectomy and may improve continence in some patients. This is performed by retracting the mobilized rectum and approximating the levators with nonabsorbable suture. Levatorplasty may be performed anteriorly, posteriorly, or both. A mechanical defect in the external anal sphincter may also be repaired at this time. The defect in the peritoneum is then closed and the bowel divided. The proximal margin should reach the anus without tension, else an ischemic stricture or anastomotic dehiscence may result. A coloanal anastomosis is then performed, either with suture or with an intraluminal circular stapler. Postoperative care is the same as for any procedure with an intestinal anastomosis. Patients have minimal discomfort, and bowel function usually returns within 3 to 5 days.

The main advantage of this procedure is avoidance of a laparotomy. However, this transperineal approach requires bowel resection with anastomosis and therefore carries a risk of stricture and anastomotic leak. Recurrence rates are less than 10%, although meaningful long-term follow-up in elderly, debilitated patients who undergo the procedure may be difficult to obtain because of comorbid illness. Thus, the choice of this procedure for young, otherwise healthy patients is controversial. Incontinence may be worsened postoperatively as a result of the loss of the rectal reservoir. However, as the neorectum undergoes adaptation, both rectal sensation and capacitance may improve. The addition of levatorplasty at the time of the rectosigmoidectomy may decrease the rate of postoperative anal incontinence. Because levatorplasty is technically straightforward and adds little morbidity, it is reasonable to perform routinely in incontinent patients.

Mucosal sleeve resection (DeLorme's procedure), originally described in 1900, was not well accepted because the technique was bloody and had a high complication and recurrence rate. Modification of the technique to include plication of the underlying muscle led to resurgence in popularity in the 1970s (Fig. 86–3). The procedure can be performed with the patient in the lithotomy position, although exposure is best and blood loss minimized with the patient in the prone/jackknife position. Regional or local anesthesia with sedation is adequate. Epinephrine-containing solutions are infiltrated into the submucosal plane to reduce hemorrhage and to lift the mucosa away from the muscle layer. A circumferential incision is made through the mucosa just above the dentate line. Dissection is carried out in the submucosal plane until the proximal extent of the prolapse is reached. The circular layer of internal sphincter muscle is then plicated in eight quadrants beginning at the apex of the dissection and ending at the distal cut edge of the mucosa just proximal to the dentate line. The stripped mucosa is resected, and a mucosal-mucosal anastomosis completes the procedure.

The advantage of the DeLorme procedure is its technical simplicity, avoidance of an abdominal procedure, and

avoidance of full-thickness bowel resection and anastomosis. Incontinence improves in 70% of the patients, possibly because the telescoped, plicated muscle cuff adds resistance at the level of the anal sphincter. However, in general, recurrence rates are higher than for perineal rectosigmoidectomy, varying between 5% and 40%. The most common complication is postoperative bleeding from the denuded muscle surface, although the technique described has reduced the incidence of significant bleeding to less than 2% overall. Avoiding tension and ischemia at the mucosal anastomosis may minimize complications such as stricture and mucosal separation. Patients with rectal prolapse that is not circumferential or does not protrude significantly beyond the anal verge may be candidates for mucosal sleeve resection. However, given the excellent results and low morbidity of perineal rectosigmoidectomy, we have found that the perineal procedure of choice for the majority of patients with rectal prolapse, usually in the older population (>60 years of age), is a perineal rectosigmoidectomy.

Extremely high operative risk patients with rectal prolapse may be considered for an *anal encirclement* procedure. Thiersch first described the original procedure in 1891. A silver wire was placed in the ischiorectal fat around the external sphincter mechanism to tighten the anal opening, thereby preventing prolapse. Currently, the encircling procedure is performed with a band of soft synthetic mesh, a silicone tube, permanent suture, or transposed gracilis muscle graft. The patient may be placed in the prone/jackknife or lithotomy position, although again we find that the prone/jackknife position provides optimal exposure. Local anesthesia with sedation is usually adequate. The rectum is irrigated with povidone iodine solution and a piece of gauze is placed into the rectum to minimize stool contamination. Two incisions are then made on opposite sides of the anus. The incisions can be placed laterally or in the anterior and posterior positions. A blunt tip clamp is passed around the anal canal outside of the external sphincter toward the opposite incision, and the encircling material is brought through the tunnel. The material is tightened with the surgeon's index finger (or number 16 or 18 Hegar dilator) in the anal canal and secured. The incisions are closed. The patient is started on a regimen of stool softeners and bulk-forming laxatives to avoid fecal impaction. Some patients require regular enemas to defecate.

The advantages of anal encirclement include a short and simple procedure with minimal trauma, repeatability, and minimal anesthetic requirement. However, anal encirclement does not cure the disease process, and the prolapse persists internally. In addition, postoperative complications occur in approximately 25% of patient, most commonly breakage, erosion, infection of the encircling material, and fecal impaction. Ten percent of patients require removal of the encirclement. Recurrence of rectal prolapse is also common, occurring in 20% to 60% of patients. Because of these limitations, anal encirclement is reserved for only the most debilitated patients with limited life expectancy.

Recurrent Rectal Prolapse

Recurrent mucosal prolapse must be differentiated from recurrent rectal prolapse in that their treatments are

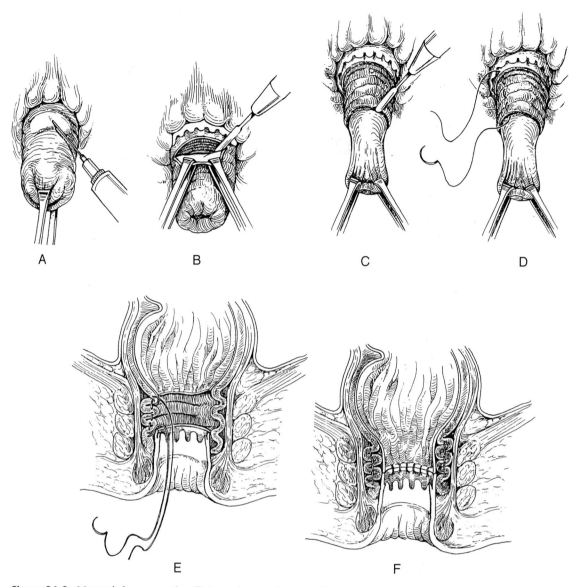

A   B   C   D

E   F

Figure 86–3. Mucosal sleeve resection (DeLorme's procedure). A dilute saline-epinephrine solution is injected submucosally to reduce bleeding and facilitate dissection *(A)*. The mucosa is separated from the underlying muscular layer *(B)*. Circumferential stripping is continued as far cephalad as is possible *(C)*. Before excision of the redundant mucosa, plicating sutures are placed in the circular muscle of the rectum *(D)*. Plication is performed *(E)*, the redundant mucosa amputated, and the mucosal anastomosis completed with absorbable suture *(F)*. (From Marcello P, Roberts P: Surgery for rectal prolapse. In Hicks T, Beck D, Opelka F, Timmcke A [eds]: Complications of Colon and Rectal Surgery. Baltimore, Williams & Wilkins, 1996:255.)

very different. Mucosal prolapse can be easily treated by rubber band ligation or by mucosal sleeve resection. Treatment of recurrent, full-thickness rectal prolapse, however, is more complicated. The selection of operative technique for recurrent prolapse depends on the original procedure performed and the medical condition of the patient (Table 86–2). Lack of attention to issues of vascular supply can have disastrous consequences.

High-risk patients who have had perineal rectosigmoidectomy should be considered for repeat perineal rectosigmoidectomy. Although the risk of re-recurrence may be substantial, the procedure is safe. Recurrence after the DeLorme procedure can be treated by perineal rectosigmoidectomy. Failure of anal encirclement can be treated by removal of the encircling material, control of

sepsis, and then repeat anal encirclement or perineal rectosigmoidectomy after the wounds have healed completely.

Low-risk patients who have undergone perineal rectosigmoidectomy may undergo repeat perineal rectosigmoidectomy or transabdominal rectopexy. Some form of imaging, however, is important to determine the cause of recurrence. If resection of the rectosigmoid is contemplated, care must be taken to ensure that adequate blood supply to the distal bowel is maintained. Low-risk patients who have undergone rectopexy alone should be considered for perineal rectosigmoidectomy or sigmoid resection, depending on the results of defecography. If defecography reveals that sacral fixation is intact, the rectum is straight, and the lead point of the prolapse is above

Table 86-2	Surgical Options for Repair of Recurrent Rectal Prolapse	

PRIMARY PROCEDURE	PROCEDURE FOR REPAIR OF RECURRENT PROLAPSE
Sigmoid resection + rectopexy	Rectopexy
	Perineal rectosigmoidectomy°
Rectopexy	Perineal rectosigmoidectomy
	Sigmoid resection ± rectopexy
Perineal rectosigmoidectomy	Perineal rectosigmoidectomy
	Rectopexy
	Sigmoid resection + rectopexy°
Mucosal sleeve resection (DeLorme's procedure)	Perineal rectosigmoidectomy
Anal encirclement	Perineal rectosigmoidectomy
	Anal encirclement

°Care must be taken to avoid creating an ischemic segment of rectosigmoid if these procedures are performed.

the rectosigmoid junction, sigmoid resection should be considered. Low-risk patients who have undergone sigmoid resection and rectopexy can be treated by repeat rectopexy or perineal rectosigmoidectomy. However, perineal rectosigmoidectomy may create an ischemic segment of bowel unless the dissection from the perineum encompasses the prior anastomosis.

Incarcerated Prolapse

If the prolapsed segment of rectosigmoid becomes incarcerated, reduction can usually be accomplished by placing the patient supine or slightly head-down, administering analgesics and anxiolytics, and gently rolling the leading edge of the prolapse into the anus. Occasionally it may be necessary to reduce the prolapse in the operating room, in which case an anal field block with local anesthetic may be helpful in achieving relaxation of the sphincter muscles. Applying sugar or other substances to the prolapsed segment to decrease edema has been described, but is rarely necessary. After reduction, surgery can then be planned on an elective basis, after inflammation has resolved.

COMPLICATIONS

In addition to the specific complications already noted, there are complications common to many of the operations used to correct rectal prolapse. Perioperative mortality rate after abdominal procedures is low (0 to 3%). Most deaths are due to comorbidity and, less often, to septic complications. Improvements in anesthetic techniques, perioperative monitoring, and utilization of perineal procedures for high-risk patients have accounted for

Pearls and Pitfalls

- Full-thickness rectal prolapse must be differentiated from hemorrhoidal prolapse preoperatively.
- Solitary rectal ulcer in the absence of procidentia may be a sign of internal intussusception of the rectum.
- Defecography is the most useful examination for detecting internal rectal intussusception and other organ prolapse through the perineum.
- Colonic evaluation with contrast enema or colonoscopy is warranted before one considers repair of rectal prolapse to exclude a tumor as the lead point of the prolapse.
- Healthy patients with constipation and rectal prolapse should be considered for sigmoid resection and rectopexy.
- High-risk patients can undergo a transperineal approach to rectosigmoidectomy.
- Fecal continence often improves in patients undergoing repair of rectal prolapse, even in the absence of anal sphincter reconstruction or levatorplasty.

the decrease in mortality rate in recent years. Perioperative mortality rate after perineal procedures remains extremely low (0 to 1%) despite the selection of higher risk patients for this approach.

Presacral hemorrhage, a potentially life-threatening complication, can occur after any procedure in which the posterior rectum is mobilized. Care must be taken during dissection in the plane between the mesorectum and the presacral fascia and during placement of rectopexy sutures. Sharp dissection with electrocautery or scissors under direct vision can be accomplished with anterior retraction of the rectosigmoid. It is often helpful to use a curved malleable blade to retract the mesorectum as the dissection proceeds to the level of the coccyx. The risk of injury to the basivertebral veins on the anterior surface of the sacrum is minimized if the urge to perform this portion of the dissection bluntly with a hand behind the mesorectum is suppressed.

SELECTED READINGS

Agachan F, Pfeifer J, Joo JS, et al: Results of perineal procedures for the treatment of rectal prolapse. Am Surg 1997;63:9.

Boccasanta P, Rosati R, Venturi M, et al: Comparison of laparoscopic rectopexy with open technique in the treatment of complete rectal prolapse: Clinical and functional results. Surg Laparosc Endosc 1998;8:460.

Eu KW, Seow-Choen F: Functional problems in adult rectal prolapse and controversies in surgical treatment. Br J Surg 1997;84:904.

Kim DS, Tsang CB, Wong WD, et al: Complete rectal prolapse: Evolution of management and results. Dis Colon Rectum 1999;42:460–466; discussion 466–469.

Oliver GC, Vachon D, Eisenstat TE, et al: DeLorme's procedure for complete rectal prolapse in severely debilitated patients. An analysis of 41 cases. Dis Colon Rectum 1994;37:461.

Sullivan E, Stranburg C, Sandoz I, et al: Repair of total pelvic prolapse: An overview. Perspect Colon Rectal Surg 1990;3:119.

Chapter 87

Ischemic Colitis

Mark D. Sawyer and Ourania A. Preventza

Ischemic colitis is the end pathophysiologic result of the interruption or diminution of blood flow to areas of the colon and represents the most common form of intestinal ischemia. Ischemic colitis was recognized as a clinical entity by Boley and colleagues in 1963, and was named by Martson and coworkers in 1966. A discrete and useful classification of this disease is difficult (Table 87–1) because there are many potential etiologic factors (Table 87–2), and the exact inciting factors underlying a clinical episode may remain uncertain. The most useful means of stratifying the disease is therefore a pragmatic determination as to which patients will respond to nonoperative therapy and which will require surgical intervention. The former group represents the great majority of these patients.

DIAGNOSIS

Clinical Presentation

The most common presenting symptoms in ischemic colitis are bloody diarrhea and abdominal pain. The typical scenario begins with abdominal pain, usually crampy in nature, followed by a strong defecatory urge, diarrhea, and a modest amount of hematochezia. Nausea and emesis may be accompanying symptoms, either resulting from the ischemia itself or resulting from a functional obstruction within the ischemic area of colon. These symptoms may progress over a few days before presentation. The natural course of the disease raises an interesting conundrum, namely, because bleeding is a manifestation of ischemia. Because many of these patients recover spontaneously (and not a few without a distinct cause identified), it may be that patients come to attention after the ischemic episode has passed—that is, the pain and hematochezia represent a reperfusion injury rather than the ischemia itself. Indeed, patients in whom an ischemic episode is documented early in its course may be expected to have an episode of hematochezia, usually self-limited, because the infarcted mucosa sloughs from the underlying reperfused tissue.

Physical Examination

A careful physical examination demonstrates tenderness over the affected area of the colon, but peritoneal signs are absent in most patients. The clinician must remember, however, that most patients with ischemic colitis are elderly and may not manifest abdominal tenderness reflective of the degree of pathology present. The presence of peritoneal irritation suggests transmural necrosis and the need for operative intervention, particularly in conjunction with signs of a systemic inflammatory response such as hypotension, fever, oliguria, altered mental status, or diffuse peritonitis.

Colonoscopy

In patients whose symptoms do not urge immediate operation, colonoscopy is the diagnostic test of choice. In addition to direct visualization, biopsies may aid in differentiating other forms of colitis or even malignancy. Flexible sigmoidoscopy may be considered in patients with left-sided pain, with the caveat that patients with ischemic colitis involving the entire colon have been described (albeit unusual). However, a normal flexible colonoscopy to the level of the mid-sigmoid does not completely exclude the diagnosis of ischemic colitis, because the ischemia may involve only segmental areas such as the cecum/ascending colon or the so-called watershed area of the splenic flexure. Colonoscopic findings depend on the severity of the ischemic insult and the point in the natural history of the disease at which the colonoscopy is performed. Areas of necrosis—blackened epithelium, shaggy with desquamation—suggest transmural necrosis, the most serious manifestation. Areas of frank necrosis may be bordered by normally perfused colon. More superficial ischemia causes patchy epithelial necrosis with sur-

Table 87–1	Various Classification Schemes for Ischemic Colitis
	Occlusive versus nonocclusive
	Gangrenous versus nongangrenous
	Acute versus chronic
	Age of the patient

Table 87–2	Etiologic Factors in Ischemic Colitis
Acute occlusive disease	
	Thromboemboli
	Atheroemboli
	Ligation of blood supply during other operations such as aortic surgery
Chronic occlusive disease	
	Atherosclerosis
	Diabetes mellitus
	Vasculitis
Low flow states	
	Dehydration
	Shock
	Vasospasm
	Cardiac failure

rounding viable mucosa. Other colonoscopic signs of ischemic colitis are more suggestive of a reperfusion phase of the injury: edema; erythema; and submucosal hemorrhage. Rarely, ischemic colitis may appear as a submucosal mass or stricture mimicking carcinoma.

Radiographic Diagnosis

Computed tomography is frequently used during the assessment of the patient with abdominal pain. Ischemic colitis appears most simply as a thickened colon wall, analogous to the "thumbprinting" seen when barium enema is the diagnostic test for the disease. More serious signs are pneumatosis coli or the even more deadly portent of gas within the portal venous system. Although not pathognomonic, the presence of air within the colon wall or the portal vein is indicative of transmural necrosis in the setting of ischemic colitis and should usually be considered an indication for urgent surgical exploration.

VASCULAR ANATOMY OF THE COLON

Normal Anatomy

In the normal state, the colon derives most of its blood supply from the superior and inferior mesenteric arteries. The superior mesenteric artery gives off the right colic artery and terminates as the ileocolic artery, which together supply the right colon, the hepatic flexure, and the proximal transverse colon. The middle colic artery arises more proximally from the superior mesenteric artery and provides the blood supply to the transverse colon. Both the right and middle colic arteries may be absent in up to one fifth of patients. The inferior mesenteric artery supplies the splenic flexure and the descending colon, and its most distal inferior branch becomes the superior rectal artery, which supplies the distal sigmoid colon and the proximal rectum. The inferior mesenteric artery can be quite small in diameter or occluded in the more elderly patients with atherosclerosis. Collateral flow between the systemic and visceral circulation takes place among small vessels joining the superior to the middle rectal arteries.

Arcing extensions of these visceral vessels course near the antimesenteric border of the colon to anastomose with each other to form the so-called marginal artery of Drummond. The continuity of this arch may be interrupted near the splenic flexure, the watershed area known as Griffith's point. A more centrifugally located analogy to the artery of Drummond is the arc of Riolan, which is an abnormal vessel that arises from a small branch off the aorta and functionally connects the aorta with the inferior mesenteric artery. In this way, the vessel provides vascular inflow to the colon and small bowel with often quite a significant chronic occlusion of the superior mesenteric artery (SMA). This vessel is usually only present with chronic occlusion of the SMA and should not be depended upon to provide circulation after a resection.

PATIENT GROUPS AND TREATMENT

Nonocclusive Ischemic Colitis in the Elderly

The majority of patients with ischemic colitis (80% to 85%) result from nonocclusive disease. No distinct causative factor can be positively implicated in up to half of these patients. This form of ischemic colitis occurs more frequently in males and most commonly involves the left colon, centered about the watershed area of the splenic flexure. The ravages of age such as atherosclerosis involving the inferior mesenteric artery, decreased cardiac output, microvascular diseases such as diabetes mellitus and vasculitis, renal failure, and the effects of various medications on blood pressure may all contribute to a transient diminution of blood flow. Minor events such as hypovolemia or vasospasm may decrease the effective blood flow to the colon below the critical point, leading to ischemia. Ischemic colitis in these patients usually responds well to optimization of hemodynamics, intravenous antibiotics, and bowel rest; in the elderly, however, the mortality rate may approach 50%.

Ischemic Colitis in Young Adults

Ischemic colitis in young adults (younger than 50 years of age) has a strikingly lower mortality rate than in elderly patients. Most patients in this age group are women, and up to half of these patients have been taking oral contraceptives. In an 8-year review of 38 patients younger than 50 years old with ischemic colitis managed at the Mayo Clinic, three fourths of the patients were successfully managed nonoperatively. In those patients requiring surgery, the most common indication was perforation.

Acute Occlusive Ischemic Colitis

The remaining 20% to 25% of patients with ischemic colitis are secondary to chronic vascular occlusive disease, which nearly always requires operative intervention. The area of gut rendered ischemic as the result of SMA thromboemboli is relative to how far from the ostium of the artery's origin the embolus lodges. The most distal branches of the SMA are the right colic and ileocolic arteries; occlusion at this level affects only the right colon. The more proximal the embolus, the larger the amount of attendant small intestinal ischemia that will be present and the more likely it is that the middle colic artery (and thus the transverse colon) will be affected as well.

Ischemic Colitis After Abdominal Aortic Reconstruction

Ischemic colitis develops in approximately 10% of patients after surgery for abdominal aortic aneurysm. This presents a difficult situation with potentially devastating sepsis in the face of recent major vascular surgery involv-

Pearls and Pitfalls

- Ischemic colitis may be a diagnosis of exclusion.
- Best diagnostic test is colonoscopy.
- Not all patients require operative intervention.
- Ischemic colitis usually presents as left-sided abdominal pain and mild hematochezia.
- One form involves women younger than 40 years old taking oral contraceptives.
- Ischemic colitis after aortic surgery is a complication in approximately 10% of patients and may require emergent operative intervention in approximately 2% of patients.

ing a new prosthetic graft. The presence of a prosthetic graft is particularly vulnerable to infection, and if it becomes infected resection and extra-anatomic bypass may be required. The ischemia in this circumstance is more akin to acute occlusive disease, precipitated by the acute loss of the inferior mesenteric artery blood supply during aortic reconstruction. The remaining blood supply to the sigmoid colon occurs via systemic collateral flow from the middle rectal arteries distally and visceral collateral flow from the middle colic artery proximally. Patients with mild ischemia (the majority) may recover with hemodynamic optimization, intravenous antibiotics, and bowel rest. In patients requiring operative intervention (overall, <2%), a primary anastomosis is to be avoided in favor of diversion to prevent life-threatening contamination of the aortic prosthesis.

Surgical Technique

Surgical treatment involves anatomic resection of all nonviable areas of colon, with care being taken to resect back to vascularized margins with viable mucosa. The amount of mesenteric fat may or may not allow easy palpation or visualization of the colonic vasculature. Aids such as a Doppler probe or intravenous fluorescein may be useful in evaluating the remaining vascular anatomy, the presence of blood flow in a particular vessel, and viability of questionable areas of colon. It is wise to reassess the surgical margins once the resection has been completed, because critical collateral blood supply may have been ablated as a consequence of the resection. The general rule in these patients is to perform a proximal diversion with a distal mucus fistula or Hartmann's pouch. It may be feasible to perform a primary anastomosis after a right hemicolectomy for limited disease without significant contamination or sepsis, but even this situation should be considered with care. The primary problem of ischemia poses grave risks for anastomotic failure, and the underlying cause of ischemia is often not alleviated by surgery performed for the symptomatic end pathology. Some consideration might also be given to a second-look procedure 12 to 24 hours later in selected patients.

Summary

Ischemic colitis represents the end pathology in a variety of factors diminishing blood flow to the colon. Typical presenting features include left-sided colon ischemia, which usually responds to intravenous fluids, antibiotics, and bowel rest after confirmation of the diagnosis with colonoscopy. Transmural necrosis should be suspected in patients with peritoneal signs or signs of sepsis, and its presence necessitates urgent surgical intervention. Operative intervention is indicated for complications of ischemic colitis such as perforation, recurrence, and strictures. When resecting the ischemic colon, the surgeon should be cognizant of the patient's vascular anatomy, particularly in patients in whom prior colectomy or aortic surgery has changed the usual collateral blood supply of the colon.

SELECTED READINGS

Boley SJ, Schwartz S, Lash J, Sterhnhill V: Reversible vascular occlusion of the colon. Surg Gynecol Obstet 1963;116:53.

Brandt L: Ischemic bowel disease: Diagnosis, management, and the role of endoscopy. Am Soc Gastrointestinal Endoscopy Clinical Update 1996;34:406.

Deana DG, Dean PJ: Reversible ischemic colitis in young women—association with oral contraceptive use. Am J Surg Pathol 1995;19:454.

Gandhi SK, Hanson MM, Vernava AM, et al: Ischemic colitis. Dis Colon Rectum 1996;39:88.

Longo WE, Ward D, Vernava AM, Kaminski DL: Outcome of patients with total colonic ischemia. Dis Colon Rectum 1997;40:1448.

Colon and Rectum: Malignant

Chapter 88
Polyps of the Colon and Rectum
Robert Fry

Because the term *polyp* refers to a projection of tissue from the inner wall of the intestine into the lumen, the term is nonspecific, and polyps can be either benign or malignant. It is most convenient and appropriate to classify polyps of the large bowel by their histology, that is, as hyperplastic, hamartomatous, inflammatory, or neoplastic (Table 88–1).

Hyperplastic (metaplastic) polyps are the most common polyps found in the large bowel but are of little clinical significance. They appear through the endoscope as small, pale, glassy mucosal nodules, usually less than 5 mm in size. Microscopic examination reveals the epithelial lining to consist of a papillary configuration, usually referred to as a "sawtooth" pattern. There is no nuclear dysplasia and no potential for malignancy. The lesions occur approximately three times more often than neoplastic polyps and are most common in the rectum and sigmoid.

Hamartomatous polyps are composed of an abnormal mixture of normal colonic tissues. Juvenile polyps are usually pedunculated, pink, and smooth polyps composed of dilated glands filled with mucus. The lamina propria

has an unusual mesenchymal appearance under the microscope. The polyps are more common in children but can also occur in adults.

Inflammatory polyps are associated with any form of severe colitis (ulcerative colitis, Crohn's disease, and ischemic colitis). These lesions are often called *pseudopolyps*, because they mimic neoplastic polyps, but they are characterized by the presence of inflammatory cells and have no malignant potential.

The *neoplastic polyp* is composed of abnormal glandular epithelium and thus they are true neoplasms. These polyps can be on a stalk (pedunculated) or flat (sessile) (Figs. 88–1 and 88–2). They are further classified according to their histologic appearance as tubular, villous, or tubulovillous (mixed) adenomas. The villous pattern is more common in large sessile lesions, whereas the pedunculated polyp is more often a tubular adenoma. The histologic abnormality of a neoplastic polyp should be further characterized according to the degree of cellular atypia or dysplasia (low, moderate, or high). An adenoma with the cytologic abnormalities of high-grade dysplasia should be considered to be just one step away from being a cancer.

Within the context of this discussion, it is important to consider a unique lesion generally referred to as the "flat adenoma." This lesion is usually small and flat, often with a central depression; because the surface does not project into the lumen of the colon, the flat adenoma may be difficult to detect even by colonoscopy (thus defying the definition of "polyp"). These lesions are usually smaller than 1 cm in diameter and may be distinguished from the adjacent normal mucosa only by subtle changes in morphology and texture. These small, innocuous lesions are important to detect because of the high incidence of carcinomas arising from them.

The main concern of the neoplastic polyp is its association with colorectal cancer. The high cancer risk of the

Table 88–1	Histology of Polyps	
POLYP	**HISTOLOGY**
Hyperplastic	Non-neoplastic mucosal nodules, "sawtooth" epithelial pattern
Hamartomatous	Abnormal mixture of endogenous tissues: juvenile polyps, Peutz-Jeghers syndrome
Inflammatory	Pseudopolyps: normal mucosal cells and inflammatory cells
	Lymphoid polyps: enlarged lymphoid follicles, often in the rectum
Neoplastic	Abnormal glands: tubular adenoma, villous adenoma, mixed adenoma

565

Colorectal Polyps

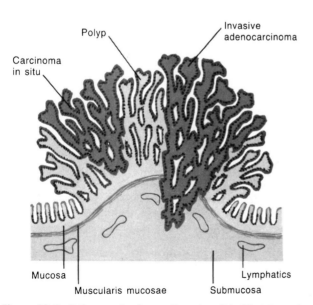

Adenocarcinoma (invades muscularis mucosae)

Carcinoma in situ (does not invade muscularis mucosae)

Polyp

Lymphatics (submucosal)

Submucosa

Muscularis mucosae

Mucosa

Stalk

Figure 88–1. Pathogenesis of a pedunculated polyp. (Modified from the Clinical Symposia Collection, vol. No. 41, plate No. 5, by Frank Netter. With permission from Novartis Pharmaceutical Corporation, East Hanover, NJ.)

		Size and Histology of Polyp Related to Possibility of Cancer

Table 88–2

	PERCENT OF POLYPS CONTAINING CANCER		
POLYP SIZE (cm)	**Tubular Adenoma (%)**	**Tubulovillous Adenoma (%)**	**Villous Adenoma (%)**
0.5–0.9	0.3	1.5	2.3
1.0–1.9	3.6	6.4	5.7
2.0–2.9	6.5	11.4	17.0
>3.0	11.0	15.0	13.1

Modified from Shinya H, Wolff WI: Morphology, anatomic distribution and cancer potential of colonic polyps: An analysis of 7000 polyps endoscopically removed. Ann Surg 1979;190:679.

stages in the development of cancer within a single polyp: normal epithelium, adenomatous tissue, dysplasia, and frank invasive cancer. Considerable circumstantial evidence supports this relationship. First, approximately half of patients with large bowel cancer have other polyps in their colon. Second, epidemiologic studies demonstrate that the incidence of colorectal polyps parallels the incidence of colorectal cancer geographically, with a high incidence in Europe and in the United States. Third, the distribution in the large bowel of polyps and cancers is similar (both occurring more frequently in the distal bowel). Fourth, reports surveying large populations reveal that the average age of patients found to have benign polyps is roughly 7 to 10 years younger than patients found to have colorectal cancer. Fifth, experimental carcinogens such as dimethylhydrazine, which is used to induce colorectal cancer in laboratory animals, first produce adenomas and only subsequently cancer.

Finally, molecular geneticists initially spearheaded by Vogelstein have provided compelling evidence for the transformation of a benign polyp into a cancer. Specific genetic alterations caused by a sequence of mutated genes, including the APC, Kras, and p53 genes, have been shown to be involved in the progression of neoplasia from a benign polyp to an invasive cancer.

CLINICAL PRESENTATION

It is important for the clinician to recognize hyperplastic, inflammatory and hamartomatous polyps for what they are and for any associated conditions. But for practical purposes, the polyp most often requiring the attention of the surgeon is the neoplastic polyp; the remainder of this discussion addresses the detection and management of neoplastic polyps arising in the large bowel.

Adenomas of the large bowel are usually asymptomatic; however, symptoms are not infrequent and include bleeding, diarrhea, passage of mucus, prolapse, and abdominal cramps. Hematochezia is the most common symptom of a polyp in the rectum or sigmoid colon. Lesions in the proximal colon may present with more altered blood in the stool and occasionally with frank hematochezia. More often, the slow blood loss associated with such lesions is not noticed, and iron deficiency ane-

flat adenoma has already been described. The risk of cancer being present in a polyp increases with the size of the polyp. Furthermore, villous tumors are more likely to be associated with cancer than tubular adenomas.

Table 88–2 demonstrates the relationship between neoplastic polyps and colorectal cancer. The most convincing evidence for this relationship, often referred to as the "polyp-cancer sequence," is the demonstration of all

Polyp

Invasive adenocarcinoma

Carcinoma in situ

Mucosa

Muscularis mucosae

Submucosa

Lymphatics

Figure 88–2. Pathogenesis of a sessile polyp. (Modified from the Clinical Symposia Collection, vol. No. 41, plate No. 5, by Frank Netter. With permission from Novartis Pharmaceutical Corporation, East Hanover, NJ.)

mia discovered during a routine medical evaluation or a stool positive for occult blood may be the only clue to the presence of the polyp. A more unusual presentation is that of a large villous adenoma secreting voluminous amounts of mucus and causing diarrhea and even fluid and electrolyte abnormalities (most notably hypokalemia). A polyp in the distal rectum may prolapse through the anus, causing the patient to confuse it with a hemorrhoid. Finally (and rarely), colonic polyps may cause a colocolonic intussusception, resulting in colicky abdominal pain.

DETECTION AND MANAGEMENT

Although polyps may arise anywhere within the colon, a significant number (especially villous adenomas) are located in the rectum and can be detected by digital rectal examination. These tumors are often soft and may be difficult to palpate, so the examination must be done with this in mind. However, even careful digital examination may fail to detect a large "carpet" villous adenoma that may occupy the entire circumference of the rectum.

Rigid sigmoidoscopy remains a useful examination tool, because most villous adenomas lie within reach of the 20-cm rigid sigmoidoscope. A cleansing enema is the only preparation necessary. This examination provides essential information to the operating surgeon concerning two issues that cannot be reliably ascertained by flexible sigmoidoscopy or colonoscopy: (1) the exact distance of the tumor from the anal verge (such measurements are notoriously unreliable because of "bowing" of the flexible endoscope); and (2) the circumferential location of the polyp. This information is critical, because if the polyp does contain a carcinoma, treatment options vary depending on the exact location of the tumor.

Flexible sigmoidoscopy is being used with increasing frequency as the first diagnostic procedure for the detection of colonic disease in patients with symptoms suggestive of a colonic neoplasm. The scope may be passed to the region of the splenic flexure and thus surveys the area at highest risk for polyps. The yield of detection of polyps is approximately three times as high for flexible sigmoidoscopy as for rigid sigmoidoscopy. The only preparation necessary for this examination is a phosphate enema. When a polyp is seen, it can be biopsied or removed by snare excision. However, the relatively unprepared bowel may contain explosive gases (methane and hydrogen), and insufflation should be by a nonflammable gas such as carbon dioxide if electrocautery is to be used. Carbon dioxide insufflation carries the advantage of rapid absorption of gas from the intestine, resulting in less colonic distention and discomfort immediately after the procedure.

Whereas polyps distal to the splenic flexure may be detected and often eliminated with the aid of a flexible sigmoidoscope, this instrument cannot reach the proximal colon. Appropriate inspection of the cecum and the ascending and transverse colon may be accomplished with acceptable accuracy either by double contrast barium enema or by colonoscopy. "Virtual" colonoscopy using three-dimensional contrast-enhanced computed tomography remains experimental and awaits confirmation of its efficacy compared with conventional colonoscopy. Only colonoscopy permits biopsy or excision of the polyp. If a polyp is detected by barium enema, then colonoscopy is still required to biopsy or excise the lesion; thus, many surgeons and gastroenterologists believe that screening of patients at high risk for polyps or malignancy may be better and more efficiently accomplished by colonoscopy. If a polyp is detected by rigid or flexible sigmoidoscopy, then the proximal colon should be examined by colonoscopy (or barium enema) because of a significant incidence of synchronous polyps. This concept is especially important if the polyp in the distal colon is greater than 1 cm in diameter, if the distal polyp has a villous component, or if multiple polyps are present. It is also important to inspect the entire colon if there is a family history of polyps or colorectal cancer.

Once a polyp has been detected, it should be removed to determine its histologic type. Exceptions to this rule are the tiny hyperplastic polyps that are obviously innocuous, and pseudopolyps in patients with inflammatory bowel disease. The method of removal depends on the size and location of the polyp. Small polyps of the rectum and sigmoid can be removed using a snare if pedunculated or by transanal excision through an operating proctoscope if the lesion is large and sessile. The removal of polyps in the more proximal colon has, like their detection, been revolutionized by introduction and widespread familiarization with the colonoscope. Even large polyps in the proximal colon may be approached initially by colonoscopy; such lesions that initially appear sessile may in fact be on a stalk that facilitates removal with endoscopic techniques. Seldom is it indicated to remove a polyp through a colotomy performed via a laparotomy. If the polyp is too large to be removed with the aid of a colonoscope, standard resection of the colonic segment and its mesentery is appropriate because of the risk of malignancy.

A common management problem arises when cancer is detected within a polyp that has been excised via the colonoscope. In such situations, careful histologic inspection of the polyp provides information essential for treatment decisions. Although there is some controversy concerning treatment recommendations in such patients, the general consensus is that the risk of operation (segmental resection of the involved colonic segment) should be weighed against the chance that the patient has been cured of the cancer by the polypectomy. Important factors to consider include the depth of penetration by the cancer (whether it invades through the musularis into the submucosa or whether it is limited to the head of a pedunculated polyp), the histologic differentiation of the tumor (well-differentiated versus poorly differentiated), the presence or absence of vascular or lymphatic invasion, and the presence or absence of cancer at the margin of resection. In addition to these factors, the opinion regarding the adequacy of resection by the endoscopist is important.

If the polyp is pedunculated and contains a focus of well-differentiated cancer confined to the head of the polyp, does not invade the musularis, has no evidence of invasion into vascular or lymphatic channels, and has been completely excised, then the chances are greater than 98% that the tumor has been completely excised, and most surgeons would not recommend further surgery. On the other extreme, if the polyp contains a poorly differentiated cancer that invades the muscularis, and there is lymphatic or vascular invasion, then the chance of lymphatic metastases is greater than the risk of mortality associated with resection of the segment of colon harboring the polyp. The same rules need to be considered for sessile polyps, but resection is more often indicated in such cases because the entire lesion cannot be excised with the colonoscope in a manner that will provide margins histologically assessable for adequate resection.

It is also important to recognize, at the time of polypectomy, the exact location of the polyp because once the polyp has been removed, identification of this location may be difficult or impossible either at repeat colonoscopy or intraoperatively. If the polyp contains a cancer that requires segmental colectomy, then the location is crucial for an appropriate operation. It is helpful to mark the site of polyps with a tattoo of India ink injected through the colonoscope into the submucosa adjacent to the polyp where the endoscopist thinks further treatment may be required. If a segmental colectomy becomes necessary, this tattoo should be readily visible to the surgeon as a black stain on the serosal surface of the bowel.

FOLLOW-UP

If a benign polyp as been completely excised, the patient should have a follow-up colonoscopy to ensure that the lesion has been completely removed, that no synchronous polyps have been missed, and that no metachronous polyps have arisen. There is considerable controversy concerning the timing of these follow-up examinations. Most surgeons would recommend repeat colonoscopy 1 year after the polypectomy, but there is evidence that a 3-year

> ## Pearls and Pitfalls
>
> - Colonic polyps are hyperplastic, hamartomatous, inflammatory, or neoplastic.
> - Neoplastic polyps include tubular, tubulovillous, and villous varieties. The risk of malignancy varies with the size and type of neoplastic polyp.
> - Polyps are usually asymptomatic but may present as hematochezia or, rarely, as diarrhea, cramps, or passage of mucus.
> - Colorectal cancer arises from polyps, which proceed to dysplasia, then carcinoma in situ, then invasive cancer.
> - Colonic polyps should be removed, and future surveillance colonoscopy should be performed.

interval may be equally safe in most patients without a polyposis syndrome.

If the polyp contains a cancer with favorable characteristics, then follow-up colonoscopy should be performed 3 to 6 months later to be sure that there is no residual tumor at the polypectomy site. Thereafter, a colonoscopy should be performed every 3 to 5 years to detect and remove any metachronous polyps.

SELECTED READINGS

Gilbertsen VA: Proctosigmoidoscopy and polypectomy in reducing the incidence of rectal cancer. Cancer 1974;34:936.

Haggitt RC, Glotzbach RE, Soffer EE, Wrible LD: Prognostic factors in colorectal carcinomas arising in adenomas: Implications for lesions removed by endoscopic polypectomy. Gastroenterology 1985;89:328.

Pollard CW, Nivatvongs S, Rojanasakul A, et al: The fate of patients following polypectomy alone for polyps containing invasive carcinoma. Dis Colon Rectum 1992;35:933.

Shinya H, Wolff WI: Morphology, anatomic distribution and cancer potential of colonic polyps: An analysis of 7000 polyps endoscopically removed. Ann Surg 1979;190:679.

Winawer SJ, Zauber AG, Ho MN, et al: Prevention of colorectal cancer by colonoscopic polypectomy. The National Polyp Study Workgroup. N Engl J Med 1993;329:1977.

Chapter 89

Colon Cancer

Andreas M. Kaiser and Robert W. Beart, Jr.

EPIDEMIOLOGY

Colorectal cancer is the third most common malignant tumor in the United States. With an estimated 130,000 new patients diagnosed each year, colorectal cancer was estimated to be responsible for almost 50,000 deaths, or 10% to 15% of cancer-related deaths, in the year 2000. The incidence of colon cancer is similar for both genders, whereas rectal cancer is more frequent in male patients (2:1). After the age of 40 years, there is an age-dependent increase with each decade, and the mean age at presentation is 70 years.

The cause of colorectal cancer is not known. However, genetic, dietary (e.g., high-fat and low-fiber), and environmental risk factors have been associated with the disease. The majority of patients have sporadic colon cancers that arise within a polyp (villous > tubulovillous > tubular adenomas). These initially benign precursor lesions may transform into precancerous dysplastic polyps and eventually into invasive cancer in a multistep process that involves mutations of several independent genes (adenoma-carcinoma sequence). A number of hereditary syndromes based on germline mutations (FAP—familial adenomatous polyposis, HNPCC—hereditary nonpolyposis colon cancer) have been recognized to predispose for the development of colon cancer at an even younger age (Table 89–1). Inflammatory bowel disease (ulcerative colitis, Crohn's disease) carries a higher incidence of colorectal carcinoma, which correlates with the duration and extent of active disease. In ulcerative colitis, the risk of colorectal cancer increases from approximately 3% in the first decade of disease to 10% to 20% in the second decade. In patients with Crohn's colitis, the disease-associated risk for colorectal cancer is also increased, but to a lesser extent. Less frequent risk factors for colorectal cancers include a history of ureterocolostomy or a previous radiation treatment.

ANATOMIC DISTRIBUTION

Approximately 25% of colorectal cancers are located in the rectum or sigmoid colon and 40% in the cecum or ascending colon; the remaining are equally distributed throughout the remaining colon. Synchronous colorectal cancers are found in 5% to 10% of patients, metachronous new primary cancers will develop in the large intestine in 20% of patients with a history of colorectal cancer, and 15% to 20% of patients have distant metastases (stage IV disease) at the time of diagnosis.

PATHOLOGY AND STAGING

Adenocarcinoma is the predominant histopathology in 90% to 95% of colorectal malignancies. Mucinous and signet cell variants account for less than 10%. Rare neoplasms include squamous and adenosquamous carcinoma, lymphomas, and carcinoids, the latter of which may develop metastatic disease if the maximal diameter of the primary lesion exceeds 1 to 2 cm.

The pattern of local growth for colorectal cancer involves circumferential and transmural invasion of the tumor through the intestinal wall into the peritoneal cavity or surrounding organ structures. Tumor dissemination occurs through lymphatic access into the locoregional lymph nodes, by hematogenous spread to distant organs (e.g., liver, lung, kidney, bone), by transperitoneal migration and seeding, and by perineural infiltration.

Modern staging classification of colorectal cancer into clinical stages I through IV follows the TNM system

Table 89–1	Comparison of Sporadic Colon Cancer, Familial Adenomatous Polyposis, Hereditary Nonpolyposis Colon Cancer, and Inflammatory Bowel Disease			
	SCC	**FAP**	**HNPCC**	**IBD**
Variants		AFAP, Gardner, Turcot	Lynch I/II	
Genetic	−	+	+	?
		Autosomal-dominant		
Number of polyps	Variable, <10	>100	<10	Inflammatory pseudopolyps
Age of onset	>40 yr, average 60–65 yr	Polyps start after age 10–20 yr, cancer in 100% at age 40 yr	Age 30–50 yr	Depends on duration/extent of active disease
Location	Left colon > right	Any location	Right colon > left	Active disease
Chemoprevention	NSAIDs? Vitamins?	NSAIDs	?	IBD suppression?
Genes	Chromosomal deletions, k-ras, DCC, p53, APC	APC	MSH2, MLH1, PMS1/2	?
Associated risks	?	Desmoids	Endometrium cancer	Extracolonic disease

FAP, familial adenomatous polyposis; HNPCC, hereditary nonpolyposis colon cancer; IBD, inflammatory bowel disease; *MSH2, MLH1,* and *PMS1/2,* genes for DNA repair enzymes; NSAID, nonsteroidal anti-inflammatory drug; SCC, sporadic colon cancer.

(Table 89–2) according to the depth of tumor invasion through the layers of the intestinal wall (T), the number of regional lymph nodes involved (N), and the presence or absence of distant metastases (M). The historical classifications (Dukes' and Astler-Coller) have largely been abandoned.

CLINICAL PRESENTATION

Symptoms of colorectal cancer are often absent before the tumor has grown to a significant size and should therefore not be considered as early signs of the tumor. Unless a patient has complications of the tumor (ileus, bleeding, perforation, fistula formation), symptoms are mostly subtle or nondiagnostic, such as weight loss, anemia, or abdominal cramps. The more distal the lesion (left side of colon or rectum), the more evident are changes in bowel habits, including bloody or mucous discharge in the stool, onset of constipation, alternating diarrhea and constipation, or a decreasing diameter of the stool. Pelvic pain may occur when a rectal cancer reaches a large size.

Because symptoms are not reliable for early detection of colorectal cancer, risk-adjusted screening programs become important. Tests for occult blood in the stool, flexible sigmoidoscopies, or colonoscopies are indicated according to the individual genetic, disease-dependent, or age-dependent risk for development of colorectal cancer.

Any large bowel obstruction, bleeding from the rectum, or passage of stool or gas through the vagina or in the urine should raise the index of suspicion for a colorectal malignancy. The differential diagnosis includes diverticulitis, Crohn's disease, benign polyps, or a postischemic stricture. Bleeding from the rectum is common with hemorrhoids, diverticular disease, or colitis, but even if such benign diseases are present, the symptoms should not automatically be attributed to them before excluding a malignant disease of the large intestine. Management of acute complications of cancer should not only include strategies to alleviate symptoms and minimize the morbidity of the complication but also to provide an oncologically adequate treatment for the tumor as its cause.

PREOPERATIVE MANAGEMENT

Operative intervention is indicated in most colorectal cancers, even in the presence of metastatic disease, unless there are overwhelming comorbidities. The aim of preoperative studies is to establish the diagnosis, to stage the disease, and to identify relevant comorbidity.

Physical Examination

The history and review of systems should include questions about changes in bowel habits, time of last stool and gas passage, weight loss, and a personal or family history of cancer, particularly of colorectal cancer. Awareness of an individual's genetic predisposition to colorectal cancer is not only of importance for the management of that patient but also for adequate counseling of potentially affected family members.

A careful physical examination aims at identifying any palpable tumor masses. The abdomen is checked for the presence of liver enlargement (for possible liver metastasis), general distention, obstructive tympanitic bowel sounds, and peritoneal signs (for possible tumor perforation). A digital rectal examination followed by a proctoscopy is necessary to determine the distance of a palpable tumor from the dentate line, the circumferential extent of disease, and the mobility of the tumor from the surrounding structures (sacrum, prostate or vagina, anal sphincter muscle), and to check for the presence of blood in the stool. A thorough physical examination is necessary to evaluate the patient's general health with regard to tolerating a major abdominal procedure under general anesthesia.

Particular attention must be paid to patients with acute symptoms in an emergency setting. Prolonged fasting, nausea, vomiting, and third spacing of fluids during a period of bowel obstruction or after a perforation rapidly cause a state of malnutrition and dehydration that requires resuscitation. Developing sepsis or acute and recurrent blood loss aggravates these symptoms and may result in a state of preshock. Volume resuscitation should parallel the clinical assessment of vital parameters. Alarming signals are tachycardia and hypotension, fever,

Table 89–2	TNM Classification and Clinical Tumor Stage		
TNM PARAMETER	**T**	**N**	**M**
0	No tumor	No lymph node (LN) metastases	No distant metastases
IS	Carcinoma in situ		
1	Tumor invades submucosa	1–3 LN metastases	Distant metastases present
2	Tumor invades muscularis propria	4 or more LN metastases	
3	Tumor invades into subserosa but not through serosa *or* invades nonperitonealized pericolic fat tissue		
4	Tumor invades through serosa *or* into contiguous organs		

Stage I: M0 + N0 → T1 or T2
Stage II: M0 + N0 → T3 or T4
Stage III: M0 + (N1 or N2) + any T
Stage IV: M1 + any N + any T

recent weight loss, poor skin turgor, dry oral mucosa, and oliguria. Acidosis and falsely high hematocrit values may reflect the effect of dehydration rather than the effect of blood loss.

Evaluation of the Large Intestine

Endoscopic and radiologic techniques are used to evaluate the colon and rectum. Regardless of the method, the goal is to document the presence and site of the malignant pathology and to exclude concomitant lesions in other segments of the large intestine.

Rigid proctoscopy and flexible sigmoidoscopy both accurately assess rectosigmoidal lesions. Particularly in an outpatient setting, these methods are considered the first-line diagnostic tests because they are rapid, and widely available and require only minimal bowel preparation (enema). The major disadvantage is that these techniques provide no information about the rest of the colon, and therefore a complementary study is needed before operation.

Colonoscopy is the method of choice because its sensitivity in detecting tumors is very high, and biopsy samples can be obtained during the procedure. Furthermore, colonoscopy allows for assessing the circumferential and longitudinal extent as well as the functional aspects (impending obstruction, bleeding source) of a colonic lesion. In addition, it provides information about the status of the remaining mucosa of the entire colon (polyps, synchronous cancer, colitis, melanosis, diverticula). Associated polyps may be removed. Limitations of colonoscopy include the inability to accurately measure the distance from the anal verge, smaller lesions may escape detection, and the cecum may, for technical reasons, not always be reached. However, if an obstructing lesion does not permit the colonoscope to be passed to inspect the proximal colon, placement of a self-expanding Wall-type stent has become a treatment option to temporarily relieve the obstruction and convert an emergency situation into an elective one.

Radiographic contrast enemas can also be used to detect colorectal cancer, most commonly by means of a double-contrast barium-air technique. However, when there is suspicion of a colonic perforation, administration of barium is contraindicated and water-soluble contrast (e.g., Gastrografin) should be used. The typical findings in colon cancer are a fixed filling defect with destroyed mucosal pattern and an annular configuration ("apple core") or an intraluminal mass or filling defect. Advantages of contrast studies are that contrast more easily passes through even severely obstructing lesions and commonly reaches the cecum; disadvantages include the inability to obtain biopsy samples and to detect small lesions. A new technique termed *virtual colonoscopy* uses computed tomography with an air-contrast enema to evaluate the colon. This technique is still largely experimental but appears to be quite sensitive.

Evaluation of Local Extent and Metastatic Dissemination

In cancer of the colon, routine imaging studies such as ultrasonography, CT, and magnetic resonance imaging (MRI) are not essential with regard to the local extent of the tumor because they do not change the local surgical approach. Although also true for mobile and circumscribed lesions of the rectum, the trend toward multimodality and neoadjuvant treatment for rectal cancer has resulted in an increasing tendency to perform more extensive preoperative imaging to stage these cancers. Endorectal ultrasonography (EUS) is highly reliable (high sensitivity and specificity) in determining an accurate T stage but is less so for determining the N stage. In patients with a large or fixed rectal mass, CT or MRI of the abdomen and pelvis may be more effective in determining the extramural extension, especially with regard to invasion of the presacral fascia and other intrapelvic organs.

Transcutaneous abdominal ultrasonography appears equally accurate for a preoperative general evaluation of the abdomen and is more rapid and more widely available than CT or MRI, provided that the radiologist is well trained in ultrasonography and the examination is adequate (minimal colonic gas). Ultrasonography identifies liver metastases, hydronephrosis, and para-aortic lymph node involvement, and it may reveal concomitant diseases such as gallstones, cysts, and ascites. Although CT and MRI provide the same information, they are more expensive and require more infrastructure.

To exclude extrahepatic metastases, a chest x-ray study in two planes is sufficient. Under special circumstances in which the presence of previously unknown tumor manifestations (e.g., recurrence versus scar tissue, solitary versus multiple liver metastases, presence of extrahepatic metastases) would have an impact on the treatment approach (operative versus nonoperative), positron emission tomography (PET) may be indicated. Routine use of PET in the primary management of colorectal cancer, however, is not recommended.

Laboratory Tests

Preoperative laboratory tests aim at providing evidence for pathophysiologic effects of the tumor and to rule out general health problems that would affect the patient's general operability (Table 89–3). A comprehensive workup includes a complete blood count, electrolytes, creatinine/blood urea nitrogen, glucose, selected liver function tests (alkaline phosphatase, aspartate aminotransferase [AST], albumin), coagulation parameters (platelet count, international normalized ratio), and the tumor marker CEA. Arterial blood gas analysis and additional tests are used according to the individual patient's risk assessment.

General Operability

Preoperative standard evaluation includes a chest x-ray study, both for cardiopulmonary assessment and to detect pulmonary metastases (see earlier text). Electrocardiographic and pulmonary function tests (forced vital capacity [FVC], forced expiratory volume in 1 second [FEV_1], residual volume [RV], and diffusion capacity) are indicated in selected patients older than 40 years of age or

Table 89–3	**Focuses of Preoperative Laboratory Tests**		
TEST FOCUS	**TEST CATEGORY**	**ITEM**	**REMARK**
Tumor/disease-specific	Complete blood count	Hct, RBC	Acute/chronic anemia? Preoperative transfusion necessary?
		WBC	Leukocytosis (tumor perforation, urinary tract infection)?
			Leukocytopenia (e.g., after chemotherapy)?
	Kidney function	Creatinine/BUN	Postrenal kidney failure (ureteral obstruction)?
			Prerenal kidney failure (dehydration/shock)?
	Liver function	Alkaline phosphatase, bilirubin	Liver metastases? Liver dysfunction (cirrhosis)?
	Electrolytes	K	Depletion in ileus, after bowel preparation?
	Urinary tract	Urine analysis	Hematuria? Infection?
	Tumor marker	CEA	Complete disappearance after surgery if preoperatively elevated?
Surgical operability	Hemostasis	Platelets	Thrombocytopenia? Dysfunction? Bleeding time? Medication (ASA)?
	Coagulation studies	Platelets, INR	Hemorrhagic diathesis? Increased bleeding risk? Medications (warfarin)?
Anesthesia	Electrolytes	Na, K	Cardiac excitability?
	Kidney function	Creatinine/BUN	Drug clearance?
	Liver function	As above	Drug metabolism?
	Drug levels	E.g., digoxin, antiepileptic medication	Cardiac stability? Interference with hepatic drug metabolism?
	Coagulation studies	As above	Contraindication for epidural anesthesia?
General	Metabolism	Glucose	Diabetes (increased risk)? Insulin and diet management?
	Kidney function	As above	Diet management? Reduced clearance of radiographic contrast?

ASA, aminosalicylic acid; BUN, blood urea nitrogen; CEA, carcinoembryonic antigen; Hct, hematocrit; INR, Interrational Normalized Ratio; RBC, red blood cell count; WBC, white blood cell count.

with a suggestive personal history. Specialized tests such as stress-electrocardiogram, echocardiogram, or interventional cardiologic studies depend on the individual patient's history and risk assessment.

Establishing a Treatment Plan

Almost all colorectal cancers are, in themselves, an indication for operative resection, unless there are contraindications from the patient's overall health status. The goal of treatment is to cure the tumor, extend survival or disease-free survival, or, in a palliative setting, to prolong symptom-free survival. Local tumor control is generally the primary treatment objective to treat local tumor complications (e.g., obstruction, bleeding, pain). Even in the presence of small-volume distant metastases (such as liver or lung metastases), resection of the primary tumor remains a reasonable priority. Because solitary or a limited number of metastases in the liver or lung can often be treated surgically by metastasectomy, with cure rates of up to 35%, their presence should not necessarily alter the surgical approach to the primary site. However, if there are extensive metastases or peritoneal carcinosis, operative cure is not a realistic goal, and alleviation of local complications by restoring the intestinal continuity is the best palliation.

The surgical and oncologic planning must consider location of the tumor, presence of synchronous lesions, underlying colonic disease, tumor stage, extent of the local procedure, and timing. After the operation has been defined, it is reasonable to consider whether the procedure is suitable for a laparotomy approach only or laparoscopy is also reasonable. Particularly in rectal cancer, the potential involvement of other pelvic organs may require preoperative consultation with other medical specialists.

A gynecologic examination or evaluation by a urologist for cystoscopy and preoperative placement of ureteral stents should be considered, and intraoperative teamwork appears to be a rational approach.

Neoadjuvant treatment (preoperative chemoradiation) may provide a benefit to certain subgroups of patients with colorectal cancer, but results from studies are contradictory. Better criteria for selecting patients need to be defined more specifically by future clinical studies. Currently, preoperative chemoradiation is recommended for locally advanced rectal cancer fixed to adjacent structures (such as the sacrum). It should be noted, though, that even if the preoperative treatment has a good response and downstages the tumor, the extent of the surgical procedure should not be altered but should still be determined by the original stage of the tumor.

Adjuvant postoperative treatment is currently recommended for stages III and IV colorectal cancer and consists of 5-fluorouracil (5FU)/leucovorin-based chemotherapy for both colon and rectal cancer, with the addition of radiation therapy for rectal cancer. Further specification of indications for different types of chemotherapy are necessary.

Getting Ready for Surgery

Bowel preparation and antibiotic prophylaxis are an integral part of the preoperative management in elective colorectal surgery to reduce postoperative wound infections or anastomotic leaks. Different regimens (orthograde cleansing alone or combined with retrograde enemas) are a matter of personal preference rather than of objective superiority. Products are based on either polyethylene glycol or sodium phosphate, the latter of which is contraindicated in patients with severe renal dysfunction. Depending on an individual patient's constitution and the degree of obstruction, the bowel cleansing should be started 1 or even 2 days before operation. The cathartic washout causes significant alterations in the patient's fluid and electrolyte balance and may result in nausea and vomiting or an orthostatic collapse. In elderly or infirm subjects, intravenous fluids and potassium, as well as monitoring of the serum electrolytes, are recommended.

Prophylactic administration of antibiotics is commonly provided intravenously, but nonabsorbable antibiotics may also be added to the bowel preparation to reduce the bacterial load. Among several intravenous regimens, a combination of a second- or third-generation cephalosporin (cefoxitin or ceftriaxone) with metronidazole is widely used; alternatively, ciprofloxacin combined with metronidazole is recommended. The optimal timing of administration is 1 to 2 hours before incision, with one dose postoperatively. In regimens for intestinal decontamination, the metronidazole may be given orally instead of intravenously, together with oral neomycin. Special considerations have to be followed for prophylaxis in patients at risk for endocarditis (e.g., patients with a mechanical heart valve).

Placement of a nasogastric tube postoperatively is not necessary on a routine basis for patients undergoing resection of the colon or rectum unless they have a complete or partial bowel obstruction. In patients who may need permanent or temporary placement of an ostomy during the surgical procedure, preoperative marking of the ideal stoma site by a stoma nurse helps to facilitate the postoperative handling by the patient.

Thromboprophylaxis is recommended in patients undergoing major surgical procedures to reduce the incidence of postoperative deep venous thrombosis and pulmonary embolism. Both pharmacologic and physical prophylaxis have proven to be effective. Low-dose unfractionated heparin or low-molecular-weight heparins reduce the development of thromboembolic postoperative complications without significant increase in bleeding complications. They are started preoperatively and continued postoperatively until full ambulation is reached. Alternatively, boots for intraoperative and postoperative pneumatic leg compression have been equally successful and lack the side effects of pharmacologic prophylaxis. Anticoagulated patients who need to be on a medication with warfarin (e.g., patients with a mechanical heart valve) perioperatively should be switched to intravenous heparin to allow for stopping the warfarin medication several days in advance. The heparin may be discontinued 4 hours before incision and resumed postoperatively with a stepwise increase of the dose.

Effective pain management is an important factor in reducing the incidence of postoperative pulmonary complications. Preoperative placement of a preemptive epidural analgesia is a valuable means which, in addition to its pain-relieving effect, promotes the earlier resumption of postoperative bowel function as a result of its suppression of sympathetic nerves. The relevant segments that need to be blocked for an abdominal incision are located at a thoracic level (Th 6 to Th 12). This epidural analgesia can be continued for up to 3 days postoperatively.

INTRAOPERATIVE MANAGEMENT

Surgical treatment for colorectal cancer aims at a wide resection of the tumor together with its vascular pedicle and the regional lymph nodes. Based on the anatomy of the colon, its blood supply, and the lymphatic drainage, a limited number of standard resections have evolved according to the location of the tumor (Table 89–4). Modifications are necessary in an emergency situation or if there is evidence of local or distant metastatic disease.

For procedures that require transanal access to carry out an intrapelvic or coloanal anastomosis or an abdominoperineal resection, the patient is placed on the operating table in a modified lithotomy position. For all other colon resections, a supine position is preferable.

Elective Resection

The optimal access is through a midline laparotomy. If the pelvis has to be exposed, the incision extends from the pubic bone to the umbilicus and may be extended above it with a circumferential incision. For all other resections, the laparotomy begins with a limited periumbilical midline incision, which may be extended on either end if necessary. The abdomen should be explored systematically to determine the extent of the local disease with regard to its resectability. Special attention is required to look for the presence of distant metastases (in the liver or peritoneum), obvious nodal disease, or additional primary lesions throughout the large intestine. Other organs are examined as well, including the gallbladder, retroperitoneum, and, in women, pelvic organs, especially the ovary, which has a predilection for metastases from colon cancer.

The tumor-bearing colon segment is mobilized from the retroperitoneum, and its vascular pedicle is isolated at its origin. Before ligating and dividing these vessels, the ureters have to be identified to ensure that they are not accidentally included in the clamp. Starting from the given landmarks, the mesentery and the major omentum are divided stepwise between pairs of clamps until the colon segment is completely isolated and may be removed. The colonic stumps on both sides are wiped with a disinfectant and anastomosed, usually end-to-end.

For cancer of the rectum, complete pelvic mobilization and a low anterior resection must be carried out, including the entire mesorectum and its lymph nodes (*total mesorectal excision*). This dissection begins with lateral mobilization of the sigmoid colon and identification of the ureters. After the peritoneal reflection is opened widely, the inferior mesenteric artery and vein are identified, divided, and ligated at the level of the left colic artery. With an attempt at preservation of the presacral nerves, the presacral space is entered at the sacral promontory and developed behind the rectum. Anteriorly, the vagina or prostate and seminal vesicles must be mobilized off the rectum using alternating sharp and gentle blunt dissection. Lateral dissection follows the side walls of the pelvis. For tumors in the upper third of the rectum, the dissection is extended at least 5 cm below the tumor, whereas for tumors in the middle or lower third of the

Table 89–4	**Standard Resections of the Colon and Rectum**			

TUMOR LOCATION	RESECTION	DESCRIPTION OF EXTENT	MAJOR BLOOD VESSEL	SAFETY MARGIN
Cecum	Right hemicolectomy	Terminal ileum to beginning of transverse colon, right flexure included	A. colica dextra A. ileocolica	5 cm
Ascending colon	Right hemicolectomy	Terminal ileum to beginning of transverse colon, right flexure included	A. colica dextra A. ileocolica	5 cm
Right colon flexure	Extended right hemicolectomy	Terminal ileum to transverse colon (proximal to left flexure)	A. colica dextra A. ileocolica A. colica media	5 cm
Transverse colon	Transverse colon resection	Transverse colon (including both flexures)	A. colica media	5 cm
Left flexure	Extended left hemicolectomy	Right flexure to descending colon (beginning of rectum)	A. colica media A. colica sinistra A. mesenterica inferior	5 cm
Descending colon	Left hemicolectomy	Left flexure to sigmoid colon (beginning of rectum)	A. colica sinistra A. mesenterica inferior	5 cm
Sigmoid colon	Rectosigmoid resection	Descending colon to rectum	A. mesenterica inferior A. rectalis superior	5 cm
Rectum >8 cm above anal verge	Low anterior rectosigmoid resection	Descending colon to rectum, double-stapling anastomosis	A. mesenterica inferior A. rectalis superior	5 cm
Rectum 3–8 cm above anal verge	Total mesorectal excision (TME)	Sigmoid colon to rectum, double-stapling anastomosis	A. mesenterica inferior A. rectalis superior	5 cm
Rectum 2–3 cm above anal verge	TME + coloanal anastomosis	Sigmoid colon to rectum, coloanal anastomosis, hand-sewn anastomosis	A. mesenterica inferior A. rectalis superior, inferior	2 cm
Rectum <2 cm above anal verge	Abdominoperineal resection	Sigmoid colon to anus, including sphincter/levator muscles, terminal colostomy	A. mesenterica inferior A. rectalis superior, inferior	

rectum the entire mesorectum is mobilized to the pelvic floor. The rectum is most easily transected with a 30-mm linear stapler, and the rectal stump is irrigated to wash out exfoliated cancer cells. The splenic flexure may require mobilization such that the sigmoid or descending colon may reach into the pelvis. The anastomosis must not be under tension and is performed either by transanally inserted circular stapler or by hand. The lower the anastomosis, the easier the technique using mechanical staplers. If there is even minimal tension, any doubt about the blood supply, or concern about anastomotic integrity, then a *protective loop ileostomy* should be created for stool diversion. Placement of one to two closed suction drains into the dependent region of the peritoneum (pelvis) is common practice for anastomoses below the peritoneal reflection.

In patients with a low rectal cancer that impinges on the anal sphincter muscle complex or is fixed to the sphincter muscle, an *abdominoperineal resection* (APR) is inevitable. The same technique is used as before, but the rectum is not transected and the anus is widely excised from below. The descending or sigmoid colon is brought out where the skin was marked preoperatively for an end colostomy.

Early and small rectal cancers (i.e., uT1N0 and possibly uT2N0, based on the endorectal ultrasonography) involving less than one third of the circumference may be treated by *transanal full-thickness excision* of the rectal wall. Because there is no lymph node sampling, there is a potential risk for undertreatment in certain patients. Because the overall risk of local recurrences is somewhat higher than that of formal resection, the place of local treatment and the role of adjuvant treatment need further clarification.

Emergency Resection

Patients requiring an emergency operation for a tumor-related complication (such as ileus, perforation, or massive bleeding) have a higher morbidity and mortality risk than persons in elective conditions. Contributing factors are lack of a mechanical bowel preparation, dehydration, a deranged metabolism, and possible preoperative sepsis. The risks for wound infections and anastomotic leakage are 3 to 6 times higher.

If the cancer is located on the right side of the colon, a resection (*right hemicolectomy* or *extended right hemicolectomy*) with a primary ileocolostomy is generally reasonable, as long as the general condition of the patient is stable and the bowel wall appears healthy. However, if the tumor is located on the left side of the colon, adjustments to the surgical approach seem prudent and include either on-table lavage or performance of a two-stage procedure instead of the elective one-stage approach. The *Hartmann procedure* is a typical example of a two-stage procedure in which the first step consists of a rectosigmoid resection with creation of an end colostomy and a blind rectal stump, which are reanastomosed in the second step, 6 weeks to 6 months later.

Alternatively, in obstructing tumors of the left side, an attempt to de-obstruct the tumor-bearing segment by colonoscopic introduction of a self-expanding metallic stent seems worthwhile. Although there is a small risk of colonic perforation, decompression of the prestenotic colon will convert an emergency situation into an elective setting by allowing several days for stabilizing the patient and performing a bowel preparation to permit primary anastomosis.

Palliation

Because colon cancer will, at some point, result in local symptoms such as large bowel obstruction, lower gastrointestinal bleeding, or tumor perforation, local tumor control is of primary importance, even in the presence of distant metastases. In contrast to the oncologically defined standard resection, a limited segmental resection of the colon is acceptable in patients with incurable metastatic disease. In particular, tumors located in the sigmoid colon or in the cecum and ascending colon are suitable for a laparoscopic or laparoscopically assisted resection because these segments are easy to mobilize to a sufficient extent to ensure a limited and safe anastomosis. If a tumor is locally too advanced to be safely resectable (e.g., infiltration of other organs) in a patient with metastatic disease, palliation may be achieved by creating a bypass such as an enterocolostomy.

Rectal cancer presenting as inoperable primary or recurrent pelvic disease may require diversion of the proximal colon. To avoid retention of mucus and formation of a mucocele in the rectum proximal to the tumor but distal to the stoma as the tumor completely occludes its distal end, a proximal mucous fistula or loop sigmoidostomy is the method of choice and may be created either by a minilaparotomy or with a laparoscopically assisted approach.

Special Situations

When synchronous cancers are present in the colon, an extended resection or even a total abdominal colectomy, with only one anastomosis, should be strongly considered. Occasionally, two separate resections (e.g., right hemicolectomy and low anterior resection) and anastomoses are preferable in elderly or infirm patients to avoid postcolectomy diarrhea. Cancer occurring in patients with an underlying pancolonic disease (e.g., ulcerative colitis, familial adenomatous polyposis [FAP]) requires a total proctocolectomy with either an ileoanal pull-through procedure or an end ileostomy. Whenever a stage II/T4 or stage III rectal cancer is suspected under these circumstances, neoadjuvant treatment is preferable to postoperative radiation of a newly created ileal J-pouch.

Unexpected intraoperative findings include locally advanced disease and presence of distant tumor spread. Liver metastases requiring a more formal resection than a simple wedge-type metastasectomy should be addressed in a second procedure unless there is clear evidence that they are not resectable. Isolated peritoneal tumor implantations should be resected if feasible, not necessarily with curative intent but rather to prevent location complications. Local primary or recurrent disease may be advanced with infiltration of the abdominal wall or adjacent organs (bladder, ureters, uterus, vagina). If the disease is not yet widespread and a complete macroscopic removal of the tumor appears achievable, an extension of the procedure may be reasonable. Even a hysterectomy, partial or complete resection of the vagina, bladder, or a ureter, or unilateral nephrectomy (pelvic exenteration) is a realistic option.

Laparoscopy for Colon Cancer

Despite the accumulating data on the use of laparoscopy for curative resections in colon cancer, concerns remain as to whether the laparoscopic technique would adversely influence the incidence or patterns of cancer recurrence. Since 1990, six randomized studies have been initiated throughout the world, the largest being a multicenter study by the National Cancer Institute. This study will eventually enroll a total of 1200 patients with stages I to III colon cancer, half of whom have already been included at publication of this book. Until the results of that study become available, we will not perform laparoscopic colon resections for cancer with a curative intent unless as part of a clinical trial. In a palliative setting, however, it is reasonable to remove the primary tumor by a laparoscopic resection.

For a laparoscopic procedure, three to four trocars are inserted. The colon should be mobilized to the same extent as during open surgery. The vascular pedicle is identified and transected. Although the technical equipment to perform an intracorporeal resection and anastomosis is available, it is questionable whether there is any advantage because, at some point, an incision must be made to retrieve the specimen. In a laparoscopically assisted technique, the mobilized segment is exteriorized through a small abdominal incision and an extra-abdominal resection and an anastomosis are performed. The anastomosis is returned to the abdomen, the fascia is closed, and the pneumoperitoneum is reestablished so the peritoneal cavity may be inspected again.

POSTOPERATIVE MANAGEMENT

Monitoring and Fluid Management

In the postoperative period, intensive care unit monitoring may be preferable in certain patients, based on advanced age, severe cardiopulmonary disease, massive overweight, emergency operation, intraoperative complications, and prolonged operative time.

Daily weighting and records of all fluids administered and of all fluid losses (blood, drains, tubes, urine, and ostomy output) should be maintained to calculate the net fluid balance. In addition, the quality of these fluids, particularly whether they are bloody, sanguineous, serosanguineous, serous, clear, or cloudy, may be a key clue to postoperative complications.

Postoperative administration of intravenous fluids is based on maintenance needs and the replacement of losses and should result in a sufficient urinary output (>0.5 mL/kg per hour).

Pain Control

Adequate pain control is of utmost importance for the patient's comfort and to reduce respiratory complications (atelectasis, pneumonia). Excellent pain control is achieved by epidural analgesia, preferably placed preoperatively with preoperative preemptive analgesia (low-dose neural blockade given before the incision) or a patient-controlled analgesia. Incentive spirometry, chest physical therapy, and bronchodilator treatment in patients at risk are part of the standard supportive care.

Thromboembolic Prophylaxis and Activity

As discussed earlier, prevention of deep vein thrombosis and pulmonary embolism requires prophylactic mechanical or pharmacologic means. These interventions should be initiated preoperatively and continued thereafter. Early ambulation must be reinforced with the patient and should be initiated postoperatively as soon as possible.

Management of Drains, Catheters, and Tubes

The epidural catheter is removed after 3 days or whenever the analgesic effectiveness is in doubt. The urinary catheter should be kept in place in men at least for the same duration because the epidural analgesia increases the likelihood of urinary retention; in women, it can be removed earlier.

Wound drains need to be specified with regard to the type of drainage (e.g., gravity, bulb suction, continuous or intermittent wall suction). Their content may indicate complications such as bleeding or fistulas. Pelvic drains are usually left in place until the first bowel movement has occurred. At that time, and if the content remains clear, they may be removed regardless of the amount of fluid drained in a 24-hour period.

A nasogastric tube is not required for colorectal procedures unless the patient had an ileus. When used, the tube is left under intermittent suction until the overall output is less than 200 to 400 mL in a 24-hour period. In the absence of nausea or vomiting, the tube may alternatively be clamped for 4- to 6-hour periods and opened to determine the residual amount per interval of gastric retention.

Diet

Patients should initially have nothing by mouth. Ice chips and oral medications taken with small sips of water are acceptable. Around the second postoperative day, oral clear liquids are allowed as tolerated and may then be advanced to full liquids. If there is no abdominal distention and the bowels start working, the diet can be advanced to a soft or regular diet.

Medications

Essential preoperative medications (particularly cardiovascular) should be resumed as needed. Prophylaxis for stress ulcer with proton pump inhibitors is almost routine for patients at risk (patients on steroids, in an intensive care unit, or who have had prolonged hypotension). True stress ulcers currently are distinctly unusual. Other medications and stool softeners should not be ordered on a routine basis but should be used selectively. Rectal suppositories or enemas are contraindicated after a low anterior resection. For promotion of bowel activity, prokinetic drugs (erythromycin, metoclopramide, neostigmine) may be used in selected patients, but they have not been shown to improve the rate of bowel function return when used routinely.

Laboratory Tests and Imaging

Postoperative evaluation includes a complete blood count and a basic electrolyte screen to determine the extent of intraoperative blood loss, to enhance electrolyte and fluid management, and to detect infective complications. The schedule should be individualized but should include one test early postoperatively (6 to 24 hours), one after 2 to 3 days, and one before discharge. Additional tests depend on the individual's course and risk. Chest radiographs or other imaging studies are ordered as needed but not on a routine basis. Contrast studies for assessment of the anastomosis are usually used only if a leak is suspected; water-soluble contrast should be used.

Clinical Management

Daily assessment of the abdomen and the bowel activity is crucial. Palpation and auscultation check for peritoneal signs and bowel sounds. The incision must be checked daily for induration, redness, dehiscence, or discharge of fluids (pus, hematoma, or serosanguineous fluids). Large amounts of serous fluids should not be mistaken for a seroma but indicate a fascial dehiscence until the contrary is proven. An ostomy should be checked for viability and for the quality and quantity of the output. The average length of stay depends on the patient's constitution but generally ranges between 5 and 7 days. Resumption of bowel movements and tolerance of a regular diet are expected before a patient is discharged. Before discharge, further treatment should be defined and should include a schedule for follow-up visits and an assumed date for the initiation of a postoperative adjuvant treatment if necessary. Chemotherapy or radiation therapy is typically not initiated before 3 weeks after operation and may be delayed if infective complications or an anastomotic leak has occurred.

COMPLICATIONS

Postoperative bleeding may occur at any time but is more frequent in the first 2 days. Complications in the early postoperative period (postoperative days 1 to 3) are more commonly related to the cardiopulmonary system and include cardiac events (e.g., arrhythmia, myocardial ischemia, or cardiac dysfunction) and pulmonary problems (e.g., atelectasis, pneumonia, aspiration, or pulmonary embolism). The latter conditions are often promoted by insufficient pain control and low-volume, inadequate respiration. High temperature in the first 2 days is more commonly related to atelectasis than to early infection.

Pearls and Pitfalls

- If a left-sided colon obstruction does not allow inspection of the rest of the colon, synchronous lesions may be missed and necessitate a second operation within a short period of time. Intraoperative colonoscopy, careful palpation of the proximal colon, or subtotal colectomy are preventive.
- Anastomosis under tension and poor blood supply may result in an anastomotic leak and cause pelvic infection and sepsis. Protective diverting ostomy does not prevent the leak as such, but its life-threatening complication. If surgery is necessary for secondary creation of an ostomy because of a leak, an attempt to close or drain the leak should be undertaken.
- Too much tension for mobilization of colon flexure can result in a tear in the splenic capsule, leading to hemorrhage. Good exposure and avoidance of too much tension are preventive.
- Injury to the presacral vein plexus can result in pelvic hemorrhage. Subtle technique and good hemostasis are preventive, and pelvic drains are recommended to avoid accumulation of pelvic hematoma, with risk of anastomotic impairment and secondary infection.
- If the ureter is not properly identified before dividing the vascular pedicle, accidental dissection of the ureter can occur and requires repair. If unrecognized intraoperatively, the ureter injury may result in a urinoma. In difficult cases (repeat operation, recurrence), preoperative placement of stents allows better identification.
- Bladder injury can result in a urinary leak. Leaks at the bladder dome should be repaired. Leaks in the bladder triangle increase the risk of ureteral damage and should therefore be repaired under direct vision after opening the bladder.
- Injury to the presacral nerve plexus may result in postoperative urinary retention and sexual dysfunction. Intraoperative identification of the nerves is preventive. The use of a nerve stimulator may be helpful.
- Tumor in the re-resection margin results an insufficient cancer operation requiring re-resection. Intraoperative frozen sections of the resection margins and stapler rings ensures cancer-free margins.
- Resection planning according to postchemoradiation stage, instead of original stage, may leave tumor islets at the original tumor margin, increasing incidence of local recurrence. Downstaging is not suitable for better resectability.

Infective complications are usually expected after the third postoperative day and may be located in the wound, urinary tract, or lungs. Workup includes bacteriologic cultures, blood and urine analysis, and a chest radiograph.

Abdominal complications include prolonged postoperative bowel dysfunction (ileus), fascial dehiscence, and anastomotic leakage, the last of which has its typical onset after postoperative days 5 to 6. Increasing abdominal pain, increasing white blood cell counts or C-reactive protein, and persistence of subdiaphragmatic air after 7 to 10 days should raise the index of suspicion; discharge of stool through drainages is sufficient proof. Management of small anastomotic leaks may be conservative, using intravenous antibiotics, whereas significant leaks require reexploration and probably proximal diversion of stool.

OUTCOMES

The operative mortality rate within 30 days is less than 1% after elective colorectal resections but increases to 20% after emergency operations. Morbidity rates include: hemorrhage, 4% to 5%; wound infections and abscess formation, 3% to 12%; sexual dysfunction after pelvic resections, 20% to 50%; and bladder dysfunction. Anastomotic complications occur in 2% to 5% of patients after colonic anastomoses and in 5% to 10% of patients after pelvic resections and low rectal anastomoses.

The 5-year survival rates after curative resection of colorectal cancer are 80% to 90% for stage I, 50% to 70% for stages II and III, and 5% to 10% for stage IV disease. The 5-year survival rate for all stages together is in the range of 50% to 60%. Aggressive resection for a local recurrence has a cure rate approaching 20% to 30% and controls symptoms in 70% of patients.

SELECTED READINGS

Beart RW: Prevention and management of recurrent rectal cancer. World J Surg 1991;15:589.

Carriquiry LA, Pineyro A: Should carcinoembryonic antigen be used in the management of patients with colorectal cancer? Dis Colon Rectum 1999;42:921.

DeHaas-Kock DF, Baeten CG, Jager JJ, et al: Prognostic significance of radial margins of clearance in rectal cancer. Br J Surg 1996;83:781.

Heriot AG, Grundy A, Kumar D: Preoperative staging of rectal carcinoma. Br J Surg 1999;86:17.

Jain SK, Peppercorn MA: Inflammatory bowel disease and colon cancer: A review. Dig Dis 1997;15:243.

Lipkin M, Reddy B, Newmark H, Lamprecht SA: Dietary factors in human colorectal cancer. Annu Rev Nutr 1999;19:545.

Nivatvongs S, Rojanasakul A, Reiman HM, et al: The risk of lymph node metastasis in colorectal polyps with invasive adenocarcinoma. Dis Colon Rectum 1991;34:323.

Ooi BS, Tjandra JJ, Green MD: Morbidities of adjuvant chemotherapy and radiotherapy for resectable rectal cancer: An overview. Dis Colon Rectum 1999;42:403.

Varma MG, Rogers SJ, Schrock TR, Welton ML: Local excision of rectal carcinoma. Arch Surg 1999;134:863.

Wallis Y, MacDonald F: The genetics of inherited colon cancer. J Clin Pathol Clin Mol Pathol 1996;49:M65.

Wheeler JM, Warren BF, Jones AC, Mortensen NJ: Preoperative radiotherapy for rectal cancer: Implications for surgeons, pathologists and radiologists. Br J Surg 1999;86:1108.

Chapter 90
Pseudomyxoma Peritonei

Stephen E. Ettinghausen and Rory R. Dalton

Pseudomyxoma peritonei (PMP) is a rare clinical condition in which mucinous material produced by an adenoma or low-grade adenocarcinoma of the appendix accumulates in the peritoneal cavity. PMP is part of a spectrum of disseminated intraperitoneal tumors that include peritoneal carcinomatosis from higher grade appendiceal and other gastrointestinal carcinomas, ovarian neoplasms, primary peritoneal mesotheliomas, peritoneal sarcomatosis, and primary peritoneal tumors. Any of these conditions may, at least initially, be mistakenly identified as PMP. Although PMP was once considered to be uniformly fatal, recent reports of improved survival outlooks with aggressive cytoreductive surgery and intraperitoneal chemotherapy have resulted in renewed interest in this fascinating condition.

PATHOGENESIS

The gelatinous material characteristic of PMP is produced by the neoplastic epithelium of an underlying appendiceal adenoma or low-grade carcinoma. This appears to be true even for some women formerly thought to have mucinous low-malignant potential tumors of the ovary with extra-ovarian spread. For PMP to occur, the mucinous material must gain access to the peritoneal cavity by obstruction and rupture or invasion through the wall of the appendix. The mucinous material is then "redistributed" throughout the peritoneal cavity in a reproducible pattern based on the normal flow of peritoneal fluid.

Cellular and mucinous material first localizes to the right lower quadrant and pelvic cul-de-sac, presumably the result of free intraperitoneal spread to dependent regions of the peritoneal cavity. Subsequently, the right subdiaphragmatic space and eventually the entire greater and lesser sacs may be filled with gelatinous material. Although in some areas the neoplastic cells may be, to varying degrees, locally invasive, the mucinous material is only loosely attached to the visceral peritoneal surfaces. The fact that acellular mucinous material may be "wiped away" from the small intestine while underlying neoplastic cells may be more adherent to the peritoneal surfaces in other areas accounts for the unique characteristics of this condition.

Varying definitions of PMP have contributed to confusion regarding the results of treatment. Recent pathologic studies have clearly demonstrated that patients with mucinous ascites from higher grade neoplasms (as determined by examination of the primary tumor or the epithelial cells disseminated throughout the peritoneal cavity) can be separated from those patients with gelatinous mucinous material and benign or "low-grade" neoplastic epithelium. The former group of patients could more properly be thought of as having "peritoneal carcinomato-

sis" and the latter as having "true" PMP. Of note, the histologic finding of a mucinous adenocarcinoma that does not produce mucus, particularly of the signet ring cell type, should not be confused with the clinical syndrome of PMP.

CLINICAL PRESENTATION

PMP may present as abdominal distention from the gelatinous material, a pelvic mass, or an abdominal wall hernia. PMP may be detected on computed tomography (CT) of the abdomen and pelvis or may be discovered at operation for presumed appendicitis, appendiceal tumor, or an inguinal hernia found to contain gelatinous material. In the absence of prior surgical procedures, a focal point of intestinal obstruction suggests a high-grade tumor and peritoneal carcinomatosis rather than PMP. If detected early, only small amounts of mucinous material may be found in the right lower quadrant and pelvic cul-de-sac. One remarkable characteristic of the patients with massive abdominal distention is the lack of a focal point of gastrointestinal obstruction; gelatinous material simply compresses the entire gastrointestinal tract. Early satiety and reflux disease develop, and patients modify their eating behavior and lose muscle mass but not weight as they reduce their intake while accumulating PMP. Usually, the process is ongoing for many months (or even years) before diagnosis.

PREOPERATIVE ASSESSMENT

Unlike serous ascites, the viscosity of the gelatinous material may prevent successful paracentesis for biochemical and cytologic examination. Barium enema examination or colonoscopy can establish an adenocarcinoma of the colon as the source of peritoneal carcinomatosis. In women, it may be impossible to distinguish ovarian cancer with peritoneal carcinomatosis from PMP before operation, and careful pathologic study of the ovaries, appendix, and the material removed from the peritoneal cavity is imperative. Almost by definition, PMP does not present with hematogenous hepatic, pulmonary, or other distant metastases.

CT of the chest, abdomen, and pelvis with intravenous and oral contrast is essential. Special techniques have been described for contrast administration to carefully evaluate the gastrointestinal tract in these patients, including the administration of up to 1200 mL of oral contrast at least 6 hours before CT. This technique allows for an accurate preoperative assessment of the involvement of the small intestine by the neoplastic process. Relative "sparing" of the small bowel demonstrated by

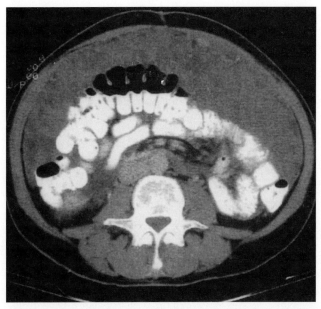

Figure 90–1. Abdominal CT demonstrating the gelatinous material characteristic of PMP. The mucinous material characteristically accumulates in and around the omentum with little material present between loops of bowel. (From Jacquet P, Jelinek JS, Chang D, et al: Abdominal computed tomographic scan in the selection of patients with mucinous peritoneal carcinomatosis for cytoreductive surgery. J Am Coll Surg 1995;181:530, with permission.)

CT suggests that complete cytoreduction may be possible (Fig. 90–1). For patients in whom CT demonstrates small bowel and mesentery surrounded by tumor (either from invasion or scarring from prior surgical procedures), complete cytoreduction is unlikely (Fig. 90–2).

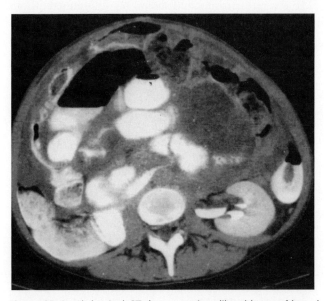

Figure 90–2. Abdominal CT demonstrating dilated loops of bowel and mucinous material between loops of bowel. This may result from the presence of higher grade invasive tumor or from adhesion formation from prior operation. (From Jacquet P, Jelinek JS, Chang D, et al: Abdominal computed tomographic scan in the selection of patients with mucinous peritoneal carcinomatosis for cytoreductive surgery. J Am Coll Surg 1995;181:530, with permission.)

NATURAL HISTORY

Until the recent descriptions of aggressive cytoreductive surgery and intraperitoneal chemotherapy, PMP was nearly uniformly fatal; one report indicated a 14% 5-year survival rate. Palliative measures such as partial cytoreduction and intestinal bypass were sometimes undertaken late in the disease process in an attempt to allow for improved gastrointestinal function. Such procedures were usually unrewarding, with only transient relief of obstruction and continued inanition and death from starvation.

CYTOREDUCTIVE SURGERY

The primary treatment of PMP is complete surgical cytoreduction. At operation, the difference between the gelatinous, relatively acellular material characteristic of PMP ("jelly belly") and the hard, fibrotic cellular material of peritoneal carcinomatosis is remarkable and clearly unforgettable. A careful abdominal exploration reveals the distribution of the mucinous material. The exploration must be extremely thorough because even small amounts of material can travel to every tiny recess of the greater and lesser sacs. The gelatinous, mucinous material will "wipe away" from the visceral and parietal peritoneal surfaces, whereas the solid cellular component is locally invasive and must be "stripped" from parietal peritoneal surfaces and may require resection of adjacent intra-abdominal structures. Use of the Cavitron ultrasonic aspirator (CUSA) for peritoneal débridement may facilitate debulking.

The technically demanding and time-consuming surgical procedures used to radically strip or excise the entire peritoneal surface have been developed and pioneered by Sugarbaker. Complete resection of the entire peritoneal surface may require splenectomy, colectomy, and, in women, hysterectomy. In some patients, the volume of intraperitoneal gelatinous material is so great that the procedure must be completed in two stages. Nasogastric suction and parenteral nutritional support may be required for up to 2 to 3 weeks in patients with large volumes of tumor who have required all of the peritonectomy procedures and have received intraoperative chemotherapy. The recurrence rate for patients after a "complete" cytoreduction is approximately 30% to 35%, with most recurrences appearing in the first 2 to 3 years.

INTRAPERITONEAL CHEMOTHERAPY

Postoperative intraperitoneal chemotherapy has been administered to patients after complete cytoreductive surgery in an attempt to prevent intraperitoneal recurrence resulting from residual microscopic disease. Intraperitoneal chemotherapy exposes residual tumor cells to greater concentrations of drug than can be achieved by intravenous infusion. When combined with cytoreductive surgery leaving either no gross evidence of disease or tumor nodules only millimeters in diameter, problems of drug diffusion are minimized. Despite the well-known effects of chemotherapy on anastomotic healing, most patients tolerate this type of intraperitoneal chemotherapy well.

Postoperative intraperitoneal chemotherapy can be administered safely to patients through indwelling peritoneal dialysis catheters and surgical drains placed at the time of cytoreduction. To prevent occlusion of these drains, the peritoneal cavity should be continuously irrigated by warmed peritoneal dialysate beginning immediately after abdominal closure. Treatment may begin 24 hours after cytoreduction. One regimen includes mitomycin C on day 1 and 5-fluorouracil on days 2 to 5. The selected volume (1000 to 1500 mL) and dose of chemotherapy is infused by gravity and allowed to remain in the peritoneal cavity for 24 hours. The fluid is drained 1 hour before instillation of the next treatment. This cycle is repeated for subsequent treatments. With a similar regimen, the morbidity rate of cytoreductive surgery and postoperative intraperitoneal chemotherapy was 37% (with no deaths). Postoperative adynamic ileus lasted a median of 21 days. A careful analysis of the patterns of recurrence in such patients concluded that the well-known problems of drug distribution within the peritoneal cavity continue to limit the effectiveness of postoperative intraperitoneal chemotherapy.

INTRAOPERATIVE HYPERTHERMIC PERITONEAL PERFUSION

Intraoperative hyperthermic peritoneal perfusion (IHPP) is a more recent technique used in the treatment of peritoneal carcinomatosis and PMP. In this setting, a closed perfusion circuit is established after the completion of cytoreductive surgery, and heated chemotherapy is cycled through the peritoneal cavity for 1 to 2 hours. Conceptually, the addition of hyperthermia (with the infusate heated to 46°C to 48°C) results in additional tumor cell kill, and the intraoperative administration of chemotherapy allows the surgeon to minimize problems of drug distribution. Studies indicate that this procedure is technically feasible with morbidity and mortality rates (35% and 5%, respectively) similar to those of cytoreductive surgery with postoperative intraperitoneal chemotherapy. Careful monitoring of patient core temperature is essential to prevent complications from hyperthermia. The mean time for cytoreductive surgery and IHPP is 11 hours (range, 5 to 19 hours). Whether the long-term outcome is truly superior to postoperative intraperitoneal chemotherapy or to complete cytoreduction alone cannot be determined with any degree of certainty because no prospective, randomized clinical trials have been published. Because of the magnitude and complexity of this treatment, this procedure is under investigation at only a few centers with extensive experience with PMP and peritoneal carcinomatosis.

RESULTS OF CYTOREDUCTIVE SURGERY AND INTRAPERITONEAL CHEMOTHERAPY

In many patients, the differentiation of PMP from higher grade tumors with peritoneal carcinomatosis cannot be made with certainty before operation. As a result, most reports contain a heterogeneous group of patients. In one careful analysis of prognostic factors done by Sugarbaker and Jablonski (1995), complete cytoreduction, low-grade tumors, appendiceal primary tumors, and absence of regional lymph node metastases predicted better outcomes. Patients with low-grade primary appendiceal tumors, no lymph node metastases, and complete cytoreductive surgery were reported to have a 99% 3-year overall survival rate. In these patients, disease-free survival would be expected to be approximately 65%. The presence of nodal metastases or higher grade tumors reduced 3-year survival rates to 65% and 66%, respectively. Patients with grossly incomplete cytoreduction were reported to have a 20% 3-year survival rate. Interestingly, a large volume of intraperitoneal tumor is not a negative prognostic factor for patients with "true" PMP but is a negative prognostic factor for patients with colon cancers and peritoneal carcinomatosis.

Several recent reports have indicated that 5- and 10-year survival rates of 53% to 75% and 34% to 60%, respectively, can be obtained with the aggressive treatment described. Few, if any, of these reports have carefully separated patients with "true" PMP from patients with peritoneal carcinomatosis. Sugarbaker has the largest personal experience and has reported an overall 5-year survival rate of 69% (in 288 patients) with a 72% overall survival rate for patients with a complete cytoreduction and a zero 5-year survival rate for patients with an incomplete cytoreduction. Although the completeness of the cytoreductive surgery appears to be an important prognostic factor, whether this is a truly independent variable or in part reflects the underlying biologic aggressiveness of the tumor remains unresolved.

Summary

PMP is a rare disorder and should be differentiated from peritoneal carcinomatosis secondary to gastrointestinal or

---

Pearls and Pitfalls

PEARLS

- Pseudomyxoma peritonei is rare: peritoneal carcinomatosis from colon cancer and ovarian cancer are more common causes of disseminated intraperitoneal tumor and represent a different disorder.
- Aggressive treatment involves an extensive surgical cytoreduction with postoperative intraperitoneal chemotherapy.
- Patients with low-grade appendiceal neoplasms and no regional lymph node metastases ("true PMP") who undergo a complete cytoreduction appear to derive the greatest benefit from this aggressive treatment plan (3-year survival rates approaching 95%).
- Carcinomatosis from adenocarcinomas without mucinous production should not be confused with pseudomyxoma peritonei.
- Because the completeness of cytoreductive surgery appears to be an important prognostic factor, these rare patients should be referred to centers that have an interest in this disease before multiple incomplete cytoreductions are performed.

ovarian primary tumors. Patients with low-grade appendiceal neoplasms and no regional lymph node metastases ("true PMP") who undergo a complete cytoreduction appear to derive the greatest benefit from this aggressive treatment plan. Because the completeness of cytoreductive surgery appears to be an important prognostic factor, these rare patients should be referred to centers with an interest in this disease before multiple incomplete cytoreductions are performed.

SELECTED READINGS

Alexander HR, Fraker DL: Treatment of peritoneal carcinomatosis by continuous hyperthermic peritoneal perfusion with cisplatin. Cancer Treat Res 1996;81:41.

Gough DB, Donohue JH, Schutt AJ, et al: Pseudomyxoma peritonei. Long-term patient survival with an aggressive regional approach. Ann Surg 1994;219:112.

Hinson FL, Ambrose NSL: Pseudomyxoma peritonei. Br J Surg 1998;85:1332.

Jacquet P, Jelinek JS, Chang D, et al: Abdominal computed tomographic scan in the selection of patients with mucinous peritoneal carcinomatosis for cytoreductive surgery [published erratum appears in J Am Coll Surg 1996;182:80]. J Am Coll Surg 1995;181:530.

Jacquet P, Stephens AD, Averbach AM, et al: Analysis of morbidity and mortality in 60 patients with peritoneal carcinomatosis treated by cytoreductive surgery and heated intraoperative intraperitoneal chemotherapy. Cancer 1996;77:2622.

Ronnett BM, Zahn CM, Kurman RJ, et al: Disseminated peritoneal adenomucinosis and peritoneal mucinous carcinomatosis. A clinicopathologic analysis of 109 cases with emphasis on distinguishing pathologic features, site of origin, prognosis, and relationship to "pseudomyxoma peritonei." Am J Surg Pathol 1995;19:1390.

Sugarbaker PH: Peritonectomy procedures. Ann Surg 1995;221:29.

Sugarbaker PH, Jablonski KA: Prognostic features of 51 colorectal and 130 appendiceal cancer patients with peritoneal carcinomatosis treated by cytoreductive surgery and intraperitoneal chemotherapy [see comments]. Ann Surg 1995;221:124.

Zoetmulder FA, Sugarbaker PH: Patterns of failure following treatment of pseudomyxoma peritonei of appendiceal origin. Eur J Cancer 1996;32A:1727.

Chapter 91
Anal Cancer

Michael P. Spencer

Anal neoplasms remain relatively rare tumors, accounting for approximately 2500 cases or less than 2% of all malignancies in the United States in 2000. Anal tumors are much less common than tumors of the colon and rectum, but the clinical significance of this diverse group of lesions exceeds that predicted by numbers alone. Given the nature of these tumors, the diagnosis is frequently delayed; additionally, anatomic constraints and increased efforts to preserve continence further restricts local surgical options. Most historical reviews have suggested a predilection of anal cancer for women in their sixth or seventh decade. More recent studies, however, particularly those from urban centers, have noted an increased incidence in young male patients. Lesions of the anal canal outnumber tumors of the anal margin overall; however, neoplasms of the anal margin are more likely to develop in men than in women. Even though numerous factors have been implicated in the etiology of anal cancer, a history of chronic inflammatory conditions and sexually transmitted disease (specifically genital warts) are associated with an increased incidence of anal cancer. Epithelial dysplasia or anal intraepithelial neoplasia (AIN) is recognized as a precursor lesion of anal cancer, and AIN has been reported with increased frequency in individuals with human papillomavirus and human immunodeficiency virus (HIV) infections.

CLINICAL PRESENTATION

Diagnosis and treatment of anal cancers is often delayed because the most common symptoms—bleeding, discharge, tenesmus, pruritus, and anal mass—are usually attributed to other benign disorders such as hemorrhoids. The presence of pain and urgency with defecation, incontinence, passage of gas or stool through a perianal or vaginal fistula portends advanced disease. Inguinal adenopathy and pain are likewise indications of metastatic involvement. On occasion, tumors are identified as an incidental finding after hemorrhoidectomy or excision of an anal tag. These patients often require re-excision to document complete removal. For these reasons, histologic evaluation, and even frozen section, should be requested of any suspicious tissues. It is imperative that both orientation and location of these lesions are well documented in case a positive margin is identified. Because anal cancers are often difficult to distinguish from benign conditions clinically, the physician must suspect neoplasia in any chronic perianal condition that has failed to respond to traditional methods. Judicious use of a punch biopsy or excisional biopsy most often confirms the diagnosis.

Histologically, the anal canal is composed of three regions. The proximal epithelium above the dentate line is columnar, whereas that below is stratified squamous epithelium but with a 6- to 12-mm intervening transitional zone, also referred as the cloacogenic region. This diversity of tissue over only a few centimeters distance gives rise to the variety of neoplasms identified in the anal canal.

PREOPERATIVE MANAGEMENT

Because cancers of the anal margin and anal canal are managed differently and have disparate outcomes, it is incumbent upon the surgeon to distinguish these lesions accurately. The literature has been inconsistent as to the classification of anal tumors, however, and this confusion has made comparisons of studies suspect and has certainly confounded outcomes. Most researchers agree on the standard definition set forth by the World Health Organization that defines anal margin tumors as those arising from the skin outside the anal verge. Anal canal tumors occur between the anal verge and the proximal aspect of the anal canal along the superior border of the sphincter complex (Fig. 91–1).

The dentate line is an additional landmark of significance for neoplasms of the anal canal. Lesions cephalad to the dentate line drain toward the superior rectal lymphatics to the inferior mesenteric nodes and laterally along the middle and inferior rectal vessels. Lesions distal to the dentate line drain toward the inguinal lymphatics,

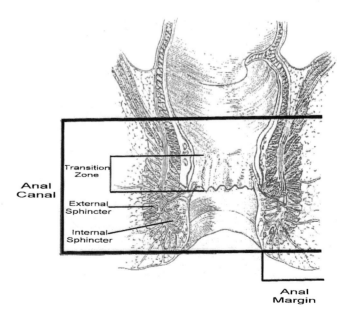

Figure 91–1. Anatomy of the anal canal, beginning at the superior border of the sphincter complex and extending distally to the hair-bearing tissue of the anal margin.

whereas neoplasms traversing the dentate line can disseminate along one or both pathways.

Accurate staging of anal cancers has obvious implications as to treatment regimens and long-term prognosis. A thorough physical examination and imaging studies, including computed tomography, magnetic resonance imaging, and endorectal ultrasonography, are useful in assessing depth of invasion and possible nodal involvement. Physical examination with emphasis on fixation, location, and possible extension to adjacent tissue is critical. Inspection of the entire perianal region for additional pathology along with abdominal examination and palpation of the groins for adenopathy is also warranted. Anoscopy, proctosigmoidoscopy, or both are useful in verifying the exact location of anal tumors relative to the dentate line but cannot provide information regarding depth of invasion. Endorectal ultrasonography is the most sensitive tool in determining the T stage or depth of involvement. Most recently, sentinel node mapping has been advocated for tumors of the distal anal canal and anal margin, purportedly optimizing identification of inguinal node involvement and minimizing the morbidity of a complete formal groin dissection.

The TNM (tumor, node, metastases) staging system for anal cancers (Table 91–1) is based on size and extent of invasion of the primary tumor as well as nodal involvement and presence of distant metastases.

OPERATIVE MANAGEMENT

Neoplasms of the Anal Canal

Epidermoid Carcinoma

Epidermoid tumors originate in the anal canal or the transitional zone and my exhibit squamous, basaloid, mucoepidermoid, or cloacogenic histology. Collectively, these tumors respond similarly and their clinical presentation, management, and prognosis parallel one another. Although etiology and presentation vary slightly with the differing histologies, the treatment options remain the same and include local excision, abdominoperineal resection (APR), and radiation plus chemotherapy (Table 91–2). A dramatic transition has occurred over the past 2 decades from radical operative excision toward local excision with sphincter preservation and maintenance of intestinal continuity. Primary APR has been associated with cure rates between 24% and 71% for node-negative patients. Because multimodality therapy provides equal or superior survival and more acceptable patient expectations, APR has been relegated to a second-line treatment reserved primarily for salvage procedures or recurrent disease. In that most patients undergoing APR are being treated for recurrent or persistent disease, they often require wider margins of resection that may necessitate reconstructive techniques to close the defect or reconstitute the vagina or pelvic floor.

Local excision for tumors confined to the mucosa and submucosa is usually curative. Lesions invading into the muscularis propria or internal sphincter are also amenable

Table 91–1	**Anal Canal Cancers: TNM Staging Classification**

Primary Tumor (T)

TX	Primary tumor cannot be assessed
T0	No evidence of primary tumor
Tis	Carcinoma in situ
T1	Tumor 2 cm or less in greatest dimension
T2	Tumor more than 2 cm, but not more than 5 cm, in greatest dimension
T3	Tumor more than 5 cm in greatest dimension
T4	Tumor of any size invades adjacent organ(s); for example, vagina, urethra, bladder—involvement of sphincter muscle(s) alone is not classified as T4

Regional Lymph Nodes (N)

NX	Regional lymph nodes cannot be assessed
N0	No regional lymph node metastasis
N1	Metastasis in perirectal lymph node(s)
N2	Metastasis in unilateral internal iliac and/or inguinal lymph nodes
N3	Metastasis in perirectal and inguinal lymph nodes and/or bilateral internal iliac and/or inguinal lymph nodes

Distant Metastasis (M)

MX	Distant metastasis cannot be assessed
M0	No distant metastasis
M1	Distant metastasis

STAGE GROUPING

0	Tis	N0	M0
I	T1	N0	M0
II	T2	N0	M0
	T3	N0	M0
IIIA	T1	N1	M0
	T2	N1	M0
	T3	N1	M0
	T4	N1	M0
IIIB	T4	N1	M0
	Any T	N1	M0
	Any T	N2	M0
	Any T	N3	M0
IV	Any T	Any N	M1

Used with permission of the American Joint Committee on Cancer Staging (AJCC), Chicago. Modified from the AJCC Cancer Staging Manual, 5th ed. Philadelphia, Lippincott-Raven, 1997.

to local excision, yet more require anoplasty for closure of the larger defect created in the anal canal. Patients with tumors of 2 cm in size or greater or with evidence of fixation or significant sphincter involvement should not be considered for local excision. If histopathologic examination after local excision demonstrates invasion into muscle or a positive margin not amenable to re-excision, postoperative chemoradiation should be considered. The dramatic results reported by Nigro and other favorable data published on combined modality therapy for anal cancer (regression, 70% to 100%; 5-year survival, rate, 82% to 87%) has greatly increased the enthusiasm for this treatment, making it the preferred course for patients with locally advanced disease not amenable to local excision. Controversy continues as to whether radiation alone or radiation plus chemotherapy provides better long-term results. Although many favor combined chemoradiation treatment, the question will not be resolved until a randomized, controlled trial is undertaken.

Table 91–2	Treatment Options for Anal Cancers		
		LOCALIZED	**ADVANCED**
Anal Canal Tumors			
Epidermoid (squamous, basaloid, mucoepidermoid)		Wide local excision	Radiation Chemoradiation APR
Adenocarcinoma		Wide local excision	Chemoradiation/APR APR
Melanoma		Wide local excision	APR ± Inguinal node dissection
Anal Margin Tumors			
Squamous cell		Wide local excision	Radiotherapy Chemoradiation Wide local excision APR ± inguinal node dissection
Verrucous (Buschke-Lowenstein)		Wide local excision	APR ± chemoradiation
Basal cell		Wide local excision with lesion mapping	APR ± radiation
Bowen's disease		Wide local excision	APR ± chemoradiation
Paget's disease		Wide local excision with lesion mapping	APR ± inguinal node dissection ± chemoradiation
Melanoma		Wide local excision ± sentinel node biopsy	APR ± sentinel node biopsy

APR, abdominoperineal resection.

Melanoma

The anal canal represents the most common site for development of melanoma within the alimentary tract, yet this remains a rare neoplasm accounting for 0.2% of all melanomas. These lesions typically present with bleeding, pain, or a mass. This neoplasm is presumed to arise from melanocytes within the anal canal; often, there is a lack of pigmentation that can make the diagnosis even more difficult. Even though the overall prognosis is grim, with 5-year survival rates of 10% or less, there is a suggestion that lesions less than 2 mm in depth and those arising in the anal canal versus the rectum have a more favorable prognosis.

No definitive evidence exists to support more aggressive surgical therapy for anal melanomas. Although the patterns of recurrence differ for local excision versus APR, long-term survival rate does not differ. In general, local excision with a 2-cm margin is advised, although some clinicians advocate sentinel node mapping for lesions in the anal canal with inguinal node biopsy in addition to local excision. Radical resection with or without inguinal lymphadenectomy is reserved for advanced disease. Adjuvant treatment with radiotherapy, immunomodulation, and other chemotherapeutic agents has been reported; however, no consistent benefit has been observed.

Adenocarcinoma

Adenocarcinoma of the anus is rare and more often represents downward extension of a primary rectal cancer. Extramucosal adenocarcinomas are thought to arise from anal ducts lining the anal canal and may be associated with fistula extending into the ischiorectal fossa or adjacent perianal skin. Wide local excision is acceptable; however, because the diagnosis is often delayed, APR is more often advised as a result of local invasion. The prognosis

is generally poor in that many patients are first seen with advanced disease. The addition of chemoradiation has shown some promise in improving local control as well as long-term survival.

Neoplasms of the Anal Margin

Squamous Cell Carcinoma

Squamous cell carcinomas throughout the body have similar histologic and clinical characteristics. These tumors infiltrate the surrounding tissues and create an ulcerated lesion that can become sizable if unattended. Metastatic disease is uncommon, and most often represents longstanding disease. Clinical presentation frequently includes itching, pain, and bleeding; late findings such as inguinal adenopathy and occasionally fistula formulation are noted with deeply infiltrating lesions. Wide local excision is the treatment of choice for early lesions, with excellent 5-year survival rates for the early lesions. Tumors greater than 5 cm are associated with a less favorable prognosis. Advanced local disease with invasion into sphincter, vagina, or regional nodes can be managed with a modified APR, including an en bloc excision of involved tissues and lymphadenectomy. Recently, sentinel node mapping has been suggested to more accurately identify nodal involvement and minimize the complications of lymphadenectomy. Chemoradiation as an adjunct to surgery has also been advocated, particularly for those patients with advanced disease not amenable to primary resection.

Verrucous Carcinoma

Verrucous carcinomas typically arise within giant condyloma acuminatum and represent a continuum in the pathologic evolution from benign condyloma to invasive squamous cell cancer. Also referred to as Buschke-

Löwenstein tumors, the etiology of this lesion is the human papillomavirus. The wartlike growths often become quite large, extending 6 cm or more beyond the anal verge; malignant transformation has been reported in up to 50% of these lesions. Distinguishing benign condyloma from the invasive cancer is often difficult. Fistulas are frequently encountered and can lead to increased problems with pain and infection. Although metastasis is not thought to occur, local recurrence is common, in up to 60% of patients in some series. Radical excision provides the best long-term prognosis; rarely, APR is required to obtain clear margins. The role of radiation and chemotherapy for primary lesions is being evaluated; thus far, it is advocated only for advanced disease.

Basal Cell Carcinoma

Basal cell carcinoma is rare, being the least common anal margin neoplasm. These lesions are usually 1 to 2 cm in size and present as a mass or ulcer. The neoplasms arise from the basal cells within the malpighian layer of the skin, producing a characteristic rolled-edge appearance with sheets of basophilic staining cells creating a chronic induration. Local excision is the treatment of choice; radical resection is uncommon because these tumors rarely extend beyond the anal canal. In the uncommon situation that these lesions do invade adjacent tissues—or in the setting of recurrence—APR is warranted.

Bowen's Disease

Bowen's disease represents an in situ intraepidermal squamous cell carcinoma that spreads in an intraepidermal manner. It is rare (less than 5%) that this lesion invades or metastasizes. The tumor produces an indurated thickening of the perinanal skin, creating fissuring or a dark, red plaque or nodule. These lesions produce few symptoms; pruritus and needle-like burning pain are the most common patient complaints. The diagnosis is often confused with other more common dermatologic conditions, and thus a high index of suspicion combined with judicious use of punch biopsies confirms the presence of large atypical cells with halved giant hyperchromatic nuclei. Bowen's disease has reportedly been associated with neoplasms elsewhere in the body; however, other studies have failed to support this view.

Wide local excision with clear margins is suggested for patients without invasion; radical surgical extirpation is needed when invasion is noted or with extensive intraepidermal extension. Topical dinitrochlorobenzene and 5-fluorouracil have also been reported as treatment options. Recurrence is noted in approximately 10% of patients; therefore, follow-up on a regular basis is warranted with biopsy as indicated.

Paget's Disease

Extramammary Paget's disease, an intraepithelial adenocarcinoma, is also a relatively rare condition. The usual appearance is that of a well-demarcated, eczematoid plaque with whitish-gray ulcerations or papillary lesions. The diagnosis is confirmed with demonstration of Paget cells on punch biopsy. Because of the frequent association of Paget's disease with underlying carcinoma of the colon, rectum, and anus, it is imperative that complete large bowel evaluation be performed before planning and initiating treatment. Local excision is recommended for simple in situ disease. More extensive involvement may require skin grafting or advancement flaps. When an associated rectal cancer is encountered, an APR is recommended. If nodal disease or concurrent advanced rectal cancer is present, adjuvant chemoradiation is indicated.

COMPLICATIONS

Altered fecal continence is perhaps the most recognized and feared complication associated with the treatment of anal cancer. Clearly, overzealous excision of superficial lesions compromising the integrity of the anal sphincter is inappropriate. In select patients, however, advanced disease or recurrent cancer may necessitate resection of a portion of the anal sphincter, potentially altering continence. Accurate preoperative assessment is imperative if the patient and the surgeon are to maximize functional results and yet maintain oncologic objectives.

Not infrequently, previously unappreciated or unsuspected neoplasms are encountered inadvertently on pathologic evaluation of presumed benign tissues. When incidental cancers are identified, these tissues are not typically oriented in a manner that will provide adequate information on depth of invasion or tumor margins. If the adequacy of resection is in doubt, then re-excision or adjuvant therapy should be considered. The surgeon must maintain a high degree of suspicion when encountering unusual findings. Preparation of the specimens in a manner that will provide useful information minimizes the need for re-excision and avoids delays in treatment or a possible compromise of outcomes.

Other frequently encountered complications associated with anorectal procedures include bleeding, impaction, urinary retention, and urgency. These problems, although common in the immediate postoperative period, are unusual long-term difficulties. Long-term complications include stricture, ectropion, and nonhealing wounds. These problems can generally be managed with conservative measures or minor surgical intervention. However, some postoperative side effects of these varied treatment approaches pose lifelong symptoms. The more aggressive measures required with advanced disease can create sexual dysfunction, chronic lymphedema, radiation proctitis, and complications associated with managing a colostomy.

Because many of the more severe and chronic complications are associated with advanced disease, attention to accurate early diagnosis is imperative. The utilization of improved diagnostic tools to provide precise assessment of the extent of disease assists the physician with accurate staging and should improve not only clinical results but also functional outcomes.

OUTCOMES

Anal cancers represent a diverse group of neoplasms with variable outcomes. In general, there has been a trend in management for most anal lesions toward sphincter preservation. Local excision remains a viable option for noninvasive neoplasms with APR currently reserved for select advanced or recurrent tumors. The 5-year survival rates reported with local excision range from 75% to 100%. Local recurrence remains a significant concern, occurring with a frequency of 20% to 78%. Many of the historical reviews of anal cancers have included multiple tumor types with inconsistent staging, making comparisons unreliable. Radical excision alone remains disappointing, with 5-year survival rates of 40% to 70%. Despite more extensive resection, the marginal results reported suggest tumor biology is the most significant factor affecting outcomes, making it difficult to justify APR alone for primary lesions.

Radiation therapy as primary treatment for anal cancers has been used for more than 50 years. Tumor response, however, has been variable, with 50% to 84% 5-year survival rates. Papillon reported a 65% disease-free survival rate in a large series of patients; however, recurrence rates and complications associated with high-dose radiation necessitated further surgical therapy in a high percentage of these patients.

Multimodality therapy popularized initially by Nigro has diminished the morbidity of high-dose radiation and radical surgery while providing superior 5-year survival rates. Nigro reported an 84% 5-year cancer-free survival rate in a large group of patients receiving chemoradiation. Numerous reports have indicated that chemoradiation provides superior oncologic results with less toxicity and better quality of life for the patient who avoids a permanent stoma; however, outcomes comparisons are difficult given the variations in chemoradiation protocols and inconsistent pathology. Currently, chemoradiation is the treatment of choice in most patients with invasive carcinoma of the anal canal. Accurate pathologic assessment and staging remain critical to the approach, care, and management of anal cancer.

Postoperative problems associated with anorectal procedures and long-term complications such as stricture, ectropion, and nonhealing wounds can generally be managed with conservative measures or minor surgical intervention. For patients with more advanced disease, chemoradiation or APR with or without groin dissection can lead to chronic lymphedema, sexual dysfunction, radiation proctitis, and stoma difficulties. Most of the more severe complications attributed to the treatment of anal cancer are associated with advanced disease. Even though these are generally amenable to treatment, more precise assessment with endorectal ultrasonography, computed tomography, and magnetic resonance imaging can assist with accurate staging and direct patients to the treatment that provides optimal clinical and functional outcomes.

Summary

Anal cancers are rare neoplasms with a diverse etiology and frequent confusion regarding the anatomic bound-

---

Pearls and Pitfalls

Diagnostic Considerations

- Suspect neoplasia with chronic or unusual anal or perianal lesions.
- Obtain a biopsy to confirm the diagnosis.
- Consider a pathologic review of routine tissues if they appear suspicious.
- Document the size, location, circumference, and orientation of the tumor.
- Obtain endoanal ultrasonography and computed tomography to assess the depth of invasion and extent of perianal disease.

Management Considerations

- Document the extent of tumor involvement, including invasion of the sphincter or adjacent structures.
- Ensure clear margins with local excision.
- Exclude metachronous tumors.
- Evaluate inguinal lymph nodes—possibly using a sentinel node approach.
- Consider adjuvant chemoradiation therapy.

---

aries of these tumors. In general, these lesions can be grouped into three distinct categories. The anal margin usually contains well-differentiated, keratinized squamous pathology and is frequently amenable to local treatment measures. Anal canal neoplasms are most often epidermoid, nonkeratinized, moderately differentiated tumors, with a histology consistent with that of the anal canal distal to the dentate line. The third group of tumors are those arising in the transitional epithelium from the rectum to anal canal; these tumors are commonly adenocarcinomas with variable degrees of differentiation. While local treatment often suffices for the majority of superficial anal canal and transition zone tumors, multimodality therapy is being used more frequently for lesions greater than 2 cm or those with more aggressive histologies. In general, the treatment plan for neoplasms of the anus and perianal skin depends on histology, extent of involvement, and invasive or metastatic nature of the tumor. The potential to offer sphincter preservation even with more advanced disease is often possible, given new treatment strategies.

SELECTED READINGS

Greenlee RT, Murray T, Bolden S, Wingo PA: Cancer Statistics 2000. CA Cancer J Clin 2000;50(1):7.

Greenall MJ, Quan SH, Stearns MW: Epidermoid cancer of the anal margin: Pathologic features, treatment, and clinical results. Am J Surg 1985;149:95.

Goldman S, Ihre T, Seligson U: Squamous-cell carcinoma of the anus: A follow-up study of 65 patients. Dis Colon Rectum 1985;28:143.

Papillon J: Current therapeutic concepts in management of carcinoma of the anal canal: Recent results. Cancer Res 1988;110:146.

Nigro ND: An evaluation of combined therapy for squamous cell cancer of the anal canal. Dis Colon Rectum 1984;27:763.

Longo WE, Vernava AM, Wade TP, et al: Recurrent squamous cell carcinoma of the anal canal: Predictors of initial treatment failure and results of salvage therapy. Ann Surg 1994;220:40.

Brady MS, Kavolius JP, Quan SHQ: Anorectal melanoma: A 64-year experience at Memorial Sloan-Kettering Cancer Center. Dis Colon Rectum 1995;38:146.

Chapter 92

Cancer of the Rectum

Martin J. Heslin and Kirby I. Bland

Colorectal cancer remains a significant problem, with approximately 140,000 new cancers diagnosed per year, of which as many as one third are located in the rectum. Current management of rectal cancer involves a multidisciplinary approach, which has resulted in significant improvements in local, regional, and distant control of disease as well as a suggestion for improvements in the surgeon's ability to preserve the anal sphincter through the use of preoperative radiation therapy. New techniques of reconstruction have minimized some of the side effects of low rectal reconstruction. Current controversies include the role of high ligation of the inferior mesenteric artery (IMA) and the role of mesorectal excision in place of radiation for earlier stage disease.

CLINICAL PRESENTATION

Clinical presentation of rectal cancer is primarily in the middle-aged patient with rectal bleeding or signs and symptoms of an obstructing mass (pain, constipation, change in the caliber of stools, tenesmus, and rectal pressure). The differential diagnosis includes other causes of rectal bleeding (hemorrhoids, diverticulosis, fissures, upper gastrointestinal [GI] source), constipation (recurrent diverticulitis with stricture), or rectal pain (fissures, thrombosed hemorrhoids, or perirectal abscesses), although especially with rectal cancer the majority of these conditions can be excluded with a complete history and physical examination. All patients with rectal bleeding should have further investigations, and the diagnosis of hemorrhoidal bleeding should be made only after the results of all tests prove negative. Baseline blood panels drawn at the time of presentation may reveal iron deficiency anemia; however, this is not present in all patients. The diagnosis of rectal cancer is not a difficult one to make, since the rectum is very accesible to digital rectal examination or proctoscopy. The potential diagnosis should be carefully formulated and diligently pursued in patients with the aforementioned signs and symptoms.

PREOPERATIVE MANAGEMENT

Preoperative management involves specific laboratory studies, radiologic studies, and endoscopic evaluations focused to achieve negative margins of resection, sphincter preservation, and preservation of bowel, bladder, and sexual function. At present, the majority of rectal cancers are managed with a multidisciplinary approach involving surgery, radiation therapy, and chemotherapy. The controversial issues relate to the order and timing of each modality. This section addresses each issue and its effect on the previously mentioned goals.

Specific preoperative laboratory studies relate to the patient's ability to safely undergo general anesthesia and postoperative follow-up of rectal cancer. Complete blood count (CBC), basic chemistry profile, and carcinoembryonic antigen (CEA) testing would be most appropriate unless other circumstances required further tests. Obtaining CEA testing preoperatively and following postoperatively is controversial, but it appears to have some benefits if the cost issue is put aside. Radiologic studies would include computed tomography (CT) of the abdomen and pelvis and a conventional chest radiograph. Evaluation of the liver and lungs for occult metastatic disease would affect the surgical management and therefore is an important test, especially with the potential morbidity associated with low rectal cancer surgery (permanent colostomy; altered bowel, bladder, and sexual function (Scoggins et al, 1999). CT evaluation of the pelvis provides important information about the local extent of the tumor with respect to pelvic sidewall invasion and ascending retroperitoneal involvement. The most important evaluation in the patient with rectal cancer is rigid proctoscopy with refinement by transrectal ultrasonography. Preoperative rigid proctoscopy by the surgeon performing the operation is a mandatory evaluation for accurately defining the distance from the anal verge, relative mobility (if the lesion cannot be reached by a finger), and location of the lesion in the lumen with respect to the urogenital organs. Transrectal ultrasonography predicts the depth of invasion with 80% to 90% accuracy and has become an important test if there is a consideration for preoperative radiation therapy (Dershaw et al, 1990); however, this test is less accurate after radiation therapy.

The patient with rectal cancer is interested primarily in avoiding a permanent colostomy, maintaining function as nearly normal as possible, and being cured of the disease. Obviously, all these issues are interrelated in the management of rectal cancer, but if a cancer cure is kept as the main priority with preservation of bowel, bladder, and sexual function, usually decisions regarding the correct operation and timing can be reached. The factors associated with decisions regarding preoperative radiation therapy and performing an operation that preserves continence, in relative order of importance, are as follows: distance from the anal verge divided into low (<7 cm), middle (7 to 11 cm), and upper (>11 cm) rectal tumors (Fig. 92–1); the gender of the patient (males having a narrow, deep pelvis and a potentially enlarged prostate, which reduces exposure); body habitus (obese patients have reduced exposure to the pelvis and thickened colonic mesentery, which may affect reconstruction); size of the tumor (bulky tumors reduce distal pelvic exposure); fixation of the tumor to surrounding structures; location of the tumor in the anterior-posterior plane (anterior tumors

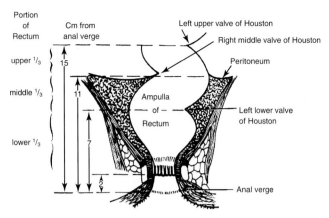

Figure 92–1. Surgical anatomy of the rectum. (From Cohen AM, Minsky BD, Schilsky RL: Cancer of the rectum. In DeVita VT Jr, Hellman S, Rosenberg SA [eds]: Principles and Practice of Oncology, 5th ed. Philadelphia, Lippincott-Raven, 1997, pp 1197–1234.)

mobilize less well than posterior tumors); and finally sphincter tone. Patients with tumors invading the anal sphincter or patients with an incontinent anal sphincter should undergo abdominoperineal resection (APR). All other patients should be considered for sphincter preservation, depending on the relative value of each of these factors. Preoperative counseling of the patient should include relative risks of permanent colostomy, reconstruction with a temporary ostomy, and reconstruction without an ostomy based on the aforementioned relative risk factors for the maintenance of continence. Local excision of rectal cancer with or without radiation therapy should be offered only in highly selected patients. Briefly, this approach should be considered in patients with well- or moderately-well-differentiated tumors without evidence of lymph node metastasis and those that are less than 8 to 10 cm from the anal verge, mobile (or <T2 by transrectal ultrasonography [TRUS]), no greater that 3 to 4 cm in diameter, and that do not take up one third of the lumen of the bowel. Relative contraindications in this subset would include an anteriorly located tumor. Further indications and the data supporting the use of local resection are beyond the scope of this chapter and are not discussed further.

Preoperative radiation therapy is a controversial subject, but it does seem to have a role in the management of middle and low rectal cancer for functional reasons, as there are few data supporting an improvement in cure or local control rates compared with postoperative treatment. At present, patients with middle or low rectal tumors that are not invading the anal sphincter but have some or all of the aforementioned poor prognostic factors for continence appear to benefit from preoperative radiation therapy with combined 5-fluorouracil (5-FU) with the goal of sphincter preservation (Minsky et al, 1995). Theoretically, the benefits include better oxygenation of the tumor during radiation, less tumor seeding, reduction in fixation of the small bowel in the pelvis, and limited or no radiation side effects on the bowel eventually used in the reconstruction. A course of radiation usually involves 6 weeks of radiotherapy, to a total dose of 4500 Gy, followed by a treatment break of 6 to 10 weeks, followed

by operation. Functional outcome seems to be decreased with a postoperative approach (Minsky et al, 1995); therefore, the patient with T3 or enlarged perirectal nodes by transrectal ultrasonography may benefit from preoperative radiation, especially if the lesion is a low-lying tumor in a male or in an obese patient who might not be a candidate for a reservoir reconstruction. Utilizing preoperative transrectal ultrasonography may also reduce the chances of overtreating patients with early-stage disease (T1/T2 N0 M0).

Utilization of enterostomal therapists preoperatively to provide in-depth patient education, and for the best possible functional results, is critically important. Our nurses meet with the patients and families to discuss temporary ileostomy or colostomy as well as the implications of permanent colostomy. The nurses provide optimal preoperative localization for an ostomy based on the gender, body habitus, and clothing habits of the patients. Postoperatively, continued education through video seminars and hands-on teaching appears to contribute to patient satisfaction and confidence with manipulation of the appliance, as well as to a potentially reduced hospital stay.

INTRAOPERATIVE MANAGEMENT

As with most complex surgical procedures, the most important factors associated with a successful operation are selection of the proper operation for the individual patient, setup of the patient in the operating room, and specific maneuvers for accomplishing the goals of cancer cure and preservation of function. The patients should be positioned in the modified lithotomy position with Allen stirrups, with right arm tucked, left arm out, and a 2-inch jellyroll or folded sheet under the pelvis to provide elevation and to rotate the pelvis forward. The initial incision should be a lower midline, with fascial division to the level of the pubic symphysis for maximal exposure. After mobilization and division of the sigmoid colon and identification of the autonomic nerve plexus at the level of the superior hemorrhoidal artery, pelvic dissection should begin.

Sharp pelvic dissection along the endopelvic fascia (or total mesorectal excision, with nerve-preserving low anterior resection) should be the technique of choice. Retrospective series have demonstrated pelvic local control far superior to traditional surgery with blunt pelvic dissection (Enker et al, 1999; MacFarlane et al, 1993), although randomized trials have not confirmed any benefit over potential risks. This technique emphasizes lateral as well as distal margins, an approach supported by pathologic evaluation of rectal cancer specimens (Quirke et al, 1986). Randomized trials are underway to evaluate its value with or without radiation therapy. The distal mucosal margin for rectal cancer has been reported to be 2 cm, although according to recent data this appears to be at least as important for the mesorectal margin as well (Reynolds et al, 1996).

The proximal extent of nodal dissection in rectal cancer has also been debated in the past. Initial data suggested that patients with positive nodes along the inferior mesenteric artery (IMA) had a worse survival, leading surgeons to believe that removal of these nodes may be associated with improved survival. Recent retrospective data from St. Mark's Hospital in London suggest that there is no survival advantage with removal of these nodes; therefore, the recommendation for ligation at the level of the aorta may be associated with increased complications and therefore is not recommended (Pezim and Nicholls, 1984) (Fig. 92–2).

APR with permanent colostomy remains the standard for tumors invading the anal sphincter and for patients with poor sphincter tone in addition to other poor prognostic factors for reconstruction. The same pelvic dissection should be utilized, as discussed earlier. Some controversies exist regarding attempts at closure of the levator sling; typically, this is not possible if an adequate resection of the muscle is performed as part of an APR.

Techniques for reconstruction of the rectum are based on the amount of native rectum remaining, in addition to the morphology of the pelvis and conduit. The use of the sigmoid colon as a conduit has specific indications and pitfalls. For low rectal anastomoses with little native rectum and especially if postoperative radiation is expected, the sigmoid colon as a straight connection is a poor choice because of overall decreased reservoir function and increased propensity for spasm. If the pelvis is small, or the mesentary of the bowel is fatty (technically precluding a J-pouch reservoir), mobilization of the splenic flexure and utilization of the descending colon is a better option. Utilization of a portion of the sigmoid, which might obviate the need for mobilization of the splenic flexure, can

be recommended for those middle or low rectal tumors that would technically allow for colonic J-pouch reconstruction (Cohen, 1993). The J-pouch colonic reservoir was developed to provide better functional outcome, which has been demonstrated to decrease the number of bowel movements and inadvertent soilages for a period of at least 2 years (Lazorthes et al, 1997).

The anastomosis is done primarily by a double-staple technique when possible, although if it is too low, a perianal hand-sewn technique becomes necessary. Prior to firing the stapler across the bowel and removing the specimen, some have advocated rectal irrigation to reduce the volume of luminal tumor cells that may get seeded in the crush of the stapler. Limited data exist to confirm or refute the benefits of this. However, the risk and time commitment are small; therefore, it is recommended. The anastomosis should be tested for air leaks by insufflation under water in the pelvis.

Proximal diversions after rectal cancer resection of low or middle rectal tumors are occasionally required. Indications include air leak during insuffflation of a double-staple anastomosis, hand-sewn perianal coloanal anastomosis, and any concern about the technical aspects of the connection, especially in a patient who would be unable to tolerate a septic episode. Obviously, the patient who has undergone anastomosis without proximal diversion who develops a significant leak requires a return trip to the operating room for diversion. Choices for diversion include ileostomy (best for the younger patient) or right-sided loop colostomy (better for older patients, in whom fluid management may become an issue). Either way, diversion is for 6 weeks to 3 months, most often with a barium study of the anastomosis to confirm no leaks or strictures, especially in the patient with intraoperative technical concerns. It is rare to obtain a barium study in patients without proximal diversion, as they can be monitored clinically during the early postoperative period.

POSTOPERATIVE MANAGEMENT

Postoperative management of the elective proctectomy patient has changed markedly in the last 10 years and, by and large, is performed with minimal intervention. Use of nasogastric tubes is for the most part historical, except in the patient with intractable nausea or vomiting during the postoperative period (<15%). In the setting of middle or low rectal cancer requiring low dissection without proximal diversion, patients are kept NPO until postoperative day (POD) 4 or 5, at which time clear fluids and crackers may be begun, with advancement as tolerated to a low-fat and low-fiber diet. Again, the historical progression through a full liquid diet prior to regular food is not recommended. With proximal diversion or with upper rectal dissection only, a clear diet may be begun as early as POD No. 2, with advancement as tolerated.

For middle or low rectal dissection, Foley catheters are left in place for 4 to 5 days to minimize pressure in the pelvis, especially if there is question about injury to the pelvic autonomic nerve system (e.g., in recurrent rectal cancer dissections where identification of these nerves is more difficult or impossible) or in the older

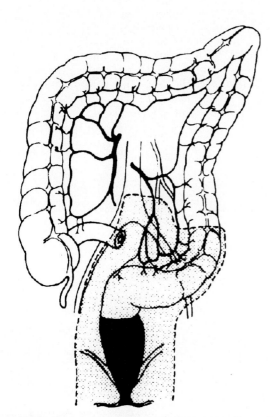

Figure 92–2. Extent of resection for rectal cancer. (From Cohen AM, Minsky BD, Schilsky RL: Cancer of the rectum. In DeVita VT Jr, Hellman S, Rosenberg SA [eds]: Principles and Practice of Oncology, 5th ed. Philadelphia, Lippincott-Raven, 1997, pp 1197–1234.)

patient with preoperative urinary dysfunction. Otherwise, they can be removed when clinically indicated. There are few data to support the use of closed suction drains in the patient with an anastomosis above the peritoneal reflection; however, we are unaware of a study comparing drain versus no drain in the patient with a middle or low rectal cancer. Installing a single closed suction drain in the pelvis, with removal after documentation of bowel function, may be done, as there are few data also to suggest that there is a significant risk with this approach.

The optimal type of prophylaxis against deep venous thrombosis (DVT) is a controversial subject. At present, all patients with operable rectal cancer carry at least two important risk factors, those being the presence of cancer and the need for pelvic surgery. Based on this, a reasonable approach would be heparin, 5000 U subcutaneously in the preoperative holding area, and then 5000 U every 8 to 12 hours starting on POD No. 1, until discharge. Some form of intermittent compression device for the intraoperative period and at least the first 48 hours postoperatively is employed to reduce the risk of extremity clot formation.

The hospital course for rectal cancer patients varies with the presence or absence of proximal diversion. For patients with proximal diversion or permanent colostomy, the usual length of the stay should be between 4 and 6 days; without proximal diversion, the hospital stay is usually between 6 and 8 days. Eliminating nasogastric tubes, early ambulation and prompt oral feeding, and a dedicated enterostomal team to help encourage learning of appliance use should reduce the length of the hospital stay.

COMPLICATIONS

The overall complication rate in these patients should be between 10% and 15%, counting both major and minor complications. Major complications include anastomotic leak, wound dehiscence, and pneumonia as well as the usual cardiopulmonary complications of the patients in this age group. Superficial wound infections, nausea, and urinary retention are the more common minor complications, which should not alter the postoperative length of stay markedly.

OUTCOMES AND ADDITIONAL THERAPY

Additional therapy for rectal cancer involves a multidisciplinary approach. Node-positive patients should receive 6 months of postoperative chemotherapy involving 5-FU and leucovorin (Fisher et al, 1988). The data supporting chemotherapy for node-negative patients are controversial. Radiation therapy is supported for use in node-positive patients (Fisher et al, 1988), although a preoperative approach has been advocated by many for the previously stated reasons in patients with T3 or node-positive disease on transrectal ultrasonography. Radiation therapy for node-negative but deeply penetrating tumors has been advocated; however, its advantages may be outweighed by a reduction in function in the patients who undergo mesorectal excision. At present, there is a Dutch

---

Pearls and Pitfalls

PEARLS

- Multidisciplinary approach, including medical oncology, radiation oncology, surgery, and enterostomal therapy nursing support
- Rigid proctoscopy performed by the operating surgeon for all operative cases
- Assessment of distance from the anal verge, gender, body habitus, sphincter tone, prostate size
- Sharp pelvic sidewall dissection, with preservation of autonomic nerves
- Adequate dissection of mesorectum a minimum of 2 cm distal to distal mucosal edge of the tumor
- Resection with proximal diversion for any question of technical problems

PITFALLS

- Lack of a combined modality approach
- Acceptance of flexible scope for measuring accurate distance from the anal verge
- Failure to recognize all factors associated with a safe, continent reconstruction
- Blunt pelvic dissection
- Inadequate dissection of mesorectum distal to the tumor
- Attempting intraoperative repair of air leak after test of anastomosis

---

trial exploring preoperative radiation therapy plus mesorectal excision versus mesorectal excision alone that may answer some of these questions.

The clinical follow-up involves CBC, liver function tests (LFTs), CEA testing, and rectal examination every 3 to 4 months for the first 2 years, and a chest radiograph every 6 months for the same time period, with a colonoscopy 1 year after resection. The recommendations for colonoscopy after cancer excision are not as well defined as those after polyp excision (Winawer et al, 1993); however, if the colon is completely cleared of polyps at the initial colonoscopy after rectal cancer excision, follow-up colonoscopy is probably safe every 2 to 3 years. Should new polyps be discovered, colonoscopy should be performed on a yearly basis until clear. The role of routine CT of the abdomen and pelvis after excision is less defined and probably does not justify the cost, unless one is investigating a physical finding or laboratory abnormality.

SELECTED READINGS

Cohen AM: Colon J-pouch rectal reconstruction after total or subtotal proctectomy. World J Surg 1993;17:267.

Dershaw DD, Enker WE, Cohen AM, Sigurdson ER: Transrectal ultrasonography of rectal carcinoma. Cancer 1990;66:2336.

Enker WE, Merchant N, Cohen AM, et al: Safety and efficacy of low anterior resection for rectal cancer: 681 consecutive cases from a specialty service. Ann Surg 1999;230:544.

Fisher B, Wolmark N, Rockette H, et al: Postoperative adjuvant chemotherapy or radiation therapy for rectal cancer: Results from NSABP protocol R-01. J Natl Cancer Institute 1988;80:21.

Lazorthes F, Chiotasso P, Gamagami RA, et al: Late clinical outcome in a randomized prospective comparison of colonic J pouch and straight coloanal anastomosis. Br J Surg 1997;84:1449.

MacFarlane JK, Ryall RD, Heald RJ: Mesorectal excision for rectal cancer [see comments]. Lancet 1993;341:457.

Minsky BD, Cohen AM, Enker WE, Paty P: Sphincter preservation with preoperative radiation therapy and coloanal anastomosis. Int J Radiat Oncol Biol Phys 1995;31:553.

Pezim ME, Nicholls RJ: Survival after high or low ligation of the inferior mesenteric artery during curative surgery for rectal cancer. Ann Surg 1984;200:729.

Quirke P, Durdey P, Dixon MF, Williams NS: Local recurrence of rectal adenocarcinoma due to inadequate surgical resection: Histopathological study of lateral tumour spread and surgical excision. Lancet 1986;2:996.

Reynolds JV, Joyce WP, Dolan J, et al: Pathological evidence in support of total mesorectal excision in the management of rectal cancer. Br J Surg 1996;83:1112.

Scoggins CR, Meszoely IM, Blanke CD, et al: Nonoperative management of primary colorectal cancer in patients with stage IV disease [see comments]. Ann Surg Oncol 1999;6:651.

Winawer SJ, Zauber AG, Ho MN, et al: Prevention of colorectal cancer by colonoscopic polypectomy. The National Polyp Study Workgroup [see comments]. N Engl J Med 1993;329:1977.

Liver: Benign

Chapter 93
Hepatitis
John J. Poterucha

Many potential agents result in liver disease, and knowledge of the more common disorders is important to the surgeon. Hepatitis viruses are among the most common causes of liver injury. Their clinical importance should be acknowledged and recognized, not only because of their propensity for liver injury but also because of the risk of transmission. The purpose of this chapter is to familiarize the surgeon with a practical approach to patients with liver disease with an emphasis on the agents causing viral hepatitis. This chapter is divided into four major sections:

• Evaluation of the patient with abnormal liver tests
• Viral hepatitis
• Postoperative liver injury
• Risk of surgery in patients with liver disease

EVALUATION OF THE PATIENT WITH ABNORMAL LIVER TESTS

The frequent use of blood tests in patient evaluation has increased the recognition of abnormal liver test results. Because these abnormalities usually indicate liver injury and are not true markers of liver function, the term "liver function tests" is best avoided. More specific markers of liver function are direct bilirubin, serum albumin, and prothrombin time.

Appropriate evaluation of patients with abnormal liver test results hinges on many clinical factors including the chief complaints of the patient, the patient's age, risk factors for liver disease, personal or family history of liver disease, medications, and findings on physical examination. Because of these multiple factors, designing a standard algorithm for the evaluation of liver test abnormalities is difficult and often inefficient. Nevertheless, with some basic information, surgeons can approach liver test abnormalities in an efficient, cost-effective

manner. To achieve this goal, this section reviews the following issues:

1. General discussion of the commonly used liver tests.
2. Differential diagnosis and discussion of diseases characterized by elevations of hepatocellular enzymes.
3. Differential diagnosis and discussion of diseases characterized by elevations of cholestatic enzymes.
4. Evaluation of the jaundiced patient.

Commonly Used Liver Tests

Serum Aminotransferases (ALT, AST)

Serum aminotransferases, also known as transaminases, are found in hepatocytes and are therefore markers of liver cell injury or hepatocellular disease. Hepatocellular injury causes these enzymes to "leak" out of liver cells. Increases in serum activities are seen within a few hours after liver injury. Aminotransferases consist of alanine aminotransferase (ALT), also known by previous terminology as serum glutamate pyruvate transaminase (SGPT), and aspartate aminotransferase (AST), also known as serum glutamate oxaloacetate transaminase (SGOT). ALT is relatively specific for liver injury, whereas AST is found not only in hepatocytes but also in skeletal and cardiac muscle and other organs. Because some automated blood tests assay only for AST, it is useful to obtain an ALT measurement before embarking on an evaluation for liver disease.

Serum Alkaline Phosphatase

Alkaline phosphatase is an enzyme found on the hepatocyte membrane that borders the bile canaliculus, the smallest branch of the biliary collecting system. Because alkaline phosphatase is also found in bone and placenta, an isolated increase of the serum enzyme activity should prompt further testing to determine whether the elevation is from liver or from other tissues. Determination of alkaline phosphatase isoenzymes is one such way; another is the determination of gamma glutamyl transpeptidase (GGT), an enzyme found largely in biliary ductules. Serum GGT is a more sensitive test for biliary disease than alkaline phosphatase. Other than to confirm the hepatic origin of an increased serum alkaline phosphatase measurement, GGT has little role in the determination of diseases of the liver because its synthesis can be induced by many medications, thereby reducing its specificity for clinically significant liver disease.

Serum Bilirubin

Bilirubin is a product of metabolism of heme taken up by hepatocytes and conjugated with glucuronic acid to form monoglucuronides and diglucuronides. Conjugation makes bilirubin water-soluble, allowing it to be excreted in bile. When bilirubin is measured in serum, there are direct (conjugated) and indirect (unconjugated) fractions. Conditions such as hemolysis or resorption of a hematoma are characterized by hyperbilirubinemia that is primarily unconjugated and less than 20% conjugated. Hepatobiliary disorders (hepatocyte dysfunction or mechanical obstruction of bile flow) produce hyperbilirubinemia that is usually much greater than 50% conjugated. Because conjugated bilirubin is water-soluble and may be excreted in urine, patients with hepatobiliary disease complicated by hyperbilirubinemia (serum bilirubin greater than 3 mg/dL) often have dark urine. In such patients, stools are lighter in color because of the absence of bilirubin pigments; with complete biliary obstruction, the stools become clay colored.

Prothrombin Time and Serum Albumin

Prothrombin time (commonly measured as INR, or International Normalized Ratio) and serum albumin are true markers of liver synthetic function. Abnormalities of prothrombin time and albumin imply severe liver disease and should prompt an immediate workup. Such patients are also at risk for decompensation after surgery. The INR is a measure of the activity of coagulation factors II, V, VII, and X, all of which are synthesized by the liver. Most coagulation factors are also dependent on vitamin K for synthesis, so deficiencies of vitamin K absorption also produce abnormalities of the INR. Vitamin K deficiency can be produced by chronic antibiotic use associated with a prolonged period of fasting and small bowel mucosal disorders such as celiac disease. In general surgical practices, however, the most common cause is related to severe extrahepatic cholestasis, leading to an inability to absorb fat-soluble vitamins, of which lack of vitamin K leads to the earliest clinical disorder. Advanced hepatocellular dysfunction resulting from acute hepatic failure or decompensated cirrhosis is characterized by an inability to synthesize clotting factors, even with adequate stores of vitamin K. A simple way to distinguish vitamin K

deficiency from liver dysfunction in a patient with a prolonged INR is to administer vitamin K. Ten milligrams of oral vitamin K for 3 days or 10 mg of subcutaneous vitamin K once normalizes the INR in a vitamin K–deficient patient, but it has little effect if the prolonged INR is due to liver disease with poor synthetic function.

Serum albumin has a half-life of 21 days, so decreases in serum albumin resulting from liver dysfunction do not occur acutely; however, serum albumin can decrease relatively quickly in a patient with a severe systemic illness such as bacteremia. These rapid decreases are likely caused by cytokine release with accelerated metabolism of albumin. An otherwise unexplained hypoalbuminemia in a patient without overt liver disease should, however, also prompt a search for albumin in the urine.

Hepatocellular Disorders

Diseases primarily affecting hepatocytes are classified as hepatocellular disorders as opposed to diseases of cholestasis and are characterized by predominant elevations of aminotransferases. The disorders are best characterized as acute (generally less than 3 months) or chronic. Acute hepatitis may be accompanied by malaise, anorexia, abdominal pain, and jaundice. Common causes of acute hepatitis are listed Table 93–1.

The absolute level and pattern of aminotransferase elevation may be helpful in the differential diagnosis. *Acute hepatitis* resulting from viruses or drugs generally produces marked elevations of aminotransferases, often in the thousands of international units (IU), and normal values are less than 30 IU. In general, the ALT tends to be more elevated than the AST. *Alcoholic hepatitis* is characterized by more modest aminotransferase elevations, always less than 400 IU and at times near normal. In addition, patients with alcoholic hepatitis usually have an AST/ALT ratio greater than 2:1. Finally, patients with alcoholic hepatitis frequently have a markedly elevated bilirubin out of proportion to the aminotransferase elevations. *Ischemic hepatitis*, which can occur in patients after

Table 93–1	**Common Causes of Acute Hepatitis**	
DISEASE	**CLINICAL CLUES**	**DIAGNOSTIC TESTS**
Hepatitis A	Exposure history	IgM anti-HAV
Hepatitis B	Risk factors	HBsAg, IgM anti-HBc
Drug-induced	Compatible medication/timing	Improvement after withdrawal from agent
Alcoholic hepatitis	History of alcohol excess, AST:ALT >2	Liver biopsy, improvement with abstinence
Ischemic hepatitis	History of hypotension	Rapid improvement of aminotransferases
Acute duct obstruction	Abdominal pain, fever	Cholangiogram

HAV, hepatitis A virus; HBsAg, hepatitis B surface antigen; AST, aspartate aminotransferase; ALT, alanine aminotransferase; anti-HBc, antibody to hepatitis B core antigen.

an episode of prolonged hypotension, can lead to marked elevations of transaminases, which improve within a few days. *Acute extrahepatic biliary* obstruction as may occur with an impacted common bile duct stone or a neoplasm may also produce very high aminotransferase levels that improve within 1 to 3 days of relief of the biliary obstruction. Any acute cause of liver inflammation may be followed by a period of hyperbilirubinemia. In general, improvement in bilirubin lags behind improvement in aminotransferases.

Chronic hepatitis exists when disease produces sustained elevations (greater than 3 months) of aminotransferases. In general, the aminotransferase elevations, usually 2 to 5 times elevated, are more modest than those seen in acute hepatitis. Patients are often asymptomatic but may complain of fatigue and right upper quadrant pain. The differential diagnosis of chronic hepatitis is lengthy; the most important and common disorders are listed in Table 93–2.

Risk factors for *hepatitis C* include a history of blood transfusions before 1990 or intravenous drug use. Patients with *hepatitis B* may give a history of illegal drug use or frequent sexual contacts. *Nonalcoholic steatohepatitis* (NASH) is a common cause of abnormal aminotransferases; these patients are often obese or have diabetes or hyperlipidemia. Genetic *hemochromatosis* is a common disorder afflicting approximately 1 in 300 people of northern European ancestry. The disease is transmitted in an autosomal recessive manner so a family history of previous liver disease or hepatocellular carcinoma may be present. Genetic hemochromatosis also causes the extrahepatic manifestations of diabetes, hypogonadism, and joint complaints. A careful history is necessary to diagnose drug-induced or alcohol-induced liver disease. *Drug-induced liver disease* may occasionally cause right upper quadrant pain mimicking biliary colic. Patients with autoimmune hepatitis may present as an acute or chronic hepatitis, and patients usually have higher aminotransferases than other disorders that cause chronic hepatitis. The presence of autoantibodies and other autoimmune disorders are helpful clues to the diagnosis.

Cholestatic Disorders

Diseases that predominantly affect the biliary system are classified as cholestatic diseases. These disorders can af-

Table 93–2	Common Causes of Chronic Hepatitis	
DISEASE	**CLINICAL CLUES**	**DIAGNOSTIC TESTS**
Hepatitis C	Risk factors	Anti-HCV
Hepatitis B	Risk factors	HBsAg
Nonalcoholic steatohepatitis	Obesity, diabetes, hyperlipidemia	Ultrasound, liver biopsy
Hemochromatosis	Arthritis, diabetes, family history	Iron studies, gene test, biopsy
Alcoholic liver disease	History, AST:ALT > 2	Liver biopsy
Autoimmune hepatitis	ALT 200–1500, usually female, other autoimmune disease	Antinuclear or anti-smooth muscle antibody, biopsy

HCV, hepatitis C virus; HBsAg, hepatitis B surface antigen; AST, aspartate aminotransferase; ALT, alanine aminotransferase.

Table 93–3	Common Causes of Cholestasis	
DISEASE	**CLINICAL CLUES**	**DIAGNOSTIC TESTS**
Primary biliary cirrhosis	Middle-aged female	Antimitochondrial antibody
Primary sclerosing cholangitis	Association with ulcerative colitis	Cholangiography (ERCP)
Large bile duct obstruction	Jaundice and pain	Ultrasonography, ERCP
Drug-induced	Compatible medication/timing	Improvement after withdrawal of agent
Intrahepatic mass lesions	History of malignancy	Ultrasonography, computed tomography

ERCP, endoscopic retrograde cholangiopancreatography.

fect the microscopic intrahepatic ducts (e.g., primary biliary cirrhosis), the large "extrahepatic" bile ducts (e.g., pancreatic cancer causing common bile duct obstruction), or both (e.g., primary sclerosing cholangitis). In general, the predominant abnormality in these disorders is an increase in serum alkaline phosphatase. Although diseases that produce elevations in serum bilirubin are often called "cholestatic," severe hepatocellular injury, such as occurs with an acute hepatitis, also produces hyperbilirubinemia because of primary hepatocellular dysfunction. Common causes of cholestasis are illustrated in Table 93–3.

Primary biliary cirrhosis is most common in middle-aged women who may complain of fatigue or pruritus. *Primary sclerosing cholangitis* (PSC) has a strong association with ulcerative colitis. Patients with PSC are usually asymptomatic but may have jaundice, fatigue, or pruritus. Extrahepatic biliary obstruction is usually due to stones or benign or malignant strictures of the large biliary ducts, either at the bifurcation of the hepatic ducts or more distally. As noted earlier, acute obstruction of the common bile duct from a stone may produce marked aminotransferase elevations. These aminotransferase elevations are less common with benign or malignant strictures that typically cause a more gradual, albeit progressive, duct obstruction. Intrahepatic mass lesions should be considered in a patient with cholestatic liver test abnormalities and a history of malignancy.

Jaundice

Efficient evaluation of the jaundiced patient is an important diagnostic skill. Jaundice is visibly evident hyperbilirubinemia and is generally recognized only when the serum bilirubin is greater than 2.5 mg/dL. As noted earlier, it may be important to note whether the bilirubin elevation is predominantly conjugated or unconjugated. A common disorder that produces an unconjugated hyperbilirubinemia is Gilbert's syndrome, in which the total bilirubin is generally less than 3.0 mg/dL and the direct bilirubin is 0.3 mg/dL or less. The bilirubin level is generally greater in the fasting state or when the patient is ill. A presumptive diagnosis of Gilbert's syndrome can be made in an otherwise well patient with unconjugated hyperbilirubinemia and a normal hemoglobin (to exclude

Table 93–4	**Comparison of the Primary Hepatitis Viruses**				
	HAV	**HBV**	**HDV**	**HCV**	**HEV**
Incubation (days)	15–50	30–160	Unknown	14–160	14–45
Jaundice	Common	Common	Common	Uncommon	Common
Course	Acute	Acute or chronic	Acute or chronic	Acute or chronic	Acute
Transmission	Fecal-oral	Parenteral	Parenteral	Parenteral	Fecal-oral
Test for diagnosis	IgM anti-HAV	HBsAg	Anti-HDV	Anti-HCV or HCV-RNA	Anti-HEV

HAV, hepatitis A virus; HBV, hepatitis B virus; HDV, hepatitis D virus; HCV, hepatitis C virus; HEV, hepatitis E virus; HBsAg, hepatitis B surface antigen.

hemolysis or resorption of a hematoma) and normal liver enzymes (to exclude liver disease). The prevalence of Gilbert's disease is 2% to 3% in the normal population.

More common in the jaundiced patient is direct hyperbilirubinemia. One good way to categorize such patients is to divide them into those with nonobstructive conditions and those with biliary obstruction. Abdominal pain, fever, and/or a palpable gallbladder are suggestive of biliary obstruction. Risk factors for viral hepatitis, a bilirubin level greater than 15 mg/dL, and persistently high aminotransferases suggest that the jaundice is due to a primary hepatocellular dysfunction, which markedly alters further diagnostic evaluation. A sensitive, specific, and noninvasive test to exclude obstructive causes of cholestasis is hepatic ultrasonography. Diseases characterized by large duct obstruction generally result in intrahepatic bile duct dilatation, especially if the bilirubin is greater than 10 mg/dL and the patient has been jaundiced for more than 2 weeks. However, if the clinical suspicion for bile duct obstruction remains strong despite a negative ultrasonography, endoscopic retrograde cholangiography should be considered.

VIRAL HEPATITIS

Viruses that cause hepatitis are important both to surgeons and surgical patients, not only because hepatitis viruses result in clinically significant liver disease but also because of the risk of transmission to health care providers. Viral infections are important causes of liver disease worldwide. There are five primary hepatitis viruses that have been identified (hepatitis A, B, C, D, and E). The designation "hepatitis F" was tentatively applied to another virus, but there has been no confirmation that this agent is a true hepatitis virus. Hepatitis G virus does not appear to cause significant liver disease.

Disorders that cause hepatitis are primarily characterized by increases in serum aminotransferase. There are other causes of hepatitis such as medications, nonalcoholic or alcoholic steatohepatitis, autoimmune hepatitis, and Wilson's disease. Other viruses, such as cytomegalovirus or Epstein-Barr virus, can also result in hepatitis as part of a systemic infection.

It is useful to divide hepatitis syndromes into acute or chronic categories. Acute hepatitis can last from weeks up to 6 months and is often accompanied by jaundice. The symptoms of acute hepatitis are similar regardless of the etiology and include anorexia, malaise, dark urine, fever, and occasionally abdominal pain. The abdominal pain accompanying hepatitis is generally located in the right upper quadrant of the abdomen. The pain is usually mild and relatively constant and should not be confused with the more severe pain associated with disorders of the biliary tract and pancreas. Chronic hepatitis is defined as the presence of hepatitis for more than 6 months. Patients with chronic hepatitis are usually asymptomatic but may complain of fatigue. Occasionally, patients have manifestations of cirrhosis (ascites, variceal bleeding, or encephalopathy) as the initial symptoms of a chronic liver disorder. Each primary hepatitis virus can cause acute hepatitis, whereas only hepatitis viruses B, C, and D result in chronic hepatitis.

This section discusses, compares, and contrasts the five most common primary hepatitis viruses. Table 93–4 compares the primary hepatitis viruses. The relative importance in terms of disease impact of these viruses is compared in Table 93–5. For each virus, general information is provided, followed by special relevance to the surgeon, especially regarding transmission.

Hepatitis A

Hepatitis A virus (HAV) causes approximately 30% of acute hepatitis in the United States. Fecal-oral (enteral)

Table 93–5	**Clinical Impact of the Hepatitis Viruses in the United States**			
	HAV	**HBV**	**HDV**	**HCV**
Acute infections (× 1000)/year	15–50	30–160	Unknown	14–160
Fulminant deaths/year	100	150	35	Rare
Total chronic infections	0	1–1.25 million	70,000	2.8–4 million
Total chronic liver disease deaths/year	0	5000	1000	10,000

HAV, hepatitis A virus; HBV, hepatitis B virus; HDV, hepatitis D virus; HCV, hepatitis C virus.

spread is the major route of transmission of hepatitis A. Groups at particularly high risk include people living in or traveling to underdeveloped countries, children in daycare centers, homosexual men, and perhaps individuals ingesting raw shellfish. Recognized common-source outbreaks from contaminated food are unusual although highly publicized. The incubation period for hepatitis A is 2 to 6 weeks.

The symptoms of acute hepatitis A infection are as described for acute hepatitis but with diarrhea also present. The most important determinant of the severity of acute hepatitis A infection is the age at which infection occurs. Those infected when younger than 6 years of age are often asymptomatic, and if symptoms are present, they rarely include jaundice. This fact accounts for why up to 40% of individuals older than 40 years of age have serologic evidence of a previous hepatitis A infection, yet neither the patient nor a parent recalls an episode of jaundice. Jaundice is more likely to develop in adults acquiring HAV than children.

The diagnosis of acute hepatitis A infection is made by the presence of IgM anti-HAV, which appears at the onset of the acute phase of the illness and disappears in 3 to 6 months. IgG anti-HAV also becomes positive during the acute phase and persists for decades. A patient with IgG anti-HAV, but not IgM anti-HAV, has had an infection in the remote past or has received hepatitis A vaccine and is considered immune.

Hepatitis A is almost always a self-limited infection, although there may be a prolonged cholestatic phase characterized by persistence of jaundice for 1 to 3 months. Rarely, acute hepatitis A infection may become fulminant and require liver transplantation. Hepatitis A infection does not result in chronic infection and should not be in the differential diagnosis of a chronic hepatitis.

Treatment of hepatitis A is supportive. Isolation of hospitalized patients is recommended, although viral titers are actually highest in the presymptomatic phase. Immunoglobulin should be administered to all household and intimate (including daycare) contacts within 2 weeks of exposure. An effective vaccine for hepatitis A has been developed and should be offered to travelers to underdeveloped countries. Widespread immunization of health care workers has not yet been recommended.

Because the HAV does not cause chronic infection, parenteral transmission (including that from needle-stick exposure) is rare. Hepatitis A infection, like any acute hepatitis, may result in jaundice, and the surgeon needs to differentiate the jaundice from acute hepatitis from that caused by obstruction.

Hepatitis B

Hepatitis B virus (HBV) is a DNA virus that causes approximately 40% of acute viral hepatitis and 15% of chronic viral hepatitis in the United States. HBV is transmitted parenterally or by sexual contact. Major risk factors in the United States are sexual promiscuity and intravenous drug use. Hepatitis B infection is also prevalent in parts of Asia and Africa where perinatal transmission is common.

Table 93–6	Hepatitis B: Serologic Markers	
TEST	**SIGNIFICANCE**
HBsAg	Marker for current infection
Anti-HBs	Marker for immunity (resolved infection or immunization)
IgM anti-HBc	Suggests recent infection
IgG anti-HBc	Marker for remote infection
HBeAg and HBV-DNA	Marker for active viral replication (high infectivity)

HBsAg, hepatitis B surface antigen; anti-HBs, antibody to hepatitis B surface; anti-HBc, antibody to hepatitis B core; HBeAg, hepatitis B e antigen; HBV-DNA, hepatitis B virus DNA.

The incubation period after HBV infection ranges from 30 days to 180 days. Acute hepatitis B in the adolescent or adult is icteric in 30%. Most patients recover after an episode of acute hepatitis B infection, although approximately 5% of infected adults have persistence of hepatitis B surface antigen (HBsAg) for longer than 6 months and are termed chronically infected. Table 93–6 is a guide to hepatitis B serologic markers. The outcome of chronic infection is also variable. Some patients have normal liver enzymes and a normal liver biopsy despite the persistence of HBsAg; these patients are termed chronic HBV carriers and have a good prognosis. Individuals with abnormal liver test results and an abnormal liver biopsy in the setting of chronic HBsAg positivity have chronic hepatitis B infection and are at much higher risk for development of cirrhosis and hepatocellular carcinoma. Spontaneous clearance of HBsAg occurs in 1% to 2% of chronically infected patients per year.

Because most acute hepatitis B infections resolve without chronic sequelae, treatment is supportive. Hepatitis B immunoglobulin should be given to household and sexual contacts of patients with acute hepatitis B infection. Chronic hepatitis B infection, if accompanied by markers of active viral replication (HBeAg), may be treated with interferon or lamivudine.

HBV is a common cause of chronic liver disease and may be transmitted by needle-stick exposure. Patients with chronic hepatitis B infection (HBsAg-positive) who are also HBeAg-positive are at greatest risk for transmitting infection. Health care workers who are exposed to needle-sticks from HBeAg-positive individuals have a 30% risk of contracting hepatitis B if they are not already immune. All surgeons and for that matter, all health care workers really should receive the hepatitis B vaccine and verify immunity (by measuring anti-HBs) 6 months after vaccination; repeat vaccination should occur every 5 years thereafter. Nonimmune surgeons who are exposed to a needle-stick from a HBsAg-positive patient should receive hepatitis B immunoglobulin as soon as possible after exposure, and they should receive the hepatitis B vaccine if they are not already immunized.

Surgeons should also be aware that hepatitis B can still rarely be transmitted by transfusion of blood products. It is estimated that 1 in every 63,000 units of blood transfused may be tainted with HBV. Surgeons may also rarely transmit hepatitis B to patients. Although routine hepatitis B testing of health care workers is not advised, the

Centers for Disease Control and Prevention states that individuals who perform exposure-prone procedures including "digital palpation of a needle tip in a body cavity or the simultaneous presence of the health care worker's fingers and a needle or other sharp instrument or object in a poorly visualized or highly confined anatomic site" are at particular risk for transmitting infection. Individuals who perform such procedures and who do not have anti-HB antibodies should know their HBsAg status and, if positive, the HBeAg status. Health care workers who are HBeAg-positive should not perform exposure-prone procedures unless they have sought counsel from an expert review panel and been advised under what circumstances, if any, they might continue to perform these procedures.

Hepatitis D

Hepatitis D virus (HDV) is a defective virus that requires the presence of HBsAg to cause disease. Consequently, there is no reason to investigate patients for HDV unless HBsAg is also present. HDV infection can occur simultaneously with HBV (coinfection) or as a superinfection in persons with established hepatitis B. Hepatitis D is diagnosed by anti-HDV antibodies and should be suspected in a patient with acute hepatitis B infection or an acute exacerbation of chronic hepatitis B infection. In the United States, intravenous drug users are the group of HBV patients at highest risk for acquiring HDV. Because hepatitis D requires the presence of HBsAg to cause disease, the general implications of hepatitis D to the surgeon are similar to the recommendations for hepatitis B.

Hepatitis C

Hepatitis C virus (HCV) is an RNA virus that infects approximately 2.8 million Americans. HCV causes 20% of acute hepatitis, 60% of chronic hepatitis, and approximately 40% of all end-stage liver disease in the United States. Clinically recognized acute hepatitis C infection is unusual, and the importance of HCV lies in its propensity to cause chronic infection. Major risk factors for hepatitis C infection are intravenous drug use and blood transfusion before 1992.

The incubation period for HCV ranges from 2 to 22 weeks. Most acute hepatitis C disease is asymptomatic and anicteric. Approximately 85% of persons with HCV infection fail to clear the virus by 6 months, and chronic infection develops. Once chronic infection occurs, spontaneous loss of the virus is rare. Up to 30% of patients chronically infected with HCV have persistently normal ALT values. Patients with chronic hepatitis C infection may have nonspecific symptoms such as fatigue and vague abdominal pain. Occasionally, patients have extrahepatic manifestations such as vasculitis associated with cryoglobulinemia. Once HCV results in cirrhosis, symptoms are more common and include fatigue or complications of end-stage liver disease.

Cirrhosis develops in approximately 20% of patients with chronic hepatitis C over a 10- to 20-year period. A long duration of infection and alcohol abuse are risk factors for the development of cirrhosis. The rate of progression of hepatitis C infection is slow, with cirrhosis generally developing after more than 15 years. Patients with cirrhosis resulting from HCV infection are at risk for development of hepatocellular carcinoma and should be screened with ultrasonography and serum alpha-fetoprotein every 6 to 12 months.

The diagnostic tests for hepatitis C are excellent. Antibody to HCV (anti-HCV) is not protective and can indicate either current or resolved infection. A guide to the interpretations of hepatitis C tests is found in Table 93–7. Anti-HCV by enzyme-linked immunoassay (EIA) is sensitive for HCV infection and is the screening test of choice in most laboratories. The specificity of the EIA is improved with the addition of the recombinant immunoblot assay (RIBA). If a patient has an abnormal ALT and risk factors for HCV acquisition, a positive anti-HCV nearly always indicates infection with hepatitis C. In someone with a normal ALT, a positive anti-HCV by EIA may represent an old, resolved infection or even a false-positive finding. The RIBA can help separate these two possibilities. A positive RIBA indicates the presence of antibodies to HCV but still could represent a resolved infection. The presence of HCV-RNA by polymerase chain reaction is diagnostic of ongoing HCV infection. HCV-RNA levels can also be obtained if therapy is being considered.

Therapy for hepatitis C infection with interferon and ribavirin results in a long-term response in approximately 40% of patients. Treatment is less likely to be effective or tolerated in patients with decompensated cirrhosis, and such patients should be considered for liver transplantation.

Hepatitis C is spread parenterally and rarely can be spread by needle-stick exposure. Prospective studies looking at seroconversion rates after a needle-stick exposure from a hepatitis C–positive patient give results varying from 0% to 11%. There is no hepatitis C vaccine available, and postexposure prophylaxis is not beneficial. After exposure to a hepatitis C–positive individual, HCV RNA should be determined in 2 to 4 weeks and anti-HCV in 3 to 6 months. In the unlikely event that hepatitis C transmission occurs, treatment with interferon and ribavirin may be offered.

There are case reports of transmission of HCV from surgeon to patients. Nevertheless, transmission is exceedingly rare, and there are currently no practice limitations for infected health care workers. Surgeons should also be

Table 93–7	**Interpretation of Anti-HCV Results**	
ANTI-HCV BY EIA	**ANTI-HCV BY RIBA**	**INTERPRETATION**
Positive	Negative	False-positive EIA, patient does not have true antibody
Positive	Positive	Patient has antibody*
Positive	Indeterminate	Uncertain antibody status

*Anti-HCV does not necessarily indicate current hepatitis C infection.
EIA, enzyme-linked immunoassay.

Table 93–8	**Acute Hepatitis: Practical Guide to Ordering Tests and Interpretation**				

TESTS TO ORDER				
IgM Anti-HAV	**HBsAg**	**IgM Anti-HBc**	**Anti-HCV**	**INTERPRETATION**
Positive	Negative	Negative	Negative	Acute HAV
Negative	Positive	Positive	Negative	Acute HBV
Negative	Negative	Positive	Negative	Acute HBV°
Negative	Positive	Negative	Negative	Chronic HBV†
Negative	Negative	Negative	Positive	Acute or chronic HCV‡
Negative	Negative	Negative	Negative	Exclude other causes

°Occasionally patients with acute HBV infection lack HBsAg.
†HBsAg without IgM anti-HBc is more suggestive of chronic HBV infection. Exclude HDV or other nonviral causes of acute hepatitis.
‡Anti-HCV may not be positive in acute hepatitis C infection and, when present, may indicate chronic infection so other causes should be excluded.
HAV, hepatitis A virus; HBV, hepatitis B virus; HCV, hepatitis C virus; HBsAg, hepatitis B surface antigen; anti-HBc, antibody to hepatitis B core.

aware that, even though blood product transfusion was a common cause of hepatitis C infection before 1990, currently the virus is only rarely spread by blood transfusion. Estimates are that only 1 in every 103,000 units of blood transfused would be infected with HCV.

Hepatitis E

Hepatitis E virus (HEV) causes large outbreaks of acute hepatitis in underdeveloped countries. Physicians in the United States are unlikely to see a case of HEV infection. A rare patient may become infected during foreign travel. Clinically, hepatitis E infection is similar to that of hepatitis A. Resolution of the hepatitis is the rule, and chronic infection does not occur.

Summary

Viral hepatitis is an important cause of morbidity and mortality in the United States. An accurate diagnosis can not only impact therapy for the individual patient but also guide passive or active immunization for individuals exposed to the index case. Ordering tests for patients with presumed viral hepatitis can be confusing; Tables 93–8 and 93–9 give a practical guide for testing for patients presenting with acute or chronic hepatitis.

POSTOPERATIVE LIVER INJURY

Mild abnormalities in liver enzymes are common after general anesthesia. Most individuals undergoing abdomi-

nal surgery have decreased hepatic blood flow, which may contribute to these mild abnormalities. A more severe acute hepatitis may occur after general anesthesia and is best described after the use of halothane but may also be seen with other general anesthetics. Postoperative jaundice may be due to liver injury, although indirect hyperbilirubinemia occasionally occurs as a result of resorption of a large hematoma. Ischemic hepatitis only occurs after a prolonged hypotensive episode and is characterized by marked elevations in aminotransferases that improve relatively quickly; however, a poorly understood jaundice may persist for several weeks.

Operations on Patients with Liver Disease

The alterations in hepatic blood flow that occur with general anesthesia can cause decompensation in patients with severe forms of liver disease. Although good data about the risks of operative intervention in patients with liver disease are lacking, it is clear that the more severe the liver disease, the more likely that decompensation will occur after surgery. The type of operation may also be important, with the highest rates of decompensation occurring after abdominal or thoracic surgery. Patients with acute hepatitis, severe alcoholic hepatitis, or cirrhosis who have evidence of decompensation are at the highest risk of postoperative liver dysfunction. In general, more severe forms of liver disease can be identified by the presence of laboratory parameters of decreased liver

Table 93–9	**Chronic Hepatitis: Practical Guide to Ordering Tests and Interpretation**	

TESTS TO ORDER		
HBsAg	**Anti-HCV**	**INTERPRETATION**
Positive	Negative	HBV
Negative	Positive	HCV
Negative	Negative	Exclude other causes

HBsAg, hepatitis B surface antigen; HCV, hepatitis C virus; HBV, hepatitis B virus.

Pearls and Pitfalls

- Surgeons should be aware of the differential diagnoses of jaundice and abnormal liver function tests.
- Markedly increased serum levels of ALT and AST usually denote hepatocellular disease but acute biliary obstruction (e.g., impacted gallstone) can also lead to an acute increase in ALT and AST.
- The hepatitis viruses are important to recognize in the surgical patient, not only for the patient but also for the health care worker.
- Health care providers should receive immunizations against hepatitis B.

Table 93–10	Child-Pugh Classification of Severity of Liver Disease		
	1 POINT	**2 POINTS**	**3 POINTS**
Encephalopathy	None	Grade 1 or 2	Grade 3 or 4
Ascites	None	Mild	Moderate or severe
Bilirubin (mg/dL)	<2	2.1–3	>3
Albumin	>3.5	2.8–3.5	<2.8
Prothrombin time (sec prolonged)	1–4	4.1–6	>6

Class A, 5–6 points; class B, 7–9 points; class C, 10–15 points.

function (hyperbilirubinemia, prolonged INR, or hypoalbuminemia) or physical examination or historical evidence of complications of portal hypertension (ascites, portal systemic encephalopathy, splenomegaly, or varices).

For patients with cirrhosis, outcomes after abdominal operations depend on the severity of liver disease as measured by the Child-Pugh score (Table 93–10). Mortality rates of 10%, 30%, and 82% have been reported with patients with Child-Pugh class A, B, and C, respectively but depend as well on the type of operation. Even patients with well-compensated cirrhosis are at significant risk for death after abdominal surgery. Decompensation of the liver disease is even more common and usually consists of the development or worsening of ascites, encephalopathy, jaundice, or bleeding. Ascites can be a

particular problem after abdominal operations, because it can compromise wound healing and puts patients with intestinal anastomoses at a markedly increased risk.

Complication rates after operations on patients with cirrhosis are high enough that nonoperative interventions are preferred if possible. When operation is required, careful monitoring of mental status and fluid status in the postoperative period is especially important. Limiting the amount of perioperative sodium-containing intravenous fluids may help prevent ascites.

SELECTED READINGS

Centers for Disease Control and Prevention: Prevention of hepatitis A through active or passive immunization: Recommendations of the Advisory Committee on Immunization Practices (ACIP). MMWR 1999;48(No. RR-12):1.
Centers for Disease Control: Immunization of health-care workers: Recommendations of the advisory committee on immunization practices and the hospital infection control practices advisory committee. MMWR 1997;46(RR-18):1.
Centers for Disease Control: Recommendations for preventing transmission of human immunodeficiency virus and hepatitis B virus to patients during exposure-prone invasive procedures. MMWR 1991;40(RR08):1.
Friedman LS: The risk of surgery in patients with liver disease. Hepatology 1999;29:1617.
Hoofnagle JH, Di Bisceglie AM: The treatment of chronic viral hepatitis. N Engl J Med 1997;335:347.
Liang TJ, moderator: Pathogenesis, natural history, treatment, and prevention of hepatitis C. Ann Intern Med 2000;132:296.
Pratt DS, Kaplan MM: Evaluation of abnormal liver-enzyme results in asymptomatic patients. N Engl J Med 2000;342:1266.
Schreiber GB, Busch MP, Kleinman SH, Korelitz JJ: The risk of transfusion-transmitted viral infections. N Engl J Med 1996;334:1685.

Chapter 94

Benign Hepatic Neoplasm

Ravi S. Chari and Mark P. Callery

Although benign tumors of the liver have been identified in approximately 1% of autopsies, the introduction of such new imaging methods as computed tomography (CT), magnetic resonance imaging (MRI), and ultrasonography (US) are considerably more sensitive and can image some kind of liver lesion in approximately 5% of patients. Benign tumors may be classified as true neoplasms, hamartomas, and pseudotumors. The *nonbiliary* neoplasms of the liver can also be classified as hepatocellular, cholangiocellular, vascular, and other nonvascular lesions (Table 94–1). This chapter discusses the optimal diagnostic and therapeutic management of the most common nonbiliary benign lesions of the liver.

HEPATIC ADENOMA

Hepatic adenomas arise in otherwise normal livers and appear as a focal abnormality or mass. The occurrence of hepatic adenoma has increased since 1960. Only eight patients with hepatic adenoma were reported between 1940 and 1960. Between 1960 and 1977, 36 patients with liver cell adenomas appeared in medical journals, and, thereafter, these benign neoplasms have been recognized frequently as a result of refinements in hepatic imaging. Although hepatic adenomas can occur in male or female adults or children, more than 90% develop in women in the third to fifth decades of life.

Because it is temporally coincident with the introduc-

Table 94–1	Histologic Classification of Benign Liver Tumors

Hepatocellular
  Hepatic adenoma (benign adenoma)
  Focal nodular hyperplasia
  Nodular regenerative hyperplasia
Cholangiocellular
  Bile duct adenoma
  Biliary cystadenoma
Vascular
  Hemangioma
  Infantile hemangioendothelioma (capillary endothelioma)
  Hereditary hemorrhagic telangiectasia
Others
  Mesenchymal hamartoma
  Leiomyoma
  Fibroma
  Lipoma
  Lymphangiomatosis
  Adrenal rest tumor
  Pancreatic heterotopia
  Inflammatory pseudotumor

From Chari RS, Meyers WC: Liver. In Levine BA, Copeland EM III, Howard RJ, et al (eds): Current Practice of Surgery. New York, Churchill Livingstone, 1994:21.

tion of oral contraceptives (OCP) in 1960, the increased incidence of hepatic adenomas in young women strongly suggests an association between oral ingestion of estrogen and development of these benign hepatocellular neoplasms. Strikingly, 90% of patients with hepatic adenomas have used oral contraceptives. Furthermore, the risk of development of hepatic adenoma increases with the ratio and strength of the OCP preparation. The annual incidence among OCP users appears to be 3 to 4 per 100,000 in users for more than 2 years. Adenomas are also associated with noncontraceptive estrogen use, androgen steroid use, diabetes mellitus, glycogen storage diseases, and iron overload.

Clinical Presentation

About half of the patients with hepatic adenomas have abdominal pain. Some experience chronic or episodic mild upper abdominal pain, whereas others have repeated acute attacks of severe pain caused by hemorrhage into the tumor or adjacent liver. Another more dramatic pain syndrome is caused by free intraperitoneal rupture, which produces hemorrhage (hemoperitoneum) and, frequently, shock. The latter syndrome occurs in 10% to 30% of patients with adenomas. Only 25% to 30% of patients sense an abdominal mass. A mass is palpable in a similar percentage. The remainder of hepatic adenomas are discovered incidentally in asymptomatic patients at autopsy, laparotomy, or during radiologic evaluation of another condition. Pregnancy is reported to stimulate growth of the adenoma and development of complications.

Preoperative Management

The imaging studies most commonly used to detect the hepatic mass are US and multiphasic helical CT. Differentiating between benign and malignant lesions may be difficult, especially if only one imaging modality is used. Therefore, a combination of imaging modalities is often recommended. On US, adenomas display a nonspecific, heterogeneous echogenic pattern. Conventional CT generally also yields little specific diagnostic information. However, multiphasic helical CT, including both arterial and portal venous phases, identifies the hypervascular adenoma quite well (Fig. 94–1). On arteriography, the lesion is typically vascular with some hypervascular regions, representing areas of hemorrhage or necrosis. Hepatic adenomas usually exhibit centripetal blood flow. Because of recent improvements and the noninvasive nature of CT and MRI technology, arteriography has become largely unnecessary in the evaluation of these lesions.

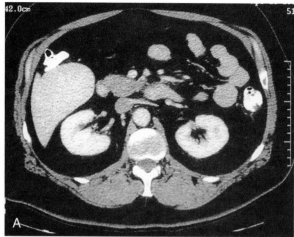

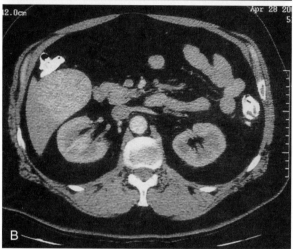

Figure 94–1. *A,* Non–contrast-enhanced computed tomography of a hepatic adenoma. *B,* After administration of contrast medium, the lesion enhances.

When radiologic studies demonstrate an inhomogeneous, hypervascular mass with internal echoes, the diagnosis of a hepatocellular tumor should be considered (particularly if there is no evidence of a primary malignancy elsewhere). MRI or erythrocyte-labeled isotope liver scan can effectively exclude the diagnosis of hemangioma. Although percutaneous needle biopsy or fine-needle aspiration for cytodiagnosis may help, even experienced pathologists have difficulty differentiating between well-differentiated hepatocellular carcinoma and adenoma, and sometimes even between adenoma and pseudotumor. For this reason, there is little or no utility of needle aspiration or biopsy in this and other hepatic lesions.

Recent work has shown that positron emission tomography (PET) is useful in differentiating malignant tumors from benign lesions. Because most malignant cells contain a relatively low level of glucose-6-phosphatase, they accumulate and trap [^{18}F] fluorodeoxyglucose (FDG) intracellularly, allowing the visualization of increased uptake. In one study, 110 patients with hepatic lesions greater than 1 cm were evaluated for potential resection and underwent PET imaging. All (100%) liver metastases from adenocarcinoma and sarcoma primaries in 66 patients and

all cholangiocarcinomas in 8 patients had an increased uptake of FDG. However, hepatocellular carcinoma had increased uptake in only 16 of 23 patients (70%), whereas all the benign hepatic lesions (n = 23), including adenoma and focal nodular hyperplasia (FNH), had poor uptake. Overall, the combination of abdominal pain, decreasing hematocrit, and a liver tumor in young female patients should strongly suggest a diagnosis of adenoma.

Histology

Hepatic adenomas are usually solitary and round but not usually encapsulated. Adenomas often bulge from the external surface of the liver and contain several large blood vessels. The cut surface is yellow or tan and has areas of hemorrhage and necrosis. Microscopically, the adenomas are composed of closely approximated cords of hepatocytes that *lack* surrounding bile ducts and have vacuolated sinusoidal borders. The hepatocytes are often paler than normal because of increased glycogen or fat content. Ultrastructurally, adenoma cells are similar to normal hepatocytes but have fewer organelles and canaliculi. Interesting, and possibly important, is the fact that up to 10% of surgically excised hepatic adenomas harbor foci of hepatocellular carcinoma.

Intraoperative Management

Hepatic adenoma most commonly presents as an undiagnosed liver mass—only a minority of patients initially present with intraperitoneal bleeding. For those patients in the latter group, the differential diagnosis includes ruptured ectopic pregnancy (less likely in women taking birth control pills), bleeding visceral artery aneurysm, and ruptured spleen. Emergency US confirms the presence of a hepatic mass, and peritoneal lavage is occasionally performed to document intraperitoneal bleed. During evaluation, the patient with suspected hemorrhage from a hepatic tumor should receive vigorous blood transfusions with hemodynamic monitoring. Operation is best performed after the initial resuscitation, while control of bleeding is usually best achieved by removal of the tumor. Nonoperative methods of managing bleeding hepatic adenomas (angiographic embolization) are usually not indicated and should be reserved for those patients who are completely unsuitable for an operative procedure.

For those patients in whom an adenoma is suspected, resection is the best treatment option for the following reasons:

1. Nonoperative discrimination between hepatic adenoma and hepatocellular carcinoma is somewhat difficult.
2. Hepatic adenomas sometimes (10%) harbor foci of hepatocellular cancer and may be premalignant lesions.
3. Hepatic adenomas may produce symptoms and sometimes life-threatening hemorrhage.

Resection can usually be performed electively with low associated morbidity and mortality risks compared with emergent resection in the hemodynamically unstable patient. Use of OCP should cease immediately with the discovery of any hepatocellular neoplasm. Several case reports document regression of liver cell tumors after discontinuation of OCP. However, cessation of OCP does *not* change the frequency of malignant transformation. Development of hepatocellular carcinoma at the site of adenoma regression has been reported. Because most patients are young and fit, laparoscopic resection may even be considered in specialized centers. In patients who are pregnant at the time of diagnosis, we recommend the removal of the adenoma electively during the second trimester.

FOCAL NODULAR HYPERPLASIA

FNH is an unusual hepatic lesion frequently confused with adenoma. No convincing evidence links use of OCP to the development of FNH. However, use of OCP may foster growth of FNH and a tendency for an established FNH to bleed. The documented incidence of FNH is increasing, probably because of the increase in abdominal imaging. Nearly 90% of FNH occurs in women, primarily in the second and third decades, but the disease also affects older women and a small number of men and children. Between 1960 and 1967, only 37 patients with FNH were described in medical journals, yet the number of patients recognized recently has increased dramatically. FNH probably represents a hyperplastic response of the hepatic parenchyma to a preexisting arterial malformation rather than a true neoplasm. FNH can occur in any portion of the liver, and approximately 10% of patients have multiple lesions.

Clinical Presentation

In contrast to hepatic adenomas, FNH is generally a benign process that does not cause symptoms. Only 10% of patients with FNH have symptoms usually consisting of mild, chronic, or intermittent abdominal pain. Acute symptoms are rare. Hemorrhage, rupture, or other problems such as malignant change are exceedingly rare.

Preoperative Management

Most imaging modalities cannot reliably establish the diagnosis of FNH. Typical CT findings for FNH include early hypodensity with subsequent isodensity and hypodensity. A central scar is a characteristic feature of FNH and may be seen on CT, US, or MRI. Arteriography is highly sensitive but lacks specificity. Of note, a central scar can also be seen in fibrolamellar hepatocellular carcinoma, hemangioma, and lymphoma. Technetium-labeled cholescintigraphy is also useful in identifying FNH. Criteria required for a diagnosis of FNH include hypoperfusion during the early phase (1 minute), no or positive contrast during the parenchymal phase, and trapping of radioactivity during the late phase (greater than 90 minutes). In 92 patients with histologic confirmation of FNH, preoperative cholescintigraphy plus US and CT led to the imaging diagnosis of FNH in 90% of patients.

Histology

FNH consists of one or more grossly viable nodules in an otherwise normal liver, most frequently formed near the surface of the liver. The nodules are usually several centimeters in size but occasionally grow to be much larger. In one series, 84% were less than 5 cm in diameter, but only 3% were larger than 10 cm. Histologically, this lesion usually has a central stellate scar, no true encapsulation is evident, and the cells, which are slightly different in color, usually blend with normal hepatic parenchyma. The ultrastructure of the hepatocytes in FNH is similar to that of normal hepatocytes. Microscopically, FNH consists of many normal hepatic cells mixed with bile ducts or ductules and divided by fibrous bands, or septa, into nodules (Fig. 94–2). The fibrous septa contain numerous bile ducts (in contrast to the absence of biliary ducts in hepatic adenoma) and a moderate lymphocytic infiltration. There is usually some evidence of mild cholestasis. The blood supply to areas of FNH is quite different from that of hepatic adenomas with most of the supply arising centrally rather than peripherally.

Intraoperative Management

Treatment of a patient with FNH depends primarily on the certainty of the diagnosis. If malignancy or an adenoma remain as possible diagnoses, the patient should undergo laparoscopy. Small superficial masses are easily removed with local excision. If FNH is conclusively diagnosed, the mass is best left undisturbed. Excisional biopsy is recommended for larger lesions even if excision requires a major liver resection. FNH occasionally occurs in the vicinity of hepatocellular carcinoma, in which case multiple biopsies may be required to avoid sampling errors. Whenever the diagnosis remains in doubt, even after biopsy, the lesion should be removed.

NODULAR REGENERATIVE HYPERPLASIA

This condition is rare, but because there is confusion between this entity and cirrhosis, its exact incidence is variable depending on the observer. Nodular regenerative hyperplasia is a noncirrhotic diffuse hepatocellular process characterized by multiple nodules and intervening areas of hepatic atrophy. It is frequently associated with portal hypertension. The primary distinction between nodular regenerative hyperplasia and cirrhosis is the absence of severe fibrosis. It is similar to FNH in that both are *not* true neoplasms. Nodular regenerative hyperplasia most likely has a variety of causes, in light of the wide variety of associated nonhepatic chronic diseases. These include myeloproliferative disorders, lymphoproliferative disorders, and collagen vascular diseases.

Clinical Presentation

The pathology of nodular regenerative hyperplasia is similar to that of lesions produced experimentally and clinically by a number of drugs including the experimental

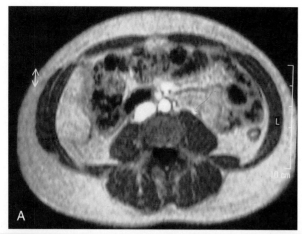

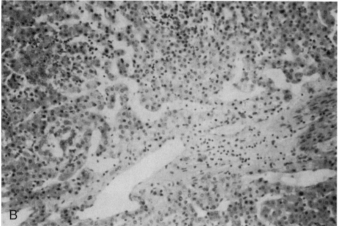

Figure 94–2. *A,* Magnetic resonance imaging demonstrating a lesion in segment 6 of the liver. This patient had persistent, dull right upper quadrant discomfort. *B,* After laparoscopic resection, pathology (× 10) confirmed the diagnosis of focal nodular hyperplasia (FNH).

carcinogens, ethionine, aflatoxin B, Thorotrast, and dimethylnitrosamine. The primary clinical effects of nodular regenerative hyperplasia are related to the underlying portal hypertension. Ascites is unusual. Occasionally, a nodule may rupture, causing hemoperitoneum similar to hepatocellular adenoma. The lesion may be discovered coincidentally at laparotomy. Treatment is usually directed toward correcting the portal hypertension. Occasional patients with advanced cirrhotic diseases and failing synthetic function are good candidates for liver transplantation.

Histology

The hepatocytes themselves are usually somewhat enlarged with pale cytoplasm. Larger nodules or groups of nodules may displace vascular structures, particularly the portal tracks. Portal hypertension probably results from obstruction of the portal venous inflow by the nodules themselves or from an independent pathophysiology.

Intraoperative Management

Treatment is usually directed toward correcting the associated portal hypertension. Occasionally, patients are good candidates for liver transplantation. In patients in whom

diagnosis is in question, biopsy or resection is appropriate to exclude the absence of malignancy.

HEMANGIOMA

Approximately 2% of autopsied livers contain cavernous hemangiomas, making this lesion the most common benign liver tumor (this is sometimes disputed because bile duct hamartomas are probably more common). Most hemangiomas are small and do not cause symptoms. However, they may be large and, when associated with diffuse hemangiomatosis, can nearly replace the liver. The lesion occurs in all age groups and is probably more common in women. The pathology is similar to that of hemangiomas in other parts of the body.

Clinical Presentation

Most hepatic hemangiomas are detected incidentally and produce no symptoms. In symptomatic patients, complaints consist of a full feeling or upper abdominal pain. Very occasionally lesions rupture as a result of trauma. Approximately 10% of patients with clinically detectable lesions are febrile. Hepatomegaly or an abdominal mass is the most common physical finding. These lesions have no malignant potential.

Preoperative Management

Radiologic imaging studies play the key role in diagnosis, although laparotomy is occasionally necessary to make the diagnosis. Percutaneous needle biopsy of suspected lesions is generally not recommended. On US, cavernous hemangiomas usually appear as well-defined, solitary, homogeneously echogenic smooth masses with faint acoustic enhancement. Although these features are fairly consistent, US rarely establishes the diagnosis definitively. In the past, hepatic angiography was considered the most accurate radiologic test for hemangiomas. Currently, time-sequenced CT obtained with a rapid intravenous injection of a radiographic contrast or gadolinium MRI permits accurate diagnosis of most hemangiomas. The primary entity in the differential diagnosis is a hypervascular malignancy. A finding of globular enhancement or areas of pooling of contrast in the periphery of the lesion is a sign that distinguishes hemangioma from hepatic metastases by helical CT. MRI with long T2 weighting and dynamic-enhanced T1 weighting are probably the most sensitive and specific modalities for the diagnosis of hemangioma.

Intraoperative Management

Most hepatic hemangiomas have a benign course. The risk of malignancy or of continued growth is negligible, and spontaneous hemorrhage is rare. Therefore, most hepatic hemangiomas should remain undisturbed by the surgeon as long as that diagnostic uncertainty can be eliminated. Surgical resection is indicated if:

1. A hemangioma produces persistent bothersome symptoms such as pain or fever.
2. Intraperitoneal or intrahepatic rupture of the lesion is suspected (extremely rare).
3. A lesion is considered large enough to be at high risk for traumatic rupture. Those lesions below the costal margin are particularly at risk for rupture.
4. Malignancy is suspected and imaging cannot definitively establish the diagnosis of hemangioma.

INFANTILE HEMANGIOENDOTHELIOMA

Infantile hemangioendotheliomas are capillary hemangiomas similar to lesions that commonly occur in infancy in skin and mucous membranes. The incidence of this neoplasm in the liver is difficult to determine because many lesions probably involute before diagnosis. The cutaneous variety is reported to occur in 0.5% of neonates. Nearly all cases occur in infancy. Incidence in girls outnumbers that in boys 2:1. Histologically, the center of the lesion is necrotic, and the periphery contains proliferating vascular channels. Some lesions appear more aggressive histologically and may be confused with angiosarcoma.

Metastases from such lesions have been reported, but rarely.

Clinical Presentation and Preoperative and Intraoperative Management

Most affected patients are asymptomatic. In most patients, the tumor is indolent and goes through various stages of proliferation, maturation, involution, and disappearance. Symptomatic patients may have high-output congestive heart failure resulting from severe arteriovenous shunting. Symptoms are associated with a 70% mortality rate as a result of congestive heart failure, hepatic failure, or rupture. Hepatic artery ligation, embolization, radiation therapy, steroids, and transplantation have been used with some success.

OTHER BENIGN SOLID TUMORS

Other benign solid tumors that may appear in the liver include lipomas, fibromas, leiomyomas, myxomas, teratomas, carcinoid tumors, and mesenchymal hamartomas. The most common benign tumors of the liver are bile duct hamartomas. These appear as small nodules on the liver surface with benign hypoplastic bile ductular epithelium on microscopic evaluation (biliary neoplasm). Carcinoid is an exceedingly rare primary, as opposed to metastatic liver tumor, and can be associated with the carcinoid syndrome. Mesenchymal hamartomas are rare but important to recognize, because they grow to an extremely large size in an infant or young child and require surgical resection. Biliary cystadenomas and bile duct adenomas are also rare and may cause pain or extrahepatic biliary obstruction (biliary neoplasms). Biliary cystadenomas are more likely than primary cysts to recur, and because there is the additional risk of malignancy, these should be resected. Other even more rare benign biliary tumors include meningioma, fibroma, and granular cell myoblastoma. Another lesion usually of little pathologic significance but which is relatively common is focal fatty change.

Some benign conditions that can be confused with hepatic neoplasms include hereditary hemorrhagic telangiectasia, peliosis hepatis, and hepatic pseudotumor. More than 50 patients with inflammatory pseudotumor have been reported; most pseudotumors are believed to arise from healed hepatic abscesses as overgrowths of chronic inflammatory tissue. Hereditary hemorrhagic telangiectasia is a diffuse telangiectatic process of the liver with numerous arteriovenous fistulas. It is rare, associated with fibrosis, and considered by some to be a form of cirrhosis. Peliosis hepatis is also a rare lesion characterized by variably sized blood lakes. The most common association is with anabolic steroid therapy, but this process has also been seen with other drugs in chronic wasting diseases. The lesion is thought to be associated with toxic damage to sinusoidal or hepatic venous endothelium. Rarely is this condition clinically important, and no intervention is required.

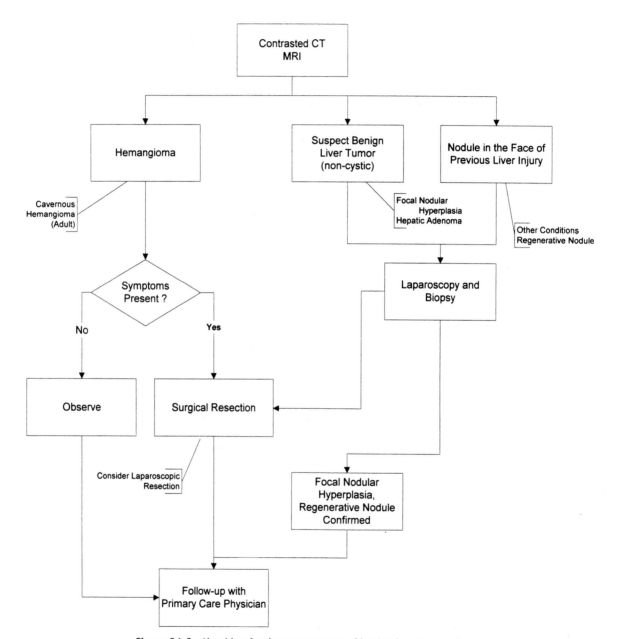

Figure 94–3. Algorithm for the management of benign hepatic neoplasms.

Pearls and Pitfalls

- Liver biopsy is seldom recommended in the evaluation of solitary liver masses that are resectable—even though the absolute risk is small, it is an unnecessary risk because it seldom modifies the management.
- Liver biopsy of solitary, resectable liver lesions can cause bleeding (possibly requiring transfusion or resulting in death) and may cause seeding of unsuspected malignancy.
- Growth and rupture of adenoma during hormonal stages of pregnancy can result in both maternal and fetal loss.
- The only way of eliminating the malignant potential of an adenoma is with complete surgical resection. Whenever possible, an adenoma should be resected (Fig. 94–3).
- Biopsy-proven adenoma can still progress to malignant transformation, even after cessation of exogenous estrogens.
- FNH can present as a symptomatic mass lesion of the liver.
- A central scar is not pathognomonic of FNH.
- Hemangiomas have negligible risk of malignant transformation or spontaneous rupture.

Postoperative Management Following Resection of Benign Hepatic Neoplasms

There are few deviations in the management of hepatic resection for benign neoplasms compared with malignant neoplasms (in the noncirrhotic patient). The operative course should be marked with judicious attention to maintaining a low central venous pressure and control of inflow vessels to minimize operative blood loss. The need for blood transfusion should be less than 5%. Drains should not be placed routinely, with a less than 10% requirement for postoperative percutaneous drainage.

We avoid nasogastric tube decompression and instead begin a regular diet in most patients on postoperative day 1. Ambulation is expected on the same day, and discharge should be planned by day 4 or 5. Hematocrit can be checked in the recovery room and on the first postoperative day and, if it is stable, another measurement is not necessary. Electrolytes and prothrombin time should be checked similarly. Complications are reflective of the operative procedure more so than the underlying pathology. Bile collection, wound infection, abscess, and pulmonary complications (effusion, atelectasis, pneumonia) have occurred in 15% to 35% of patients. Most of these complications do not lengthen postoperative stay.

OUTCOMES

When pathology has confirmed the benignity of the lesion and there is no reason to believe that there is residual disease, there is no requirement for postoperative imaging. Outcome is generally good with operative mortality rates of less than 1%. Risk of recurrence for most of these lesions is negligible, and routine surveillance is not necessary.

SELECTED READINGS

Chari RS, Meyers WC: Liver surgery. In Levine BA, Copeland EM III, Howard RJ, et al (eds): Current Practice of Surgery, 1st ed. New York, Churchill Livingstone, 1994.
Gordon S, Reddy R, Livingstone A, et al: Resolution of a contraceptive-steroid-induced hepatic adenoma with subsequent evolution into hepatocellular carcinoma. Ann Intern Med 1986;105:547.
Delbeke D, Martin W, Sandler M, et al: Evaluation of benign vs malignant hepatic lesions with positron emission tomography. Arch Surg 1998;133:510.
Kerlin P, Davis G, McGill D, et al: Hepatic adenoma and focal nodular hyperplasia: Clinical, pathologic, and radiologic features. Gastroenterology 1983;84:994.
Weimann A, Ringe B, Klempnauer J, et al: Benign liver tumors: Differential diagnosis and indications for surgery. World J Surg 1997;21:983.

Chapter 95
Hepatic Abscess
Hiram C. Polk, Jr., and Benjamin D. Tanner

Hepatic abscesses can be broadly classified as either pyogenic or amebic, depending on the underlying pathogen. Pyogenic liver abscesses are the most common type in the United States and are usually caused by gram-negative bacteria. Amebic abscesses, on the other hand, are exclusively caused by infection with the parasite *Entamoeba histolytica*. The prevalence of pyogenic hepatic abscesses in recent studies is 13 to 22 per 10,000 hospitalized patients, which is not dissimilar to the number reported by Ochsner and DeBakey in the preantibiotic era of 1938. Excluding patients who are intravenous drug abusers and those who are positive for human immunodeficiency virus (HIV), there has, however, been an upward shift in the age distribution of the disease, presumably secondary to the increased use of antimicrobials as well as the underlying etiologies. Early in the last century, the usual cause was pyelophlebitis resulting from acute appendicitis in the younger population. With antibiotics, the distribution has shifted to an older, more debilitated group of patients with a greater range of etiologies. Currently, biliary tract disease represents the most common factor in the pathogenesis of pyogenic hepatic abscess.

Treatment of bacterial liver abscesses has changed during recent decades as well. Before the advent of modern antibiotics, the mortality rate was more than 75%. Currently, standard treatment includes some form of external drainage with antibiotic therapy. Newer diagnostic methods, including ultrasonography and computed tomography (CT) with the possibility of noninvasive treatment, have not only given the surgeon an alternative to open surgical drainage but also substantially reduce the morbidity and mortality rates in patients with a pyogenic liver abscess.

PYOGENIC LIVER ABSCESS

Clinical Presentation

The most common cause of pyogenic hepatic abscess is biliary tract disease. The underlying pathology may be from obstruction, malignant or benign, or from direct extension of some infected source such as a gangrenous gallbladder. Most studies indicate that biliary tract disease causes hepatic abscesses in about 40% of patients. Other causes include (1) pyelophlebitis (appendicitis, diverticulitis), (2) systemic bacteremia (intravenous drug abuse, endocarditis), (3) cryptogenic etiology, (4) malignancy (hematologic, colonic), and (5) trauma (Table 95–1). Most hepatic abscesses are solitary and located in the right lobe of the liver. Approximately 20% of patients have bilobar involvement, with a minority having only left-sided disease. The predilection for the right lobe is attributed both

to its size and preferential flow of blood from the superior mesenteric vein via the portal vein during bacterial seeding. Multiple, small abscesses are found in 40% of patients and arise without antecedent biliary tract disease, usually from systemic bacterial seeding, as in the case of intravenous drug abuse or endocarditis.

Patients with hepatic abscesses have a variable clinical presentation, depending on the underlying etiology. However, some symptoms appear to be common to the disease process. Most patients have right upper-quadrant pain, fever, and general malaise as the usual symptoms, but this is highly variable; indeed, less than one third of patients with hepatic abscess have this complete triad of symptoms on presentation. Other symptoms include rigors, nausea and vomiting, anorexia, and night sweats. Physical examination may reveal abdominal tenderness, hepatomegaly, jaundice, or a right subpulmonic effusion, or right lower lobe rales.

Laboratory examination of the patient with possible hepatic abscess should consist of a complete blood count (with differential) and comprehensive metabolic panel including liver function tests. Although the most consistent abnormality found by laboratory tests is leukocytosis, its absence does not exclude the possibility of hepatic abscess. Depending on the duration of the illness, anemia may also be evident. Liver function test results are usually abnormal, but they do little to differentiate the patient with an abscess from someone with underlying hepatobiliary disease not associated with hepatic abscess. Increased alkaline phosphatase with hyperbilirubinemia is frequently encountered because of the high association of biliary tract disease in this group of patients. It is important to note that the laboratory examination should only support the surgeon's clinical diagnosis of hepatic abscess. No single abnormality, or lack thereof, unequivocally establishes the diagnosis.

Radiographic imaging has become the standard means of diagnosing a hepatic abscess. Plain chest radiographs may show nonspecific abnormalities that are helpful in

Table 95–1	Etiology of Pyogenic Liver Abscess	
ETIOLOGY	**PERCENTAGE OF PATIENTS**
Biliary tract	34
Portal vein	18
Cryptogenic	18
Bacteremia	9
Direct extension	8
Tumor	7
Trauma	6

From Bowers ED, Doberneck RC: Pyogenic liver abscess and splenic abscess. In Fry DE (ed): Surgical Infections. Boston, Little Brown and Company, 1995:297–301, with permission.

608

suspecting the diagnosis. Elevation of the right diaphragm and right-sided lower lobe atelectasis or effusion is occasionally present. CT and ultrasonography have emerged as the most specific and sensitive modalities available in the diagnosis of a liver abscess. Ultrasonography is the preferred initial imaging choice because of its low cost, availability, ability to image biliary lithiasis and intrahepatic biliary obstruction, and nearly nonexistent incidence of complications. It is most useful for differentiating between the cystic contents of an abscess versus the solid tissue of a neoplasm. CT offers a higher diagnostic yield and has the attractive advantage of potentially revealing the underlying cause of the hepatic abscess. Figure 95–1 shows the typical appearance of a solitary pyogenic liver abscess. The diagnostic sensitivities of ultrasonography and CT are approximately 86% and 100%, respectively. An additional benefit of these imaging studies is the potential for simultaneous therapeutic intervention using percutaneous aspiration and avoidance of surgical drainage.

Preoperative Management

Once the diagnosis of pyogenic hepatic abscess is suspected, broad but defined parenteral antibiotics should be instituted. *Escherichia coli* is the most frequently encountered organism causing hepatic abscess. Other bacteria cultured from hepatic abscesses are listed in Table 95–2. The preponderance of these organisms are aerobic gram-negative pathogens, with anaerobic bacteria involved either in combination or as single isolates; anaerobes are more common in the cryptogenic hepatic abscesses. In this setting, ceftazidime or aztreonam are appropriate choices. Aminoglycosides should be avoided because they are generally not needed, and their avoid-

Table 95–2	Bacteriology of Pyogenic Liver Abscess	
BACTERIA		**PERCENT CULTURES**
Aerobes		76
Enteric gram-negative rods		39
Escherichia coli		20
Others		19
Nonenteric gram-negative rods		7
Gram-positive cocci		30
Streptococcus sp.		11
Enterococcus sp.		10
Staphylococcus sp.		8
Anaerobes		24
Gram-negative rods		11
Gram-positive cocci		10
Gram-positive rods		3

From Bowers ED, Doberneck RC: Pyogenic liver abscess and splenic abscess. In Fry DE (ed): Surgical Infections. Boston, Little Brown and Company, 1995:97–301, with permission.

ance will prevent renal and auditory toxicities. If antistaphylococcal coverage is clinically necessary, then nafcillin can be added, while reserving vancomycin for the methicillin-resistant organisms. In treating hepatic and amebic abscesses, metronidazole is important because it is active against anaerobes as well as *Entamoeba histolytica*. (Amebic hepatic abscesses are discussed in detail in the next section.) Once bacterial isolates are obtained, whether from blood or abscess culture, antibiotic therapy should be altered as directed by diagnostic sensitivities and narrowed as appropriate.

CT or ultrasound-guided percutaneous aspiration has become the mainstay for obtaining hepatic abscess aspirates. In some highly select patients, aspiration with appropriate antibiotics may effectively treat these abscesses. However, most surgeons consider placement of percutaneous drains, along with parenteral antibiotics, as the treatment of choice in management of hepatic abscesses caused by bacteria. The catheter should be 7 French to 10 French and may even be appropriate for multiple, small abscesses located close together. These procedures are associated with minimal morbidity and low recurrence rates. Success rates in excess of 80% have been achieved, thus avoiding operative intervention.

In addition to treatment of the hepatic abscess, a comprehensive evaluation of the abdominal cavity is warranted to determine the underlying cause. The value of this investigation is the ability to direct further therapeutic interventions. As previously stated, biliary tract disease is the most likely source of hepatic abscess. However, underlying colonic malignancy, diverticulitis, and Crohn's disease may also have abscess formation as their initial manifestation. CT of the abdomen may be helpful in detecting sources other than the pancreaticobiliary tract. Other studies, such as barium enema, colonoscopy, and gastrointestinal studies with oral contrast, may also aid the surgeon in identifying the primary disease process and determining therapy. Treatment of the underlying cause not only decreases the chance of recurrent hepatic abscess but also prevents progression of the patient's inciting illness.

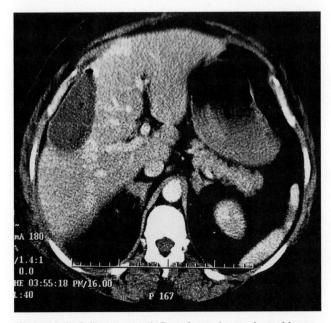

Figure 95–1. Solitary pyogenic liver abscess in a patient with metastatic colon cancer.

Operative Management

Operative intervention for hepatic abscess may be necessary when conservative management with antibiotics and percutaneous drainage fail. In addition, open surgical evacuation may be pursued if the patient's primary disease necessitates operative management. The approach depends on the size, number, and location of the abscess, as well as the need for access to treat the underlying cause. Traditionally, a posterior approach through the bed of the 12th rib was used for fear of intraperitoneal spread of the infection. This method is currently only recommended for high-lying posterior abscesses. Currently, either a subcostal or midline approach may be used.

After a thorough examination of the entire abdominal cavity for other abscesses, the liver is isolated from the other viscera with laparotomy pads. If the abscess is not readily apparent on inspection, then needle aspiration may be used to define the location. Intraoperative ultrasonography may be useful to locate a deep-seated abscess or multiple, small collections. Aspiration using trocar suction helps avoid unnecessary spillage of purulence. After evacuation of the contents, the abscess cavity should be unroofed and any loculations disrupted to allow free access to the entire cavity. Multiple biopsy specimens of the abscess wall should be sent for pathologic evaluation to ensure that malignancy is not the causative agent. Culture of the aspirate is analyzed for aerobic and anaerobic bacteria, fungus, and amebic trophozoites. Placement of soft suction drains prevents recurrence and allows resolution of the cavity. Drains should always be brought out through separate stab incisions in the skin. Multiple abscesses may require several drains to provide adequate egress of fluid and prevent recurrence.

Postoperative Management

The duration of antibiotic treatment of hepatic abscesses resulting from bacterial infection is of major controversy in the surgical literature. Historically, antibiotics were continued for 6 weeks after drainage. More recent data leave this matter unclear. It may be that high-dose intravenous antibiotics should be continued when the abscesses are multiple, such as those associated with intravenous drug abuse or impaired immune states, or both. Whether there is a place for oral antibiotics after a 1- or 2-week course of parenteral drug therapy is both a cost and efficacy issue that remains to be clarified. Clinical resolution of infection appears to be the most reliable indicator of duration of therapy rather than any set amount of time.

Drains, whether percutaneous or surgically placed, need to be continuously monitored for amount and character of effluent. The decision to remove them is based on the condition of the patient as well as a reduction in the output of these drains. Generally, a contrast study of a drain is a method to objectively assess resolution of a hepatic abscess cavity. Once the cavity has resolved, slowly withdrawing the catheter per day until it is completely out is a good way to allow the drain tract to heal and avoid a chronic fistula.

Complications

Most problems associated with treatment of hepatic abscesses arise from percutaneous drainage. Patients with coagulopathies or ascites are generally better served with an open surgical procedure. Abscesses located in the left lobe or near vital vascular or biliary structures may make percutaneous access difficult and potentially dangerous for the patient. Either percutaneous or open drainage can be associated with sepsis, and the astute surgeon should be ready for this in the postprocedure period. Septicemia is the most common complication after treatment and carries an increased mortality rate.

The underlying disease process associated with hepatic abscess may also be a source of complications. Prolonged ileus, pneumonia, pulmonary embolus, and pleural effusion are just a few of the possible complications that can arise during treatment of the patient with hepatic abscess. Currently, abscesses present in a population of older patients who have an array of associated comorbidities that must be addressed during treatment or else become exacerbated.

Outcomes

The mortality rate for pyogenic hepatic abscesses remains approximately 50%. Solitary abscesses have a much lower mortality rate than multiple abscesses because of the high association of underlying malignant biliary obstruction with the latter. The mortality rate is virtually 100% in all reviews for hepatic abscess when adequate drainage is not possible. Factors that influence mortality are age, severity of underlying disease, associated malignancy, and presence of shock. Hypoalbuminemia and hyperbilirubinemia, indicative of impaired liver function, also correlate with poor survival outlook.

Most surgeons favor initial treatment with a trial of percutaneous aspiration and drainage, in addition to antibiotics. Bertel and associates (1986) achieved successful results in 80% of patients, with a morbidity rate of 20% in a series of patients treated in this fashion. Open surgical drainage should be undertaken early in patients with inadequate drainage or when the patient's clinical condition does not improve. Hepatic pyogenic abscess caused by an identifiable abdominal source can be treated in one of two ways. Initial percutaneous drainage can be used as a temporizing measure in the critically ill patient before definitive operative laparotomy to correct the inciting pathology. Some patients can also undergo open drainage of the abscess and treatment of the underlying disease in a combined approach, if their condition allows. Treatment failures with the percutaneous route are commonly caused by inadequately drained multiple abscesses and by not addressing a correctable cause of the abscess. In addition, left-sided hepatic abscesses are difficult to approach percutaneously and often require surgical drainage for resolution.

AMEBIC HEPATIC ABSCESS

Clinical Presentation

Amebic hepatic abscesses are caused by the parasite *Entamoeba histolytica*. This pathogen exists in two forms, a cyst and the invasive trophozoite. Colonic infestation is common in tropical and subtropical locations around the world. With increased immigration from these areas, amebiasis is becoming more prevalent, and asymptomatic infestation involves 5% to 10% of the population, especially in the Southwest United States. In addition, travelers to these areas may become infected by ingesting the cystic stage of the parasite as it is commonly passed in a fecal-oral manner.

The cyst matures into the invasive trophozoite, which resides in the large intestine and can cause colitis. If the trophozoite invades colonic tissue, then it may pass through mesenteric venules and eventually take up residence in the liver. Thrombosis and liquefactive necrosis occur, later forming the abscess cavity. The material collected from these cavities has a characteristic appearance described as "anchovy paste," which results from the mixture of blood and necrotic hepatic parenchyma.

Patients with amebic hepatic abscesses differ epidemiologically from those with pyogenic abscesses. These patients tend to be younger, are usually men, and are immigrants or have a history of travel to an endemic area. The onset of presentation may be closely related to recent travel or may appear years later. Immigrants from Mexico comprise the largest percentage of patients with an amebic hepatic abscess in the United States.

The hepatic abscess may be preceded by intestinal manifestations; however, concomitant hepatic abscess is found in only one third of those patients with amebic colitis. Diarrhea occurs in more than half of patients with an abscess but is not by itself diagnostic. Right upper quadrant pain, fever, nausea, vomiting, and anorexia may be present. As mentioned earlier, these symptoms can also be found in association with pyogenic abscesses and do not definitively discriminate between the two types of collections. Physical examination may show abdominal tenderness, particularly in the right upper quadrant and associated hepatomegaly.

A complete blood count and liver function tests should always be ordered when the diagnosis of any type of hepatic abscess is considered. A nonspecific increase in serum transaminases is seen in more than 50% of these patients, along with a mild increase in the alkaline phosphatase. Hyperbilirubinemia is seldom observed with an amebic hepatic abscess, although hypoalbuminemia is not uncommon. Leukocytosis and anemia are usually evident.

The confirmation of infection by *Entamoeba histolytica* is best made with the indirect hemoagglutination test. Titers of 1:128 are suggestive of hepatic abscess. Several studies indicate 100% seropositivity in patients with documented amebic liver abscess. The major limitation of serologic studies is the time required for completion. It is prudent to begin empirical therapy while waiting for the results of such tests. Stool cultures and rectal biopsies may be helpful to diagnose amebiasis, but these studies do not definitively define hepatic involvement and have

been negative, even in the face of abscess formation and intestinal invasion.

Ultrasonography is the initial radiologic test of choice in diagnosing amebic hepatic abscess. It is highly accurate, noninvasive, and can detect small (less than 2 cm) abscesses. CT can be used when ultrasonography is negative and the diagnosis is still in question. It may also be indicated after failed amebicidal therapy and in those with suspected complications (i.e., perforation or erosion into adjacent structures). Chest radiography may include findings such as elevated diaphragm, effusion, and atelectasis, which are common to hepatic abscess despite the etiology.

Management

Options for treatment of amebic hepatic abscess do not differ from those for pyogenic abscess. In general, amebicidal agents and drainage, whether surgical or percutaneous, are the standards of care. Metronidazole is the agent used most widely in the United States and is started at a dose of 750 mg orally three times per day while awaiting confirmation by serologic testing. It has a low cost and minimal side effects and its efficacy is greater than 90%. Symptoms usually abate within 72 hours of initiation of treatment. The total duration of therapy is 4 to 6 weeks. For patients not responsive to metronidazole or in those with recurrences, iodoquinol or dehydroemetine should be used. Amebicidal therapy alone without concomitant drainage is curative in more than 75% of patients with amebic hepatic abscess.

Occasionally, aspiration of the abscess may become necessary. It should be reserved for patients with uncertain diagnoses, failed medical therapy, or possible sus-

---

Pearls and Pitfalls

- Pyogenic hepatic abscess is the most common type of hepatic abscess in the United States.
- Gram-negative bacteria are the most common cause of pyogenic abscess.
- The most common etiologies include biliary tract disease, intravenous drug abuse, endocarditis, diverticulitis, and cryptogenic (source never found).
- Antibiotics and a drainage procedure, whether percutaneous or operative, are the standard of care for pyogenic abscess.
- Empirical treatment of pyogenic abscess should usually include agents against anaerobic bacteria.
- Failure to diagnose and treat the underlying source of pyogenic abscesses is associated with recurrence.
- High-dose parenteral antibiotics are warranted for patients with impaired immunity and when multiple abscesses associated with intravenous drug abuse are present.
- *Entamoeba histolytica* is the cause of amebic hepatic abscess.
- Indirect hemoagglutination is the key diagnostic test for an amebic abscess.
- Treatment with metronidazole alone results in successful outcome in about 90% of patients with an amebic hepatic abscess.

pected secondary bacterial infection. In the latter case, appropriate antibacterial agents to cover gram-negative species should be started and modified based on results of diagnostic sensitivities. Aspiration may also be required in large left-lobed abscesses to prevent erosion into adjacent pleural or pericardial structures. Drainage by percutaneous or surgical routes is not usually necessary and may only promote bacterial seeding of the abscess. Open surgical drainage via midline or subcostal incision may become necessary when free perforation of the abscess occurs to allow for débridement of necrotic hepatic tissue and washout of the abdomen.

Complications

Therapy with metronidazole is associated with minimal side effects that include nausea, vomiting, headache, and rashes. Unlike many amebicidal drugs, cardiac toxicity is not encountered with its use. The most dreaded complication of amebic hepatic abscesses is rupture into the adjacent pleural or pericardial spaces. Intrapericardial rupture is observed in less than 2% of all patients but carries a high mortality rate. Thoracic involvement occurs as pulmonary amebic abscess, bronchobiliary fistula, or empyema. This is the most common complication associated with hepatic amebic abscess and occurs in 4% to 7% of patients. Tube thoracostomy or lung resection, or both, may be necessary to resolve these problems.

Outcomes

More than 90% of patients with amebic hepatic abscess become symptom-free after 3 days of therapy with metronidazole. In 75% of these patients, this treatment successfully resolves the abscess without further management. Secondary bacterial infection or resistant parasites that require the addition of a second amebicidal agent to eradicate the abscess can cause failure of this regimen. The mortality rate is generally less than 1% when disease is confined to the liver. Patients with thoracic involvement have a mortality rate of 6%, whereas those with pericardial extension or free intraperitoneal perforation carry a mortality rate that approaches 50%.

SUGGESTED READINGS

Basile JA, Klein SR, Worthen NJ, et al: Amebic liver abscess: The surgeon's role in management. Am J Surg 1983;146:67.
Bertel CK, van Heerden JA, Sheedy PF: Treatment of pyogenic hepatic abscesses. Arch Surg 1986;121:554.
Gerzof SG, Johnson WC, Robbins AH, Nabseth DC: Intrahepatic pyogenic abscesses: Treatment by percutaneous drainage. Am J Surg 1985;149:487.
Huang CJ, Pitt HA, Lipsett PA, et al: Pyogenic hepatic abscess: Changing trends over 42 years. Ann Surg 1996;223:600.
Nordestgaard AG, Stapleford L, Worthen FS, Klein SR: Contemporary management of amebic liver abscess. Am Surg 1992;58:315.

Chapter 96
Portal Hypertension
Stuart J. Knechtle and Layton F. Rikkers

Surgical management of portal hypertension has been refined radically by the recent developments of alternative therapies, including endoscopic sclerotherapy, transjugular intrahepatic portosystemic shunt (TIPS), and liver transplantation. Surgical shunts for the management of variceal hemorrhage are consequently being performed less commonly but, when indicated, have improved outcomes in a more select patient population. Surgical decision making within the context of a multidisciplinary approach to portal hypertension is discussed in this chapter, with particular emphasis given to patient selection for surgery.

CLINICAL PRESENTATION

In the United States, the most common cause of portal hypertension is underlying chronic liver disease caused by alcohol abuse, hepatitis B infection, hepatitis C infection, or autoimmune diseases (sclerosing cholangitis, primary biliary cirrhosis, and autoimmune hepatitis). In children, biliary atresia represents the most common cause. Extrahepatic portal vein occlusion or hepatic vein occlusion (Budd-Chiari syndrome) may cause portal hypertension in the absence of intrinsic liver disease. In contrast, the most common cause of portal hypertension internationally is schistosomiasis. Because etiology determines the course of treatment, it is crucial to determine the underlying cause of portal hypertension and the severity of liver disease.

Stigmata of portal hypertension on physical examination include splenomegaly, a prominent venous pattern on the abdomen, ascites, and portosystemic encephalopathy. Indicators of underlying liver disease include spider angiomata, palmar erythema, gynecomastia, and jaundice. Initial laboratory evaluation should include a complete blood count, hepatitis serology, measures of hepatic synthetic function (serum albumin and prothrombin), measures of hepatic excretory function (serum bilirubin, alkaline phosphatase, and gamma-glutamyltranspeptidase), and indicators of hepatocellular injury or necrosis (AST, ALT). Percutaneous liver biopsy can be helpful in assessing the cause of liver disease and determining its activity. The Child-Pugh classification still remains the most useful measure of hepatic functional reserve (Table 96–1). A serum alpha-fetoprotein level should be obtained to assess the potential presence of hepatocellular carcinoma.

Biphasic computed tomography (CT) is helpful in assessing the presence of ascites, heterogeneity of the hepatic parenchyma compatible with cirrhosis, and a space-occupying liver lesion that could represent a hepatocellular carcinoma. Duplex ultrasonography is useful in assessing the patency and direction of blood flow in the portal vein and hepatic veins. Before considering a surgi-

cal shunt, however, visceral angiography should be done to more precisely define the splanchnic venous anatomy. The results of this examination often dictate both the course of treatment and the choice of surgical procedure.

The presence of underlying portal hypertension is most commonly manifested by one of its complications: gastrointestinal bleeding; ascites; encephalopathy; or hypersplenism. The most life-threatening of these complications is hemorrhage from esophageal or gastric varices or portal hypertensive gastropathy. The diagnosis is best made by endoscopic visualization of the bleeding varices or by the presence of large varices in a patient who has recently bled in the absence of other lesions. As discussed later, endoscopy can also be therapeutic when combined with sclerotherapy or band ligation of varices. Approximately 90% of patients with portal hypertension in whom upper gastrointestinal hemorrhage develops bleed from varices or portal hypertensive gastropathy; the remaining 10% of patients, however, bleed from other sources such as Mallory-Weiss tears or peptic ulcer disease. Variceal bleeding is usually of esophageal origin (80%) and more rarely from gastric varices (20%). Occasionally, varices in other sites such as the duodenum, colon, or an ileostomy stoma may be the source of bleeding. Endoscopic diagnosis is therefore essential before proceeding with treatment and is facilitated by first evacuating blood from the esophagus and stomach. Only one third of patients with varices eventually bleed from them, but once hemorrhage has occurred, the likelihood of a recurrent episode is greater than 80%. The nonoperative and operative treatment of variceal bleeding is discussed later.

Ascites resulting from portal hypertension is caused by altered hepatic and splanchnic hemodynamics, resulting in transudation of fluid into the interstitial space and eventually into the peritoneal cavity when lymph drainage capacity of the liver is exceeded. Ascites commonly develops after resuscitation from a variceal hemorrhage but may also develop spontaneously. Medical therapy consisting of dietary salt restriction and diuretics effectively

Table 96–1	Child-Pugh Criteria for Hepatic Functional Reserve		
	A	B	C
Serum bilirubin (mg/100mL)	<2.0	2.0–3.0	>3.0
Serum albumin (g/100 mL)	>3.5	2.8–3.5	<2.8
Prothrombin time (↑ sec)	1–3	4–6	>6
Ascites	None	Slight	Moderate
Neurologic disorder	None	Minimal	Advanced, "coma"

613

resolves or manages ascites in more than 90% of patients. The diuretic of choice is spironolactone in doses of 100 to 400 mg per day, but a more potent diuretic, such as furosemide, is sometimes necessary as well. Development of ascites refractory to medical management portends a poor prognosis, with a 1-year survival rate generally less than 50% without aggressive surgical intervention.

Options for treatment of medically intractable ascites include intermittent, large volume paracentesis, a surgically placed peritoneovenous shunt, TIPS, and a nonselective portosystemic shunt. Although all are effective to some degree, all have significant disadvantages. Repeated paracentesis may result in inadvertent puncture of the bowel and result in peritonitis, peritoneovenous shunts commonly occlude or become infected, and either TIPS or surgically created nonselective shunts may be complicated by encephalopathy. None of these options prolong survival, although quality of life may be enhanced. Presently, the most commonly used intervention for medically intractable ascites in the United States is TIPS.

Portosystemic encephalopathy may manifest in a variety of ways, including an altered level of consciousness, intellectual deterioration, personality change, and the presence of asterixis on physical examination. Although encephalopathy may develop spontaneously in patients with chronic liver disease, it most commonly develops as a result of one or more precipitating factors such as gastrointestinal bleeding, dehydration, infection, excess dietary protein, surgical portosystemic shunt, or TIPS. The pathogenesis of encephalopathy has not been completely elucidated, but one or more cerebral toxins, such as blood ammonia, likely play a role. The high ratio of plasma aromatic to branched chain amino acids present in patients with liver failure has been hypothesized to result in false neurotransmitters in the central nervous system and the subsequent development of encephalopathy. The high frequency of encephalopathy after surgical or radiologic portosystemic shunts is presumably secondary to cerebral toxins that originate in the intestines, bypassing the first-pass metabolic capacity of the liver.

Treatment of encephalopathy is directed at eliminating the responsible precipitating factors. This approach includes restriction of dietary protein, treatment of infections, evacuation or increased transit of blood from the intestine, and avoidance of pharmacologic sedation. Patients with clinically significant encephalopathy of a chronic or recurring nature can be treated with lactulose or neomycin. Lactulose given in a dose of 30 g four times a day or until a cathartic effect is noted is the most effective treatment of chronic encephalopathy. Orally administered neomycin in a dose of 1.5 g every 6 hours is generally used only in the acute setting. Lactulose combined with mild protein restriction (60 to 80 g per day) is the recommended treatment for chronic intermittent encephalopathy.

Although thrombocytopenia or leukopenia resulting from splenic sequestration is commonly associated with portal hypertension, clinically significant hypersplenism (platelet count less than 50,000 or white blood cell count less than 1500) occurs rarely. Hypersplenism is generally improved by portal decompression with a surgical shunt

or TIPS but almost never represents the sole indication for such a procedure.

TREATMENT OF VARICEAL BLEEDING

Management of esophageal varices can be separated into three phases: (1) prophylaxis, (2) treatment of the acute bleeding episode, and (3) prevention of recurrent bleeding. There is a large variety of nonoperative and operative treatments available. No single therapy is ideal for all circumstances; rather, the overall treatment plan should be individualized for optimal results. Sequential therapies are often necessary. Because the only definitive treatment for patients with chronic liver disease who bleed from varices is liver transplantation, the appropriate candidates and timing for this operation need to be considered.

Prophylaxis

Because only one third of patients with varices eventually bleed, the disadvantages of most prophylactic therapies outweigh their benefits. Early shunt trials in the 1960s showed no benefit of these operations in patients with varices who had not previously bled. Likewise, most trials of endoscopic therapy in the prophylactic setting have also shown no benefit. Nonselective beta blockade has proved efficacious for prophylaxis in patients with varices that are likely to bleed (large varices with red color signs on them). A meta-analysis of multiple randomized, controlled trials shows that beta blockade results in a 20% reduction in likelihood of hemorrhage.

Treatment of the Acute Bleeding Episode

Endoscopic treatment of varices with either sclerosis or band ligation and pharmacotherapy with infusion of either octreotide or vasopressin combined with nitroglycerin represent the mainstays of emergency treatment. Occasionally, extrinsic tamponade with a Sengstaken-Blakemore tube is necessary when exsanguinating hemorrhage develops. When these nonoperative treatments fail, TIPS is the portal decompressive procedure of choice in most institutions. Because many patients with acute variceal bleeding have decompensated hepatic function caused by hypotension, they tend to be at high risk for emergency surgical intervention. There are a few remaining surgical advocates of emergency portal systemic shunts, but the mortality rate associated with these procedures is generally high in this population of patients. More effective nonoperative treatments (endoscopic therapy, pharmacotherapy, and TIPS) have made emergency surgery unnecessary in most circumstances.

Prevention of Recurrent Bleeding

In most centers, serial endoscopic treatment (sclerosis, banding), sometimes in combination with nonselective beta-blockade, is the preferred initial therapy for prevention of recurrent variceal bleeding. Portal decompressive procedures, either TIPS or operative shunts, are reserved for failures of endoscopic treatment and for patients in whom initial endoscopic therapy is not indicated. Prospective, controlled trials of endoscopic therapy and of pharmacotherapy with nonselective beta-blockade reveal that more than 50% of patients will eventually rebleed from varices, and that up to one third of patients will eventually fail these relatively noninvasive treatments. Evidence suggests that band ligation of esophageal varices is preferable to sclerosis, because complications are less and fewer treatment sessions are required to eradicate varices. In some controlled investigations, rebleeding is less likely after band ligation than after variceal sclerosis. In contrast, endoscopic therapy has been less effective for gastric varices and portal hypertensive gastropathy than for esophageal varices. Patients bleeding from these gastric sites may require portal decompression by means of a TIPS or an operative shunt earlier in their course than patients with esophageal varices.

Thus, operative procedures have a more limited role in the management of patients with portal hypertension than in the past. The key indication for a shunting operation currently is a patient with good hepatic functional reserve (Child-Pugh class A or B +) who has failed nonoperative therapy. Patients with advanced hepatic dysfunction (Child-Pugh class B − and C) are best served by

liver transplantation if they are candidates for this procedure (nonalcoholic cirrhotics and abstinent alcoholic cirrhotics). Individuals with advanced liver disease who are not candidates for liver transplantation and who fail nonoperative means of controlling their bleeding are probably best served by a TIPS procedure with frequent post-TIPS surveillance for TIPS occlusion.

PORTAL SYSTEMIC SHUNTS

Distal Splenorenal Shunt

Indications and General Aspects

The distal splenorenal shunt (Warren shunt) (Fig. 96–1) was developed for the purpose of selectively decompressing esophageal varices while simultaneously preserving portal blood flow to the liver and portal venous hypertension. The distal splenic vein, when anastomosed to the left renal vein, decompresses selectively the splanchnic veins draining the stomach, spleen, and part of the pancreas. Ligation of the coronary and gastroepiploic veins separates the high-pressure superior mesenteric venous system from the gastrosplenic venous system, at least temporarily. The pressure in the superior mesenteric vein

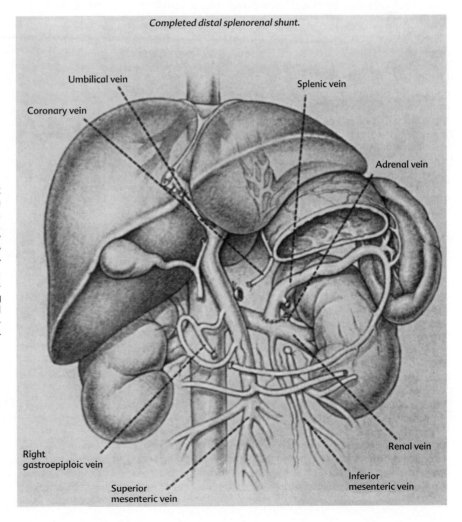

Completed distal splenorenal shunt.

Umbilical vein

Coronary vein

Splenic vein

Adrenal vein

Right gastroepiploic vein

Superior mesenteric vein

Inferior mesenteric vein

Renal vein

Figure 96–1. The distal splenorenal shunt provides selective variceal decompression through the short gastric veins, spleen, and splenic vein to the left renal vein. Hepatic portal perfusion is maintained by interrupting the umbilical vein, coronary vein, gastroepiploic vein, and any other prominent collaterals. (From Rikkers LF: Distal splenorenal shunt for portal hypertension. Surgery Illustrated 1988. Drawing by William B. Westwood. Courtesy of LTI Medica and the Upjohn Company. Copyright 1988 by Learning Technology Incorporated.)

remains high and venous blood flow continues to perfuse the liver. Prograde hepatopetal portal flow is maintained in most patients with nonalcoholic cirrhosis and noncirrhotic portal hypertension, collateral flow from the portal venous system to the shunt often develops in patients with alcoholic cirrhosis. If the coronary vein is not ligated, hepatopetal portal flow is lost early. Nevertheless, over time after a distal splenorenal shunt, collaterals gradually develop through a pancreatic network called the *pancreatic siphon.*

The distal splenorenal shunt is contraindicated in patients with moderate or severe ascites because lymphatics are transected during the dissection of the left renal vein, and the liver continues to have elevated sinusoidal pressure. Hence, the shunt may worsen rather than relieve ascites.

The controlled trials comparing distal splenorenal to nonselective shunts have demonstrated no survival advantage to either procedure. However, selective shunts were associated with less encephalopathy in four of the seven trials; the remaining three trials showed no difference in encephalopathy rates. One trial showed a higher rate of rebleeding associated with the distal splenorenal shunt, but the remaining studies showed no difference in rebleeding.

Any patient being considered for a surgical shunt, especially a distal splenorenal shunt, should undergo visceral angiography. The distal splenorenal shunt requires a patent splenic vein at least 6 to 8 mm in diameter. Patients with a previous splenectomy or a thrombosed splenic vein are not candidates for the procedure. Moreover, the angiogram shows the anatomic proximity of the splenic and renal vein.

Comparison of the distal splenorenal shunt to repeated endoscopic therapy has shown that rebleeding is less frequent with a selective shunt, but that endoscopic treatment more effectively maintains hepatic portal perfusion. Encephalopathy rates were not different. Based on these studies, endoscopic therapy is recommended for effective control of an initial bleed and when possible, as the definite procedure of choice. However, patients who fail endoscopic treatment should promptly undergo surgery or a TIPS procedure. Finally, another group of patients who may benefit from a distal splenorenal shunt are patients with variceal hemorrhage who live in a remote area with poor access to emergency endoscopic therapy. Because endoscopic therapy generally involves multiple visits and less reliably prevents recurrent bleeding, surgical shunts may be preferable in selected patients.

Technique

A transverse upper abdominal incision is used, and the liver is biopsied. To expose the splenic vein, dissection is begun along the generally avascular inferior border of the pancreas after taking down the gastrocolic ligament. Dissection of the splenic vein out of the bed of the pancreas can be challenging, particularly if the pancreas is fibrotic. The splenic vein needs to be dissected for an adequate length so that it can be anastomosed to the left renal vein without sharp angulation or kinking of the vein.

However, dissection does not need to be carried all the way to the hilum of the spleen (splenopancreatic disconnection) in an attempt to prevent future development of the pancreatic siphon.

If identification of the left renal vein is particularly difficult, as in a very obese patient, intraoperative ultrasonography may be useful. After dissecting the left renal vein, the splenic vein is divided where it joins the superior mesenteric vein. The distal end of the splenic vein is anastomosed end-to-side to the left renal vein. Once the distal splenorenal shunt is completed, Doppler ultrasonography can be used to follow shunt patency intraoperatively and postoperatively thereafter.

Nonselective Shunts

Indications and General Aspects

The end-to-side portacaval shunt (Fig. 96–2) has been compared in randomized controlled trials with conventional medical management for the treatment of portal hypertension. In these trials, no survival advantage was demonstrated for shunt patients, although all four studies were biased in favor of medical management because medical failures crossed over to surgical therapy. Bleeding was controlled effectively by surgical shunts (<3%) whereas 70% of medically treated patients re-bled. Encephalopathy complicated the course of 20% to 40% of shunt patients, some of whom had severe encephalopathy.

A controlled trial evaluating end-to-side versus side-to-side portacaval shunts showed no significant difference between the two procedures. The direct side-to-side portacaval shunt has also been compared with the interposition mesocaval shunt, also a nonselective shunt. No significant hemodynamic or clinical differences were demonstrated in this study. An advantage of the mesocaval shunt (see later text) is that it avoids dissection in the porta hepatis, an important consideration in patients who may be future candidates for liver transplantation. A scarred porta hepatis from a previous surgical shunt adds substantially to the technical difficulty of liver transplantation; for this reason, portacaval shunts should be avoided in patients who will likely be candidates for liver transplantation.

Indications for a nonselective shunt currently include the following: (1) an emergency shunt for variceal hemorrhage in a patient not responding to medical therapy or attempted TIPS, (2) an elective shunt in the presence of significant ascites, and (3) the Budd-Chiari syndrome. In patients in whom endoscopic therapy has failed and who are not candidates for a selective shunt because of technical considerations, a nonselective shunt may serve as a long-term bridge to liver transplantation. However, in this setting, initial TIPS may be preferable, reserving an operative nonselective shunt for TIPS failure. Patients who re-bleed following TIPS or have significant TIPS complications and who are not candidates for a selective shunt, should be considered for a surgical nonselective shunt. Clearly, the role for nonselective shunts has become narrow in the current era.

The Budd-Chiari syndrome when complicated by se-

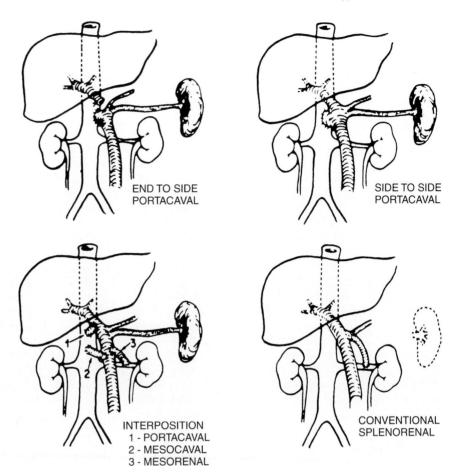

Figure 96–2. Nonselective shunts completely divert portal blood flow away from the liver. (From Rikkers LF: Portal hypertension. In Moody FG, et al [eds]: Surgical Treatment of Digestive Disease. Chicago, Year Book, 1986:409–424.)

vere ascites, abdominal pain, and portal hypertension, is an appropriate indication for a side-to-side portacaval shunt. The shunt serves as the major efferent conduit draining blood from the liver. If fulminant liver failure or cirrhosis has developed from longstanding hepatic vein occlusion, liver transplantation should be done. The Budd-Chiari syndrome often is associated with an underlying hypercoagulable state, and anticoagulation may be necessary to prevent shunt thrombosis. Family members should be screened for an inheritable disorder of coagulation (see Chapter 98).

Technique of Mesocaval Shunt

When performing a mesocaval shunt, an attractive material for the conduit between the superior mesenteric vein and the inferior vena cava is the autologous jugular vein. The left internal jugular vein is generally of adequate length and diameter for this purpose and avoids the use of prosthetic material and its accompanying risk of thrombosis. The patient is positioned with the head turned to the right and the shoulder rolled to allow for neck extension. The neck is prepped as for a carotid endarterectomy at the same time that the chest and abdomen are prepped. Once the superior mesenteric vein and inferior vena cava are dissected free and the necessary length of graft measured, a left-sided neck incision is made and the left internal jugular vein procured. Care should be taken to orient the vein correctly in its C-

shaped direction of flow when it is placed in the abdomen. The graft needs to be positioned such that the duodenum does not compress or kink it. The vein graft is anastomosed to the side of the superior mesenteric vein and its distal end to the inferior vena cava. An externally supported ringed PTFE (polytetrafluoroethylene) graft may be used instead of a vein graft.

Technique for Side-to-Side Portacaval Shunt

Via a transverse upper abdominal incision, the porta hepatis is exposed. The common bile duct and hepatic artery are retracted medially, allowing exposure of the portal vein. Adequate length of the portal vein must be dissected to allow approximation of portal vein to the vena cava. The infrahepatic inferior vena cava is exposed. The vena cava and portal vein are partially clamped with side-biting vascular clamps and approximated for the anastomosis.

When doing a portacaval shunt for Budd-Chiari syndrome, one should anticipate that the caudate lobe may be enlarged. In some situations, the caudate lobe extends inferiorly over the inferior vena cava, making it technically difficult to perform a side-to-side portacaval shunt. In such situations, either a mesocaval shunt can be performed as an effective alternative or a prosthetic graft can be interpositioned between the portal vein and vena cava.

Recently, there has been some interest in the use of narrow diameter (<10 mm) portacaval shunts that act as "partial" shunts. These grafts are easier to construct because the length of portal vein and vena cava that needs to be exposed is shorter, only enough to allow a side-biting vascular clamp. These small-diameter shunts effectively decrease portal pressure but do not completely shunt portal flow; thus, hepatopetal flow continues to a great extent.

Devascularization Operations

Esophagogastric devascularization is considerably less effective than shunt procedures for preventing future variceal bleeding. Re-bleeding rates in Western series have ranged from 25% to 50% after these operations. In our practice, indications for a devascularization operation are a thrombosed distal splenorenal shunt and diffuse splanchnic venous thrombosis, often in noncirrhotic individuals with a hypercoagulable syndrome. Many of these patients bleed from gastric rather than esophageal varices, making esophageal transsection a nonessential component of the operation. Devascularization technically involves splenectomy and devascularization of the distal 7 cm of the esophagus and proximal two thirds of the stomach through an abdominal incision. Although re-bleeding eventually develops in many of these patients, it tends to be more manageable with pharmacotherapy and endoscopic therapy.

Liver Transplantation

Liver transplantation has emerged as the preferred treatment for patients with advanced liver failure (Child-Pugh B or C). Variceal bleeding is the most common clinical manifestation of portal hypertension prompting evaluation for liver transplant. Thus, the majority of patients with portal hypertension associated with end-stage liver failure currently undergo liver transplantation rather than a surgical shunt or TIPS. These patients are managed with endoscopic therapy or pharmacotherapy, or both, until transplantation can be done; TIPS is done for failure of these treatments. Nevertheless, because liver transplantation is itself associated with significant morbidity and risk of mortality and because the supply of donor livers is limited, Child-Pugh A or early B liver disease may be treated appropriately with surgical shunts as a long-term bridge to liver transplantation. However, many of these patients may never require liver transplantation either because the portosystemic shunt is effective or because they die of some other cause.

Another consideration is that most liver transplant programs in the United States require at least 6 months of abstinence from alcohol before liver transplantation. Therefore, an active alcoholic with cirrhosis and variceal hemorrhage may benefit from an elective surgical shunt. This group of patients is at increased risk of progressive liver failure after shunt surgery as a result of active alcoholism and this approach also selects those patients unable to stop drinking.

A final group of patients who may benefit from a surgical shunt are those who have undergone a previous liver transplantation complicated by late portal vein thrombosis. These patients generally maintain good liver function but stigmata of portal hypertension develop, including gastrointestinal bleeding.

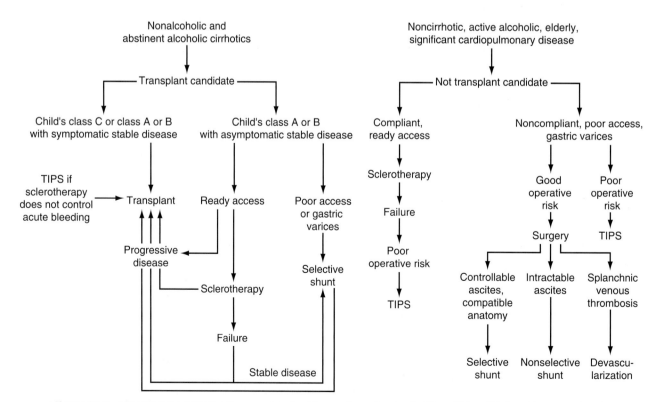

Figure 96–3. Algorithm for definitive therapy of variceal hemorrhage (see text). (From Rikkers LF: Portal hypertension. In Levine BA, et al [eds]: Current Practice of Surgery, vol. 3, New York, Churchill Livingstone, 1995.)

Whereas surgical shunts have been mentioned as a long-term bridge to liver transplantation, the more common short-term bridge to liver transplantation is TIPS. By improving hemodynamics, relieving ascites, and preventing bleeding, TIPS may actually improve a patient's Child-Pugh classification. TIPS may therefore salvage some patients for liver transplantation who would otherwise not survive until a liver was available.

SELECTION OF THERAPY

An algorithm summarizing current decision making in the management of variceal hemorrhage is shown in Figure 96–3. Patients are divided into those potentially eligible to receive a liver transplant versus patients who are not transplantation candidates. The sequential use of various modalities is illustrated. The current use of procedures performed for variceal hemorrhage suggests that, although sclerotherapy and banding continue to be used frequently, the use of TIPS has dramatically increased in frequency, as has liver transplantation. Nonselective shunts are rarely used, whereas selective shunts are still performed but only in a highly select group of patients.

OUTCOMES

While liver transplantation is applied to most patients with advanced liver failure and TIPS is performed in patients who are either poor surgical candidates or are advanced in age, the outcomes achieved in a selected population of patients undergoing surgical portosystemic shunts are greater than 90% 1-year survival and greater than 70% 5-year survival. Long-term survival in this patient population is generally limited by progression of liver disease or development of hepatoma in patients with hepatitis B or C. However, most patients with Child-Pugh class A cirrhosis who undergo portosystemic shunting maintain adequate liver function long term and avoid the need for liver transplantation.

Pearls and Pitfalls

- Pharmacologic therapy (beta-blockers) and endoscopic treatment (sclerotherapy, banding) are the first-line therapies for most patients who bleed from esophagogastric varices.
- Endoscopic variceal ligation is more effective than endoscopic sclerotherapy in preventing rebleeding and is associated with fewer complications.
- Because of the effectiveness of endoscopic therapy and TIPS (for failure of endoscopic therapy), emergency shunts are infrequently required.
- TIPS is an effective short-term bridge to liver transplantation when endoscopic treatment fails to control variceal bleeding.
- Shunts are preferred to TIPS for endoscopic treatment failures with good hepatic functional reserve (Child-Pugh class A and B) or noncirrhotic portal hypertension.
- Shunts are preferred to long-term endoscopic treatment for noncompliant patients and for those living long distances from tertiary medical care.
- The selective distal splenorenal shunt decompresses the esophagogastric varices but preserves hepatic portal perfusion in many patients and thus results in a better quality of life than do nonselective shunts.

SELECTED READINGS

Knechtle SJ, D'Alessandro AM, Armbrust MJ, et al: Surgical portosystemic shunts for treatment of portal hypertensive bleeding: Outcome and effect on liver function. Surgery 1999;126:708.

Laine L, Cook D: Endoscopic ligation compared with sclerotherapy for treatment of esophageal variceal bleeding: A meta-analysis: Ann Intern Med 1995;123:280.

Ochs A, Rossle M, Haag K, et al: The transjugular intrahepatic portosystemic stent shunt for refractory ascites. N Engl J Med 1995;332:1192.

Papatheodoridis GV, Goulis J, Leandro G, et al: Transjugular intrahepatic portosystemic shunt compared with endoscopic treatment for prevention of variceal rebleeding: A meta-analysis. Hepatology 1999;30(no. 3):612.

Rikkers LF: The changing spectrum of treatment for variceal bleeding. Ann Surg 1998;228:536.

Rikkers LF, Jin G, Langnas AN, Shaw BW Jr: Shunt surgery during the era of liver transplantation. Ann Surg 1997;226:51.

Spina GP, Henderson JM, Rikkers LF, et al: Distal spleno-renal shunt versus endoscopic sclerotherapy in the prevention of variceal rebleeding: A meta-analysis of 4 randomized clinical trials. J Hepatol 1992;16:338.

Chapter 97
Cystic Diseases of the Liver
Florencia G. Que

Cystic lesions of the liver are commonly encountered in clinical practice with the use of modern imaging techniques. The vast majority of these lesions are asymptomatic simple cysts. Most simple cysts can be diagnosed reliably on the basis of radiographic imaging features and do not require therapeutic intervention. When symptoms occur, they develop insidiously as a consequence of cyst expansion and adjacent organ compression. Vague upper abdominal pain or fullness occurs in one third of patients. Jaundice is rare but may develop from bile duct compression. This chapter describes the etiology, pathology, diagnosis, and management of noninflammatory cystic lesions of the liver.

Cystic lesions of the liver can be broadly divided into four groups: congenital; inflammatory; neoplastic; and traumatic. Congenital cysts of the liver are most common and include simple cysts and polycystic liver disease (PLD). Inflammatory cysts of the liver are generally related to infectious etiologies and are not discussed here. Primary cystic neoplasms are the rare cystadenomas and the rarer cystadenocarcinomas. Traumatic cysts arise from an injury to the liver, which causes either a subcapsular hematoma or a transected biliary duct.

CONGENITAL CYSTS

Congenital cysts of the liver are dilatations of the biliary tree lined with biliary epithelium. Simple cysts usually lack continuity with the biliary ductal system. Patients with signs and symptoms associated with these cysts can present a variety of ways. The overwhelming majority of patients with hepatic cysts remain asymptomatic.

Etiology and Pathogenesis

Simple cysts and PLD reputedly arise from aberrations of the normal development of the intrahepatic bile ducts. Around the third week of fetal development, the hepatobiliary system develops from a solid proximal endodermal anlage that gives rise to the hepatocytes and small intralobar ductal cells. The distal anlage is the origin of the gallbladder and the main biliary ductal cells. Moschowitz in 1906 postulated that aberrant ducts are formed during embryogenesis and result in cysts. Later, von Meyenberg suggested an excess development of intralobular bile ducts that become dilated over time. The biliary epithelium secretes fluid that accumulates and forms cysts. These cysts enlarge over time, become dilated, and fill with fluid. The cysts enlarge because they lack biliary drainage. Experimental evidence in mice has challenged the previously postulated etiologies. Defective production of the basement membrane in bile ducts has been hypoth-

esized. The basement membrane of the bile duct heaps up on itself and causes dilatation of the proximal ducts. The enlarged bile ducts eventually compress the communication with other bile ducts. Fluid rapidly accumulates within the obstructed biliary segment, and macroscopic cysts arise. Histologically, simple cysts are lined by a cuboidal epithelium. These lesions are small clusters of bile ducts surrounded by fibrous portal tracts. As the cysts enlarge, the epithelium flattens and becomes fibrotic.

Simple cysts can be single or multiple. They are distributed randomly throughout the liver and vary widely in size from a few millimeters to greater than 20 cm. Only about 10% of patients with simple cysts will be symptomatic. Complications of cysts other than pain are uncommon but include hemorrhage, infection, and biliary obstruction. Hemorrhage, the most frequent complication, is usually heralded by sudden onset of acute abdominal pain. Hypotension is unusual unless the cyst is huge or a hemorrhage becomes uncontained by cyst rupture.

Serum liver function tests offer little diagnostic aid. Although the diagnosis can be made incidentally at surgery in most patients, abdominal imaging by ultrasonography (US) or computed tomography (CT) should usually be diagnostic. US shows an anechoic lesion with posterior enhancement. Similarly, CT shows a low attenuation lesion with discrete borders (Fig. 97–1A). Other imaging techniques have little value because they lack anatomic detail. Simple cysts are circular to ovoid, lack septations, and have uniformly thin walls. Uncommonly, a simple cyst may have incomplete septations, although a common wall of adjacent cysts may mimic complete septations. Current, state-of-the-art US, CT, and magnetic resonance imaging are equivalent and approach 98% diagnostic accuracy for simple cysts 1 cm or larger in diameter. Any mural nodularity or irregular thickening, multiple septations, or a fluid level within a cystic mass should alert the clinician to diagnostic alternatives other than a simple cyst, and further diagnostic studies are indicated. Signs and symptoms of sepsis accompany cyst infection and jaundice with bile duct obstruction.

Treatment

The indications for treatment of simple cysts are symptoms related to cyst size, complications, growth, or imaging studies suggestive of malignancy. Operative management is elective, and the surgical treatment of choice is complete cyst excision. Several caveats regarding cyst excision warrant comment. First, simple cysts grow by expansion but not by invasion. Consequently, the parenchyma immediately adjacent to the cyst atrophies or becomes attenuated, and the major vasculature and ducts are splayed around the cysts. Second, the interface be-

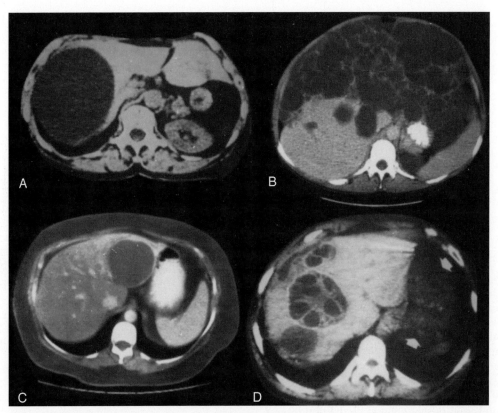

Figure 97–1. Cystic lesions in liver. *A,* Simple cyst. *B,* Polycystic liver disease. *C,* Cystadenoma. *D,* Echinococcal cyst. (From Sarr MG: Cystic disease of the liver. In Cameron JL [ed]: Current Surgical Therapy, 5th ed. St. Louis, Mosby–Year Book, 1995, pp 265–270.)

tween the cyst and the parenchyma or ducts remains discrete. These features allow development of a plane of dissection immediately between the cyst and the liver parenchyma and even between major vessels and bile ducts. Provided that excessive risk is avoided, complete excision is advised. Cyst decompression before resection is avoided because complete excision is precluded or made technically complicated by decompression. Any inadvertent entry into the cyst during excision is closed, and dissection is completed. If the cyst wall is densely adherent to major intrahepatic vasculature or bile ducts, the cyst wall adherent to these structures is maintained to avoid potential damage, but the remainder of the cyst wall is excised. Any residual epithelium can be ablated by electrocautery, laser, or alcohol to reduce the risk of recurrence. The recurrence rate is related to the amount of residual cyst wall epithelium after excision. Bile-stained contents or cholangiotomies should prompt identification of the exact site of bile leak and ligation of the individual ductal defect. Roux-en-Y cystenterostomy is virtually never indicated for simple cysts regardless of the size or complication. A total or near-total excision with intraperitoneal marsupialization can always be performed with less risk of recurrence or complication than with a cystenterostomy. Drainage of the cyst excision site externally using a suction catheter prevents any perihepatic accumulation and controls any transient bile leaks. Cyst fenestration can be performed either laparoscopically or via laparotomy. The laparoscopic approach has proven to be as effective as open laparotomy in selected patients with

symptomatic anterior cysts, provided the majority of this external cyst wall is excised. Regardless of the approach, wide excision of the superficial cyst wall is an important technical factor in reducing recurrence. This operative technique permits continual resorption of the cystic secretions by the peritoneum. Infected cysts should be treated as hepatic abscesses. Percutaneous external drainage is preferred. If operative drainage is required, a portion of the cyst wall should be excised to provide complete drainage. Omental packing of the excision site is usually unnecessary.

Percutaneous aspiration alone has limited efficacy because the recurrence rate approaches 100%. Its role may be to determine if a cyst is the cause of symptoms or to function as a temporizing measure before definitive therapy. Initially, diagnostic cyst aspiration is performed to confirm whether the cyst is symptomatic and to exclude biliary communication. If the presence of a simple cyst is confirmed by a nonpurulent, nonbilious aspirate, the cyst contents are completely aspirated. Although recurrence after aspiration alone is almost certain, symptomatic recurrence is not. If symptoms do recur, either repeat aspiration with alcohol ablation or excision can be employed. If ablation is preferred, the cyst is intubated percutaneously and aspirated completely. Percutaneous sclerosis after aspiration is performed to ablate the secretory epithelial lining of liver cysts in an attempt to reduce recurrence rates. The cyst is aspirated, and if blood or bile is encountered, the procedure is aborted because sclerosants may cause irreparable bile duct or vascular injury. Alcohol is injected temporarily through a drainage catheter, and the patient's position is altered to ensure exposure of the entire epithelial surface to alcohol; the alcohol is aspirated, and the drainage catheter is removed. When this procedure is successful, the epithelium is ablated, and the cyst is obliterated gradually by fibrous contraction. Most smaller (<10 cm) simple cysts will respond to aspiration with alcohol ablation. Although repeated intervention may be necessary in some patients, reported complications are few.

POLYCYSTIC LIVER DISEASE

Etiology and Pathogenesis

Unlike simple cysts, PLD is inherited either as an autosomal recessive trait associated with congenital hepatic fibrosis in infancy or childhood or as an autosomal dominant trait presenting in adulthood. PLD progresses insidiously over years and is associated with polycystic renal disease and progressive renal insufficiency. However, liver failure is uncommon. Indeed, even with marked hepatosplenomegaly and portal hypertension, liver function may be normal. PLD in adults may also be associated with multiple cysts of the pancreas, spleen, ovaries, and lungs.

Symptoms and signs develop late in the natural history of PLD and are related to increased liver volume and adjacent visceral compression. The most common complaints are increasing abdominal girth, chronic abdominal pain, satiety, weight loss, respiratory compromise, physical disability, and descensus. Ascites can be prominent, although other stigmas of chronic liver disease are rare. Physical examination reveals a large nodular liver. Abdominal tenderness is uncommon. Liver function tests are commonly normal or only mildly abnormal. Although the diagnosis of PLD is readily confirmed by US or CT, CT most clearly defines the extent of liver and adjacent organ involvement (see Fig. 97–1B).

Treatment

Surgical intervention is reserved for selected patients who exhibit significant impairment of clinical performance secondary to a massively enlarged liver or for patients experiencing complications of rupture, infection, or hemorrhage. The choice of treatment is dictated by the extent of liver involvement and by the complication. For patients with a few dominant cysts, percutaneous aspiration with alcohol ablation may provide prolonged symptomatic relief. For patients with diffuse involvement, operative management becomes more formidable. Cyst fenestration with intraperitoneal marsupialization or resection has been the mainstay of surgical therapy. Resection poses a significant risk of biliary ductal injury, vasculature compromise, and liver insufficiency owing to cystic distortion of the intrahepatic anatomy. Although cyst decompression by fenestration avoids these risks, decompression is often limited technically by the number and size of cysts and the bulky liver mass. Fenestration with intraperitoneal marsupialization has provided temporary symptomatic re-

lief, but long-term reduction in abdominal girth has rarely been documented. Anatomic hepatic resection in combination with cyst fenestration has been employed successfully in selected symptomatic patients, but careful patient selection is required. Candidates for combined resection and fenestration should have at least two adjacent liver segments relatively spared of cystic involvement, near-normal liver function, significant impairment of clinical performance status owing to increased liver mass, and no significant cardiopulmonary compromise. At operation, anatomic resection is preceded by lobar vascular isolation without inflow occlusion. The transection plane is developed by sequential cyst fenestration. Intraseptal vessels and bile ducts are suture ligated. Cholecystectomy is performed to eliminate potential confounding diagnostic problems postoperatively.

Data on the natural history of PLD suggest that progression of cystic disease is slow and that patients are provided with prolonged benefits from this approach. Liver transplantation is indicated for (1) patients with progressive PLD after resection and fenestration, (2) patients with liver failure with or without renal failure, or (3) severely symptomatic patients with diffuse PLD without segmental sparing.

NEOPLASTIC CYSTS

Etiology and Pathogenesis

Cystadenomas and cystadenocarcinomas are rare neoplasms that constitute fewer than 5% of hepatic cysts. A review of the literature reveals that 80% of these patients are women who present with abdominal pain or a mass. A multiloculated or thick-walled cyst with solid intracystic components identified by abdominal CT or US should suggest a cystic neoplasm (see Fig. 97–1C). Hypervascularity of the cyst wall is suggestive of a cystadenocarcinoma. Cystadenomas are characterized histologically by moderate to dense cellular supporting stroma and a cuboidal or columnar, mucus-producing epithelium with papillary projections. A cystadenocarcinoma shows similar stromal composition with papillary adenocarcinoma lining the cysts and invasion of the cyst wall. Importantly, a cystadenocarcinoma may involve the cyst wall only focally. Therefore, numerous histologic sections are required to exclude malignancy. Because of the risk of unpredictable malignant progression and the more practical risk of recurrence after partial excision, cystadenomas should be resected completely. Excision of cystadenomas can be accomplished with enucleation. Only rarely is an anatomic resection required because of size or location. Cystadenocarcinomas are considered malignant degeneration of cystadenomas, similar to the progression in mucinous cystic diseases of the pancreas and ovary. The pathogenesis of a cystadenoma to a cystadenocarcinoma has been documented. Cystadenocarcinomas should be approached as for any primary hepatic neoplasm and should be resected widely by standard hepatic resection and not enucleation. The 5-year survival for patients with cystadenocarcinoma is 25%; this rate is similar to the survival rate obtained with resection of other primary hepatic malignancies.

TRAUMATIC CYSTS

Etiology and Pathogenesis

Traumatic cysts occur after significant trauma to the liver with disruption of intrahepatic bile ducts or formation of a subcapsular hematoma. These cysts are rare and constitute fewer than 0.5% of liver cysts. Because these cysts do not have an epithelial lining, they actually represent hepatic pseudocysts. The contained rupture usually presents as a cystic mass filled with old blood or bile. Clinical presentation is similar to that of simple cysts of the liver. The indication and treatment options are also similar. Occasionally, these lesions resolve spontaneously; therefore, a period of observation for potential resolution is preferred unless the severity of the symptoms precludes observation. Because the cyst lining is nonsecretory, partial excision is adequate.

MISCELLANEOUS CYSTIC LESIONS

Other cystic-like lesions can masquerade as true cysts. Infective lesions appear cystic. Echinococcal cysts occur within the liver in regions endemic to echinococcus (see Fig. 97–1D). Similarly, hepatic abscesses of bacterial or parasitic (e.g., amebic) etiology also resemble cystic lesions, although the clinical scenario differs.

Pearls and Pitfalls

- Simple hepatic cysts usually require no treatment.
- Rule out an infective etiology (bacterial, amebic).
- If a nodule is found on the inner lining of a cyst, it should be considered a cystic neoplasm.
- Simple unroofing a simple cyst without cyst wall excision results in a near-total recurrence rate.
- Understanding of the intrahepatic vascular and biliary anatomy is essential for the surgical treatment of PLD owing to distortion of the anatomy by the cysts.
- If the pathologist determines that a cyst is a cystadenoma, be sure to remove the entire cyst wall in the event that a cystadenocarcinoma is found on permanent section.

SELECTED READINGS

Jeyarajah DR, Gonwa TA, Testa G, et al: Liver and kidney transplantation for polycystic disease. Transplantation 1998;66:529.

Koperna T, Vogl S, Satzinger U, Schulz F: Nonparasitic cysts of the liver: Results and options of surgical management. World J Surg 1997;21:850.

Montorsi M, Torzilli G, Fumagalli U, et al: Percutaneous alcohol sclerotherapy of simple hepatic cysts: Results from a multicentre survey in Italy. HPB Surg 1994;8:89.

Que FG, Nagorney DM, Gross JB Jr, Torres VE: Liver resection and cyst fenestration in the treatment of severe polycystic liver disease. Gastroenterology 1995;108:487.

Sarr MG: Cystic disease of the liver. In Cameron JL (ed): Current Surgical Therapy, 5th ed. St. Louis, Mosby–Year Book, 1995, pp 265–270.

Zacherl J, Scheuba C, Imhof M, et al: Long-term results after laparoscopic unroofing of solitary symptomatic congenital liver cysts. Surg Endosc 2000;14:59.

Chapter 98
Budd-Chiari Syndrome

Andrew S. Klein and John L. Cameron

Budd-Chiari syndrome (BCS) is a rare, often fatal form of portal hypertension caused by hepatic venous outflow obstruction. The syndrome, as described originally by Budd in 1859 and later by Chiari in 1899, was attributed to an inflammatory process at the level of the hepatic venules, similar in its histopathologic description to an entity now classified as veno-occlusive disease of the liver. Two distinct forms of BCS, unrelated to veno-occlusive disease of the liver, predominate among patients in Western and Asian countries, respectively. The "Western" form of BCS is caused by thrombotic occlusion of the major hepatic veins, whereas the "Eastern" form occurs secondary to occlusion of the suprahepatic vena cava and/or the hepatic veins by membranous intraluminal webs. The therapeutic management strategies of these three disease entities (hepatic vein thrombosis, membranous venous webs, and veno-occlusive disease of the liver) are quite different. The following discussion focuses exclusively on the Western form of BCS caused by hepatic vein thrombosis.

A variety of predisposing factors have been linked to the thrombotic form of this disease, including polycythemia rubra vera, factor V Leiden mutation, estrogen usage, paroxysmal nocturnal hemoglobinuria, pregnancy, cirrhosis, viral hepatitis, trauma, parasitic infections of the liver, and visceral malignancy. The patient's family should also be screened for an underlying coagulopathy that may require treatment as well. The clinical presentation of BCS is variable. A minority of patients develop chronic liver dysfunction, and BCS is not recognized until the patients present with end-stage hepatic cirrhosis, ascites, and portal hypertension. At the opposite end of the clinical spectrum, but also involving a minority of patients, is presentation as fulminant hepatic failure, characterized by massive hepatocellular necrosis, encephalopathy, and synthetic dysfunction. Most patients, however, have an acute or subacute illness typified by the classic triad of abruptly appearing ascites, right upper quadrant pain, and hepatomegaly. The rapid development of ascites, by far the most prominent component of BCS, is noted in the vast majority of patients. Other symptoms and signs include splenomegaly (22%), jaundice (19%), gastrointestinal bleeding (13%), and encephalopathy (4%). A striking percentage (76%) of patients with BCS are women.

Surprisingly, most patients with BCS have minimal biochemical evidence of liver dysfunction. Except in the acute, fulminant presentation, serum transaminase, bilirubin, alkaline phosphatase, and prothrombin time are usually normal or only mildly deranged. Consequently, these tests are not particularly useful in establishing the diagnosis, nor are they helpful in predicting the clinical course. Serum albumin, often low in these patients owing to protein loss in the ascites, should not be misinterpreted as a sign of synthetic dysfunction.

PREOPERATIVE MANAGEMENT

A variety of noninvasive diagnostic procedures have been suggested to establish the diagnosis of hepatic vein thrombosis, including pulsed duplex ultrasonography, technetium colloid or gallium scintiscans, magnetic resonance imaging, and computed tomography. The "gold standard" for confirming the diagnosis of BCS is hepatic venography; the classic finding is a "spider web" appearance of partially recanalized hepatic veins (Fig. 98–1). Caval compression related to caudate lobe hypertrophy or owing to pericaval fibrosis is common, and thus inferior vena cava (IVC) venography with direct imaging of the suprahepatic, retrohepatic, and infrahepatic IVC, combined with venous pressure measurements at these locations, is an important adjunct to hepatic venography. Three patterns of IVC involvement may be recognized: (1) total occlusion, (2) patency of the IVC with a reduction (>75%) in the luminal diameter or a pressure gradient (>20 mm Hg) between the right atrium and the infrahepatic IVC, or (3) patency of the IVC with no significant caval obstruction or pressure gradient. For patients to be treated operatively, the results of the venogram are important for selecting the procedure most appropriate for each individual (Fig. 98–2). For patients with massive ascites and portal hypertension, many physi-

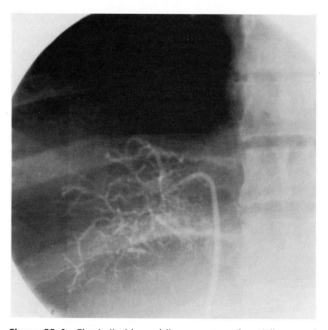

Figure 98–1. Classic "spider web" appearance of partially recanalized hepatic veins. (From Klein AS: Budd-Chiari syndrome. In Cameron JL [ed]: Current Surgical Therapy, 5th ed. St. Louis, Mosby–Year Book, 1995, p 325.)

624

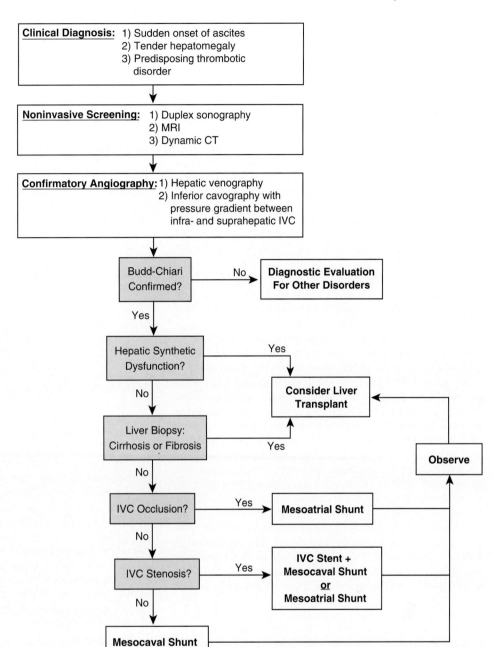

Figure 98–2. Diagnostic and therapeutic algorithm for patients with acute Budd-Chiari syndrome.

cians have been reluctant to perform a percutaneous liver biopsy as part of the work-up of the BCS. However, this procedure can be performed with a very low incidence of complications. Centrolobular congestion dominates the histologic picture, but its spectrum ranges from mild sinusoidal dilatation with erythrocyte extravasation to cellular atrophy and loss of central venous hepatocytes. The degree of venous thrombosis and subsequent parenchymal pathology can vary between hepatic lobes, and thus *bilobar* biopsies are indicated. Most worrisome is the finding of severe hepatic fibrosis or cirrhosis, a poor prognostic indicator for patients being evaluated for porto-mesenteric-systemic decompression.

Once the diagnosis of BCS has been established, some form of definitive treatment should be instituted without delay. Medical treatment of the acute form of BCS con-

sists of diuretics, anticoagulation, and treatment of underlying disorders (e.g., withdrawal of estrogens, phlebotomy for patients with polycythemia). Although anecdotal reports of successful therapy with urokinase or streptokinase have appeared, most patients present too late (>1 month after symptoms began) for thrombolytic agents to be successful. The Nd:YAG laser and balloon angioplasty have been used to obliterate venous webs responsible for the congenital form of BCS predominant in Asian countries, but those techniques are not helpful in managing the thrombotic Western form of this disease.

INTRAOPERATIVE MANAGEMENT

The management approach focuses on conversion of the portal vein from an inflow vessel to an outflow tract to decompress the congested liver. A variety of portal-systemic or mesenteric-systemic shunts have been proposed. Our group has chosen the superior mesenteric vein (SMV) as our access to the portal system because it can be isolated rapidly and safely, well away from the large, congested liver. For noncirrhotic patients with no evidence of IVC compression or obstruction, a synthetic graft connecting the SMV and the IVC (mesocaval "C shunt") is preferred (Fig. 98–3). Other groups prefer a direct side-to-side portocaval shunt whenever possible; an advantage of this latter approach is that avoidance of a prosthetic graft decreases the chance of thrombosis of the shunt. Noncirrhotic patients with total IVC occlusion are treated with a long externally supported, "ringed" prosthesis that bypasses the obstructed IVC and connects the SMV directly to the right atrium (mesoatrial shunt). If the IVC is patent, but flow through the liver is impeded in a patient without histologic evidence of cirrhosis, two options are available: (1) mesoatrial shunt or (2) insertion of a metallic stent to widen the narrowed segment of IVC, followed by a mesocaval shunt.

Operative management of portal hypertension is an increasingly uncommon strategy, given the availability of endoscopic and radiologic procedures to treat variceal bleeding and the option of orthotopic liver transplantation as definitive therapy for patients with end-stage liver disease. Some technical caveats are worth noting. A bilateral subcostal incision approach affords excellent exposure to the mid- and upper abdomen and is the same incision that would be used for a liver transplantation, should one be required later. The classic findings of BCS are massive ascites and a firm, distended liver that often appears purplish in color. To perform the mesocaval shunt, the transverse colon is retracted superiorly and the SMV is identified through the base of the colonic mesentery and dissected for a distance of 5 to 6 cm. The dissection is carried superiorly to expose the SMV as it passes over the third portion of the duodenum and under the neck of the pancreas. The caliber of the vein is usually widest

at this point, has few (if any) branches, and is the ideal site for the shunt. The SMV does *not* need to be dissected circumferentially; only anterior exposure of the vein is necessary to allow safe placement of a side-biting clamp. Division of one or more small branches off the SMV may be required. Occasionally, a small tributary from the superior mesenteric artery may cross the SMV and can be ligated after trial occlusion and confirmation of collateral blood flow to the portion of the bowel supplied by this vessel. The IVC is exposed inferiorly and laterally along the third portion of the duodenum. For most adult patients, a 14- to 16-mm, low-porosity Dacron graft is appropriate. The IVC anastomosis is performed first, and the graft is navigated in a gentle "C" curve around the duodenum. The planes of the IVC and the SMV are not parallel; thus, the marking lines on the graft will rotate from the IVC to the SMV position. Another approach involves a direct side-to-side portacaval anastomosis, which usually does not require a prosthesis. This area of the portal vein may be difficult to approach surgically because of the swollen liver. Mobilization of the portal vein down to the duodenum will be necessary to allow a tension-free anastomosis to the IVC.

POSTOPERATIVE MANAGEMENT

At the completion of the mesenteric-systemic shunt, immediate reduction in the congested appearance of the liver is often noted. Adequate decompression of the portal venous system should be documented, measuring the pressures in the portal circulation and the right atrium. A successful shunt will reveal a substantial decrease in pressure within the mesenteric venous system, approaching that of the IVC. All shunted patients are anticoagulated immediately after the operation. In most patients, heparinization can be initiated the night of surgery with continuous intravenous infusion at 700 to 1000 U per hour. Lifelong anticoagulation is maintained with warfarin. Shunt patency is confirmed postoperatively with duplex ultrasonography or magnetic resonance imaging. Encephalopathy is very unusual in this patient population.

COMPLICATIONS

Other types of portasystemic shunts have been suggested for patients with BCS. The side-to-side portacaval shunt is not appropriate for all patients with BCS. The caudate lobe, which drains directly into the IVC, is often hypertrophic in these patients and may render a side-to-side portacaval shunt technically difficult. A second factor that may render the portacaval shunt less attractive than the mesocaval shunt is the potential need for a liver transplantation in the future. Surgical operations that involve dissection of the portal vein increase the morbidity and mortality for a subsequent liver transplantation.

Success with the transjugular intrahepatic portosystemic shunt (TIPS) in portal hypertension and variceal hemorrhage has prompted some to attempt this procedure in patients with BCS. TIPS may be considered when one of the major hepatic veins is uninvolved in the thrombotic process or when the orifice of a major vein can

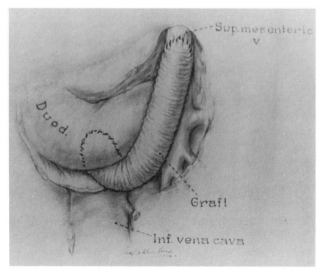

Figure 98–3. Mesocaval C-type shunt. (From Klein AS: Budd-Chiari syndrome. In Cameron IL [ed]: Current Surgical Therapy, 5th ed. St Louis, Mosby-Year Book, 1995, pp 323–331.)

be cannulated. There are anecdotal reports of successful management with TIPS, but long-term follow-up information is insufficient. Given the need for frequent TIPS revision documented in other patient populations, TIPS is best viewed as a bridge to another form of therapy such as liver transplantation. Incorrect placement of the TIPS can lead to disastrous complications during a subsequent liver transplantation. Migration of the metallic stent into the suprahepatic vena cava or right atrium will interfere with control of the IVC at the time of hepatectomy. Placement of the stent too far distally into the main portal vein can lead to similar difficulties in controlling vascular inflow to the liver. Over time, the TIPS becomes incorporated into the vessel wall and cannot be removed without risk of tearing the portal vein, which could result in uncontrollable hemorrhage. Accurate placement of the TIPS, however, allows total excision of the stent at the time of hepatectomy. These are strong arguments that favor limiting TIPS insertions to radiology teams familiar with the potential consequences of misplacement, who have readily available, on-site transplantation surgical consultation, if needed.

Patients with severe fibrosis or cirrhosis do poorly after mesenteric-systemic shunting, and definitive therapy in the form of liver transplantation is a better option. Transplantation may be the only option for fulminant hepatic failure, "unshuntable" vascular anatomy (e.g., portal vein thrombosis), or previous attempts at operative decompression. Several precautions are in order. Extension of the thrombotic process superiorly into the suprahepatic IVC, as well as pericaval fibrosis common in BCS, often increases the technical difficulty of a liver transplantation. Also, the adult-to-adult living donor liver transplantation, in which the right hepatic lobe is removed from a healthy volunteer donor and implanted into the recipient, leaving the IVC intact, may not be appropriate for BCS patients with caval involvement.

OUTCOMES

The 1-year and 5-year survival rates in our series of 43 patients treated with mesocaval or mesoatrial shunting were 83% and 75%, respectively. The long-term survival for liver transplantation is equal to or superior to that expected for mesenteric-systemic shunts. The 5-year post-transplantation survival rate has been reported to be 80%. Improved survival with liver transplantation has been attributed to several factors, including lifelong anticoagulation or antiplatelet therapy in patients with identifiable hypercoagulable states. Nevertheless, a more selective use of transplantation is mandated by (1) the widening gap between the increasing number of patients in need of liver replacement and the relatively static pool of organs available for transplantation, (2) the unpredictable availability of donor organs, (3) the need for and consequences of lifelong immunosuppression, and (4) the dramatically higher cost of transplantation versus nontransplantation therapies.

In conclusion, early diagnosis and decompression of the portomesenteric venous system can provide excellent survival for the majority of patients with BCS. Patients

---

Pearls and Pitfalls

- BCS should be suspected in patients, especially women, who present with the sudden onset of ascites and tender hepatomegaly.
- Patients with the acute form of BCS generally have minimal biochemical evidence of liver dysfunction.
- The gold standard for making the diagnosis of BCS is hepatic venography.
- Bilobar liver biopsy should be performed in patients with BCS to avoid sampling errors.
- Thrombolytic therapy, unless instituted early in the course of BCS, is generally not useful and may result in a delay of administration of appropriate therapy.
- Most noncirrhotic patients with BCS are best managed with surgical portosystemic decompression, not with TIPS.
- A surgical shunt offers a better long-term solution than a TIPS offers.
- Mesocaval or mesoatrial shunts are preferred operations for most of these patients.
- The choice of surgical shunt is based in large measure on the presence or absence of vena cava obstruction.
- Side-to-side portacaval shunts should be avoided in BCS patients with cirrhosis both for technical reasons and because subsequent liver transplantation is associated with increased morbidity and mortality.
- Exquisite care must be taken in the dissection of the SMV, which tends to be relatively thin-walled and delicate in these patients, who have not been exposed to longstanding portal hypertension.
- Liver transplantation is the procedure of choice for BCS patients with fulminant failure, histologic evidence of cirrhosis, unshuntable vascular anatomy, or failed shunts.
- Surgical management of BCS is successful in 75% to 85% of patients.
- TIPS should be viewed as a bridge to transplantation or as a therapeutic option for patients who are not candidates for surgical decompression.
- TIPS should be performed only by radiologists familiar with the consequences of inaccurate TIPS placement.

---

with histologic evidence of hepatic cirrhosis or with anatomic complications that preclude mesenteric-systemic shunting should be considered for orthotopic liver transplantation.

SELECTED READINGS

Bismuth H, Sherlock S: Portasystemic shunting versus liver transplantation for the Budd-Chiari syndrome. Ann Surg 1991;214:581.

Ganger DR, Klapman JB, McDonald V, et al: Transjugular intrahepatic portosystemic shunt (TIPS) for Budd-Chiari syndrome or portal vein thrombosis: Review of indications and problems. Am J Gastroenterol 1999;94:603.

Hemming AW, Langer B, Grieg P, et al: Treatment of Budd-Chiari syndrome with portosystemic shunt or liver transplantation. Am J Surg 1996;171:176.

Orloff M: Budd-Chiari syndrome: Shunt or transplant? HPB Surg 1998;11:136.

Ryu RK, Durham JD, Krysl J, et al: Role of TIPS as a bridge to hepatic transplantation in Budd-Chiari syndrome. J Vasc Interv Radiol 1999;10:799.

Wang Z, Zhu Y, Wang S, et al: Recognition and management of Budd-Chiari syndrome: Report of one hundred cases. J Vasc Surg 1989;10:149.

Zeitoun G, Escolano S, Hadengue A, et al: Outcome of Budd-Chiari syndrome: A multivariate analysis of factors related to survival including surgical portosystemic shunting. Hepatology 1999;30:84.

Chapter 99
Hemangioma

James V. Sitzmann

Hepatic hemangiomas occur in approximately 7% of the population and thus represent the most common benign tumor of the liver. Hemangiomas clinically are noted most frequently in the third to fourth decade of life, but the tumor can be evident at any time in life from the neonatal to geriatric periods. The incidence of hemangioma is two to three times more common in women. The female predominance suggests an association with estrogen. The occurrence of hemangiomas in women is greater during their reproductive years, especially with the use of oral contraceptives, and hemangiomas often exhibit rapid growth during pregnancy. Direct causal links between estrogen and the growth or development of hemangiomas, however, has not been proved.

Hemangiomas are classified pathologically as cavernous hemangiomas, sclerous or sclerosing hemangiomas, or as infantile or adult hemangiomatosis. On gross examination, hemangiomas appear as red, blue, or gray, soft ballotable tumors with the color variant dependent on the degree of sclerosis. The gross tumor has a somewhat thin capsule and a friable texture. A clear plane is usually evident between the lesion and normal hepatic parenchyma with isolated feeder vessels entering from the normal parenchyma at numerous points. On microscopic examination, dilated cystic vascular spaces are lined with endothelial cells showing varying degrees of sclerosis and fibrosis. Most hemangiomas are small tumors with diameters between 1 and 3 cm, but they can grow to gigantic proportions in excess of 10 to 20 cm (i.e., cavernous hemangioma) (Fig. 99–1).

Hemangiomatosis of the liver is rare and predominantly affects children in the first year of life, although adults also can have hemangiomatosis. Most patients are diagnosed within 6 months of birth. With hemangiomatosis, hemodynamically significant shunt can occur because of increased blood flow through the tumor; similar changes may occur on occasion with giant cavernous hemangiomas. This shunt results in audible bruits in a small percentage of patients and congestive heart failure. The development of infantile hemangiomatoses in children can also be associated with the Kasabach-Merritt syndrome, which consists of thrombocytopenia and hypofibrinogenemia, which leads to coagulopathy in conjunction with congestive heart failure.

CLINICAL PRESENTATION

Most hemangiomas are asymptomatic and are discovered during routine abdominal imaging using computed tomography (CT), magnetic resonance imaging (MRI), or ultrasonography for nonrelated reasons. Symptoms are present in only a minority of patients and are most often associated with a large size or, in the case of hemangio-matosis, numerous lesions. The most common presenting symptom is early satiety with left lobe lesions or, in right lobe lesions, a dull right upper quadrant pain. Intratumoral bleeding or spontaneous intraperitoneal rupture has been reported but is rare. If lesions reach a massive size, such as in the case of cavernous hemangiomas, or if substantial replacement of the liver occurs because of widespread hemangiomatosis, high-output heart failure can occur.

Laboratory examination usually is not informative but, on occasion, thrombocytopenia or hypofibrinogenemia can occur. There have been anecdotal reports of escalating biliary pigment crystal formation in patients with large hemangiomas, which is thought to be related to an increase of blood flow through the lesion and increased red blood cell trapping and subsequent breakdown.

DIAGNOSIS

The diagnosis of hemangioma often is made at operation. If a hepatic tumor is encountered during an operation, it can be identified, in most patients, without biopsy by the typical bluish red appearance and soft ballotable texture. Most hemangiomas, however, are diagnosed by radiographic techniques. The imaging modalities to definitively diagnose a hemangioma include Doppler ultrasonography, CT, MRI, technetium 99m–labeled red cell scintigraphy, and angiography. Ultrasonography is the least expensive, most commonly used modality that often diagnoses hemangiomas. The hemangioma is most often noted incidentally during the course of abdominal ultrasonography for

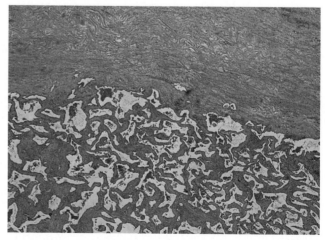

Figure 99–1. Low-power micrograph of a cavernous hemangioma (computed tomography appearance is depicted in Figure 99–2). Classic sharply defined margins with large cavernous vascular spaces characterize this lesion.

other disorders. Findings indicate a hyperechoic mass sharply demarcated from the adjacent hepatic parenchyma. Blood flow directly into the lesion can be detected on occasion, and feeder vessels also can be identified. Ultrasonography is most effective with larger lesions, but in smaller lesions (less than 1 to 2 cm), the sensitivity of ultrasonography declines precipitously. Overall, ultrasonography has a poor sensitivity (approximately 60%), and the hemangioma can be confused with other hyperechoic lesions, such as hepatic adenoma, focal nodular hyperplasia, hepatocellular carcinoma, or even a solitary metastasis.

CT is the modality most widely used to confirm the diagnosis of hemangioma. Contrast and postcontrast studies must be obtained for CT to definitively diagnose hepatic hemangioma (Fig. 99–2). The noncontrast findings show a hypodense, well-demarcated lesion in the liver parenchyma. Postcontrast images show the classic signs of a peripheral zone of enhancement around the lesion associated with a corrugated inner margin. The center of the lesion remains hypodense and reflects large venous pooling. The size of the lesion remains constant throughout the study. CT can lead to misdiagnosis of a hemangioma if the lesion "fills in" during the contrast administration and, as a consequence, is missed. This substantiates the need for both precontrast and postcontrast views. Small lesions (less than 2 cm) are difficult to discern because of loss of resolution of the corrugated inner margin and the peripheral "rim" effect during contrast administration. Hemangiomas that are sclerosed or hyalinized fail to enhance because of abundant fibrous stroma. Hemangiomas can be confused on CT with other lesions, especially hypervascular metastases or focal fatty infiltration.

A dynamic, spiral CT is the preferred examination. The dynamic, spiral CT is obtained during the contrast administration. This technique is the most accurate, low-cost screening test for hemangioma and has a sensitivity of 75% to 80% and a specificity of 80% to 88%.

An alternative imaging modality with a high sensitivity and specificity is MRI. T1- and T2-weighted images are typically obtained. The T1 image shows the mass as distinct from the hepatic parenchyma, and the T2 images should be isodense to hyperintense. Use of intravenous MRI contrast, especially gadolinium enhancement (flash sequence), significantly improves lesion detection. Peripheral rim enhancement with or without lesion enhancement is typical with gadolinium contrast. The accuracy of MRI in defining hemangioma is equal to or better than CT (approximately 90%). Overall sensitivity has been reported at 80% with specificity as high as 99%. However, because MRI is more expensive than CT and much less readily available, it is usually used only in selected situations. For small lesions suspected to be hemangiomas that cannot be characterized even by state-of-the-art CT or MRI, hepatic scintigraphy may be useful. Scintigraphy, which involves the injection of technetium-99m sulfur colloid, was a traditional screening procedure for the evaluation of space-occupying hepatic disease before the advent of CT and MRI. The test involves injection of 3 to 6 mCi of radioisotope attached to .1- to 2-μm sulfur colloid particles. The hepatic Kupffer cells and macrophages extract 90% of the particles as they pass through the liver. Scintigraphy is reported to have greater sensitivity than ultrasonography or CT in detection of this type of space-occupying lesion (86% versus approximately 75%). However, scintigraphy has low specificity (79%) when compared with ultrasonography or CT (82% and 91%, respectively). Scintigraphy can be augmented to improve its specificity by using technetium 99m–labeled red blood cells. The tagged red blood cell study increases the specificity of hepatic scintigraphy. Hemangiomas most often show up as a "cold spot" in conventional scintigraphy and as a "hot spot" after the injection of labeled red blood cells. Increased uptake is seen because of the pooling of red blood cells in the central venous lakes of the tumor. Hemangiomas smaller than 2 cm, which are thrombosed or have significant hyalinization or sclerosis, produce false-negative scintigraphic images and appear "cold" on tagged red blood cell screening. Lesions located deep within the confines of the liver can be obscured by overly-

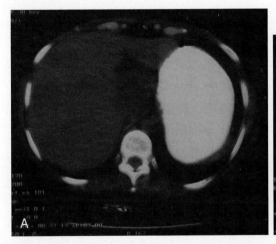
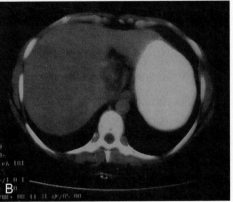

Figure 99–2. Pre– and post–contrast-enhanced computed tomography of hemangioma in the caudate lobe and right lobe of the liver. The pre–contrast-enhanced view (A) shows a well-defined hypodense lesion. The post–contrast-enhanced view shows the classic peripheral filling with the lesion becoming isodense. The central "mottled" appearance (B), which represents late venous filling, is diagnostic of hemangioma.

ing hepatic parenchyma and may cause a false-negative report.

Angiography has no current use in the treatment or management of hemangioma and is mentioned only for historical interest in the diagnosis of hemangioma. Typical findings demonstrate normal hepatic arterial vessels with pooling of contrast medium in the center of the lesion. An intense vascular blush often gives rise to a classic "cotton wool" appearance. This fluffy vascular blush is characteristic of hemangiomas but is usually seen only in larger lesions. Not only is angiography invasive, but it is also not as accurate as CT or MRI, and it is more costly. Thus, angiography is not used currently for either staging, diagnosis, or operative planning.

Hemangiomas are increasingly diagnosed using combined modality evaluations. This approach involves ultrasonography with CT or MRI, with scintigraphy being used in a "triage" or "staged" fashion. Doppler ultrasonography is used for initial screening and diagnosis. Dynamic, contrast-enhanced spiral CT or MRI is used to characterize the lesions and then, in the small group that is left uncharacterized, technetium 99m–labeled red blood cell scanning is performed in conjunction with hepatic scintigraphy. This approach has proved to be 91% accurate in the evaluation of hepatic hemangioma; overall sensitivity is 86% with a specificity of nearly 100%. The positive predictive value is almost 100%, whereas the negative predictive value is 81%. Other clinicians have suggested using MRI in addition to CT in place of tagged red blood cell studies in order to increase the accuracy to 92%.

The role of biopsy requires special comment. Percutaneous biopsy of hepatic lesions is a popular modality among radiologists, but it has no role in the diagnosis or management of hemangiomas or most other single hepatic masses. Biopsy carries a significant risk of bleeding and rarely produces enough tissue for definitive diagnosis of the lesion. In fact, the sample often produces normal liver cells or an abundant amount of blood. Fine-needle biopsy limits the ability of the pathologist to interpret the pathognomonic architecture of the hemangioma because of the small sample size. Core biopsies of hyalinized or sclerosed lesions, which can be seen as solid masses on radiographic evaluation, can be misdiagnosed as sarcomas or fibrous metastatic tumors and could lead to the inappropriate resection of benign lesions. It is preferable to repeat the CT or MRI within a short period of time (6 weeks to 3 months) in patients in whom there is an indeterminate diagnosis. If there is change in the size of the lesion that would lead to the conclusion that it is not a hemangioma, the clinician should proceed with other diagnostic modalities such as laparoscopic inspection and biopsy, open biopsy, or resection.

NATURAL HISTORY

The natural history of hemangiomas is usually a benign one. Several authors have reported large series of patients in whom hemangiomas were found incidentally on abdominal imaging. Most patients followed for periods of 2 to 10 years had minimal to no change in size of the hemangioma. Approximately 10% of patients followed for almost 9 years experienced some growth in their hemangiomas, and new hemangiomas developed in 12%. Exceptions to the normally benign course include the rare patients with intratumoral bleeding or with large hemangiomas that rupture as a result of trauma.

TREATMENT

The benign natural history of most hemangiomas and the high percentage of asymptomatic lesions have led to controversy over appropriate aggressiveness of treatment. Treatment alternatives include conservative observation, resection (enucleation, or lobar or segmental resection), hepatic transplantation, cryoablation or thermal ablation, arterial embolization, or medical therapy with steroids. There is general agreement among most surgeons that, if a hemangioma is discovered incidentally, the hemangioma is less than 4 cm in diameter, and there are fewer than three lesions on diagnostic imaging, then the patient can most likely be discharged from any further formal follow-up. It is important that the diagnosis be accurate; this level of confidence may involve sequential imaging over a period of time. Most patients with small hemangiomas can be reassured that this lesion will not lead to further symptoms or result in substantive risk.

Conservative observation consists of repeat physical examinations and radiographic imaging (dynamic CT) in patients with asymptomatic lesions between 4 and 7 cm in size (giant cavernous hemangiomas) or when more than three lesions are present. Observation can be suggested initially for larger lesions with repeat CT or ultrasonography at 6-month intervals and then, subsequently, at annual intervals with ultrasonography.

Resection is the most controversial and the most definitive therapy available. The indications for resection include symptomatic hemangiomas, intratumoral bleeding, and uncertainty in diagnosis or enlargement on serial observation. Size alone is not itself an indication for resection of hemangiomas.

Debate continues about which technique of resection affords the best results. Hepatic resections are based on lobar or segmental hepatic anatomy. However, hemangiomas can be selected for enucleation because of their benign nature and the distinct anatomic pathology that distinguishes a clear plane between the tumor and normal parenchyma. Hemangioma is, in fact, the only hepatic tumor that can be enucleated safely with little risk of recurrence. Comparative studies of enucleation versus resection have demonstrated that the operative time and the estimated blood loss are less when enucleation is performed. Because the length of hospitalization is equivalent and the risk of complications is less, most hepatic surgeons use enucleation whenever possible in the management of giant hemangioma. Hepatic transplantation has been reported in fewer than 20 patients. The indications for hepatic transplantation in the management of hemangioma are rare but important, and include patients with multiple hemangiomatoses, giant cavernous hemangioma in which there is greater than 70% hepatic replacement, or the combination of hemangiomas and multiple adenomatoses. The results of surgical therapies are good, and, in most series, there is no mortality, and the complication rate is less than 10%.

Interarterial therapies have been advocated in the treatment of hemangiomas in selected situations. These interarterial therapies include hepatic arterial ligation, embolization, or interarterial pharmacologic therapy with either selective vasospastic agents or ethanol. The indications for hepatic arterial therapy are extremely rare but include uncontrolled hemorrhage, high-output congestive heart failure, or Kasabach-Merritt syndrome with disseminated intravascular coagulation and hypofibrinogenemia or thrombocytopenia. Selective intra-arterial treatment with vasopressin has not proved successful. Interarterial therapy with ethanol also has not demonstrated beneficial effects and has a significant potential for toxicity. The therapy most widely accepted is embolization. Embolization has not consistently led to any decrease in the size of the lesion, and there are only rare reports of a definitive resolution of symptoms. Arterial therapy should be viewed, therefore, as a transition to surgical therapies, such as resection for giant hemangioma, stabilization of hemorrhage from a hemangioma, and transplantation in patients with hemangiomatosis, congestive heart failure, or disseminated intravascular coagulation.

Medical therapy is rarely used in the management of hemangioma and has only been described for infantile hemangiomatosis. Steroid administration may be of benefit to patients with hemangioma-associated coagulopathy. There is no documented benefit to lesion size or long-term control of symptoms.

Cryoablation and thermal ablation are newer techniques of hepatic tumor control that have been developed in the past decade. There are only anecdotal reports of the use of cryoablation or thermal ablation in the therapy of hemangiomas. These modalities have limited utility because of the consequences of tumor blood flow, which lessens their therapeutic effect. When performing cryoablation, the rapid tumor blood flow warms the probe and prevents the necessary core cooling. With thermal ablation, the blood acts as a coolant and prevents the heat-induced coagulation. There is a significant risk of coagulopathy associated with large hemangiomas, which can increase the potential of complications during puncture of the lesion by the thermal or cryoprobe. Neither cryoablation nor thermal ablation is recommended for lesions larger than 3 to 6 cm. Most hemangiomas are at least 6 cm in size before they are associated with symptoms. The lesion size is, therefore, a limiting factor in the use of these modalities.

Summary

Hemangioma is the most common benign neoplasm of the liver, and ranges in size from a single, small lesion to

Pearls and Pitfalls

- Hemangiomas are the most common tumors of the liver.
- The natural history of hepatic hemangiomas is a benign one; only the very large cavernous hemangiomas may cause symptoms.
- Intratumoral hemorrhage or free intraperitoneal rupture with hemorrhage is rare.
- Diagnosis involves ultrasonography, CT, MRI, red blood cell–tagged scintigraphy, or some combination of these tests.
- Treatment of the rare symptomatic patient usually involves resection of the lesion by enucleation; formal anatomic resection is usually not necessary.
- Follow-up depends on size and number of lesions. If smaller than 4 cm, no specific follow-up is necessary. For lesions larger than 6 cm or for more than three lesions, surveillance imaging is suggested, usually with ultrasonography.

large tumors in excess of 10 cm, or it may present as multiple lesions throughout the liver. In most patients, no specific follow-up is needed for asymptomatic lesions smaller than 4 cm in size or fewer than three in number. Careful follow-up is recommended for asymptomatic lesions greater than 4 cm or in patients with more than three to four lesions. In most patients, the definitive therapy for symptomatic lesions is resection.

SELECTED READINGS

El-Desouki M, Mohamadiyeh M, al-Rashad R, et al: Features of hepatic cavernous hemangioma on planar and SOECT Tc-99m–labeled red blood cell scintigraphy. Clin Nucl Med 1999;24:585.

Gedaly R, Pomposelli JJ, Pomfret EA, et al: Cavernous hemangioma of the liver: Anatomic resection vs enucleation. Arch Surg 1999;134:407.

Hosten N, Puls R, Lemke AJ, et al: Contrast-enhanced power Doppler sonography: Improved detection of characteristic flow patterns in focal liver lesions. J Clin Ultrasound 1999;27:107.

Leifer DM, Middleton WD, Teefey SA, et al: Follow-up of patients at low risk for hepatic malignancy with a characteristic hemangioma at US. Radiology 2000;214:167.

Moreno EA, Del Pozo RM, Vincente CM, et al: Indications for surgery in the treatment of hepatic hemangioma. Hepatogastroenterology 1996;43:422.

Pietrabissa A, Giulianotti P, Campatelli A, et al: Management and follow-up of 78 giant haemangiomas of the liver. Br J Surg 1996;83:915.

Russo MW, Johnson MW, Fair JH, et al: Orthotopic liver transplantation for giant hepatic hemangioma. Am J Gastroenterol 1997;92:1940.

Suzuki H, Nimura Y, Kamiya J, et al: Preoperative transcatheter arterial embolization for giant cavernous hemangioma of the liver with consumption coagulopathy. Am J Gastroenterol 1997;92:688.

Yu JS, Kim MJ, Kim KW, et al: Hepatic cavernous hemangioma: Sonographic patterns and speed of contrast enhancement on multiphase dynamic MR imaging. AJR Am J Roentgenol 1998;171:1021.

Liver: Malignant

Chapter 100

Hepatocellular Carcinoma

Roger L. Jenkins and Anne L. Lally

Hepatocellular carcinoma (HCC) represents the most common solid tumor of the gastrointestinal tract worldwide and accounts for more than a million deaths annually. Its incidence varies considerably with geographic regions because of marked differences in causative factors around the globe. In regions of the world where hepatitis B and C is endemic, HCC is found with the highest incidence, demonstrating the critical importance of viral infection as a major causative agent. Except in Africa where concomitant cirrhosis is present in only 60% of patients, approximately 90% of patients with HCC have underlying cirrhosis. The presence of cirrhosis of any etiology should be considered an important risk factor for the development of HCC. This association points out the importance of continued periodic surveillance in the cirrhotic population. In the United States where the etiology of cirrhosis is more diverse, the incidence of HCC is less than 4 per 100,000 of the general population and accounts for less than 1% of all cancer deaths. The recent emergence of hepatitis C as a public health concern afflicting almost 4 million individuals will undoubtedly lead to a much higher incidence of HCC in patients with cirrhosis who are antigen-positive for the hepatitis C virus (HCV).

CLINICAL PRESENTATION

Hepatocellular Carcinoma *Without* Cirrhosis

The presence or absence of underlying cirrhosis is one of the key elements affecting modes of presentation and dictating diagnostic strategy. Only approximately 10% of patients with HCC have an otherwise normal liver. Although some studies have suggested a significant role for estrogens in the pathogenesis of some of these neoplasms, the number of cases attributable to hormonal agents is exceedingly small compared with the number of women using estrogen-based oral contraceptive agents. Usually these patients have few, if any, risk factors and may first come to attention with abdominal or shoulder pain, a palpable upper abdominal mass, or hepatomegaly on physical examination. In these patients, there are no stigmata of chronic liver disease unless the tumor has advanced to the point of major vascular invasion. Radiographic evaluation typically demonstrates a large mass, which surprises patients and their families that a mass could achieve such size before discovery. Rarely, a tumor undergoes necrosis, intralesional hemorrhage, and free intra-abdominal bleeding before presenting as an acute medical emergency. Unlike HCC that develops in the background of cirrhosis where surveillance programs allow observation of growth rates, little information is available on growth rates of noncirrhotic HCC. This small noncirrhotic group has the greatest potential for surgical cure. Although survival rates with noncirrhotic HCC are better than those with cirrhotic HCC, it is probably not a less malignant lesion; instead this group reflects the potential treatment bias introduced by a greater functional hepatic reserve in the setting of liver resection.

A disproportionate amount of attention has been paid to an unusual variant of HCC known as the fibrolamellar variant of HCC. Representing no more than approximately 5% to 10% of noncirrhotic HCC, this lesion occurs in younger patients and is associated with a better prognosis. This better prognosis of fibrolamellar HCC reflects the often well-circumscribed nature of the tumors, the absence of coexisting cirrhosis, the young age of the patients, and the relative ease of resection. Grossly and radiologically, these lobulated tumors often contain a central scar and may be confused radiologically for focal nodular hyperplasia. Histologically, these lesions are characterized by broad lamellar bands of collagen separating large polygonal tumor cells with abundant eosinophilic cytoplasm. Many of these lesions present at an advanced stage because of the paucity of symptoms. Bulky nodal disease is not unusual in patients with more advanced disease but should not dissuade the surgeon from considering resection. These nodal metastases may be removed with a portal lymphadenectomy at the time of hepatic resection (Fig. 100–1). Although the classic fibrolamellar lesion is generally considered to confer better outcome with radical resection, many of these lesions are of mixed histology with the prognosis linked to the nonfibrolamellar characteristics of the carcinoma.

The development of jaundice, ascites or gastrointestinal bleeding should be considered as ominous signs. Jaundice in this population usually reflects biliary obstruction by either extrinsic compression or direct intraluminal extension of the tumor, although parenchymal replacement may occur in very late stages. HCC has a propensity for thrombotic extension into branches or even the main trunk of the portal vein, resulting in portal hypertension, ascites formation, and variceal collateral development. Extension into the hepatic veins, suprahepatic vena cava, and atrium may present with a clinical picture consistent with the Budd-Chiari syndrome.

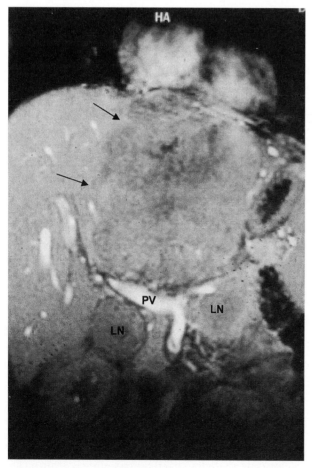

Figure 100–1. Massive fibrolamellar HCC in a 30-year-old man with extensive nodal involvement. The tumor (*arrows*) was resected by an extended left hepatic lobectomy along with excision of all nodal disease. LN, lymph node; PV, main trunk of portal vein.

Hepatocellular Carcinoma *with* Cirrhosis

In the patient with cirrhosis, signs and symptoms of cirrhosis may overshadow the presence of an underlying neoplasm. Any patient with cirrhosis with clinical deterioration manifesting as new onset bleeding, ascites, wasting, or jaundice should be evaluated for development of HCC. This presentation reflects the impact of tumor progression superimposed upon compromised hepatic reserve in the cirrhotic liver and accounts for why HCC has a reputation as a rapidly progressive fatal tumor. With more aggressive screening regimens (ultrasonography, serum alpha-fetoprotein [AFP] levels) and the existence of an increasingly large number of patients who are followed up while awaiting liver transplantation, the discovery of HCC at a relatively small size is becoming more common. Occasionally, HCC can be a relatively slow-growing tumor with a high degree of variability in behavior within a particular patient. The clinician needs to consider this variable growth rate when designing treatment regimens, particularly when considering the morbidity associated with operative resection applied to the cirrhotic patient. Although resection of these lesions still represents the treatment standard, the degree of hepatic impairment by cirrhosis limits the surgical options to fewer than 25% of cirrhotic patients harboring HCC. Improved understanding of the behavior of HCC in cirrhosis has reawakened interest in the use of liver transplantation as the primary treatment of carefully selected patients. Several reports have suggested that, when liver transplantation is carried out for cirrhotic HCC smaller than 3 cm in diameter, survival rates are equivalent to those with non-neoplastic cirrhotic diseases. Although the role of timely transplantation in HCC has been severely limited by cadaveric donor organ availability, evolving methods of organ allocation, more widespread introduction of split liver grafts, and the recent introduction of adult living donor liver transplantation will undoubtedly spur renewed interest in this aggressive surgical option. Meanwhile, operative or percutaneous techniques of liver ablation have assumed increasingly important roles in the treatment of the mild or moderately impaired cirrhotic patient with HCC.

Evaluation

Evaluation of the patient with a liver mass should always start with a careful history to look for underlying risk factors for tumor and to rule out the possibility of a metastatic recurrence of a nonhepatic malignancy. Laboratory and radiologic studies are directed toward assessing underlying liver disease, ruling out metastatic origin or extension, and determining anatomic feasibility of resection. Measurements of "liver function tests" are essential. Increases in serum hepatocellular enzyme activities (AST [aspartate aminotransferase], ALT [alanine transaminase]) imply an ongoing ischemic or hepatitic process, whereas an increased alkaline phosphatase activity implies an element of biliary obstruction. Increase in serum bilirubin concentration in the absence of major bile duct obstruction or liver replacement suggests derangement of hepatic synthetic function from an underlying acute or chronic liver disorder. Prolongation of the prothrombin time, which is not correctable with vitamin K is a relatively accurate indicator of poor hepatic reserve. Decrease in the serum albumin level concentration may reflect impaired synthesis, nutritional deficiencies, or septic stress. Thrombocytopenia may indicate hypersplenism as a manifestation of underlying portal hypertension.

Increases in serum AFP greater than 20 ng/mL occurs in 60% to 75% of patients with HCC. Serum concentrations may fluctuate considerably, particularly in the patient with HCV infection in whom increases as high as 400 ng/mL may reflect ongoing inflammation and regeneration of hepatocytes mass. Even so, all patients with HCV disease and an increasing serum AFP level should undergo imaging studies in search of an early HCC. AFP is increased in fewer than 25% of patients with the fibrolamellar variant of HCC. Even in the absence of obvious stigmata of chronic liver disease, all patients with a liver tumor should undergo serologic studies for hepatitis B surface antigen (HB$_s$Ag), hepatitis B core antibody (HB$_c$Ab), and HCV antibody. Although radiologic studies may suggest a benign lesion within the liver, serologic evidence of hepatitis B virus (HBV) or HCV infection or increases in serum AFP should make the clinician suspicious of HCC.

Critical to the evaluation and management of the patient with a liver mass is the logical use of existing imaging technologies. In younger patients, the differential diagnosis is often a benign process such as cavernous hemangioma, focal nodular hyperplasia, hepatic adenoma, or an unusual malignant process. In older patients, the differential diagnosis most commonly includes metastases from a known or occult extrahepatic malignancy. The role of ultrasonography is more important for the patient with small tumors than for the large masses typically seen in the noncirrhotic patient. Even though this versatile tool is largely operator dependent, it can suggest the presence of cirrhosis or fatty infiltration, ascites, portal hypertension (splenomegaly or varices), characteristics of the tumor (solid versus cystic), or vascular involvement (portal or hepatic veins). The entire liver should be imaged in an organized fashion to rule out the possibility of multiple lesions. No study is complete without assessment of the portal vein and hepatic veins. One drawback, however, is that the images produced by ultrasonography do not readily translate into precise anatomic constructs for most surgeons.

Computed tomography (CT) has the advantages of examiner-independent reproducibility and the ability to better portray the relationship of a tumor to the liver and surrounding anatomic structures. Thus, CT should play an early role in the process of staging disease and planning surgical strategy. A carefully performed CT, both with and without intravenous contrast, is helpful in highlighting lesions that may be otherwise isodense with the surrounding liver. Of critical importance however, is assessing the proximity of any tumor to major hepatic venous structures. Many of the larger tumors expand to compress or distort the inferior vena cava, the main portal vein, or one of its major trunks, yet they are still readily resectable. A tumor thrombus may be seen lying within the lumen of the portal vein with contrast enhancement

or may be suggested by the presence of decreased attenuation of an entire hepatic lobe (Fig. 100–2). This finding generally implies a poor outlook even with technically successful resection. Most important is determining whether one or more major hepatic veins can be preserved to allow adequate hepatic recovery from the planned resection. Planning the extent of liver resection is almost invariably based more on hepatic vein anatomy than on portal vein, hepatic artery, or biliary anatomy.

Magnetic resonance imaging (MRI) provides an alternative tool for evaluation of a patient with a liver tumor without radiation exposure. In terms of diagnostic sensitivity, MRI provides little benefit over good quality triphasic CT in most centers. However, angiographic or biliary sequences can demonstrate tumor relationships to vascular and biliary structures and may be useful in patients who cannot undergo quality CT imaging because of contrast hypersensitivity. Because of the sophistication of enhanced CT and MRI images, arteriography is rarely used for diagnosis or in planning resection. In general, arteriography is reserved for those nonresectable cases that are to be treated by hepatic artery chemoembolization techniques.

The use of percutaneous biopsy of a liver tumor should be limited strictly to situations in which the result would alter treatment strategy. Patients who are otherwise candidates for resection are not going to benefit from biopsy, regardless of the histology of the lesion. The decision to operate is a clinical decision that does not rely on a tissue diagnosis. In instances of suspected but unproved associated cirrhosis, biopsy of an uninvolved portion of the liver may be more important to treatment planning than biopsy of the tumor itself.

Special consideration must be given to the patient with more advanced cirrhosis (Childs B or C) in whom a new lesion develops that is suspicious for HCC. This scenario is common in the patient with HCV disease awaiting liver transplantation as well as in the patient newly referred with cirrhosis of any etiology. Resection is usually not an option for these patients because of limited hepatic re-

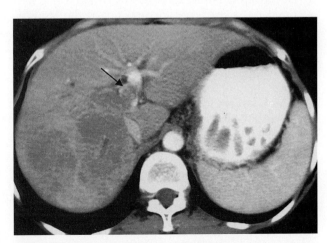

Figure 100–2. A 48-year-old HBV-positive woman with large right lobe HCC and tumor thrombus extending into the left portal vein (*arrow*). Despite right lobectomy and tumor thrombectomy with portal vein reconstruction, she died of disseminated hepatic disease 4 months later.

serve. Ablative techniques may provide local tumor control as a bridge to transplantation, or ablation may become the primary treatment in patients who are not candidates for transplantation.

PREOPERATIVE MANAGEMENT

The requirements of preoperative management vary depending on whether the patient with a tumor has coexisting cirrhosis. Usually the history, initial laboratory evaluation, and the configuration of the uninvolved portion of the liver as seen on CT assist the clinician in determining the presence of background cirrhosis. For the patient without cirrhosis, the most important studies are related to proper imaging of the tumor in relationship to intrahepatic anatomy. Resectability is essentially defined by the ability to remove the tumor with adequate margins and leave enough uninvolved liver to sustain life until hepatic regeneration has occurred. The importance of remnant size and regeneration has focused occasional attempts to embolize branches of the portal vein to the involved portion of the liver in order to stimulate preoperative hypertrophy of the uninvolved segment. Although this technique may have a role in rare situations, it is generally not required and adds complexity to the average plan for resection. The configuration of the hepatic venous outflow tracts in relation to the tumor is the most important determinant of resectability. Even massive tumors are resectable if there is adequate venous outflow of an appropriately sized remnant liver. This is not to say that the importance of portal venous and hepatic arterial structures can be ignored, but control and reconstruction of these latter two structures arc often possible even in seemingly ominous situations. Therefore, accurate CT or MRI with adequate visualization of vascular structures is the most important diagnostic study. Because most HCC lesions remain localized within the liver and surrounding nodal tissue, we do not obtain bone scans or a CT of the chest unless symptoms indicate their need or unless liver transplantation is being considered.

The patient harboring an HCC in a cirrhotic liver may be considered a candidate for resection if the lesion is conveniently located and small enough to allow removal of relatively limited amounts of the cirrhotic liver (Table 100–1). Thus, the focus of information obtained at the time of imaging is directed toward defining the limits of a segmental or multisegmental resection that includes the tumor with at least a 1-cm margin and preserves overall functional liver mass. Just as important as the quality of the imaging studies is the examination of physical and

Table 100–1	**Criteria for Resectability in Cirrhotic Hepatocellular Carcinoma**

Bilirubin <2.0 mg/dL
Serum albumin >3.0 mg/dL
International normalized ratio (INR) <1.8
Absence of ascites
Absence of encephalopathy
Sublobar resection potential

laboratory parameters that determine whether a patient should be a surgical candidate. Jaundice (bilirubin > 2.0 mg/dL) or ascites should preclude surgical consideration, and an international normalized ratio (INR) greater than 1.7 or a serum albumin concentration less than 3 g/dL indicate excessive risk with resection attempts. The literature is replete with techniques of hepatic function such as indocyanine green clearance devised to more accurately predict hepatic reserve and operative risk. Although many of the techniques have become more accurate, the availability of varied treatment options for cirrhotic patients with HCC should limit the reliance of the surgeon on these methods. Patients who are poor candidates for operative resection are probably best served by percutaneous or laparoscopic radiofrequency ablation (RFA). Ablative techniques may not achieve complete tumor destruction, but when used with overlapping zones of necrosis, these techniques appear to be viable options for the patient at too high a risk for resection.

Operative resection or ablative procedures are major operations that introduce considerable physiologic stress to the patient, both intraoperatively and postoperatively. Older patients with underlying cardiac disease should be screened preoperatively to assess perioperative risk. Age alone should not be a determinant of surgical candidacy, because patients well into their 80s may tolerate resection of a major portion of the liver without difficulty.

Depending on the urgency of surgical intervention and the amount of time available preoperatively, patients are requested to donate 1 to 2 units of autologous blood, which is made available the day of surgery. Approximately 80% of all liver resections can be accomplished without the need for blood transfusion or using only autologous blood. Even so, each patient is typed and cross-matched for at least 4 units of blood preoperatively.

INTRAOPERATIVE MANAGEMENT

Anesthesia Preparation

Preparation for the potential for unexpected significant blood loss dictates the extent of intravenous access obtained. Generally, at least one large-bore intravenous cannula is inserted peripherally for rapid blood administration. Central venous access with a large-bore cannula is obtained following induction of anesthesia. A broad-spectrum antibiotic is administered just before entry into the operating room to reduce the incidence of wound infection. Compression boots are applied to the lower extremities for prophylaxis against venous thrombosis. Avoidance of dangerous levels of hypothermia during long operations is accomplished by raising the ambient temperature of the room or by application of lower or upper extremity pneumatic warming devices. Although an intraoperative blood-salvaging system is not used in every instance, it should be readily available just outside the room to be set up within 5 minutes if excessive blood loss is anticipated or occurs.

Operative Preparation

The patient is positioned supine on the operating table with both arms extended perpendicular to the trunk on well-padded arm boards. For patients with centrally located tumors or where the use of total vascular isolation is anticipated, the entire anterior chest and both groin areas are prepped into the sterile operative field to allow insertion of cannulas for venovenous or portosystemic bypass (see later text). Because there may be concern about the presence of advanced cirrhosis or unexpected hepatic metastases not visible on imaging studies, diagnostic laparoscopy is usually suggested after induction of anesthesia. The camera port is inserted in the periumbilical region using an open technique and a pneumoperitoneum is established. A brief inspection of the abdomen with particular attention to the uninvolved portion of the liver is then carried out. Biopsy sample of the tumor may be obtained under direct vision if a decision is made not to perform formal resection. Additional ports may be placed to allow the introduction of a laparoscopic ultrasonography probe for direct imaging of the liver parenchyma and vascular structures. Occasionally, this technique may define more extensive disease than expected, altering the operative decision, but its greatest utility is in guidance for laparoscopic ablative techniques.

Ablative Techniques

Although anteriorly situated tumors may be amenable to ablation by alcohol injection, cryosurgery, or RFA with probes placed under direct laparoscopic vision, the depth of ablation cannot be accurately gauged without the use of ultrasonographic imaging. All three ablative techniques, when used as a single application, are practically limited to lesions less than 6 cm in diameter that do not abut major vascular structures. Multiple applications in overlapping concentric zones may achieve destruction of lesions larger, although these techniques are somewhat limited by the amount of necrotic tissue produced and the operative time required for multiple ablations. Although ablation may be accomplished under laparoscopic or open laparotomy control by the surgeon in situations in which

planned surgical resection is aborted, the patient is better served by ultrasonographic or CT-guided percutaneous ethanol (PEI) or RFA if they are not good operative candidates, thus avoiding the morbidity of an open celiotomy. Alcohol ablation has the advantage of low cost and ease of use and induces coagulative necrosis of injected tissues within a few days. The margin of alcohol infiltration may be difficult to gauge even under ultrasonographic guidance, and one cannot always be sure of encompassing the entire lesion. We typically reserve this technique for the ablation of small suspicious lesions found during intraoperative ultrasonography when the lesions cannot be encompassed by modification of the resection plane or when they are in deep or strategically poor locations where separate resection is not feasible. Cryosurgical ablation has the advantage of convenient monitoring of the advancing ice sphere by ultrasonography, but the cannulas and equipment are more cumbersome. More recently, advancements in the equipment for RFA have made this technology currently the preferable option for most surgeons and most patients. Probe placement under ultrasonographic guidance is straightforward, and the equipment is amenable to using operative, laparoscopic, or percutaneous approaches (Fig. 100–3). All three ablative techniques suffer from the uncertainty of complete destruction of the lesion and require significant dedication on the part of the operator. For this reason, resection is still the preferred treatment method for primary or metastatic liver tumors.

Operative Exposure

Operative exposure is one of the keys to safe hepatic surgery. Although right thoracotomy with extension across the costal margin combined with abdominal incision may be indicated on rare occasion, modern fixed table retraction devices allow the vast majority of resections to be performed using only an abdominal incision. Complex tumors involving vascular structures in the region of the

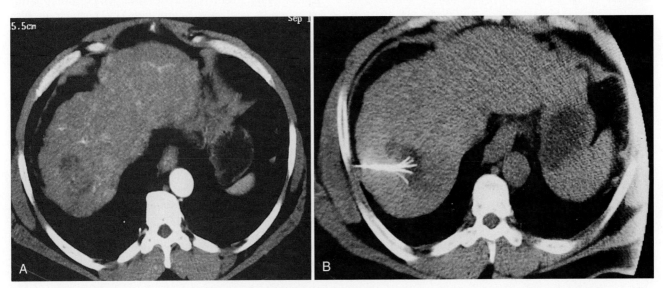

Figure 100–3. *A,* A 56-year-old HCV-positive man with local recurrence of HCC in the right lobe of the liver 2 years after ethanol ablation. *B,* Percutaneous ablation of recurrent HCC with radiofrequency probe under CT guidance.

suprahepatic vena cava are sometimes best approached by a midline sternotomy and extending the incision downward to the umbilicus. This approach allows intrapericardial control of the vena cava above the liver with relative ease. The more typical operative exposure, however, is obtained by a right subcostal incision that can be extended to the left of midline as needed for the type of resection planned. An additional upward extension in the midline toward the xiphoid can further improve exposure at the level of the suprahepatic vena cava. Excision of the round ligament and division of the falciform ligament up to the level of the suprahepatic vena cava is performed before placement of the abdominal wall retractor. We prefer a fixed retractor secured to the rail on the left side of the operating table. An extension bar available as an accessory allows the large round split ring to be suspended several inches above the incision. A series of blades on angled ratchets are used to elevate the costal margin in both the cephalad and ventral directions. Additional blades may be added inferiorly to retract the stomach or duodenum caudally. This configuration optimizes the space available to the surgeon for extensive medial rotation of the right lobe of the liver when necessary.

Intraoperative ultrasonography (IOUS) is an essential tool for the liver surgeon and is performed after placement of the retraction device and liver mobilization. IOUS permits the surgeon to visualize the deeper margins of the tumor and the relationships to important vascular structures. It is particularly valuable for mapping the course of the middle hepatic vein, which plays a major role in many lobar resections. The course of important vessels can be marked on the surface of the liver with cautery to serve as a guide during parenchymal transection. Familiarity with the segmental anatomy of the liver is important in planning single or multisegmental resections that are not based on formal lobar anatomy.

Techniques to Control Blood Loss

Division of the liver parenchyma can be attended by significant blood loss typically from hepatic venous structures. A number of techniques are used to reduce blood loss during the period of parenchymal division. Because the source of most bleeding during liver division is the hepatic venous system, the most convenient technique to use is the maintenance of a low central venous pressure, which lowers pressure in the inferior vena cava and the hepatic veins. Preliminary division and ligation of portal vein and hepatic artery branches to the involved segments or lobe reduces the component of blood loss from inflow structures. This maneuver requires enough dissection in the hepatic hilum to have adequately identified the appropriate structures. The surgeon should be familiar with the common variations in hepatic artery anatomy such as a replaced right hepatic artery originating from the superior mesenteric artery, nestled between the bile duct and posterior to the portal vein on the right side of the hilum, and a replaced left hepatic artery arising from the left gastric artery and lying in the hepatogastric ligament. When possible, the hepatic vein outflow vessels to the involved portion of the liver should be controlled before

parenchymal transection to minimize back bleeding. In the case of right hepatic lobectomy, division of the right triangular ligament and rotation of the liver from right to left exposes numerous small hepatic vein branches draining from the right lobe into the inferior vena cava. Sequential division of these vessels allows the liver to be separated from the vena cava upward toward the right hepatic vein. The right hepatic vein can then be encircled for later division by suture or stapling device. It is important not to divide the hepatic vein structures until inflow structures have been controlled or else the liver will become congested. Similarly, the left hepatic vein or the confluence of the left and middle hepatic veins can be encircled before major left lobe or extended left lobe resections. After division of the left triangular and hepatogastric ligaments, the left lateral segment of the liver is rotated left to right. The fibrous plane between the upper extent of the caudate lobe and the left lateral segment of the liver is opened at the level of the suprahepatic vena cava to allow entry into the space between the IVC and the left hepatic vein. Downward retraction of the entire liver then allows exposure of the anterior aspect of the suprahepatic vena cava. The crevice between the right and middle hepatic veins can usually be exposed and widened and often one can actually identify the space between the left and middle hepatic veins by the same maneuver. One can then encircle the confluence of left and middle hepatic veins or, with a bit more effort, the left hepatic vein alone.

Another technique to reduce blood loss is the use of temporary hilar inflow occlusion (Pringle maneuver). A tourniquet or vascular clamp is placed across the entire hepatoduodenal ligament for periods of up to 45 minutes without major consequence in the noncirrhotic patient. Need for longer periods of occlusion is best handled by intermittent release of the inflow occlusion, rather than by maintaining a prolonged total occlusion of more than 45 minutes. Periods of less than 15 minutes are recommended for cirrhotic livers. The authors do not use this technique routinely but only when bleeding from the cut surface of the liver appears excessive. An extension of this technique is total vascular isolation (TVI), which involves temporary occlusion of both the suprahepatic and infrahepatic vena caval segments in conjunction with hilar inflow occlusion. Encirclement of the infrahepatic vena cava is relatively simple, whereas encirclement of the IVC at the diaphragm requires more preparation. First, one must divide both left and right coronary ligaments and the hepatogastric ligament. Dissection behind the IVC at the level of the diaphragm can be carried out as the liver is rotated from right to left and the plane between the IVC and the diaphragmatic crus is opened. A tape can then be placed around the IVC to facilitate subsequent clamp placement. TVI has the potential to induce significant hypotension through stagnation of blood in the abdominal viscera and lower extremities. Stability of the patient during TVI may be improved using a venovenous bypass circuit. Venovenous bypass is a technique originally developed for the anhepatic phase of liver transplantation that allows bypass of blood from the infrahepatic vena cava and intestinal mesenteric veins back to the superior vena cava. Size 15-French heparin-bonded cannulas may be introduced rapidly into the femoral and subclavian veins using percutaneous techniques with blood flow facilitated by a centrifugal force pump. An additional cannula may be inserted into the inferior mesenteric vein to allow decompression of the portal system. The advantage of this bypass system is the hemodynamic stability afforded by return of lower extremity and splanchnic blood flow to the patient during prolonged periods of portal and caval interruption. In more recent years, we have used this technique more sparingly, preferring to use intravenous volume loading and short periods of portal and caval clamping instead. Most patients tolerate this technique well, and their tolerance may be assessed by temporary hand compression of the hepatic hilum and vena cava before committing to a technique.

The assistant plays a major role in reducing blood loss during parenchymal transection by applying upward traction of the liver and firm manual compression. Both of these maneuvers compress the intrahepatic venous structures. The use of cautery, the ultrasonic dissector (CUSA), and particularly the argon beam coagulator (ABC), is important in reducing blood loss from the cut margin of the liver, both during and after resection. The ABC uses electrical current along a stream of inert argon gas and can coagulate broad portions of the liver. When properly used, the ABC can seal veins up to 4 or 5 mm in size along the cut surface. Finally, the use of commercially available fibrin sealants can assist in controlling hemorrhage, particularly within crevices along the site of transection.

Parenchymal Division

The technique used for division of the liver parenchyma varies with the consistency of the liver and the preferences of the surgeon. The most common method of liver transection is by finger or instrument fracture. Bridging biliary and vascular structures are divided with right angles and individually ligated or sutured. More controlled transection can be accomplished either with the harmonic scalpel or the CUSA. These devices obliterate the parenchymal elements in the plane of division while exposing the more fibrous vascular elements for controlled ligation. The method used, however, is less important if attention has been paid to the principles of controlling blood loss discussed earlier. After completion of the transection, pressure is applied to the cut surface of the liver for several minutes to allow a coagulum to form. Any persistent bleeders may be suture-ligated or cauterized with the ABC. After irrigation with saline, a careful search is made for any bile leaks. Omentum, if available, can be brought up against the cut margin of the liver, and a single closed suction drain is often placed alongside the cut margin of the liver, although many surgeons do not routinely place drains after an uncomplicated hepatic resection.

Most unexpected findings during planned liver resection relate to unexpectedly extensive disease or intraoperative bleeding. Tumor extension to the diaphragm or pericardium should be managed by en bloc resection of parts of these structures as necessary to achieve an adequate surgical margin and an R_o resection. Even large defects in the diaphragm can be repaired by simple suture closure with minimal reduction in lung capacity. A polytetrafluoroethylene patch can be used to bridge pericardial defects.

Uncontrolled bleeding is the nemesis of the liver surgeon and occasionally occurs even in the best of hands. Almost invariably, the source of the bleeding is the middle hepatic vein or its tributaries that are injured during misdirection of the parenchymal transection plane. If upward traction and compression of the liver cannot control such bleeding, then TVI may be required to safely repair the vein and complete the resection. Getting the surgical specimen out as expeditiously as possible without causing additional injury should be a major goal because this allows direct pressure on the site of injury and a more controlled direct suture repair. The surgeon should never be hesitant to firmly pack the resection bed with laparotomy pads when persistent venous bleeding cannot be controlled surgically. Re-exploration with pack removal is often all that is necessary 24 to 48 hours later.

POSTOPERATIVE MANAGEMENT

Patients are extubated in the operating room or recovery room according to conventional anesthetic criteria. An assessment of function of the remnant liver is most easily obtained by measurement of the INR. It is not unusual for the INR to go as high as 1.8 after major resection of a noncirrhotic liver. In the absence of blood from the surgical drain, fresh-frozen plasma is not administered so that the trend in the INR can be followed. The hematocrit is monitored immediately in the recovery room and then once or twice over the next 24 hours as indicated. Pain control after hepatic resection is most easily accomplished using an epidural catheter placed before anesthetic induction or subsequently in the recovery room. In the absence of an epidural catheter, parenterally administered narcotics should be carefully administered. Patients undergoing resection of more than 50% of their liver or patients with compensated cirrhosis are extremely sensitive to the sedating effects of systemically administered narcotics.

Patients ambulate and resume a regular diet on the first postoperative day. The drain is removed by the fourth postoperative day but is left in place at the time of discharge if the drainage contains bile. The patient is discharged 5 to 7 days after surgery.

COMPLICATIONS

A full set of liver function tests is obtained within the first 24 hours after surgery. Increase in the serum bilirubin level to 5 mg/dL is not unusual within the first 48 hours after major resection in an otherwise normal liver and returns to baseline rapidly. Cirrhotic patients even undergoing very limited resections are more likely to have delayed and persistent increases in serum bilirubin concentrations as a result of intrahepatic cholestasis. Persistently increasing serum bilirubin concentrations within the first week after major hepatic resection should be evaluated by endoscopic retrograde cholangiopancreatography (ERCP) to rule out surgically induced biliary obstruction. A small amount of bile staining in the suction drain is not unusual and usually clears within 3 to 5 days after surgery. Drainage of more concentrated bile in quantities greater than 100 mL per day suggests a more significant biliary injury. The source of the majority of bile leaks is small biliary radicals on the cut surface of the liver, and spontaneous closure usually occurs within 2 weeks of surgery. Occasionally, however, a major biliary radical injured at the hilar plate or along the cut surface of the liver persists in draining. The key principles in managing a major biliary leak after liver resection include ensuring adequate local drainage by drains left at the time of surgery or placed radiologically. An ultrasonography or CT demonstrating a fluid collection in the presence of persistent biliary leakage suggests the need for placement of an additional percutaneous drain. Large volumes of drainage of greater than 300 mL for more than 2 weeks or in the presence of acholic stools should prompt ERCP to rule out injury to the remnant central ductal system. In addition to delineating the site of injury, a sphincterotomy and stent may be placed to bridge a stricture and reduce impedance to flow out the ampulla. If the bile duct is completely obstructed, the surgeon must assume major surgical injury and proceed to percutaneous biliary imaging to determine the site of injury. Surgical revision with conversion to Roux-en-Y hepaticojejunostomy is necessary in such patients.

Infective complications after liver resection are more common in patients with coexisting cirrhosis or in patients with persistent bile leaks. Fever within the first 2 or 3 days after liver resection should prompt a search for the most common causes such as pulmonary, urinary, wound, or intravenous catheter–related sources. Fever more than 3 days after hepatic resection suggests an infected perihepatic collection in the absence of an obvious wound source. Antibiotic therapy and percutaneous drainage of any intra-abdominal collection is indicated. Prompt treatment of infection is important, because sepsis appears to delay hepatic regeneration after hepatic resection.

Patients with cirrhosis who appear to have tolerated a limited liver resection well for the first few days after surgery may still have significant complications over the next few weeks. The development of anasarca and ascites may not occur within the initial 5- to 7-day hospitalization period but can appear in a delayed fashion a week or two later. Salt restriction in conjunction with the administration of spironolactone and furosemide usually leads to resolution over a few weeks. An ultrasonography study of the portal vein should be considered because postoperative thrombosis of the portal vein may be the culprit. Spontaneous thrombosis of the portal vein is seen occasionally in patients with cirrhosis without antecedent surgery, and the management is expectant without the use of anticoagulants.

Perioperative mortality rates for resection of HCC should be less than 10% if patients are selected properly. Judicious use of ablative techniques in the poor and marginal patients will likely contribute to a further decline in operative mortality rates.

OUTCOMES

A number of characteristics of the tumor influence the potential for recurrence, including multiple lesions or bilobar involvement, size greater than 5 cm, gross or microscopic vascular invasion, positive surgical margins, an infiltrative growth pattern, and advanced tumor, node, metastasis (TNM) stages (Table 100–2). The attainment of an adequate surgical margin (>1 cm) is the only prognostic factor the surgeon can control.

Continued surveillance of the patient undergoing liver resection or ablation for HCC is crucial to the early detection and treatment of disease recurrence. Patients are imaged by CT at 3- to 4-month intervals the first year, 6-month intervals the second year, and annually thereafter. Serum AFP measurement is another useful parameter in patients who had an increased AFP measurement preoperatively. Recurrence, in most instances, is within the liver. The fibrolamellar variant of HCC may recur as bulky disease within regional lymph nodes and may be resectable in patients with a long disease-free interval. The clear cell variant of HCC has a propensity for pulmonary and osseous metastases as well as liver metastases, although recurrent disease may not be detectable for several years after resection. Limited recurrence of HCC within the liver after liver resection may be amenable to percutaneous RFA or alcohol ablation. More widespread hepatic recurrence may be controlled for variable periods by hepatic artery chemoembolization, while systemic chemotherapy is reserved for extrahepatic disease.

Three- and 5-year survival rates after surgical resection of HCC vary depending upon the proportion of patients with coexisting cirrhosis, but range from 30% to 70% and 25% to 50%, respectively. Most deaths are from recurrent intrahepatic tumor or progressive cirrhosis and liver failure. A number of investigators have reported 3-year survival rates after alcohol ablation of cirrhotic HCC that are similar to results obtained with surgical resection. This observation should temper the enthusiasm for overly aggressive attempts to resect small lesions in cirrhotic patients.

For patients with massive HCC in an otherwise normal liver, aggressive resection remains the treatment of choice. When resection of such lesions is not possible, hepatic artery chemoembolization or systemic chemotherapy may be feasible. The very high recurrence rates after total hepatectomy and liver transplantation in such patients make this option foolhardy unless carried out as part of an investigational adjuvant therapy protocol. Recurrence in a cirrhotic liver after either resection or

Table 100–2	**Poor Prognostic Factors in HCC**
	Multiple lesions
	Bilobar involvement
	Vascular invasion
	Positive surgical margins
	Infiltrative growth pattern
	Size >5 cm diameter
	Advanced TNM stages

Overall Survival

% survival

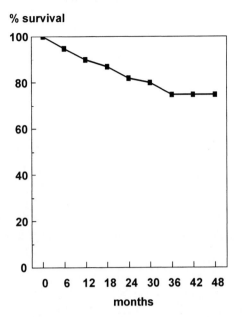

Recurrence-Free Survival

% survival

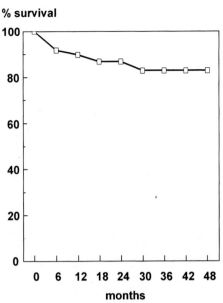

Figure 100–4. Patient survival after liver transplantation for cirrhosis and HCC. Patients were selected if they had solitary tumors less than 5 cm in diameter or three or fewer lesions all less than 3 cm in diameter. (Adapted from Mazzaferro V, Regalia G, Doci R, et al: Liver transplantation for the treatment of small hepatocellular carcinomas in patients with cirrhosis. N Engl J Med 1996;334:693.)

ablation of an HCC may occur locally because of positive margins or more distantly as a de novo lesion arising in a diffusely abnormal liver. The propensity for new lesions to develop in patients with cirrhosis who are under observation has prompted a more aggressive use of liver transplantation as a more durable treatment option. Results of liver transplantation for the treatment of cirrhotic HCC less than 5 cm in diameter are encouraging, with survival rates approaching those of patients undergoing liver transplantation for cirrhosis of viral etiology (Fig. 100–4). Indeed, those results would appear to extend even to patients with three or fewer lesions as long as the maximum size of the largest lesion does not exceed 3 cm.

CONCLUSION

Surgical resection remains the gold standard for the management of HCC in the normal liver and the small HCC

in the compensated cirrhotic liver. Knowledge of hepatic segmental anatomy and adherence to the principles of control of blood loss have improved the safety of even the more extensive liver resections. Nonsurgical methods, such as alcohol ablation, cryotherapy, or RFA, are emerging as reasonable treatment alternatives to resection for the cirrhotic HCC patient with limited functional reserve. The increased potential for recurrent or de novo tumor formation in HBV- and HCV-positive patients after resection or ablative therapy has focused more attention on the role of liver transplantation as a more viable option for carefully selected patients. With the limits placed upon liver transplantation by the availability of donor organs, ablative techniques are becoming increasingly important in local tumor control while awaiting transplantation. Live donor liver transplants are likely to play a prominent role in the timelier implementation of transplantation for HCC.

SELECTED READINGS

Adam R, Akpinar E, Johann M, et al: Place of cryosurgery in the treatment of malignant liver tumors. Ann Surg 1997;225:39.

Bismuth H, Chiche L, Adam R, et al: Liver resection versus transplantation for hepatocellular carcinoma in cirrhotic patients. Ann Surg 1993;218:145.

Bismuth H, Chiche L, Castaing D: Surgical treatment of hepatocellular carcinomas in noncirrhotic liver: Experience with 68 liver resections. World J Surg 1995;9:35.

Fong Y, Sun RL, Jarnagin WR, Blumgart LH: An analysis of 412 cases of hepatocellular carcinoma at a western center. Ann Surg 1999;229:790.

Schwartz ME, Sung M, Mor E, et al: A multidisciplinary approach to hepatocellular carcinoma in patients with cirrhosis. J Am Coll Surg 1995;180:596.

Stevens WR, Johnson CD, Stephens DH, Nagorney DM: Fibrolamellar hepatocellular carcinoma: Stage at presentation and results of aggressive surgical management. AJR Am J Roentgenol 1995;164:1153.

Vauthey JN, Klimstra D, Franceschi D, et al: Factors affecting long-term outcome after hepatic resection for hepatocellular carcinoma. Am J Surg 1995;169:28.

Pearls and Pitfalls

- Surgical resection remains the optimal treatment for HCC in the noncirrhotic patient.
- Resectability is determined by the tumor's relationship to hepatic venous structures on triphasic CT or MRI.
- Adequate surgical margin is one of the few risk factors under surgeon control.
- Limited resection is feasible in cirrhotic patients with adequate hepatic reserve.
- Ablative techniques are emerging as effective treatments for cirrhotic HCC.
- Liver transplantation may be the most effective treatment of cirrhotic HCC smaller than 5 cm.

Chapter 101

Metastatic Cancer of the Liver

Jeffrey D. Wayne and Jean-Nicolas Vauthey

SURGICAL TREATMENT OF COLORECTAL LIVER METASTASES

More than 130,000 patients with colorectal cancer are diagnosed in the United States each year. Even though 85% of patients have tumors amenable to resection for cure, the cancer recurs in half of these patients within 5 years. Approximately 20% of cases of recurrent disease involve metastases only in the liver, and one third to one half involve resectable disease. Without treatment, median length of survival is 12 to 15 months, with a 5-year survival rate of 3% or less. In an effort to prolong survival, many treatment modalities have been employed, but surgical resection remains the only method by which long-term survival may be achieved. Numerous studies document the safety and efficacy of hepatectomy in the treatment of metastatic colorectal cancer with an operative mortality rate of less than 5% and a 5-year actuarial survival rate of up to 37%. Thus, surgical therapy is the preferred treatment of recurrent colorectal cancer confined to the liver.

NATURAL HISTORY

Several retrospective studies have defined the natural history of untreated disease. Two studies specifically looked at patients with resectable disease who did not undergo resection. One group reported 5-year survival rates of 3% and 0%, respectively, for patients with either solitary or multiple metastases. Scheele and colleagues analyzed 62 patients with "resectable" tumors who did not undergo resection and found a median survival rate of 14 months, with no 5-year survivors.

Scheele and colleagues defined the impact of surgical resection of hepatic colorectal metastases in a large, single-institution prospective series spanning more than 2 decades. Three hundred fifty patients who underwent curative resection (negative microscopic margins) had 5- and 10-year survival rates of 39% and 24%, respectively. Those with microscopic or macroscopic residual disease had a median length of survival of only 14 months. If patients remained tumor-free at 5 years, 88% were still tumor-free at 10 years (Fig. 101–1). This is the best presumptive evidence that surgery has a direct impact on the natural history of the disease.

INDICATIONS AND CONTRAINDICATIONS TO SURGERY

The only true contraindications to resection are the presence of extrahepatic disease and the inability to achieve complete resection (Table 101–1). The absolute number of metastases no longer contraindicates resection. Several series have reported long-term survival rates in patients with more than four metastases. Similarly, bilobar disease is also no longer considered a contraindication to operative intervention.

Although the inability to achieve a negative margin remains an absolute contraindication to resection, patients with surgical margins of less than 1 cm have 5- and 10-year survival rates of 37% and 21%, even with margins of 1 to 9 mm. Thus, although associated with a decreased survival outlook, a close resection margin (1 to 9 mm) does not constitute an absolute contraindication to resection.

PREOPERATIVE EVALUATION

No universally accepted or definitive guidelines exist regarding the intensity of surveillance after treatment of primary colorectal cancer. This apparent anomaly is because regimens that use frequent follow-up have failed to result in improved overall or disease-free survival. Even though patients assigned to more frequent follow-up had recurrences diagnosed earlier and underwent more operations, this earlier diagnosis failed to translate into improved overall or cancer-specific survival. Most of these studies, however, did not include monitoring of carcinoembryonic antigen (CEA) levels.

CEA may be important in that 75% to 90% of patients with hepatic colorectal metastases have an elevated CEA measurement. In a meta-analysis from seven studies describing 3283 patients, 5-year survival rate was improved by 9% when follow-up included CEA monitoring. Furthermore, in a large, single-institution experience published by Rosen and colleagues, recurrent cancer diagnosed by CEA elevation was associated with a 5-year actuarial survival rate of 34%, versus 17% if liver metastases were diagnosed by symptoms and 0% if diagnosed by physical examination or liver enzyme elevation.

IMAGING STRATEGIES

Computed tomography (CT) is the test most widely used to diagnose liver metastases. CT is readily available and allows assessment of both intrahepatic and extrahepatic sites of recurrence. A recent advancement has been the development of CT arterial portography (CTAP). During CTAP, contrast material injected into the superior mesenteric artery is delivered to the liver via the portal vein. Because metastases derive their blood supply from the hepatic artery, they appear as hypodense lesions. Unfortunately, CTAP is invasive, technically demanding, and expensive. With the advent of helical CT and magnetic

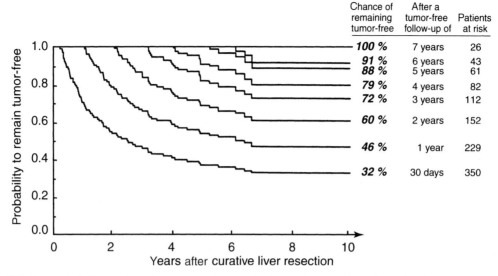

Chance of remaining tumor-free	After a tumor-free follow-up of	Patients at risk
100 %	7 years	26
91 %	6 years	43
88 %	5 years	61
79 %	4 years	82
72 %	3 years	112
60 %	2 years	152
46 %	1 year	229
32 %	30 days	350

Figure 101–1. Survival after curative liver resection. Increase in the probability of remaining free from recurrence after a disease-free follow-up of 1 to 7 years. (From Scheele J, Stangl R, Altendorf-Hofmann A, Paul M: Resection of colorectal liver metastases. World J Surg 1995;19:59, with permission.)

resonance imaging (MRI), the superiority of CTAP has come into question. The authors favor a quadruple-phase (precontrast, arterial, portal, and delayed) helical CT with rapid intravenous contrast injection (3 to 5 mL per second) and 5-mm cuts through the liver.

In patients with a history of colorectal cancer and an indeterminate lesion on CT, MRI may be useful to distinguish metastatic from benign disease. Lesions such as cysts, hemangiomas, focal steatosis, focal nodular hyperplasia, and hepatic adenoma all mimic metastases. MRI delineates vascular and biliary anatomy and may facilitate surgical planning. Cell-specific contrast agents such as superparamagnetic iron oxide or manganese-pyridoxal diphosphate (Mn-PDP) have improved the sensitivity of MRI in the detection and characterization of hepatic metastases. Recent studies have shown MRI with these agents to be as sensitive as CTAP in detecting liver metastases.

Positron emission tomography (PET) has recently been used to image liver tumors. PET appears to have a higher accuracy than CT (93% versus 76%). However, a formal comparison between PET and triple-phase helical CT has not been performed, and the overall additional benefit provided by PET remains to be delineated.

All patients who are candidates for surgery should undergo preoperative CT of the abdomen and pelvis and chest radiographic study. In addition, all require a full colonoscopy to exclude local recurrence or metachronous colorectal cancer. Recurrent extrahepatic disease is an

absolute contraindication for hepatic surgery because these patients derive no benefit from surgical resection. Patients should undergo standard pulmonary and cardiac workup, if indicated by history or symptoms. The patient's baseline hepatic function should be determined. Resections of up to 75% can be safely performed, as long as concurrent liver disease does not compromise the hepatic remnant.

TECHNIQUES OF RESECTION

Current techniques of resection are based on the liver's functional anatomy, as described by Couinaud. Commonly performed anatomic resections with the various nomenclatures used to describe these procedures are shown in Figure 101–2.

Resection of hepatic colorectal metastases begins with a laparotomy, usually through a bilateral subcostal incision, with a full exploration for evidence of extrahepatic disease. Suspicious nodules are biopsied, and frozen sections are obtained. If the exploration is negative, the liver is mobilized by dividing all supporting ligaments. The liver is palpated to identify lesions not seen on preoperative imaging. Intraoperative ultrasonography is a valuable adjunct at this point to identify nonpalpable lesions and to define vascular anatomy. This technique aids in the decision to proceed with a segmental or more traditional resection. The goal is complete resection with negative margins. Under intermittent vascular inflow occlusion, the hepatic parenchyma is divided with an ultrasonic dissector (Pringle's maneuver). Small vessels are controlled with electrocautery, while larger vessels and biliary radicals are individually sutured and ligated. The argon beam coagulator may also be useful to obtain final hemostasis.

Preoperative laparoscopy, with or without laparoscopic ultrasonography, has been advocated to decrease the number of nontherapeutic explorations. In one recent

Table 101–1	**Absolute Contraindications to Resection of Hepatic Colorectal Metastases**

Extrahepatic tumor except for local recurrence, direct invasion of adjacent structures, isolated lung metastases
Lymph node metastases at the liver hilum
Anticipated incomplete resection

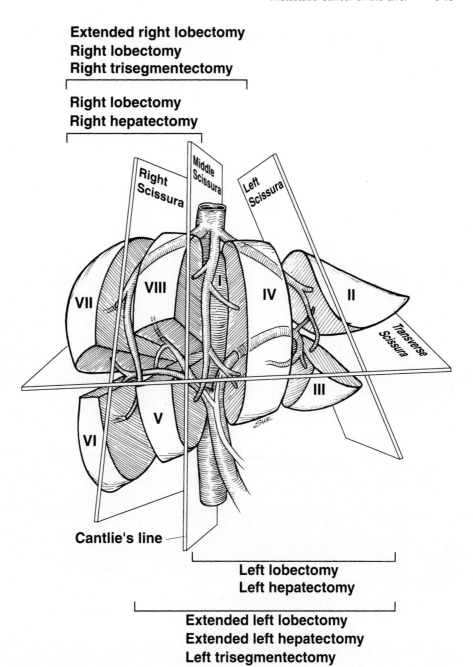

Figure 101–2. Functional anatomy of the liver. Resection lines for extended and nonextended resections with alternative nomenclatures. (Modified from Vauthey JN: Liver imaging: A surgeon's perspective. Radiol Clin North Am 1998;36:445, with permission.)

study, 6 of 23 cancers thought to be resectable by conventional imaging studies were found to be unresectable by the combination of diagnostic laparoscopy and laparoscopic ultrasonography; thus, the patients were spared unnecessary laparotomy. Jarnagin and colleagues prospectively analyzed a group of patients with primary and secondary hepatobiliary cancers deemed resectable by conventional studies; 83% of patients subjected to laparotomy after an initial staging laparoscopy underwent a potentially curative resection, compared with only 66% of those not staged laparoscopically. However, because these studies were not randomized and did not include state-of-the-art imaging (thin-cut quadruple-phase helical CT) preoperatively, the ultimate role for laparoscopy in the management of hepatic colorectal metastases has yet to be defined.

Perioperative Results

In experienced hands, liver resection is safe, carrying a 0% to 5% mortality rate (Table 101–2). The most common cause of death is perioperative hemorrhage or liver failure. In a prospective, single-institution series of 469 patients studied over 30 years, the overall 30-day mortality rate was 4%. Mortality rate was higher during the first 2 decades (12%) and decreased to 3% during the 1980s. Fong and coworkers reported a perioperative mortality rate of 2.8% for 1001 consecutive resections.

The most common perioperative complication associated with liver resection was infection. The rate of perihepatic abscess ranged from 1% to 9%, whereas wound infections were reported in 3% to 6% of patients and postoperative pneumonia was found in 4% to 8%. Postop-

Table 101–2	Results of Resection for Colorectal Cancer Liver Metastases				
STUDY	**NUMBER OF PATIENTS**	**OPERATIVE MORTALITY RATE (%)**	**OPERATIVE MORBIDITY RATE (%)**	**5-YEAR SURVIVAL RATE (%)**	**MEDIAN SURVIVAL DURATION (MONTHS)**
Schlag, 1990	122	4	38	30	32
Doci, 1991	100	5	35	30	28
Gayowski, 1994	204	0	—	32	33
Scheele, 1995	469	4	16	33	40
Nordlinger, 1996	1568	2	23	28	—
Jamison, 1997	280	2	—	27	32
Ambiru, 1999	168	4	30	26	23
Fong, 1999	1001	3	—	37	46

erative hepatic failure occurred in 4% to 5%. Significant hemorrhage was unusual (1% to 2% of all patients undergoing hepatectomy). Overall, most patients can be discharged less than 2 weeks after hepatic resection. A combination of proper patient selection and meticulous surgical technique contributes to the reduction of major complications.

Long-Term Survival and Results of Re-resection

Two large multicenter studies have analyzed the results of hepatic resections. One multi-institutional experience that included 859 patients with potentially curative liver resections had an actuarial 5-year patient survival rate of 33%. Another study, from the French Association of Surgery involving 1818 patients from 85 centers, had actuarial survival rates of 84% at 1 year, 40% at 3 years, and 25% at 5 years. Several other large series from the past decade are listed in Table 101–2. Five-year survival rates in these series ranged from 25% to 37%, with a median survival expectation of 28 to 46 months.

Factors affecting survival are presented in Table 101–3. The factors most consistently associated with recurrence are positive resection margin, liver metastasis synchronous with the primary tumor, and positive lymph node status of the primary tumor. Other factors that increase the risk of recurrence after liver resection include symptomatic disease, presence of satellitosis (metastases around the main metastatic nodule within the same segment or within 2 cm), and high preoperative serum CEA

level. Most patients with positive hilar lymph nodes do not benefit from hepatectomy for colorectal metastases.

Finally, the performance of an anatomic resection is a significant factor related to overall and tumor-free survival. Performance of an anatomic resection resulted in a lower incidence of positive margins (2% versus 16%) when compared with wedge resection. Furthermore, segmental resection resulted in a longer median length of survival (53 versus 38 months) than that with wedge resection.

The most common sites of recurrence after resection of hepatic colorectal metastases are the liver and the lung. Several groups have reported successful repeat liver resection. In one series of 170 consecutive patients undergoing repeat hepatic resection, median length of survival was 34 months and 5-year survival rate was 32%. After resection of isolated metastases in both the liver and the lung, median actuarial survival expectation was 3.8 years; there were 30% actual 5-year survivors.

Follow-Up

After resection of colorectal metastases, follow-up is mandatory, because many patients with recurrences are amenable to further treatment with curative intent. A preoperatively increased serum CEA measurement should return to normal after 6 weeks. Office visits with liver function studies, serum CEA level, abdominal and pelvic CT, and chest radiograph studies should be repeated every 4 to 6 months. A colonoscopy is suggested in the first year after colon resection and every 3 years thereafter

Table 101–3	Predictors of Recurrence after Hepatic Resection of Colorectal Metastases					
STUDY	**POSITIVE MARGIN**	**SYNCHRONOUS TUMOR**	**NODE-POSITIVE PRIMARY**	**SIZE >10 CM**	**NUMBER OF METASTASES**	**BILOBAR DISEASE**
Gayowski, 1994	Yes	Yes	Yes	No	Yes	Yes
Scheele, 1995	Yes	Yes	Yes	Yes	No	No
Jamison, 1997	No	—	No	No	No	—
Jenkins, 1997	Yes	Yes	—	—	No	—
Ambiru, 1999	Yes	—	Yes	—	Yes	—
Fong, 1999	Yes	—	Yes	—	Yes	No

if the baseline colonoscopy is normal. This schedule should be continued for up to 7 years, based on long-term follow-up data of disease-free survival after liver resection (see Fig. 101–1). With repeat liver resection providing an option for cure, such follow-up is clearly justified.

Adjuvant Systemic Chemotherapy

Even after curative liver resection, recurrent disease develops in 65% to 75% of patients, with half of the recurrences occurring in the liver alone or as a component of systemic disease. With hopes of improving survival rates, systemic chemotherapy has been applied in the adjuvant setting for these patients who have undergone curative liver resection. Several retrospective studies used a 5-fluorouracil (5-FU)–based regimen, and median length of survival (30 to 60 months) was not prolonged in the groups receiving adjuvant chemotherapy compared with those undergoing surgery alone.

Regional Chemotherapy

Hepatic Artery Access

Because of the poor response rate to systemic chemotherapy, surgeons and oncologists have explored the use of hepatic artery chemotherapy (HAC) in patients with resectable and unresectable metastatic colorectal cancer. The rationale for regional chemotherapy is that direct delivery should lead to an increase in response rate while limiting systemic toxicity. Initially delivered via percutaneous catheters or subcutaneous ports, HAC was markedly improved by the development of implantable infusion pumps in the 1980s. This new delivery system allowed patients greater freedom of movement and ensured accurate and reliable delivery of chemotherapeutic agents.

Arterial anatomy is defined preoperatively with selective angiography of the celiac axis and superior mesenteric artery. The abdomen is explored to rule out extrahepatic disease. The vascular anatomy is then exposed and confirmed. With standard anatomy, the catheter is placed in the gastroduodenal artery, which is ligated distally. A cholecystectomy is performed in all patients to prevent chemotherapy-induced cholecystitis. The pump is placed in a subcutaneous pocket through a separate transverse skin incision. Vascular isolation is confirmed using fluorescein dye injection and a Wood lamp. An additional baseline evaluation of the pump is obtained 3 to 4 days postoperatively with a hepatic arterial infusion scintigraphy obtained via the pump side-port.

Adjuvant Hepatic Artery Chemotherapy

Four randomized trials using HAC have been reported. In one study, the addition of HAC to surgery alone increased mean disease-free survival expectation from 9 to 32 months. However, there was no difference in 3-year survival rates between the two groups. Similarly, another multicenter, prospective randomized trial of resection

plus HAC with 5-FU versus resection alone also failed to show an improvement in survival rate.

Kemeny and colleagues published a single-center, randomized study comparing patients receiving regional floxuridine (FUDR) and dexamethasone via an implantable pump and systemic 5-FU and leucovorin (LV) (combined therapy) with patients receiving systemic 5-FU and LV alone (monotherapy) after liver resection. A significant difference was observed in 2-year survival rates (86% versus 72%, $P = .03$) and hepatic disease-free survival (90% versus 60%, $P < .001$) when comparing combined therapy with monotherapy. The Eastern Cooperative Oncology Group prospective, randomized trial compared 56 patients randomized to hepatic resection alone with 53 patients randomized to hepatic resection followed by HAC with FUDR for four cycles and systemic 5-FU for 12 cycles. Preliminary analysis showed the 3-year recurrence-free rate was 34% for the patients receiving surgery alone and 58% ($P < .05$) for the patients receiving adjuvant chemotherapy. Five-year survival rate, however, was not different. These trials showed a trend toward increased survival rates in patients receiving adjuvant HAC. Of note, these studies did not include use of newer agents (irinotecan [CPT-11] and oxaliplatin) that appear to be more effective in the treatment of advanced metastatic colorectal carcinoma.

Hepatic Artery Chemotherapy for Unresectable Metastases

Six randomized studies have compared systemic chemotherapy with HAC for unresectable metastases. All six studies compared sustained-release FUDR delivered via implantable pumps with systemic 5-FU or FUDR. All showed a greater response rate to HAC than to systemic chemotherapy. HAC was associated with longer median survival expectation than was systemic therapy, but the difference was statistically significant in only three studies. Even though HAC appears to be a valuable treatment option for the management of unresectable colorectal cancer metastases, none of the studies to date has been large enough to support a valid conclusion. Furthermore, none of the current studies used the current standard chemotherapy for colorectal cancer (5-FU plus LV) as systemic treatment. At the University of Texas M. D. Anderson Cancer Center, HAC is currently used in patients with unresectable hepatic colorectal metastases on protocol for those who fail to respond to systemic therapy.

SURGICAL TREATMENT OF NONCOLORECTAL METASTASES

Whereas surgical resection of colorectal metastases to the liver has gained widespread acceptance, the role of hepatic resection for noncolorectal liver metastases is less clear. Until recently, there were no large series to guide clinical decision making. In fact, it was suggested that resection of metastases from many noncolorectal primaries, specifically breast, sarcoma, and upper gastrointestinal adenocarcinomas, is not indicated and may be associated with significant morbidity. However, the reduction in operative morbidity and mortality rates with major hepatic resections has allowed for a reexamination of the role of surgery in the treatment of noncolorectal liver metastases.

Liver Metastases from Carcinoid Tumors

Resection of liver metastases from carcinoid tumors has become part of the standard of care for patients with malignant carcinoid syndrome because of the indolent nature of these tumors, which are often slow-growing. The mean survival expectation of patients with carcinoid tumors metastatic to the liver from the onset of symptoms is 8.1 years. Resection and hepatic artery embolization were initially proposed as a means of palliating the profoundly symptomatic patients. Soreide and colleagues reported a retrospective review of 75 patients who underwent aggressive surgical management of their advanced abdominal carcinoid tumors. Forty-eight percent underwent interventions directed at metastatic disease in the liver, consisting of resection, hepatic artery ligation, and/or embolization. Median length of survival in this group was 216 months, compared with 48 months for patients who did not undergo hepatic intervention ($P < 0.001$). Que and coworkers from the Mayo Clinic reviewed 75 patients, most of whom underwent hepatic resection for symptomatic metastatic neuroendocrine tumors. Fifty (75%) of these tumors were carcinoids. Resections included 38 formal lobectomies or extended resections and 38 nonanatomic resections. Perioperative mortality rate was 2% and morbidity rate was 24%. Four-year survival rate was 73%, but, perhaps more importantly, symptomatic response was achieved in 90% of patients, with a mean duration of response of 19 months.

In another series of 38 patients with liver-only metastases from neuroendocrine tumors, the 5-year survival rate was 73% for the 15 patients who were able to undergo complete resection of their disease but only 29% for the 23 patients with a similar tumor burden but whose cancer was thought to be unresectable. Although not randomized, this small series suggests that hepatic resection may not only palliate these highly symptomatic patients but may also improve survival.

Finally, orthotopic liver transplantation has been suggested as an alternative therapy for selected patients with neuroendocrine hepatic metastases. Le Treut and associates reported a 4-year survival rate of 69% for 15 patients undergoing orthotopic liver transplantation for metastatic carcinoid tumors. This is in contrast to an 8% 4-year survival rate reported for 16 patients with noncarcinoid neuroendocrine tumors. Further long-term studies are needed to clarify the role of transplantation in the treatment of hepatic metastases from neuroendocrine tumors. Given the scarcity of organ donors and limited resources, it is unlikely that organ transplantation will be available to many patients with metastatic carcinoid tumors in the near future.

Non-neuroendocrine Metastases

The role of hepatic resection for metastases from non-neuroendocrine primaries is even less well defined. Most studies are anecdotal and include patients with widely varied tumor types. Recently, several institutions have published their experience with noncolorectal non-neuroendocrine metastases, providing some guidelines as to the selection of patients who will benefit from hepatic resection. Tuttle and coworkers from M.D. Anderson Cancer Center at the University of Texas reported a 5-year actuarial survival rate of 44%, with a median survival expectation of 54 months for 45 patients undergoing resection of noncolorectal liver metastases. Similarly, Harrison and associates reported a 5-year overall survival rate of 37% for 96 patients undergoing liver resection for noncolorectal non-neuroendocrine metastases. Most of these tumors were genitourinary or soft-tissue primaries. By multivariate analysis, the only predictors of increased survival rate were disease-free interval of less than 36 months before discovery of liver metastases, curative resection, and primary tumor type (genitourinary was greater than soft tissue, which was greater than gastrointestinal). These results confirm other findings that long-term survival was possible for patients with liver metastases from renal tumors (particularly Wilms' tumors), but not for those with soft-tissue or gastrointestinal (noncolorectal, non-neuroendocrine) primaries.

Thus, even though recent survival data for patients undergoing resection of noncolorectal non-neuroendocrine metastases are encouraging, most of these cancers will eventually recur. Whereas mortality rate is low at centers with experience in liver resection, procedure-related morbidity is not negligible. Patient selection is critical when opting for resection, and resection should only be considered in the context of a multimodality treatment plan at specialized hepatobiliary centers.

NOVEL TREATMENT APPROACHES

Surgical resection remains the most effective treatment for hepatic colorectal metastases. Not every patient qualifies as a surgical candidate for "curative" liver resection because there may be too large a primary tumor mass, multicentricity, or direct invasion of hepatic vasculature. For these patients, some form of in situ ablative therapy may be appropriate. The most popular ablative techniques are cryosurgery and radiofrequency ablation (RFA). These relatively new techniques have allowed a greater proportion of patients with liver metastases to undergo potentially curative treatment when combined with resection. Alternatively, when used as part of a multimodality approach, they may offer prolonged palliation of advanced or unresectable disease. For those who cannot undergo surgery because of insufficient parenchymal reserve, preoperative portal vein embolization is currently being investigated.

Cryotherapy

Cryotherapy is a local ablative technique for treating unresectable metastatic disease to the liver. This method uses a vacuum-insulated cryoprobe, cooled by liquid nitrogen, to rapidly freeze and thaw the liver tumor. The cryoprobe is inserted into the tumor under visualization with intraoperative ultrasonography. During repeated freeze–thaw cycles, intracellular and extracellular ice formation causes tumor cell death. Freezing is usually continued until the "iceball" visualized under ultrasonography extends at least 1 cm beyond the tumor. Normal liver parenchyma is spared, and blood loss is usually minimal.

As with other forms of therapy, patient selection is critical. Patients must be able to tolerate general anesthesia and the physiologic stress of cryosurgery. Cryosurgery is contraindicated in the presence of extrahepatic malignancy or if the whole tumor cannot be ablated safely. Cryosurgery is rarely beneficial as a palliative procedure.

A number of studies have demonstrated the safety of this technique with mortality rates ranging from 0% to 4%. Morbidity, however, can be significant. Procedure-related complications include hypothermia, biliary fistula, intrahepatic and subphrenic abscess, coagulopathy, and pyrexia.

Seifert and Morris analyzed 85 patients who underwent complete cryoablation of colorectal liver metastases over a 7-year period. At a median follow-up of 22 months, local recurrence at the cryosite was observed in 33%, liver recurrence in 65%, and extrahepatic recurrence in 56%. Size of metastasis greater than 3 cm was a factor associated with local recurrence. This phenomenon may be due to inability to achieve an adequate decrease in temperature away from the cryoprobe. Other factors associated with a favorable outcome include low presurgical serum CEA measurement, absence of extrahepatic disease, absence of nodal involvement, complete cryoablation, and differentiation of the primary tumor. Median survival expectation was 26 months, with a 5-year survival rate of 13%.

Cryotherapy has also been used in conjunction with surgery when the resection margin is involved or suboptimal (<1 cm). With a median follow-up of 19 months, cryotherapy of the resection edge in 44 patients after liver resection for colorectal liver metastases with an involved or inadequate resection margin resulted in 16 of 44 patients being alive and disease-free. Recurrence involving the liver developed in 19 patients, but only five of these recurrences were at the resection edge (9%).

Radiofrequency Ablation

RFA is the newest technique for local ablation of tumors not amenable to resection. RFA can be performed percutaneously, laparoscopically, or as part of a formal laparotomy. An RF electrode is placed within the substance of a tumor under ultrasonographic or CT guidance. The array is deployed, and thermal (RF) energy is generated. Cellular protein undergoes coagulative necrosis as local temperatures exceed 40°C to 50°C (Fig. 101–3).

Early results with RFA are encouraging. Curley and colleagues reported on 123 patients with primary or metastatic hepatic malignancies treated with RFA. Sixty-one (50%) of the tumors treated were hepatic colorectal metastases. Small (<3 cm) peripheral tumors in 31 patients were treated by percutaneous RFA, and the remaining tumors were treated during an open operative procedure. There were no treatment-related deaths, and the morbidity rate was 2%. With a median follow-up of 15 months, only 2% of tumors had recurred at the RFA site; however, 28% of cancers recurred at distant sites.

One advantage of RFA over cryosurgery is that the procedure may be performed percutaneously, thus avoiding laparotomy. Other distinct advantages include the ease of the procedure and the low incidence of complications. Further study is needed, however, to assess the impact of RFA on long-term survival.

Portal Vein Embolization

Portal vein embolization is performed preoperatively in selected patients when there is potential for an inadequate volume of functional hepatic parenchyma after a major resection. The rationale for this technique is to induce hypertrophy of the future liver remnant. This technique was first reported in 1986 in 21 patients with hepatocellular carcinoma. Postembolization CT and operative findings demonstrated that the nonembolized liver increased in size.

A variety of different substances have been used for embolization, including absolute alcohol, ethiodized oil

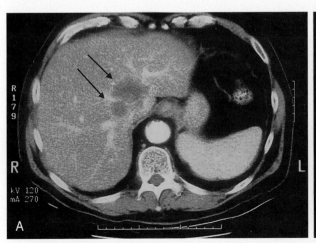
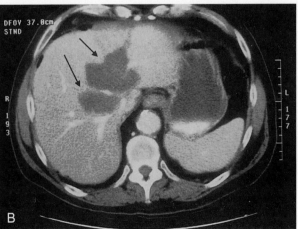

Figure 101–3. Radiofrequency ablation (RFA) of a liver metastasis. Computed tomography of liver metastasis before (*A*) and 3 months after RFA (*B*).

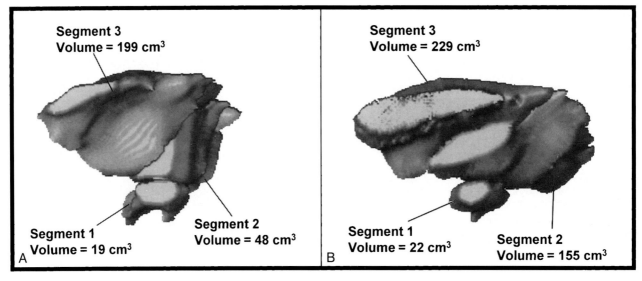

Figure 101–4. Portal vein embolization. Volume of future liver remnant (FLR) before (*A*) and after (*B*) portal vein embolization. (From Vauthey JN, Chaoui A, Do KA, et al: Standardized measurement of the future liver remnant prior to extended liver resection: Methodology and clinical associations. Surgery 2000;127:512, with permission.)

and cyanoacrylate, and gelatin particles with metal coils. No one substance has been found to be superior in terms of safety, ease of use, or results. Portal vein embolization is most commonly performed via percutaneous puncture of a portal vein radicle under ultrasonographic guidance. Portal vein embolization is well tolerated and, in the absence of chronic liver disease, induces a 25% to 80% increase in the absolute volume of the nonembolized liver (Fig. 101–4). Two to four weeks are usually required to enable adequate hypertrophy. After this period, surgical resection can be planned. Complications with this technique are rare and include bleeding, hemobilia, and possible propagation of the thrombus.

General indications for portal vein embolization are based on the size of the future liver remnant and the extent of the proposed procedure. Currently, there is no consensus as to a safe minimal size. In the 2000 series by Vauthey and coworkers, the volume of the future liver remnant was calculated in 20 patients before extended right lobectomy. In 12 patients who underwent preoperative portal vein embolization, there was a significant increase in the future liver remnant (26% versus 36%, $P <$ 0.01). In the 15 patients who underwent the anticipated resection, a future liver remnant of less than or equal to 25% was associated with an increased duration of hospital stay and an increase in postoperative complications. In another study with long-term follow-up after portal vein embolization, the overall 5-year survival rate was 29% in 27 patients with metastases from colorectal cancer deemed unresectable without portal vein embolization.

Pearls and Pitfalls

- Without treatment, median survival outlook with hepatic metastases from colorectal carcinoma is only 12 to 15 months with a 5-year survival rate of less than 3%.
- Selected patients with colorectal metastases to the liver after previous curative colorectal surgery are candidates for curative surgical resection.
- Operative mortality rate is less than 5% with a 5-year survival rate of 27% to 37% in major series.
- Contraindications include uncontrolled primary disease, hilar metastases, and inability to remove all known disease.
- Helical (quadruple-phase) CT is the initial radiologic study of choice. MRI is useful to rule out benign disease and better define vascular and biliary anatomy.
- The role of chronic hepatic artery infusion of chemotherapy for unresectable colorectal liver metastases is as yet unproven.
- Close follow-up after hepatic resection is mandatory for up to 7 years because re-resection may provide cure.
- Hepatic resection may be indicated for palliation or cure in selected patients with functional and nonfunctional neuroendocrine liver metastases.
- Cryotherapy or RFA may be useful in selected patients with otherwise unresectable metastases confined to the liver.
- Percutaneous portal vein embolization increases the size of the anticipated liver remnant preoperatively.
- The number of patients with advanced metastatic liver cancer who are candidates for major hepatic resection may be increased by preoperative portal vein embolization.

Although a final role for portal vein embolization has yet to be defined, continued experience with this emerging technology should be pursued at specialized centers.

SELECTED READINGS

Curley SA, Izzo F, Delrio P, et al: Radiofrequency ablation of unresectable primary and metastatic hepatic malignancies: Results in 123 patients. Ann Surg 1999;230:1.

Fong Y, Fortner J, Sun RL, et al: Clinical score for predicting recurrence after hepatic resection for metastatic colorectal cancer: Analysis of 1001 consecutive cases. Ann Surg 1999;230:309.

Harrison LE, Brennan MF, Newman E, et al: Hepatic resection for noncolorectal, nonneuroendocrine metastases: A fifteen-year experience with ninety-six patients. Surgery 1997;121:625.

Jarnagin WR, Bodniewicz J, Dougherety E, et al: A prospective analysis of staging laparoscopy in patients with primary and secondary hepatobiliary malignancies. J Gastointest Surg 2000;4:34.

Kemeny N, Huang Y, Cohen AM, et al: Hepatic arterial infusion of chemotherapy after resection of hepatic metastases from colorectal cancer. N Engl J Med 1999;341:2039.

Le Treut YP, Delpero JR, Dousset B, et al: Results of liver transplantation in the treatment of metastatic neuroendocrine tumors. A 31-case French multicentric report. Ann Surg 1997;225:355.

Que FG, Nagorney DM, Batts KP, et al: Hepatic resection for metastatic neuroendocrine carcinomas. Am J Surg 1995;169:36.

Rosen CB, Nagorney DM, Taswell HF, et al: Perioperative blood transfusion and determinants of survival after liver resection for metastatic colorectal carcinoma. Ann Surg 1992;216:493.

Scheele J, Stangl R, Altendorf-Hofmann A, Paul M: Resection of colorectal liver metastases. World J Surg 1995;19:59.

Seifert JK, Morris DL: Indicators of recurrence following cryotherapy for hepatic metastases from colorectal cancer. Br J Surg 1999;86:234.

Soreide O, Berstad T, Bakka A, et al: Surgical treatment as a principle in patients with advanced abdominal carcinoid tumors. Surgery 1992;111:48.

Tuttle TM: Hepatectomy for noncolorectal liver metastases. In: Curley SA (ed): Liver Cancer. New York, Springer, 1998:201–211.

Vauthey JN, Chaoui A, Do KA, et al: Standardized measurement of the future liver remnant prior to extended liver resection: Methodology and clinical associations. Surgery 2000;127:512.

Biliary: Benign

Chapter 102

Postcholecystectomy Syndrome

Frank G. Moody and Karen Kwong

The majority of patients (>80%) who undergo cholecystectomy for the complications of gallstones suffer no long-term ill effects from the procedure. Unfortunately, about 20% of patients operated on in the open cholecystectomy era experienced symptoms, over time, similar to those for which the patients originally underwent cholecystectomy. Whether laparoscopic cholecystectomy will be associated with a similar outcome is not yet known, because this less invasive approach has been used only since 1990. However, patients with such symptoms have been seen even at this early date of follow-up. Keep in mind that it took 50 years for the condition termed *postcholecystectomy syndrome* to be defined as a clinical entity, and to this day skeptics deny its existence. The following discussion is mostly speculative but is diced with facts and observations from experience that suggest that, in its severest form, postcholecystectomy syndrome is a relatively rare but real entity and will continue to occur even when the gallbladder is removed through the laparoscope.

CLINICAL PRESENTATION

Differential Diagnosis

The typical patient with postcholecystectomy syndrome is a middle-aged woman who, months or years after cholecystectomy (average duration of 60 months), presents with recurrent episodes of midepigastric or right upper quadrant abdominal pain. This pain may occur day or night, is usually not related to meals, and requires a trip to the emergency department for injection of a narcotic analgesic. The pain usually subsides after a day or two, only to recur months later. The intervals between episodes often decrease over time, and the relief from narcotic analgesics becomes addictive. When this type of painful episode occurs early after cholecystectomy in asso-

ciation with jaundice and elevation of liver enzymes, its usual cause is a retained common duct stone. A bile duct stricture from injury may also present with painful jaundice in the presence of a reformed stone. A stone retained or reformed within a long cystic duct remnant or retained gallbladder may also present weeks or months after cholecystectomy. There is ample evidence in the literature that a long cystic duct, per se, is not a source of postcholecystectomy pain. This is fortunate, because the cystic duct is purposefully left long to avoid bile duct injury when a laparoscopic cholecystectomy is performed. It is important to recognize that a stone left in the cystic duct may provoke episodes of pain and that the duct itself may be a stone-forming organ if it is sufficiently large. Biliary causes of postcholecystectomy syndrome are listed in Table 102–1. Of the entities on this list, biliary dyskinesia remains mysterious and unyielding to even the marvels of endoscopic manometry. A retained gallbladder, an uncommon cause of the syndrome, results when the organ is inadvertently only partially removed in patients with advanced acute cholecystitis.

In our age of sophisticated diagnostic technology, it is unlikely that one would overlook a nonbiliary source of symptoms before cholecystectomy. Peptic ulcer, reflux esophagitis, and nongallstone pancreatitis represent some of the more common entities that masquerade as gall-

Table 102–1	Biliary Sources of Postcholecystectomy Syndrome
Common duct stones	Cystic duct remnant
Retained gallbladder	Stenosing papillitis
Traumatic stricture	Biliary dyskinesia

From Moody FG: Postcholecystectomy syndrome. In Moody FG (ed): Surgical Treatment of Digestive Disease. Chicago, Year Book, 1986, p 296.

653

Table 102–2	Nonbiliary Sources of Postcholecystectomy Pain

Irritable bowel syndrome	Coronary artery disease
Peptic ulcer	Intra-abdominal adhesions
Reflux esophagitis	Intercostal neuritis
Nonbiliary pancreatitis	Wound neuroma
Liver disease	

From Moody FG: Postcholecystectomy syndrome. In Moody FG (ed): Surgical Treatment of Digestive Disease. Chicago, Year Book, 1986, p 297.

stone disease (Table 102–2). Irritable bowel syndrome can also mimic the pain of biliary colic and is known to be associated with an increased incidence of gallstones. This is an elusive clinical problem that can persist after cholecystectomy. Intercostal neuralgia is also difficult to distinguish from biliary colic before or after cholecystectomy. A neuroma formation within the divided right intercostal nerve in the lateral aspect of a right subcostal incision may be a trigger point for episodic pain, but this entity can be excluded as the source of biliary- or pancreatic-type pain by a simple local nerve block.

Stenosing papillitis, a relatively rare disease of the papilla of Vater, requires special consideration because it is one of the most elusive pathologic entities in patients with the severe, chronic, painful form of postcholecystectomy syndrome. Since the mid-1970s, attempts have been made to understand the pathogenesis of this complex problem, leading to the conclusion that this disorder is due to chronic passage of gallstones, instrumentation of the papilla of Vater, or—rarely—cholesterolosis of the latter structure. The typical patient is a middle-aged woman who has undergone a cholecystectomy after years of recurrent episodes of biliary colic. Many referred patients did not have gallstones within the gallbladder at the time of cholecystectomy but did have cholesterolosis of the gallbladder, suggesting that they were chronic stone passers. Several patients also had cholesterolosis of the papilla of Vater confirmed by histologic examination.

Diagnostics

A careful history is the key to ascribing a precise etiology for postcholecystectomy problems. Knowledge of the symptoms that led to the original cholecystectomy is important, as are the details of the operative and pathologic findings. A review of preoperative and intraoperative imaging studies is also important because it may provide a clue as to why the patient has symptoms that are often similar to those he or she had preoperatively. Unfortunately, in the typical patient, neither the history nor the physical examination reveals why the patient has pain. The laboratory approach to such a patient is structured around the working diagnosis and initially includes an analysis of liver function, serum amylase and lipase measurement, and hemogram. These results are usually normal with stenosing papillitis, but they may be diagnostic in patients with a retained stone and/or acute or chronic pancreatitis. A normal physical examination and normal serum chemistries present a dilemma in terms of how

best to proceed in diagnosing and treating a patient who is often in desperate need of resolution of the problem. Making a diagnosis in a cost-effective manner with entities that may or may not even exist is the challenge. Our philosophy is to do the least invasive (and often least expensive) tests first and to stretch them out to allow time to better know the patient. We have the patient keep a pain diary during this period.

When the patient is first seen in the emergency department, the imaging should begin with plain films and ultrasonography of the abdomen. The former may show calcification within the biliary tree, pancreas, or kidney, whereas the latter may demonstrate a dilated biliary tree or an abnormality within the pancreas. If the patient is first seen in the office, we usually proceed with whatever test appears to be appropriate in light of the imaging studies that have already been done. Most patients have had an extensive work-up, including ultrasonography, computed tomography (CT), endoscopic cholangiopancreatography, endoscopic examination of the upper gastrointestinal tract, and even magnetic resonance cholangiopancreatography and cholescintigraphy. Although these studies may occasionally reveal an enlarged bile or pancreatic duct or delayed emptying of the bile duct on cholescintigraphy, most often these tests do not reveal abnormalities that suggest a diagnosis. Even in the presence of advanced stenosing papillitis, diagnostic test results are positive in only 25% of patients. Imaging studies, however, may demonstrate biliary stones, strictures, acid-peptic disorders, or pancreatic disease, and thus reveal something that is recognizable and treatable. The problem is what to do when all the results are negative, which is often the case in patients with postcholecystectomy pain. In fact, even endoscopic biliary manometry has a relatively low yield in this population, but it has been used successfully in identifying a small subset of patients with stenosing papillitis. The problem is that it is not readily available in most communities, is difficult to perform and interpret, and may itself induce an episode of acute pancreatitis in about 5% of patients. We rely on endoscopic examination of the upper gastrointestinal tract, endoscopic cholangiopancreatography, and CT to rule out or "rule in" the entities discussed earlier. If we become convinced over time, during the course of our relationship with the patient, that the patient is likely harboring stenosing papillitis, we examine the papilla of Vater by a direct, open, transabdominal approach and perform a procedure called *transduodenal sphincteroplasty and transampullary septectomy*. Since the 1970s, we have performed this operation on 131 highly selected patients suspected of having stenosing papillitis. This represents only a small fraction of patients referred with this diagnosis who, on careful review, were found to have other reasons for their postcholecystectomy pain. Included in our study were several patients who had a previous endoscopic sphincterotomy for postcholecystectomy pain. As discussed later, sphincterotomy done endoscopically or by the transduodenal route has a low success rate because the problem is related to narrowing of the duct of Wirsung, which is not corrected by anterior sphincterotomy alone. However, Geenen and associates (1989) at the Medical College of Wisconsin have reported success with endoscopic sphincterotomy in a group of patients with increased pressures within the papilla of Vater as identified by endoscopic manometry. This study has the power of a randomized controlled trial, and its success was likely related to the identification of a subset of patients whose pain was from the biliary component of the vaterian complex.

PREOPERATIVE CONSIDERATIONS

The indications for an operative approach in patients with postcholecystectomy syndrome have been more clearly defined by both advances in biliary imaging and lessons learned from trial and error. For example, we no longer recommend removal of a long cystic duct remnant unless it contains a gallstone, and exploration is not recommended for patients with pancreas divisum unless they have an enlarged dorsal duct. Retained common duct stones and biliary strictures with and without stones can be effectively treated by endoscopic extraction and dilatation, although we prefer a direct surgical approach to benign strictures. At issue is what to do for the patient who has often severe episodes of upper abdominal pain and who is suspected of having stenosing papillitis. Even in the absence of any objective criteria attributable to the cause of postcholecystectomy pain, some surgeons will perform a sphincteroplasty and septectomy based on the patient history and on one or more objective signs of an abnormality in pancreatic biliary function. The rationale for the procedure, which includes widening of the ostia of the duct of Wirsung, is shown schematically in Figure 102–1.

The operation is performed transabdominally by opening the duodenum over the papilla of Vater. The ampulla is divided along its anterior surface for a distance of 2 cm to fully expose the transampullary septum, the fold of tissue that separates the duct of Wirsung from the bile duct within the papilla of Vater. This tissue is usually thickened and fibrotic to the extent that it markedly narrows the pancreatic duct to a pinpoint opening. Only more recently have some endoscopists been able to safely divide the band of scar tissue, although stenting of the orifice has become routine. We do not recommend pancreatic ductal stenting because it may contribute to more fibrosis of the septum and may induce a deeper stricture within the duct of Wirsung that cannot be easily treated even by an open approach. It is important to ascertain before surgery whether the patient is addicted to narcotic analgesics, because if he or she is addicted, you must deal with the issue up front and inform the patient that he or she will have to be detoxified after the procedure. Preoperative consultation with pain specialists before the operation is important so that they will be available for pain management in the postoperative period. Early in our experience, we tried to preoperatively detoxify addicted patients suffering from postcholecystectomy pain, with little success. However, we have had a very high success rate (>70%) with detoxification after surgery.

PERIOPERATIVE CONSIDERATIONS

Patients are operated on the day they are admitted. Wound prophylaxis is provided with a single dose of a second-generation cephalosporin antibiotic. Pneumatic sequential compression devices are applied to the lower extremities for antithrombosis. The abdomen is entered through the incision used previously for the original cholecystectomy or through a midline incision if the cholecystectomy was performed laparoscopically. After careful examination, the pancreas is explored through the lesser sac, and the biliary tree is examined after mobilizing the duodenum (Kocher's maneuver). It is important to visualize and palpate the cystic duct and bile duct. If a stone is felt, we deal with it in the usual fashion. In the presence or the absence of a stone, we make a small opening in the cystic duct and pass a small filiform or biliary Fogarty catheter through the papilla to facilitate its identification after making a small (2 cm) lateral longitudinal duodenotomy at a point where it enters the duodenum. Placing a 5-0 silk suture into the substance of the papilla at the 3-o'clock and 9-o'clock positions facilitates elevation of the papilla from its posterior position. Kocher's maneuver is essential to allow anterior elevation of the duodenum. Grasping the exposed tip of the filiform also helps bring the papilla into the center of the duodenotomy, where an incision can easily be made on its anterior surface at the 11-o'clock position. We start this with iris scissors, maintaining hemostasis with short bursts of electrocautery. As the bile duct mucosa separates from the duodenal mucosa, we secure each margin of the papilla with interrupted absorbable 5-0 sutures of polyglycolic acid. Do not handle or grasp the papilla with instruments because this will cause bruising and bleeding. Take a generous sliver biopsy at this point for histologic examination. After the opening is enlarged to a centimeter or more, the transampullary septum will come into view. The opening of the duct of Wirsung may not be immediately identifiable because of scar tissue and inflammation. We recommend use of a headlight and ×5 magnification to facilitate identification of the dimple on the posterior lip of the papilla where the opening of the duct of Wirsung should be. The insertion of the smallest lacrimal probe into this opening and the passage of larger probes along its side often allow identification of the duct beyond this point of constriction. Again using iris scissors, we divide the septum into the duct for a distance of a centimeter or more. Approximation of the epithelium of the duct of Wirsung to the bile duct mucosa with interrupted 7-0 absorbable sutures provides a relatively large and smooth opening into the duct of Wirsung, which now will admit a 3-mm or larger probe. A biopsy should also be taken of the septum during the course of the procedure. Once the septum is divided, the anterior sphincteroplasty is completed for a distance of at least 2 cm, with care being taken to approximate the full circumference of the papillary mucosa to that of the duodenum. At this point, the bile duct should easily admit a 5-mm probe, and the duct of Wirsung should enter the duodenum through a separate opening (Fig. 102–2). The duodenotomy is then closed in a two-layer longitudinal fashion, the filiform is removed, and the cystic duct is secured by ligation and excision of its tip. A soft, closed suction drain is placed in the superior aspect of the right lumbar space well away from the duodenotomy.

Several precautions must be carefully taken. The most

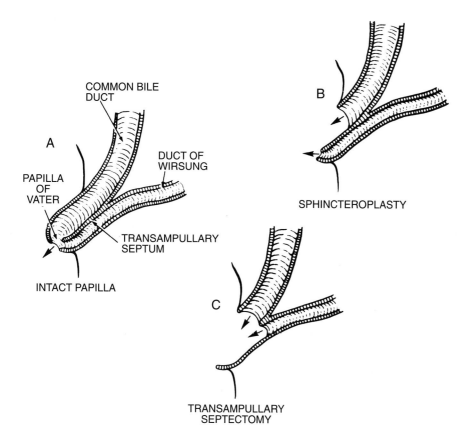

COMMON BILE
DUCT

A

PAPILLA
OF
VATER

DUCT OF
WIRSUNG

TRANSAMPULLARY
SEPTUM

INTACT PAPILLA

B

SPHINCTEROPLASTY

C

TRANSAMPULLARY
SEPTECTOMY

Figure 102–1. This schema of the components of the papilla of Vater is designed to emphasize the location and functional role of the transampullary septum. Note that it serves to separate the flow of pancreatic juice from the bile as they traverse the papilla to enter the duodenum *(A)*. Anterior sphincteroplasty leaves the septum intact *(B)*. We have hypothesized that injury to the septum from the chronic passage of gallstones leads to inflammation and fibrosis of the septum and gradual narrowing of the opening, or the duct of Wirsung. In the schema, resistance to the outflow of pancreatic juice is the source of episodic pain in this population of patients. Transampullary septectomy *(C)* removes this point of resistance within the pancreatic ductal system. (From Moody FG, Berenson M, McClosky D: Transampullary septectomy for abdominal pain. Ann Surg 1977; 186:415.)

Figure 102–2. This is a schematic view of the papilla of Vater after completion of a transduodenal sphincteroplasty and a transampullary septectomy. Note that the openings of the bile and pancreatic ducts now enter separately in the lumen of the duodenum and that all epithelial surfaces have been carefully approximated. The sphincteroplasty and the septectomy are extended into their respective ducts for a distance that ensures that a maximal opening has been obtained. This is at least 2 cm for the anterior sphincteroplasty and 1 cm for the septectomy. (From Moody FG, Becker JM, Potts JR: Transampullary septectomy for postcholecystectomy pain. Ann Surg 1983;197:630.)

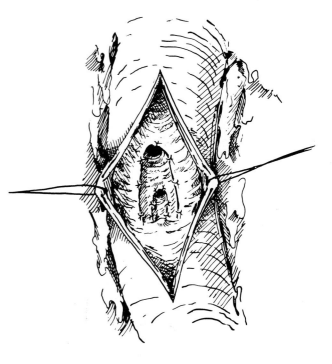

serious complication that can occur is a leak from the duodenal closure. We have not encountered this problem, and we take great pains to obtain a secure closure of the duodenotomy (with an inner row of 4-0 absorbable suture and a reinforcing row of 4-0 silk sutures in interrupted fashion). In addition, we sew a piece of omentum over the closure to ensure that it will not come in contact with the drain. Pancreatitis is a problem we have encountered. Most patients have a transient hyperamylasemia. Eight of 131 patients who underwent sphincteroplasty and septectomy had clinical manifestations of postoperative pancreatitis that prolonged their hospital stay; one patient with severe necrotizing pancreatitis died from multiple organ failure. Intraoperative pancreatograms are not indicated because they may also contribute to postoperative pancreatitis.

POSTOPERATIVE MANAGEMENT

A nasogastric tube placed at the time of induction of anesthesia is left in place for 48 hours, or longer if the patient has an ileus. Early removal of the nasogastric tube may be associated with emesis as a result of duodenal atony or pancreatitis. After removal of the nasogastric tube, the patient is started on ice chips and sips of water. If these feedings are tolerated, the patient is advanced to six small feedings of a bland diet. Pharmacologic acid suppression is employed throughout the hospital course. Early ambulation and aggressive pulmonary toilet are essential to an uncomplicated recovery. The mechanical compression devices are kept in place until the patient is fully ambulated. We do not use minidose heparin or antiplatelet therapy in these patients. The drain, which usually drains very little, is removed on the fifth day when the patient is eating. Discharge usually occurs on the 7th to 10th day when the patient is fully ambulatory and eating a soft diet. This is a very conservative program, but it is consistent with the fact that many of these patients come to us on large dosages of narcotic analgesics; it is our goal to have them off injectable narcotics and on mild to moderate, less addictive medications at the time of discharge. Managing this problem in its addictive phase is not for the faint of heart, but precise surgery, compassion, and a disciplined detoxification program will rehabilitate a large percentage of these patients.

COMPLICATIONS

The common complications in 96 postcholecystectomy patients who underwent transduodenal septectomy and transampullary septectomy are listed in Table 102–3. The most common, and serious, complication was pancreatitis that was mild in most patients but lethal in one patient. A 55-year-old woman with a well-documented history of pancreatitis developed necrotizing pancreatitis that, unfortunately, was lethal despite intensive management. The location of her papilla within a duodenal diverticulum and the prior episodes of pancreatitis made the septectomy portion of her operation very difficult. The manipulation required to gain entrance into the duct of Wirsung may have contributed to the severity of her pancreatic

Table 102–3	**Complications of Transduodenal Sphincteroplasty and Transampullary Septectomy in 93 Postcholecystectomy Patients**

COMPLICATION	NO. OF PATIENTS
Pancreatitis	7
Ileus	4
Atelectasis	3
Cholangitis	3
Pneumonia	3
Pulmonary embolism	2
Others*	

*Bile drainage, 3; gastrointestinal bleeding, 1; wound infection, 1.
From Moody FG, Becker JM, Potts JR: Transduodenal sphincteroplasty and transampullary septectomy for postcholecystectomy pain. Ann Surg 1983; 197:627.

inflammation. We doubt that this complication was due to inexperience, because her procedure was done late in the series. The unusual papillary anatomy and prior episodes of pancreatitis likely contributed to the complication. Obviously, we have avoided operating on such patients since that time.

OUTCOMES

The best follow-up we can provide derives from Frank Moody's work in Salt Lake City, Utah, where he was able to follow up 83 patients from 1 to 10 years (Table 102–4). These 83 patients included all comers, including some patients with chronic pancreatitis (3) or pancreas divisum (8) and several whose gallbladders were in place at the time of the procedure. About three fourths had a satisfactory result after sphincteroplasty and septectomy, with marked improvement in pain control. Half were relieved of their painful attacks. Unfortunately, about 25% of patients gained no benefit. The worst results were in postcholecystectomy patients with chronic pancreatitis and in those with pancreas divisum; we believe that these patients should no longer be candidates for the procedure.

Table 102–4	**Results from 83 Postcholecystectomy Pain Patients Followed Up for 1 to 10 Years**

FINDINGS	RESULTS		
	Good	Fair	Poor
Papillitis	15	16	9
Septitis	17	10	9
Dysfunction	4	1	2
Overall (%)	36 (43)	27 (33)	20 (24)
Prior sphincteroplasty	9	3	3
Papillary cholesterolosis	3	5	2
Anomaly	2	1	1
Concomitant cholecystectomy	2	6	6

From Moody FG, Becker JM, Potts JR: Transduodenal sphincteroplasty and transampullary septectomy for postcholecystectomy pain. Ann Surg 1983;197:627.

Pearls and Pitfalls

PEARLS

- After cholecystectomy, about 20% of patients will have some element of postcholecystectomy syndrome. Severe pain, however, is rare.
- Differential diagnosis includes retained stones, biliary strictures, biliary dyskinesia, stenosing papillitis, and other gastrointestinal disorders, such as duodenal ulcer and irritable bowel disease.
- Investigation should include ultrasonography, CT, biliary scintigraphy, upper gastrointestinal endoscopy, and, possibly, biliary manometry, if available.
- When no obvious cause can be determined, stenosing papillitis, a diagnosis evident only at operation, should be considered.

- Treatment of suspected stenosing papillitis involves an operative transduodenal biliary sphincteroplasty and a ductal septectomy. Good results are obtained in 75% of patients.
- Patients should be selected with great care, and no promises should be made as to outcomes.
- It is best to avoid alcoholics and those with chronic pancreatitis in selecting candidates for surgery.
- Beware of pancreas divisum when the dorsal duct is normal.
- Remember that the majority of these patients are addicted to analgesics and must enter a formal detoxification program for success.

Also, patients for whom alcohol consumption appeared to play a role in their pain syndrome did less well.

Some helpful hints follow on approaching patients who have severe, debilitating upper abdominal pain of obscure origin after cholecystectomy. Because we do not have firm criteria for identifying which patients have an inflamed or scarred papilla of Vater (stenosing papillitis) except at operation, the surgical approach is empirical. The patients must be fully informed of the uncertainty as to whether enlargement of the openings of the bile and pancreatic duct will relieve them of their pain, and they must understand that the treatment includes postoperative narcotic detoxification. We have been pleasantly surprised that a large number of patients were helped for a long time, and look forward to when advances in knowledge and technology will render this severe, incapacitating, but—fortunately—rare postcholecystectomy pain a thing of the past. Possibly, earlier removal of the gallbladder in

chronic stone passers through the use of laparoscopic cholecystectomy will accomplish this end.

SELECTED READINGS

Geenen JE, Hogan WJ, Dodd WJ, et al: The efficacy of endoscopic sphincterotomy after cholecystectomy in patients with sphincter-of-Oddi dysfunction. N Engl J Med 1989;320:82.

Moody FG: Postcholecystectomy problems. In Cameron JL (ed): Current Surgical Therapy, 6th ed. St. Louis, Mosby, 1998, pp 424–428.

Moody FG, Becker JM, Potts JR: Transduodenal sphincteroplasty and transampullary septectomy for postcholecystectomy pain. Ann Surg 1983;197:627.

Moody FG, Berenson MM, McClosky D: Transampullary septectomy for postcholecystectomy pain. Ann Surg 1977;186:415.

Nausbaum MS, Warner BW, Sax HC, Fischer JE: Transduodenal sphincteroplasty and transampullary septectomy for primary sphincter of Oddi dysfunction. Am J Surg 1989;157:38.

Stephens RU, Burdick GE: Microscopic transduodenal sphincteroplasty and transampullary septoplasty for papillary stenosis. Am J Surg 1986;152:621.

Chapter 103

Lithotripsy of Gallstones
Gustav Paumgartner

The treatment of gallstones without surgery has long been a goal of medical therapy. Oral bile acid dissolution therapy has been such an option for selected patients with gallstones, but it is limited by stone size and stone composition and usually requires a relatively long duration of treatment. To overcome these difficulties, extracorporeal shock-wave lithotripsy was introduced by Sauerbruch and associates in 1986 as a noninvasive treatment modality for selected patients with cholelithiasis. Its goal, like that of cholecystectomy, is to prevent pain, morbidity, and mortality from gallstone disease. After considerable and wide interest in extracorporeal shock-wave lithotripsy soon after its introduction, its use for the treatment of gallbladder stones dramatically declined with the introduction of laparoscopic cholecystectomy. It will be a task of this millennium to assign extracorporeal shock-wave lithotripsy of gallbladder stones, and perhaps more advanced developments of this treatment modality, its proper place in the armamentarium of gallstone therapy. In contrast to the very restricted use of extracorporeal shock-wave lithotripsy for gallbladder stones, this new treatment modality continues to be well accepted for treatment of difficult bile duct stones.

Shock waves are high-pressure waves that obey the laws of acoustics, but they differ from sound waves and conventional ultrasound waves by being highly distorted from the normal representation of sinusoidally varying acoustic pressure waves. They are characterized by a positive pressure pulse of short duration with an extremely short rise time. The positive pressure pulse is followed by a negative pressure pulse of much lower amplitude but longer duration. Because most human tissues have an acoustic impedance approximately equal to that of water, shock waves can be transmitted into the body with little attenuation. The shock waves are focused to create a limited area of high pressure at the location of the stone while keeping the pressure in the surrounding tissue relatively low. This keeps tissue damage outside the focal area to a minimum.

Lithotripters from different manufacturers vary with respect to the mechanisms used for shock-wave generation, focusing, and targeting. Shock waves can be generated by use of an underwater spark gap (electrohydraulic principle), piezoelectric crystals, or an electromagnetic membrane. Spark-gap lithotripters are focused by an ellipsoidal metal reflector. To focus piezoelectrically generated shock waves, the piezoelectric crystals are mounted on a spherical dish. Electromagnetically generated shock waves are usually focused by acoustic lenses, but a metal reflector can also be used.

In all types of lithotripters, the shock waves are generated under water. They travel through the water with little loss of energy and are transmitted into the human body through a compressible water-filled bag interfaced with the skin by an ultrasonic coupling gel or by various types of water basins. The shock-wave pulse travels practically unimpeded through the water and the soft tissues of the body. When it hits the anterior surface of the stone and again when it leaves the posterior surface, the changes of acoustic impedance lead to the liberation of compressive and tensile forces. In addition, cavitation phenomena occur at the anterior surface of the stone. Together, these effects result in the fragmentation of the stone. The size as well as the microcrystalline structure and the architecture of the stone, rather than its chemical composition, determine its fragmentability.

SHOCK-WAVE LITHOTRIPSY OF GALLBLADDER STONES

Before the appropriate therapeutic approach can be chosen, the stage of gallstone disease must be defined. There are three stages of cholelithiasis: (1) the asymptomatic stage; (2) the symptomatic stage without complications; and (3) the symptomatic stage with complications such as acute cholecystitis, choledocholithiasis, biliary pancreatitis, gallbladder cancer, and gallstone ileus.

The natural history of asymptomatic gallstones is generally benign; therefore, expectant management is indicated in most patients with asymptomatic gallbladder stones, which are usually detected during routine ultrasonographic examinations. Patients with a history of biliary colic are at a substantially higher risk for recurrent biliary pain and complications than are patients with asymptomatic stones. A therapeutic intervention should, therefore, be recommended for most patients with symptomatic gallstones. The complicated forms of cholecystolithiasis usually require prompt and invasive therapy.

Surgeons and physicians agree that laparoscopic cholecystectomy is the standard treatment of symptomatic gallstone disease. It can be performed irrespective of type, number, and size of the stones. However, some patients are reluctant to undergo surgery or general anesthesia despite the small risks involved. Often, the patient insists on the least invasive treatment to eliminate the gallstones and the symptoms. In a subset of patients, nonsurgical therapy may be suitable when there is a high operative risk. The pros and cons of the different treatment modalities need to be discussed with the patient. Therefore, proper counseling of the patient requires that the physician be familiar with the different treatment options for gallstones and their respective selection criteria.

Extracorporeal shock-wave lithotripsy is aimed at clearing the gallbladder of stones by two mechanisms. As an adjunct to oral bile acid dissolution therapy, it increases the surface-to-volume ratio of the stones and thereby enhances dissolution of cholesterol stones. By creating small stone fragments that can pass into the duodenum, it achieves clearance of stone material without prior dissolution. An analysis of stone fragments in the feces of patients who underwent extracorporeal shock-wave lithotripsy showed that 3-mm fragments can pass into the intestine without causing symptoms.

Preinterventional Management

Careful evaluation of the patient with regard to symptoms and general criteria, stone characteristics, and gallbladder function is necessary to determine whether the patient is eligible for shock-wave treatment.

SYMPTOMS AND GENERAL CRITERIA. In general, patients with asymptomatic gallbladder stones should not undergo shock-wave lithotripsy. Selected patients with symptomatic gallbladder stones may be considered for shock-wave lithotripsy if they want to avoid surgery or general anesthesia or are unfit for open surgery or laparoscopic cholecystectomy. Patients must have a history of either biliary pain or complications of gallstone disease. Biliary pancreatitis is a contraindication because with lithotripsy of the stone, the small stone fragments generated can lead to another episode of gallstone pancreatitis (Table 103–1). Because of the risk of hematoma, patients with coagulopathy or those receiving anticoagulants must be excluded. Pregnancy must be ruled out by a laboratory test.

STONE CHARACTERISTICS. Efficacy of shock-wave lithotripsy decreases with the increasing number and size of stones and with the presence of calcifications. To ensure a sufficiently high efficacy of treatment, shock-wave lithotripsy should be limited to solitary radiolucent stones with a maximum diameter of 20 mm (see Table 103–1). Some investigators have suggested that exclusion of patients with stones exhibiting more than 50 Hounsfield units on computed tomography improves results with regard to the rate of stone clearance and time required for stone clearance, but this approach has not gained wide acceptance. Certain sonographic echo patterns that suggest a pure cholesterol stone are valuable criteria for selection of optimal candidates for shock-wave lithotripsy.

GALLBLADDER FUNCTION. Patency of the cystic duct must be documented by oral cholecystography or by ultra-sonography. Gallbladder emptying is a major determinant of stone clearance. About two thirds of the patients with solitary stones up to 20 mm in diameter and gallbladder ejection fractions of more than 60% cleared all their fragments from the gallbladder within 3 months after a lithotripsy. In contrast, less than 30% with ejection fractions of less than 60% cleared their fragments within the same time period. Therefore, it is advisable to determine gallbladder emptying induced by a test meal and to select for extracorporeal shock-wave lithotripsy only patients who exhibit gallbladder emptying of more than 60% of the fasting volume.

When patients ask for a noninvasive treatment of gallstones, such as extracorporeal shock-wave lithotripsy, we use the algorithm shown in Figure 103–1. This algorithm is based on the selection and exclusion criteria for oral bile acid dissolution therapy, shock-wave lithotripsy, and cholecystectomy and also on their ranking with regard to invasiveness.

Interventional Management

Patients with gallbladder stones are usually treated in the prone position. In this position, the gallbladder is closest to the abdominal wall, with no interposition of intestinal gas, and is most distant from the right costal margin. With lithotripters equipped with an overhead shock-wave generator, a supine oblique position is used. Ultrasonography is used for stone imaging and targeting and for monitoring the process of fragmentation.

Use of an electrohydraulic lithotripter and a high energy per shock wave pulse usually causes pain, and intravenous analgesics are needed. Piezoelectric lithotripters, in general, do not cause pain, and their use does not require analgesia, but a higher number of shock-wave discharges per treatment session and multiple treatment sessions are required to achieve similar results. An electromagnetic lithotripter that transmits the shock-wave energy over a larger body surface area also causes less pain and requires intravenous analgesia in only a small percentage of patients. A new strategy, commonly called "the pulverization strategy," applies a higher number of shock waves, in repeated sessions if necessary, to obtain very fine fragments. This method results in higher stone-free rates, especially in the first 3 months after lithotripsy.

Often, stone fragments are retained in the gallbladder even if they are small enough (2 to 3 mm) to pass through the cystic duct. A study that did not achieve optimal fragmentation in a high percentage of patients used adjuvant bile acid treatment with ursodeoxycholic acid to improve the results of lithotripsy. However, complete clearance of stones can also be achieved by biliary lithotripsy without adjuvant bile acid therapy when the fragments are very small (<2 mm, or sludge) and the gallbladder contracts well.

Outcomes

CLEARANCE OF STONES. Complete clearance of gallbladder stones is determined by the degree of fragmentation and gallbladder emptying. The degree of fragmenta-

Table 103–1	Selection Criteria for Extracorporeal Shock-Wave Lithotripsy of Gallbladder Stones

Stage of Gallstone Disease
Symptomatic stage without complications
Gallbladder
Opacification on oral cholecystogram or sonographic evidence of patency of cystic duct (gallbladder contraction after a test meal)
Gallbladder emptying >60% of fasting volume
Stones
Radiolucency on radiograph
Only 1 stone
Stone diameter ≤20 mm

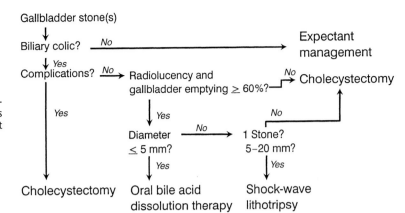

Figure 103–1. Algorithm for management of gallbladder stones, if the least invasive approach that is possible and that can be justified from a medical point of view is chosen.

tion depends on quantitative (size and number of the stones) and qualitative (structure, calcifications) stone characteristics and on the shock-wave dose (energy of shock waves, number of shock waves administered per session, number of treatment sessions). Adjuvant bile acid therapy has been shown to be a determinant of outcome when fragments are larger than 3 mm, but it appears to play no significant role when a particularly fine disintegration (pulverization) to fragments smaller than 2 mm, or to sludge, is achieved.

The largest study (711 patients) with the longest follow-up after extracorporeal shock-wave lithotripsy and adjuvant bile acid therapy (5 years) was reported by Sackmann and colleagues in 1991. The greatest success was obtained in patients with a radiolucent, solitary stone less than 20 mm in diameter; 68% and 84% of patients were stone free at 6 and 12 months after lithotripsy, respectively. These results can be improved if only patients with gallbladder emptying of more than 60% of the fasting gallbladder volume are selected. The stone-free rate decreased with increases in the number and size of the stones, with the presence of a calcified rim, and with diminished gallbladder emptying. Other groups reported complete gallstone clearance of radiolucent solitary gallbladder stones up to 20 mm in diameter in about 60% of patients 6 months after lithotripsy and in about 75% of patients 12 months after lithotripsy. In a group of patients with stones up to 20 mm in diameter and gallbladder emptying of more than 60%, Sauter and associates improved fragmentation by repeated lithotripsy sessions. Under these conditions, rates of complete stone clearance 6 months after initial treatment with and without adjuvant bile acid therapy were 63% and 77%, respectively.

COMPLICATIONS. Only few minor complications were directly related to the application of the shock waves. After electrohydraulic shock-wave lithotripsy, petechiae of the skin occurred at the site of shock-wave entry in 8%, transient gross hematuria occurred in 4%, and liver hematoma occurs very rarely. Neither short-term nor long-term post-treatment liver function values differed from pretreatment values. About one third of patients experienced one or more episodes of biliary colic related to the presence of stone fragments. About 2% developed mild biliary pancreatitis, and 1% developed transient cholestasis. These events were not directly related to the

application of shock waves but rather to the passage of stone fragments, and they usually occurred during the first weeks after lithotripsy. Endoscopic sphincterotomy to remove stone fragments from the common bile duct was necessary in only about 1% of patients. Cystic duct obstruction, generally without symptoms and resolving spontaneously, was observed in 5% of patients. Elective cholecystectomy was performed because of persistence of fragments and symptoms in approximately 3% of patients. In published trials of several thousands of patients, no fatalities attributable to lithotripsy were reported.

RECURRENCE OF STONES. Patients whose gallbladder stones have been cleared by extracorporeal shock-wave lithotripsy are at risk for stone recurrence. Gallstone recurrence after successful lithotripsy was 7% after 1 year and increased to 31% after 5 years. The lower recurrence rate compared with that after oral bile acid dissolution therapy can be explained by the fact that 90% of patients initially had a solitary stone and that the majority of patients initially had good gallbladder emptying. Studies of oral bile acid dissolution therapy show that the risk of gallstone recurrence is lower in patients who had a solitary stone. Incomplete emptying of the gallbladder is a risk factor for stone recurrence. Recurrent stones are usually small (mean diameter of 6 mm) at the time of detection, are multiple in 60% of patients, and cause recurrent biliary pain in 60% of patients.

SHOCK-WAVE LITHOTRIPSY OF BILE DUCT STONES

Extracorporeal shock-wave lithotripsy is a rapid, safe, and effective nonsurgical option to overcome failures of routine endoscopic measures in the treatment of difficult bile duct stones. In a small percentage of patients with bile duct stones, endoscopic sphincterotomy and endoscopic techniques such as mechanical lithotripsy fail because the stones are too large or too numerous or are impacted. Laser lithotripsy and contact electrohydraulic lithotripsy have been introduced to intracorporeally disintegrate bile duct stones. These techniques require the lithotripter probe to be brought close to or in direct contact with the bile duct stone under endoscopic or fluoroscopic guidance. These procedures are technically difficult, especially with bile duct stenosis or intrahepatic stones. Often, the stones are not accessible by any of these techniques, especially if they are located intrahepatically. In these situations, extracorporeal shock-wave lithotripsy has been very useful for the disintegration of bile duct stones. Since this treatment was first reported in 1985, many trials have shown it to be highly effective when endoscopic measures and mechanical lithotripsy fail. The method is safe and easier to perform than are intracorporeal techniques.

Preinterventional Management

Before extracorporeal shock-wave lithotripsy, patients must undergo a complete work-up, including endoscopic cholangiography. Shock-wave treatment is indicated if routine endoscopic measures fail to remove bile duct stones, if access to the bile ducts has been established by nasobiliary tube or transhepatic catheter, and if the orifice of the common bile duct into the duodenum is large enough for spontaneous passage or extraction of fragments. Patients with coagulopathy and those taking medication with anticoagulant effects must be excluded.

Interventional Management

Fluoroscopy is necessary for stone location. Therefore, a kidney lithotripter with a fluoroscopic system for stone location is preferable to a lithotripter with ultrasonic stone location only. For visualization of the stones, a contrast medium is instilled into the common duct via a nasobiliary tube. About three fourths of treatments require general anesthesia, and 25% can be performed with intravenous sedation with analgesia. Prophylactic antibiotics are recommended. The gallbladder of patients with cholangitis should be drained with a nasobiliary tube before shock-wave lithotripsy. If the first session of shock-wave lithotripsy fails, the treatment can be repeated within approximately 1 week.

Outcomes

STONE CLEARANCE. The bile ducts can be cleared of all stones in 70% to 90% of patients. Repeated sessions are required in about one third of patients. Endoscopic extraction of fragments is necessary in 70% to 90% of patients because the fragments are usually larger than are the fragments after lithotripsy of gallbladder stones.

COMPLICATIONS. No mortality directly related to the procedure has been reported. In the 1992 study of Sauerbruch and colleagues, 30-day mortality was 1% (one patient died of biliary pancreatitis after endoscopic sphincterotomy). Thus, shock-wave lithotripsy compares

Pearls and Pitfalls

- Lithotripsy can be an effective nonsurgical means of clearing the gallbladder of gallstones.
- Laparoscopic cholecystectomy has almost replaced gallstone lithotripsy except in selected situations (e.g., nonoperative candidates, patients who refuse anesthesia).
- Best results are achieved with solitary stones with a diameter of ≤20 mm and a gallbladder ejection fraction of >60%.
- Oral ursodeoxycholic acid may help clear stone fragments remaining in the gallbladder.
- Complications are rare but include biliary colic (30%), biliary pancreatitis (2%), and transient cholestasis (1%).
- Recurrence of stones after successful treatment is about 30% at 5 years.
- Lithotripsy is a well-accepted method of clearing common bile duct stones not amenable to other interventional techniques.

favorably with open surgery in this group of usually elderly, high-risk patients. Mild and transient hemobilia was observed in fewer than 10%. Further complications directly caused by the shock waves include hematoma of the liver and gross hematuria. The most important complication after extracorporeal shock-wave lithotripsy was cholangitis, in 4% of patients, thus mandating antibiotic prophylaxis.

For patients with major comorbidity and/or failure of standard methods of endoscopic or surgical removal of bile duct stones, extracorporeal shock-wave lithotripsy facilitates stone clearance in up to 90%, with very low morbidity and mortality. It is expected that the use of extracorporeal shock-wave lithotripsy in the treatment of these patients will increase.

SELECTED READINGS

Boscaini M, Piccinni-Leopardi M, Andreotti F, et al: Gall stone pulverisation strategy in patients treated with extracorporeal lithotripsy and follow up results of maintenance treatment with ursodeoxycholic acid. Gut 1994;35:117.

Pauletzki J, Sailer C, Klüppelberg U, et al: Gallbladder emptying determines early gallstone clearance after shock-wave lithotripsy. Gastroenterology 1994;107:1496.

Paumgartner G: Extracorporeal shock-wave lithotripsy. Eur J Gastroenterol Hepatol 1994;6:867.

Sackmann M, Niller H, Klüppelberg U, et al: Gallstone recurrence after shock-wave therapy. Gastroenterology 1994;106:225.

Sackmann M, Pauletzki J, Sauerbruch T, et al: The Munich Gallbladder Lithotripsy Study: Results of the first 5 years with 711 patients. Ann Intern Med 1991;114:290.

Sauerbruch T, Holl J, Sackmann M, Paumgartner G: Fragmentation of bile duct stones by extracorporeal shock-wave lithotripsy: A five-year experience. Hepatology 1992;15:208.

White DM, Correa RJ, Gibbons RP, et al: Extracorporeal shock-wave lithotripsy for bile duct calculi. Am J Surg 1998;175:10.

Chapter 104

Asymptomatic Gallstones

Robert V. Rege and Daniel B. Jones

Most patients with gallstones are asymptomatic, remain so, and do not know that they have them. In Western society, gallstones are found, by ultrasonography, in about 10% of women and about 5% of men younger than age 50 years. Gallstone prevalence increases with age, reaching as high as 50% of women and 15% of men age 60 years or older. Gallstones are more likely to develop in patients with a family history of gallstones, ethnic groups such as Native Americans, obese men and women, diabetic patients, patients with ileal disease, individuals who lose weight rapidly or who receive parenteral nutrition, and women with multiple pregnancies. Approximately 50% of patients remain asymptomatic throughout their lifetime, and as a general rule they do not require operation or medical therapy.

Symptoms attributable to gallstones develop in 1 million people in the United States annually, and complications of gallstones or symptoms requiring cholecystectomy develop in approximately 500,000 of these patients each year. The number of cholecystectomies performed per year has increased since the introduction of laparoscopic cholecystectomy, possibly because physicians and patients alike are more willing to consider a minimal-access operation. The indications for laparoscopic surgery should not differ from those for open cholecystectomy, especially because it is not clear that early operation decreases the risk of either long-term morbidity or mortality.

CLINICAL PRESENTATION

Natural History of Gallstones

In most patients with gallstones, symptoms never develop, and gallbladder stones frequently remain silent for years. For this reason, elective operation is currently not recommended for patients with asymptomatic (silent) gallstones. In 1982, Gracie and Ransohoff reported 123 faculty members with silent gallstones at the University of Michigan who had a very low rate of problems over 15 years of observation. Conversion from asymptomatic to symptomatic gallstones occurred in only 10% of patients by 5 years, 15% by 10 years, and 18% by 15 years. Other studies subsequently have shown rates of conversion from asymptomatic to symptomatic disease ranging from essentially the same to no more than twice as high. Symptoms requiring cholecystectomy appear to develop in only approximately 1% to 2% of asymptomatic patients per year, and the majority of patients do not require operation during periods of observation as long as 20 years. Symptoms usually develop before serious complications, and serious complications, such as acute cholecystitis or gallstone pancreatitis, occur at a rate of only 1% in asymptomatic patients per year. Treatment of patients with complications is almost as safe as elective operation. The slight increases in mortality and morbidity rates in these patients are counterbalanced by the cost and complications of prophylactic cholecystectomy, which would occur in the larger number of patients with asymptomatic gallstones in whom problems would never develop.

The risk of observation of patients with asymptomatic gallstones is less than or equal to the risk of operation (Table 104–1). Therefore, asymptomatic gallstones should be observed, with cholecystectomy being reserved for patients in whom symptoms or complications develop and those at increased risk. Despite this recommendation, operations are still performed frequently for asymptomatic gallstones. Although this is often due to a misunderstanding of the fate of silent gallstones, some groups of patients with gallstones may be at higher risk for development of symptoms or complications. This chapter focuses on prophylactic cholecystectomy in select patients with silent gallstones (Table 104–2).

In contrast, recurrent episodes of biliary colic develop in patients with symptomatic gallstones; these patients are at increased risk for development of complications of their gallstone disease (see Table 104–1). Sixty-nine percent of the symptomatic patients in the National Cooperative Gallstone Study experienced recurrent episodes of pain within 2 years, and 44% required biliary tract surgery within 6 years. In the GREPCO study, serious complications of gallstone disease developed in 7% of symptomatic patients by 10 years, and cholecystectomy was more likely to be performed in these patients than in asymptomatic patients (45% versus 24%). Patients with symptomatic disease are likely to require cholecystectomy and are at higher risk for development of complications of gallstones.

Gallstones do not always cause specific symptoms. Many patients have episodes of mild, transient abdominal pain, nausea, dyspepsia, and flatulence. These symptoms are not specific for gallstones in that other gastrointestinal diseases, including peptic ulcer disease, gastroesophageal reflux, and irritable bowel disease, also cause them. Patients with mild, nonspecific symptoms are classified in the literature as "mildly symptomatic." Discrepancies in the literature often are due to a failure to classify patients

Table 104–1	The Natural History of Gallstones	
	SYMPTOMS REQUIRING CHOLECYSTECTOMY	COMPLICATIONS OF GALLSTONES
Asymptomatic	1%–2%/yr	1%–2%/yr
Mild symptoms	6%–8%/yr	1%–3%/yr
Symptomatic	5%–30%/yr	7%/yr

Table 104–2	**Potential Indications for Prophylactic Cholecystectomy**

Congenital hemolytic anemia
Cirrhosis
Immunosuppression
Nonfunctioning gallbladder
Gallstones greater than 2.5 cm in diameter
Children with gallstones
Porcelain gallbladder
Bariatric surgery
Incidental gallstones found during intra-abdominal operation
No access to medical care

with gallstones appropriately. Patients with mild symptoms require operation more frequently than do asymptomatic patients, but less frequently than symptomatic patients. Cholecystectomy is required only in a minority (6% to 8% per year) of these mildly symptomatic patients, and the rate of development of serious complications is low, approximately 1% to 3% per year (see Table 104–1). Thus, mildly symptomatic patients are generally not candidates for cholecystectomy because they act more like asymptomatic than symptomatic patients. Moreover, many of the 5% of patients with persistent symptoms after cholecystectomy arise from the group of patients with atypical or nonspecific symptoms. If symptoms increase in frequency or interfere with lifestyle, and if the patient understands the distinct possibility that cholecystectomy may not solve the problems, then cholecystectomy should be considered.

In summary, patients with symptomatic gallstones should be offered elective laparoscopic cholecystectomy. In general, the risk of operation is low compared with the risk and suffering associated with observation alone. On the other hand, patients with asymptomatic gallstones and those with mild symptoms are at low risk for development of serious complications. Symptoms will develop in a minority of patients and can be treated safely. Analyses of cost-effectiveness and life expectancy show no advantage of prophylactic cholecystectomy over observation of asymptomatic gallstone patients; thus, operation is not indicated in these groups of patients.

Prophylactic Cholecystectomy

Selected patients with asymptomatic gallstones may be at increased risk for development of symptoms or complications. If such a group could be identified, prophylactic cholecystectomy might be reasonable, depending on their level of risk. Historically, diabetic patients with gallstones were considered to have a higher incidence of gallstones, a greater risk of complications, and increased morbidity and mortality rates for emergent operation; many surgeons advocated prophylactic cholecystectomy in diabetics with silent gallstones. Recent studies have addressed this issue by documenting the natural history of gallstones in diabetic patients. Symptoms developed in approximately 15% of diabetic patients with asymptomatic gallstones by 5 years, compared with 48% of symptomatic diabetic patients. These data are comparable to those

observed in nondiabetic patients with gallstones. Most importantly, the morbidity and mortality risks associated with biliary tract operations performed on diabetic patients were similar or only slightly higher than in nondiabetic patients. However, diabetic patients with an episode of acute cholecystitis were more likely to fail medical therapy and require emergent operation; furthermore, gangrene was more likely to develop. Overall, the morbidity and mortality rates associated with the treatment of diabetic patients were only minimally higher than those of nondiabetic patients; thus, prophylactic cholecystectomy in diabetic patients with asymptomatic gallstones probably should no longer be recommended routinely.

Cirrhotic patients have an increased incidence of gallstones, and the morbidity and mortality rates associated with cholecystectomy increase as cirrhosis becomes more advanced. In a study of 58 cirrhotic patients with gallstones, 23 were observed, and symptoms did not develop in any of those patients. Morbidity and mortality rates in the cirrhotic patients who underwent cholecystectomy were acceptable in Child A and B patients; no patient died and significant complication developed in only one patient. However, all patients required blood transfusion, a significant finding because blood transfusion is only rarely needed in noncirrhotic patients undergoing cholecystectomy. In contrast, in 10 Child C patients, one died and significant complications developed in four others. Thus, symptoms develop infrequently in cirrhotic patients with gallstones, but when symptoms or complications develop in Child class C patients, morbidity and mortality risks of operative and nonoperative therapy are high. Watchful waiting is reasonable with silent stones. Early intervention is warranted in Child A and B patients but probably only after symptoms develop.

Biliary symptoms may develop in patients with asymptomatic gallstones after they undergo an operation for unrelated intra-abdominal problems. Comparison of incidental cholecystectomy in 195 gallstone patients undergoing elective colonic surgery with 110 patients who did not have their gallbladder removed revealed that the cholecystectomy added no morbidity or mortality risk to colectomy. Postoperatively, 12% and 22% of patients who did not have cholecystectomy required surgery for symptomatic gallstone disease by 2 and 5 years, respectively. More recently, other researchers reported that postoperative symptoms developed eventually in 54% of 156 patients undergoing abdominal surgery with asymptomatic gallstones left in situ, and 22% required cholecystectomy within 30 days of operation or within the same hospitalization. Concomitant cholecystectomy is thus usually safe and should be performed for patients whose condition is stable if the cholecystectomy can be done with little technical difficulty and if the risk of proceeding with a second procedure is acceptable.

Some selected groups have clear indications for prophylactic cholecystectomy. Prophylactic cholecystectomy is indicated in patients with congenital hemolytic anemia. These patients continue to form gallstones, usually of the pigment type, and, eventually, symptoms or complications develop from their gallstones. Cholecystectomy in obese patients in whom gallstones have already developed and who undergo bariatric surgery is indicated because in a large number of these patients symptoms develop that are difficult to separate from symptoms caused by complications of their primary operation. Moreover, in 36% of patients who require gastric bypass operations for morbid obesity who did not have gallstones previously, gallstones developed within 6 months of their operation during the period of rapid weight loss. Even more remarkable is the fact that symptoms develop in 40% of these patients and 28% require cholecystectomy during the first year after operation. Prophylactic cholecystectomy adds minimal morbidity and mortality risks to most bariatric operations and is clearly indicated in patients with gallstones. Many surgeons perform cholecystectomy during bariatric procedures in lieu of medical therapy even if no gallstones are detected.

Current data do not yet indicate whether other patients with more than one risk factor benefit from prophylactic cholecystectomy. Some surgeons have suggested that patients with large gallstones (>2.5 cm) are at increased risk for development of complications. Children with gallstones, in general, should have their gallbladders removed because they are expected to live more than 20 years with their gallstones. Patients with calcified gallbladders should also undergo cholecystectomy because of the increased risk of gallbladder cancer in a "porcelain gallbladder." Refinements in treatment of gallstones in selected patients require a deeper understanding of the natural history of gallstones in subgroups of patients with silent gallstones who may be at higher risk for subsequent operation or complications. Studies are still needed to predict the risk factors for conversion of asymptomatic to symptomatic gallstones and the groups of patients at high risk for development of gallstone complications. Currently, only selected patients with asymptomatic gallstones should undergo prophylactic cholecystectomy.

PREOPERATIVE MANAGEMENT

Preparation of asymptomatic patients for prophylactic cholecystectomy is the same as for symptomatic patients. Patients fast from midnight before the operation and are admitted to the hospital the morning of the operation. Preoperative sedatives, an H_2-receptor antagonist, and a single dose of intravenous cephalosporin are administered. When the patient arrives in the operating room, sequential compression stockings are often used on both legs to avoid pooling of blood in the lower extremities caused by the reverse Trendelenburg position. After induction of general anesthesia, an orogastric tube may be placed to decompress the stomach and a urinary catheter may be placed if the patient did not void before arrival in the operating room. Laparoscopic cholecystectomy is then performed according to the usual technique.

COMPLICATIONS

Cholecystectomy has several associated complications. Bile duct injury is a devastating complication of laparoscopic cholecystectomy. Injuries to the bile ducts occur in approximately 0.5% of laparoscopic cholecystectomies, several times the rate of injury with open cholecystec-

Pearls and Pitfalls

- Most gallstones occur in asymptomatic patients.
- The incidence of gallstones increases directly with age. In women older than the age of 60 years, the incidence is approximately 50%; in men older than 60 years, the incidence is approximately 15%.
- Conversion of asymptomatic to symptomatic gallstones occurs in approximately 10% of patients by 5 years, 15% by 10 years, and 18% by 15 years.
- The risks associated with observation of patients with asymptomatic gallstones appear to be less than the risks associated with prophylactic cholecystectomy.
- Selected patient groups with asymptomatic gallstones may be appropriate candidates for "prophylactic" cholecystectomy.

tomy. The most common cause of bile duct injury during laparoscopic cholecystectomy is misidentification of a major bile duct as the cystic duct. Causes for misidentification are usually technical and result from superior traction of the gallbladder aligning the cystic duct and common bile duct. The common duct may be "tented up" because of too vigorous superior and lateral traction placed on the gallbladder, making it susceptible to injury during placement of clips. Meticulous dissection of the hepatocystic triangle should expose the "critical view" of the structures surrounding the neck of the gallbladder and decrease these types of injuries. A cholangiogram may also be helpful if the anatomy is in doubt. If it does not avoid injury, it will recognize the problem immediately so that it can be addressed promptly.

OUTCOMES

Currently, laparoscopic cholecystectomy may be performed safely, and most patients benefit from less postoperative pain, early hospital discharge, and rapid recuperation. However, the indications for cholecystectomy should not change in the era of laparoscopic cholecystectomy. Recent studies suggest that symptoms develop in fewer than 20% of individuals with asymptomatic gallstones and that the risk of "prophylactic" operation outweighs the potential benefit of surgery. For selected patients with asymptomatic cholelithiasis, cholecystectomy may be recommended. As with other elective procedures, morbidity should be minimal.

SELECTED READINGS

Attili AF, DeSantis A, Capri R, et al: The natural history of gallstones: The GREPCO experience. Hepatology 1995;21:656.

Bragg LE, Thompson JS: Concomitant cholecystectomy for asymptomatic cholelithiasis. Arch Surg 1989;124:460.

Del Favero G, Caroli A, Meggiato R, et al: Natural history of gallstones in non–insulin-dependent diabetes mellitus: A prospective 5-year follow-up. Dig Dis Sci 1995;39:1704.

Diehl AK: Epidemiology and natural history of gallstone disease. Gastroenterol Clin North Am 1991;20:1.

Friedman GD: Natural history of asymptomatic and symptomatic gallstones. Am J Surg 1992;165:399.

Gracie WA, Ransohoff DF: The natural history of silent gallstones. The innocent gallstone is not a myth. N Engl J Med 1982;307:798.

Hooper KD, Landis JR, Meilstrup JW, et al: The prevalence of asymptomatic gallstones in the general population. Invest Rad 1991;26:939.

Ishizaki Y, Bandai Y, Shimomura K, et al: Management of gallstones in cirrhotic patients. Surg Today 1993;23:36.

Juhasz ES, Wolff BG, Meagher AP, et al: Incidental cholecystectomy during colorectal surgery. Ann Surg 1994;219:467.

Landau O, Deutsch AA, Kott I, et al: The risk of cholecystectomy for acute cholecystitis in diabetic patients. Hepatogastroenterol 1992;39:437.

Menegaux F, Dorent R, Tabbi D, et al: Biliary surgery after heart transplantation. Am J Surg 1998;175:320.

Orozco H, Takahashi T, Angel M, et al: Long-term evolution of asymptomatic cholelithiasis diagnosed during abdominal operations for variceal bleeding in patients with cirrhosis. Am J Surg 1992;168:232.

Schwesinger WH, Diehl AK: Changing indications for laparoscopic cholecystectomy. Stones without symptoms and symptoms without stones. Surg Clin North Am 1996;76:493.

Shiffman ML, Sugerman HJ, Kellum JM, et al: Gallstone formation after rapid weight loss: A prospective study in patients undergoing gastric bypass surgery for treatment of morbid obesity. 1991;86:1000.

Chapter 105

Cholecystolithiasis

Mark A. Talamini and Catherine L. Stanfield

The prevalence of gallstones is high in most western countries. In the United States, approximately 10% of men and 20% of women will have cholelithiasis by age 65 years, with the total cases exceeding 20 million. The precise incidence is unknown because many individuals with gallstones are asymptomatic, but cholelithiasis develops in approximately 1 million patients each year. Rapid weight loss in the obese, and obesity itself, particularly in women, increase the risk of gallstone formation. Gallstones develop in approximately one third of patients with Crohn's disease with inflammatory involvement of the terminal ileum. Diabetes mellitus, cirrhosis, and pregnancy also are associated with an increased risk of cholelithiasis and of symptomatic gallbladder disease.

ETIOPATHOGENESIS

Gallstones are crystalline structures, concretions, or accretions of normal or abnormal bile constituents. They can be divided into three major types: cholesterol; pigment; or mixed stones. In the West, cholesterol or mixed stones account for 80% of the total, with pigment stones comprising the remaining 20%. In contrast, in Asia, 80% are pigment stones, with the balance being cholesterol or mixed, obviously indicative of different etiologies. Mixed and cholesterol gallstones contain approximately 70% cholesterol monohydrate plus an admixture of calcium salts, bile acids, bile pigments, proteins, fatty acids, and phospholipids. Pigment stones are comprised primarily of calcium bilirubinate, with less than 2% cholesterol.

Obesity, high-calorie diets, or certain medications can increase biliary secretion of cholesterol, in turn supersaturating the bile with cholesterol and increasing the lithogenicity of bile. Impaired hepatic synthesis of bile salts or conditions affecting the enterohepatic circulation of bile salts may lead to decreased hepatic secretion of bile salts and phospholipids, thereby lowering the solubilization of cholesterol and increasing the lithogenicity of bile. Other conditions such as pregnancy or heritable disorders of biliary constituents (e.g., in Native American Pima Indians) can lead to bile supersaturated with cholesterol. Thus, an excess of biliary cholesterol in relation to bile acids and phospholipids may be due to hypersecretion of cholesterol, hyposecretion of bile acids, or both.

In addition to primary cholesterol gallstones, pigment stones represent a different pathogenesis. Abnormalities in the amount or type of biliary pigments excreted can lead to crystallization of pigment stones. For instance, hemolysis pigment is excreted in the bile; disorders of hemolysis such as hereditary spherocytosis are associated with pigment gallstones. For poorly understood reasons, cirrhosis has a higher rate of pigment stones. In the Orient, bacteriobilia with organisms containing β-glucu-

ronidase may deconjugate bile salts leading to development of pigment gallstones.

CLINICAL PRESENTATION

Cholelithiasis is often asymptomatic and may be discovered incidentally during the course of a routine radiographic study, operation, or autopsy. When symptoms are present, patients typically complain of epigastric or right upper quadrant discomfort, heartburn, flatulence, and food intolerance, particularly to fats and cabbage. Pain, frequently referred to as biliary colic (a true misnomer), develops in 10% to 25% of patients with gallstones and is believed to be precipitated by the lodging of one or more stones in the neck of the gallbladder or in the cystic duct. An alternative explanation for the pain is that the gallbladder contracts down upon a large stone or a large number of stones, contacting the inner wall of the gallbladder. Characteristically located in the right upper quadrant and radiating to the right shoulder or mid back, the pain is steady, with a crescendo-decrescendo pattern of severe intensity lasting for 1 to 4 hours. Often the patient tries many different positions (unsuccessfully) to relieve the pain. The patient may complain of a residual mild ache or soreness in the right subcostal region for the following 24 hours. Frequently, nausea and vomiting accompany these episodes. This pain begins almost invariably in the evening, 30 minutes to 1 hour after the evening meal or in the early hours of the night, awakening the patient from sleep. Onset of biliary colic in the morning or early afternoon should lead the clinician to question the diagnosis. In addition, the classic-quoted phrase that biliary colic tends to follow a fatty meal is attractive in theory, but is probably more of "an old wives' tale" than a reliable finding. Jaundice may occur if a stone migrates from the gallbladder into the common bile duct causing biliary obstruction. When symptoms do not abate, but rather progress to include unrelenting severe pain with fever and leukocytosis, the diagnosis is usually that of acute cholecystitis representing acute inflammation of the wall of the gallbladder. The differential diagnosis should always include cholangitis, pancreatitis, and peptic ulcer disease.

DIAGNOSIS

A diagnosis of symptomatic gallstones or chronic cholecystitis may be made based on history and physical examination, with studies such as abdominal ultrasonography or radionuclide scans (for acute cholecystitis) done for confirmation. On physical examination, a positive Murphy's sign (pain on inspiration produced with right upper quadrant palpation, without comparable pain in left upper quadrant) suggests either acute cholecystitis or significant ongoing inflammation. Usually patients with only intermittent biliary colic have a normal physical examination between episodes. A palpable, nontender gallbladder under the right costal margin (Courvoisier's sign) is due to an enlarged gallbladder, usually from chronic extrahepatic biliary obstruction, representing a more sinister etiology such as pancreatic cancer and is usually associated with jaundice. Rarely, a palpable gallbladder represents a hydrops of the gallbladder resulting from chronic complete obstruction of the cystic duct with so-called "white bile"; this represents reabsorption of the intraluminal bile salts with replacement by uninfected mucus. Oral cholecystography, which is rarely used, is 98% accurate (negative when the gallbladder opacifies, positive when it does not) when compliance is assured, the contrast agent is absorbed, and liver function is normal. Ultrasonography is currently the gold standard for the evaluation of cholelithiasis because of its high sensitivity and accuracy in detecting gallstones and biliary dilatation. Because ultrasonography depends on interfaces of different tissue densities, the contrast between stone and tissue density is usually easily seen. Stones as small as 2 mm in diameter can be identified confidently within the gallbladder. Acoustic "shadowing" of opacities or stones within the gallbladder lumen, which change when the patient moves, are indicative of cholelithiasis. Biliary sludge, which has a low echogenic profile, typically forms a layer in the most dependent portion of the gallbladder. This layer shifts with postural changes but characteristically does not produce acoustic shadowing. Ultrasonography is also effective in detecting thickening of the gallbladder wall and the presence of pericholecystic fluid, which are both signs of inflammation. Radionuclide studies are not able to "see" stones and do not provide much anatomic detail; however, they are able to detect occlusion of the cystic duct or the common bile duct and can therefore confirm a diagnosis of acute cholecystitis or cholangitis resulting from significant ductal obstruction.

MANAGEMENT

Overview

A decision to proceed with cholecystectomy is based on communication of the clinical issues for that patient, along with a discussion of the risks and benefits to the patient. Each person's presentation, the patient's physical examination, and the radiologic evaluation should create an estimate of the likelihood that the presenting complaints are indeed caused by the gallstones. Many organs and conditions, including the gallbladder, can contribute to a variety of symptoms along the "sixth dermatome" of referred pain, many of which can mimic gallbladder-type pain. In the setting of acute cholecystitis, the patient gains relief when the gallbladder is removed. However, most patients with gallstones and symptoms strongly suggestive of biliary colic are far less clear-cut. The wise surgeon makes it clear to patients with chronic symptoms that there is at least some chance that the symptoms are *not*

related to the gallstones, and thus cholecystectomy may not resolve their symptoms. In addition, the risks of operation also vary. Patients with multiple previous abdominal procedures, cirrhosis, or serious cardiopulmonary disease are at increased risk even from a laparoscopic cholecystectomy. Controversy regarding patients with gallstones but without symptoms (silent asymptomatic gallstones) has not changed in the past 50 years. There is widespread agreement that cholecystectomy is indicated in a patient with symptoms resulting from calculous disease, but data supporting cholecystectomy for asymptomatic patients are lacking.

Since its introduction in the United States in 1989, laparoscopic cholecystectomy has clearly become the operative approach of choice. Compared with open cholecystectomy, laparoscopic cholecystectomy is less invasive, leads to fewer wound infections and incisional hernias, requires a shorter hospital stay, offers the patient a rapid recovery back to work or normal daily activities, and dramatically decreases postoperative pain. The progression of open cholecystectomy to overnight stay after laparoscopic cholecystectomy to an outpatient laparoscopic cholecystectomy initiated a study reviewing nursing and patient opinions. We investigated patients' desire and ability to be discharged successfully on the day of operation and to support a safe and comfortable postoperative course at home without direct medical intervention. In this study, 70% of patients rated their pain as a 7 or greater (on a scale of 1 to 10) and 50% or more suffered nausea and vomiting. These findings led us to alter our anesthetic regimen, adding antiemetics and administration of a local anesthetic, leading to a much more successful program of outpatient laparoscopic cholecystectomy in appropriate patients.

Preoperative Management

Patients scheduled for laparoscopic cholecystectomy usually require a minimal preoperative workup. History, physical examination, anesthesia evaluation, and laboratory screen (hemoglobin, electrolyte panel, liver function tests) complete the basic evaluation. Barring any abnormalities in this workup, patients are told to take nothing by mouth after midnight the day before operation, except for any necessary medications the morning of surgery. Patients with acute cholecystitis usually are already receiving intravenous hydration, antibiotics (such as a second-generation cephalosporin), and a nasogastric tube if there is persistent vomiting from associated ileus. These patients with acute cholecystitis should undergo cholecystectomy within the first few days of their illness before the inflamed tissues become too severely indurated; if the diagnosis is delayed for 5 to 7 days, some consideration should be given to delaying cholecystectomy for 6 weeks after the inflammation has subsided. In the intervening period, a laparoscopic cholecystectomy is less likely to be successful, and even open surgery can be difficult.

Intraoperative Management

Laparoscopic cholecystectomy is clearly the standard means of surgically removing the gallbladder and is well described. The key step is identification and safe dissection of the gall bladder–cystic duct junction. The safest way to approach this challenge is to begin the dissection on the gallbladder, a structure easily identified, and then dissect down toward the cystic duct–gallbladder junction. An additional maneuver that may help is to open the plane between the gallbladder and the liver on both sides of the cystic duct by incising the peritoneal covering and to retract the infundibulum of the gallbladder both anteriorly and laterally to the patient's right–not rostrally. These maneuvers allow clearer identification. If identification of the junction cannot be accomplished with these maneuvers, it may be best to convert to an open procedure rather than to persist and risk complication. During dissection of the gallbladder from the liver, the hook cautery is most often used. By placing the hook behind the tissue to be divided, the hook can be seen through the tissue. If the hook cannot be seen, division of the tissue will often result in a hole in the gallbladder or dissection into the liver. For additional postoperative comfort, bupivacaine is injected into all wounds, and an analgesic is administered toward the end of the operation. An antiemetic can be given during the operation as well to reduce the incidence of postoperative vomiting.

The issue of the need for routine versus selective intraoperative cholangiography was controversial before laparoscopic cholecystectomy, and it continues to be so. Some surgeons contend that routine cholangiography reduces at least the severity of common bile duct injury and perhaps the incidence of bile duct injury. The surgeon should be prepared to deal with the information revealed by intraoperative cholangiography. If stones are found, they can be removed via laparoscopic common duct exploration, conversion to open common duct exploration, or postoperative endoscopic papillotomy and stone extraction.

Postoperative Management

Most patients after laparoscopic cholecystectomy probably can be discharged the same day, as long as they are reliable and meet certain criteria. Conditions at home must be acceptable. After laparoscopic cholecystectomy, there is often substantial initial pain, which begins to subside rather quickly. If pain persists or increases, the patient should be evaluated immediately. If there is fever, jaundice, or any condition impeding rapid recovery, the patient should be evaluated immediately. After open cholecystectomy, hospitalization is required, often just for a few days, for pain control and until bowel function returns.

Complications

The most potentially dangerous complications associated with laparoscopic cholecystectomy fall into two categories: access complications and bile duct injuries. Access complications occur during either the insertion of the Veress to establish pneumoperitoneum or the insertion of trocars to provide abdominal access. Any time that placement of a Veress needle or the initial trocar is difficult, damage to

intra-abdominal organs must be suspected, necessitating a careful and complete examination of the abdominal cavity with the laparoscope once it is placed. If the laparoscopic view reveals potential organ damage, the site must be thoroughly examined laparoscopically, and if any doubt exists, through an open incision. Expansion of a retroperitoneal hematoma or damage to a loop of bowel deep in the abdomen may not be visible and can go undetected. All subsequent trocars should be placed under complete laparoscopic vision and therefore should be safe.

Bile duct injuries are the "Achilles heel" of laparoscopic cholecystectomy. Multiple studies confirm that the incidence of this problem is increased when the gallbladder is removed laparoscopically as opposed to during open cholecystectomy. To avoid this injury, the surgeon must stubbornly refuse to clip and cut any structure before it is clearly and confidently identified. The surgeon should display a willingness to convert to an open procedure if the cystic duct–gallbladder junction cannot be clearly identified—it is not a sign of weakness but rather maturity.

Postoperatively, patients should have rapid resolution of pain. Any deviation should be viewed with suspicion as the first sign of possible trouble. A report of severe pain, fever, jaundice, or vomiting within hours to a few days after cholecystectomy should lead to a priority review by the surgical staff. If there is suspicion of duct injury, computed tomography is a good first test. The presence of a bile collection may be a biliary leak from a dislodged cystic duct clip, the bed of the liver, or a major duct injury. A dilated biliary tree is almost always a sign of trouble. These finding need to be pursued aggressively with specific imaging of the biliary tree via endoscopic retrograde cholangiopancreatography, transhepatic cholangiography, or magnetic resonance cholangiopancreatography. Repair of a major bile duct injury is best performed by surgeons experienced in this type of operation, with a team accustomed to managing the support services necessary; best results are obtained at a center of excellence (and experience). Full disclosure to the patient and family with rapid transfer to a larger, experienced center may *avoid* a medicolegal investigation.

Medical Management

An alternative treatment to cholecystectomy might be the administration of certain medications to dissolve gallstones in selected patients. Chenodeoxycholic acid (CDCA) can partially or completely dissolve cholesterol gallstones, whereas ursodeoxycholic acid (UDCA), which is structurally similar to CDCA, is less toxic to hepatocytes and does not cause as much diarrhea as CDCA. Patients must, however, have a functioning gallbladder with radiolucent stones less than 15 mm in diameter; in this select group of patients (approximately 15% to 20% of all patients with gallstones), complete dissolution can be achieved in 50% to 60% of patients within 2 years with the use of UDCA. The highest success rate occurs in patients with radiolucent floating stones less than 5 mm in diameter. There are many drawbacks and limitations of dissolution therapy. Less than 20% of patients with symptomatic cholelithiasis are good candidates for this treatment, and stones tend to recur (30% to 50% in 3 to 12 years of follow-up) because the chemical consistency of the bile that predisposed them to formation of gallstones originally has not changed. Most patients, when offered the risk–benefit option, elect cholecystectomy rather than to take pills and wait for their bothersome symptoms to resolve.

Gallbladder Lithotripsy

Just as the option of ultrasonic fragmentation of kidney stones took the urologic world by storm in the 1980s and has persisted so, gallstone lithotripsy offered a similar possibility. Many lithotriptors were ordered, protocols were started, clinics were marketed, and everyone was interested. However, few, if any, centers still offer this as a viable option for symptomatic gallstones for several reasons: once fragmented and cleared with adjuvant use of UDCA, the gallstones tend to recur; fragmentation therapy requires an anesthetic and may need to be repeated; fragmentation may precipitate biliary colic, acute cholecystitis, or gallstone pancreatitis; and, finally, the advent of a minimally invasive procedure to remove the cause of the gallstones and the chance of recurrence has virtually relegated gallstone lithotripsy to the annals of surgical history as a theoretically attractive but impractical treatment.

Outcomes

Since laparoscopic cholecystectomy created a paradigm shift in the world of general surgery, outcomes studies abound with its widespread adoption. One early study examined the shift from open to laparoscopic cholecystectomy by collecting data harvested from all inpatient hospitals in Maryland. The first laparoscopic cholecystectomy in the state was performed in late 1989; by 1991, well over 75% of cholecystectomies in the state were performed laparoscopically. The data also suggested that the laparoscopic operation had lower mortality and morbidity rates than open cholecystectomy. Another large outcomes study examined the medical records of 3448 cholecystectomy patients in Minnesota. Postoperative functional status was evaluated by a questionnaire that was sent to all patients 6 months after their procedure. A laparoscopic technique was performed in 2490 patients (72%), of which, 195 (8%) operations were converted to an open cholecystectomy. These latter patients were out of work longer, requiring an average of 31 days, as opposed to 15 days after laparoscopic surgery. In the areas where laparoscopic cholecystectomy was available, no significant increase in total numbers of cholecystectomies occurred. A "learning curve" did, however, appear to exist, with fewer operative and general complications occurring for surgeons with increasing experience with the laparoscopic approach. With laparoscopic procedures entrenched in modern surgical training programs, this learning curve for the routine procedures has disappeared.

Pearls and Pitfalls

- The prevalence of gallstones far surpasses the prevalence of symptomatic gallstones.
- Ultrasonography remains the gold standard of diagnosis.
- Most episodes of biliary colic occur in the evening; the concept of symptoms following a fatty meal may be "an old wives' tale."
- When identification of cystic duct–gallbladder junction is difficult, dissect from gallbladder *toward* cystic duct.
- A cystic duct packed with stones requires both milking of the stone back up into the gallbladder *and* an intraoperative cholangiogram.
- Spilled gallstones in the peritoneum require retrieval; otherwise abscesses may occur.
- Surgeons should discuss the possibility of conversion to an open cholecystectomy with *all* patients and family members *preoperatively*.
- It is not a failure to convert from a laparoscopic to an open cholecystectomy if the anatomy is not clear—this ultimately is safer for the patient (and the surgeon!).
- When a common or hepatic bile duct injury occurs during laparoscopic cholecystectomy, the surgeon should place a drain and discuss the situation immediately with family members and the patient. The patient should be transferred to a center of excellence (and experience). The situation should be discussed with legal counsel. Full, honest, immediate disclosure with patient and family will do more to prevent a lawsuit than anything else.

Laparoscopic cholecystectomy has become entrenched and large volumes of data allow clinicians to provide patients with reasonably accurate numbers regarding the risks of laparoscopic cholecystectomy. In patients without previous upper abdominal surgery and without acute cholecystitis, there is a conversion rate to open cholecystectomy of 4% and a bile duct injury rate of 0.20% to 0.33%. In the current legal environment, many consider it wise to write these numbers on the operative consent form in addition to discussing them with the patient.

SELECTED READINGS

Ido K, Isoda N, Suzuki T, et al: Confirmation of a "safety zone" by intraoperative cholangiography during laparoscopic cholecystectomy. Surg Endosc 1996;10:798.

Memon MA, Deeik RK, Maffi TR, Fitzgibbons RJ Jr: The outcome of unretrieved gallstones in the peritoneal cavity during laparoscopic cholecystectomy: A prospective analysis. Surg Endosc 1999;13:848.

Shea JA, Berlin JA, Bachwich DR, et al: Indications for and outcomes of cholecystectomy: A comparison of the pre and post laparoscopic eras. Ann Surg 1998;227:343.

Steiner CA, Bass EB, Talamini MA, et al: Surgical rates and operative mortality for open and laparoscopic cholecystectomy in Maryland. N Engl J Med 1994;330:403.

Talamini MA, Coleman J, Sauter P, et al: Outpatient laparoscopic cholecystectomy: Patient and nursing perspective. Surg Laparosc Endosc Percutaneous Techniques 1999;9:333.

Talamini MA, Gadacz TR: Gallstone dissolution. Surg Clin North Am 1990;70:1217.

Chapter 106

Choledocholithiasis

Attila Nakeeb

Prior to the early 1990s, the management of choledocholithiasis was straightforward. Common bile duct (CBD) stones were diagnosed by intraoperative cholangiography during open cholecystectomy, and any stones found were removed by an open CBD exploration. However, with the advent of laparoscopic cholecystectomy in 1989, the approach to CBD stones has changed. Options now include preoperative endoscopic retrograde cholangiography (ERC) with endoscopic sphincterotomy and stone extraction, laparoscopic transcystic common bile duct exploration (LTCBDE), laparoscopic choledochotomy and bile duct exploration, open CBD exploration, or postoperative ERC with endoscopic sphincterotomy. The approach to managing choledocholithiasis needs to be individualized for each patient and depends on such factors as the clinical condition of the patient, institutional expertise in ERC with endoscopic sphincterotomy, the surgeon's laparoscopic ability, and the availability of the proper equipment to perform laparoscopic CBD exploration.

CLASSIFICATION AND ETIOLOGY

CBD stones can be classified as being either primary or secondary. Primary duct stones develop de novo within the bile ducts, whereas secondary stones develop in the gallbladder and subsequently fall into the CBD. In the United States more than 85% of all bile duct stones are secondary. Primary duct stones typically occur in patients with benign biliary strictures, sclerosing cholangitis, choledochal cyst disease, or sphincter of Oddi dysfunction. These conditions are all associated with bile stasis, which promotes the overgrowth of bacteria in bile. Bacterial enzymes then lead to the deconjugation of bilirubin and the breakdown of biliary lipids, which results in the formation of brown pigment stones. Secondary bile duct stones have a composition similar to that of gallbladder stones. Approximately 75% are cholesterol stones that form as the result of the supersaturation of cholesterol in bile, and 25% are black pigment stones that form as the result of excess bilirubin excretion into bile. The classification of CBD stones into primary or secondary is of therapeutic importance, because primary stones require removal of the stones and a biliary drainage procedure (choledochoenterostomy or sphincteroplasty), whereas secondary stones can be treated by removal of the stones and cholecystectomy. In general, CBD stones discovered less than 2 years after cholecystectomy are considered to be secondary stones, and those discovered after 2 years are classified as primary stones.

CLINICAL PRESENTATION

CBD stones are often asymptomatic and discovered only during cholangiography at the time of cholecystectomy.

CBD stones are present in 8% to 15% of patients with symptomatic cholecystolithiasis. The incidence varies with age and is approximately 5% in younger patients and more than 20% in older patients with gallstones. Patients with symptomatic choledocholithiasis will present with biliary colic, noncomplete extrahepatic biliary obstruction, cholangitis, or pancreatitis. Obstruction of the CBD results in right upper quadrant pain and jaundice. Typically, the pain and jaundice associated with CBD stones are more intermittent and transient than when the biliary obstruction is due to a malignancy. Cholangitis develops if obstruction to bile flow occurs in the presence of infected bile. Indeed, bacteriobilia is present in 85% of patients with choledocholithiasis. Cholangitis presents with Charcot's triad of fever, right upper quadrant pain, and jaundice. A small percentage of patients with cholangitis develop severe shock, with hypotension and mental status changes, and require urgent biliary decompression. Gallstone pancreatitis can develop from transient obstruction of the ampulla of Vater by CBD stones. Most patients with gallstone pancreatitis experience a mild, self-limited attack from which they recover within a few days. However, some patients will progress to develop severe pancreatitis with peripancreatic necrosis, infection, or pseudocyst formation.

PREDICTORS OF COMMON BILE DUCT STONES

No single clinical or laboratory variable is completely accurate in predicting the presence of choledocholithiasis. Therefore, the results of a detailed history and physical examination, laboratory evaluation, and diagnostic imaging tests must be taken together when assessing the likelihood that a patient has CBD stones. Serum liver function tests (bilirubin, alkaline phosphatase, and transaminases) can be useful in predicting common duct stones. If any one value of the liver profile is elevated, the risk of CBD stones approaches 20%. With two elevated values, the risk increases to nearly 40%; with three or more, nearly half the patients will have a CBD stone. However, about 5% of patients with no liver function abnormalities will have CBD stones identified by cholangiography at the time of cholecystectomy. A recent meta-analysis has shown the presence of cholangitis, CBD stones identified on ultrasonography, and jaundice to be the strongest indicators of CBD stones. A patient with any one of these indicators has at least ten times the risk of having CBD stones compared with a patient without any risk factor (Table 106–1).

DIAGNOSTIC STUDIES

ULTRASONOGRAPHY. Transabdominal ultrasonography is usually the first test performed when evaluating patients

Table 106–1	**Predictive Values of Preoperative Indicators of Common Bile Duct Stones**			
INDICATOR	**POSITIVE LIKELIHOOD RATIO**	**NEGATIVE LIKELIHOOD RATIO**	**SENSITIVITY**	**SPECIFICITY**
Cholangitis	18.3	0.93	0.11	0.99
CBD stones on ultrasound	13.6	0.70	0.38	1.00
Preoperative jaundice	10.1	0.69	0.36	0.97
Elevated bilirubin	4.8	0.77	0.69	0.88
Elevated alkaline phosphatase	2.6	0.65	0.57	0.86
Pancreatitis	2.1	0.96	0.10	0.95
Cholecystitis	1.6	0.94	0.50	0.76
Amylase	1.5	0.99	0.11	0.95

Adapted from Abboud BA, Malet PF, Berlin JA, et al: Predictors of common bile duct stones prior to cholecystectomy: A meta-analysis. Gastrointest Endoscopy 1996;44:450–459.

with biliary disease. Ultrasonography is very sensitive for the diagnosis of gallstones within the gallbladder. Unfortunately, its sensitivity for the detection of CBD stones is only 15% to 30%, but when seen, the specificity is quite high. However, ultrasonography can identify CBD dilation, which suggests choledocholithiasis. If the diameter of the extrahepatic bile duct is less than 3 mm, CBD stones are exceedingly rare, whereas a diameter greater than 10 mm in a jaundiced patient predicts CBD stones more than 90% of the time. Advantages of ultrasonography include its low cost, widespread availability, lack of ionizing radiation, and noninvasive nature.

MAGNETIC RESONANCE IMAGING. Magnetic resonance cholangiopancreatography (MRCP) has recently been developed as another noninvasive means of imaging the biliary tract. Several studies have shown that MRCP can diagnose CBD stones with a sensitivity of 90%, a specificity approaching 100%, and an overall diagnostic accuracy of 97%. The main advantage of MRCP is that it allows for the direct imaging of the biliary tract without the need for an intravenous or intrabiliary contrast agent or for an invasive procedure. Disadvantages include its high cost, the lack of general availability, and the lack of any therapeutic capacity. MRCP may become more popular as costs are reduced and surgeons become more skilled with laparoscopic techniques for managing CBD stones.

PREOPERATIVE CHOLANGIOGRAPHY. Cholangiography is the gold standard for diagnosis of CBD stones. Both endoscopic retrograde cholangiography (ERC) and percutaneous transhepatic cholangiography (PTC) can be used to directly visualize the biliary tree. Since ERC can be both therapeutic and diagnostic, it is the preferred approach for patients suspected of having CBD stones. Skilled endoscopists can successfully cannulate the CBD in approximately 90% of patients. ERC may be unsuccessful in patients with previous gastric surgery (Bilroth II reconstruction), periampullary diverticula, or tortuous biliary ducts. PTC may be used to image the bile ducts if ERC is unsuccessful; however, if there is no biliary dilatation, PTC is successful in only 60% to 70% of patients. It is especially useful in patients with extensive intrahepatic stone disease or biliary sepsis.

INTRAOPERATIVE CHOLANGIOGRAPHY. Debate continues over the need to perform *routine* intraoperative cholangiography at the time of cholecystectomy. Advocates of routine intraoperative cholangiography argue that asymptomatic CBD stones are identified and biliary injuries prevented by performing routine intraoperative cholangiography. Critics of this approach suggest that the incidence of retained stones is no greater when cholangiography is performed selectively, based on high risk and predictive clinical and laboratory criteria. Indications for cholangiography during open cholecystectomy include (1) a dilated CBD, (2) a wide cystic duct, (3) palpable CBD stones, (4) increased serum liver function levels or bilirubin, and (5) a history of pancreatitis. The indications for intraoperative cholangiography during laparoscopic cholecystectomy should be similar. If these criteria are adhered to strictly, approximately 30% of patients will require intraoperative cholangiography at the time of cholecystectomy. Intraoperative cholangiography can identify the size, number, and location of CBD stones in addition to defining biliary anatomy. This information is critical in choosing the most appropriate treatment for CBD stones.

Laparoscopic intraoperative cholangiography can be accomplished successfully in more than 95% of patients. After dissecting out the gallbladder–cystic duct junction, the cystic duct is clipped distally near the junction. A small incision is then made in the anterior wall of the cystic duct. A 4- or 5-French cholangiocatheter is inserted into the cystic duct either percutaneously or via a right upper quadrant trocar. Upward and lateral traction on the gallbladder can facilitate the cannulation. If the valves of Heister prevent passage of the catheter, a hydrophilic "glidewire" can be placed across the cystic duct and the cholangiocatheter advanced over the wire. The catheter is then fixed to the duct with a hemoclip or a cholangioclamp. Dilute (<50%) contrast medium should be used for cholangiography so that small stones will not be obscured by the dye. The cholangiogram should be carefully evaluated for filling defects within the ducts, the presence of contrast material entering the duodenum, and the intrahepatic biliary anatomy. If contrast medium fails to enter the duodenum, spasm of the sphincter of Oddi due to opiate administration may be responsible. Intravenous administration of naloxone or glucagon may be helpful to relieve sphincter spasm. If contrast material does not fill the intrahepatic ducts, the patient should be placed in the Trendelenburg position to favor flow of the contrast material into the hepatic ducts.

INTRAOPERATIVE ULTRASONOGRAPHY. Intraoperative ultrasonography can identify CBD stones at the time of cholecystectomy. In experienced hands, intraoperative ultrasonography is comparable to intraoperative cholangiography for diagnosis of CBD stones. Laparoscopic ultrasonography is performed with a high-frequency (7.5- to 10-mHz) probe, and the bile duct is imaged in the transverse and longitudinal planes. The distal bile duct can be visualized 95% of the time.

MANAGEMENT

Currently several options are available to the surgeon for the treatment of CBD stones. In choosing the most appropriate approach for an individual patient, factors such as the local endoscopic expertise, the surgeon's laparoscopic skill, and the patient's clinical condition must be considered. A potential algorithm for the management of CBD stones is shown in Figure 106–1.

PREOPERATIVE ENDOSCOPIC RETROGRADE CHOLANGIOGRAPHY (ERC)

ERC with endoscopic sphincterotomy is an effective treatment for CBD stones. Stones can be removed from the CBD in 90% of patients. After sphincterotomy, most stones smaller than 1 cm in diameter will pass spontaneously. A balloon catheter or stone basket can also be used to retrieve stones if needed. If endoscopic clearance is incomplete, an endoscopic stent can be placed into the CBD to maintain drainage and prevent cholangitis.

Preoperative ERC and endoscopic sphincterotomy is the preferred management option for CBD stones in several conditions. In the setting of acute suppurative cholangitis, morbidity and mortality are markedly decreased if preoperative biliary decompression and stone removal are accomplished before cholecystectomy. Patients with severe gallstone pancreatitis (Ranson criteria >3) or with significant deterioration of their clinical condition have also been shown to benefit from early ERC and stone clearance. Cholecystectomy can then be performed after the pancreatitis has resolved. In patients with a dilated CBD (>8 mm) shown on ultrasonography and jaundice, an ERC should also be performed to rule out a malignancy or biliary stricture that would alter the surgical management. In patients who are high operative risks, ERC and endoscopic sphincterotomy can be performed to remove CBD stones, and the gallbladder can be left in place. Finally, preoperative ERC and endoscopic sphincterotomy may be performed if the surgeon is not able to perform a laparoscopic bile duct exploration and when there is a high suspicion of CBD stones.

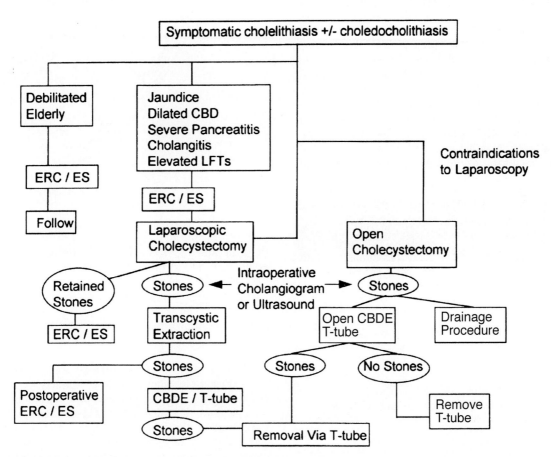

Figure 106–1. An algorithm for the management of cholelithiasis. CBD, common bile duct; CBDE, common bile duct exploration; ERC, endoscopic retrograde cholangiography; ES, endoscopic sphincterotomy; LFTs, liver function tests. (From Jones DB, Soper NJ: Common duct stones. In Cameron JL (ed): Current Surgical Therapy, 5th ed. St. Louis, CV Mosby, 1995, pp 337–342.)

Endoscopic sphincterotomy is contraindicated in patients with a coagulopathy or a long distal CBD stricture. When endoscopic sphincterotomy is combined with ERC, the morbidity rate approaches 10%. Potential complications include bleeding (2% to 3%), duodenal perforation (1%), pancreatitis (2%), and cholangitis (1% to 2%). The mortality rate after endoscopic sphincterotomy is 1%.

LAPAROSCOPIC TECHNIQUES

The two approaches for laparoscopic CBD exploration are laparoscopic transcystic common bile duct exploration (LTCBDE) or laparoscopic choledochotomy (Table 106–2). The indications for transcystic duct exploration are filling defects noted on cholangiography (CBD stones), stones less than 9 mm in diameter, stones below the cystic duct entrance to the bile duct, and fewer than six stones. Contraindications to LTCBDE are a small, friable cystic duct, more than 8 stones in the CBD, common hepatic duct stones, and stones larger than 1 cm. Laparoscopic choledochotomy can be performed if LTCBDE fails or is contraindicated, if stones are present above the cystic duct, or if there are multiple stones. The only contraindication to laparoscopic choledochotomy is a small CBD (<6 mm) that might be narrowed during its closure.

LAPAROSCOPIC TRANSCYSTIC DUCT BILE DUCT EXPLORATION.
The success rate for LTCBDE is about 85%. This technique involves blunt dissection of the cystic duct down to its junction with the CBD. A cystic ductotomy is made approximately 1.5 cm from the common duct, and a hydrophillic glidewire is inserted into the CBD. A cholangiocatheter can then be advanced over the glidewire into the CBD and saline irrigated through the catheter in an attempt to flush small stones out of the duct. If the stones in the CBD are larger than the lumen of the cystic duct, the cystic duct can be dilated with a balloon catheter. A radial balloon dilating catheter with an outer diameter the size of the largest stone but smaller

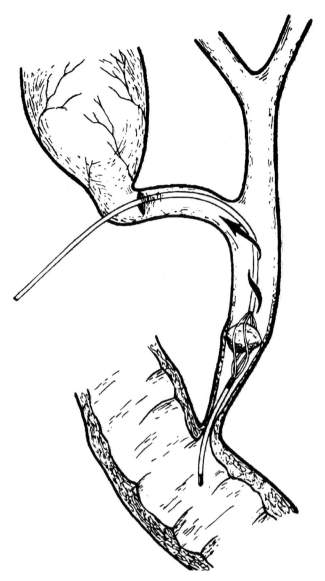

Figure 106–2. Laparoscopic transcystic bile duct exploration with a helical stone basket. (From Crawford DL, Phillips EH: Laparoscopic common bile duct exploration. World J Surg 1999;23:343–349.)

than the size of the CBD should be used to dilate the cystic duct. Stone retrieval baskets can be inserted over the glidewire and stones extracted under fluoroscopic guidance (Fig. 106–2). Helical 4- to 5-French baskets with flexible leaders should be used to avoid injuring the CBD. Approximately 75% of CBD stones can be successfully cleared with fluoroscopic wire basket techniques.

Many surgeons prefer flexible choledochoscopy via the cystic duct, which allows for stone extraction under direct vision. Success rates greater than 95% have been reported for bile duct clearance using choledochoscopy when the CBD can be successfully cannulated. After dilation of the cystic duct, a flexible choledochoscope with an outer diameter of between 2.7 mm and 3.2 mm and a working channel of at least 1.2 mm is inserted into the CBD. Stones can then be visualized directly. A stone basket can

Table 106–2	**Laparoscopic Transcystic Common Bile Duct Exploration Versus Laparoscopic Choledochotomy**

	TRANSCYSTIC	CHOLEDOCHOTOMY
Stones		
Number	<8	Any
Size	<9 mm	Any
Location	Distal to cystic duct	Entire duct
Bile duct size	Any	>6 mm
Drain	Optional cystic duct tube	T-tube
Contraindications	Friable cystic duct	Small-diameter duct
	Intrahepatic stones	Inability to suture
	Multiple large stones	laparoscopically
Advantages	No T-tube	T-tube for postoperative
	Short hospital stay	access

Adapted from Phillips EH, Korman JE: Laparoscopic management of common bile duct stones. In Cameron JL (ed): Current Surgical Therapy, 6th ed. St. Louis, CV Mosby, 1998.

be advanced past the stone and the stone captured (Fig. 106–3). The choledochoscope, basket, and stone are then removed from the cystic duct as one unit. Multiple passes of the scope are made until the duct is clear. To document stone clearance, a completion cholangiogram should be performed. A cystic duct drainage tube can be left in place if findings on the cholangiogram are equivocal. This tube can be used postoperatively for cholangiography and later for percutaneous radiographic treatment of retained stones if necessary. The cystic duct stump should be ligated—rather than clipped—for added security.

LAPAROSCOPIC CHOLEDOCHOTOMY. Laparoscopic choledochotomy is an excellent approach to CBD stones when the diameter of the CBD is 6 mm or greater. The anterior wall of the CBD is dissected bluntly and a longitudinal choledochotomy made in the anterior wall below the cystic duct. The choledochotomy should be made at least as long as the diameter of the largest stone. Two stay sutures placed in the CBD can be used to tent up the anterior wall to facilitate the incision. A larger choledochoscope (3.3 mm, 2.4-mm working channel) can then be placed into the CBD and stones extracted with baskets or balloon catheters (Fig. 106–4). The choledochotomy is then closed over a T-tube with 4-0 absorbable suture.

Advantages of laparoscopic choledochotomy over LTCBDE include the ability to remove larger stones (>1 cm), to remove stones from the proximal hepatic ducts, to remove multiple stones, and to use biliary lithotripsy to fragment impacted stones. The disadvantages of laparoscopic choledochotomy are that it requires a T-tube and considerable laparoscopic suturing skill to close the choledochotomy.

POSTOPERATIVE ERC OR CBD EXPLORATION

If CBD stones are seen on an intraoperative cholangiogram, the surgeon must decide how the stones should be managed. The options include immediate laparoscopic or open CBD exploration or referral for postoperative ERC. Postoperative ERC and endoscopic sphincterotomy is successful in about 90% of patients, provided a skilled interventional gastroenterologist is available. However, postoperative ERC is associated with the same risks as preoperative ERC, including bleeding, perforation, pancreatitis, and cholangitis. If ERC is not successful in retrieving a retained stone, the patient will require either an open procedure to clear the bile duct or an attempt at PTC with a transhepatic approach at stone retrieval. A recent prospective randomized trial has shown that in the hands of an experienced laparoscopist, laparoscopic CBD exploration at the time of laparoscopic cholecystectomy is equally as effective as ERC at achieving stone clearance. The procedure-related complication rates are similar with both approaches, but the laparoscopic bile duct exploration is associated with a significantly shorter length of hospital stay (Table 106–3).

OPEN COMMON BILE DUCT EXPLORATION

Open CBD exploration is the gold standard for removal of CBD stones. Since open CBD exploration is no longer commonly performed in our era of laparoscopic cholecystectomy, the technique is described briefly here. The first step is to fully Kocherize the duodenum so that a hand can be placed behind the head of the pancreas, allowing the distal CBD to be palpated. Occasionally, it may be possible to milk impacted stones proximally. The supraduodenal CBD is then exposed and two stay sutures placed in the CBD below the cystic duct. The anterior wall of the bile duct is then elevated with the stay sutures and a longitudinal choledochotomy made near the duodenum. The bile duct can then be explored for stones. Rigid instruments should not be used to extract stones, because they can injure the delicate ductal epithelium or perforate the distal, intrapancreatic portion of the CBD. A soft

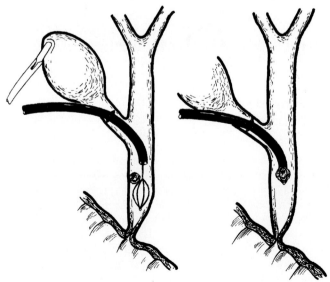

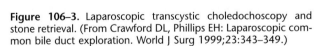

Figure 106–3. Laparoscopic transcystic choledochoscopy and stone retrieval. (From Crawford DL, Phillips EH: Laparoscopic common bile duct exploration. World J Surg 1999;23:343–349.)

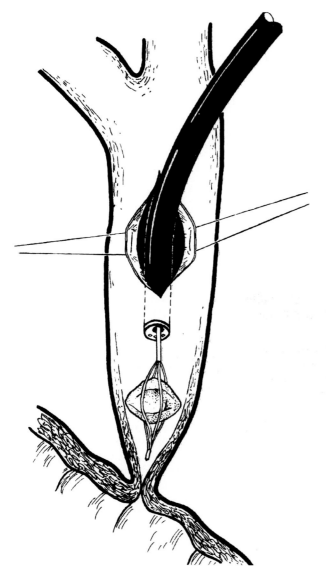

Figure 106–4. Laparoscopic choledochotomy with stone removal by choledochoscopy. (From Crawford DL, Phillips EH: Laparoscopic common bile duct exploration. World J Surg 1999;23:343–349.)

rubber irrigating catheter can be used to gently flush out any stones or debris. Balloon-tipped catheters can be passed proximally and distally into the ducts to retrieve stones.

Adequate clearance of the duct should be confirmed visually with flexible choledochoscopy. Remaining stones can be removed by irrigation with stone forceps, wire baskets, or balloon catheters. A T-tube should be placed in the bile duct and the choledochotomy closed with 4-0 absorbable suture. Completion cholangiography is performed before closing the abdomen to rule out the presence of retained stones or a bile leak around the T-tube. Postoperatively, a T-tube cholangiogram is performed 3 to 7 days after the exploration. If the cholangiogram is normal, the tube can be clamped and the tube pulled 6 weeks later. If retained stones are detected, the tract is allowed to mature, and percutaneous extraction can be performed by an interventional radiologist under fluoro-

scopic control in 4 to 6 weeks. Open CBD exploration can be accomplished with almost no mortality in patients under 60 years but has a mortality of up to 4% in elderly patients, in large part related to comorbidity and associated cholangitis.

DRAINAGE PROCEDURES

TRANSDUODENAL SPHINCTEROPLASTY. Patients with a stone impacted at the ampulla of Vater that cannot be removed with a CBD exploration or with multiple stones in a nondilated CBD may require a transduodenal sphincteroplasty to allow retrieval in retrograde fashion. A sphincteroplasty is also indicated in the presence of an ampullary stenosis or a choledochocele. The first step in a sphincteroplasty is again to perform a Kocher maneuver. A small longitudinal duodenotomy is made in the lateral aspect of the duodenum at the level of the ampulla; a common mistake is to make the duodenectomy anterior in the duodenal wall, making visualization and transampullary manipulation very difficult. Two stay sutures are placed on each side of the ampulla to elevate it. A small incision is made at the 10 to 11 o'clock position in the sphincter, taking care to avoid the pancreatic duct, which is found at the 4 o'clock position. The sphincterotomy is extended through the sphincter (approximately 1.5 cm), and the impacted stone is removed. The bile duct and duodenal mucosa are then reapproximated with interrupted 4-0 absorbable sutures. The duodenotomy can be closed transversely to prevent narrowing of the lumen.

CHOLEDOCHOENTEROSTOMY. Patients with grossly dilated bile ducts (greater than 2 cm), multiple stones (more than 5), intrahepatic stones, primary CBD stones, or a distal biliary stricture should be considered for a biliary drainage procedure. The two options are a choledochoduodenostomy or a Roux-en-Y choledochojejunostomy. The choledochoduodenostomy can be performed in either a side-to-side or an end-to-side fashion. Advantages of a choledochoduodenostomy are that it can be performed rapidly, requires only one anastomosis, and the bile duct can still be accessed endoscopically. However, a side-to-side anastomosis leaves the distal CBD in continuity and can very rarely lead to the CBD "sump syndrome." In this situation, food and debris from the duodenum enter the distal limb of the CBD and obstruct the anastomosis or the pancreatic duct orifice, leading to cholangitis or pancreatitis, respectively. Roux-en-Y choledochojejunostomy, also an excellent option for biliary drainage, is performed by a side-to-side anastomosis of the Roux-en-Y limb to the CBD or by dividing the CBD and creating an end-to-end anastomosis to a 60-cm Roux limb. Since an end-to-end choledochojejunostomy is completely diverting, the development of the sump syndrome is usually not a concern for cholangitis but can still lead to pancreatitis. For these reasons many surgeons prefer a transduodenal sphincteroplasty.

INTRAHEPATIC STONES

Intrahepatic stones are uncommon in Western countries. However, they are prevalent in Asia and represent a

Table 106–3	**Comparison of Laparoscopic Bile Duct Exploration with Postoperative Endoscopic Retrograde Cholangiography for Bile Duct Stones Identified During Laparoscopic Cholecystectomy**				
	N	PRIMARY DUCT CLEARANCE (%)	SECONDARY DUCT CLEARANCE (%)	MORBIDITY (%)	MEAN HOSPITAL LENGTH OF STAY (DAYS)
Laparoscopic CBD exploration	40	75	100	18	1.0
Postoperative ERC and endoscopic sphincterotomy	40	75	93	15	3.5

Adapted from Rhodes M, Sussman L, Cohen L, Lewis MP: Randomized trial of laparoscopic exploration of common bile duct versus postoperative endoscopic retrograde cholangiography for common bile duct stones. Lancet 1998;351:159–161.

common but difficult management problem. Intrahepatic stones are primarily brown pigment stones. In Western countries, intrahepatic stones occur in association with diseases characterized by prolonged partial bile duct obstruction, such as sclerosing cholangitis, benign and malignant biliary strictures, choledochal cysts, and Caroli's disease. In Asia, intrahepatic stones, or Oriental cholangiohepatitis, often occurs secondary to biliary parasites.

Cholangiography, either endoscopic or percutaneous, is the most valuable technique in the evaluation of patients with intrahepatic stones. The transhepatic percutaneous approach is preferable in most patients, because it allows for direct repeated access to the intrahepatic bile ducts for therapeutic interventions. Transhepatic biliary drainage catheters can be inserted and gradually upsized to a 16-French size. The tract is then allowed to mature for 5 to 6 weeks, after which the stones are removed with the use of steerable stone retrieval baskets under fluoroscopic guidance or with percutaneous choledochoscopy.

Although some patients with intrahepatic stone disease can be managed nonoperatively, many patients require surgical intervention. A Roux-en-Y hepaticojejunostomy is usually constructed, with intraoperative choledochoscopy used to clear the bile ducts of stones. Large-bore transhepatic stents can be placed intraoperatively to provide later or chronic access to the biliary tree for percutaneous stone extraction or the treatment of strictures postoperatively. Using this approach, a stone clearance rate of greater than 90% can be expected (Table 106–4). Another option for management of intrahepatic stones is the creation of a hepaticocutaneous jejunostomy. This technique involves creating a side-to-side Roux-en-Y hepaticojeju-

Pearls and Pitfalls

- Common duct stones are either primary duct stones (brown pigment, earthy stones) that form secondary to bile stasis from bacterial sources, or secondary duct stones that originated in the gallbladder.
- Choledocholithiasis may be asymptomatic or present with a spectrum of signs involving Charcot's triad (right upper quadrant pain, fever, jaundice).
- Suspicion of choledocholithiasis is based on signs and symptoms and other predictors, such as abnormal serum liver function tests, a recent history of pancreatitis, and a CBD greater than 6 mm.
- Diagnosis may include preoperative ultrasonography, ERC, PTC, or MRCP or may be made at the time of operation via intraoperative cholangiography.
- Management of preoperatively diagnosed choledocholithiasis involves either ERC with endoscopic sphincterotomy or CBD exploration via an open or laparoscopic technique.
- Management of intraoperatively diagnosed choledocholithiasis involves immediate open or laparoscopic CBD exploration or postoperative ERC with endoscopic sphincterotomy.
- Primary common duct stones should be treated not only by clearance of the duct but also by some form of biliary drainage procedure: sphincteroplasty, choledochoduodenotomy, or choledochojejunostomy.

nostomy with a longer than usual Roux limb and extending the blind end of the Roux limb beyond the anastomosis up to the anterior abdominal wall. The limb is then marked with metal wire or clips that allow an easy percutaneous access to the biliary system if needed. If the intrahepatic stone disease is isolated to a single lobe or segment of liver and is associated with significant intrahepatic biliary strictures or atrophy, a hepatic resection may be the best approach to the treatment of the stone disease.

SELECTED READINGS

Abboud BA, Malet PF, Berlin JA, et al: Predictors of common bile duct stones prior to cholecystectomy: A meta-analysis. Gastrointest Endosc 1996;44:450.

Crawford DL, Phillips EH: Laparoscopic common bile duct exploration. World J Surg 1999;23:343.

Cuschieri A, Lezoche E, Morino M, et al: E.A.E.S. multicenter prospective

Table 106–4	**Treatment of Intrahepatic Stone Disease at the Johns Hopkins Hospital**
Patients	54
Percutaneous treatment only	26%
Surgical treatment	74%
Postoperative percutaneous treatment	33%
Mean follow-up	60 mo
Successful stone clearance	94%
Patients symptom free	87%
Recurrent stones or stricture	20%

Adapted from Pitt HA, Venbrux AC, Coleman JA, et al: Intrahepatic stones: The transhepatic team approach. Ann Surg 1994;219:527–537.

randomized trial comparing two-stage vs. single-stage management of patients with gallstone disease and ductal calculi. Surg Endosc 1999;13:952.

Freeman M, Nelson D, Sherman S, et al: Complications of endoscopic biliary sphincterotomy. N Engl J Med 1996;335:909.

Pitt HA, Venbrux AC, Coleman JA, et al: Intrahepatic stones: The transhepatic team approach. Ann Surg 1994;219:527.

Rhodes M, Sussman L, Cohen L, Lewis MP: Randomized trial of laparoscopic exploration of common bile duct versus postoperative endoscopic retrograde cholangiography for common bile duct stones. Lancet 1998;351:159.

Rosenthal RJ, Rossi RL, Martin RF: Options and strategies for the management of choledocholithiasis. World J Surg 1998;22:1125.

Tierney S, Pitt HA: Choledocholithiasis and cholangitis. In Bell RH, Rikkers LF, Mulholland MW (eds): Digestive Tract Surgery: A Text and Atlas. Philadelphia, Lippincott-Raven, 1996, pp 407–431.

Chapter 107
Choledochal Cyst

Jennifer R. Curry and Raymond J. Joehl

Choledochal cysts have typically been described as an affliction of infancy and childhood. However, the diagnosis of choledochal cyst disease is becoming a more frequent occurrence for adults. Cystic disease of the biliary tree is an uncommon problem that is often confused with benign biliary tract or pancreatic disease. Choledochal cysts are congenital dilations of the extrahepatic and/or intrahepatic bile duct. As a result of improved imaging technology, the diagnosis and, therefore, the known incidence of choledochal cysts has increased. Complications of cystic biliary disease include cholangitis, cystolithiasis, jaundice, and cholangiocarcinoma. Cyst excision is imperative for both treatment and prevention of malignancy.

ETIOPATHOGENESIS

The pathogenesis of choledochal cysts remains obscure. It is unclear whether choledochal cysts are truly congenital or whether they may be acquired early in life. The classic embryologic theory suggests that cystic abnormalities result from inequality in the proliferation of epithelial cells at the stage when the primitive biliary ducts are still solid. If the cellular proliferation is increased at the hepatic portion compared with the duodenal portion of the bile duct during epithelial occlusion, then at canalization the hepatic portion will become abnormally dilated. The distal bile duct remains normal in size or becomes narrowed or stenotic. The distal stenosis may cause increased proximal pressure, which further weakens the proximal common duct and leads to its dilation.

In 1969, Babbit proposed that an abnormal junction of the pancreaticobiliary system was the basis of biliary ductal cyst development. Normally, the common channel of the pancreatic and bile ducts is shorter than 10 mm in adults. However, most patients with choledochal cysts have a much longer common pancreaticobiliary channel (>20 mm). This anomalous junction results in loss of the normal sphincteric mechanism. Because secretory pressure in the pancreas is greater than hepatic and common bile duct pressure, pancreatic juice may reflux into the biliary tree, which may, in turn, result in inflammation and degradation of the ductal wall with subsequent dilation. However, this abnormal choledochopancreatic junction has also been found in patients with no evidence of biliary ductal cysts. Moreover, not all patients with biliary tree dilations have an abnormal junction. Therefore, the role of anomalous duct anatomy as the cause of choledochal cyst disease is unclear.

ANATOMIC CLASSIFICATION AND PATHOLOGY

In 1959, Alonso-Lej and colleagues reviewed the world literature on biliary duct disease and proposed the first widely used classification system of choledochal cysts. In 1977, Todani and associates modified that classification to the currently accepted classification, which includes intrahepatic ductal disease (Table 107–1).

Type I cysts are the most common and compose 60% to 80% of all patients with choledochal cysts. Of the three subtypes of type I, the cystic variety is the most common, followed by the fusiform type. The focal subtype is the least frequent. Type I cysts tend to be large, involve the entire common bile duct, and may extend from the porta hepatis into the intrapancreatic bile duct. The common bile duct usually narrows distal to the cyst, and the ampulla may be compressed by the large cyst, causing obstructive jaundice.

Type II cysts are isolated diverticula of the common bile duct; they account for less than 3% of all choledochal cysts. Type III cysts, also known as choledochoceles, are characterized by dilation of the intraduodenal portion of the common bile duct and account for 2% to 6% of choledochal cysts. In these type III cysts, the cystic dilation may also be intrapancreatic, causing obstructive jaundice and episodes of pancreatitis. Typically, both the common bile duct and the main pancreatic duct enter the choledochocele separately. The choledochocele, in turn, communicates with the duodenal lumen through a separate opening. Choledochoceles have no potential for malignancy because the cyst walls are lined with normal duodenal mucosa. Type IVa disease (combined intrahepatic and extrahepatic biliary dilation) occurs in 20% to 40% of patients with choledochal cysts, whereas isolated intrahepatic cysts (type IVb) are relatively rare.

With the exception of choledochocele, histopathology is similar for all these cysts. Normal biliary epithelium is either absent or replaced by an abnormal columnar epithelium. Glandular cavities may be found in the mucosal layer, associated with a chronic inflammatory cell infiltrate. The wall of the cyst is usually thickened with dense collagenous tissue within the strands of smooth muscle.

Table 107–1 | **Anatomic Classification of Cystic Disease of the Biliary Tree (Choledochal Cysts)**

Type I, cystic dilation of the common bile duct (extrahepatic biliary tree); type Ia, cystic; type Ib, focal; type Ic, fusiform

Type II, saccular diverticulum of the common bile duct (extrahepatic biliary tree)

Type III, choledochocele—dilation of the common bile duct within the duodenum (extrahepatic biliary tree)

Type IVa, multiple dilations of the intrahepatic and extrahepatic biliary tree

Type IVb, multiple extrahepatic cysts

Type V, Caroli's disease—dilation confined to the intrahepatic biliary tree

Infants and young children have less evidence of inflammatory changes, whereas adults typically have more inflammation extending to adjacent structures, such as the portal vein. In most patients with choledochal cyst disease, there are no abnormalities in liver histology. However, there may be minor periportal fibrosis and evidence of chronic biliary obstruction, especially in adult patients. Although calculi may be found within the cysts, they are bilirubinate pigment stones and are due to biliary stasis.

CLINICAL PRESENTATION

The incidence of choledochal cysts ranges from 1:100,000 to 1:150,000. More than one third of all reported patients are Japanese. There is a 3:1 female-to-male predominance. Approximately 60% of patients are diagnosed before the age of 10 years. However, with the advances in diagnostic imaging, more adults are being recognized with choledochal cyst disease.

The classic triad of jaundice, right upper quadrant mass, and episodic abdominal pain is present in only a minority of patients (5% to 30%). Most children have two of the three classic findings. Jaundice is more likely present in children than in adults. A palpable abdominal mass is also a finding more common in children. Adults tend to have nausea and vomiting in association with abdominal pain. Pancreatitis and a history of cholecystectomy for biliary symptoms are also more common in adults.

CASE STUDY

A 20-year-old female college student presented with several days of anorexia, lethargy, nausea, vomiting, chills, fever, and upper abdominal pain. Physical examination demonstrated mild distress, slight scleral icterus, tenderness in the right upper quadrant and midepigastrium, and no abdominal masses. Serum total bilirubin was 2.8 mg, and alkaline phosphatase was 212 U/L (normal <110 U/L); other laboratory studies were normal. Ultrasonography showed cholecystolithiasis with a moderately dilated common bile duct. At laparoscopic cholecystectomy, the surgeon found unusual anatomy and converted to an "open" procedure. The gallbladder was removed, and a T tube was inserted into a dilated common bile duct. After transfer of the patient to a university center, a cholangiogram demonstrated a fusiform choledochal cyst involving the common hepatic duct, and the common bile duct was saccular. A very narrow distal common bile duct stricture was evident (Fig. 107–1). One week after the initial operation, excision of the extrahepatic bile duct system and the choledochal cyst was performed with Roux-en-Y hepaticojejunostomy. The pathology report showed a benign choledochal cyst. The patient's bilirubin level normalized, and she was discharged 5 days postoperatively. Six months later, she resumed college.

PREOPERATIVE MANAGEMENT

The diagnosis of choledochal cyst disease depends on accurate imaging rather than on physical examination or

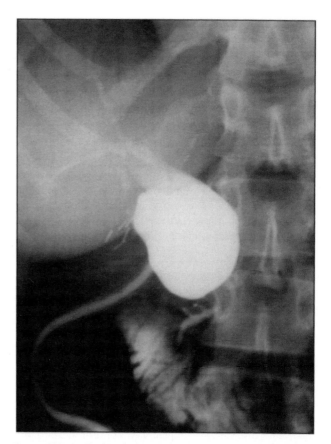

Figure 107–1. T-tube cholangiogram in patient with choledochal cyst 1 week after cholecystectomy. A fusiform choledochal cyst involves the common hepatic duct, whereas the common bile duct is saccular. A narrow, distal common bile duct stricture is visible.

laboratory values. Laboratory evaluation may demonstrate mildly abnormal liver function or amylase values, but it is often not helpful in establishing the diagnosis. Plain radiographs may suggest a right upper quadrant mass or a calcified cyst, or they may be normal. Upper gastrointestinal contrast studies may be useful for larger cysts, which displace the duodenum anteromedially.

Cholangiography is the most essential tool in the diagnosis and delineation of biliary cyst disease. Endoscopic retrograde cholangiopancreatography best visualizes the pancreaticobiliary junction but may not fully define the intrahepatic extent of the cysts. Percutaneous transhepatic cholangiography is complementary because, by visualizing the proximal ductal system, it helps define type IV and type V cysts. A cholangiogram excludes other causes of dilated common bile duct, such as tumor or stone, and establishes the anatomic relations necessary to formulate an operative plan. The use of cholangiography increased preoperative diagnosis of choledochal cysts from less than 40% of patients in the 1970s to more than 80% of patients in the 1990s.

Other diagnostic resources include ultrasonography and computed tomography (CT). Ultrasonography can accurately determine size, contour, and location. CT also delineates the size, location, and extent of intrahepatic and extrahepatic biliary dilation. Magnetic resonance imaging may prove useful in the noninvasive diagnosis and definition of choledochal cysts.

OPERATIVE MANAGEMENT

When the diagnosis is made, choledochal cysts should be excised, with reconstruction by Roux-en-Y hepaticojejunostomy. Exception to this standard practice involves treatment of Caroli's disease and type III cysts. External drainage of choledochal cysts is indicated as a treatment only in patients severely ill from sepsis or cholangitis. Although enteric drainage without resection was the mainstay of therapy in the 1950s, long-term follow-up revealed the rate of reoperation and postoperative morbidity to be 30% to 50%. A high incidence of anastomotic stricture associated with cholangitis and stone disease occurred when cyst walls were not completely excised but were instead used as sites for biliary enteric anastomosis. Moreover, the risk of malignancy in retained choledochal cysts is unacceptably high, indicating the need for total cyst excision whenever possible. From the 1970s to the present, complete excision of the cyst with Roux-en-Y hepaticojejunostomy became standard practice; it is associated with a decreased incidence of stricture, cholangitis, and malignancy.

Operative Technique

Preoperative placement of biliary catheters may be necessary to decompress the biliary system and may facilitate identification of the bile ducts. The ascending colon and hepatic flexure are reflected inferiorly and medially, and an extensive Kocher's maneuver is performed, providing exposure of the entire biliary tree. The gallbladder and the cystic duct are mobilized, and the right hepatic artery is identified. Whenever a choledochal cyst operation is performed, the gallbladder is removed. Once the gallbladder is removed, the anterior wall of the cyst is identified in the porta hepatis and is mobilized to where the common bile duct passes behind the posterior aspect of the pancreas. The anterior wall of the distal common bile duct is divided transversely, and preoperatively placed stents are mobilized through the opened duct.

The posterior wall of the cyst is then divided, and the defunctionalized distal common bile duct is oversewn. The cyst is reflected anteriorly in a cephalad direction and dissected free from the portal vein and hepatic artery until a normal-caliber common hepatic duct is located. In most patients, the bifurcation of the hepatic ducts is uninvolved with cystic dilation, and an anastomosis between the proximal-most common hepatic duct and a Roux-en-Y limb of jejunum is performed. If dilation extends to the bifurcation, the hepatic duct is divided just distal to the bifurcation.

Reconstruction is accomplished using a 60-cm, retrocolic, Roux-en-Y loop of jejunum. An end-to-side hepaticojejunostomy is created using a single layer of monofilament absorbable or long-lasting absorbable sutures. Transhepatic stents can be placed through the hepatic ductal anastomosis and into the Roux limb, especially if the hepatic duct is small (<7 mm). These transhepatic catheters should be left in place for 4 to 8 weeks to decompress and protect the anastomosis and to provide access for postoperative cholangiography.

When serious inflammation and scar are encountered around the cyst, the posterior or medial aspect of the cyst wall can be left intact to avoid injury to the portal vein and hepatic artery during efforts to excise the cyst. The anterior, lateral, and medial walls of the cyst should be completely excised, but the posterior wall should be divided into a thick inner layer and a thin outer layer. The inner layer is removed by blunt dissection, and the outer layer is left adherent to the portal vessels (a modification described by Lilly in 1979). This procedure has some risk of subsequent malignant degeneration of the retained posterior outer layer of the choledochal cyst.

COMPLICATIONS AND OUTCOMES

Many complications have been associated with choledochal cyst disease. The most commonly reported is cystolithiasis. Choledocholithiasis coexists in 8% of patients and is believed to be due to biliary stasis, which explains the predominance of pigment stones. Jaundice, recurrent cholangitis, pancreatitis, and cholecystitis are other common complications. However, the second most common complication is development of cholangiocarcinoma. Cholangiocarcinoma may involve the gallbladder, duodenum, and intrahepatic ducts as well as the cyst itself. The average age at diagnosis is 32 years, which is much younger than the age at which primary cholangiocarcinoma occurs. The age at diagnosis of a choledochal cyst appears to be related to the later development of carcinoma. In patients who have choledochal cysts discovered at 10 years of age or younger, the risk of developing cholangiocarcinoma is approximately 1%, whereas the risk increases to 15% for patients older than 20 years. Not only is age at diagnosis related to risk of carcinoma, but treatment is an important factor as well. In 1977, Todani and associates reported a higher incidence (17.5%) of carcinoma arising within choledochal cysts that had been previously treated with cyst bypass. The higher incidence and young age at diagnosis of cholangiocarcinoma may be related to the anomalous pancreaticobiliary junction resulting in reflux of pancreatic enzymes into the biliary tree. Rare complications include secondary biliary cirrhosis with portal hypertension, cyst rupture with diffuse peritonitis, and hepatic fibrosis.

Postoperative complications after choledochal cyst excision and biliary reconstruction are relatively uncommon. Typically, the postoperative length of hospitalization is 7 to 10 days. Anastomotic leak may occur and is usually recognized by the presence of bile in an operatively placed drain. Cholangiography can be used to confirm the presence of a biliary-enteric anastomotic leak. Most patients heal these leaks with percutaneous external biliary drainage. Occasionally, anastomotic narrowing or stenosis may occur (<10% incidence). In addition, pancreatitis may develop if distal dissection of the cyst was too extensive or if sutures were placed that subsequently occluded pancreatic ductal flow.

CAROLI'S DISEASE

In 1958, Caroli and colleagues described congenital dilations of intrahepatic bile ducts involving a segment, a sector, a lobe, or both halves of the liver. This disease is also known as type V choledochal cyst disease. Caroli's disease is a rare entity divided into a simple type and a periportal fibrotic type. Simple Caroli's disease, although complicated by recurring inflammation, infection, and pain, is not associated with hepatic fibrosis and portal hypertension. The periportal fibrotic type tends to present in childhood, whereas the simple type presents later in life as fluctuating episodes of symptoms and infections.

The etiology of Caroli's disease is unknown, but it is thought to be hereditary. Stenosis and dilations of the bile ducts give rise to biliary stasis and, secondarily, to intrahepatic biliary lithiasis and biliary infection. Clinically, patients suffer from intermittent episodes of right upper abdominal pain and fever. Patients also experience asymptomatic periods for years between episodes. However, the normal course of Caroli's disease is dominated by recurrent or persistent biliary infection consisting of suppurative cholangitis, septicemia with gram-negative organisms, and intrahepatic as well as subphrenic abscesses. Caroli's disease may also be associated with nephrospongiosis or Cacchi-Ricci disease.

Diagnosis is made by radiologic examination of the biliary system (as well as the urinary tract). Cholangiography will demonstrate abnormal dilations of the intrahepatic bile ducts. CT is helpful in visualizing dilations of the biliary system, calculi within the ducts, and renal malformations. Ultrasonography may be useful in demonstrating intracystic vascular tracts (Marchal's sign), which are pathognomonic for type V choledochal cyst disease. Intravenous urography should be considered because of the frequent association with nephrospongiosis.

The treatment of patients with Caroli's disease depends on anatomic characteristics, presence or absence of associated liver disease, and extent of infection. Localized forms that involve one lobe of the liver (almost always the left lobe) are potentially curable by resection. Therefore, unilobular type V disease is best treated with a hepatic lobectomy. Bilateral ductal dilation can be managed with the insertion of long-term indwelling transhepatic catheters that are used to flush the ducts and allow access to the biliary tree for cholangioscopy. In patients with severe cirrhosis secondary to hepatic fibrosis or recurring cholan-

---

Pearls and Pitfalls

- Symptoms and signs of a choledochal cyst mimic biliary colic, cholecystitis, or choledocholithiasis.
- The best diagnostic tests include direct ductal imaging procedures.
- With improvements in imaging, more adults with choledochal cysts are being recognized.
- Todani's classification system describes the anatomic location of the cystic changes.
- The best treatment involves complete excision of the entire choledochal cyst, not biliary-enteric drainage of the cyst wall.
- Patients with choledochal cysts have an increased risk of developing cholangiocarcinoma, not only within the cyst but also throughout the rest of the biliary tree.
- Risk of cholangiocarcinoma varies directly with age at diagnosis.

---

gitis, orthotopic hepatic transplantation should be considered.

The prognosis associated with unilobular disease amenable to resection is good. However, prognosis for patients with bilateral intrahepatic cysts is poor. Caroli's disease is associated with development of cholangiocarcinoma with a risk as high as 7%. Therefore, aggressive surgical treatment for unilobular disease and the option of transplantation for bilobular intrahepatic disease are necessary for a favorable outcome in patients with type V cyst disease.

SELECTED READINGS

Lenriot J, Gigot JF, Segol P, et al: Bile duct cysts in adults. Ann Surg 1998;228:159.

Lilly JR: Total excision of choledochal cysts. Surg Gynecol Obstet 1979;146:254.

Lipsett P, Pitt HA, Colombani PM, et al: Choledochal cyst disease: A changing pattern of presentation. Ann Surg 1994;220:644.

Nagorney D, McIlrath D, Adson M: Choledochal cysts in adults: Clinical management. Surgery 1984;196:656.

Rossi R, Silverman ML, Braasch JW, et al: Carcinomas arising in cystic conditions of the bile duct. Am Surg 1987;205:377.

Todani T, Watanabe Y, Narusue E, et al: Bile duct cysts: Classification, operative procedures, and review of 37 cases including cancer arising from choledochal cyst. Am J Surg 1977;134:263.

Chapter 108

Biliary Dyskinesia

James Toouli

Motility disorders of the gastrointestinal tract are common. Biliary motility disorders are also known as *biliary dyskinesia*; this term refers to a spectrum of acalculous disorders of either the gallbladder or the sphincter of Oddi. Patients present clinically in one of three ways: with gallbladder dyskinesia, with sphincter of Oddi dysfunction of the bile duct sphincter, or with sphincter of Oddi dysfunction of the pancreatic sphincter.

GALLBLADDER

Abdominal pain is the most common symptom associated with a motility disorder of the gallbladder. The pain is usually felt in the epigastrium or in the right upper quadrant. This pain occurs in episodes and is quite severe, often lasting 2 to 3 hours or until it is relieved by analgesics. It may radiate to the back and under the tip of the right scapula. The pain may follow a high-fat meal and may be associated with nausea and vomiting. Occasionally, the pain wakes the patient in the early hours of the morning and is not relieved by changing posture or taking antacids.

Examination during an episode of pain reveals tenderness under the right costal margin, and there may be localized guarding, but this is usually absent. The temperature is usually normal, and there are no changes in white blood cell count or in liver function or serum amylase. Although these symptoms occur most commonly in women aged 35 to 55 years, they are also recognized in younger or older patients of either sex.

The diagnosis of gallbladder disease owing to gallstones is usually made during the presentation described earlier, and thus the most appropriate first investigation is biliary ultrasonography. In these patients, the typical findings are of a normal gallbladder, with no sludge and no bile duct dilation. When other possible causes of upper abdominal pain (e.g., peptic ulcer, irritable bowel syndrome, nonulcer dyspepsia) have been excluded, options include a second ultrasonography or an oral cholecystogram.

In patients for whom the suspicion of biliary tract disease remains strong, further investigation should be pursued. Endoscopic retrograde cholangiopancreatography (ERCP) or, more recently, magnetic resonance cholangiopancreatography is sometimes useful to eliminate the presence of a small stone in the bile duct and may be combined with endoscopy to exclude any gastric or duodenal pathology.

At the end of the endoscopic procedure, gallbladder contraction may be produced by intravenous injection of cholecystokinin octapeptide (CCK-OP), 40 ng/kg over 3 minutes. Gallbladder bile, which flows into the bile duct and duodenum, can then be aspirated through the ERCP catheter and examined for the presence of cholesterol crystals. This technique provides a "pure" sample of bile. The finding of cholesterol crystals in gallbladder bile is strongly associated with the presence of small calculi in the gallbladder or cholesterolosis. Such patients usually benefit from cholecystectomy. In patients for whom ERCP has not been performed, bile from the gallbladder can be obtained for examination for crystals by placing a catheter in the duodenum and aspirating bile through the tube after the administration of CCK-OP.

Provocation tests have been used to reproduce pain in patients with suspected gallbladder motility disorders. These investigations, which involve an infusion over 3 minutes of CCK-OP to determine if patients have reproduction of their typical pain, lack objectivity and are not recommended. A more objective investigation uses technetium 99m–labeled iminodiacetic acid or its derivatives to study the volume of the hepatobiliary system via gamma camera and computer analysis (called a hepato-iminodiacetic acid [HIDA] scan) (Fig. 108–1). The gallbladder ejection fraction (GBEF) may be derived by use of the following formula:

$$\text{GBEF (\%)} = \frac{\text{change in gallbladder activity}}{\text{baseline gallbladder activity}} \times 100$$

The normal gallbladder empties more than 50% of its volume in response to a standard meal or a 45-minute intravenous infusion of CCK-OP (20 ng/kg per hour). An abnormal GBEF has a value of less than 40%. The patient should not experience pain during the performance of this investigation, although mild cramping and nausea are common.

The timing of the CCK-OP–stimulated HIDA scan, however, is important. The CCK-OP infusion is begun only *after* the gallbladder has filled with the biliary excretion agent; this usually takes 30 to 60 minutes. The CCK-OP infusion is *not* begun before or at the time of intravenous administration of the biliary excretion agent. Also, CCK-OP should be given as an infusion rather than as a bolus; the latter method can stimulate false-positive tests.

The appropriate treatment for patients with identified gallbladder dyskinesia is cholecystectomy. Its efficacy was evaluated in 24 patients with an abnormal GBEF. Patients were randomized prospectively to either cholecystectomy or noninterventional follow-up. All but one of the patients having cholecystectomy were cured of biliary symptoms at 3 years after the operation. Histologic examination of the gallbladders removed at operation revealed features of chronic cholecystitis such as increased gallbladder wall thickness, fibrosis, and chronic inflammatory cells. None of the patients had gallstones. Those patients who did not have cholecystectomy continued to have symptoms, and three patients subsequently developed gallstones.

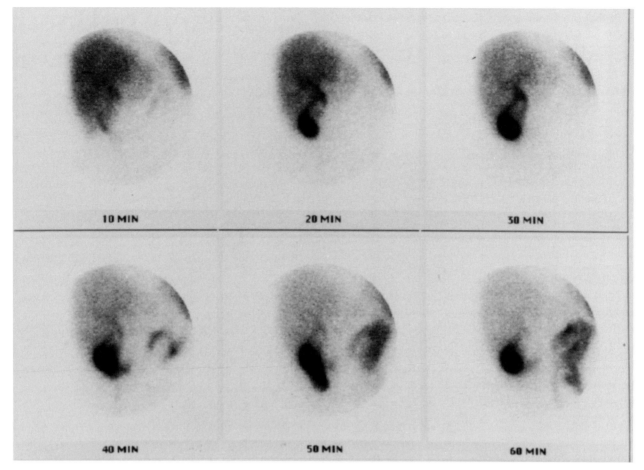

10 MIN   20 MIN   30 MIN

40 MIN   50 MIN   60 MIN

Figure 108–1. Gallbladder scintigraphy, illustrating an abnormal gallbladder ejection fraction in response to infusion of cholecystokinin octapeptide.

Consequently, patients with symptoms suggestive of gallbladder dyskinesia who have a GBEF of less than 40% should undergo laparoscopic cholecystectomy.

SPHINCTER OF ODDI

In the late 1800s, Rugero Oddi proposed that the sphincter he had recently identified could malfunction, resulting in clinical symptoms. This motility disorder of the biliary tract is known as sphincter of Oddi dysfunction.

The pathogenesis of dysfunction of the sphincter of Oddi is unknown. One possibility is the existence of primary disorders of local or systemic smooth muscle contractility, perhaps related to defects in the enteric nervous system. Secondary disorders also seem likely, either from direct damage to the sphincter (e.g., passage of a gallstone, postinflammatory stenosis) or from indirect effects of humoral factors that modulate motility on the sphincter.

The sphincter of Oddi is a smooth muscle structure of approximately 1 cm in length situated at the junction of the bile duct, the pancreatic duct, and the duodenum. Its function has been characterized by manometric techniques that allow direct measurement of pressure changes within the sphincter using a small catheter directed into either the bile duct or the pancreatic duct—so-called manometry.

The sphincter normally produces high-pressure phasic contractions that are superimposed on a modest basal pressure. The pressure changes produce a resistance to flow while at the same time propelling small volumes of bile or pancreatic juice into the duodenum. Most flow occurs between the phasic contractions, but the contractions also serve to keep the sphincter segment empty. The sphincter does not serve as a pump, but rather as a low-pressure resistor. An increase in flow and a decrease in resistance across the sphincter occur when there is a fall in basal pressure and a decrease in the amplitude and frequency of phasic contractions. These changes in resistance are normally produced by neural stimuli via local reflexes from the duodenum or by circulating hormones such as cholecystokinin. Thus, increases in delivery of bile into the duodenum occur from a decrease in pressure across the sphincter.

Clinically, patients who present with sphincter of Oddi dysfunction can be divided into two broad groups. The majority of patients have symptoms that are mainly referable to the biliary tract, whereas a smaller group present with symptoms that are referable to the pancreas.

The majority of patients with sphincter of Oddi dysfunction are women who have had a cholecystectomy for treatment of presumed symptomatic gallstones. The operation usually results in improvement in symptoms, but pain recurs after 2 to 10 years. The pain generally occurs in episodes that last for up to several hours or until relieved by analgesics. These episodes may occur at intervals of weeks or months. Some patients also describe discomfort in the upper abdomen that is more frequent, possibly occurring every day. In addition, symptoms consistent with irritable bowel syndrome may coexist with episodic biliary-type pain. Some patients are aware that their symptoms can be precipitated or aggravated by opioid analgesics, including codeine. Indeed, the first episode of pain may have been experienced after taking opiate medication, usually for an unrelated procedure.

Physical examination during an acute episode of pain reveals a distressed but afebrile patient who often moves on the examination couch to find the most comfortable position. Abdominal examination is usually noncontributory beyond revealing mild to moderate tenderness in the epigastrium or right upper quadrant. Signs of local or general peritonitis are *not* associated with this condition.

Blood screens reveal a normal white blood cell count, but 20% of patients show increases in serum concentrations of liver transaminases (particularly in blood specimens that are taken 3 to 4 hours after the onset of pain), occasionally accompanied by increases in serum bilirubin and alkaline phosphatase. In a subgroup of patients, the serum amylase may be increased either solely or in conjunction with changes in liver enzymes. These patients' affliction is often given the clinical label of idiopathic recurrent pancreatitis.

Patients who present with significant postcholecystectomy biliary- or pancreatic-type symptoms should be evaluated by ERCP. The majority of patients will have a cause other than sphincter of Oddi dysfunction to explain their symptoms—most commonly, bile duct stones. During ERCP, it is important to correctly position the patient to adequately screen the bile and pancreatic ducts. It should also be noted whether pain is produced on manipulating the sphincter of Oddi with the ERCP catheter. The rate of drainage of contrast material from the bile duct after the procedure may also be important. Pain reproduction and delayed flow from the bile duct have low sensitivity and specificity for sphincter of Oddi dysfunction; however, they are supportive of the diagnosis in the setting of symptoms and radiologic signs such as duct dilation. A number of studies have now shown that significant bile duct dilation (more than 2 to 3 mm) does *not* occur after cholecystectomy and that dilation of the bile duct suggests a relative stenosis of the sphincter of Oddi.

Flow across the sphincter of Oddi may be evaluated in postcholecystectomy subjects using cholescintigraphy after the injection of a technetium 99m–labeled iminodiacetic acid derivative, which is excreted into bile from the liver. This is a minimally invasive investigation that may provide useful data regarding flow dynamics across the sphincter of Oddi. Unfortunately, methodologic problems, including difficulty with the clear separation of liver, bile duct, and duodenum and errors induced by bile duct

dilation, make this investigation one of low sensitivity for sphincter of Oddi dysfunction. However, delay in flow of radionuclide from the bile duct into the duodenum suggests an increased resistance to flow that could be due to sphincter of Oddi dysfunction.

Techniques to measure pressure across the sphincter of Oddi have enhanced our understanding of the normal physiology of the human sphincter of Oddi and have also defined with accuracy and reproducibility the presence of manometric disorders of the sphincter. Miniaturized manometry catheters, made of either polyethylene or Teflon, are used for pressure measurement and have three lumens. The outer diameter measures 1.5 mm or 1.7 mm, and the catheter has three side holes on its recording tip at 2-mm intervals, starting 10 mm from the distal tip. Thus, the three lumens record across a length of 5 mm from within the sphincter of Oddi complex. The catheter is connected to transducers in series. The catheter is perfused with water, and the whole system is capable of accurately recording pressure changes of up to 300 mm Hg/sec.

Sphincter of Oddi manometry is carried out using a side-viewing duodenoscope, as for ERCP. The manometry catheter is inserted through the biopsy channel. The catheter is passed into either the bile duct or the pancreatic duct to record the duct pressure. It is then withdrawn so that all three recording ports are positioned within the sphincter segment (Fig. 108–2). Baseline recording from the sphincter is made for approximately 3 to 5 minutes. The response to an intravenous bolus dose of CCK-OP, 20 ng/kg, is then assessed. Catheter position in either the pancreatic duct or the bile duct may be assessed by injecting contrast medium (<1 mL) through the most distal port while screening by fluoroscopy.

Endoscopic sphincter of Oddi manometry is the most objective of all available investigations for determining the characteristics of sphincter of Oddi motility (Table 108–1). Furthermore, when the procedure is done by

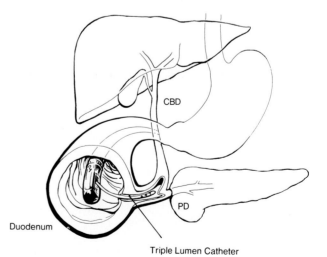

Figure 108–2. Endoscopic sphincter of Oddi manometry. The triple-lumen catheter is passed through the biopsy channel of a duodenoscope and inserted into either the bile duct or the pancreatic duct so that the three ports record from the sphincter.

Table 108–1	**Characteristics of Sphincter of Oddi Manometry**

| | NORMAL VALUES | | |
CHARACTERISTICS	Median	Range	ABNORMAL VALUES
Basal pressure (mm Hg)	15	3–35	>40
Amplitude (mm Hg)	135	95–195	>300
Frequency (n/min)	4	2–6	>7
Sequences			
Antegrade (%)	80	12–100	
Simultaneous (%)	13	0–50	
Retrograde (%)	9	0–50	>50
CCK, 20 ng/kg	Inhibits		Contracts

CCK, cholecystokinin.

staff with experience in performing biliary manometry, the diagnosis is reproducible and appears to differentiate normally functioning sphincters from abnormally functioning ones. Manometrically, the sphincter of Oddi is characterized by regular phasic contractions superimposed on a modest basal pressure (Fig. 108–3). The majority of the contractions are oriented in an antegrade direction, but simultaneous and retrograde contractions can be recorded in control subjects. However, the decision to proceed with endoscopic manometry should not be taken lightly because as many as 5% to 8% of subjects will develop postprocedural acute pancreatitis.

Manometric abnormalities have been identified in patients with clinically suspected sphincter of Oddi dysfunction. Using these manometric findings, sphincter of Oddi dysfunction has been subdivided, irrespective of whether the symptoms are primarily biliary or pancreatic, into two major groups (Table 108–2): sphincter of Oddi stenosis and sphincter of Oddi dyskinesia. This manometric division has allowed the targeting of specific therapies for

patients in whom diagnosis of sphincter of Oddi dysfunction is made.

Sphincter of Oddi Stenosis

Manometrically, these patients have an increased basal pressure of more than 40 mm Hg within the sphincter of Oddi (Fig. 108–4). Patients with manometric stenosis of the sphincter of Oddi may have a dilated bile duct at ERCP and increases of liver enzymes during episodes of pain. However, the correlation is not strong; thus, these signs alone cannot be used to determine sphincter stenosis.

The finding of sphincter of Oddi stenosis may involve the bile duct sphincter, the pancreatic duct sphincter, or both sphincters. Stenosis in the pancreatic duct sphincter is associated with pancreatic sphincter of Oddi dysfunction, and treatment of these patients requires division not only of the bile duct portion of the sphincter of Oddi but also of the septum between the bile duct and the pancre-

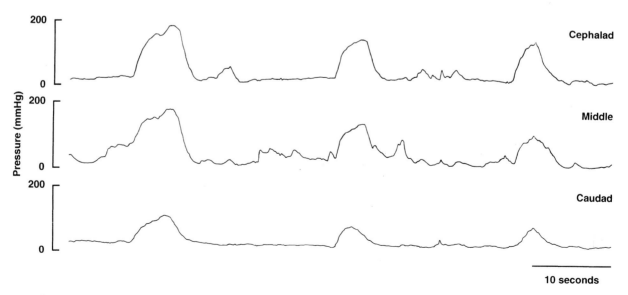

Figure 108–3. Manometric recording from the sphincter of Oddi. Prominent phasic contractions are superimposed on a modest basal pressure.

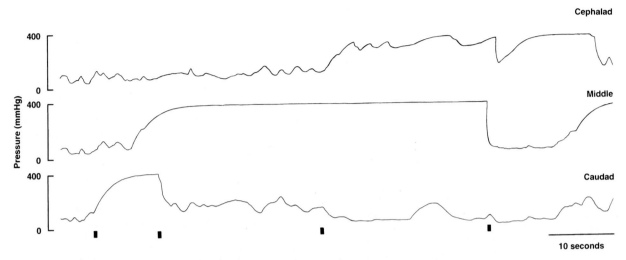

Figure 108–4. Manometric tracings illustrating sphincter of Oddi stenosis characterized by a high basal pressure. The black squares illustrate a stepwise withdrawal of the triple-lumen catheter across a narrow stenosis.

atic duct to effectively relieve the relative obstruction to the flow of pancreatic juice.

Sphincter of Oddi Dyskinesia

In this group are placed a number of manometric abnormalities that have been described in patients with suspected sphincter of Oddi dysfunction, as follows.

RAPID PHASIC CONTRACTIONS. These represent spontaneously occurring bursts of rapid phasic contractions similar to the effects of morphine. They have been called tachyoddia.

INTERMITTENT EPISODES OF ELEVATED BASAL PRESSURE. An intermittent elevation of the basal pressure may sometimes be noted in association with tachyoddia.

EXCESSIVE RETROGRADE CONTRACTIONS. In normal subjects, the majority of sphincter of Oddi contractions are orientated in an antegrade direction. However, an excess of simultaneous and retrograde contractions may reflect an abnormally functioning sphincter, which may impair bile flow.

Table 108–2	Sphincter of Oddi Dysfunction	
Stenosis	Basal pressure > 40 mm Hg	
Dyskinesia	Frequency > 7/min	
	Intermittent increases in basal pressure	
	Retrograde contractions > 50%	
	Paradoxical CCK-OP response	

CCK-OP, cholecystokinin octapeptide.

PARADOXICAL RESPONSE TO CHOLECYSTOKININ. The normal response of the human sphincter of Oddi to the administration of cholecystokinin is inhibition of phasic contractions and decrease in basal pressure. A paradoxical response is recorded when cholecystokinin has no effect on the sphincter contractions or produces an increase in contraction frequency, an increase in basal pressure, or both.

The options for management of sphincter of Oddi dysfunction are either division of the sphincter or pharmacotherapy. In the past, uncertainty regarding the diagnosis of sphincter dysfunction has been associated with uncertainty regarding therapy. However, the development of sphincter manometry and the recognition of abnormal motility have led to the identification of individuals who may be cured by targeted treatment.

In two prospective studies, patients with biliary-like pain were randomized into groups who received either an endoscopic sphincterotomy or a sham procedure. Patients with manometric evidence of stenosis of the sphincter of Oddi treated by sphincterotomy were more likely to show improvement in symptoms than were patients with sphincter stenosis who had the sham procedure. If the manometric diagnosis was dyskinesia, significant differences were not observed, although there was a trend toward improvement with sphincterotomy. These studies led to the conclusion that patients with significant sphincter of Oddi dysfunction, as characterized by an increased basal pressure (stenosis), should be treated by division of the sphincter of Oddi.

In many patients with idiopathic recurrent pancreatitis, biliary manometry reveals sphincter stenosis of the pancreatic ductal sphincter. Pancreatic duct stenosis may also be found in patients who have had a biliary sphincterotomy for the treatment of recurrent pancreatitis. Thus, endoscopic sphincterotomy is often ineffective for recurrent pancreatitis, and treatment must specifically include division of the pancreatic sphincter. This is achieved by an operative transduodenal approach with division of the septum between the bile duct and the pancreatic duct (pancreatic septectomy), which creates a wide opening for both ducts.

The effectiveness of this operation in producing symptomatic relief in patients with recurrent pancreatitis depends on the selection of patients. Approximately 70% of patients with abnormally increased basal pressure are improved by sphincteroplasty and pancreatic septoplasty (septectomy). Lack of improvement may be related to the fact that many of these patients have been treated for years with a variety of analgesics, including opiates, and that some have developed dependence on medication.

The role of pharmacotherapy in sphincter of Oddi dysfunction is limited because there are no drugs that are specific, long-acting, and free of side effects. Buscopan (hyoscine butylbromide) may be helpful for acute episodes of pain. However, its action is short lived, and it cannot be taken prophylactically. The calcium channel blocker nifedipine has also been used with some success to relieve pain, but it may be associated with cardiovascular side effects. Long-acting nitrates may also benefit some patients.

Patients with sphincter of Oddi dysfunction, either biliary or pancreatic in type, should undergo manometry to determine whether stenosis is present. The patients with unequivocal stenosis proceed to division of the sphincter. This division is achieved by the endoscopic approach in patients with biliary-type symptoms, whereas division is achieved by an open operation in patients with pancreatic symptoms.

Pearls and Pitfalls

- Think of biliary dyskinesia in patients with signs and symptoms of biliary colic, but with no stones on ultrasonography.
- There are two forms of biliary dyskinesia: gallbladder and sphincter of Oddi.
- Gallbladder dyskinesia requires documentation by a CCK-OP–stimulated HIDA scan to quantitate GBEF.
- Documented gallbladder dyskinesia responds well to cholecystectomy.
- Sphincter of Oddi dysfunction may involve stenosis of the sphincter, abnormal retrograde contractions, and a paradoxical hyperresponse to CCK-OP.
- Selected patients with sphincter of Oddi dysfunction respond well to endoscopic sphincterotomy.

SELECTED READINGS

Geenen JE, Hogan WJ, Dodds WJ, et al: The efficacy of endoscopic sphincterotomy in post-cholecystectomy patients with sphincter of Oddi dysfunction. N Engl J Med 1989;320:82.
Toouli J, Di Francesco V, Saccone GTP, et al: Division of the sphincter of Oddi for treatment of dysfunction associated with recurrent pancreatitis. Br J Surg 1996;83:1205.
Toouli J, Roberts-Thomson I, Dent J, Lee J: Sphincter of Oddi manometric disorders in patients with idiopathic recurrent pancreatitis. Br J Surg 1985;72:859.
Toouli J, Roberts-Thomson I, Dent J, Lee J: Manometric disorders in patients with suspected sphincter of Oddi dysfunction. Gastroenterology 1985;88:1243.
Toouli J, Roberts-Thomson I, Kellow J, et al: Manometry based randomised trial of endoscopic sphincterotomy for sphincter of Oddi dysfunction. Gut 2000;46:98.
Yap L, McKenzie J, Wycherley A, Toouli J: Gallbladder ejection fraction for acalculous gallbladder pain. Gastroenterology 1991;101:786.

Chapter 109

Primary Sclerosing Cholangitis

Steven A. Ahrendt and Henry A. Pitt

Primary sclerosing cholangitis (PSC) is an idiopathic inflammatory disease resulting in multifocal intrahepatic and extrahepatic biliary strictures, chronic cholestasis, and eventually biliary cirrhosis. Since the 1980s, management of patients with PSC has undergone considerable evolution. Before the mid-1980s, a variety of surgical procedures were used to manage patients with PSC, often with rather poor results. During the 1980s, liver transplantation became established as a viable option for managing patients with end-stage liver disease, and it has since developed into the only appropriate therapeutic option for PCS patients once cirrhosis has developed. PCS is currently the fourth leading cause of liver failure leading to liver transplantation in the United States. However, the appropriate management of PSC patients early in the course of their disease remains controversial. Since the mid-1980s, a wide variety of surgical, endoscopic, and medical therapies have been introduced into practice without any clear-cut evidence that these treatment modalities can slow the progression of PSC to cirrhosis.

CLINICAL PRESENTATION

Clinical Setting and Symptoms

In 1998, Ahrendt and colleagues reported that two thirds of patients with PSC are men and that the mean age at diagnosis is 45 years. Although PSC has been diagnosed at all ages, the majority of patients are between 30 and 60 years of age, and the majority have inflammatory bowel disease. The most common symptoms at the time PSC is diagnosed include jaundice, pruritus, fever, abdominal pain, fatigue, and weight loss.

The symptoms of PSC follow a highly variable course. Although more than 50% of patients with PSC are diagnosed from abnormal serum biochemistries while they are asymptomatic, the majority of patients eventually develop symptoms. However, the symptoms of pain, pruritus, and fever are each present less than 20% of the time in most patients. In addition, most symptomatic episodes involve only one of these symptoms at a time, and the episodes often resolve in 2 or fewer days. Fever and chronic fatigue are the most troublesome symptoms of PSC. The symptom variability makes it difficult to evaluate the efficacy of a given treatment or intervention.

Natural History

The median survival of patients with PSC from the time of diagnosis ranges from 10 to 12 years. Patients with no symptoms at the time of diagnosis have a longer survival than do patients presenting with symptoms. Several factors have been identified that correlate with survival or with the need for liver transplantation in PSC. These variables include patient age, serum bilirubin, and evidence of portal hypertension such as splenomegaly or variceal hemorrhage, as well as degree of hepatic fibrosis on liver biopsy (histologic stage).

Associated Diseases

Approximately 70% of patients with PSC also have inflammatory bowel disease. In addition, patients with PSC are at increased risk of developing cholangiocarcinoma and colon cancer. With the improved results of liver transplantation for managing the complications of end-stage liver disease in PSC, cancer has become the leading cause of death in these patients.

PSC will be diagnosed in about 5% of patients with inflammatory bowel disease. Most patients (87%) with PSC and inflammatory bowel disease have ulcerative colitis. The activity and course of each of these two diseases act independently, and operative management of the inflammatory bowel disease does not alter or affect the course of the PSC. PSC has been shown to be an independent risk factor for colon cancer in patients with ulcerative colitis. The incidence of dysplasia within colonic biopsies from patients with ulcerative colitis and PSC is higher than that in patients with ulcerative colitis. Thus, colonoscopy is warranted in all patients with PSC, either for exclusion of the diagnosis of inflammatory bowel disease in patients without a prior history or for surveillance in patients with ulcerative colitis or Crohn's disease.

PSC is also a well-known risk factor for cholangiocarcinoma. Cholangiocarcinoma is common (30% to 42% incidence) in autopsy series of patients with PSC and has been diagnosed in 5% to 10% of patients undergoing liver transplantation despite an extensive preoperative evaluation to exclude this diagnosis. Cholangiocarcinoma is often diagnosed early in the clinical course of PSC, with more than 50% of patients in one series being diagnosed within 1 year of onset of biliary symptoms. Most patients developing cholangiocarcinoma in the setting of PSC do not yet have established cirrhosis. Cytologic examination of biliary brushings and biopsies has a low sensitivity of diagnosing cholangiocarcinoma. Despite early optimism that the serum tumor marker carbohydrate antigen 19-9 (CA 19-9) would be useful for diagnosing cholangiocarcinoma in the setting of PSC, prospective studies have documented a high false-positive rate and a sensitivity of only 50%.

DIAGNOSTIC EVALUATION

Laboratory Evaluation

Liver function studies support the diagnosis of PSC and are essential for monitoring the course of the disease. A cholestatic pattern is most common with increases in serum alkaline phosphatase and gamma glutamyl transferase and with smaller elevations in aminotransferases. The serum bilirubin can fluctuate in PSC. CA 19-9 may be increased in patients with PSC and cholangiocarcinoma, but sensitivity and specificity are unsatisfactory.

A liver biopsy is crucial and necessary to determine disease stage and to guide therapeutic decisions. Four histologic stages have been identified in PSC and include portal inflammation (stage I), portal and periportal fibrosis (stage II), bridging fibrosis (stage III), and cirrhosis (stage IV). These histologic findings are nonspecific and support rather than make this diagnosis. More than 90% of patients with stage II PSC will progress to stage III or stage IV over 5 years, and 50% of patients with stage III PSC will develop cirrhosis over a 5-year period.

Imaging Studies

The diagnosis of PSC is made from the cholangiographic appearance of the biliary tract in the appropriate clinical setting. Typical cholangiographic findings of PSC include multifocal biliary strictures and diverticular outpouchings in the major bile ducts (Fig. 109–1). Both the intrahepatic and the extrahepatic ducts are involved in more than 85% of patients, although the disease is occasionally limited to either the intrahepatic or the extrahepatic biliary tract. Traditionally, endoscopic retrograde cholangiography has been used to make the diagnosis of PSC. More recently, magnetic resonance cholangiography has demonstrated accuracy comparable to that of endoscopic retrograde cholangiography in diagnosing PSC. Visualization of the entire biliary tree is critical to avoid missing a cholangiocarcinoma, and transhepatic cholangiography may be required if endoscopic retrograde cholangiography is unsuccessful.

Differential Diagnosis

The differential diagnosis of a patient presenting with pruritus, jaundice, right upper quadrant pain, or fatigue

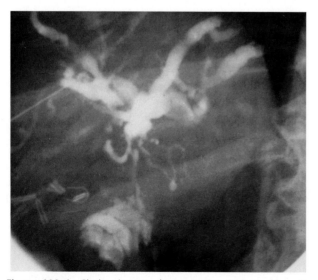

Figure 109–1. Cholangiogram demonstrating PSC involving the extrahepatic biliary tract.

includes the different causes of extrahepatic biliary obstruction and chronic liver disease. Cholangiography demonstrating the typical features of the disease is necessary to make the diagnosis of sclerosing cholangitis. Before the diagnosis of PSC can be established, the common causes of secondary sclerosing cholangitis must be excluded. Recurrent episodes of bacterial cholangitis secondary to choledocholithiasis or a benign biliary stricture can produce multiple biliary strictures. Acquired immunodeficiency syndrome (AIDS) and intra-arterial chemotherapy with floxuridine may also lead to a cholangiographic picture similar to that of PSC. In patients with focal biliary strictures, especially of the extrahepatic biliary tree, the diagnosis of cholangiocarcinoma needs to be considered and may be extremely difficult to differentiate from localized PSC with currently available diagnostic modalities. In asymptomatic patients with inflammatory bowel disease and biochemical evidence of cholestasis, the diagnosis of PSC should be strongly considered and cholangiography performed. Similarly, in children as well as teenagers with inflammatory bowel disease, pruritus and jaundice may be less pronounced, and the clinical and biochemical picture may be more suggestive of autoimmune hepatitis. However, cholangiography will confirm the diagnosis of PSC.

SELECTION OF THERAPY

Multiple therapeutic options exist for patients with PSC, which suggests that none of the options is ideal. In general, asymptomatic patients should not be treated. No currently available medical therapy has demonstrated any effect on disease progression, and these patients should be treated only in clinical trials. Symptomatic patients with persistently increased liver function test results, pruritus, pain, or fatigue, evidence of significant extrahepatic or hilar strictures, and liver biopsy demonstrating absence of cirrhosis are candidates for an endoscopic or operative approach to improve biliary drainage. In addition, patients with dominant biliary strictures suggesting cholangiocarcinoma should undergo surgical exploration and resection of the extrahepatic bile ducts rather than prolonged efforts to establish a tissue diagnosis. When patients develop cirrhosis, liver transplantation is the only reasonable therapy.

OPERATIVE MANAGEMENT

Surgical Resection

In appropriately selected patients, resection of the extrahepatic biliary tract and hepatic duct bifurcation may provide lasting relief from jaundice, exclude or make the diagnosis of cholangiocarcinoma in a dominant biliary stricture, and postpone the need for liver transplantation. The hepatic duct bifurcation is frequently involved with a dominant stricture and is included in the resection in 80% of patients (Fig. 109–2). Therefore, percutaneous stents are placed into the right and the left hepatic ducts preoperatively, both to aid in the dissection of the hepatic duct bifurcation and to stent the hepaticojejunostomies.

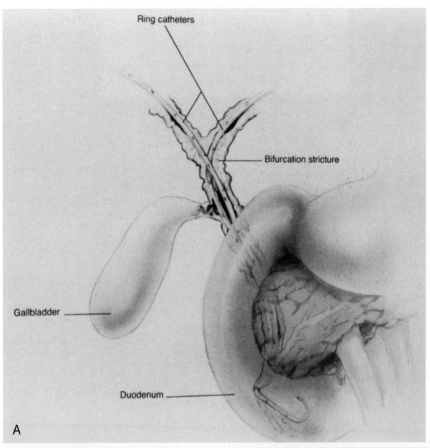

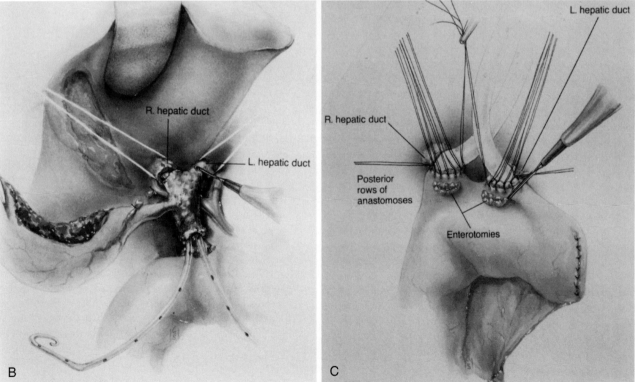

Figure 109–2. *A,* Resection of extrahepatic bile ducts and gallbladder in a patient with PSC. Note the preoperatively placed transhepatic stents. *B,* The extrahepatic bile duct and hepatic duct bifurcation are removed by dividing the distal common bile duct, the left hepatic duct, and the right hepatic duct. *C,* Bilateral hepaticojejunostomies with transhepatic stents.

Illustration continued on following page

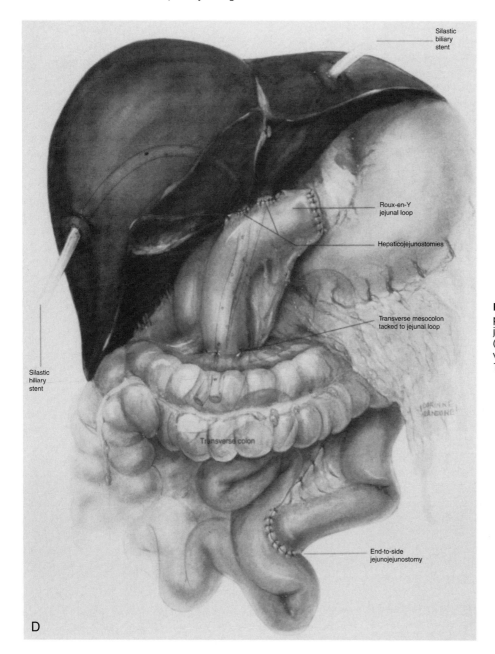

Silastic biliary stent

Roux-en-Y jejunal loop

Hepaticojejunostomies

Transverse mesocolon tacked to jejunal loop

Silastic biliary stent

Transverse colon

End-to-side jejunojejunostomy

Figure 109–2 *Continued. D,* Completed retrocolic Roux-en-Y hepatico-jejunostomies with stents in place. (From Cameron JC: Atlas of Surgery, vol. 1. Philadelphia, BC Decker, 1990.)

D

Prophylactic antibiotics are selected based on preoperative bile culture and sensitivities. An upper midline incision provides adequate exposure to the right upper quadrant for extrahepatic biliary resection and reconstruction or for hepatic resection should a cholangiocarcinoma be encountered; this incision also allows ideal placement of transhepatic stents on the anterior abdominal wall.

For extrahepatic biliary resection, a cholecystectomy is performed if the gallbladder is still in place, and the common bile duct is divided at the level of the superior edge of the pancreas. The common bile duct is dissected proximally off the portal vein up to the level of the bifurcation. The right and left hepatic ducts are divided just above the hepatic duct bifurcation, and frozen sections are taken of each margin and of any suspicious areas to exclude cholangiocarcinoma. Our technique is to replace the preoperatively placed stents with larger Silas-

tic catheters. Hepaticojejunostomies are then created over the stents between both hepatic ducts and a Roux-en-Y limb of jejunum. The stents are brought out through the abdominal wall below the costal margin to minimize patient discomfort; moreover, these stents allow subsequent ductal intubation and decompression. Closed suction drains are placed at the exit sites of the two catheters from the liver and adjacent to the hepaticojejunostomies.

Liver Transplantation

The technical aspects of liver transplantation for PSC are similar to those of liver transplantation for other causes of end-stage liver disease with several important exceptions. The native bile duct is resected to the superior edge of the pancreas to remove as much biliary epithelium as possible, thereby decreasing the risk of cholangiocarcinoma. The biliary tract is reconstructed with a Roux-en-Y choledochojejunostomy instead of the standard choledochocholedochostomy.

POSTOPERATIVE MANAGEMENT

Surgical Resection

Management of patients undergoing biliary tract reconstruction during the early postoperative period is similar to that of patients undergoing other major abdominal procedures. Early ambulation is encouraged. Pneumatic compression devices are preferred over anticoagulation for thromboembolism prophylaxis because of the increased risk of bleeding in patients with jaundice and hepatic dysfunction. Perioperative antibiotics are continued postoperatively until patients are afebrile for 24 hours because of the frequent occurrence of cholangitis after the intraoperative manipulation of the transhepatic stents, which all have bacterobilia. The transhepatic biliary stents are connected individually to bile bags and placed for gravity drainage. The stents are flushed twice daily with 10 mL of saline to maintain patency. An oral diet is resumed once the postoperative ileus has resolved. A transhepatic cholangiogram is obtained between the fifth and seventh postoperative days to evaluate for an anastomotic leak. If no leak is demonstrated, the stents are capped, converting to internal biliary drainage. The closed suction drains are left in place for an additional 24 hours; if the drainage remains nonbilious, they are removed. The mean length of hospitalization after a Roux-en-Y hepaticojejunostomy for PSC should be 10 to 14 days.

Liver Transplantation

Management of patients with PSC undergoing liver transplantation is similar to that of other patients undergoing this procedure. The mean postoperative length of stay after liver transplantation is several days longer for PSC than for hepaticojejunostomy.

COMPLICATIONS

Endoscopic Therapy

The overall complication rate after endoscopic biliary dilation and/or stenting is 15%. The most common complications are pancreatitis, which is usually mild, and radiologically detectable perforations of the intrahepatic or extrahepatic biliary tract, which usually resolve without formation of a biloma or abscess. Technical success at dilating or stenting dominant extrahepatic or hilar strictures is achievable in approximately 90% of patients. Less common complications include acute cholecystitis or hydrops of the gallbladder from cystic duct obstruction.

Surgical Resection

The overall morbidity rate after Roux-en-Y hepaticojejunostomy is at least 35%. Common complications include cholangitis, hemobilia, bile leak, and wound infection. Rarely, hepatic arterial bleeding related to the transhepatic stent has required embolization for control. In a series of 40 noncirrhotic patients undergoing biliary reconstruction, the operative mortality rate was 3%.

Liver Transplantation

Common complications after liver transplantation include acute rejection, intra-abdominal hemorrhage, hepatic artery thrombosis, and infection. The overall morbidity rate is approximately 50%. Hospital mortality after liver transplantation for PSC ranges from 3% to 19%.

OUTCOMES

Medical Therapy

Ursodeoxycholic acid has been studied in several prospective, randomized, placebo-controlled trials in patients with PSC. This drug consistently lowers serum bilirubin and transaminases but has failed to provide either a clinically detectable reduction in symptoms or a measurable delay in the progression of the disease. Other drugs, including penicillamine, methotrexate, colchicine, cyclosporine, and pentoxifylline, have been examined in clinical trials and have also not been found to be effective. A pilot study reported by Schramm and colleagues in 1999 suggests that combined therapy with azathioprine, prednisolone, and ursodeoxycholic acid has demonstrated improved liver histology in 60% of patients, as well as persistent biochemical improvement. These results have yet to be confirmed in a controlled trial.

Endoscopic Therapy

Several centers have reported their results with endoscopic management of dominant extrahepatic biliary strictures in PSC. Short-term reductions in serum bilirubin and cholestatic symptoms have been noted. As reported by Ponsioen and associates in 1999, a single short period of endoscopic stenting produced symptomatic relief in 83% of 44 patients with PSC and at least one dominant extrahepatic stricture. Further endoscopic therapy was required in 40% of patients within 3 years of the initial period of endoscopic stenting. However, the disease is characterized by fluctuations in symptoms and degree of cholestasis, and, to date, no controlled data exist demonstrating that endoscopic therapy alters the natural history of the disease. One additional concern among patients managed endoscopically is the risk of delayed diagnosis of cholangiocarcinoma. Up to 9% of patients with dominant strictures managed endoscopically are ultimately diagnosed with cholangiocarcinoma.

Surgical Resection

Ahrendt and colleagues reported in 1998 that resection of the extrahepatic biliary tree, although used less frequently

Table 109–1	**Survival in Noncirrhotic Patients with Primary Sclerosing Cholangitis by Treatment Method**

OVERALL SURVIVAL IN YEARS (%)

Procedure	Number	Risk Score*	1 Year	3 Years	5 Years
Resection	40	3.36 ± 0.12	95	92	85
ES/BD	26	3.13 ± 0.27	88	72†	58†
Percutaneous stenting	17	3.59 ± 0.28	87	79	63
Combined nonoperative	43	3.27 ± 0.21	87	74‡	59‡

TRANSPLANT-FREE SURVIVAL IN YEARS (%)

Procedure	Number	Risk Score*	1 Year	3 Years	5 Years
Resection	40	3.36 ± 0.12	95	92	82
ES/BD	26	3.13 ± 0.27	83	56†	42†
Percutaneous stenting	17	3.59 ± 0.28	87	64†	51‡
Combined nonoperative	43	3.27 ± 0.21	85	59†	46†

*Multicenter risk score.
†$P < 0.01$ versus resection; ‡$P < 0.05$ versus resection. Overall survival includes patients undergoing liver transplantation.
ES/BD, endoscopic sphincterotomy plus balloon dilation.
Adapted from Ahrendt SA, Pitt HA, Kalloo AN, et al: Primary sclerosing cholangitis: Resect, dilate, or transplant? Ann Surg 1998;227:412.

Pearls and Pitfalls

- Patients with PSC usually have inflammatory bowel disease and are at increased risk for developing colon cancer and cholangiocarcinoma.
- 30% to 50% of patients with PSC and cholangiocarcinoma present within 1 year of the diagnosis of PSC.
- Failure to appreciate that cholangiocarcinoma may present early in the course or may be the initial presentation of PSC will cause some patients to be overlooked.
- Biliary brushings and cytology have very low (50% to 60%) sensitivity for diagnosing cholangiocarcinoma, particularly in the setting of indwelling endoprostheses, and are unreliable for excluding the diagnosis of cancer.
- Patients with PSC but without an antecedent history of inflammatory bowel disease still require surveillance colonoscopy at appropriate intervals.
- Liver transplantation is the procedure of choice for PSC patients with cirrhosis.
- Selected patients with PSC and predominant extrahepatic biliary strictures may benefit from operative resection of the extrahepatic biliary tree; liver transplantation may be delayed.

since the early 1990s, may delay or, more rarely, prevent the need for liver transplantation in highly selected patients. In a series of 50 patients followed up for more than 5 years, the overall 1-year, 3-year, and 5-year survival rates after bile duct resection were 86%, 84%, and 76%, respectively. Patients without cirrhosis fared even better, with 1-year, 3-year, and 5-year survival rates of 95%, 92%, and 85%, respectively (Table 109–1). Furthermore, overall survival for noncirrhotic patients managed with bile duct resection was significantly longer than that for a group of 35 concurrent noncirrhotic patients managed with endoscopic balloon dilation. The majority of patients

were managed with chronic indwelling transhepatic biliary catheters, and only one patient (2%) required a second operation for focal extrahepatic biliary obstruction and cholangitis. Moreover, none of these patients developed cholangiocarcinoma with long-term follow-up, perhaps as a result of resection of the highest-risk hilar biliary epithelium.

Seven of these 50 patients (14%) underwent liver transplantation an average of 63 months after bile duct resection. Two subsequently died. Survival free of liver transplantation for the 40 patients who did not have cirrhosis at the time of PSC diagnosis was 95%, 92%, and 82% at 1, 3, and 5 years after resection (see Table 109–1). Transplant-free survival was significantly longer for the

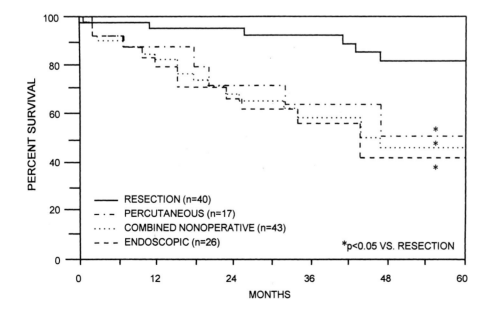

Figure 109–3. Transplant-free survival for noncirrhotic patients with PSC. Transplant-free survival for resected patients was longer than that for patients managed with endoscopic dilation ($P < 0.01$), percutaneous stenting ($P < 0.05$), or both nonoperative techniques ($P < 0.01$). (From Ahrendt SA, Pitt HA, Kalloo AN, et al: Primary sclerosing cholangitis: Resect, dilate, or transplant? Ann Surg 1998;227:412.)

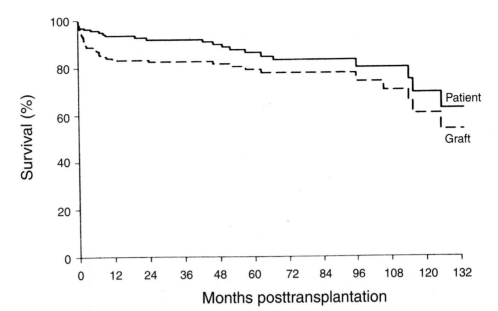

Figure 109–4. Actuarial patient and graft survival in PSC patients undergoing liver transplantation. (From Graziadei IW, Wiesner RH, Marotta PJ, et al: Long-term results of patients undergoing liver transplantation for primary sclerosing cholangitis. Hepatology 1999;30:1121.)

noncirrhotic patient managed with biliary resection than for the noncirrhotic patients with PSC managed with endoscopic balloon dilation (Fig. 109–3). Serum bilirubin levels have also been monitored after biliary resection and nonoperative management of patients with PSC. Only biliary resection significantly reduced serum bilirubin levels at 1, 2, and 3 years after surgery when compared with pretreatment levels.

Liver Transplantation

The operative mortality and long-term results of liver transplantation for PSC continue to improve. One-year and 5-year patient survival after liver transplantation for PSC at several high-volume centers ranges from 90% to 94% and 80% to 86%, respectively (Fig. 109–4). Actuarial 5-year graft survival ranges from 60% to 79%. The most common causes of liver failure leading to retransplantation are hepatic artery thrombosis, chronic rejection, primary nonfunction, and recurrent PSC. Chronic ductopenic rejection occurs in 10% of patients an average of 5 months after liver transplantation. Both patient and graft survival are markedly reduced (25% at 5 years) in patients with chronic rejection. Nonanastomotic biliary strictures are more common after liver transplantation for PSC than for other causes of chronic liver disease (18% versus 1%). Cholangiographic evidence of PSC (nonanastomotic biliary strictures in the intrahepatic or extrahepatic biliary tract with beading and irregularity) is present in 18% of transplanted livers at a mean length of 421 days after transplantation.

In summary, although medical therapy can improve liver function test results, it has not been proven to delay progression of PSC, including need for liver transplantation, development of cholangiocarcinoma, or survival.

Thus, patients managed medically should be included in clinical trials. Similarly, balloon dilation and stenting of dominant strictures have not been proven to improve survival and may, in fact, delay the diagnosis of cholangiocarcinoma. Surgical resection of hilar and extrahepatic strictures in noncirrhotic patients may postpone or prevent the need for transplantation and the development of cholangiocarcinoma in carefully selected patients. Nevertheless, liver transplantation remains the treatment of choice for patients with PSC and cirrhosis. Liver transplantation, however, has significant short-term and long-term morbidity and should not be employed too early in the natural history of the disease.

SELECTED READINGS

Ahrendt SA, Pitt HA, Kalloo AN, et al: Primary sclerosing cholangitis: Resect, dilate, or transplant? Ann Surg 1998;227:412.

Ahrendt SA, Pitt HA, Nakeeb A, et al: Diagnosis and management of cholangiocarcinoma in primary sclerosing cholangitis. J Gastrointest Surg 1999;3:357.

Angulo P, Larson DR, Thernau TM, et al: Time course of histological progression in primary sclerosing cholangitis. Am J Gastroenterol 1999;94:3310.

Angulo P, Lindor KD: Primary sclerosing cholangitis. Hepatology 1999;30:325.

Cameron JC: Atlas of Surgery, vol. 1. Philadelphia, BC Decker, 1990.

Graziadei IW, Wiesner RH, Marotta PJ, et al: Long-term results of patients undergoing transplantation for primary sclerosing cholangitis. Hepatology 1999;30:1121.

Hultkrantz R, Olsson R, Danielsson A, et al: A three-year prospective study on serum tumor markers used for detecting cholangiocarcinoma in patients with primary sclerosing cholangitis. J Hepatol 1999;30:669.

Kornfeld D, Ekbom A, Ihre T: Survival and risk of cholangiocarcinoma in patients with primary sclerosing cholangitis. Scand J Gastroenterol 1997;32:1042.

Lee JG, Schutz SM, England RE, et al: Endoscopic therapy of sclerosing cholangitis. Hepatology 1995;21:661.

Ponsioen CY, Lam K, van Milligen de Wit AWM, et al: Four years experience with short-term stenting in primary sclerosing cholangitis. Am J Gastroenterol 1999;94:2403.

Schramm C, Schirmacher P, Helmreich-Becker I, et al: Combined therapy with azathioprine, prednisolone, and ursodiol in patients with primary sclerosing cholangitis. Ann Intern Med 1999;131:943.

Biliary: Malignant

Chapter 110
Cholangiocarcinoma
Jonathan B. Koea and Leslie H. Blumgart

Cholangiocarcinoma is a rare malignancy that accounts for up to 2% of all cancer diagnoses in the United States. This tumor has an overall annual incidence of 1.2 in 100,000, and incidence increases with age, with two thirds of all patients being older than 65 years. Perhaps because of its rarity, the diagnosis and management of this tumor remain a challenge for general and gastrointestinal surgeons.

Cholangiocarcinoma can develop anywhere along the biliary tree from the intrahepatic bile ducts to the ampulla of Vater. Intrahepatic cholangiocarcinoma (peripheral cholangiocarcinoma) is a rare neoplasm accounting for 6% to 10% of all cholangiocarcinomas and is managed with hepatic resection. The extrahepatic bile ducts are roughly divided into thirds by the insertion of the cystic duct and the superior border of the duodenum (Fig. 110–1). Tumors of the upper third, or hilar tumors, are those located proximal to the cystic duct up to and including the bifurcation into right and left hepatic ducts. These lesions account for 56% of all cholangiocarcinoma and often require hepatic resection as well as bile duct resection to obtain tumor clearance. Middle-third tumors account for 17% of cholangiocarcinomas, are located between the upper border of the duodenum and the cystic duct junction, and can often be managed with biliary resection alone. Lower-third or distal bile duct tumors account for 17% of cholangiocarcinomas, arise between the ampulla of Vater and the upper border of the duodenum, and are usually managed with pancreaticoduodenectomy.

This chapter reviews the clinicopathologic features and management strategies necessary for both intrahepatic and extrahepatic cholangiocarcinoma.

Cholangiocarcinomas are of three types: intrahepatic (peripheral) cholangiocarcinomas, hilar cholangiocarcinomas, and distal biliary cholangiocarcinomas. These three types (see Fig. 110–1) present differently and thus will

be discussed separately. This chapter addresses these three forms after discussing general etiopathogenesis.

GENERAL ETIOPATHOGENESIS

Regardless of the site of origin within the biliary tree, cholangiocarcinomas share similar etiologic factors. Pathologic conditions resulting in acute or chronic biliary

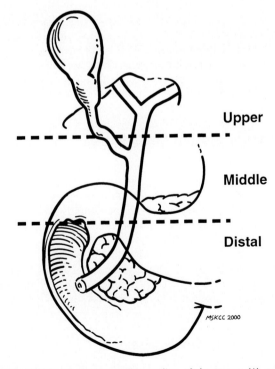

Figure 110–1. Cholangiographic outline of the upper (A), middle (B), and lower (C) thirds of the extrahepatic bile ducts.

epithelial injury predispose to tumor development within the biliary tree.

Biliary Infection

Common in southeast Asia, recurrent pyogenic cholangio-hepatitis, or oriental cholangiohepatitis, results from chronic portal bacteremia and portal inflammation, which predisposes to intrahepatic pigment stone formation. Bile duct obstruction leads to recurrent episodes of cholangitis and stricture formation, and up to 10% of these patients will develop cholangiocarcinoma.

Hepatic infestation with *Clonorchis sinensis, Ascaris lumbricoides,* and *Opisthorchis viverrini* also serves as a risk factor for cholangiocarcinoma in endemic areas. These parasites enter the portal circulation via the duodenum and migrate to the intrahepatic and extrahepatic bile ducts. Adult flukes cause biliary obstruction, periductal fibrosis, and hyperplasia, which probably represents premalignant lesions. Other infectious agents implicated in development of cholangiocarcinoma are hepatitis C and the chronic typhoid carrier state.

Cystic Disease of the Biliary Tree

Patients with cystic biliary abnormalities have up to a 28% incidence of subsequent cholangiocarcinoma, most often involving the extrahepatic biliary tree. The risk of carcinoma is related to age; more than 75% of the cholangiocarcinomas associated with choledochal cysts present in adults. The risk of cholangiocarcinoma developing within an unresected choledochal cyst is as high as 17% in some series (lower in others) by age 20 years, and it continues to climb with increasing age. In contrast, when cysts are recognized in childhood and are resected, the risk decreases markedly but does not return to zero, suggesting a generalized defect across the biliary epithelia. The high entry of the pancreatic duct into the extrahepatic bile duct in patients with choledochal cysts suggests that reflux of pancreatic secretion onto bile duct epithelium may cause malignant transformation in conjunction with bile stasis and stone formation, inflammation, and chronic infection.

Primary Sclerosing Cholangitis

Sclerosing cholangitis is a chronic inflammatory disease affecting both intrahepatic and extrahepatic bile ducts and resulting in multiple benign strictures. Up to 80% of patients with primary sclerosing cholangitis have ulcerative colitis, and, like ulcerative colitis, sclerosing cholangitis is probably autoimmune in etiology, with 60% of patients having serum antibodies that cross-react with bile ductules. Cholangiocarcinoma occurs in 40% of patients dying of sclerosing cholangitis and in 20% of patients undergoing orthotopic liver transplantation for this condition.

Inflammatory Bowel Disease

Cholangiocarcinoma is also associated with ulcerative colitis. The incidence ranges from 0.1 to 1%, and cholangio-carcinomas typically develop in the fifth decade of life. In general, patients with cholangiocarcinoma have pancolitis and a long duration of disease. Definitive surgical treatment of colonic disease does not completely remove the risk of developing biliary malignancy.

Chemical Carcinogens

A number of chemical agents and drugs have been implicated in the development of cholangiocarcinoma, including asbestos, dioxin, nitrosamines, and polychlorinated biphenyls. Drugs that have been suggested as contributing to the pathogenesis of cholangiocarcinoma are isoniazid, methyldopa, and oral contraceptives.

Radionuclides

Thorium dioxide as a 25% solution was used as a radio-contrast agent for approximately 30 years until the late 1950s. Thorium dioxide emits alpha particles and has a biologic half-life of 200 years. After intravenous injection, the thorium dioxide was retained within the reticuloendothelial system for the duration of the patient's life. The average latent period for development of thorium dioxide–associated cholangiocarcinomas is at least 25 years; these neoplasms tend to be in the intrahepatic biliary tree.

PERIPHERAL CHOLANGIOCARCINOMA

Pathology

On gross examination, peripheral cholangiocarcinomas are gray, scirrhous masses that are never encapsulated. Growth is infiltrative, and the tumor edge is poorly defined. Histopathologically, the tumor is usually a poorly differentiated adenocarcinoma (Fig. 110–2). Mucus secretion is demonstrable in the majority of tumors, but bile production is never observed. The minority show different patterns with focal areas of papillary carcinoma with mucus production, signet ring cells, and squamous cell, mucoepidermoid, and spindle cell variants. Cholangiocarcinomas stain for carcinoembryonic antigen (CEA), and many also stain for the tumor markers carbohydrate antigen (CA) 50 and CA 19-9. K-*ras* oncogenes are detectable in 70% of intrahepatic cholangiocarcinomas.

Thirty percent of patients with peripheral cholangiocarcinoma will have peritoneal or hepatic metastases at presentation, and many will not be detected until staging laparotomy or laparoscopy is undertaken. More than three quarters of patients dying of cholangiocarcinoma have metastases in regional lymph nodes, hepatic parenchyma, or peritoneal cavity, and 10% have pulmonary or bone metastases.

Clinical Features

Patients with peripheral cholangiocarcinoma may present with malaise and abdominal pain; fever is uncommon. Jaundice is present in one third of patients. Rarely, pe-

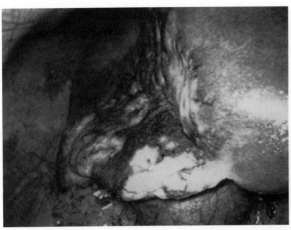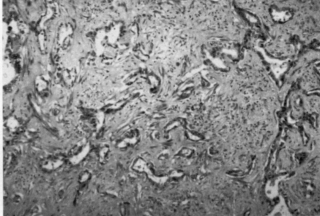

Figure 110–2. Intraoperative photograph of a large, peripheral cholangiocarcinoma arising in segment V *(left)*. Biopsy demonstrated a poorly differentiated carcinoma *(right)*.

ripheral cholangiocarcinoma may invade the central biliary tree and cause obstruction. In contrast, obstructive jaundice dominates the clinical presentation of hilar and extrahepatic cholangiocarcinomas.

Differential Diagnosis

Patients present with radiologic evidence of a solitary, intrahepatic, soft-tissue mass. Percutaneous needle biopsy will demonstrate adenocarcinoma. Patients, therefore, should be investigated for both upper and lower gastrointestinal primary tumors and should also have hepatitis serology and serum α-fetoprotein levels tested to rule out a poorly differentiated hepatocellular carcinoma. In the absence of any primary gastrointestinal tumor, patients with biopsy-proven adenocarcinoma in the liver should be considered to have a peripheral cholangiocarcinoma.

Laboratory Data

Laboratory investigations are nonspecific in peripheral cholangiocarcinoma, although increases of alkaline phosphatase and γ-glutamyltransferase may be seen. Patients may be hypoalbuminemic and mildly anemic, but white blood cell counts may be raised or within the normal range. Carcinoembryonic antigen and α-fetoprotein are usually within normal limits, and hepatitis serology is usually negative. However, levels of CA 19-9 may be elevated.

Radiologic Investigations

Radiographic studies show a characteristically avascular soft-tissue mass in the liver without biliary or gallbladder dilation. Magnetic resonance imaging (MRI) shows a hypodense or isodense lesion on T_1-weighted images and a hyperdense lesion on T_2-weighted images (Fig. 110–3*A*), whereas computed tomography (CT) usually shows an avascular soft-tissue mass (see Fig. 110–3*B*). MRI is useful in assessing intrahepatic biliary tumors for defining the extent of disease and vascular proximity. Duplex ultrasonography may aid in defining the extent and nature of

vascular involvement and may detect small satellite lesions not seen with other modalities.

Management

Patients with peripheral cholangiocarcinoma should be considered for surgical exploration and resection if they are medically fit. The presence of bilobar metastases or extrahepatic disease, however, is a contraindication to hepatic resection.

Perioperative antibiotics (a cephalosporin or a combination of clindamycin and an aminoglycoside in penicillin-allergic patients) should be ordered to cover both gram-negative and gram-positive organisms.

The abdomen should be shaved from the level of the nipples to the anterior superior iliac spines. Exploration should commence with a laparoscopy. The liver should be inspected for hepatic metastases, and any suspicious lesions should be biopsied and sent for frozen section. Bimanual palpation of the left and right lobes can also be carried out using biopsy forceps to gain an appreciation of the hepatic parenchyma; deeper metastases are often palpable in this manner. The peritoneum should be inspected for metastatic deposits. In some centers, the lesser sac is opened and the celiac and para-aortic lymph nodes inspected. Laparoscopic ultrasonography can also be used to more clearly define the intrahepatic ducts, the involvement of the hepatic parenchyma, and the presence of both nodal and hepatic metastases. If the laparoscopy is negative, the operation proceeds with a subcostal incision. A midline extension may be required to facilitate access to the suprahepatic vena cava. A thorough laparotomy should then be performed. The caudate lobe should also be formally assessed for involvement. After Kocher's maneuver is performed, the retroduodenal and retropancreatic lymph nodes are inspected and biopsied if suspicious. Intraoperative ultrasonography is performed at this time. If the decision is made to proceed with resection, then central venous pressure should be kept below 5 mm Hg to minimize blood loss.

Partial hepatectomy can be undertaken. Inflow control is obtained by ligation and transection of the ipsilateral portal vein and hepatic artery. The ipsilateral hepatic vein

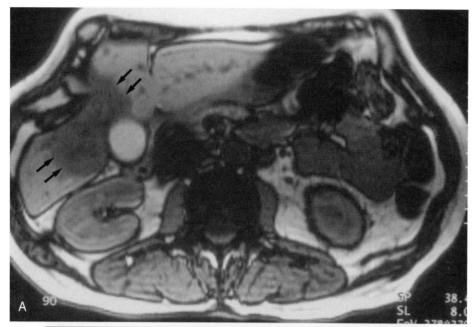

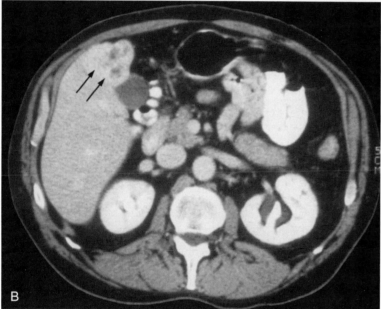

Figure 110–3. Peripheral cholangio-carcinoma. *A,* T1-weighted magnetic resonance imaging demonstrating a hypovascular peripheral cholangio-carcinoma in segment V *(arrows). B,* Computed tomography with intravenous contrast enhancement demonstrating a hypovascular peripheral cholangiocarcinoma in segment IV *(arrows).*

may be isolated and divided before parenchymal division. Parenchymal division is undertaken by sequentially crushing hepatic parenchyma or by use of the Cavitron Ultrasonic Surgical Aspirator to expose the intrahepatic vascular and biliary structures, which can then be controlled with titanium clips or absorbable ligatures. Once transection has been carried out and hemostasis has been verified, the abdomen can be closed in layers. Routine use of a surgical drain is not necessary.

Postoperative Management

Postoperatively, we use 5% dextrose with half-normal saline and 15 mEq of potassium phosphate per liter. The prothrombin time and phosphate level should be checked at least twice daily in patients after major hepatic resec-

tion. Plasma phosphate levels should reach a nadir 48 hours after hepatic resection as liver parenchymal regeneration takes place. Increases in prothrombin time of 16 seconds or more (International Normalized Ratio [INR] of 1.6) should be treated with fresh-frozen plasma. Oral feeding is generally commenced when bowel function returns. As soon as the patient can tolerate a regular diet, intravenous fluids and analgesia may be discontinued and oral agents begun. The average hospital stay is 8 days after a standard hepatectomy.

COMPLICATIONS

Hemorrhage

Postoperative hemorrhage following liver resection is now fortunately rare, and fewer than 1% of liver resections require urgent return to the operating room for blood loss. Most commonly, the site of hemorrhage is from the hepatic veins arising from the vena cava or intrahepatic branches. The risk of bleeding can be minimized by careful mobilization and control of these veins before parenchymal division. Low central venous pressure anesthesia greatly assists this dissection, causing the vena cava to fall away from the liver.

Liver Failure

The risk of postoperative liver failure is negligible in patients after resection of extrahepatic bile ducts alone. However, there is a small but significant risk in patients undergoing hepatic resection in addition to biliary resection. In the noncirrhotic liver, the risk of hepatic failure after resection of less than 50% of the parenchyma is approximately 1%. However, if more than 50% of the functioning parenchyma is removed, then this risk climbs to 10% and even higher with underlying cirrhosis.

Biloma

Postoperative bilomas are due to either a biliary leak from a major duct or leakage from a small bile duct in the hepatic parenchyma. Most commonly, these present 5 to 7 days postoperatively with increasing serum bilirubin. Most infected collections after hepatic resection are infected bilomas and will present similarly, but with signs of sepsis. Patients in whom a biloma is suspected should be initially investigated with a CT and drained percutaneously.

Coagulopathy and Thromboembolic Disease

After hepatic resection, some degree of coagulopathy is common, accompanied by prolonged prothrombin times. Patients should receive prophylactic vitamin K and fresh-frozen plasma if the prothrombin time increases to more than 16 seconds (INR > 1.6). This coagulopathy, coupled with early ambulation, makes thromboembolic disease rare in patients after hepatic resection. Thromboembolic prophylaxis with low-molecular-weight heparin should be instituted in the perioperative period if the patient has recognized risk factors (previous thromboembolic disease, obesity, smoking).

Hypophosphatemia

Hypophosphatemia is common in patients after major hepatic resection. In general, plasma phosphate concentrations begin to decrease within 12 hours after surgery owing to increased metabolic activity in the remaining liver and synthesis of adenosine triphosphate. Phosphate levels reach a nadir 48 hours postoperatively; however, continuing phosphate supplementation may be required after this time as well.

Pulmonary

Pulmonary complications are related to use of an upper abdominal incision, poor analgesia, and resulting hypoventilation. Emphasis should be placed on adequate analgesia and early ambulation. We use incentive spirometry at the patient's bedside, and preoperative teaching focuses on the importance of deep breathing, adequate cough, and early ambulation. Epidural analgesia postoperatively also aids pain control and thus ambulation and respiratory function.

OUTCOMES

Resection and Transplantation

Only 20% of patients with intrahepatic cholangiocarcinomas have resectable lesions at presentation, usually due to late clinical diagnosis. After complete resection, 5-year survival is approximately 40%. Vascular invasion and satellite lesions are adverse prognostic factors.

Orthotopic liver transplantation has been used with median survival of up to 18 months in node-negative patients; however, no node-positive patients have survived beyond 2 years. For patients with small, node-negative tumors, a 3-year survival rate of 64% can be expected. For the vast majority of patients, transplantation is not an option, and resection, when possible, should be considered the treatment of choice.

Chemotherapy and Radiation Therapy

The use of chemotherapy alone using fluorouracil or other agents does not improve survival, either as adjuvant therapy after resection or in patients with unresectable lesions. Radiation therapy has been extensively investigated, using external beam radiation, intraoperative radiation, and brachytherapy. There have been no prospective trials defining a role for radiation, and no retrospective investigation has shown improved survival with its use. In addition, 10% of patients have treatment-related complications with duodenal obstruction and bleeding. Whether adjuvant chemotherapy, radiation therapy, or both after curative resection is of any benefit remains unknown.

HILAR CHOLANGIOCARCINOMA (KLATSKIN'S TUMOR)

Pathology

Extrahepatic cholangiocarcinomas can be divided into three types based on their macroscopic appearance. *Sclerosing tumors,* the most common, are characterized by an annular thickening of the bile duct with an associated desmoplastic reaction. The ductal mucosa is often intact, and symmetrical luminal narrowing is a feature (Fig. 110–4). These lesions are most common at the hepatic hilus. *Nodular tumors* are characterized by a nodule of tumor that projects into the lumen of the bile duct, causing an eccentric luminal obstruction. Both these tumor types are distinguished by longitudinal spread of tumor within the duct wall and periductal tissues. Extensive submucosal tumor spread may occur beneath an

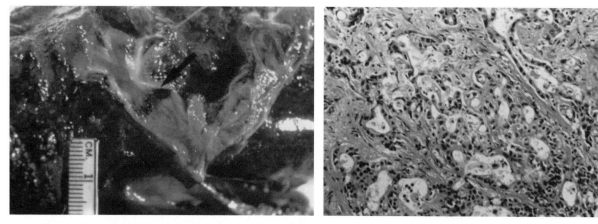

Figure 110–4. Scirrhous cholangiocarcinoma. Pathologic specimen after resection of a hilar cholangiocarcinoma. Concentric narrowing of the proximal common hepatic duct is illustrated *(left; arrow)*. Histopathologic examination demonstrated adenocarcinoma with a significant fibrous stroma *(right)*.

intact epithelium and often into other bile ducts at points of bifurcation, especially at the hepatic hilus where tumor extension into caudate ducts can occur. Most importantly, the full extent of tumor may not be appreciated endoscopically, with radiologic investigation, or with intraoperative palpation, making frozen section analysis mandatory. *Papillary tumors* account for 10% of cholangiocarcinomas and occur most commonly in the distal bile duct. These polypoid lesions expand rather than constrict the bile duct (Fig. 110–5). Because they often have a narrow stalk with minimal invasion, they are frequently confined within the bile duct and can be resected, despite their growth to a large size. Papillary tumors have a more favorable prognosis than do nodular or sclerosing subtypes.

Clinical Presentation

The early symptoms of hilar cholangiocarcinoma are subtle. Abdominal pain, nausea, and weight loss occur but are nonspecific. Often, the diagnosis is not evident until patients develop jaundice or until abnormal liver function test results have been noticed. Unfortunately, jaundice can be a relatively late feature, and many patients will already have developed segmental ductal obstruction with ipsilateral lobar atrophy. Pruritus in the absence of a defined dermatologic disorder often precedes the jaundice and is an important complaint that should mandate investigation. Jaundice may also be intermittent in the papillary tumors secondary to fragmentation of the polypoid tumor with embolic obstruction of the distal bile duct. Pedunculated tumors may also act as ball valves within the biliary system, causing transient obstruction.

Evaluation of patients with hilar cholangiocarcinoma should focus on their overall state of health and their cardiopulmonary reserve. Prominent collateral venous channels on the abdominal wall suggest portal venous obstruction and advanced disease. The liver edge may be palpable and firm owing to chronic biliary obstruction. The gallbladder should be decompressed and not palpable.

In spite of a 30% incidence of bacterobila in patients with hilar cholangiocarcinoma, cholangitis at presentation is rare. Endoscopic and percutaneous instrumentation increase the incidence of bacterial contamination to at least 60%, and cholangitis in these patients is not uncommon. *Enterococcus, Klebsiella, Streptococcus,* and *Enterobacter* are the most common offending organisms.

Diagnosis

LABORATORY INVESTIGATIONS. Liver function testing demonstrates an obstructive picture with increased total

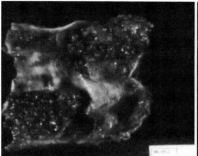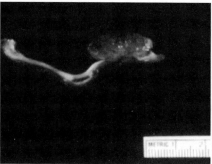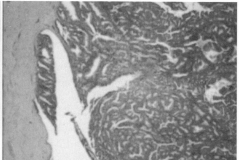

Figure 110–5. Papillary cholangiocarcinoma. Gross pathologic specimen demonstrating a papillary lesion lying within the opened common hepatic duct *(left)* and the predominantly polypoid growth *(middle)*. Histopathologic examination showed a papillary tumor with no evidence of malignancy *(right)*.

serum bilirubin and alkaline phosphatase levels. Aspartate transaminase may be normal or only mildly elevated. Coagulation studies should be checked, and a prolonged prothrombin time should be treated with vitamin K injections (10 mg subcutaneously daily for 3 days). The serum albumin level represents the patient's nutritional status and the synthetic function of the liver. Hepatitis B and hepatitis C status should be verified.

The diagnosis of hilar cholangiocarcinoma is usually made on the basis of obstructive jaundice and the presence of an obstructing lesion at the hepatic hilus. Radiologic evaluation is important in both diagnosis and staging of the tumor to define management strategy. Histologic confirmation of malignancy can be difficult to obtain and is not mandatory before operative exploration. Endoluminal brush biopsies are positive in only 25% of patients. In the absence of previous biliary surgery or radiation, a focal lesion within the biliary tract is indicative of a cholangiocarcinoma, and further investigations should be undertaken to define the extent and resectability of the lesion rather than its histopathology.

CHOLANGIOGRAPHY. Percutaneous or endoscopic cholangiography is crucial. Percutaneous transhepatic cholangiography (PTC) outlines biliary anatomy proximal to the obstructing lesion and is necessary for operative planning. Endoscopic retrograde cholangiography (ERC) can be limited by demonstrating only the distal extent of the biliary obstruction, which may not permit operative planning.

COMPUTED TOMOGRAPHY. CT is both widely available and useful. The pattern of ductal dilation will provide clues to the site and extent of hilar obstruction. A mass may be visible (Fig. 110–6A). In addition to providing information about intrahepatic metastases, CT may make extrahepatic disease in the peritoneum and celiac and portal lymph nodes evident. Portal lymphadenopathy must be interpreted with caution in patients with biliary stents because benign lymphadenopathy is common. The

most important finding on CT is lobar atrophy, which implies portal vein obstruction or long-standing biliary obstruction.

DUPLEX ULTRASONOGRAPHY. This investigation is indispensable in the evaluation of hilar cholangiocarcinoma. Ultrasonography can define involvement of the portal vein and extent of biliary and parenchymal involvement (see Fig. 110–6B). Duplex ultrasonography predicts portal vein involvement accurately in 90% of patients. The presence of papillary tumors may also be demonstrated (Fig. 110–7A).

MAGNETIC RESONANCE CHOLANGIOPANCREATOGRAPHY. This noninvasive mode of biliary imaging may replace PTC and ERC in the preoperative evaluation of hilar obstruction. Magnetic resonance cholangiopancreatography (MRCP) provides relatively high-resolution images of the intrahepatic and extrahepatic biliary tree. Obstructed segmental ducts can be demonstrated that may not be imaged on PTC or ERC (see Fig. 110–7B). MRCP is also able to define vascular involvement, and it images hepatic metastases, portal lymphadenopathy, and lobar atrophy (Fig. 110–8). Unlike PTC and ERC, MRCP is not associated with increased incidence of bacterobilia.

Differential Diagnosis

Stricture at the hilus and jaundice are virtually pathognomonic of cholangiocarcinoma. However, other causes account for approximately 10% of patients with these findings. Focal benign strictures may masquerade as cancer in 5% of patients with hilar strictures. These lesions often cause smooth, symmetrical strictures on cholangiography and have a soft, rubbery consistency on intraoperative palpation. Similarly, a dominant stricture occurring in the setting of sclerosing cholangitis may also have radiologic and clinical features suggestive of malignancy. It is usually not possible to differentiate benign from malignant stric-

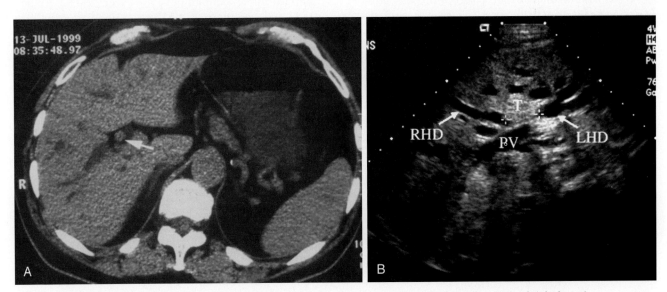

Figure 110–6. *A,* Computed tomography demonstrating a mass lesion *(arrow)* involving the proximal right hepatic duct. *B,* Transabdominal ultrasonography showing tumor (T) at the confluence of the right (RHD) and left (LHD) hepatic ducts. The portal vein (PV) is also shown and is not involved by tumor.

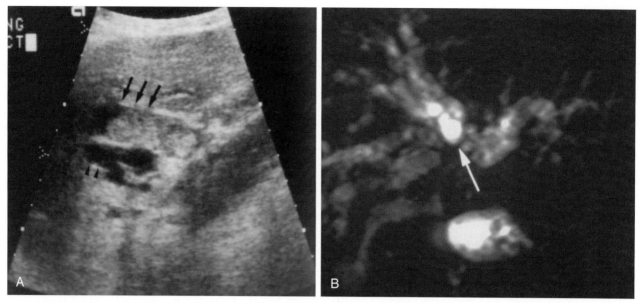

Figure 110–7. Papillary cholangiocarcinoma. *A,* Transabdominal ultrasonography demonstrating a papillary tumor expanding the right hepatic duct *(large arrows).* The portal vein is shown beneath the tumor *(small arrows). B,* Magnetic resonance cholangiocreatography showing a narrowing at the hepatic hilus *(arrow)* with intrahepatic ductal dilation.

tures until the lesion is resected. Other benign causes of hilar or hepatic duct obstruction include Mirizzi's syndrome resulting from the impaction of a gallstone within the neck of the gallbladder. Gallbladder carcinoma can obstruct the common hepatic or right hepatic duct because of invasion into either the lesser omentum or segments IV and V of the liver.

Preoperative Management

The evaluation of the patient with suspected cholangiocarcinoma has four objectives: (1) assessment of the extent and level of biliary tract and portal vein involvement, (2) assessment of the liver for evidence of lobar atrophy or concomitant liver pathology, (3) evaluation of nodal and/or distant metastases, and (4) assessment of the patient's performance status.

Patients with hilar cholangiocarcinoma should be considered for operative exploration and resection if they are medically fit. Ipsilateral lobar atrophy is not a contraindication to resection provided the contralateral branch and main trunk of the portal vein are patent. A summary of contraindications to operative exploration in hilar cholangiocarcinoma is presented in Table 110–1.

Staging

The two most commonly used staging systems are the American Joint Committee on Cancer (AJCC) tumor, nodes, and metastasis (TNM) system and the modified

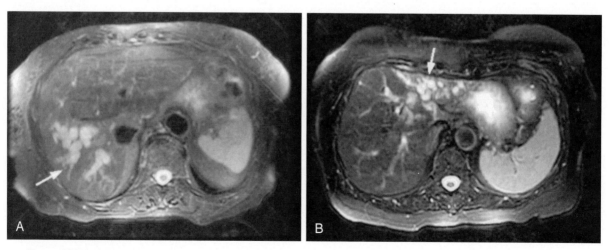

Figure 110–8. Magnetic resonance imaging demonstrating lobar atrophy. *A,* Right lobar atrophy with crowding of the ducts *(arrow)* and hypertrophy of the left lobe. *B,* Left lobar atrophy with crowding of the ducts *(arrow)* and hypertrophy of the right lobe.

Table 110–1	Contraindications to Operative Exploration in Patients with Hilar Cholangiocarcinoma

Medically unfit patient
Extrahepatic metastases (peritoneum, lung, bone)
Metastases to celiac, portocaval, and para-aortic lymph nodes
Intrahepatic metastases
Involvement to second-order ducts bilaterally
Encasement of both right and left portal veins
Encasement of the main portal vein

Table 110–3	Modified Bismuth-Corlette Classification for Hilar Cholangiocarcinoma

Type I	Below the biliary confluence
Type II	Confined to the biliary confluence
Type IIIa	Extension into right hepatic duct
Type IIIb	Extension into left hepatic duct
Type IV	Extension into right *and* left hepatic ducts

Bismuth-Corlette classification for hilar cholangiocarcinoma (Tables 110–2 and 110–3). Both systems emphasize the extent of tumor involvement within the hepatic ductal system while ignoring potential tumor involvement of the hepatic artery and portal vein, as well as the functional status of the underlying liver. In an attempt to improve the clinical and prognostic utility of the AJCC TNM staging system, we have proposed a new clinical tumor staging system that takes into consideration both vascular involvement by local tumor extension and the presence or absence of liver atrophy (Table 110–4).

Preoperative Preparation

BILIARY DECOMPRESSION. Biliary instrumentation is associated with an increased incidence of positive bile cultures for enteric organisms. Patients with endoscopic stents have a 100% incidence of bacterobilia, whereas those with percutaneous stents have positive bile cultures in 65% of patients. The rate of postoperative infective complications in stented patients is increased, and usually the organism responsible is the same as that cultured from bile. Therefore, our policy is not to perform biliary stenting for high bile duct obstruction alone; moreover,

Table 110–2	AJCC Staging System for Cholangiocarcinoma

Stage 0	Tis	N0	M0
Stage I	T1	N0	M0
Stage II	T2	N0	M0
Stage III	T1, T2	N1, N2	M0
Stage IVA	T3	Any	M0
Stage IVB	Any	Any	M1

Tis   Carcinoma *in situ*
T1   Tumor invades subepithelial connective tissue (T1a) or fibromuscular layer (T1b)
T2   Tumor invades perifibromuscular connective tissue
T3   Tumor invades adjacent structures: liver, pancreas, duodenum, stomach, gallbladder, colon, or stomach
N0   No lymph node metastases
N1   Metastasis in the cystic duct, pericholedochal, and/or hilar lymph nodes
N2   Metastasis in the peripancreatic (head only), periduodenal, periportal, celiac, superior mesenteric, and/or posterior pancreaticoduodenal lymph nodes
M0   No distant metastases
M1   Distant metastases

From AJCC Cancer Staging Manual, 5th ed. Philadelphia, Lippincott-Raven.

endoscopic stents are often ineffective at relieving jaundice in very proximal obstructions. We reserve preoperative stenting for patients with cholangitis who require biliary decompression, and we prefer a percutaneous approach with drainage of both lobes, using two stents if necessary.

NUTRITIONAL SUPPORT. Many patients with hilar cholangiocarcinoma are nutritionally depleted by the time they present for operative intervention. Fortunately, most have a functioning gastrointestinal tract. Total parenteral nutrition is usually not needed; however, preoperative enteral nutritional support is frequently employed either with a nasojejunal feeding tube or, more frequently, with high-protein dietary supplements. If indicated, enteral feeding can be continued postoperatively via a jejunal feeding tube.

PREOPERATIVE MANAGEMENT. Patients with jaundice should be admitted preoperatively for intravenous rehydration. Vitamin K should be administered, and fresh-frozen plasma should be considered if prothrombin time is prolonged. Perioperative antibiotics should cover both gram-negative and gram-positive organisms. In patients with a biliary stent in place, an amoxicillin–clavulanic acid combination or clindamycin in penicillin-allergic patients should be used in addition to an aminoglycoside. In unstented patients, an intravenous cephalosporin is sufficient. Mechanical bowel preparation is usually not indicated in patients with hilar cholangiocarcinoma.

INTRAOPERATIVE MANAGEMENT. Exploration should commence with a laparoscopy. In a prospective evaluation of diagnostic laparoscopy, 40% of patients with unresectable cholangiocarcinomas were identified with laparos-

Table 110–4	Proposed Modified T Stage Criteria for Hilar Cholangiocarcinoma

T1   Tumor confined to the confluence and/or right or left hepatic duct without portal vein involvement or liver atrophy
T2   Tumor confined to the confluence and/or right or left hepatic duct with ipsilateral liver atrophy. No portal vein involvement demonstrated.
T3   Tumor confined to the confluence and/or right or left hepatic duct with ipsilateral portal vein branch involvement with or without associated ipsilateral lobar liver atrophy. No main portal vein involvement (occlusion, invasion, or encasement)
T4   Either of the following:
      Tumor involving both the right and the left hepatic duct up to the secondary biliary radicals bilaterally
      Main portal vein encasement

copy; the remainder proved unresectable owing to advanced local disease. If laparoscopy is negative, we prefer a subcostal incision; a midline extension may be required to access the suprahepatic vena cava. A thorough laparotomy should also assess the caudate lobe for involvement. After Kocher's maneuver, the retroduodenal and retropancreatic lymph nodes are inspected and biopsied if metastases are suspected. Intraoperative ultrasonography is also performed at this time. Intrahepatic metastases or metastases in the celiac, retroduodenal, and portocaval lymph nodes preclude resection, and these patients should be considered for palliative biliary bypass.

An initial dissection will define the extent of tumor and the chances of resectability. The peritoneum over the gastrohepatic omentum is incised, and the common bile duct and hepatic artery are exposed. All lymphatic structures should be clipped and divided. The lymph nodes overlying the common hepatic artery should be removed en bloc. The common bile duct is encircled at the upper border of the duodenum and divided, oversewing the distal end. By elevating the proximal end, the extrahepatic bile ducts and portal lymph nodes can be retracted superiorly and the portal vein and hepatic arteries skeletonized. The proximal extent of the tumor is assessed by palpation, and portal vein involvement is assessed by palpation posterior to the biliary system. Segmental bile duct resection without hepatectomy can be undertaken if at least a 0.5-cm length of hepatic ducts can be exposed proximal to the tumor and if there is no parenchymal invasion. If the tumor extends into secondary biliary radicals, or if there is ipsilateral portal venous involvement, then a concomitant hepatic resection is needed. If a short segment of the main or contralateral portal vein is involved, portal venous reconstruction can be considered, but the risk to the patient increases. If the tumor extends to the left to involve the caudate ducts, caudate resection should also be performed. Partial hepatectomy requires inflow control by ligation and transection of the ipsilateral portal vein and hepatic artery; the ipsilateral hepatic vein can be isolated and divided before parenchymal division. The remaining bile duct can then be reconstructed with a 70-cm Roux-en-Y loop of jejunum. The anterior row of interrupted absorbable sutures should be placed first and the needles left on. A posterior row, taking both jejunal serosa and bile duct, should then be placed. Once this row is complete, the jejunum can be "railroaded" into the hilus and the sutures tied. The jejunal component of the anterior wall can then be completed.

If a segmental bile duct resection must be carried out, multiple hepatic ductal orifices may require reconstruction. In general, the side walls of adjacent ducts should be approximated with absorbable sutures and then anastomosis carried out in a technique similar to that used after hepatic resection. A surgical drain should be placed behind the anastomosis, and the abdomen is then closed.

POSTOPERATIVE MANAGEMENT. Postoperatively, patients are managed as described previously for peripheral cholangiocarcinoma if they have undergone a hepatectomy. Perioperative antibiotics should be continued until intraoperative bile cultures are negative or for 5 days postoperatively. Surgical drains are monitored for the presence of bile. It is not unusual for bilious drainage to occur in the initial postoperative period. This is usually of low volume (<100 mL per day), and it resolves without further intervention. High-volume leaks are indicative of a significant biliary fistula and require further management. If the drainage resolves, drains can be removed after feeding is begun. In general, the average length of stay after resection of hilar cholangiocarcinoma is 10 days for those patients requiring hepatic resection and 8 days for segmental bile duct resection alone.

COMPLICATIONS. In addition to the complications of hepatectomy, there are several complications that are unique to this type of procedure.

Hemorrhage. Bleeding may be from the hepatic veins or their branches, as in the case of surgery for peripheral cholangiocarcinoma. However, postoperative blood loss may also occur from structures at the hilus, particularly the portal vein and its branches. This can be minimized by careful attention to dissection and control of all venous branches with nonabsorbable sutures or staples.

Infection and Sepsis. Postoperative collections usually present with an increase in serum bilirubin and are due to a bile leak from a major or, more commonly, a minor duct. When sterile, they can be managed with percutaneous drainage. However, superinfection of these collections is more serious and will present as signs of sepsis. Infected postoperative collections should also be drained percutaneously and the patient treated with appropriate antibiotic therapy.

Biliary Fistula. A persistent biliary fistula after biliary enteric anastomosis generally suggests a technical error such as suture-line disruption or failure to incorporate a significant bile duct within the anastomosis. Fistulae may present as postoperative collection or bilious drainage from a drain. The initial management is directed at controlling the leak. Cholangiography, fistulography, or biliary radionuclide scintigraphy should define the origin of the fistula, the adequacy of drainage, and the presence of biliary-enteric continuity. Hilar fistulae are treated with prolonged drainage. Most fistulae close spontaneously, but usually with development of a stricture. Once a stricture has occurred, surgical correction is generally necessary.

Portal Vein Thrombosis. Although a rare complication, this generally occurs in patients in whom a venous resection with reconstruction has been performed. In the immediate postoperative period, portal vein thrombosis may manifest as tachycardia unresponsive to fluids. When portal vein thrombosis occurs later in the postoperative course, the sudden development of ascites, often in association with signs of liver failure, should alert the clinician to the diagnosis. Urgent operative intervention and thrombectomy may be successful in reestablishing flow; however, once thrombosis is established, treatment is primarily supportive. This can be a lethal complication.

OUTCOME. The only potential cure for hilar cholangiocarcinoma is resection. However, only about a third of patients with hilar cholangiocarcinoma are candidates for curative resection, and among this group, only those with

Table 110–5	**Contemporary Series of Surgical Resection for Hilar Cholangiocarcinoma**					
FIRST AUTHOR	**NUMBER RESECTED**	**% LIVER RESECTION**	**% NEGATIVE MARGIN**	**% POSITIVE MARGIN**	**3-YEAR SURVIVAL MARGIN* (%)**	**PERIOPERATIVE MORTALITY (%)**
Madariaga (1998)	28	100	50	50	40	14
Figueras (1998)	16	50	63	37	43	0
Nagino (1998)	138	90	78	22	43	6
Miyasaki (1998)	76	86	75	25	40	5
Burke (1998)	30	73	83	17	56†	6

*Figures reflect median survival.
†Figures reflect 5-year survival rates.

a negative histologic margin will attain long-term survival. Several contemporary series of patients with hilar cholangiocarcinoma managed with resection are presented in Table 110–5. Most groups are now performing liver resection for hilar cholangiocarcinoma in 50% to 100% of patients. Using this approach, a negative histologic margin was able to be achieved in more than half the patients, with a trend toward increased survival in all studies. Madariaga and colleagues, who perform liver resection in 100% of hilar cholangiocarcinomas, reported in 1998 the highest operative mortality of 14%. These authors pursued an extremely radical approach with 9 of 27 patients undergoing vascular reconstruction of the portal vein, the hepatic artery, or both in an attempt to get tumor clearance. The four operative deaths occurred in the nine patients requiring vascular reconstruction. Evidence in support of such an aggressive approach to hilar cholangiocarcinoma is reflected in the 40%-to-60% 3-year survival rates reported in series for which this strategy is followed.

A more controversial approach to the management of hilar cholangiocarcinoma is orthotopic liver transplantation (OLT). OLT has been performed for both resectable and unresectable hilar cholangiocarcinoma; however, the high incidence of lymph node metastases associated with this disease has markedly limited adoption of this approach. In 1996, Pichlmayr and associates reported a series of 249 patients with hilar cholangiocarcinoma of whom 125 underwent resection and 25 underwent OLT. Resection yielded equivalent or superior 5-year survival (27% versus 17%) at all stages of disease. Klempnauer and colleagues had similar results as reported in 1997. These results suggest that radical resection offers the best possibility of prolonged survival with a good quality of life.

PALLIATIVE AND ADJUVANT TREATMENT. When advanced local disease or distant metastases are identified, therapeutic intervention should be directed toward relief of biliary obstruction and associated symptoms. Endoscopic stenting for hilar cholangiocarcinoma is associated with a high failure rate, whereas percutaneous biliary drainage can be placed in almost all patients. We prefer metallic wall stents to plastic stents for long-term palliative relief of malignant biliary obstruction. These stents are completely internal, require no catheter care, and have a longer duration of patency than do plastic stents (6 to 8 months). In the absence of infective symptomatology, the entire liver need not be drained, because it has been shown that only 30% of the functioning hepatic mass needs to be decompressed for relief of jaundice and pruritus.

If patients are identified as unresectable at laparotomy, we favor performing an intrahepatic bilioenteric bypass to the segment III hepatic duct. The procedure provides excellent palliation, eliminates the need for stent change, and can be performed with low operative morbidity and mortality. In a series of 20 patients, there was no operative mortality, and a 1-year patency rate of 80% was observed. Other palliative options include placement of transhepatic stents with or without transtumoral extension into the gut.

ADJUVANT THERAPY. There is no effective adjuvant therapy for cholangiocarcinoma. Patients with hilar cholangiocarcinoma have been treated with 2000 cGy delivered via intraductal brachytherapy catheters afterloaded with iridium followed by 5000 cGy of external beam radiation over 5 to 6 weeks. Mean survival was 14 months, with all patients surviving for 6 months. Similar promising

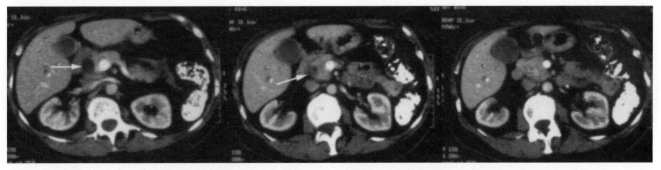

Figure 110–9. Sequential computed tomography taken 0.5 cm apart. A dilated common bile duct is demonstrated *(left; arrow)*. The next scan demonstrates an irregular filling defect in the common bile duct *(middle; arrow)*. The last scan shows a nondilated common bile duct *(right)*.

results using external beam radiotherapy alone and neo-adjuvant chemoradiotherapy have been reported; however, all approaches are considered investigational.

Currently, there is no effective chemotherapeutic agent for cholangiocarcinoma. A single study reported one complete response with a partial response (PR) rate of 20% using a regimen of fluorouracil, leucovorin, and carboplatin. In most reports, however, minimal response and PR rates far less than 20% are observed.

Photodynamic therapy has been studied in the palliative management of hilar cholangiocarcinoma. Unresectable patients treated intravenously with a hematoporphyrin derivative, followed 2 days later by intraluminal cholangioscopic photoactivation, have shown a precipitous fall in serum bilirubin and a subjective improvement in quality of life. No procedure-related morbidity or mortality was reported. Median survival was 14 months. Although this new modality appears promising, validation of these results awaits further investigation.

DISTAL CHOLANGIOCARCINOMA

These tumors include those that arise in the middle third of the extrahepatic bile ducts and true cholangiocarcinomas arising in the distal common bile duct. Most tumors are adenocarcinomas; however, papillary tumors are relatively more common in the distal bile duct than at the hilus.

Clinical Presentation

Symptomatic presentation of distal bile duct cancer is similar to that of hilar lesions. Up to 90% of patients present with progressive, painless jaundice, and one third will complain of abdominal pain, weight loss, or fever. Examination usually demonstrates a jaundiced patient with a palpable gallbladder. Distal cholangiocarcinomas are usually misdiagnosed as adenocarcinoma of the pancreatic head. Usually there is no mass lesion present on cross-sectional imaging with CT or MRI (Fig. 110–9).

ERC or MRCP will show a stricture of the distal common bile duct, usually with a normal pancreatic duct as the key to identifying this as cholangiocarcinoma and not pancreatic adenocarcinoma. Solitary strictures of the middle third are usually indicative of cholangiocarcinoma; however, gallbladder carcinoma may also give rise to malignant strictures in this location.

Histologic confirmation of malignancy is also unnecessary for lesions affecting the distal bile duct. Benign strictures in the absence of chronic pancreatitis do occur in the distal bile duct but are very rare.

PREOPERATIVE MANAGEMENT. This is similar to that for hilar tumors. Jaundiced patients should be admitted the day before surgery for intravenous hydration. Preoperative biliary drainage should be considered in patients with symptoms and signs of cholangitis. Coagulopathy should be managed with vitamin K and fresh-frozen plasma. Perioperative antibiotic therapy is important. The patient should consent to possible extrahepatic bile duct excision alone, possible pancreaticoduodenectomy, or palliative biliary bypass if the tumor proves unresectable.

INTRAOPERATIVE MANAGEMENT. Operative exploration begins with a diagnostic laparoscopy. If the laparoscopy is negative, we prefer a bilateral subcostal incision. The principal decision is whether a pancreaticoduodenectomy must be performed to obtain tumor clearance, depending on the relationship of the lower extent of the tumor to the superior border of the duodenum. If the tumor lies adjacent to the duodenum or is retroduodenal, a pancreaticoduodenectomy will be required. If bile duct excision alone is being performed, a portal lymphadenectomy should be carried out with division of the common bile duct in its retroduodenal portion. Biliary reconstruction is carried out with a Roux-en-Y limb. If pancreaticoduodenectomy is required, our practice is to perform a standard resection without sparing the pylorus.

Pearls and Pitfalls

- The most common location of cholangiocarcinoma is at the hepatic hilus.
- Conditions that predispose to acute or chronic biliary epithelial injury are associated with tumor development, including hepatolithiasis, parasitic infestation, sclerosing cholangitis, inflammatory bowel disease, and choledochal cysts.
- Peripheral cholangiocarcinomas are rare. They present as a hypovascular mass in the liver and when possible are managed with hepatic resection.
- Extrahepatic cholangiocarcinomas are divided into papillary, nodular sclerosing, and diffuse types.
- Papillary tumors, which account for about 10% of cholangiocarcinomas, are more common in the distal extrahepatic ducts and have a more favorable prognosis.
- Nodular sclerosing tumors compose 90% of hilar cholangiocarcinomas and narrow the ductal bifurcation.
- Lobar atrophy with crowding of the ducts and contralateral hypertrophy is indicative of chronic biliary obstruction or ipsilateral portal venous involvement.
- Biliary stent placement should not be undertaken for hyperbilirubinemia alone but rather for cholangitis. Infective stent-related complications are less frequent if the stent has been placed percutaneously rather than endoscopically.
- For hilar cholangiocarcinoma, the critical intraoperative decision is whether to perform a hepatic resection or a segmental bile duct resection; tumors that involve the left biliary system may require a caudate resection.
- Suspicious portal and celiac lymph nodes should be biopsied for metastatic disease before the common bile duct is divided.
- For hilar cholangiocarcinoma, portal vein involvement is the most important predictor of resectability, whereas negative margins are the most important predictor of survival.
- Ninety percent of distal cholangiocarcinomas present with jaundice. Endoscopic biopsies are often unhelpful, and treatment is by surgical resection with either bile duct excision alone or pancreaticoduodenectomy. Positive lymph nodes are predictive of adverse outcome.

POSTOPERATIVE MANAGEMENT. Perioperative antibiotics should be continued until intraoperative bile cultures are found to be negative. For patients who have undergone a pancreaticoduodenectomy, we administer 100 μg of octreotide subcutaneously twice daily when the pancreas is of soft consistency and the pancreatic duct is of small caliber, because these patients are most at risk of postoperative pancreatic leak.

COMPLICATIONS. After extrahepatic bile duct resection and pancreaticoduodenectomy, patients can develop the same complications as those seen in patients after hilar resections; however, several specific complications should be mentioned. Postoperative hemorrhage can occur after pancreaticoduodenectomy from the stump of the gastroduodenal artery or the pancreatic or gastric anastomoses. Other common sites of hemorrhage are the jejunal mesenteric arcade and the region of the ligament of Treitz. A pancreatic leak may occur at the site of the pancreaticojejunostomy. If possible, pancreatic leaks should be controlled with percutaneous drain placement and managed with parenteral nutrition and octreotide, because their natural history is to heal without requiring further operative intervention.

OUTCOMES. In a series of 45 patients with completely resected distal cholangiocarcinoma at Memorial Sloan-Kettering Cancer Center, New York, median survival was 33 months, and 5-year actuarial survival was 27%. Patients treated with stent placement alone had a 1-year survival of 37%, and there were no 2-year survivors. Only positive lymph node status was predictive of adverse prognosis in a multivariate model. The most common sites of disease recurrence were the tumor bed and the liver. Systemic metastatic disease is rare.

SELECTED READINGS

Burke E, Jarnagin WR, Hochwald SN, et al: Hilar cholangiocarcinoma patterns of spread, the importance of hepatic resection for curative operation, and a presurgical clinical staging system. Ann Surg 1998;228:385.

Figueras J, Llado-Garriga L, Lama C, et al: Resection as elective treatment of hilar cholangiocarcinoma (Klatskin tumor). Gastroenterol Hepatol 1998;21:218.

Fong Y, Blumgart LH, Lin E, et al: Outcome and treatment for distal bile duct cancer. Br J Surg 1996;83:1712.

Harrison LE, Fong Y, Klimstra DS, et al: Surgical treatment of 32 patients with intrahepatic cholangiocarcinoma. Br J Surg 1998;85:1068.

Jarnagin WR, Burke E, Powers C, et al: Intrahepatic biliary enteric bypass provides effective palliation in selected patients with malignant obstruction at the hepatic duct confluence. Am J Surg 1998;175:453.

Klemphauer J, Ridder GJ, Werner M, et al: What constitutes long-term survival after surgery for hilar cholangiocarcinoma? Cancer 1997;79:26.

Madariaga JR, Iwatsuki S, Todo S, et al: Liver resection for hilar and peripheral cholangiocarcinomas: A study of 62 cases. Ann Surg 1998;227:70.

Miyazaki M, Ito H, Nakagawa K, et al: Aggressive surgical approaches to hilar cholangiocarcinoma: Hepatic or local resection? Surgery 1998;123:131.

Nagino M, Nimura Y, Kamiya J, et al: Segmental liver resection for hilar cholangiocarcinoma. Hepatogastroenterology 1998;45:7.

Pichlmayr R, Weimann A, Klempnauer J, et al: Surgical treatment in proximal bile duct cancer: A single-center experience. Ann Surg 1996;224:628.

Chapter 111
Cancer of the Gallbladder

Sandeep Malhotra and Yuman Fong

Gallbladder cancer is an aggressive malignancy associated with a poor clinical outcome. This cancer spreads early by direct invasion of adjacent structures, as well as via lymphatic and hematogenous routes. Shed or spilled gallbladder cancer cells also have a remarkable ability to grow on all surfaces; consequently, peritoneal implants, abdominal wound implants, or recurrences at the laparoscopic port or needle biopsy site are encountered frequently. Thus, this cancer usually presents with advanced disease, and the 5-year survival rate in most large series is less than 5%, with a median survival outlook of less than 6 months. Surgical excision represents the only effective therapy, and extensive procedures are usually necessary for a complete excision of the neoplasm. This chapter reviews the natural history, biology, staging, and surgical treatment of gallbladder cancer with an emphasis on surgical decision making.

ANATOMIC CONSIDERATIONS

The gallbladder lies on segments IVB and V of the liver, and these segments are involved early in tumors arising in the fundus and body of the gallbladder. Tumors of the infundibulum or cystic duct readily obstruct the common bile duct and produce jaundice. The hepatic artery and portal vein are also in close proximity to the infundibulum, and invasion of these vascular structures is often the reason for their being unresectable. In addition, the proximity of the duodenum and the transverse colon to the gallbladder makes these adjacent organs possible sites for direct tumor extension (Fig. 111–1).

CLINICAL PRESENTATION

The duration of symptoms does not seem to provide any clues as to the presence of tumor. The clinical presentation of gallbladder cancer is difficult to distinguish from that of biliary colic or chronic cholecystitis. Right upper quadrant or epigastric discomfort is the most common symptom. Jaundice occurs in up to one third of patients. Weight loss tends to be a sign of advanced disease.

In some symptomatic patients, preoperative diagnostic imaging establishes the diagnosis of gallbladder cancer and further treatment is definitive for that disease. In other patients, however, symptoms are attributed to gallstone disease, and they are subjected to cholecystectomy for presumed benign gallstone disease. The gallbladder carcinoma is found incidentally at surgery or only after pathologic analysis of the cholecystectomy specimen. The strategy for definitive care is discussed here for both these situations.

Laboratory Examinations

Routine blood chemistry tests are nonspecific for gallbladder cancer. Increased alkaline phosphatase activity or serum bilirubin concentrations are often seen but can easily be attributed to associated gallstone disease. If gallbladder cancer is suspected, serum levels of the tumor markers carcinoembryonic antigen (CEA) or carbohydrate antigen 19-9 (CA 19-9) may be helpful. A CEA level greater than 4 ng/mL is more than 90% specific for the diagnosis of gallbladder cancer when an imaging test suggests a

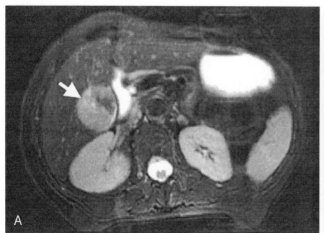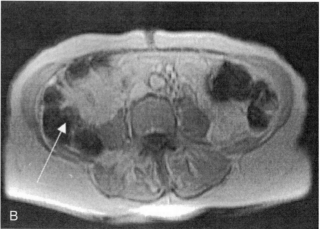

Figure 111–1. Magnetic resonance imaging demonstrating typical appearance of gallbladder cancer. *A,* The origins of the tumor in the gallbladder appearing as a sessile large polyp. *B,* Extension of this tumor inferiorly to involve the transverse mesocolon and right colon. Resection was accomplished with an en bloc liver resection, portal lymphadenectomy, and right colectomy.

gallbladder cancer, but it is only 50% sensitive. Ca 19-9 in this clinical setting is a better serum marker for gallbladder cancer; levels greater than 20 units/mL have a 79% sensitivity and 79% specificity.

Radiologic Diagnosis

Before the routine use of computed tomography (CT) and ultrasonography, the preoperative diagnosis of gallbladder carcinoma was evident in only 10% of patients. In the 1980s, CT and real-time ultrasonography increased the preoperative diagnosis rate to about 80%. The most common finding on ultrasonography is an inhomogeneous mass replacing all or part of the gallbladder (see Fig. 111–1). More than 90% of patients with gallbladder cancers also have gallstones, and approximately 1% of all patients undergoing cholecystectomy for stones are found to have an incidental gallbladder cancer. Therefore, vigilance should be exercised when examining the ultrasonography for patients under evaluation for gallstones, especially if polyps, eccentric wall thickening, or any generalized systemic symptoms (weight loss, malaise, or constant right upper quadrant pain) are present.

If gallbladder cancer is suspected on ultrasonography, or if the patient is found incidentally on pathologic analysis of an excised gallbladder to have cancer, additional imaging to stage the disease (see Staging Systems) is indicated, the goals of which are to rule out unresectable disease. The major sites of disease that would render the lesion unresectable are peritoneal disease, discontiguous liver disease, retropancreatic or celiac lymphatic metastases, and local vascular (portal vein or hepatic artery) encasement. Current generation helical CT or magnetic resonance imaging can often define unresectable disease and are the next tests of choice. On occasion, angiography may be necessary for definitive demonstration of suspected vascular encasement. For the jaundiced patient in the past, endoscopic or percutaneous cholangiograms were necessary for defining the extent of biliary involvement by tumor and for surgical planning. Recent advances in ultrasonography and magnetic resonance cholangiopancreatography (MRCP) allow noninvasive substitutes that reduce the morbidity of perioperative workup and decrease the chance of biliary sepsis.

Preoperative Pathologic Diagnosis

If a gallbladder cancer is suspected, percutaneous biopsy should be undertaken only if the lesion is clearly unresectable and if palliative treatment requires histologic confirmation. Gallbladder cancer has a great propensity for growth in needle biopsy tracts and in the peritoneum if spilled. All effort should be made to attempt complete en bloc resection of gallbladder cancer if possible. At open surgery, if diagnostic doubt remains and a diagnosis is necessary to justify a radical resection, the gallbladder can be completely excised and sent for frozen section analysis. Alternatively, bile cytology is a good way of securing a diagnosis. In recent studies, the sensitivity of bile cytology alone for the diagnosis of gallbladder cancer

was approximately 65%. The false-positive rate was less than 1%.

STAGING SYSTEMS

Multiple staging systems have been described for gallbladder cancer, taking into account pathologic and clinical characteristics with prognostic significance. The main staging systems referred to in the literature over the past 5 years include the modified Nevin system, the Japanese Biliary Surgical Society system, and the AJCC/UICC TNM staging system (Table 111–1). These staging systems differ mainly in the relative weight placed on nodal metastases. The modified Nevin system seems to be the best supported by Western data, and it is likely that the AJCC staging system will soon be modified accordingly.

OPERATIVE MANAGEMENT

Preoperative Preparation

Medical evaluation and selection of patients for surgery is as for other major liver surgery. Because most patients undergoing surgery for gallbladder cancer are elderly, it is prudent to optimize their cardiac and pulmonary status. Coagulation defects should be sought and corrected, especially if there is preoperative jaundice. Laxatives and enemas are administered; colonic preparation is particularly important for patients with large tumors that may invade the transverse colon (see Fig. 111–1). Prophylactic antibiotics are directed at biliary tract flora or specifically at the biliary microbiology results, if available. There is no known or accepted indication for neoadjuvant chemotherapy or radiation therapy.

Intraoperative Management

Whether a cholecystectomy has already been performed before the gallbladder cancer is recognized will have significant influence over operative conduct. The most important criterion dictating extent of resection, however, is extent of disease as predicted by stage and as found at the time of exploration. The most practical way of approaching gallbladder cancer is to consider the disease according to T stage (Fig. 111–2).

T1 tumors are confined within the muscular layer of the gallbladder. There is general agreement that simple cholecystectomy is sufficient. Most series document a long-term survival rate of greater than 90% with simple cholecystectomy. Most of these tumors are found incidentally during pathologic analysis after previous cholecystectomy (Fig. 111–3). The pathology should be reviewed to ensure that there is no extension of tumor to the margins, including the cystic duct margin. If all margins are negative, no further operative therapy is indicated.

T2 tumors have transgressed the muscular layer of the gallbladder but not the serosa. It might be initially thought that a simple cholecystectomy would suffice. However, there is convincing data that effective surgical therapy for T2 gallbladder cancer should consist of a

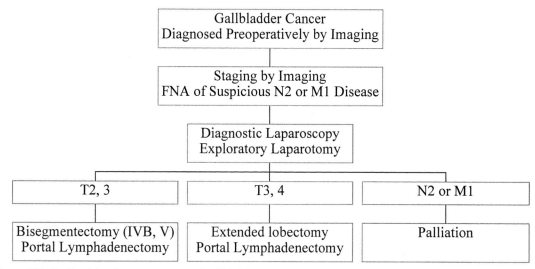

Figure 111–2. Algorithm for management of gallbladder cancer found as a suspicious mass or thickening on preoperative imaging. T1 lesions will most likely not be recognized until after cholecystectomy. If there is a strong suspicion of a T1 papillary lesion, then a simple cholecystectomy should be performed with a pathologic frozen section for examining depth of invasion and the cystic duct margin.

Table 111–1	**Summary of Most Commonly Used Staging Systems**			
STAGE	**TNM**	**MODIFIED NEVIN**	**JAPANESE***	**PROPOSED NEW STAGING**
I	Mucosal or muscular invasion (T1N0M0)	In situ carcinoma	Confined to gallbladder capsule	Mucosal or muscular invasion (T1N0M0)
II	Transmuscular invasion, within serosa (T2N0M0)	Mucosal or muscular invasion	N1 lymph nodes; minimal liver or bile duct invasion	Transmural invasion within serosa (T2N0M0)
III	Liver invasion <2 cm; lymph node metastasis (T3N0–1M0)	Transmural direct liver invasion	N2 lymph nodes; marked liver or bile duct invasion	(A) Liver invasion <2 cm (T3N0M0) (B) Liver invasion >2 cm (T4N0M0)
IV	(A) Liver invasion >2 cm (T4N0M0, T4N1M0) (B) Distant metastasis (TxN2M0, TxNxM1)	Lymph node metastasis	Distant metastasis	(A) Nodal metastases (TxN1M0) (B) Distant metastases (TxN2M0, TxNxM1)
V	—	Distant metastasis	—	—

*Japanese Biliary Surgery Society.

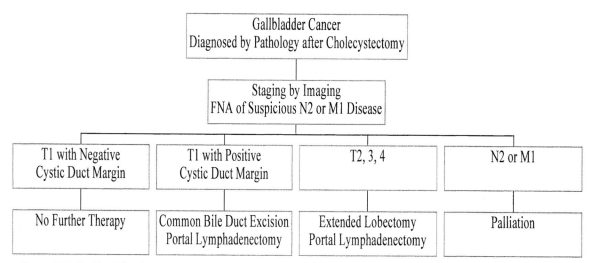

Figure 111–3. Algorithm for management of gallbladder cancer found incidentally on pathologic examination of a cholecystectomy specimen.

radical resection, including resection of adjacent liver and portal lymphadenectomy. The plane of dissection for a simple cholecystectomy along the liver is usually in the subserosal plane of the perimuscular connective tissues and may violate a T2 tumor. In addition, approximately one third of patients with T2 gallbladder cancer have regional lymph node metastases. Thus, it is not surprising that a number of clinical series have demonstrated that radical resection, even after prior simple cholecystectomy, is associated with significantly better long-term outcome than simple cholecystectomy.

The usual presentation of T2 gallbladder cancer is also during pathologic analysis of a simple cholecystectomy specimen (see Fig. 111–3). The patient should be staged by imaging to rule out unresectable disease. Treatment should then be re-exploration, liver resection, and portal lymphadenectomy.

T3 and T4 tumors have extended beyond the serosa of the gallbladder to involve liver or adjacent organs. T3 tumors extend less than 2 cm into the liver, whereas T4 tumors extend greater than 2 cm. Recent data reporting actual long-term disease-free survival after resection of bulky gallbladder cancers support use of aggressive radical resections as therapy for selected patients with these tumors (Table 111–2). T4 tumors have a much lower resectability rate than T3 lesions, because of a higher incidence of distant metastases, including peritoneal dissemination. However, if resected, the long-term outcomes of T3 or T4 tumors are similar. Resection usually requires a major liver resection (lobectomy or trisegmentectomy) combined with a portal lymphadenectomy.

Patients with Prior Cholecystectomy

Many patients, particularly those with early stage lesions, are seen for definitive therapy after prior cholecystectomy. Several series support repeat laparotomy and radical resection for appropriately selected patients who previously underwent an open cholecystectomy. Recent data also support radical re-resection after prior laparoscopic cholecystectomy. Some differences in operative conduct are appropriate for these patients compared with patients who are first seen for initial surgery. Scars from the recent surgery can easily be confused with tumor. Not only are the procedures longer, but more extensive liver resections are also generally needed. Stage for stage, peritoneal dissemination of tumor is more common. Previous incisions and all laparoscopic port sites should also be excised, because wound site recurrences are common.

Patients seen for primary surgery for suspected gallbladder cancer should have laparoscopic staging before open laparotomy. As many as 50% of patients with unresectable disease are identified by laparoscopy, and the morbidity of an unresectable laparotomy can be avoided. If the disease appears resectable, laparotomy should then be undertaken with initial evaluation of peritoneum, liver, and regional nodes. The lesser sac is entered early, and the celiac lymph nodes and caudate lobe are assessed. A generous Kocher maneuver facilitates assessment of peripancreatic lymph nodes. Extent of liver resection is dictated by the bulk of tumor, extent of scarring from previous surgery, and vascular involvement by tumor. The vessels at greatest risk are the right portal vein and right hepatic artery. Proximity of tumor or actual involvement of these vessels is the reason that the majority of T3 and T4 neoplasms require a right hepatic lobectomy. Patients with a T2 tumor and some patients with T3 cancer can often undergo an extended cholecystectomy, including resection of liver segments IVB and V (see Fig. 111–2). Patients with prior cholecystectomy and patients with T3 or T4 tumors usually require a lobectomy for an R0 resection of tumor (see Fig. 111–3).

A complete portal lymphadenectomy is reasonable because nodal metastases occur in more than one third of patients with T2, T3, or T4 cancers. Except in the thinnest of patients, a thorough lymphadenectomy requires excision of the common bile duct, because nodal tissues can be adherent. Patients with prior cholecystectomy almost always require common duct excision, because scarring in the porta hepatis further obscures planes for dissection. Finally, patients with right portal vein or hepatic artery involvement by tumor should also have resection of the common bile duct, because transection of the bile duct allows for much safer dissection of the vasculature in this area, particularly if the junction of the right and left portal vein requires dissection. If the common duct is resected, biliary continuity should be reestablished using a 70-cm Roux-en-Y loop of jejunum.

POSTOPERATIVE CARE

Postoperative care is similar to that for other hepatobiliary resections. A nasogastric tube is used if a biliary anastomosis is performed to prevent distention of the Roux-en-Y loop that may compromise the anastomosis. Early ambulation is encouraged. Abdominal drains are also used if a biliary anastomosis is performed, particularly if endoscopic or percutaneous biliary drains were placed preoperatively. Such preoperative biliary manipulation leads to bacteriobilia, which predisposes to postoperative infections. If a major liver resection has been performed, a coagulation profile should be monitored and fresh-frozen plasma used when appropriate. Phosphorus supplementation is also necessary during the initial period of liver regeneration. The hospital stay is usually between 10 and 14 days.

Table 111–2	Survival After Extended Resection for Gallbladder Cancers		
PRIMARY AUTHOR	**N**	**% STAGE III/IV**	**5-YR SURVIVAL (%)**
Nakamura, 1989	15	86	25
Donohue, 1990	42	78	33
Ogura, 1991	982	48	42
Shirai, 1992	40	52	45
Ouchi, 1994	36	47	38
Todoroki, 1999	123	84	36
Fong, 2000	100	63	38

RESULTS

Operative Morbidity and Mortality

An important consideration in the recommendation for radical surgery is the operative complication rate. Most patients undergoing treatment for gallbladder cancer are in their seventh decade of life and are at increased operative risk because of medical comorbidity. Consequently, postoperative complications are reported in up to 50% of patients, and mortality rate remains in the 5% range. Perioperative deaths are usually due to hepatic failure or pulmonary complications and occur mainly in the patients subjected to major liver resection (Table 111–3).

Long-term Results After Resection

There remains no doubt that resection has a major influence on outcome. In a multi-institutional review, Ogura and colleagues (1991) recently reported a 51% 5-year survival rate for 984 patients undergoing radical resection versus 6% for 702 patients undergoing more conservative management. These results are echoed by our results from the Memorial Sloan-Kettering Cancer Center where resection was associated with a 38% 5-year survival rate, but nonoperative therapy resulted in only a 4% 5-year survival rate. Even for advanced local disease, data are accumulating to support surgical resection (summarized in Table 111–2). In our data, surgical resection is associated with a 67% actuarial 5-year survival rate for patients with completely resected stage III and 33% 5-year survival for patients with completely resected stage IV tumors.

Table 111–3	Intraoperative Pitfalls, Danger Points, and Postoperative Complications Associated with Extended Cholecystectomy and Liver Resections for Gallbladder Cancer

INTRAOPERATIVE DANGER POINTS	POSTOPERATIVE COMPLICATIONS
Hemorrhage from hepatic or portal veins or hepatic arteries	Ascites
	Biliary fistula
	Biliary obstruction
Air embolism form hepatic venous injury	Coagulopathy
	Hemorrhage
Injury to biliary ductal system, with postoperative obstruction or fistula	Hypophosphatemia
	Intra-abdominal infection
	Liver failure
Portal or hepatic vein compromise with subsequent ischemia or postsinusoidal portal hypertension	Pneumonia
	Respiratory compromsie from pleural effusion
Proloned vascular inflow occlusion leading to refractory liver injury	
Injury to diaphragm, inferior vena cava, or intestine	

ADJUVANT THERAPY

There are no data documenting utility of adjuvant therapy for gallbladder cancer. Nevertheless, many patients, particularly those with documented lymph node metastases, often undergo treatment with chemotherapy using 5-fluorouracil (5-FU) or gemcitabine combined with external beam radiation therapy.

PALLIATIVE MANAGEMENT

Only a minority of patients subjected to evaluation for gallbladder cancer are candidates for resection. Most have unresectable disease, and the chance of surviving 1 year is only 15%. The poor overall course of gallbladder cancer needs to be considered, especially when deciding upon palliative management. The main goals of palliation should be relief of pain, jaundice, and bowel obstruction. Palliation should be accomplished as simply as possible given the aggressive nature of this disease. Biliary bypass for obstruction can be difficult because of advanced disease in the porta hepatis. Therefore, the surgical bypass of choice is a segment III bypass. In the patient with a dilated biliary tree who is found at laparotomy to have unresectable cancer, such a bypass is reasonable. If the preoperative diagnosis is advanced, unresectable gallbladder cancer in the jaundiced patient, a noninvasive radiologic approach to biliary drainage is preferred to avoid the morbidity and recovery time of a laparotomy with surgical bypass.

Numerous chemotherapies have been evaluated in treatment of gallbladder cancer, including 5-FU, Adriamycin (doxorubicin), and nitrosoureas; however, tumor responses occur in only a minority of patients. Radiation therapy has also been used as palliation for gallbladder cancer, but with no clear documentation of utility. If these therapies are attempted, the patient should be closely monitored and therapies stopped as soon as there are any signs of tumor progression.

GALLBLADDER POLYPS

Gallbladder polyps are a common problem faced by the general surgeon. Approximately 5% of the general population have gallbladder polyps. The most important issue in care of the patient with a gallbladder polyp is the differentiation between benign polyps, premalignant lesions, and gallbladder cancer. The majority of polyps are benign, and most are cholesterol polyps. These are pseudotumors that consist histologically of submucosal lipid-laden macrophages. Other benign polyps include epithelial tumors (adenoma), mesenchymal tumors (fibroma, lipoma, hemangioma) or other pseudotumors (inflammatory polyps, adenomyoma). Of these, the only type of lesion thought to be precancerous is the adenoma. None except adenomas need treatment unless symptomatic.

Cholesterol polyps, which make up greater than 90% of benign lesions, are usually multiple (>3), small, and have an intact mucosa. Malignant lesions are significantly more likely to be found in patients older than 50 years of

Pearls and Pitfalls

- Clinical presentation of gallbladder cancer usually mimics that of cholelithiasis.
- With current state-of-the-art imaging, most patients with gallbladder cancer can be recognized preoperatively.
- Staging of gallbladder cancer usually is best accomplished by helical CT and preoperative staging laparoscopy.
- Operative therapy includes a radical resection of liver parenchyma and portal lymph nodes in patients with T2–T4 lesions.
- For T1 lesions (disease confined to mucosa without invasion of muscularis), cholecystectomy alone is sufficient.
- For fully resected gallbladder cancer, 5-year survival rates approach 35%.
- Palliative resection for gallbladder cancer should be reserved for selected patients.
- There is no good evidence that chemotherapy or radiation therapy is effective, even though these therapies are used commonly.

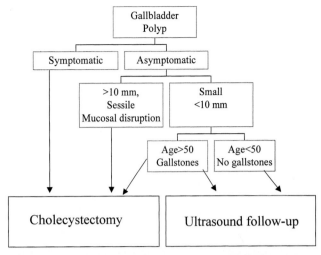

Figure 111–4. Algorithm for treatment of gallbladder polyps. (Modified from Boulton and Adams, Lancet 349:1032, 1997.)

age and are more likely to be present as a solitary lesion, sessile in character, and greater than 1.0 cm in diameter. Ultrasonography is the most practical test for evaluating polypoid lesions of the gallbladder, having a sensitivity of 90% and a specificity of 94% in making the diagnosis. For symptomatic polyps, cholecystectomy is recommended (Fig. 111–4). For patients with gallbladder polyps and other reasons for cholecystectomy, such as cholelithiasis, cholecystectomy should be performed. For polyps suspicious for cancer (size greater than 1 cm, less than three lesions, eroded mucosa), cholecystectomy should be performed. Other patients should be followed up with ultrasonography every 6 months, and cholecystectomy should be performed if any change is noted. Some investigators have advocated cholecystectomy for patients with fewer than three polyps regardless of size, but with polyps smaller than 1 cm, the vast majority are benign.

Because of the poor prognosis of gallbladder cancer and the low morbidity of a cholecystectomy, any suspicion of cancer should prompt cholecystectomy. Open cholecystectomy is recommended if cancer is even remotely suspected to decrease the risk of gallbladder rupture and spillage of tumor. In addition, the surgeon should be prepared to perform a definitive radical resection if invasive cancer is proven by frozen section histology.

SELECTED READINGS

Boulton RA, Adams DH: Gallbladder polyps: When to wait and when to act [published erratum appears in Lancet 1997;349:1032]. Lancet 1997;349:817.

Donohue JH, Nagorney DM, Grant CS, et al: Carcinoma of the gallbladder. Does radical resection improve outcome? Arch Surg 1990;125:237.

Drouard F, Delamarre J, Capron J: Cutaneous seeding of gallbladder cancer after laparoscopic cholecystectomy. N Engl J Med 1991;325:1316.

Fong Y, Heffernan N, Blumgart LH: Gallbladder carcinoma discovered during laparoscopic cholecystectomy: Aggressive reresection is beneficial. Cancer 1998;83:423.

Fong Y, Jarnagin W, Blumgart LH: Gallbladder cancer: Comparison of patients presenting initially for definitive operation with those presenting after prior non-curative intervention. Ann Surg 2000;233:557.

Nevin JE, Moran TJ, Kay S, King R: Carcinoma of the gallbladder: staging, treatment, and prognosis. Cancer 1976;37:141.

Ogura Y, Mizumoto R, Isaji S, et al: Radical operations for carcinoma of the gallbladder: Present status in Japan. World J Surg 1991;15:337.

Shirai Y, Yoshida K, Tsukada K, Muto T: Inapparent carcinoma of the gallbladder: An appraisal of a radical second operation after simple cholecystectomy. Cancer 1988;62:1422.

Spleen: Benign

Chapter 112
Splenectomy
Richard T. Schlinkert

Splenectomy is a relatively straightforward procedure. However, immunologic consequences and postsplenectomy sepsis may be life threatening, and caution should be exercised when deciding to proceed with the operation. Splenic surgery is indicated in select patients with trauma, sequestration and destruction of hematologic elements by the spleen, lymphoma, myeloproliferative diseases, cysts or masses, wandering spleen, and symptomatic sinistral (left-sided) portal hypertension. This chapter addresses nontraumatic diseases of the spleen that may warrant surgical intervention. Close collaboration of surgeon and hematologist can aid in proper selection of the patient for splenectomy, accurate timing of surgery, adequate preoperative preparation of the patient, and effective management of postoperative complications.

DESTRUCTION OF HEMATOLOGIC ELEMENTS

Thrombocytopenia

Thrombocytopenia may result from decreased platelet production, altered distribution of platelets, and increased platelet breakdown. Decreased platelet production may be seen in rare hereditary conditions or may be acquired secondary to viral infection, nutritional deficiencies, neoplasm involving the bone marrow, and presence of drugs or toxins. Splenectomy will not benefit these patients. Patients with altered platelet distribution, such as those with portal hypertension, usually have splenomegaly but only moderate thrombocytopenia (platelet count of 30,000 to 100,000/mm³). Symptoms of bleeding are generally absent unless another condition exists. The absolute platelet count may be normal, and splenectomy is not indicated. Thrombocytopenia secondary to increased platelet destruction may be related to immune factors, consumption of platelets, and clotting factors (e.g., disseminated intravascular coagulation) or to platelet aggregation in the microvasculature (e.g., thrombotic thrombocytopenic purpura). Therapeutic splenectomy is limited to patients with certain immune thrombocytopenias.

Immune Thrombocytopenic Purpura

Immune thrombocytopenic purpura (ITP) is the most common cause of nontraumatic elective splenectomy. Patients present with bruising and report that they bleed easily. Constitutional symptoms should lead one to consider other diagnoses. The spleen is of normal size or is, at most, slightly enlarged. A palpable spleen should call the diagnosis into question. The spleen appears to be a source of antiplatelet antibody production, as well as the major site of platelet destruction in most patients. The liver also acts as a site of platelet destruction in certain patients. Despite the fact that the disease is believed to be related to antiplatelet antibodies, detection of platelet antibodies is unreliable and not currently useful for diagnosis. Rather, the diagnosis rests on the finding of thrombocytopenia without other detectable cause. The mean platelet volume is increased. Bone marrow biopsy may not be necessary, but when it is obtained, it shows a normal to increased number of megakaryocytes. Patients should have a negative human immunodeficiency virus (HIV) screen and an otherwise normal peripheral smear and should be taking no offending medications.

Initial treatment is with corticosteroids. A subset of patients will respond to steroids, and the thrombocytopenia will not recur when the steroids are discontinued. Others, however, will continue to fail chronic treatment with high doses of steroids or may not respond at all to steroid therapy. These subsets of patients should be

Table 112–1	Indications for Splenectomy in Hemolytic Anemias

RED CELL PATHOLOGY	INDICATIONS FOR SPLENECTOMY
Red cell membrane defects	
Hereditary spherocytosis	All°
Hereditary elliptocytosis	Severe hemolysis only
Hereditary stomatocytosis	Probably all
Rh-null syndrome	Hemolytic episodes and splenomegaly
Red cell metabolic defects	Individualized to defect
Sickle cell disease	Acute splenic sequestration
β-Thalassemia	Excessive transfusions required
Autoimmune hemolytic anemia	Failure or complications of steroids

°When the patient is an adolescent, if possible.

considered for laparoscopic splenectomy. Approximately 90% of patients will respond rapidly to splenectomy, with long-term success of 65% to 80%. Accessory spleens should be specifically and methodically looked for and removed at the time of splenectomy because these are found in 10% to 15% of patients and may be the cause of failure of splenectomy to resolve the thrombocytopenia.

ITP may occur during pregnancy. Intervention is usually reserved for platelet counts of fewer than 50,000/mm³. Glucocorticoids are the first line of therapy. Splenectomy, when required, should be undertaken during the second trimester if medical therapy fails.

HIV-Related Immune Thrombocytopenia

HIV-related immune thrombocytopenia presents in a fashion similar to that of ITP. Immune complexes, rather than platelet antibodies, may be more important mediators of this disease. There appears to be decreased production of platelets despite a normal to increased number of megakaryocytes in the bone marrow. Thrombocytopenia is unrelated to the stage of HIV infection and does not portend an early progression to acquired immunodeficiency syndrome. Platelet counts may improve spontaneously, and thus splenectomy should be reserved for the symptomatic patient. Splenectomy does not cause progression of the underlying disease.

Hemolytic Anemia

Hemolytic anemia responsive to splenectomy may be related to genetic defects of the red blood cells or to autoimmune processes. Genetic defects include abnormalities of the red blood cell membrane (e.g., hereditary spherocytosis) and defects in red blood cell metabolism. The more common hemolytic anemias are listed in Table 112–1 along with general indications for splenectomy with each disease. In general, if these diseases present in childhood, delaying splenectomy until after the immune system matures is preferable.

Lymphoma

HODGKIN'S DISEASE. Hodgkin's disease is defined by the characteristic Reed-Sternberg cell. Histologic sub-

types include lymphocyte predominant, nodular sclerosis, mixed cellularity, and lymphocyte depleted. Radiotherapy may be used to treat localized disease, and chemotherapy has shown dramatic cure rates for disseminated disease. The increased use of chemotherapy has caused a decreased demand for staging laparotomy. The only current indication for staging laparotomy, then, is to determine if a patient might be treated with radiotherapy alone. In general, patients with B-symptoms (night sweats, fever, weight loss) will receive chemotherapy and are not considered for staging. At many institutions, even early-stage Hodgkin's disease is treated with combined chemotherapy and radiation, negating the need for staging. Patients with clinical stage IA disease with involvement of a node high in the neck may be treated with radiotherapy and might not require staging. Selected patients with stage IIA or stage IIIA disease may benefit from staging, if radiotherapy alone is planned or desirable.

NON-HODGKIN'S LYMPHOMA. Most patients with non-Hodgkin's lymphoma do not require splenectomy. However, selected patients may benefit from splenic removal. The primary indications for splenectomy in non-Hodgkin's lymphoma include diagnosis (when disease is limited to the spleen), predominance of splenic disease, serious symptoms of splenomegaly, and cytopenias limiting additional treatments. The decision to proceed with splenectomy depends on the subtype of non-Hodgkin's lymphoma, the overall condition of the patient, the degree of impairment secondary to symptoms, and the need to continue chemotherapy. Collaboration with a hematologist is imperative in patient selection.

Myeloproliferative Disease

Myeloproliferative diseases exist on a spectrum that can be divided based on the presence or absence of a genetic translocation between chromosomes 9 and 22 known as the Philadelphia chromosome (Table 112–2). Philadelphia chromosome–negative proliferative diseases include a spectrum of essential thrombocytosis, polycythemia vera, and agnogenic myeloid metaplasia (essential megakaryocytic granulocytic metaplasia). Splenectomy is of no benefit in the first two conditions, but it may be considered in selected patients with highly symptomatic agnogenic myeloid metaplasia (Table 112–3). Splenectomy in this group of patients, however, carries significant risks intraoperatively because of the size of the spleen and the

Table 112–2	Classification of the Spectrum of Myeloproliferative Disorders

PHILADELPHIA CHROMOSOME [t(9;22)] NEGATIVE

Essential thrombocytosis
Polycythemia vera
Agnogenic myeloid metaplasia
Atypical chronic myeloproliferative diseases

PHILADELPHIA CHROMOSOME [t(9;22)] POSITIVE

Chronic myelocytic leukemia

Table 112–3	Indications for Splenectomy in Agnogenic Myeloid Metaplasia

Mechanical discomfort owing to splenic size
Thrombocytopenia unresponsive to medical treatment
Hypercatabolic state
Forward-flow portal hypertension

vascular adhesions that may develop, as well as postoperatively related to thrombosis, to hemorrhage secondary to the underlying coagulopathy, and to the overall poor condition of many of these patients. Operative mortality approaches 10%.

Chronic myelocytic (myelogenous) leukemia represents Philadelphia chromosome–positive myeloproliferative disease. Splenectomy has been shown to be of no use in the early management of this disease. Patients who enter the accelerated phase of this disease (blast crisis) have, in at least one study, shown benefits from splenectomy, including pain control, reversal of thrombocytopenia, and decreased transfusion requirements. Others, however, have not supported this approach, and thus splenectomy remains controversial.

Cysts, Abscesses, and Tumors

True *epithelial cysts,* as well as pseudocysts, have been reported in the spleen. In general, if these are asymptomatic and small, no therapy is required. If the cysts cause symptoms, then treatment ranging from extensive unroofing of a peripheral epithelial cyst to partial or total splenectomy may be indicated; unroofing is associated with a recurrence rate of 10% to 20%.

Abscesses of the spleen may be difficult to diagnose but should be considered in patients with undefined febrile illnesses, particularly if there is left upper quadrant pain, thrombocytosis, or a left pleural effusion. Isolated, single splenic abscesses may be drained percutaneously. Certain fungal infections and small bacterial abscesses with susceptible organisms may be managed medically. The remaining splenic abscesses, however, will require splenectomy.

Hemangioma represents the most common benign neoplasm of the spleen. Older series suggested that splenectomy should be performed on all patients because the diagnosis remained in question. However, with newer, better methods of imaging, the diagnosis is obtained preoperatively. Newer data suggest that many of these lesions are small and may never cause symptoms. In general, if the lesion is large or symptomatic, then resection is indicated. Smaller lesions may be observed and followed up with ultrasonography to be certain that they are not enlarging.

Hamartomas also occur in the spleen, and again resection is reserved for symptomatic lesions or situations in which malignancy cannot be excluded. Indications for resection of *lymphangiomas* are similar. *Peliosis* is a rare condition marked by perifollicular, blood-filled cavities. This condition may present with splenic rupture, and thus splenectomy appears warranted based on the limited data.

Angiosarcoma is the primary malignancy involving the spleen. This malignancy is rare, with only 6 patients diagnosed in a 51-year period at the Mayo Clinic in Minnesota. This is an aggressive tumor, and the patient may present with splenic rupture. Resection is indicated.

Wandering Spleen

Occasionally, the spleen may float freely in the abdominal cavity, suspended by hilar attachments. Patients present with abdominal pain and a palpable mass, which is frequently in the right lower quadrant. Acute torsion and infarction of the spleen may occur, as may congestive splenomegaly. Splenopexy is indicated if the spleen is viable and hypersplenism is not present. Splenectomy is otherwise curative.

Sinistral Portal Hypertension

Sinistral portal hypertension, or left-sided portal hypertension, is caused by thrombosis or obstruction of the splenic vein. The spleen enlarges, and gastric varices develop via the short gastric veins, which represent the primary venous drainage of the spleen. Although esophageal varices may also be present, gastric varices predominate. Venous obstruction may be documented by a number of imaging procedures, including Doppler ultrasonography, contrast-enhanced computed tomography, magnetic resonance imaging, and angiography. Although splenectomy is curative, it carries a much greater operative morbidity because of the large perigastric and perisplenic varices. Blood loss requiring transfusion is not unusual, primarily because of the associated diseases leading to splenic venous thrombosis (e.g., chronic pancreatitis, thrombotic disorders). Splenectomy should probably be reserved for those patients with symptomatic sinistral portal hypertension (gastric variceal hemorrhage). Only about 25% of patients become symptomatic.

Surgical Technique

Splenectomy may be performed by either an open or a laparoscopic approach. The advantages of the laparoscopic approach have been well documented for spleens of normal to mildly increased size. Regardless of the approach, the steps of the operation are essentially the same. The ligamentous attachments of the spleen are sequentially divided to mobilize the spleen, and the hilar vessels are secured and transected. Accessory spleens should be carefully sought during operations for splenic hyperfunction.

PREOPERATIVE PREPARATION. Patients should receive pneumococcal and *Haemophilus influenzae* vaccines. Patients exposed to meningococcus or those who are immunosuppressed should be vaccinated against these organisms as well. More commonly, all patients are receiving all three immunizations. These vaccines are especially important for children and immunosuppressed adults. Associated coagulopathies should be corrected, if feasible. Many of these patients will have hypercoagulable states, and prophylaxis against deep venous thrombosis is warranted.

OPEN SURGERY. The abdomen is entered through an upper midline or left subcostal incision. After a search for accessory spleens, the spleen is mobilized by dividing the splenorenal and splenophrenic ligaments. Blunt dissection is carried medially in a plane posterior to the pancreas. This maneuver allows the surgeon to deliver the spleen up and out of the abdomen from the depths of the left upper quadrant. The splenocolic ligament and the gastrosplenic ligament are then divided. Ties on the short gastric veins must be secure and not incorporate the gastric wall. Finally, hilar vessels are divided and are either doubly ligated or suture ligated.

LAPAROSCOPIC SURGERY. The patient is positioned in the right lateral, semidecubitus position. Four trocars are placed about the left costal margin, with a fifth trocar placed more inferiorly for camera placement. First, the splenocolic ligament is divided, followed by the gastrosplenic ligament, including the short gastric vessels. The harmonic scalpel markedly simplifies these maneuvers. The spleen is then reflected anteriorly, and the splenorenal and splenophrenic ligaments are divided. Careful dissection allows exposure of the posterior aspect of the splenic hilum. The spleen is reflected posteriorly and, if possible, a ligature or vascular stapler is secured about the splenic artery. The spleen is then elevated toward the diaphragm, and the hilar vessels are divided with a stapling device. The spleen is placed into a bag and retrieved through a trocar site. For the less experienced laparoscopic surgeon, the hand-assisted technique may be used.

Splenomegaly

Large spleens have been removed laparoscopically; however, data regarding the safety and efficacy of the laparoscopic approach for these spleens are not yet conclusive. Truly massive spleens, such as those in agnogenic myeloid metaplasia, should, at present, be approached only by open technique. These and other similarly enlarged spleens pose unique challenges to the surgeon. Exposure of the splenic hilar vessels and even, at times, of the main splenic artery may be difficult; vascular adhesions may be

present between the spleen and the surrounding structures, such as the diaphragm. The splenic vein may be massively enlarged, requiring division and oversewing or stapling.

Pearls and Pitfalls

Elective splenectomy may be indicated for
- Unresponsive ITP or HIV-related thrombocytopenia;
- Lymphoma (with or without staging laparotomy);
- Myeloproliferative disorders;
- Cysts, abscesses, and neoplasms;
- Wandering spleen; and
- Symptomatic sinistral portal hypertension.
- Splenectomy for myeloproliferative disorders carries a high morbidity (and mortality) and should be undertaken selectively.
- A minimal access (laparoscopic) approach is feasible in selected patients without severe splenomegaly.
- Before splenectomy, the patient should receive pneumococcal, *H. influenzae,* and possibly meningococcal immunizations, especially if the patient is younger than 15 years or is immunosuppressed.

SELECTED READINGS

Bouvet M, Babiera GV, Termuhlen PM, et al: Splenectomy in the accelerated or blastic phase of chronic myelogenous leukemia: A single-institution, 25-year experience. Surgery 1997;122:20.

Brodsky J, Abcar A, Styler M: Splenectomy for non-Hodgkin's lymphoma. Am J Clin Oncol 1996;19:558.

Coon WW: Surgical aspects of splenic disease and lymphoma. Curr Probl Surg 1998;35:547.

de Bree E, Tsiftsis D, Christodoulakis M, et al: Splenic abscess: A diagnostic and therapeutic challenge. Acta Chir Belg 1998;98:199.

Johnson JR, Samuels P: Review of autoimmune thrombocytopenia: Pathogenesis, diagnosis, and management in pregnancy. Clin Obstet Gynecol 1999;42:317.

Katkhouda N, Hurwitz MB, Rivera RT, et al: Laparoscopic splenectomy: Outcome and efficacy in 103 consecutive patients. Ann Surg 1998;228:568.

Lord RVN, Coleman MJ, Milliken ST: Splenectomy for HIV-related immune thrombocytopenia. Arch Surg 1998;133:205.

Michiels JJ, Kutti J, Stark P, et al: Diagnosis, pathogenesis and treatment of the myeloproliferative disorders essential thrombocythemia, polycythemia vera and essential megakaryocytic granulocytic metaplasia and myelofibrosis. Neth J Med 1999;54:46.

Rutherford CJ, Frenkel EP: Thrombocytopenia: Issues in diagnosis and therapy. Med Clin North Am 1994;78:555.

Schlinkert RT, Teotia SS: Laparoscopic splenectomy. Arch Surg 1999;134:99.

Tefferi A: The Philadelphia chromosome negative chronic myeloproliferative disorders: A practical overview. Mayo Clin Proc 1998;73:1177.

Chapter 113

Cyst and Abscess of the Spleen
Donald E. Fry

Lesions of the spleen have traditionally been viewed as quite rare in the absence of prior trauma. However, the liberal use of abdominal computed tomography (CT) and ultrasonography (US) for patients with nonspecific abdominal complaints has resulted in an increased incidence of recognition of cystic lesions in or around the spleen. Many of these cystic lesions are not necessarily related to the symptoms that initiated the diagnostic CT or US. Nevertheless, the surgeon must be cognizant of the diagnostic possibilities of these infrequently encountered cystic lesions, so that appropriate therapy may be initiated.

EPIDERMOID CYSTS

Epidermoid cystic lesions, although quite uncommon, represent the most common nonparasitic cysts of the spleen. These cysts are true cysts and thus are lined by a squamous epithelium. The vast majority of patients will have a solitary cyst. These cysts are unilocular in 80% of patients, with the remainder having internal septations or multiloculations. Calcifications of the cyst wall are present in about 10% of patients.

The natural history of these cysts remains unknown. Symptomatic cysts are most commonly seen in the second or third decade of life (Table 113–1) and are usually larger than 10 cm. Signs and symptoms usually consist of poorly defined left upper quadrant or left flank pain. Diaphragmatic irritation may cause apical left shoulder pain or even hiccoughs. Large cystic lesions that compress the stomach may lead to abdominal fullness or early satiety. Lesions smaller than 8 cm in diameter are usually asymptomatic. It is unclear what the natural history of the small cyst will be. Some resolve spontaneously. Since few cysts present as symptomatic lesions after age 30, it is generally accepted that the asymptomatic lesion smaller than 8 cm does not increase in size and does not pose a symptomatic problem later in life.

Large lesions may occasionally rupture and present clinically as an acute abdomen. Rupture may be spontaneous or secondary to mild trauma. Rupture and hemorrhage into the peritoneal cavity, or hemorrhage into the cyst cavity, is also known to occur. Hemorrhage is usually seen with centrally located cystic lesions that erode into the large hilar vessels of the spleen. Rarely, a splenic cyst becomes infected, as identified by acute or chronic exacerbation of prior symptoms with left upper quadrant tenderness, fever, and leukocytosis. Differentiation of an infected cyst versus a splenic abscess cannot be clearly defined until splenectomy is performed.

Symptomatic cysts, or those larger than 10 cm, should be managed surgically. Eccentrically located cysts at either pole of the spleen may be managed with hemisplenectomy, particularly when the patient is an adolescent.

In contrast, patients with large, centrally located lesions require splenectomy. Splenectomy is the treatment of choice in all patients older than age 30, given the limited risk of postsplenectomy sepsis in this age group. Both open or percutaneous drainage procedures and open marsupialization are associated with a high recurrence and are not viable treatment options. Laparoscopic techniques may be employed in unroofing procedures, but an extensive unroofing is necessary to prevent recurrence. In symptomatic pediatric patients, sclerosis of the cyst cavity has been advocated, with some success.

PERITONEAL AND CONGENITAL CYSTS

These cystic lesions of the spleen are clinically very similar to the epidermal cyst. Pathologically, they demonstrate a cuboidal epithelial lining that appears analogous to the peritoneum. These primary cysts are uniformly unilocular, and patients rarely have more than one cyst of the spleen. The clinical presentation is similar to epidermal cysts of the spleen, and differentiation is made only by pathologic assessment. Management is the same as for epidermal cysts.

DERMOID CYSTS

Cystic dermoid lesions of the spleen are exceedingly unusual. These lesions are differentiated from epidermal cysts by having epidermal elements, or from peritoneal cysts by having epidermoid elements (e.g., hair, rarely teeth) within the cyst. Dermoids may have an increased potential for malignancy, although this is difficult to discern from the limited number of published reports of patients with this disorder. Treatment probably should be by splenectomy.

PARASITIC CYSTS

Parasitic cysts of the spleen are uncommon, and especially so in the United States. Echinococcal cysts are the most

Table 113–1	Symptoms in Patients with Large Cystic Lesions of the Spleen
SYMPTOM	**REASON**
Left upper quadrant pain	Capsular distention of the spleen; pressure on adjacent organ structures
Early satiety	Displacement and compression of the patient's stomach
Apical shoulder pain	Compression and irritation of the diaphragm that results in referred pain to the shoulder
Shortness of breath	Enlarged spleen or splenic mass interferes with excursion of the diaphragm

Table 113–2	**Tests Employed to Establish the Diagnosis of Echinococcal Disease**

Casoni skin test: uses antigen to detect reactivity of the patient
Immunoelectrophoresis: antigen detection from the microbe
Enzyme-linked immunosorbent assay: antibody detection
Complement fixation: antibody detection
Hemagglutination: antibody detection
Latex agglutination: antibody detection
Polymerase chain reaction: detection of microbial DNA

common. In the United States, echinococcal cysts are rare but are more often seen in the Southwest and should be part of the differential diagnosis of any splenic lesion. The liver is the most common site of echinococcal cysts, with only about 5% of patients who have liver involvement having an associated splenic echinococcal cyst. These splenic cysts are usually unilocular and very commonly have calcifications of the cyst wall.

Signs and symptoms are usually nonspecific with left upper quadrant tenderness, but diagnosis may be incidental to the evaluation of patients with disease that is coexistent in the liver. Rupture of the splenic cyst with release of the scolices of the *Echinococcus granulosus* into the free peritoneal cavity may result in the patient presenting with hypotension secondary to anaphylaxis. Various serologic tests are available to confirm the clinical diagnosis (Table 113–2).

Treatment is splenectomy. Extreme care must be taken to avoid disruption of the cyst during splenectomy to avoid the possibility of anaphylaxis. Large cysts and those which have expanded through the splenic capsule to involve adjacent organs should have hypertonic sodium chloride (15% to 30%) injected into the cyst cavity, followed by careful evacuation 10 minutes later. Evacuation is best achieved with a large-bore suction trocar to minimize spillage of the cyst contents even after hypertonic therapy. Formalin has been used for intracystic injection, but it is a more toxic alternative than hypertonic sodium chloride. Percutaneous drainage of echinococcal cysts is not appropriate because of the possibility of intraperitoneal spillage of the cyst content. Partial splenectomy is seldom feasible because of the size of the lesions.

SPLENIC PSEUDOCYSTS

Splenic pseudocysts are the most common mass-occupying lesion of the spleen. Splenic pseudocysts (to be distinguished from pseudocysts of pancreatic origin) are usually the consequence of antecedent trauma after resorption of intra- or extrasplenic hematomas or areas of splenic necrosis. The increased use of nonoperative management of splenic injuries in both adults and children has made these lesions more common than in the past. Pseudocysts are unilocular in more than 70% of patients, and have irregular but smooth-appearing walls to the cyst. Mural calcifications are present in about half of the patients with chronic long-present pseudocysts. Clinical signs and symptoms of splenic pseudocysts usually consist of left upper quadrant pain, but referred shoulder pain may be present secondary to diaphragmatic irritation.

Management of splenic pseudocysts depends on the patient's signs and symptoms and the temporal relationship to the traumatic event. Increased nonoperative management of splenic trauma results in patients undergoing sequential CT imaging. Pseudocysts recognized within the first 3 months after injury, especially when asymptomatic, should be observed because many will spontaneously resolve. Long-standing symptomatic pseudocysts from remote trauma that have thick walls and calcification require splenectomy. Some have been treated successfully with percutaneous drainage, while others have been unroofed operatively without splenectomy via a minimally invasive approach. Partial splenectomy is seldom feasible.

SPLENIC ABSCESS

Splenic abscesses occur more commonly than true cysts of the spleen. Splenic abscesses require some form of injury or impairment of the spleen. Experimental splenic abscesses developed in rabbits after intravenous injection of staphylococcal bacteria only after ischemia or infarction of splenic tissue; abscesses of the spleen did not occur in normal spleens. Splenic abscess usually requires the presence of preexistent sickle cell disease, intravenous drug abuse, bacterial endocarditis, or splenic trauma (Table 113–3). Large hematomas and infarcted tissue within the spleen make this complication a potential concern in the nonoperatively managed trauma patient who has major postinjury infective complications.

The patient with splenic abscess usually presents with fever and leukocytosis. Nontrauma patients with the aforementioned risk factors may have poorly localized left upper quadrant abdominal pain and tenderness, and some will have referred pain to the left shoulder. In patients with endocarditis or the patient with intravenous drug abuse, the organism most commonly involved is *Staphylococcus aureus*. In the trauma patient, complaints of abdominal pain or left upper quadrant tenderness may not be present. A high index of suspicion should be maintained for splenic abscess in the patient with suspected or documented splenic trauma.

The diagnosis is established with abdominal CT. Ultra-

Table 113–3	**Patient Groups and Reasons for Development of Splenic Abscess**

RISK FACTOR FOR ABSCESS	RATIONALE
Sickle cell disease	Microinfarction of the spleen allows any interval bacteremia event to seed the spleen
Intravenous drug abuse	Embolization of the spleen with contaminated particulate matter
Bacterial endocarditis	Embolization of the spleen with infected vegetations from the infected heart valve
Splenic trauma	Hematoma and/or necrotic splenic tissue becomes a pabulum for a subsequent bacteremia event

sonography or the traditional radionuclide liver-spleen scan may on occasion be useful. However, the patient being evaluated for a possible splenic abscess needs assessment of other potential sources of infection within the abdomen (e.g., synchronous hepatic abscess); thus, contrast-enhanced CT is the most cost-effective diagnostic test. Identification of extrasplenic extension of the abscess may be useful when one is planning treatment.

The best treatment for splenic abscess is splenectomy. Percutaneous drainage may be attempted in selected patients with a well-defined single focus but commonly proves inadequate because of multiloculation of the abscess cavity; high recurrence rates are common from incomplete drainage. Extrasplenic extension of the abscess is also a hazard for injury to the stomach, colon, and small bowel with percutaneous drainage.

Operative splenectomy may on occasion be a formidable procedure in these patients. A laparoscopic approach may not be prudent unless all the abscess or abscesses are well visualized to be small and intrasplenic. Ideally, control of the splenic artery may be desirable as the initial technical maneuver. Evacuation of the abscess cavity may be required after dearterialization to avoid injury to adjacent structures and to facilitate removal of the friable, inflamed spleen itself. A "rind" of abscess wall is commonly left after splenectomy on the surfaces of the adjacent stomach, diaphragm, colon, pancreas, and small bowel. Left upper quadrant drainage with closed suction catheters is desirable in this circumstance. Because of the extension of inflammation outside of the spleen, partial resection of the spleen for abscess is seldom a viable consideration.

The microbiology of splenic abscess can include virtually any organism and requires culture documentation at the time of drainage or splenectomy. Immediate Gram stain of the abscess will provide important evidence of the pathogen. *Staphylococcus aureus* is the most common agent. Antibiotic therapy for staphylococcal abscess should be continued for a minimum of 10 days in the hope of minimizing the secondary consequences of endocarditis. Some patients may have antecedent endocarditis or may demonstrate evidence of endocarditis at the time of diagnosis of splenic abscess; these patients will require much longer courses of antibiotic therapy. Nafcillin and oxacillin remain the antibiotic choices for methicillin-sensitive *Staphylococcus* species. Methicillin-resistant staphylococci require vancomycin therapy. Gram-negative bacteria and even fungi (*Candida albicans*) may be seen and need antimicrobial therapy addressed to the specific

> ## Pearls and Pitfalls
> - Cystic lesions of the spleen may involve primary cysts (epidermoid, peritoneal, or dermoid), parasitic cysts, post-traumatic pseudocysts, and splenic abscesses.
> - Pancreatic pseudocysts may mimic a primary splenic cyst.
> - Primary cysts or pseudocysts usually require intervention only when symptomatic.
> - Parasitic cysts are echinococcal in origin and require careful operative planning.
> - Splenic abscesses occur in the setting of endocarditis, intravenous drug abuse, or secondary infection of the traumatized spleen.
> - Splenic abscesses are best treated with splenectomy.

pathogen. The duration of antibiotic therapy for the more unusual pathogens should be extended, based on the patient's clinical response. Gut anaerobes (e.g., *Bacteroides fragilis*) are infrequently seen in splenic abscesses but may occur if the patient sustains a mixed intra-abdominal infection from colonic sources.

Since splenectomy is often the treatment of choice for patients with splenic cysts, pseudocysts, and abscess, the surgeon must be cognizant of the potential for postsplenectomy sepsis. Postsplenectomy sepsis is seen on occasion in patients younger than 30 years of age and most commonly among patients within 3 years of splenectomy. Patients with medical indications for splenectomy have rates of postsplenectomy sepsis higher than those of patients with splenectomy for cysts, pseudocysts, and abscess. All patients after splenectomy should receive vaccination for pneumococcus, meningococcus, and *Haemophilus influenzae*. Patients and family should be fully informed of the potential risks so that prompt medical attention can be sought at the onset of suspicious symptoms.

SELECTED READINGS

Fry DE, Richardson JD, Flint LM: Occult splenic abscess: An unrecognized complication in heroin abuse. Surgery 1978;84:650.
Fry DE: Parasitic infections: Echinococcal disease. In Fry DE (ed): Surgical Infections. Boston, Little, Brown, 1995, pp 629–633.
Moir C, Guttman F, Jequier S, et al: Splenic cysts: Aspiration, sclerosis, or resection. J Pediatr Surg 1989;24:646.
Sinha PS, Stoker TA, Aston NO: Traumatic pseudocyst of the spleen. J R Soc Med 1999;92:450.
Yavorski CC, Greason KL, Egan MC: Splenic cysts: A new approach to partial splenectomy: Case report and review of the literature. Am Surg 1998;64:795.

Spleen: Malignant

Chapter 114
Malignant Diseases of the Spleen
Steven C. Gross and William G. Cance

Splenic malignancies are relatively uncommon. Despite the spleen's high blood flow and filtering function, the spleen is a rare site of metastatic disease. These observations have led to the hypothesis that the lymphoid tissue within the spleen is somehow protective, which could explain why the majority of malignancies involving the spleen come from lymphoproliferative and myeloproliferative disorders that have aberrant hematologic function. Surgery has had a limited role in management of the splenic malignancy and is rarely a primary therapy. However, surgical treatment can be important in diagnostic staging, palliation, and improved survival outlook in selected patients.

CLINICAL PRESENTATION

Splenomegaly and Hypersplenism

Splenomegaly is the most common presentation of splenic malignancy, but most patients with splenomegaly do not have cancer. Suspicion of malignancy should be aroused in patients with fever, night sweats, weight loss, adenopathy, weakness, or malaise. A complete blood count with differential and peripheral smear along with a bone marrow biopsy can help investigate concerns for hematologic malignancy. Splenomegaly requires a minimum splenic weight of 500 g as opposed to the normal weight of 150 to 250 g. Massive splenomegaly, noted at weights greater than 1000 g and where the spleen may be palpable below the costal margin, can cause early satiety from pressure on the stomach or marked pain as a result of splenic infarcts, visceral peritoneal stretch, or subcapsular hematoma.

Most clinical situations that require palliation involve hypersplenism. Hypersplenism is a condition defined by four requirements: (1) profound anemia, thrombocyto-

penia, or leukopenia; (2) bone marrow hyperplasia; (3) splenomegaly; and (4) clinical improvement after splenectomy. The pathophysiology of hypersplenism revolves around splenic hyperactivity, resulting in increased consumption of blood cells. Clinical consequences of hypersplenism include anemia refractory to transfusion and medical therapy, low white blood count with resulting immunosuppression that increases infections, and a low platelet count leading to increased risk of hemorrhage. Splenectomy offers significant palliation for these clinical and laboratory manifestations of hypersplenism and splenic discomfort.

Lymphoproliferative Disorders
(Table 114–1)

Hodgkin's disease (HD) is a potentially curable lymphoma diagnosed by the presence of Reed-Sternberg cells on biopsy. Traditionally, noninvasive methods of detection of HD within the spleen have not been adequate; surgery has been used to diagnose the presence of subdiaphragmatic disease, because HD typically spreads in the abdomen first to the spleen. Numerous studies have reported the usefulness of fine-needle or core biopsies of the spleen with a low incidence of complications, such as mild to moderate pain, decreasing hematocrit necessitating transfusion, and splenectomy. However, such biopsies obtain a limited sample that may not be diagnostic because a negative result does not exclude splenic malignancy, and persistent concerns of safety exist.

Staging laparotomy upstages 25% to 35% and downstages 10% to 15% of patients, resulting in an approximately 40% chance of altering the stage of a patient and possibly altering therapy. If staging is negative for abdominal involvement, radiotherapy may be an appropriate single therapy. If HD involves the spleen or both

Lymphoproliferative disorders
    Non-Hodgkin's lymphoma (NHL)
    Hodgkin's disease (HD)
    Chronic lymphocytic leukemia (CLL)
    Hairy cell leukemia
    Waldenström's macroglobulinemia
    Acute lymphoblastic leukemia
    Plasmacytoma
Myeloproliferative disorders
    Chronic myelogenous leukemia (CML)
    Myelofibrosis (agnogenic myeloid metaplasia)
    Polycythemia vera
    Essential thrombocythemia
Primary tumors
    Hemangiosarcoma
    Kaposi's sarcoma
    Lymphangiosarcoma
    Malignant fibrous histiocytoma
    Fibrosarcoma
    Leiomyosarcoma
    Malignant teratoma
Metastatic tumors
    Melanoma
    Breast
    Colon
    Testicular

sides of the diaphragm, chemotherapy is usually the main mode of therapy. Indications for operative staging in HD are limited to clinical stage I (single lymph node group) or stage II (more than one lymph node group or extralymphatic site, all on the same side of the diaphragm) disease, wherein, in the absence of subdiaphragmatic disease, the patient would receive radiation alone. In clinical stage I or II, there is a 30% to 50% chance of concomitant splenic involvement; in 50% of patients, the spleen is the only abdominal site of HD.

However, surgical staging has fallen out of favor with most medical oncologists for several reasons:

1. Development of nonsurgical prognostic factors predictive of the need for systemic therapy (e.g., age older than 40 years, male gender, high erythrocyte sedimentation rate, histology, tumor bulk, number of involved sites) or low risk (<10%) of subdiaphragmatic disease (e.g., stage I female or male with lymph predominant histology, stage II in female younger than 27 years of age).
2. Concerns of operative cost, morbidity, and mortality from open splenectomy, especially the lifetime risk of overwhelming postsplenectomy infection (OPSI).
3. Advances in radiologic imaging to detect subdiaphragmatic disease (positron emission tomography shows some promise).
4. More liberal use of chemotherapy.

In general, oncologists consider staging laparotomy only if prognostic factors are not conclusive, and surgery alone can decide the need for chemotherapy versus radiation therapy alone. In argument for surgery, more accurate staging can better determine appropriate therapy, help minimize dosage, and decrease long-term complications. Laparoscopic surgery shows promise in offering less morbidity yet allow accurate assessment of subdiaphrag-

matic disease. However, as radiologic studies become more sensitive, surgery may become unnecessary.

Non-Hodgkin's lymphoma (NHL) is a cancer of the lymphoreticular system, involving the spleen in 35% to 80% of patients. Patients with NHL usually do not require splenectomy for staging, because the disease is systemic, and therapy involves multiagent chemotherapy. In patients refractory to medical therapy, splenectomy can be beneficial for palliation of pain, hypersplenism, and excessive tumor burden.

Lymphocytic leukemias benefit from splenectomy only in limited situations. *Chronic lymphocytic leukemia* (CLL) is a slowly progressive leukemia affecting people in their sixth or seventh decade of life with worsening lymphocytosis, fatigue, lymphadenopathy, and organomegaly. Splenectomy is performed for massive splenomegaly or hypersplenism refractory to chemotherapy and splenic radiation. *Hairy cell leukemia* predominantly affects middle-aged and older men with splenomegaly or hypersplenic complications; characteristic "hairy cells" are found within blood, marrow, or other tissues. Traditionally, splenectomy was the primary therapy and offered a 90% response rate, but chemotherapy has since become first line therapy. New drugs such as alpha-interferon, pentostatin, and 2-chlorodeoxyadenosine offer equivalent to improved remission rates without any surgical morbidity. Splenectomy is reserved for patients with disease refractory to chemotherapy or who have splenic rupture. In patients with *Waldenström's macroglobulinemia* (IgM hyperviscosity syndrome, lytic bone lesions, hypercalcemia, anemia, and Bence Jones proteinuria), splenectomy is reserved for disease unresponsive to chemotherapy.

Myeloproliferative Disorders

Myelofibrosis (agnogenic myeloid metaplasia) results in relentless fibrosis of bone marrow and other viscera that leads to massive splenomegaly and, on occasion, hypersplenism. Severe anemia can result, and initial therapy involves steroids and danazol. Although it was thought to make anemia worse in the past, splenectomy has been shown to help correct problems of hypersplenism such as anemia refractory to frequent transfusions. Splenic irradiation may be a safer option for poor operative candidates.

Whereas patients with acute myelogenous leukemia gain no palliation from splenectomy, surgery can palliate patients with hypersplenism related to *chronic myelogenous leukemia* (CML). However, splenectomy is reserved for patients refractory to bone marrow transplantation, chemotherapy, and splenic irradiation. Surgery offers no better survival outlook, nor does it stop progression of disease, although it does improve the quality of life. However, the operative morbidity and mortality rates for splenectomy in these patients are much greater.

Primary and Metastatic Tumors

Primary cancers of the spleen are rare. *Hemangiosarcoma* is an aggressive cancer of the spleen that presents with anemia and a rapidly growing abdominal mass. There is a 30% risk of rupture. Life expectancy is 6 months regardless of medical or surgical treatment, and no cures have been reported. *Kaposi's sarcoma* of the spleen has been documented but is rare even in patients with acquired immunodeficiency syndrome.

Metastases to the spleen are uncommon (4% to 7% in autopsies for carcinoma) and are associated with several types of primary malignancies, most commonly melanoma, breast, lung, ovary, and testicle. Half of the lesions come from melanoma, which is usually widespread at diagnosis. In fact, most patients with clinically obvious splenic involvement have widely metastatic disease. Most patients remain relatively asymptomatic.

Even though radiologic techniques are improving in evaluation and staging of lymphoma and leukemia, CT and lymphangiography detect subdiaphragmatic disease in only 75% of patients. Gallium scans are of poor quality below the diaphragm. Most leukemic or lymphomatous infiltration of the spleen is uniform in echogenicity (ultrasound), density (CT), and signal (magnetic resonance imaging) unless metastases are greater than 1 cm and can therefore be detected. Such studies are often limited in that only splenomegaly (>500 g) is suggestive of splenic malignancy. However, one third to one half of patients with lymphoma and splenomegaly have no pathologic involvement of the spleen; conversely, one third of patients with lymphoma and normal-appearing spleens have pathologic involvement. Splenectomy for pathologic evaluation still offers the best means of determining malignancy within the spleen.

PREOPERATIVE MANAGEMENT

Vaccination against *Pneumococcus, Meningococcus,* and *Haemophilus influenzae* should be administered preoperatively to reduce the risk of OPSI. Administration ideally should be more than 10 days in advance; but, if not done before surgery, vaccination should be performed postoperatively at least 1 week *after* surgery. A single dose of preoperative antibiotic is usually given. If the patient has had a prolonged course of steroids within the past year, 100 mg of intravenous hydrocortisone should also be administered preoperatively.

It is important to type blood and blood products in advance of the operation; many patients are difficult to crossmatch because antibodies have developed from numerous prior transfusions. Ideally, the patient's hematocrit should be greater than 30. Preoperative transfusion of packed cells may be needed. The products should be warmed properly to avoid hemolysis by cold agglutinins found occasionally in patients with lymphoma or CLL. Platelets should be available with thrombocytopenia (<50,000), and *transfusion after splenic artery ligation* is the best means to prevent splenic consumption of platelets. Preoperative embolization of the splenic artery decreases operative blood loss and may facilitate safer dissection of massive spleens in some patients.

In myeloproliferative disorders (especially myelofibrosis or CML) with preoperative thrombocytosis, the risk of splenic or superior mesenteric venous thrombosis is significant. No hard data exist for preoperative prophylaxis, but anticoagulation with aspirin or low-dose subcutaneous heparin may lower the risk of thrombotic events.

Some surgeons advocate alkylating chemotherapy or platelet phoresis to reduce the preoperative platelet count to less than 200,000.

INTRAOPERATIVE MANAGEMENT

An orogastric tube is placed to decompress the stomach and facilitate the ligation of short gastric blood vessels. Choice of incision often depends on the size of the spleen. Although most surgeons perform open splenectomy, laparoscopic splenectomy is increasing in popularity.

Open Splenectomy

A left subcostal incision offers optimal splenic exposure, but an upper midline incision is preferred when access to the entire abdomen is needed, such as in HD staging, in the severely thrombocytopenic patient, or when a massive spleen is present. To perform splenectomy, first, the lateral and posterior retroperitoneal attachments are released with sharp dissection, and the spleen is mobilized into the wound. Then the short gastric blood vessels are divided with care away from the stomach wall to ensure gastric wall viability. Finally, the hilar blood vessels are ligated, taking care to not traumatize the pancreatic tail. In very large spleens or expected difficult dissection, some surgeons advocate early ligation or preoperative embolization of the splenic artery. Early intraoperative ligation of the splenic artery also may allow some autotransfusion of blood out of the spleen back into body circulation before splenic vein ligation.

With hypersplenism, accessory splenic tissue must be sought and removed to minimize recurrence. Locations in order of decreasing frequency include the splenic hilum, ligamentous attachments, tail of pancreas, transverse mesocolon, greater omentum, small bowel mesentery, reproductive organs, and presacral space. Re-inspection of the diaphragm, greater curvature of the stomach, and hilum must be done to ensure hemostasis. Routine use of a drain is not advocated because recent randomized prospective trials have shown that closed drainage does not decrease (and may increase) the risk of infection. Concerns of pancreatic injury is an exception, necessitating a short period of closed drainage.

Although decreasing in frequency, staging laparotomy for HD remains a reason for splenectomy. In open staging procedures, a midline incision is preferred, and the surgeon should perform needle biopsies of both lobes of the liver, a wedge biopsy of the left liver lobe, splenectomy, and biopsies of hepatoduodenal, para-aortic, pelvic, and any other suspicious lymph nodes before splenectomy. If there is obvious disease in the liver or lymph nodes, splenectomy should not be performed, because the surgery is a staging procedure, not a therapeutic one. In women, oophoropexy is important to preserve fertility by moving the ovaries out of para-aortic radiation fields.

Laparoscopic Splenectomy

Techniques in laparoscopy are improving and have been applied successfully to splenectomy. In idiopathic thrombocytopenic purpura (ITP), laparoscopic splenectomy is

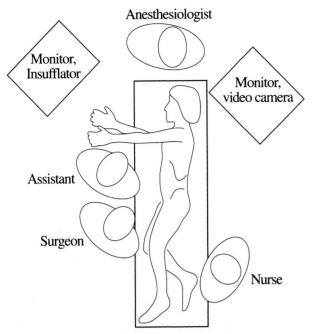

Figure 114–1. Positioning of equipment and personnel for laparoscopic splenectomy. (Adapted from Walsh RM, Heniford BT: Laparoscopic splenectomy for non-Hodgkin lymphoma. J Surg Oncol 1999;70:116–121.)

considered the standard of care by most surgeons. Staging laparotomy is suited ideally for a laparoscopic approach. The patient is positioned with the right side down (Fig. 114–1) and port sites are chosen:

The first is placed near the midline and 4 cm below the spleen tip using an open technique.
The next is positioned near the tip of the eleventh rib along the posterior axillary line.
The last is a middle port placed halfway between the other two along the anterior axillary line (Fig. 114–2).

The positions may vary according to spleen size and a fourth port may be needed. The order of dissection is

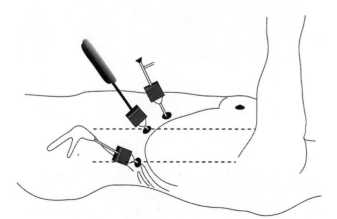

Figure 114–2. Trocar placement for laparoscopic splenectomy. The surgeon places the most medial port near the midline using open technique, the most lateral port is near the tip of the eleventh rib, and the middle port is placed in between, at least 2 cm below the costal margin. (Adapted from Walsh RM, Heniford BT: Laparoscopic splenectomy for non-Hodgkin lymphoma. J Surg Oncol 1999;70:116–121.)

similar to the open technique. The harmonic scalpel is used for takedown of the lateral peritoneal attachments for obtaining biopsy samples, and for ligating the short gastric vessels (Fig. 114–3). Endostapling devices with vascular staples can be used to ligate and divide the short gastric vessels (Fig. 114–4) and especially for the splenic artery and vein (Fig. 114–5). Removal of the spleen is performed with placement into a retrieval bag; the spleen is excised in chunks with ringed forceps, or a port site is enlarged to facilitate removal. Although usually the operative time is longer, laparoscopic splenectomy is associated with less ileus, earlier toleration of diet, shorter hospitalization, less pain, and overall less hospital expense.

POSTOPERATIVE MANAGEMENT

Traditionally, nasogastric decompression has been used to prevent gastric distention and to decompress the short gastric blood vessels postoperatively, but no such complications have been reported in laparoscopic cases in which the nasogastric tube is removed in the operating room. If the platelet count increases to more than 1 million, the patient is hydrated adequately, and antiplatelet therapy such as aspirin is started. If on steroids for hypersplenism, the patient should be placed on a gradual steroid taper. With upper abdominal dissection and incisions, patients are at risk for pneumonia and other pulmonary complications, so adequate pain control, chest physiotherapy, incentive spirometry, and early ambulation are important.

COMPLICATIONS

The incidence of postoperative morbidity and mortality in splenectomized patients is higher for the subgroup of

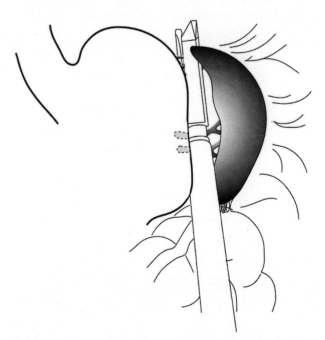

Figure 114–3. A harmonic scalpel removes ligamentous attachments to the spleen and takes down peritoneal attachments in a lateral to medial fashion. (Adapted from Walsh RM, Heniford BT: Laparoscopic splenectomy for non-Hodgkin lymphoma. J Surg Oncol 1999;70:116–121.)

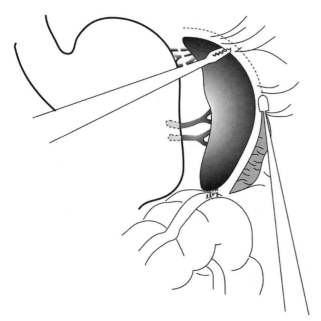

Figure 114–4. An endostapler with a vascular staple clip ligates and divides the short gastric blood vessels. (Adapted from Walsh RM, Heniford BT: Laparoscopic splenectomy for non-Hodgkin lymphoma. J Surg Oncol 1999;70:116–121.)

patients with malignancy as opposed to nonmalignant indications. Data conflict whether an increase in splenic size increases complications. Complications of splenectomy include hemorrhage, thrombosis, infection, pancreatic fistula, and death. Operative mortality rate from staging laparotomy is less than 0.5%. Even though open splenectomy improves quality of life, it has not been shown to improve survival in myelofibrosis with 7% to 18% postoperative mortality and 40% morbidity rates. Complications for splenectomy in CLL were as high as 30%, but response rates were greater than 85% in two series. Splenectomy for chronic myeloproliferative disorders carries a very high mortality risk and should be chosen only after a careful consideration of the risk–benefit ratio.

Postoperative bleeding occurs in as many as 4% to 16% of patients, depending on the reason for splenectomy. Coagulopathies should be corrected with transfusion of platelets or fresh-frozen plasma. Hemodynamic instability or a rapid decrease in hematocrit warrants urgent re-exploration. Thrombosis and thromboembolic events occur in 2% of patients; the risk is greatest (5%) in patients with myeloproliferative disorders. Treatment involves anticoagulation with heparin and eventually long-term warfarin.

Infections are a concern in splenectomized patients, because the immunologic contribution of the spleen is removed, and many patients are later exposed to immunosuppressing steroids or chemotherapy. Respiratory complications and subphrenic abscesses account for half of infective complications. Persistent left lower lobe infiltrate or other unexplained slow recovery should raise suspicion of pancreatic injury, fistula, or subphrenic fluid collection. Routine closed drains do not change the 1% to 5% risk of subphrenic fluid collections. Most subphrenic

abscesses are due to inadequate hemostasis or injury to the pancreas, and percutaneous drainage may be necessary. Re-exploration to rule out hollow viscous injury or to evacuate undrainable collections should be considered if the patient's condition does not improve rapidly after percutaneous drainage. Continued bladder catheterization causes urinary tract infections, which account for 2% to 6% of septic complications.

OPSI is a rare complication but has a grave prognosis. Half of the cases occur within a year of splenectomy. Data on incidence were largely collected before routine preoperative immunization, but most studies show a rate of 1% to 3% with a subsequent mortality rate ranging from 50% to 80%. The risk is greater in children and patients receiving resection for hematologic malignancy. Immunized patients appear to have less risk of OPSI compared with unimmunized patients. Controversy exists over the use of chronic prophylactic oral antibiotics postoperatively in children younger than 15 years old to prevent OPSI. Daily oral penicillin (or erythromycin in those who are allergic to penicillin) is required for high-risk patients such as the immunocompromised and children younger than 4 years of age who cannot communicate reliably when they are sick. Physicians must warn patients and their families that *any* "minor" infection may lead to serious and potentially fatal illness and must be evaluated by a doctor *immediately*. A medical bracelet noting asplenia is recommended.

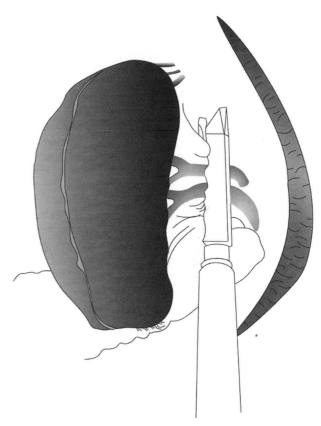

Figure 114–5. An endostapler with a vascular staple clip ligates and divides the hilar blood vessels. (Adapted from Walsh RM, Heniford BT: Laparoscopic splenectomy for non-Hodgkin lymphoma. J Surg Oncol 1999;70:116–121.)

Pearls and Pitfalls

- Most malignancies of the spleen are due to lympho-proliferative and myeloproliferative disorders.
- One third to one half of patients with lymphoma and splenomegaly have no pathologic involvement of the spleen; conversely, one third of patients with lymphoma and normal-appearing spleens have pathologic involvement of the spleen.
- Staging laparotomy for Hodgkin's disease is limited to stage I or II disease, wherein subdiaphragmatic pathology changes therapy (chemotherapy versus radiation alone).
- Splenectomy in treatment of malignancy is usually for palliation of hypersplenism or symptomatic splenomegaly refractory to medical therapy.
- Vaccination against *Pneumococcus, Meningococcus,* and *H. influenzae* before splenectomy is important in minimizing the lifetime risk of OPSI.
- Laparoscopic splenectomy offers less morbidity and costs less than open splenectomy.
- Splenectomy for myeloproliferative disorders has a high morbidity and mortality association—the decision to undergo splenectomy should not be made lightly.

OUTCOMES

More than 75% of cytopenias are improved after splenectomy in HD, NHL, and CLL. In hairy cell leukemia with hypersplenism, 5-year survival rates approach 65% to 75%. Isolated reports of metastasis solely to the spleen have shown survival long term from splenectomy followed by adjuvant therapy. Whereas data show an increased risk of a secondary leukemia in HD patients undergoing a specific regimen of chemotherapy (MOPP), patients who underwent staging splenectomy had an even higher risk. In other malignancies (CLL, CML, myelofibrosis), splenectomy is potentially palliative but offers no prolonged survival benefit and has high morbidity and mortality.

SELECTED READINGS

Abeloff MD: Clinical Oncology. New York, Churchill Livingstone, 2000.

Advani RH, Horning SJ: Treatment of early-stage Hodgkin's disease. Semin Hematol 1999;36:270.

Aisenberg AC: Problems in Hodgkin's disease management. Blood 1999;93:761.

Baccarani U, Carroll BJ, Hiatt JR, et al: Comparison of laparoscopic and open staging in Hodgkin disease. Arch Surg 1998;133:517–21; discussion 521–522.

Bowdler AJ: The Spleen: Structure, Function, and Clinical Significance. London, Chapman and Hall, 1990.

Brigden ML, Pattullo AL: Prevention and management of overwhelming postsplenectomy infection: An update. Crit Care Med 1999;27:836.

Carde P, Hagenbeek A, Hayat M, et al: Clinical staging versus laparotomy and combined modality with MOPP versus ABVD in early-stage Hodgkin's disease: The H6 twin randomized trials from the European Organization for Research and Treatment of Cancer Lymphoma Cooperative Group. J Clin Oncol 1993;11:2258.

Cuschieri A, Forbes CD: Disorders of the Spleen. Oxford, England, Blackwell Scientific, 1994.

Decker G, Millat B, Guillon F, et al: Laparoscopic splenectomy for benign and malignant hematological diseases: 35 consecutive cases. World J Surg 1998;22:62.

Donini A, Baccarani U, Terrosu G, et al: Laparoscopic vs open splenectomy in the management of hematological diseases [in process citation]. Surg Endosc 1999;13:1220.

Hiatt JR, Phillips EH, Morgenstern L: Surgical Diseases of the Spleen. New York: Springer, 1997.

Jox A, Sieber M, Wolf J, Diehl V: Hodgkin's disease: New treatment strategies toward the cure of patients. Cancer Treat Rev 1999;25:169.

Walsh RM, Heniford BT: Laparoscopic splenectomy for non-Hodgkin lymphoma. J Surg Oncol 1999;70:116.

Walsh RM, Heniford BT: Role of laparoscopy for Hodgkin's and non-Hodgkin's lymphoma. Semin Surg Oncol 1999;16:284.

Williams RS, Littell RD, Mendenhall NP: Laparoscopic oophoropexy and ovarian function in the treatment of Hodgkin disease. Cancer 1999;86:2138.

Pancreas: Benign

Chapter 115
Necrotizing Pancreatitis

Karen D. Libsch and Michael G. Sarr

Necrotizing pancreatitis is the most severe form of acute pancreatitis and accounts for as many as 3% to 5% of all patients with acute pancreatitis in tertiary referral centers. Necrotizing pancreatitis has a common origin in the pancreatic parenchymal inflammation that characterizes milder forms of acute pancreatitis, but with necrotizing pancreatitis the inflammation rapidly progresses to necrosis, which involves both the pancreatic parenchyma, the adjacent tissues, or both. Necrosis, liquefaction, and subsequent superinfection may involve not only the necrotic pancreas and its immediate surrounding tissues but also extrapancreatic retroperitoneal fatty tissue of the small and large bowel mesentery and the retroperitoneal, paracolic, and retrocolic compartments. Although this degree of severity of disease is seen in a minority of patients, it accounts for the vast majority of morbidity and mortality resulting from acute pancreatitis. The mechanisms that trigger the necrotizing process are poorly understood—whereas the etiology of pancreatitis appears to have little bearing on severity, excessive upregulation of inflammatory pathways, the amount of parenchymal and peripancreatic necrosis, and the development of subsequent bacterial infection affect severity both of local inflammation and of systemic complications. Currently, necrotizing pancreatitis carries a mortality risk of 15% to 40% and a morbidity rate of approximately 80%.

DIAGNOSIS

Diagnosis of necrotizing pancreatitis is based on clinical suspicion. Early indicators of prognosis include the severity of the initial presentation and response to initial treatment. Ranson developed criteria that represented the first staging system to distinguish between the milder edematous and the more severe necrotizing forms of acute pancreatitis. These criteria involved a combination of 11 clinical and laboratory parameters gathered during the first 48 hours after the onset of disease. A need to evaluate disease severity and response to treatment early into the disease has spawned multiple newer staging systems. Recently, the Acute Physiology and Chronic Health Evaluation (APACHE) II grading system has been used successfully to stage severity of disease. In addition, there has been intense experimental interest in developing a laboratory-based, quantitative marker for necrotizing pancreatitis. Proposed blood tests measure levels of proinflammatory markers such as C-reactive protein, lactate dehydrogenase, polymorphonuclear neutrophil elastase, phospholipase A_2 catalytic subunit, and cytokines such as interleukin (IL)-1 and IL-6. Although initial results are promising, these laboratory evaluations are presently available only at research centers. Contrast-enhanced computed tomography (CT), which is widely available, is the most reliable method to diagnose necrotizing pancreatitis. CT has an overall clinical accuracy for the detection of necrosis of approximately 95%. However, the decision to obtain a CT scan should be based on clinical assessment and suspicion of a complication of the pancreatitis, not just to confirm a suspected diagnosis of necrotizing pancreatitis. In patients in whom severe disease such as shock or hypoxemia develops, who do not improve after 3 to 4 days of treatment, whose condition deteriorates after treatment, or in whom a complication is suspected, a CT scan should be obtained.

CLINICAL MANAGEMENT

Initial management of necrotizing pancreatitis first requires recognition that the patient has this severe form of acute pancreatitis, not just self-limited edematous pancreatitis. Use of the Ranson criteria or the APACHE II scoring system aids in making this important decision.

731

Once the patient is identified as having necrotizing pancreatitis, fluid and electrolyte resuscitation should be undertaken aggressively with close hemodynamic monitoring in an intensive care unit (ICU) setting.

Before the mid-1990s, no further adjuvant therapy had been shown to be of benefit, including antibiotics, agents used to suppress pancreatic exocrine secretion, or agents used to inhibit the action of pancreatic enzymes. Recently, however, at least four studies have shown a decrease in superinfection of pancreatic necrosis with the use of certain antibiotics that penetrate well into pancreatic parenchyma, such as imipenem. Although the practice is still controversial, many centers use high-dose imipenem for 10 days to 2 weeks in patients with necrotizing pancreatitis.

Another primary consideration is nutritional support. Total parenteral nutrition should be instituted early in the hospital course, converting to enteral nutrition as soon as is feasible. Enteral nutrition is safer, less expensive, and may help preserve the gut mucosal barrier, thereby also decreasing superinfection of the pancreatic necrosis by gut-derived organisms translocating across the mucosa.

CT findings guide further clinical management. Decreased enhancement of the pancreatic parenchyma seen on dynamic contrast-enhanced CT imaging (Fig. 115–1) and peripancreatic fluid collections delineate the extent

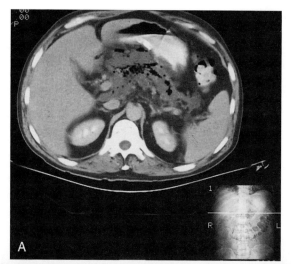

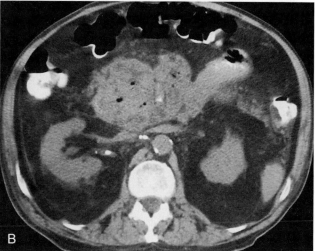

Figure 115–2. Computed tomography of infected necrotizing pancreatitis showing extraluminal gas.

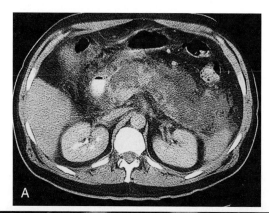

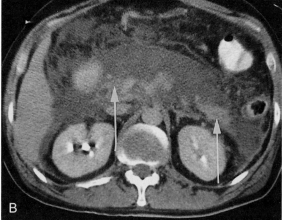

Figure 115–1. Contrast-enhanced computed tomography of necrotizing pancreatitis. *A,* Patchy enhancement of body, tail, and head of the gland. *B,* Enhancement only of a small segment of the head and tail of the gland (*arrows*).

of pancreatic and peripancreatic disease. The extent of pancreatic parenchymal necrosis observed on CT imaging directly correlates with expected mortality risk. The retrocolic, paracolic, and retroperitoneal tissue reaction defines the extent of extrapancreatic necrosis, the presence of which doubles mortality rate. In a few patients, CT delineates extraluminal gas (Fig. 115–2), which is pathognomonic of infection with a gas-producing organism, and is sufficient to diagnose infected pancreatic necrosis. More commonly, CT-guided percutaneous fine-needle aspiration of pancreatic or peripancreatic fluid is necessary to prove infection.

Infection complicates the course of approximately 30% of patients with necrotizing pancreatitis. Bacteriologic analysis reveals a predominance of gram-negative enteric bacteria, the origin of which has been thought to be bacterial translocation from gut. A recent increase in gram-positive bacteria may be secondary to use of antibiotic prophylaxis against gram-negative organisms. In a recent series at our institution, operative cultures of 55 patients with infected necrotizing pancreatitis grew gram-positive cocci in 11 patients (20%), gram-negative rods in

20 patients (36%), mixed infections (including anaerobes and fungi) in 20 patients (36%), and pure fungal growths in 4 patients (7%). The risk for infection increases with the extent of pancreatic or peripancreatic necrosis, as well as the duration of the acute disease course. Despite current state-of-the-art therapy, the mortality rate among patients with infected necrosis is higher than among patients with noninfected necrotizing pancreatitis. Currently, more than 80% of deaths among patients with acute pancreatitis are caused by septic complications as a consequence of pancreatic infection. Thus, the presence of infected necrotizing pancreatitis is an absolute indication for surgical intervention.

The management of sterile necrosis is more controversial. Acute necrotizing pancreatitis refractory to maximal supportive therapy is considered a relative indication for surgery. Most surgeons recommend aggressive treatment focusing on treating the systemic manifestations of the disease by maximizing intravenous fluid therapy, mechanical ventilation, hemofiltration or hemodialysis, nutritional support, and, especially, administration of broad-spectrum antibiotics to prevent superinfection. Response to treatment should be reflected in a decreasing APACHE II score. Even in the presence of organ dysfunction, however, as long as the necrosis remains sterile, many advocate at least 3 to 6 weeks of maximal medical treatment to optimize comorbidities as well as to allow demarcation of necrosis before surgical therapy.

SURGICAL MANAGEMENT

The rationale for surgical débridement in necrotizing pancreatitis is to remove the necrotic pancreatic and peripancreatic tissues (necrosectomy) to both evacuate necrotic material (that is or may become infected) and to stop progression of the necrotizing process. Furthermore, removal of infected necrotic material helps to abort some of the inflammatory drive related to release of bacterial toxic compounds into the circulation, which is responsible for remote organ failure. This concept has led most pancreatic surgeons to advocate an extensive, complete necrosectomy complemented by various techniques to allow for adequate drainage, not only of the ongoing residual infection and resolving suppuration, but also of pancreatic exocrine secretions extravasating from injured pancreatic parenchyma. Although timing of surgical intervention remains controversial in sterile necrosis, most surgeons agree that necrosectomy ought to be performed as soon as bacterial infection is diagnosed.

Necrosectomy

Careful necrosectomy is the basic principle in surgical management of necrotizing pancreatitis. The goal is to identify and remove all areas of necrosis and infection while ensuring external drainage of persistent suppuration, weeping of denuded tissues, and extravasation of pancreatic exocrine secretion. A recent preoperative CT scan serves as the crucial anatomic guide to locate all areas of necrosis.

Inspection

We prefer a midline incision. Upon entrance to the abdominal cavity, a systematic and comprehensive manual and visual exploration is conducted of the entire pancreas and surrounding tissues. Access to the retroperitoneal peripancreatic space is obtained via the gastrocolic ligament. Manual and blunt dissection is the technique of choice. When trying to expose the necrosis in the lesser sac via the gastrocolic ligament, the cavity containing the necrosis can almost always be found by probing bluntly with a finger. Once found, the cavity can then be more fully exposed and unroofed in a controlled fashion, using the surgeon's fingers to provide a safe guide to the plane between the stomach and the colon. In this fashion, usually the entire pancreas (except for the uncinate process) can be visually and manually inspected. If there is difficulty inspecting the head and uncinate area of the pancreas from this approach, it can be reached through the right transverse mesocolon or via a plane posterior to the second and third portion of the duodenum. Exploration then proceeds to delineate the extent of extrapancreatic necrosis. Routine intraoperative exposure, unroofing, and both visual and manual inspection of both paracolic gutters, the mesocolon, the tissue surrounding the superior mesenteric vessels at the base of the small bowel mesentery, as well as the subdiaphragmatic region needs to be undertaken. Palpation by itself can be deceiving as to the presence or absence of fat necrosis, especially in the obese patient. An indurated area in the retroperitoneum signifies fat necrosis and should be visually inspected by unroofing the overlying peritoneum.

Débridement

Manual and blunt débridement is the technique of choice to remove necrotic material. Gentle scooping out of the putty-like material is sufficient in most patients. All devitalized tissue amenable to blunt débridement should be removed. However, special care should be taken when necrotic tissue remains adherent to apparently viable tissue. Blunt avulsion or sharp dissection away from the viable tissue may cause bleeding that is difficult to control. Similarly, bridges or septa that persist across an area of débrided necrosis may represent still-patent blood vessels. Because of concerns about future hemorrhage from the site of ligature, we prefer to leave these untouched rather than ligating them. Débridement should be sufficiently extensive to remove the main necrotic areas, but it should be done carefully to avoid damage to surrounding structures, especially major vessels or the small or large bowel. After débridement, affected areas should be irrigated to remove devitalized tissue, inflammatory exudate, and residual bacteria.

External Drainage

Controversy surrounds the technique of external peripancreatic drainage. Open packing with repeated wound pack changes, closed wide peripancreatic drainage, continuous postoperative peripancreatic lavage, and planned, repeated operative débridements with delayed primary wound closure over drains are the most well-accepted techniques developed to provide a controlled route of egress for ongoing evacuation of retroperitoneal debris produced by the necrotizing process and the extravasated pancreatic secretions.

Open Packing with Repeated Wound Pack Changes

After débridement and irrigation, omentum is interposed at the inferior wound edge (bilateral subcostal incision) and the colon to reduce fistula formation from the bowel and to compartmentalize the pancreatic bed from the general peritoneal cavity. The wound is left fully open as a "laparostomy." A nonadherent dressing such as Silastic sheeting or Adaptic (Johnson & Johnson, Kalamazoo, MI) gauze is also placed over exposed viscera and vessels. Moistened gauze is then packed into the cavities resulting from débridement. Daily wound pack changes are performed, at first in the operating room and subsequently, after formation of early granulation tissue, at bedside. During pack changes, packing is gently removed, the area is irrigated, and new moistened gauze packing is replaced. Wound packing continues until the suppurative process has completely resolved, and clean granulation tissue begins to cover débrided surfaces. Then the packing is removed, and the wound is allowed to heal by second intention.

Closed Wide Peripancreatic Drainage

After necrosectomy, the cavities resulting from débridement are packed with 3/4 inch Penrose drains stuffed with gauze, in addition to placing a soft, silicone-rubber closed-suction drain in each major extension of the cavity. The drains are brought out through separate stab wounds and sutured to the skin. Beginning 6 to 10 days after surgery, the stuffed Penrose drains are removed, one at a time, on sequential days, to allow the cavity to collapse. The closed suction drains are the last to be removed and are not withdrawn until their output is minimal. If a pancreatic fistula results, the drain tract is allowed to mature and then the drain is gradually withdrawn to allow the fistula to close behind it.

Continuous Postoperative Peripancreatic Lavage

Surgical débridement is followed by extensive intraoperative lavage with 6 L to 12 L of isotonic saline to clear the pancreatic bed. Large single-lumen and double-lumen catheters are placed in the lesser sac for postoperative lavage. On the left side, the drain is positioned behind the large bowel, below the spleen and in front of the kidney; on the right side, the tube is placed in the infrahepatic space. In patients with extensive extrapancreatic necrosis, additional tubes can be placed as necessary for complete evacuation of debris and exudate. After this procedure, the gastrocolic and duodenocolic ligaments

are sutured to form a closed compartment. This compartment is lavaged postoperatively in the ICU at a rate of 2 L per hour with hyperosmolar, potassium-free dialysis fluid. When ascites is also present, lavage of the lesser sac can be combined with short-term peritoneal lavage. As the patient improves and signs of systemic sepsis resolve, the volume of lavage is gradually reduced. The drains can be removed when no more necrotic material is present in the lavage fluid and there is no evidence of a pancreatic fistula.

Planned, Repeated Operative Débridements with Delayed Primary Wound Closure

After the original necrosectomy, if areas of questionable viability are noted or necrotic tissue remains adherent to viable areas, the decision is made to return to the operating room in 2 days for repeat exploration and necrosectomy. With this approach, the débrided areas are packed with moistened sponges; if exposed, the splenic or superior mesenteric vessels are protected by interposition of a layer of nonadhesive dressing such as Adaptic gauze or a thin layer of Silastic sheeting. Antibiotic-soaked gauze is used for packing if the exudate from the retroperitoneum is especially thick and purulent. Soft, closed-suction drains are positioned on top of the gauze packing to evacuate free fluid. Abdominal wall closure proceeds with a zipper sewn to the fascia. Reoperation is planned for 48 hours later and proceeds as at the initial necrosectomy. The zipper is opened and the abdomen fully explored in a systematic fashion. Additional necrosectomy is performed as needed. The process is repeated every 2 days until there is no more suppuration or necrosis. The average number of reoperations is about two.

Once the surgeon has decided that further débridement is not necessary, soft, closed-suction peripancreatic drains are placed, at least one individual drain in each separate anatomic area of necrosis, and the wound is closed definitively. Drains are removed when output is minimal.

Comparison of Drainage Techniques

There have been no prospective, randomized trials comparing techniques. Each technique has its advantages and drawbacks. In open packing, although it is clear that the wound pack changes offer adequate débridement, the daily pack changes risk repeated trauma to exposed colon, vascular structures, and pancreas. The open wound allows loss of fluid, proteins, and electrolytes and leads to abdominal wall failure with subsequent development of hernias that can be extremely difficult to repair. In contrast, the closed techniques are associated with a higher incidence of recurrent intra-abdominal abscesses, possibly the result of incomplete initial necrosectomy or débridement or perhaps from inadequate clearing of necrotic tissue by the drainage systems used. Postoperative closed lavage involves a prolonged ICU course with concomitant increased demand of technical equipment and cost. Planned reoperations increase the stress on the patient. Although we prefer the technique of scheduled, repeated necrosectomy, reported experiences conclude that all these methods achieve similar results, as long as all necrotic material and fluid collections are removed and reoperation is performed promptly if there is evidence of ongoing sepsis.

Complications of Surgical Intervention

Recurrent Intra-abdominal Abscess

Recurrent intra-abdominal abscess prolongs hospitalization and increases morbidity and mortality. This complication should be suspected in patients with signs and symptoms of ongoing infection (fever, pain, leukocytosis, bacteremia, hemodynamic instability with increased fluid requirements). Diagnosis is confirmed by subsequent CT. Percutaneous drainage should be attempted if the abscess involves only a single region. Reoperation, guided by CT, may be necessary for definitive treatment, especially if there are multiple areas of abscess or a large, multilocular complex abscess. Repeat necrosectomy should be performed following the same operative principles as previously described.

The incidence of recurrent intra-abdominal abscess requiring reoperation is 25% to 40% in most series. The likely etiology of this complication is an "incomplete" initial necrosectomy, a problem well-demonstrated when repeated wound pack changes are practiced; with each subsequent pack change, ostensibly "new" areas of necrosis are found. More likely, these areas of necrosis were overlooked or not fully appreciated during the initial necrosectomy. The technique of repeated scheduled necrosectomy decreases the incidence of recurrent intra-abdominal abscess, but, because the decision to end repeated trips for necrosectomy is based on surgical judgment, which is affected by experience and individual surgical style, this technique decreases but does not eradicate this complication.

Pancreatic and Gastrointestinal Fistulas

Pancreatic and enterocutaneous fistulas remain a frequent complication of necrotizing pancreatitis and its management. Pancreatic fistulas (approximately 25%) are invariably associated with pancreatic parenchymal necrosis (as opposed to peripancreatic tissue necrosis alone) and develop secondary to disruption of ductal continuity within the necrotic pancreas. Enzyme-rich fluids and inflammatory products dissect throughout retroperitoneal tissues and into the transverse mesocolon where they may involve and injure the vascular supply to the colon with subsequent vascular thrombosis. This mechanism or direct autodigestion of the wall of adjacent organs by these secretions gives rise to enteric fistulas. Too aggressive operative débridement and poorly positioned drains causing pressure necrosis on adjacent hollow viscera are additional iatrogenic causes of fistulization.

Pancreatocutaneous fistula should be treated conservatively, because two thirds will resolve spontaneously. Indications for operative intervention are persistence of the pancreatocutaneous fistula for more than 3 to 6 months,

formation of a symptomatic pseudocyst, presence of a proximal ductal stricture not amenable to endoscopic intervention, and communication with an enterically and anatomically isolated segment of the pancreas. One third of patients with pancreatocutaneous fistulas ultimately require operative closure for their fistula.

Upper gut fistulas (stomach, duodenum, small bowel) also tend to resolve spontaneously, as long as there is no distal obstruction. Duodenal fistulas, in particular, are occasionally recognized at the time of the initial necrosectomy and present challenges in management. Appropriate placement of drains during necrosectomy or under radiographic guidance is essential to management. Regardless of initial management challenges, the majority close with conservative means, and they do not affect outcome.

In contrast to proximal gut fistulas, colonic fistulas often require operative intervention and do increase mortality risk, suggesting a more fulminant course of necrotizing pancreatitis. Colonic involvement in necrotizing pancreatitis may present either early in the form of colonic necrosis or, more commonly, as a colocutaneous fistula later in the course. If colonic necrosis is recognized at the initial operation, colectomy and proximal diversion should be performed. Asymptomatic, low-output, well-controlled colocutaneous fistulas, noted by the presence of a communication with the colon on radiographic sinogram, are usually of no clinical significance and usually close spontaneously. In contrast, uncontrolled or high-output fistulas should be managed by proximal diversion and colectomy. The high incidence of colonic complications with necrotizing pancreatitis, ranging from 20% to 64%, and the higher associated mortality rate has led some centers to suggest routine use of prophylactic diverting loop ileostomy during initial necrosectomy, the role of which has yet to be defined.

Hemorrhage

Intra-abdominal hemorrhage requiring operative intervention is not an uncommon complication and is seen in as many as 20% of patients with necrotizing pancreatitis. The pathogenesis appears to be similar to that of fistulas—extension of the necrotizing process and proteolytic enzymes to involve blood vessel walls. Erosion of drains and a too aggressive or traumatic operative technique represent other causes. Hemorrhage is more frequently venous than arterial. Angiography for localization and potentially for definitive therapy may be considered, but prompt surgical intervention is quick, safe, and effective. Appropriately and timely diagnosed, hemorrhage itself does not usually lead to death. However, even when hemorrhage is controlled, the mortality rate in this group of patients is higher, suggesting the necrotizing process is more aggressive in patients in whom postoperative bleeding develops. The frequent coexistence of fistulas and hemorrhage, reflecting increased locoregional severity of the necrotizing pancreatitis, supports this concept.

Incisional Hernia

Ventral hernias more often develop in patients treated with open packing because such wounds close by secondary intention. Conversely, hernias develop less often in patients whose treatment included closed drainage after necrosectomy. Using the technique of planned, repeated necrosectomy with temporary closure with zipper and attempted delayed primary abdominal wall closure, incisional hernias developed in 27% of our patients. The loss of abdominal wall, the repeated abdominal explorations, and coexisting fistulas make repair of these hernias a challenging prospect; almost half our patients required mesh or tissue expanders to close the defect.

LONG-TERM SEQUELAE OF NECROTIZING PANCREATITIS

Because necrotizing pancreatitis is a life-threatening disease, survival has been the main criterion for successful treatment in most studies. Only recently have efforts been made to evaluate the late outcome of patients who survive the disease.

Pancreatic Insufficiency

Risk of pancreatic insufficiency closely correlates with amount of pancreatic parenchymal necrosis. Endocrine pancreatic insufficiency, usually the first sign of pancreatic dysfunction to develop, has been reported in 39% to 92% of patients after successful treatment of necrotizing pancreatitis. Overt diabetes mellitus develops in 13% to 50% of patients, whereas abnormal glucose tolerance tests may be seen in an additional 26% to 60%. Development of endocrine pancreatic insufficiency is more common among patients with alcohol-induced necrotizing pancreatitis, probably related to preexisting damage of the pancreatic parenchyma caused by chronic ingestion of alcohol. There is conflicting evidence regarding the natural history of endocrine pancreatic insufficiency—whereas some investigators have demonstrated that improvement in glucose tolerance may occur, others have suggested that endocrine function deteriorates with time.

Incidence of exocrine insufficiency is generally more than endocrine insufficiency. The incidence of exocrine insufficiency is estimated to be 38% to 46%. Clinically significant steatorrhea, seen in 16% to 20% of surviving necrotizing pancreatitis patients, is much less common. As with pancreatic endocrine insufficiency, exocrine insufficiency is more common in patients with alcoholic pancreatitis. Once established, pancreatic insufficiency appears to persist.

Recurrent Pancreatitis

Recurrent pancreatitis occurs in 13% to 30% of patients who have survived necrotizing pancreatitis, but appears to occur almost exclusively in patients who not only have a history of alcohol abuse but who also continue alcohol consumption. Recurrent pancreatitis rarely develops in patients with a nonalcoholic etiology. Recurrent abdominal pain without hyperamylasemia, dyspeptic symptoms without steatorrhea, or typical pancreatic pain resembling mild episodes of subclinical acute pancreatitis may occur

in 10% to 16% of patients. Such episodes generally resolve quickly.

Quality of Life

Few studies have investigated whether survivors of necrotizing pancreatitis achieve a satisfactory quality of life after recovery from their illness. Broome and colleagues followed up 22 survivors and reported a satisfactory quality of life, comparable to the quality of life of age-matched control subjects, using the Short Form-36 Health Survey (SF-36). SF-36 includes questions relating to physical and mental well-being; 70% of respondents had returned to work. In another study, no patient needed regular medical or nursing care as a result of their necrotizing pancreatitis, and self-assessment of quality of life demonstrated satisfaction in 77% of patients. In our own experience with 44 patients followed up for a mean of 5 years, we found that performance status (measured by the Eastern Cooperative Oncology Group status) worsened in 9%, related principally to recurrent pain or severe steatorrhea. These patients had higher APACHE-II scores on admission for necrotizing pancreatitis compared with those who maintained the same performance status after recovery from the illness. Similarly, 23% of patients were unable to return to work because of complications related directly to the necrotizing pancreatitis. These patients also had higher APACHE-II scores on admission. Overall, however, these preliminary results appear to indicate that most survivors can expect a return to productivity and a satisfactory quality of life.

Summary

Necrotizing pancreatitis is a serious, life-threatening form of acute pancreatitis. Diagnosis of necrotizing pancreatitis remains primarily a clinical diagnosis, although contrast-enhanced CT has improved diagnostic accuracy. Initial management of the patient with necrotizing pancreatitis should be conservative, managing systemic complications of the disease and administering prophylactic imipenem. Surgical intervention is indicated for those patients whose

---

Pearls and Pitfalls

- Necrotizing pancreatitis represents approximately 3% to 5% of all episodes of acute pancreatitis.
- Treatment should involve aggressive fluid and electrolyte resuscitation, 10 days to 2 weeks of imipenem, and nutritional support (preferably enteral feeding).
- In approximately 30% of patients, infected necrosis develops, which requires operative treatment.
- Operative treatment involves necrosectomy and provision for external drainage of the peripancreatic region; mortality rate is approximately 20%.
- Potential morbidity of necrosectomy includes hemorrhage, pancreatic fistulas, and gastrointestinal fistulas (duodenal, small bowel, or colonic).
- Long-term effects of necrotizing pancreatitis include endocrine and exocrine insufficiency (approximately 30% to 50%).

necrosis becomes infected. A relative indication for surgery is the case of sterile necrosis that fails to improve with maximal medical treatment. Before operative management is pursued, adequate time (4 to 6 weeks) should pass to allow necrosis to demarcate internally. Surgical management consists of a careful, thorough débridement and then some method of postoperative drainage. Various methods of drainage are preferred by pancreatic surgeons, all of which have similar outcomes as long as the initial débridement is thorough and there is no hesitation to return to the operating room if signs of clinical decompensation develop. Postoperative complications include recurrent intra-abdominal abscess, fistula, and hemorrhage, all of which can potentially affect mortality risk. Colonic fistulas and hemorrhage indicate a more severe course of disease. Longer term complications of surgical treatment include ventral hernias and pancreatic insufficiency. Only rarely does recurrent pancreatitis complicate recovery in the nonalcoholic patient. Given the severity of necrotizing pancreatitis and the associated morbidity and mortality risks, it is encouraging that preliminary studies on survivors' quality of life demonstrate a return to premorbid conditions of productivity and satisfaction.

SELECTED READINGS

Beger HG, Isenmann R: Surgical management of necrotizing pancreatitis. Surg Clin North Am 1999;79:783.

Bradley EL III, Allen K: A prospective longitudinal study of observation versus surgical intervention in the management of necrotizing pancreatitis. Am J Surg 1991;161:19.

Broome AH, Eisen GM, Harland RC, et al: Quality of life after treatment for pancreatitis. Ann Surg 1996;223:665.

Buchler P, Reber HA: Surgical approach in patients with acute pancreatitis: Is infected or sterile necrosis an indication—in whom should this be done, when, and why? Gastroenterol Clin North Am 1999;28:661.

Fernandez-del Castillo C, Rattner DW, Makary MA, et al: Debridement and closed packing for the treatment of necrotizing pancreatitis. Ann Surg 1998;228:676.

Mier J, Leon EL, Castillo A, et al: Early versus late necrosectomy in severe necrotizing pancreatitis. Am J Surg 1997;173:71.

Murr MM, Tsiotos GG, Sarr MG. Operative management of necrotizing pancreatitis by repeated planned necrosectomy and delayed primary closure of the abdominal wall. In Sarr MG (ed): Problems in General Surgery. New York, Lippincott-Raven, 1996.

Tsiotos GG, Luque-de Leon E, Sarr MG: Long-term outcome of necrotizing pancreatitis treated by necrosectomy. Br J Surg 1998;85:1650.

Tsiotos GG, Luque-de Leon E, Soreide JA, et al: Management of necrotizing pancreatitis by repeated operative necrosectomy using a zipper technique. Am J Surg 1998;175:91.

Tsiotos GG, Sarr MG: Complications of surgical treatment of necrotizing pancreatitis. In Sarr MG (ed): Problems in General Surgery. New York, Lippincott-Raven, 1996.

Chapter 116
Acute Pancreatitis
Michael G. Sarr, Oscar Joseph Hines, and Howard A. Reber

Acute pancreatitis is a nonbacterial inflammatory process of the pancreas resulting from intrapancreatic activation, release, and digestion of the organ by pancreatic enzymes. Most episodes of acute pancreatitis are mild, and patients usually recover quickly. However, 10% of episodes of acute pancreatitis are severe and may be complicated by infection, multiple organ system failure, and death. Acute pancreatitis is characterized clinically by acute abdominal pain and increased serum activities of pancreatic enzymes. Patients may experience single or multiple episodes of this disease.

ETIOLOGY

The most common causes of acute pancreatitis are alcohol abuse and gallstones. The relative incidence of these etiologies depends on the geographic location; gallstone pancreatitis is more common in rural areas, whereas alcohol-induced acute pancreatitis predominates in the inner city. Other causes of acute pancreatitis include endoscopic retrograde cholangiopancreatography (ERCP) postoperatively, and hyperlipidemia (types I and V). Several drugs have definitely been implicated, including azathioprine, valproic acid, and several of the drugs effective against human immunodeficiency virus (HIV). Several others are suspect, including thiazide diuretics. Much less common etiologies include ischemia, viral disorders, hypercalcemia, and a hereditary form related to germline mutations in the trypsinogen gene.

PATHOGENESIS

The formerly popular theories of intraductal activation of pancreatic enzymes in the pancreas, bile reflux into the pancreatic duct, pancreatic ductal rupture, and intraparenchymal activation of pancreatic enzymes all have been disproved as pathogenic mechanisms. Most pancreatic physiologists now believe that the common pathway by which multiple etiologies induce acute pancreatitis is through a disruption of receptor-mediated secretion of pancreatic enzymes at the apical surface of the acinar cell. Normally, most pancreatic enzymes are synthesized and packaged as inactive proenzymes (e.g., trypsinogen) in the Golgi apparatus as condensing vacuoles. These vacuoles migrate toward the apical membrane and, in so doing, become so-called zymogen granules. Exocrine stimuli cause the zymogen granules to fuse with the apical cell membrane, thereby releasing these *proenzymes* into the pancreatic duct as inactive precursors. When the secretions enter the duodenum, the duodenal enzyme enterokinase cleaves a peptide off the trypsinogen molecule, which activates trypsin. Trypsin then autoactivates

the other proenzymes. By this and other mechanisms, the pancreas protects itself from autodigestion.

During acute pancreatitis, this mechanism is disrupted. The fusing of zymogen granules with the apical membrane of the acinar cell is disrupted; zymogen granules build up in the acinar cell and fuse with lysosomes within the cell. This fusion process allows the acid hydrolases within the lysosome to activate these proenzymes, which then overwhelms the cell and leads to cell death. This theory of "colocalization" appears to explain almost all the experimental models of acute pancreatitis. Thus, in summary, acute pancreatitis occurs from a primary cell death of the acinar cell, rupture of the cell with intraparenchymal release of activated digestive enzymes, and autodigestion of the pancreas and surrounding parenchyma. Exactly how the multiple etiologies, including alcohol, partial ductal obstruction (gallstones), and ERCP, cause activation of this common pathway remains under active investigation.

Several points should be made concerning alcohol-induced acute pancreatitis. Exactly how ethanol induces the cellular injury is unknown, but recent evidence suggests that intrapancreatic metabolism of alcohol leads to buildup of metabolites via an alternative pathway. Susceptible patients develop acute pancreatitis early in their life, and not after a long history of years of drinking, as occurs with cirrhosis or chronic pancreatitis. Thus, most patients with acute alcoholic pancreatitis are in their late teens or twenties, and not older than age 40. Thus, alcohol as an etiology in a 50-year-old patient with his or her first episode of acute pancreatitis can be reliably excluded.

CLINICAL PRESENTATION

Acute pancreatitis begins with severe and persistent epigastric or upper abdominal pain that may radiate to the back. The attack may be temporally related to the ingestion of a large meal or alcohol. Patients may also experience nausea and persistent vomiting. The symptoms are the same regardless of the etiology, even when an episode of acute pancreatic inflammation occurs in a patient with chronic pancreatitis. The pain may be less severe with edematous pancreatitis compared with the necrotizing form of the disease, but this characteristic is not invariable. Examination may reveal signs of dehydration and decreased blood volume, with tachycardia and hypotension. The often-referred-to findings of a bluish color (ecchymosis) around the umbilicus (Cullen's sign), or in the flanks (Grey Turner's sign), are exceedingly rare and are of little practical value. Palpation reveals abdominal tenderness most marked in the epigastrium but sometimes present throughout the abdomen. The bowel sounds are decreased or absent. Usually, no masses are palpable, but when an upper abdominal mass or fullness is present, it most often represents a swollen pancreas, pseudocyst, or abscess. With necrotizing pancreatitis, the abdomen may be distended with intraperitoneal fluid or dilated small and large bowel secondary to ileus. The temperature is only mildly elevated (100°F to 101°F) in uncomplicated cases. There may also be evidence of a pleural effusion, especially on the left side.

Other intra-abdominal diseases can present in a similar manner, including perforated gastric or duodenal ulcer, acute cholecystitis, and small bowel obstruction. Therefore, acute pancreatitis is largely a diagnosis of exclusion. The clinical findings should be confirmed by laboratory investigation. If doubt remains about the diagnosis, a laparotomy may be indicated for diagnosis (<2% of patients), since the diseases with which acute pancreatitis is most likely to be confused can be lethal if not treated surgically.

Laboratory findings may include an increased hematocrit if dehydration is marked or, *very rarely,* a low hematocrit resulting from pancreatic or retroperitoneal hemorrhage. In the absence of suppurative complications, a white blood cell count over 12,000/mm³ is unusual. Liver function tests are usually normal, but mild increases in the serum bilirubin concentration (<4 mg/dL) may be seen. This mild jaundice is probably due to partial obstruction of the intrapancreatic portion of the common bile duct by the swollen head of the pancreas. The serum amylase activity rises to more than 2.5 times normal (and usually 8 to 20 times normal) within 6 hours of the onset of an acute episode and usually remains elevated for several days. Values above 1500 IU/dL are characteristic (but not diagnostic) of biliary pancreatitis; lower values are more typical for acute alcoholic pancreatitis. The sensitivity of serum amylase in diagnosing pancreatitis ranges from 55% to 80%. In patients with abdominal pain and hyperamylasemia, 70% are found to have pancreatitis. Serum amylase activity may be increased in other diseases, including perforated ulcer, gangrenous cholecystitis, and small bowel obstruction. The level of the serum amylase activity does not correlate with the severity of the episode of pancreatitis, however. Indeed, the serum amylase activity may rarely be normal in patients with acute pancreatitis owing to increased urinary clearance of the enzyme, in patients with hyperlipidemia, and in patients with chronic pancreatitis.

Serum lipase activity may be a more sensitive and specific test than amylase to diagnose acute pancreatitis. Serum lipase has a longer half-life than amylase, which makes it a better test for patients who present later in the course of the disease. Lipase may also be increased in other diseases including cholecystitis and perforated viscus, however. If a cutoff of three times the upper level of normal lipase is used for the diagnosis of acute pancreatitis, the sensitivity and specificity are close to 100%. Serum trypsin and elastase activities also are increased in acute pancreatitis and may be used for diagnosis; however, these tests are not yet available clinically.

Radiologic studies are sometimes useful in confirming the diagnosis but are not routinely needed. However, computed tomography (CT) should be performed in all patients whose illness has not begun to resolve within several days or whenever complications are suspected. The possible findings include pancreatic edema, a mass of inflamed pancreatic and peripancreatic tissues, pancreatic and/or peripancreatic fluid collections, abscess, and pancreatic necrosis. Extension of the inflammation from the pancreas to other tissue planes (retrocolic, perinephric) implies a more serious prognosis. The adequacy of pancreatic vascular perfusion of the pancreas should be estimated on the CT during the arterial phase of an intravenous contrast-enhanced bolus. Viable pancreas enhances as the contrast material flows through it, while the lack of enhancement correlates with pancreatic necrosis. Patients with more than 50% of the pancreas that is nonperfused (infarcted) are more likely to develop pancreatic infection and to require surgical intervention.

Other less useful radiologic studies include plain abdominal films and ultrasonography. The most frequent finding on a plain abdominal film is the so-called sentinel loop, which represents dilatation of an isolated loop of intestine (duodenum, jejunum, or transverse colon) adjacent to the pancreas. In patients with biliary pancreatitis, a plain abdominal film may show radiopaque gallstones in the region of the gallbladder (10% to 15% of the time). However, ultrasonography is the best way of confirming the presence of gallstones when biliary pancreatitis is suspected. Ultrasonography may also reveal an edematous, swollen pancreas or acute peripancreatic fluid collections, but this study is often inconclusive because overlying bowel gas prevents a complete examination. Serial ultrasonography studies may be useful in following the clinical course of patients with protracted or complicated pancreatitis or fluid collections.

PREOPERATIVE MANAGEMENT

The treatment of uncomplicated acute pancreatitis should be nonsurgical. Initial management is directed toward restoration of fluid and electrolyte balance, avoidance of secretory stimulation of the pancreas, and pain relief. With these simple interventions, uncomplicated pancreatitis usually resolves within 4 to 5 days. The 10% of patients with severe acute pancreatitis need intensive care and aggressive fluid resuscitation and may eventually require surgery. Central venous pressure should be monitored, and electrolytes should be serially checked and replaced appropriately. The amount of crystalloid and colloid (albumin, blood) given should be sufficient to maintain an adequate hematocrit, circulating blood volume, and urine output. Renal failure from inadequate replacement is a frequent finding in patients who die early in the course of this disease. Moreover, the pancreatitis itself may become more severe from the impaired pancreatic perfusion that can accompany the shock state. For these reasons, the most important aspect of early resuscitation is adequate, aggressive fluid replacement. Hypocalcemia can occur in patients with severe pancreatitis and must be treated urgently with parenteral calcium to protect against cardiac arrhythmias. Hypomagnesemia is also common, particularly in alcoholic patients, and the magnesium should be replaced. Ventilatory support may be required, and renal function must be maintained. Oral

Table 116–1	Utility of Peritoneal Lavage in Acute Pancreatitis				

STUDY	TREATMENT	n	COMPLICATIONS (%)	DEATHS (%)
Teerenhovi et al	Control	12	50	17
	Lavage—7 days	12	73	36
Ihse et al	Control	20	30	5
	Lavage	19	42	21
Mayer et al	Control	46	28	35
	Lavage—3 days	45	27	38
Ranson et al (1974)	Lavage—2 days	15	40	20
	Lavage—7 days	14	22	0

intake should be withheld until the ileus has resolved, and pain is absent. Nasogastric suction should be instituted in patients with severe pain or those who are vomiting.

Currently, there are no specific drugs effective in treating pancreatitis. Many approaches have been evaluated. Attempts at decreasing pancreatic exocrine secretion by nasogastric suction, antacids, or inhibition of acid secretion, all designed to prevent release of the pancreatic stimulatory hormone secretin in reaction to the presence of acid in the duodenum, proved to be not helpful. Similarly, infusion of antiproteases intravenously in an attempt to neutralize extravasated exocrine secretions also proved unsuccessful. More recently, clinical and experimental studies suggest that platelet-activating factor antagonists and related anti-inflammatory cytokine agents may eventually have a role. For example, in limited trials, lexipafant, a platelet-activating factor antagonist, reduced the severity of organ failure in patients with severe disease. Prophylactic antibiotics, such as imipenem, which penetrate pancreatic parenchyma, and possibly antifungal agents should be given in patients with severe disease to decrease the incidence of superinfection of necrotic pancreas. The most common infecting organisms are enteric bacteria, including *Escherichia coli* (~35%), *Klebsiella pneumoniae* (~24%), *Enterococcus* spp. (~24%), and various fungal species. Other less frequently isolated organisms are *Staphylococcus* (~14%), *Pseudomonas* spp. (~11%), *Proteus* (~8%), aerobic *Streptococcus* (~7%), *Enterobacter* (~7%), and *Bacteroides* (~6%).

Parenteral nutrition has no specific beneficial effect on the course of pancreatitis. It should be used as in any other patient when oral intake must be withheld for prolonged periods and when enteral nutrition is not possible. Elemental diets delivered proximal to the ligament of Treitz are not indicated, since they do not avoid pancreatic stimulation; however, early enteral feeding distal to the ligament of Treitz may help maintain the gut mucosal barrier and minimize sepsis. Peritoneal lavage has been used in patients with severe acute pancreatitis to remove "toxins" and various metabolites from the peritoneal cavity and minimize their systemic absorption. Although controlled trials failed to show that this decreased mortality rates (Table 116–1), there was some evidence that the incidence of cardiopulmonary complications was lessened. For this reason, and because there are anecdotal reports in which patients rapidly improved during lavage therapy, peritoneal lavage may still be considered in se-

lected patients who are deteriorating during the first several days of onset of disease.

Endoscopic intervention may be lifesaving in some patients with severe biliary pancreatitis. Endoscopic sphincterotomy should be seriously considered when a patient with pancreatitis is known to have gallstones, when the serum bilirubin concentration is elevated above 2 to 4 mg/dL, when the alkaline phosphatase level is elevated, *and* when the clinical course does not improve within 24 to 36 hours. At least four randomized studies have evaluated the utility of urgent sphincterotomy and stone extraction (Table 116–2). If a skilled endoscopist is available, endoscopic retrograde cholangiography (without pancreatography) with endoscopic sphincterotomy to remove the stone may abort the severity of the attack.

If infection is suspected, a percutaneous fine-needle aspirate of collections of fluid or poorly perfused pancreatic tissue on CT or ultrasonography as a guide should be undertaken. The material should be sent for Gram stain and bacterial and fungal culture. Proof of infection is an indication for laparotomy and surgical débridement of the infected and necrotic material.

INTRAOPERATIVE MANAGEMENT

For most patients with mild pancreatitis, surgery directed toward the pancreas itself is not necessary. However, in patients with mild to moderate severity biliary pancreatitis (caused by gallstones), a laparoscopic cholecystectomy

Table 116–2	Early ERC and Endoscopic Sphincterotomy (ES) in Acute and Severe Gallstone Pancreatitis		

STUDY	TREATMENT	COMPLICATIONS (%)	DEATHS (%)
Neoptolemos et al (1998)	ERC/ES	19	0
	Conservative	63	13
Nowak et al	ERC/ES	14	1
	Conservative	34	11
Fan et al	ERC/ES	20	3
	Conservative	76	18
Folsch et al (1997)	ERC/ES	17	5
	Conservative	14	3

should be performed during the same admission when the pancreatitis and pain resolves, usually within 3 to 4 days after admission. This operation can be done safely, and it avoids the recurrent pancreatitis that occurs in as many as 30% of patients in the first 6 months after the initial episode if a cholecystectomy is not performed. Any stones noted in the bile ducts should also be removed. The elderly patient who is a high anesthetic risk may be better treated, not by a laparoscopic cholecystectomy, but rather by an endoscopic sphincterotomy. Although this approach does not prevent formation of gallstones or the development of cholecystitis, sphincterotomy should prevent further episodes of acute pancreatitis.

If the patient develops severe acute pancreatitis from gallstones with a large inflammatory peripancreatic reaction or frank necrotizing pancreatitis, early cholecystectomy is not indicated and should be postponed until the peripancreatic reaction has resolved (about 3 to 6 months). Some consideration should be given to performing an endoscopic sphincterotomy to protect the patient from recurrent gallstone pancreatitis in the interim.

For patients with severe necrotizing pancreatitis and infection, surgical intervention is indicated. The goals are to remove infected and devitalized pancreatic and peripancreatic tissue, to drain pus and other fluid collections, and to leave drains behind which will control drainage of extravasated pancreatic exocrine secretions from areas of pancreatic parenchymal necrosis. Wide exposure is required for a thorough exploration of the peripancreatic and retroperitoneal tissues. The CT provides a "road map" to the areas that require drainage, so that uninvolved tissue planes do not need to be opened and unnecessarily contaminated. Viable pancreatic parenchyma should be preserved. Hemostasis may require suture ligation of bleeding vessels, but significant bleeding usually suggests that the surgeon should limit further dissection in that area. Once most of the necrotic material has been removed and all of the fluid collections have been drained, several large drains are placed in the most involved areas. Further discussion of the surgical management of necrotizing pancreatitis and its postoperative complications can be found in Chapter 115.

POSTOPERATIVE MANAGEMENT

Most patients who have undergone laparoscopic cholecystectomy for mild gallstone pancreatitis can be discharged within 24 hours. Patients with severe disease need continued intensive care management and prophylactic intravenous antibiotics. An abdominal CT obtained at weekly intervals will help guide further therapy and document improvement during the postoperative course. Many weeks are usually required before patients are well enough to be discharged from the hospital.

Pancreatic Pseudocyst

A pancreatic pseudocyst is a collection of fluid that develops in association with a leak of pancreatic fluid from the inflamed parenchyma or from a disrupted duct. The wall of the pseudocyst is composed of fibrous, nonepithelialized tissue and is usually found in close proximity to the pancreas. Occasionally, a pseudocyst may present at great distance from the pancreas (e.g., thorax, groin), when the fluid dissects through tissue planes. As many as 30% of patients with acute pancreatitis form acute fluid collections around the time of the acute attack. These fluid collections are not associated with extravasation of exocrine secretion, but rather with an inflammatory reaction. The majority of these acute fluid collections resolve without intervention, and, therefore, these should be managed expectantly. In about 5% of these patients, the acute fluid collection actually represents extravasated exocrine secretions that will go on to develop into a chronic pseudocyst, which *may* require treatment. Asymptomatic pseudocysts up to 5 to 6 cm in diameter can be observed safely, and their progress is usually followed with either serial ultrasonography or CT. Larger pseudocysts of any size that are symptomatic require treatment.

Pancreatic pseudocysts most often present with pain or gastrointestinal obstruction when the cyst distorts the stomach or duodenum. Serious complications can also occur, although they are uncommon (<10% of patients). These complications include hemorrhage into the cyst, perforation, and infection of the cyst. Hemorrhage may be suspected with the acute onset of abdominal pain and with the usual systemic signs of decreased blood volume. An abdominal CT may show the cyst with the contained blood, which is of a density different from that of the usual cyst fluid. Angiography confirms the diagnosis, and the interventional radiologist should be called on to embolize the bleeding vessel. If not, emergency surgery with ligation of the vessel or resection of the cyst is required. Spontaneous perforation of a pseudocyst is a surgical emergency characterized by the sudden onset of intense abdominal pain with peritonitis. Patients require urgent operation with external cyst drainage. Infection of a pseudocyst should be suspected if signs of sepsis develop. Diagnosis by CT and treatment with percutaneous cyst drainage are usually effective. In the absence of these life-threatening complications, elective surgery of pseudocysts is usually delayed for 4 to 6 weeks until the cyst has developed a mature wall that will hold sutures at the time of repair. Most of these patients can eat and be discharged from the hospital during the interval of cyst maturation.

Pseudocysts may be treated surgically, endoscopically, or by radiologic-guided drainage. Endoscopic methods require the placement of several double-pigtail stents through the stomach or duodenal wall into the adjacent cyst. The stents are eventually removed, and in about 80% of patients the cyst is permanently eradicated. These endoscopic techniques require an expertise that has become widely available recently. Radiologic approaches consist of percutaneous external drainage of the cyst with eventual removal of the drainage catheter weeks later. Many of these pseudocysts will recur. Surgical treatment usually consists of drainage of the cyst internally into either the stomach (cystogastrostomy) or the duodenum (cystoduodenostomy) or into a Roux-en-Y limb of jejunum (cyst jejunostomy). Both are safe and effective, with recurrence rates less than 10%. If the pseudocyst is in the tail of the pancreas, a distal pancreatectomy with excision of the cyst may be best (see Chapter 119).

Table 116–3	**Ranson Criteria**

At Admission or Diagnosis
Age >55 yr
White blood cell count >16,000/mm³
Blood glucose >200 mg/dL
Serum lactic dehydrogenase >350 IU/L
Serum glutamic oxaloacetic transaminase >250 U/dL
During the Initial 48 Hours
Hematocrit fall >10%
Blood urea nitrogen rise >5 mg/dL
Serum calcium <8 mg/dL
Arterial Po_2 <60 mm Hg
Base deficit >4 mEq/L
Estimated fluid sequestration >6 L

OUTCOMES

The majority of patients with acute pancreatitis have a self-limited course and an excellent outcome. A minority of patients (10%) have severe disease with necrosis of the pancreas and the complications discussed earlier. Ranson's criteria, determined during the first 48 hours after disease onset (Table 116–3), have been used widely to establish the severity and likelihood of death from pancreatitis. The APACHE II score may be more useful, since it can be used at any time during the course of disease. Serum markers also may be used to determine severity and estimate prognosis; these include C-reactive protein, interleukin-6, and neutrophil elastase. Contrast-enhanced CT provides the most objective information about the extent of the inflammatory process, the degree of pancreatic necrosis, and the presence of infection, all of which affect the treatment and the prognosis.

SELECTED READINGS

Folsch UR, Nitsche R, Ludtke R, et al: Early ERCP and papillotomy compared with conservative treatment for acute biliary pancreatitis. The German Study Group on Acute Biliary Pancreatitis. N Engl J Med 1997;336:237.

Pearls and Pitfalls

- Etiologies of acute pancreatitis depend on patient demographics; in urban locations, alcohol predominates, while in more rural settings, gallstones predominate.
- Patients older than 40 years of age who are experiencing their first episode of acute pancreatitis virtually never have acute alcoholic pancreatitis.
- Acute pancreatitis is largely a diagnosis of exclusion; increased amylase and lipase levels only support the clinical diagnosis.
- Most episodes (85%) of acute pancreatitis resolve within 2 to 4 days.
- Specific treatment for acute pancreatitis is lacking except for prophylactic intravenous antibiotics in necrotizing pancreatitis.
- Mild gallstone pancreatitis is best treated with same admission laparoscopic cholecystectomy; cholecystectomy should be delayed in patients with severe gallstone pancreatitis.
- Older or infirm patients who have gallstone pancreatitis but who do not have a history of biliary colic may be best treated solely with an endoscopic sphincterotomy.
- Acute peripancreatic fluid collections during an episode of acute pancreatitis usually resolve and require no treatment.
- Asymptomatic pancreatic pseudocysts can be managed expectantly unless they are very large.

Frey CF, Bradley EL III, Beger HG: Progress in acute pancreatitis. Surg Gynecol Obstet 1988;167:282.

McFadden DW, Reber HA: Indications for surgery in severe pancreatitis: State of the art. Int J Pancreatol 1994;15:83.

Neoptolemos JP, Carr-Locke DL, London NJ, et al: Controlled trial of urgent endoscopic retrograde cholangiopancreatography and endoscopic sphincterotomy versus conservative treatment for acute pancreatitis due to gallstones. Lancet 1988;2:979.

Ranson JHC, Rifkind KM, Roses DF, et al: Prognostic signs and the role of operative management in acute pancreatitis. Surg Gynecol Obstet 1974;139:69.

Steer ML: The early intraacinar cell events which occur during acute pancreatitis. Pancreas 1998;17:31.

Chapter 117

Chronic Pancreatitis: Endotherapy First, Then Surgery

L. William Traverso

Any discussion of chronic pancreatitis and its therapy must first acknowledge our improved understanding of the natural history of this disease through modern techniques of imaging. Imaging is crucial for patient selection in order to make treatment decisions for chronic pancreatitis. Modern imaging allows the surgeon to determine almost all of the anatomy preoperatively and then, using that knowledge, predict the likelihood for successful treatment. With follow-up studies, these results based on the anatomy ensure adequate patient selection.

In general, in order for a patient to be a candidate for any type of surgery directed at chronic pancreatitis, the patient must have specific anatomic changes, and all forms of more conservative treatment must have failed, including endotherapy. Surgery is the last resort after all forms of nonsurgical treatment have failed. In properly selected patients, surgery then improves their condition such that the vast majority will be free of their preoperative symptoms.

In addition to having the proper anatomy, the patient must also have had the origin of his or her chronic pancreatitis removed (e.g., cholecystectomy for gallstones, endoscopic papillotomy for ampullary stenosis, or termination of alcohol abuse). If the patient has not stopped drinking alcohol, he or she should not be considered a candidate for surgery. One of the most critical members of a chronic pancreatitis multidisciplinary team is the professional who treats alcohol abuse. In a patient who is currently drinking alcohol, the change in the anatomy is a dynamic process, and an operation that may be appropriate on one day would not be the choice of treatment later.

PREOPERATIVE WORKUP AND OPERATIVE CRITERIA

Modern Imaging to Define the "Composite Pancreas"

Every patient undergoing surgery for chronic pancreatitis will have had at least computed tomography (CT) studies and endoscopic retrograde cholangiopancreatography (ERCP). Some also require visceral arteriography. Currently, the role of magnetic resonance cholangiopancreatography (MRCP) is being evaluated. Intraoperatively, fluoroscopic pancreatography and ultrasonography are frequently used. After the specimen has been removed or the drainage procedure has been accomplished, the surgeon adds his or her observations to the data of preoperative modern imaging. Frequently, even modern im-

aging is found to have limitations when verified by the observations during surgery or dissection of the operative specimens. Therefore, combining preoperative imaging with observations during surgery yields a *composite view* of the pancreatic ductal system and parenchyma that cannot be obtained using just imaging techniques. This "composite pancreas" represents the anatomic picture that must be then compared with the outcomes of the procedures. An accurate composite pancreas compared with short- and long-term surgical outcomes will yield reliable selection criteria for patients in the future. In this chapter, the composite pancreas findings are compared with the long- and short-term outcomes after pylorus-preserving pancreaticoduodenectomy. This comparison generates reliable selection criteria.

CLINICAL PRESENTATION—SYMPTOMS AND ANATOMY

Almost every patient seen for medical treatment of chronic pancreatitis has abdominal pain. When the pain becomes disabling, it is due to progressive disease documented by anatomic changes varying from ductal disruption, partial obstruction, or complete obstruction. Disabling abdominal pain is difficult to define. Traverso and colleagues found that 94% of patients undergoing any form of surgical treatment for chronic pancreatitis had abdominal pain and that pain had been present for an average of 5.6 years before surgery (range 1 month to 35 years). The pain was described as continuous in half the patients and as intermittent chronic relapsing pancreatitis in the other 50%. The frequency of exacerbating episodes was every 5.3 months, and alcohol was the etiology in most patients.

Once the clinician has determined that the patient has disabling abdominal pain, then the clinical diagnosis of "chronic pancreatitis" must be confirmed. The Marseilles classification of 1963 contains a preliminary definition of chronic pancreatitis, that is, chronic pancreatitis represents "residual pancreatic damage either anatomical or functional that persists even if the primary cause or factors are eliminated." Once this general definition of the disease has been met, then anatomic changes are assessed. Candidates for surgery must have the "marked" variety of anatomic changes according to the Cambridge Image Severity scale (Table 117–1); the six items in the footnote denote "abnormal" findings associated with the "marked" stage on the scale. Roman numerals have been assigned to the scale in Table 117–1 that are not in the original reference. Any one of the six items classify the

Table 117–1	Cambridge Classification of Image Severity	

CAMBRIDGE CLASS*	MAIN PANCREATIC DUCT	ABNORMAL SIDE BRANCHES
I. Normal	Normal	None
II. Equivocal	Normal	<3
III. Mild	Normal	≥3
IV. Moderate	Abnormal	>3
V. Marked	Abnormal†	>3

*Roman numerals are assigned by the author and were not used in the original article.

†Marked abnormalities of main pancreatic duct are
1. Main pancreatic duct (MPD) terminates prematurely (abrupt, tapering, or irregular)
2. Multiple MPD strictures
3. MPD dilated >10 mm
4. Ductal filling defects (stones)
5. "Cavities" intrapancreatic or extra-pancreatic
6. Contiguous organ involvement (common bile duct, duodenum, arterial venous fistula)

patient into the Cambridge Class V stage of "marked" image severity. A schematic showing all the possibilities that could be seen on the "composite" view of the pancreas is depicted in Fig. 117–1.

SEQUENCE OF THERAPY FOR CHRONIC PANCREATITIS—TRY ENDOTHERAPY FIRST

The first criterion for interventional treatment is the presence of abdominal pain, which is present in 98% of

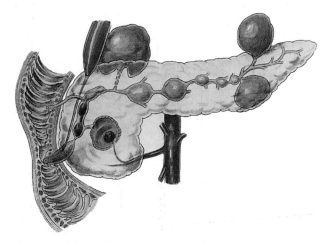

Figure 117–1. Possible complications of chronic pancreatitis encountered when one plans surgical therapy. The combination of all findings yields the "composite pancreas." From left to right, the following complications are depicted: duodenal stenosis, common bile duct stricture, main pancreatic duct stricture (with ductal stones), intrapancreatic pseudocyst with contained pseudoaneurysm (arterial venous connection), ductal disruption at the genu with extrapancreatic pseudocyst formation, chain-of-lakes ductal dilatation, distal pancreatic duct disruptions with focal extrapancreatic pseudocyst collections. (From Traverso LW: The surgical management of chronic pancreatitis: The Whipple procedure. In Cameron JL [ed]: Advances in Surgery, vol 32. St. Louis, Mosby, 1999, pp 23–39, with permission.)

patients. In an asymptomatic patient, there are essentially no indications for interventional or surgical treatment other than to surgically treat a persistent external pancreatic fistula. Therefore, the sequence of therapy is to treat abdominal pain by approaching the predisposing anatomy. Conservative medical therapy is essentially that as described by Ammann and colleagues—removal of the etiology, analgesics as necessary, and support of exocrine or endocrine insufficiency. Exacerbation of chronic pain is associated with local complications, mainly ductal disruption anatomically expressed as a pseudocyst. Medical therapy is usually abandoned when something beyond symptoms is added to the clinical history. These additional complications are usually an escalation of the pain associated with anatomic changes, such as development of a pseudocyst, pancreatic duct stricture (with or without pancreatic duct stones), biliary stenosis, or duodenal stenosis.

Endotherapy is the next option with this escalation of pain. This procedure begins with ERCP to visualize the main pancreatic duct (MPD). The anatomy derived from ERCP classifies the patient into one of three potential anatomic findings: MPD stones, MPD strictures, or MPD disruption. To allow endoscopic intervention within the MPD, a pancreatic sphincterotomy is required; therefore, all patients have an MPD stent left in place after the sphincterotomy to ensure adequate MPD decompression. In the postmanipulation period, the stent avoids postprocedure pancreatitis or ductal blowout because of transient edema at the sphincterotomy site. The transampullary MPD stent is temporary because a stricture can result if the stent is left in place longer than 4 to 6 weeks. Endotherapy is an evolving concept that should only be used in centers with extensive ERCP experience and where proficient management of complicated pancreatitis is already practiced. In addition, endotherapy must be practiced where a "multidisciplinary team" provides the additional modalities of conventional surgery, interventional radiology, anesthesia in the fluoroscopy suite, and extracorporeal shock wave lithotripsy (ESWL). Endotherapy decisions revolve around the status of the MPD, that is, whether this duct is obstructed with stones or stricture. MPD obstruction is caused either by stones alone or, more commonly, by a stricture (with or without stones). Endotherapy can be definitive by itself. Alternatively, the use of endotherapy is complementary to operative therapy, allowing for resolution of inflammation or infection because of ductal decompression.

Case examples are useful to illustrate how endotherapy and surgery interrelate in three scenarios: (1) MPD obstruction caused by stones, (2) MPD obstruction caused by MPD stricture with or without stones, and (3) MPD disruption with pseudocyst formation. A decision tree based on ductal anatomy is provided in Table 117–2.

In a symptomatic patient, suppose the MPD in the pancreatic head is obstructed by stones without major stricture (middle section of Table 117–2). This anatomic pattern is uncommon (<10%) but occasionally occurs. There are no stones or stricture in the MPD of the body or tail, but the duct in the body of the pancreas is "dilated" (>5 mm as per the Cambridge classification). Endotherapy is the first therapy and is therefore desig-

Table 117–2	Decision Tree Based on Ductal Anatomy in Order of Application, A to D					
STATUS OF MAIN DUCT	**ENDOTHERAPY**	**PUESTOW ± EHL**	**FREY**	**PPW**	**DISTAL**	**NO TREATMENT**
Head MPD—no obstruction Body/tail MPD: Normal						A
Dilated°†		A				
Stricture					B	A†‡
Head MPD—obstructed by stones° Body/tail MPD: Normal	A		B			
Dilated†	A	B	C			
Stricture	A					B‡

*Head MPD—obstructed by
  stricture ± stones*
Body/tail MPD:
  Normal
	A		B	C		

Dilated†	A	B	C	D		
Stricture	A		C¶	D¶		B‡

"A" is the first treatment consideration in each row, additional letters indicate the sequence if A fails.
°Uncommon anatomic pattern (<10%)
†MPD dilation defined by the Cambridge report is 6.5 mm in the head and 5.0 mm in body
‡Consider current use of alcohol and, if so, any surgery is contraindicated
¶Avoid total pancreatectomy and the 44% incidence of marginal ulceration, "Puestow" the duct through the stricture in the body or tail
EHL, electrohydraulic lithotripsy; PPW, pylorus-preserving Whipple; MPD, main pancreatic duct.

nated "A" in Table 117–2. Endotherapy attempts to remove the stones using baskets and wires via the transampullary approach. ESWL may be necessary to develop smaller stone fragments, allowing their extraction. With short-term follow-up, approximately half of the patients benefit; however, many still go on to operative therapy.

In patients without MPD stricture in the head of the gland, if endotherapy fails to break the chronic pancreatitis-associated pain cycle, then a Puestow-like ductal drainage procedure is indicated if the duct is dilated (designated "B" in the middle row of Table 117–2). Failure of endotherapy is usually the result of further stone formation in the MPD after stent removal or repetitive clogging of the MPD stent. During a Puestow procedure, the MPD is opened longitudinally in the neck of the gland extending into the pancreatic tail. If MPD stones deep in the head of the gland cannot be removed from the lateral pancreatic duct incision of the Puestow procedure, we incorporate electrohydraulic lithotripsy (EHL) delivered through intraoperative pancreatoscopy. The goal is to ensure that the pancreatic duct is open into the duodenum. If this cannot be accomplished with EHL, then a ventral pancreatic head resection (Frey) procedure may be used (designated "C" in Table 117–2). If ventral head resection does not appear to be an option because of concomitant complications, such as duodenal or biliary stenosis, then a pylorus-preserving Whipple (PPW) procedure is used (designated "D" in the sequence of therapy of Table 117–2).

A more common anatomic pattern is MPD stricture (with or without stones) and the treatment used is de-

picted in the last section of Table 117–2. A short-term transampullary stent provides ductal decompression upstream from the stricture. The endoscopist may be able to remove some or all of the stones through the stricture with or without ESWL. Balloon dilatation may be used. Operation is necessary if these endotherapy maneuvers followed by short-term transampullary MPD stenting fail to break the pain cycle by relieving an inflammatory stricture in the MPD *or if the appearance of the stricture suggests neoplasm*; PPW is then used.

Endotherapy is also applied to the ductal disruptions of chronic pancreatitis that result in pseudocysts, either intrapancreatic or extrapancreatic. These pseudocysts were termed "cavities" in the Cambridge classification. Endotherapy methods for treating ductal disruptions include transenteric or transampullary drainage of the pseudocyst with concomitant placement of double pigtail stents. The method of choice is guided by the anatomy. This type of drainage procedure is only applicable to a pseudocyst and is contraindicated for a fluid collection related to resolving peripancreatic necrosis. These latter cavities contain a significant amount of debris and are not amenable to drainage through the small diameter stents or drains used with endotherapy. These smaller stents cannot be exchanged or upsized as readily as percutaneous drains placed by interventional radiology. Because of clogged or small diameter stents or drains, the cavities with debris will be inadequately drained by endotherapy, resulting in a peripancreatic abscess. A true non–debris-containing pseudocyst can be drained transenterically through a transgastric or transduodenal route, or if the ductal disruption can be demonstrated to connect to the pseudocyst, then through a transampullary approach through the MPD. In the latter case the stent is placed through the MPD obstruction into the cavity.

SURGICAL THERAPY FOR CHRONIC PANCREATITIS

Even though endotherapy may have failed to be definitive by itself, during the process the patient benefited because the operation was facilitated in the following ways: pain was relieved by ductal or cyst decompression, portal venous congestion was decompressed with cyst decompression, time allowed nutrition to be optimized, biliary decompression allowed obstructive jaundice or cholangitis to be reversed, and peripancreatitis from ductal disruption was relieved. All of these benefits result in less morbidity (e.g., less blood loss or sepsis) during or after operation.

In summary, resection or drainage procedures are reserved for patients who have all of the following criteria: disabling pain, chronic pancreatitis, severe anatomic changes (class V of the Cambridge Image Severity scale), failed endotherapy, and removal of the etiology for the chronic pancreatitis. In our experience, the majority of these patients (60%) require pancreaticoduodenectomy because the "pacemaker" for chronic pancreatitis appears to reside within the head of the pancreas. Outcome studies indicate that removing the head terminates the problem. The remaining patients receive a drainage procedure, such as the Puestow (10%), or a distal pancreatectomy (30%). Caution should be exercised if a distal pancreatectomy is suggested by the anatomic findings. Only approximately half of these patients receive adequate pain relief, probably because the disease involves the entire gland, is still in progress, or the patient is currently abusing alcohol. Distal pancreatectomy is best reserved for a truly isolated mid-ductal stricture secondary to trauma or after an episode of recrotizing pancreatitis in a nonalcoholic.

A series of images are used to present a case in which endotherapy facilitated subsequent resectional therapy (Figs. 117–2 and 117–3). In this patient, after many years of alcohol ingestion, severe abdominal pain and biliary obstruction developed as a result of necrosis of the pancreatic head. He underwent exploratory laparotomy at another hospital where the surgeon found a huge "tumor" in the pancreatic head and referred him to our institution. A CT showed that the pancreatic head had been replaced by a fluid collection that was displacing and compressing both the superior mesenteric artery and superior mesenteric vein and obstructing the biliary system. The common bile duct was also markedly dilated (see Fig. 117–2). An ERCP showed that only a 1-cm remnant remained of the MPD between the major ampulla and the cyst. This short segment of MPD emptied directly into the huge pseudocyst. An endoscopic papillotomy was performed, and the pseudocyst was drained into the duodenum via a transampullary pigtail stent. In addition, just downstream from the ampulla, an endoscopic transduodenal incision was made into the pseudocyst and double pigtail stents

were placed into the cyst cavity. Finally, the patient's common bile duct stenosis was stented with a transampullary common bile duct stent. At the end of this procedure, the patient had one common bile duct stent and three stents into the pseudocyst. One month later, the pseudocyst and the biliary tree were nicely decompressed (see Fig. 117–3). Several months later, a PPW was performed. One year later, the patient was pain-free, eating a regular diet, and not taking pain medicines.

OUTCOME ANALYSIS OF PYLORUS-PRESERVING WHIPPLE PROCEDURE FOR CHRONIC PANCREATITIS

In 1997, we summarized our experience with 57 consecutive patients who met the criteria mentioned previously and underwent pancreaticoduodenectomy for chronic pancreatitis. Most (97%) of these patients underwent PPW. The remaining 3% of patients, who had a previous antrectomy for peptic ulcer disease, could not undergo reconstruction with pylorus preservation and received a Kausch-Whipple procedure. Hospital and 30-day operative mortality rates were zero, and 98% of patients were available for follow-up after a mean of 42 months. All patients had intractable preoperative abdominal pain and chronic pancreatitis according to the Marseilles 1963 classification. All patients had the Cambridge Class V or "marked" image severity; 96% had MPD obstruction, and the 4% without MPD obstruction were patients with intrapancreatic "cavities" (or pseudocysts) in the head connected to the MPD (as in the patient illustrated in Figs. 117–2 and 117–3). All patients had multiple elements of the Cambridge Classification listed at the bottom of Table 117–1 to support head resection. Patient characteristics included 63% male, 75% alcohol etiology, 56% pancreatic pseudocyst ("cavities") in the head, 23% previous pancreatic operations such as pseudocyst or main ductal drainage procedures, and 33% diabetic preoperatively. All received ERCP and CT to develop a composite pancreas image, and 100% of the gross specimens were dissected by the surgeon with the pathologist to draw the "composite pancreas."

Mesenteric angiograms were obtained in 77% of the patients; 47% were abnormal with 26% having hepatic artery anomalies that might have been difficult to determine because of the chronic inflammation. In addition, 12% had splenic vein thrombosis, and 9% had arteriovenous fistulas (primarily off the gastroduodenal artery in the wall of a pseudocyst) as illustrated in Figure 117–4. The role of endotherapy is prominent in these patients because 65% had common bile duct obstruction, 47% had undergone preoperative common bile duct stenting, 96% had pancreatic duct obstruction, 39% had documented MPD disruption, and 35% required MPD stenting. Percutaneous drainage was required in 19% for peripancreatic fluid collections.

The 5-year actuarial survival rate was 93% and, in the patients who were not diabetic preoperatively (n = 37), the actual 5-year occurrence rate of diabetes was 32%. This diabetes was not a consequence of the resection because no patient became diabetic sooner than 12

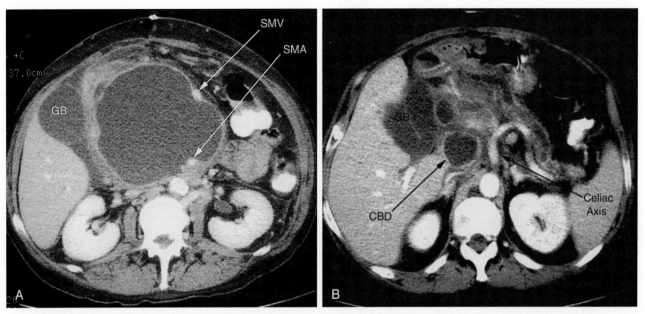

Figure 117–2. *A,* Preoperative computed tomography (CT) shows a giant pseudocyst replacing the head of the pancreas. The final "composite pancreas" after including data from an ERCP indicated that drainage from the body and tail entered the pseudocyst and then drained into the duodenum through a remaining 1-cm segment of main pancreatic duct. Note the compressed superior mesenteric vein (SMV) as the cyst displaces the SMV away from the superior mesenteric artery (SMA). GB, gall bladder. *B,* In a CT slice more cephalad through the area of the celiac axis, note how extrinsic compression by the cyst has resulted in marked common bile duct (CBD) dilation.

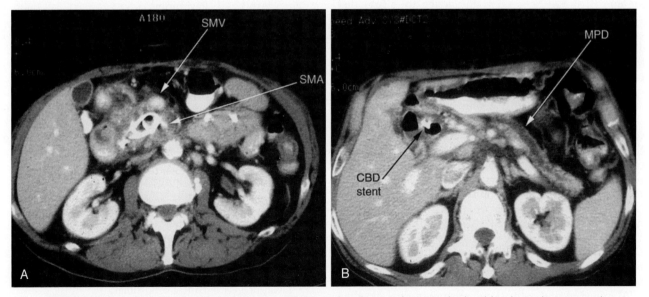

Figure 117–3. *A,* One month after endotherapy, CT shows that the pseudocyst in the head has been decompressed around the transampullary and transduodenal stents. The portal venous system (SMV) has returned to its usual location closer to the SMA. *B,* Note the decompressed common bile duct with indwelling endostent in this cut more cephalad than view *(A)* and the atrophied pancreatic tail and body around a dilated main pancreatic duct.

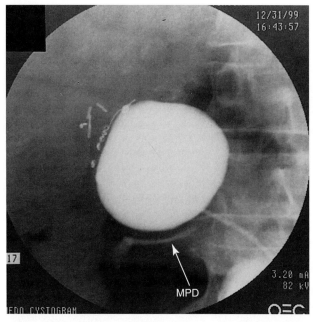

Figure 117–4. Intraoperative injection of contrast medium through a needle and tubing (entering at a right angle at 4 o'clock to the cyst) into a large pseudocyst in the head of the gland. Preoperatively, the gastroduodenal artery (GDA) has been embolized to stop a leaking arteriovenous fistula in the cyst wall—note the coils in the GDA from 9 to 11 o'clock on the wall of the cyst. The main pancreatic duct (MPD) was visualized at 4 o'clock to the cyst *(arrow)* with contrast material flowing to the left into the duodenum (at 7 o'clock to the cyst). This intraoperative fluoroscopic pseudocystogram showed that the cyst connected to the main pancreatic duct, confirming that a ductal disruption was present.

months after the operation, indicating that the criteria for operation had been accurate enough to ensure that nonfunctional pancreatic tissue had been excised.

Patients with a follow-up of greater than 1 year (n = 43) had a mean follow-up of 4½ years. When asked if they still had pain and, if so, whether it was still disabling, every patient indicated that he or she had a "good" response and that the pain was no longer disabling. In addition, 76% indicated that they were free of all pain. What about the 24% of patients who still had some residual discomfort (although no longer disabled)? Recall that the majority of these patients had alcohol-induced chronic pancreatitis. The psychologic makeup of these patients became evident because the incidence of patients resuming alcohol intake was also 24%.

In regard to activity, 93% returned to work, school, or full activity. All maintained their preoperative weight, and none complained of dumping or significant diarrhea. Diarrhea was noted by 14% of patients if they failed to take supplemental exocrine enzymes, whereas 77% of the patients were taking exocrine enzymes.

Marginal ulceration or occult gastrointestinal bleeding occurred in 6 of these 43 patients (14%). Four had undergone total pancreatectomy, an operation that used to be used more liberally in patients with severe chronic pancreatitis who were diabetic preoperatively. There was a statistically significant correlation of total pancreatectomy with peptic ulceration, that is, 44% of those patients with total pancreatectomy had peptic ulceration, whereas

peptic ulceration or occult gastrointestinal bleeding subsequently developed in only 6% of pancreaticoduodenectomy patients. These data suggest that surgeons should avoid total pancreatectomy; it is rarely required from the composite anatomy and strongly related to postoperative gastrointestinal bleeding.

CONCLUSION

A schema is developed that outlines criteria to consider for patients with severe pancreatitis in whom disabling abdominal pain develops. If the symptomatic patient has severe chronic pancreatitis that reaches the Cambridge Class V "marked" stage of image severity, then endotherapy is indicated. If endotherapy fails, then surgery is

---

Pearls and Pitfalls

- Appropriate evaluation of patients with chronic pancreatitis first requires appropriate imaging of the parenchyma and ductal system—CT and ERCP.
- After conservative therapy (oral pancreatic enzymes, analgesics), endotherapy should be tried—stone extraction with ESWL if needed, stenting of ductal stricture, or drainage of pseudocysts.
- Even if endotherapy only buys time, it may facilitate surgical treatment.
- Surgical intervention involves ductal drainage (if the duct is dilated more than 5 mm) with or without parenchymal resection; if the ductal system is not dilated, pylorus-preserving proximal pancreatoduodenectomy has good results.

Criteria for Resection—Pain Must Be Associated with Pathology

- Abdominal pain must be disabling.
- Pathology of at least the Cambridge Image Severity scale of "marked" must be present.
- Conservative treatment (medical therapy, endotherapy) has failed.
- Etiology has ceased or been removed—alcohol or gallstones.

If Resection Is Necessary, then Prevent Morbidity and Blood Loss

- Allow inflammation to subside with endotherapy for jaundice or enlargening pseudocysts and by embolizing pseudoaneurysms. Look for them around a pancreatic head cyst from the gastroduodenal artery or its branches.
- Know dangerous anatomy, such as replaced right or common hepatic arteries from the superior mesenteric artery and occluded portal venous or splenic vein systems.
- Always consider cancer a possibility.

Head Resection Is Required in the Majority of Cases

- If anatomy suggests that distal resection is needed, more imaging is necessary, or the patient may be continuing to drink alcohol and current anatomy will change.

indicated. Usually these patients have pathologic changes centered in the pancreatic head, and a pylorus-preserving pancreaticoduodenectomy (PPW) is performed. After an average follow-up of at least 4 years, PPW provided either good to excellent relief of disabling abdominal pain. These patients were highly selected using the anatomic profile of the composite pancreas. Long-term follow-up, which has never been available with cancer patients after the Whipple procedure, showed few gastrointestinal side effects from PPW without predisposition for diabetes other than that from the continued parenchymal destruction from smoldering chronic pancreatitis in the pancreatic remnant. Total pancreatectomy should be avoided in these patients, even if the patient is already diabetic. From this personal experience using anatomic criteria and close follow-up, the long-term outcomes of pain relief in virtually all patients after PPW will represent a benchmark for results after procedures that employ less resec-tion. Therapy should be based on reliable imaging criteria to select patients. Then the outcomes of new and promising procedures such as lithotripsy and limited head resections can be compared with the benchmarks derived after PPW.

SELECTED READINGS

Ammann RW, Muellhaupt B, Zurich Pancreatitis Study Group: Natural history of pain in alcoholic chronic pancreatitis. Gastroenterology 1999; 116:1132.

Axon ATR, Classen M, Cotton PB, et al: Pancreatography in chronic pancreatitis: International definitions. Gut 1984;25:1107.

Mathews K, Correa RJ, Gibbons RP, et al: Extracorporeal shock wave lithotripsy for obstructing pancreatic duct calculi. J Urol 1997;158:522.

Sarles H: Proposal adopted unanimously by the participants of the symposium. In Sarles H (ed): Pancreatitis. Symposium, Marseilles April 25 and 26, 1963. Basel, S. Karger, 1963, pp VII–VIII.

Traverso LW, Kozarek RA: Pancreatoduodenectomy for chronic pancreatitis. Anatomic selection criteria and subsequent long-term outcome analysis. Ann Surg 1997;226:429.

Chapter 118
Pancreas Divisum

Andrew L. Warshaw

The human pancreas is formed from dorsal and ventral embryonic anlagen, which fuse so that most or all of the pancreatic secretions empty via the ventral duct (Wirsung) through the papilla of Vater. Approximately 20% of ductal systems retain the dorsal duct (Santorini) communication to the minor (or accessory) papilla. The term *pancreas divisum* was devised to describe conditions in those patients (10% of Western populations) in whom the two duct systems do not fuse, leaving the dorsal duct obligated to drain all or part of the body and tail of the gland via the accessory papilla (Fig. 118–1). The ventral duct in these patients may (5% to 7%) or may not (2% to 4%) be separately present. In an equal number of persons, the communication between the dorsal and ventral ducts may be filamentous and functionally unimportant (incomplete pancreas divisum). Each of these variations shares a dependence on the accessory papilla as the major outflow tract for the pancreas, leading to the term *dominant dorsal duct*. The prevalence of these circumstances appears to be lower in Asian populations.

The possible pathogenesis of clinical disorders attributed to pancreas divisum has only been postulated since the widespread application of endoscopic pancreatography. The controversy includes a relation to recurrent acute pancreatitis, chronic pancreatitis, and syndromes of chronic abdominal pain. Inasmuch as the anatomic circumstances are far more prevalent than any possible clinical associations, it is assumed that a cofactor, possibly insufficiency or stenosis of the accessory papilla, must be required to convert pancreas divisum from just a harmless anatomic variant to a causative etiology. Either a dominant dorsal duct or accessory papilla stenosis alone would have no significant impact on pancreatic secretory pressure because secretions could exit unimpeded by one orifice or the other. However, if the two factors coexist, there is inescapable impedance to dorsal duct emptying, potentially leading to hypertension in the dorsal duct distribution, at least at times of active secretion such as during stimulation by meals. Dorsal duct hypertension and impaired emptying has been demonstrated indirectly by ultrasonographic imaging of the duct after secretin stimulation and directly by ductal pressure measurement in normal persons (11 ± 1 mm Hg) versus symptomatic patients with pancreas divisum (24 ± 1 mm Hg). In this treatise, the terms pancreas divisum and dominant dorsal duct syndrome, used interchangeably, presume that a mechanical or functional accessory papilla stenosis is also part of the pathogenesis.

CLINICAL PRESENTATION

Most people with dominant dorsal duct anatomy have no symptoms, and none ever develop. Most instances are found incidentally during pancreatography. The discovery is of potential importance only when a cause is being sought for recurrent pancreatitis or for an unexplained abdominal pain syndrome. Pancreas divisum anatomy has been found to be significantly more common among patients being investigated for unexplained pancreatitis than for biliary conditions. Pancreas divisum may actually be protective against gallstone-induced pancreatitis by separating the bile duct from the principal pancreatic channel.

It has come to be widely accepted that pancreas divisum and other dominant dorsal duct anatomic variants associated with accessory papilla stenosis can cause recurrent attacks of acute pancreatitis, proven by increases in serum amylase and lipase and by inflammatory changes seen by ultrasonography (US), computed tomography (CT), or magnetic resonance imaging (MRI). Most series are composed of a majority of women (3:1 over males) with an average age of 34 years at diagnosis. Whether this indicates a hormonal or genetic contribution to the pathogenesis is unknown. Whereas the dominant dorsal duct anatomy is congenital, it is also unknown whether the accessory papilla stenosis is congenital or acquired. Reports of symptomatic pancreas divisum in childhood are appearing, perhaps because of the greater awareness of the condition and better access to endoscopic retrograde cholangiopancreatography (ERCP) in children.

The association with established chronic pancreatitis is less clear or perhaps less frequent. Statistical analyses have not established a greater incidence of pancreas divisum in patients with chronic pancreatitis, but there are striking and indisputable examples of severe acinar loss and fibrosis confined to the dorsal duct segment. Perhaps the dorsal duct hypertension is not sufficient, either because of degree or intermittency, to cause chronic parenchymal injury in most patients.

A syndrome of epigastric and back pain consistent with a pancreatic origin and without other demonstrable cause has also been attributed to pancreas divisum. The absence of objective correlates such as hyperamylasemia naturally engenders skepticism. The inability to exclude unrelated pathology, including psychopathology, has led to a much higher rate of treatment failure (when surgically directed at accessory duct sphincteroplasty; see later text) than when there is a confirmed history of acute pancreatitis. Nonetheless, because a significant number of patients with only a pain syndrome respond to accessory papilla sphincteroplasty, the causal relation between pancreas divisum and "hypertensive pancreatopathy" should not be lightly dismissed. Longitudinal observations in these patients often indicate infrequent attacks of pancreatitis initially, perhaps only every year or two, but with increasing frequency in the passage of time. Similarly, pain may be sporadic at first but becomes daily and eventually continuous. Hyperamylasemia may be documented early

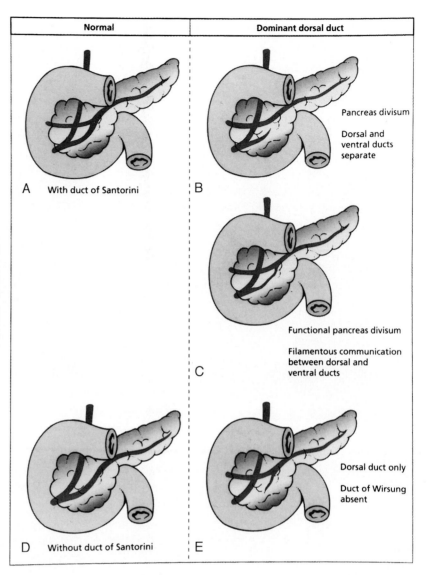

Normal	Dominant dorsal duct

A With duct of Santorini

B

Pancreas divisum

Dorsal and
ventral ducts
separate

C

Functional pancreas divisum

Filamentous communication
between dorsal and
ventral ducts

D Without duct of Santorini

E

Dorsal duct only

Duct of Wirsung
absent

Figure 118–1. Variants of pancreatic duct anatomy. *A,* Complete, conjoined dorsal and ventral duct system ("normal"). *B,* Pancreas divisum, noncommunicating dorsal and ventral ducts. *C,* Incomplete or functional pancreas divisum. *D,* Absent dorsal duct segment leading to accessory papilla. *E,* Absent ventral duct segment leading to major papilla. (Each of the variants *B, C,* and *E* is characterized by the necessity of all or most pancreatic secretions to egress through the accessory papilla.)

on but ceases to occur later, thus obscuring the objective diagnosis.

The attacks of pancreatitis in most patients tend to be mild. Pancreatic necrosis, pseudocysts, or other life-threatening complications have been exceedingly rare. Similarly, progression to diabetes, exocrine insufficiency, or calcification also appears to be quite unusual. Fear of these consequences, therefore, need not precipitate intervention if symptoms are otherwise not compelling. Conversely, we have not observed the spontaneous subsidence of symptoms and consequently cannot advise a noninterventional approach in order to await "burn-out."

DIAGNOSIS

The diagnosis of pancreas divisum can only be made by pancreatography inasmuch as the parenchyma is intact; only the duct system servicing the ventral and dorsal segments differs from a "normal" or complete communicating collecting system. For the past 25 years, ERCP has been the means used to delineate the pancreatic duct system, and ERCP still provides the most detailed pan-

creatograms (and associated cholangiograms), showing not only the map of channels but also a more certain discrimination between congenital discontinuity and acquired disruption (tumor, pancreatitis), very small communicating branches, and inflammatory changes in secondary branches. Recently, the quality of magnetic resonance cholangiopancreatography (MRCP) has improved to the point that an accurate diagnosis of pancreas divisum or dominant dorsal duct without a ventral duct can be made by MRCP alone, although subtle changes in secondary branches may not be evident.

Typically, the ventral duct in pancreas divisum extends proximally only 2 to 4 cm from the major ampulla. It is formed from the confluence of fine tapered secondary branches that service a part of the head and the uncinate process, but do not extend to the midline (Fig. 118–2). This foreshortened ventral duct must not be confused with a ventral duct truncated by neoplasm (Fig. 118–3) or by stricture or obstruction acquired by scarring as a consequence of fibrosis in chronic pancreatitis or the parenchymal destruction from necrosis in acute pancreatitis. The morphology of this acquired ventral duct termina-

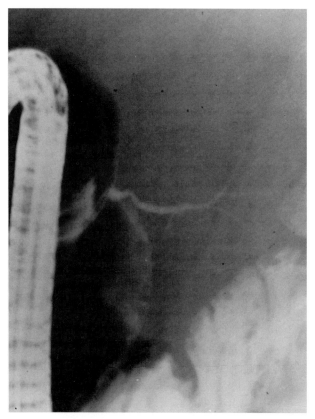

Figure 118–2. Pancreas divisum (ventral pancreatogram). The ventral duct (of Wirsung) is foreshortened but tapers peripherally into secondary branches without abrupt termination.

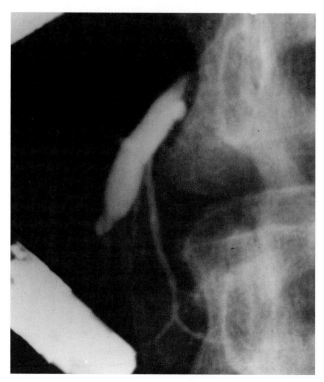

Figure 118–3. "False" pancreas divisum (ventral pancreatogram). The ventral duct terminates abruptly in this patient obstructed by cancer.

tion, called false pancreas divisum, is easily differentiated from the congenital anomaly in that the visualized portion of the main ventral duct is wider, may be longer, and terminates abruptly as a cutoff, rather than tapering peripherally into its branch ducts.

Inability to locate a ventral duct at the major papilla should raise the suspicion that the dorsal duct, emptying into the minor papilla, represents the entire pancreatic drainage system. Failure to appreciate this phenomenon has led to underestimation of the prevalence of dominant dorsal ducts and to potentially missed diagnostic possibilities. Cannulation of the dorsal duct via the accessory papilla is necessary to confirm the anatomy (Fig. 118–4) and to assess for chronic obstructive and inflammatory changes. Cannulation of the dorsal duct can be accomplished by experienced endoscopists in more than 90% of patients.

The dorsal duct, despite the typically small orifice of the accessory papilla, generally has a normal, nondilated appearance. Significant dilation has been exceptional, and true fibrotic chronic pancreatitis has been noted in only 3 of 200 pancreatograms in the author's series of symptomatic patients. Pancreatography is routinely performed in the fasting, unstimulated state. Dilation may occur after secretin stimulation, and this change may provide diagnostic and prognostic information.

Visual estimation of the presence or absence of accessory papilla stenosis by the endoscopist has been unreliable, as has been the difficulty or ease of cannulation.

Manometry through this tiny channel has proved difficult and of poor predictive value in selecting patients for endoscopic or surgical treatment.

We described the use of ultrasonography during secretin stimulation to uncover functional papillary stenosis. The concept is based on a limited egress of pancreatic secretions, which may be inapparent at the typical baseline low-flow state but are obvious during stimulated high flow. The author observed prolonged dilation of the pancreatic duct (for 20 to 30 minutes) in accessory papilla stenosis, in contrast to the brief 1 to 3 minutes seen

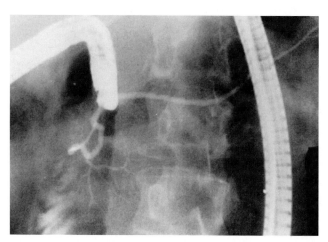

Figure 118–4. Pancreas divisum (dorsal pancreatogram via the accessory papilla). The dorsal duct serves most or all (as in this example) of the pancreas.

normally. This dilation and more constant delayed emptying ostensibly mimics the effect on the pancreas of a meal and may indicate the pathogenic mechanism for "hypertensive pancreatopathy" and pancreatitis. The author's studies indicate an 80% to 90% positive predictive value for successful amelioration of recurrent acute pancreatitis and even of chronic pancreatic pain in patients with a positive ultrasound-secretin test. More recently endoscopic ultrasonography (EUS) and MRCP have also been used to monitor pancreatic duct size during secretin stimulation. Catalano et al. (1998) reported that the EUS-secretin test predicted success of endoscopic therapy directed at the accessory papilla in 81% of patients.

Caution is warranted when there is evidence of chronic duct dilation or fibrosis. The duct does not dilate in chronic pancreatitis, probably because the secretory capacity of the gland and compliance of the duct (ability of the duct to change size in a fibrotic bed) are greatly reduced.

A therapeutic trial of dorsal duct stenting has been proposed to determine whether relief of the presumed ductal hypertension will relieve symptoms. If symptoms are frequent or continuous, a response could be apparent in a short time. If the pattern of the disease is one of occasional attacks, much longer periods of observation would be required, possibly confounded by placebo effect and risking stent-induced injury to the ducts.

Wehrmann et al. (1999) injected botulinum toxin into the minor papilla during outpatient endoscopy. Four of five patients had relief of episodes of abdominal pain and hyperamylasemia for up to 10 months. Two responded to needle-knife sphincterotomy upon relapse. These investigators suggest botulinum toxin injection may help select patients for other forms of sphincter therapy.

THERAPY

Varshney and Johnson have proposed five categories of symptomatic pancreas divisum, which have utility in selecting a treatment program: (1) minimal symptoms; (2) recurrent acute pancreatitis or recurrent pain without other apparent cause; (3) proven chronic pancreatitis; (4) chronic pain without evidence of chronic pancreatitis; and (5) other complications (e.g., pseudocyst, hemorrhage, abscess). Although there is no proven benefit to any noninterventional therapy for symptomatic pancreas divisum, dietary and pharmacologic approaches are warranted first, especially in minimally symptomatic patients. These include a low-fat diet, high-dose pancreatic enzymes, and possibly long-acting somatostatin analogues (perhaps especially as new drugs with a 30-day duration of effect become available), although firm data upon which to base these suggestions are lacking. Chronic analgesics, particularly narcotics, should be used with caution.

ENDOSCOPIC THERAPY

Endoscopic approaches to the accessory papilla have evolved from dilation to long-term stenting, endoscopic sphincterotomy, and finally a combination of sphincterotomy and short-term stenting. The last is the currently

accepted preference because the prior approaches induced too much pancreatitis and did not produce lasting benefit (sphincterotomy alone), induced irreversible stent-induced injury to the duct, and required frequent stent replacement for occlusion by debris. Nonetheless, a randomized (unblinded) trial of long-term stent therapy by Lans et al. (1992) showed a 90% benefit to stenting (>50% reduction in pain, reduced emergency department visits and hospitalizations) versus 11% among control subjects over a mean follow-up of more than 2 years. The study lends credence to therapy directed at relieving obstruction at the accessory papilla.

Several investigators have reported successful use of a combination of sphincterotomy and short-term (2 weeks) stenting. Lehman et al. (1993) reported significant reduction in pain and hospital days per month in 13 of 17 (76%) patients with recurrent acute pancreatitis, 3 of 11 with chronic pancreatitis, and 6 of 23 with chronic pain. However, even with short-duration stenting, 50% had dorsal duct changes at the time of stent removal. Kozarek and colleagues (1995) reported good results in 11 of 15 (73%) patients with recurrent acute pancreatitis, 6 of 19 with chronic pancreatitis, and 1 of 5 with chronic pain; 20% of their patients had procedure or stent-related pancreatitis and 12% had restenosis of the accessory papilla.

SURGICAL THERAPY

The operative approach to patients with dominant dorsal duct syndrome parallels that of endoscopic sphincterotomy and stenting but has the potential advantages of greater long-term patency and assured entry into the accessory papilla. The operation has been applied with success to symptomatic patients without changes of chronic pancreatitis.

Surgical enlargement of the accessory papilla is accomplished by sutured sphincteroplasty through a transverse duodenotomy (Fig. 118–5). The technique requires identification of the accessory papilla anterior and 2 to 3 cm proximal to the major papilla (with the aid of secretin stimulation), incision in its anterosuperior lip to eliminate the mucosal cap on the end of the duct, and sutured approximation of the pancreatic and duodenal mucosae with fine absorbable synthetic sutures to control bleeding and promote healing with minimal scar. A 5-French pediatric feeding catheter, left in the duct and brought out through the duodenum and abdominal wall, ensures unimpeded drainage during recovery and is removed in 2 weeks.

The author's current experience of 165 patients mirrors our prior long-term analysis of 88 patients treated by

Table 118–1	Chance of Beneficial Outcome After Accessory Papilla Sphincteroplasty	
ULTRASOUND SECRETIN TEST	**RECURRENT ACUTE PANCREATITIS**	**CHRONIC PAIN ONLY**
Positive	90% (19/21)	94% (15/16)
Negative	64% (7/11)	21% (3/14)

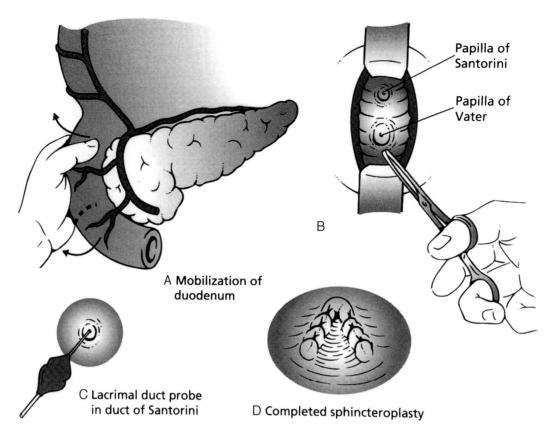

Figure 118–5. Technique of accessory papilla sphincteroplasty. *A,* A transverse incision is made in the duodenum just proximal to the major papilla after wide duodenal mobilization. *B,* The minor papilla is located 2 to 3 cm proximal and 1 to 2 cm anterior to the major papilla. If it is not readily seen, localization can be aided by palpation and by intravenous secretin (1 U/kg). *C,* The accessory papilla is cannulated with a fine probe and an incision is made in its anterosuperior lip. *D,* The incised edges of the duodenal and pancreatic-duct mucosae are joined with interrupted, fine, synthetic, absorbable sutures.

accessory papilla sphincteroplasty. At a mean follow-up of 53 months, 70% were significantly improved: 85% of those judged at operation to have a stenotic papilla; 82% of those with documented recurrent acute pancreatitis; and 92% of those with a positive ultrasound-secretin test (Table 118–1). The experience of other surgical investigators has been consistent (Table 118–2).

Mortality rates in published series have been less than 1% and the complication rates approximately 4%. Endoscopic therapy or repeat sphincteroplasty for restenosis is efficacious about half the time, but the author and coworkers have resorted (successfully) to pancreaticoduode-

nectomy for severe restenosis after failed endoscopic or surgical treatment in seven patients. Although abnormalities in the sphincter of Oddi, as indicated by manometric measurements, have been reported to accompany pancreas divisum anatomy in some patients, the author and colleagues found no difference in outcomes whether or not choledochal sphincteroplasty is added to accessory papilla sphincteroplasty.

Accessory papilla sphincteroplasty is inadequate and unsuccessful when there is established chronic fibrotic pancreatitis, calcification, or markedly dilated ducts, with or without a "chain-of-lakes." Whether the chronic pan-

Table 118–2	Outcomes of Accessory Papilla Sphincteroplasty for Dominant Dorsal Duct Syndromes (Pancreas Divisum)					
AUTHOR	**TOTAL PATIENTS (NO.)**	**RECURRENT ACUTE PANCREATITIS**		**CHRONIC PAIN SYNDROME**		**RESTENOSIS (%)**	**MEAN FOLLOW-UP (MO)**
		No.	**% Success**	**No.**	**% Success**		
Warshaw et al.	88	43	82	45	56	7	53
Madura	30	11	82	19	77	—	31
Keith et al.	21	13	100	8	75	5	53
Bradley and Stephan	31	31	84	—	—	6	76

Pearls and Pitfalls

- Pancreas divisum is found in approximately 10% of the population.
- A subset of these patients have recurrent acute pancreatitis, a chronic pain syndrome, or, rarely, chronic pancreatitis.
- Symptomatic pancreas divisum is believed to be related to mechanical or functional stenosis of the accessory (minor) papilla.
- Sphincterotomy (endoscopic or surgical) has best results (approximately 80% success) in well-established recurrent acute pancreatitis.

creatitis in such patients was caused by accessory papilla obstruction or is pathogenetically unrelated and coincidental is moot and of no importance to choice of therapy. Chronic pancreatitis and its complications in patients with pancreas divisum are treated like those of any causation: longitudinal duct drainage (modified Puestow procedure) if the main duct is sufficiently dilated, pancreaticoduodenectomy or duodenum-sparing pancreatic head resection if it is not.

As pancreas divisum becomes recognized and treated more frequently in childhood, the evolving principles of the therapeutic choices are the same as in adults. Rarely a patient is found to have advanced chronic pancreatitis of the body and tail of the pancreas with sparing of the head of the gland, possibly caused by a malformed, stenotic junction of the dorsal and ventral ducts; distal pancreatectomy relieves the associated pain.

There are several reports of isolated ventral chronic pancreatitis in patients with pancreas divisum. The pathogenesis of this condition is not understood, but successful relief of pain has been reported after sphincteroplasty of the major papilla and pancreatolithotomy or pancreaticoduodenectomy.

SELECTED READINGS

Bradley EL, Stephan RN: Accessory duct sphincteroplasty is preferred for long-term prevention of recurrent acute pancreatitis in patients with pancreas divisum. J Am Coll Surg 1996;183:65.

Catalano MF, Lahoti S, Alcocer E, et al: Dynamic imaging of the pancreas using real-time endoscopic ultrasonography with secretin stimulation. Gastrointest Endosc 1998;48:580.

Guelrud M: The incidence of pancreas divisum in children. Gastrointest Endosc 1996;43:83.

Keith RG, Shapero TF, Saibil FG, Moore TL: Dorsal duct sphincterotomy is effective long-term treatment of acute pancreatitis associated with pancreas divisum. Surgery 1989;106:660.

Kozarek RA, Ball TJ, Patterson DJ, et al: Endoscopic approach to pancreas divisum. Dig Dis Sci 1995;40:1974.

Lans JI, Geenen JE, Johanson JF, Hogan WJ: Endoscopic therapy in patients with pancreas divisum and acute pancreatitis: A prospective, randomized, controlled clinical trial. Gastrointest Endosc 1992;38:430.

Lehman GA, Sherman S, Nisi R, Hawes RH: Pancreas divisum: Results of minor papilla sphincterotomy. Gastrointest Endosc 1993;39:1.

Madura JA: Pancreas divisum: Stenosis of the dorsally dominant pancreatic duct: A surgically correctable lesion. Am J Surg 1986;151:742.

Neblett WW III, O'Neill JA Jr: Surgical management of recurrent pancreatitis in children with pancreas divisum. Ann Surg 2000;231:899.

Warshaw AL, Cambria RP: False pancreas divisum: Acquired pancreatic duct obstruction simulating the congenital anomaly. Ann Surg 1984;200:595.

Warshaw AL, Simeone J, Schapiro RH, et al: Objective evaluation of ampullary stenosis with ultrasonography and pancreatic stimulation. Am J Surg 1985;149:65.

Warshaw AL, Simeone JF, Schapiro RH, Flavin-Warshaw B: Evaluation and treatment of the dominant dorsal duct syndrome (pancreas divisum redefined). Am J Surg 1990;159:59.

Wehrmann T, Schmitt T, Seifert H: Endoscopic botulinum toxin injection into the minor papilla for treatment of idiopathic recurrent pancreatitis in patients with pancreas divisum. Gastrointest Endosc 1999;50:545.

Chapter 119
Pancreatic Pseudocyst
Gerard V. Aranha

Pancreatic inflammation may be associated with a variety of enzyme-rich pancreatic fluid collections. These fluid collections may be acute or chronic, localized or generalized, and sterile or infected. The term *pseudocyst* has been used for all forms of localized fluid collections.

Strictly, however, a pseudocyst is a localized collection of extravasated pancreatic juice surrounded by a wall of fibrous tissue arising as a consequence of pancreatic inflammation from a variety of etiologies. This chapter deals with the presentation, diagnosis, surgical treatment, postoperative management, complications, outcomes of surgery, and alternatives to surgical treatment of pseudocysts.

CLINICAL PRESENTATION AND DIAGNOSIS

Pancreatic pseudocyst is a well-recognized complication of acute and chronic pancreatitis, occurring in 2% to 10% of patients. Most frequently, pseudocysts are a result of pancreatitis initiated by alcohol abuse. Other etiologic factors include biliary tract disease, trauma, operative injury, pancreatic cancer, and unusual causes of pancreatitis such as hyperlipidemia, familial pancreatitis, drugs, and hypercalcemia. Patients with pancreatic pseudocyst may be asymptomatic or have upper abdominal or back pain. If there is gastric outlet obstruction, patients may have early satiety, nausea, and vomiting. Pruritus and jaundice caused by obstruction of the common duct by pseudocyst is a rare presentation, as is edema of the legs and weight gain resulting from compression or obstruction of the inferior vena cava. Other rare forms of presentation may be alteration in bowel habits and crampy abdominal pain caused by colonic obstruction by the pseudocyst. Rarely, variceal bleeding resulting from obstruction of either the splenic or portal vein may occur; similarly, arterial hemorrhage into a cyst resulting from formation of a pseudoaneurysm in the adjacent visceral vessels can be a devastating complication and a dramatic presentation. Finally, patients with infected pseudocyst have signs of sepsis, including high temperature, elevated white blood cell count, chills, and hemodynamic instability. On physical examination, a fullness or a mass may be present on abdominal examination. A persistently elevated serum amylase is also present in about 60% of patients. The aforementioned findings may suggest the presence of a pancreatic pseudocyst, but the diagnosis can only be confirmed by radiologic studies. Ultrasonography (US) and computed tomography (CT) can accurately identify the presence of one or more masses in the pancreas and delineate whether the mass is cystic or solid.

We have used US to determine the nature and cause of cystic pancreatic lesions at our institution. Seventy patients underwent serial US examinations over a period of 6 weeks. Twenty-four (34%) had spontaneous resolution of their peripancreatic fluid collections. Forty-six (66%) had persistent cysts and needed surgery. The mean diameter of the cystic collection in those who had spontaneous resolution was 4.2 cm, whereas in those in whom the fluid collections persisted, the diameter was 8.7 cm. Thus, cysts greater than 6 cm are unlikely to resolve and many surgeons would suggest operative intervention; a waiting period of 4 to 6 weeks would be desirable to allow the cyst wall to mature. Our data reflected the experience of Bradley et al. (1979) on the natural history of pancreatic pseudocyst. These data, combined with the reported 30% to 50% rate of serious complications for unoperated pseudocysts, led to the recommendation for operative drainage of most pseudocysts in the late 1970s and the 1980s.

With the advent of more sophisticated imaging studies, including CT, pseudocysts are discovered more often in association with acute pancreatitis. CT allows precise documentation of the size, location, number, and thickness of the wall of pancreatic pseudocyst. Yeo and colleagues (1990) reviewed 75 patients with pancreatic pseudocyst as documented by CT. Operative management was used only for patients with persistent abdominal pain, enlargement, or complications of pseudocyst. Approximately one half of the patients were managed nonoperatively, and the remainder were treated operatively. The patients undergoing nonoperative treatment were asymptomatic. At a mean follow-up of 1 year, 60% had complete resolution of the pseudocyst and 40% had pseudocysts that remained stable or decreased in size. Only one pseudocyst complication developed in the nonoperative group. In this study also, the size of the pseudocyst was a significant predictor of the need for operative drainage. Pseudocysts greater than 6 cm in diameter required surgical treatment 67% of the time, whereas, in pseudocysts smaller than 6 cm, only 40% of the patients required operative treatment. Yeo and colleagues concluded that a large proportion of pancreatic pseudocysts without specific indications for operative treatment can be safely managed nonoperatively with careful clinical and radiologic follow-up. More recent data from Vitas and Sarr (1992) support a nonoperative approach in selected patients with pseudocyst. In their study, 68 patients with asymptomatic pseudocysts were initially treated expectantly. In only six patients (9%) did a severe complication occur, and in only 24 patients (35%) was operative treatment required. One patient with intracystic hemorrhage underwent angiographic embolization. Forty-three patients (63%) were successfully treated without any form of intervention. Once again, pseudocyst diameter correlated with resolution and the need for eventual operative treatment (Table 119–1). In conclusion, with good clinical and radiologic follow-up, conser-

Table 119–1	**Relationship of Size to Resolution of Pseudocyst**			
AUTHOR	**TEST**	**SIZE (cm)**	**RESOLUTION (%)**	
Vitas and Sarr, 1992	CT	<5	83	
		>5	50	
Yeo et al., 1990	CT	<6	60	
		>6	37	
Aranha et al., 1983	Ultrasound	<5	90	
		>5	15	

vative treatment of pseudocysts appears to be appropriate in asymptomatic patients without evidence of complications. These cysts are usually less than 5 cm in diameter. For pseudocysts greater than 5 cm, if the underlying pancreatitis is resolved, a low-fat oral diet may be resumed. If the underlying pancreatic inflammation is not resolved, an interval of bowel rest with parenteral nutrition for 4 to 6 weeks is recommended. Failure of medical therapy or complications of the pseudocyst initially or during conservative management usually requires appropriate intervention.

SURGICAL MANAGEMENT

Preoperative management of patients undergoing surgery for pseudocyst includes restoration of fluid and electrolyte balance, correction of nutritional deficiencies, bowel prep, and prophylactic antibiotics to cover gram-negative aerobes. The elective management of pancreatic pseudocyst has changed markedly in the past few years. Surgery is no longer the only option for treatment, and alternatives such as percutaneous and endoscopic drainage have been offered as suitable alternatives. Additionally, the presence of an asymptomatic pseudocyst may be treated expectantly. The surgical treatment of pancreatic pseudocyst may be broadly classified into three categories: (1) internal drainage, (2) resection, and (3) external drainage.

Internal Drainage

Enteric drainage of a pseudocyst into the stomach, duodenum, or jejunum is possible, depending on which organ is contiguous to the pseudocyst. Drainage of a pseudocyst into the stomach and duodenum is undertaken only if the two organs together form a conjoined part of the pseudocyst wall. Otherwise, a Roux-en-Y cyst jejunostomy is indicated. For drainage into the stomach or duodenum, an anterior gastrotomy or duodenotomy is made, respectively. The cyst is localized with a needle attached to a 10-mL syringe. After this maneuver, an 11-blade knife is used to cut along the needle tract to enter the cyst. The cyst contents are evacuated and cultured if necessary. A biopsy sample of the cyst wall is obtained to rule out a cystic neoplasm. An opening of at least 3 to 4 cm is made between the cyst and the stomach or duodenum. The opening is then oversewn with a running suture (Fig. 119–1); this technique avoids bleeding and leakage of cyst contents postoperatively. For cysts drained into the

jejunum, a Roux-en-Y limb of 60 cm is used. The cyst is once again located in the dependent position with a syringe and needle, and entry into the cyst is made with an 11-blade knife. A generous opening of 3 to 4 cm is made, and a single layer anastomosis is made side-to-side between the cyst and the Roux limb (Fig. 119–2). Table 119–2 summarizes the recent surgical data of the internal drainage of pseudocysts. Note that, in the most recent series, no deaths have been reported for internal drainage.

Resection

Resection of a pseudocyst requires removal of the attached pancreas (Fig. 119–3). Because the walls of pancreatic pseudocyst often consist of adjacent viscera, it is sometimes impractical to resect the cyst itself. Although a resection is effective in eliminating the pseudocyst, there may be substantial morbidity and mortality risk. Consideration for resection of a pseudocyst should be reserved for those pseudocysts located in the distal pancreas that do not have an associated inflammatory reaction. In addition, if a major vascular communication (usually a pseudoaneurysm) with a pseudocyst has occurred, internal or external drainage with "oversewing" of the vessel is associated with high risk of postoperative bleeding from the cyst. In these patients, a resection is indicated, sometimes even requiring a pancreaticoduodenectomy. Resection is also indicated when a cystic neoplasm cannot be excluded.

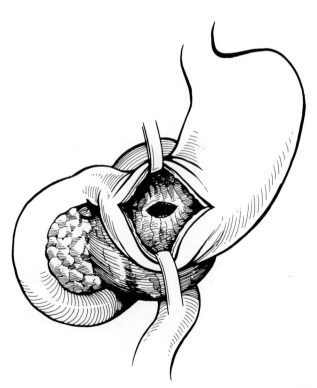

Figure 119–1. Cystogastrostomy used for internal drainage of pseudocysts posterior to the stomach in which the anterior cyst wall becomes adherent to the posterior wall of the stomach.

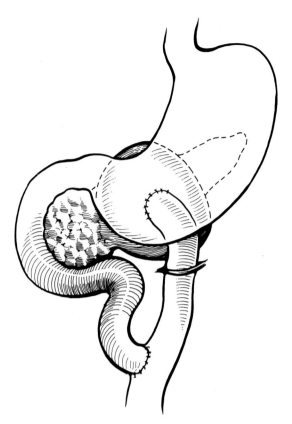

Figure 119–2. Internal drainage into a Roux-en-Y loop of jejunum for those cysts not adherent to the posterior gastric or duodenal wall.

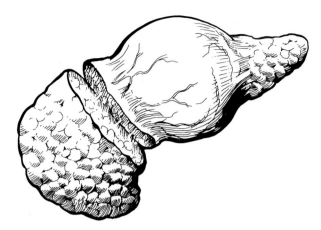

Figure 119–3. Resection of body and tail of pancreas reserved for those patients in whom a cystic neoplasm cannot be ruled out.

External Drainage

External drainage is used for infected pseudocysts and for those cysts that do not have a mature wall at the time of exploration. The reported experience suggests that external drainage is associated with a high rate of morbidity and mortality. Because 60% of pseudocysts may have a ductal communication, a persistent fistula may be anticipated in a certain percentage of patients who undergo external drainage.

SPECIAL CIRCUMSTANCES

Surgeons treating pancreatic pseudocyst may encounter several situations that need special attention. These in-

clude (1) multiple pseudocysts, (2) cysts in the head of the pancreas associated with common bile duct or duodenal obstruction, (3) cysts that cannot be differentiated from cystic neoplasms, and (4) cysts that recur after prior internal or external drainage.

Multiple Pseudocysts

Some authors have suggested resection of the body and tail for multiple pseudocysts. However, our experience is that multiple pseudocysts can still be treated with internal drainage, with a combination of cystogastrostomy and a Roux-en-Y cystojejunostomy. Alternatively, multiple cysts may be converted into one large cyst for a single anastomosis, usually a Roux-en-Y cystojejunostomy. In the circumstance of multiple pseudocysts, we liberally use intraoperative ultrasonography to make sure that all cysts have been drained.

Common Bile Duct and Duodenal Obstruction

In our experience, pseudocysts causing common bile duct or duodenal obstruction do not require treatment by pancreaticoduodenectomy. These cysts are usually readily amenable to internal drainage, either Roux-en-Y cystojejunostomy or cystoduodenostomy with relief of the obstruction. If the obstruction is not relieved because of

Table 119–2	Results of Surgical Internal Drainage of Pseudocysts (Selected Series)				
AUTHOR, YEAR	**NO. OF PROCEDURES**	**INTERNAL DRAINAGE**	**SUCCESS NO. (%)**	**COMPLICATIONS NO. (%)**	**MORTALITY RATE NO. (%)**
Shatney and Lillehei, 1981	114	58	51 (94)	7 (29)	4 (6.8)
Aranha et al., 1982	81	59	52 (88)	5 (8.5)	4 (6.7)
Warshaw and Rattner, 1985	39	31	NA	2 (6.5)	0
Yeo et al, 1990	39	30	NA	NA	0
Vitas and Sarr, 1992	46	26	23 (88)	5 (20)	0
Heider et al., 1999	66	42	25 (83)	24 (36)	0

NA, not available.

fibrosis or inflammatory changes that continue to obstruct the bile duct or duodenum, then our preference is for a biliary enteric bypass or a gastrojejunostomy, which are safer procedures. Biliary obstruction is usually relieved by a choledochoduodenostomy or a Roux-en-Y hepaticojejunostomy. A duodenum-preserving subtotal resection of the pancreas may also be an alternative in this circumstance.

Cysts That Cannot Be Differentiated from Cystic Neoplasms

Occasionally, it is difficult to differentiate a cystic neoplasm from a pseudocyst. Patients with cystic neoplasms usually do not have a prior history of pancreatitis or gallstones and are predominately female. CT in patients with cystic neoplasms reveals internal septa and solid intracystic components often with calcification within the cyst or its wall and a hypervascular stroma. If the cyst fluid is aspirated, cystic neoplasms are likely to have a high level of carcinoembryonic antigen, a positive mucin stain, and occasionally a positive cytology, whereas pseudocysts have a high concentration of amylase. If the clinical setting and laboratory and radiologic investigation suggest the presence of a cystic neoplasm, then resective therapy, either pancreaticoduodenectomy for lesions in the head or distal pancreatectomy for lesions of the body and tail, is mandatory. Internal drainage of cystic neoplasms leads only to recurrence of the cyst and continued symptoms.

Pseudocysts That Recur after Prior Internal or External Drainage

The most common reasons for pseudocysts to recur after prior drainage are the following: (1) cysts drained externally that have a communication with the main pancreatic ductal system recur or form a pancreaticocutaneous fistula; (2) inadequate anastomotic opening made at surgery between the cyst cavity and the stomach or the jejunum; (3) pseudocysts missed at first operation; (4) pseudocysts associated with chronic pancreatitis; and (5) cystic neoplasms mistaken for pancreatic pseudocysts.

If a pseudocyst recurs after prior external drainage, then internal drainage is indicated. If a pancreaticocutaneous fistula has resulted because of external drainage, Roux-en-Y pancreaticojejunostomy is indicated. When an inadequate opening is made between the cyst cavity and the stomach or the jejunum, we create an opening of at least 4 cm in diameter; larger is safe. In addition, we oversew the common wall between the cyst cavity and the intestine. For pseudocysts missed at the time of the first operation, the pancreas and the surrounding tissue are carefully examined after an internal drainage procedure using intraoperative US. For pseudocysts associated with chronic pancreatitis, continued or recurrent abdominal and back pain after pseudocyst drainage is another problem encountered. Most frequently, this is a manifestation of underlying chronic pancreatitis. In patients whose pseudocyst develops in the setting of chronic pan-

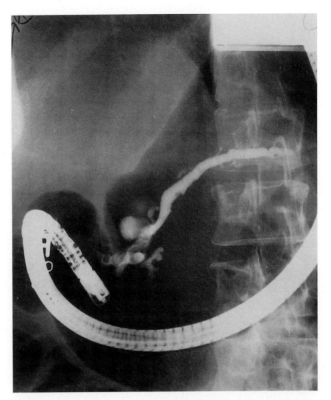

Figure 119–4. Endoscopic retrograde cholangiopancreatography showing a dilated duct and associated pseudocyst in a patient with chronic pancreatitis.

creatitis, we obtain endoscopic retrograde cholangiopancreatography (ERCP) (Fig. 119–4). If the pancreatic duct is dilated, we believe it should be decompressed at the time of cyst drainage by incorporating drainage from the unroofed pancreatic duct and the pseudocyst into the same Roux-en-Y jejunal limb (Fig. 119–5). Combined drainage of pancreatic duct and pseudocyst can be performed with no increase in morbidity or mortality risk. In patients who have continued or recurrent pain after

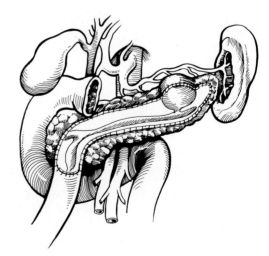

Figure 119–5. Roux-en-Y jejunal limb used to drain a dilated pancreatic duct and associated pseudocyst in a patient with chronic pancreatitis.

pseudocyst drainage, the pancreatic duct is evaluated by ERCP. Lateral pancreaticojejunostomy is performed if the duct is dilated. If cystogastrostomy has been performed previously, this is taken down, and the entire open pancreatic duct including the previous site of drainage into the stomach is incorporated into the side-to-side pancreaticojejunostomy. Any remaining defect in the posterior wall of the stomach is closed primarily. If the initial operation was a cystojejunostomy, the same Roux limb can be used to drain the adjacent opened pancreatic duct. Almost always, sufficient redundancy of the jejunal limb is present to permit this.

ALTERNATIVES TO SURGICAL THERAPY

Percutaneous Drainage

Percutaneous drainage of pseudocysts has been reported for more than 2 decades. Percutaneous drainage consists of two varieties, either therapeutic aspiration alone or percutaneous catheter drainage of the pseudocyst. We use percutaneous aspiration when there is clinical suspicion of infection in a pseudocyst, such as with fever and a white blood cell count greater than 18,000 per mm^3. Percutaneous aspiration without catheter drainage is fraught with high recurrence rates and should not be used as primary therapy. On the other hand, the placement of percutaneous catheter drainage has many supporters; however, there has not been a prospective, randomized study comparing percutaneous catheter drainage with operative drainage of pseudocysts. Percutaneous catheter drainage is indicated mostly for treatment of infected pseudocysts when laparotomy for external drainage will not add any significant benefit. Percutaneous drainage avoids the morbidity and mortality risks of operative external drainage. The long-term use of percutaneous catheter drainage has the potential of creating a pancreaticoenteric fistula, which necessitates operative management. Table 119–3 summarizes recent data on percutaneous drainage of pseudocysts. Several problems associated with percutaneous drainage include inability to completely evacuate the cyst, inability to percutaneously drain a recurrent cyst, and the need to intervene operatively to resolve the cyst completely.

Endoscopic Therapy

Endoscopic approaches to treatment of pseudocysts include two basic approaches: *transmural* (gastric or duode-

nal) *entry* into the cyst with internal stent placement or *transpapillary-transductal cyst drainage*. In the former, the cyst needs to intimately compress the gut lumen to permit creation of a safe communication between the posterior gastric wall and the cyst cavity. In this technique, a point in the posterior gastric or duodenal wall devoid of vascular structures and revealing an adherent cyst wall no greater than 1 cm away is punctured with a precut knife through the endoscope. The opening is then cannulated with a guide wire followed by a sphincterotome catheter to enlarge the cyst enterostomy to 1.5 cm in length. Contrast is injected to ensure both opacification of the cyst and adequate drainage. In the transpapillary-transductal cyst drainage, the pancreatic cyst must communicate with the pancreatic duct. A stent is placed and left for 6 to 8 weeks or until CT shows cyst resolution. Features that make pseudocysts ideal candidates for endoscopic therapy are those cysts greater than 5 cm in size that have gut compression, are single and mature, and are not associated with a disconnected segment of pancreatic duct. Multiple cysts, adjacent severe inflammation, a disconnected pancreatic duct segment, portal hypertension, and significant necrosis or debris within the pancreatic pseudocyst are contraindications for endoscopic therapy. Table 119–4 summarizes recent data on endoscopic drainage of pseudocysts. Endoscopic therapy, although successful initially, often needs to be combined with operative intervention for complete resolution of pancreatic pseudocysts.

Laparoscopic Management of Pancreatic Pseudocyst

There are no large published series on the laparoscopic treatment of pseudocysts. However, there is no reason to doubt that the same procedure done in an open fashion can be done laparoscopically. The goals of laparoscopic drainage would be identical: adequate internal drainage of the pseudocyst; biopsy of the wall to confirm a benign nature; dependent drainage; and follow-up imaging to make sure that pseudocysts and other cysts are completely drained.

THE ROLE OF ERCP IN THE TREATMENT OF PSEUDOCYST

In recent years, ERCP has been given an increasing role in the management of pancreatic pseudocysts to predict

Table 119–3	Results of Percutaneous Drainage of Pseudocysts (Selected Series)					
AUTHOR, YEAR	NO. OF PATIENTS	DURATION OF DRAINAGE (DAYS)	SUCCESS NO. (%)	FAILURE NO. (%)	RECURRENCE NO. (%)	COMPLICATIONS
Freeny et al., 1988	23	29	15 (65.2)	8 (34.8)	2 (8.7)	3 (13)
Adams, 1991	52	42.1	NA	NA	10 (19)	10 (19)
Criado et al., 1992	42	20	9 (21)	26 (78)	7 (21)	7 (16.6)
Heider et al., 1999	66	51 ± 15	28 (42)	38 (58)	11 (16.6)	61 (92)

NA, not available. Failure included technical failure, inability to evacuate cyst completely, and need for surgery.

| Table 119–4 | **Results of Endoscopic Treatment of Pseudocysts (Selected Series)** |

| AUTHOR, YEAR | METHOD OF PSEUDOCYST TREATMENT | | | SUCCESS NO. (%) | COMPLICATIONS NO. (%) | DEATH NO. (%) |
	Transpapillary No.	Cystogastrostomy No.	Cystduodenostomy No.			
Smits et al., 1996°	16	8	7	31 (83)	6 (16)	0
Binmoeller et al., 1995°	31	6	10	47 (88)	6 (11)	0
Catalano et al., 1995°	21	0	0	16 (76)	0	0
Vitale et al., 1999°	9		27	24 (83)	1 (3)	0

°Combination therapy; that is, endoscopy + surgery in several patients.

the success of surgical versus percutaneous or endoscopic treatment. Ahearne and colleagues (1992) have recommended that ERCP before treatment of the pseudocyst may help determine optimal treatment. If ERCP demonstrates a connection to the main pancreatic duct, obstruction of the pancreatic duct, or evidence of chronic pancreatitis, then surgical treatment is desired. However, if these findings are not present, percutaneous drainage may suffice. This study was retrospective, and no prospective study has been done to compare surgical treatment with percutaneous treatment using ERCP guidelines. One of the potential problems of using preoperative ERCP is the chance of creating an infected pseudocyst or inducing pancreatitis as a result of the procedure. If ERCP is to be used in the decision making as to the treatment of a pseudocyst, it should be done within 24 hours of the operative procedure. We see no role for ERCP in acute pancreatitis unless it is to dislodge an impacted stone at the distal common bile duct in a patient with gallstone pancreatitis. However, in an established pseudocyst, if clinical and other indicators suggest the presence of chronic pancreatitis, we use ERCP to guide our decision-making process toward the appropriate operative procedure.

COMPLICATIONS OF PSEUDOCYSTS

The complications of pancreatic pseudocysts include cyst infection, bile duct and duodenal obstruction, cyst hemorrhage, acute intraperitoneal rupture, pancreatic ascites, gastrointestinal or biliary fistula, and mediastinal dissection of the pseudocyst. Pseudocyst infection, bile duct obstruction, and duodenal obstruction have already been addressed.

Hemorrhage

Cyst hemorrhage can be a devastating complication. Hemorrhage may occur before or after drainage of the pseudocyst. If bleeding develops, selective visceral angiography is a crucial diagnostic and potentially therapeutic maneuver. Angiography can demonstrate a pseudoaneurysm, which is the most common cause for significant hemorrhage in patients with pseudocysts. Transcatheter embolization should be considered for control of bleeding in this situation. Using embolization whenever possible is important, because it is frequently difficult to reach and

control the site of bleeding or to obtain proximal and distal arterial control. Distorted anatomy from the pseudocyst, its associated peripancreatic inflammation, and postoperative changes resulting from recent operation make operative control hazardous at best. Nevertheless, emergency celiotomy should be undertaken once the diagnosis has been proved angiographically and embolization is either unsuccessful or inappropriate. If the patient has exsanguinating hemorrhage, emergency operation is necessary without preoperative arteriography. No one preset or routine approach will always meet the challenge of exsanguinating hemorrhage from a pseudocyst. Several maneuvers may be necessary to control the bleeding, including manual tamponade, packing of the pseudocyst, digital compression of the bleeding vessel, and intraluminal arterial occlusion using a balloon catheter. Once initial control is established and volume resuscitation obtained, a more deliberate and careful resection for definitive control is undertaken. Anterior gastrotomy, lateral duodenotomy, splenectomy, or even major gastric resection may be required to obtain adequate operative exposure and ensure definitive control of the bleeding point. Extensive proximal and distal arterial ligation and intracystic suture ligation are the preferred methods for a nonresective operative control of hemorrhage. Intracystic suture ligation alone is associated with a high rebleeding rate of 50% to 75% and should be augmented by extracystic ligation of the feeding vessel whenever possible. A distal pancreatectomy can be used for bleeding arising from the body and tail. Bleeding sources in the head of the pancreas are often lethal; a pancreaticoduodenectomy to control bleeding in unstable patients will carry an extremely high mortality risk and should be reserved for use when all other measures have failed. In contrast, under pseudo-elective conditions, this procedure may be the best choice.

Pancreatic Ascites

Pancreatic ascites results from an internal pancreatic fistula to the peritoneal cavity that results from disruption of the main pancreatic duct or a leaking pseudocyst into the free intraperitoneal cavity. The differentiation of internal pancreatic fistula from other conditions as a source of the ascites can be accomplished easily and rapidly by demonstration of a markedly elevated amylase content in the peritoneal fluid. Most physicians choose an initial period of nonoperative treatment once the diagnosis of

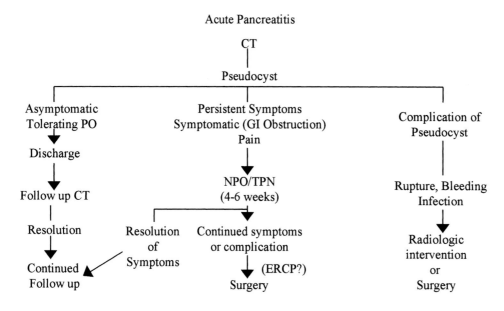

Figure 119–6. Algorithm for treatment of a pseudocyst associated with an attack of acute pancreatitis.

pancreatic ascites has been confirmed. Management includes no oral intake, reducing the ascitic volume by repeated paracentesis, and total parenteral nutrition. Octreotide may be useful in decreasing the pancreatic exocrine secretion and insertion of an intraductal pancreatic stent may prove successful as well. Surgery is indicated if nonoperative therapies are unsuccessful after a period of 2 weeks. Before surgery, an ERCP allows delineation of the site of the rupture of the main duct. If the fistula is in the tail, a distal pancreatectomy may be performed. If the ERCP reveals a direct leak from the pancreatic duct in the head or body, then anastomosis between the site of ductal rupture and Roux-en-Y loop of jejunum usually controls the situation.

Gastrointestinal or biliary fistulas are initially treated conservatively by "resting" the gut (and pancreas), eliminating oral intake, and instituting nasogastric suction. Nutritional support is provided by the parenteral route. Most important, adequate drainage of the fistula prevents and controls sepsis. Most often, these fistulas close; occasionally, however, surgical treatment is necessary.

Mediastinal Dissection of a Pseudocyst

In this situation, many strategies have been employed. For asymptomatic cysts, watchful waiting has been successful. Treatment of symptomatic cysts by external drainage or by cyst-enteric anastomosis has been reported. With a mediastinal pseudocyst, there is often a connection to the main pancreatic duct. In those patients in whom the cyst is symptomatic, drainage of the cyst with decompression of the main pancreatic duct by means of a lateral pancreaticojejunostomy, especially if the patient has chronic pancreatitis and a dilated duct, would be most appropriate.

TREATMENT APPROACH

For pseudocysts developing during an episode of acute pancreatitis, the treatment algorithm is depicted in Figure 119–6. In contrast, treatment of a presumed pancreatic pseudocyst discovered either incidentally or when suspected by vague symptoms is outlined in Figure 119–7.

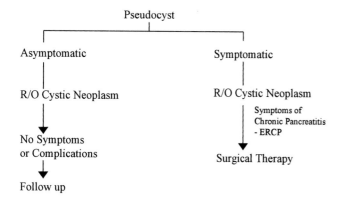

Figure 119–7. Algorithm for treatment of pseudocyst discovered incidentally.

> **Pearls and Pitfalls**
>
> - In the past, spontaneous resolution of pseudocyst was thought to be uncommon and pseudocysts developing complications were reported in 50% of patients.
> - With newer methods of imaging (CT, US), recent evidence suggests that spontaneous resolution of pseudocysts may approach 50% and complications occur much less frequently than was once observed.
> - Patients who are asymptomatic are treated nonoperatively, whereas those with symptoms are treated interventionally (surgery, percutaneous drainage, or endoscopic internal drainage).

SELECTED READINGS

Ahearne PM, Baillie JM, Cotton PB, et al: An endoscopic retrograde cholangiopancreatography (ERCP)–based algorithm for the management of pancreatic pseudocysts. Am J Surg 1992;163:111.

Aranha GV, Prinz RA, Esquerra AC, Greenlee HB: The nature and course of cystic pancreatic lesions diagnosed by ultrasound. Arch Surg 1983; 118:486.

Aranha GV, Prinz RA, Freeark RJ, et al: Evaluation of therapeutic options for pancreatic pseudocysts. Arch Surg 1982;117:717.

Binmoeller KF, Seifert H, Walter A, Sohhendra N: Transpapillary and transmural drainage of pancreatic pseudocysts. Gastrointest Endosc 1995;42:219.

Bradley EL, Clements JL Jr, Gonzalez AC: The natural history of pancreatic pseudocysts: A unified concept of management. Am J Surg 1979; 137:135.

Catalano ME, Geenen JE, Schmalz MJ, et al: Treatment of pancreatic pseudocysts with ductal communication by transpapillary pancreatic duct endoprosthesis. Gastrointest Endosc 1995;42:214.

Criado E, DeStefano AA, Weiner T, Jaques PF: Long term result of percutaneous catheter drainage of pancreatic pseudocysts. Surg Gynecol Obstet 1992;175:293.

Freeny PC, Lewis GP, Traverso LW, Ryan JA: Infected pancreatic fluid collections: Percutaneous catheter drainage. Radiology 1988;147:435.

Heider R, Meyer AA, Galanko JA, Behrns KE: Percutaneous drainage of pancreatic pseudocysts is associated with a higher failure rate than surgical treatment in unselected patients. Ann Surg 1999;229:781.

Shatney CH, Lillehei RC: The timing of surgical treatment of pancreatic pseudocysts. Surg Gynecol Obstet 1981;152:809.

Smits ME, Rauws EAJ, Tytgat GNJ, Huibregtse K: The efficacy of endoscopic treatment of pancreatic pseudocysts. Gastrointest Endosc 1996;42:202.

Vitale GC, Lawhon JC, Larson GM, et al: Endoscopic drainage of pancreatic pseudocyst. Surgery 1999;126:616.

Vitas GJ, Sarr MG: Selected management of pancreatic pseudocysts: Operative versus expectant management. Surgery 1992;11:123.

Warshaw AL, Rattner DW: Timing and drainage for pancreatic pseudocyst. Ann Surg 1985;202:720.

Yeo CJ, Bastidas JA, Lynch-Nyhan A, et al: The natural history of pancreatic pseudocysts documented by computed tomography. Surg Gynecol Obstet 1990;170:411.

Chapter 120
Obstructive Jaundice: Preoperative Evaluation

Gregory G. Tsiotos

Jaundice, when noticed by the patient, can be a dramatic and alarming symptom that generally leads the patient to seek prompt medical advice. When hematologic and hepatic conditions have been excluded based on history, findings on peripheral blood smear, and serologic and liver function test results, the diagnosis of obstructive jaundice is made. Although in the majority of patients, obstructive jaundice is related to benign conditions (i.e., gallstones and their complications), the suspicion of malignancy involving the biliary tract should be raised very early and should be considered a probability until definitively proven otherwise. Because malignancies are generally aggressive, intervention at the earliest possible stage is of paramount importance if an improved outcome is to be obtained. Thus, patients with obstructive jaundice should be referred promptly to a surgeon or a gastroenterologist familiar with hepatobiliary diseases and surgery, whether operative treatment is needed or not.

Despite the previous tendency toward pessimism regarding resection, the past few years have been marked by a tremendous decrease in morbidity and mortality rates after major pancreatic and hepatic resections. Currently, in centers of excellence with a major interest in pancreatic and liver surgery, the mortality rate after major hepatic or pancreatic resection is consistently less than 5%. In addition, morbidity is substantially decreased, and 5-year survival after such operations for malignancy has also increased. This definite improvement has shifted the attitude of experienced physicians and surgeons. It also explains why patients with obstructive jaundice should undergo evaluation and operation in centers with dedication to and a proven record in hepatobiliary and pancreatic surgery.

With these provisions in mind, this chapter (1) discusses the initial evaluation of patients with obstructive jaundice and the distinction between benign and malignant causes, (2) analyzes the role of the various diagnostic and staging modalities in the definitive work-up of and operative planning for a patient with a tumor involving the biliary tree and suggests an algorithm based on efficacy, safety, and cost, and (3) discusses the role of preoperative biopsy and biliary decompression in patients undergoing surgery for tumor-related obstructive jaundice.

CLINICAL PRESENTATION

Initial Work-up

When a careful history is taken, obstructive jaundice is rarely the sole presenting symptom; the jaundice generally accompanies a constellation of other *acute* or *chronic* symptoms. It is crucial to recognize this distinction as early as possible for correct, timely, and effective triage. Acute symptoms such as fever, acute abdominal pain, tenderness on examination, and chills generally reflect gallstone-related disease (e.g., choledocholithiasis or cholangitis). Chronic symptoms, usually a nonspecific spectrum involving weight loss, fatigue, anorexia, vague abdominal or back pain, and recent onset of diabetes mellitus, generally reflects the presence of a neoplasm. Obviously, most patients with obstructive jaundice, especially if younger than 50 years of age, belong to the former group; this explains why physicians in nonreferral centers may tend to generalize and to manage mostly all patients with obstructive jaundice as if complicated gallstone disease is present.

With this approach, diagnosis and management of a possible tumor are often delayed. Gallstones may very well coexist, especially in older patients, and are often assumed to be the cause of the biliary obstruction. Not infrequently, patients undergo other surgical procedures directed at the gallstones (e.g., laparoscopic cholecystectomy, common bile duct exploration, T-tube placement) that only prolong the time to diagnosis and complicate subsequent definitive surgery. Chronic symptoms often tend to be overlooked at the primary care level. Vague abdominal or back pain may be attributed to musculoskeletal disorders, gastroesophageal reflux, cholelithiasis, or peptic ulcer disease, which may in fact coexist. Valuable time elapses during which various treatments prove fruitless, symptoms worsen, and the tumor grows. The lesson is that jaundice in anyone older than the age of 40 years should be assumed to be caused by extrahepatic biliary obstruction until proven otherwise. Obstructive jaundice secondary to gallstone disease can be ruled in or out relatively easily based on careful history-taking alone. The nature, location, and pattern of coexisting pain and the presence of fever and chills may translate to choledocholithiasis; recent (laparoscopic) cholecystectomy may allude to the presence of an iatrogenic bile duct–obstructing injury.

"Painless jaundice" with a palpable gallbladder (Courvoisier's sign) has classically been associated with pancreatic cancer; this clinical presentation refers to the absence of right upper quadrant pain, as in gallstone disease, and the enlargement of the gallbladder due to outflow obstruction. (Patients with chronic cholecystitis have thickened gallbladders that do not dilate with obstructing choledocholithiasis.)

Most laboratory findings are not diagnostic except for an increased white blood cell count with possible left shift, alluding to an acute (usually gallstone-related) cause. Liver function tests demonstrating a cholestatic pattern (i.e., increased levels of alkaline phosphatase, bilirubin, and γ-glutamyltransferase and increased prothrombin time) are highly suggestive of biliary tract obstruction but are not specific for an obstructing stone or a tumor. This profile in a patient older than 40 years of age should, however, immediately prompt an aggressive search for a malignant cause of biliary obstruction.

Ultrasonography

After history-taking, the patient, who is usually still being cared for by the primary care provider, generally undergoes abdominal ultrasonography (US), a readily available, cheap, rapid, and sensitive screening test for presumed biliary obstruction and the most sensitive test for gallstone disease. In general, US will usually be able to define the anatomic level of the obstructing lesion (proximal or distal bile duct) as well as signs of acute inflammation (thickened bile duct wall with intramural [pericholecystic] fluid). If an obstructing stone is not identified (and not all stones in the bile duct are able to be seen on US), a soft tissue mass is the logical alternative, although often this cannot be demonstrated because of overlying duodenal and colonic gas.

At this point, complicated gallstone disease can usually be ruled in or out very reliably. If the condition turns out to be gallstone-related obstructive jaundice, the work-up is now practically complete, and the appropriate management is initiated (described in detail in other chapters). If, however, an obstructing tumor is suspected, a *critical point* in the evaluation, but not the final step, has been reached. One may continue with further tests—usually nondefinitive, sometimes not appropriate, and generally time consuming—during which no definitive management plan exists, time elapses, and the tumor grows, or the patient may be referred to a center with a special interest in hepatobiliary disease, where further evaluation will be dictated by specific guidelines based on modern, state-of-the-art principles.

Definitive Work-up

In the past, the suspicion of the presence of a tumor causing obstructive jaundice would initiate a battery of tests aimed at pinning down the precise diagnosis (i.e., "What is this tumor?"). Today, with the decreasing morbidity and mortality rates (<5%) associated with major hepatobiliary-pancreatic surgery, the attitude of experienced surgeons has shifted toward a willingness to undertake major pancreatic and liver resections. Thus, today's experienced hepatobiliary surgeon approaches a periampullary or a hilar tumor in a much more aggressive and confident way. There is no longer a hesitation to operate or an unwillingness to embark on pancreatectomy or hepatectomy without tissue diagnosis. In addition, the routine exhaustion of every possible diagnostic method in an attempt to rule out conditions that would not absolutely necessitate resection (i.e., chronic pancreatitis, periampullary adenoma) is now a thing of the past. When faced with a patient with a mass causing obstructive jaundice, today's surgeon is more willing to resect the mass without an objective tissue diagnosis and an extensive work-up to identify its pathologic nature; rather, he or she is much more concerned whether this mass is indeed resectable. This is very important to recognize because the question of the past, "What is this mass?" (i.e., precise diagnosis), is now replaced by the question, "Can I take it out?" (i.e., preoperative clinical staging). Consequently, the way in which various tests are used has also changed.

Resectability and *operative planning* are the concepts that should dominate the preoperative evaluation, and diagnostic and staging modalities should be chosen with these specific principles firmly in mind. Tumors causing obstructive jaundice are conceptually categorized into three groups: hilar; mid-duct; and periampullary. At each location, resectability and operative planning depend on different but very specific imaging findings; thus, each diagnostic or staging test should be pursued to address specific questions. This is the framework in which we discuss the definitive work-up for tumors causing obstructive jaundice.

HILAR TUMOR

When US reveals intrahepatic biliary tract dilatation but nondilated normal extrahepatic bile ducts, the suspicion of a proximal obstructing tumor is raised, usually a cholangiocarcinoma or a perihilar hepatocellular carcinoma. US is not reliable in demonstrating the obstructing lesion itself, because US is highly operator dependent, and there may be overlying duodenal or colonic gas obscuring the view. Moreover, many of these neoplasms are quite small. Diagnostic and staging tests should aim at excluding distant disease (metastases) and defining proximal (along the bile duct) as well as radial extension of the lesion. Precise definition of the proximal extension in relation to the hepatic duct bifurcation is critical, because it clarifies whether one or two bilioenteric anastomoses are needed after resection, whether a hemihepatectomy is required as part of a curative operation, or whether the tumor involves the contralateral ductal system and, if so, to what extent. (Extensive involvement of the contralateral ductal system would make the tumor unresectable.) Knowledge of the presence of radial extension to the hepatic artery proper and the portal vein or to their main branches is also crucial, because involvement by tumor of the contralateral hepatic artery and the portal vein or main portal vein thrombosis makes the tumor unresectable.

Dynamic contrast-enhanced computed tomography (CT) should be performed first. CT will often demonstrate the obstructing tumor and the extent of periductal hepatic parenchymal involvement and will reliably reveal signs of extrabiliary and extrahepatic metastatic disease. Although CT provides information on the proximal and distant extent of the tumor along the hepatic ducts, a direct biliary imaging study is required to delineate ductal anatomy in detail. The relationship of the tumor to the surrounding blood vessels can also be inferred but not absolutely defined by CT, because the fat plane between the duct, hepatic artery, and the portal vein (especially at the level of the liver hilum) is normally very thin (unlike the normally thicker fat plane between the portal vein and the head of the pancreas, for example). A good-quality CT will demonstrate occlusion of the artery, the vein, or branches but will not reliably reveal perivascular infiltration of the wall by the tumor.

Next, the anatomy of the biliary system and the pattern of its involvement with tumor must be defined as accurately as possible. Of the two possible luminal imaging studies—percutaneous transhepatic cholangiography (PTC) and endoscopic retrograde cholangiography (ERC)—the former yields the most information by far. ERC is more widely available, easier to perform, and less uncomfortable for the patient and demonstrates the luminal distortion and the distal extent of the tumor. It may not demonstrate accurately the ductal anatomy *proximal to* the lesion, however, which is what the surgeon must know to assess resectability and to form an operative plan. PTC (after correction of the prothrombin time) is the best imaging test for demonstration of these important anatomic parameters of staging and resectability. PTC provides the following information: (1) the relationship of the proximal extent of the tumor to the hepatic duct bifurcation, which alludes to the number of bilioenteric anastomoses that the surgeon should be prepared to perform after resection (at least a 1-cm margin beyond the tumor is required); (2) the level of extension of tumor along one of the hepatic ducts, which indicates the need for ipsilateral hemihepatectomy for curative resection; (3) the possible extension along the contralateral hepatic duct, which may indicate the need for an intrahepatic contralateral bilioenteric anastomosis (after ipsilateral hemihepatectomy) if the extension is limited, or which may define unresectability if the tumor extends further inside the contralateral side; (4) precise delineation of the relationship of the right posterior ductal system to the right anterior ductal system and to the main hepatic duct (often, the former drains directly into the main hepatic duct, which is very important in planning the resection and the reconstruction); and (5) the presence of a diffuse ductal condition (not caused by tumor), such as primary sclerosing cholangitis.

After ductal anatomy has been defined, the possibility of vascular involvement should be investigated (reflected by the presence of obstruction, stenosis, or stricture). Hepatic arteriography followed by a splanchnic venous phase is currently the test of choice. Tumor thrombosis of the main portal vein, infiltration by tumor of the hepatic artery proper and the portal vein, and involvement of the contralateral hepatic artery and the portal vein—regardless of whether the ipsilateral (to the tumor) counterparts are involved—are very significant findings and define unresectability. Angiography also reveals an aberrant left or right hepatic artery (each present in about 20% of patients), which is also essential knowledge in the appropriate planning of a major curative hilar or liver resection. With the ever-improving quality of and experience with dynamic CT, most of the information yielded by angiography can be extracted from CT; however, no prospective study has yet compared each test's efficacy in predicting vascular involvement with the operative find-

ings or with each other. Angiography is still performed in almost all patients with hilar tumors in whom resection is contemplated, but it should not necessarily be considered the gold standard for vascular involvement, because possible infiltration of the adventitia of a vessel with preservation of its internal luminal circumference and contour will probably be missed. The predictive value of CT in such circumstances has not yet been studied prospectively.

With the information gathered from these three tests (performed in the stated order), all issues relevant to resectability and operative planning should be sufficiently addressed, and a complete management plan can be implemented. PTC and angiography carry some risk of complications (approximately 5% together). Being invasive, both are associated with hemorrhage (especially in patients with coagulopathy), infection, cholangitis (due to insertion of bacteria into a biliary tree with stasis), and pseudoaneurysm formation. Magnetic resonance imaging (MRI), supplemented by magnetic resonance cholangiopancreatography (MRCP) and magnetic resonance angiography (MRA), seems to be an ideal diagnostic and staging modality for hilar tumors, because in theory it can replace all three previously mentioned tests. Indeed, there is good evidence that it may yield all the information required. MRI has shown excellent results in anecdotal reports and small retrospective studies. Currently, there are several prospective studies under way to define the accuracy of MRI in operative planning in comparison with operative findings (the gold standard), CT, PTC, and angiography. In the future, with improving technology and increasing diagnostic experience with magnetic resonance modalities, MRI in conjunction with MRCP and MRA may very well replace all currently used staging procedures. Such a development would not only protect patients from the small but existing risks of two invasive tests but also prove to be cheaper and faster, which are important factors in today's era of cost- and resource-containment.

In patients with hilar tumors requiring hemihepatectomy or a lesser liver resection, assessment of liver function, usually based on Childs-Pugh classification, is of paramount importance. Hepatic parenchymal function is the most significant determinant of not only the operative risk associated with hepatectomy but also the volume of parenchyma that can be removed without risk of insufficiency and failure of the remaining portions of the liver.

MID-DUCT TUMOR

Preoperative evaluation of a mid-duct tumor is very similar to that of a hilar tumor, because the criteria for resectability and operative planning are essentially the same. A mid-duct tumor is suspected when US demonstrates dilatation of the intrahepatic and a portion of the extrahepatic biliary tract. As with hilar tumors, the same diagnostic and staging issues need to be addressed. First, CT is used to demonstrate the mass and its relation (distance) to the head of the pancreas and to identify possible distant disease. The direct ductal imaging procedure required may be ERC because exhaustive information regarding the ductal anatomy cephalad to the bifurcation is not as essential; in addition, ERC is more readily available and generally safer than PTC in most institutions, especially in this patient population. The extent of the tumor along the duct and the distance between its proximal margin and the ductal bifurcation need to be accurately defined.

Angiography is focused on involvement of the hepatic artery proper and the main portal vein, the level of their respective bifurcations, and the possible presence of an aberrant left or right hepatic artery. Because the fat plane between the bile duct and the vascular structures is thicker at this level than at the hilum, CT can more accurately predict vascular involvement. Although small retrospective studies support this concept, no firm data are available. MRI, MRCP, and MRA, performed all in one setting, may also replace the combination of CT, ERC, and angiography in the evaluation of these patients.

PERIAMPULLARY TUMOR

When US reveals intrahepatic *and* extrahepatic biliary tract dilatation, a periampullary mass should be suspected. In this clinical scenario, resectability and operative planning depend on a different set of issues: (1) presence of distant disease (metastasis to liver, lungs, or distant lymph nodes or ascites); (2) relation of the tumor to the peripancreatic blood vessels (superior mesenteric artery and vein, portal vein); and (3) presence of peritoneal implants (as in pancreatic cancer). Thus, a well-organized algorithm is needed to address these issues, and the choice among the various diagnostic and staging modalities should be based on the efficacy of each, its risk, and *whether the test will yield information that will directly affect the management of the patient or the evaluation plan.*

Spiral or helical CT (rapid scanning with very thin sections during bolus intravenous contrast agent injection) is currently the accepted gold standard. Not only does it delineate the presence of a periampullary mass (often as a hypodense lesion), but it also provides information about liver metastases, peripancreatic nodal spread, ascites, and involvement or obstruction of the superior mesenteric–portal vein confluence. Areas of periampullary fullness or enlargement, even in the absence of a discrete mass, should increase suspicion and should prompt further investigation. The sensitivity of CT in demonstrating liver metastases depends on their size. Most lesions (approximately 90%) 2 cm in diameter or greater are evident as less-dense defects in the hepatic parenchyma; metastases smaller than 1 cm are usually not evident and are missed. This concept has been the strongest argument for preoperative staging laparoscopy. Detection of nodal metastases is much less accurate.

Although enlarged peripancreatic lymph nodes, especially along the common hepatic artery, are often evident, it is virtually impossible to determine whether they are nodal metastases or just enlarged, reactive nodes so commonly seen with established extrahepatic biliary obstruction. Peritoneal metastases are rarely imaged directly, but their presence may be inferred by the presence of ascites.

If ascites is present, this should precipitate percutaneous aspiration cytologic testing; if the results are negative, a laparoscopic examination should be performed in an attempt to confirm peritoneal metastases and thereby avoid nontherapeutic celiotomy.

If distant disease is ruled out by findings on spiral CT, the next important factor is possible vascular involvement by the tumor. Again, spiral CT can accurately evaluate the normally present "fat" plane between the superior mesenteric artery–portal vein and the head-uncinate region of the pancreas. Preservation of this plane strongly suggests lack of direct invasion or abutment of the primary neoplasm against these veins. Preservation of the superior mesenteric vein–portal vein contour throughout its extent with loss of the fat plane is an indeterminate finding. Most surgeons in the United States would agree that occlusion of the superior mesenteric vein–portal vein junction, especially with the presence of collateral vessels, is an absolute sign of unresectability and should preclude abdominal exploration and attempts at resection. Compression of these veins with loss of the smooth contrast column is consistent with, but not necessarily diagnostic of, tumor involvement.

Recently, grading systems (0 to 4) based on the degree of impairment of CT-assessed vascular contour and the circumferential contiguity of tumor to vessel have been suggested and tested; they seem to predict resectability and unresectability very accurately. Lower grades (0 or 1; preserved perivascular fat plane or loss of fat plane with smooth displacement of the vessel, respectively) are associated with resectability close to 100%, and higher grades (3 or 4; encased narrowed vessel greater than 50% of the circumference or occluded vessel, respectively) correlate with unresectability in 90% to 95% of patients. The middle grade (2; irregularity of one side of the vessel less than 50% of its circumference) is associated with resectability in 40% of patients. This approach provides for much more rational and objective vascular involvement by CT criteria and supports the argument that formal angiography as a routine staging modality is not necessary (see later). Currently, one cannot reliably base the decision to operate on angiographic findings, and angiography adds little to a good-quality, contrast-enhanced CT, especially the more sensitive spiral CT.

Another argument for preoperative angiography is that it can demonstrate important vascular anomalies (aberrant right hepatic artery originating from the superior mesenteric artery; aberrant left hepatic artery originating from the left gastric artery) in 30% of patients, so that injury to these vessels may be prevented. These anomalies, however, should be readily apparent to the experienced pancreatic surgeon; the replaced right hepatic artery is appreciated as an arterial pulse palpable in the posterior aspect of the hepatoduodenal ligament, and the replaced left hepatic artery is an arterial vessel traversing the lesser omentum. The surgeon exploring a periampullary tumor with intent to resect should be familiar with the normal anatomy of the region and its variations and should not depend on angiography ("road mapping") to identify the individual patient's peripancreatic vascular anatomy.

After tumor delineation, absence of distant disease, and relation of the periampullary tumor to the major peripancreatic vessels have been sufficiently addressed by means of spiral CT, the last crucial issue is the possible presence of peritoneal and small liver metastases (implants), which are features of unresectability and are usually not evident even on the best spiral CT. These micrometastases are usually multiple, widespread, and almost uniformly quite small (1 to 3 mm). Because they can be present in 10% to 20% of patients with cancer of the head of the pancreas, and survival of such patients does not exceed 6 months, it becomes crucial to identify this substantial subgroup accurately before noncurative celiotomy is performed.

Many surgeons consider staging laparoscopy with inspection of liver, peritoneal, and omental surfaces and biopsy of suspicious lesions to be a routine preoperative staging procedure for otherwise clinically resectable periampullary tumors. This minimally invasive procedure can be performed on an outpatient basis, can identify the patients in whom palliative endobiliary stenting is all that is needed, and can improve the quality of the remaining life of these unfortunate patients. There is preliminary evidence that peritoneal cytologic examination during laparoscopy may reveal yet another subgroup in whom celiotomy and resection will not add any survival benefit.

Endoscopic retrograde cholangiopancreatography (ERCP) is often performed automatically in nonreferral centers after obstructive jaundice is diagnosed. Although ERCP is very sensitive in showing irregular strictures of the pancreatic or the bile duct, or both ("double duct" sign), the current sophistication of spiral CT questions the necessity for ERCP as well as its routine practice. There is a definite role for ERCP when the diagnosis is equivocal (e.g., in patients with obstructive jaundice in whom no mass is evident on CT or in patients with known chronic pancreatitis in whom development of a pancreatic neoplasm is suspected). Generally, for the good-risk patient with new-onset obstructive jaundice in whom CT clearly shows a periampullary tumor, ERCP offers no further therapeutically useful information; in addition, it subjects the patient to a small risk because it is an invasive procedure.

Other sophisticated diagnostic and staging modalities have also been suggested. Endoscopic US in patients with obstructive jaundice and a mass evident on CT appeared to be promising in assessing peripancreatic vascular involvement, but four prospective studies, each with a similar number of patients, had contradictory results regarding whether it was cost effective or added therapeutically important data. MRI, which has the advantage of lacking ionizing radiation, depicts the tumor, the peripancreatic vessels, and the biliary tree, but no study has adequately compared it with spiral CT. Tumor markers (e.g., CA 19-9, CA 242) and molecular biologic techniques (e.g., detection of K-*ras*, p53, and *DCC* mutations), although potentially useful in screening high-risk groups, do not generally contribute to the definitive diagnosis, but they may produce statistically significant differences in a large patient population. Their practical use in the *individual* patient remains questionable, however. Very few, if any, hepatobiliary surgeons would rely on the results of any of them to determine the need for definitive

invasive procedures except under very specific, select conditions.

PREOPERATIVE BIOPSY

Once a hilar or a periampullary mass causing obstructive jaundice is demonstrated on CT, traditionally there has been an urge to obtain tissue diagnosis, usually by means of CT- or US-guided fine needle aspiration biopsy or endoscopically obtained tumor brushings. Although this is a common practice in nonreferral centers, there are many problems associated with this "knee-jerk" reaction and thus many reasons to resist it. First, although the specificity and the positive predictive value of these techniques are virtually 100%, the sensitivity and the negative predictive value are generally only 70%, and malignancy cannot be excluded with certainty. Second, although percutaneous biopsy is generally quite safe, several potentially serious complications can occur (approximately 1% of the time), including hemorrhage, pancreatitis, fistula, abscess, and, rarely, death. Third, and of more concern, are several reports of tumor seeding along the subcutaneous track of the needle or intraperitoneally. Thus, *preoperative biopsy has little or no role in the evaluation of the good-risk patient with a clinically resectable* hilar or periampullary mass. A biopsy with negative results will not prevent operative exploration and resection. If the results of the percutaneous biopsy will not alter management, there is no reason to perform it.

There is a definite place for preoperative biopsy *when resection is not possible*. This includes poor-risk patients who are not able to tolerate a major hepatic, biliary, or pancreatic resection but who are candidates for palliative chemoradiation therapy and need tissue confirmation.

PREOPERATIVE BILIARY DECOMPRESSION

Endoscopic stent placement to relieve obstructive jaundice is another often automatic response just after a hilar or a periampullary mass is diagnosed, often even before consultation with a surgeon. This invasive procedure usually takes place before the resectability of the tumor has been assessed and has been adopted by many as part of the initial work-up and preparation of the patient with a presumed malignant stricture of the biliary tree.

Realistically, the major reason for this practice is that it quickly and relatively safely palliates the most dramatic symptom (pruritus) and its associated discomfort (altered appearance). Also, it generally reflects pessimism regarding the feasibility of definitive treatment, because it is commonly believed that this palliative measure may be the only procedure that most patients will ever need. For the few who will undergo exploration for palliation or resection, placement of a biliary stent does not burn any bridges and may decrease postoperative morbidity and operative mortality. Another important factor, often underappreciated, is the small but not insignificant risk of complications (bile duct or duodenal perforation, hemorrhage, pancreatitis) that may delay definitive therapy and compromise the final outcome. The true benefits of preoperative biliary decompression, however, are related to reversal of jaundice-induced immunosuppression (allegedly decreasing perioperative morbidity and mortality) and improvement in postoperative liver function. Based on today's evidence, the rational criterion for preoperative biliary decompression is *whether a major hepatectomy will be a part of the planned curative resection* of the mass; this is not a pertinent question for a distal bile duct obstruction.

For a hilar tumor involving the bifurcation and extending toward one of the hepatic ducts—for which a *hemihepatectomy should be performed*—the functional status of the remaining half of the liver is of paramount importance. Hemihepatectomy reduces by around 50% the amount of available parenchyma, which needs to be at its optimal functional status. Also, patients with profound jaundice due to proximal cholangiocarcinoma are more prone to develop portal and peripheral endotoxemia with compromise of renal function. For these reasons, patients in whom liver resection is planned should undergo preoperative biliary decompression, because this will improve the function of the remaining hepatic parenchyma and will decrease the risk of postoperative hepatic and renal failure and sepsis.

When *hemihepatectomy is not part of the intended curative operation* (e.g., for hilar tumor up to but not beyond the bifurcation or for mid-duct or periampullary tumors), preoperative biliary decompression offers no advantage because the available liver parenchyma remains intact. On the contrary, in addition to the risk of complications (as stated previously), preoperative biliary stents convert a sterile biliary system to a colonized one with bacterobilia, increasing the risk of cholangitis and possibly postoperative infections. In a recent large study of 567 patients undergoing pancreaticoduodenectomy, it was demonstrated that preoperative stenting was associated with significantly higher rates of wound infection and pancreatic fistula and offered no benefit (Sohn et al, 2000).

In the good-risk patient in whom the tumor causing obstructive jaundice is deemed resectable with no need for hepatectomy based on the appropriate staging, preoperative biliary decompression *has no place*. Some have suggested that a stent can be helpful during bile duct dissection, serving as an intraoperative guide. It is doubtful, though, whether an experienced hepatobiliary surgeon needs a biliary stent to identify and dissect the bile duct safely. Moreover, the intraluminal foreign body incites an inflammatory reaction in the hepatoduodenal ligament, making dissection more difficult. A dilated bile duct makes for an easier bilioenteric anastomosis, a finding not as prominent after decompression.

In patients with *unresectable hilar or mid-duct tumors*, biliary stenting may be the only intervention needed; chemoradiation therapy may be added in some instances. In those patients with *unresectable periampullary tumors*, the presence or the absence of gastric outlet obstruction as well as life expectancy should be considered. Gastric outlet obstruction dictates operative gastrojejunostomy. A proximal, wide, and durable hepaticojejunostomy should be constructed. Preoperative biliary stenting would be of no benefit. On the contrary, in patients with a short

life expectancy (less than 6 months, such as with liver metastases) without duodenal obstruction, biliary stenting may be the ideal palliative measure. The same is true for patients with serious comorbid conditions making them unsatisfactory candidates for potential resection. This subgroup will have the best quality of life with endoscopic palliation. In summary, preoperative biliary decompression should be used selectively and not routinely in patients with biliary obstruction. This decision often requires the experience and judgment of a referral center with a special interest in pancreatic disease.

Summary

The role of the primary care physician is crucial in the optimal management of patients with obstructive jaundice. Increased awareness and a low threshold of suspicion are the most important means of decreasing the delay in diagnosis of an obstructing tumor. Triage is equally important; patients with obstructive jaundice not due to gallstone disease (based on absence of acute symptoms and US findings) should undergo final evaluation and operation by experienced surgeons with dedication to and a proven record of low morbidity and mortality in hepatobiliary and pancreatic surgery. In such a setting, where operative resection is so safe, precise preoperative pathologic diagnosis of a tumor causing obstructive jaundice is less important than appropriate clinical staging. US indicates the rough location of an obstructing tumor

---

Pearls and Pitfalls

- For patients older than 40 years, jaundice should first be assumed to be due to biliary duct obstruction (rather than primary hepatopathy) and requires aggressive work-up.
- Although US is usually the first screening test ordered, in patients with chronic symptoms, CT may be a better test.
- Further diagnosis and staging depend on the location of obstruction (hilar, mid-duct, or periampullary).
- Hilar lesions are best evaluated by means of CT, PTC, and angiography.
- Mid-duct lesions are best evaluated by means of CT, ERCP, and angiography.
- Periampullary masses require only CT; direct ductal imaging (PTC, ERCP) provides no useful therapeutic information.
- In general, preoperative biopsies are of no help for resectable lesions.
- In general, preoperative biliary decompression (endoscopic biliary stents) are of no benefit unless (1) the lesion is unresectable, (2) the serum bilirubin level is greater than 20 mg/dL, or (3) major hepatectomy is planned (e.g., hilar cholangiocarcinoma extending up a major hepatic duct).
- Staging laparoscopy may prevent a nontherapeutic laparotomy.
- Pessimism regarding major hepatic or pancreatic resection because of a presumed operative mortality rate of 20% or more is no longer warranted; current operative mortality rates of less than 5% are seen in centers of excellence.

based on the level of bile duct dilatation and decompression. Consequently, a very organized algorithm should be implemented to assess resectability accurately and to develop the operative plan.

- If a hilar tumor is suspected, spiral CT, PTC, and arteriography with venous phase address all pertinent issues.
- For a mid-duct tumor, spiral CT, ERC, and arteriography with venous phase are the tests required.
- For a periampullary tumor, spiral CT addresses distant metastasis and the relationship to the peripancreatic vasculature, and laparoscopy identifies peritoneal implants.
- ERCP, although not indicated when a periampullary tumor is evident on CT, is important when the cause of obstructive jaundice cannot be demonstrated on CT.
- Preoperative biopsy is indicated when the tumor is clinically unresectable; it is not indicated when the tumor is clinically resectable.
- Preoperative biliary decompression is indicated when

hemihepatectomy is part of the intended curative procedure. It is not indicated when the liver will remain intact after tumor resection (e.g., periampullary and mid-duct tumors, hilar tumors not requiring hepatectomy).

SELECTED READINGS

Balthazar EJ, Chako AC: Computed tomography of pancreatic masses. Am J Gastroenterol 1990;85:343.

Fernandez-del Castillo C, Rattner DW, Warshaw AL: Further experience with laparoscopy and peritoneal cytology in the staging of pancreatic cancer. Br J Surg 1995;82:1127.

Luque-de Leon E, Tsiotos GG, Balsiger B, et al: Staging laparoscopy for pancreatic cancer should be used to select the best means of palliation and not only to maximize the resectability rate. J Gastrointest Surg 1999;3:111.

Makary MA, Warshaw AL, Canteno BA, et al: Implications of peritoneal cytology for pancreatic cancer management. Arch Surg 1998;133:361.

Sohn TA, Yeo CJ, Cameron JL, et al: Do preoperative biliary stents increase post-pancreaticoduodenectomy complications? J Gastrointest Surg 2000;4:258.

Tsiotos GG, Sarr MG: Diagnosis and clinical staging of pancreatic cancer. In Howard JM, Idezuki Y, Ihse I, et al (eds): Surgical Diseases of the Pancreas, 3rd ed. Baltimore, Williams & Wilkins, 1998, pp 497–513.

Chapter 121

Cystic Neoplasms of the Pancreas

George H. Sakorafas and Michael G. Sarr

Although pancreatic pseudocysts are by far the most commonly recognized peripancreatic cystic lesions, primary cystic neoplasms of the pancreas have received considerable interest recently, mainly because of the improvement in and the wide availability of the newer modalities of pancreatic imaging. With the resulting increase in recognition of these lesions (especially in asymptomatic patients), considerable interest has been focused not only on the preoperative differentiation of cystic neoplasms from benign cystic conditions but also on the differentiation of various forms of cystic neoplasms, because their management differs radically. This chapter summarizes our current state of knowledge regarding the histopathology, clinical presentation, diagnosis, management, and prognosis of pancreatic cystic neoplasms.

HISTOPATHOLOGIC CLASSIFICATION

The vast majority of primary cystic neoplasms of the pancreas are classified into one of two groups: serous or mucinous. Acinar cell cystadenocarcinomas, cystic islet cell neoplasms (both nonfunctioning and functioning, such as cystic insulinomas), cystic choriocarcinomas, cystic teratomas, and angiomatous neoplasms represent extremely rare types of cystic neoplasms of the pancreas and are not discussed further in this chapter (Table 121–1). In 1978, Compagno and Oetel made a significant contribution to the understanding of these neoplasms based on their histopathology (serous vs. mucinous) by defining the tumor biology, the natural history, and the malignant potential of cystic neoplasms. Thus, we now understand the crucial importance of defining the cell type of the lining epithelium—serous neoplasms are uniformly benign, whereas mucinous neoplasms carry a latent (or an overt) malignant potential. Therefore, the distinction between serous cystadenomas and their malignant or premalignant counterparts, mucinous cystic neoplasms, is especially critical.

Serous Cystadenomas

The gross appearance of serous cystadenoma is a cluster of small cysts (<2 cm). The overall size of these neoplasms varies from a few centimeters to as large as 25 cm (mean, 6 to 10 cm). They have a thin, almost translucent wall that usually easily separates from surrounding structures without inflammatory or fibrous adherence, as would be expected of a postinflammatory pancreatic pseudocyst. Cystic fluid is usually clear and notably without mucin. Although there is no obvious anatomic predilection within the pancreas, serous cystadenomas tend to be located in the head of the pancreas, as opposed to mu-

cinous cystadenomas, which are more frequently found in the body and the tail regions. Their epithelium does not express mucin production and is without cellular characteristics of atypia or dysplasia. The stroma separating these microcystic areas is a fibrous connective tissue that is quite vascular (on angiography) and may even be calcified; this unique calcification gives rise to a characteristic sunburst, radial, or stellate scar pattern on computed tomography (CT) (Fig. 121–1A).

Studies using electron microscopic and immunohistochemical techniques have suggested that the cell of origin is the centroacinar cell, possibly explaining the peripheral anatomic location of these cells within the pancreatic parenchyma. Specific stains for mucin, chromogranin, regulatory entero- or neuroendocrine peptides, and carcinoembryonic antigen (CEA) are routinely negative, adding further credence to the hypothesis that these neoplasms do not arise from ductal epithelium. Malignant transformation of serous cystadenoma is distinctly uncommon; indeed, fewer than 10 patients with a biopsy-proven malignant form of serous cystadenoma have been reported. Therefore, all serous cystic neoplasms of the pancreas should be considered benign lesions with essentially nonmalignant potential.

Table 121–1	Cystic Tumors of the Pancreas

Cystic Neoplasms

Serous cystadenoma
Mucinous cystadenoma/cystadenocarcinoma spectrum
Acinar cell cystadenocarcinoma
Papillary-cystic epithelial neoplasm
Cystic teratoma
Cystic choriocarcinoma
Angiomatous neoplasm (angioma, lymphangioma, hemangiothelioma)

Acquired Cysts

Parasitic cyst
  Echinococcal (hydatid) cyst
  Taenia solium cyst
Postinflammatory cystic fluid collection
  Pancreatic pseudocyst
  Pancreatic pseudopseudocyst (inflammatory exudative collection)
  Pancreatic sequestrum (postnecrotic)

Congenital True Cysts

Single true cysts
  Polycystic disease of the pancreas without related anomalies
  Pancreatic macrocysts associated with cystic fibrosis
  Polycystic disease of the pancreas associated with cerebellar tumors and retinal angiomata (von Hippel-Lindau disease)
  Pancreatic cysts associated with polycystic disease of kidneys
Enterogenous cysts
Dermoid cysts
Endometriosis

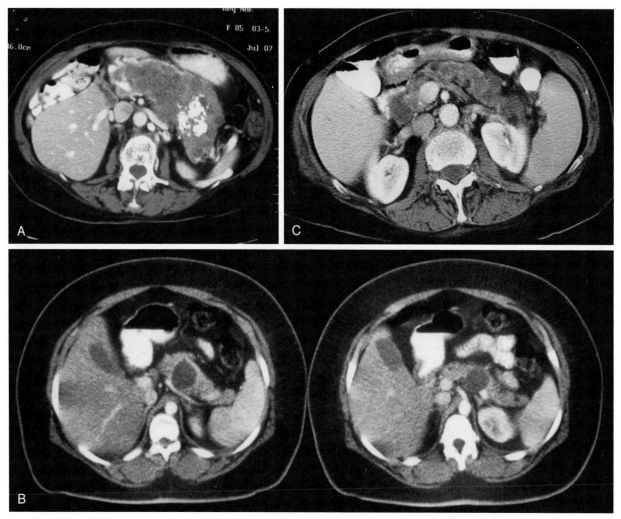

Figure 121–1. Computed tomography of cystic neoplasms of the pancreas. *A,* Typical serous cystadenoma. Note central starburst calcification and multiple small cysts. *B,* Mucinous cystic neoplasm. Note larger cyst and lack of peripancreatic or pericystic inflammation. *C,* Intraductal papillary mucinous tumor. Note markedly dilated main pancreatic duct.

Spectrum of Mucinous Cystadenoma and Cystadenocarcinoma

In contrast to benign serous cystadenomas, mucinous cystic neoplasms represent a more diverse, broader, heterogeneous spectrum ranging from benign cystadenomas, with a latent but real potential for malignant transformation, to the much less common overt cystadenocarcinomas, with frank tissue invasion and aggressive metastatic potential. For these reasons, some pathologists have suggested that all these lesions should be considered to be at least a grade 1 cystadenocarcinoma, even in the absence of documented invasion, thus warranting routine resection. The gross appearance of mucinous cystic neoplasms is often different from that of their microcystic serous counterparts. The individual cystic areas are larger (usually 2 cm or larger, and occasionally up to 25 cm; mean size, 8 to 10 cm) and generally contain fewer than six separate cysts. Rarely, the neoplasm has just one macrocyst. Typically, the cysts are not unilocular but have septa within them and may have an eccentric solid component. As with serous neoplasms, the surrounding tissues

lack an inflammatory pericystic reaction except when malignant transformation and tissue invasion have occurred.

Mucinous cystic neoplasms contain columnar epithelium that expresses mucin. The intracystic fluid is thicker and more viscous than in serous cystadenomas and contains mucus. The epithelial cells may also stain for carcinoembryonic antigen and serotonin, suggesting an origin from ductal or stem cells. Papillary invaginations are common, and on occasion multiple discontinuous areas of atypia, dysplasia, carcinoma in situ, and overtly invasive carcinoma may occur within the same neoplasm. In as many as one third of tumors, there may even be limited areas of a cuboidal-appearing epithelium resembling serous cystadenoma.

These neoplasms are notorious for containing multiple areas of discontinuous epithelium. Incomplete, denuded epithelium may be found in 70% of mucinous cystadenomas and cystadenocarcinomas, with a mean of 40% (but as great as 98%) of the cyst wall being devoid of an epithelial lining. Thus, one can understand how the unwary surgeon can confuse mucinous cystadenocarcinomas for mucinous cystadenomas or even for pancreatic pseudocysts, especially if the diagnosis is based on a single frozen-section biopsy of the cystic wall. For these reasons, complete histopathologic evaluation should involve multiple sections from all areas of the tumor mass, especially in areas of papillary excrescence.

Intraductal Papillary Mucinous Tumors

Intraductal papillary mucinous tumor (IPMT) of the pancreatic ducts is a new and increasingly reported entity that represents a variant in the spectrum of mucinous cystic neoplasms of the pancreas. This entity has a variety of names, including mucinous ductal ectasia, mucin-producing tumor, mucin hypersecreting tumor, ductectatic cystadenoma or cystadenocarcinoma, intraductal mucin-hypersecreting neoplasm, mucinous villous adenomatosis, intraductal papillary neoplasm, and intraductal papillary mucinous neoplasm, or IPMT. IPMT is the favored term because it seems to best represent this disorder.

Intraductal papillary mucinous tumors are less well appreciated than mucinous cystic neoplasms and present differently, with a more nonlocalized abnormality on diagnostic imaging tests. IPMT contains dysplastic lesions that are frequently diffuse and are often associated with copious mucin production; often, mucus can be seen extruding from a bulging papilla of Vater. Pancreatic ductal dilatation varies from generalized dilatation of the main pancreatic duct for all or part of its extent to more segmental dilatation of the ducts involving a major segment of the gland. It is unknown whether dilatation of the pancreatic duct is due to partial obstruction by mucin or to abnormal ductal dysplastic epithelium. The dysplastic epithelium may be flat, micropapillary, or grossly papillary. It may contain segments of simple tall columnar cells and may have other areas demonstrating the spectrum of changes from mucinous hyperplasia to severe dysplasia to carcinoma. In situ or invasive cancer is present in about 30% to 50% of patients at diagnosis. IPMT is commonly associated with episodic pancreatic-like pain.

There is no evidence of a relationship between IPMT and serous cystic neoplasms of the pancreas because the latter are lined by nonmucinous, glycogen-rich, nondysplastic epithelium. In contrast, there may be a relationship between IPMT and mucinous cystic neoplasms of the pancreas. Cysts may coexist in patients with IPMT; the epithelia are cytologically identical, and both conditions are potentially or overtly malignant. Classically, mucinous cystic neoplasms are cystic and dysplastic lesions that do not communicate with the ductal system.

The natural history of IPMT or the presence of an associated malignant focus cannot be predicted based on preoperative features (e.g., ductal obstruction at endoscopic retrograde cholangiopancreatography), findings on endoscopic ultrasonography, or cytologic examination of molecular alterations (e.g., K-*ras* mutations) detected in the pancreatic juice or in the stool. Thus, the natural history of IPMT is difficult to assess without histologic examination of the tissue because malignancy cannot be reliably excluded preoperatively. The prolonged course of many of these patients suggests that the dysplastic component may remain in situ for many years. The out-

come for patients, however, is predictable based on the histopathologic findings at operation. The presence of invasive carcinoma within IPMT connotes a dismal prognosis.

Unusual Cystic Disorders

Rare cystic disorders that masquerade as cystic neoplasms include the exceedingly rare primary pancreatic cysts, the cysts of von Hippel-Lindau disease, the associated pancreatic cysts of the polycystic kidney, liver, and pancreas spectrum, and the peripancreatic cysts arising from the spleen, the left adrenal gland, the kidney, the mesentery, or the retroperitoneum.

CLINICAL PRESENTATION

There are no symptoms or signs pathognomonic of cystic neoplasms. Many patients (up to 40%) will be truly asymptomatic, with the cystic mass discovered only incidentally. When the patient is symptomatic, the presentation is nonspecific and is related to the mass effect of the neoplasm. A history of acute or chronic pancreatitis is absent except in the rare patient in whom the cystic neoplasm causes an episode of acute pancreatitis, presumably from partial duct obstruction. Although many of these neoplasms occur in the body and the tail of the pancreas, they do not invade the retroperitoneal nerves (causing back pain) or involve the fourth portion of the duodenum (causing distal duodenal obstruction) despite their often large size. A complaint of abdominal fullness, often with a component of early satiety, is most common. Unlike in ductal pancreatic adenocarcinoma, jaundice is unusual. Therefore, the absence of jaundice in the presence of a large cystic mass in the proximal pancreas should raise the suspicion of a cystic neoplasm. IPMT may present differently from other cystic neoplasms. Because of the functional pancreatic ductal obstruction due to mucin hypersecretion, pancreatic exocrine insufficiency may prompt further evaluation.

DIAGNOSIS

Except in the patient with a palpable abdominal mass, most cystic neoplasms are found only after diagnostic imaging. Because most peripancreatic cystic masses are not cystic neoplasms, the clinician needs to maintain a high index of suspicion, especially in patients without a history of acute or chronic pancreatic disease. An objective diagnosis relies on the finding of a cystic pancreatic mass on diagnostic imaging as well as an appropriate clinical setting.

Abdominal Ultrasonography and Computed Tomography

Most cystic neoplasms will be identified as such with abdominal ultrasonography and CT in conjunction with the clinical history. The differentiation between serous and mucinous cystic neoplasms as well as between neoplasms and pancreatic pseudocysts can usually be obtained with reasonable assurance. Mucinous neoplasms are usually composed of fewer than six cysts of larger size (generally greater than 2 cm), explaining the descriptive term macrocystic (see Fig. 121–1*B*). Serous cystadenomas are multicystic masses (usually more than six individual cysts) consisting of cysts smaller than 2 cm (microcystic) (see Fig. 121–1*A*). Overall, size is of no discriminative value. About 15% of serous cystadenomas will have central calcification, giving a "sunburst" appearance on CT. Although 20% of mucinous cystadenomas will have some calcification, it tends to be patchy and peripheral; when it has an eggshell appearance, the likelihood of mucinous cystadenocarcinoma increases. Pseudocysts rarely have calcified walls. In the absence of distant metastases, CT and ultrasonography are unable to differentiate between benign and malignant mucinous cystadenomas. Ductal adenocarcinoma can mimic a cystic neoplasm by causing symptomatic or asymptomatic localized ductal obstruction resembling a cystic neoplasm or by manifesting central necrosis. Other imaging tests (magnetic resonance imaging or angiography) are of little added benefit.

On CT or ultrasonography, IPMT appears as a markedly dilated pancreatic duct (see Fig. 121–1*C*). Variants include unusual segmental lesions that involve only one branch of the pancreatic ductal system, usually the uncinate lobe. Many of these potentially malignant mucinous neoplasms were treated as chronic pancreatitis in the past. The mucinous globules or the areas of malignant transformation may appear as filling defects within the ductal system.

Endoscopic Retrograde Pancreatography

Endoscopic retrograde pancreatography has little to offer in the evaluation of serous or mucinous cystic neoplasms of the pancreas because these neoplasms do not communicate with the pancreatic ductal system. Endoscopic retrograde pancreatography may be helpful in the differentiation between pancreatic pseudocysts and cystic neoplasms, however. In contrast, in IPMT, endoscopic retrograde pancreatography reveals a markedly dilated main pancreatic duct, which may contain filling defects related to mucinous concretions or duct-based neoplastic proliferation. The endoscopist will often note the copious egress of mucin from a bulging papilla.

Percutaneous Fine-Needle Aspiration of the Cystic Fluid

Recent interest has centered on the analysis of intracystic fluid to differentiate among cystic disorders of the pancreas. Fine-needle aspiration may be indicated in other potentially difficult clinical situations, such as the presence of an asymptomatic, presumed cystic neoplasm in the head of the pancreas that would require proximal pancreatectomy in an elderly or a high-risk patient. The ability to confirm the presence of a serious cystadenoma confidently or, more important, to exclude the presence of a mucinous cystadenoma or cystadenocarcinoma would

enable the surgeon to select a nonoperative approach in selected high-risk patients.

FINE NEEDLE CYTOLOGY. Experience with fine needle cytology remains relatively limited. Aspiration as a definitive diagnostic test has several pitfalls, including sample error, lack of characteristic cystic contents, and a small risk of complications (e.g., pancreatitis or tumor seeding along the needle track by carcinoma). Although occasionally cytologic analysis may reveal malignant cells, its sensitivity and its specificity are low. A large concentration of amylase strongly suggests that the cyst is a pancreatic pseudocyst; the only exception is IPMT, in which the neoplasm involves the epithelial cellular lining of the main pancreatic ductal system. The presence of increased viscosity (mucin) appears to be quite specific for mucinous lesions. Increased concentrations (350 mg/dL or more) of the tumor marker carcinoembryonic antigen may be both sensitive and specific in the differentiation between mucinous and serous neoplasms. This differentiation may be most important in an elderly patient with a cystic mass in the head of the pancreas, which would require pancreatoduodenectomy if it were a mucinous cystic neoplasm.

MANAGEMENT

Most surgeons agree that all mucinous cystic neoplasms of the pancreas should be removed because of the risk of latent or overt malignancy. Although cystic neoplasms of the body or the tail region of the pancreas are readily managed with the less risky distal pancreatectomy, cystic lesions in the head of the pancreas pose a more difficult and controversial problem, especially in the high-risk or elderly patient. Is resection necessary or warranted in all such patients? What about cyst enucleation, palliative biliary bypass, or cystoenteric drainage? Is there a role for adjuvant chemotherapy and radiation therapy? Because most pathologists believe that IPMT involving the main pancreatic duct is a premalignant condition jeopardizing the entire ductal system, should all patients with IPMT undergo total pancreatectomy?

Serous Cystadenoma

In the past, the prevailing therapeutic philosophy was that judicious observation was warranted, and resection was unnecessary. The recent decline in mortality rate after major pancreatic resections (including pancreatoduodenectomy), the accumulating number of complications of serous cystadenomas, including the rare possibility of malignant transformation, complications related to preoperative diagnostic procedures, and, most important, the inability to differentiate confidently between serous and mucinous neoplasms have changed the therapeutic philosophy of most surgeons to one of a more aggressive approach in the younger, good-risk patient.

When these neoplasms involve the body or the tail of the pancreas, most surgeons suggest resection. Complete resection ensures cure. Controversy exists regarding asymptomatic lesions in the head of the pancreas, espe-

Table 121–2	Differential Diagnosis Between Cystic Neoplasms and Pseudocysts	
FACTOR	**CYSTIC NEOPLASM**	**PSEUDOCYST**
Age	Older	Younger
Sex	Male << female	Male > female
Recent/past medical history	Normal	Pancreatic disease
Imaging findings	Multiple cysts, no adjacent inflammation	Single cyst, pancreatic/peripancreatic inflammation
Endoscopic retrograde cholangiography	Normal	Ductal changes, communication with the cyst (>50%)
Serum amylase	Normal	Increased (50%–70%)
Cyst fluid amylase	Normal	Increased
Gross appearance	Thin wall; clear fluid; cystic mass not adherent to adjacent structures	Thick wall; dirty fluid; cyst adherent to stomach, mesocolon, and so forth

cially in the frail or the elderly patient. Confirming these lesions confidently as benign serous neoplasms (vs. premalignant mucinous counterparts) would allow a nonaggressive therapeutic approach (observation) in the asymptomatic patient, given the known slow progression of these lesions over many years.

Whenever a nonresectional approach is contemplated, the surgeon and the patient must acknowledge the small risk of mistaking a mucinous for a serous cystic neoplasm. Other potential technical approaches, such as enucleation, cystoenterostomy, or percutaneous external drainage or percutaneous intracystic sclerosis (as used for simple hepatic cysts), are generally to be condemned.

Mucinous Cystic Neoplasms

The appropriate management of mucinous cystic neoplasms, whether in the proximal or the distal pancreas and whether symptomatic or not, is complete resection because of the latent (or overt) risk of malignancy. Enucleation is not indicated because of the malignant potential, which raises concern about an incomplete resection, and the tendency of these lesions to be more centrally located, risking injury to a main duct with a resultant pancreatic fistula. With curative resection in the absence

of invasion, 5-year survival is 100%. These lesions tend to push adjacent structures aside rather than to invade them; despite their often large size, this should not be a contraindication to exploration. Because of the less aggressive natural history of these lesions (when compared with ductal adenocarcinoma), aggressive resection is indicated when necessary (i.e., superior mesenteric vein resection, lymphadenectomy, or en bloc resections of adherent structures). The role of chemotherapy or radiation therapy in mucinous cystic neoplasms of the pancreas remains undefined, but these modalities should be strongly considered despite curative resection.

Intraductal Papillary Mucinous Tumors

The appropriate management of IPMT is undefined. IPMT manifests a greater latent or overt malignant potential than do other cystic neoplasms of the pancreas. The difficulty is that except in the unusual patient with localized segmental disease, probably all of the pancreatic duct epithelium is at risk of malignant transformation; thus, the appropriate operation appears to be total pancreatectomy. Total pancreatectomy necessitates complete endocrine and exocrine insufficiency, which represents a significant long-term morbidity. Pancreatoduodenectomy is a reasonable option for segmental lesions involving the proximal pancreatic duct, provided that the distal pancreatic duct is histologically spared. Similarly, distal pancreatectomy is reasonable for segmental IPMT involving only the distal gland.

DIFFERENTIAL DIAGNOSIS

With improvements in imaging, a number of cystic lesions are being recognized with increasing frequency and must be considered clinically in the differential diagnosis of cystic neoplasms of the pancreas. General guidelines on the differentiation between cystic neoplasms of the pancreas and pseudocysts are presented in Table 121–2.

SELECTED READINGS

Johnson CD, Stephens DH, Charboneau JW, et al: Cystic pancreatic tumors: CT and sonographic assessment. Am J Radiol 1988;151:1133.
Loftus EV Jr, Olivares-Pakzad BA, Batts KP, et al: Intraductal papillary-mucinous

---

Pearls and Pitfalls

- Cystic neoplasms of the pancreas should be considered in patients with peripancreatic "cysts" when there is no history of previous inflammatory pancreatic disease.
- Differentiation between mucinous and serous neoplasms is crucial because mucinous neoplasms are potentially malignant.
- Modern imaging will be able to differentiate between mucinous and serous neoplasms about 95% of the time.
- Serous cystadenomas can be followed expectantly if they are asymptomatic.
- Mucinous cystic neoplasms should be excised.
- The management of IPMT requires selective judgment.
- Complete resection of noninvasive mucinous cystic neoplasms is curative.

tumors of the pancreas: Clinicopathologic features, outcome, and nomenclature. Members of the Pancreas Clinic, and Pancreatic Surgeons of Mayo Clinic. Gastroenterology 1996;110:1909.

Pyke CM, van Heerden JA, Colby TV, et al: The spectrum of serous cystadenoma of the pancreas: Clinical, pathological, and surgical aspects. Ann Surg 1992;215:132.

Sarr MG, Carpenter HA, Prabhakar LP, et al: Clinical and pathological correlation of 84 mucinous cystic neoplasms of the pancreas: Can one reliably differentiate benign from malignant (or premalignant) neoplasms? Ann Surg 2000;231:205.

Warshaw AL, Rutledge PL: Cystic tumors mistaken for pancreatic pseudocysts. Ann Surg 1987;205:393.

Yeo CJ, Sarr MG: Cystic and pseudocystic diseases of the pancreas. Curr Probl Surg 1994;31:165.

Pancreas: Malignant

Chapter 122
Pancreatic Carcinoma
Marina E. Jean and Douglas B. Evans

BACKGROUND

Natural History and Patterns of Treatment Failure

Pancreatic cancer, the fourth leading cause of cancer-related death in adults, accounted for approximately 28,000 deaths in the year 2000 in the United States. Because of the frequent inability to diagnose pancreatic cancer while it is still both localized and surgically resectable and the lack of effective systemic therapies, incidence rates virtually equal mortality rates. Exocrine pancreatic cancer is characterized both by early vascular dissemination and spread to regional lymph nodes. Subclinical liver metastases are present in the majority of patients at the time of diagnosis, even when findings of imaging studies are normal. Patient survival depends on the extent of disease and the performance status at diagnosis. Clinical staging using physical examination, chest radiography, and computed tomography (CT) of the abdomen can accurately define the extent of disease, which is best categorized as resectable, locally advanced, or metastatic.

Patients who undergo surgical resection for localized nonmetastatic adenocarcinoma of the pancreas have a long-term survival rate of approximately 10% to 20% and a median survival of 16 to 24 months. Duration of survival appears to be superior in those patients who receive either preoperative or postoperative chemotherapy and external-beam radiation therapy (chemoradiation). Disease recurrence after "curative" pancreaticoduodenectomy remains common; however, after surgery alone, local recurrence occurs in up to 75% of patients, peritoneal recurrence occurs in 25%, and liver metastases occur in 50%. When surgery and adjuvant chemoradiation are used to maximize local and regional tumor control, liver metastases become the dominant form of recurrence.

Patients with locally advanced nonmetastatic but nonresectable disease have a median survival of 6 to 10 months. A survival advantage has been demonstrated when these patients are treated with chemoradiation compared with no treatment or radiation therapy alone. Patients with distant metastatic disease have a short survival (3 to 6 months), the length of which depends on the extent of disease and the performance status of the patient. For patients with metastatic pancreatic cancer who have good performance status, systemic chemotherapy is appropriate, and treatment with gemcitabine (a deoxycytidine analogue) appears to be the standard in the United States.

Epidemiology

The risk of developing pancreatic cancer is low in the first three or four decades of life but increases sharply after the age of 50 years, and most patients are between 60 and 80 years of age at diagnosis. Pancreatic cancer occurs more frequently in men, but the incidence and the mortality appear to be increasing in women, probably secondary to the increased use of tobacco. It has been estimated that about 10% of pancreatic cancers occur in families with a first- or second-degree relative who also has had pancreatic cancer. Incidence rates for pancreatic cancer are highest in industrialized societies and western countries, particularly in native Hawaiians, African Americans, and Korean Americans. Mortality rates for pancreatic cancer in African Americans are higher than for any other ethnic group in the United States and are considerably higher than the rates observed in African blacks, suggesting an environmental contribution to increased risk.

Cigarette smoking is the most firmly established risk factor associated with pancreatic cancer. Pancreatic malignancies can be induced in animals through long-term administration of tobacco-specific nitrosamines or through parenteral administration of other N-nitroso compounds. These carcinogens are metabolized to electrophiles, which readily react with DNA, leading to miscoding and activation of specific oncogenes such as K-*ras*. The current estimates suggest that approximately 30% of pancreatic cancers are due, in part, to cigarette smoking. Recent studies have shown that the risk of pancreatic cancer increases as the amount and the duration of smoking increase and that long-term smoking cessation (>10 years) reduces risk by 30% relative to the risk of current smokers. Data regarding the effect of consumption of coffee and excessive alcohol appear conflicting, but the majority of studies conducted over the past 10 years have failed to demonstrate consistently an increased risk of pancreatic cancer.

Diabetes mellitus is thought to be both an early manifestation of and a predisposing factor for pancreatic carcinoma. Pancreatic adenocarcinoma of duct cell origin can induce peripheral insulin resistance. This has been shown in recent studies, which have demonstrated that after a recent diagnosis of diabetes, the nonobese adult has an increased risk of developing pancreatic cancer. This risk decreases with the duration of diabetes and appears limited to those with non–insulin-dependent diabetes or to patients whose disease was diagnosed at or after the age of 40 years.

The incidence of pancreatic adenocarcinoma is also increased in patients with hereditary pancreatitis. Molecular data suggest that mutations in the cationic trypsinogen gene play a crucial role in hereditary and possibly acquired forms of pancreatitis and increase the risk of pancreatic cancer. In hereditary pancreatitis, a single amino acid substitution inactivates the cationic trypsin cleavage site, causing uncontrolled trypsin activation and pancreatic autodigestion. Hereditary pancreatitis has an autosomal dominant transmission with 80% penetrance. An association with sporadic acute pancreatitis (induced by alcohol or recurrent biliary disease) is not established; if the patient has chronic pancreatitis, however, there is a definite increased incidence of pancreatic cancer. As stated earlier, as many as 10% of pancreatic cancers have some form of familial predisposition.

Pathology

The normal pancreas contains acinar cells, which account for 80% of the cells and the volume of the gland; duct cells make up 10% to 15%, and islet cells account for about 1% to 2%. The pancreatic architecture is markedly altered in pancreatic carcinoma; the predominant histologic feature is dense collagenous stroma with atrophic acini, remarkably preserved islet cell clusters, and a slight-to-moderate increase in the number of ducts, both normal-appearing and cancerous. Ninety-five percent of malignant neoplasms of pancreatic origin arise from the exocrine portion of the gland. The diagnosis of ductal adenocarcinoma rests on the identification of mitoses, nuclear and cellular pleomorphism, discontinuity of ductal epithelium, and evidence of perineural, vascular, or lymphatic invasion. Much more infrequent are tumors arising from the islets of Langerhans (endocrine) cells of the pancreas. Primary nonepithelial tumors of the pancreas (e.g., lymphomas or sarcomas) are extremely rare.

Molecular Biology of Pancreatic Cancer

Pancreatic cancer is characterized by specific point mutations at codon 12 of the K-*ras* oncogene on chromosome 12p13 in 75% to 90% of pancreatic adenocarcinomas. The ras protein is an important signal-transduction mediator for receptor protein tyrosine kinases. The mutated *ras* oncogene is not able to convert GTP to inactive GDP, resulting in a constitutively active ras protein, unregulated cellular proliferation signals, and susceptibility to transformation. All ras proteins are produced in the cytoplasm as biologically inactive precursors and must undergo posttranslational enzymatic modification to allow the membrane localization necessary for biologic activity of the protein product. Farnesyl protein transferase, an enzyme, catalyzes the first of a series of steps necessary for ras to localize to the cell membrane. Inhibitors of farnesyl protein transferase are being investigated as possible anticancer agents in patients with pancreatic cancer.

Loss of the function of the tumor suppressor gene *p53* occurs in 50% to 70% of human pancreatic adenocarcinomas and also contributes to unregulated cell growth. The *p53* gene, located on chromosome 17p13, is critical to normal cellular function. p53 protein levels increase with DNA damage. p53 is important because it has a dual role: It can halt cell cycle progression at the G_1-S checkpoint in response to DNA damage, and it can induce apoptosis if DNA damage is beyond repair.

Allelic deletions involving *p16* have been found in 85% of human pancreatic tumors. The *p16* gene on chromosome 9p21, a class of cyclin-dependent kinase inhibitory genes, inhibits the cyclin D_1–*Cdk*-4 complex that normally phosphorylates the retinoblastoma protein. This phosphorylation releases transcription factors, which turn on genes that allow cell cycle progression. Inactivation of *p16* therefore leads to unregulated cell growth.

The newly discovered tumor suppressor *DPC4* (*Smad4*), on chromosome 18q21, is an important component of the transforming growth factor beta signaling pathway, which normally downregulates the growth of epithelial cells, stimulates differentiation, and promotes apoptosis. *DPC4* was found to be homozygously deleted in 30% of pancreatic carcinomas and was inactivated in another 20% of patients studied. Loss of this important growth regulatory pathway also appears to contribute to unregulated cell growth.

The aggressiveness of pancreatic cancer also correlates with factors that regulate growth (epidermal growth factor receptor), angiogenesis (vascular endothelial growth factor), invasion (type IV collagenase genes), and multidrug resistance. Targeting molecular alterations may lead to novel treatment strategies as well as improving our understanding of the relative roles of these changes in pancreatic cancer biology.

CLINICAL PRESENTATION

The majority of pancreatic cancers develop in the head of the pancreas or the uncinate process. Adenocarcinoma of the body or the tail of the pancreas is less common and is usually metastatic at the time of diagnosis; the lack of obvious or pathognomonic clinical signs and symptoms delays diagnosis in most patients. Jaundice is present only in patients in whom the tumor arises in close proximity to the intrapancreatic portion of the bile duct. Small tumors of the pancreatic head, especially in the periampullary region, may obstruct the bile duct and cause the patient to seek medical attention when the tumor is still localized and potentially resectable. In the absence of biliary obstruction, few patients present with potentially resectable disease because patient complaints are nonspecific, as are clinical signs on physical examination.

The pain typical of locally advanced pancreatic cancer is dull and fairly constant and is of visceral origin, localized to the middle and upper back owing to tumor invasion of the celiac and the mesenteric plexuses. This pain can often be well managed by means of percutaneous or endoscopic celiac plexus block, using a neurolytic agent to destroy the nerves around the celiac plexus. Vague, intermittent epigastric pain occurs in some patients; its cause is less clear. Fatigue, weight loss, and anorexia are common even in the absence of mechanical gastric outlet obstruction. Pancreatic exocrine insufficiency due to obstruction of the pancreatic duct may result in an element of malabsorption and steatorrhea, but diarrhea or gross steatorrhea occurs infrequently. Glucose intolerance is present in the majority of patients with pancreatic cancer. Although the exact mechanism remains unclear, altered β-cell function and impaired tissue insulin sensitivity are present.

PREOPERATIVE MANAGEMENT

Diagnostic Imaging

Current technology should allow physicians to stage the extent of disease (resectable, locally advanced, metastatic) accurately before surgery. There is rarely a need for exploratory surgery in the management of patients with biopsy-proven or suspected pancreatic or periampullary cancer. Our current algorithm for diagnosis and treatment of patients with presumed or biopsy-proven adenocarcinoma of the pancreatic head or periampullary region is illustrated in Figure 122–1. Helical CT with intravenous and oral contrast material is the initial study of choice for determining whether a patient has potentially resectable, locally advanced, or metastatic disease. A non–contrast-enhanced CT is obtained through the liver and pancreas at 10-mm thicknesses and at a 10-mm interval to identify liver metastases and to localize the pancreas. Intravenous contrast agent enhancement is achieved with nonionic contrast material administered by an automatic injector at a rate of 3 to 5 mL/second for a total of 150 mL. At least two phases of pancreatic scanning are performed. First, the pancreatic parenchyma phase, which employs 3- to 5-mm thicknesses, starts 30 to 40 seconds after the

delivery of intravenous contrast material; this phase is the best for detection of pancreatic neoplasms. The second phase, which is done at 5- to 7-mm thicknesses to detect liver and peritoneal metastases, begins 60 to 65 seconds after the start of contrast agent injection to cover the entire liver and upper abdomen.

For a mass in the pancreatic head, the CT criteria for tumor resectability include (1) the absence of extrapancreatic disease, (2) no direct tumor extension to the celiac axis or the superior mesenteric artery (SMA), and (3) a patent superior mesenteric–portal vein (SMPV) confluence (Fig. 122–2). Patients whose tumors do not meet these CT criteria are not considered candidates for pancreaticoduodenectomy. We do not consider surgical resection in patients with clear evidence of arterial encasement on preoperative CT. Because the accuracy of CT in predicting unresectability is well established, the majority of patients with disease determined to be unresectable on CT can be spared laparotomy; biliary decompression, when necessary, can be performed using endoscopic or laparoscopic methods.

Patients with extrahepatic biliary obstruction in the absence of a mass in the pancreas undergo endoscopic retrograde cholangiopancreatography and endoscopic ultrasonography (EUS). EUS may identify an occult pancreatic mass, making possible fine needle aspiration biopsy. The more widespread use of EUS-guided fine needle aspiration biopsy will allow the frequent application of preoperative (neoadjuvant) chemoradiation. If there is no tissue diagnosis of malignancy, patients who have clinical and radiologic findings suggesting a pancreatic or a periampullary neoplasm undergo pancreaticoduodenectomy. Such patients often have a neoplastic stricture of the intrapancreatic portion of the common bile duct on endoscopic retrograde cholangiopancreatography in the absence of a mass seen on CT or EUS.

Over the past decade, laparoscopy has been suggested in patients with radiographic evidence of localized pancreatic cancer to detect extrapancreatic metastases not seen on CT and thereby prevent nontherapeutic celiotomy. CT-occult extrapancreatic disease is relatively uncommon (10% to 15% of patients) when the primary tumor is judged resectable by means of high-quality CT images. Therefore, many believe that it is difficult to justify the expense of laparoscopy as a separate staging procedure; however, laparoscopy immediately before laparotomy during the same period of anesthesia is reasonable in patients with potentially resectable pancreatic cancer when a decision has been made to proceed with pancreaticoduodenectomy if no peritoneal or liver metastases are noted at laparoscopy.

Tumor Markers

Identification of a tumor marker specific for pancreatic cancer would make possible screening, early diagnosis, determination of prognosis, and post-treatment monitoring for tumor recurrence. Unfortunately, the sensitivity and the specificity of currently available tumor markers for pancreatic cancer are inadequate for screening of the general population. The incidence of pancreatic carci-

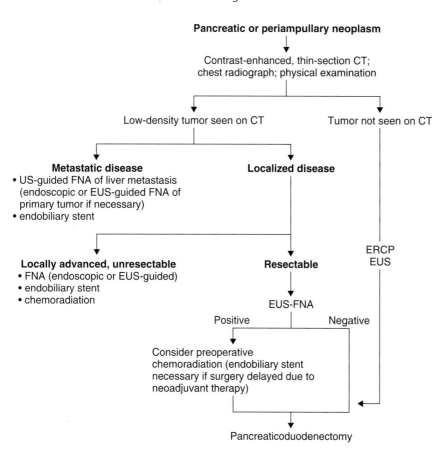

Figure 122–1. Management of patients with suspected or biopsy-proven adenocarcinoma of the pancreatic head or the periampullary region. When there is no obvious mass or pretreatment biopsies are nondiagnostic, patients who have clinical and radiologic findings suggesting a pancreatic or a periampullary neoplasm undergo pancreaticoduodenectomy. CT, computed tomography; ERCP, endoscopic retrograde cholangiopancreatography; EUS, endoscopic ultrasonography; FNA, fine needle aspiration; US, ultrasonography.

noma in adults older than the age of 50 years is approximately 50 in 100,000, and currently available tumor markers have a maximal sensitivity of 90% and a specificity of 95%. Therefore, for every 100,000 people screened, there would be 45 true-positive cases and 5000 false-positive cases. Furthermore, attempts to limit screening to high-risk populations is hindered by the difficulty in precisely defining high-risk groups.

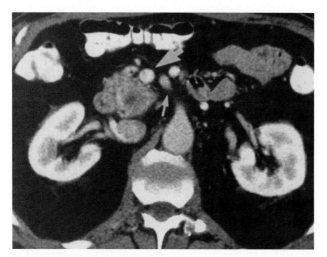

Figure 122–2. Contrast-enhanced computed tomography demonstrating a resectable adenocarcinoma of the pancreatic head. Note the normal fat plane between the low-density tumor and the superior mesenteric artery (*small arrow*) and the superior mesenteric vein (*large arrow*).

The carbohydrate antigen CA 19-9 is the most commonly used tumor marker for pancreatic cancer. Elevated levels of CA 19-9 can be detected in the serum of patients with pancreatic cancer. Using a cutoff value of 37 U/mL, the sensitivity of CA 19-9 in diagnosing pancreatic cancer ranges from 68% to 93%, and the specificity ranges from 68% to 98%. The higher the level of CA 19-9, the greater the specificity and positive predictive value. Serum levels of CA 19-9 appear to correlate with extent of disease; serum levels greater than 1000 U/mL are associated with a 96% chance of being unresectable. CA 19-9 levels of 5000 to 10,000 U/mL are suggestive of disease that has already spread to the liver or the peritoneum. The sensitivity of CA 19-9 in the diagnosis of small pancreatic tumors (<4 cm) is only 57%, however. Some patients with large tumor burdens have normal CA 19-9 levels. One possible explanation for such false-negative results is that 5% of the population is Lewis blood type A negative and thus unable to synthesize the CA 19-9 antigen. After pancreaticoduodenectomy, CA 19-9 levels decline, and a normal CA 19-9 level is associated with improved survival.

Circulating serum levels of CA 19-9 are also influenced by cholestasis and jaundice, with elevated levels observed in patients with cholangitis or cirrhosis. The elevation of CA 19-9 levels in patients with benign biliary disease is the result of insufficient hepatic metabolism of CA 19-9. The level of CA 19-9 can also be elevated in patients with other solid tumors, including adenocarcinoma of the stomach, colon, and esophagus, and hepatocellular carcinoma.

Several other glycoproteins (CA 50, DUPAN-2, CA

125) and oncofetal antigens (carcinoembryonic antigen, alpha-fetoprotein) have been investigated, but their sensitivity and specificity have not been high enough to provide additional diagnostic information beyond that achieved with CA 19-9. Pancreatic enzymes (e.g., elastase, trypsin, amylase) have also been considered potential tumor markers, but their low specificity for pancreatic cancer makes them of no diagnostic value. Current investigations have focused on the possible use of assays to detect both mutations of K-*ras* and p53 antibodies in peripheral blood or K-*ras* mutations in pancreatic or duodenal juice or stool.

INTRAOPERATIVE MANAGEMENT

Selected patients with cardiopulmonary disease receive a pulmonary artery catheter before anesthesia. Because of the length of the operative procedure and the frequent requirement for large volumes of intraoperative and postoperative fluid, we use invasive monitoring liberally in the acute postoperative period. We prefer combined general and epidural anesthesia during surgery; the epidural catheter is used for postoperative pain control for 72 hours. A short course of perioperative antibiotic coverage is employed, but prolonged postoperative antibiotic use in the absence of documented or suspected infection is discouraged.

Pancreaticoduodenectomy

The standard surgical treatment for adenocarcinoma of the pancreatic head is pancreaticoduodenectomy, as described by Whipple in 1935. In 1946, Waugh and Clagett modified the one-stage procedure to its current form. The goals of surgical therapy outlined by Waugh and Clagett have not changed in the past 50 years: (1) There should be reasonable opportunity for cure; (2) the risk of death should not outweigh the prospects for cure; and (3) the patient should be left in as normal a condition as possible. Pancreaticoduodenectomy, as performed today, involves removal of the pancreatic head, the duodenum, the gallbladder, and the bile duct with or without removal of the gastric antrum.

Our recommended technique for pancreaticoduodenectomy uses a bilateral subcostal or a midline incision. The abdomen is carefully explored to exclude extrapancreatic metastatic disease. The liver and the peritoneal surfaces are examined; intraoperative ultrasonography of the liver is used selectively when preoperative CT findings are indeterminate, suggesting possible hepatic metastasis. We would not proceed with tumor resection in the presence of biopsy-proven liver or peritoneal metastases. The issue of performing lymph node biopsy for frozen-section analysis remains controversial. Positive lymph nodes are a prognostic factor (along with poorly differentiated histology and microscopically positive resection margins) predictive of decreased duration of survival. Importantly, the majority (60% to 90%) of resected specimens contain microscopic metastases in regional lymph nodes, however. In a good-risk patient with localized resectable pancreatic cancer, we currently do not view lymph node metastases

(within the resection) as an absolute contraindication to pancreaticoduodenectomy when the latter is performed as part of a multimodality approach to pancreatic cancer. Therefore, we do not perform random lymph node sampling for frozen-section analysis at the time of pancreaticoduodenectomy. Positive lymph nodes outside the resection margins (e.g., celiac axis, para-aortic, base of small bowel mesentery) usually imply advanced incurable disease, and a pancreaticoduodenectomy would not be performed. Each patient should be considered individually; for example, in a high-risk patient (due to medical comorbidity or oncologic concerns) with suspicious adenopathy, a positive regional lymph node may be viewed as a contraindication to proceeding with pancreaticoduodenectomy.

In the absence of extrapancreatic metastatic disease, one can proceed directly with tumor resection; in our practice, intraoperative maneuvers to assess local tumor resectability are unnecessary if adequate preoperative imaging with high-quality CT has been performed. The assessment of local tumor resectability preoperatively rather than intraoperatively is a major innovation in the surgical management of localized pancreatic cancer. Traditionally, two intraoperative maneuvers were used by the surgeon to determine if the primary tumor is resectable. First, a Kocher maneuver was performed to enable the surgeon to determine the relationship of the tumor to the SMA (Fig. 122–3). It is often difficult or impossible to assess accurately this critical tumor-vessel relationship after a Kocher maneuver, especially for larger tumors, for those containing significant peritumoral fibrosis, or in reoperative cases. The relationship of the tumor to the right lateral wall of the SMA is the most critical aspect of the *pre*treatment staging evaluation.

The second maneuver traditionally performed to assess resectability was to develop a plane of dissection between the anterior surface of the SMPV confluence and the neck of the pancreas to exclude tumor involvement, which in the opinion of most surgeons precludes resection. The rationale for this maneuver is also unclear, however, be-

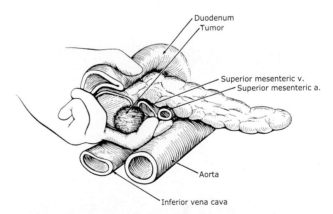

Figure 122–3. Palpation of the relationship of the tumor to the mesenteric vessels after the Kocher maneuver; it is often impossible to assess this critical relationship accurately. Preoperative thin-section contrast-enhanced computed tomography is the imaging modality of choice to assess this relationship. a., artery; v., vein. (From Cusack JC Jr, Fuhrman GM, Lee JE, Evans DB: Managing unsuspected tumor invasion of the superior mesenteric-portal venous confluence during pancreaticoduodenectomy. Am J Surg 1994;168:352–354.)

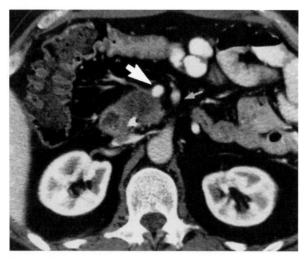

Figure 122–4. Contrast-enhanced computed tomography demonstrating tumor involvement of the posterolateral wall of the superior mesenteric vein *(large arrow)*. Pancreaticoduodenectomy will likely require segmental resection of the superior mesenteric vein. Note the normal fat plane between the low-density tumor and the superior mesenteric artery *(small arrow)*.

cause the anterior wall is rarely involved. Preoperative contrast-enhanced CT can often alert the surgeon to the possibility of isolated tumor invasion of the superior mesenteric vein (SMV) or the SMPV confluence (Fig. 122–4). Venous involvement is frequently an unexpected finding at the time of laparotomy despite good-quality preoperative imaging. Surgeons who perform pancreaticoduodenectomy should have the technical ability to perform partial or segmental venous resection.

The surgical resection as performed by the authors is divided into six clearly defined steps (Fig. 122–5). The most difficult and oncologically important part of the operation is step 6. After traction sutures are placed on the superior and the inferior borders of the pancreas, the pancreas is transected (usually with electrocautery) at the level of the portal vein. If there is evidence of tumor

adherence to the portal vein or the SMV, the pancreas can be divided at a more distal location in preparation for segmental venous resection. The specimen is separated from the SMV by ligation and division of the small venous tributaries to the uncinate process and the pancreatic head. Exposure of the SMA is necessary for direct ligation of the inferior pancreaticoduodenal artery. The specimen should be removed from the right lateral wall of the SMA under direct vision.

The soft tissue adjacent to the proximal 3 to 4 cm of the SMA represents the retroperitoneal margin (Fig. 122–6). A grossly positive retroperitoneal margin should not be seen if high-quality preoperative imaging has been performed. A microscopically positive retroperitoneal margin will occur in 10% to 20% of patients; margin positivity results from the tendency of pancreatic cancer to spread along perineural sheaths, not always from direct extension of the primary tumor.

Pancreatic, Biliary, and Gastrointestinal Reconstruction

Reconstruction after pancreaticoduodenectomy begins by bringing the proximal jejunum through a defect in the transverse mesocolon (retrocolic) to allow creation of a pancreaticojejunal anastomosis (Fig. 122–7). The pancreatic remnant is mobilized from the retroperitoneum and the splenic vein for a distance of 2 to 3 cm. In our practice, a two-layer, end-to-side, duct-to-mucosa pancreaticojejunostomy is performed over a small Silastic stent. If the pancreatic duct is dilated, a stent is not employed. The pancreatic anastomosis is followed by a single-layer biliary anastomosis; a stent is rarely used in the construction of the hepaticojejunostomy. The biliary anastomosis is followed by an anticolic, end-to-side gastrojejunostomy (two-layer anastomosis) or a duodenojejunostomy (one-layer anastomosis) if a pylorus-preserving technique is used (see later). Two closed-suction drains are placed before abdominal closure—one anterior to the pancreatic anastomosis and one in the right upper quadrant. A gas-

Pancreaticoduodenectomy

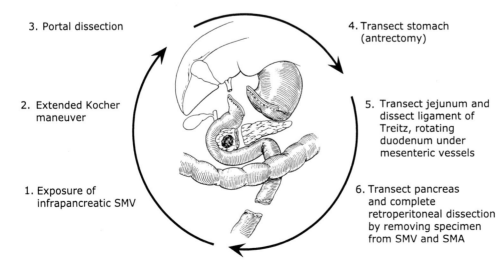

3. Portal dissection

2. Extended Kocher maneuver

1. Exposure of infrapancreatic SMV

4. Transect stomach (antrectomy)

5. Transect jejunum and dissect ligament of Treitz, rotating duodenum under mesenteric vessels

6. Transect pancreas and complete retroperitoneal dissection by removing specimen from SMV and SMA

Figure 122–5. Six surgical steps of pancreaticoduodenectomy as performed at The University of Texas M.D. Anderson Cancer Center. The operation is performed in a clockwise direction beginning at 6 o'clock. The final step in tumor resection is when the specimen is removed from the right lateral wall of the superior mesenteric artery (SMA). SMV, superior mesenteric vein.

complications of parenteral nutrition in patients who require prolonged hospitalization because of perioperative or postoperative complications. The most common complication associated with pancreaticoduodenectomy is poor gastric emptying, resulting in inadequate nutritional support; placement of an 18-French gastrostomy tube and a 10-French jejunal feeding tube for postoperative alimentation prevents needless patient morbidity.

Pylorus Preservation

Preservation of the antrum and the pylorus in combination with pancreaticoduodenectomy was first described by Traverso and Longmire in 1978. Since then, increasing numbers of pancreatic surgeons have employed this modification of the procedure. Proponents claim that preservation of the pylorus improves long-term upper gastrointestinal function and the nutritional profile. Non-proponents argue that nutritional improvements are modest, come at the expense of an increase in early postoperative delayed gastric emptying, and may compromise oncologic margins of resection and peripyloric lymphadenectomy. Published data have yielded mixed results. Despite the controversy, most pancreatic surgeons would agree that pylorus preservation should not be performed in patients with bulky tumors of the pancreatic head, duodenal tumors involving the first or the second portions of the duodenum, or lesions associated with grossly positive pyloric or peripyloric lymph nodes.

Tumors of the Pancreatic Body and the Tail

Because adenocarcinomas of the pancreatic body and the tail do not cause obstruction of the common bile duct or other pathognomonic symptoms, early diagnosis is rare; virtually all patients have locally advanced or metastatic disease at the time of diagnosis. CT provides an excellent assessment of the relationship of the tumor to the celiac axis and the origin of the SMA; arterial encasement is present in the majority of patients. In the rare patients who appear to have resectable disease, staging laparoscopy will identify occult metastatic disease in 50% and will prevent nontherapeutic celiotomy. Multimodality therapy is preferred owing to the short survival reported for most patients following surgery alone.

POSTOPERATIVE MANAGEMENT AND COMPLICATIONS

In the authors' practice, all patients who undergo pancreaticoduodenectomy receive a standardized approach to postoperative care (critical pathway). Included in the critical pathway is drain management. The lateral subhepatic drain is removed on the second postoperative day if there is no bile in the drainage fluid and the output is less than 150 mL/24 hours. The amylase level in the medial drain (placed near the pancreatic anastomosis) is checked on the third postoperative day. If the amylase level is normal and the drain output is less than 200 mL/24 hours, the medial drain is removed on the fourth postoperative day.

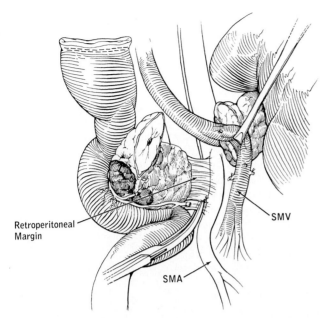

Figure 122–6. The final step in tumor resection during pancreaticoduodenectomy. Medial retraction of the superior mesenteric–portal vein confluence facilitates dissection of the lateral wall of the proximal superior mesenteric artery (SMA); this site represents the retroperitoneal margin (also referred to as the mesenteric margin) and should be identified and inked for the pathologist. The inferior pancreaticoduodenal artery (or arteries) is identified at its origin from the SMA, is ligated, and is divided. SMV, superior mesenteric vein.

trostomy tube and a jejunostomy tube are used. A gastrostomy tube prevents prolonged nasogastric tube placement and facilitates independent patient care. Enteral feeding via the jejunostomy tube prevents the expense and the

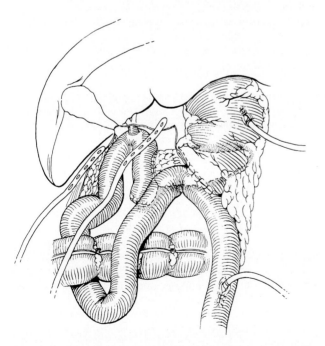

Figure 122–7. The completed reconstruction of the pancreas, the bile duct, and the stomach after pancreaticoduodenectomy. Note gastrostomy tube, jejunostomy tube for enteral feeding, and two closed suction drains.

Postoperative fevers commonly develop, but those occurring after the third or fourth postoperative day demand careful evaluation. Potential sources include those common to all types of major abdominal surgery (e.g., pneumonia, deep venous thrombosis, central line sepsis, urinary tract infection, and wound infection). Complications specific to pancreaticoduodenectomy usually involve the pancreaticojejunostomy, which is the anastomosis at greatest risk for leak (including about 15%). Because leaks from either the biliary or the gastric anastomosis are uncommon, intra-abdominal sepsis is considered to be due to a pancreatic anastomotic leak until proven otherwise. The study of choice for evaluation of presumed intra-abdominal sepsis is CT. A localized fluid collection near the pancreaticojejunostomy with or without an air-fluid level should prompt CT-guided aspiration. Percutaneous catheter drainage is indicated if the fluid appears infected on gross examination. After pancreatectomy, it is common to see nonloculated ascitic fluid on postoperative CT; this finding rarely represents infection or anastomotic leak and does not require aspiration or drainage unless clinical signs of sepsis persist and another source of infection has not been identified. Anastomotic leaks at the pancreaticojejunostomy generally close once adequate drainage has been established. Octreotide is often used to treat established pancreatic anastomotic leaks that required percutaneous drainage.

Postoperative gastrointestinal or drain tract bleeding should prompt immediate evaluation with arteriography. Although uncommon, an arterioenteric fistula from a pseudoaneurysm may occur 10 days to a few weeks after pancreaticoduodenectomy. The most common cause is a pancreatic anastomotic leak resulting in inflammation, infection, and blowout of the ligated stump of the gastroduodenal artery. Gastrointestinal or drain tract bleeding represents a true emergency; the only patients likely to survive are those in whom the diagnosis is made immediately. Arteriography with embolization of the hepatic artery is the treatment of choice. Reoperation and attempted surgical control of hemorrhage from the stump of the gastroduodenal artery are exceedingly difficult and, in our opinion, carry a mortality rate higher than that associated with hepatic artery embolization.

Patients are ready for discharge when they are afebrile, are able to tolerate gastrostomy tube clamping without nausea or vomiting, and have adequate caloric intake from oral feeding or a combination of oral and jejunostomy feedings. Medical management of poor gastric emptying with erythromycin is attempted if the period of delayed emptying is greater than 2 weeks. Patients are discharged with instructions to follow a regimen of pancreatic enzyme replacement and administration of an H_2 histamine receptor antagonist.

ADJUVANT THERAPY AND OUTCOMES

Preoperative and Postoperative Chemoradiation

The Gastrointestinal Tumor Study Group (GITSG) performed the first prospective randomized study of adjuvant chemoradiation (500 mg/m²/day of 5-fluorouracil for 6 days and 40 Gy of radiation) versus observation after curative pancreaticoduodenectomy. This study demonstrated a survival advantage with multimodality therapy compared with resection alone (20 months vs. 11 months). Similar results have been reported from Johns Hopkins Hospital, where 120 patients were reviewed who underwent pancreaticoduodenectomy for adenocarcinoma of the pancreatic head during a 4-year period. The median survival was 19.5 months for patients receiving adjuvant therapy, compared with 13.5 months for the group who received surgery alone. In 1987, the European Organization for Research and Treatment of Cancer initiated a prospective, randomized, multi-institutional trial comparing adjuvant chemoradiation after curative pancreatectomy with surgery alone. Between 1987 and 1995, 218 patients with periampullary cancers of all types were randomly assigned to receive either chemoradiation (40 Gy in a split course and 5-fluorouracil given as a continuous infusion at a dose of 25 mg/kg/day during external-beam radiation therapy) or no further treatment. In the 114 patients with pancreatic cancer, the median duration of survival was 17 months with adjuvant treatment versus 13 months without treatment.

This apparent survival benefit with postoperative chemoradiation, combined with the growing interest in preoperative therapy for other solid tumor malignancies, has prompted several institutions to initiate studies exploring the value of chemoradiation delivered before pancreaticoduodenectomy (*neo*adjuvant therapy). Potential advantages of preoperative versus postoperative chemoradiation include the following: (1) Because chemotherapy and radiation are given first, delayed postoperative recovery has no effect on the delivery of multimodality therapy; (2) the frequency of pancreaticojejunal anastomotic leaks is decreased in patients who receive preoperative chemoradiation; (3) the high frequency of resection with histologically positive margins (approximately 20%) suggests that surgery alone is inadequate local therapy; and (4) patients who develop disseminated disease (seen on restaging studies) after chemoradiation will not be subjected to laparotomy.

Whenever possible, pancreaticoduodenectomy should be performed as part of a multimodality treatment program (protocol-based, if possible) to include either preoperative or postoperative chemoradiation.

Outcomes

Recent advances in surgical technique, anesthesia, and critical care have resulted in a 30-day in-hospital mortality rate of less than 4% for pancreaticoduodenectomy performed at major referral centers by experienced surgeons. These low mortality rates appear to be a function of the volume of pancreatic surgery performed by the individual surgeon and the institution. For example, Birkmeyer and colleagues at Dartmouth Medical School studied 7229 Medicare patients older than 65 years of age who underwent pancreaticoduodenectomy at 1772 hospitals between 1992 and 1995. The study population was divided into quartiles according to hospital volume, with high-

Pearls and Pitfalls

PEARLS

- Pancreatic cancer is an aggressive disease in need of more effective therapies.
- In the absence of major innovations in the treatment of metastatic pancreatic cancer, the greatest opportunity to improve the length and the quality of patient survival lies in the direct control of the primary care provider and the general surgeon.
- Certain subgroups are at higher risk for developing pancreatic cancer, including patients with chronic pancreatitis, patients with hereditary pancreatitis, and non-obese adults older than 40 years of age with recent-onset diabetes mellitus.
- Use of high-quality imaging studies allows accurate pretreatment staging and can prevent unnecessary surgery (and its mortality and morbidity) in patients with unresectable pancreatic cancer.
- Nonresectable pancreatic cancers can be palliated with biliary stents and celiac plexus blocks for pain.
- In patients without extrapancreatic disease whose primary tumor fulfills the CT criteria for resectability, pancreaticoduodenectomy should be performed in an organized, methodical series of steps, with a resulting in-hospital mortality rate of 4% or less.
- All patients with pancreatic cancer should be offered participation in clinical studies, when available, evaluating new and innovative treatment strategies, including adjuvant or neoadjuvant chemoradiation.
- New molecular techniques may allow earlier diagnosis or even screening in high-risk subsets.
- In patients with locally advanced or metastatic disease, do not consider the use of chemotherapy or radiation therapy without cytologic or histologic confirmation of invasive carcinoma.

PITFALLS

Common Errors in Preoperative Evaluation

- Misinterpretation of CT findings is possible. The relationship between the low-density tumor and the SMA and the SMV should be clearly delineated.
- The operative plan should be specific and clearly conveyed to the patient.

Common Errors in Intraoperative Management

- Local tumor resectability should be established preoperatively; there is no role for extensive dissection to assess resectability once the abdomen has been opened.
- The portal dissection (step 3, Fig. 122–5) and the retroperitoneal dissection (step 6) are the two most difficult steps in performing pancreaticoduodenectomy. During portal dissection, overly aggressive dissection at the origin of the gastroduodenal artery can result in intimal dissection of the hepatic artery. During retroperitoneal dissection, failure to mobilize the SMPV confluence fully risks injury to the SMA and also may result in a positive margin owing to incomplete removal of the uncinate process and the mesenteric soft tissue adjacent to the SMA.

volume centers defined as those that performed five or more pancreaticoduodenectomies per year. The 40 high-volume hospitals (2% of all hospitals) performed 1541 (21%) of the 7229 pancreaticoduodenectomies. The hospital mortality rate was 11% overall, 4% in high-volume hospitals, and 10% to 16% in medium-volume (two to five Whipple procedures per year) and very low-volume (less than one Whipple procedure per year) hospitals. These data show a definite relationship between surgical volume and outcome. A significant level of experience with major pancreatic resection is thus necessary to achieve low levels of surgical morbidity and mortality. These studies support the concept of patient referral to centers of high volume for potential curative surgery in pancreatic cancer.

SELECTED READINGS

Birkmeyer JD, Finlayson SR, Tosteson AN, et al: Effect of hospital volume on in-hospital mortality with pancreaticoduodenectomy. Surgery 1999;125:250.

Breslin TM, Hess KR, Harbison DB, et al: Neoadjuvant chemoradiation for adenocarcinoma of the pancreas: Treatment variables and survival duration. Ann Surg Oncol 2001;8:123.

Evans DB, Abbruzzese JL, Willett CG: Cancer of the pancreas. In DeVita VT, Hellman S, Rosenberg SA (eds): Cancer: Principles and Practice of Oncology, 6th ed. Philadelphia, Lippincott Williams & Wilkins, 2001, pp 1126–1161.

Evans DB, Lee JE, Pisters PWT: Pancreaticoduodenectomy (Whipple operation) and total pancreatectomy for cancer. In Nyhus LM, Baker RJ, Fischer JF (eds): Mastery of Surgery, 3rd ed. Boston, Little Brown, 1997, pp 1233–1249.

Evans DB, Pisters PWT, Lee JE, et al: Preoperative chemoradiation strategies for localized adenocarcinoma of the pancreas. J Hepatobiliary Pancreat Surg 1998;5:242.

Leach SD, Lee JE, Charnsangavej C, et al: Survival following pancreaticoduodenectomy with resection of the superior mesenteric-portal vein confluence for adenocarcinoma of the pancreatic head. Br J Surg 1998;85:611.

Lillemoe KD, Cameron JL, Hardacre JM, et al: Is prophylactic gastrojejunostomy indicated for unresectable periampullary cancer? A prospective randomized trial. Ann Surg 1999;230:322.

Lin PW, Lin YJ: Prospective randomized comparison between pylorus-preserving and standard pancreaticoduodenectomy. Br J Surg 1999;86:603.

Porter GA, Pisters PWT, Mansyur C, et al: Cost and utilization impact of a clinical pathway for patients undergoing pancreaticoduodenectomy. Ann Surg Oncol 2000;7:484.

Regine WF, John WJ, Mohiuddin M: Evolving trends in combined modality therapy for pancreatic cancer. J Hepatobiliary Pancreat Surg 1998;5:227.

Spitz FR, Abbruzzese JL, Lee JE, et al: Preoperative and postoperative chemoradiation strategies in patients treated with pancreaticoduodenectomy for adenocarcinoma of the pancreas. J Clin Oncol 1997;15:928.

Traverso LW, Longmire WP Jr: Preservation of the pylorus in pancreaticoduodenectomy. Surg Gynecol Obstet 1978;146:959.

Yeo CJ, Cameron JL, Sohn TA, et al: Six hundred fifty consecutive pancreaticoduodenectomies in the 1990s: Pathology, complications, and outcomes. Ann Surg 1997;226:248.

Chapter 123
Nonfunctional Islet Cell Neoplasms

Said Elshihabi and Alexander R. Miller

Islet cell neoplasms of the pancreas constitute a rare clinical entity. Nonfunctional islet cell neoplasms are subtler in presentation than their functional counterparts, often resulting in delayed or missed diagnoses. If the clinician does not consider these lesions in the differential diagnosis of pancreatic masses, errors will be made in the diagnostic evaluation as well as in planning appropriate therapy. This concept is clinically relevant because of the uniformly better prognosis associated with this group of pancreatic neoplasms compared with more common ductal adenocarcinomas of the pancreas. Islet cell neoplasms warrant a more aggressive surgical approach, even in the setting of locally advanced disease. The assumption that a locally advanced pancreatic mass represents ductal adenocarcinoma will deny potentially curative surgery to selected patients. For these reasons, differentiation of islet cell neoplasms from other pancreatic masses is critical.

Nonfunctioning islet cell neoplasms were originally defined as lesions that do not display clinical symptoms related to the release of a regulatory hormone. The development of specific radioimmunoassays and monoclonal antibodies used for immunohistochemical staining has facilitated the detection of clinically silent islet cell tumors in patients considered to have "nonfunctional" pancreatic neoplasms. The use of these methods combined with advanced imaging techniques has forced reconsideration of the definition of nonfunctional and has resulted in a greater number of clinically silent intra-abdominal masses being diagnosed incidentally. Although a number of these neoplasms demonstrate immunohistochemical staining for certain hormones, the absence of associated symptoms remains the diagnostic standard for their designation as nonfunctional.

CLINICAL PRESENTATION

Islet cell neoplasms are present in only a small proportion of patients with pancreatic neoplasms. These neoplasms occur in fewer than 1 in 100,000 people per year. The subset of nonfunctioning islet cell tumors within this group accounts for approximately 1 in 5 million patients. Estimates of the proportion of nonfunctioning islet cell tumors (as a numerator of all islet cell neoplasms) range from 15% to 65%. The average age of presentation is in the fifth to sixth decade of life.

In comparison with ductal adenocarcinoma, islet cell neoplasms are characterized by slower growth and more gradual development of symptoms. They tend to be relatively large (2 cm or greater) with a significant chance (30% to 60%) of metastasis at the time of diagnosis. The complaints of patients typically include nausea, vomiting, and abdominal and back pain. Larger tumors may produce dyspepsia, early satiety, extrahepatic biliary obstruc-

tion, gastrointestinal bleeding, and obstruction. Unlike ductal adenocarcinoma of the pancreas, islet cell tumors often do not obstruct the common bile duct. Anorexia, weight loss, and malaise are more prevalent with malignant neoplasms. Constipation and steatorrhea may be present but are more common with typical pancreatic adenocarcinomas.

The primary determinant of the clinical presentation is the anatomic location of the neoplasm. Although less frequently than with ductal adenocarcinomas, nonfunctional islet cell neoplasms in the head of the pancreas may cause biliary obstruction, resulting in jaundice, or may invade intrapancreatic nerves, causing back pain. Neoplasms located in the body and the tail of the gland may present as palpable masses and may also cause back pain. Unfortunately, gastroduodenal symptoms occur late in the course of left-sided pancreatic tumors. Although the odds of identifying and diagnosing these masses continue to improve, 10% to 15% of nonfunctional islet cell neoplasms continue to be diagnosed inadvertently during radiologic imaging or surgical exploration.

PREOPERATIVE MANAGEMENT

Clinical Assessment

A crucial aspect of the evaluation of a patient suspected of having a pancreatic neoplasm is determining whether an islet cell neoplasm should be included in the differential diagnosis. Patients should be queried about duration of symptoms, clinical performance status, and family history of similar problems or familial diseases predisposing to islet cell neoplasms (i.e., multiple endocrine neoplasia type 1, von Hippel-Lindau disease, tuberous sclerosis, or von Recklinghausen's disease). Ruling out a functional islet cell neoplasm is facilitated by inquiring about symptoms such as hyperglycemia (glucagonoma, somatostatinoma), hypoglycemia (insulinoma), peptic ulcer disease (gastrinoma), and severe diarrhea (gastrinoma, watery diarrhea hypokalemia acidosis [WDHA] syndrome). Physical examination should include assessment of nutritional status, skin condition (jaundice or skin disease such as migratory necrolytic erythema occurs with glucagonomas), lymph node basins, abdomen, rectum, and lower extremities.

There are four hormone-related reasons why a nonfunctional islet cell tumor may appear clinically silent.

1. Neoplasms may not produce sufficient serum hormone concentrations to cause clinical symptoms.
2. The hormone(s) may be produced but not released into the systemic circulation.
3. The hormone may remain in its inactive or proform.

4. The hormone may not produce symptoms despite large amounts in the circulation (e.g., pancreatic polypeptide, neurotensin).

A serum screen for peptides associated with nonfunctional islet cell neoplasms (e.g., pancreatic polypeptide, substance P, and neurotensin) may be beneficial if an islet cell tumor is suspected, but it is not routinely recommended outside the context of a clinical protocol because the yield will be low. About 10% of patients with clinically diagnosed nonfunctioning islet cell tumors have increased serum levels of related peptides (e.g., somatostatin, vasoactive intestinal polypeptide, gastrin, glucagon, and calcitonin). Laboratory evaluation should include serum electrolyte analysis, complete blood cell count, coagulation studies, and hepatic enzyme analysis.

Radiologic Assessment

A variety of imaging techniques have been used in the preoperative evaluation of pancreatic neoplasms, and radiologic clues may allow one to assign priority to clinical suspicion regarding the differential diagnosis of observed neoplasms. Ultrasonographic evaluation of pancreatic tumors includes transabdominal (transcutaneous), endoscopic, and intraoperative. Transabdominal ultrasonography allows identification of larger tumors (>2 cm in diameter). The ultrasonic appearance is affected by hyalinized stroma, hemorrhage, and, occasionally, cystic degeneration. Although accuracy rates in localizing nonductal tumors in the pancreas range from only 20% to 70%, ultrasonography is helpful in identifying metastatic disease to the liver. The echogenicity of metastatic lesions may vary. Hyperechogenic lesions suggest islet cells, whereas hepatic metastases from pancreatic adenocarcinoma are typically hypoechoic. Endoscopic ultrasonography (EUS) has become a favored diagnostic tool as experience with this modality has increased. EUS can visualize the entire pancreas and the surrounding structures and is particularly useful in detecting smaller lesions, with

sensitivity rates ranging from 77% to 100%. A recent study reported EUS-based detection of islet cell neoplasms as small as 5 mm. This study verified EUS and intraductal ultrasonography as being safe and useful procedures in detecting small tumors and differentiating neoplastic from focally inflammatory pancreatic disease.

A final mode of evaluation is intraoperative ultrasonography, a technique extremely useful for localizing small intrapancreatic lesions. Although this modality is more useful for patients suspected of having functional islet cell neoplasms (potentially amenable to enucleation), intraoperative evaluation of nonfunctional tumors may detect occult hepatic metastases or resolve unclear anatomic relationships. The sensitivity ranges from 75% to 100%.

Computed tomography (CT) is currently the optimal and most practical imaging tool for the evaluation of pancreatic masses. CT has a sensitivity rate of greater than 90% in detecting pancreatic neoplasms 2 cm or larger, particularly with dual-phase helical scanners and 3- to 5-mm sections through the pancreas. The viable hypervascular portions of an islet cell tumor usually appear hyperdense relative to the uninvolved adjacent parenchyma after intravenous contrast administration (Figs. 123–1 and 123–2). These findings are in contrast to the appearance of pancreatic ductal adenocarcinomas, which are typically hypodense on contrast-enhanced images. A major benefit of this imaging modality is its ability to detect areas of necrosis, calcification, and cystic degeneration. Owing to the hypervascular state of these tumors, they are prone to internal necrosis and may demonstrate nonenhanced regions of low attenuation. Dystrophic calcification, indicative of the chronic nature of most nonfunctioning islet cell neoplasms, has been reported in 20% to 25% of patients. CT features that are relatively uncommon in ductal adenocarcinomas but are frequently associated with islet cell neoplasms include large tumor size, hyperenhancement with intravenous contrast material, major cystic degeneration occasionally mimicking a unilocular cystic neoplasm, and calcification. These characteristics are also observed in metastatic lesions.

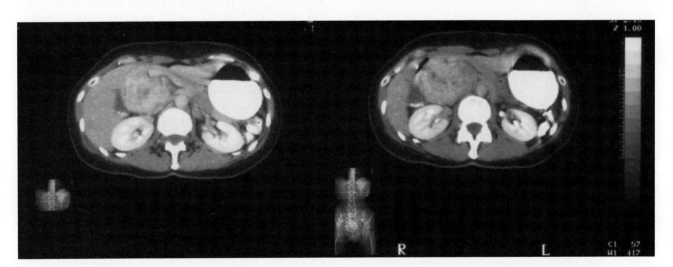

Figure 123–1. Computed tomography performed with intravenous and oral contrast agents, demonstrating a large hyperdense mass in the head of the pancreas that displaced the superior mesenteric artery and vein. This nonfunctional islet cell neoplasm was completely resected without the need for venous replacement, and the patient is alive more than 6 years postoperatively.

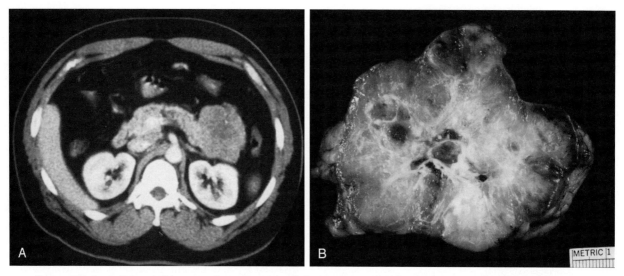

Figure 123–2. *A,* Computed tomography performed with intravenous and oral contrast agents, illustrating a large mass in the tail of the pancreas. This nonfunctional islet cell neoplasm was completely resected with distal pancreatectomy and splenectomy. *B,* Bisected gross specimen of the same neoplasm. This tumor demonstrates typical pathologic features, including pale color and surrounding areas of fibrosis generating a desmoplastic reaction within the pancreatic parenchyma.

The ability of magnetic resonance imaging to be an effective tool in the diagnosis and the evaluation of pancreatic masses has recently been enhanced by faster image acquisition and angiographic visualization. Pancreatic masses generally have very high intensity on T2-weighted images and fat-suppressed inversion-recovery images. T1-weighted images are more variable but are often of intermediate or low intensity. Moreover, magnetic resonance imaging with gadolinium is more sensitive to tumor vascularity than CT with intravenous contrast material. Dynamic gadolinium-enhanced images improve the accuracy of identification and differentiation of islet cell tumors from pancreatic adenocarcinomas. Magnetic resonance imaging of hepatic metastases employing mangofodipir, a novel contrast agent, has demonstrated T1-weighted image enhancement of metastases from nonfunctional islet cell tumors. The newest generation of magnetic resonance software will more accurately define characteristics of islet cell neoplasms.

Another modality for localization of clinically occult neuroendocrine neoplasms involves the radioisotope-labeled somatostatin analogue octreotide. Somatostatin receptor imaging with octreotide (Octreoscan) allows scintigraphic detection of lesions that possess somatostatin receptors. These receptors have been reported in most islet cell tumors regardless of functional status. Using ^{111}In-labeled octreotide, tumor localization with a total body scanner (preoperatively) or an intraoperative gamma counter may assist in diagnosis and subsequent tumor resection. Another advantage of this imaging tool is the ability to detect occult or distant metastases, especially those arising from nonfunctional islet cell tumors. One drawback of scintigraphic tumor detection is that uptake of the tracer is theoretically based on the number of somatostatin receptors rather than on the size of the neoplasm. Therefore, large tumors with few receptors may be undetected.

INTRAOPERATIVE MANAGEMENT

Within the surgical community, a more aggressive operative approach is well justified for islet cell neoplasms, in contrast to the management of ductal adenocarcinomas. The very nature of islet cell masses as "displacers" rather than "invaders" of local (vascular) anatomy warrants consideration of resection despite the presence of what appears to be locally advanced or even metastatic disease. There have been isolated reports of patients in whom the superior mesenteric vein has appeared virtually occluded, with development of collateral circulation, owing to a nonfunctioning islet cell tumor. At exploration, some neoplasms are completely resectable, with no need for venous resection or replacement because they externally compress but do not invade the superior mesenteric vein (see Fig. 123–1). Therefore, in the absence of known metastatic disease, the size or the local anatomy of the primary tumor should not necessarily preclude an attempt at curative resection.

The anatomic site of the primary lesion directs the type of resection. Because nonfunctioning islet cell neoplasms are typically larger and have a significant incidence of metastasis and, therefore, malignant potential, a simple enucleation procedure is usually not appropriate. A formal pancreatectomy should be performed unless there is a small pancreatic mass in a patient with significant comorbidity, which is rare. Nonfunctioning neoplasms in the body and the tail of the pancreas are best treated with distal pancreatectomy and splenectomy and not simple enucleation as for an insulinoma (see Fig. 123–2). Adjacent involved organs, including the transverse mesocolon, the stomach, the left adrenal gland, and Gerota's fascia, may all be removed en bloc. For masses involving the neck, the head, or the uncinate process of the pancreas, pancreatoduodenectomy is justified. Either a pylorus-preserving resection or a classic Whipple-type procedure is appropriate, depending on the surgeon's preference. Though displacement of mesenteric vessels appears to be more common than invasion, one should always be prepared to perform venous resection and replacement if preoperative imaging suggests loss of the normal fat plane between the superior mesenteric vein and the pancreas. Nodal metastases outside the usual field of resection (i.e., hepatoduodenal ligament, common hepatic artery, celiac plexus, or superior mesenteric artery) should not preclude an attempt at curative resection and should be included with the specimen.

Owing to the favorable course of these neoplasms, surgeons responsible for patients with a nonfunctioning islet cell neoplasm must not take a nihilistic approach toward their management. Obviously, treatment plans are individualized, but an aggressive approach is justified in a low-risk patient. Furthermore, palliation and cytoreduction are important considerations when evaluating symptomatic patients. Owing to tumor hypervascularity, severe gastrointestinal hemorrhage secondary to local invasion of the stomach or the duodenum can be an indication for palliative pancreatectomy and noncurative resection. A similar situation occurs in patients with obstructive jaundice secondary to a locally unresectable islet cell neoplasm. An operative biliary bypass is warranted, because this has been shown to be superior to an endoscopically placed biliary endoprosthesis for patients with the expectation of extended survival. Duodenal bypass via gastrojejunostomy should also be considered for patients with gastroduodenal obstruction.

Although most hepatic metastases from islet cell neoplasms are multiple and bilobar, the rare patient with resectable metastases should be given the chance for curative resection if the primary neoplasm can be controlled. If bulky residual disease outside the liver has been identified, hepatic resection is not warranted, because hepatic metastases themselves rarely cause local problems in patients with nonfunctional islet cell neoplasms.

POSTOPERATIVE MANAGEMENT

Postsurgical Care

The immediate postoperative management of patients with nonfunctional islet cell neoplasms of the pancreas is identical to that provided to patients undergoing pancreatic resection for other indications. Meticulous attention to cardiorespiratory status and fluid balance is paramount. Nutrition is critical, but controversy exists regarding the appropriate means of administration. Within 48 hours, the gut should be able to tolerate enteral feedings. Therefore, surgeons who place oral or jejunal feeding tubes may initiate low-volume hypotonic feedings in the early postoperative period. As is the case for most gastroenterologic surgical procedures, a milestone in postoperative care is the commencement of bowel function, which allows an oral diet to be initiated as well as consideration of transition from parenteral to oral medications. Attention to endocrine and exocrine pancreatic function is warranted; this is accomplished by monitoring serum glucose and by

clinical assessment of fecal fat for steatorrhea (oily, foul-smelling, floating stools). Insulin administration or pancreatic enzyme replacement may be required either temporarily or for long-term management.

Oncologic Follow-Up and Systemic Therapy

Oncologic surveillance of surgically treated patients involves regular clinical and radiologic assessment on an outpatient basis. A baseline evaluation is suggested 3 to 4 months after resection, and CT should be considered 4 to 6 months after resection. Clinical examinations are typically scheduled every 4 to 6 months for the first 5 years and annually thereafter. CT and chest radiographs are appropriately performed on an annual basis. If an elevation of serum peptide level was noted preoperatively, follow-up with serial analyses is appropriate, but this is rare.

Chemotherapy for nonfunctioning islet cell carcinomas is of unclear benefit but may be useful in selected patients with favorable performance status. Patients with nonfunctioning neoplasms derive little survival or symptomatic benefit from octreotide unless diarrhea is a symptom. Patients receiving long-term octreotide therapy must be monitored for the development of gallstones, which are known to occur in approximately 50% of treated individuals. The primary chemotherapeutic agents used against nonfunctioning islet cell neoplasms include streptozotocin and 5-fluorouracil. In contrast to ductal adenocarcinoma of the pancreas, in which adjuvant chemoradiation appears to increase survival, no similar data have been obtained in regard to islet cell neoplasms.

Recent studies have evaluated the role of chemoembolization therapy for liver metastases from pancreatic endocrine and neuroendocrine tumors. Coil embolization is combined with regional (via hepatic artery) delivery of chemotherapy. Observations of increased overall survival, reduction in tumor bulk, and diminished hormone levels have been reported.

Another form of palliation of hepatic metastases includes ablative therapy. Various approaches have been described for the treatment of hepatic metastases (primarily from colorectal carcinoma) and have recently been used in patients with refractory neuroendocrine tumors. Both cryosurgery and radiofrequency ablation have dramatically relieved symptoms, with significant reduction in the occurrence of tumor markers.

COMPLICATIONS

Pancreatic resections are fraught with complications, but recent data suggest that excellent outcomes may be achieved in centers experienced in the management of such procedures. The most common complication associated with pancreaticoduodenectomy is leakage of the pancreaticojejunostomy site. Randomized studies evaluating the use of octreotide in patients undergoing pancreatic resection have yielded equivocal results. Our current approach is to provide octreotide (150 μg subcutaneously three times a day) to patients undergoing pancreatic re-

---

Pearls and Pitfalls

PEARLS

- Include islet cell neoplasms in the differential diagnosis of pancreatic masses.
- Locally advanced lesions on CT imaging are often resectable; every possible attempt at curative resection should be explored.
- Treat these patients more aggressively than patients with ductal adenocarcinoma of the pancreas.
- There is a role for palliative debulking and resection of (symptomatic) metastatic disease.
- Chemotherapeutic options include 5-fluorouracil and streptozotocin.

PITFALLS

- The term *nonfunctional* refers to the lack of a definable symptom complex related to oversecretion of a hormone.
- Do not assume poor outcome; median survival is 3 to 5 years.
- Do not assume that mesenteric vessel compromise means that the tumor has invaded the vessel; islet cell neoplasms may displace or compress externally without invasion. Be prepared to perform venous resection or contiguous organ resection if the tumor is locally advanced.
- Histologic differentiation between benign and malignant islet cell neoplasms is difficult; metastatic disease or contiguous organ involvement provides a clear demonstration of malignancy.

---

section who are clinically identified to have "soft" or normal pancreatic parenchyma. Pancreatic leaks are suspected based on postoperative temperature elevation or leukocytosis, often beginning 5 or more days after resection. If a drain has been left near the anastomosis, alteration of the output and the character of the drain effluent will be noted. Indeed, one may sample the drain fluid before considering drain removal to assess amylase content; concentrations of amylase of more than 500 to 1500 U/L are indicative of anastomotic leak. If a drain is not in place at the time of leak recognition, percutaneous drainage can typically be accomplished with interventional radiologic assistance. Reoperation is rarely necessary, except for postoperative bleeding. If bleeding occurs at the pancreaticojejunostomy site, jejunotomy just distal to the anastomosis should be considered to allow suture control of hemorrhage without anastomotic disruption.

CONCLUSION

Nonfunctioning pancreatic islet cell neoplasms remain difficult to diagnose owing to their clinically subtle presentation and rarity. Despite the frequent presence of hepatic and nodal metastases, the evaluation and assessment of these neoplasms must be aggressive because surgical treatment may offer substantial benefit to the patient. With more advanced imaging and diagnostic modalities, the detection of such masses has become more

sensitive and accurate. Along with contemporary imaging modalities, novel forms of nonsurgical therapy may soon show promise in treating hepatic metastases and therefore further improve survival rates associated with these neoplasms.

SELECTED READINGS

Broder LE, Carter SK: Pancreatic islet cell carcinoma. Clinical features of 52 patients. Ann Intern Med 1973;79:101.

Cheslyn-Curtis S, Sitaram V, Williamson RC: Management of non-functioning neuroendocrine tumors of the pancreas. Br J Surg 1993;80:625.

Dial PF, Braasch JW, Rossi RL, et al: Management of nonfunctioning islet cell tumors of the pancreas. Surg Clin North Am 1985;65:291.

Eckhauser FE, Cheung PS, Vinik AI, et al: Nonfunctioning malignant neuroendocrine tumors of the pancreas. Surgery 1986;100:978.

Eelkema EA, Stephens DH, Ward EM, Sheedy PF II: CT features of nonfunctioning islet cell carcinoma. AJR Am J Roentgenol 1984;143:943.

Evans DB, Skibber JM, Lee JE, et al: Nonfunctioning islet cell carcinoma of the pancreas. Surgery 1993;114:1175.

Legaspi A, Brennan MF: Management of islet cell carcinoma. Surgery 1988;104:1018.

Lo CY, van Heerden JA, Thompson GB, et al: Islet cell carcinoma of the pancreas. World J Surg 1996;20:878.

Prinz RA, Badrinath K, Chejfec G, et al: "Nonfunctioning" islet cell carcinoma of the pancreas. Am Surg 1983;49:345.

Schwartz RW, Munfakh NA, Zwqeng TN, et al: Nonfunctioning cystic neuroendocrine neoplasms of the pancreas. Surgery 1994;115:645.

Thompson GB, van Heerden JA, Grant CS, et al: Islet cell carcinomas of the pancreas: A twenty-year experience. Surgery 1988;104:1011.

White TJ, Edney JA, Thompson JS, et al: Is there a prognostic difference between functional and nonfunctional islet cell tumors? Am J Surg 1994;168:627.

Yeo CJ, Wang BH, Anthone GJ, Cameron JL: Surgical experience with pancreatic islet cell tumors. Arch Surg 1993;128:1143.

Hernia

Chapter 124

Femoral Hernia

Jeffrey T. Landers and David Krusch

A femoral hernia is a protrusion of preperitoneal or intraperitoneal tissue through the femoral canal, medial to the femoral vein, and into the femoral triangle. Femoral region hernias can also occur in external femoral (Hasselbach's), prevascular (Teale's), retrovascular (Serafini), pectineal (Callison-Cloquet), and lacunar ligament (de Laugier) positions (Fig. 124–1).

HISTORY

Guy de Chauliac (c. 1298–1368 AD), in his *Chirurgia Magna*, was the first known author to differentiate between femoral and inguinal hernia. Repair from below the inguinal ligament was described originally by Lawrence (1818) and later by Astley Cooper (1827), Socin (1879), Dubreuil (1880), Wood (1885), Cushing (1888), and Bassini (1894). The Lawrence method involved closing the femoral canal as high as possible by suturing Poupart's ligament to the pectineal fascia and had about a 10% recurrence rate (Tanner, 1964). The approach from below the inguinal ligament was later modified so that the inguinal ligament was sutured to Cooper's ligament (Skandalakis, 1993). Gilbert's (1991) mesh plug has also been used in femoral hernia repair from below the inguinal ligament.

Femoral hernia repair from above the inguinal ligament was first described by Annandale (1876). Suturing of the inguinal ligament to Cooper's ligament from above was first described by Ruggi (1892), and Lotheissen (1898) sutured the conjoined tendon to Cooper's ligament. Koontz (1964) proposed a rectus sheath–relaxing incision to release the tension caused by suturing the conjoined tendon to Cooper's ligament, but other authors (e.g., Nyhus, 1964) denied the need for a relaxing incision.

CLINICAL PRESENTATION AND DIAGNOSIS

Femoral hernias often present as a typical inguinal hernia with symptoms of discomfort or, on occasion, an intermittent lump or straining. They are more common in women, especially thin women. The unwary surgeon will be surprised later when he or she opens an access into the inguinal canal and does not find a hernia. Other common presentations are those of a mass, presumed to be an "inguinal node" or a bowel obstruction of unknown cause. On physical examination, any nonreducible mass in the femoral triangle should be considered an incarcerated femoral hernia until proved otherwise. Similarly, the femoral triangle should also be examined for a small mass in all patients with a small bowel obstruction. The diagnosis of a femoral hernia is a clinical one.

PRACTICAL ASPECTS OF FEMORAL HERNIA REPAIR

All femoral hernias should be repaired owing to the relatively high incidence of incarceration and strangulation of the hernia contents because of the often narrow neck of the sac at the femoral canal. The basic concept behind all of the listed repairs is twofold: (1) reduction of the hernia contents from the femoral canal, and (2) obliteration of the canal to prevent future herniation. Reduction of the sac contents can be as simple as manual reduction, or complex enough to require division of the inguinal ligament with potential bowel resection via an opening of the floor of the inguinal canal. Likewise, there have been numerous techniques described for obliteration of the canal. The simplest repair has utilized a "plug" of prosthetic material inserted into the canal, usually a self-made, rolled-up polypropylene plug, but the more tradi-

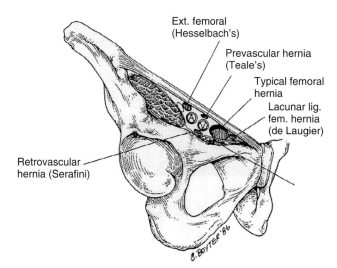

Figure 124–1. Anatomy of right inguinal hernia defects, as seen anteriorly. Note femoral canal just medial to the external iliac vein as it passes under the inguinal ligament to form the femoral vein. ext., external; fem., femoral; lig., ligament. (From Skandalakis JE: Surgical Anatomy and Technique: A Pocket Manual. New York, Springer-Verlag, 1995.)

tional repair has been suture approximation of the conjoined region to Cooper's ligament. Described in the following are the four most common repair techniques used in a modern surgical practice (infrainguinal repair, anterior transinguinal repair, posterior preperitoneal repair, and laparoscopic repair).

INFRAINGUINAL REPAIR

This approach involves the following steps. Incise transversely over the femoral swelling (femoral triangle) and with careful, sharp dissection expose the hernia sac. Open the sac and inspect the contents. If contents are viable, reduce carefully into the abdominal cavity. Infarcted preperitoneal fat should be resected. An infarcted loop of bowel usually cannot be resected with reanastomosis performed through the hernia defect, but a counterincision via either a preperitoneal approach or a formal celiotomy is necessary.

If the hernia cannot be reduced into the peritoneal cavity, incise the inguinal ligament to widen the hernia ring. With the sac contents reduced, ligate the hernia sac with 2-0 silk suture, excise the sac, and reduce the remainder into the peritoneal cavity. Suture the inguinal ligament to Cooper's ligament with 2-0 Prolene (Fig. 124–2). An alternative is to insert a mesh plug and secure it to the pectineus fascia posteriorly, inguinal ligament anteriorly, and Cooper's ligament (if possible) with interrupted 2-0 Prolene sutures.

ANTERIOR (TRANSINGUINAL) REPAIR

Femoral hernias can be repaired via the typical inguinal hernia approach. To do this, the inguinal canal is entered through the transversalis fascia, and the cord mobilized. However, because a femoral hernia occurs posterior to

the inguinal floor, exposure of the orifice requires creation of a complete direct inguinal hernia by transecting the transversalis fascia from the medial edge of the inferior epigastric vessels at the internal ring to the pubic tubercle. This then exposes the preperitoneal space, and with careful blunt dissection the femoral canal (and hernia sac) is relatively easily exposed. Repair of the defect is completed by a McVay repair of Cooper's ligament, with approximation of the transversalis and conjoint tendon (if present) to Cooper's ligament with a transition stitch up to the inguinal ligament at the medial edge of the external iliac vein as it passes under the inguinal ligament. This maneuver obliterates the femoral canal. If the defect is big or there is too much tension at the repair, a sheet of prosthetic mesh (usually polypropylene) can patch the defect, being sewn to Cooper's ligament and then draped rostrally *under* the transversalis fascia.

POSTERIOR (PREPERITONEAL) REPAIR

Many surgeons believe this approach to be the most versatile because it gives the best visualization of femoral hernias. The incision begins several finger breadths rostral to the inguinal ligament and at least 2 cm rostral to the internal ring. The incision is sharply carried through external oblique fascia, internal oblique muscle, and transversalis fascia. A light touch is necessary to avoid entrance into the peritoneum. Careful, preperitoneal sweeping with a finger allows exposure of the femoral hernia neck under the abdominal wall caudal to the incision. If the femoral hernia is not incarcerated, the hernia may be reduced without inspection of contents. With an index finger around the hernia neck, push the sac with the opposite index finger and reduce the hernia through the femoral canal into the inguinal canal. If incarcerated, the sac should be opened and the contents inspected. Fluid may be sent for culture and cytology. If the neck of the defect is too tight, it can be incised medially through the lacunar ligament—*not laterally*—because the

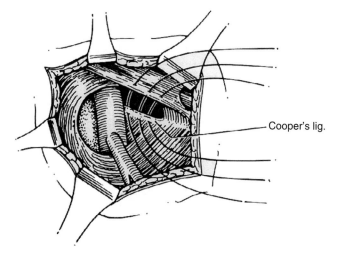

Cooper's lig.

Figure 124–2. Posterior view of a left femoral hernia. Note approximation of transversalis fascia and remnants of lacunar ligament to Cooper's ligament (lig.). (From Skandalakis JE: Surgical Anatomy and Technique: A Pocket Manual. New York, Springer-Verlag, 1995.)

lateral wall is composed of the femoral vein. Resect infarcted tissue or bowel and perform bowel reanastomosis if viable ends are accessible via the defect (and gross, colonic stool spillage has not occurred). A lower, abdominal midline incision is rarely necessary because viable bowel for reanastomosis is usually accessible via the hernia ring. Gross colonic stool spillage or infarcted colon is safely managed with resection and colostomies; subsequent hernia repair is done without mesh. With the femoral hernia sac reduced, the repair proceeds by approximating the anteromedial transversalis fascia and lacunar ligament to Cooper's ligament to obliterate the defect. A panel of mesh can be used if the defect is large.

LAPAROSCOPIC REPAIR OF THE FEMORAL HERNIA

The totally extraperitoneal approach (TEPA) for laparoscopic hernia repair can be modified from a direct or indirect inguinal hernia repair to an approach for femoral hernia repair. The femoral hernia sac can be reduced by blunt, laparoscopic dissection, and the femoral canal space covered with a panel of mesh stapled in place to

---

Pearls and Pitfalls

- Think "incarcerated hernia" when asked to see a patient with acute inguinal adenopathy.
- Occult femoral hernias can cause small bowel obstruction.
- Repair can be by an anterior infrainguinal approach, a typical anterior transinguinal approach, a posterior preperitoneal approach, or a laparoscopic technique.

---

cover both the femoral canal and the posterior aspect of the inguinal canal, where direct inguinal hernias tend to occur. Care must be taken to avoid femoral vein injury or constriction.

SELECTED READINGS

Sabiston D Jr, Lyerly HK (eds): Textbook of Surgery: The Biological Basis of Modern Surgical Practice, 15th ed. Philadelphia, WB Saunders, 1997, pp 1227–1229.

Stoppa R: Hernia Healers. Paris, Arnette, 1999, pp 16, 110–111, 114.

Zinner MJ, Schwartz SI, Ellis H (eds): Maingot's Abdominal Operations, 10th ed. Stamford, CT: Appleton & Lange, 1997, pp 527–528.

Chapter 125

Inguinal Hernias

John B. Martinie and A. Gerson Greenburg

A textbook chapter cannot serve as an encyclopedic reference, nor can it condense every aspect of the field of hernia surgery into a few pages. This chapter provides a brief, flexible algorithm representing a surgical approach to inguinal hernias. The approach and the algorithm reflect our preferences for the management of adult groin hernias.

A plethora of hernia repairs is currently used in clinical practice, and all are well described. It appears that all have achieved excellent clinical results. Different techniques can consistently produce good results; thus, there is no *best* way to repair a hernia. This concept is contrary to the proposal put forth by many hernia "specialists" that all inguinal hernias can be repaired by the same technique. Inguinal hernias *are not* all the same. A consistent feature of groin hernias is their anatomic variation. A surgical approach based on individualization of repair is predicated more on an appreciation of the precise anatomic defect but takes into account other factors as well, such as patient age, recurrence, bilaterality, and comorbidity. The hernia classification system of Nyhus attempts to address this problem and proposes techniques best suited to each type. We are proponents of the philosophy of individualization of hernia repairs based on the particular defect and discuss a logical, algorithmic approach to the clinical problem of hernias.

CLINICAL PRESENTATION AND DIAGNOSIS

With all the advances in medicine over the past century, little has changed in the diagnosis of hernias, which remains strongly rooted in the history and the physical examination. Despite the myriad of diagnostic tools developed for other medical problems, the surgeon's hands still diagnose most groin hernias. Although a hernia is often an obvious diagnosis, it takes an experienced clinician to detect early or occult hernias or to differentiate them from other ailments (e.g., acute hydrocele, epididymitis, and inguinal adenopathy). Often, a patient will present to his or her physician complaining of a bulge or a lump in the groin. Sometimes this will be a new occurrence, but often the lump will have been present for some time, the patient not deeming it worthy of a visit to the doctor. Occasionally, the reason for the visit is the commonly associated pain and discomfort from the herniation or the increasing size of the lump. The report of a groin mass becoming more and more difficult to reduce is a red flag for the physician, and expeditious repair should be performed. Pain or discomfort of varying characteristics and intensities is common with groin hernias. The clinician must consider the details of this complaint to differentiate a hernia from other groin and inguinal disorders

(e.g., testicular torsion, which is accompanied by steady, excruciating pain, or a pulled groin muscle, which is characterized by a constant, deep ache exaggerated with movement). Frequently, patients will report a sensation of something "popping out" when they are lifting or straining; the lump suddenly disappears after lying down.

The history and the physical examination should focus on the patient's complaints, yet examination must also include a global assessment of the patient's current health condition, including past medical and surgical history. History of previous hernia surgery is an often-overlooked clue to the presence of recurrence. Herniorrhaphy during childhood may have been forgotten by the patient. History of respiratory problems (e.g., heavy smoking, chronic cough, emphysema, or chronic obstructive pulmonary disease), prostatism, or chronic constipation should alert the physician to the probability of a direct hernia in patients with such conditions. Obscure conditions affecting connective tissue or chronic malnutrition would also predispose one to the development of hernias. Any information about the activity that produces or exacerbates the lump or its associated symptoms should be sought.

A patient with a known hernia that has been either neglected or simply followed owing to a lack of symptoms will often present with a large mass in the groin that is no longer reducible. The duration of this incarceration should be determined, as well as any symptoms suggestive of bowel obstruction or strangulation. The natural history of incarceration and the well-known inability to differentiate incarceration from strangulation have led to the generally accepted belief in immediate repair. Indeed, a not-infrequent scenario facing clinicians is the patient who does not have a painful groin mass but, rather, complains of generalized abdominal discomfort and distention, nausea, and vomiting. If the physician is not careful to examine the groin (including the area of the femoral triangle), incarceration or strangulation may be missed.

The examination of a patient with complaints of groin pain or a mass in the groin should focus on the inguinal, the rectal, and the abdominal regions. Any scars or obvious masses should be noted. The external genitalia, particularly the scrotum and the testes in men, should be inspected. Asymmetry, irregularity, or swelling of the testes should be noted. Either the physician should have male patients stand and cough, or the Valsalva maneuver can be performed, placing the index finger gently into the region of the external inguinal ring by invaginating the scrotum. This allows for the evaluation of both direct and indirect hernias as well as the general condition of the floor of the inguinal canal. If an obvious inguinal hernia is present when the patient is examined lying down, insertion of a finger into the inguinal canal is unnecessary and often quite uncomfortable. ("Turn your head and cough" is quite uncomfortable and usually unnecessary!) Female patients should also be asked to stand and cough while the examiner places his or her fingers over the area of the inguinal and the femoral canals. An enlarged external ring is not diagnostic of a hernia, and the distinction between types of hernias based on digital examination alone is often imprecise. Rectal and bimanual vaginal examination should also be performed if indicated. If there is a palpable bulge or fullness, one should determine whether it enlarges with coughing or the Valsalva maneuver or is reducible by having the patient lie down.

If the physician is unable to detect a hernia or is unable to distinguish a groin mass from another entity, there are several diagnostic tools available. Ultrasonography is a quick, noninvasive, and relatively inexpensive test that can usually distinguish between solid masses and hollow or fluid-filled structures, such as bowel or hydroceles. It has little sensitivity in the detection of occult hernias. Computed tomography (CT), if performed with an oral contrast agent, can detect small hernias, but only if the hernia contents have not been fully reduced into the abdominal cavity during the CT. The sensitivity of CT is increased if the radiographer has the patient perform the Valsalva maneuver during the examination. Herniography is a modality used more frequently in Europe to diagnose occult hernias in patients with groin symptoms but no findings on examination. Although an exquisitely sensitive test for such hernias, herniography has not gained popularity in the United States, perhaps because of its invasive nature, discomfort, and user-dependent technique.

The differential diagnosis of a groin mass should include hernias, hydroceles, testicular neoplasms, epididymitis, inguinal adenopathy (of both infective and neoplastic origin), and lipomas. Lymphoma often presents as a nonpainful lump in the groin. Inguinal pain alone should broaden the differential diagnosis to include various musculoskeletal disorders, lumbar disk problems, pulled groin muscles, and osteochondritis as well as certain sexually transmitted diseases, including lymphogranuloma venereum and chancroid.

MANAGEMENT

Indications for Surgery

For the past century, surgeons have argued that the presence of a hernia is of itself an indication for surgical intervention. To avoid the potential complications of incarceration and strangulation, generally all groin hernias should be repaired. Although this is a widely held view, this concept has been challenged recently. At this time, an ongoing randomized prospective study is under way to evaluate immediate elective repair versus a "wait and watch" approach for asymptomatic groin hernias.

Several factors must be considered before determining the appropriateness and the timing of surgery. The goal of hernia repair should be the restoration of the normal anatomic relationships in the area with elimination of fascial defects, which could serve as a focal point for incarceration of abdominal contents. Treatment of large defects, direct hernias, and hernias of long standing is less urgent owing to the lower likelihood of incarceration. Smaller defects and indirect and femoral hernias are more likely to become incarcerated and should be repaired without delay. The increased morbidity and mortality associated with emergency repair of an incarcerated or a strangulated hernia, especially in the elderly patient, justify this aggressive approach to hernia repair.

Most hernias are not acutely incarcerated, are associated with minimal discomfort, and can be managed on an elective basis, which allows for better operative planning as well as preoperative evaluation of patients who are at risk of comorbid conditions. The older patient with significant cardiopulmonary disease or other systemic illness (e.g., hepatic insufficiency or ascites) with a relatively asymptomatic hernia may not be a suitable candidate for surgery. Hernias that are causing pain, numbness, intermittent bowel symptoms, or genitourinary discomfort require repair. Attributing abdominal pain and discomfort to the presence of a groin hernia must be done with caution. Not all hernias are associated with pain, and not all pain is related to a hernia. Indeed, pain out of proportion to that expected from an inguinal hernia should alert the wary physician to another disorder or to the possibility of the pain persisting after repair of the hernia. This should be discussed with the patient preoperatively in depth to minimize the possibility of a medicolegal action postoperatively should the pain persist.

Acutely incarcerated hernias usually present as painful, nonreducible groin masses. If it is determined during history-taking that the hernia has been "stuck out" for more than a few hours, or if there are signs of strangulation or obstruction, no attempts at reducing the hernia should be made. Rather, the patient should be taken immediately to the operating room for exploration of the hernia, reduction and possible bowel resection, and repair of the hernia defect. A preperitoneal approach in this situation allows excellent and often superior visualization of the hernia sac, its contents, and the inguinal anatomy, as well as allowing for a definitive procedure in the event that a bowel resection is indicated.

Preoperative Evaluation

The preoperative work-up for a patient undergoing herniorrhaphy depends not only on the patient's medical condition and risk factors but also on the type of anesthesia to be used. A young, otherwise healthy patient with no preexisting medical conditions will usually require only an initial screening history and physical examination. Some hospitals require a hematocrit and a platelet count or other laboratory tests, but for American Society of Anesthesiologists class I and II patients, these are often unnecessary. If the patient is older than 40 years of age, electrocardiography is usually required. Tests for electrolytes, renal function, and coagulation should be done only if the patient's history and examination warrant them. A preoperative chest radiograph should be obtained for all patients with a history of smoking or cardiopulmonary disease or who are older than the age of 50 years.

The type of anesthesia to be used should be chosen after discussions among the surgeon, the anesthesiologist, and the patient. The surgeon's and patient's preference for a particular type of anesthesia plays a major role in this decision. For patients undergoing general anesthesia, the cardiopulmonary risks are increased, and more thorough preoperative evaluation is required. The incidence of myocardial infarction after inguinal hernia repair is extremely low. For patients with preexisting cardiopulmonary disease, the preoperative evaluation may include a cardiac stress test. Some surgeons believe that it is easier to perform the procedure with the patient under mild intravenous sedation with local or spinal anesthesia. For the patient with significant cardiac disease, general anesthesia and full monitoring may be required. Regional anesthesia may offer no benefit to these patients because of the associated difficult-to-regulate vasodilatation; these techniques are often (unjustifiably) thought to present fewer risks for cardiac patients, quicker recovery times, and equal or better analgesia. For most anterior repair techniques, all forms of anesthesia are acceptable, including local, spinal or epidural, and general. Posterior and laparoscopic repairs require general anesthesia to attain full relaxation of the abdominal wall musculature.

Intraoperative Management

Repair of primary hernias has changed dramatically since 1990, with ongoing controversy regarding the best method of repair. Classic anterior approaches that use musculoaponeurotic tissue for the repair were associated with recurrence rates of 15% to 30%. The multilayered repairs of Bassini, Shouldice, and Cooper have generally given way to anterior tension-free mesh repairs, preperitoneal repairs, and, more recently, laparoscopic techniques. The philosophy of individualization of hernia repairs based on the precise anatomy of the defect was initially set forth by Nyhus, who proposed a classification system for groin hernias. Different approaches and the use of prosthetic material were indicated for different classes of hernias. An elaborated classification of hernia anatomy was later proposed by Robbins and Rutkow (1998), who described their experience using a tension-free mesh plug repair. Contrary to Nyhus and many others, however, Rutkow proposes that his method is suitable for all types of groin hernias—primary, recurrent, simple, and complex. The authors recognize the excellent results achieved by both philosophical camps.

We question whether the technique of mesh plug repair can be extrapolated to the general practice surgeon. The critical factor in achieving good results is not so much the approach to the repair as it is the skill of the surgeon and the creation of a tension-free repair. Because of the considerable anatomic variations of hernias, Shahinian and Greenburg (1993) proposed an algorithm for surgical management (Fig. 125–1). This approach takes into account several factors, including the elective or emergent nature of the situation, the type and the size of the hernia, and whether incarceration or strangulation is involved. We have been proponents of the philosophy of Nyhus, who bases the type of repair on the anatomic defect. An organized, algorithmic approach to groin hernias allows establishment of an orderly sequence of evaluation and matches the repair to the situation.

Of the many techniques developed and adapted over the past 100 years, three major categories remain: anterior repairs with and without mesh, posterior repairs, and laparoscopic repairs. Anterior repairs consist of techniques that correct the defect by opening the external oblique aponeurosis and approaching the internal inguinal ring and the floor of the canal from the "front." These types of repairs include simple high ligations of the hernia sac and closure of the internal ring—the Marcy repair—and more complicated reconstructions: Shouldice repair, modified Shouldice repair, and Bassini and Cooper ligament repairs. Tension-free or Lichtenstein repairs using mesh in the reconstruction are also classified as anterior. The mesh plug repair, the hernia-mesh plug system, and the Kugel patch system are unique in that they are an anterior approach and dissection, but they base durability on posterior buttress physiology.

Posterior repairs, which are approached through a higher transverse incision (situated rostral to the internal ring), gain access to the preperitoneal space through the abdominal wall musculature. This approach affords a superior view of the internal inguinal ring and the floor of the canal as well as the hernia sac and contents. It is analogous to viewing the inguinal anatomy from behind. This allows better visualization of the defect, easier reduction of incarceration, and definitive care of potential strangulation. The posterior repair also avoids dissection around the neurovascular structures and should reduce the incidence of nerve and testicular injuries, already less than 0.05%. This approach is of particular importance in recurrent hernias, when the normal virgin anterior anatomy has been lost owing to a previous anterior repair.

Laparoscopic repairs are similar to posterior repairs in that they allow visualization of the inguinal anatomy and the hernia defect from the posterior aspect. The operative plan for hernia repairs begins once the diagnosis is made and a decision for surgery has been entertained. Next to consider is whether the situation is elective or emergent. If the hernia is incarcerated and strangulation is possible, the open preperitoneal approach may be preferred provided that the surgeon is familiar with this approach. If the hernia is reducible and the operation is elective, the approach chosen depends on several factors. The surgeon's and the patient's preferences notwithstanding, a recurrent hernia is usually preferably repaired via the preperitoneal approach. Proponents of laparoscopic techniques have also claimed an advantage in recurrent hernia repairs. In addition, bilateral hernias and the need to return early to work, exercise, or professional sports have been touted as indications for laparoscopic repair.

After the general approach has been determined, the specific anatomic abnormality must be considered during the procedure: Is the hernia direct, indirect, or both? Is it a femoral hernia? Is there a lipoma present? What are the conditions of the internal ring and the posterior floor of the canal? What is the condition of the remaining native tissues, and are they suitable for use in the repair?

Specific Defects and Presentations

The simple indirect inguinal hernia with an intact floor and a nondilated internal ring is a common finding in the

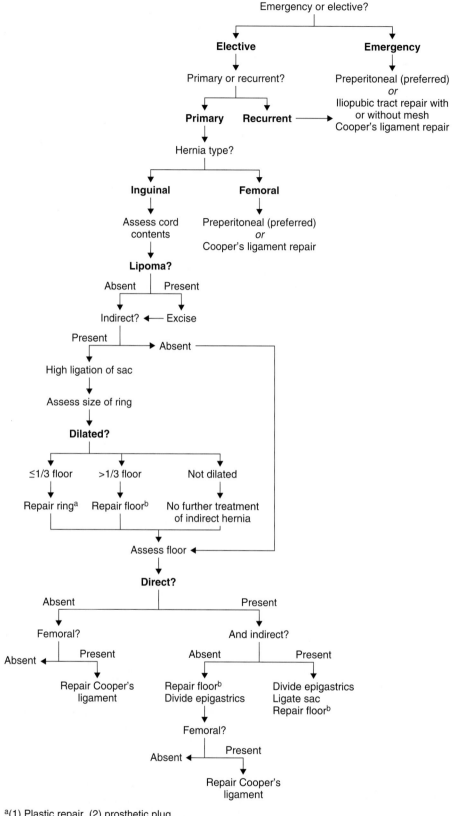

Figure 125–1. Management of hernia repair. (From Levine BA, Copeland EM III, Howard RJ, et al: Current Practice of Surgery. New York, Churchill Livingstone, 1993.)

very young patient and can be managed with most anterior hernia repairs. Dissection and high ligation of the hernia sac and excision of cord lipoma are usually all that is required. Some surgeons secure the neck of the sac to the fascia transversalis. If the internal ring allows passage of no more than the tip of a standard Kelly clamp, no further action needs to be taken. Placing sutures into an inguinal floor that is anatomically and functionally normal in an attempt to prevent later development of a direct inguinal hernia as an adult appears to be counterproductive and risks injury to the cord and the cord structures. This concept is not accepted by all surgeons, many of whom also place a sheet of mesh anterior to the floor of the inguinal canal.

If there is dilatation of the internal ring associated with an indirect hernia, repair of this defect is indicated. This can be done by suturing the medial transversus abdominis aponeurosis to the lateral iliopubic tract, starting medially and moving laterally until the internal ring is tightened sufficiently to allow only a Kelly clamp to pass (modified Marcy repair). Some surgeons advocate placement of onlay mesh and a mesh plug to repair this anatomic defect of the internal ring. If the enlarged internal ring is markedly dilated and blends medially with a weakness in the floor of the canal such that greater than one third of the distance from the pubic tubercle to the lateral aspect of the internal ring is widened, complete repair of the floor is indicated.

A pantaloon hernia is present when a direct and an indirect component coexist, with the inferior epigastric vessels between the two. Dividing the inferior epigastric vessels to facilitate a single repair of this defect, in a fashion similar to that used for an isolated direct hernia, is advisable.

When a direct hernia is present, the surgeon needs to assess carefully the quality and the quantity of strong native tissue (Table 125–1). If both the fascia transversalis and the transversus abdominis aponeurosis are of good quality and can reach the iliopubic tract or the shelving edge of the inguinal ligament without tension, an anterior suture repair using these tissues is recommended. This repair uses running nonabsorbable sutures to distribute the tension along the length of the tissues and is a modification of the Shouldice repair. If the native tissues are inadequate (which is more common), or if there is concern about tension, a tension-free or Lichtenstein repair is most appropriate. There have been many modifications of this technique since its inception, but the basic principle is to secure a prosthetic mesh material over the inguinal floor. The original procedure called for running nonabsorbable sutures to fasten the mesh to the pubic tubercle medially, the shelving edge of the inguinal ligament inferiorly, and the conjoined tendon superiorly. Many authors have abandoned this practice, using only a few tacking sutures to keep the mesh in place until fibrosis and ingrowth of native tissue into the mesh occur.

A femoral hernia, if diagnosed preoperatively, can be most easily corrected by using a posterior approach. This approach may involve either the preperitoneal or the laparoscopic technique. Because a femoral hernia lies deep to the inguinal ligament and the floor of the inguinal canal, the fascia transversalis must be divided to gain access to the femoral hernia from an anterior approach. Both the preperitoneal and the laparoscopic techniques allow superior visualization of the femoral defect and ease of repair by permitting exposure of Cooper's ligament. This type of hernia can be repaired either by using interrupted sutures to bring the fascia transversalis to Cooper's ligament or by placing a mesh onlay patch over the defect.

Laparoscopic Repair

Significant progress has been made in laparoscopic hernia repair since the early 1980s. Initial results were saddled with recurrence rates as high as 20% to 30%. Many recurrences occurred in the immediate postoperative period, sometimes in the recovery room. There was also an unacceptably high complication rate, and vascular and hollow viscous injuries occurred. The addition of increased cost and length of the procedure made for a doubtful future. Cost remains a factor because reimbursement has not been at the level needed to meet expenses. Traditional open hernia techniques are relatively quick, inexpensive outpatient procedures with low complication rates and excellent results. The actual benefit of laparoscopic inguinal hernia repair is difficult to justify on a cost basis. Proponents of the laparoscopic method claim reduced postoperative pain and earlier return to normal activity as specific advantages, but these putative advantages have not been widely accepted.

POSTOPERATIVE MANAGEMENT

The evolution of surgery has transformed the techniques for hernia repair and the postoperative management of these patients. In the past, patients were admitted to the hospital for 3 to 7 days after hernia repair, were placed on bed rest, and were instructed to minimize physical activity. Months of slow recuperation followed before physical activity could be resumed. Today, more than 95% of hernia surgeries are performed in outpatient surgical settings, where the patient arrives the morning of surgery and leaves the same day. Admission after hernia repair occurs occasionally, but the admission is closely scrutinized by insurance agency case managers.

Patients are instructed to begin walking immediately and to start light activity. A motivated individual who performs mostly light duty may return to work a few days after surgery. Patients who perform strenuous activity and

Table 125–1	Hernia: The "Good Stuff"

Inguinal ligament
Lacunar ligament (Gimbernat's)
Pectineal ligament (Cooper's)
Iliopubic tract
Anterior femoral sheath
Fascia transversalis°
Conjoined fascial "area"
Arch of the internal oblique and transabdominal aponeurosis
Prostheses (mesh plugs and patches)

°In the absence of a direct hernia.

heavy lifting are commonly instructed to wait 2 weeks before resuming their normal duties. Men are instructed to wear supportive, brief-type underwear or an athletic supporter for comfort. Patients should be instructed to avoid the use of any nonsteroidal or aspirin products for 1 week and to rely on an acetaminophen-opiate combination for postoperative pain. On the second postoperative day, the patient may be allowed to shower and should be instructed to remove the surgical dressing. The postoperative visit in the surgeon's office is usually scheduled 2 weeks after surgery; the patient should be instructed to call if any signs of infection develop.

COMPLICATIONS

Preoperative complications of hernias are the impetus for repair. Misdiagnosis of a groin hernia may occur more frequently with femoral hernias. Incarceration is a common result with a neglected or an undiagnosed hernia, particularly indirect or femoral. The incarceration can contain small bowel, colon, bladder, or omentum and occurs when the contents of the hernia sac become irreducible. Some surgeons attempt manual reduction and, if successful, delay elective repair of the hernia. This procedure risks possible reduction of strangulated or infarcted bowel into the peritoneal cavity, albeit rare. Intestinal obstruction is another sequela of an incarcerated hernia and results in a significant increase in morbidity and mortality. Finally, strangulation and visceral infarction are often the natural end points of a neglected incarcerated hernia and represent the ultimate complication.

The incidence of intraoperative complications and technical errors is low in groin hernia surgery; some types of repairs have higher rates than others. In addition, certain classes of repairs (e.g., laparoscopic) have unique complications. Hemorrhage is always a possibility, especially during "re-do" and emergent surgery. The most common sources of significant major bleeding are the inferior epigastric vessels and the external iliac or femoral vein; however, bleeding requiring hospitalization and transfusion should be exceedingly rare. Transection of the inguinal cord or the cord structures is also a low-frequency event and can result in the loss of the testicle in male patients. Damage to the ilioinguinal, the iliohypogastric, and the genitofemoral nerves is relatively common (approximately 5%) and may result in a sensory deficit in the inguinal region or even a chronic pain syndrome or neuralgia. This can be caused by complete or partial transection of the nerve, traction or electrocautery injury, or suture entrapment of the nerve. If the neuralgia is of significant duration and severity, exploratory surgery may be indicated in an attempt to resect the involved neuroma. Ischemic orchitis, testicular atrophy, and testicular infarction are potential complications resulting from devascularization of the testes or, more commonly, obstruction of venous drainage. The testes have a rich blood supply from collaterals, however, and division of the testicular vessel alone does not always result in loss of the testicle unless the testicle has been fully mobilized out of the scrotum, a maneuver rarely indicated in inguinal hernia surgery.

Division of the vas deferens is an uncommon event in routine primary hernia repair. The incidence increases with recurrent and large incarcerated hernias when normal anatomy is distorted. If the patient wishes to retain reproductive ability, immediate urosurgical consultation for repair should be considered. Injury to the intestines is also a possibility if there is bowel in the hernia sac or if bowel comprises part of the sac, as in sliding hernias. Careful dissection should prevent such events, but if one is encountered, primary repair of the injury is usually sufficient. Another rare complication in a sliding hernia is injury to the urinary bladder, which can comprise the medial wall of a large sliding hernia. Bladder injury should be repaired with two layers of absorbable suture material, and a urinary catheter should be left in place for several days to decompress the bladder.

Postoperative complications of groin hernia surgery include urinary retention, scrotal and groin ecchymosis and hematoma, testicular atrophy, hydrocele, and wound infection. It is both surprising and encouraging that the incidence of infections after repair using prosthetic mesh has been reported to be less than 0.1%. Hernia recurrence—which has plagued surgeons for centuries and has driven the search for better techniques—has fortunately decreased significantly with modern techniques.

Complications of laparoscopic hernia repair are the same as for laparoscopy in general and are also related to the specific type of repair. Bleeding from the abdominal wall trocar site usually involves the inferior epigastric arteries and occurs in about 3% of patients. Hernias occur in about 1% of 10-mm trocar sites if not repaired; thus, all 10-mm sites should be closed. Injury to the bowel, the bladder, or a major vascular structure from either a sharp trocar or a sharp instrument also occurs in less than 1% of repairs; this can be avoided by using an open laparoscopic Hasson technique for creation of the pneumoperitoneum. Hypercapnia, intestinal ileus, and adhesions are all reported complications of pneumoperitoneum creation for laparoscopic repair. Groin neuralgia after laparoscopic

---

Pearls and Pitfalls

- Most hernias cause some discomfort, but beware of the patient with severe pain. Search for another cause.
- Not all groin masses are hernias, and not all lumps in the femoral triangle are inguinal nodes. Beware the incarcerated femoral hernia.
- Not all inguinal hernias should be repaired.
- Acutely incarcerated inguinal hernias that are unable to be reduced require immediate repair; those able to be reduced should be repaired semi-urgently.
- There is no one best operation but rather several operations depending on type of hernia, age of patient, and local tissue available.
- The "good stuff" in hernia repair includes the inguinal ligament, the lacunar ligament (Gimbernat's), the pectineal ligament (Cooper's), the iliopubic tract, the anterior femoral sheath, the fascia transversalis, the conjoined fascial area, the arch of the internal oblique and transabdominal aponeurosis, and the prosthetic material (mesh plugs and patches).

repair is the most common problem, perhaps more so than after anterior repairs, and results from placing staples on the mesh in the lateral infrainguinal area, the location of the majority of nerves. This problem can best be avoided by not placing any staples below the inguinal ligament laterally and by keeping the total number of staples to a minimum. The incidence of cord and testicular problems appears to be low with this method of repair, as is the incidence of hydrocele, seroma, and hematoma of the groin or the scrotum. The incidence of wound infections and infections associated with use of prosthetic mesh also appears to be extremely low with laparoscopic techniques but always remains a concern with the routine placement of a foreign material into the body.

RESULTS OF HERNIA REPAIRS

The ultimate test of a hernia repair, and perhaps the one most important to the patient, is the rate of recurrence. Over the years, recurrence rates have decreased with the introduction of new repair methods, such as tension-free, prosthetic, and laparoscopic techniques. Enthusiasm for the use of prosthetic mesh plugs and for tension-free repairs is supported by reports from Rutkow and Robbins, Wantz, and others, who have demonstrated recurrence rates of 1% to 2% as well as diminished postoperative complication rates. The higher rates of recurrence seen with older, suture-based, "tissue-to-tissue" repairs may be due to the use of weakened, attenuated tissue placed under tension. If tissue of adequate durability can be found and can be approximated without tension, results equal to those seen with the use of mesh can be achieved. To support this, Nyhus, Greenburg, and Patino have all demonstrated recurrence rates of 1% to 2% with the preperitoneal approach, using mesh only where inadequate tissue exists.

Review of the literature on laparoscopic repairs demonstrates a recurrence rate of 0% to 5%. Since 1990, there has been significant improvement in the techniques, instrumentation, and operative skills of surgeons performing this procedure. Indeed, the learning curve for laparoscopic hernia repair appears to be about 20 procedures, significantly less than for laparoscopic cholecystectomy. The MRC Laparoscopic Groin Hernia Trial Group recently published the results of a randomized prospective trial in the United Kingdom and Ireland. At 1-year follow-up of 928 patients, there were seven recurrences in the laparoscopy group and none in the open repair group (2% vs. 0).

SELECTED READINGS

Greenburg AG: Preperitoneal repair of recurrent groin hernias. Perspect Gen Surg 1991;2:43.

Laparoscopic versus open repair of groin hernia: A randomized comparison. The MRC Laparoscopic Groin Hernia Trial Group. Lancet 1999;354:185.

Nyhus LM, Condon RE (eds): Hernia. Philadelphia, JB Lippincott, 1995.

Robbins AW, Rutkow IM: Mesh plug repair and groin hernia surgery. Surg Clin North Am 1998;78:1007.

Ryberg A, Lund R, Filip C, Fitzgibbons R Jr: Laparoscopic hernia procedure. In Ponsky J (ed): Complications of Endoscopic and Laparoscopic Surgery. Philadelphia, Lippincott-Raven, 1997.

Shahinian TK, Greenburg AG: Hernias. In Levine BA, Copeland EM III, Howard RJ, et al: Current Practice of Surgery. New York, Churchill Livingstone, 1993.

Chapter 126

Incisional Hernia

John M. Clarke

Incisional hernias of the abdominal wall are among the commonest conditions requiring surgical intervention. As increasing numbers of abdominal operations are being performed—many of them on less fit and more obese patients—it is not surprising that incisional hernias are being seen in increasing numbers. Many repairs will ultimately prove to be failures. This chapter considers the reasons for failure of what seem to be straightforward surgical procedures for incisional hernia. Somewhat more complex approaches with more promise for long-term success are also offered. Thankfully, lessons have been learned from earlier poor results, and fresh approaches to this frustrating problem are being reported as our understanding of physiology and anatomy increases. For this we are indebted to the French surgeons and their tradition of research and expertise in surgery of the abdominal wall, to Wantz, who popularized their ideas in this country and added his own experience, and to many plastic surgeons, who taught us to understand the components of the abdominal wall.

CLINICAL PRESENTATION

An incisional hernia presents as a bulge or a lump in the abdomen, usually beneath the scar but sometimes off to one side of the incision. The bulge or the lump may or may not be painful, depending on the size of the defect and what the hernia contains. A hernia may originate in the immediate postoperative period but not be recognized, representing occult dehiscence. More often, after a period of months or years, the patient notices the lump and seeks advice or is found on routine surveillance to have an asymptomatic hernia. Initial presentation with incarceration or strangulation is unusual but is more frequent in the obese patient, although adhesional intestinal obstruction in association with an incisional hernia is not rare. Back pain may be a major chronic complaint, especially with larger and long-standing hernias, probably related to the exaggerated lordosis that occurs as these patients lose their abdominal domain. History-taking and physical examination are usually sufficient to demonstrate and define an incisional hernia, but in the obese or difficult patient, imaging with computed tomography may be necessary for diagnosis. Computed tomography may also demonstrate unsuspected multiple defects and can define the contents of the hernia, but imaging is not usually necessary for diagnosis or preoperative planning.

PATHOPHYSIOLOGY AND PREVENTION

A number of factors may contribute to the development of an incisional hernia including obesity, chronic cough, wound infection, postoperative ileus, ventilator therapy, ascites, and a poor nutritional state. Several studies have suggested that patients who develop an incisional hernia have both defects in collagen formation and increased activity of certain metalloproteinases that serve to break down collagen. Technical factors during the initial operation, especially suture techniques, may play a role. "Mass closure" of the popular midline incision has markedly reduced the incidence of abdominal wound disruption in the early postoperative period, but incisional hernias eventually occur in at least 10% of patients.

One accepted technique of primary abdominal closure is well established. Monofilament suture material is placed with wide bites encompassing both layers of the rectus sheath and part of the rectus muscle. The sutures are placed about 1 cm apart and, most important, without undue tension. The surgeon (and especially the assistant) must resist the urge to pull a continuous suture too tightly and thereby produce undesired tissue effects. The old adage, "Approximation, not strangulation," remains appropriate. Wounds that are obviously contaminated should be managed with mass closure as described previously as well as open packing of the subcutaneous tissues and skin. This approach should markedly reduce the chances of deep wound infection, consequent fascial dissolution, and ultimately herniation.

Although use of full-thickness external retention sutures is popular in some practices, there is no evidence that this technique is more effective than mass closure, and external retention sutures have the additional disadvantages of interfering with open care of the contaminated wound and causing significant pain at the sites of insertion.

The pathophysiology of ventral incisional hernias is unique in that as the defect enlarges, dynamic changes evolve. These have important implications with regard to operative correction of the problem. With the more familiar inguinal hernia, the primary forces acting on the defect are gravitational and unidirectional. With midline ventral hernias, however, the lateral or "belt" muscles exert a dynamic cephalolateral pull against the edges of the hernial defect, widening the defect and eventually causing contraction of these lateral muscles. The lateral muscles may be thought of as having their insertion at the linea alba, by way of the rectus sheath. When they are separated from their point of insertion, contracture is the result, just as would be the case with an extremity muscle separated from its insertion on bone. Furthermore, without the tendinous insertion at the midline, the abdominal wall is impaired from a functional standpoint and loses the dynamism necessary for the overall well-being of the patient.

With large incisional hernias (>10 cm of separation), these changes may seriously affect other systems. The concept of eventration disease explains respiratory insufficiency, which may cause significant postoperative problems in a minority of patients. In such patients, usually with massive and long-standing hernias, an external abdominal cavity forms and the intra-abdominal pressure increases with breathing, resulting in reduced diaphragmatic excursion. The function of the diaphragm becomes less efficient, and eventually the true abdominal cavity becomes relatively smaller. This pathophysiology may produce severe respiratory insufficiency when the hernia is reduced and the defect is closed. Rarely, postoperative abdominal compartment syndrome may occur, manifested by decreased venous return as well as pulmonary compromise.

PREOPERATIVE MANAGEMENT

A small percentage of ventral incisional hernias may remain asymptomatic and show minimal enlargement over long periods of time. These may be managed nonoperatively, especially in the high-risk patient. In most instances, however, the natural history of incisional hernia is one of gradual enlargement, mandating operative repair. Ideally, the corrective surgery should be done before the hernia produces the anatomic and physiologic changes that occur after years of neglect. Preoperative management must be guided by an understanding of the pathophysiology of ventral hernia (outlined earlier) and of the specific problems created as these hernias develop.

Meticulous attention to preoperative skin care is important. Patients with redundant folds of skin with chronic dermatitis should be treated with topical antibacterial, antifungal, and drying agents. Nonhealing ulcers may have an ischemic cause and may resist all forms of therapy other than excision. Patients should also be advised that it may be necessary to resect varying amounts of skin and subcutaneous tissue and that they may lose the umbilicus. Weight loss is usually desirable and advised but is seldom achieved.

Optimization of pulmonary status is of paramount importance and should include cessation of smoking, incentive spirometry, and administration of bronchodilators or mucolytics, if indicated. In addition to the usual general medical evaluation and the stabilization of chronic conditions, it is appropriate preoperatively to administer intravenous antibiotics and sequential compression devices to reduce venous stasis. Bowel preparation similar to that used for colon surgery may be indicated if there is significant concern regarding the need for intraperitoneal dissection in a patient with known severe adhesions. Indwelling bladder catheters are used if an operation of longer than 1 hour is expected. The need for nasogastric intubation and central venous catheterization must be individualized.

In the unusual patient in whom eventration disease is evident or suspected, or if the size of the hernia is such that primary closure is in doubt, preoperative therapeutic creation of a pneumoperitoneum (provided that a peritoneal cavity is present) may be helpful in restoring diaphragmatic function and stretching the abdominal muscles to facilitate closure of the primary defect. The

technique is straightforward. With the patient under local anesthesia, a catheter is inserted into the peritoneal cavity with or without radiographic imaging. Many different catheters have been used, including the Veres needle, peritoneal dialysis catheters, venous catheters, and a thoracentesis catheter. The latter comes with a pressure-activated valve within the drainage tubing, which obviates the need to turn a stopcock as each syringe of air is injected. (To accomplish this, however, the tubing must be arranged with an adapter in reverse so that the valve injects rather than withdraws, as it was designed to do.) Once the peritoneal cavity has been entered, air is injected until the patient complains of shoulder pain or abdominal discomfort. The amount of air that will be tolerated at the first sitting may be 500 to 1500 mL. The catheter may be withdrawn and a suture placed in the defect, or the catheter may be left indwelling.

Repeat punctures are much easier because an air interface was established with the first insufflation; 500 to 1000 mL may be injected at subsequent visits. The procedure is repeated every 2 or 3 days for 2 to 3 weeks, at which time the lateral flank areas should feel less tense on palpation. Application of an abdominal binder during this period of time may increase the effectiveness of the pneumoperitoneum, but it is not always well tolerated by the patient and should be used selectively. It should be emphasized that therapeutic pneumoperitoneum is necessary in only a small percentage of patients and that the technique is best suited to the hospitalized patient.

INTRAOPERATIVE MANAGEMENT

The choice of an operative technique for repair of an incisional hernia depends on the size of the defect, previous procedures, and the general condition of the abdominal wall. Small defects of 5 cm or less may often be repaired primarily, but even in the simplest case, the presence of obesity or abnormal tissues may necessitate special measures. In most patients, general anesthesia with good muscle relaxation is essential.

Three acceptable operative techniques for large incisional hernias are described, but it is obvious that the choice of technique has to be individualized and that personal preference is often the deciding factor. All acceptable operative procedures share common steps, as follows:

1. Reconstruct the linea alba to close the defect without tension.
2. Reattach the tendinous insertions of the lateral "belt" muscles, usually with prosthetic material.
3. Restore normal abdominal pressure to avoid diaphragmatic dysfunction.
4. Excise redundant or devitalized skin and subcutaneous tissue, including the umbilicus in many instances.

With any of the following operative procedures, the choice of incision depends on the abdominal wall configuration and the location of old incisions. A midline technique is usually easiest, and it is often best to start with excision of skin and subcutaneous tissue in the shape of an ellipse around the hernia. This allows the sac to be approached from its lateral margins and makes the dissection easier. Approaching the defect in this manner saves time and reduces the risk of injury to viscera within the sac. Because there is almost always redundant skin to be excised, a lateral approach to the sac also facilitates this step.

ACCEPTABLE TECHNIQUES

Retromuscular Prosthesis (Stoppa Technique)

This is a very popular and widely used of the sound techniques for large incisional hernia repair internationally. Minimal subcutaneous flaps are raised, the sac is separated from the muscular defect, and the posterior sheath of the rectus is incised. This may be done either by incising the anterior sheath first or by approaching the posterior sheath directly through the midline. In either case, sac and peritoneum should be saved to close over the viscera. A definite peritoneal-posterior sheath layer is necessary to prevent contact between the retromuscular mesh and the viscera. If sac and peritoneum are insufficient to accomplish this, then absorbable mesh may be interposed between the abdominal viscera and the permanent prosthetic mesh. Examples of absorbable mesh include polyglactin 910 and polyglycolic acid.

The retrorectus space is developed laterally past the entrance point for the neurovascular structures. Permanent mesh is then inserted, preferably 6 to 10 cm lateral to the midline on each side. Either interlocked polyester or polypropylene may be used. This retromuscular mesh is held with traction sutures of heavy absorbable material (Fig. 126–1A). The traction sutures may be placed with the Reverdin needle, a threadable needle on a handle that acts as a suture passer (see Fig. 126–1B). The traction sutures anchor the mesh laterally, passing through the oblique muscles, and are tied subcutaneously through small buttonhole skin incisions. The advantage of these traction sutures is that they not only fix the mesh in a taut configuration but also have the effect of relieving tension on the midline and facilitating reconstruction of the linea alba.

If the midline fascia still cannot be approximated, then some form of relaxing incision in the anterior rectus sheath may be used. A number of techniques are available, but most surgeons who use a relaxing incision prefer multiple staggered vertical incisions. These have been described as quincuncial because they may be viewed as a series of four slits forming a rectangle, with an additional slit in the center. Because the flaps are raised at the deep level, there is less need for skin and subcutaneous resection with this technique. Suction drains beneath and superficial to the rectus are suggested (see Fig. 126–1C).

Medial Reflection of the Rectus Sheath and Anterior Mesh Placement (Chevrel Technique)

With the Chevrel technique, wider subcutaneous flaps are raised. The midline fascia is reconstructed by first

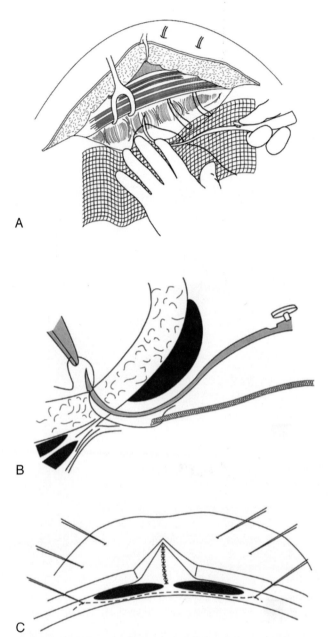

A

B

C

Figure 126–1. Retromuscular mesh placement and suture fixation (Rives-Stoppa technique). *A,* The dissection extends lateral to where the neurovascular structures enter the rectus muscle. The peritoneum and the posterior sheath must be closed to avoid contact between the mesh and the viscera. Absorbable mesh (polyglactin 910) may be necessary to accomplish this. *B,* Use of Reverdin needle to pass traction sutures to hold the mesh in a taut position. The suture is tied to itself through a buttonhole skin incision. *C,* Cross-sectional view of the retromuscular mesh (*dotted line*) and lateral traction sutures. The linea alba is closed primarily, with use of rectus sheath relaxing incisions as necessary. (*A* to *C* from Wantz GE: Atlas of Hernia Surgery. New York, Raven Press, 1991.)

closing the attenuated linea alba, then making long vertical incisions in the anterior rectus sheath, reflecting each edge medially and suturing each edge to another with an overlapping technique (Fig. 126-2A and B). Three layers of nonabsorbable sutures are used for this "wrapover." (In less challenging cases, this may be modified by using multiple small incisions in the rectus sheath, as described

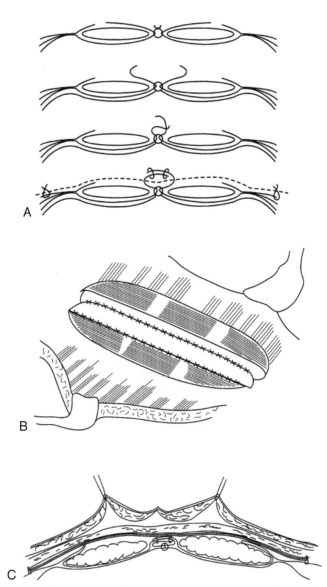

Figure 126–2. Midline reconstruction by means of fascial plasty and anterior mesh reinforcement (Chevrel technique). *A,* Cross-sectional view of the first step. The rectus fascia is incised on each side, and flaps are folded medially to be sutured together (overlapped) after closure of the linea alba. Mesh (*dotted line*) is placed anteriorly to cover the bare rectus muscle and is held in place with lateral sutures and fibrin glue. *B,* Anterior view with defect closed before mesh is placed. *C,* Cross-sectional view of abdominal wall after repair has been completed. (*A* and *B* from Chevrel JP, Rath AM: The use of fibrin glues in the surgical treatment of incisional hernias. Hernia 1997;1:11; *C* from Wantz GE: Incisional hernia, the problem and the cure. J Am Coll Surg 1999;188:439.)

previously.) Once the midline has been reconstructed, the large, bare rectus muscle area, which results from medial reflection of the rectus sheath, is covered with polypropylene mesh. The mesh is then sutured to the external oblique fascia and is also made to adhere to the abdominal wall with fibrin glue sealant (see Fig. 126–2C). Early fixation is therefore the rule, and the prevention of sub-prosthetic seromas may add to the early strength of this technique. Fibrin sealant (Tisseel VH Kit; Baxter International, Deerfield, Ill) has only recently become commercially available in the United States and is still not widely

used, perhaps because of fear of transmission of viral or other infectious agents in products made from human plasma. Studies suggest that this risk is small. The Chevrel technique may be preferable for epigastric defects, in which a retromuscular prosthesis is less effective (as are lateral traction sutures) because of the narrow space and the fixation of the musculature to the costal arch. Also, if infection occurs, mesh placed anterior to the musculofascial layer is easier to manage than it would be in a deep retromuscular location.

Fascial Partition and Primary Midline Reconstruction with Anterior Tensioned Mesh (Ramirez Technique)

The Ramirez technique, which has been described by a number of plastic surgeons, has been modified by the author. It is derived from the "components separation" technique, which in turn is based on the anatomic fact that the external oblique muscle and the aponeurosis may be incised and separated from the deeper abdominal wall muscles to produce a sliding myofascial flap. Because the neurovascular elements pass deep to the internal oblique muscle, little physiologic damage is done. Defects as large as 20 cm have been closed primarily with this technique.

Extensive subcutaneous flaps are raised, recognizing that blood supply to the skin edges will be compromised, and the skin will require trimming. The external oblique aponeurosis is then incised vertically or "parasagittally" 1 or 2 cm lateral to the rectus muscle. (Gentle cautery stimulation of the rectus muscle will identify this point, which may be obscure on simple inspection or palpation.) The lateral cut edge of the external oblique is then picked up with an Allis forceps and is bluntly mobilized from the deeper internal oblique, thus separating the components of the abdominal wall. As this is done, the vertical incision in the external oblique is extended to the costal margin above and to the inguinal canal below. The incision should curve medially toward its inferior part. Lateral mobilization extends to the lumbodorsal fascia and the iliac fossa. After this has been accomplished bilaterally, midline closure may be done with nonabsorbable sutures and a standard mass closure technique. Minimal tension should be required. In the unusual case in which the defect is very large, it is also possible to incise the posterior rectus sheath to add more length to the sliding myofascial flap created by the maneuvers mentioned earlier. The epigastric area may pose a problem owing to the relative fixation of the musculofascial tissues within the costal arch. If necessary, the epigastric midline can be strengthened and closed by medial reflection of the rectus sheath and wrapover, as described for the Chevrel technique.

As with the other techniques, handling of the sac is individualized. It may be inverted, opened, or partly resected. Because no mesh is placed between the peritoneum and the muscle, a separate peritoneal closure is not critical in this method, and midline reconstruction may be done as a single layer. Once the midline has been closed, there will be a wide gap between the cut lateral edge of the external oblique and the cut medial edge where it was severed near the lateral border of the rectus.

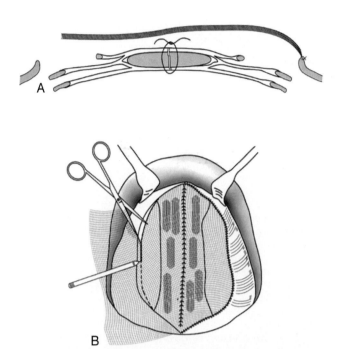

Figure 126–3. Fascial partitioning and midline reconstruction with anterior mesh under tension (Ramirez technique). *A,* Cross-sectional view showing lateral mobilization of the external oblique (fascial partition), permitting tension-free midline reconstruction. Anterior mesh is placed under tension between the lateral cut edges of the external oblique. This provides strain relief for the midline closure and effectively restores the insertion of the lateral belt muscles. *B,* Anterior view showing the mesh being placed under tension and cut before being sutured to the remaining lateral external oblique. (*A* and *B* from DiBello JN, Moore JH: Sliding myofascial flap of the rectus abdominis muscles for the closure of recurrent ventral hernias. Plast Reconstr Surg 1996;98:466.)

This deficiency, although not likely of great structural importance, may leave the patient with some lateral bulging. It is the author's preference to suture polypropylene mesh under moderate tension between the cut right and left lateral edges of the external oblique muscle and the aponeurosis (Fig. 126–3A).

The mesh is cut to fit the curved edge of the lateral leaf of the external oblique and is sutured to it with polypropylene. After one edge has been sutured, the mesh is drawn across the entire abdominal wall, and the point where it will be tailored to fit snugly when attached to the opposite lateral cut edge of the external oblique is marked (see Fig. 126–3B). This has the effect of reattaching the tendinous insertion of the external oblique muscle and at the same time removing tension from the midline closure, like a subcutaneous binder. The mesh is tailored to cover the epigastrium. Tacking sutures of absorbable material are placed to eliminate dead space, but fibrin glue may eliminate the need for this in future trials. Two suction drains are placed, and liberal skin and subcutaneous trimming is done. Routine closure of the remaining layers completes the operation.

UNACCEPTABLE OPERATIVE APPROACHES

Two other techniques are mentioned here but are not recommended. The first is simple bridging of the defect with prosthetic material by suturing mesh to the edges of the defect. Although some have reported good results with this technique, many surgeons with interest in this field would be skeptical of uniformly good results except for very small hernias. This common technique may appear to have corrected the bulge in the abdominal wall, especially in the early postoperative period, but physiologically it leaves much to be desired. Such "gap bridging" does not recreate a dynamic abdominal wall, does not restore the normal abdominal pressure, and does not reattach the tendinous insertions of the lateral muscles. The best that one may hope for with this technique is what Read has called controlled diastasis, which will inevitably enlarge as the lateral muscles, deprived of their midline insertion, continue to retract.

The same arguments may apply to laparoscopic techniques, which are enjoying enthusiastic acceptance for obvious reasons. Early good results must be viewed with caution for the reasons outlined previously. Differences of opinion about these results may actually represent a degree of semantic dissonance. Some would say that there can be no meaningful estimation of recurrence with laparoscopic placement of a prosthesis, especially in the early stages of follow-up, because the hernial defect was not effectively repaired in the first place. Newer materials notwithstanding, this technique also violates the principle of avoiding contact between prosthetic material and the viscera.

The good results of endoscopic repair of inguinal hernias should not be extrapolated to the physiologically more complex situation that exists when hernias occur higher in the abdominal wall. For all these reasons, skepticism about the long-term results of laparoscopic repair seems justified at this stage in its development.

PROSTHETIC MATERIALS

For practical purposes, there are two types of permanent mesh recommended for incisional hernia repair. European surgeons generally prefer interlocked polyester mesh (Dacron or Mersilene) for retromuscular repairs. Its advantage is that it is more supple and less apt to be noticed by the patient. The other type of mesh, polypropylene (Marlex or Prolene mesh), is more popular in the United States, possibly because of a perception that it tolerates infection better, although this is not borne out either by the European studies or by Wantz's extensive experience. Polypropylene is indeed much stronger and should be used for techniques in which the mesh is placed anterior to the fascia. Both of these meshes are macroporous (having pores larger than 75 microns) and therefore allow penetration by fibroblasts, with resultant tissue ingrowth. Although expanded polytetrafluoroethylene, or PTFE has been used extensively, it is less desirable for incisional hernia repair because of its microporous nature (pores less than 10 microns) and consequent lack of tissue incorporation. From anecdotal reports, PTFE also seems unlikely to support secondary healing in the presence of infection. This would be expected, because the pores are too small to allow entrance of neutrophils and macrophages.

POSTOPERATIVE MANAGEMENT

There are no exceptional postoperative management issues for most patients with incisional hernias. Routine orders for abdominal procedures will suffice, except that extra attention must be paid to respiratory status, especially with more extensive repairs. Chest radiographs are often necessary for these patients, and oxygen saturation and cardiac monitoring are helpful in the early diagnosis of respiratory insufficiency. Incentive spirometry is encouraged as soon as the patient has recovered from the anesthesia and is continued at least 48 hours. Antibiotic prophylaxis should be brief (perioperative), and early ambulation (with abdominal support) is encouraged. Some patients will require nasogastric suction; it is better to decompress the stomach if there is any doubt about the development of distention due to adynamic ileus. Once peristalsis is effective, diet is advanced as tolerated. Drains are removed as soon as drainage is minimal (less than 30 to 50 mL/24 hours), but this may take 3 to 10 days. In the absence of complications, most patients may be discharged within 3 to 6 days.

Many surgeons recommend external abdominal support in the form of a binder, which may be placed in the operating room after the dressings are applied. Patients are advised to wear it when ambulatory for 6 to 12 weeks. This binder is for patient comfort and does nothing to prevent recurrence. Constipation is to be avoided for obvious reasons, and the use of stool softeners and stimulant laxatives on a preventive basis is strongly emphasized to patients and family members at the time of discharge.

COMPLICATIONS

Most early postoperative complications involve the respiratory system, with atelectasis and pneumonia being seen most commonly. Adynamic ileus and adhesional obstruction are no more frequent than with any other abdominal procedure. An external fistula may occur (rarely) in complex reconstructions and will eventually require mesh removal. Complications specific to incisional hernia surgery usually involve the skin and the subcutaneous tissue flaps. Minor skin sloughs are common and usually of no consequence. If the eschar is dry, débridement may be delayed to avoid premature exposure of any anteriorly placed mesh. Superficial exposed mesh may be trimmed locally to avoid the need for complete removal. Seromas occurring after drain removal are usually managed with percutaneous aspiration. The aspirate should be cultured, but a culture with positive results does not always mean that major intervention is indicated. Often, these problems respond to systemic antibiotic therapy, drainage, and local wound care. Edema and diffuse cellulitis require aggressive parenteral antibiotic therapy. Major skin breakdowns with exposure of mesh are unusual and may require trimming of the exposed mesh with later secondary closure or skin grafting.

OUTCOMES

1. The retromuscular mesh technique (Rives-Stoppa) has been the most widely used of the acceptable methods

---

Pearls and Pitfalls

PEARLS

- Attend to preoperative medical, respiratory, and skin care.
- Verify that the proper equipment is available (e.g., mesh, Reverdin needle).
- Prepare the bowel, administer intravenous antibiotics, insert a Foley catheter, and employ deep venous thrombosis prophylaxis.
- Excise the skin ellipse, and approach the sac from its lateral borders.
- Choose retromuscular, Chevrel, or fascial partitioning technique.
- Save the sac for peritoneal closure if the retromuscular approach is chosen.
- If there is insufficient peritoneum with the retromuscular method, use absorbable (Vicryl) mesh.
- Use Mersilene or polypropylene for the retromuscular method, but use only polypropylene anteriorly.
- Reconstruct the midline and the linea alba, if at all possible.
- Recognize that the epigastrium may present with tissue loss and inability to mobilize enough length by lateral fascial incisions. Use rectus sheath reflection techniques or wide retromuscular mesh.
- Consider creation of a preoperative pneumoperitoneum if midline approximation is doubtful.
- Resect redundant skin and subcutaneous tissue generously, including the umbilicus.
- Use closed suction drains.

PITFALLS

- Do not extrapolate the "tension-free" theory of inguinal hernia repair to the dynamically different defect in incisional hernias.
- Do not simply patch an incisional hernial defect with prosthetic material.
- Do not allow permanent prosthetic material to assume an intraperitoneal position.
- Do not assume that newer materials allow this rule to be violated.
- Do not be rigid about a particular technique.
- Do not underestimate the magnitude of surgery for large ventral hernias.
- Do not underestimate the time that it will take to do this surgery properly.
- Do not be quick to accept simplistic approaches to a complex problem.

---

for incisional hernia repair. Large series both from this country and from abroad have now been published. In the hands of those experienced in the technique, recurrence rates in the range of 5% to 8% are reported, with complication rates of less than 10% and mortality rates of less than 1%.

2. The rectus sheath reflection–overwrap repair with anterior mesh placement (Chevrel technique) is largely the work of one investigator, but excellent results have been reported. Mortality rate in the latest series was 0%; wound complications occurred in 10% of patients, and recurrences were documented in 5%.

3. Much smaller series are reported for the "plastic"

operation of fascial partitioning and midline closure, but recurrence risk appears to be in the same general range of 10% to 15%. The addition of anterior mesh under tension, attached to the lateral cut edges of the external oblique musculoaponeurotic layer, has produced very satisfying results in the author's relatively small series. Time and further experience are necessary before we will know whether this technique produces results comparable to those described earlier.

These results are extraordinary when one considers that many patients included in these series were obese, poor-risk individuals who had complex and recurrent defects. Good results with any technique for incisional hernia repair depend on adherence to principles established by clinical and experimental studies, briefly outlined earlier. For a deeper understanding of these important principles, the reader is referred to "Selected Readings."

Summary

- Incisional hernias involve dynamic processes within the abdominal wall leading to inevitable gradual enlargement of the defect; therefore, repair is usually indicated.
- Preoperative risk factors for incisional hernia include obesity, chronic obstructive pulmonary disease, malnutrition, cancer, and steroid treatment.
- Principles of repair include reconstruction of the linea alba, reattachment of the insertions of the lateral belt muscles, restoration of normal abdominal pressure, and excision of redundant or devitalized skin.
- Accepted surgical procedures include retrorectus pros-

thetic repair, medial reflection of the rectus sheath with anterior mesh repair, fascial partitioning, primary midline reconstruction, and use of anterior mesh under tension.
- Simple patching of hernia defects with mesh is to be discouraged.
- Postoperative care should stress pulmonary management.
- Recurrence rates for these large incisional hernias after accepted repairs should be 5% to 15%.

SELECTED READINGS

Amid PK: Classification of biomaterials and their related complications in abdominal wall hernia surgery. Hernia 1997;1:15.

Chevrel JP, Rath AM: The use of fibrin glues in the surgical treatment of incisional hernias. Hernia 1997;1:9.

DiBello JN, Moore JH: Sliding myofascial flap of the rectus abdominis muscles for the closure of recurrent ventral hernias. Plast Reconstr Surg 1996;98:464.

Neihardt JPH, Chevrel JP, Flament JB, Rives J: Defects of the abdominal wall. In Chevrel JP (ed): Hernias and Surgery of the Abdominal Wall. New York, Springer-Verlag, 1998, pp 111–169.

Ramirez O, Ruas E, Lee A: "Components separation" method for closure of abdominal wall defects: An anatomic and clinical study. Plast Reconstr Surg 1990;86:519.

Ramirez O: Abdominal herniorrhaphy [letter]. Plast Reconstr Surg 1994;93:660.

Stoppa R, Ralaimiaramanana F, Henry X, Verhaeghe P: Evolution of large ventral incisional hernia repair. The French contribution to a difficult problem. Hernia 1999;3:1.

Thomas WO, Parry SW, Rodning CB: Ventral/incisional abdominal herniorrhaphy by fascial partition/release. Plast Reconstr Surg 1993;91:1080.

Voeller G, Ramshaw B, Park AE, Heniford BT: Incisional hernia [letter]. J Am Coll Surg 1999;189:635.

Wantz G: Incisional hernioplasty with Mersilene. Surg Gynecol Obstet 1991;172:129.

Wantz GE, Chevrel JP, Flament JB, et al: Incisional hernia: The problem and the cure. J Am Coll Surg 1999;188:429.

Chapter 127
Uncommon Abdominal Wall Hernias

Kamal M. F. Itani

Spigelian and lumbar hernias are the most common of the unusual abdominal wall hernias. Although an obturator hernia is classified as pelvic (together with perineal and sciatic hernias), it is by far the most common of this group and the most likely to be encountered by a general surgeon. With the boom in minimally invasive surgery, a new form of abdominal wall hernia, postlaparoscopy trocar hernia, is being recognized with increasing frequency. A Richter's hernia can occur within any type of abdominal wall or pelvic hernia, but the most common location is at the site of a femoral hernia. Fewer than 1000 of each of these types of hernia have been reported in the English literature.

Preoperative preparation of patients for elective repair of these types of hernia should be no different from that for inguinal or incisional hernias. When performed electively, these procedures can be done on an ambulatory basis. One dose of antibiotic covering the usual skin flora is recommended preoperatively, especially if prosthetic mesh may be used in the repair. In patients with incarceration with signs and symptoms of bowel obstruction, the patient should be properly resuscitated with fluids and should have a nasogastric tube placed for decompression. Patients presenting with fever, elevated white blood cell count, or other signs of bowel strangulation require broad-spectrum antibiotics, which should probably be continued postoperatively for several days if prosthetic material is used.

Intraoperatively, any segment of bowel with visible signs of irreversible ischemia or necrosis should be resected. Great care should be applied to avoid spillage or gross contamination, especially if the use of prosthetic material is unavoidable. Postoperatively, gastric decompression and support with intravenous fluids are continued in patients with incarcerated or strangulated organs until return of bowel function. Patients are immediately ambulated and are advised to return to specific activities as soon as they feel up to them. Return to heavy weight-bearing may be dependent on the type of hernia and the technique of repair. In patients requiring repair of a pelvic hernia, as well as in all those undergoing laparoscopic repair or a repair necessitating accurate monitoring of fluid status, it may be advisable to place a Foley catheter.

SPIGELIAN HERNIA

Most spigelian hernias occur in the area between the level of umbilicus and the level of the arcuate (semicircular) line, where the spigelian fascia is widest and weakest. The hernias occur particularly at the point where the semilunar and the arcuate lines meet, because it is at this point that all the fibers of the transversus abdominis muscle pass in front of the rectus muscle.

Patients usually complain of nonspecific abdominal pain, palpable resistance in the anterior abdominal wall over the hernia, or evidence of intestinal obstruction. Physical findings that facilitate diagnosis are a palpable hernia or a palpable hernial orifice. These hernias can be notoriously difficult to diagnose on physical examination, although patients usually have distinct tender points over the hernial orifice in the spigelian fascia (Table 127–1).

The diagnosis of spigelian hernia remains difficult be-

Table 127–1	**Uncommon Abdominal Wall Hernias**			
TYPE OF HERNIA	**LOCATION**	**SIGNS°**	**ADJUNCTIVE DIAGNOSTIC TESTS†**	**SURGERY‡**
Spigelian	Junction of arcuate and semilunar lines	Tenderness, bulge	Ultrasonography, CT	Primary repair Mesh occasionally
Lumbar	Superior or inferior lumbar space	Bulge, back pain	Ultrasonography, CT	Primary repair Mesh occasionally
Postlaparoscopy trocar	Abdominal wall	Tenderness, bulge	Ultrasonography, laparoscopy	Primary repair
Obturator	Obturator foramen	Howship-Romberg sign	CT, laparoscopy	Intra-abdominal or retroperitoneal approach; avoid neurovascular bundle
Richter's	Abdomen or pelvis	Tenderness, bowel obstruction	Ultrasonography, laparoscopy	Careful bowel inspection; repair is site dependent

°All patients might present with various degrees of bowel obstruction.
†Adjunctive test can be used if the diagnosis is in doubt.
‡Laparoscopic repair with mesh has been described for all these hernias.
CT, computed tomography.

cause few physicians consider this possibility, either because of a lack of knowledge or because of the rarity of this type of hernia. In addition, the symptoms are not characteristic, and the hernia often develops intramurally (i.e., between the fascial layers of the abdominal wall); thus, both the hernia sac and the orifice may be difficult to detect on palpation.

For these reasons, additional investigation may be necessary. Imaging by means of ultrasonography is the best, the easiest, and the most reliable test for diagnosing spigelian hernia. Thin-section computed tomography will also confirm the presence of this condition, especially when the diagnosis is elusive or other intra-abdominal conditions are suspected (Fig. 127–1).

A transverse or an oblique skin incision is made over the lump at the point of maximum tenderness, marked preoperatively. A subcutaneous hernia will immediately reveal itself, but more commonly the hernia is interstitial (or intramural), and the external oblique aponeurosis must be split to demonstrate the sac. The sac is opened, and the visceral content is inspected. The sac may be excised or inverted. The defect in the fascia of the transversus abdominis and the internal oblique, if small, is closed with a monofilament suture. The slit in the external oblique is repaired similarly. If the defect is large or the tissues are attenuated, prosthetic mesh reinforcement may be indicated (see Table 127–1).

Recurrence rate with this technique should be less than 1%. Laparoscopy with mesh repair is gaining momentum in the diagnosis and the repair of these hernias. In anecdotal reports, the laparoscopic technique is described as involving less dissection and prompt recovery.

LUMBAR HERNIA

Lumbar hernias are quite rare. They are subdivided into hernias of the superior (Grynfeltt-Lesshaft) or the inferior (Petit's) lumbar space (Fig. 127–2). The literature suggests that the superior lumbar space is more commonly involved. Lumbar hernias can be congenital or acquired.

It is extremely unusual to find bowel in a lumbar

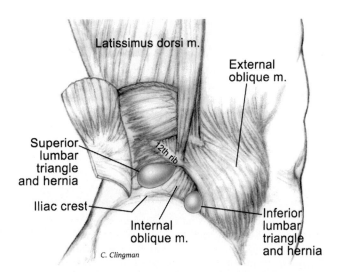

Figure 127–2. Location of superior (Grynfeltt-Lesshaft) and inferior (Petit's) lumbar spaces, with hernias protruding through the lumbodorsal fascia. m., muscle.

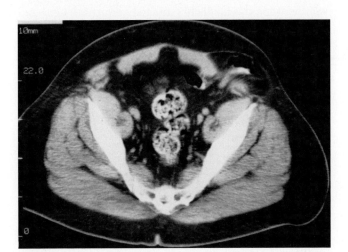

Figure 127–1. Computed tomography of the lower abdomen, showing a large left spigelian hernia.

herniation because the retroperitoneal tissues are most commonly herniated. If the hernia is tender to palpation, pain may be referred through the lumbar nerves to the leg, the thigh, or the scrotum, confusing the diagnosis. Lumbar hernia as a cause of low back pain is not well recognized, however. Most lumbar hernias present as a mass or a bulge that is visible on standing. They tend to enlarge and may reach quite significant proportions, overhanging the iliac crest. When the diagnosis is elusive, ultrasonography or computed tomography may be useful. Numerous complicated procedures involving muscle transfers and muscle or fascial flaps and grafts have been described for repair of the hernia. They should be abandoned in favor of simpler repairs, however (see Table 127–1).

With the patient lying on his or her side, an oblique skin crease incision is made over the area of the hernia, and the sac is dissected down to its neck and opened. After inspection of the contents, these are reduced. The empty sac can be simply inverted or excised. When good tissue is present and the defect is small, it can be closed with a monofilament suture. When the defect is large and the tissues are poor, the hernia is best repaired with a large sheet of prosthetic nonabsorbable mesh. After being laid in the preperitoneal space between the peritoneum and the abdominal wall muscles, the mesh is fixed around its periphery with a series of monofilament synthetic nonabsorbable sutures passed through the full thickness of the abdominal wall. Alternatively, laparoscopic repair through a transperitoneal route has been described, with prosthetic mesh used to patch the defect.

POSTLAPAROSCOPY TROCAR HERNIA

With the increasing number of laparoscopic procedures being performed (both general and gynecologic) as well as the use of larger and larger trocars (>12 mm in diameter), more postoperative hernias can be expected. Most are Richter's hernias without peritoneal lining and contain small or large intestine or omentum. The incidence has been reported to be around 1% but appears to be rising with increasing size of the trocar. About one fourth of these hernias are umbilical; the rest are extraumbilical. Patients typically present within 2 weeks of laparoscopic surgery with nausea, vomiting, and a painful abdomen with tenderness at the site of herniation (see Table 127–1). In some instances, however, the clinical course can be protracted, with an "ileus" or a partial small bowel obstruction occurring up to 1 year after the original laparoscopic procedure. Prevention is essential in avoiding and reducing the incidence of these hernias. Recommendations for avoiding these hernias include fascial closure every time a 10-mm or larger trocar is used, ensuring by direct visualization that intraperitoneal tissue is not drawn into the trocar canal when the probes are removed, and the use of cone-shaped noncutting rather than sharp cutting trocars. When this condition has been diagnosed, the fascial edge and the complete extent of the hernial defect should be defined. Any incarcerated bowel should be reduced after proper inspection. The defect should then be closed as a formal herniorrhaphy with nonabsorbable sutures and a synthetic patch, if necessary (see Table 127–1).

OBTURATOR HERNIA

Obturator hernias occur along the obturator canal, which is the portion of the obturator foramen through which the obturator nerve and vessels exit the pelvis. The defect is usually located anterior and medial to the neurovascular bundle that traverses the obturator canal (Fig. 127–3). Normally, it is a closed space except for the point of exit of the neurovascular bundle.

Patients with obturator hernias are usually elderly, thin females who present acutely. Many patients have acute symptoms that become progressively more severe, and many have experienced previous attacks that resolved spontaneously. The presenting complaints are usually abdominal pain and vomiting, whereas the most common signs are abdominal distention and constipation, which result in a diagnosis of mechanical obstruction. The next most common symptom is pain extending down the medial aspect of the thigh to the knee. Flexion of the thigh usually exacerbates the pain. This pain pattern, known as the Howship-Romberg sign or obturator neuralgia, occurs in approximately 50% of patients. In the absence of this pain, correct preoperative diagnosis is rare. Approximately 20% of patients will have a palpable mass just lateral to the adductor longus tendon in the proximal part of the thigh (see Fig. 127–3). This mass is best palpated with the patient supine and the thigh flexed, abducted, and externally rotated. Vaginal and rectal examinations might be helpful when a laterally situated mass is detected. The value of computed tomography or laparoscopy in the diagnosis of this condition has not been established, but these tests may be helpful (see Table 127–1).

Operative repair of obturator hernias has been performed through various approaches. The abdominal approach—open or laparoscopic—is preferred when compromised bowel is suspected. The retropubic (Cheatle-

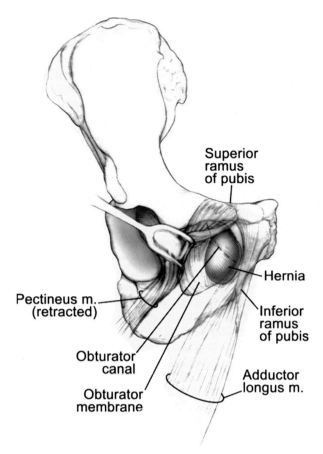

Figure 127–3. Obturator canal, where hernia occurs most frequently medially and anteriorly and protrudes into the thigh lateral to the adductor longus muscle. m., muscle.

Henry) and the inguinal approaches, both retroperitoneal, offer the advantage of staying outside the peritoneal cavity; they can be performed if a diagnosis is obtained preoperatively. The contents of the sac should be inspected and reduced, and the sac should be resected or inverted. Occasionally with the retroperitoneal approach, a counterincision in the femoral triangle is required to decompress the sac, which presents medial to the femoral vein between the medially retracted adductor longus and the pectineus muscle (which can be divided) (see Fig. 127–3). Numerous methods have been described for clo-

---

Pearls and Pitfalls

- Unusual abdominal wall hernias include spigelian, lumbar, obturator, postlaparoscopy trocar, and Richter types.
- Appropriate diagnosis requires a high index of suspicion and knowledge of the existence of these hernias.
- Richter's hernias often are not associated with a formal bowel obstruction if the entire circumference of the incarcerated bowel is not involved; nevertheless, the incarcerated part of the bowel may be ischemic and at risk for necrosis.
- Repairs may require prosthetic mesh and may often be possible through a laparoscopic approach.

sure of the defect, including the use of synthetic plugs, Marlex mesh, or Teflon cloth as well as the use of omental or costal cartilage plugs. The defect can also be repaired by suturing the pectineal muscle to the periosteum of the obturator canal.

RICHTER'S HERNIA

For a hernia to be considered a Richter hernia, the antimesenteric border of the intestine must protrude into the hernia sac but not to the point of involving the entire circumference of the intestine. The symptoms and the clinical course vary widely depending on the degree of obstruction, which is related to the amount of bowel circumference involved (see Table 127–1). Richter's hernias have received increased attention with the increased use of the laparoscope through small-diameter trocar incisions.

Repair of a Richter hernia is based on location. Critical to the repair is an adequate evaluation of the viability of the intestine. In some situations, it is impossible to assess or treat the compromised bowel adequately through the incision for hernia repair. In these cases, an additional midline incision or enlargement of the original trocar incision may be indicated to allow an adequate exploratory laparotomy. Diagnostic laparoscopy can be used as an alternative to laparotomy to evaluate the intestine (see Table 127–1).

SELECTED READINGS

Kadirov S, Sayfan J, Friedman S, Orda R: Richter's hernia: A surgical pitfall. J Am Coll Surg 1996;182:60.
Lajer H, Widecrantz S, Heisterberg L: Hernias in trocar ports following abdominal laparoscopy: A review. Acta Obstet Gynecol Scand 1997;76:389.
Light HG: Hernia of the inferior lumbar space: A cause of back pain. Arch Surg 1983;118:1077.
Orcutt TW: Hernia of the superior lumbar triangle. Ann Surg 1971;173:294.
Spangen L: Spigelian hernia. Surg Clin North Am 1984;64:351.
Yip AW, AhChong AK, Lam KH: Obturator hernia: A continuing diagnostic challenge. Surgery 1993;113:266.

Gastrointestinal Bleeding

Chapter 128

Upper Gastrointestinal Hemorrhage: Diagnosis and Treatment

John Maa and Kimberly S. Kirkwood

Upper gastrointestinal (UGI) bleeding is defined as hemorrhage proximal to the ligament of Treitz. UGI bleeding accounts for more than 300,000 hospitalizations and 15,000 to 30,000 deaths annually. The mortality rate of 6% to 10% has remained unchanged over the past 50 years, and death is often attributable to the serious comorbid conditions prevalent in this patient population. Between 5% and 25% of patients with UGI bleeding are already hospitalized for treatment of another illness.

Among all patients with GI hemorrhage, bleeding from the esophagus, the stomach, and the duodenum occurs in about 80%. The colon is the site of bleeding in the majority of the remaining patients, whereas bleeding from the small intestine is rare, occurring in only about 1% of patients.

The epidemiology of UGI bleeding has changed since 1985. Widespread use of nonsteroidal anti-inflammatory drugs has contributed to an increased incidence of gastric and duodenal ulcers. UGI bleeding is twice as common in men, and the incidence increases 30-fold from the third to the ninth decade of life.

Approximately 80% of patients with UGI bleeding will be successfully managed with endoscopic or supportive therapy. Recent advances in interventional radiology have added complexity to the treatment algorithms for the remaining 20%. Rapid evaluation and triage continue to be critical first steps to ensure a favorable outcome.

CLINICAL PRESENTATION

HISTORY AND DIFFERENTIAL DIAGNOSIS. Only about 60% of patients with previously documented UGI bleed-ing will be bleeding from the same site on subsequent presentation. Even patients with known esophageal varices will be bleeding from other sites 30% of the time. The history should focus on those factors that suggest a cause and on clinical features that predict outcome. The source of bleeding may be suggested by the nature and the duration of blood loss, the presence of comorbid medical conditions (cirrhosis, renal failure, connective tissue disorders), and the use of medications (nonsteroidal anti-inflammatory drugs, salicylates, or anticoagulants). The patient should be questioned regarding alcohol intake, which may suggest gastritis, and possible caustic ingestion, which may point to esophagitis. A history of previous gastric surgery raises the question of bleeding from recurrent peptic or anastomotic ulcer. Patients with (even small) aortic aneurysms, especially those who have undergone previous aortic surgery, are at risk of development of aortoduodenal fistula. Such individuals may present with a sentinel bleed (i.e., a brief episode of hematemesis followed hours or days later by massive hemorrhage). Hematemesis after vomiting or retching or after blunt abdominal trauma suggests a Mallory-Weiss tear. Burns, trauma, sepsis, or recent major physiologic stress can lead to the development of stress ulcers (Curling's ulcers in the duodenum after burns or Cushing's ulcers in the stomach after head trauma).

Overall, peptic ulcer, acute gastritis, esophageal varices, esophagitis, and Mallory-Weiss tears account for more than 90% of causes of UGI hemorrhage. Less common causes of UGI bleeding include occult neoplasms, stress ulcers, portal gastropathy, Dieulafoy's lesions, lesions related to acquired immunodeficiency syndrome

814

(lymphoma, tuberculosis, *Mycobacterium avium-intracellulare* infection, cytomegalovirus, Kaposi's sarcoma), and iatrogenic causes.

PATTERN OF BLEEDING. The magnitude and the rate of bleeding are important determinants of outcome. The pace of the diagnostic evaluation and of the therapeutic intervention hinges on the pattern of bleeding.

Several terms are commonly used to estimate the rate of bleeding. *Massive* UGI bleeding refers to the loss of blood so rapid that it causes hypotension or shock. *Significant* bleeding in an adult implies a loss of at least 800 mL of blood with a decrease in blood hemoglobin of 2 mg/dL or a drop in hematocrit of 6% to 8%. *Hematemesis* may range in color from bright red to the shade of coffee grounds. The latter, which occurs when blood remains in the stomach long enough for gastric acid to convert hemoglobin to methemoglobin, suggests an esophageal or a gastric source. The passage of black, tarry, nonformed stools, or *melena*, reflects the oxidation of heme by intestinal and bacterial enzymes to produce the dark product, hematin. Melena is seen with the loss of at least 100 to 500 mL/day of blood. Although melena usually results from bleeding in the UGI tract, it can, on rare occasion, result from colonic or small intestinal bleeding sources. Conversely, although *hematochezia* is usually associated with lower gastrointestinal bleeding, it can reflect a UGI source if intestinal transit is rapid enough during brisk bleeding that bright red or maroon blood is passed unchanged in the stool. *Occult* bleeding refers to blood loss that is suggested by iron deficiency anemia or by evidence of blood in the stool on guaiac or Hemoccult testing. Healthy people lose 2.5 mL/day of blood in their stools. Tests for occult blood should detect 10 to 50 mL/day. False-positive results may occur owing to the presence of dietary hemoglobin, myoglobin, or peroxidases of plant origin. Iron or bismuth ingestion can cause black stools, but these elements do not cause false-positive reactions.

PHYSICAL EXAMINATION. A major goal of the physical examination is to determine the presence and the severity of shock. Patients with a heart rate (HR) of greater than 100 beats per minute or a systolic blood pressure (SBP) of less than 100 mm Hg have an increased mortality rate. Additional signs of shock include the following: a reduced level of consciousness; cool, clammy, mottled skin; tachypnea; flat jugular veins; and oliguria. Of the frequent causes of UGI bleeding, only portal hypertension is associated with diagnostic clues on physical examination. The stigmata of liver disease that may be present include hepatosplenomegaly, jaundice, ascites, spider angiomas, palmar erythema, and large hemorrhoidal veins. Among patients with UGI bleeding, abdominal tenderness is extremely uncommon and should initiate an aggressive search for some other related condition, such as bowel ischemia, infarction, or perforation. A careful rectal examination should be performed to look for hemorrhoids, fissures, gross blood, or melena. Direct examination of a stool specimen is an important bedside diagnostic test that provides valuable information for risk stratification.

NASOGASTRIC ASPIRATION. Evaluation of the nasogastric aspirate is a direct extension of the physical examina-

tion and remains an important diagnostic maneuver. After local anesthetic has been applied, an 18-French nasogastric tube (NGT) is passed into the stomach, and 50 to 100 mL of tap water is instilled and aspirated. The presence of red blood in the aspirated fluid indicates active bleeding and is associated with increased risk of complications and death, whereas a clear aspirate identifies patients at lower risk. The presence of bilious nonbloody fluid suggests a lower gastrointestinal source; however, a nonbloody aspirate is seen in 15% of patients with a true upper site of bleeding. There is no benefit to large-volume lavage, which can contribute to pulmonary aspiration. The NGT should remain in place until the patient undergoes endoscopy, because it helps to keep the stomach decompressed and serves as an indicator of rebleeding.

LABORATORY TESTING. Laboratory testing should be used to evaluate the extent of blood loss, to determine the presence of coagulopathies, and to corroborate the presence of comorbid conditions (e.g., underlying liver or renal disease). Initial laboratory tests should include complete blood count, prothrombin time, partial thromboplastin time, and measurement of levels of transaminases, electrolytes, blood urea nitrogen, and creatinine. Blood should also be sent for typing and cross-matching; usually 2 to 4 units of packed cells should be made available. An initial hematocrit of less than 30 or the presence of coagulopathy is a marker of poor outcome. Azotemia, or a blood urea nitrogen/creatinine ratio of greater than 36, suggests a UGI source. (A ratio of less than 36 is not helpful diagnostically.) The azotemia seen in UGI bleeding results from gut absorption of nitrogen from blood proteins combined with volume depletion. Azotemia usually clears 3 days after cessation of bleeding. With chronic blood loss, the mean corpuscular volume may be low, signifying iron deficiency anemia.

An electrocardiogram (ECG) should be performed for any patient older than 40 years of age with chest or epigastric pain or known cardiovascular or pulmonary disease. It is also useful to obtain a baseline ECG in the face of significant bleeding because ECG changes may guide the need for transfusion.

PREOPERATIVE MANAGEMENT

INITIAL TRIAGE AND RESUSCITATION. On presentation, patients with UGI bleeding are stratified according to their risk of imminent death. *Active bleeding* is usually apparent clinically by the finding of ongoing hematemesis, hematochezia, or melena and is confirmed by passage of the NGT. Patients with UGI bleeding and hypotension (SBP of less than 100 mm Hg, or 30 mm Hg less than a previous baseline value) regardless of HR are at high risk and require immediate resuscitation. Isotonic fluid should be administered via large-bore intravenous catheters, usually in the antecubital fossa. Placement of central lines should usually be deferred to the intensive care unit setting unless no other access is available. Monitoring should include continuous ECG, oxygen saturation surveillance, urinary catheterization, and measurement of blood pressure every 2 to 5 minutes. Endotracheal intubation should be considered in the vomiting or semiconscious patient. Those patients who fail to respond rapidly to isotonic fluid should be transfused to achieve hemodynamic stability (see later). It is helpful to consult both gastroenterologic and surgical specialists early in the evaluation.

Patients who present with normal blood pressure and tachycardia (HR > 100 beats per minute) fall into the moderate risk category. Isotonic fluids are administered until the vital signs are normal. In these patients, the decision to transfuse is usually based on serial hematocrit values—rather than hemodynamic instability—in conjunction with the finding of active bleeding in the nasogastric aspirate. Continuous ECG, oxygen saturation, and blood pressure should be monitored every 15 minutes. A gastroenterologist should be consulted promptly.

Patients with normal vital signs are at low risk of dying as a result of GI bleeding. An intravenous line is placed, and vital signs are measured every 30 minutes. Consultation with a gastroenterologist may be deferred until the results of the nasogastric aspirate analysis and hematocrit are known.

BLOOD TRANSFUSION. In patients with UGI bleeding, there may be several scenarios in which transfusion of blood products is appropriate. The patient with clinical evidence of active bleeding and shock who fails to respond rapidly to crystalloid requires transfusion. Therapy should not be delayed to await initial hematocrit results because these may be falsely high before plasma equilibration. Packed red blood cells should be given to achieve hemodynamic stability. If cross-matched blood is not available, type-specific or type O blood may be substituted. Patients with stable blood pressure and clinical evidence of active bleeding should be transfused with packed red cells to keep the hematocrit in the range of 25 to 30, depending on comorbid factors such as cardiopulmonary disease.

BLEEDING DISORDERS. Cirrhotic patients may present with both thrombocytopenia and a prolonged prothrombin time. Actively bleeding patients with thrombocytopenia should receive platelets to keep their counts greater than 50,000. Platelets may also be considered in patients with platelet dysfunction due to recent aspirin use (within 3 days). Fresh frozen plasma should be given to actively bleeding patients with a prolonged prothrombin time. Uremic patients with UGI bleeding and platelet dysfunction may derive initial benefit from 1-deamino(8-D-argi-

nine) vasopressin (DDAVP; 0.3 μg/kg intravenously every 12 to 24 hours) and subsequent benefit from conjugated estrogen (0.6 mg/kg per day intravenously for 5 days).

TRIAGE IN THE EMERGENCY ROOM. During the first hour in the emergency room, history-taking and physical examination are performed, the nasogastric aspirate is obtained, the stool is examined, the laboratory results are made available, and the initial response to resuscitation becomes apparent. A reassessment is then performed based on the patient's predicted risk of further bleeding or death (Table 128–1). Patients with ongoing hemodynamic instability should be transferred to the intensive care unit without delay for continued resuscitation and for placement of arterial and possibly central venous lines. Esophagogastroduodenoscopy (EGD) should be performed in the intensive care unit once the blood pressure has stabilized. Endotracheal intubation will often be required to protect the airway adequately during both EGD and gastric lavage (if necessary). Patients with ongoing tachycardia after initial resuscitation with clinical evidence of active bleeding requiring more than 2 units of blood, or with significant comorbid conditions, should be admitted to a regular hospital bed. EGD in the endoscopy unit should be performed once the patient is stable. Healthy patients whose vital signs normalize after initial resuscitation and who have no evidence of active bleeding may be transferred to the endoscopy unit before admission because many will be found to have lesions amenable to outpatient management.

ENDOSCOPY. Endoscopy is the primary *diagnostic* tool for patients with UGI bleeding. The sensitivity of upper endoscopy is greater when the procedure is performed early (within 24 hours of the onset of bleeding). Although in the majority of patients, only one bleeding site will be identified, two or more sites are seen in 15% of patients. Lesions that may be prone to rebleeding include those that are actively bleeding at the time of EGD, those that have adherent clot, and those that have a "visible vessel" at the base of an ulcer. The therapeutic repertoire of the endoscopist has expanded greatly in the past 20 years. *Therapeutic* modalities can be divided into thermal methods and injection therapy. Thermal methods can be further subdivided into contact (e.g., monopolar electrocoagulation, bipolar-multipolar electrocoagulation, heater probe) and noncontact methods (e.g., laser therapy). Endoscopic sclerotherapy of variceal bleeding achieves he-

Table 128–1	Triage of Patients with Upper Gastrointestinal Bleeding in the Emergency Department		
PARAMETERS FOR TRIAGE	**ENDOSCOPY UNIT**	**REGULAR BED**	**ICU BED**
Vital signs	Normal SBP *and* HR	HR > 100 *and* SBP > 100	SBP < 100°
Clinical features	No active bleeding *and* ≤2 units of blood *and* no active comorbidity	Clearing NG aspirate *or* >2 units of blood *or* active comorbidity	Actively bleeding *or* requires intubation *or* severe comorbidity
Resuscitation	IV access ± blood	IV fluids, vital signs every 15 minutes ± blood	IV fluids, vital signs every 2–5 minutes, blood ± intubate
Goal	Immediate EGD Possible discharge	Early EGD	EGD in ICU, once stable

°Or 30 mm Hg less than prior baseline value.
EGD, esophagogastroduodenoscopy; HR, heart rate; ICU, intensive care unit; IV, intravenous; NG, nasogastric; SBP, systolic blood pressure.

mostasis in the majority of patients and has greatly reduced the need for emergency surgical portosystemic shunts. When combined with these therapeutic techniques, early endoscopy is associated with shorter hospital stays and improved outcome.

From the surgeon's viewpoint, the specificity in localization of bleeding sites achieved with endoscopy (approximately 90%) is clearly superior to that achieved with contrast radiography (approximately 50%). The sensitivity of endoscopy is 70% to 85%; this may be improved with repeated examinations, particularly if visibility is impaired by blood clots or ingested food within the stomach.

ANGIOGRAPHY. There are several clinical settings in which selective angiography can be useful in the diagnosis or the treatment of patients with UGI bleeding. If endoscopy fails to localize the bleeding site owing to impaired visibility as a result of active bleeding and blood clots in the stomach, celiac arteriography will often identify the site of hemorrhage. Diagnostic success is likely only when the rate of bleeding is greater than 0.5 mL/minute, as it often is when bleeding is of a large enough quantity to interfere with endoscopic visibility. Infusion of vasoconstrictors (e.g., vasopressin) through the angiographic catheter or embolization of the bleeding vessel with Gelfoam may halt bleeding in special cases so that diagnostic endoscopy may be used to evaluate or treat the lesion. In patients in whom bleeding is due to severe diffuse gastritis, embolization of the left gastric artery or other contributing branches may reduce bleeding. Embolization is usually not useful for bleeding duodenal ulcers in which the gastroduodenal artery is the primary vessel because this high-flow arcade with multiple collateral feeders is refractory to angiographic control. Diagnostic arteriography and embolization are usually definitive therapy for bleeding from pseudoaneurysms, such as may accompany severe or chronic pancreatitis. Aortography is the best means of identifying patients with aortoduodenal fistulas. Finally, the transjugular intrahepatic portosystemic shunt (TIPS) procedure is effective for patients with recurrent variceal bleeding and may provide a valuable bridge to liver transplantation.

OTHER RADIOGRAPHIC STUDIES. There is little role for the use of *plain abdominal radiographs* in the localization of UGI bleeding unless abdominal pain, peritoneal signs, or marked distention are present. UGI *barium studies* have no role in the initial evaluation of active bleeding when endoscopy is available. Barium studies may identify mucosal lesions but cannot confirm active bleeding from a suspected site. Furthermore, barium contrast will interfere with subsequent endoscopic, arteriographic, or computed tomographic studies.

PHARMACOTHERAPY. In patients with suspected portal hypertension and variceal bleeding, the somatostatin analogue *octreotide* has been shown to reduce the magnitude of bleeding, presumably via its effects on decreasing overall splanchnic blood flow. Octreotide (100 μg bolus followed by 50 μg/hour) can be initiated early after presentation of such patients to the emergency department. Controlled clinical trials have shown no benefit from the administration of H_2 *histamine receptor antagonists* or *proton pump inhibitors* to control UGI bleeding. The efficacy of these agents in reducing the incidence of recurrent hemorrhage during hospitalization of patients with UGI bleeding also remains unproved. It is appropriate to include these agents as part of the planned therapy for peptic ulcer once such a diagnosis is made.

INTRAOPERATIVE MANAGEMENT

THE DECISION TO OPERATE. The decision to operate for control of UGI bleeding depends more on *rate*, *duration*, and *magnitude* of blood loss than on the specific cause. The need for transfusion should be continually monitored. An ongoing dialogue between the endoscopist and the surgeon greatly facilitates decision making. It is often helpful for the surgeon to observe endoscopy in high-risk patients, because subtle features of the anatomic location and the nature of the bleeding may guide strategic planning.

Every effort should be made to *localize* the site of bleeding preoperatively. Repeated endoscopy or angiography is sometimes necessary to avoid nontherapeutic laparotomy. The most common cause of rebleeding after operation for UGI bleeding is inadequate preoperative localization.

Preoperative resuscitation is essential to avoid serious anesthetic complications. Ideally, SBP, HR, and urine output are normal following resuscitation; however, this goal is not always achievable in the setting of rapid bleeding. In some patients, the safest course of action is to complete the resuscitation in the operating room after the bleeding has been controlled and, it is hoped, before the patient develops coagulopathy. Patients older than 60 years of age tolerate continued blood loss less well than younger patients. The threshold for operation should, therefore, be lower in elderly patients to avoid secondary cardiovascular, pulmonary, or renal complications.

Intraoperatively, resuscitation efforts continue concurrently with the surgical procedure. The actively bleeding patient should be given a warming blanket, a blood warmer, and a warm room to keep the core body temperature higher than 35°C. An upper midline incision usually provides good exposure and retains flexibility. Access to a bleeding peptic ulcer can generally be achieved via a pyloroplasty incision, which allows for immediate digital control of the bleeding site. The proximal stomach is easily accessed via a high anterior gastrotomy incision. Placement of narrow deep retractors or stay sutures facilitates exposure and excision or ligation of bleeding sites. Branches of the left gastric artery that may feed proximal bleeding points can be ligated either from inside the stomach lumen or at the serosal surface where the vessel enters the gastric wall along the lesser curvature.

POSTOPERATIVE MANAGEMENT

Following successful control of UGI bleeding, postoperative management focuses on supportive therapy to allow organ systems to recover from preoperative hypovolemic hemorrhagic shock. Elderly patients are at especially high risk of renal insufficiency, myocardial infarction, and adult respiratory distress syndrome from hypoperfusion and massive transfusions. Hematocrit should be checked every 6 hours initially to be certain that bleeding has stopped. It is useful to leave an NGT for a day or so postoperatively if there is any question of ongoing hemorrhage. Any sign of rebleeding warrants immediate investigation, usually by repeat EGD to localize and characterize the source, or possibly operative intervention, depending on the original findings (e.g., large ulcer with a visible vessel).

COMPLICATIONS

Among patients with UGI bleeding, the primary complication of treatment is *rebleeding*. In 85% of patients, bleeding stops within a few hours of admission. About 25% of patients rebleed once bleeding has stopped, and these episodes tend to occur within the first 2 days of admission. Many patients who rebleed will require surgical control, most commonly for peptic ulcer. The mortality rate, despite treatment, is 30% in patients who rebleed versus 3% in those who do not. Death is uncommon when fewer than 7 units of blood are required, and the mortality rate increases progressively thereafter. The mortality rate is higher in the elderly and in patients already in the hospital for other illnesses; these latter patients are often quite ill from their preexistent comorbidity. It is relatively uncommon for patients to die as a result of exsanguination per se; rather, they die of multisystem organ failure, shock, dilutional coagulopathy, and the sequelae of massive transfusions.

OUTCOMES AND PROGNOSIS

Several clinical features associated with a low risk of serious bleeding in patients who present with UGI bleeding have been identified. These include the following:

1. Age of less than 75 years.
2. Absence of unstable comorbid disease.
3. Absence of ascites on physical examination.
4. A normal prothrombin time.
5. SBP of greater than 100 mm Hg within 1 hour of admission.
6. NGT aspirate free of blood.

Such patients may be managed expediently with early endoscopy and, in some cases, outpatient follow-up.

In contrast, factors associated with a high risk of rebleeding and death include the following:

1. Rapid bleeding
2. Hematemesis
3. Hypotension on admission
4. A transfusion requirement of more than 4 units of blood or more than 1 unit every 8 hours
5. Elevation in the level of serum fibrin degradation products

COMMON PROBLEMS

The major difficulty that confronts surgeons caring for patients with UGI bleeding is the decision to operate. To some extent, it is possible to predict which patients are at higher risk of rebleeding or are likely to require operative intervention. Several questions summarized in Table 128–2 can be used to guide the process of decision making. Patients with nonvariceal hemorrhage with *active* bleeding at the time of presentation, particularly those with hypotension, are more likely to require surgery. Preoperative localization of the bleeding source is critical, because some forms of even massive hemorrhage (e.g., from esophageal varices or diffuse gastritis) are better treated nonsurgically. Particularly in the setting of rapid bleeding, blood clots in the stomach obscure the endoscopist's view, making localization difficult. It is worth the effort to intubate the airway to protect against aspiration, to place a large-bore (32-French) tube in the stomach to lavage and clear it, and to repeat endoscopy.

Rebleeding following endoscopic or surgical control warrants prompt reevaluation via endoscopy to determine the nature of the problem and the possible need for (repeat) operation if the patient is stable. The elderly patient with cardiorespiratory comorbidity who has already received 4 to 6 units of blood but rebleeds may be better treated with operative intervention rather than a second or a third attempt at definitive endoscopic treatment. Significant rebleeding after endoscopic control usually warrants surgical intervention. Bleeding following surgery may be due to mucosal erosions or may be anastomotic, which often responds to endoscopic techniques; in contrast, recurrent bleeding due to gastric or duodenal ulcers may warrant reoperation.

Pearls and Pitfalls

- In 80% of patients, GI bleeding originates from a UGI source.
- Bright red blood per rectum can be from a UGI source if the bleeding is brisk enough.
- With acute hematochezia, the nasogastric aspirate should be tested for blood, because the evaluation will then be directed at a UGI source.
- Patients with GI bleeding should be screened for coagulopathy via evaluation of platelets, prothrombin time, and partial thromboplastin time.
- Initial triage to assign the patient to semi-elective endoscopy, hospitalization, or the intensive care unit depends on HR, SBP, and presence of comorbidity.
- Provided the patient is relatively stable, attempts to localize the source of bleeding should be made before operative intervention. It may be difficult or impossible in the operating room to determine whether the bleeding is from esophagus, stomach, or duodenum.
- One of the hardest decisions is when to operate. The elderly patient with significant cardiorespiratory comorbidity who has already received 4 to 6 units of blood may be better served by immediate operation rather than a second or a third attempt at endoscopic control.

Table 128–2	Common Problems in Caring for Patients with Upper Gastrointestinal Bleeding		
QUESTION	**EVALUATION**	**GOAL**	

Is there *active* bleeding?	Hematemesis
	NGT
	Hematochezia
	Serial hematocrit
		Determine:
		    Pace of intervention
		    Likelihood of surgery	

What is the bleeding *rate*?	SBP, HR Pattern of bleeding Serial hematocrit	Risk stratification	
What if blood obscures the endoscopist's view?	Lavage° and repeat EGD Consider angiography	Determine if lesion amenable to surgery Preoperative localization	
What if bleeding *recurs* after endoscopic or surgical control?	Repeat EGD	Define anatomic site Determine need for surgery	

°Airway protection is afforded by airway intubation *before* lavage
EGD, esophagogastroduodenoscopy; HR, heart rate; NGT, nasogastric tube; SBP, systolic blood pressure.

Summary

Upper gastrointestinal bleeding is defined as hemorrhage proximal to the ligament of Treitz. Overall, peptic ulcer, acute gastritis, esophageal varices, esophagitis, and Mallory-Weiss tears account for more than 90% of UGI hemorrhages. The magnitude and the rate of bleeding determine the pace of the diagnostic evaluation, the therapeutic intervention, and, ultimately, the outcome. Criteria are provided to facilitate risk stratification of patients at the time of presentation and to guide resuscitation. Upper endoscopy is the mainstay of diagnosis and therapy. The decision to operate for acute UGI bleeding depends on rate, duration, and magnitude of blood loss and should follow adequate resuscitation and localization whenever possible. Figure 128–1 summarizes the diagnostic and the therapeutic strategies in the management of patients with UGI bleeding.

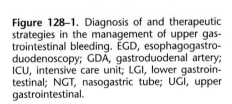

Figure 128–1. Diagnosis of and therapeutic strategies in the management of upper gastrointestinal bleeding. EGD, esophagogastroduodenoscopy; GDA, gastroduodenal artery; ICU, intensive care unit; LGI, lower gastrointestinal; NGT, nasogastric tube; UGI, upper gastrointestinal.

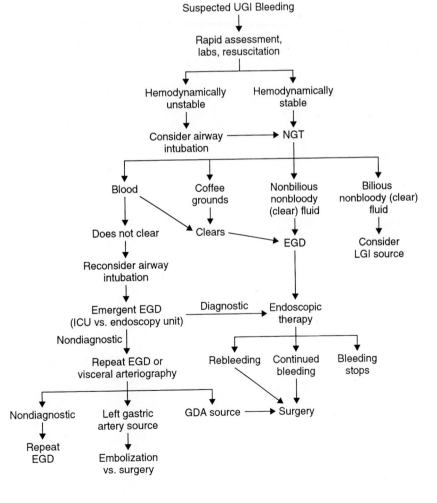

SELECTED READINGS

Besson I, Ingrand P, Person B, et al: Sclerotherapy with or without octreotide for acute variceal bleeding. N Engl J Med 1995;333:555.

Kankaria AG, Fleischer DE: The critical care management of nonvariceal upper gastrointestinal bleeding. Crit Care Clin 1995;11:347.

Katschinski B, Logan R, Davies J, et al: Prognostic factors in upper gastrointestinal bleeding. Dig Dis Sci 1994;39:706.

Peter DJ, Dougherty JM: Evaluation of the patient with gastrointestinal bleeding: An evidence based approach. Emerg Med Clin North Am 1999;17:239.

Rockall TA, Logan RF, Devlin HB, Northfield TC: Risk assessment after acute upper gastrointestinal haemorrhage. Gut 1996;38:316.

Terdiman JP: Update on upper gastrointestinal bleeding. Basing treatment decisions on patients' risk level. Postgrad Med 1998;103:43.

Chapter 129

Lower Gastrointestinal Bleeding

Nadine L. Duhan and Theodore J. Saclarides

INTRODUCTION

Massive lower gastrointestinal (GI) bleeding requiring emergent surgery constitutes approximately 1.5% of all surgical emergencies. Defined as a blood loss of recent onset occurring distal to the ligament of Treitz and resulting in hemodynamic instability or anemia or requiring blood transfusion, it often presents solely as hematochezia. Although 80% to 85% of patients with lower GI bleeding stop spontaneously, surgery may ultimately be required in the instances in which bleeding continues or hemodynamic instability persists. Efforts are directed at localizing the site of bleeding and, with the use of endoscopy and angiography, at identifying and often effectively controlling the bleeding without surgery. Approximately 10% to 20% of patients will have no identified source of bleeding. Urgent surgery without a localized source offers a particular challenge to the surgeon.

CLINICAL PRESENTATION

Acute versus chronic bleeding can be distinguished by a history that assesses onset of symptoms, recent changes in stool character, and other risk factors. The risk factors include aspirin, nonsteroidal anti-inflammatory drugs (NSAIDs), anticoagulant use, or comorbidities including renal failure and cirrhosis that may lead to coagulopathies. A history of GI disease (e.g., peptic ulcer, inflammatory bowel disease, or anorectal disorders) can help focus the direction of the evaluation. Associated symptoms, such as dyspepsia, hematemesis, abdominal pain, and recent changes in bowel habits, should be elicited. Characteristically, the patient with lower GI bleeding presents with hematochezia, whereas the patient with an upper GI bleed presents with melena. Melena involves a black, tarry, *nonformed* stool in the absence of medications that turn the stool black (oral iron, several over-the-counter medications containing bismuth). *Melena* is a very specific term and does not just mean blood in the stool or an uncharacteristic dark stool. Only 250 mL of blood is required to form melenotic stool, and melena can persist for several days after the bleed has resolved. When accompanied by hematemesis, melena is usually indicative of an upper GI source, whereas melena alone may rarely involve a source distal to the ligament of Treitz. Hematochezia, defined as liquid blood mixed with clots and stool, is indicative of a lower GI source. Its color may range from maroon to bright red, indicating how vigorous a bleed. However, owing to the cathartic nature of blood, a vigorous upper GI bleed can also present with hematochezia; therefore, nasogastric lavage should always be performed to exclude an upper GI source.

Eighty-five percent of the instances of massive lower GI bleeding are attributable to colonic sources. Most commonly identified are diverticula and angiodysplastic lesions; other causes include ischemia, inflammatory bowel disease, neoplasms, and polypectomy sites. Anorectal disease rarely causes massive lower GI bleeding, but in the cirrhotic or coagulopathic patient, hemorrhoids, anorectal varices, and fissures can cause significant bleeding. Occasionally, one may encounter radiation-induced hemorrhagic proctitis and rectal ulcers in the patient who is having significant bleeding. Approximately 5% will have a small bowel lesion as the source (Table 129–1).

Patients require surgical resection for ongoing, recurrent, or hemodynamically unstable GI bleeding that cannot be controlled endoscopically or angiographically. Localization is essential for ensuring that the bleeding portion of bowel is removed, while limiting the extent of resection if possible. If the patient is stable and an adequate initial colonoscopy, angiography, or nuclear medicine scan does not identify the lesion, enteroclysis can be performed to exclude a source in the distal small bowel. At times, the bleeding source cannot be identified endoscopically, often because of the inability to cleanse the bowel of retained blood and stool or because of bleeding that has stopped spontaneously without an identifiable source. Also, arteriovenous malformations and diverticula are comorbidities in the elderly that are often seen endoscopically, but are not definitely identified as the bleeding

Table 129–1	Causes of Acute Lower GI Bleeding

Diverticular disease (15%–55%)
Angiodysplasia (3%–37%)
Neoplasia (8%–36%)
Colitis (6%–22%)
  Ischemic
  Infectious
  Inflammatory bowel disease
  Radiation proctoscopy
Polypectomy sites (0.1 to 4%–11%)
Anorectal causes (3%–9%)
  Hemorrhoids
  Varices
Upper GI sources (10%–15%)
  Gastric ulcer
  Duodenal ulcer
  Esophageal varices
Small bowel sources (5%)
  Crohn's disease
  Vascular ectasia
  Meckel's diverticulum
  Neoplasms

Data from Billingham RP: The conundrum of lower gastrointestinal bleeding. Surg Clin North Am 1997;77:241; Zuccaro G Jr: Management of the adult patient with acute lower GI bleeding. Am J Gastroenterol 1998;93:1202; and Zuckerman GR, Prakash C: Acute lower intestinal bleeding. Part II: Etiology, therapy, and outcomes. Gastrointest Endosc 1999;49:228–238.

source unless an active bleed or clot is seen in association with the lesion.

The methods used to localize lesions are also limited. Angiography will localize the bleed if it is actively bleeding at the time of the procedure or if there is a site of abnormal blood vessels. Similarly, technetium-labeled red blood cell scans require active bleeding, but delayed (6 to 12 hours later) scans may pick up intermittent bleeding. Localization by technetium scans may also be skewed by shunting of the tagged red blood cells away from the bleeding site. When preoperative evaluation has been inconclusive, intraoperative maneuvers for cleansing the bowel and endoscopically localizing the bleeding source can aid the surgeon at the time of operation. Rarely, a patient will require "blind," segmental or subtotal colectomy without having the bleeding source identified. Radical blind colectomy does not guarantee that the patient will not rebleed from an unidentified lesion in a more proximal portion of the bowel.

INITIAL MANAGEMENT OF ACUTE, MASSIVE GASTROINTESTINAL BLEEDING

The initial examination should include overall assessment of hemodynamic stability. With massive GI bleeding, large-bore peripheral intravenous access should be obtained, and fluid resuscitation and supplemental oxygen should be administered. If the patient is hypotensive, one can assume a minimal loss of 15% of blood volume. Patients presenting in shock are more likely to develop further complications (i.e., renal ischemia and acute tubular necrosis [ATN]), and aggressive resuscitation should be implemented. Indications for transfusion depend on the initial hemoglobin-to-hematocrit ratio and hemodynamic stability as well as whether the patient is still actively, briskly bleeding. For a patient with cardiac comorbidities, the threshold for transfusion is lower. For the patient with coagulopathies, transfusion of fresh-frozen plasma, platelets, and cryoprecipitate as well as vitamin K should be given as indicated.

Essential initial laboratory tests include a complete blood count, coagulation studies, and a crossmatch for blood transfusion. Electrolyte panels help assess the level of dehydration and may also help in grossly localizing the source of the bleeding lesion. A ratio of blood urea nitrogen (BUN) to creatinine greater than 36 is generally indicative of an upper GI source, whereas a ratio less than 20 is suggestive of a lower GI source; this decreased ratio is related to reabsorption of blood products.

For the stable patient, nasogastric lavage should be performed to exclude an upper GI source. If coffee-ground material or bright red blood is present in the lavage, upper endoscopy should be performed. Proctosigmoidoscopy should always be done to exclude anorectal lesions. With accessible lesions, banding or cautery can be performed at the bedside prior to colonoscopy.

About 85% of lower GI bleeding is self-limited and will resolve spontaneously; however, 10% will be ongoing and severe enough to require intensive care. These patients should be monitored carefully with serial hemoglobin and coagulation studies. For patients with blood loss

greater than 1500 mL within a 24-hour period, 85% ultimately require definitive surgery. Patients in whom bleeding resolves spontaneously can be managed nonoperatively with observation, and the evaluation can be approached in a nonurgent manner. Overall, 10% to 25% will rebleed, depending on the type of lesion; therefore, identification of the bleeding source is essential.

Diagnostic Evaluation

One of the challenges facing the investigation of a patient with lower GI bleeding is that there is no universally agreed on algorithmic approach to the evaluation. The decision to perform colonoscopy, nuclear medicine scans, or angiography should be tailored to each patient, based on risk factors, rate of bleeding, and known etiologies and comorbidities. A briskly bleeding source may render colonoscopy impractical, and a slow bleed may not be detectable on a bleeding scan or angiogram. The availability of resources, and the skills of the operator, vary at each institution and should be taken into account (Fig. 129–1).

Colonoscopy

A total of 90% of colonoscopies are successful in establishing a diagnosis and 50% are therapeutic; thus, colonoscopy should be the first diagnostic approach in most situations. Identification of the bleeding source is suggested by seeing fresh blood localized to one location and confirming no blood proximal to the area. An adherent clot is also indicative of the source. Often potential sources, such as diverticula and angiodysplasia (Fig. 129–2), are identified. However, if bleeding or clot is not visualized, then it cannot be considered the active source with certainty. In the event that no active bleeding or clot is recognized, there is a 10% to 25% chance of misdiagnosing a potential site as the source of bleed. Even if a source is identified, it is advisable to repeat the colonoscopy in a less acute setting after a good bowel preparation, so that coexisting lesions are not missed, especially in the case of polyps or neoplasms. Of note, when a patient has had a recent colonoscopic polypectomy and the polyp site is the probable source of bleeding, repeat colonoscopy and the additional use of electrocoagulation should be undertaken cautiously because of the risk of inducing perforation.

When a bleeding source is identified, several methods are available by which to endoscopically achieve hemostasis. Commonly, injection sclerotherapy with sodium tetradecol or ethanolamine oleate is employed, particularly for angiodysplasia. In one small study of 15 patients, an injection of a 3.3% solution of ethanolamine at a tangential angle to the lesion (4-mm needle) in 2- to 3-mL quantities (2 to 3 injections per lesion) led to a 75% success rate. There were no complications except for scarring at the injection sites and rebleeding (25% at 2 years).

Monopolar cautery applied in short bursts or the better controlled bipolar electrical current (BICAP) can be applied; however, the surgeon must exercise care to avoid full-thickness, transmural burns. Heater-probe thermal

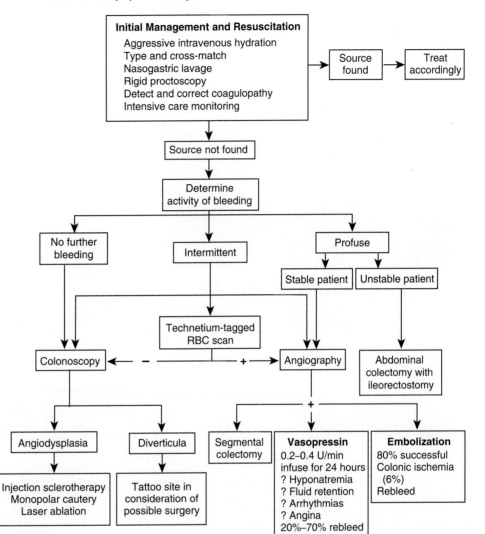

Lower Gastrointestinal Hemorrhage
80%–85% have a colonic source
80%–85% stop spontaneously

Figure 129–1. Algorithm for approach to lower GI bleeding.

cautery is best utilized directly over small angiodysplastic lesions. When a large vessel is visualized during colonoscopy, an endoclip can be used to control the bleeding.

Lasers can also be used as a nonsurgical approach to the treatment of the bleeding patient, although their use is not always practical. Nd:YAG lasers are the most appropriate, as they have better coagulation properties and a more flexible fiber, allowing passage through a colonoscope. It is important to have a well-prepared colon to enhance visibility, making this a less practical option in the acute setting. Also, many colonoscopies for emergent lower GI bleeding are done portably at the bedside; thus, the nonportable Nd:YAG laser is usually not available. Utilized primarily for angiodysplastic lesions, this laser was shown in one series to have an 82% success rate at 18 months follow-up. Complications included perforation (4%), penetrating laser ulcer (2%), and recurrent bleeding within 2 years of follow-up. Most of the recurrences were attributed to missed lesions or incompletely treated patients.

For the patient in whom resection may be indicated, tattooing the bowel near the lesion at the time of endoscopy can assist the surgeon in locating the source of bleeding at the time of surgery. This is particularly useful when other potential bleeding sources are present (e.g., diverticulosis) or when the lesion will be difficult to identify from the serosal surface.

Controversy exists as to the best time to perform colonoscopy. Immediate colonoscopy offers the advantage of identifying the lesion while it may be actively bleeding, but this approach has the disadvantage of potentially inadequate visualization. Delay of colonoscopy in the stable patient permits an adequate bowel preparation, but at an increased chance that the source of bleed may not be identified. In the presence of skilled operators, however, colonoscopy is usually the most efficient means by

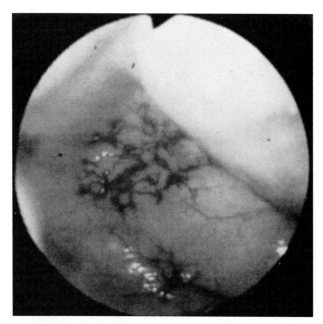

Figure 129–2. Angiodysplastic lesion of the cecum seen through the colonoscope. (From Gordon PH, Nivatvongs S: Principles and Practice of Surgery for the Colon, Rectum and Anus, 2nd ed. St. Louis: Quality Medical Publishing, 1999.)

which to both diagnose and treat the source of bleeding, and this approach has been shown to effectively treat lower GI bleeding in approximately 25% of cases.

Nuclear Medicine Scans

Technetium 99m–labeled red blood cell scintiscans are an accurate, noninvasive method of localizing GI bleeding that offers several advantages over angiography. With a sensitivity of approximately 93% and a specificity of 95%, technetium scans are able to identify *active bleeding* at a rate as low as 0.1 to 0.5 mL/min. These nuclear medicine scans offer the advantage of not requiring a radiographic contrast agent and, therefore, of avoiding the complications and reactions associated with contrast dyes. These scans are also less expensive than angiography and appear to be cost-effective as a screening study prior to angiography in the appropriate clinical situation. Eighty-three percent of localized hemorrhages will be identified within 90 minutes; delayed imaging is possible if the bleeding is intermittent or not immediately identifiable.

Two types of Tc 99m studies are available. Tc 99m sulfur colloid can detect active bleeding as slow as 0.05 to 0.1 mL/min, and it is considered the most sensitive of tests. Sequential static or dynamic images are taken for up to 20 minutes, with increasing intraluminal activity indicative of a positive result. This type of scan is most appropriate in the unstable patient with active bleeding when rapid localization is necessary or when labeled red blood cell scanning is not feasible. Because the sulfur colloid label is cleared rapidly by the reticuloendothelial system, intermittent or later bleeding is not evaluated well.

Tc 99m–labeled red blood cells (Fig. 129–3) is the

study of choice when intermittent bleeding occurs, and can detect a bleeding rate as slow as 0.1 to 0.2 mL/min. The labeling takes approximately 30 minutes, so this should be reserved for hemodynamically stable patients. Initial flow images should be obtained followed by sequential static or dynamic images for 60 to 90 minutes or until a source is localized. Delayed films can be taken up to 48 hours after initial infusion. Technetium-tagged red blood cell scanning is an excellent method of distinguishing left-sided sources from right-sided ones, is most sensitive for slower and intermittent bleeds, and can help screen for which patients should undergo angiography and which should undergo prompt surgery. The major limitation of scintiscans is that they are strictly a localizing procedure, and are neither diagnostic nor therapeutic. If the source of bleeding is in the middle small bowel, exact localization is difficult at best.

Angiography

Angiography, unlike scintigraphy, is capable of localizing, diagnosing, and potentially treating the source of a lower GI bleed. Angiography requires vigorous bleeding (>0.5 mL/min) that must be active during the 20-second window of infusion and imaging. Angiography is the most accurate localizing technique in the emergent setting, successfully identifying the bleed in 70% to 90% of patients. Results are best if all three mesenteric vessels are cannulated. The superior mesenteric artery should be injected first, since the bleeding source is most likely to occur within its distribution, followed by the inferior mesenteric artery and the celiac axis. If there is no active bleeding at the time of examination, provocative measures, such as thrombolytics or heparin at the time of

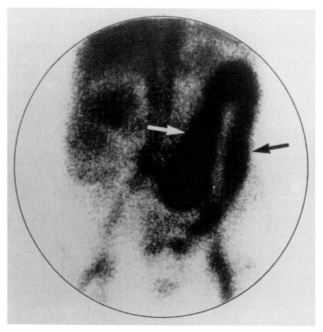

Figure 129–3. 99m Tc-labeled red blood cell scan showing accumulation in the left transverse, splenic flexure and descending colon. (Courtesy Michael McKusick, M.D., Rochester, Minn.)

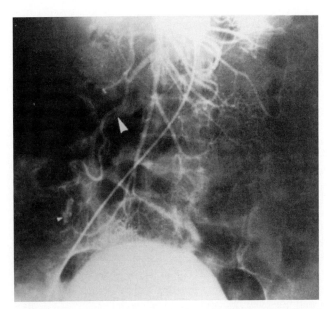

Figure 129–4. Angiodysplastic lesion identified by mesenteric angiography. Note the vascular tuft in the right colon *(small arrowhead)* and the early filling vein *(large arrowhead)*. (Courtesy Michael McKusick, M.D., Rochester, Minn.)

contrast injection, can unmask the lesion: however, this should be undertaken with caution. Angiography can be diagnostic in 50% to 75% of the patients, and it can distinguish between an angiodysplastic lesion (Fig. 129–4) and a bleeding diverticulum (Fig. 129–5). The disadvantages of angiography include complications from its invasiveness, including bleeding, thrombosis, or dissection of the cannulated vessels. Similar to the case with scinti-

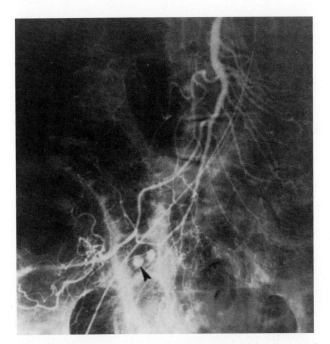

Figure 129–5. Diverticular bleeding demonstrated by mesenteric angiography. Note the extravasation of contrast medium in the lumen of the transverse colon. (Courtesy Michael McKusick, M.D., Rochester, Minn.)

scans, effective angiography requires active bleeding; however, with angiography, only arterial or capillary bleeding is detectable, and the sensitivity of angiography decreases with bleeding rates less than 1 mL/min. In contrast, angiography will show the presence of abnormal collections of blood vessels even in the absence of active bleeding. Angiography also requires an available interventional radiologic team, and the accuracy of results will be operator dependent.

Once the lesion is localized angiographically, several therapeutic options exist, including most commonly the infusion of vasoconstrictors. Vasopressin at a rate of 0.2 U/min is initially infused for approximately 20 to 30 minutes into the localized vessel and titrated up to 0.4 U/min. If bleeding stops, the catheter should remain in place and the infusion continued for 6 to 12 hours. If bleeding is controlled, the rate can be decreased by 50% for another 6 to 12 hours; then the vasopressin should be stopped and saline infused for an additional 6 to 12 hours. Prior to removing the catheter, a repeat angioscan should be performed to confirm cessation of bleeding. A total of 60% to 100% of lesions will stop bleeding, and short-term control will be achieved until a more definitive procedure can be performed. While reports vary, complications occur in as many as 40% of patients, with roughly 50% having recurrence of bleeding. Minor morbidities include complications, such as fluid retention, hyponatremia, transient hypertension, sinus bradycardia, and transient arrhythmias (i.e., premature ventricular contractions [PVCs], atrial fibrillation). About 10% develop severe complications, including pulmonary edema, arrhythmia, myocardial infarction, mesenteric thrombosis, and intestinal ischemia or infarction. Contraindications for vasopressin infusion include severe coronary artery disease (CAD) and peripheral vascular disease, although patients with cardiac risk factors can have simultaneous intravenous nitroglycerin infusion if needed.

Transcatheter embolization can be used to control lower GI bleeding. Embolization is most often used when the patient is a poor surgical candidate and comorbidities (i.e., CAD) contraindicate the use of vasoconstrictors. Embolic substances include Gelfoam, microcoils, polyvinyl alcohol particles, and, rarely, detachable balloons. Frequent side effects (15%) include abdominal pain, fever, ischemia, and infarction of the bowel. One group treated 17 bleeding episodes in 16 patients using transcatheter arterial embolization. Embolization successfully stopped the bleeding in 14 of 17 patients (82%); in one instance in which embolization failed, a repeat attempt proved successful. One patient rebled (6%), and two patients required surgery emergently, one for colonic necrosis (6%) and one for persistent bleeding after an unsuccessful embolization. Mild complications included fever, leukocytosis, abdominal pain, and rash.

The choice to perform angiography versus a nuclear medicine scan will be influenced by multiple considerations, including an index of suspicion for a specific pathology, the results of prior colonoscopy, the availability of resources, the briskness and intermittent behavior of the bleeding, patient stability, and comorbid conditions. The urgency of localization and the desire to treat the bleeding nonsurgically must be balanced against the risks of angiography and its treatment modalities. Controversy still exists over the risks of ischemic bowel when embolization is attempted, and the skill of the operator must be taken into account when one determines the risk-benefit ratios. For the more stable patient, one may use a bleeding scan to determine the activity of the bleed, and then use angiography if a treatment or more accurate localization is desired.

TREATMENT

When the cause of the bleed is known, treatment should be determined by the type of lesion as well as the stability and comorbidity of the patient. Visualized angiodysplastic lesions identified with colonoscopy are treated with low-power electrocautery or laser photocoagulation to obliterate the circumference and feeder vessels first. This approach is 90% effective but carries up to a 6% risk of bowel perforation. Sclerosing agents, as previously described, are also effective for selected angiodysplastic lesions. If the bleeding source is identified angiographically and embolization is chosen, the most distal vessels should be cannulated so as to direct the embolization toward the lesion without damaging unnecessary bowel. Of note, *angiodysplastic lesions will not respond to intra-arterial vasopressin.* If nonsurgical management of bleeding from angiodysplasia fails, the exact location and determination of additional coexisting lesions should be determined if possible prior to surgical intervention. If a bleeding diverticulum is identified endoscopically, bipolar electrocautery or topical epinephrine can stop the acute bleeding. Again, care taken to avoid perforation is essential.

About 20% of massive bleeds are caused by malignant lesions. Polypectomy or biopsy should be performed if hemostasis is not in jeopardy, and, if possible, resection should be performed electively at a later time. Polypectomy sites have a 0.1% to 0.4% risk of significant GI bleeding, but 70% will resolve spontaneously. For those that do not stop bleeding, cautery and again using a snare to remove the growths can successfully control the bleeding, with care taken to avoid perforation. Some advocate angiography and vasopressin infusion as a more efficient method of treating postpolypectomy bleeding: this approach may avoid the delay caused by bowel preparation, and the risk of perforation from colonoscopy and endoscopic treatments.

It is rare (3% to 5%) for massive bleeding to occur in inflammatory bowel disease. If the patient is unstable, emergent resection is indicated; otherwise, medical management may be successful. Bleeding from ischemic bowel, especially the nonocclusive variety, is evaluated with early angiography to selectively vasodilate the affected vessel with papaverine, thrombolytics, or stenting when appropriate. If peritonitis is present, prompt surgery is indicated. The high mortality associated with ischemic bowel (up to 60% to 100%) mandates a high index of suspicion for this disease.

The need for urgent surgery for acute lower GI bleeding is determined by multiple factors, including the ability to resuscitate the patient and to keep up with ongoing blood loss. Whether or not a known source is identified, the threat to the patient of recurrent bleeding must be balanced against the overall morbidity of an urgent or planned surgery. Accepted indications for operative intervention include transfusion requirements greater than 4 to 6 U in 24 hours, 10 U overall, or recurrent bleeding during the same hospitalization. If a patient is too unstable for diagnostic procedures, if the evaluation is nondiagnostic and the bleeding continues, or if the patient has severe repeated episodes of bleeding after endoscopic or angiographic attempts to control bleeding, emergent resection is indicated. Intraoperatively, the bowel should be palpated to identify possible masses, cecal thickening, or abnormal serosal vessels. Intraoperative "on-the-job" lavage with concomitant intraoperative endoscopy may be performed if preoperative localization studies were nondiagnostic. Intraoperative endoscopy offers the advantage of the surgeon's being able to guide the endoscope through the bowel and identify lesions that may be in the small bowel or not previously visualized secondary to poor bowel cleansing.

When a source is not identified, a decision as to the extent of the resection must be made. If fresh blood is in the right colon and abnormal serosal vessels or cecal thickening suggests a right-sided bleed, a right hemicolectomy may be sufficient. When localization is made preoperatively, a directed segmental colectomy can be performed. Otherwise, a subtotal colectomy with ileorectal anastomosis may be necessary. When there is an *identified source*, as many as 14% of patients undergoing limited segmental resections will experience rebleeding. Any resection *without a localized source* carries the risk of rebleed from an unidentified, unresected lesion, with an incidence of rebleeding of 42% in some series.

Pearls and Pitfalls

- Most episodes of massive lower GI bleeding are colonic in origin (85%), and most stop spontaneously (80% to 85%).
- Diagnostic evaluation is determined by patient stability, rate of bleeding, and institutional practices. For the stable patient, colonoscopy is the first test ordered and can be therapeutic. For the unstable patient with life-threatening hemorrhage, surgery is usually required.
- Angiography is chosen for the patient whose bleeding is brisk and ongoing, whose vital signs fluctuate according to the extent of blood loss, and in whom resuscitation is able to keep the patient hemodynamically stable.
- If a bleeding source is identified angiographically, a decision must be made whether to proceed with selective infusion of vasoconstrictors or embolization. Colonic necrosis (6%) and rebleeding (6%) are recognized complications of embolization. Complications of vasopressin can be expected in 40% of patients.
- For the patient whose bleeding is slow and ongoing, nuclear medicine scanning, angiography, or colonoscopy can be chosen. Colonoscopy offers the opportunity to treat some lesions at the time of examination.

SELECTED READINGS

Bemvenuti GA, Jülich MM: Ethanolamine injection for sclerotherapy of angiodysplasia of the colon. Endoscopy 1998;30:564.

Billingham RP: The conundrum of lower gastrointestinal bleeding. Surg Clin North Am 1997;77:241.

Gunderman R, Leef JA, Lipton MJ, Reba RC: Diagnostic imaging and the outcome of acute lower gastrointestinal bleeding. Acad Radiol 1998;5(suppl 2):S303.

Gutierrez C, Mariano M, Vander Laan T, et al: The use of technetium-labeled erythrocyte scintigraphy in the evaluation and treatment of lower gastrointestinal hemorrhage. Am Surg 1998;64:989.

Luchtefeld MA, Senagore AJ, Szomstein M, et al: Evaluation of transarterial embolization for lower gastrointestinal bleeding. Dis Colon Rectum 2000;43:532.

Rutgeerts P, Van Compel F, Geboes K, et al: Long-term results of treatment of vascular malformations of the gastrointestinal tract by neodymium:YAG laser photocoagulation. Gut 1985;26:586.

Schwartz, et al: Principles of Surgery, 7th ed. New York, McGraw-Hill, 1999, pp 1061–1067.

Thomas MG: Obscure lower gastrointestinal bleeding. Br J Surg 1999;86:579.

Zuccaro G Jr: Management of the adult patient with acute lower gastrointestinal bleeding. Am J Gastroenterol 1998;93:1202.

Chapter 130

Gastrointestinal Bleeding of Obscure Origin

Mark D. Duncan and Thomas H. Magnuson

Obscure gastrointestinal (GI) bleeding, defined as recurrent or persistent bleeding without a diagnosed source after initial endoscopic survey, represents both a diagnostic and a therapeutic challenge to the general surgeon. Obscure bleeding may be the manifestation of several conditions, the hallmark of which is recurrent hemorrhage from sites within the GI tract that are not able to be detected with routine endoscopic studies, including esophagogastroduodenoscopy (EGD) and colonoscopy. Bleeding is often very slow or intermittent, contributing to the difficulty in identifying the lesion. Obscure bleeding may be either overt, with recurrent passage of visible blood, or occult. Although often used in relation to undiagnosed bleeding, the term *occult bleeding* is best used to describe the initial presentation of a positive fecal occult blood test or iron deficiency anemia in the absence of visible blood in the stool.

The surgical management of obscure GI bleeding initially involves invasive and noninvasive approaches to identifying the lesion or the source of bleeding. The interventional approach requires a diagnostic algorithm tailored to the clinical presentation and to available endoscopic and radiographic expertise. When this challenge is met, the surgeon can most appropriately treat the bleeding.

The management of acute, severe upper and lower GI bleeding is not usually considered together with the management of obscure bleeding and is not reviewed here. This chapter outlines the diagnostic steps recommended in the identification of the site of obscure GI bleeding in the nonacute or the stabilized patient.

CLINICAL PRESENTATION

In perhaps 5% of patients, GI bleeding qualifies as being obscure, often involving passage of visible blood per rectum. It is difficult to describe the incidence of obscure bleeding by anatomic location or causative lesion, because these will vary depending on the choice of secondary diagnostic techniques and the thoroughness of the initial endoscopic observations (EGD and colonoscopy). The cause of obscure bleeding remains undetected despite extensive investigation in 50% of patients. In patients for whom a source is identified, the majority will have bleeding due to angioectasia (also termed angiodysplasia) or arteriovenous malformation (AVM), with a smaller number of patients having neoplasms (e.g., GI stromal tumors, previously termed leiomyomas, lymphoma, carcinoid, or other lesions). Table 130–1 lists common and uncommon lesions of the upper GI tract and the small bowel that

cause obscure GI bleeding. The incidence of angiodysplasia as a cause of obscure bleeding increases with age. Conversely, small bowel tumors are more often associated with younger patients; 14% of patients younger than 50 years of age with obscure bleeding had small bowel tumors, compared with 3% of patients older than 50.

For overt lower GI bleeding, in addition to colonoscopy, the standard initial evaluation includes tagged red-cell studies followed by angiography. Bleeding from diverticula or angiodysplasia is intermittent and recurrent. Diverticula are readily evident on colonoscopy or contrast enema study. Although this diagnosis may not account for all bleeding that is attributed to it, diverticulosis is nonetheless rarely listed as a source of obscure bleeding. Radioisotope bleeding scans can demonstrate the site of bleeding when the rate exceeds 0.1 mL/minute. Angiography more precisely localizes the site of bleeding and allows possible embolization but requires a bleeding rate of 0.5 to 1.0 mL/minute. Most clinical centers use angiography only after a bleeding scan with positive results, which targets surgical therapy (usually hemicolectomy). A

Table 130–1	Etiology of Obscure Gastrointestinal Bleeding

Common
   AVMs (angioectasias or true AVMs)
   Tumors
      Gastrointestinal stromal tumors
      Adenocarcinoma
      Lymphoma
      Carcinoid
Uncommon
   Lipoma
   Jejunoileal diverticulosis
   Small bowel ulcer or erosion
   Dieulafoy's lesions
   Cameron's erosion (in a large hiatal hernia)
Rare
   Nevus lesion
   Kaposi's sarcoma
   Polyposis syndrome
   Meckel's diverticulum
   Tuberculosis
   Wirsungorrhagia (hemosuccus pancreaticus)
   Hemobilia
   Foreign body
   Varices
   Crohn's disease
   Celiac sprue
   Vasculitis
   Aortoenteric fistula

AVMs, arteriovenous malformations.

recently suggested alternative to conventional angiography is the use of helical computed tomography with intra-aortic catheterization, which allows identification of the majority of angiographically discernible bleeds without the need for selective visceral arterial cannulation. In selected patients, precipitated angiography after administration of anticoagulants or vasodilators may improve the diagnostic yield. This must be weighed against the obvious consequences of precipitating hemorrhage. When the aforementioned algorithm is followed and a source remains undetected, the bleeding is considered obscure, and a small bowel source is suspected.

A number of imaging modalities are available to assist in the localization of obscure GI bleeding. This second line of investigation includes enteroscopy, small bowel follow-through contrast studies, enteroclysis, and visceral angiography (Table 130–2).

IMAGING

Enteroscopy

Push enteroscopy, in which a long enteroscope (Olympus SIF-100; Olympus America, Melville, NY) is advanced orally, has been suggested by some to be the standard approach for evaluating the small bowel as a source of obscure bleeding. Sonde enteroscopy, so named for the ability to sound the depths of the intestine, is unavailable at most centers, has long procedure times, causes patient discomfort, and permits no therapy. A source of bleeding will be identified in about 50% of patients via push enteroscopy. The most common lesions discovered with enteroscopy are AVMs of the small bowel. In one report, about one third of examined patients had AVMs, and 6% had small bowel tumors. In a recent series, Zaman and colleagues (1999) studied 95 patients; sources of bleeding were found in 35, and 25 of the lesions were within reach of EGD. Although enteroscopy was developed to evaluate lesions beyond the second portion of duodenum, a significant number of upper GI tract lesions within reach of standard EGD ("missed lesions") were found with this procedure. The diagnostic yield of enteroscopy exceeds that of small bowel radiography. Significant complications of enteroscopy are uncommon but include abdominal pain, pancreatitis, and GI mucosal tears.

If enteroscopy is unavailable or unrevealing, small bowel follow-through or enteroclysis is recommended, although the diagnostic yield is only about 10%. Enter-

oclysis is the better choice for radiographic examination because it permits a more concentrated barium study of the small intestine without obscuring the view with overlapping gastric contrast material. The low yield reflects the fact that both of these tests are able to demonstrate tumors but are poor at detecting the more common AVMs. Furthermore, it was shown at surgery that false-positive results occurred in up to one fifth of lesions reported on small bowel radiography. Although commonly employed to search for obscure bleeding sites, barium contrast studies should be reserved for use after enteroscopy with negative findings. In addition, if such equipment or expertise is not available, enteroclysis remains the preferred method.

Missed Lesions

Any series of patients with obscure or unexplained GI bleeding includes a high incidence of individuals with gastroduodenal or colonic lesions that were not appreciated at the initial study. These abnormalities include typical sources of upper GI bleeding (e.g., peptic ulcer disease) as well as the less common but perhaps more frequently missed AVM of the stomach or the proximal duodenum, Cameron's erosion within a large hiatal hernia, and Dieulafoy's lesion (i.e., an arteriole presenting through a small mucosal defect, typically in the proximal stomach). Most data come from series in which enteroscopy was used; bleeding sites within reach of standard EGD were found in about 20% of patients. Such "missed" lesions accounted for about 50% of identified bleeding sources. Repeated upper endoscopy, either as a second EGD or as part of a dedicated enteroscopy, is justified, particularly in patients in whom the bleeding is not overt.

In the colon, angiodysplasia and tumors account for most missed lesions, reflecting their relative frequency in detected causes of bleeding. Visceral angiography may be performed in patients for whom the previously mentioned investigations prove to be unrevealing. Even in the absence of active bleeding, a typical blush appearance may be demonstrated with AVMs of the small bowel or the colon. The diagnostic yield of angiography has been reported to be as high as 40% but is probably much lower in most centers.

Intraoperative Endoscopy

If the second line of investigations has not yielded a bleeding source, consideration should be given to exploratory laparotomy with intraoperative endoscopy. At this point, it is appropriate to reconsider the relative risks and benefits that further intervention poses compared with a strategy of observation and possible intermittent transfusion on a case-by-case basis. Operative therapy is appropriate for patients with an ongoing need for transfusion for a bleeding site that remains undiagnosed despite extensive evaluation. Traditionally, this encompasses open abdominal exploration plus operative "hands-on" assisted enteroscopy using a standard colonoscope. The enteroscope can be inserted perorally and can be manually guided through the small bowel. As the endoscope is

Table 130–2	**Diagnostic Options in Evaluation of Obscure Gastrointestinal Bleeding**

Repeat EGD	Enteroclysis
Repeat colonoscopy	Meckel's scan
Tagged red blood cell scan	Push enteroscopy
Angiography	Sonde enteroscopy
Helical CT angiography	Intraoperative enteroscopy
Precipitated angiography	Laparoscopic enteroscopy
Small bowel follow-through	

CT, computed tomography; EGD, esophagogastroduodenoscopy.

advanced, the jejunoileum is pleated over the instrument. Because this maneuver causes small abrasions or tears in the mucosa, it is recommended that the primary viewing and examination be during insertion rather than during withdrawal to avoid misinterpreting such iatrogenic lesions as being the cause of the obscure bleeding. Alternatively, the endoscope may be introduced via one or multiple enterotomies to diminish the potential trauma to the small bowel mucosa or the mesentery. Intraoperative endoscopy permits both abdominal exploration and guidance of small bowel endoscopy. These approaches also have the advantage of permitting operative or endoscopic therapy in the same setting.

When a specific lesion has been identified, the involved segment of bowel is resected. If multiple AVMs are detected that are not isolated to a single segment, it is better to cauterize the visible angioectasias (or to use laser ablation), to forgo resection, and to consider postoperative medical therapy. By following an intraoperative endoscopic protocol, a lesion was found in 70% of patients in a Mayo Clinic series, but some patients rebled despite resection of the identified lesion; ultimately, only 41% of patients undergoing the combined procedure had no further bleeding. This likely reflects the multicentricity of AVMs. More recently, minimally invasive techniques have been applied to the problem of obscure bleeding. Percutaneous transabdominal (laparoscopic) enteroscopy can be performed, as well as laparoscopically assisted peroral enteroscopy. The diagnostic yield for a combined surgical and endoscopic technique is reported to be anywhere from 52% to 93%, but these are highly selected patients.

Significant morbidity, including serosal tears or mesenteric venous tears requiring resection, has been reported to be associated with operative-assisted enteroscopy. We have had experience with one patient in whom iatrogenic bleeding from an upper GI mucosal tear required early postoperative transfusion. Published morbidity rates are 2% to 42%; death is rare but was reported to occur in up to 11% of patients in one study.

MANAGEMENT

The management of the primary disorder in obscure GI bleeding is dictated by both the lesion itself and the manner in which it was detected. At the time of endoscopy, AVMs may be directly cauterized or obliterated by means of laser therapy. Separate recent studies demonstrate that enteroscopic electrocauterization decreases the subsequent need for transfusion, but the majority of patients still bleed, and only one third have no further bleeding. Angiographically localized lesions may undergo embolization or may be infused with vasopressin; however, these applications are limited by potential local effects (e.g., bowel infarction) and systemic effects (e.g., as in coronary artery disease); moreover, vasopressin therapy is transient and of benefit only during an acute bleed.

In many instances, the goal of diagnosis and localization is to permit targeted operative therapy to remove the segment of bowel from which the obscure bleeding emanates. Certainly, tumors warrant resection; vascular malformations, when localized preoperatively or intraoperatively, are well managed with resection, with acceptable rebleeding rates. Recurrent bleeding episodes in patients undergoing segmental bowel resection reflect the multicentricity often seen with AVMs. The creation of colostomies or enterostomies for the purpose of localizing GI bleeding, although reported, is seldom necessary and is not therapeutic.

Medical therapy is reserved for multiple vascular lesions, for persistent bleeding after endoscopic or surgical treatment, or for patients in whom no source of bleeding

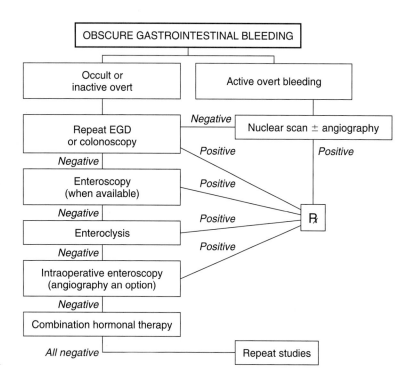

Figure 130–1. Algorithm for the management of obscure gastrointestinal bleeding. EGD, esophagogastroduodenoscopy.

Pearls and Pitfalls

- About 5% of all patients with GI bleeding fall into the category of obscure bleeding (i.e., there is no obvious source after EGD and colonoscopy).
- About 20% of patients with obscure GI bleeding have lesions that will be detectable on repeat EGD or colonoscopy.
- Angioectasias (AVMs) account for most patients with obscure bleeding.
- Enteroscopy is better than enteroclysis, which is in turn better than small bowel follow-through, at detecting obscure sites.
- During intraoperative enteroscopy, the small bowel should be viewed during insertion rather than withdrawal to avoid misinterpreting iatrogenic mucosal injury.
- Only about 40% of patients subjected to abdominal exploration and intraoperative enteroscopy are cured of GI bleeding.

is found despite complete evaluation. We can infer from detectable lesions that recurrent obscure bleeding has a reasonable likelihood of emanating from small bowel AVMS and may be amenable to medical therapy. Several reports have demonstrated the efficacy of combined hormonal therapy with norethindrone and mestranol. In one study by Barkin and Ross (1998), 0 of 38 patients (25 known AVMs and 18 patients with bleeding of obscure cause) rebled after a mean of 2½ years follow-up. Combined hormonal therapy has been proposed for all patients in whom multiple (>5) AVMs have been identified.

An algorithm for evaluation and management of obscure GI bleeding is presented in Figure 130–1. When obscure bleeding is recurrent and active, the standard work-up (i.e., nuclear scan with tagged red blood cells followed by angiography) is indicated. When a bleeding site is detected, appropriate therapy is instituted. When no site is detected, the same pathway is followed as for nonovert obscure bleeding. Repeat routine and extended EGD or colonoscopy, depending on clinical indication, is next performed to exclude missed lesions. If no bleeding site is identified, push enteroscopy can be considered when local expertise is available, followed by enteroclysis. If these studies fail to localize a source of significant persistent or recurrent bleeding, intraoperative enteroscopy is considered. Although we do not routinely use visceral angiography in patients without overt bleeding, others feel strongly that angiography and screening computed tomography are of potential help. Finally, for patients in whom no lesion is detected after operation, empirical combination hormone therapy is recommended.

SELECTED READINGS

American Gastroenterological Association medical position statement: Evaluation and management of occult and obscure gastrointestinal bleeding. Gastroenterology 2000;118:197.

Barkin JS, Ross BS: Medical therapy for chronic gastrointestinal bleeding of obscure origin. Am J Gastroenterol 1998;93:1250.

Lopez MJ, Cooley JS, Petros JG, et al: Complete intraoperative small-bowel endoscopy in the evaluation of occult gastrointestinal bleeding using the sonde enteroscope. Arch Surg 1996;131:272.

Ress AM, Benacci JC, Sarr MG: Efficacy of intraoperative enteroscopy in diagnosis and prevention of recurrent, occult gastrointestinal bleeding. Am J Surg 1992;163:94.

Szold A, Katz LB, Lewis BS: Surgical approach to occult gastrointestinal bleeding. Am J Surg 1992;163:90.

Zaman A, Sheppard B, Katon RM: Total peroral intraoperative enteroscopy for obscure GI bleeding using a dedicated push enteroscope: Diagnostic yield and patient outcome. Gastrointest Endosc 1999;50:506.

Zuckerman GR, Prakash C, Askin MP, Lewis BS: AGA technical review on the evaluation and management of occult and obscure gastrointestinal bleeding. Gastroenterology 2000;118:201.

Minimally Invasive GI Procedures

Chapter 131
Laparoscopic Colectomy
Bernardo Tisminezky and Heidi Nelson

Laparoscopic colon resection involves a spectrum of procedures performed under video surveillance, enabling a surgeon to excise or repair a segment of the colon with a minimal-access (minimally invasive) technique. The majority of these procedures are laparoscopically assisted, which means that part of the operation (most often, resection and anastomosis) is performed extracorporeally. Less often, surgeons perform total laparoscopic colectomy. The benefit of the latter is not yet clearly determined. This chapter therefore describes the laparoscopically assisted procedure.

PREOPERATIVE MANAGEMENT

Preoperative evaluation and preparation of the patient for laparoscopic colon surgery should generally be the same as for conventional surgery. Routine bowel preparation is performed the day before surgery. Prophylaxis against deep venous thrombosis is provided by the application of sequential compression devices, and prophylactic antibiotics are administered at the induction of anesthesia. To avoid the risk of injury to the stomach and the bladder during surgery, a nasogastric tube and a urinary catheter are inserted. Patients who are likely to need a temporary or a permanent stoma are marked before surgery by a stoma therapist.

PREOPERATIVE PREPARATION

Owing to the anatomy and the size of the colon, laparoscopic colorectal procedures are more complex and technically more challenging than laparoscopic cholecystec-

tomy. The basic technical aspects of colorectal laparoscopy should follow the same operative principles applied in a conventional open procedure; therefore, a familiar concept can be applied. A team approach must be emphasized early in the educational process, because without a skilled team (surgeon, assistant, and nursing staff), colorectal laparoscopy will remain difficult. The same personnel involved in open surgery should be trained in minimal-access surgery. The tools used for laparoscopic colectomy should include not only standard general laparoscopic equipment but also instruments specific to colorectal surgery. The minimum basic equipment needed for laparoscopic colectomy includes (1) trocars and cannulas (10 to 12 mm), with stability threads and adapters; (2) grasping devices, such as alligator graspers and Babcock clamps; and (3) disposable cautery scissors.

INDICATIONS AND CONTRAINDICATIONS

Laparoscopic colectomy may be considered whenever resection of a segment of colon is required, particularly for benign conditions (Table 131–1). With regard to the treatment of colon cancer, the laparoscopic approach is still controversial. At present, patients undergoing laparoscopic colectomy for carcinoma should be enrolled in prospective randomized trials. Contraindications to laparoscopic colon resection can be divided into absolute and relative, depending on patient or disease-related factors (see Table 131-1). A large bulky tumor, a large phlegmonous mass (in Crohn's disease), and acute disease complications (e.g., obstruction, ileus, and perforation

833

Table 131–1

Indications and Contraindications

INDICATIONS	CONTRAINDICATIONS
Colon polyps (not amenable to endoscopic resection)	**Absolute**
Crohn's disease	Patient-related
Volvulus	Major cardiac disease
Diverticulitis	Severe pulmonary disease
Rectal prolapse	Liver disease with portal hypertension
Colonic diversion (ileostomy or colostomy creation)	Coagulopathy
Colon carcinoma (controversial)	Pregnancy
	Disease-related
	Tumor infiltration into adjacent structures (T4)
	Large phlegmon mass
	Colovesical fistula
	Acute complications: obstruction, perforation, and ileus
	Relative
	Patient-related
	Morbid obesity
	Multiple previous abdominal surgeries "Prohibitive adhesions"
	Disease-related
	Large mass (>8–10 cm)
	Primary tumor with resectable liver metastasis
	Transverse colon cancer
	Carcinomatosis

with diffuse peritoneal contamination) are contraindications to laparoscopic surgery. Dilatation of the small or the large bowel can obstruct the surgeon's view inside the abdominal cavity. These factors, plus overdistention and the relative fragility of the bowel, increase the risk of perforation.

Most absolute contraindications are based on medical conditions. Pneumoperitoneum has the potential to cause dramatic changes in the physiology of the cardiovascular and the pulmonary systems; hence, patients who present with marginal cardiac or respiratory reserve or major vascular disease should not be considered for this type of surgery. Liver disease with portal hypertension is an absolute contraindication. Coagulopathy that cannot be corrected is generally a contraindication to any kind of surgery. This is especially true in laparoscopic surgery, where constant oozing from dissected tissues will impair visualization of the intra-abdominal cavity, increasing the risk of inadvertent damage to important structures.

INTRAOPERATIVE MANAGEMENT

The patient should be positioned on the operating table with both arms (tucked, padded, and protected) at the sides. It is imperative that the patient be secured on the operating table with beanbags or ankle straps if the supine position is used or with Allen stirrups if the modified lithotomy position is used. Once the patient is positioned, the cords from the video camera, the light source, the insufflator, and cautery should be arranged in a convenient configuration so as not to interfere with the operative field. Minor adjustments of the monitor in the cephalad or the caudad direction can fine-tune these alignments

when the dissection moves from the upper to the lower abdomen. The monitor is placed on the side of the disease.

RIGHT HEMICOLECTOMY

Right hemicolectomy is performed in a five-step procedure. Cannula insertion uses a three-trocar (all 10 to 12 mm) approach. The abdomen is insufflated with carbon dioxide to create a pneumoperitoneum of 12 to 14 mm Hg. The camera (laparoscope) can be introduced in the supraumbilical port, and the other two cannulas can be inserted under direct visualization. Inserting cannulas over scars should be avoided when possible; usually, the left upper quadrant is scarless.

Step two involves the exploratory phase, when the feasibility of the procedure is determined. Indications for early conversion to an open procedure include massive abdominal adhesions, small bowel–pelvic adhesions, unanticipated findings, and altered anatomy. Proceeding under these conditions has a higher probability of causing injury, which in the end will adversely affect operative and postoperative recovery and will increase the amount of morbidity and the length of hospital stay. In patients with Crohn's disease, it is imperative to "run" the entire small bowel by a hand-over-hand technique using two alligator clamps, always kept under direct vision.

Step three involves mobilization of the cecum. The patient is positioned in steep Trendelenburg's position with the left side down to allow the small bowel to fall out of the operative field. The 30-degree laparoscope is removed from the supraumbilical site and is placed through the left upper paramedian cannula. The surgical assistant controls the laparoscope, while the surgeon identifies the terminal ileum and the base of the cecum and then proceeds to grasp the peritoneum of the ileocecal junction. Grasping the bowel itself (especially with Babcock clamps) is to be avoided. Once this is done, the surgeon incises the peritoneum with cautery or scissors. The dissection commences along the peritoneum of the terminal ileum, where the appropriate plane can be readily identified, and progresses toward the hepatic flexure, following the white line of Toldt's membrane (Fig. 131–1).

Step four includes mobilization of the hepatic flexure and the transverse colon (Fig. 131–2). Once the colon is mobilized to the level of the hepatic flexure, the laparoscope is moved to the lower cannula in the midline. The operating surgeon and the assistant change positions, and the operating table is repositioned to head up (reverse modest Trendelenburg's) with the left side kept down. The assistant holds the camera and provides visualization of the operative field. Meanwhile, the surgeon grasps the cephalad part of the hepatic flexure at the peritoneal attachment, elevating the tissues (using an upward force) toward the abdominal wall and directing them caudad toward the left hip. Mobilization of the colon at the hepatic flexure should start along the free lateral peritoneal edge; retraction of the ascending and the transverse colon inferomedially allows the omentum to be freed from the hepatic flexure. If small vessels are found, they

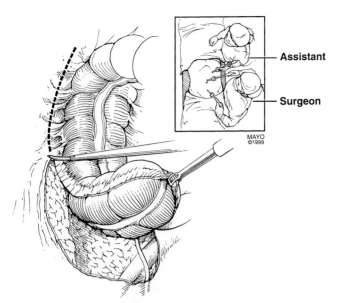

Figure 131–1. Mobilization of the cecum. Cannula positioning for right hemicolectomy employs a three-trocar approach (*inset*). Two are inserted through the midline: One is inserted at the supraumbilical site, and the other is placed in the lower midline approximately 8 cm caudad to the first trocar. The third cannula is introduced into the left upper quadrant below the rib cage in the midclavicular line. With the patient in Trendelenburg's and left-side-down positioning, countertraction of the ileocecal junction toward the left shoulder raises the cecum, achieving transperitoneal visualization of the ureter and the iliacs and facilitating dissection of the cecum. (Reprinted with permission of Mosby and Mayo Foundation. Tisminezky B, Nelson H: Laparoscopic approach to colon cancer. In Cameron JL, Balch CM, Langer B [eds]: Advances in Surgery, Vol 34. St Louis, Mosby, 2000, pp 67–119.)

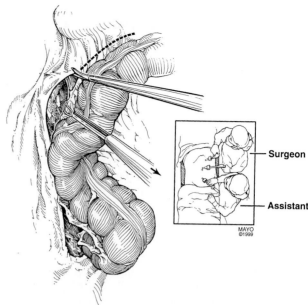

Figure 131–2. Mobilization of the hepatic flexure. The surgeon and the assistant operator change positions (*inset*), and the operating table is repositioned to reverse modest Trendelenburg's (head up) position with the left side kept down. Mobilization of the ascending colon at the hepatocolic flexure should start along the free lateral peritoneal edge; next, the hepatocolic ligament is divided, and hemostasis is obtained by means of electrocautery or clips. Mobilization of the hepatocolic flexure should provide visualization of both the duodenum and the right ureter. (Reprinted with permission of Mosby and Mayo Foundation. Tisminezky B, Nelson H: Laparoscopic approach to colon cancer. In Cameron JL, Balch CM, Langer B [eds]: Advances in Surgery, Vol 34. St Louis, Mosby, 2000, pp 67–119.)

should be secured with a grasper, cauterized twice, and then divided; as an alternative, vascular clips can be used, but they are only rarely required. Mobilization of the hepatic flexure should provide visualization of both the duodenum and the right ureter.

The dissection of the transverse colon should extend to at least the level of the gallbladder, preferably beyond. The colon is elevated to expose the mesentery of the superior mesenteric, the ileocolic, the right colic, and the middle colic vessels, all of which can be visualized. Applying moderate tension on the junction of the ileum and the cecum readily displays the ileocolic vessels and facilitates intracorporeal ligation. Mesenteric windows are created within the avascular planes, and the vascular pedicle is then secured using hemoclips, endoloops, or a linear vascular stapler (Fig. 131–3).

Step five involves the processes of exteriorization, resection, and anastomosis. To exteriorize the right colon, the incision at the supraumbilical port is enlarged vertically around the umbilicus for about 4 to 6 cm, depending on the size of the patient and the specimen. It is important to maintain mesenteric orientation at all times for proper creation of the anastomosis. When small incisions are used, it is easy to become disoriented. When this is in doubt, the mesenteric edges of resection verify proper orientation.

Next, resection of the diseased segment is performed in a standard manner, respecting appropriate proximal and distal margins. An anastomosis is then executed in a

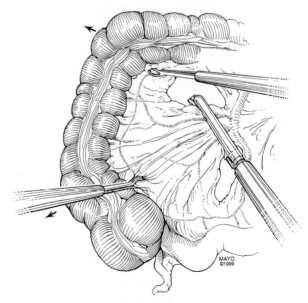

Figure 131–3. Intracorporeal vascular ligation. Vascular pedicle ligation of the ileocolic and the right colic arteries is accomplished using a 30-mm linear stapler. The vascular structures should be swept free of critical retroperitoneal structures, such as the ureter, before they are ligated. Full cecal and hepatic flexure mobilization followed by intracorporeal vascular pedicle ligation facilitates the extracorporeal delivery of the right colon (described in the text). (Reprinted with permission of Mosby and Mayo Foundation. Tisminezky B, Nelson H: Laparoscopic approach to colon cancer. In Cameron JL, Balch CM, Langer B [eds]: Advances in Surgery, Vol 34. St Louis, Mosby, 2000, pp 67–119.)

standard mechanical or hand-sewn fashion. The mesenteric defect is closed or is left open, depending on the anatomy and the extent of resection. The bowel is returned to the peritoneal cavity, and the abdominal wound is closed. The operative and the dependent fields within the abdominal cavity are irrigated thoroughly. With a pneumoperitoneum reestablished, the laparoscope is reinserted to inspect the operative field for hemostasis. The cannulas are removed under direct visualization to ensure hemostasis. All 10-mm or greater fascial defects are closed; caution should be exercised to avoid injury to the underlying bowel. The skin is closed with absorbable subcuticular suture.

LEFT HEMICOLECTOMY

Resection of the left colon is essentially the reverse of resection of the right colon. The same five-step approach can be applied to resection of the descending colon. Exteriorization, resection, and anastomosis are performed as described for resection of the right colon.

SIGMOIDECTOMY

The patient is placed in a synchronous position (legs up) for abdominal and perineal exposure. Step one includes port site selection and creation of a pneumoperitoneum. Next, the laparoscope is introduced, and the rest of the cannulas are inserted under direct visualization. A total of three or four cannulas (three 10- to 12-mm and one 5-mm) are placed (1) supraumbilically, (2) below the umbilicus, (3) in the right lower quadrant, (4) optionally,

in the left lower quadrant (5-mm port, for exteriorization of the colon). Once these ports are placed, the abdominal cavity and the pelvis can be inspected to judge the best sites for the additional one or two ports.

Step two involves sigmoid mobilization. The patient is placed in a steep Trendelenburg's (right side down) position to displace the small bowel toward the right upper quadrant, leaving the sigmoid mesentery exposed. The cephalad assistant operates the laparoscope, and the caudad assistant, using a grasping instrument introduced through the lower quadrant cannula, grasps the pericolic mesentery and retracts it toward the right side of the patient (Fig. 131–4). Conversion to an open procedure is necessary if the ureter cannot be identified confidently. Care should be taken to ensure that the ureter is swept down and away from the mesenteric structures so that it is not inadvertently injured during ligation of the vascular pedicle. Once the sigmoid colon is mobilized, the dissection is continued caudad toward the presacral space. With the sigmoid retracted cephalad and to the patient's right, the presacral window on the patient's left can be opened, the iliac vessels can be easily identified, and the presacral space can be defined. The dissection should continue until the proximal to middle rectum is free along the left margin.

With the sigmoid retracted in the opposite manner (toward the patient's left side), the presacral window on the right is next opened. The superior hemorrhoidal and sigmoid vessels are visualized as the sigmoid colon and the proximal rectum are brought under tension by means of caudal traction.

Step three involves ligation of the vascular pedicle. Elevating the dissected colon exposes the mesenteric ves-

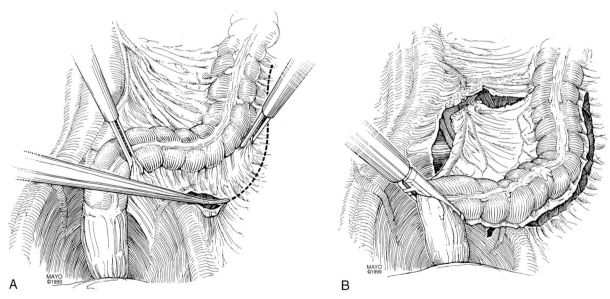

Figure 131–4. Intracorporeal sigmoid dissection and rectal transection. *A,* The assistant's grasper and the surgeon's Babcock clamp achieve two-point traction on the sigmoid's lateral peritoneal attachment. The surgeon uses a scissors to incise the peritoneal attachment. Mobilizing the sigmoid colon should allow visualization of the left ureter. *B,* After pedicle ligation, the sigmoid and the proximal rectum become fully mobilized. Next, a linear stapler positioned at the distal margin of the mobilized rectum is fired to divide the rectum. (Reprinted with permission of Mosby and Mayo Foundation. Tisminezky B, Nelson H: Laparoscopic approach to colon cancer. In Cameron JL, Balch CM, Langer B [eds]: Advances in Surgery, Vol 34. St Louis, Mosby, 2000, pp 67–119.)

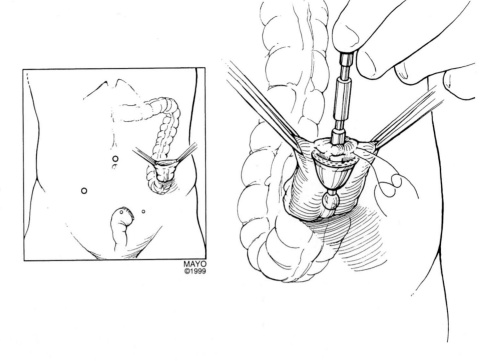

Figure 131–5. Laparoscopically assisted sigmoidectomy. The left inferior quadrant cannula site is extended into a 4-cm transverse incision (*inset*). The sigmoid is delivered extracorporeally, and the proximal margin is identified. The bowel is resected, and a purse-string suture is placed to secure the anvil of a circular stapler. Next, the descending colon is returned to the abdominal cavity. (Reprinted with permission of Mosby and Mayo Foundation. Tisminezky B, Nelson H: Laparoscopic approach to colon cancer. In Cameron JL, Balch CM, Langer B [eds]: Advances in Surgery, Vol 34. St Louis, Mosby, 2000, pp 67–119.)

sels, and two incisions are made in the avascular planes on both sides of the vessels. The superior hemorrhoidal vessels and the sigmoid arteries are isolated; ligation of the vascular pedicle at the level of the aortic bifurcation is executed using vascular staplers, clips, or endoloops. After ligation is achieved, the sigmoid becomes more mobile for anastomotic purposes. If necessary, the descending colon can be dissected further cephalad, including the splenic flexure. Dissecting techniques are equivalent to those described for dissection of the splenic flexure during left colectomy.

Step four involves stapling and division of the proximal rectum (see Fig. 131–4). The dissection is accomplished by working side-to-side along the rectal wall (right to left). The rectum is divided using a linear cutting stapler.

Step five is the exteriorization phase (Fig. 131–5). The incision for the left inferior quadrant cannula site is extended. The specimen is delivered extracorporeally, and the proximal margin is identified. The bowel is cleared of mesentery and is resected proximal to the tumor, usually at the junction of the sigmoid and the descending colon. The peritoneal cavity is irrigated and is checked for blood, and the fascial defects are closed.

Step six, the anastomosis, commences with reinsufflation of the abdomen. The anvil is attached to the shaft of the stapling device, which has been introduced through the anus and advanced across the staple line (Fig. 131–6). The stapling device can be closed to approximate the bowel ends and is then fired. A proctoscope is used to examine the anastomosis for hemostasis and integrity. The cannulas are removed under direct visualization, and the fascial defects and the skin are closed.

An alternative approach, as alluded to previously, is to perform a hand-sewn anastomosis through a small lower midline incision. A low midline incision of 5 to 6 cm is made, and the bowel is exteriorized, cleared of mesentery,

and divided. The specimen is excised, and an end-to-end anastomosis is performed, taking care that proper mesenteric alignment is fulfilled. The colon is returned to the peritoneal cavity, the abdominal cavity is irrigated, and the fascial layer is closed. This approach is most applicable in cases of benign disease, in which the sigmoid colon is redundant and easily exteriorized.

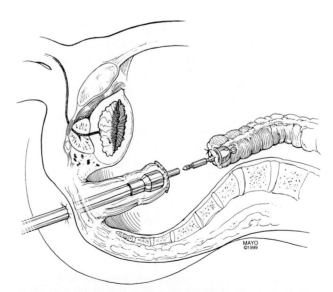

Figure 131–6. Intracorporeal colorectal anastomosis. Sagittal view showing the shaft of the stapler in the rectum and the circular anvil in the descending colon. Both ends are connected, maintaining proper mesentery orientation. Next, the stapler is fired. A proctoscope is then used to examine for hemostasis and anastomosis integrity. (Reprinted with permission of Mosby and Mayo Foundation. Tisminezky B, Nelson H: Laparoscopic approach to colon cancer. In Cameron JL, Balch CM, Langer B [eds]: Advances in Surgery, Vol 34. St Louis, Mosby, 2000, pp 67–119.)

POSTOPERATIVE MANAGEMENT

Postoperative care after laparoscopic colectomy varies little from that after open surgery except that recovery time is usually shorter. The nasogastric tube and the Foley catheter are removed once the procedure is concluded or on the first postoperative day. Patients are offered clear liquids the same day as surgery or the following day; essentially, the diet is progressed according to the patient's degree of hunger and tolerance. Patients are encouraged to walk soon after surgery, which is often done with minimal discomfort. Antibiotic therapy does not vary from that used for conventional colectomy. Patients are usually dismissed between day 3 and day 6 postoperatively on a regimen of oral analgesics once a regular diet is tolerated.

COMPLICATIONS

Treatment of benign disorders such as inflammatory bowel disease is associated with inherent technical difficulties that may result in a greater risk of development of complications. An inflammatory mass with greater vascularization is difficult to dissect, planes are not easily visualized, and the risk of bleeding and bowel perforation is increased. In regard to malignancies, neoplasms larger than 8 to 10 cm in diameter are technically difficult to manage laparoscopically. Furthermore, removing a tumor of this magnitude in one piece through a small 4- to 6-cm incision is not feasible.

Bleeding can occur as a result of either direct injury of blood vessels secondary to unrecognized coagulopathy or failure of hemostasis during the procedure. Excessive traction placed on the mesentery of the bowel may tear small vessels, resulting in hemorrhage. Bleeding can be controlled directly with clips, cautery, or endoloops as well as laparoscopic suturing. A surgeon should never apply clips or sutures blindly; if it is not possible to stop the bleeding or to get appropriate exposure, conversion to an open procedure should be done.

Perforation of the small bowel, the colon, or the ureter is the most common visceral injury reported during laparoscopic colectomy. Excessive traction placed on the bowel is one cause of such injuries, and inadvertent cautery is another. Injury to the small and the large bowel may result in iatrogenic enterotomy or colotomy. To prevent these injuries, attention to the details of tissue handling and avoidance of laparoscopic surgery in patients with complete obstruction are encouraged. Depending on the degree of bowel injury, intraperitoneal contamination, and technical ability, the enterotomy or the colotomy can be repaired intracorporeally via an assisted technique or, if necessary, via conversion to an open procedure.

During laparoscopic colectomy, identification of the ureter in the operative field is essential. Before the incision in the peritoneum is made, the ureter can often be visualized as it courses over the bifurcation of the iliac artery. Once peristalsis of the ureter is demonstrated, the peritoneum can be safely incised (away from the ureter), and, before the tissues are stained with blood, the ureter can be seen directly and can be bluntly teased down so that the vascular pedicles can be transected safely.

OUTCOMES

Laparoscopic colectomy to date is associated with low morbidity and mortality rates. These excellent outcomes may occur because most of the published studies represent the experience of highly accomplished laparoscopic surgeons. A morbidity rate of approximately 15% has been reported, involving intraoperative or postoperative complications. Bleeding and iatrogenic bowel injury during the laparoscopic procedure have been recorded as intraoperative complications; they were more often reported in the early experience with laparoscopic colectomy. The incidence of certain postoperative complications (e.g., wound infections and adhesions) has been reported to be decreased with laparoscopic surgery. According to some, but not all, authors, the frequency of wound infections may be reduced by up to 50% with laparoscopic colorectal procedures. It has been reported that the frequency of reoperative surgery for small intestinal obstruction has decreased owing to adhesive obstructions after laparoscopic colectomy.

Operative time for laparoscopic bowel resection is longer than for conventional open surgery. Almost every series noted high variability with regard to the slope of the learning curve, however. The average operative time was 189 minutes; early in a surgeon's experience, operative times can average 246 minutes, whereas after some experience (10 to 20 laparoscopic resections), mean operative time decreases to 155 minutes. In general, as the reported number of patients has increased, operating times have decreased.

There is an average incidence rate of 24% for conversion of laparoscopic colectomy to open conventional laparotomy. Reasons for conversion most frequently described are unclear anatomy, adhesions, bleeding, and bowel perforation. Conversion rates tend to decrease as a result of increased surgeon proficiency and improvement in judgment with respect to patient and disease selection.

CONTROVERSIES REGARDING THE LAPAROSCOPIC APPROACH TO COLON CANCER

Is this new technology appropriate for the treatment of colorectal cancer? Issues that have concerned surgeons the most regarding the use of laparoscopic procedures for colon cancer include adequacy of laparoscopic intraoperative staging, adequacy of resection, and local recurrence of tumor in port sites. Because palpation is not feasible during laparoscopic procedures and evaluation is limited to visual inspection, a problem is created during intraperitoneal staging of the disease. This disadvantage can likely be compensated for by combining preoperative abdominal computed tomography or ultrasonography with laparoscopic visual inspection of the abdominal cavity. The same accuracy can be obtained with this combination as with intraoperative bimanual palpation. Intraoperative laparoscopic ultrasonography appears to be accurate and sensitive in identifying liver metastasis from colorectal cancer. With regard to the adequacy of the extent of the resection and the number of nodes harvested after

---

Pearls and Pitfalls

Prevention of Technique-Related Complications

- To prevent perforation of the colon or the small bowel, use atraumatic instruments, exert traction on the peritoneal attachments, not on the bowel, and employ gentle manipulation.
- To prevent splenic injury, ensure that the table is in reverse Trendelenburg's position, and place gentle traction on the splenic flexure.
- To prevent ureteral injury, make sure that the ureter has been properly identified, avoid cautery in the ureter field, and use ureteral stents as necessary for difficult cases.
- To prevent bladder injury, employ catheter decompression of the bladder.
- To prevent mesenteric bleeding, create mesenteric windows in avascular planes, and use the double-clip technique for major vessels or, if needed, suture ligation.
- To prevent an anastomotic leak, ensure proper bowel alignment, avoid tension, check for good vascularization of proximal and distal ends, and employ proper suturing or stapling techniques.
- To prevent wound or trocar site infection, use adequate bowel preparation and antibiotic prophylaxis, irrigate and ensure hemostasis of the trocar site, and use a bag for tissue extraction.
- To prevent trocar site recurrence, protect the port site during manipulation of the specimen, use a bag for specimen extraction, avoid the chimney effect, and irrigate and ensure hemostasis of the cannula site.

Management of Technique-Related Complications

- Management of perforation of the colon or the small bowel includes laparoscopic repair, if technically feasible, or conversion to open exploration.
- Management of splenic injury includes control of capsular bleeding, electrocautery or a topical hemostatic agent, splenectomy if necessary, or conversion.
- Management of ureteral injury is conversion to open exploration and repair over a stent.
- Management of bladder injury includes laparoscopic repair, if technically feasible, or conversion.
- Management of mesenteric bleeding includes laparoscopic clip or suture control or conversion.
- Management of anastomotic leak includes laparoscopic repair (intraoperative recognition), conversion, or open procedure and diversion (postoperative recognition).
- Management of wound or trocar site infection includes open drainage of the infected site or débridement.
- Management of trocar site recurrence includes excision of metastasis, systemic chemotherapy, and evaluation for systemic metastasis.

---

laparoscopic colectomy, many reviews and studies have reported no differences in the length of bowel excised, the presence of tumor-free margins, and the number of lymph nodes retrieved when compared with conventional open surgery.

A major concern in treating colon cancer with a laparoscopic approach is the altered pattern of recurrence that has been reported in a few patients. Although the incidence of port site recurrence was high (up to 15%) in early reports, recent studies with larger samples have demonstrated a decline in the incidence rates. This fact suggests that the learning curve may have played an important factor in the pattern of altered implantation. A confident answer to the question regarding wound tumor implants will come only after properly constructed, prospective randomized trials (e.g., the current ongoing multicenter trial of laparoscopic colectomy for malignancy sponsored by the National Institutes of Health) have been completed.

CONCLUSION

Laparoscopic colectomy has gained generalized acceptance as a safe, efficient, and beneficial option for the treatment of benign colonic diseases as well as for palliation of advanced malignant disease. There are strong indications that a laparoscopic approach to colon cancer

will be an optimal alternative treatment in selected patients. Prospective randomized trials are under way to demonstrate the feasibility and the safety of the procedure and the long-term survival.

SUGGESTED READINGS

Bouvet M, Mansfield PF, Skibber JM, et al: Clinical, pathologic, and economic parameters of laparoscopic colon resection for cancer. Am J Surg 1998;176:554.

Fielding GA, Lumley J, Nathanson L, et al: Laparoscopic colectomy. Surg Endosc 1997;11:745.

Franklin ME Jr, Rosenthal D, Abrego-Medina D, et al: Prospective comparison of open vs. laparoscopic colon surgery for carcinoma. Five-year results. Dis Colon Rectum 1996;39:S35.

Goletti O, Celona G, Galatioto C, et al: Is laparoscopic sonography a reliable and sensitive procedure for staging colorectal cancer? A comparative study. Surg Endosc 1998;12:1236.

Hoffman GC, Baker JW, Fitchett CW, Vansant JH: Laparoscopic-assisted colectomy. Initial experience. Ann Surg 1994;219:732.

Lord SA, Larach SW, Ferrara A, et al: Laparoscopic resections for colorectal carcinoma. A three-year experience. Dis Colon Rectum 1996;39:148.

Lumley JW, Fielding GA, Rhodes M, et al: Laparoscopic-assisted colorectal surgery. Lessons learned from 240 consecutive patients. Dis Colon Rectum 1996;39:155.

Marchesa P, Milsom JW: Laparoscopic techniques for inflammatory bowel disease. Semin Laparosc Surg 1995;2:246.

Nelson H, Weeks JC, Wieand HS: Proposed phase III trial comparing laparoscopic-assisted colectomy versus open colectomy for colon cancer. J Natl Cancer Inst Monogr 1995;19:51.

Senagore AJ, Luchtefeld MA, Mackeigan JM: What is the learning curve for laparoscopic colectomy? Am Surg 1995;61:681.

Stocchi L, Nelson H: Laparoscopic colectomy for colon cancer: Trial update. J Surg Oncol 1998;68:255.

Chapter 132
Laparoscopic Appendectomy
Sareh Parangi and Richard Hodin

GENERAL

Appendectomy is one of the most common procedures performed by general surgeons, and has classically been accomplished through a right lower quadrant muscle-splitting incision. However, laparoscopic surgical procedures have revolutionized the care of surgical patients over the last 11 years, and one of the first such procedures described was the laparoscopic appendectomy (Semm, 1983). Interestingly, although some general surgeons find laparoscopic appendectomy easier to perform, it has not shared the same widespread acceptance as certain other laparoscopic procedures, such as cholecystectomy, Nissen fundoplication, and adrenalectomy. A reluctance to routinely perform laparoscopic appendectomies has been based on several factors: (1) unwillingness to insufflate an abdomen that potentially harbors purulence, (2) lack of clear-cut time, or cost saving, or both, and (3) performance of many appendectomies at night when staff experienced in the use of laparoscopic equipment may not be available. In addition, many surgeons already consider an open appendectomy performed through a small muscle-splitting incision as "minimally invasive" surgery. Despite these issues, laparoscopic appendectomy has been embraced by many in the surgical community, and occasionally patients will request this approach. As such, laparoscopic appendectomy should probably be part of the armamentarium of the capable general surgeon.

INDICATIONS FOR SURGERY

The indications for surgery are the same as those for open appendectomy, and all patients with suspected appendicitis are potential candidates for laparoscopic appendectomy. Patients who may especially benefit from the laparoscopic approach include the following: (1) obese patients in whom a larger than normal incision would be required for an open approach, (2) female patients in whom the diagnosis is unclear, and (3) patients who are extremely concerned about cosmesis or faster recovery, or both.

Potential Advantages

One of the most important advantages of a laparoscopic approach is realized in patients in whom the diagnosis is not clear-cut. For example, premenopausal females with lower abdominal tenderness and equivocal signs and symptoms may benefit from early laparoscopy performed to prevent delays in diagnosis. Many of the gynecologic etiologies of pain can be fully taken care of through the laparoscope, with the surgeon thereby avoiding an unnecessary laparotomy. With laparoscopic appendectomy, the entire abdominal cavity can be thoroughly explored, something that is not possible through a right lower quadrant incision. This videoscopic exploration can lead to the accurate diagnosis of pelvic inflammatory disease, ovarian torsion, ovarian cyst, Meckel's diverticulum, perforated duodenal ulcer, infarcted omentum, cholecystitis, and perforated diverticulitis. A recent surge in preoperative computed tomography (CT) in patients with suspected appendicitis may obviate some of the advantages of laparoscopy listed earlier.

Laparoscopic appendectomy may also offer advantages, including a decrease in postoperative pain and analgesic use, a reduction in hospital stay, and a more rapid return to normal activities and work, although this is still controversial. In addition, most patients perceive a cosmetic advantage to laparoscopic appendectomy compared with the standard open operation.

Potential Disadvantages

Potential disadvantages of laparoscopic appendectomy include increased operative time and overall cost, as reported in some series. In addition, laparoscopy is associated with a few rare but unique complications, such as trocar injuries.

CURRENT ANALYSIS OF OPEN VERSUS LAPAROSCOPIC SURGERY

A number of prospective randomized studies have compared laparoscopic and open appendectomy, and two large meta-analyses have also been performed. Since the published studies were carried out in a variety of different institutions and countries, the conclusions should be applicable to the general population. Overall, laparoscopic appendectomy appears to take approximately 30% longer to perform than open appendectomy. This difference may disappear as surgeons gain more experience with the laparoscopic approach; in fact, more recent studies demonstrate marked decreases in operating time, with overall operating-room times being slightly decreased in laparoscopic cases. Analgesic requirements are less with laparoscopic appendectomy, and differences in hospital stay have reached statistical significance in favor of laparoscopic appendectomy. However, factors such as the hospital setting and the underlying pathologic process may have a greater influence on the length of stay than the operative approach. The meta-analyses have revealed that wound infection rates are higher after open appendectomy than after laparoscopic appendectomy, with a pooled odds ratio of 2.6 ($P = 0.003$). Most studies have found in favor of a shorter convalescence and somewhat earlier return to work for laparoscopic appendectomy (Table 132–1). It is important to recognize, however, that none of the studies blinded the patients or health care providers, and it is clear that preconceived notions on the part of health care staff can greatly influence the use of analgesia and the duration of hospitalization. Generally, laparoscopic appendectomy is considered a safe operation in the setting of acute or gangrenous appendicitis. Decision making in patients with perforated appendicitis must be individualized. One large retrospective study points to a larger number of postoperative abscesses in patients with perforated appendicitis who were treated laparoscopically versus those who underwent open appendectomies. However, multiple other studies, including large prospective studies and meta-analyses, point to no increases in rates of postoperative intra-abdominal abscess formation in patients with perforated appendicitis who undergo laparoscopic appendectomies. In fact, multiple studies have demonstrated that the incidence of wound infections and the length of hospitalization are clearly reduced in patients with perforated appendicitis who undergo laparoscopic appendectomy.

DIAGNOSIS AND OPERATIVE TECHNIQUE

Essential Equipment and Personnel

Laparoscopic appendectomy is generally performed with the use of a 30-degree angled laparoscope, one 5- to 11-mm trocar, one 5-mm trocar, bipolar cautery, atraumatic grasping forceps, atraumatic reticulating dissector (dolphin or blunt-tipped), and a laparoscopic stapling device (e.g., the EndoGIA, U.S. Surgical Corp) with vascular and gastrointestinal cartridges. A laparoscopic clip applier (1 cm), looped suture (e.g., Endoloop, Ethicon, Inc), and specimen retrieval bag may be used in some situations. The surgical team should be fully trained with regard to intracorporeal suturing, and the use of laparoscopic stapling devices. Given the high incidence of appendicitis, laparoscopic appendectomy can be an important operation to be used in the training of surgical residents.

Patient Preparation and Positioning

A complete history and physical examination, along with appropriate laboratory tests, are required prior to laparoscopic appendectomy. A pregnancy test should generally be performed in premenopausal females. Laparoscopic appendectomy is not contraindicated in pregnancy, but the knowledge that the patient is pregnant may alter port placement and the pressure of the pneumoperitoneum established. Additionally, in patients with prolonged symptoms (i.e., more than 5 days), the possibility of a perforated appendicitis with abscess or phlegmon should be considered. These patients may be better treated with antibiotics and CT-guided drainage with subsequent interval laparoscopic appendectomy. Some patients with perforated appendicitis may be treated with open appendectomies, depending on the surgeon's preference and experience. Previous abdominal operations and scars should be taken into consideration, as they may change the location of trocars.

Broad-spectrum antibiotics should be given just prior to incision. The patient should be positioned supine on the operating table, with arms at the sides. A Foley catheter and orogastric tube may be used during the operation, but they can generally be removed at the end of the case. If suspicion of a gynecologic etiology is high, a lithotomy position should be considered to allow better access for manipulation of the uterus. Either subcutaneous heparin or sequential compression devices on the lower extremities can be used for prophylaxis against deep venous thrombosis.

Trocar Placement

As with all laparoscopic operations, care should be taken with regard to trocar placement. Three trocars are usually needed for the operation (Fig. 132–1A). The camera is generally placed in the infraumbilical position, and a 5-mm port in the right lower quadrant to grasp the appendix. An 11-mm port is placed in the suprapubic or left lower quadrant region to be used for dissection and for stapling or other devices. Alternative trocar placements have been described, but the underlying principle is to allow triangulation of the ports, so that instruments are not placed along the path of the camera.

Operative Procedure

With the patient under general anesthesia, the infraumbilical camera port is inserted with the use of a closed or open approach. Injection of a long-acting local anesthetic

Table 132–1	Meta-analyses of Prospective Randomized Trials Comparing Laparoscopic and Open Appendectomies				
	OPERATIVE TIME (min)	HOSPITAL DAYS	RECOVERY DAYS	WOUND INFECTION	POSTOPERATIVE ABSCESS
Number of trials analyzed	17	17	12	15	15
Laparoscopic appendectomy	63	3.1	11.4	2.9%	1.8%
Open appendectomy	48	3.5	17	7.2%	0.8%
Significant difference (P < 0.001)	Yes	No	Yes	Yes	No

Data obtained from meta-analysis of Chung RS, Rowland DY, Li P, Diaz J: A meta-analysis of randomized controlled trials of laparoscopic versus conventional appendectomy. Am J Surg 1999;177:250–256.

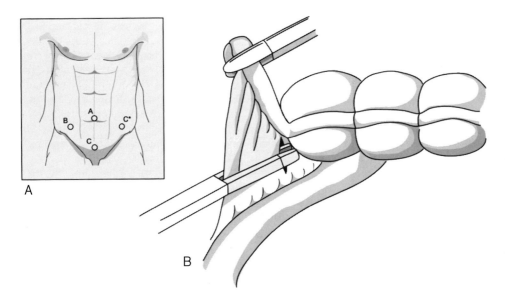

Figure 132–1. *A,* The camera is placed in the infraumbilical position (A), and a 5-mm port (B) is placed in the right lower quadrant to grasp the appendix. An 11-mm port is placed in the suprapubic (C) or left lower quadrant region (C*) to be used for the stapling devices, the clip applier, and the possible passage of sutures. *B,* The appendix is retracted toward the anterior abdominal wall, and an endostapler is used to divide the mesoappendix. Another firing of the stapler is then used to divide the base of the appendix.

in all incisions is desirable. The authors prefer using the open approach, which allows direct visualization of entry into the peritoneal cavity, thereby reducing the risk of intestinal or vascular injury. The abdomen is insufflated with carbon dioxide to a pressure of 12 to 15 mm Hg, the camera is inserted, and a thorough visualization of the abdominal contents is performed. Special attention is paid to both paracolic gutters, the pelvis, the gallbladder, the liver, and the peritoneal surfaces. The presence or absence of pus in the peritoneal cavity is noted. The operating ports are then inserted under direct vision and instruments used to manipulate the cecum and visualize the appendix.

Placement of the patient in the Trendelenburg position with the left side down can often aid in moving the omentum and small bowel away from the right lower quadrant. If the inflamed appendix is located in the retrocecal position, dissection of the lateral peritoneal reflection may be required and can be done either bluntly or with sharp dissection using electrocautery. In the case of severe inflammation in this region, it is best to use blunt dissection and stay close to the cecal wall, in order to avoid injury to the ureter or iliac vessels. The appendix is grasped and traced to where it joins the cecum (see Fig. 132–1*B*). The inflamed appendix can be quite rigid, making manipulation somewhat difficult. If the appendix cannot be grasped easily, a looped suture or an endoloop can be secured to the tip to allow for easier manipulation. If further manipulation of the appendix is required and cannot be obtained with the use of the standard three ports described earlier, this loop of suture can be inserted through a 14-gauge intravenous catheter placed in the right lower quadrant. The appendix should be retracted so as to expose the mesoappendix and the base of the appendix. The mesoappendix can be taken down in a retrograde fashion, starting at the attachments near the tip of the appendix (see Fig. 132–1*B*). The mesoappendix is most easily controlled by creating a window at the base of the appendix through which the tip of the EndoGIA can be positioned (with the use of a vascular cartridge with 2-mm staples). Before firing the stapler, care must

be taken to ensure that the tip of the stapler is free from other structures. Although clips have also been used to control the mesoappendix, this requires the added cost of the clip applier. If there is severe inflammation of the mesoappendix, an antegrade dissection may be used. In such a situation, the appendix may be divided at the base first, and then dissection of the mesoappendix is begun, starting at the base of the appendix and moving toward the tip.

Once the mesoappendix is divided, attention is turned to the appendix itself. The junction of the base of the appendix and the cecum needs to carefully dissected, and the appendix divided with the use of the stapling device introduced through the 11-mm port. If the base of the appendix is severely inflamed, one needs to be certain that healthy tissue is included in the staple line. Once divided, the stump of the appendix should be inspected for bleeding or leaks and should not be manipulated or cauterized, since injury can result from sparking onto the staple line. The appendiceal stump need not be inverted, since simple ligation has been shown to be perfectly safe. In the presence of severe inflammation at the base of the appendix, conversion to open appendectomy is advised, allowing for stump inversion into the cecal wall. This degree of inflammation of the appendiceal base should be assessed as early as possible during the operation, so that the decision to convert to an open procedure can be made early on during laparoscopy.

Once the appendix is free, it should be removed without contaminating the fascial or subcutaneous tissues. This can be accomplished either by placing the appendix in a bag prior to removal or by retracting the appendix into the larger port and pulling out the entire port. If needed, the port can then be washed and reinserted back into the peritoneal cavity. Irrigation of the right lower quadrant, and even the entire peritoneal cavity, is easily accomplished via laparoscopy. Port sites larger than 10 mm should be closed with absorbable fascial sutures. The skin is closed with subcuticular sutures in most cases.

If a normal appendix is found at laparoscopy and no other intra-abdominal pathology is discovered, the authors recommend removal of the appendix. This recommendation is based on the fact that subtle inflammatory changes of the appendix may be difficult to detect, and the morbidity of removing a normal appendix is negligible. If an explanation of the patient's signs and symptoms has been found, such as perforated ulcer, pelvic inflammatory disease, cholecystitis, or diverticulitis, there is no need to remove the normal appendix. The patient must, however, be specifically made aware of whether or not the appendix was removed.

POSTOPERATIVE MANAGEMENT

When orogastric tubes and Foley catheters are used, they can be removed while the patient is still in the operating room. The patient's diet can be advanced in a liberal fashion after operation, and patients can usually be discharged safely within 24 hours, requiring minimal narcotics and tolerating a regular diet. In the case of simple appendicitis, no further antibiotics are administered, but in gangrenous or perforated appendicitis a more prolonged course of intravenous antibiotics (2 to 5 days) is generally recommended.

Possible Complications

Laparoscopic appendectomy carries most of the same risks as open appendectomy, as well as risks associated with laparoscopy. Reported complications of laparoscopic appendectomy include wound infection, ileus, abscess formation, stump leak with fecal soilage, hemorrhage, and urinary tract infection (see Table 132–1). Other more serious complications such as pulmonary embolus and death have also been reported for laparoscopic appendectomy, as they have been for open appendectomies.

SPECIAL CONSIDERATIONS

Laparoscopic Appendectomy during Pregnancy

Laparoscopic appendectomy during pregnancy has not been well studied. Reviews of the combined experience with laparoscopic appendectomy and cholecystectomy seem to indicate that laparoscopy is well tolerated by mother and fetus. Initial trocar placement for the pneumoperitoneum needs to performed via an open technique, with special attention paid to the position of the gravid uterus, depending on the stage of pregnancy. The patient's obstetrician should be involved in operative planning, and intra-abdominal pressures should not exceed 14 mm Hg.

Interval Laparoscopic Appendectomy

Interval laparoscopic appendectomies after initial nonoperative treatment of a periappendiceal abscess can be

Pearls and Pitfalls

- Laparoscopic appendectomy should be considered in all patients with appendicitis. Patients who may especially benefit include obese patients, female patients with an unclear diagnosis, and patients who are strongly concerned about cosmesis.
- Meta-analyses of large, randomized studies have shown that laparoscopic appendectomies take longer than open appendectomies, but analgesic requirements and hospital stay are shorter. Operative times are reduced in laparoscopic appendectomies performed by surgeons with greater experience.
- Generally, laparoscopic appendectomy is considered a safe operation in the setting of acute or gangrenous appendicitis.
- In perforated appendicitis, the decision to intervene laparoscopically needs to be individualized.
- Once the base of the appendix is divided with the stapler, the stump should not be manipulated or cauterized because sparking injury can result. There is no need to invert the stump.

performed safely and easily. At operation, there is usually very little residual inflammation, making manipulation of the appendix easy, considerably reducing operative time. Patients undergoing interval appendectomies are usually able to go home on the same day that surgery was performed, resulting in a decrease in hospital stay compared with open interval appendectomies.

Tumors Discovered during Laparoscopic Appendectomy

There is not much published on the proper algorithm to follow when a tumor of the appendix is discovered during a laparoscopic appendectomy. Some authors recommend conversion to an open procedure for fear of causing diffuse peritoneal carcinomatosis, as has been reported for a mucinous adenocarcinoma of the appendix.

SELECTED READINGS

Chung RS, Rowland DY, Li P, Diaz J: A meta-analysis of randomized controlled trials of laparoscopic versus conventional appendectomy. Am J Surg 1999;177:250.

Gonzalez Moreno S, Shmookler BM, Sugarbaker PH: Appendiceal mucocele: Contraindication to laparoscopic appendectomy. Surg Endosc 1998;12:1177.

McCall JL, Sharples K, Jadallah F: Systematic review of randomized controlled trials comparing laparoscopic with open appendicectomy. Br J Surg 1997;84:1045.

Nezhat FR, Tazuke S, Nezhat CH, et al: Laparoscopy during pregnancy: A literature review. J Soc Laparoendosc Surg 1997;1:17.

Nguyen DB, Silen W, Hodin RA: Appendectomy in the pre- and postlaparoscopic eras. J Gastrointest Surg 1999;3:67.

Nguyen DB, Silen W, Hodin RA: Interval appendectomy in the laparoscopic era. J Gastrointest Surg 1999;3:189.

Ortega AE, Hunter JG, Peters JH, et al: A prospective, randomized comparison of laparoscopic appendectomy with open appendectomy. Laparoscopic Appendectomy Study Group. Am J Surg 1995;169:208–212; discussion 212–213.

Paik PS, Towson JA, Anthone GJ, et al: Intra-abdominal abscesses following laparoscopic and open appendectomies. J Gastrointest Surg 1997;1:188.

Semm K: Endoscopic appendectomy. Endoscopy 1983;15:59.

Chapter 133

Laparoscopic Small Bowel Resection

Goodluck Eze and Steven D. Wexner

Advances in laparoscopic surgery not only have drastically modified the thinking of most surgeons but also have helped to change the approach to many disease processes in the last decade. Laparoscopic surgery has gained widespread acceptance because of the many perceived advances over open laparotomy, such as decreased postoperative pain, shorter hospitalization, faster return to normal activity, reduced complications, and improved cosmesis.

As more experience is gained with simpler procedures, larger and more complex operations such as gastric, colorectal, and small bowel surgery have been successfully completed laparoscopically. Previous abdominal surgery and suspected intestinal adhesions were, until recently, considered relative contraindications against laparoscopy, owing to the risk of bowel injury and limited visualization. Increasing surgical experience and refinement of surgical instrumentation, optics, and video monitoring equipment all have facilitated advances with these procedures.

INDICATIONS FOR A LAPAROSCOPIC APPROACH

The indications for laparoscopic small bowel surgery are the same as those for traditional small bowel resection with laparotomy. The use of this technology should not, in any way, compromise surgical techniques or alter traditional, sound judgment. If at any time during the laparoscopic procedure the surgeon thinks that the desired efficacy and safety of the procedure cannot be attained, the procedure should be converted to open laparotomy. The current potential indications for and contraindications against laparoscopic small bowel resection are outlined in Table 133–1.

CLINICAL FINDINGS

A thorough history and physical examination are important in evaluating patients scheduled for small bowel resection. Most patients with small bowel obstruction manifest abdominal pain, nausea and vomiting, obstipation, and abdominal distention. Distention can be mild or severe but is often absent in proximal bowel obstruction. Bowel sounds are high-pitched and active and may be accompanied by visible peristalsis in asthenic patients. Abdominal tenderness tends to be diffuse and may be localized to a single quadrant in strangulation obstruction. The stool is usually free from blood unless bowel ischemia has supervened. Evidence of dehydration is commonly seen, with tachycardia, postural hypotension, and oliguria.

Incarceration of the small bowel from either an inguinal or a ventral hernia is usually evident on physical examination. The diagnosis of femoral hernia, obturator hernia, and diaphragmatic hernia, however, may be challenging, particularly in obese individuals. Primary small bowel lesions, such as carcinoma, carcinoid, lymphoma, and benign and malignant soft tissue tumors, which often present with obstruction, may be appreciable as a mass on physical examination of the abdomen. Palpation of an intra-abdominal mass may indicate malignancy possibly not amenable to curative resection. Malignant lymphoma often presents as a palpable mass, localized to a resectable segment of small intestine. Most palpable masses are mobile unless there is invasion into the surrounding structures; masses caused by intussusception are generally benign. Signs of intestinal perforation, including abdominal distention, peritoneal irritation, hypoactive bowel sounds, or a silent abdomen, are usually associated with malignant lymphomas or adenocarcinomas of the small intestine.

LABORATORY FINDINGS

Laboratory tests may be normal in the early stages of small bowel obstruction. However, with progression of obstruction, leukocytosis, abnormalities in electrolytes, and hemoconcentration may become more pronounced. Hyperamylasemia can accompany bowel distention or infarction, with leakage of intestinal amylase into the peritoneal cavity and eventual peritoneal absorption. The presence of marked metabolic acidosis and increased white blood cell counts of more than 15,000/mm^3 suggest bowel ischemia or strangulation. There are no specific laboratory findings that accompany Crohn's disease. The severity of

Table 133–1	Indications and Contraindications of Laparoscopic Small Bowel Surgery

Indications
  Adhesive small bowel obstruction
  Inflammatory diseases of the small bowel, Crohn's disease, tuberculous enteritis, typhoid enteritis, etc.
  Benign tumors of the small bowel
  Irreducible intussusception with or without associated polyps
  Selected mesenteric-based masses or lymphadenopathy
  Arteriovenous malformation localized to the small bowel
  Small bowel diverticula including Meckel's diverticulum
  Stricture
  Malrotation of the small bowel
  Stenosis or congenital atresia of the small bowel
  Metastatic malignant lesions
Contraindications
  History of radiation
  Fecal peritonitis
  Hemodynamic instability
  Active intraabdominal hemorrhage
  Lack of surgeon's experience
  Potentially curable malignant lesions

disease, and the presence of complications such as abscess or fistula, may lead to an increased sedimentation rate, hypoalbuminemia, anemia, and steatorrhea.

RADIOLOGIC FINDINGS

A mass, suspected small bowel obstruction, unexplained diarrhea, malabsorption, intestinal bleeding, and abdominal pain warrant supine and upright plain abdominal films. In small bowel obstruction, a ladderlike pattern of dilated small bowel loops with fluid or air levels, or both, confirm small bowel obstruction. These features may be absent in proximal obstruction, early obstruction, or closed loop obstruction, or, in some patients, when fluid-filled loops contain little gas. Opaque gallstones and air in the biliary tree should be excluded in patients with a history of gallstone disease. Certain radiologic findings such as edema or thickening of the small bowel wall and loss of a mucosal pattern suggest strangulation.

Patients with intestinal bleeding that cannot be localized by upper gastrointestinal endoscopy and colonoscopy should undergo a radionuclide bleeding scan or angiography. Two scans are used in radionuclide bleeding scan: the technetium sulfur colloid scan and the ^{99m}Tc pertechnetate–labeled red blood cell scan. The technetium sulfur colloid scan is rarely used currently, owing to the short half-life of the radionuclide, which makes detection of a bleeding site possible only if there is active bleeding during the examination. The more commonly used ^{99m}TC pertechnetate–labeled red blood cell scan labels autologous red blood cells from the patient in vitro with the technetium marker; the cells are then reinfused into the patient. Images are obtained every 5 minutes for 30 to 60 minutes, then every 10 minutes for another 30 to 60 minutes, and then again at 2 to 4 hours for 24 hours; the scan can detect bleeding rates as low as 0.1 mL/min.

Angiography is a useful modality for patients with acute bleeding and negative endoscopic procedures or a negative radionuclide scan. Vascular lesions, such as angiodysplasia, aortoenteric fistula, and hemangioma, account for most of the diagnostic abnormalities that can be definitely diagnosed with angiography. Diagnostic evaluation with contrast-enhanced studies (barium or Gastrografin) is indicated for patients with no indication of perforation or peritonitis and when there is no clinical suspicion of partial obstruction on plain abdominal radiographs. In such patients, contrast-enhanced studies confirm the presence, severity, and possible etiology of obstruction. In a gasless abdomen, ultrasonography may provide valuable information by demonstrating distended, fluid-filled bowel. Computed tomography is also useful in the diagnosis of small bowel obstruction when one assesses patients with abdominal malignancy or those with an acute abdomen complicated by sepsis. Its utility, however, in patients with intermittent obstruction has not yet been established.

PREOPERATIVE MANAGEMENT

The preoperative management of small bowel obstruction is directed by a clinical history and physical examination,

as the operative procedure may be either elective or urgent. In urgent operative intervention, decompression of the stomach is mandatory with a nasogastric tube. These patients require careful monitoring of blood pressure, pulse rate, central venous pressure, temperature, and urine output. A complete blood count and determination of serum electrolytes, blood urea nitrogen, creatinine, and amylase should be obtained. If the hematocrit is greater than 50%, rapid administration of lactated Ringer's solution should be immediately administered to lower the value into a normal range. Deficiencies of sodium, potassium, and chloride should also be promptly corrected by 0.9% intravenous sodium chloride; potassium chloride is added once a satisfactory urine output has been established.

Preoperative preparation for elective surgery is the same as for any elective bowel resection. All patients are given broad-spectrum oral and parenteral antibiotics and a standard mechanical cathartic bowel preparation of 90 mL of sodium phosphate (Fleet's Phospho-Soda, C. B. Fleet Co., Lynchburg, VA) 24 hours prior to surgery.

PATIENT POSITIONING AND OPERATING ROOM SETUP

The patient is placed in the modified supine position in Allen stirrups (Allen Medical, Bedford Heights, OH). A bladder catheter and nasogastric tube are used to decompress the bladder and stomach, respectively; general endotracheal anesthesia is utilized. The operating table should be electronic to be easily maneuverable to various positions required for maximizing laparoscopic exposure. At least two monitors should be used, preferably with one directly opposite the surgeon and one facing the line of view of the telescope (Fig. 133–1).

TROCAR POSITIONING

The first laparoscopic trocar is placed in the periumbilical region for patients who have not undergone previous abdominal surgery. For patients who have undergone one or more previous incisions, the trocar should be placed in the left upper quadrant as this area of the abdomen is less likely to develop adhesions. Furthermore, the jejunum is covered with the omentum and thus protected from adhesions. Regardless of the site selected, the open technique is preferred for patients undergoing laparoscopic surgery for bowel obstruction or enterolysis or who have had a prior laparotomy. Direct visualization of the peritoneal cavity permits periumbilical takedown of any adhesions near the site of trocar placement under direct visual control or before actually "blindly" inserting the trocar.

The laparoscope is inserted into the abdominal cavity and all other subsequent trocars are placed under direct visual guidance. The number of trocars placed depends on the anatomy and the surgeon's preference. In general, a maximum of three to four ports are required to perform a complete enterolysis.

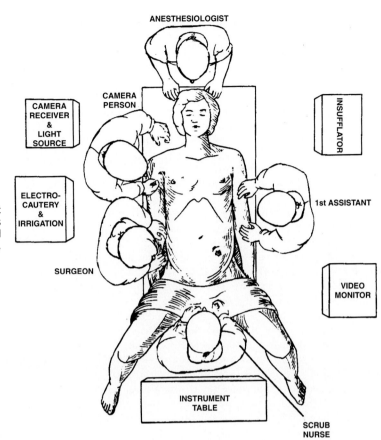

Figure 133–1. Positioning of monitors for laparoscopic small intestinal surgery. (From Luchtefeld MA: Hartmann's takedown. In Wexner SD [ed]: Laparoscopic Colorectal Surgery [Protocols in General Surgery Ser.]. New York, Wiley-Liss, 1999, pp 213–222.)

LAPAROSCOPIC TECHNIQUE

Once the first trocar is placed, pneumoperitoneum of 15 mm Hg is established, during which there is careful observation of the hemodynamic status of the patient. If any abnormalities are noted or if the patient becomes unstable, the intra-abdominal pressure should be decreased. Once the camera is in the peritoneal cavity, an initial general inspection is performed; the authors generally prefer two to four 10-mm ports, as a port of this diameter permits placement of the camera through any site. Subsequent port placement is directed by pre-existing adhesions; points for trocars that will facilitate lysis of adhesions are chosen. Careful inspection of the entire small bowel starts at the ileocolic junction; this landmark is the easiest to find along the small intestine when one starts at the appendix. The bowel should be gently manipulated with an atraumatic clamp, with frequent repositioning of the operating table to facilitate retraction. Extreme care is necessary when one inspects the bowel, as traumatic iatrogenic myotomies or enterotomies can occur if too much traction or pull is exerted by the grasping forceps, especially in thin, acutely obstructed bowel. When adhesions are encountered, they should be carefully lysed with scissors under direct vision, thereby avoiding thermal injury to the adjacent bowel (Fig. 133–2). Abnormalities requiring small bowel resection should prompt a laparoscopic-assisted procedure. The small bowel is then gently grasped with a Babcock clamp through a 10-mm periumbilical port and delivered through an enlarged umbilical incision.

In general, the rate-limiting step for the size of the incision is the size of the specimen. A large or benign tumor or an inflamed mesentery may dictate a larger incision. The specimen should not be delivered until the wound has been protected with some type of plastic drape. After delivery, the mesentery can be scored. Vessels can then be clamped, divided, and suture-ligated. After the bowel is circumferentially cleared of fat at the desired resection margins, each end can be divided with a 75-mm linear cutting device. A handsewn or stapled

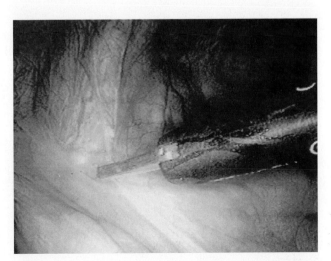

Figure 133–2. Sharp dissection of filmy adhesions with the use of the Harmonic Scalpel. (Ethicon Endosurgery, Inc., Cincinnati, OH.)

anastomosis can then be fashioned in the usual manner, along with closure of the mesenteric defect. After verification of luminal patency and anastomotic hemostasis, the anastomosis can be returned to the peritoneal cavity. After irrigation, the entire small bowel length can be inspected through this incision by the operator's delivering any additional areas. This maneuver is particularly helpful in patients with Crohn's disease in whom concomitant stricturoplasty or additional resections can be performed. Ultimately, after irrigation, all port sites and their incisions are closed with interrupted, absorbable sutures. Subcutaneous layers are irrigated and verified for meticulous hemostasis.

The biggest debate is the extent to which enterolysis should be performed. Some surgeons advocate performing a limited lysis of adhesions directed either by preoperative radiographic or by clinical findings (point tenderness) or intraoperative findings (proximal dilatation with distal decompression). The authors prefer complete enterolysis from either the ileocecal junction or the prior ileocolic anastomosis, proceeding proximally to the duodenal-jejunal flexure. After enterolysis, the entire small bowel must be carefully inspected to ensure that no enterotomies or myotomies have been made. After all of the adhesions have been carefully and successfully lysed in a laparoscopic manner and any myotomies or enterotomies have been identified, a decision must be made as to whether to enlarge the umbilical port for extracorporeal repair or to perform an intracorporeal repair. Such a decision must be made, based on the available equipment and the expertise of the surgical team as well as the extent and location of the injury. If a bowel resection has been performed through a limited incision, any additional injured or diseased sites can be treated through this same incision in an expeditious and cost-effective manner. Similarly, if an incision has been made, the authors would utilize the opportunity to place Seprafilm (Genzyme Corporation, Cambridge, MA), a compound of sodium hyaluronate and carboxymethylcellulose, under the incision. A prospective randomized, surgeon-blinded trial was undertaken that included 183 patients who underwent restorative proctocolectomy. Seprafilm resulted in significant decreases in the incidence, extent, and severity of adhesions. Several additional trials with similar conclusions have subsequently been performed.

Results of enterolysis for small bowel obstruction are difficult to judge, as some of the publications emanate from the gynecologic literature, with chronic pelvic pain as the primary symptom. In this population, "success" is often judged by a reduction in pain, rather than bowel obstruction. Similarly, issues of fertility that are germane to the gynecologic literature have not been addressed in the general or colorectal surgical studies. Therefore, Table 133–2 focuses on "success" as relief of obstructive signs and symptoms and also morbidity.

SMALL BOWEL TUMORS

Although Table 133–1 lists many potential reasons for laparoscopic small bowel surgery, small bowel tumors are rare. Concerns have been raised over the adequacy of laparoscopy for the treatment of potentially curable colorectal carcinoma. Specifically, port site implantation has been raised as a concern. Accordingly, while the authors would advocate laparoscopic resection of any preoperatively identified metastatic small bowel tumor, they still prefer an open laparotomy for potentially curable lesions. Unfortunately, many small bowel malignancies are discovered only during laparotomy or laparoscopy. In these instances, we would continue as originally planned. As an example, if the patient had already been scheduled for a laparoscopy for bowel obstruction, and a small bowel carcinoma was identified, an inspection would be undertaken. If metastatic disease was noted, laparoscopy-assisted resection would be performed, as discussed earlier. Alternatively, if no metastatic disease was noted, the procedure would be converted to an open laparotomy for a resection. If a preoperatively known benign small bowel neoplasm was the indication for surgery, a laparoscopic-assisted resection, as outlined earlier, would be performed.

Besides adhesions and very rare benign tumors, more common indications for laparoscopic small bowel proce-

Table 133–2	Results of Laparoscopy for Small Bowel Obstruction				
AUTHOR	**n**	**INDICATION**	**OPERATIVE TIME MEAN (RANGE, MIN)**	**LENGTH OF HOSPITALIZATION MEAN (RANGE, DAYS)**	**CONVERSION RATE (%)**
Keating, 1992	5	Acute SBO	NS	3	0
Freys, 1992	58	Chronic abdominal pain	80 (25–195)	5 (2–11)	2 (34)
Francois, 1994	52	Acute SBO = 17	95 (20–240)	3 (1–10)	3 (5.7)
		Chronic abdominal pain obstructive symptoms = 35			
Franklin, 1994	23	Acute SBO	70 (20–120)	2.5 (1–14)	3 (13)
Luque de Leon, 1998	14	Acute intermittent SBO	108 (55–160)	2.9 ± 0.7	14 (35)
	12	Acute intermittent SBO	135 (80–185)	5.4 ± 0.17	
Bailey, 1998	31	Acute SBO	64 (15–180)	3.1 (1–15)	9 (13)
	15	Acute SBO	83 (25–160)	NS	
Strickland, 1999	40	Acute SBO	68	3.6	16 (40)

NS, not stated; SBO, small bowel obstruction.

Table 133–3	Indications for Laparoscopic Fecal Diversion

Perianal Crohn's disease	Fecal incontinence
Colonic pseudo-obstruction	Rectourethral fistula
Radiation proctitis	Rectal carcinoma

dures are related to inflammatory bowel disease. There are basically three groups of patients. The first group includes individuals who have undergone a total abdominal colectomy and are desirous of, and candidates for, takedown of the ileostomy and anastomosis to the rectum as an ileoproctostomy. This procedure can be performed laparoscopically, although it is beyond the scope of this chapter to discuss laparoscopy-assisted Hartmann's reversal. The only caveats appropriate at this juncture are the utilization of intraoperatively placed bilateral ureteric catheters. After stomal mobilization and placement of the anvil, a laparoscopic enterolysis would be performed, followed by anastomosis and verification of anastomotic integrity.

The second group is composed of patients scheduled to undergo a diverting loop ileostomy, generally for peri-anal Crohn's disease. This group may be trying to avoid a permanent ileostomy after proctocolectomy, but they may also have hopes of improving their perianal status by temporary fecal diversion. Other individuals may require loop ileostomy for a variety of reasons, including repeat repairs of rectovaginal fistulas, sphincter lacerations, other anorectal trauma, and a variety of other indications (Table 133–3). As previously reported, the results with laparoscopically constructed loop ileostomy compare quite favorably to those achieved with laparotomy and ileostomy or, even, to trephine stoma (Table 133–4). Figure 133–3 illustrates the authors' technique of laparoscopic loop ileostomy creation. The patient is marked preoperatively by an enterostomal therapist for a location in the right iliac fossa away from the epigastric vessels, any pre-existing scars, the costal margin, the anterosuperior iliac spine, the pubis, and the umbilicus. Stomas are generally created with two ports, one in the supraumbilical midline and one through the stoma site. The most important facet here is to ensure appropriate orientation of the small bowel limb during maturation of the stoma. A variety of options exist, including intracorporeal marking with clips, sutures, or cautery, or a combination of extracorporeal and intracorporeal verification by sliding an instrument along the limb for verification. Figure 133–4 demon-

Table 133–4	Results of Laparoscopic Intestinal Stoma

AUTHOR	n	PROCEDURE	OPERATIVE TIME MEAN (RANGE, MIN)	LENGTH OF HOSPITALIZATION MEAN (RANGE, DAYS)	CONVERSION (%)	POSTOPERATIVE MORBIDITY (%)
Fuhrman, 1994	19	Abdominoperineal resection = 7 Loop colostomy = 6 Loop ileostomy = 2 Loop sigmoid colostomy = 7	NS	NS	2 (11)	2 (11)
Almqvist, 1995	18	Loop ileostomy = 6 Loop colostomy = 12	47 (45–115) 50 (42–102)	NS	2 (11)	0
Ludwig, 1996	24	Loop ileostomy = 16 Sigmoid loop colostomy = 1 End colostomy = 6 Transverse colostomy = 1	60 (20–120)	6 (2–28)	1 (4)	1 (4.7)
Kini, 1996	7	Loop ileostomy = 1 Loop colostomy = 6	NS	NS	0	0
Oliveira, 1997	32	Loop ileostomy/colostomy = 29 End colostomy = 3	76 (30–210)	6.2 (2–13)	5 (15.6)	2 (6)
Hollyoak, 1998	55	NS	54.3	7.4	2 (5)	7 (12.7)
Young-Fadok, 1998	19	End colostomy = 18 End ileostomy = 1	176 (115–270)	12.7 (3–55)	3 (16)	4 (21)
Schwander, 1998	42	Loop ileostomy = 7 Loop sigmoid colostomy = 32 End sigmoid colostomy = 3	74 (30–200)	13 (6–47)	1 (2.4)	4 (9.5)
Bemelman, 1997	10		62	8.8	0	NS
Roe, 1994	4	Loop ileostomy = 1 Loop colostomy = 3	NS	9.5 (6–14)	0	0
Lyerly, 1994	4	Loop ileostomy = 1 Loop colostomy = 3 End colostomy = 1	NS	NS	NS	NS
Lange, 1991	1	Loop colostomy	100	12	0	0
Romero, 1992	1	End colostomy	NS	NS	0	0
Khoo, 1993	1	Loop ileostomy	60	3	0	0

NS, not stated.

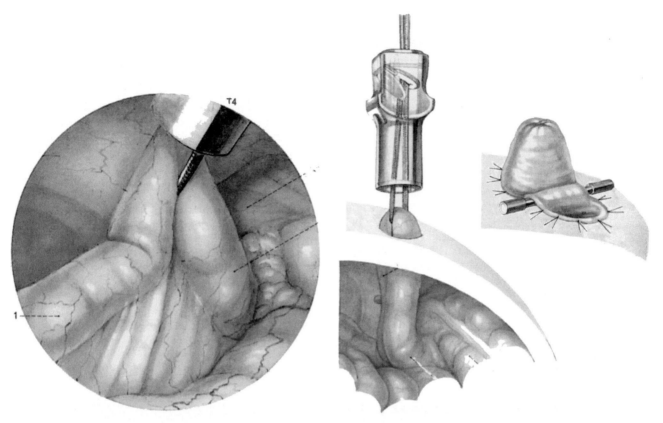

Figure 133–3. Laparoscopic stoma creation. (From Kockerling F: Anlage einer Loop-ileostomie. In Kremer K, Lierse W, Platzer W, et al [eds]: Chirurgische Operationslehre: Minimal-Invasive Chirurgie [in German]. Stuttgart, Thieme, 1995, pp 248–253.)

strates port positioning for stoma creation. After the stoma loop has been delivered above the skin, it can be divided and matured as an end or a loop stoma (see Fig. 133–3).

The third group of patients, probably the most frequent, are the individuals with either primary or recurrent ileal Crohn's disease. In this group of patients, preoperative evaluation must include thorough examination of the colon with biopsy even of normal-appearing areas to exclude colonic Crohn's disease. A small bowel series or preferably an enteroclysis should be performed to exclude proximal synchronous disease. The authors have, on occasion, noted proximal strictures missed radiographically that were treated during a laparoscopic-assisted procedure by synchronous stricturoplasty. A computed tomography should also be obtained to exclude any phlegmons. The authors do not consider enteroenteric, enterovesical, enterocolic, or enterovaginal fistulas or the presence of a phlegmon as contraindications to this surgery. However, enterocutaneous fistulas may mitigate against a laparoscopic procedure.

The operation begins as outlined previously. The position of the operating surgeon between the legs is quite useful for performing hepatic flexure mobilization and also to allow transanal access for any intraoperative colonoscopy, as necessary. Two monitors should be utilized, oriented near the patient's shoulders. In general, the authors use a single periumbilical 10-mm port with a 10-mm left lower quadrant and a 10-mm left paraumbilical port. With the patient in Trendelenburg position with the left side down, the dissection commences by utilizing a 10-mm Babcock clamp to gently retract the right colon in a medial direction. The line of Toldt is incised with the scissors and ultrasonic scalpel up to and around the hepatic flexure to the midtransverse colon to the left of the middle colic vessels. The surgeon divides the gastrocolic omentum along its avascular plane with the ultrasonic scalpel, taking care not to injure the gastroepiploic vessels. The right ureter and duodenum are identified and reflected posteriorly out of harm's way. The endpoints of the dissection are the superior mesenteric vessels, the duodenum and head of the pancreas, and the middle colic vessels along with the right ureter. After full mobilization, specimen delivery, resection, and anastomosis are effected, as already outlined.

The results of ileocolic resection for Crohn's disease are documented in Table 133–5. Every series in which laparoscopy has been compared with laparotomy for the treatment of distal ileal Crohn's disease has favored laparoscopy. Advantages have been noted, including decreased morbidity, shorter hospitalization, and improved cosmesis, as noted in a study by Dunker and colleagues (1998). An added benefit is the possibility of a decreased incidence of adhesions and perhaps a decreased rate of small bowel obstruction during follow-up.

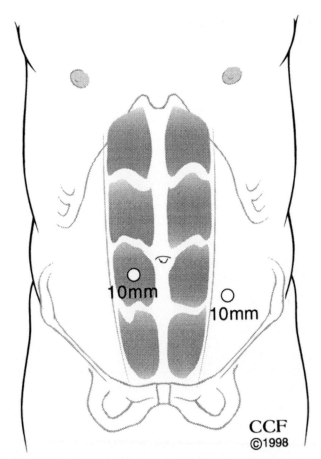

Figure 133–4. Port site placement for laparoscopic stoma creation. (From Ludwig KA, Strong S: In Wexner SD [ed]: Laparoscopic Colorectal Surgery [Protocols in General Surgery Ser.]. New York, Wiley-Liss, 1999, pp 213–222.)

POSTOPERATIVE MANAGEMENT

In general, the nasogastric tube is removed in the operating room. The bladder catheter is removed the morning after surgery. Parenteral broad-spectrum cephalosporin antibiotics are administered for 24 hours unless antibiotics are required in the therapeutic mode because of spillage of intestinal contents or peritonitis. Patients are allowed fluids ad libitum, commencing the evening of surgery, and patients are advanced to a solid diet when flatus is passed. Patients are discharged when a bowel movement has occurred, often 2 or 3 days after a completely laparoscopic enterolysis and 6 to 7 days after a laparoscopic-assisted ileocolic resection for Crohn's disease. Patients who have undergone a laparoscopically constructed ileostomy often require 6 or 7 days in hospital, not because of failure of the bowel to function but because of the need to receive adequate education about enterostomal care and maintenance. Prophylaxis for deep venous thrombosis is maintained until the patient has been discharged from the hospital, with the use of a combination of subcutaneous heparin and sequential compression device stockings. Patients are permitted to return to full activity as soon as 1 week.

The most common complications of laparoscopic small

bowel procedures are hemorrhage and enterotomy. Both of these morbidities are usually due to inadequate visualization. Thus, it is critical that at all phases of the procedure, optimal visualization be maintained. Meticulous attention to detail, including hemostasis, is essential. The failure to adequately visualize an area should prompt the surgeon to reorient the laparoscope or the view, perhaps by adding additional ports, or to reorient the patient on the operating table. The failure to proceed in a timely manner despite these alterations should lead to conversion to a laparotomy. In this instance, conversion should not be reviewed as failure, but rather as exercising sound judgment to prevent any deleterious effect on the patient. If conversion to an open operation is undertaken as a preemptive prophylactic procedure, rather than because a complication has occurred, the patient should not undergo any permanent sequelae. Conversely, if the surgeon persists in a maneuver despite a lack of visualization or if the surgeon performs alternative maneuvers and fails to achieve that visualization, the probability of a suboptimal outcome is higher. The surgeon thus should exercise sound judgment.

All of the usual potential complications of a laparotomy are also possible after a laparoscopic approach, including anastomotic leakage, postoperative ileus, bowel obstruction, deep venous thrombosis, myocardial infarction, transient ischemic attack, and other problems.

CONCLUSION

Laparoscopic small bowel surgery can be advantageous relative to cosmesis, return of bowel function, resumption of normal activity, and decreased disability. The most common indications are ileal Crohn's disease and adhesive intestinal obstruction. Neither of these procedures is recommended to the neophyte laparoscopist, as both are potentially challenging. However, when performed by an appropriately skilled team with adequate instrumentation and well-selected patients, the results can be gratifying.

Pearls and Pitfalls

- The indications for a laparoscopic approach to small bowel abnormalities should be the same as those for open laparotomy.
- The most common disorders amenable to a laparoscopic approach include selected patients with small bowel obstruction, Crohn's disease, or the need for a diverting stoma.
- An open procedure is preferred for a potentially curable or resectable small bowel neoplasm.
- A laparoscopic approach offers less pain, shorter hospital stay, and earlier return to full function.
- Laparoscopic small bowel resection, with or without ascending colectomy, or enterolysis requires advanced laparoscopic skills.
- Enterotomies from too vigorous traction on grasping forceps may occur, especially if visualization is not satisfactory.
- The surgeon should not feel a sense of failure because of having to convert to an open operation.

Table 133–5	Results of Laparoscopic Resection for Crohn's Disease

AUTHOR	n	PROCEDURE	OPERATIVE TIME MEAN (RANGE, MIN)	LENGTH OF HOSPITALIZATION MEAN (RANGE, DAYS)	CONVERSION (%)	POSTOPERATIVE MORBIDITY (%)
Liu, 1995	5	Ileocectomy = 3 Sigmoid colectomy = 1 Stricturoplasty = 1	175 (120–235)	7 (6–13)	0	1 (20)
Thibault, 1995	3	Total proctocolectomy with end ileostomy	441	10	0	2 (66)
Reissman, 1996	51	Ileocolic resection = 32 TAC + IRA = 6 IRA post TAC/end ileostomy = 3 Gastrojejunostomy = 3 TAC and end ileostomy = 1	2.4 (0.6–4.5)	5.1 (3–18)	7 (14)	8 (14)
Bauer, 1996	25	Ileocolic resection = 24 Ileal resection = 1	NS	6.5	6 (24)	NS
Jess, 1996	8	Ileocolic resection	145	5	1 (12)	3 (37.5)
Bemelman, 1997	7	Ileocolic resection = 7 Stoma formation = 10	150	5.2	1 (14)	1 (14)
Wu, 1997	46	Ileocolic resection	144 (75–300)	4.5 (2–8)	5 (11)	3 (20)
Singh, 1998	24	Right colectomy = 5 Fistula division = 5 Ileocolic resection = 4 Ileostomy = 3 Stricturoplasty = 3 Small bowel resection = 2 Miscellaneous = 2	NS	9 (5–40)	2 (8)	7 (29)
Dunker, 1998	11	Ileocolic resection	NS	5.5 (4–8)	0	1 (9)
Canin-Endres, 1999	94	Ileocolic resection = 70 Small bowel resection = 13 Right hemicolectomy = 3 Subtotal colectomy = 3 Anterior rectal resection = 2 Sigmoid resection = 3	183 (96–400)	4.2 (3–11)	1 (1)	12 (12.7)
Milsom, 1993	9	Ileocolic resection	170	7	0	0
Kreissler-Haag, 1994	20	Ileocolic resection/small bowel resection	NS	NS	0	0
Ludwig, 1996	31	NS	248 (20–380)	6 (2–21)	6 (19)	1 (3.2)

NS, not stated; TAC, total abdominal colectomy; IRA, ileorectal anastomosis.

SELECTED READINGS

Bailey IS, Rhodes M, O'Rourke N, et al: Laparoscopic management of acute small bowel obstruction. Br J Surg 1998;85:84.

Becker JM, Dayton MT, Fazio VW, et al: Prevention of postoperative abdominal adhesions by a sodium hyaluronate–based bioresorbable membrane: A prospective, randomized, double-blind multicenter study. J Am Coll Surg 1996;183:297.

Dunker MS, Stiggelbout AM, van Hogezand RA, et al: Cosmesis and body image after laparoscopic-assisted and open ileocolic resection for Crohn's disease. Surg Endosc 1998;12:1334.

Joo JS, Agachan F, Wexner SD: Laparoscopic surgery for benign gastrointestinal fistulas. Surg Endosc 1997;11:116.

Oliveira L, Reissman P, Nogueras J, Wexner SD: Laparoscopic creation of stomas. Surg Endosc 1997;11:19.

Reissman P, Salky BA, Pfeifer J, et al: Laparoscopic surgery in the management of inflammatory bowel disease. Am J Surg 1996;171:47.

Chapter 134

Laparoscopic Common Bile Duct Exploration

Craig C. Chang and Gregory G. Tsiotos

The advent of laparoscopic cholecystectomy has in many respects been "dissociated" from other adjunct procedures performed concomitantly at the time of cholecystectomy, such as intraoperative cholangiography and common bile duct (CBD) exploration. In the era of open cholecystectomy, these related procedures were performed more liberally at the time of cholecystectomy. However, in the minimally invasive era, other minimally invasive approaches to possible or proven choledocholithiasis outside the operating room have become more popular, such as the liberal use of preoperative endoscopic retrograde cholangiography (ERC) or postoperative ERC with stone extraction.

In this context, laparoscopic common bile duct exploration (LCBDE) should be considered an "advanced" laparoscopic procedure. The surgeon must be very comfortable with laparoscopic dissection, suturing, and handling of instruments and be able to work with both hands laparoscopically, as with open surgery. LCBDE is not a simple "resectional" laparoscopic procedure (i.e., cholecystectomy, appendectomy) in which simple dissection and transection of certain connective tissue or vascular structures is all that is needed; in contrast, LCBDE is a "reconstructive" procedure in which more advanced laparoscopic skills are required. The ability and comfort level needed by a surgeon to perform LCBDE depends on his or her frequency and level of comfort, of performing intraoperative cholangiograms. Generally, surgeons who rarely perform intraoperative cholangiograms, or who collaborate with gastroenterologists skilled in ERC and endoscopic stone extraction techniques, are less likely to achieve a high comfort level and success rate with LCBDE. Realistically, a prerequisite to becoming proficient in LCBDE is the *liberal* or *routine use* of intraoperative cholangiography. This chapter discusses the indications of LCBDE, elaborates on the techniques available, and outlines potential or frequent pitfalls.

INDICATIONS

A positive intraoperative cholangiogram or a preoperative ERC that demonstrates CBD stones unable to be removed endoscopically should prompt CBD exploration. Routine intraoperative cholangiography identifies CBD stones in as many as 10% of patients undergoing laparoscopic cholecystectomy; most are unsuspected. The incidence of choledocholithiasis increases significantly when liver function tests and levels of pancreatic enzymes are abnormal or when ultrasonography shows dilated bile ducts (>5 to 6 mm). Such features, if known preopera-

tively, are strong indications for intraoperative cholangiography or possibly for preoperative ERC, which will successfully clear the CBD in approximately 85% of patients when standard stone extraction techniques are combined. However, as previously mentioned, the liberal use of preoperative ERC, or only *selective* performance of intraoperative cholangiography when choledocholithiasis is highly probable, will not allow the surgeon to move along the learning curve of this technically demanding procedure. On the contrary, the liberal use of intraoperative cholangiography during laparoscopic cholecystectomy will help the interested surgeon to become proficient in LCBDE.

The most significant contraindication to LCBDE is the surgeon's inability to perform or inexperience in safely performing the maneuvers necessary for LCBDE. Other contraindications include the failure to progress with the procedure, patient instability, and uncontrolled bleeding. Previous upper abdominal surgery or inflammation (i.e., cholecystitis or cholangitis) may be relative contraindications for the less experienced surgeon. In such settings, more meticulous and careful dissection and precise identification of anatomic structures are required.

TECHNIQUE

Overview

The two approaches to LCBDE are transcystic and via a direct choledochotomy. Either is performed with the patient in reverse Trendelenburg position and rotated to the left to optimize exposure of the hepatoduodenal ligament. Port sites are the same as for laparoscopic cholecystectomy. Either a 0 degree or 30 degree laparoscope, placed through the umbilical port, can be used. After ligation and transection of the cystic artery, and distal ligation of the cystic duct, the confluence of the cystic duct and the common hepatic duct is carefully dissected, and the cystic duct is partially transected. Care must be taken to avoid complete transection of the cystic duct, because this greatly hampers subsequent duct manipulation, exposure, and instrumentation, which is essential for LCBDE. Fluoroscopic cholangiography is obtained, and the presence, number, and location of common duct stones are noted. When the expertise is present, laparoscopic ultrasonography may be used in place of cholangiography.

LCBDE is greatly facilitated by appropriate preparation of the surgical team. A special "LCBDE cart" containing all the possible necessary pharmacologic agents, instruments, devices, and sutures should be prepared

Table 134–1	Indications for Laparoscopic CBD Exploration with a Transcystic Approach or via Choledochotomy	
FACTOR	**TRANSCYSTIC**	**CHOLEDOCHOTOMY**
One stone	+	+
Multiple stones	+	+
Stones ≤6 mm in diameter	+	+
Stones >6 mm in diameter	–	+
Intrahepatic stones	–	+
Diameter of cystic duct <4 mm	–	+
Diameter of cystic duct ≥4 mm	+	+
Diameter of CBD <6 mm	+	–
Diameter of CBD ≥6 mm	+	+
Cystic duct entrance—lateral	+	+
Cystic duct entrance—posterior	–	+
Cystic duct entrance—distal	–	+
Inflammation—mild	+	+
Inflammation—marked	+	–
Suturing ability—poor	+	–
Suturing ability—good	+	+

From Petelin J: The SAGES Manual. New York, Springer-Verlag, 1999, p 168.

carefully and kept sterile and ready for use. Each of the two operative approaches (transcystic or via direct choledochotomy) is better suited for certain properties of the CBD stones, the CBD itself, anatomic and physiologic characteristics of the patient, and factors associated with the individual surgeon who performs the procedure; these are outlined in detail in Table 134–1. Surgeons who perform LCBDE should be experienced with the techniques and able to change from one to the other. Several techniques, applicable to either approach, are available for stone extraction (i.e., simple flushing, baskets, choledochoscopy); they differ in the degree of complexity and invasiveness. In principle, one should start with the technique that is the easiest, least invasive, and least potentially traumatic to the CBD and, if it is not successful, proceed to the next. Generally, transcystic LCBDE should be attempted prior to choledochotomy, because it is highly successful in the majority of cases, is less invasive, and does not require experience with laparoscopic suturing techniques. After LCBDE, completion choledochoscopy or cholangiography should always be obtained to confirm successful clearance of the CBD. Although postprocedure decompression of the biliary tree has been performed traditionally after open CBD exploration by inserting an internal stent, T-tube, or transcystic drainage catheter, there has been increasing experience recently with successful primary duct closure without T-tube placement (see later).

Transcystic LCBDE

This approach is the simplest technique and is more likely to succeed when the stones are small (<6 mm), and when

the cystic duct is >4 mm and enters the CBD via a relatively straight lateral course. Lateral retraction of the gallbladder straightens the cystic duct and aligns it with the CBD, thereby facilitating instrumentation through the same cystic duct defect used for the cholangiogram. Insertion of instruments through the cystic duct defect is ensured by the coordinated movement of the instrument itself (guided by a grasper) and the proper alignment of the biliary tree (Fig. 134–1).

Saline flushing is the first and simplest technique employed to clear stones. Use of 1 to 2 mg of glucagon (1 or 2 ampules) intravenously will relax the sphincter of Oddi such that flushing of the cystic duct with 50 to 500 mL of saline may allow the stones to empty into the duodenum. This simple technique alone can clear choledocholithiasis at least 50% of the time but is less successful when there are multiple stones larger than 6 mm. If simple flushing is not successful, the balloon technique can be used; typically a 4-French biliary Fogarty catheter is passed through a 14-gauge sleeve used for cholangiography, passed via the cystic duct and CBD into the duodenum through the papilla, and inflated. The balloon catheter is withdrawn with the balloon inflated, thus raking the CBD stones and debris retrograde and out the cystic duct. One potential problem is that stones and debris may be displaced proximally into the common hepatic duct. These stones and debris can be maneuvered back into the CBD with irrigation or with passage (if possible) of the balloon retrograde into the common hepatic duct.

The use of transcystic baskets is a third method. The size of the cystic duct is critical; if the luminal diameter is less than 2.5 mm, it may not dilate enough to allow insertion of instruments or stone withdrawal. Dilatation of the cystic duct is performed by several methods. First, successive dilatation with mechanical, over-the-wire dilators can be used with or without fluoroscopy; although

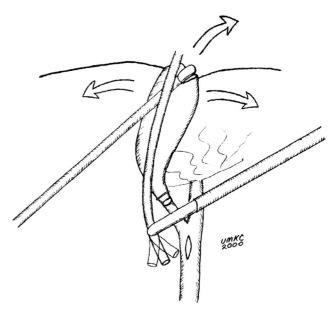

Figure 134–1. Alignment of the axis of the choledochoscope and the axis of the CBD by coordinated rotational movements of the tip of the choledochoscope (using its rotational controls and an atraumatic grasper) and the body or fundus of the gallbladder.

inexpensive, these dilators exert a shear force on the cystic duct mucosa that may dissect into the CBD and cause biliary obstruction. Second, pneumatic dilators can be passed over a wire exerting a radial force that enlarges the cystic duct. Third, a longitudinal incision can be made on the cystic duct to enlarge the opening into the CBD. A variety of baskets can be used. Typically, the 4.5-mm Dormia or ureteric stone baskets are inserted under fluoroscopic or choledochoscopic control, opened, and withdrawn after engaging the stone. Several models of cholangiocatheters allow repeat injection of contrast medium during basket extraction, with no need for catheter change. The surgeon should be continuously aware of the risks of capturing the papilla with these baskets or perforation of the bile duct with overly aggressive attempts to bring stones through the cystic duct.

Choledochoscopy is the last resort. Although it can be used via a transcystic approach, realistically it is used more often via choledochotomy and will be discussed in detail below. Completion cholangiography, which should be performed routinely, will confirm CBD clearance. The cystic duct is then doubly clipped or ligated; if the duct has torn or been cut to involve the CBD, the defect needs to be sutured with an absorbable suture material. A drain is not routinely placed.

LCBDE via Choledochotomy

If the transcystic approach is unsuccessful or not technically possible, or if the stones are large or located in the common hepatic duct (see Table 134–1), a direct choledochotomy is performed. The CBD should be larger than 6 mm in diameter and preferably more than 8 mm because subsequent healing and fibrosis may cause stricture of a narrow CBD. Choledochotomy allows removal of large stones, exploration of the proximal biliary tree, and insertion of larger instruments, but it also requires significant expertise at laparoscopic suturing. Gross dilatation of the CBD (>2.5 cm) with multiple brown stones indicates the diagnosis of primary duct stones. Consideration should then be given to some form of a definitive biliary drainage procedure (i.e., transduodenal sphincteroplasty, choledochoduodenostomy) to prevent recurrent stone formation.

Exposure of the CBD for the choledochotomy is relatively straightforward. Maintaining continuity of the cystic duct with the CBD provides traction and exposure. The peritoneum overlying the CBD anteriorly is divided distal to the cystic duct–common duct confluence. A 1-cm choledochotomy is created with low-voltage cutting cautery, scissors, or a sheathed knife; this size choledochotomy can stretch to accommodate removal of 1.5-cm stones. A larger choledochotomy is usually not necessary and would require a longer suture line with a higher risk of CBD stricture. Stone extraction involves one of the techniques already mentioned in transcystic LCBDE. In addition, stones may be milked toward the choledochotomy by applying external compression with atraumatic graspers. Once at the choledochotomy, the stone is grasped and removed.

Choledochoscopy has been used increasingly for LCBDE, mainly via choledochotomy. The transcystic approach only allows the scope to move distally in the CBD; visualization of the proximal biliary system (common hepatic duct) is possible less than 10% of the time. The typical choledochoscope has a diameter of 3.3 mm (10-French) with a 1.2-mm working channel, but smaller sizes facilitate the transcystic approach. The choledochoscope is inserted via the anterior abdomen near the mid-clavicular line through a fifth port. For most surgeons, choledochoscopy appears an unduly complex and demanding procedure unless certain principles are strictly followed. *First,* the entire choledochoscopy setup should be sterile, kept on a separate cart in the operating room, and ready for use. Ancillary personnel should be familiar with and in-serviced in its use. *Second,* a second camera can be attached to the choledochoscope and, with the use of readily available video-mixing technology, two images should appear on the screen, one from the laparoscope and one from the choledochoscope ("screen-on-screen" technique). With this imagery, the surgeon can look at *the same screen* to have simultaneously an "outside" view of the pathway of the choledochoscope and an "inside" view of the bile duct lumen. This technique tremendously facilitates safe and coordinated work and prevents wasting of time and frustration. *Third,* insertion of the scope into the CBD is facilitated by the coordinated moves of the tip of the scope (guided by atraumatic forceps and its own rotational controls) and appropriate rotation and traction of the cystic duct so that the distal 2 cm of the scope and the CBD are aligned (see Fig. 134–1). Care should be taken to avoid grasping the very end of the scope with the forceps, because damage of this fragile and expensive instrument is very likely. *Fourth,* after insertion, the scope should be continuously flushed with saline, as this provides the viewing medium, facilitates distention, and clears the lumen of debris. *Fifth,* the lumen of the CBD should be always kept in the center of the viewing scope. The failure to follow these two last principles results in a fuzzy, reddish picture without orientation and with a poor image. The scope may need to be pulled back, allowing the irrigation to restart; this maneuver allows the tip to be rotated until the CBD lumen comes into view at the center of the screen again.

Once the stone or stones are visualized, several options exist for extraction. First, after administration of glucagon, the scope can be used to push the stone out of the CBD and into the duodenum (less likely with larger stones and papillary edema). Second, wire baskets can be inserted through the working channel; the capture of each stone can be viewed on the screen. The choledochoscope and wire basket are then removed from the duct as a unit, and the stone is deposited on the omentum for later retrieval. Using these two methods, CBD clearance can be achieved more than 90% of the time in experienced hands. Third, for large impacted stones, lithotripsy can be utilized with either electrohydraulic or laser lithotripters, although the latter are prohibitively expensive. The lithotripsy probes are inserted through the working channel and, under direct choledochoscopic vision, placed *directly on* the stone to fragment it and facilitate subsequent removal either by flushing or by wire basket. Injury to the CBD is a well-recognized complication when the probe tip is applied to the duct; thus, care is necessary.

After stone extraction, a completion cholangiogram is obtained, and the choledochotomy is closed (see later).

Biliary Drainage

In the early experience of transcystic LCBDE, a transcystic drainage tube would have been left in place (secured into the cystic duct stump with an absorbable loop suture) and removed 1 to 2 weeks postoperatively. With increasing experience and especially when post-LCBDE cholangiography excludes the possibility of a retained stone, transcystic biliary drainage offers little if any benefit; currently, this practice is not favored. Biliary drainage after choledochotomy (usually via a T-tube choledochostomy) has been a routine. The crossbar of the T-tube is shortened to 2 cm, its back half removed, and the tube positioned at the inferior end of the choledochotomy, which is then closed with interrupted 4-0 absorbable sutures placed 2 mm apart. Although a T-tube allows decompression and subsequent instrumentation, other means of biliary drainage, such as antegrade sphincterotomy and internal stenting have been used as well. Antegrade sphincterotomy requires that a duodenoscope be inserted to check the position and depth of the sphincterotomy; however, this technique is associated with several logistic and technical difficulties and has not gained widespread acceptance. Internal stenting should be reserved for patients with cholangitis or sludge to ensure adequate and prolonged drainage of the biliary system. Currently, routine post-CBDE biliary drainage is not dogma. There is increasing interest and success in simple choledochotomy closure in carefully selected patients. The choledochotomy can be closed safely without a T-tube in patients with a large CBD (>6 mm), especially when choledochoscopy or any other kind of CBD instrumentation has been uneventful, when there has been minimal manipulation of the incised CBD edges, and when no doubt remains concerning complete clearance of the CBD. With increasing expertise and the appropriate selection of patients, the routine use of tube choledochoscopy is expected to decrease in the next few years. Finally, a closed-suction drain is placed in the right upper quadrant to control a possible bile leak.

Potential Complications

1. *Inability to Clear the Duct via Transcystic Approach because of Multiple Stones.* Conversion to choledochotomy greatly enlarges the options for instruments and allows larger stones to be removed. One should first extract the stones closest to the choledochotomy. The surgeon should acknowledge where he or she is on the learning curve of laparoscopic suturing (remember, a choledochotomy can always be closed through a subcostal incision!). Certainly, it is better to convert to an open approach than to have an inadequate closure or stricture of a CBD closed laparoscopically. Completion cholangiography is essential in verifying duct clearance, the absence of bile leak, and CBD stenosis.
2. *Impacted Stone or Stones at the Ampulla.* Impacted stones may be very difficult to remove even with open CBD exploration and may occasionally require transduodenal sphincteroplasty. Laparoscopic lithotripsy may prove to be very helpful in this setting. The equipment is available in several operating rooms, but its use requires training and may also require credentialing.
3. *Perforation of the CBD with Baskets.* To prevent this complication, the basket should be opened as soon as its tip passes into the CBD. The use of forceps through the medial epigastric port facilitates advancement of the open basket into the distal portion of the CBD. The closed basket should be withdrawn slowly. Incomplete closure heralds stone capture. Completion cholangiography is the best diagnostic tool for excluding CBD perforation. Remember, when perforation occurs inadvertently, the patient's best chance of an uncomplicated recovery is if the injury is recognized at the time of surgery and an appropriate repair is performed.
4. *Inadequate Visualization of the CBD with Choledochoscopy.* To maximize visualization, one requires continuous irrigation via the scope to distend the CBD. If a choledochotomy is performed, gathering the edges of the CBD together around the scope forms a seal and allows distention. Otherwise, the scope should be reoriented with rotational moves of its tip guided by its controls.

It cannot be overemphasized that if LCBDE does not progress as planned or an inadvertent CBD injury is suspected, the surgeon should be prepared to change the plan to an open approach. This decision depends largely on the environment in which one is practicing. If endoscopic expertise is available locally, consideration should be given to closing the cystic duct or CBD defect, and submitting the patient to postoperative ERC and stone extraction. However, it is always a wise and a definite sign of surgical maturity to convert to an open operation and complete the CBD exploration with traditional means. As with all other laparoscopic procedures, conversion to an open approach should not always be considered a complication or failure, but rather a sign of mature judgment that serves the patient's best interests.

OUTCOME

Open CBD exploration and laparoscopic cholecystectomy with postoperative ERC and endoscopic sphincterotomy are the established standards against which LCBDE must be compared. Mortality resulting from open CBD exploration is almost nil in younger patients but approaches 4% in patients older than 60 years of age. The morbidity and mortality rates of endoscopic sphincterotomy in the context of laparoscopic cholecystectomy are 7% (primarily secondary to pancreatitis and bile duct perforation) and 1% to 2%, respectively. Morbidity associated with endoscopic sphincterotomy may further increase up to 10% with CBD diameters less than 10 mm. The morbidity and mortality rates of LCBDE are 6% to 18% and 1%, respectively; the success rate is well above 90% in the experienced laparoscopist, and conversion to open operation may occur 5% to 10% of the time. More specifically, transcystic LCBDE is successful about 80% of the time

Pearls and Pitfalls

- LCBDE is an evolving technique.
- In experienced hands, LCBDE is successful in more than 90% of patients.
- Routine use of postexploration intraoperative cholangiography is a prerequisite for performing LCBDE safely and successfully.
- An approach either via the cystic duct or via a choledochotomy may be necessary; when possible, the former is faster and has fewer potential complications.
- Laparoscopic CBD clearance can be accomplished in a manner similar to open CBD exploration with the use of prograde flushing, basket extraction choledochoscopic techniques, or catheter-based lithotripsy.
- When LCBDE is unsuccessful, the need for conversion to open CBD exploration or for ERC with endoscopic sphincterotomy the next day should not be considered a complication or failure when it is in the patient's best interest.

experienced hands. This approach offers the advantage of a single anesthetic for the treatment of CBD stones and cholecystectomy. The following general principles should be kept in mind:

- Liberal (preferably routine) use of intraoperative cholangiography during laparoscopic cholecystectomy is a prerequisite for a surgeon's performing LCBDE safely, successfully, and in a timely manner.
- Based on the characteristics of the bile duct, the stone or stones, and the surgeon's expertise, the transcystic or the choledochotomy approach can be used. The former is easier, often successful, and less invasive. However, larger and multiple stones are usually successfully managed only via choledochotomy.
- From the variety of methods available for clearing the CBD (e.g., flushing, balloon, basket), one should employ the easiest and least invasive first.
- Completion cholangiogram is essential, but postexploration biliary drainage is not necessarily required under the appropriate circumstances.

(some experts suggest >95%) and has a morbidity rate of 4% to 10%, and the incidence of retained stones is 1% to 6%. As one might expect, the success rate for LCBDE via choledochotomy is somewhat higher (88% to 100%), but morbidity is higher as well (5% to 18%) with the incidence of retained stones varying between 0 and 5%. Overall, it seems that today LCBDE, compared with endoscopic sphincterotomy, is at least equally effective in clearing CBD stones and is associated with a shorter hospital stay, a decreased total operative time, and an equal or lower morbidity rate; it also has the additional benefit of lower cost, a factor of increasing importance in today's era of cost containment.

Summary

LCBDE is an evolving technique which allows successful clearance of CBD stones in 90% to 95% of patients in

SELECTED READINGS

Heili MJ, Wintz NK, Fowler DL: Choledocholithiasis: Endoscopic versus laparoscopic management. Am Surgeon 1999;65:135.

Liberman MA, Phillips EH, Carroll BJ, et al: Cost-effective management of complicated choledocholithiasis: Laparoscopic transcystic duct exploration or endoscopic sphincterotomy. J Am Coll Surg 1996;182:488.

Martin IJ, Bailey IS, Rhodes M, et al: Towards T-tube free laparoscopic bile duct exploration. Ann Surg 1998;228:29.

Memon MA, Hassaballa H, Memon MI: Laparoscopic common bile duct exploration: The past, the present, and the future. Am J Surg 2000;179:309.

Petelin JB: Laparoscopic common bile duct exploration: Transcystic duct approach. SAGES manual: Fundamentals of Laparoscopy and GI Endoscopy. New York, Springer-Verlag, 1999, pp 167–177.

Petelin JB: Tools of the trade: The common bile duct stone cart. J Gastrointest Surg 2000;4:336.

Rhodes M, Sussman L, Cohen L, Lewis MP: Randomized trial of laparoscopic exploration of common bile duct versus postoperative endoscopic retrograde cholangiography for common bile duct stones. Lancet 1998;351:159.

Chapter 135
Advanced Gastrointestinal Laparoscopic Procedures

Michael G. Sarr, Tonia M. Young-Fadok, and Troy M. Duininck

Laparoscopic, minimally invasive, or minimal access techniques have revolutionized many aspects of the surgical world, not just in general surgery but also with multiple applications in urologic, orthopedic, gynecologic, and cardiovascular surgery as well. We have all heard the often quoted phrase, "Every operation can be accomplished (in gastrointestinal surgery) laparoscopically." While probably true in theory, whether every operation *should* be performed with minimal access techniques currently is definitely not appropriate, and in the future, whether this prediction proves true will depend on many variables—equipment, individual expertise versus global surgeon expertise, refinements in technology, and, most of all, experience. For instance, what is possible globally to the gastrointestinal (GI) surgeon in 2001 was not possible just 5 years ago. For example, laparoscopic splenectomy has matured over the last 5 years into an accepted, if not the preferred, approach in many patients. Similarly, although laparoscopic Nissen fundoplication was certainly uncommon in most general surgeons' practice 10 years ago, this advanced laparoscopic technique has become an almost routine operation in the general GI surgeons' armamentarium. Whether laparoscopic colectomy, gastric bypass, gastrectomy, and so on will gain equal global utilization awaits future developments.

Moreover, we currently do not fully appreciate or understand all the potential benefits of a minimal access technique. Everyone recognizes the cosmetic advantages of smaller incisions and usually the decrease in postoperative pain—these concepts drive the public pressure on our profession—e.g., witness the *unparalleled growth*, development, and training of board-certified surgeons in laparoscopic cholecystectomy in the early 1990s; clearly this advance was indicated. But, in contrast, the purported but often unsubstantiated advantages claimed of a minimal access approach in decreasing the postoperative stress response (decrease in catecholamines, interleukins, cytokines, stress hormones) have not been demonstrated consistently. Similarly, minimal access approaches do not always decrease postoperative hospitalization, e.g., laparoscopic appendectomy or inguinal herniorrhaphy.

Other considerations also apply. Is a minimal access approach justified if it is inordinately more expensive or if the complication rate is considerably greater? Who should award credentials in advanced techniques to surgeons? How many operations under direct supervision (again by whom?) are necessary before the surgeon is allowed to carry out this or that advanced procedure? Should advanced procedures be regionalized and performed only in centers of excellence by *laparologists*? All these are difficult questions with no current answers

acceptable to all—surgeons, patients, third party payers, government regulators, the American Board of Surgery, etc.

This chapter does not attempt to answer all these questions. Similarly, a technical discussion of all the "advanced" laparoscopic techniques is beyond the scope of this chapter and the capability of most practicing general surgeons. The aim of this chapter is to catalog and briefly discuss advanced techniques as applied to GI disorders and to demonstrate the spectrum of minimally invasive procedures, at least within the realm of laparoscopy and thoracoscopy as applied to the gut.

BASIC PRINCIPLES OF ADVANCED LAPAROSCOPIC SURGERY

Three basic principles have controlled the development and application of advanced laparoscopic procedures—expertise, experience, and technology.

Expertise

Advanced techniques require a different set of operative technical skills that must be learned anew by the already trained surgeon. Laparoscopic cholecystectomy utilizes basic skills of cautery dissection and clip application but very few in the realm of bowel mobilization, intracorporeal knot tying, or suturing. Similarly, mesenteric dissection, intestinal transection and anastomosis, organ dissection from connective tissue, and gastrointestinal transposition are not techniques that are facile without special training and experience. Even in the spectrum of general surgery training programs currently, many of these advanced skills have not yet become part of the basic core curriculum, and, thus, the interest in and need for laparoscopic fellowships has blossomed.

Experience

Some procedures that are currently approached laparoscopically at centers of excellence address disorders that the typical general surgeon sees rarely in his or her practice. For instance, adrenalectomy is readily amenable to a laparoscopic approach, yet only tertiary referral centers can enjoy a large enough experience with these disorders to allow (and to justify) adequate training in a minimally invasive approach. Similar arguments may be put forth for other disorders amenable to a laparoscopic approach, such as esophageal achalasia, islet cell neoplasms of the pancreas, common bile duct exploration, total colectomy with ileo-pouch-anal reconstruction, and so on.

Technology

Many laparoscopic procedures necessarily awaited the technologic advancements required both to facilitate the operation and to allow its safe conduct. For instance, the harmonic scalpel, the endoscopic GI staplers, and even the development of hand-assisted, minimally invasive techniques radically expanded the breadth of many GI operations at least potentially amenable to the advanced laparoscopist. Currently, the concept of robotics appears to be the next horizon to reach in facilitating the advanced procedures *both* for the advanced laparoscopist and, it is hoped, for the remainder of the GI surgeons who are not currently laparologists.

SPECTRUM OF MINIMAL ACCESS GASTROINTESTINAL SURGERY

The following discussion attempts to address the state-of-the-art in minimal access approaches for GI diseases. For a more in-depth review, see the reference by Young-Fadok, Smith, and Sarr (2000).

Esophagus (Table 135–1)

Secondary only to gallbladder disease, a minimally invasive approach to esophageal disorders, specifically gastroesophageal reflux disease (GERD), has grown exponentially over the last decade to become the accepted gold standard (see Chapter 44). Laparoscopy has led to the rebirth of antireflux surgery; indeed, a laparoscopic Nissen fundoplication involves no resection or anastomosis, and it should be (and was) an ideal prototype laparoscopic challenge. This procedure became a natural focus for a disorder affecting 15% to 30% of our population to a variable extent. The previous need for a formal celiotomy (or in many institutions, a left thoracotomy) was replaced by a minimally invasive approach. Introduction of a 1-day hospitalization, minimal convalescence, and absence of the pain and morbidity due to the celiotomy or thoracotomy has actually changed the *indications* for operative treatment of GERD, in both the public's eye and that of the physician, surgeon and internist alike. Currently, laparoscopic antireflux surgery *is* the gold standard. Certain laparoscopic experts have even successfully approached selected patients laparoscopically after the failure of previous antireflux surgery.

Other esophageal disorders, although amenable to a minimally invasive approach, are less readily treated outside of centers of excellence because of their rarity and need for more advanced technical skills. Paraesophageal hiatus hernias introduce a greater complexity in their mobilization and choice of repair, yet many such patients should be readily approachable laparoscopically. Again, this is the approach of choice for those surgeons with experience. Similarly, motility disorders such as achalasia and other spastic disorders of the esophageal smooth muscle can be approached either laparoscopically or thoracoscopically depending on the location of the disorder. The basic tenets of open operation can be transferred to minimally invasive instruments. Similar arguments are applied to esophageal diverticula.

Neoplasms of the esophagus currently represent the new frontier. Leiomyomas appear readily amenable to thoracoscopic enucleation. In contrast, esophageal malignancies (adenocarcinoma and squamous carcinoma), which require formal resections (with or without lymphadenectomy) and reconstruction, add an additional quantum of necessary complexity. Currently, a thoracoscopic esophageal mobilization is not uncommon, but a fully minimally invasive resection and reconstruction remains in the developmental stage and will need to be compared critically with the open approach in terms of morbidity and survival. Clearly, this group of procedures will require focused expertise.

Stomach (Table 135–2)

Although the concept was good, early speculation of a minimally invasive approach toward peptic ulcer disease has not really materialized (i.e., laparoscopic highly selective vagotomy), because indications and need for elective operative intervention are exceedingly rare. Intractability of duodenal ulcer disease has virtually disappeared with introduction of potent antisecretory agents and our understanding of the etiology of duodenal ulcer disease (*Helicobacter pylori*). Probably the most applicable indications are (or will be?) for perforation and obstruction.

Although percutaneous endoscopic gastrostomy (PEG) has all but replaced open gastrostomy tube placement, certain patients are not candidates for PEG placement because of previous oropharyngeal surgery, anatomic abnormalities, intra-abdominal adhesions, or a high-lying

Table 135–1	**Laparoscopic Surgery of Esophageal Disorders**
INDICATIONS	**PROCEDURE**
Gastroesophageal reflux disease (GERD)	
Normal esophageal peristalsis	Laparoscopic Nissen (360-degree fundoplication)
Decreased esophageal peristalsis	Laparoscopic Toupet (270-degree fundoplication)
Shortened esophagus	Laparoscopic Collis or Nissen
Paraesophageal hiatus hernia	Repair, gastropexy, ± fundoplication
Motility disorders	
Achalasia	Laparoscopic Heller esophagogastric myotomy
Diffuse spasm	Thoracoscopic esophageal myotomy
Neoplasms	
Leiomyomas	Thoracoscopic resection
Carcinomas	Resection, reconstruction
Diverticula	
Zenker's	Transoral diverticulostomy or diverticulectomy or myotomy
Epiphrenic	Thoracoscopic diverticulectomy ± esophageal myotomy

Table 135–2	**Laparoscopic Surgery of Gastric Disorders**

INDICATIONS	PROCEDURE
Peptic ulcer disease	
Intractability	Laparoscopic parietal cell vagotomy or hemigastrectomy or reconstruction
Perforation	Laparoscopic closure of perforation
Pyloric obstruction	Laparoscopic gastrojejunostomy ± vagotomy
Anastomotic ulcer	Thoracoscopic truncal vagotomy
Decompression or feeding	Laparoscopic gastrostomy
Neoplasms	
Leiomyoma	Laparoscopic enucleation or wedge resection
Carcinoma	Laparoscopic resection, reconstruction, and lymphadenectomy
Morbid obesity	Laparoscopic Roux-en-Y gastric bypass, vertical banded gastroplasty, and gastric banding

stomach. Laparoscopic placement of a tube gastrostomy (or tube jejunostomy) is readily available with current industry-developed kits.

Currently, selected gastric neoplasms are amenable to a minimally invasive approach. Stromal tumors (leiomyomas and selected leiomyosarcomas) can be removed either by "enucleation" if benign or by stapler-facilitated wedge resections. Adenocarcinoma introduces more controversy, not only because of need for a wider gastric mobilization, but also because of the necessity for resection, reconstruction of gastrointestinal continuity, and lymphadenectomy. Minimally invasive surgery for gastric cancer is still in its developmental stage and should be considered experimental.

Surgery for morbid obesity (bariatric surgery) is now established as a viable treatment for medically complicated obesity. Although technically very challenging, many centers have developed expertise in a minimally invasive approach to Roux-en-Y gastric bypass and vertical banded gastroplasty. Hospitalization is shortened, and the risk of ventral hernia (which is 15% to 20% after open bariatric surgery) is avoided. It is important that the laparoscopic approach should not compromise the choice of the appropriate procedure, i.e., the "easier" vertical banded gastroplasty versus the more technically challenging but more effective Roux-en-Y gastric bypass procedure. Laparoscopic gastric "banding" using an "adjustable" external silicone band has become very popular in Europe and Central and South America; although theoretically attractive, believable results concerning acute morbidity, and especially long-term success, are lacking and must await the future.

Small Intestine and Appendix (Table 135–3)

SMALL INTESTINE. Selected patients with adhesive small bowel obstruction are amenable to laparoscopic adhesiolysis, especially if the adhesions are expected to be mini-

mal (e.g., previous appendectomy, cholecystectomy, hysterectomy, and so on). A laparoscopic approach not only allows quicker recovery with less pain than open celiotomy, it may also decrease further adhesion formation. Crohn's disease has become a major disorder able to be approached laparoscopically. Currently, most procedures utilize a laparoscopy-assisted approach, with laparoscopic mobilization of the small bowel and right colon and exteriorization of the bowel with extracorporeal resection and hand-performed anastomosis, after which the bowel is "dropped" back intraperitoneally. This is one procedure for which formal cost analysis has demonstrated significant cost savings with a laparoscopic approach. Other less common applications include placement of a feeding jejunostomy, full-thickness bowel biopsy for unexplained malabsorption, therapeutic adhesiolysis for congenital rotational disorders (e.g., malrotation), and intestinal resection for selected benign and malignant neoplasms.

APPENDIX. Laparoscopic appendectomy, although no longer an advanced procedure, nevertheless remains controversial (see Chapter 64). Of all the GI laparoscopic procedures, laparoscopic appendectomy appears to be the one most subject to surgeon preference. When the preoperative diagnosis of appendicitis proves incorrect at the time of laparoscopy, a complete intra-abdominal exploration should be carried out to look for some other etiology; indeed, a laparoscopic approach to Meckel's diverticulitis and other selected disorders can be accomplished laparoscopically and should be considered part of the surgeon's armamentarium.

Colon and Rectum (Table 135–4)

Colonic disorders probably represent the second largest group of disorders (other than the biliary tree) that are most amenable in theory and most prevalent in incidence to a laparoscopic approach (see Chapters 74, 76, and 89). Diverticulitis limited to the sigmoid colon is currently accepted as an appropriate indication for laparoscopic colectomy. Use of transanally inserted intraluminal circular staplers markedly facilitates the restoration of colonic continuity since the colocolostomy just above the peritoneal reflection is not amenable to a laparoscopist-assisted extracorporeal hand-sewn approach. Laparoscopic polypectomy with preoperative tattooing of the polyp via co-

Table 135–3	**Laparoscopic Surgery of the Small Intestine and Appendix**

INDICATIONS	PROCEDURE
Small bowel obstruction	Adhesiolysis
Crohn's disease	Small bowel resection or anastomosis
Enteral feeding	Tube jejunostomy
Malabsorption	Full-thickness biopsy
Malrotation	Ladd procedure
Neoplasm	
Benign	Wedge resection
Carcinoma or carcinoid	Resection or reconstruction
Appendicitis	Appendectomy, Meckel's diverticulectomy

Table 135–4	Laparoscopic Surgery of the Colon and Rectum

INDICATIONS	PROCEDURE (ALL LAPAROSCOPIC)
Diverticulitis	Sigmoid colectomy or reanastomosis
Colonic polyp	Segmental colectomy
Polyposis syndromes (FAP, HNPCC)	Proctocolectomy and ileal pouch–anal anastomosis or total abdominal colectomy and ileorectal anastomosis
Colon cancer	Right colectomy, left colectomy
	Anterior resection, abdominoperineal resection
Inflammatory bowel disease	
Ulcerative colitis	Proctocolectomy, ileal pouch–anal anastomosis
Crohn's disease	Colectomy, bypass
Rectal prolapse	Anterior resection, rectopexy
Hirschsprung's disease	Colectomy, reconstruction
Colonic dysmotility (slow transit constipation)	Total abdominal colectomy and ileorectal anastomosis
Colonic diversion	Ileostomy or colostomy

FAP, familial adenomatous polyposis; HNPCC, hereditary nonpolyposis colon cancer.

lonoscopy and takedown of a temporary colostomy after a previous Hartmann's procedure are natural extensions of this approach as well.

The use of laparoscopic techniques for colonic resection of colon cancer remains controversial. Although technically feasible, with data supporting adequate margins and a comparable lymphadenectomy, controversy centers on the adequacy of lymphadenectomy as well as the potential risk of wound implantation and alterations in the biology of the colon cancer secondary to the carbon dioxide pneumoperitoneum. It is surprising that these controversies still exist, thus laparoscopic colectomy for colon cancer is not yet fully accepted. Currently, a large multicenter trial funded by the National Institute of Health (NIH) is exploring this issue definitively. Patient accrual should be completed by the end of 2001, but the trial still needs several years to mature.

Inflammatory bowel disease is a maturing field for advanced laparoscopic techniques. Patients with ulcerative colitis are amenable to laparoscopic mobilization of the intra-abdominal colon and even the rectum down to the levator muscles. Several groups have developed the skills necessary for creation of an ileal pouch and the ability either to perform a mucosectomy and sew it to the anus from below, or to use a stapler to create the anastomosis. For Crohn's colitis, a laparoscopic abdominal colectomy with ileorectal anastomosis or proctocolectomy with Brooke's ileostomy is possible.

Other conditions able to be managed laparoscopically with the use of techniques previously developed for simple colectomy include management of rectal prolapse by either anterior resection or rectopexy and colectomy and reconstruction of colorectal or coloanal continuity for Hirschsprung's disease.

Biliary and Hepatopancreatic System
(Table 135–5)

BILIARY. In addition to the widely applied laparoscopic cholecystectomy for increasingly difficult cholecystectomies, the advanced laparoscopist has been able to carry out common bile duct explorations entirely through the laparoscope. Laparoscopic common duct explorations can be performed in either of two ways. The first and easiest technique (transcystic approach) is through a large cystic duct with the use of either wire baskets and balloon catheters with the help of fluoroscopic control or a small ureteroscope (3.2 mm) with a working channel (1.2 mm) for insertion of delicate wire stone baskets. This technique is best applied when the cystic duct is of a large diameter, stones are small (<6 mm), and stones are not in the common hepatic duct or in an intrahepatic location. The second technique (direct choledochotomy) involves dissecting the common bile duct, creating a choledochotomy, and inserting a choledochoscope for direct, visually monitored ductal clearance; this approach requires a larger duct, is used for larger or more proximally based stones, and, most importantly, requires laparoscopic suturing skills for inserting a T-tube after ductal exploration.

LIVER. Most liver-based laparoscopy currently is used for direct inspection of the liver surface (see later section on staging of intraperitoneal malignancies) or for a directed liver biopsy. Symptomatic simple hepatic cysts are usually fairly easily amenable to peritoneal marsupialization by

Table 135–5	Laparoscopic Surgery of the Hepatopancreatobiliary System

INDICATIONS	PROCEDURE (ALL LAPAROSCOPIC)
Biliary Tree	
Cholecystolithiasis	Cholecystectomy
Acute cholecystitis	Cholecystectomy
Choledocholithiasis	Common bile duct exploration
Liver	
Directed biopsy	Liver biopsy
Hepatic cyst	Cystectomy, marsupialization
Neoplasm	
Benign	Wedge resection
Malignant	Wedge resection, lobectomy*
Pancreas	
Neoplasm	
Benign	Enucleation, distal pancreatectomy
Malignant	
Resection	Distal pancreatectomy, pancreatoduodenectomy†
Palliation	Cholecystojejunostomy, gastrojejunostomy
Inflammatory diseases	
Pseudocyst	Cystoenteric drainage‡
Localized pancreatic necrosis	Necrosectomy or drainage
Chronic painful pancreatitis	Thoracoscopic splanchnicectomy

*Left lateral lobectomy.
†Yes, at least two pancreatoduodenectomies have been performed—this use of minimally invasive techniques is questionable.
‡Combined endoluminal laparoendoscopic approach.

excising the exposed cyst wall (not just incising it) and *widely* exposing the cyst cavity; laser or argon-beam coagulation of the intracystic lining minimizes recurrence. Laparoscopic hepatectomy remains in its developmental stage, limited primarily by lack of technical aids in controlling hemorrhage. Wedge excisions can be carried out, and limited lobectomy of the left lateral segment (segments II and III) is possible, but formal lobectomy or formal segmental excisions are in the realm of only a few highly skilled individuals and await advances in technology.

PANCREAS. As with the liver, most pancreas-directed laparoscopies are for staging of pancreatic malignancies, rather than for therapy. Centers of excellence have carried out directed enucleations of insulinomas or other benign islet cell tumors; distal pancreatectomies have also been performed with success for benign neoplasms. For malignant neoplasms, a few distal pancreatectomies have been reported. One exceptionally gifted laparologist has carried out two formal pancreatoduodenectomies; while undoubtedly pushing the envelope, this type of tour-de-force is clearly premature (at least currently)! The concept of laparoscopic palliation of extrahepatic biliary and duodenal obstruction from a nonresectable pancreatic cancer is attractive in avoiding a full celiotomy; both bile duct and duodenum can be bypassed with creation of a loop cholecystojejunostomy and gastrojejunostomy.

Selected aspects of inflammatory disease of the pancreas are currently approachable via minimally invasive techniques. Pancreatic pseudocysts may be drained enterically either via a laparoscopic suturing technique or as a laparoendoscopic technique in conjunction with an endoscopic approach; whether this offers any benefit over a purely endoscopic internal drainage is questionable. Localized, organized pancreatic or, preferably, peripancreatic necrosis appears amenable to a laparoscopic débridement under vision, rather than a purely percutaneous drainage; insertion of a laparoscope into the cavity allows direct, visually controlled "necrosectomy" and cavity débridement. Finally, for patients with painful chronic pancreatitis not amenable to pancreatic resection or drainage, a primary neurectomy can be accomplished thoracoscopically via a lesser and least bilateral splanchnicectomy, thereby avoiding the morbidity of formal thoracotomy.

Staging of Intra-abdominal Malignancies
(Table 135–6)

The use of minimally invasive techniques in an attempt to prevent a nontherapeutic laparotomy has received considerable attention, primarily with upper gut neoplasms. Laparoscopic staging of presumed pancreatic ductal cancer will avoid a nontherapeutic celiotomy in 10% to 15% of patients with "clinically resectable" periampullary neoplasms and about 40% of patients with body/tail cancers. Extensive experience in staging pancreatic cancers has spread to the evaluation of esophageal, gastric, hepatic, and primary biliary neoplasms as well, again directed at attempting to avoid a nontherapeutic, nonpalliative celiotomy. The use of laparoscopic ultrasonography adds

Table 135–6	Laparoscopic Staging of Intra-abdominal Malignancies	
SITE OF NEOPLASM	**TYPE**
Distal esophagus	Adenocarcinoma or squamous carcinoma
Stomach	Adenocarcinoma
Liver	Hepatoma
Biliary tree	Cholangiocarcinoma
Pancreas	Pancreatic carcinoma
Lymphoma	Hodgkin's, other

other important data concerning liver metastases, proximity to vascular structures, and so on. This approach is useful when another type of less invasive palliation is possible (e.g., endoscopic or percutaneous biliary stent, laser relief of esophageal obstruction). Staging of selected patients with Hodgkin's disease, including splenectomy, is also possible.

THE FUTURE

As our skills and technology improve, procedures now currently beyond the envelope will undoubtedly become possible. We need to keep an open mind and be prepared

---

Pearls and Pitfalls

- Advanced laparoscopic procedures are here to stay.
- Just the fact that an operation *can be performed* laparoscopically does not mean it *should be*. In contrast, keep an open mind—surgery is changing.
- Advanced laparoscopy requires *expertise* (intracorporeal suturing, bowel mobilization, intestinal transection or reanastomosis), *technologic advances* (endostapling, harmonic scalpel, suturing devices), and *experience* (volume of specialized cases, referral practice, indepth understanding).
- Advanced esophageal procedures address GERD, paraesophageal hiatus hernias, motility disorders (achalasia), and selected neoplasms.
- Advanced gastric procedures address peptic ulcer disease, selected neoplasms, morbid obesity, and gastrostomy placement.
- Advanced small bowel procedures can treat adhesive small bowel obstruction, Crohn's disease, selected neoplasms, and appendicitis.
- Advanced colonic procedures deal with colectomies for diverticulitis, colon cancer, and inflammatory bowel disease or management of rectal prolapse.
- Advanced procedures in the hepatopancreatobiliary tree include common bile duct explorations, biliary bypasses for obstructing cancers, hepatic cystectomies, limited hepatic resections, and selected pancreatic resections and enucleations. Some postinflammatory disorders of the pancreas are amenable to minimally invasive procedures (pseudocysts, organized pancreatic necrosis).
- Laparoscopic staging of upper gut malignancies (esophagogastric, hepatic, biliary, and pancreatic) will prevent unnecessary and nontherapeutic celiotomies.

to develop new skills as the technology improves. We also must be careful to acknowledge the importance of educating the public on the pros and cons of a minimally invasive approach. Just because it *can* be done laparoscopically does not mean it *should* be done. On the other hand, we need to remain open-minded and to accept new minimally invasive approaches, retrain ourselves in new technical skills, and support technologic ingenuity.

SELECTED READINGS

Alverdy J, Vargish T, Desai T, et al: Laparoscopic intracavity debridement of peripancreatic necrosis: Preliminary report and description of the technique. Surgery 2000;127:112.

Ascencio F, Aguilo J, Salvadore JL, et al: Video-laparoscopic staging of gastric cancer; A prospective multicenter comparison with non-invasive techniques. Surg Endosc 1997;11:1153.

Bannon MP, Zietlow SP, Harmsen WS, et al: A prospective randomized comparison of laparoscopic appendectomy with open appendectomy. Surgery 2001;129:390.

Bennett CL, Stryker SJ, Ferreira R, et al: The learning curve for laparoscopic colorectal surgery: Preliminary results from a prospective analysis of 1194 laparoscopic-assisted colectomies. Arch Surg 1997;132:41.

Bradley EL III, Reyhout JA, Peer GL: Thoracoscopic splanchnicectomy for "small duct" chronic pancreatitis: Case selection by differential epidural anesthesia. J Gastrointest Surg 1998;2:88.

Clinical Outcomes of Surgical Therapy (COST) Study Group: Fleshman JW, Nelson H, Peters WR, et al: Early results of laparoscopic surgery for colorectal cancer: Retrospective analysis of 372 patients treated by Clinical Outcomes of Surgical Therapy (COST) Study Group. Dis Colon Rectum 1996;39:S53.

Conlon KC, Dougherty E, Klimstra DS, et al: The value of minimal access surgery in the staging of patients with potentially resectable peripancreatic malignancy. Ann Surg 1996;223:134.

Dorman JP, Franklin ME Jr, Glass JL: Laparoscopic common bile duct exploration by choledochotomy: An effective and efficient method of treatment of choledocholithiasis. Surg Endosc 1998;12:926.

Fernandez del Castillo C, Rattner DW, Warshaw AL: Further experience with laparoscopy and peritoneal cytology in the staging of pancreatic cancer. R J Surg 1995;82:1127.

Horgan S, Eubanks TR, Jacobsen G, et al: Repair of paraesophageal hernias. Am J Surg 1999;177:354.

Jarnagin WR, Bodniewidcz J, Dougherty E, et al: A prospective analysis of staging laparoscopy in patients with primary and secondary hepatobiliary malignancies. J Gastrointest Surg 2000;4:34.

Katkhonda N, Hurwitz M, Gugenheim J, et al: Laparoscopic management of benign solid and cystic lesions of the liver. Ann Surg 1999;229:460.

Luque-de León E, Metzger A, Tsiotos GG, et al: Laparoscopic management of small bowel obstruction: Indications and outcome. J Gastrointest Surg 1998;2:132.

Sardinha TC, Wexner SD: Laparoscopy for inflammatory bowel disease: Pros and cons. World J Surg 1998;22:370.

Schlinkert RT, Sarr MG, Donohue JH, et al: General surgical laparoscopic procedures for the "non-laparoscopist." Mayo Clin Proc 1995;70:1142.

Young-Fadok TM, Sgambati SA, Nelson H: Post-operative benefits of laparoscopic resection for Crohn's disease: A case-matched series. Surg Endosc 1999;13(suppl):S90.

Young-Fadok TM, Smith CD, Sarr MG: Laparoscopic minimal-access surgery: Where are we now? Where are we going? Gastroenterology 2000;118:S148.

Wittgrove AC, Clark GW: Laparoscopic gastric bypass, Roux-en-Y experience of 27 cases, with 3–18 months follow-up. Obesity Surg 1996;6:54.

Thoracic

Chapter 136
Infections of the Pleural Cavity
Alberto L. de Hoyos and Alex G. Little

Infections of the pleural cavity usually start as parapneumonic effusions. Strictly speaking, a parapneumonic effusion is any pleural effusion associated with bacterial pneumonia, lung abscess, or bronchiectasis. Parapneumonic effusions can be simple effusions, complicated effusions, or empyemas. Simple parapneumonic effusions are uninfected, free-flowing pleural fluid collections; complicated parapneumonic effusions are early infected fluid collections, while thoracic empyemas are well-established collections of pus within the pleural cavity.

Although parapneumonic effusion develops in 36% to 57% of patients with pneumonia, fewer than 5% progress to empyema. Parapneumonic effusion (40% to 60%), prior thoracic surgery (15% to 30%), and thoracic trauma (10%) are responsible for most patients with empyema. The morbidity and mortality rates of patients with parapneumonic effusion are higher than those of patients with pneumonia alone owing in part to inadequate management of the pleural effusion. Mortality from empyema ranges from 1% to 19%. The prognosis is worse in the elderly, in patients with coexistent cardiac, pulmonary, or renal disease, and in patients with hospital-acquired or culture-positive empyema, especially those involving gram-negative bacteria or multiple pathogens.

PATHOPHYSIOLOGY AND CLASSIFICATION

The diagnosis and treatment of infections of the pleural cavity are best considered in relation to the altered anatomy and physiology of the pleura. The formation of a pleural effusion is determined by the relationship between hydrostatic and oncotic pressures, by the permeability of the pleural membrane, and by the efficiency of lymphatic drainage of the pleural space (Starling's forces). The pleural space is normally sterile yet is readily suscep-

tible to colonization once fluid has accumulated. After deposition of microorganisms into subpleural air spaces, migration and adherence of polymorphonuclear leukocytes to the adjacent endothelium results in endothelial injury and increased capillary permeability. The excess extravascular lung water increases the interstitial-pleural pressure gradient and drives fluid from the interstitium into the pleural space, resulting in an effusion if the rate of fluid production exceeds lymphatic drainage reabsorption. The resulting parapneumonic effusion serves as a rich culture medium that allows bacteria to float away from phagocytic cells and to multiply relatively unimpeded, reaching concentrations as high as 10^{10} bacteria per milliliter of infected fluid. Furthermore, infected pleural fluid is deficient in the opsonins and complements required for optimal phagocytic function; moreover extremes of acidity and hypoxia that develop further impair local neutrophil function and antibiotic activity.

In 1962, The American Thoracic Society classified pleural cavity infections into three stages, based on the natural history of the disease: (1) exudative; (2) fibrinopurulent; and (3) organizational. These stages are not sharply defined but rather represent a spectrum. Once infection of the pleural space is established, the pathologic stage reached in the sequential progression from an acute process to a chronic state dictates the treatment strategies. Errors made in this assessment lead to inadequate intervention and result in a more prolonged illness.

CLINICAL PRESENTATION

The clinical manifestations vary, depending on the underlying pulmonary process, the responsible organism, the quantity of bacteria and fluid in the pleural space, the stage of the disease, and the host defense mechanisms. The clinical presentation can range from an absence of symptoms to a severe febrile illness with toxemia and shock. In general, it is difficult to distinguish patients with infected pleural effusions from those with sterile parapneumonic effusions on the basis of the history and physical examination because of the underlying pulmonary process. The clinical manifestations include fever, dyspnea, chest pain, and cough with mucopurulent sputum. Infected pleural effusions due to aerobic organisms usually manifest acutely, whereas in anaerobic pleuropulmonary infections the time course is usually more protracted. Factors predisposing to aspiration such as alcoholism, unconsciousness, and periodontal disease are common in patients with anaerobic infections. Occasionally, an empyema or a complicated effusion is manifested by failure of response or worsening of the clinical condition despite adequate antibiotic therapy for pneumonia. A sudden expectoration of a large amount of purulent sputum or hemoptysis suggests the development of a bronchopleural fistula.

The physical examination usually reveals decreased breath sounds, dull percussion, and restricted respiratory excursions. Although rales from an associated pneumonia may be heard, the presence of a pleural friction rub is not distinctive. With chronicity, an empyema can erode the chest wall and present as a spontaneously draining subcutaneous abscess, known as empyema necessitatis. Other manifestations of chronic empyema include chondritis and osteomyelitis of the ribs, pericarditis, mediastinal and vertebral abscesses, disseminated infection, and multiple organ system failure. Anemia and leukocytosis may be present but are nonspecific.

MICROBIOLOGY

The bacteriology of pleural infections has changed considerably in the past 50 years. In the preantibiotic era, *Streptococcus pneumoniae* accounted for 50% to 70% of patients. The introduction of antibiotics in the mid-1940s led to a shift in microbial populations; anaerobic organisms are now the most common bacteria, being identified in 75% of patients, either alone (35%) or in combination with aerobic organisms (41%). Aerobes alone are recovered in only 24% of patients. The most frequent anaerobic isolates are *Fusobacterium, Prevotella* species (previously known as *Bacteroides melaninogenicus*), *Peptostreptococcus, Bacteroides fragilis,* and *Lactobacillus* and *Clostridium* species. The most commonly encountered aerobic organisms are alpha-hemolytic streptococci (*S. viridans*), group D nonenterococcal streptococci, coagulase-negative staphylococci, and the gram-negative organisms *Pseudomonas aeruginosa, Escherichia coli,* and *Klebsiella pneumoniae.*

Staphylococcus aureus is a relatively common cause of empyema in otherwise healthy adults and children, and in patients who have had sustained chest trauma or undergone surgery, whereas alcoholic males are particularly susceptible to infection with *Klebsiella pneumoniae.*

PLEURAL FLUID ANALYSIS

Thoracentesis plays a critical role in the evaluation of pleural effusions, and in 90% of adult patients yields useful information. Thoracentesis should be performed when: (1) the fluid is anatomically accessible and adequate in volume; (2) a microbiologic diagnosis is necessary; or (3) pulmonary function is compromised by the effusion. The appropriate site of diagnostic thoracentesis is selected by examination of the chest radiographs, computed tomography (CT), or ultrasonography (US). An 18- or 19-gauge needle is utilized. Approximately 20 to 50 mL of fluid is removed into a heparinized syringe, its odor and color noted, and aliquots prepared for measurement of pH, glucose, lactate dehydrogenase (LDH), protein, and cell count.

An exudate is defined by any of the following: (1) a pleural fluid–to–serum protein ratio greater than 0.5; (2) a pleural fluid LDH–to–serum LDH ratio greater than 0.6; or (3) a pleural fluid LDH more than two thirds of the upper normal limit for serum. A transudate does not meet any of the aforementioned three criteria. If the patient has a transudative effusion, no further laboratory tests on the pleural fluid are indicated. If the patient has an exudative pleural effusion, the remaining pleural fluid is sent for white blood cell count and differential, cytologic examination, Gram stain, and cultures for aerobic and anaerobic bacteria, mycobacteria, and fungi. Aspiration of frank pus from the pleural space establishes the diagnosis of empyema and requires no additional diagnostic studies beyond Gram stain and culture. If the initial Gram stains are negative, the pleural fluid should be centrifuged and the sediment stained. In stage 1 or the exudative stage, the pleural fluid is a thin exudate with a white blood count (WBC) less than 1000 cells/mm³, LDH below 500 to 1000 U/L, pH greater than 7.20, and a glucose level greater than 40 mg/dL. This is also called a simple parapneumonic effusion. Stage 2, or the fibrinopurulent or transitional stage, is characterized by infection of the pleural fluid. The fluid becomes turbid and contains bacteria and cellular debris. The pleural fluid glucose is usually less than 40 mg/dL, the LDH greater than 1000 U/L, the WBC greater than 5000/mm³, and the pH less than 7.20. Fibrin is deposited parallel to the pleural surfaces and as the stage progresses, fibrinopurulent membranes partition the pleural space into two or more loculations. As the fluid thickens, amorphous gelatinous masses adhere to the pleural surfaces, compromising lung expansion. This is also termed a complicated parapneumonic effusion. If the condition goes untreated, the fluid becomes frankly purulent, giving rise to an empyema. During this stage, loculations prevent extension of the infective process but make evacuation of the pleural cavity by nonsurgical means progressively difficult. In Stage 3, the chronic or organizing stage, fibroblasts migrate into the pleural cavity and produce an inelastic membrane called the pleural peel or cortex, entrapping the lung and markedly altering lung function.

A pH greater than 7.30 on admission virtually always predicts a good outcome with antibiotic treatment of the pneumonia only. Patients with a pleural fluid pH between 7.20 and 7.30 require close observation with further diagnostic testing, such as repeat thoracentesis or CT, if clinically indicated, before a decision is made concerning drainage of the pleural space. If determined properly, the pH value correlates best with the extent and stage of the inflammatory process.

IMAGING

PLAIN RADIOGRAPHS. The posteroanterior and lateral chest radiographs are the best initial diagnostic modalities. When the patient is upright, free pleural fluid accumulates in the lowest part of the hemithorax in the posterior costophrenic angles. Lateral decubitus views allow detection of 50 to 100 mL of fluid and the presence of loculation if the fluid fails to layer-out along the dependent chest. In the decubitus view with the involved side upright, the free fluid forms layers against the mediastinum, and one can assess how much of the radiodensity is due to the fluid and how much is due to a parenchymal infiltrate. In the view with the involved side dependent, the amount of free pleural fluid can be semiquantitated by measuring the distance from the chest wall to the outside of the lung. If the thickness of fluid exceeds 10 mm, a diagnostic thoracentesis is indicated. However, it is not necessary to tap all parapneumonic effusions if the volume of fluid remains small, the patient is doing well, the fluid moves freely, or the radiograph is improving.

The typical radiographic appearance of parapneumonic effusions or empyemas is shown in Figure 136–1. When the effusion is loculated and is not freely flowing, it appears in a posterolateral location on a lateral radiograph with the corner border toward the hilum, as shown in Figure 136–1*B*. Effusions can also be multiloculated, with

areas of consolidation of the adjacent lung, and can reach a considerable size and even opacify an entire hemithorax, causing deviation of the mediastinum toward the unaffected side. The observation of an air-fluid level in the plain film suggests a lung abscess, perforated viscus, concomitant pneumothorax, a bronchopleural fistula, or an infection with gas-forming organisms.

COMPUTED TOMOGRAPHY (CT). Computed tomography is of great value in the overall evaluation of parapneumonic effusions and should be done early in the assessment of patients with complex parapneumonic effusion or empyema. Computed tomography is helpful in (1) differentiating pleural fluid from peripheral parenchymal infiltrates or pleural thickening, (2) evaluating parenchymal disease, (3) determining loculation, (4) characterizing the pleural surfaces, and (5) guiding and assessing therapy.

Complicated effusions and empyemas are frequently associated with nearby pulmonary consolidation and can be mistaken for a lung abscess. A lung abscess usually presents as a poorly defined, roughly spherical mass surrounded by consolidated but noncompressed lung. An empyema is usually elongated, conforms to the shape of the chest wall, and compresses the adjacent lung. Its wall is thin and uniform, and the interface angle with the chest wall is obtuse. The margins of the empyema cavity are composed of inflamed visceral and parietal pleura that enhances after administration of intravenous contrast medium. The visceral and parietal layers are separated by

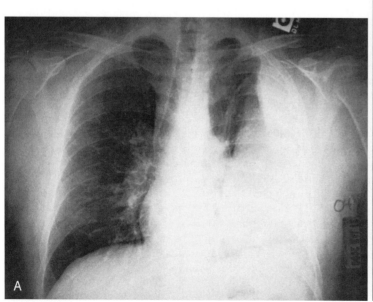
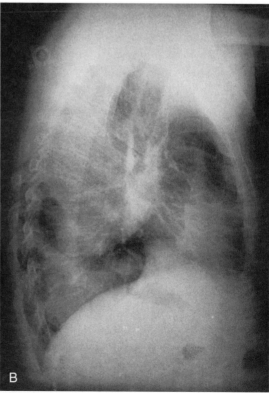

Figure 136–1. Typical appearance of a parapneumonic effusion. *A,* Posterior-anterior radiograph of the chest demonstrating a left-sided effusion. *B,* Lateral radiograph of the chest demonstrating a posterior D-shaped opacity.

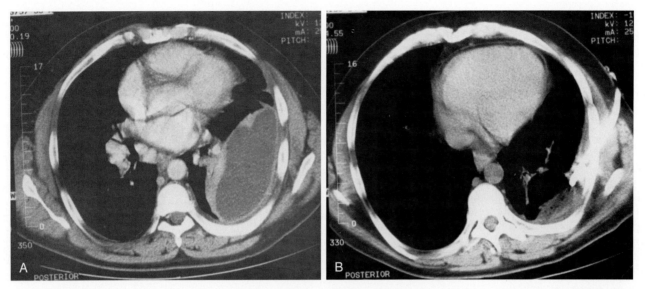

Figure 136–2. *A,* CT demonstrating a left-sided empyema and the enhanced visceral and parietal pleural surfaces, the so-called "split pleural sign." *B,* CT of the same patient after VATS débridement.

the interposed empyema fluid, giving rise to the "split pleura sign" (Fig. 136–2).

ULTRASONOGRAPHY (US). Ultrasonography is widely available, provides guidance for thoracentesis or pleural catheter placement, and can be transported to the bedside. US is particularly useful in sampling fluid that does not freely form layers on decubitus films, and can distinguish solid from liquid pleural abnormalities better than chest radiography. The presence of discrete pleural septations has prognostic importance because loculated collections require drainage for their resolution. Computed tomography, however, gives additional information not obtained by US.

MANAGEMENT

The therapeutic armamentarium for parapneumonic effusion or empyema consists of antibiotic therapy, thoracentesis, tube thoracostomy, radiologic-guided percutaneous catheter drainage, intrapleural fibrinolytic agents, and a variety of surgical drainage procedures including video-assisted thoracic surgery (VATS) and open thoracotomy. Table 136–1 gives an overview of the classification, diagnostic criteria, and treatment options of parapneumonic effusions.

The initial diagnostic challenge is to distinguish pleural effusions that will respond to antimicrobial therapy alone from collections that require tube thoracostomy or surgi-

Table 136–1	Classification and Therapy for Parapneumonic Effusions and Empyema	
CLASS	**DIAGNOSTIC CRITERIA**	**TREATMENT**
Insignificant effusion	Small (<10 mm) fluid collection on a lateral decubitus film	Antibiotics Thoracentesis usually unnecessary
Parapneumonic effusion	Fluid collection >10 mm thick on lateral decubitus film	Antibiotics plus Thoracentesis
Borderline complicated effusion	pH 7–7.2 and/or LDH value > 1000 IU/L; glucose level >40 mg/dL; negative Gram stain and culture	Antibiotics Tube thoracostomy usually necessary
Simple complicated effusion	pH <7 and/or glucose value <40 mg/dL and/or positive Gram stain or culture	Antibiotics and tube thoracostomy
Complex complicated effusion	Above characteristics plus multiple loculi	Antibiotics plus Tube thoracostomy ± fibrinolytics VATS
Simple empyema	Single loculus of pus or free-flowing fluid	Tube thoracostomy ± VATS plus Antibiotics
Complex empyema	Multiple loculi of pus	VATS or Thoracotomy plus Antibiotics
Chronic empyema	Thick pleural peel; trapped lung	Decortication plus Antibiotics

Modified from Bartlett JG: Empyema. In Gorbach SL, Bartlett JG, Blacklow NR (eds): Infectious Diseases, 2nd ed. Philadelphia, WB Saunders, 1992, pp 639–644.

cal drainage for their resolution. The clinical presentation, imaging characteristics, and pleural fluid analysis are the keys to guide the choice of therapy as shown in Figure 136–3.

Uncomplicated parapneumonic effusions usually require no specific therapy. Treatment of the underlying pnemonia is the basis of therapy. Thoracentesis or, rarely, tube thoracostomy drainage of the pleural fluid is indicated for large fluid collections causing respiratory compromise by compression of the adjacent lung. Once the diagnosis of a complicated parapneumonic effusion or empyema has been established, treatment follows the traditional guidelines for managing any abscess: (1) antibiotic therapy for controlling the underlying infection; (2) adequate drainage; and (3) obliteration of the dead space. Infected pleural effusions should be approached and treated with the same urgency as an intra-abdominal abscess or as any collection of pus in any body cavity.

ANTIBIOTICS. Early antimicrobial therapy for pneumonia minimizes the development of parapneumonic effusion and aborts the progression of uncomplicated effusion to complicated effusion or empyema. Antimicrobial agents able to penetrate the pleural compartment in sufficient quantities to achieve and exceed the minimal inhibitory concentration include penicillins, cephalosporins, aztreonam, clindamycin, and ciprofloxacin. Aminoglycosides are less capable of entering the empyema collection, and, more importantly, they are inactivated by the acidic pH of the pleural fluid environment. The development of an empyema after a penetrating wound to the chest is related to the contamination of the pleural space at the time of the injury. Studies indicate that prophylactic antibiotics have a role in the prevention of empyema in patients undergoing closed-tube thoracostomy for traumatic hemothorax or pneumothorax. The most important factor, however, in preventing empyema remains the complete evacuation of any hemothorax.

Empirical therapy using combinations of agents against aerobes and anaerobes is recommended. A positive Gram stain of pleural fluid is utilized to guide initial antibiotic therapy, which may need to be adjusted according to the patient's clinical course and the results of the pleural fluid

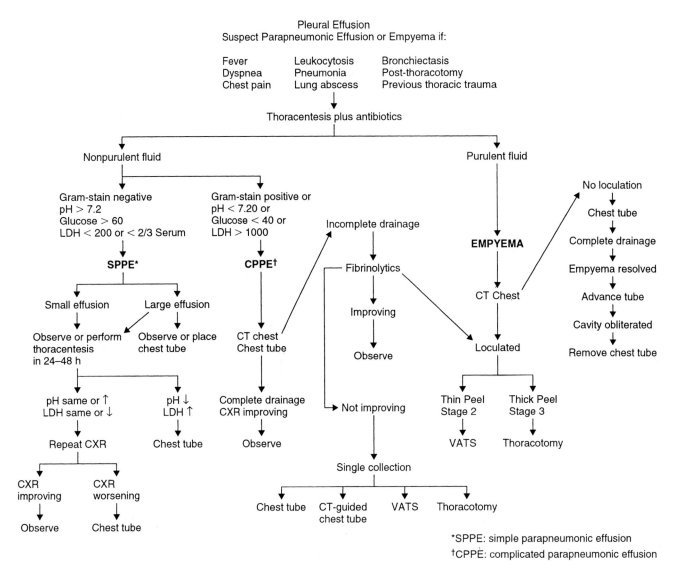

Figure 136–3. Algorithm demonstrating an approach for the treatment of parapneumonic effusion.

cultures and sensitivities. Often, several weeks of therapy are necessary to achieve satisfactory resolution.

ULTRASONOGRAPHIC SUCTION DRAINAGE. This technique involves the introduction of a 20-French to 24-French catheter into the pleural cavity under US guidance. With suction up to 100 mm Hg, the catheter is directed into the most dependent of the regions of the infected cavity, allowing removal of thin septations and drainage of fluid. This is a theoretically attractive technique for effusions in the early stage in debilitated patients, although the authors have no personal experience with it.

TUBE THORACOSTOMY. The decision to institute tube thoracostomy is based on the characteristics of the pleural fluid and the absence of multiple loculations demonstrated by plain films or CT. The indications for tube thoracostomy include complicated parapneumonic effusion and empyema, as indicated by gross pus in the pleural space, organisms on Gram stain of the pleural fluid or culture, pleural fluid glucose less than 40 mg/dL, LDH greater than 1000 U/L, or pleural fluid pH below 7.20. If the CT demonstrates a multiloculated effusion, tube thoracotomy will be inadequate, and the pleural space infection should be approached by VATS or open thoracotomy.

A 26-French to 36-French thoracostomy tube should be utilized. The chest tube must be positioned at the most dependent level and must enter the fluid collection. If there is a single loculation, precise definition of the size and shape of the space to be drained can be achieved with US or CT. A preliminary thoracentesis to localize the fluid collection with certainty helps in selecting the optimal site for chest tube insertion. In the presence of a bronchopleural fistula, an additional tube at a higher and more anterior level should be considered. It is also important to utilize tubing and connections of maximal diameters throughout the whole system, as narrowing at any site increases resistance to flow and hampers drainage.

Adequate drainage of an early complicated parapneumonic effusion is usually achieved with simple tube thoracostomy. Success rates deteriorate to 35% with empyema. Failures occur mainly as the result of incomplete drainage because of loculated or inaccessible collections, improper tube positioning, or high fluid viscosity. Successful drainage by tube thoracostomy of a complicated parapneumonic effusion is associated with rapid clinical and radiologic improvement. If no significant improvement occurs over 24 to 48 hours, incomplete drainage or inappropriate antibiotic therapy should be suspected and investigated with repeat CT or review of microbial sensitivities. If CT demonstrates a single remaining loculation, a second chest tube should be inserted or a catheter placed under CT guidance. The chest tubes are left in place until the pleural cavity is obliterated by expansion of the lung, pleural fluid is serous and less than 50 to 100 mL/day, infection is controlled, and any bronchopleural fistula is sealed. Fibrinolytic agents or a more extensive surgical procedure such as VATS is required if closed thoracostomy drainage fails to achieve resolution. In patients with an established empyema, when there are no remaining

signs of infection and the lung is stuck to the chest wall, the chest tubes are opened to the atmosphere and slowly advanced from the pleural space over a period of several weeks to allow resolution of the infection and obliteration of any residual cavity.

Although uncommon, complications associated with tube thoracostomy may occur, including subcutaneous emphysema, chest wall hematoma, hemothorax, lung laceration, chylothorax, and injury to mediastinal structures, diaphragm, or intra-abdominal viscera.

INTRAPLEURAL FIBRINOLYTIC AGENTS. Enzymatic débridement of the pleural space with the use of fibrinolytic agents such as streptokinase (SK) or urokinase (UK) facilitates chest tube drainage of loculated or viscous early-stage fibrinopurulent collections. SK or UK are administered as a solution of 250,000 U in 100 mL of sterile normal saline via chest tubes or catheters. The chest tubes are clamped, and patients are encouraged to change their positions at regular intervals to enhance distribution of the instilled agent. After 4 to 6 hours, the chest tubes are unclamped and placed back on suction. This procedure can be repeated daily until clinical improvement is achieved, radiographic resolution is obtained, or significant pleural fluid drainage ceases. Success rates for fibrinolytic agents vary between 70% to 90% and are influenced by the appropriate selection of patients. A good outcome is usually obtained in complicated effusions and early empyemas.

Operative Treatment

ANESTHETIC MANAGEMENT. A double-lumen endotracheal tube for contralateral lung ventilation is essential for a VATS and may be very helpful for open thoracotomy in selected patients. In the presence of a bronchopleural fistula, it helps avoid contamination of the normal dependent lung. Postoperative pain control is essential for the unrestricted breathing and coughing necessary for maintenance of adequate ventilation and clearance of pulmonary secretions. Epidural analgesia is ideally suited for this purpose. Early ambulation with portable suction devices, incentive spirometry, and chest physiotherapy should be instituted routinely. All patients receive heparin subcutaneously and/or are fitted with sequential compression devices for prophylaxis against deep venous thrombosis.

VIDEO-ASSISTED THORACIC SURGERY (VATS). VATS is gaining popularity in the management of patients with complex parapneumonic effusions or early empyema and is competitive with open thoracotomy. Timely management and patient selection are critical for its success. VATS is particularly useful during the fibrinopurulent stage of empyema. At this stage, empyemolysis is achieved with complete breakdown of all loculations and drainage of the gelatinous exudate from the pleural cavity. Early fibrin membranes or thin peels can usually be removed from the visceral pleura to allow re-expansion of the lung. A unilocular space and full lung expansion must be achieved at the completion of the procedure. Before closure, a chest tube or tubes are placed for postoperative drainage of the pleural space. The tubes are removed when there are no remaining signs of infection, and drainage is serous and less than 50 to 100 mL/day.

Once the empyema has progressed to the organized state, VATS is often unsuccessful due to the thicker and more adherent pleural peel entrapping the lung, and an open procedure becomes mandatory. In borderline cases, VATS can be used as an initial step. Some of these early organizing empyemas can be dealt with by VATS, while in more advanced cases VATS can assist in identifying the most appropriate site for thoracotomy incision to approach the empyema.

THORACOTOMY. Samson and Buford proposed early thoracotomy for evacuation of pleural space infections during stage 2 and the initial part of stage 3 when the pleural surfaces are covered by amorphous gelatinous fluid collections, but a true fibrous peel has not formed. Blunt finger dissection usually suffices to disrupt the fibrinous septations and allows access to all other areas of the pleural cavity. Total elimination of fibrin membranes from the lung, diaphragm, and parietal pleura facilitates immediate and full lung re-expansion. Thoracostomy tubes are placed anteriorly and posteriorly; additional chest tubes or other closed suction drains may be utilized to drain more inaccessible areas. The earlier the drainage procedure is performed, the better the outcome, provided that the underlying pulmonary process is adequately addressed and completely resolved with antibiotic therapy. This time-honored surgical technique is being supplanted by VATS for most patients.

Special Situations

POSTPNEUMONECTOMY EMPYEMA. Infection of the pleural space after pneumonectomy is a potentially life-threatening process. Flooding of the remaining lung may occur if a bronchopleural fistula develops. An early postpneumonectomy empyema declares itself within a few days or up to 1 to 2 weeks. Recognition is based on a characteristic clinical syndrome: (1) expectoration of frothy, pink sputum; (2) a falling air-fluid level on chest radiograph; (3) persistent low-grade fever; and (4) persistent clinical complaints. Predisposing factors include a technically difficult closure with jeopardy of the blood supply to the bronchial stump, preoperative radiation, a long bronchial stump with bronchitis at the site of closure, and contamination of the pleural space. Management involves tube thoracostomy and reopening of the chest for meticulous débridement. The bronchopleural fistula is closed and protected with an intercostal or diaphragmatic muscle graft. Empyema should be suspected in the absence of a detectable bronchopleural fistula when there is loculation of the pleural fluid, spiking fever, or persistent or worsening systemic complaints. Thoracentesis is required for culture and sensitivity testing. Antibiotics are initiated, and reoperation is performed. Coverage of the bronchial stump may be required, depending on the operative findings. A chest wall window to allow irrigation and packing is usually employed for an established empyema.

Late postpneumonectomy empyema is often associated with a peribronchial abscess in the vicinity of a stitch with rupture into the pleural space. The bronchopleural fistula

is usually smaller, and the onset of symptoms is more insidious than in acute empyemas. The fistula is usually on the side of the bronchial stump, rather than at the end of the stump, as is the case in early postpneumonectomy empyema. Since it is more difficult to sterilize these chronically infected spaces, reoperation with wound closure is unlikely to be successful. Consequently, a chest wall window is usually constructed. Secondary closure may be performed when the space is free from infection and granulation tissue covers the wound. If a bronchopleural fistula is detected, closure and protection of the stump is warranted. In poor-risk patients, permanent drainage is usually well tolerated, provided a coexisting fistula does not result in impaired gas exchange. An epithelialized tract is required and can be performed at the time of the original thoracotomy by using a Clagett window or an Eloesser full-thickness skin flap.

CHRONIC EMPYEMA. Chronicity develops as the result of (1) a delay in diagnosis, (2) inadequate drainage in the acute stage, (3) continuing reinfection from a bronchopleural fistula, (4) a retained hemothorax, and (5) specific infections, such as tuberculosis and fungal infections.

In the early chronic stage, rib resection and open drainage remain the treatment of choice, particularly in the poor-risk elderly or debilitated patient. The lung is usually able to expand through the still stretchable visceral peel. However, this process may be lengthy and entails open wound care and frequent dressing changes. Once the residual sinus tract has closed, there is usually a remarkable resolution of the pleural thickening, so that permanent and disabling fibrothorax is unlikely to persist. Indeed, if this radiologic and functional improvement does not occur, one must suspect the presence of an undrained infection. If the chronic infection does not resolve over time, the pleural space becomes obliterated by the formation of a fibrous peel or cortex. This space-occupying lesion is the target of a decortication.

DECORTICATION. The major indications for decortication are the formation of a fibrous peel or cortex owing to chronic empyema, a chronic organized hemothorax, and tuberculous pleuritis with lung entrapment. The goals of therapy are to limit morbidity and mortality, shorten hospital stay, and return pulmonary function to baseline. The principles for successful decortication include the following: (1) removal of the fibrin membranes overlying the visceral pleura to promote complete re-expansion of the collapsed lung; (2) adequate wide exposure; (3) development of a proper plane of cleavage between the peel and the visceral pleura; (4) removal of the peel by blunt dissection, with a finger or with gauze; (5) complete freeing of the lung to achieve circumferential mobilization and re-expansion; (6) closure of bronchopleural fistulas; (7) adequate hemostasis, and (8) wide drainage by placing two or more chest tubes or other drainage devices to ensure complete evacuation and obliteration of any potential space.

MUSCLE TRANSPOSITION. Indications for muscle transposition in empyema include obliteration of a persistent pleural space and reinforcement of the bronchial stump after closure of a bronchopleural fistula. The two most common techniques are (1) use of multiple muscular flap transpositions to fill and obliterate the postpneumonectomy space, and (2) use of a single muscular flap to close a persistent bronchopleural fistula and subsequent management of the remaining empyema cavity by a modified Clagett procedure. The extracostal muscles most commonly utilized are the latissimus dorsi, the serratus anterior, the pectoralis major, the pectoralis minor, and the rectus abdominis. The technique of standard muscular transfers entails the following steps: (1) appropriate antibiotics; (2) débridement of the empyema cavity; (3) closure of any bronchopleural fistula; (4) transposition of the muscular flap or flaps; (5) total obliteration of the empyema cavity; (6) pleural tube drainage; and (7) primary closure of the wound. When a remaining cavity is present, open pleural drainage is performed in the most dependent area of the thorax in the form of a modified Clagett procedure. Wet dressings of diluted povidoneiodine solutions (0.001%) are packed into the thorax and changed three or four times daily. When healthy granulation tissue is present throughout the cavity, secondary closure of the chest is done after the residual cavity has been filled with an antibiotic solution.

TUBERCULOSIS OF THE PLEURA. Tuberculous effusions are rare, but their incidence may increase with the increase in pulmonary tuberculosis in inner city areas, and with the acquired immunodeficiency syndrome (AIDS) epidemic. Pleural involvement may occur during the primary parenchymal lung infection when subpleural foci rupture into the pleural space or during the post–primary infection period when adhesions occur between the two pleural surfaces, and extension of the infection results in granulomatous involvement of the pleura. As pleural fluid accumulates, progressive deposition of fibrous tissue occurs along the pleural surfaces entrapping the underlying lung. In later stages, fibrosis and calcification of the fibrous peel may occur with contraction of the hemithorax. In some patients, a bronchopleural fistula develops, and secondary contamination of the pleural space results in a mixed tuberculous-pyogenic infection. A loculated pyopneumothorax may result. In this setting, extensive tuberculous and pyogenic infection of the lung is common, sometimes destroying an entire lobe or lung. Most patients with pure pleural tuberculosis respond to treatment with thoracentesis, nutritional support, and antituberculous chemotherapy. Tube thoracostomy is usually not recommended even in the presence of a pH lower than 7.20 or a glucose level less than 40, since most of these effusions respond favorably to antituberculous medications.

Patients with pleural and parenchymal disease should receive medical therapy for 6 to 12 months directed toward the underlying parenchymal cavities and infiltrates. Once the parenchymal disease clears or is under control, the pleural process can be approached surgically if necessary. Careful assessment is made of the ability of the underlying lung to re-expand. Antituberculous drugs, adequate host immunity, complete obliteration of any residual space, and complete excision of infected tissue contribute to ultimate success.

Patients with mixed pyogenic and tuberculous pleural infections in association with parenchymal tuberculosis frequently have a bronchopleural fistula, severe cavitary disease, advanced bronchiectasis, and destruction of a lobe or an entire lung. Initial therapy consists of antituberculous drugs in association with antibiotics to address the pyogenic component. Simple decompression of the pleural space is often not possible and has little potential in promoting lung expansion. Surgical intervention requires major resection as well as decortication of the pleural space in the form of pleuropneumonectomy. Alternatively, lung resection or pneumonectomy can be done through the empyema space, and the residual space is dealt with an Eloesser or Clagett procedure, muscle transfers, or thoracoplasty.

Pearls and Pitfalls

- A parapneumonic "pleural" effusion is any pleural effusion associated with lung infection.
- A simple parapneumonic effusion is a free-flowing, uninfected fluid collection that requires no specific therapy.
- A complicated parapneumonic effusion is an infected fluid collection prone to developing loculations that requires drainage.
- A thoracic empyema is a collection of frank pus within the pleural cavity.
- Parapneumonic effusions progress through defined stages: exudative, fibrinopurulent, and organizational.
- The clinical manifestations of parapneumonic effusion or empyema vary, depending on the underlying pulmonary process, the responsible organism, the amount of bacteria and fluid in the pleural space, the stage of the disease, and host defense mechanisms.
- Pleural cavity infections due to aerobic organisms usually present acutely, whereas anaerobic infections have a more subacute course.
- Anaerobic organisms are the most common cause of parapneumonic pleural space infections.
- Computed tomography identifies any pleural fluid loculations.
- The initial diagnostic challenge is to recognize pleural effusions that require drainage, but clinical presentation, imaging characteristics, and pleural fluid analysis guide therapy.
- Indications for chest tube thoracostomy include an unilocular fluid collection, aspiration of gross pus, organisms on Gram stain or culture, pleural fluid pH below 7.20, glucose below 40 mg/dL, or LDH greater than 1000 U/L.
- VATS or thoracotomy is required for patients with complicated parapneumonic effusion or empyema requiring surgical débridement, but open thoracotomy is necessary for entrapped lung.
- Any residual pleural cavity must be obliterated or drained, and any associated bronchopleural fistula repaired and protected with vascularized tissue.
- Tuberculous pleural effusions may present during the primary infection or during reinfection.
- Tube thoracostomy is usually not indicated in tuberculous effusion that is not complicated by bronchopleural fistula.
- Surgical treatment of a tuberculous pleural space infection should be preceded by a course of antituberculous medications.

SELECTED READINGS

Andrews NC, Parker EF, Shaw RR, et al: Management of nontuberculous empyema: A statement of the subcommittee on surgery. Am Rev Resp Dis 1962;85:935.

Bartlett JG: Empyema. In Gorbach SL, Bartlett JG, Backlow NR (eds): Infectious Diseases, 2nd ed. Philadelphia, WB Saunders, 1992, pp 639–644.

Bryant RE, Salmon CJ: Pleural empyema: State-of-the-art clinical article. Clin Infect Dis 1996;22:747.

Deschamps C, Pairolero PC, Allen MS, Trastek VF: Management of early postpneumonectomy empyema and bronchopleural fistula. Chest Surg Clin North America 1996;19:519.

Fry W: Surgical management of empyema. In Kaiser L, Kron IL, Spray TL (eds): Mastery of Cardiothoracic Surgery. Philadelphia, Lippincott-Raven, 1998, pp 247–256.

Gharagozloo F, Trachiotis G, Wolfe A, et al: Pleural space irrigation and modified Clagett procedure for the treatment of early postpneumonectomy empyema. J Thorac Cardiovasc Surg 1998;116:943.

Kinasewitz GT: Pleural fluid dynamics and effusions. In Fishman AP (ed): Pulmonary Disease and Disorders. New York, McGraw-Hill, 1998, pp 1389–1410.

Landreneau RJ, Keenan RJ, Hazelrigg SR, et al: Thoracoscopy for empyema and hemothorax. Chest 1995;109:18.

Lee-Chiong TL, Matthay RA: Current diagnostic and medical management of thoracic empyema. Chest Surg Clin North Am 1996;19:419.

Light RW, Rodriguez RM: Management of parapneumonic effusions. Clin Chest Med 1998;19:373.

Magovern CJ, Rusch VW: Parapneumonic and post-traumatic pleural space infections. Chest Surg Clin North Am 1994;17:561.

Mouroux J, Maalouf J, Padovani B, et al: Surgical management of pleuropulmonary tuberculosis. J Thorac Cardiovasc Surg 1996;111:662.

Shields TW: Decortication of the lung. In Shields TW (ed): General Thoracic Surgery, 4th ed. Malvern, PA, Williams & Wilkins, 1994, pp 710–713.

Thurer RJ: Decortication in thoracic empyema: Indications and surgical technique. Chest Surg Clin North Am 1996;19:519.

Wain JC: Management of late post-pneumonectomy empyema and bronchopleural fistula: Empyema, spaces and fistula. Chest Surg Clin North Am 1996, p 519.

Chapter 137

Lung Abscess

Henning A. Gaissert and Leonard A. Mermel

Bacterial lung abscess in developed countries has seen marked declines both in incidence (about 10-fold) and mortality (from 40% to 10%) during the past four decades. The general surgeon no longer encounters this disease, except perhaps when practicing in an area remote from thoracic specialists. A bacterial lung abscess may be a concomitant finding in a patient with another surgical problem, or the abscess may occur as a postoperative complication or as a consequence of surgical therapy (e.g., in a transplant patient). The purpose of this chapter is to provide a general perspective on the pathogenesis and treatment of bacterial lung abscess.

CLINICAL PRESENTATION

The classic bacterial lung abscess is caused originally by aspiration of oropharyngeal contents. The typical patient lacks temporary or permanent protection of the airway; for example, as the result of alcoholism or dental work. Table 137–1 lists the important settings predisposing to lung abscess. Cough, fever, and chest pain ensue from days to weeks after the initiating event, often accompanied by putrid sputum. If the abscess persists, hemoptysis, inanition, and weight loss develop. Some or all of these symptoms may be absent. For example, patients with postobstructive pneumonia and abscess may have a nonproductive cough. The history may then only become evident when a chest radiograph suggests the diagnosis.

The organisms found in bacterial lung abscesses usually reflect the resident flora of the gingival crevice. The abscess contains a polymicrobial mix of anaerobic or microaerophilic bacteria. It is noteworthy that this entity is rare among edentulous patients or those with good oral hygiene. Consequently, a high incidence of bronchogenic carcinoma is found in such patients who develop a lung abscess. An increase in the population of immunosuppressed individuals has changed the clinical presentation in two important respects. The initial symptoms are subdued or abolished by immunosuppression, and the organisms found in the culture may be unusual, such as *Nocardia* and *Rhodococcus*. In developing countries, parasitic infections such as paragonimiasis cause pulmonary abscesses. Causative organisms are listed in Table 137–2.

The typical lung abscess is located in the periphery of the lung. If it is close to the pleura, the visceral and parietal layers adhere to each other. Gravitational flow and patient position at the time of aspiration determine the location of the cavity. Most aspirations occur into the right lung owing to the vertical axis of the right mainstem bronchus. When the patient is supine, aspiration is expected to occur into the posterior segment of the upper lobes or superior and posterobasal segment of the lower

lobes; when aspiration occurs in the lateral position, an abscess will develop in the anterior or posterior segment of the upper lobes. When the patient is prone, aspiration will occur into the middle lobe, and when he or she is upright, it will find its way into the basal segments of the lower lobes. If, in contrast, a cavity is encountered where aspiration is unusual (e.g., in the apical segment), a bacterial origin other than tuberculosis should be questioned and malignancy suspected.

The possibilities in the differential diagnosis of lung abscess include a variety of malignant and benign conditions. *Lung cancer* may lead to abscess formation, owing to secondary infection of necrotic tumor or obstruction of a larger bronchus. Airway obstruction may not be visible on bronchoscopy. In developed countries, the incidence of lung cancer is higher than that of bacterial lung abscess. Any abscess should therefore be followed with lingering suspicion of malignancy until radiographic abnormalities resolve. *Lobar gangrene* is a more extensively destructive process that leads to multiple small cavities within the same segment or lobe. *Empyema* is a localized infection of the pleural space. Empyemas coexist in approximately one third of abscesses. *An infection of a pre-existing cavity* (i.e., a bulla) is often located in the apex of the lung and, in contrast with an abscess, has a sharp demarcation from the surrounding lung. A *pneumatocele*, occurring more commonly in children, is a lucency within the lung resulting from air entrapment distal to a bronchus injured by infection. A pulmonary sequestration or bronchogenic duplication may also become infected, forming a type of lung abscess in a nontypical location. Lung abscess may also occur from hematogenous spread; for example, in drug users with right-sided endocarditis.

Table 137–1	Conditions Associated with Aspiration and Anaerobic Lung Abscess

Dental disease
  Periodontal abscess
  Tooth extraction
Failure of glottic closure
  Tracheotomy
  Endotracheal intubation
Dysphagia or failure of upper or lower esophageal sphincters
  Esophageal motility disorders
  Carcinoma of the esophagus
  Nasogastric intubation
  Zenker's diverticulum
Neurologic impairment
  Alcohol intoxication
  General anesthesia
  Seizure disorder
  Bulbar paralysis

Table 137–2	**Microbial Causes of Lung Abscess**

Bacteria
  Anaerobes **C** or **D**
    Peptostreptococcus
    Bacteroides
    Fusobacterium
    Actinomyces
  Gram-negative aerobes
    Klebsiella **C** or **D**
    Escherichia coli **C** or **D**
    Burkholderia pseudomallei (meliodosis) **U**
    Legionella **D**
  Gram-positive aerobes
    Staphylococcus aureus **C** or **D**
    Rhodococcus equi **D**
  Miscellaneous aerobes
    Nocardia **D**
Fungi
  Aspergillus **D**
  Blastomyces dermatitidis **C** or **D**
  Coccidioides immitis **C** or **D**
  Cryptococcus neoformans **D**
  Histoplasma capsulatum **C** or **D**
  Rhizopus sp. (mucormycosis) **D**
  Paracoccidioides **U**
  Sporothrix **C** or **D**
  Mycobacterium **C** or **D** or **U**
Parasites **U**
  Entamoeba histolytica
  Echinococcus
  Paragonimus

Predominantly affected population indicated by **C** for immunocompetent hosts, **D** for immunodeficient hosts, and **U** for patients in underdeveloped countries.

They usually present as multiple abscesses and are often due to *Staphylococcus aureus*.

DIAGNOSIS

The chest radiograph usually demonstrates a rounded, peripheral opacity. When abscess drainage has occurred (e.g., following spontaneous internal drainage into the bronchial tree), a cavity with an air-fluid level is seen. Computed tomography (CT) should be obtained in every patient to further define the abscess, to look for other abscesses as well, to detect bronchial obstruction, and to look for an underlying mass lesion (malignancy) proximal to the abscess. In contrast with localized pleural empyema, a lung abscess contacts the chest wall at acute angles. In empyema, the angle with the chest wall is obtuse; parietal and visceral pleura are inflamed and enhance the interface between lung and empyema fluid (split pleura sign). Other radiographic studies are not helpful in separating benign from malignant disease. Hemoptysis is common, and persistent abscess may lead to anemia.

Even in a typical bacterial lung abscess, an attempt should be made to obtain material for culture. Conversely, in immunosuppressed patients, a culture of the abscess is mandatory, owing to the potentially wide spectrum of unusual pathogens. Expectorated sputum is contaminated with oral pathogens and therefore is often not useful.

Acceptable specimens are a transtracheal aspirate, a transthoracic needle aspirate, and a bronchoscopy-derived specimen, preferably using a protected brush. Specimens of abscess fluid derived from bronchoscopy or needle aspiration are preferred.

Specimens should be submitted for aerobic and anaerobic cultures; stains and cultures for fungi and *Nocardia* should be requested in immunocompromised patients. Submit cultures for acid-fast specimens, especially in high-risk patients (e.g., patients from highly endemic countries) and those with upper lobe involvement. Again, the importance of aggressive evaluation of immunocompromised patients is emphasized, even if the patient does not appear to be ill at presentation.

THERAPY

Standard antibiotic therapy for a lung abscess in the nonimmunosuppressed adult consists of clindamycin, 600 to 900 mg every 8 hours intravenously. Unfortunately, recently recognized resistance to clindamycin among streptococci can have an adverse impact on therapy, and all streptococci should be tested for susceptibility against the antimicrobial agent used. Other antibiotics are probably effective; however, no clinical data exist. Two large, prospective studies of antibiotic therapy found clindamycin to be superior to penicillin G with regard to treatment failure, relapse, and duration of fever. Anaerobic bacteria have increasingly expressed β-lactamase activity, and antibiotics such as ampicillin-sulbactam should be considered in patients with clindamycin-resistant streptococci. The duration of intravenous therapy is until fever resolves, usually 4 to 6 days. Oral therapy is continued until the chest radiograph shows complete resolution of the cavity, usually after 6 to 12 weeks.

The need for drainage is infrequent. Most lung abscesses establish spontaneous drainage into a bronchus, and surgical interventions are reserved for patients with a fulminant course or persistent fevers in the presence of an undrained fluid collection. An empyema should always be drained. Historically, surgical drainage of lung abscess through the chest wall was established by rib resection and incision once adherence of parietal and visceral pleura had occurred. Currently, percutaneous catheter drainage is often preferred for this purpose. Bronchopleural fistula and empyema are complications of this procedure when proximal bronchial obstruction, by a tumor, for example, prevents drainage of the abscess. Rigid bronchoscopy can be employed to resect the obstruction, and an obstructing malignant tumor can be reduced by radia-

Table 137–3	**Indications for Pulmonary Resection**

Coexisting malignancy
Lobar gangrene
Massive hemoptysis
Abscess within destroyed lung, bullae, or cysts

Pearls and Pitfalls

- Lung abscess is a potentially life-threatening disease especially in the immunocompromised patient. Evaluation and treatment should be conducted without delay, no matter how stable the patient appears.
- In immunosuppressed patients, every effort must be made to identify the causative organism. This may require transcutaneous aspiration or bronchoscopy with a protected brush.
- A lung cancer may be missed if there is failure to follow a lung abscess until radiographic stability is reached. Computed tomography is suggested for patients presenting with lung abscess.
- Surgical treatment is rarely indicated except for coexistent obstructing malignancy, severe hemoptysis, lobar destruction, or destroyed, nonfunctional parenchyma.

tion. Sudden bronchoscopic relief of obstruction carries the risk of contaminating uninfected lung owing to spillage of pus.

At one time, resection of a lung abscess by lobectomy was acceptable treatment, because antibiotic therapy was less advanced, and resection reliably removed the focus of infection. The indications for any operation have undergone extensive refinement in the patient without an underlying malignancy or other source of bronchial ob-

struction, particularly since a lung resection in a patient during or shortly after a severe infection is associated with substantial morbidity. Current surgical indications include coexistent malignancy, lobar gangrene, massive hemoptysis, or the presence of nonfunctional lung parenchyma containing bullae or cysts (Table 137–3).

OUTCOME

Early institution of intravenous antibiotics leads to resolution of the abscess in most patients. Surgical intervention is required infrequently. Lung abscess is associated with the highest mortality among immunodeficient individuals who are already weakened by their underlying illness. Growing tourism, globalization of trade, and changing patterns of antibiotic resistance are expected to influence the future presentations of this disease.

SELECTED READINGS

Bartlett JG: Anaerobic bacterial infections of the lung and pleural space. Clin Infect Dis 1993;16:S248.
Brook I: Lung abscess and pleural empyema in children. Adv Pediatr Infect Dis 1993;8:159.
Conces DJ: Bacterial pneumonia in immunocompromised patients. J Thorac Imaging 1998;13:261.
Pohlson EC, McNamara JJ, Char C, Kurata L: Lung abscess: A changing pattern of the disease. Am J Surg 1985;150:97.
Wiedemann HP, Rice TW: Lung abscess and empyema. Semin Thorac Cardiovasc Surg 1995;7:119.

Chapter 138

Hemoptysis in Benign Disease

Robert J. Cerfolio

Hemoptysis is defined as the coughing up of blood from the lungs or bronchial tree. It is a sign caused by a wide variety of pathologic conditions that span a spectrum of disorders and prognoses. Hemoptysis may herald a life-threatening event or may merely be a sign of mild bronchitis. The underlying cause may be malignant or benign. As the title of this chapter indicates, the author focuses on the latter.

Many authors have arbitrarily divided hemoptysis into several categories to help readers understand its etiology and treatment. It has been described as scant or massive, intermittent or continuous, and bright red or dark blue. For the most effective review of the management of hemoptysis, however, it is best to divide it into categories of massive or nonmassive. Massive hemoptysis is defined as the coughing of blood from the lungs or airways of more than 600 mL per day. In reality, this textbook definition is not clinically practical. Most patients have sputum and saliva mixed with their hemoptysis, and it is almost impossible to accurately quantify the amount. Yet, an estimate of the amount of blood is important in providing direction for identification of the cause, evaluation of the patient, treatment, and prognosis. The clinician must be concerned about not only the amount but also the potential for the blood to impede ventilation and oxygenation.

The patient with intermittent episodes of blood-stained sputum may have a bronchogenic malignancy. Although the underlying disease may be life-threatening, the hemoptysis can usually be managed with an elective outpatient evaluation. The patient who presents to the emergency room with episodes of recurrent hemoptysis that is "bright red and fills up a half a cup at a time" may have benign disease. Although the underlying disease itself may not be life-threatening, the hemoptysis represents a true surgical emergency and a significant risk to life. This chapter deals with the latter type of patient.

DEFINITION

The physician must first ensure that the blood the patient is "spitting up" actually started in the lungs or airway. Hematemesis, bleeding from the nasopharynx, and even epistaxis should be considered and excluded. The former two conditions not uncommonly masquerade as hemoptysis and lead the clinician down the wrong diagnostic and therapeutic path. If there is any question as to the etiology of spit-up blood, panendoscopy of all the appropriate systems (nasal, pharyngeal, tracheobronchial, and esophagogastric endoscopy) should be performed. Once the bleeding source has been correctly identified (usually by bronchoscopy), a full diagnostic evaluation of the cause of hemoptysis should be undertaken.

CLINICAL PRESENTATION

The most common cause of non–life-threatening hemoptysis is bronchitis. These patients are usually smokers. Because of their risk factors for bronchogenic carcinoma, they should have a chest radiograph, bronchoscopy, and computed tomography (CT) of the chest. Even if the patient is receiving an anticoagulant, the bleeding should not be attributed to the anticoagulant, and the evaluation should still be performed. If these studies and the sputum cytology are unrevealing, the patient should be reassured. Antibiotics may be prescribed if the epithelium of the airway is inflamed. However, it is probably more important to counsel the patient on the importance of stopping smoking and/or the need for lifelong surveillance to help diagnose an early cancer, rather than to treat the bronchitis with antibiotics. *If the bleeding is from a malignant source, the treatment options are discussed elsewhere in this book* and include surgical resection, radiation therapy, chemotherapy, photodynamic therapy, or, less advisedly, brachytherapy.

The patient with "significant recurrent" hemoptysis (more than half a cup or more than once per day) should be admitted into the hospital. When the hemoptysis is this large, the physician should resist the temptation to intubate the patient. If the patient is awake, alert, and adequately protecting his or her airway, with good arterial oxygen saturations and stable hemodynamics, he or she is more safely managed without an endotracheal tube. Once intubated, even a large No. 9 endotracheal tube does not offer the same size lumen that the patient's own hypopharynx affords. Moreover, suctioning should be used to clear the lumen, instead of the patient independently clearing the airway. However, if the patient desaturates or has hypotension, the airway must be protected. These patients are best initially treated by rigid bronchoscopy. If a chest radiograph has been performed or previous radiographs from prior admissions implicate one side as the most likely source of the bleeding, that side should be turned down, with the nonbleeding side up. This maneuver may protect the nonbleeding lung from being flooded with blood.

DIAGNOSIS AND MANAGEMENT OF THE PATIENT WITH SIGNIFICANT HEMOPTYSIS

The diagnostic and therapeutic procedure of choice in a patient with significant hemoptysis is rigid bronchoscopy. Rigid bronchoscopy by an experienced bronchoscopist is easy to perform and there are few, if any, patients who cannot be safely intubated with a rigid bronchoscope.

The rigid bronchoscope, in contrast with the flexible bronchoscope, affords the surgeon the opportunity to evacuate large amounts of blood and clot, while adequately ventilating and oxygenating the patient. In contrast, flexible fiberoptic bronchoscopy via an endotracheal tube compromises both ventilation and oxygenation. Moreover, it is often difficult, time-consuming, and, at times, impossible to completely evacuate large clots from the airway.

Surgical Technique

We perform rigid bronchoscopy by first placing a toothguard on patients who have upper teeth. The patient's head is placed at the end of the table, the neck extended, and the scope inserted through the vocal cords under direct vision. The author has found that a hand-held laryngoscope in one hand, and the bronchoscope in the other, helps aid insertion by elevating the tongue and epiglottis. This technique, along with appropriate suction, is especially helpful for insertion if the hypopharynx is filled with blood. One should always be prepared to convert to laryngoscopy and suspend the laryngoscope on a stand as well.

Once intubated, the author's preference for ventilation is jet ventilation. By jetting through a side channel of the scope, the surgeon has ample room to work while still oxygenating the patient simultaneously. Ventilation occurs via the open end of the scope. A tank of oxygen with appropriate connectors and tubing should be available at all times in the bronchoscopy suite. If this is not available (and the author strongly recommends that it should be), one can place conventional tubing on the end of the scope. Once the airway is protected, blood should be evacuated with large-bore suckers placed down the rigid bronchoscope under direct vision.

The patient should be resuscitated and stabilized, and clotting factors administered if the patient is coagulopathic. Flexible fiberoptic bronchoscopy can then be performed through the rigid scope to assess the distal tracheobronchial tree. The residual blood should be irrigated with saline and removed. A bleeding source should be identifiable. If the source is in the trachea, mainstem bronchi, or bronchus intermedius and is a segmental or focal area of tissue or a mass, it can usually be controlled with carbon dioxide laser, YAG laser, ice-cold saline lavage, or topical epinephrine. Although the surgeon should rightfully be careful in biopsying a mass that has caused massive hemoptysis and might necessitate an emergency operation, biopsy should be performed nonetheless for several reasons. First, bleeding from the biopsy is more easily managed once the airway has been controlled and the lesion is in view. Second, a malignant mass requires an evaluation and treatment strategy different from that for a benign one. For these reasons, the authors perform frozen-section analysis, even if this means having to call the pathologist into the hospital in the middle of the night. Tissue confirmation may very well be helpful in the immediate management of the patient. Prior to biopsy, one should ensure that the laser is functioning and that an ampule of diluted epinephrine in ice-cold saline is available to squirt over the lesion after biopsy as needed.

If the offending lesion is distal to the mainstem bronchi and the bronchus intermedius, the application of carbon dioxide laser via the rigid bronchoscopy is usually impossible. In some large patients, usually males taller than 6 feet, a rigid bronchoscope can be inserted into the lower lobes. However, in general, even a No. 7 rigid scope is too large or cannot negotiate the turns to get consistent access to the lower lobe bronchi. In this situation and always for the left upper lobe, different techniques are required. YAG laser via a flexible scope may be used. However, the authors recommend caution with the use of the YAG laser for left upper lobe lesions; in this setting the authors prefer photodynamic therapy or surgical resection.

If an offending lesion cannot be identified, the surgeon should try to ascertain which side of the bronchial tree, the right or left, had the most or freshest blood in it. Then, a thorough evaluation of each lobe and its subsegments should be undertaken. Often, it is necessary to place the flexible scope just inside the opening of each lobe and to let it remain there patiently. This approach ensures that one has not missed a slow oozing from each lobe. This technique should be performed sequentially, starting at the lower lobes and working cephalad, eliminating each segment and lobe one at a time as the source of bleeding.

Photodynamic therapy, a relatively new technique, may even be useful acutely. Although it is currently thought that the photosensitizing agent must be given 48 to 72 hours prior to activation, it may work acutely. Intravenous Photofrin (2 mg/kg) is given in the operating room, and the KTP laser can be shone onto the lesion. Photodynamic therapy, the most effective treatment of recurrent hemoptysis in a nonacute setting in our hands for malignant lesions, has become our treatment of choice for patients with recurrent significant hemoptysis from malignant disease who have stage IV lung cancer and/or endobronchial metastases who are not candidates for surgical resection.

If the bleeding source is identified and cannot be controlled, a final option is to exclude or block that part of the airway. This option, which is usually not needed, should be reserved for the rare lesion that cannot be controlled with the techniques described previously. If repeated attempts to stop the bleeding fail or if the bleeding is coming from a subsegmental bronchus that cannot be intubated and thus treated with a laser or scope, that part of the airway should be excluded from the rest of the bronchial tree. A small Fogarty catheter can be placed, first down through a single-lumen endotracheal tube and then down into the segment in question. Care should be taken not to inflate too much air in the balloon, so bronchial ischemia is prevented. The patient should be stabilized, coagulopathy corrected, fluid status normalized, elective radiographic evaluation performed, pulmonary function evaluated, and elective surgical resection or percutaneous embolization performed. Keys to surgical resection in this setting, *discussed elsewhere in this textbook,* include double-lumen endotracheal tubes or blockers, early division of the bronchus, and buttressing of the bronchus if the patient had inflammatory disease with a muscle or autogenous tissue.

If the bleeding is from a proximal lobar segment and the entire lung needs to be blocked, a double-lumen endotracheal tube should *not* be placed for several reasons. First, although it is easy to place electively, it is difficult to place in a bloody airway. A double-lumen tube requires a pediatric bronchoscope, and suctioning significant amounts of blood through this instrument is difficult. Second, it is difficult to suction a double-lumen tube later in the intensive care unit. Third, it may cause pressure necrosis or ischemia if left in place for more than 24 hours. Fourth, if dislodged in the middle of the night in a blood-filled airway, it requires specially trained personnel to reposition it, who may not be available acutely.

DIAGNOSIS AND MANAGEMENT IN THE PATIENT WITH NONSIGNIFICANT HEMOPTYSIS

In the patient who does not require urgent bronchoscopy, the authors prefer that chest radiography, pulmonary function testing, and chest CT be performed prior to bronchoscopy. Pulmonary function testing itself may exacerbate hemoptysis. Ventilation-perfusion scans should also be performed if a large mass, obstructed lung, or poorly perfused lung is suspected, and the patient has compromised pulmonary function, to evaluate whether pneumonectomy is an option. Arteriography may also be indicated not only to aid in localizing the site but, more importantly, to embolize enlarged bronchial arteries that lead to the offending lesion.

Arteriographic embolization is especially useful in the patient with granulomatous disease, characterized by enlarged lymph nodes or bronchiectasis. The blood vessels that supply these lymph nodes are branches off of the bronchial artery and can become quite large. Some examples of these disorders are tuberculosis, cystic fibrosis, cystic sarcoidosis, or other diseases that can lead to bronchiectasis. Embolizations may also be used therapeutically in the patient with hemoptysis who has an arteriovenous malformation.

Computed tomography of the chest is extremely important in guiding treatment. Based on its findings, along with the other diagnostic studies mentioned, different treatment strategies can be developed. In general, the treatment options available are surgical resection, bronchial artery embolization, and medical therapy for treating the underlying cause. Often, these latter two options are best used as a bridge to surgery. They can slow down bleeding and allow the surgeon the opportunity to stabilize the patient, clear the airway, improve oxygenation, correct coagulopathies, and then perform an elective surgical resection with less risk than that with an emergent operation. Although it is impossible to identify all the salient features that lead one to choose one specific treatment strategy over another given the scope of this chapter, some basic guidelines can be offered.

In general, the therapeutic decision depends on the underlying pulmonary function, extent, and anatomic dis-

tribution of disease, surrounding pulmonary parenchyma and the etiology of the bleed. If CT reveals enlarged calcified lymph nodes, usually from fungal disease such as histoplasmosis or tuberculosis, surgical treatment is difficult. These nodes cause hemoptysis by eroding into the bronchus or the pulmonary artery. If the lymph nodes are large and focal and if bronchoscopy confirms this area as the site of bleeding, thoracotomy and surgical incision and curettage of the nodes may be the best option. This operation is difficult and risky because the nodes distort the normal anatomy, and they are plastered to the pulmonary artery. If the nodes are multiple and small, surgical resection with curettage should be avoided, and embolization should be employed.

If CT shows a peripheral abscess cavity, surgical resection is best. Aspergilloma cavities in nondiseased lung can usually be easily resected. Operation should be performed electively to reduce the risk. After any pulmonary resection for hemoptysis, bronchoscopy should be performed at the end of the operation to remove residual blood from the tracheobronchial tree. If the patient has invasive *Aspergillus* and the surrounding lung is severely involved or diseased (i.e., bronchiectasis), surgical resection carries a high mortality. These patients are usually ill and have poor pulmonary function. All attempts at medical management and arteriographic embolization should be exhausted prior to surgery.

If the CT with contrast enhancement shows an arteriovenous fistula, management depends on whether it is single or focal, ruptured, or contained and its location. For fistulas that are single and subpleural, surgical resection is best, since rupture can lead to exsanguination into the free pleural space. If the patient is pregnant, management depends on the stage of her pregnancy and

---

Pearls and Pitfalls

- Hemoptysis can be from malignant or benign disease.
- First, one must ascertain that bleeding is from the tracheal bronchial tree, not the nose or stomach.
- If hemoptysis is massive, one should perform immediate rigid bronchoscopy for diagnostic and therapeutic reasons.
- If hemoptysis is nonmassive, perform chest radiography, chest CT, and elective bronchoscopy.
- Most acute bleeding can be controlled with carbon dioxide or YAG lasers, ice-cold saline lavage, and/or topical epinephrine.
- If one cannot control bleeding (which is rare), identify the exact source, block off that part of the airway, to prevent blood from filling the rest of the airway.
- Resuscitate the patient, correct underlying coagulopathy, perform radiographs, obtain pulmonary function tests, and ventilation-perfusion scans. Use arteriography if the patient is still bleeding or is unstable for operation, or in isolated cases if anatomy is better treated with embolization (i.e., patients with bronchiectasis from cystic sarcoidosis or tuberculosis, or patients with multiple arteriovenous fistulas).
- Once the patient is stabilized, if the bleeding source is focal or if there is a cavitary lung mass or nodule, resect electively.

the location of the fistula. Often, arteriovenous fistulas are present during pregnancy because of the hypervolemic state and the smooth muscle dilation caused by the hyperprogesterone state. The prolonged periods of fluoroscopy required for multiple embolizations in the pregnant patient need to be weighed into the risk/benefit ratio even with the uterus shielded. If the patient has Osler-Weber-Rendu disease, the fistulas are often multiple and best handled by embolization.

Pulmonary emboli may also present with significant hemoptysis and the usual treatment of anticoagulation cannot be used. The patient should have a caval filter placed and treated expectantly. Other rare causes of hemoptysis include mitral stenosis and vascular-bronchial or tracheal fistulas. The latter, although uncommon, seem to be increasing in frequency as more patients have repair of ascending aortic aneurysms, and more patients live to be older. The synthetic thoracic aortic graft can erode into the left mainstem bronchus, the pulmonary artery, or into the left upper or left lower lobe. The authors have treated three patients with this problem. The aneurysm itself prior to repair may also erode into the lung, the airway, or surrounding vessels. A tracheal-innominate fistula is another situation that requires careful planning and intraoperative management; ligation of the innominate artery is usually required.

In conclusion, hemoptysis, although usually scanty and intermittent, can often be massive and continuous. Successful treatment depends on carefully planned algorithms. For massive hemoptysis, early rigid bronchoscopy to aid in diagnosis and to treat the various underlying causes is required.

SELECTED READINGS

Haponik EF, Chin R: Hemoptysis: Clinicians' perspectives. Chest 1990;97:541.

Conlan AA, Hurwit SS, Krige L, et al: Massive hemoptysis. J Thorac Cardiovasc Surg 1983;85:120.

Faber LP, Jensik RJ, Chamla SK: The surgical implications of broncholithiasis. J Thorac Cardiovasc Surg 1975;70:779.

Guimaraes C: Massive hemoptysis. In Pearson FG et al (ed): Thoracic Surgery. 2nd ed. New York, Churchill Livingstone, 1998, pp 581–596.

Stedman's Medical Dictionary, 24th edition, Williams & Wilkins, 1982.

Trastek VF, Pairolero PC, Ceithaml EL: Surgical management of broncholithiasis. J Thorac Cardiovasc Surg 1985;90:842.

Wedzicha JA, Pearson MC: Management of massive haemoptysis. Resp Med 1990;84:9.

Chapter 139

Spontaneous Pneumothorax and Lung Volume Reduction Surgery

M. Bulent Tirnaksiz, Antonio L. Visbal, and Claude Deschamps

SPONTANEOUS PNEUMOTHORAX

Entry of air into the pleural space is secondary to a disruption in the continuity of the pleural membrane, whether it is parietal, visceral, or mediastinal. Spontaneous pneumothoraces can be classified as primary, in which there is no identifiable pathology, and secondary, usually associated with chronic obstructive pulmonary disease (COPD). Catamenial pneumothoraces, which occur at the time of menstruation, are rare. Traumatic pneumothoraces include not only those seen with thoracic injuries but also pneumothoraces complicating positive-pressure mechanical ventilation or invasive monitoring techniques, such as Swan-Ganz catheterization. Pneumothorax complicates transthoracic needle biopsy in about 20% of patients.

Primary Spontaneous Pneumothorax

Primary spontaneous pneumothorax occurs predominantly in young, healthy men. The overall incidence is estimated at 5 to 10 cases per 100,000 per year, but it can be as high as 1 in 500 young men. Most primary spontaneous pneumothoraces are caused by rupture of subpleural blebs (Fig. 139–1) in lungs that are otherwise normal. Air escape occurs when the distending pressure in the bleb exceeds the elastic strength of its wall and causes it to rupture intrapleurally. The pathogenesis of these apical blebs is unknown, although spontaneous pneumothoraces occur most often in tall, thin individuals who are often smokers; they may be associated with connective tissue disorders such as Marfan's syndrome. It is postulated that, in the tall and thin, the rapid growth

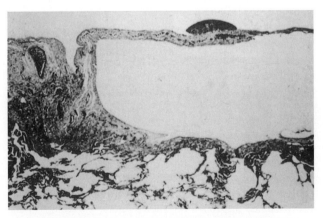

Figure 139–1. Photomicrograph of a subpleural bleb.

rate of the lung relative to pulmonary vasculature causes ischemia and bleb formation at the apex, farther away from the main arterial supply of the pulmonary hilum. It is also postulated that higher transpulmonary pressures at the apex in tall individuals lead to greater alveoli distending pressures.

DIAGNOSIS. The predominant symptom of pneumothorax in young people is an acute pleuritic chest pain, which often subsides over 24 hours. Physical exertion is rarely related to the occurrence of pneumothorax. Although the extent of collapse can best be quantified by measuring the diameters of the lung and hemithorax on chest radiograph, most physicians estimate pneumothoraces without actual measurements, which might result in an underestimation of the pneumothorax. If the diagnosis is suspected but cannot be confirmed by a routine chest radiograph, a chest film taken during expiration may accentuate the pneumothorax.

MANAGEMENT OF FIRST EPISODE—UNCOMPLICATED. Patients with less than a 20% collapse, minimal symptoms, and no radiologic evidence of progression can be observed. Roentgenographic lung volume studies can identify that the rate of air absorption from the pleural space is relatively constant at 1.25% per day when the leak has sealed. Activities should be restricted, and 2 to 3 days of in-hospital observation may be needed to ensure that no complications develop. The main argument for more aggressive management is that the duration of therapy can be shortened considerably by surgery. Absolute indications for tube drainage include a more than 20% collapse shown on the first chest film, tension pneumothorax, disease of the contralateral lung, symptoms, or progression of the pneumothorax on successive chest film.

CHEST TUBE INSERTION. The preferred site of insertion of the chest tube is at the fourth or fifth interspace in the midaxillary line, rather than the second interspace in the midclavicular line. The former is more cosmetically acceptable, and the technique of insertion is easier. There are no chest wall muscles to go through, and the risk of puncturing the internal mammary artery is avoided. In addition, when inserted through the axilla, the tube has a natural tendency to slide upward along the lateral chest wall. There are two accepted techniques: the *trocar method* is popular but is more likely to injure the lung or other intrathoracic structure; *blunt dissection* with a Kelly hemostat clamp is safer and has largely replaced the trocar method. Although water-seal suction drainage has no documented advantage, most surgeons believe that a high negative intrapleural pressure promotes sealing of the leak against the parietal pleura and secondary pleural symphysis. One-way flutter valves like the Heimlich valve allow the pleural space to be evacuated without the inconvenience of a water-seal system. Outpatient management with a flutter valve can be safe and cost effective.

MANAGEMENT OF FIRST EPISODE COMPLICATED BY TENSION. Although most primary spontaneous pneumothoraces are uncomplicated, such problems as tension, hemorrhage, persistent air leak, failure to expand, or recurrence may force the surgeon to change the treatment plan. Tension pneumothorax requires immediate action. It occurs when a tear in the lung produces a one-way valve that opens during inspiration (and air flows into the pleural space) but closes during exhalation. As tension increases, the mediastinum shifts toward the contralateral side. Tension pneumothorax interferes with ventilation, venous return, and ultimately cardiac output. Tension may develop at any time, and its onset is often sudden and dramatic.

HEMOPNEUMOTHORAX. Pleural effusion reportedly occurs in 20% of patients with pneumothorax, but frank hemothorax occurs in less than 5%. In general, the bleeding is arterial and secondary to a torn adhesion between visceral and parietal pleurae. The bleeding point is nearly always on the chest wall side of the adhesion. The onset is often insidious, and the diagnosis can be delayed if a small chest catheter has been used to drain the space. When lung expansion successfully tamponades the bleeding site, as is often the case, treatment can be conservative. Some of these individuals may need surgical intervention for control of the bleeding and removal of blood clots.

Specific Situations

Although most air leaks have already sealed when the chest is drained or stop within the first 12 to 24 hours, 3% to 4% of patients will develop a persistent fistula after several days of drainage. When this problem occurs, chest tube drainage for more than 10 days is inadvisable, and operative treatment should be considered to close the fistula and obliterate the space. Despite proper tube placement and adequate suction, the lung may show only partial expansion on postdrainage chest radiograph. Management requires direct operative closure of the fistula or decortication of the lung or both. Spontaneous pneumothorax may be associated with a pneumo-mediastinum. Air is thought to dissect into the mediastinum along the bronchi or the vascular sheaths of pulmonary vessels. This finding has no clinical consequence, although compression of the great vessels has been reported in children. Simultaneous bilateral pneumothorax is rare. Subcutaneous emphysema always indicates that drainage is inadequate. The chest tube may be malpositioned or obstructed, or one of the side holes might have slipped outside the pleural cavity. In other patients, the drainage system is not working properly, or the amount of suction is inadequate for a large leak.

RECURRENCE. Primary spontaneous pneumothorax tends to recur. The risk of recurrence is about 20%, but this risk increases to 60% to 80% in patients who have suffered more than one previous episode. Risk factors include more than one previous episode, smoking, COPD, air leak for more than 48 hours during the first episode, and large air cysts seen on the chest film or computed tomography. The significance of the method of treatment used during the first episode and the duration of pleural intubation are unknown. Some investigations have suggested that leaving the tube for 3 to 4 days induces an inflammatory reaction and reduces the chances of recurrence.

MANAGEMENT. To prevent recurrences, the pleural space should be obliterated and the disease site resected. Pleural space obliteration can be accomplished by chemical pleurodesis, mechanical abrasion, or parietal pleurectomy, and resection is by suture closure, wedge resection, or electrocoagulation. The surgeon should look actively for other blebs or bullae likely to be in the apical area of the upper lobe or the superior segment of the lower lobe. Failure to identify a bleb is an independent predictor of recurrence rate in patients with spontaneous primary pneumothoraces. Intrapleural instillation of chemical agents starts an inflammatory reaction of the pleural mesothelium, with adhesion and fibrosis formation. The main inconveniences of these techniques are their toxicity, which consists of a painful febrile reaction and pleural effusion, the nonuniformity of pleural adhesions, which also tend to form over mediastinal and diaphragmatic surfaces, and the variability of results.

Tetracycline and talc are the two chemicals most often used for pleurodesis. Scarification of the pleura with dry gauze is effective in preventing recurrences, especially when combined with bleb excision. Regardless of the instrument used to create pleurodesis, the surgeon should aim at causing enough inflammation to cause capillary bleeding. The reported results have been consistently good, with minimal operative trauma and morbidity. This technique has the advantage of preserving an extrapleural plane if a future thoracotomy is needed. Parietal pleurectomy creates an inflammatory surface that promotes fixation of the lung to the endothoracic fascia. Many surgeons have described pleurectomy as the most secure procedure to obtain permanent pleurodesis. Because the disease is nearly always limited to the lung apex, an apical pleurectomy, combined with bleb excision, is recommended for definitive control of recurrences.

OPERATIVE APPROACHES. Surgery for pneumothorax can be performed through a formal lateral thoracotomy, axillary thoracotomy, or most appropriately a video-assisted thoracoscopic (VATS) approach. A formal thoracotomy is rarely indicated nowadays because of the resulting pain and disability. Adequate exposure to the apex with minimal discomfort can be achieved with both the axillary thoracotomy (Fig. 139-2) and VATS (Figs. 139-3 to 139-5) approaches. Advantages of the VATS approach include better visualization of the entire pleural space and possibly a shorter hospital stay. The recurrence rate has been reported to vary between 3% and 6%. Benefits of the axillary approach are the cosmetic advantage of the

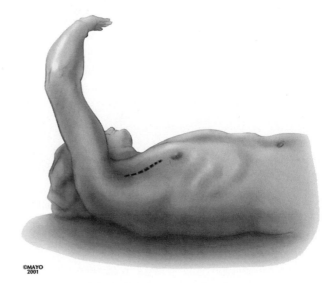

Figure 139–2. Axillary approach for the surgical treatment of a spontaneous recurrent pneumothorax.

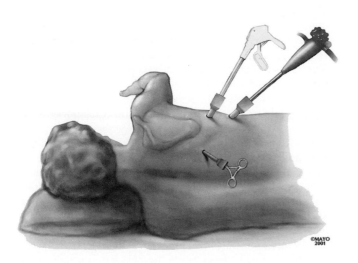

Figure 139–3. VATS approach for the surgical treatment of a spontaneous recurrent pneumothorax.

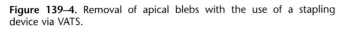
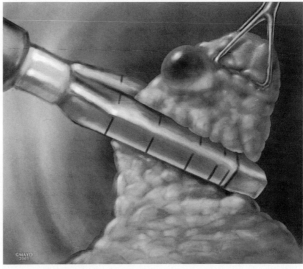

Figure 139–4. Removal of apical blebs with the use of a stapling device via VATS.

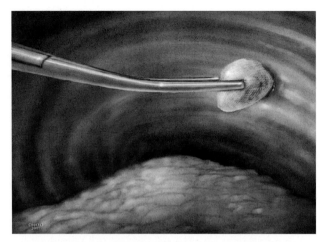

Figure 139–5. Mechanical pleurodesis with a dry gauze via VATS.

hidden scar and possibly a lower recurrence rate than with the VATS approach. Postoperative complications occur in 5% to 20% of patients and include prolonged air leak, bleeding, loculated pleural space problems, and recurrent pneumothoraces.

CONCLUSION. Recurrent pneumothoraces can be surgically approached with VATS or a transaxillary incision. These two approaches are safe, morbidity is minimal, and results are acceptable.

LUNG VOLUME REDUCTION SURGERY

In the late 1950s, Brantigan proposed that the removal of lung tissue would increase the circumferential pull on small airways and thereby relieve bronchial obstruction and dyspnea. Although many patients reported benefit, he made no attempt to document improvements in lung function. Because of an 18% perioperative mortality, the Brantigan procedure was not widely accepted, and the concept was viewed as ill-conceived by authorities of the time. The contemporary version of lung volume reduction surgery (LVRS) by open surgical resection was championed by Cooper and colleagues (1996). Their experience grew from observations made in patients undergoing lung transplantation for COPD. In their early experience with 20 patients, LVRS by median sternotomy produced an impressive 82% improvement in FEV_1 6 months after surgery.

Indication for Lung Volume Reduction Surgery

Typically, patients who have undergone LVRS in recent years have suffered from end-stage emphysema. Such patients exhibit severe obstruction and hyperinflation, and such patients are limited by severe dyspnea at rest or with mild exertion. Historically, indications and exclusion criteria for the procedure reflect physiologic reasoning and anecdotal experience, and these criteria have varied from center to center. Inclusion criteria often have limited

the procedure to patients with an FEV_1 of less than 40% of predicted, a total lung capacity greater than 120% predicted, and age less than 75 years old. Pulmonary hypertension, left ventricular dysfunction, hypercapnia, and other significant co-morbidities have all been considered relative exclusion criteria. Much emphasis has been placed on the regional distribution of emphysema as an important selection criterion. The distribution of emphysema is usually assessed with computed tomography as it guides the surgeon to "target areas" of more extensive disease. The prevailing view is that patients with upper lobe predominant emphysema are better surgical candidates than those with a more homogeneous distribution of disease.

Rationale

The emphysematous destruction of lung tissue causes a loss of elastic recoil, with a number of important consequences. First, airways tethered to lung parenchyma lose their support so that their diameter at any given lung volume is reduced. This mechanism contributes to the increase in specific airway resistance and reduced maximal expiratory flow. Second, the volume at which the lungs and chest cavity operate increases because the outward recoil of the chest wall is opposed to a lesser extent by the inward recoil of the lungs and because reduced expiratory flows cause dynamic hyperinflation. Dynamic hyperinflation, in turn, has important consequences on respiratory muscle activity and energetics and undoubtedly affects hemodynamics. Having to operate at high volumes not only places the inspiratory muscles at a mechanical disadvantage but also increases their elastic load from inadvertent positive end-expiratory pressure. Compounding the mechanical consequences of emphysema are the impaired gas exchange function of the lung and the propensity for limitations in cardiovascular exercise. Ventilation-perfusion mismatch, through its effect on physiologic dead space, raises the ventilatory requirement of patients. Hypoxemia complicating mismatch, hypoventilation, and sleep disordered breathing in turn promote pulmonary vasoconstriction, pulmonary hypertension, cor pulmonale, and right-sided heart failure. The success of LVRS in selected patients implies that these patients were limited by mechanical constraints on the respiratory system. After LVRS, the smaller remaining lung exerts a greater retractive force on the small airway by improving elastic recoil.

Surgical Technique

MEDIAN STERNOTOMY. Before the operation, while the patient is still awake, a thoracic epidural catheter is inserted for intraoperative and postoperative analgesia. Initially, a 6- to 8-ml bolus of 0.25% bupivacaine and 75 to 100 μg of fentanyl are injected in the epidural catheter, followed by a continuous infusion of 0.075% bupivacaine and 5 μg/ml of fentanyl at a rate of 8 to 10 ml/hr. A double-lumen tube is used for selective ventilation. The vertical skin incision is made shorter than the sternotomy

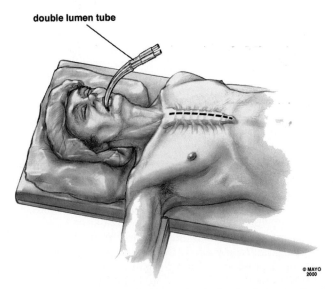

double lumen tube

© MAYO
2000

Figure 139–6. Median sternotomy incision (*broken line*) starts 2 cm below the edge of the manubrium and ends at the level of the xiphoid process. Note that the patient is intubated with a double-lumen tube.

to minimize the risk of postoperative sternal infection, in case a tracheostomy would be required during the postoperative period (Fig. 139–6). A small sponge is placed on a ring forceps, inserted under the xiphoid process, and used gently to sweep the pleura laterally on each side. Ventilation is temporarily stopped during the actual sternotomy. These maneuvers decrease the odds of penetration of the pleural space when the sternum is divided with the saw. The sternum is handled delicately, with hemostasis achieved with the electrocautery. Pads are placed on the sternal edges to minimize potential damage by the retractor, which can be standard or an internal mammary retractor. Ventilation is resumed on one side, while the procedure starts on the contralateral, deflated side, usually the side of the most affected lung. After 5 to 10 minutes, the areas of the lung with the most

perfusion will be deflated, while the areas most affected by emphysema will remain inflated.

The pleura is opened carefully to avoid damage to the adjacent lung. At the beginning of our experience, we were routinely attempting to bring down a portion of the apical parietal pleura to achieve a pleural tent, hoping to decrease the postresection residual pleural space. More often than not, the fragility of the tissue resulted in fenestrated parietal pleura that defeated the purpose, and we have since abandoned this fruitless exercise. The pleural space is inspected, and the lung is palpated delicately to search for unexpected pathology. When present, adhesions are meticulously divided with the electrocautery as far from the lung itself as possible, to avoid tears in the pulmonary parenchyma. Manipulations and electrocautery are avoided in the neighborhood of the phrenic nerve. Then, the inferior pulmonary ligament is divided under direct vision with the electrocautery to favor optimal postoperative re-expansion. Although this maneuver can cause hypotension, it is usually transient and well tolerated. The pleural cavity is then half filled with saline solution to elevate the lung in the wound. This maneuver minimizes manipulation of the fragile emphysematous lung and decreases chances of prolonged air leak or pulmonary contusion.

The areas of intended resection are usually identified prior to operation by computed tomography and perfusion scan. Usually the disease is worst in the apices. The lung to be resected is grasped with several Duvall clamps (Fig. 139–7), and the resection consists of removing approximately 50% of the upper lobe, using three to five applications of a linear 90-mm stapling device with 4.8-mm staples. The stated goal of LVRS is to remove 20% to 30% of each lung, yet it is unclear exactly how this number was adopted. The resection follows an inverted U shape to avoid significant mismatch between the contour of the new apex and the chest wall. The staple line is buttressed with bovine pericardial strips (Peri-strips Dry, Bio-Vascular, St. Paul, MN) or polytetrafluoroethylene (PTFE) to minimize postoperative air leaks. If pleu-

Figure 139–7. Several Duvall clamps are gently applied along the area to be resected. The stapling device is oriented in a manner so as to effect an inverted U shape excision of the parenchyma.

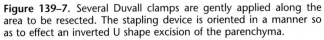

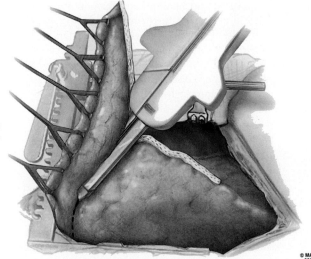

© MAYO
2000

ral adhesions are too dense in the area of intended resection, *extra*pleural dissection is recommended, and the parietal pleura adherent to the lung should be included in the resected specimen. When the disease is worst in the lower lobe, as in α_1-antitrypsin deficiency, the resection follows the curve of the underlying diaphragm.

The lung is then gently re-expanded under saline solution to look for air leaks. Although minimal leaks are tolerated, every effort is made to address a significant leak with either reapplication of the stapler, careful suturing of the parenchyma with nonabsorbable sutures, or, ideally, application of one of the recently FDA-approved lung sealant products (FocalSeal, Focal, Inc, Lexington, MA). The saline solution is suctioned, hemostasis is verified, and the pleural space is drained with a single 32-French chest tube, inserted laterally with the tip positioned at the apex. No specific effort is made to close the pleura since it is rarely possible to achieve a hermetically sealed closure. The contralateral side is then deflated, and the procedure is repeated in a similar fashion.

Throughout the operation, optimal communication with the anesthesiologist is of the utmost importance. The timing of the re-expansion of the lung, the maximal airway pressure (less than 25 cm H_2O), and the timing of extubation (usually in the operating room after the skin closure) are key points at which coordination between the surgical team and the anesthesiologist is vital.

A variety of other different techniques are available to perform lung volume reduction surgery. Laser ablation of pulmonary tissue is still promoted by some, but most surgeons have abandoned this procedure. Plication without resection of lung parenchyma has also been used but has not met with great enthusiasm.

Other Techniques

Surgeons who use a sternotomy route for lung reduction surgery generally perform bilateral reductions. Bilateral procedures result in greater improvements in lung function, but there may be a role for unilateral parenchymal reduction in selected patients. Surgeons who perform lung reduction by a thoracoscopic approach (VATS) have used both unilateral and bilateral approaches. When unilateral LVRS is indicated, posterolateral thoracotomy should be considered only if VATS is contraindicated. Anterior bilateral thoracotomies through the clamshell approach may allow a better exposure of the lower lobes and the posterior lung field. However, there is little justification to use this approach instead of the more simple, less painful midline sternotomy. There is no consensus whether LVRS via median sternotomy or via VATS is superior. Some have suggested that this depends upon surgeon preference. Several non-randomized studies have suggested that equivalent results are achieved.

Postoperative Care

The patient is extubated in the operating room, observed in the postanesthesia recovery unit, and then transferred for overnight stay in the intensive care unit. Postoperative

acidosis and hypercapnia, which are common in the first 12 to 24 hours, usually improve with time, as the effects of anesthesia gradually disappear and better pain control is achieved. Postoperative pain management consists of thoracic epidural analgesia supplemented by patient-controlled intravenous morphine analgesia and nonsteroidal anti-inflammatory agents.

A cephalosporin antibiotic is administered preoperatively and continued until the last chest tube is removed. We have a low threshold for empiric treatment with broad spectrum antibiotics when a new infiltrate is noted on the daily chest radiograph or when a change occurs in the appearance of the sputum. Oxygen saturation is monitored continuously and kept above 90% at all times. In patients using inhaled bronchodilators preoperatively, that medication is resumed on the first postoperative day. Rarely, parenteral steroids will be required to manage an acute exacerbation of bronchospasm. Chest tubes should not be removed before any air leaks have stopped and drainage is less than 300 mL over 24 hours. In the presence of a prolonged air leak (greater than 7 days), a Heimlich valve can be used to allow for dismissal home, provided the lung remains expanded while on water-seal. Early ambulation is encouraged, and an exercise bike or treadmill is prescribed two to four times a day, as tolerated, starting on the second postoperative day.

Outcome of LVRS

Most case series of LVRS focus on changes in FEV_1 as an important surrogate outcome for shortness of breath. Short-term improvements range from 30% to 99% of baseline. However, it is not uncommon to encounter patients with remarkable improvements in exercise performance despite minimal changes in FEV_1. The initial estimates of doubling FEV_1 with surgery have not withstood the test of time. The first report indicated a 99% increase in the FEV_1 (range 64% to 200%) in eight patients who underwent bilateral LVRS by median sternotomy. A more recent update by Cooper and colleagues (1996) on 150 bilateral LVRS procedures indicated an average improvement in FEV_1 of 51% at 6 months. Results for bilateral staple LVRS by VATS are similar. It remains unclear whether improvements from LVRS in pulmonary mechanics can be sustained or whether LVRS is followed by an accelerated decline in function. Other potential benefits from LVRS include decrease of supplemental oxygen dependence ("oxygen liberation"), decrease of exogenous corticosteroid dependence ("corticosteroid liberation"), and improvement in the quality of life.

Morbidity and Mortality of Lung Volume Reduction Surgery

Postoperative complications occur in as many as 50% of patients. Persistent air leak (>7 days) is the most commonly reported complication and occurs in 30% to 54% of patients. Reoperation has been necessary in up to 15% and tracheostomy in 13% of patients. Postoperative

Pearls and Pitfalls

- Spontaneous pneumothorax is most common in tall young men.
- Recurrence rates are about 20% but increase with a history of previous episodes.
- Some small, stable spontaneous pneumothoraces may be treated conservatively without a chest tube.
- Recurrence usually prompts operative treatment by thoracoscopic resection of blebs and pleurodesis.
- Lung volume reduction surgery (LVRS) is a recent technique for resecting space-occupying but non-functional emphysematous lung tissue to improve residual lung function.
- Candidates must be carefully selected.
- Operative approaches include a thoracoscopic approach or access via a median sternotomy.
- Although symptomatic improvements are common, morbidity and mortality are high.

pneumonia occurs in about 10% of patients. As might be expected, postoperative cardiac arrhythmias have been reported in about 15% of patients, and gastrointestinal complications, including cecal perforation, prolonged ileus, colitis, and peptic ulcer disease, are also reported, possibly related to the increased use of corticosteroid in this patient population. The mean length of hospital stay for patients undergoing LVRS ranges from 13 to 22 days and tends to fall with experience. The Heimlich valve has been useful in reducing total hospitalization in selected patients. Discharge to intermediate care or rehabilitation hospitals is required in 25% of patients for short-term rehabilitation.

In-hospital mortality varies between 5% and 10%. Long-term survival rates are difficult to ascertain from the literature, but mortality at 1 year has been as high as 25%. Considerable uncertainty remains about the natural history of COPD, making it difficult to place LVRS mortality figures into an appropriate context.

CONCLUSION

Despite the initial enthusiasm for LVRS for the treatment of patients with emphysema, it is imperative that the safety and efficacy of the procedure be established. The existing literature demonstrates that a largely undefined group of patients with emphysema appear to benefit from LVRS for an unknown period of time. As many as 30% of patients who have undergone LVRS do not appear to have benefited from surgery, and many more have been excluded from consideration based on hypothetical constructs that may not withstand the rigor of a carefully designed clinical trial. Several questions persist, including the long-term risk of surgery vs. medical therapy, the optimal selection criteria, the best measures of efficacy, the mechanisms of improvement (or lack of improvement), the duration of benefit, the procedure's cost effectiveness, and the optimal surgical technique. Until such basic questions are answered, it will remain difficult to advise patients regarding the best management of their emphysema. The National Emphysema Treatment Trial has the potential to answer many of these questions and should be welcomed by all who deal with patients who have this difficult problem.

SELECTED READINGS

Cooper JD, Patterson GA, Sundaresan RS, et al: Results of 150 consecutive bilateral lung volume reduction procedures in patients with severe emphysema. J Thorac Cardiovasc Surg 1996;112:1319.

Kim KH, Kim HK, Han JY, et al: Transaxillary minithoracotomy versus video-assisted thoracic surgery for spontaneous pneumothorax. Ann Thorac Surg 1996;61:1510.

Shrager JB, Kaiser LR, Edelman JD: Lung volume reduction surgery. Curr Probl Surg 2000;37:290.

Utz JP, Hubmayr RD, Deschamps C: Lung volume reduction surgery for emphysema: Out on a limb without a NETT. Mayo Clin Proc 1998;73:552.

Waller DA: Video-assisted thoracoscopic surgery for spontaneous pneumothorax: A 7-year learning experience. Ann R Coll Surg Engl 1999;81:387.

Waller DA, Forty J, Morritt GN: Video-assisted thoracoscopic surgery versus thoracotomy for spontaneous pneumothorax. Ann Thorac Surg 1994;58:372.

Chapter 140

The Thymus

Kirsten Bass Wilkins, Nora Malaisrie, Leon Schlossberg,
and Gregory B. Bulkley

INTRODUCTION

Mediastinal Anatomy

The mediastinum comprises the space in the chest between the pleural cavities and contains all the viscera of the chest except the lungs and the trachea. It is bordered by the thoracic inlet superiorly and the diaphragm inferiorly, the sternum anteriorly, the thoracic spine posteriorly, and the medial parietal thoracic pleurae bilaterally. Conventionally, the mediastinum is divided into four subdivisions: inferior, middle, anterior, and posterior mediastinum (Fig. 140–1). These divisions are based on both their content and the corresponding medical disorders that may arise within them (Table 140–1).

The anatomy of the mediastinum accounts for the clinical presentation of the pathologic conditions that develop within it. The contents of the mediastinum are invisible externally and are surrounded by bony struc-tures; thus, lesions arising within this structure are often asymptomatic until they have advanced sufficiently to cause a local mass effect. The treatment of diseases arising within the mediastinum is largely surgical, with radiation therapy and chemotherapy also playing a role.

Thymic Anatomy

The thymus is an organ in the anterosuperior mediastinum embryonically derived from the third and fourth pairs of pharyngeal pouches. During development, the resulting left and right thymic lobes descend into the superior and anterior mediastinum and fuse to form a single gland connected by a ventral isthmus. Smaller bilateral cervical horns extend into the neck (Fig. 140–2). Not infrequently, the inferior parathyroid glands may be located within the thymic capsule, challenging the parathyroid surgeon.

The arterial blood supply of the thymus derives from

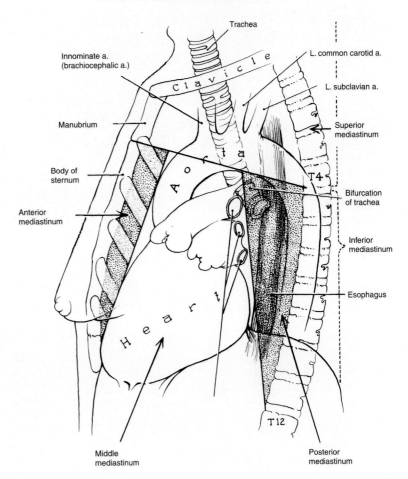

Figure 140–1. Gross anatomy of the human mediastinum, lateral view. (From Bulkley GB: The mediastinum and the thymus gland. In Zuidema GD [ed]: The Johns Hopkins Atlas of Human Functional Anatomy. Baltimore, The Johns Hopkins University Press, 1997. Used with permission.)

Table 140-1	**Anatomic Regions of the Mediastinum**

ANATOMIC REGION	CONTENTS	MASSES (TUMORS)
Superior mediastinum Inferior mediastinum Anterior mediastinum	Great vessels, vagus, phrenic and recurrent laryngeal nerves, thymus, lymph nodes (thyroid, parathyroid)	Thymomas, lymphomas, germ cell tumors, goiter, parathyroid adenomas, metastatic carcinomas
Middle mediastinum	Heart, pericardium	Pericardial cysts, cardiac myomas, metastatic carcinomas
Posterior mediastinum	Esophagus Aorta Inferior vena cava Thoracic duct, lymph nodes Thoracic intercostal nerve roots	Esophageal carcinoma Esophageal and bronchial cysts Duplications, rests, and diverticula Aortic aneurysms Metastatic carcinoma, neural tumors

several small thymic arteries, which arise from the internal thoracic (mammary) and inferior thyroid arteries. The two to six major thymic veins drain into the innominate, left brachiocephalic, internal thoracic, and inferior thyroid veins (Fig. 140–3).

Jaretzki's anatomic and histologic study (1991) discovered an extensive (normal) distribution of ectopic or accessory thymic tissue in the neck as well as in the anterior and even posterior mediastinum. Such ectopic thymic tissue in the mediastinum may be indistinguishable grossly from fat, even to the eye of an experienced surgeon (Fig. 140–4).

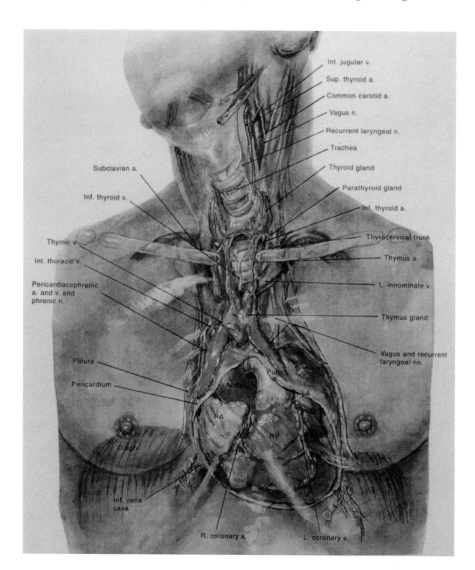

Figure 140–2. Gross anatomy of the human thymus gland within the mediastinum, anterior view. (From Bulkley GB: The mediastinum and the thymus gland. In Zuidema GD [ed]: The Johns Hopkins Atlas of Human Functional Anatomy. Baltimore, The Johns Hopkins University Press, 1997. Used with permission.)

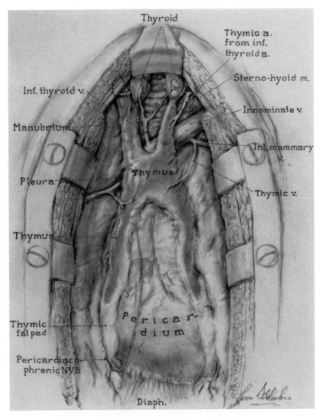

Figure 140–3. Gross (visible) anatomy of the human thymus. Immediately after median sternotomy, a typical, somewhat hyperplastic, thymus of a young patient with myasthenia gravis is depicted as it appears grossly to the eye of the operating surgeon. (From Bulkley GB, Bass KN, Stephenson GR, et al: Extended cervicomediastinal thymectomy in the integrated management of myasthenia gravis. Ann Surg 1997;226:324–335. Used with permission.)

The thymus is normally at its absolute largest in childhood, between the ages of 10 and 15 years, when it achieves a maximal weight of 25 to 50 g. As the child ages, the thymus decreases in size, and starting in the second decade the cellular elements of the thymus are replaced gradually by fatty infiltration. This process of fatty involution is usually complete by age 60 years, at which time the normal gland has decreased in size by 50% or more. Congenital thymic agenesis or hypoplasia is associated with lethal neonatal immunodeficiency. The congenital absence of the thymus as well as of the parathyroid glands is referred to as DiGeorge's syndrome, the human equivalent of the "nude" mouse.

The lobes of the thymus are divided into numerous lobular follicles, each of which are composed of a cortex and a medulla containing epithelial cells and lymphocytes. *Thymic follicular hyperplasia* refers to the appearance of lymphoid follicles within the thymus when the thymus itself may be normal in weight or slightly enlarged. This condition is most commonly encountered in patients with myasthenia gravis and is present in as many as 85% of these patients. In the absence of myasthenia, it is not considered a disease entity, and the "tissue windows" of modern computed tomography (CT) and magnetic resonance imaging (MRI) equipment allow its discrimination from thymic neoplasm with 90% accuracy.

THYMOMA

Thymoma is the most common primary anterior mediastinal tumor and accounts for 15% to 20% of all mediastinal masses. Thymomas are derived from thymic *epithelial* cells, thus distinguishing them from thymic lymphomas, germ cell tumors, and carcinoid tumors. Thymomas are classified into benign and malignant types, based on the presence or absence of capsular invasion and/or cellular atypia at presentation. Malignant thymomas are additionally divided into type I and type II. Type I malignant thymomas show invasion without evidence of cytologic atypia. These tumors tend to recur locally or by the formation of pleural implants. Type II malignant thymomas (thymic carcinomas) display cytologic atypia, with or without evidence of capsular invasion. Thymic carcinomas are uncommon, tend to be more locally aggressive, and are capable of lymphatic and hematogenous metastasis.

Several histologic classifications of thymomas have been proposed (Table 140–2). Thymomas are divided into predominantly epithelial, predominantly lymphocytic, or mixed lymphoepithelial types. More recently, thymomas have been graded on the basis of their differentiation toward normal thymic cortical epithelium or medullary epithelium.

Clinical staging of thymoma at presentation is shown in Table 140–2. Stage I tumors are completely encapsulated, both grossly and microscopically. This staging system then advances sequentially, with increasing degrees of invasion and spread, to stage IVb (metastatic) disease.

Clinical Presentation

Although thymomas are relatively rare neoplasms, they account for one third of all anterior mediastinal masses. The differential diagnosis for anterior mediastinal masses includes thymoma, lymphoma, substernal thyroid gland, and metastatic neoplasms including germ cell tumor. The exact incidence of thymomas is unknown, but most large series report 100 to 200 patients over approximately 30 years with an equal sex distribution. Although rare in childhood, thymomas may occur at any age, with a peak incidence in the fifth and sixth decades.

Thirty percent of patients are asymptomatic at the time of diagnosis. The thymoma is usually discovered incidentally during routine chest radiography, during CT, or at cardiac surgery. The remaining 70% are symptomatic at the time of presentation. Local symptoms are related to a mass effect in the anterior mediastinum and include chest pain (often described as "pressure"), dyspnea on exertion, cough, pneumonia, hoarseness, or hemoptysis. Systemic signs may include weight loss, fatigue, superior vena cava syndrome, or paraneoplastic syndromes, including myasthenia gravis, pure red cell aplasia, hypogammaglobulinemia, collagen vascular diseases, and aplastic anemia.

Myasthenia gravis is by far the most common associated disorder, occurring in 15% to 40% of patients with thymoma. Conversely, 15% to 30% of myasthenic patients have an associated thymoma. In a recent review of 136 thymoma patients seen at the Johns Hopkins Hospital,

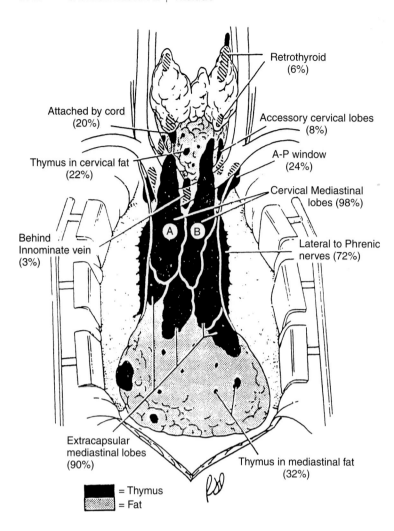

Retrothyroid
(6%)

Attached by cord
(20%)

Accessory cervical lobes
(8%)

A-P window
(24%)

Thymus in cervical fat
(22%)

Cervical Mediastinal
lobes (98%)

A B

Behind
Innominate vein
(3%)

Lateral to Phrenic
nerves (72%)

Extracapsular
mediastinal lobes
(90%)

Thymus in mediastinal fat
(32%)

■ = Thymus
▒ = Fat

Figure 140–4. Distribution of thymic tissue. This illustration is modified by Jaretzki from his classic description of the location of thymic tissue in 50 consecutive patients operated on by maximal thymectomy for myasthenia gravis. The digits on the figure represent the percentage (of those 50 patients) that had thymic tissue at that particular site. This classic study provides the rationale for the use of extended cervicomediastinal, or maximal, thymectomy for the treatment of myasthenia gravis. (From Jaretzki, A: Thymectomy for myasthenia gravis: Analysis of the controversies regarding technique and results. Neurology 1997;48[suppl 5]:S52–S63. Used with permission.)

Table 140–2	**Clinical Staging and Pathologic Classification of Thymomas**			
	OVERALL 5-YEAR SURVIVAL RATE (%)	**MASAOKA STAGE**	**LATTES/BERNATZ PATHOLOGIC CLASS**	**MÜLLER-HERMELINK PATHOLOGIC CLASS**
I	85–100	Macroscopically encapsulated and no microscopic capsular invasion	Lymphocytic: 2/3 of cells are lymphoid	Cortical: epithelial cells are large and pale, with vesicular nuclei
II	60–80	Macroscopic invasion into adjacent tissue (fatty or mediastinal pleura) or microscopic capsular invasion	Mixed: both lymphocytic and epithelial, with 1/3 or 2/3 of cells lymphoid	Medullary: epithelial cells are spindled with oval or fusiform nuclei
III	50–75	Macroscopic invasion into adjacent organ(s)	Epithelial: 2/3 of cells are epithelial	Mixed: both cortical and medullary features, with predominating feature reported as such
IVa	40–60	Pleural or pericardial dissemination	Spindled: 2/3 of cells are epithelial and elongated (fusiform)	WDTC: tightly packed epithelial cells with cytologic atypia and frequent mitotic figures
IVb	40–60	Lymphogenous or hematogenous metastasis	Thymic carcinoma: cytologically malignant cells	Thymic carcinoma: cytologically malignant cells

27% of patients presented with an independent second primary malignancy at some point in their course (Table 140–3). Although it is not surprising that such an association exists, given the role of the thymus in immune function, the mechanism of this relationship is unclear. However, the fact that thymomas are associated frequently with secondary neoplasms should heighten the physician's clinical suspicion and facilitate the earlier diagnosis of other tumors in patients with thymomas.

Preoperative Management

Radiologic Studies

A total of 50% to 60% of thymomas are visible on routine posteroanterior and lateral plain radiographs of the chest.

Table 140–3	Thymus: General Concepts

Thymoma
Differential diagnosis. Anterior mediastinal mass: thymoma, substernal goiter, lymphoma, metastatic carcinoma
70% present symptomatically, 30% radiographically
Anesthesia induction can be dangerous
Clinical (Masaoka) stage guides therapy and predicts prognosis
  Stage I, Resect
  Stage II, Resect and adjuvant radiotherapy
    Stage III, Radiate, resect, radiate
    Stage IV, Resect
      IVa + intrapleural ^{32}P } Reresect
      IVb + observation } prn
Only *independent predictor* of long-term prognosis = completeness of resection.
Prolonged, indolent course: patient survival
  5 yr ~70%
  10 yr ~55%
  15 yr ~38%
  20 yr ~35%
Patient twice as likely to die from other causes
30% of thymomas associated with myasthenia gravis
High incidence of associated disparate neoplasms
Myasthenia Gravis
Must have chest imaging (CT or MRI): 30% have thymomas
For generalized MG or severe, debilitating MG, thymectomy should be considered:
  early
  electively—MG under good control
  never during MG crisis
The *normal distribution* of thymic tissue includes extensive rests beyond the visible thymic capsule throughout the soft tissue of the neck and anterior mediastinum
Response to thymectomy is proportional to the completeness of resection of all thymic tissue
Response to anterosuperior cervicomediastinal exenteration (ASCME): 86% improve at least 1 Drachman grade
  Median improvement = 2 grades (of 5)
  Given ASCME, response is not predictable
  Response is delayed, maximal 3 to 12 months postoperatively
  Response is permanent, not transient
  There is *no* measurable associated systemic immunosuppression
  Other associated autoimmune diseases do *not* improve
Postoperative analgesia with epidural morphine improves pulmonary function significantly
During the perioperative period, serial FVCs are followed as a vital sign indicating, primarily, adequate analgesia and, secondarily, control of myasthenia
Even mild infections (e.g., UTI, sinus, viral URI) can precipitate MG crisis even in patients with otherwise mild disease; perioperative control of infection and atelectasis is critical to success

The thymoma appears as an anterior mediastinal mass, usually best visualized on the lateral view (Fig. 140–5).

Chest CT or MRI should also be obtained, each being more sensitive (65% to 90%) for the discrimination of thymic enlargement from hyperplasia versus thymoma. The CT appearance of the normal thymus gland is as a bilobed or, more often, triangular density situated just anterior to the aortic arch, with extensions from the left brachiocephalic vein down to the root of the great vessels (Fig. 140–6). On chest CT, the degree of local invasion by a thymoma may be assessed to some degree, including involvement of vascular structures and the presence of pleural implants or invasion of lung parenchyma (Fig. 140–7).

Biopsy

If on CT or MRI, an anterior mediastinal mass can clearly be identified as a thymoma, routine transthoracic biopsy by either fine-needle aspiration (FNA) or core-needle biopsy is neither helpful nor recommended before surgical resection. However, FNA, core-needle biopsy, or open biopsy may be helpful in stage III and stage IV disease if neoadjuvant chemotherapy or radiation is planned *prior* to surgical resection, or if the mass is not clearly identifiable as a thymoma and must be differentiated from a lymphoma, metastatic seminoma, or another condition that would be treated other than by primary resection.

Preoperative Radiotherapy

Thymomas that are clearly, by preoperative imaging, too extensive or massive to allow complete resection should undergo confirmative biopsy, preoperative radiation with about 40 to 45 Gy, followed by exploration for resection about 3 to 4 weeks after the last treatment. Many of these tumors are rendered resectable, or at least more amenable to effective debulking.

Intraoperative Management

Surgical Resection

Surgical resection is the mainstay of treatment for thymoma. In fact, the only variable that is an *independent predictor* of decreased thymoma-related death is complete surgical resection. Median sternotomy provides the best operative exposure for thymic resection. Even for small, well-encapsulated thymomas, complete surgical resection of the thymus, all associated fatty areolar tissue, and adequate soft tissue and pleural margins is indicated. This approach decreases local recurrences. Interestingly, resection of thymoma alone, without the adjacent thymic tissue, has been associated with the later development of myasthenia gravis. To ensure complete resection, the authors utilize an anterosuperior cervicomediastinal exenteration (ASCME; "maximal thymectomy") (see later).

Most stage I and stage II thymomas can be completely resected utilizing this ASCME. However, in the setting of stage III thymomas, resection of the tumor as well as

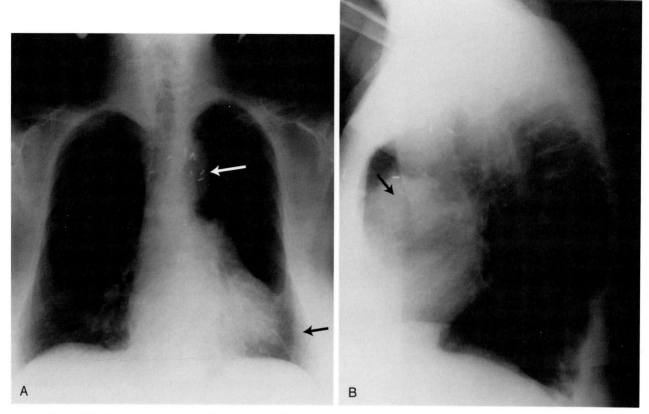

Figure 140–5. Posteroanterior and lateral chest radiographs in a patient with myasthenia gravis and a recurrent thymoma. *A,* Posteroanterior chest radiograph revealing an obvious mediastinal mass *(large arrow).* Note the pleural effusion that is associated with metastatic pleural implants *(small arrow). B,* On the lateral view, it is clear that the mass is in the *anterior* mediastinum *(arrow).* (From Wilkens KB, Bulkley GB: Thymectomy in the integrated management of myasthenia gravis. In Cameron J [ed]: Advances in Surgery. St. Louis, Mosby, 1999. Used with permission.)

of involved adjacent organs should be undertaken if clinically feasible. This may require resection of invaded pericardium, lung, innominate vein, and/or diaphragm. It is not unusual for thymomas to encase the phrenic neurovascular bundles (especially on the left side), making it necessary and appropriate to resect a single phrenic nerve if this will achieve a negative surgical margin. This aggressive approach to resection is based on the knowledge that complete resection is an independent predictor of survival.

With ASCME, a majority of patients are able to undergo complete resection. However, with very advanced disease, complete resection may be impossible, and in these situations some authors advocate partial resection (debulking), citing that partial resection improves survival compared with biopsy alone. Surgical clips are left along the margins of resection to aid the radiation oncologist during adjuvant radiation therapy.

Finally, repeat surgery is often undertaken for the resection of local recurrences within the chest, including the mediastinum, pleural implants, or segments of lung parenchyma. This is usually part of a multimodality therapy, including radiation and/or chemotherapy. Long-term survival can often be achieved even in patients with locally recurrent disease when this aggressive multimodality approach is used.

Anesthetic Considerations

Large anterior mediastinal masses may be associated with an increased risk of severe cardiopulmonary complications during general anesthesia. Superior vena cava obstruction may be exacerbated and extrinsic airway compression may occur because of the loss of negative intrathoracic pressure and of bronchial smooth muscle tone. Patients with a history of superior vena cava syndrome, severe dyspnea, or unrecognized myasthenia gravis are at increased risk for these complications. In such patients, several approaches, such as use of fiberoptic intubation with the patient awake, use of longer endotracheal tubes to allow passage beyond obstructed areas, avoidance of muscle relaxants, and use of standby cardiopulmonary bypass, may be helpful.

Postoperative Management

Analgesia

The use of adjuvant epidural morphine is of small benefit intraoperatively, but it is of great benefit postoperatively. In a randomized, prospective, double-blind, placebo-controlled trial, patients undergoing thymectomy for myasthenia gravis who received epidural morphine not only

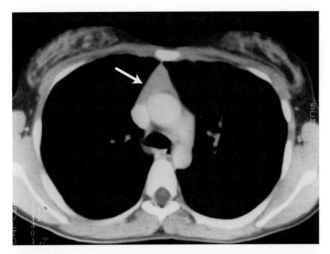

Figure 140–6. Computed tomography (CT) of the normal thymus in a 16-year-old girl. The CT appearance of the normal thymus gland *(arrow)* is as a bilobed or, more often, as shown here, a triangular density situated just anterior to the aortic arch, with extensions from the left brachiocephalic vein down to the root of the great vessels. (From Wilkens KB, Bulkley GB: Thymectomy in the integrated management of myasthenia gravis. In Cameron J [ed]: Advances in Surgery. St. Louis, Mosby, 1999. Used with permission.)

experienced less pain but also had much better pulmonary function postoperatively.

Radiation Therapy

Since thymomas are radiosensitive, radiation therapy is often used as adjuvant therapy after surgical resection. Stage I tumors rarely recur, making adjuvant therapy unnecessary. In patients with stage II and stage III disease, 40 to 45 Gy are routinely administered to the mediastinum in an attempt to decrease local recurrence rates. One series in stage II and III disease patients showed

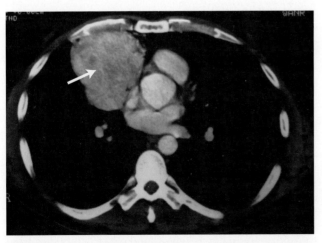

Figure 140–7. Computed tomography revealing the presence of a large but well-encapsulated thymoma *(arrow).* (From Wilkens KB, Bulkley GB: Thymectomy in the integrated management of myasthenia gravis. In Cameron J [ed]: Advances in Surgery. St. Louis, Mosby, 1999. Used with permission.)

5-year recurrence rates of 0 versus 53% in the patients who did not undergo adjuvant radiation therapy.

Neoadjuvant (preoperative) radiation therapy may be necessary in patients with stage III disease considered unresectable at the time of presentation because of invasion into the heart, pulmonary hilum, or great vessels. Radiation often effects regression of the tumor to the extent that complete resection can be accomplished. Radiation therapy may be used also for palliating patients with stage III or IV disease with significant symptoms, such as superior vena cava syndrome or airway compromise. Many patients experience rapid relief of symptoms, with an increase in both quality of life and duration of survival.

Radiation therapy may also have a major role in treating recurrent disease. Patients may require repeat surgical excision of local recurrences within the chest cavity. Postoperative radiation may be of use if they have not previously received a maximal dose of radiation. The complications associated with radiation therapy include transverse myelitis, radiation pneumonitis, and cardiomyopathy.

Chemotherapy

While the treatment of thymoma is based predominantly on surgical resection and adjuvant radiation, some centers are utilizing multiagent chemotherapy combined with surgery and radiation for the treatment of unresectable, locally advanced, and metastatic disease. Cisplatin is commonly used, along with other chemotherapeutic agents, and most studies report at least partial regression of tumor. Interestingly, the use of glucocorticoids has also been associated with tumor regression or lack of progression in patients with advanced disease. A similar association was noticed in some patients receiving steroids for control of myasthenic symptoms. Somatostatin-like agents have also been reported to be effective. However, at this time, the effect of chemotherapy on overall survival is unknown.

Complications

Operative mortality for thymectomy in most series should be less than 1%. Operative morbidity is also quite low. The most common complications include cardiac dysrhythmias and pleural effusions. As mentioned earlier, occasionally the phrenic nerve is intentionally sacrificed if it is involved with a tumor. Inadvertent permanent injury to either the phrenic or the recurrent laryngeal nerves occurs 1% of the time, while transient nerve dysfunction occurs in 2% to 3% of patients. Thoracic duct injury with consequent lymphothorax is seen about 1% of the time. In about half of these patients the fistula from the thoracic duct closes spontaneously following prolonged pleural damage, while half will require reoperative repair.

Outcomes

Tumor stage at initial presentation and the extent of surgical resection predict prognosis (see Table 140–2). In a recent review of 136 thymoma patients seen at Johns Hopkins, the *overall* patient survival rates were 71%, 56%, 44%, 38%, and 33% at 5, 10, 15, 20, and 25 years, respectively. Median survival was 12 years. In this study, about 35% of the deaths were related directly to thymoma or its treatment, and 60% were unrelated. The overall thymoma-related mortality rate was 14%, and the nonthymoma-related mortality rate was 26%. Thus, patients with thymomas were almost twice as likely to die from causes unrelated to the thymoma itself, reflecting the indolent nature of most of these neoplasms. Indeed, the thymoma-related survival rate was 87% at 5 years, 85% at 10 years, and 80% at 15 years. Independent predictors of improved overall survival were complete resection, presence of myasthenia gravis, age less than 57 at the time of diagnosis, and presence of lymphocytic, mixed, or spindle cell tumors. In contrast, the only clinical indicator that proved to be an *independent predictor* of improved thymoma-related survival was complete surgical resection.

MYASTHENIA GRAVIS

Myasthenia gravis is a neuromuscular disorder characterized by apparent weakness and fatigue of voluntary muscles associated with circulating antibodies against the neuromuscular acetylcholine receptor. Myasthenia gravis affects 1 in 75,000 people. There are two peaks in incidence: the first, which affects predominantly women (about 2:1), occurs during the second and third decades; the second occurs in the sixth and seventh decades and affects men more often.

Although it is clear that myasthenia gravis is an autoimmune disease, the origin of this autoimmune response remains unclear. In the search for an etiology, the thymus has been a logical focus; approximately 75% of myasthenic patients have some thymic abnormality. About 15% to 30% of patients with myasthenia gravis have a thymoma, whereas approximately 70% have rests of lymphoid follicular hyperplasia. Many myasthenic patients also have other autoimmune disorders, including thyroiditis (often manifested as hypothyroidism), Grave's disease, collagen vascular diseases, and rheumatoid arthritis.

Clinical Presentation

The characteristic signs and symptoms of myasthenia gravis are weakness and fatigability of the skeletal muscles exacerbated by repetitious activity and improved by rest. Impairment of extraocular muscles, manifested as ptosis or diplopia, is frequently the initial presentation. In approximately 15% of patients, the disease remains symptomatically localized to the extraocular and eyelid muscles. However, in most patients, weakness of facial and bulbar muscles develops, as well as generalized somatic weakness. Because of the facial and bulbar distribution of the weakness, the patient may present with a flattened smile, nasal voice, slurred speech, or difficulty in swallowing or chewing. Patients may cough after swallowing or may show other signs of aspiration. Generalized limb weakness is often proximal in distribution, and patients may complain of difficulty in climbing stairs, rising from

chairs, or elevating their arms for prolonged periods. Diaphragmatic and chest wall involvement reduces tidal volume as well as the strength and volume of the cough, predisposing the patient to lower respiratory infection. Patients are said to be in crisis when respiratory or bulbar symptoms become so severe that they cannot adequately sustain their own ventilation. The clinical spectrum of the disease as classified by Drachman is summarized in Table 140–4.

Preoperative Management

Diagnosis

On physical examination, neurologic dysfunction is limited to the motor nervous system, with sparing of sensory involvement. The Tensilon (edrophonium) test is used as an initial confirmatory test. Tensilon inhibits the enzyme acetylcholinesterase, which results in a transient buildup of acetylcholine at the neuromuscular junction, potentiating transmission and resulting in enhanced muscle strength in the myasthenic patient. Repetitive nerve stimulation studies should be done; a rapid decrement in the amplitude of the evoked muscle action potential is considered a positive response. In patients with questionable results, this test should be repeated with measured responses to stimulation of a single fiber. Antiacetylcholine receptor antibodies are assessed by radioimmunoassay, but only 85% of myasthenic patients have detectable increases in antibody levels.

The patient should be screened for associated autoimmune disorders. In particular, thyroid testing is performed, as both hyperthyroidism and hypothyroidism may exacerbate the symptoms of myasthenia gravis and, if undiscovered, can substantially increase operative risk. Thymoma is frequently associated with myasthenia gravis; thus, mediastinal imaging should consist of posteroanterior and lateral plain films as well as CT or MRI of the chest.

Medical Management

Anticholinesterase agents are widely used as the first-line of treatment in myasthenic patients. Mestinon (pyridostigmine) is most commonly used. When anticholinesterase agents are not adequately effective at managing the myasthenic symptoms, systemic, non–antigen-specific immunosuppressive agents, including corticosteroids, azathioprine, cyclosporin A, and cyclophosphamide, have been used as a means of reducing the immune response to the acetylcholine receptor. This approach is in contrast with the goal of thymectomy, which is to induce functional improvement by what appears to be, effectively, a more antigen-specific immunosuppression. Plasmapheresis is particularly effective in inducing rapid but short-term, nonspecific systemic immunosuppression via removal of the antiacetylcholine receptor (and other) antibodies from the circulation. It is often used as a means of optimizing the patient's medical condition quickly, albeit transiently, during the perioperative period. The detailed medical management of the patient with myasthenia gravis should

					FORWARD ARM ABDUCTION	MUSCLE GROUP	
CLASS	FUNCTIONAL IMPAIRMENT (ADLs)	OCULAR (PTOSIS/ DIPLOPIA)	FACIAL MUSCLE WEAKNESS	BULBAR MUSCLE WEAKNESS	TIME	STRENGTH (0–5)	FVC (%)
D1	Minimally independent ADLs	Intermittent	Mild	Normal	>3 min	5	>80
D2	Mildly independent ADLs	Constant	Significant	Mild, intermittent	>3 min	5−	>80
D3	Moderately independent ADLs	Constant	Significant	Significant, continuous	<3 min >90 sec	4 4+	<80 >50
D4	Moderately severe assisted ADLs	Constant	Significant	Severe, not debilitating	<90 sec >30 sec	4−	<80 >50
D5	Severely dependent crisis	Constant	Significant	Severe, debilitating	≤30 sec	≤3+	≤50

Table 140–4 · **Drachman Classification for Functional Status of Myasthenia Gravis**

ADLs, activities of daily living; FVC, forced vital capacity.

be supervised by a neurologist experienced with this disease.

Perioperative Management

The patient's medical condition should be optimized prior to thymectomy. This may be by the use of anticholinesterase agents alone or with the use of corticosteroids or plasmapheresis, or both. A patient should never undergo thymectomy while in myasthenic crisis. It is illogical to rush the patient to the operating room in an attempt to induce acute clinical improvement, as there is a lag of 3 months to 1 year before the beneficial effects of thymectomy become apparent.

General anesthesia can be performed safely, but myasthenic patients are particularly sensitive to nondepolarizing muscle relaxants. Therefore, although some anesthesiologists prefer to use depolarizing muscle relaxants, the authors avoid them, as they are not needed for a sternotomy. As discussed earlier, epidural morphine is recommended as a postoperative adjunct to thymectomy, unless there is a specific contraindication.

Operative Management

Thymectomy

In 1912, Sauerbruch reported remission of myasthenia gravis after the removal of the thymus gland in a woman with Graves' disease and myasthenia gravis. In 1939, Alfred Blalock reported the striking and sustained improvement of the symptoms of myasthenia gravis in a young woman 3 years after the removal of a cystic mass in the thymus gland. In 1944, Blalock reported the results of 20 trans-sternal thymectomies in myasthenic patients who experienced remarkable improvement in their myasthenic symptoms. Since then, thymectomy has been used with increasing success in achieving palliation and remission in patients with a wide spectrum of disease symptoms. In recent years, extensive but uncontrolled data clearly indicate that the results of thymectomy are so much better

than those of medical management alone that few patients with generalized myasthenia gravis are treated without early surgery.

Trans-sternal Thymectomy

A conventional trans-sternal thymectomy entails resection of the intracapsular cervical and mediastinal thymus gland via a full median sternotomy. Masaoka and colleagues (1996) have used a more extensive resection called a trans-sternal extended thymectomy, which includes en bloc resection of the thymus along with the extracapsular mediastinal fat. They found that the highest palliation rates (88%) were seen after trans-sternal extended thymectomy. These results were significantly better than those achieved with the use of either the trans-sternal simple resection (84%) or the transcervical simple resection (50%), suggesting that the more thymic tissue removed, the more probable the patient was to achieve functional improvement.

Anterosuperior Cervicomediastinal Exenteration (ASCME)—Maximal Thymectomy

Jaretzki's proposed "maximal" approach to thymectomy is based on his anatomic findings that thymic tissue is normally distributed extensively in both the neck and the mediastinum, outside of the capsular confines of the mediastinal lobes and their cervical extensions (see Fig. 140–4). Jaretzki uses a midcervical collar incision, separate from, and in addition to, a full median sternotomy. The mediastinal dissection entails bilateral mediastinal pleural excisions from the level of the thoracic inlet to the diaphragm (and 1 cm anterior to the phrenic nerves). The posterior mediastinal pleura is then carefully elevated (with the adherent phrenic neurovascular bundle) from the underlying thymic tissue. An en bloc dissection from diaphragm to innominate vein and from hilum to hilum is undertaken via sharp dissection directly on the pericardium. All thymic tissue and mediastinal fat, as well as the medial visceral mediastinal pleurae, are removed. The phrenic neurovascular bundles are preserved. Also included in the mediastinal dissection are the anterior pericardiophrenic fat pad, the fatty tissue in the sulcus between the superior vena cava and the aorta, and the fatty and lymphoid tissue in the aortopulmonary window. The intact specimen is then separated from the innominate vein by ligation and division of the thymic veins. The cervical dissection is then undertaken to the level of the hyoid. Care is taken to avoid injury to the recurrent laryngeal nerves. Pretracheal fat is removed en bloc with the cervical lobes of the thymus, which are followed to their termination in fibrous cords, or, not uncommonly, into accessory thymic lobes. The thyroid lobes are then mobilized, and any thymic tissue superior or posterior to the thyroid is removed (Fig. 140–8). Care is taken to distinguish parathyroid tissue. Jaretzki estimates that 98% to 100% of all thymic tissue is removed in this fashion.

Jaretzki warns that while trans-sternal extended resection has the potential to be comparable to his "maximal" procedure, the neck dissection during extended thymec-

tomies is frequently limited to the cervical extensions of the cervical-mediastinal lobes; accessory cervical lobes, retrothyroid thymus, and microscopic thymus in cervical fat may be overlooked. As a result, the trans-sternal extended thymectomy cannot provide maximal removal of thymic tissue. This view is supported by reports of, and the authors' own experience with, patients with thymic hyperplasia requiring re-exploration after initial transcervical or even trans-sternal resection, with the subsequent removal of residual thymic tissue finally affecting prolonged remission.

The authors use an operative technique similar to that of Jaretzki. However, instead of using a cervical incision, in these patients, who are often young females, access to the neck and the thyroid are obtained via elevation of a cervical flap from the cephalad end of the vertical sternotomy incision to the cricoid cartilage. This is facilitated by midline division of the platysma from beneath the skin, without dividing the skin.

Transcervical Thymectomy

Most advocates of transcervical thymectomy use an extended transcervical approach that involves a curved collar incision made between the sternocleidomastoid muscles. In the neck, the dissection is limited to the cervical lobes of the intracapsular thymus gland, but the accessory lobes, retrothyroid thymus, and pretracheal thymic fat are not resected. Once the neck dissection is complete, a special retractor is placed beneath the sternal notch. Upward traction is applied to the sternum to allow direct visualization of the anterior mediastinum, facilitating removal of the mediastinal thymic lobes and the anterior mediastinal fat. Cooper and colleagues (1988) have used this approach, with low morbidity, an excellent cosmetic result, favorable rates of improvement (95% of the patients followed had improved by at least one Osserman class, and 86% had improved by at least two classes), and a remission rate of 52%. It is unlikely, however, that complete resection accomplished with ASCME can be completed with the use of this transcervical approach. For example, complete resection of the epiphrenic fat pads, or of the tissue in the aortopulmonary window, may be difficult via a small neck incision. To date, no randomized trial has compared techniques. In the authors' opinion, ASCME remains the gold standard against which less invasive techniques must be measured with meticulous follow-up.

Postoperative Management

Although some surgeons prefer to discontinue oral anticholinesterase medication the night before surgery, the authors continue this medication until the time of surgery. Patients with persistent weakness may be supplemented with a continuous infusion of a cholinesterase inhibitor started at the time the mediastinum is closed. Usually, the dose of intravenous neostigmine, in milligrams, required as a continuous infusion over a 24-hour period is equal to the total daily dose of Mestinon, in milligrams, divided by 60. For the hourly dose, this value obviously

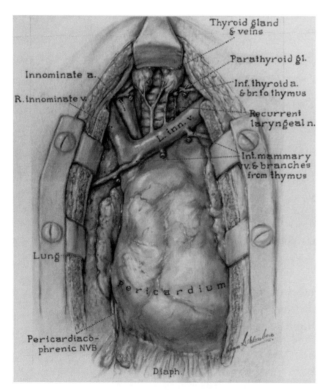

Figure 140–8. Anterosuperior cervicomediastinal exenteration (ASCME) as practiced at Johns Hopkins. This illustration depicts the mediastinal anatomy of a patient after ASCME as described. All fibrofatty connective tissue anterior to the pericardium, great vessels, trachea, and thyroid gland has been removed between the jugular veins and the (medial) parietal mediastinal pleura, from the diaphragm to the superior poles of the thyroid. Although not shown here, the dissection is carried to the superior poles of the thyroid gland, and to the hyoid bone. Thus, all evident fibrofatty connective tissue is removed from the anterior mediastinum, the diaphragm, and the superior mediastinum and neck, sparing only the great vessels and their branches, the internal thoracic vessels, the phrenic neurovascular bundles, and the recurrent laryngeal nerves. (From Bulkley GB, Bass KN, Stephenson GR, et al: Extended cervicomediastinal thymectomy in the integrated management of myasthenia gravis. Ann Surg 1997;226:324–335. Used with permission.)

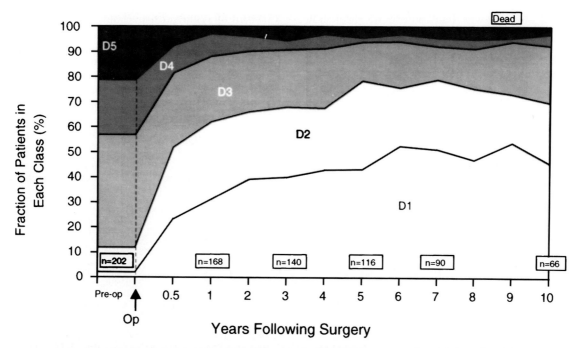

Figure 140–9. Response to therapy for all patients. This depicts the proportion of patients within each Drachman class (D1 to D5) before ASCME and at regular intervals after surgery for 10 years. Whereas only 12% of patients were class D2 or better before surgery, 86% and 83% of these patients were in this category after 5 and 10 years, respectively. The major increment of improvement appears within the first 6 months to a year but not immediately after surgery. These apparent differences in the distribution of disease severity are highly significant ($P < 0.001$) at each of the postoperative intervals. Only those who have died *from myasthenia gravis* are shown in the DEAD classification. (From Bulkley GB, Bass KN, Stephenson GR, et al: Extended cervicomediastinal thymectomy in the integrated management of myasthenia gravis. Ann Surg 1997;226:324–335. Used with permission.)

must be divided again by 24. The authors usually start this infusion at half this rate and assess the response thereafter.

Complications

The complications of thymectomy in patients with myasthenia gravis are the same as those described for thymoma. However, there is an increased risk of respiratory insufficiency that may require prolonged intubation or reintubation in these patients.

Outcomes

Before thymectomy was routinely performed in myasthenic patients without thymoma, the mortality from the disease approached 30% over 5 years. Today, with thymectomy as part of the integrated management of myasthenia gravis, this mortality rate has decreased to well below 5%. There is now a consensus that most patients with generalized myasthenia gravis, as well as those with debilitating ocular symptoms not controlled by anticholinesterase agents, should undergo elective thymectomy.

Pearls and Pitfalls

- The differential diagnosis of anterior mediastinal masses includes thymoma, lymphoma, substernal thyroid, and germ cell tumors.
- Thymomas, which account for about one third of anterior mediastinal masses, are often asymptomatic or manifest symptoms related to a local mass effect (cough, hoarseness, and pneumonia).
- Surgical resection is the mainstay for thymoma, but preoperative radiation therapy may convert locally advanced, unresectable thymomas to resectable lesions.
- Postoperative adjuvant radiation therapy is indicated even after "curative" resection; 5-year survival rates are stage-dependent but, overall, approach 70%.

- Myasthenia gravis is an autoimmune disorder of autoantibodies against the acetylcholine receptor at the skeletal motor end-plate.
- Diagnosis of myasthenia gravis is by the Tensilon (edrophonium) test or repetitive nerve stimulation with measurement of evoked muscle action potentials.
- Most of the patients with symptomatic myasthenia gravis should undergo thymectomy, not only because of the risk of thymoma (approximately 15% to 30%) but because symptomatic improvement occurs in roughly 85%.

Among 72 patients who had undergone Jaretzski's "maximal" thymectomy (without thymoma) reported in 1988, 96% showed some clinical improvement, 46% had no symptoms, and 33% were in remission at the time of last follow-up (6 months to 89 months). More than 200 patients (including patients with associated thymoma) have undergone thymectomy for myasthenia gravis since 1969 at Johns Hopkins. Only the last 127 patients in this series underwent this extended cervicomediastinal thymectomy, whereas the previous patients had undergone a more conventional trans-sternal thymectomy. In these 127 patients, there was no perioperative mortality, and morbidity was low. Patient improvement was quantified objectively with the use of the Drachman classification. The percentages of patients who sustained improvement over time are shown in Figure 140–9. By multivariate analysis, males, non-African-Americans, and patients who had not received preoperative plasmapheresis had an increased likelihood of improvement. However, the variable most predictive of improvement was having undergone the extended cervicomediastinal, as opposed to conventional trans-sternal, thymectomy. This increased the odds of improvement by 2.5 fold. The preoperative duration of symptoms, pathologic diagnosis (even the presence of thymoma), and age at surgery were not predictive of improvement. While ASCME is not a cure for myasthenia, it has a major effect in the majority (86%) of patients. Most are relieved of a major debilitating, potentially lethal disease, and are left with symptoms that constitute little more than a minor nuisance.

SELECTED READINGS

Bulkley GB, Bass KN, Stephenson GR, et al: Extended cervicomediastinal thymectomy in the integrated management of myasthenia gravis. Ann Surg 1997;226:324.

Cooper JD, Al-Jilaihawa AN, Pearson FG, et al: An improved technique to facilitate transcervical thymectomy for myasthenia gravis. Ann Thorac Surg 1988;45:242.

Drachman DB: Myasthenia gravis. N Engl J Med 1994;330:1797.

Jaretzki A: Transcervical/trans-sternal "maximal" thymectomy for myasthenia gravis. In Shields T (ed): Mediastinal Surgery. Philadelphia, Lea & Febiger, 1991, pp 372–376.

Masaoka A, Monden Y, Nakahara K, Tanioka T: Follow-up study of thymomas with special reference to their clinical stages. Cancer 1981;48:2485.

Masaoka A, Yamakawa Y, Niwa H, et al: Extended thymectomy for myasthenia gravis patients: A 20-year review. Ann Thorac Surg 1996;62:853.

Wilkins KB, Bulkley GB: Thymectomy in the integrated management of myasthenia gravis. Adv Surg 1999;32:105.

Wilkins KB, Sheikh E, Green R, et al: Clinical and pathologic predictors of survival in patients with thymoma. Ann Surg 1999;230:562.

Chapter 141

Mediastinal Masses
Sudish C. Murthy and Malcolm M. DeCamp, Jr.

THE MEDIASTINUM

The mediastinum defines that space located between the thoracic outlet and the diaphragm and is bounded laterally by the pleura, anteriorly by the sternum, and posteriorly by the spine and ribs. Structures in the mediastinum include much of the aerodigestive tract, the heart and great vessels, thymus, thoracic duct and associated lymphatic structures, major components of the autonomic nervous system, and, occasionally, ectopic endocrine glands. The intricate arrangement of tissues within the mediastinum contributes, in part, to the varied pathology found within this space and mandates a thorough knowledge of embryology and anatomy for surgeons who treat mediastinal disease processes.

Although the anatomy of the mediastinum is well defined, little consensus exists regarding compartmental subdivision of this complex space. This becomes germane when one considers the localization, safe biopsy, and treatment of primary mediastinal tumors. Several schemes have been proposed, and each has some merit. For this discussion, the division of the mediastinum has been simplified to encompass three major compartments (Fig. 141–1). It should be appreciated that a large mass in one compartment can easily encroach on another, and thus at some level the lines of division are not of critical importance.

The *anterosuperior mediastinum* extends from the manubrium and first rib superiorly to the diaphragm inferiorly. This compartment is bounded by the sternum anteriorly and by the ventral aspect of the upper thoracic vertebrae posteriorly. Within this compartment are the thymus and associated lymphatic tissues, the arch vessels, and the trachea and paratracheal lymph nodes. Ectopic parathyroid tissue may occasionally be found in this compartment, owing to the shared embryonic ancestry with the thymus. Thyroid masses may also descend into the anterosuperior mediastinum by direct extension.

The *middle mediastinum* extends from the pericardial reflection on the ascending aorta to the diaphragmatic surface of the pericardium. The heart and proximal ascending aorta, pericardium, carina and lymph nodes, and pulmonary hila are within this compartment. The superior vena cava (SVC) is located in the middle mediastinum as well, but it is often involved by compression or direct invasion from anterosuperior mediastinal masses.

The *posterior mediastinum* is bounded superiorly by the first thoracic vertebral body and inferiorly by the diaphragm. The ventral aspect of the upper thoracic vertebral bodies serves as the anterior border of this compartment above the atria, while the posterior pericardium limits the anterior extent in the caudal portion of this space. Posteriorly, the articulation of thoracic ribs with the vertebral bodies functions as the boundary. The posterior mediastinum contains the costovertebral sulci, associated segmental nerve roots, the sympathetic chain, azygos vein, and descending aorta. Several structures course through all compartments (e.g., the esophagus, thoracic duct, vagus nerve, phrenic neurovascular bundle), thereby precluding their assignment to any one anatomic space.

DISTRIBUTION AND INCIDENCE

Although the mediastinum is a common site of metastasis for some malignancies (lung, esophageal, gastric, hematologic), primary tumors and cysts are relatively rare. Primary mediastinal masses account for only 3% of the tumors within the chest, and between 25% and 50% are found to be malignant. The distribution and histology of mediastinal tumors vary greatly between adult and pediatric populations (Table 141–1). Almost two thirds of all masses are found within the anterosuperior mediastinum in adults, and more than 50% of masses in this compartment are malignant. Contrast this with mediastinal masses in children, in whom more than one half arise in the posterior mediastinum. The histologic distribution of primary mediastinal masses is summarized in Table 141–2. As might be expected from the anterosuperior mediastinal predominance in adults, thymic, lymphomatoid, and germ

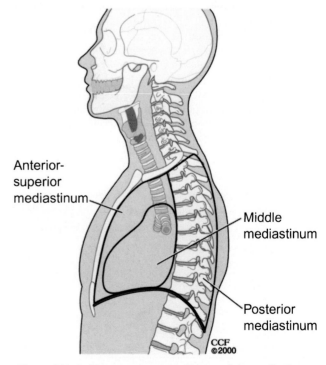

Figure 141–1. Three-compartment division of the mediastinum.

Table 141–1	Primary Mediastinal Masses in Adult and Pediatric Populations

COMPARTMENT	ADULT (% malignant)	PEDIATRIC (% malignant)
Anterosuperior	64% (56)	38% (25)
Middle	10% (16)	10% (17)
Posterior	26% (18)	52% (34)

Table 141–3	Most Common Invasive Primary Mediastinal Masses in Adults

HISTOLOGY	LOCATION*	PERCENT	5-YR SURVIVAL (%)
Lymphoma	A/M	42	54
Thymoma	A	26	60**
Germ cell	A	14	51
Neurogenic	P	14	56
Mesenchymal	A/M/P	9	33

*A, Anterosuperior; M, middle; P, posterior.
**For Stages II–IV.

cell origins are most common. In contrast, in children neurogenic tumors, arising primarily within the posterior mediastinum, are most common.

Longitudinal, population-based studies have suggested an increasing rate of malignancy found within primary mediastinal masses from 1960 to 1990 in both adult and pediatric groups. This increasing incidence involves lymphomas in adults and malignant neurogenic tumors in children. Increased use and availability of computed tomography (CT) in the management of other diseases frequently identifies unrelated incidentalomas, many of which turn out to be early mediastinal cancers.

Even with advances in the treatment of lymphoma, the prognosis of patients with primary mediastinal malignancy is not particularly optimistic. In adults, the overall 5-year survival rate is 33% to 60% for invasive mediastinal malignancies (Table 141–3). Lymphoma is the most common pathology, and it represents more than 40% of invasive malignancy in adults. Mediastinal mesenchymal tumors, primarily sarcomas, are the most lethal cancers, but, fortunately are quite rare.

SIGNS AND SYMPTOMS

The compact clustering of structures within the mediastinum leaves little space for asymptomatic enlargement of a solid mass. Consequently, it is not surprising that even when constitutional symptoms are discounted, as many as 75% of adults will present with symptoms attributable to their mediastinal malignancy. These signs and symptoms result from compression or frank invasion of adjacent structures and usually portend an ominous outcome. Benign lesions are symptomatic in only 30% of adults. Respiratory complaints include dyspnea, cough, hemoptysis, and, rarely, hoarseness (Table 141–4). Large anterosuper-

ior mediastinal masses may compress the airway when the patient is recumbent; thus, induction of general anesthesia for surgical biopsy must be carefully monitored, and fiberoptic intubation with the patient awake may be necessary if the airway appears tenuous. Dyspnea is occasionally caused by diaphragmatic palsy secondary to phrenic nerve invasion, and, rarely, a recurrent nerve may be involved, causing ipsilateral vocal cord dysfunction and hoarseness.

Posterior mediastinal involvement of the nerve roots, spinal cord, or sympathetic chain can lead to intercostal neuralgia, cord compression, or Horner's syndrome. Esophageal compression produces dysphagia and may predispose to aspiration. Very rarely, atrial arrhythmias can be precipitated by a large posterior mediastinal mass impinging on the posterior pericardium and left atrium.

Superior vena cava (SVC) syndrome occurs when the SVC becomes completely obstructed or compressed by large anterosuperior mediastinal masses. This symptom complex includes facial and upper extremity swelling, respiratory compromise from upper airway and tongue edema, headache, nausea and vertigo from cerebral venous hypertension, and development of superficial chest venous varicosities. Treatment is initially designed to rapidly debulk the mediastinum either with chemotherapy, radiation, and/or surgery.

The physical examination identifies definitive mediastinal pathology in only 40% of patients. Horner's syndrome (ptosis, myosis, anhydrosis) and the SVC syndrome should not escape detection by an astute clinician. On chest examination, a unilateral wheeze may signify mainstem compression, or decreased diaphragmatic excursion might suggest phrenic nerve paralysis. Masses may be detected

Table 141–2	Primary Mediastinal Masses in Adult and Pediatric Populations

ADULT		PEDIATRIC	
Thymic	26%	Neurogenic	43%
Lymphoma	17%	Lymphoma	18%
Germ cell	14%	Cystic	15%
Neurogenic	14%	Germ cell	8%
Cystic	13%	Thymic	7%
Mesenchymal	9%	Mesenchymal	5%
Other*	7%	Other*	4%

*Other includes endocrine masses.

Table 141–4	Clinical Presentation of Adults with Primary Mediastinal Tumors

SYMPTOM	PERCENT
Respiratory	26
Chest or neck pain	23
SVC syndrome	5
Dysphagia	1
Other	4
Constitutional	11
Asymptomatic	30

in the low neck as they emerge from the thoracic outlet. Both tracheal deviation and SVC syndrome suggest large anterosuperior mediastinal masses. Moreover, a general survey of the patient may identify signs consistent with a previously unsuspected endocrine anomaly, such as an ectopic parathyroid adenoma and mediastinal pheochromocytoma.

DIAGNOSTIC EVALUATION

Because of the low-yield of the physical examination in the evaluation of a mediastinal mass, clinicians must rely on a variety of diagnostic modalities to help define the disease process. Serum levels of beta-human chorionic gonadotropin (β-HCG) and alpha-fetoprotein (AFP) are useful in the diagnosis of germ cell tumors, while LDH levels assist in lymphoma evaluation. Radiographic imaging studies, however, are the mainstay of diagnosis.

CHEST RADIOGRAPH. All patients presenting with clinically significant respiratory or chest pain symptoms should have posteroanterior and lateral chest radiographs as part of their evaluation. Not only will these help to demonstrate a nonmediastinal etiology of the symptoms (e.g., pneumonia, pleural or pericardial effusion, hiatal hernia, rib fracture), but more than 95% of patients referred for management of a mediastinal mass will have the lesion identified by a plain radiograph. Chest tomography has been replaced largely by cross-sectional imaging techniques.

COMPUTED TOMOGRAPHY (CT). Chest CT has rapidly become the most popular diagnostic technique for mediastinal masses. With the advent of high-resolution spiral techniques, enormous information regarding the composition, position and relation to other vital structures, regional spread, and resectability of a mediastinal lesion can be obtained in minutes. Moreover, a high-quality CT proves invaluable in directing percutaneous, endoscopic, or open biopsy techniques.

OTHER IMAGING STUDIES. Magnetic resonance imaging (MRI) is most useful in the characterization of neurogenic lesions, vascular anomalies, and tumors involving the aortic arch, arch vessels, or brachial plexus. MRI offers detailed views in sagittal and coronal planes, in addition to axial imaging, thus permitting greater characterization of masses abutting the spinal canal and neural foramina or the brachial plexus. Angiography and ultrasonography have been supplanted by MRI and CT. Transesophageal ultrasonography and ultrasound-directed biopsy of mediastinal masses may prove useful in the future. Radionuclide studies (gallium) are occasionally employed in staging lymphomas and germ cells tumors.

Tissue Procurement Techniques

Although radiographic characterization of a mediastinal mass may be sufficient to preclude the necessity for tissue diagnosis, this policy should be followed only for obviously benign and asymptomatic mediastinal lesions. The majority of symptomatic mediastinal masses require an invasive

technique for tissue procurement. The location of the mass and radiographic appearance, general health of the patient, and expertise at the institute determine the most appropriate procedure. The goal of tissue biopsy is two fold: first, for diagnosis; and second, depending on the diagnosis, for further characterization of the mass (e.g., lymphoma typing).

Percutaneous needle biopsy is frequently used for diagnosis, especially in poor operative candidates. A success rate of 85% can be expected, either with an aspirate for cytology or a core-needle biopsy for histology. Complications such as pneumothorax and bleeding occur at a rate of about 5% at skilled centers. One limitation of this approach is that only small amounts of tissue can be recovered, often precluding use when lymphoma is suspected. Moreover, many lesions are inappropriate for the technique because of their anatomic location (e.g., juxtaposed to the pulmonary artery). Finally, many surgeons believe that capsular breach in order to make a diagnosis of early-stage thymoma is unwise.

Less-invasive surgical approaches for tissue procurement include mediastinoscopy, anterior mediastinotomy (Chamberlain procedure), and transbronchial biopsy. Mediastinoscopy can access the middle mediastinum and the posterior aspect of the anterosuperior mediastinum but is of limited utility, since few primary mediastinal masses present in these areas. Anterior mediastinotomy provides excellent access to the anterosuperior mediastinum. A transverse parasternal incision positioned over the appropriate intercostal space can be easily extended laterally, and/or proximal rib cartilage can be resected should better operative visualization be required. Most pathologists require a 1 cm³ amount of tissue for appropriate lymphoma typing; this amount of tissue can easily be garnered through this approach. A Wolf mediastinoscope can be introduced through a small mediastinotomy incision to facilitate biopsy of masses in the anterosuperior compartment. The surgeon must be wary of crush artifact and sampling error when employing this variation.

Video-assisted thoracoscopic surgery represents a new and useful tool in the management of mediastinal disease. A detailed survey of all mediastinal compartments from one side of the chest is easily obtained. Malignancies can be accurately staged and safely biopsied with a 100% diagnostic accuracy and a less than 4% complication rate.

With these less-invasive techniques, sternotomy or thoracotomy is rarely required for diagnosis. These approaches are best reserved for excisional biopsy or extirpative attempts.

ANTERIOR MEDIASTINAL MASSES

In adults, the most common primary neoplastic disorders of the anterior superior mediastinum are thymoma (45%), lymphoma (20%), germ cells tumors (15%), ectopic endocrine neoplasms (15%), and mesenchymal tumors (<5%). In pediatric and adolescent populations, lymphoma predominates, and thymic neoplasms are seldomly encountered.

THYMOMA. Thymoma is an epithelial malignancy arising in the thymus. Although the majority of thymomas appear histologically benign, some have the capacity for aggressive behavior (Fig. 141–2). While other malignancies employ the TNM classification, thymoma staging is based on another scheme. The Masaoka clinical staging system requires a postoperative histologic examination of the tumor because capsular invasion represents a critical component of the staging system. Thymomas are classified into noninvasive (stage I), minimally invasive (stage II), extensively invasive (stage III), and metastatic (stage IV). Although there are multiple histologic staging systems, prognosis appears more dependent on clinical stage.

The peak incidence of thymoma occurs between the fourth and the sixth decades. As many as 50% of patients are asymptomatic at the time of presentation, often fortuitously diagnosed during evaluation for an unrelated intrathoracic problem. Common signs and symptoms include those listed in Table 141–4. Unique to the symptom complex of thymoma are parathymic syndromes, the most

well documented of which is myasthenia gravis (MG). Myasthenia gravis complicates 30% to 50% of patients with thymoma, although only 15% of patients with MG have thymoma. Because of this association, all patients with suspected thymoma should have MG excluded to prevent an unexpected myasthenia crisis following elective thymectomy. Other parathymic syndromes include hypogammaglobulinemia (10% of thymoma patients), pure red cell aplasia (5% of patients), and numerous autoimmune diseases. Although parathymic syndromes cause significant morbidity and mortality, they often herald the existence of a thymoma prior to capsular invasion.

Thymomas confined to the thymus are best approached surgically. Many argue that biopsy prior to resection should be avoided to prevent capsular disruption and local dissemination of tumor. The most common surgical approach is through a median sternotomy, although cervical and video-assisted approaches have been

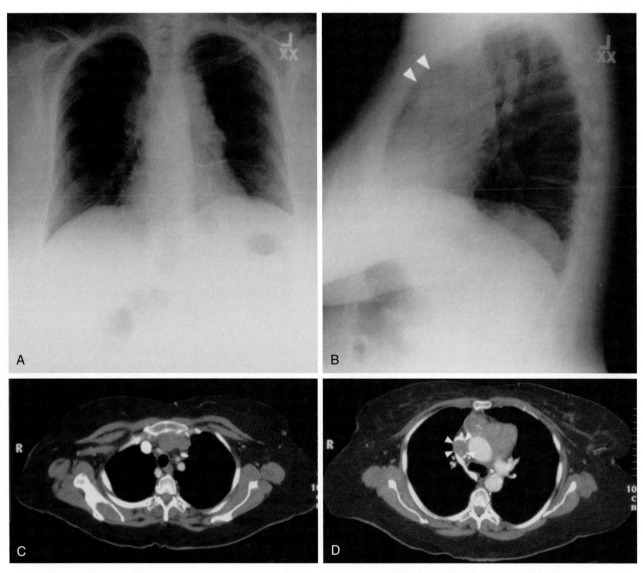

Figure 141–2. Radiographic staging of a patient with invasive thymoma. Posteroanterior chest radiograph *(A)* demonstrates widened mediastinum, and lateral chest radiograph *(B)* shows involvement of anterosuperior mediastinum *(arrows)*. CT of the upper chest *(C)* demonstrates replacement of thymus with tumor, and an image at the level of the carina *(D)* identifies tumor-embolus causing near-complete SVC obstruction *(arrows)*.

employed with arguably similar results. Even when gross invasion is present, en bloc exenteration of the thymus and adjacent structures provides survival benefit. Thymectomy for MG results in a 75% response rate, although only 10% to 20% achieve a drug-free remission.

For stage I (noninvasive) thymoma, the low risk of recurrence (<5%) and excellent long-term prognosis (>90% 10-year survival) do not justify the use of adjuvant therapy. However, when capsular invasion is present, the local recurrence rate is greater than 30%. Consequently, most surgeons suggest adjuvant radiotherapy for stage II disease. Platinum-based chemotherapy regimens are employed as primary therapy for more advanced thymoma and as salvage therapy for recurrence after surgery. Trials of multimodality therapy and octreotide for advanced disease are ongoing.

A very rare primary anterosuperior mediastinal malignancy, thymic carcinoma, is a disease entity different from invasive thymoma. The two most common cell types are squamous and lymphoepithelioma-like. Thymic carcinoma is a locally aggressive neoplasm and, unlike thymoma, frequently metastasizes to regional lymph nodes and distant sites. Combination chemoradiotherapy is the accepted therapy, and a 5-year survival rate of 30% is expected.

Thymic carcinoid may be mistaken for thymoma preoperatively. This lobulated tumor may exhibit areas of hemorrhage and necrosis on chest CT. Histologically identical to carcinoid tumors at other sites, 50% of patients present with endocrine-type syndromes. Cushing syndrome, from ectopic ACTH production, is the most common. The classic carcinoid syndrome is seldom seen, and therapy is complete surgical resection.

LYMPHOMA. Secondary mediastinal involvement by lymphoma presenting in extrathoracic sites occurs commonly in both Hodgkin's (>60%) and non-Hodgkin's (>20%) subtypes. However, presentation of lymphoma as a primary mediastinal tumor represents fewer than 5% of supradiaphragmatic Hodgkin's and non-Hodgkin's disease. Nonetheless, lymphoma is still the most common invasive mediastinal malignancy in adults and children. The nodular sclerosing histology is the most common type of Hodgkin's lymphoma, while large cell lymphoma and lymphoblastic lymphoma are the most frequent non-Hodgkin's types.

Symptoms and signs typically include cough and chest pressure, especially when bulky disease is present. Symptomatic SVC compression is observed more frequently with large cell and lymphoblastic lymphoma (30% to 60%). Systemic B-type lymphoma symptoms, fever, night sweats, and weight loss often accompany pain and respiratory complaints, and all symptoms are more common in the pediatric population. Interestingly, mediastinal lymphoma is perhaps the most frequently encountered mediastinal tumor presenting as a diagnostic emergency, attributable to airway compromise from rapidly proliferating neoplasms.

The role of surgery in primary mediastinal lymphoma is restricted to tissue procurement for diagnosis and accurate lymphoma subtyping. Seldom will needle aspiration or core-needle biopsy provide sufficient material for complete pathologic analysis. Superficial extrathoracic nodal disease (cervical, axillary, inguinal) should serve as a surrogate biopsy site if present. Moreover, bone marrow biopsy may prevent the need of an invasive mediastinal biopsy. For disease restricted solely to the mediastinum, one of the previously described biopsy techniques is chosen, depending on the anatomic location of the pathology.

Treatment options for mediastinal lymphoma include radiotherapy, chemotherapy, or combination therapy, as directed by cell-type and stage of the primary tumor. Occasionally, thymic lymphoma is discovered during resection of a suspected thymoma. In this scenario, complete resection simplifies postoperative therapy aimed at local control.

Castleman's disease is a rare lymphoproliferative disorder that can present as isolated mediastinal adenopathy. Complete excision or close observation is warranted if Castleman's disease is encountered, as there are reports of lymphomatous transformation.

GERM CELL TUMORS. Primary mediastinal germ cell tumors represent a heterogeneous group of benign and malignant neoplasms originating from ectopic primitive gonadal tissue. The histologies of primary mediastinal tumors are identical to their gonadal counterparts, and the anterosuperior mediastinum is the most common extragonadal site. Patients are usually young (<30 years) with an overwhelming male predominance (>90%) in malignant tumors. The evaluation of a suspected mediastinal germ cell tumor must include a complete physical examination with testicular ultrasonography to exclude a gonadal primary.

TERATOMA. Also known as dermoid cysts, these benign neoplasms are the most common primary mediastinal germ cell tumors. Histologic diagnosis is based on the recovery of at least two of three embryonic layers from the mass. The lesions are more commonly diagnosed incidentally in adults than in children, in whom cough, pain, and dyspnea are part of the symptom complex. A chest CT is often sufficient for diagnosis, and complete surgical excision provides excellent long-term results. Teratocarcinoma involves malignant transformation down seminomatous, embryonal, choriocarcinoma, or endodermal sinus cell lineages. Fortunately, these are extremely rare.

SEMINOMA. Seminomas constitute the majority of malignant mediastinal germ cell neoplasms. This diagnosis should prompt an active investigation for a testicular primary, as well as CT assessment of the abdomen, retroperitoneum, and pelvis for metastatic diseases. Therapy and survival are stage-dependent. Only 10% of pure seminoma tumors will be mildly positive for β-HCG, and thus, finding significantly elevated serum levels of either β-HCG and/or alpha fetoprotein (AFP) should arouse the suspicion of a mixed lesion. Surgery is restricted to tissue procurement for diagnosis and as salvage therapy in chemotherapy failures.

NONSEMINOMATOUS GERM CELL TUMORS. Teratocarcinoma, choriocarcinoma, embryonal carcinoma, and endodermal sinus tumors are much less common than are seminomas and are rarely found in the mediastinum.

Serum markers document the response to therapy and relapse, as more than 90% of patients will have elevations in either AFP or β-HCG pretherapy. Combination platinum-based chemotherapy yields a 50% 5-year survival. Extirpative surgery is reserved for salvage situations. Surprisingly, of patients operated on for presumed residual disease after chemotherapy, only 25% have viable germ cells in the resected specimen, whereas 70% of specimens demonstrate necrosis or therapy-induced teratoma.

Other Anterior Mediastinal Tumors

MESENCHYMAL TUMORS. Mesenchymal tumors, 50% of which are malignant, account for only a small percentage of primary mediastinal tumors. They are randomly distributed within the mediastinal compartments, with symptomatology dependent on location and size. Benign tumors are universally amenable to complete resection and cure, while the prognosis for malignant lesions is poor.

PARATHYROID ADENOMA. Ten percent of parathyroid adenomas are ectopic and as many as one half occur in the anterosuperior mediastinum adjacent to the thymus. Pathologically, a mediastinal parathyroid adenoma behaves like its cervical counterpart and is usually suspected when hyperparathyroidism persists after cervical parathyroidectomy. Radiographic localization is critical. To this end, ^{99m}Tc-sestamibi scintigraphy and MRI are utilized. Once the adenoma is successfully located, transcervical, thoracoscopic, or trans-sternal approaches may be employed for excision and cure.

MEDIASTINAL GOITER. Encroachment of an enlarged thyroid gland into the anterosuperior mediastinum is often mistaken as a primary mediastinal mass. Most patients are asymptomatic women with a palpable cervical goiter. Primary intrathoracic goiter without a cervical component is exceptionally rare. Therapy is instituted only if symptoms of airway compromise or dysphagia exist. Most mediastinal goiters can be approached surgically through a low cervical incision. Occasionally, a partial sternal split is required.

MIDDLE MEDIAL MASSES

Aside from lymphoma, very few primary malignancies arise in the middle mediastinum. However, benign cysts of foregut and pericardial origin are commonly encountered in this locale. Foregut cysts are epithelium-lined structures and are classified histologically as bronchogenic, enterogenous, neuroenteric, and nonspecific types.

BRONCHOGENIC CYSTS. These lesions are the most frequently observed mediastinal cystic masses and account for 50% to 60% of all foregut cysts. They are commonly located in the subcarinal region and cause symptoms by compression or direct rupture into the lung and/or central airways. Complete surgical resection is indicated.

ENTEROGENOUS CYSTS. These cysts, also known as esophageal duplication cysts, are lined by some form of alimentary tract epithelium and as many as 60% contain gastric mucosa. They rarely communicate with the true esophageal lumen. The cyst wall is characterized by two well-developed smooth muscle layers and a myenteric plexus. The majority of esophageal duplication cysts are found in children, as only 25% remain asymptomatic and are diagnosed in adult years. As with bronchogenic cysts, enterogenous cysts are prone to infection, and consequently resection is warranted. The existence of gastric mucosa predisposes to spontaneous hemorrhage as well. These cysts are termed *neuroenteric* when accompanied by a vertebral anomaly.

PERICARDIAL CYSTS. Commonly found at the cardiophrenic angles, these simple cysts are seldomly symptomatic and infrequently require resection. Pericardial cysts are filled with clear serous fluid and are often referred to as spring water cysts.

POSTERIOR MEDIASTINAL MASSES

Neurogenic tumors are the most common posterior mediastinal mass. More than 90% of neurogenic neoplasms are located in the posterior mediastinum, and they collectively constitute 80% of all primary posterior mediastinal tumors. Neurogenic tumors occur twice as frequently in children and as many as 80% are benign in both adult and pediatric populations. Neurogenic neoplasms are classified into one of three categories according to tissue of origin—peripheral nerves, sympathetic ganglia, or paraganglionic tissues. Although most are asymptomatic, those compressing the spinal cord or somatic nerve roots will lead to specific syndromes dependent on the cord level or dermatome involved. To this end, an MRI is extremely helpful in planning operative therapy (Fig. 141–3).

PERIPHERAL NERVE TUMORS. Schwannomas and neurofibromas represent the most common mediastinal neurogenic tumors (see Fig. 141–3). These benign neoplasms usually arise from nerve roots, although any intrathoracic nerve may be involved. Schwannomas develop from the nerve sheath, are encapsulated, and are homogeneous. They are composed solely of Schwann cells without nerve or collagen fibrils. In contrast, neurofibromas are heterogeneous, well-localized lesions that are not encapsulated and result from a disorganized proliferation of all neural elements (i.e., Schwann cells, myelinated and unmyelinated nerve fibers, and fibroblasts). Hereditary neurofibromatosis accounts for 40% of patients with neurofibroma. Multiple neurogenic tumors or a single plexiform neurofibroma heralds this syndrome.

Radiographically, both tumor types present as sharply demarcated, rounded, paraspinal masses. As many as 50% produce benign pressure deformity of adjacent ribs, although clinically only a small percentage of patients experience paresthesia or pain from local compressive effects. A small percentage of lesions have spinal canal extension and present as dumbbell or hourglass configurations; thus, screening with MRI is indicated.

Malignant tumors of nerve sheath origin (MTNSO) are rare sarcomatous counterparts of schwannomas and neurofibromas. Although sporadic occurrence is observed,

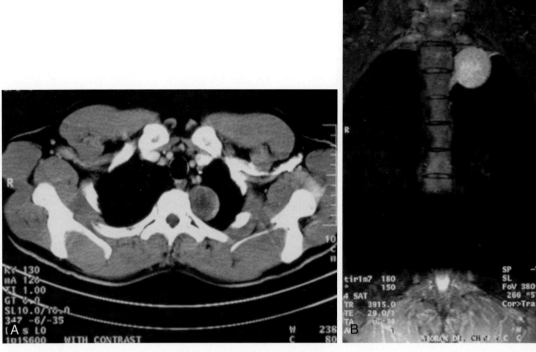

Figure 141–3. Axial image of CT *(A)* and sagittal section of MRI *(B)* of a posterior mediastinal neurogenic tumor. MRI suggests a nerve root origin of the tumor.

most MTNSO present in the setting of neurofibromatosis. They are difficult to distinguish radiographically from schwannoma and neurofibroma unless evidence of local invasion is demonstrated.

Treatment for all these neoplasms is complete surgical resection. Occasionally, adjuvant therapies are employed for MTNSO. Combined neurosurgical and thoracic surgical approaches are used for dumbbell tumors. Local recurrence for schwannoma and neurofibroma is less than 5% and is attributable to incomplete resection.

GANGLIONIC TUMORS. These neural neoplasms represent a spectrum ranging from benign (ganglioneuroma) to malignant (ganglioneuroblastoma) to highly malignant (neuroblastoma) variants. They originate from nerve cells in sympathetic ganglia and adrenal glands and constitute as many as one third of posterior mediastinal neurogenic tumors.

Ganglioneuromas are benign neoplasms of mature ganglion cells clustered in a bed of dense stromal tissue. These tumors occasionally have dumbbell-like features and are best characterized by MRI. When present, symptoms usually arise from intraspinal extension or local compression. Cure is effected by complete resection.

Mixed tumors of ganglioneuroma and neuroblastoma elements are termed *ganglioneuroblastoma*. The degree of malignant behavior varies widely, depending on the proportion of mature ganglion cells and immature neuroblastoma cells in the lesion. Tumor staging is the same as for neuroblastoma.

Neuroblastoma is primarily a malignancy of young children. Fifty percent of neuroblastomas originate in the adrenal glands, but the posterior mediastinum is the most common extra-adrenal site (20% of patients). Neuroblastomas can elaborate catecholamines and cause systemic symptoms similar to those of pheochromocytoma. Consequently, detection of catechol breakdown products in the urine (VMA) may assist in the preoperative evaluation. The staging of neuroblastoma (and ganglioneuroblastoma) is predicated on local extension, lymphatic spread, and detection of occult metastasis. Stage I represents a noninvasive, ipsilateral tumor. Ipsilateral involvement of

---

Pearls and Pitfalls

- Mediastinal masses are being recognized with increasing frequency owing to modern imaging.
- Symptoms and signs are vague, including dyspnea, cough, hoarseness, or, on occasion, the SVC syndrome.
- Anterior mediastinal masses include thymomas, lymphoma, germ cell tumors, and endocrine tumors (thyroid, parathyroid).
- Middle mediastinal tumors are rare but include lymphoma, bronchogenic and duplication cysts, and pericardiac cysts.
- Posterior mediastinal masses are usually (90%) of nerve cell origin—schwannomas, neurofibromas, ganglioneuromas, and paraganglionomas.
- Diagnosis is best obtained with CT or MRI, but a conventional chest radiograph is very helpful.
- The best treatment for most of these tumors is surgical excision except for lymphoma.

adjacent soft tissues, bone, spinal canal, or regional lymph nodes is classified as stage II. Stage III tumors extend across the midline and with contralateral lymph node spread. Stage IV disease is characterized by disseminated metastases. Treatment for stage I disease is surgical. For more advanced presentations, neoadjuvant or adjuvant strategies are often employed. Negative prognostic factors include older age at diagnosis, large tumor size, advanced stage, and extra-adrenal primary.

PARAGANGLIONIC TUMORS. Paraganglia act as chemo-receptors and store catecholamine granules. The most common sites for paraganglionic tumors include the glo-mus jugulare, carotid bodies, aortic arch, and abdominal aorta. Within the chest, tumors arise within the aortico-sympathetic paraganglia in the costovertebral sulcus (mediastinal pheochromocytoma) and in the aortic body of the middle mediastinum (chemodectomas). The malig-nant potential of mediastinal pheochromocytoma is slightly greater than its abdominal counterpart, while its catechol production is slightly less. Regardless of location, 10% of pheochromocytomas are familial. Associated ge-netic syndromes include familial pheochromocytoma, multiple endocrine neoplasia (MEN II A and B), neuro-fibromatosis, and von Hippel–Lindau syndrome. Com-plete surgical resection is the best therapy.

CONCLUSION

The complex anatomic and histologic arrangement of tis-sues within the mediastinum invariably accounts for the variety of pathology within the compartment. Although specialty training in thoracic surgery may be necessary for the management of many primary mediastinal masses, an understanding of both the anatomy of the mediastinum and the etiology of primary mediastinal masses is critical for the general surgeon.

SELECTED READINGS

Bacha EA, Chapelier AR, Macchiarini P, et al: Surgery for invasive primary mediastinal tumors. Ann Thorac Surg 1998;66:234.

Lara PN: Malignant thymoma: Current status and future directions. Cancer Treat Rev 2000;26:127.

Roviaro G, Varoli F, Nucca O, Vergani C, Maciocco M: Videothoracoscopic approach to primary mediastinal pathology. Chest 2000;117:1179.

Shields TW: Mediastinal Surgery. Philadelphia, Lea & Febiger, 1991.

Strollo DC, Rosado-de-Christenson ML, Jett JR: Primary mediastinal tumors. Part II. Chest 1997;112:1344.

Strollo DC, Rosado-de-Christenson MLR, Jett JR: Primary mediastinal tumors. Part I. Chest 1997;112:511.

Whooley BP, Urschel JD, Antkowlak JG, Takita H: Primary tumors of the mediastinum. J Surg Oncol 1999;70:95.

PEDIATRIC

Chapter 142

Neonatal Bowel Obstruction
Thomas F. Tracy, Jr.

Many level II and level III nurseries are sometimes faced with the complex problems associated with neonatal intestinal obstruction. General surgeons responsible for covering these areas need to have an understanding of the basic etiologies of newborn small and large bowel obstruction in order to stabilize babies with these conditions or, in fact, to perform definitive treatment. This chapter presents the diagnostic steps that can be taken to rapidly arrive at a diagnosis and subsequently to direct prompt surgical intervention or take further steps at stabilization and transfer of the patient to a pediatric surgical center. Malrotation and midgut volvulus is an important consideration and common cause of bowel obstruction in newborns; therefore, it is presented in a separate chapter.

PATHOPHYSIOLOGY

The specific embryonic and fetal etiologies of both intrinsic and extrinsic bowel obstruction in the newborn are complex and are just beginning to be understood. The failure of canalization of the small bowel within the duodenum has been cited as one of the possible events leading to duodenal atresia and stenosis. However, this mechanism does not clearly explain conditions, such as annular pancreas, that have the same impact and clinical presentation. On the other hand, the obstruction that is caused by intestinal duplication cannot be easily put in the same framework as failure of canalization. Stenosis and intestinal atresia are thought to also result from intrauterine vascular incidents that cause disruption of the fetal mesenteric blood supply to the developing intestine. This disruption results in degrees of obstruction ranging from stenosis to atresia and complete absence of large segments of the mesentery.

Bowel obstructions resulting from distal mechanical and functional bowel obstruction are more clearly understood when one considers meconium ileus and Hirschsprung's disease. The former is found in patients with inspissated meconium, usually due to cystic fibrosis. A variant of this is known as meconium plug syndrome, and although it may present in a similar fashion, it is not related to cystic fibrosis. It is, however, associated with a similar entity, known as small left colon syndrome, found in infants of diabetic mothers as well as mothers with eclampsia. Hirschsprung's disease is due to the failure of ganglion cells to migrate into the colon, commonly into the distal rectosigmoid area. Alternatively, some investigators have demonstrated a failure of differentiation in the myenteric plexus of the distal rectosigmoid. Obstruction of the anorectum is due to abnormal fusion of the cloaca or division of the urogenital septum. It is probable that the "high" and "low" forms of imperforate anus have different embryonic etiologies and will require further study for complete elucidation of all the features of each.

CLINICAL PRESENTATION

The clinical presentation of neonatal bowel obstruction is dependent on the level of intestinal obstruction and typically evolves in an infant with progressive abdominal distention, vomiting, or failure to pass meconium. Clear prenatal clues to a proximal obstruction should be considered with a history of polyhydramnios. An ever-increasing number of newborns are delivered with a fetal diagnosis of duodenal or other suspected bowel atresia, based on prenatal ultrasound performed during the evaluation of polyhydramnios. The classic "double bubble" of duodenal atresia demonstrated by gastric and duodenal air seen on plain abdominal radiographs can also be found on prenatal ultrasound. Instead of air, two cystic spaces are found side by side, representing a dilated stomach and duodenum secondary to obstruction from duodenal atresia, intraluminal duodenal webs, or annular pancreas.

The more distal obstructions rarely lead to polyhydramnios except late in pregnancy. More commonly, prenatal ultrasound reveals dilated fluid-filled loops of intestine. The presentation of bowel dilatation and complex cystic structures within the fetal abdomen is an ominous sign of meconium ileus with perforation. This late gestational event, representing giant cystic meconium peritonitis, results in significant peritoneal inflammation and peritoneal calcifications.

None of these prenatal presentations of bowel obstruction should prompt any alteration in the timing or the method of delivery. They should, however, prompt a prenatal surgical consultation with the family. This is an important time to present an initial set of differential diagnoses, to establish a basis for continued prenatal follow-up, and to introduce the family to surgical or transfer options in a nonemergent, nonthreatening setting.

When postnatal visceral distention is coupled with any element of newborn respiratory disease, it can produce significant changes in ventilation and, subsequently, oxygenation. Bilious vomiting can be an early presentation in higher forms of jejunal atresia; however, it is usually a late feature of distal obstruction. Nonbilious vomiting results from obvious preampullary obstruction. The failure to pass meconium is a classic sign for entities such as meconium ileus, meconium plug, or Hirschsprung's disease. The usual "rule of thumb" is that meconium should be passed within the first 48 hours. The failure to pass meconium has also been noted in more distal bowel atresias. Colonic stenosis and Hirschsprung's disease can present late in the neonatal course and may be associated with explosive diarrhea, heralding enterocolitis. The etiology of enterocolitis associated with Hirschsprung's disease is not well defined; however, it does relate to colonic stasis and bacterial overgrowth during the first 72 hours of life. Selective immunoglobulin deficiencies have been sought, and, occasionally, identified in a cohort of patients with Hirschsprung's disease.

Erythema of the abdominal wall, and rectus muscle rigidity, are relatively late findings of active peritonitis. They are normally present only in patients in whom the degree of visceral distention has led to ischemia and perforation, or in patients in whom segmental mesenteric defects have allowed for localized volvulus, resulting in either ischemia or infarction.

DIAGNOSIS OF BOWEL OBSTRUCTION IN THE NEWBORN

Several general diagnostic possibilities should be considered before the surgeon considers the individual etiologies of bowel obstruction in the newborn. The prenatal and perinatal historical details of polyhydramnios and bilious versus nonbilious vomiting have been presented and are important considerations. Simple observation of the baby and inspection of the abdomen can give excellent clues to the diagnosis. A visible upper abdominal bubble differentiates a proximal obstruction from a more distal obstruction in which numerous visible loops are found underneath the thin newborn abdominal wall. An imperforate anus or cloacal abnormality is readily evident on physical examination. Rectal examination after 48 hours of failure to pass meconium will stimulate a bowel movement, prompting the consideration of Hirschsprung's disease.

The mainstay of the work-up of the newborn with bowel obstruction is plain radiographs of the abdomen. Air is an excellent contrast material, and the majority of diagnoses are relatively apparent (Fig. 142–1). Following plain radiographs, upper abdominal or lower gastrointestinal (GI) contrast studies are often used. In most cases, pediatric radiologists favor the use of water-soluble contrast medium for these studies. This is a valuable agent for both diagnosis and treatment in the case of meconium plug and in many cases of meconium ileus.

After contrast studies, abdominal ultrasound can be very informative. Pediatric ultrasonographers have extended the well-known ultrasound diagnosis of pyloric stenosis and intussusception to malrotation, duodenal atresia or webs, intestinal duplications or atresia, meconium ileus or peritonitis, and even Hirschsprung's disease. In Hirschsprung's disease, pediatric radiologists have demonstrated the ganglion cell transition zone within the rectosigmoid with extreme accuracy. Ultrasound is also an important modality for the evaluation of associated genitourinary anomalies, especially with "midline defects," such as duodenal atresia and imperforate anus.

PREOPERATIVE MANAGEMENT

The basic principle of gastrointestinal decompression via an orogastric or nasogastric tube is essential. The place-

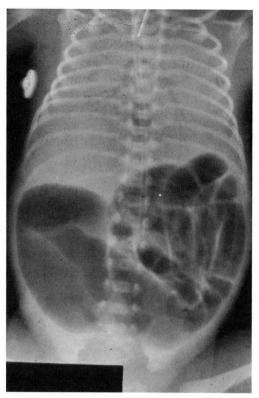

Figure 142–1. Plain x-ray film of the abdomen in the newborn with ideal atresia. Note the excellent contrast enhancement provided by air and the clear evidence of bowel obstruction due to the atresia.

ment of this tube depends on whether the infant is endotracheally intubated. Sump suction is continuously applied, and gastric fluid is replaced with 0.45N saline. Resuscitation from prolonged obstruction is mandatory in achieving urine outputs of 1 to 2 ml/kg per hour. Boluses of cystaloid of 10 to 20 ml/kg are often required. Maintenance fluids of 100 to 150 ml/kg per day should be initiated. The use of pressors, such as dopamine, is discouraged in the setting of intestinal ischemia until adequate volume restoration has been accomplished. Appropriate goals in a newborn are to obtain a mean arterial blood pressure of 45 mm Hg or greater and to achieve capillary refill less than 4 seconds. Antibiotics (ampicillin and gentamicin) are customary, and vitamin K is administered. Typing and cross-matching are performed on packed red blood cells in all neonates, pending abdominal exploration.

OPERATIVE MANAGEMENT

Extreme care for neonatal respiratory and cardiac support should be provided by a pediatric anesthesiologist. The main concern of these sections, however, is emergent care required by the newborn and performed by general surgeons. Appropriate intravenous access should have already been established. Temperature support in a heated operating room or by a convection warmer must be supplied. Urine output is monitored with special Foley catheters carefully inserted into the bladder. Packed red blood cells are always available.

Operative exploration for the majority of bowel obstructions is accomplished through a supraumbilical transverse incision. The use of a fine-pointed cautery minimizes blood loss as the abdominal layers are divided. The falciform ligament should be doubly ligated and divided to prevent traction on the neonatal liver. The only contraindication to division of this ligament should be the infant with an umbilical vein line for resuscitation. This circumstance requires that the structure remain carefully intact. Extreme care must be directed to the neonatal liver throughout the entire procedure. Too small an incision or an errant retraction can lead to fatal liver lacerations. As always, adequate exposure and careful retractor placement will prevent this complication.

Neonatal bowel anastomoses are generally performed with 4-0 or 5-0 silk in a single layer fashion. Some pediatric surgeons prefer absorbable polyglactin suture. Emergency decompression with ostomies for any of the described conditions can never be faulted when one is faced with complications, such as perforation or ischemia and peritonitis. In these cases, stomas should be generous and tacked with simple sutures to the fascia and skin. Full maturation of stomas is a waste of time and may lead to ischemia in these emergent situations. Abdominal wounds are closed with running or interrupted absorbable suture. Pressure dressings should not be applied to fragile stomas, and these can simply be painted with neomycin or bacitracin jelly to allow for adequate stomal arterial perfusion and venous return. Specific diagnostic and management concerns will be presented for the major causes of neonatal bowel obstruction, from proximal to distal.

Duodenal Obstruction

The three main causes of duodenal obstruction are duodenal atresia, annular pancreas, and duodenal webs, sometimes referred to as a "wind sock abnormality." All these present with a relatively scaphoid abdomen and upper abdominal distention of the stomach. Plain x-ray films of the abdomen show the classic "double bubble" of complete duodenal obstruction. A contrast-enhanced study is not required. Operative exploration is accomplished through a right supraumbilical transverse incision to expose the duodenum. A large duodenal bulb is usually encountered and both duodenal atresia and annular pancreas is readily evident from external inspection. No attempt should be made to dissect the annular pancreas in any fashion, and both can be repaired with a duodenoduodenotomy or duodenojejunostomy. The preferred method of repair is to mobilize a small segment of duodenum just distal to the point of stenosis or annular pancreas to allow its mobilization up to the large proximal duodenal bulb (Fig. 142–2). A transverse incision is made across the large duodenal bulb, and a longitudinal incision is then made down the distal segment. A suture is then taken from the midportion of the inferior lip of the transverse incision to the uppermost portion of the lower longitudinal incision. Likewise, the midpoint of the upper incision

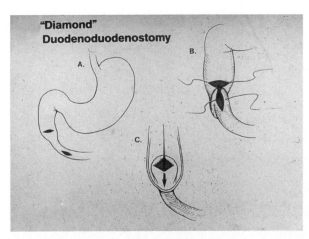

Figure 142–2. Duodenal atresia. This figure depicts the arrangement of the proximally dilated duodenum and distally collapsed duodenum in duodenal atresia or annular pancreas. *A,* A transverse incision is made in the upper duodenal portion, and a longitudinal incision is made in the lower duodenal portion. *B,* Suture placement is depicted for closure, with the upper portion of the longitudinal segment brought to the midportion of the transverse incision. *C,* Following the appropriate alignment, interrupted sutures were placed to allow for a "diamond" anastomotic opening.

is sutured to the most distal segment of the longitudinal lower incision. Interrupted sutures are then placed in between to allow for a "diamond-shaped" anastomosis, which allows for maximal patency and rapid refeeding. Occasionally, these infants require a course of parenteral nutrition until GI function returns.

For infants with internal duodenal webs, the external duodenal caliber is relatively uniform. A duodenotomy reveals a web, which must be carefully excised. The mucosal edges are very superficially oversewn by running a fine absorbable suture. Special care is taken not to obstruct the ampulla.

Small Intestinal Atresia

These atresias can occur anywhere from the proximal jejunum to the distal ileum. They present usually with abdominal distention and bilious vomiting. Plain x-ray films reveal a variable number of air-filled loops in the proximal intestine (see Fig. 142–1). With more distal atresias, a significant number of air-filled loops develop. In order to accurately diagnose distal atresias, some radiologists prefer to perform a water-soluble contrast enema to identify the presence of a microcolon through noting failure of contrast material to reflux into the small bowel. This study also serves to rule out a distal obstruction from some other cause, such as meconium ileus or plug.

Exploration for jejunoileal atresia can be accomplished through a supraumbilical transverse incision. The proximal atresias usually present in a straightforward manner with a dilated proximal jejunum that usually is 6 to 10 times the diameter of distal segments (Fig. 142–3). Careful inspection for multiple distal atresias is required with all small bowel atresias and is usually accomplished by a combination of passage of fine 8- or 10-French red rubber

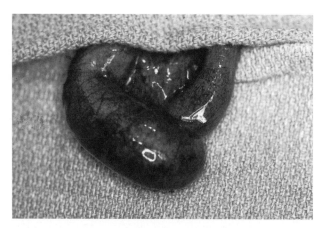

Figure 142–3. Jejunal atresia. This intestine demonstrates the significant dilatation of the proximal segment that will require tapering enteroplasty to arrive at a caliber comparable to that of the distal segment. A primary end-to-end anastomosis will allow for restoration of intestinal continuity.

catheters or saline infusion via the same catheters. Multiple atresias have often been identified in this manner. The proximal dilated segments may require tapering, performed via the antimesenteric application of several lengths of the GIA stapler. This procedure decreases intestinal caliber and provides for an appropriate size match for a primary anastomosis. With distal atresias, extreme care must be taken in the identification of associated meconium ileus, which can present as an atresia with inspissated concretions of meconium distally and in segments between atretic segments. These concretions will require evacuation at a later date, and with this finding an ostomy would be preferred for infants with meconium ileus.

Apart from the aforementioned considerations, end-to-end anastomoses can be accomplished with fine 4–0 or 5–0 silk. It is of primary importance that multiple small intestinal segments not be resected. Short bowel syndrome will be the unfortunate outcome unless multiple anastomoses are performed. In any cases in which there is a question, proximal decompression would be preferable to errant resection and loss of important small bowel. Mesenteric defects that are often seen with these abnormalities can be closed with simple tacking with fine suture, and care must be taken to preserve the vascular arcade.

A special consideration should be made for the "Christmas tree," or "apple peel," deformity of intestinal atresia. In this case, a long central mesenteric vessel supports the entire small bowel or remnants of small bowel (Fig. 142–4). Kinking of this vessel can cause immediate mesenteric ischemia; in such a case, again, decompression and referral to a pediatric surgical center may be lifesaving.

Intestinal Duplication

Intestinal duplications involve all three layers of the intestine and can occur in any area from the stomach through the rectum. The most common location of intestinal duplications is ileal, with the anomaly arising as a solitary cyst from the mesenteric border of the intestine. These duplications may present as intestinal obstruction in the newborn. Generally, they present later as the cyst expands and the lumen becomes depressed or, alternatively, as a mass palpitated on physical examination. In infants who present later in life, intermittent obstructive signs or symptoms may have been part of the history. With small cystic duplications, resection and reanastomosis is usually all that is required. Long tubular duplications have been extensive and need special care, with resection of the mucosa of the duplication and closure of the connection to the normal bowel lumen. These surprisingly also are noted quite late in life.

Meconium Ileus

With cystic fibrosis, inspissated meconium can obstruct the distal small bowel. Meconium adheres tenaciously to the bowel wall and requires special agents for dissolution. Infants present with distended loops of visible bowel. Plain x-ray films show a "soap-bubble" appearance, and may show intraperitoneal calcifications and pseudocysts if there has been perforation in utero. For infants with uncomplicated meconium ileus, a contrast enema with water-soluble contrast medium not only provides a diagnosis but also can provide the hydroscopic solution necessary for loosening the meconium and beginning to evacuate it. For infants who are well decompressed from above, it is safe to perform as many as three attempts at fluoroscopic-guided irrigation of inspissated meconium by reflux of the contrast material into the terminal ileum. This procedure clearly requires the assistance of pediatric radiologists. At no time should the water-soluble contrast medium be injected under pressure, as this will most certainly lead to perforation. The contrast enema will also show a diagnostic microcolon, as seen with ileal atresia.

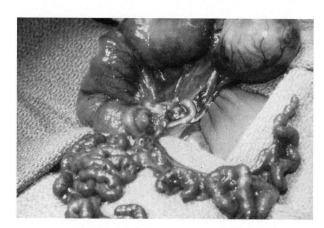

Figure 142–4. Multiple small bowel atresias, including an "apple-peel" deformity. These multiple segments must be individually spliced together, occasionally over a silicone catheter, to allow for intestinal continuity and to prevent short bowel syndrome. Most of these segments become functional. Occasionally, subsequent enteroplasties have to be performed. This is an extremely complex anomaly and requires significant expertise for reconstruction.

If these maneuvers fail to relieve the obstruction, exploration can be achieved through a supraumbilical or infraumbilical transverse abdominal incision. The obstructing meconium is usually evident, and at this point it is the surgeon's option either to perform a loop ostomy for decompression or to perform evacuation of the meconium via a small enterotomy. In meconium ileus that appears to have relatively loose meconium, a simple needle injection of irrigants has been described. A 3% solution of *N*-acetylcysteine (Mucomyst) has been the solution of choice for separating meconium from the mucosa. Distal irrigation with mobilization should allow for appropriate evacuation, and the enterotomy can simply be closed. Some surgeons prefer to leave a small T-tube within the lumen of bowel that is fashioned to be removed soon after intestinal patency has been documented. Additionally, this conduit can be used to infuse Mucomyst into the distal bowel prior to removing the T-tube. Numerous special stomas have been described for meconium ileus; however, generally these are not necessary, and they are reserved for complicated cases with distal atresias, which are subsequently referred to expert pediatric surgeons.

As mentioned previously, meconium ileus can result in a complicated problem following in utero perforation. Intra-abdominal meconium incites an intense peritoneal reaction, with a widespread serositis. Giant pseudocysts are formed adjacent to perforations, and quite often during operative exploration no specific bowel loops are discernible. The most appropriate management at this time is decompression via the most available and mobilizable piece of intestine (Fig. 142–5). The remainder of the intestine will require reconstruction after the resolution of peritonitis. Drains should be placed, and the abdomen should be irrigated with warm saline to flush out the remainder of the meconium. The abdomen should not be irrigated with Mucomyst. Re-exploration should not be considered for 4 to 6 weeks, once the infant has been nutritionally stabilized after this newborn insult.

Colonic Obstruction

Meconium Plug Syndrome

This fairly common condition results in progressive abdominal distention, prompting plain x-ray films that show distal obstruction. The same Gastrografin enema required for meconium ileus and jejunal atresia will demonstrate a small left colon with several meconium plugs. In the absence of such a finding, a small left colon can be seen in the newborns who are infants of diabetic mothers or mothers who have had eclampsia. The water-soluble contrast medium is therapeutic in the case of meconium plug.

Hirschsprung's Disease

Hirschsprung's disease is also a common distal bowel obstruction that follows failure of ganglion cells to develop or migrate into the colon. With the absence of ganglion cells, there is a failure of colonic relaxation and there is proximal dilatation of the normal ganglionic bowel. The usual segment of aganglionosis is in the rectosigmoid, where there is a transition zone from contracted aganglionic bowel to dilated normal bowel (Fig. 142–6). In the newborn, this can sometimes be seen on plain x-ray films, but most often it is a contrast enema that shows a transition zone from abnormal colon to relaxed, dilated normal colon in the rectosigmoid. The absence of ganglion cells on rectal biopsy is diagnostic. Rectal biopsy can be performed with a suction apparatus, which, in expert hands, has an excellent yield. This type of specimen can also be provided by an excisional biopsy of rectal mucosa and submucosa. Expert pathology support must be present for accurate diagnosis. In the meantime, the infant should be decompressed both from above and from a rectal tube placed at the time of performance of the contrast enema. Warm saline irrigations will decompress the colon in the majority of babies, and this procedure can maintain the child in an acceptable condition until he or she can be transferred to a pediatric surgical center. In emergent situations or in situations in which definitive treatment is necessary, a simple end-colostomy just above the transition zone will establish decompression and will allow for transition through the neonatal period (see Fig. 142–6). Although neonatal endorectal pull-throughs are

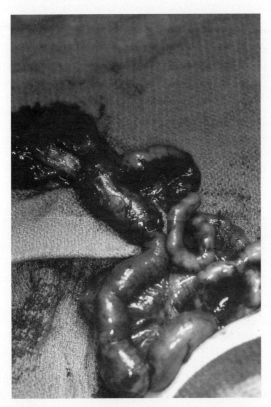

Figure 142–5. Meconium ileus with prenatal perforation. Significant meconium peritonitis with staining of the serosal surfaces is evident on the extended bowel, toward the top of the picture. This is a relatively mild reaction compared with some cases. The bowel was easily mobilized in this case for a stoma to be performed prior to irrigations into the remainder of the intestine. Intestinal continuity can be re-established after 4 to 6 weeks.

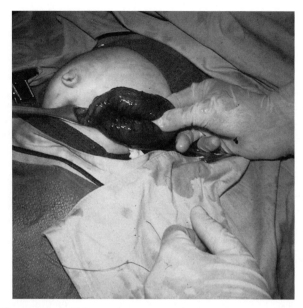

Figure 142–6. This case demonstrates the transition zone of Hirschsprung's disease. The proximally dilated bowel in the surgeon's hand is the ganglionic segment of the sigmoid colon. The distal decompressed end is aganglionic. At the level of dilatation, a biopsy should be performed to confirm the presence of ganglion cells. Occasionally, there is a transition zone, and the surgeon must be able to discern a clear demarcation of ganglion cells prior to performing an ostomy at that level.

now commonplace, an ostomy allows growth prior to definitive anorectal reconstruction by one of several endorectal reconstructive methods. The goal of all Hirschsprung's reconstruction is to bring ganglionic bowel down to the anus either by removal of the aganglionic segment or by an endorectal pull-through. Surgeons should take care to ascertain that biopsies are taken from the endcolostomy, ensuring that an adequate number of ganglion cells are present. If no ganglion cells are present, decompression cannot be achieved. A more proximal ostomy should then be performed at the level of ganglion cells; hence, the term *leveling colostomy*. Of course, infants born with total-colon Hirschsprung's disease require an ileostomy, and in this rare condition extensive reconstruction is required.

During the immediate postoperative period, surgeons should take extreme care to watch for enterocolitis. High fever and watery diarrhea-like output can occur, even in the presence of a colostomy, especially in children who have Hirschsprung's disease associated with trisomy 21. The exact etiology is unknown, but antibiotics, stomal decompression, and adequate hydration must be provided during periods of enterocolitis.

Imperforate Anus

The final major obstruction that occurs in newborns is imperforate anus. A significant description of all the types and associated malformations is precluded in this chapter; however, distal bowel obstruction and the absence of an anus should prompt consideration for decompression via colostomy. The most important consideration is the recog-

---

Pearls and Pitfalls

PEARLS

- Polyhydramnios is highly suggestive of proximal small bowel obstruction.
- Plain x-ray films of the abdomen are usually diagnostic.
- Water-soluble contrast enemas are therapeutic for meconium plug and meconium ileus.
- Divided colostomies in imperforate anus prevent urosepsis due to urinary contamination from rectourethral or vesicle fistulas.

PITFALLS

- Jejunal atresias may require tapering enteroplasty for adequate peristaltic function and anastomotic size match.
- An annular pancreas must not be dissected prior to duodenoduodenostomy.
- Multiple atresias must undergo segmental anastomosis to prevent short bowel syndrome.
- Transverse colostomy, rather than sigmoid colostomy, is preferred for cloacal abnormalities.

---

nition of associated urogenital anomalies. In patients who have a cloacal abnormality, the colon may be required for vaginal reconstruction. Therefore, a transverse colostomy would be the treatment of choice. For all others, a diverting, divided sigmoid colostomy will allow for adequate decompression of the large bowel. This procedure will also prevent any contamination of the urinary tract that results in urosepsis in males, in whom there is usually a rectourinary fistula to the urethra or bladder in higher anomalies. Definitive correction of imperforate anus is extremely complex and requires an important understanding of the pelvic anatomy and associated abnormalities of the urogenital sinus. A thorough work-up should be carried out in a pediatric surgical center following decompressive colostomy.

Summary

The majority of neonatal bowel obstructions are diagnosed in a straightforward manner by simple radiographic examination. The key for general surgeons who are asked to see infants with this condition is that their safety is provided for by gastrointestinal decompression with adequate resuscitation, which generally allows for transfer to a specialized center. Should there be catastrophic problems with perforation or any other associated complications, the approaches outlined in this chapter should provide for safe operative neonatal care and subsequent transition of the patient to a higher level nursery.

SELECTED READINGS

Bailey PV, Tracy TF, Connors RH, et al: Congenital duodenal obstruction: A 32-year review. J Pediatr Surg 1993;28:92.
Berrocal T, Lamas M, Gutieerrez J, et al: Congenital anomalies of the small intestine, colon, and rectum. Radiographics 1999;19:1219.

Corteville JE, Gray DL, Langer JC: Bowel abnormalities in the fetus—correlation of prenatal ultrasonographic findings with outcome. Am J Obstet Gynecol 1996;175:724.

Dalla Vecchia LK, Grosfeld JL, West KW, et al: Intestinal atresia and stenosis: A 25-year experience with 277 cases. Arch Surg 1998;133:490–496; discussion 496–497.

Fortuna RS, Weber TR, Tracy TF, et al: Critical analysis of the operative treatment of Hirschsprung's disease. Arch Surg 1996;131:520–524; discussion 524–525.

Kimura K, Tsugawa C, Ogawa K, et al: Diamond-shaped anastomosis for congenital duodenal obstruction. Arch Surg 1977;112:1262.

Mak GZ, Harberg FJ, Hiatt P, et al: T-tube ileostomy for meconium ileus: Four decades of experience. J Pediatr Surg 2000;35:349.

Pena A: Posterior sagittal approach for the correction of anorectal malformations. Adv Surg 1986;19:69.

Pena A, Hong A: Advances in the management of anorectal malformations. Am J Surg 2000;180:370.

Stern LE, Warner BW: Gastrointestinal duplications. Semin Pediatr Surg 2000;9:135.

Sullivan PB: Hirschsprung's disease. Arch Dis Child 1996;74:5.

Wilcox DT, Bruce J, Bowen J, Bianchi A: One-stage neonatal pull-through to treat Hirschsprung's disease. J Pediatr Surg 1997;32:243–245; discussion 245–247.

Zia-ul-Miraj M, Madden NP, Brereton RJ: Simple incision: A safe and definitive procedure for congenital duodenal diaphragm. J Pediatr Surg. 1999;34:1021.

Chapter 143
Anomalies of Bowel Rotation: Malrotation and Midgut Volvulus

Christopher K. Breuer, Donald L. Sorrells, and Thomas F. Tracy, Jr.

INTRODUCTION

Mall, Professor of Anatomy at Johns Hopkins University, wrote the first meaningful description of the embryology of bowel rotation in 1898. He was able to describe the rotation and fixation of the bowel through the use of reconstructed embryos. Subsequently, another paper, "Anomalies of intestinal rotation: Their embryology and surgical aspects," was published in 1923 by Dott. This classic paper correlated clinical observations to embryology. In 1936, Ladd wrote the key article on the treatment of this condition. Ladd's description of the release of the duodenum and placement of the cecum in the left upper quadrant remains the definitive surgical treatment for nonrotation with midgut volvulus.

EMBRYOLOGY. Normal bowel rotation is achieved by the end of the first trimester of pregnancy. An understanding of this process is imperative to understanding anomalies of bowel rotation. Snyder and Chaffin demonstrated in an article in 1954 a clear description of the anomalies of rotation. The embryology of malrotation was compared with the twisting of a loop of rope around a fixation point that represented the superior mesenteric vessels.

The intestinal tract develops as a single tube consisting of the foregut, midgut, and hindgut. Two processes are required for normal bowel rotation. The duodenojejunal loop and the distal cecocolic loop rotate and become fixed in the retroperitoneum.

The duodenojejunal loop lies above or anterior to the superior mesenteric artery. This loop first rotates counterclockwise 90 degrees to the right of the artery and then another 90 degrees under the artery. Finally, the loop rotates another 90 degrees across the spine and upward. This establishes the position of the duodenojejunal junction on the left side of the spine, level with the duodenal bulb. This junction, of course, becomes the ligament of Treitz.

The cecocolic loop originally hangs beneath the superior mesenteric artery. Rotation also occurs in a counterclockwise direction. First, the loop moves to the left of the artery approximately 90 degrees. Then the loop proceeds above the artery 90 degrees. A final movement to the right and downward 90 degrees establishes the typical inverted U-shaped configuration of the colon.

Whereas rotation of the bowel occurs by the end of the third month of gestation, fixation to the retroperitoneum occurs gradually until term. Normal fixation to the retroperitoneum results in a wide mesenteric base from the ligament of Treitz to the cecum. This wide mesenteric base is resistant to volvulus. The duodenojejunal loop achieves fixation to the retroperitoneum shortly after rotation. The cecocolic loop is fixed to the retroperitoneum in a much slower time course, extending to near term. This embryology explains the observation of infants with a mobile or high cecum.

CLASSIFICATION OF ABNORMALITIES OF INTESTINAL ROTATION. A large spectrum of abnormalities of intestinal rotation exists. Malrotation refers to all these abnormalities of intestinal rotation and attachment. More specifically, nonrotation refers to lengthening of the bowel on the superior mesenteric artery (SMA) axis with essentially no rotation. Incomplete rotation occurs when there is some rotation of the bowel about the SMA axis but not complete rotation. Both nonrotation and incomplete rotation are susceptible to midgut volvulus. Duodenal obstruction and reverse rotation (internal hernia) are seen with incomplete rotation. Incomplete fixation, on the other hand, refers to a failure of descent of the cecum and fixation of mesenteries. Internal hernia (mesocolic) and cecal volvulus are associated with incomplete fixation.

ASSOCIATED ANOMALIES. Associated anomalies are seen in as many as 50% of patients with malrotation. Duodenal atresia is one of the more common findings, and partially obstructing duodenal webs must not be overlooked in infants with malrotation. Frequently, these infants will have a double bubble on plain radiograph.

Congenital diaphragmatic hernias, omphaloceles, and gastroschises all have obligate varying degrees of nonrotation depending on the extent of intestinal displacement outside the abdomen. Malrotation associated with congenital diaphragmatic hernia, gastroschisis, or omphalocele is generally not corrected at the time of operation for these defects. Various other associations have been made with malrotation, including mesenteric cysts, intestinal atresias, Hirschsprung's disease, and intussusception. There are even some reports of an increased incidence of malrotation in patients who require operation for gastroesophageal reflux. Malrotation is a ubiquitous anomaly with many frequent associations.

CLINICAL PRESENTATION

ACUTE MIDGUT VOLVULUS. The majority of patients presenting with acute midgut volvulus are infants. In the first week of life, 30% will present; over 50% will present within the first month of life. Vomiting is present in 95% of cases. The vomitus is almost always bilious but can be bloody with intestinal necrosis. Abdominal distention is present in 56% of patients, and stools have gross blood in 28%. Pain and tenderness are frequently present, especially with bowel ischemia. Neonates generally appear ill, with decreased capillary refill in the extremities and grunting respirations. The infant will rapidly progress to dehydration, lethargy, and profound shock.

Plain abdominal radiographs may reveal a gasless abdomen or dilated bowel suggesting obstruction. Unfortunately these films may be deceiving and look relatively normal (Fig. 143–1). Occasionally there may be evidence of duodenal obstruction with a double bubble sign. The constellation of clinical symptoms (bloody stools, bilious vomiting, lethargy and peritoneal findings), along with plain films that do not show pneumatosis indicating necrotizing enterocolitis, necessitates immediate laparotomy to prevent the loss of significant amounts of bowel. If the diagnosis is in doubt or there are no signs of bowel ischemia, then most pediatric surgeons would proceed with an upper gastrointestinal series to demonstrate duodenal obstruction or failure of duodenal rotation across the midline with fixation by the ligament of Treitz.

CHRONIC MIDGUT VOLVULUS. Presentation is generally marked by intermittent partial intestinal obstruction. In infants and children older than 1 month of age, intermittent bilious vomiting is present in 30%, with colicky abdominal pain in 20%. Some of these patients present with failure to thrive, chronic malabsorption, and diarrhea.

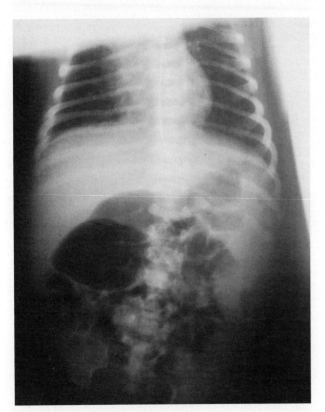

Figure 143–1. Infant with malrotation and midgut volvulus. This plain film of the abdomen shows variably dilated small and large bowel loops with no evidence of ascites. There is no characteristic picture of obstruction; however, at exploration total intestinal ischemia was found, indicating the lack of radiographic features often associated with malrotation and midgut volvulus.

A history of bilious emesis demands an immediate upper gastrointestinal series. However, in patients without bilious emesis, an upper gastrointestinal series is usually obtained as part of a work-up for chronic abdominal pain or failure to thrive. Surgery is indicated in all patients with the findings of malrotation, and a significant number of these patients will have postoperative resolution of symptoms.

ASYMPTOMATIC MALROTATION. The finding of malrotation on radiography or at surgery in the asymptomatic patient poses an interesting question. There has been some historical controversy on this indication for a Ladd's procedure. However, the current consensus is that corrective surgery is indicated at any age, but particularly in asymptomatic infants younger than 2 years of age.

At the time of appendectomy for acute appendicitis, there may be evidence of malrotation. Generally, the appendectomy should be performed and a follow-up formal upper gastrointestinal series performed after recovery from emergency surgery. If the upper GI study demonstrates malrotation, then corrective surgery should be undertaken.

Reverse Rotation. In this rare anomaly, the duodenum and colon rotate in the reverse direction in relation to the superior mesenteric vessels. The transverse colon passes posteriorly through a tunnel formed by these vessels. The duodenum passes anterior to these vessels. The transverse colon is obstructed by the anterior passage of the superior mesenteric vessels. Surgical correction involves mobilizing the duodenum and underlying mesenteric vessels anteriorly and laterally off the transverse colon.

MESOCOLIC HERNIAS. Mesocolic hernias occur secondary to a lack of fixation of the mesentery of the right or left side of the colon and the duodenum. The bowel becomes entrapped in these mesenteric pouches. The right mesocolic hernia can be identified on upper gastrointestinal series by the appearance of the entire small bowel on the right side of the abdomen. Embryologically, the prearterial duodenojejunal loop fails to rotate around the superior mesenteric artery, and the small bowel is surrounded by the mesentery of the ascending colon. Surgically, the lateral peritoneal attachment of the right colon is incised, and the colon is reflected toward the left.

Left mesocolic hernias form in a sac of the left colonic mesentery. The inferior mesenteric vein forms the neck of the hernia. The cecum is in its normal position in the right lower quadrant. Frequently, the small intestine can be manually reduced from the hernia, and then the inferior mesenteric vein is tacked to the retroperitoneum, obliterating the orifice of the hernia. Sometimes reduction of the hernia requires careful mobilization of the inferior mesenteric vein, followed by retroperitoneal fixation of the vein.

IMAGING. An upper gastrointestinal series is definitive and demonstrates the sweep of the duodenum. Contrast should proceed from the duodenal bulb across the spine and then downward. The third portion of the duodenum should cross back to the left side of the spine, making the duodenal C-loop. The fourth portion of the duodenum should ascend to the level of the greater curve of the stomach. This is the ligament of Treitz, and it is frequently at approximately the same level as the duodenal bulb. Any deviation from this radiologic appearance suggests a possible rotational abnormality. More overt diagnostic findings are obstruction of the duodenum, abnormal right-sided position of the ligament of Treitz, and the filling of jejunal loops on the right side of the abdomen.

Plain abdominal x-ray films are often nondiagnostic. However, sometimes the double bubble sign of duodenal obstruction can be seen. Volvulus of the midgut is often characterized by a gasless abdomen.

Ultrasound is a very rapid diagnostic test for defining vascular flow through the superior mesenteric vessels. There is a characteristic "whirlpool" flow pattern of the superior mesenteric vessels with volvulus. A fluid-filled duodenum and dilated thick bowel loops are also indicators of malrotation with volvulus. Experienced ultrasonographers can exclude malrotation by demonstrating normal rotation of the C-loop relative to the superior mesenteric artery and vein. A barium enema is generally not helpful in the diagnosis of malrotation and midgut volvulus and may add harmful delay. The cecum may appear to be in the right lower quadrant while the small bowel is not normally rotated and fixed retroperitoneally.

PREOPERATIVE MANAGEMENT

Infants and children with a significant vomiting history are frequently at least 10% to 15% dehydrated. Rapid resuscitation with crystalloid is indicated. Temperature regulation is essential. Nasogastric tube decompression should be started, and a Foley catheter should be placed. Broad-spectrum antibiotics are given. Ultimately, survival of the patient is dependent upon expeditious laparotomy. Strong consideration should be given to an anticipated period of postoperative ventilatory management. Central venous pressure monitoring and arterial lines will aid in resuscitation. However, they should not delay movement to the operating room and initiation of the laparotomy.

INTRAOPERATIVE MANAGEMENT

INITIAL EXPLORATION. The standard operative approach is through a right upper quadrant transverse incision (Fig. 143–2). A midline laparotomy can be used in older patients (Fig. 143–3). Appearance of the small bowel at first, instead of the omentum and colon, is the first indication of malrotation. The first step is to eviscerate the bowel through a generous incision and inspect for volvulus. With a volvulus, the gut is derotated in a counterclockwise fashion. If there is ischemic gut, warm saline sponges should be packed around the bowel. After an adequate period of time, bowel viability should be assessed with both Doppler and infused fluorescein if necessary. Situations with clearly demarcated intestinal necrosis require sound surgical judgment and may include bowel resection, stomas, or a second-look operation (Fig. 143–4). The guiding principle in questionable bowel viability is the preservation of maximal bowel length. With significant ischemia and reperfusion, the small bowel may

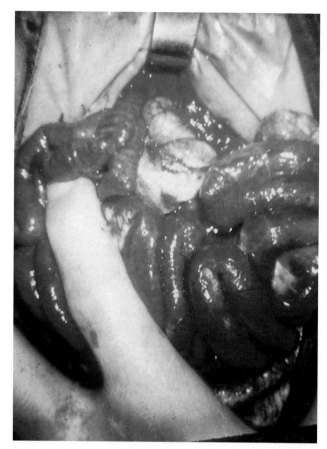

Figure 143–2. The abdomen is opened through a transverse abdominal incision. Immediately, ischemic small bowel presents prior to the omentum and colon. This is indicative of malrotation and midgut volvulus. The next step is appropriate detorsion of the base of the mesentery with a counterclockwise turn.

swell and ascites may develop, leading to abdominal compartment syndrome (Fig. 143–5). The end-result is further compression of recovering bowel or marginally ischemic bowel. Significant attention must be directed to this potential complication, and judgment at the time of closure should prompt a construction or placement of a Silastic silo in infants and a temporary mesh closure in older patients.

LADD'S PROCEDURE. If the bowel is viable, then Ladd's procedure and appendectomy should be performed. The essential steps of the procedure are based on the division of all abnormal "bands," or adhesions, that extend from the retroperitoneum across the duodenum and the proximal mesentery. To begin the procedure, the small intestine is spread out over the lower abdominal wall to allow maximum splaying of the mesentery. The duodenum and ascending colon are usually found parallel to each other. The mesenteric vessels are located posterior to these structures. Between the cecum, ascending colon, duodenum, and right lateral gutter, there are peritoneal folds called Ladd's bands. These bands are carefully incised along the medial aspect of the duodenum. The underlying tissue of the anterior leaf of the mesentery is divided, exposing the superior mesenteric artery. This allows the ascending colon and duodenum to be separated, widening

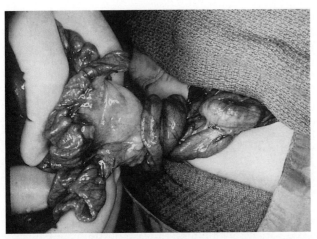

Figure 143–3. A slightly older patient with chronic evidence of malrotation and midgut volvulus. This patient presented to her local physician with abdominal pain and bilious vomiting on four separate occasions. Finally, with complete obstruction, the patient was referred, and a laparotomy was performed. Successful detorsion and fixation of the gut was accomplished.

the base of the mesentery. Eventually, with complete lysis, the cecum and ascending colon lie in the left upper abdomen. The duodenum and proximal jejunum should now lie in a straight line down the right gutter, and the ileocecal junction should be placed on the opposite side of the abdomen, with the small bowel resting below in a U shape. The mesentery should be free from any constricting bands at its base.

A standard or inversion appendectomy is performed. Without appendectomy, the appendix is in the left upper quadrant and presents an unnecessary, potential diagnos-

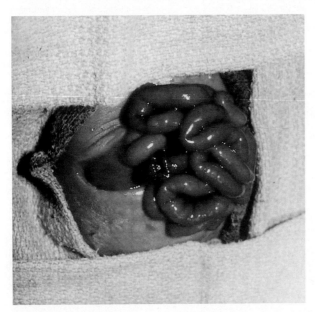

Figure 143–4. Significant ischemia noted after detorsion of this entire small bowel. A second-look laparotomy was performed, and a moderate segment of jejunum required resection with placement of stomas. Reanastomosis was accomplished 8 weeks later, and the patient was weaned from total parenteral nutrition 2 months postoperatively.

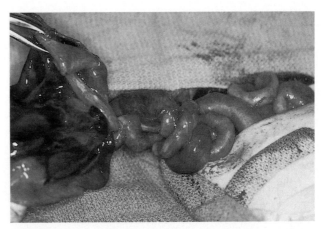

Figure 143–5. Total midgut volvulus associated with an apple peel deformity of intestinal atresia.

tic challenge with the onset of appendicitis. Duodenal and colonic fixation sutures are no longer recommended. The incidence of recurrent volvulus is 5% to 8%.

DUODENAL OBSTRUCTION. If the work-up demonstrates duodenal obstruction (i.e., double bubble sign, cut-off of contrast material), an intrinsic duodenal obstruction must be ruled out at the time of surgery. A gastrotomy should be performed and a Foley or red rubber catheter passed through the duodenum into the proximal jejunum. If there is no obstruction, the balloon should be inflated in the proximal jejunum and pulled through the duodenum in a retrograde manner. This maneuver prevents the physician's missing a partially obstructing duodenal web. Findings of obstruction require repair of the duodenal obstruction as described in Chapter 142, on a newborn intestinal obstruction.

POSTOPERATIVE MANAGEMENT

As mentioned previously, several important postoperative considerations must be focused on. The first is that, following significant midgut volvulus, edema of the small intestine will gradually lead to significant swelling due to interstitial fluid losses, as well as the development of ascites secondary to extravascular third space losses intra-abdominally. All efforts for intestinal decompression should be maintained. Strong consideration should be given to abdominal closure with either a silo or temporary mesh. Intestinal viability can be continuously checked through both these methods. Prompt re-exploration of the abdomen, with resection of compromised or clearly ischemic intestine, should be performed at second-look procedures within the first 48 hours. Small bowel anastamoses may not be feasible, and, not infrequently, multiple stomas will need to be formed through or adjacent to an open abdominal wall. Again, maintenance of total intestinal continuity is the foremost consideration when the risk of short bowel syndrome is significant.

With assured intestinal viability and resolution of the inflammatory response and secondary edema, abdominal closure can be considered. With either primary or delayed abdominal closure, decompression of what may be com-

Pearls and Pitfalls

PEARLS

- Normal bowel rotation is achieved by the end of the first trimester of pregnancy.
- Malrotation refers to a wide spectrum of abnormalities of intestinal rotation, which include nonrotation, incomplete rotation, duodenal obstruction, and reverse rotation. In addition, associated congenital abnormalities such as duodenal atresia, congenital diaphragmatic hernias, omphaloceles, gastroschisis, mesenteric cysts, intestinal atresias, and duplications may all have elements of malrotation or nonrotation, predisposing to volvulus. Surgery is indicated in all patients with findings of malrotation.
- Patient survival depends on expeditious laparotomy and the usual counterclockwise detorsion of any volvulus.
- The guiding principle with questionable bowel viability is preservation of maximum bowel length; second-look procedures are often necessary. "Silo" abdominal wall closure to prevent mesenteric compression or postoperative abdominal compartment syndrome may be life-saving.

PITFALLS

- Plain abdominal radiographs are often nondiagnostic. Expeditious upper GI evaluation is mandatory with any suspicion of malrotation.
- Barium enema is generally not helpful in diagnosis of malrotation and midgut volvulus and may cause harmful delay.
- Rapid resuscitation of infants and children with a vomiting history is imperative.
- Lysis of ALL obstructing retroperitoneal bands crossing the duodenum and mesentery must follow detorsion.
- Lysis of medial and lateral adhesions will allow expansion of the base of the mesentery and complete freedom for the duodenum. Duodenal and colonic fixation sutures are no longer recommended.

promised intestine with ischemia or reperfusion injury will be critical. This may be a condition where jejunal tube feeding may be limited and should not be tested. Transmural ischemia of the intestine will lead to mucosal sloughing, resulting in decreased barrier function, translocation, and progressive sepsis with attempted enteral feeding. The unfortunate but life-saving need for total parental nutrition early in the postoperative course may be the only choice. Certainly for those infants, children, and older patients who have no significant ischemia, abdominal closure can proceed. Following appropriate return of GI function, feedings can be initiated.

With long-standing duodenal obstruction, significant duodenal dysmotility can complicate the postoperative course. Prolonged decompression may be necessary during a period of parenteral re-feeding, as for superior mesenteric artery syndrome. No doudenal tapering should be undertaken at the time of the initial operation; however, this consideration may require significant evaluation prior to being performed, even at a later date. For the most part, most patients resolve this dysmotility, and progression of enteral feeding can be normal.

Adhesive bowel obstruction is not unheard of. Those patients who have not had an appropriate extension or widening of the mesentery remain at risk for recurrent volvulus. For patients with obligate malrotation—that is, congenital diaphragmatic hernia, gastroschisis, or omphalocele—all clinicians should remain vigilant for volvulus at any time. Segmental volvulus has been described as caused by adhesions or alterations in the mesentery of those patients with atresia associated with malrotation.

OUTCOMES

Surgery is very successful, with only a 5% or lower chance of recurrent volvulus or bowel obstruction. Failure is usually not on the basis of any failures of intestinal fixation, and therefore plicating sutures have been largely abandoned. Failure does occur from a lack of complete expansion of the mesentery or through an inappropriate dissection of the duodenum with subsequent inaccurate placement of the intestine. Of course, an appropriate appendectomy should be performed so as not to confuse the future diagnosis of acute appendicitis on variable abdominal pain in the left upper abdomen.

SELECTED READINGS

Bailey PV, Tracy TF Jr, Connors RH, et al: Congenital duodenal obstruction: A 32-year review. J Pediatr Surg 1993;28:92.

Brennom WS, Bill AH: Prophylactic fixation of the intestine for midgut nonrotation. Surg Gynecol Obstet 1974;138:181.

Dott NM: Anomalies of intestinal rotation: Their embryology and surgical aspects with report of five cases. Br J Surg 1923;11:251.

Fukuya T, Brown BP, Lu CC: Midgut volvulus as a complication of intestinal malrotation in adults. Dig Dis Sci 1993;38:438.

Haymond HE, Dragstedt LR: Anomalies of intestinal rotation. Surg Gynecol Obstet 1931;53:316.

Ladd WK: Surgical diseases of the alimentary tract in infants. N Engl J Med 1936;215:705.

Mall FP: Development of the human intestine and its position in the adult. Bull Johns Hopkins Hosp 1898;9:197.

O'Neill JA, Rowe MI, Grosfeld JL, et al: Pediatric Surgery, 5th ed. St. Louis, CV Mosby, 1998, pp 1199–1213.

Philippart AI, Farmer D: Congenital pyloric stenosis and duodenal obstruction. In Nyhus LM, et al [eds]: Mastery of Surgery, 3rd ed. Boston, Little, Brown, 1997, pp 926–927.

Powell DM, Otherson HB, Smith CD: Malrotation of the intestine in children: The effect of age in presentation and therapy. J Pediatr Surg 1989;24:777.

Rescorla FJ, Shedd FJ, Grosfeld JL, et al: Anomalies of intestinal rotation in childhood: Analysis of 447 cases. Surgery 1990;108:710.

Rowe MI, O'Neill JA, Grosfeld JL, et al: Essentials of Pediatric Surgery. St. Louis, CV Mosby, 1995, pp 492–500.

Simpson AJ, Leonidas JC, Krasna IH, et al: Roentgen diagnosis of midgut malrotation: Value of upper gastrointestinal radiographic study. J Pediatr Surg 1972;7:243.

Snyder WH, Chaffen L: Embryology and pathology of the intestinal tract: Presentation of 40 cases of malrotation. Ann Surg 1954;140:368.

Chapter 144

Abdominal Wall Defects: Omphalocele and Gastroschisis

Thomas F. Tracy, Jr.

Abdominal wall defects are some of the most dramatic newborn congenital disorders that are potential encounters for general surgeons. These defects in development are triggered by chromosomal, environmental, or teratogenic alterations. Pediatric surgeons have found that the management and care of these defects remain surgical challenges during the newborn period and are a significant diagnostic and therapeutic concern for prenatal fetal management.

The largest epidemiologic studies have found that generally omphalocele occurs in 1 in 4000 births, and gastroschisis in 1 in 6000 to 10,000 births. Both occur in males and females equally. Abdominal wall malformations are presented together topically because of the common clinical presentation of a ventral abdominal defect and the common surgical treatment goal of closure of that defect. Distinctions between gastroschisis and omphalocele have been generated only through general anatomic and embryologic definitions.

Omphalocele is a central abdominal defect through which both hollow and solid abdominal viscera can pass. These defects are uniformly covered by a membrane of amnion externally and peritoneum internally. The umbilical cord inserts into the membrane. The central defect can extend for a few centimeters in diameter or can present as defects that extend to the lower chondral margins. These latter defects, known as giant omphaloceles, contain liver, small and large bowel, and, occasionally, other organs. Smaller defects may have only a few loops of bowel and can be more realistically viewed as hernias of the umbilical cord.

In gastroschisis, the ventral defect is uniformly small (≤4 cm) and is found to the right of an intact, central umbilical cord. There have been rare reports of left-sided defects. The external appearance of uncovered loops of bowel may be either clearly discerned or hidden owing to shortening of the bowel. In many cases, there is an extensive reactive inflammatory peel on the bowel serosa. The liver and other solid organs remain within the abdomen, but the stomach and gonads may also be found externally. These are clearly two distinct definitions of the pathology of both ventral defects.

PATHOPHYSIOLOGY

The physiologic impact of an omphalocele is directly related to its size and, more significantly, to any associated anomalies. Pulmonary hypoplasia can accompany giant omphalocele. One would anticipate that a large ventral defect, which could be considered the reverse of a congenital diaphragmatic hernia, would therefore not interfere with lung development. The presence of a large defect does appear to direct the development of a globular liver that conforms to its extracoelomic position, rather than its normal lobular architecture. To date, no specific alterations in the fetal intestine have been determined microscopically. Only in cases of ruptured omphalocele has there been any evidence of serosal inflammation. Normal motility and function have been almost universally observed, and surprisingly there have been few cases of delayed complications from associated malrotation. In contrast with the absence of any detrimental effects on the fetal gut by an omphalocele, gastroschisis results in severe abnormalities of fetal bowel function. The current hypothesis is that fetal intestinal injury with abdominal wall defects is related to amniotic fluid exposure and partial intestinal obstruction in utero. Villous atrophy has been identified as the structural basis for the clinical problem of altered nutrient uptake in the newborn.

ASSOCIATED ANOMALIES

It is key to recognize that few associated abnormalities are found in infants with gastroschisis compared with those in infants with omphalocele. Obligate malrotation occurs as with all the defects of the abdominal wall, including congenital diaphragmatic hernia. Intestinal atresia, polyhydramnios, and Meckel's diverticulum represent 75% of the associated problems in patients with gastroschisis. Only 21% of cases of gastroschisis, however, had an associated malformation. In contrast, 54% of patients with omphalocele had associated malformations. Fetal studies have demonstrated that more than 40% of fetuses with omphalocele had karyotypic abnormalities, compared with no fetuses with gastroschisis. As expected, abnormal karyotypes were encountered in fetuses with multiple anomalies compared with isolated defects. Abnormal karyotypes include trisomy 18, 13, and 21, as well as Turner syndrome and Klinefelter syndrome. As many as 72% of patients with omphalocele have anomalies within the cardiovascular, genitourinary, and central nervous systems. The most common cluster of abnormalities is found in Beckwith-Wiedemann syndrome, composed of omphalocele, macroglossia, and pancreatic hyperplasia resulting in hypoglycemia along with other elements of visceromegaly, and craniofacial abnormalities. This syndrome has been mapped to chromosome 11p15.5.

Gastroschisis is associated primarily with jejunoileal atresia. The most disturbing complication of the malformation is the potential for in utero midgut volvulus. This catastrophic complication can also occur postnatally owing to the failure to recognize a fragile, compromised vascular pedicle to the extruded gut. As many as 30% of newborns with gastroschisis have significant growth retardation. Most newborns with gastroschisis are below the 50th percentile in weight and commonly have low serum levels of albumin, immunoglobulin G, transferrin, and total serum proteins. It appears, however, that intrauterine growth retardation does not negatively affect outcome.

PRENATAL DIAGNOSIS

The ability to diagnose most abdominal wall defects through prenatal ultrasound has immediate consequences for subsequent treatments. The diagnosis of omphalocele or gastroschisis can be made after 14 weeks' gestation, when the fetal midgut has normally returned to the abdominal cavity. If an abdominal wall defect is identified on screening maternal ultrasound, a follow-up examination should be done, with special emphasis on the search for associated malformations, especially in cases of omphalocele. Serial ultrasound examinations should concentrate on the appearance of eviscerated bowel in gastroschisis, noting the presence of bowel dilation and the development of a fibrotic peel. Both are late gestational manifestations of bowel atresia or constriction at the point of the abdominal wall defect and exposure of the gut to amniotic fluid. In clinical studies of the development of gut dilation, there is a good correlation with fetal distress, but no correlation with surgical outcome. The presence of a bowel diameter greater than 18 mm may be associated with a delay in oral feeding and a high likelihood of bowel resection. The clinical significance of a finding of bowel dilation in a fetus with an abdominal wall defect is not yet clear. It is premature to initiate or alter fetal or obstetric therapy on the basis of these findings in infants with gastroschisis.

Fetal markers have had some usefulness in the diagnosis of ventral defects. The most studied and understood marker has been the presence of elevated maternal α-fetoprotein (AFP) in serum, indicating either a neural tube or a ventral defect. Ninety percent of cases of omphalocele and 100% of gastroschisis cases are associated with elevated AFP. Screening for elevated maternal AFP is the most direct indication for a fetal ultrasound examination to determine the presence of a ventral defect.

PRENATAL MANAGEMENT

General surgical consultants may not have the opportunity to be involved with the prenatal diagnosis, as more centers have found that this is a critical time for the resources of a fetal management team or multidisciplinary perinatal center. Decisions incorporating medical, ethical, moral, and religious data need to be made regarding the termination of pregnancy in cases of defined and confirmed lethal anomalies. Counseling about ventral abdominal defects and any identified associated anomalies must begin once the specific diagnoses have been made. One approach has been to introduce families at the point of diagnosis to all the components of a fetal management group, including the high-risk perinatal center, the newborn intensive care unit, neonatologists, the pediatric surgical staff, and clinical nurse specialists. Based on the diagnosis of gastroschisis or omphalocele, the exact nature of the defect, pathophysiology, expected fetal course, and potential complications are first introduced. The parents are familiarized with the individual events and physicians. As discussed previously, the associated conditions of growth retardation, respiratory distress, and potential preterm delivery prompt important follow-up and delivery at a complete perinatal center. For gastroschisis, studies have demonstrated a greater rate of primary closure, with significantly less postoperative assisted ventilation for prenatally transferred newborns. Trends toward earlier enteral feeding and discharge have been noted.

In infants with omphalocele it has become apparent that the morbidity and mortality are directly related to associated congenital anomalies. In infants with giant omphalocele, cesarean section may become necessary in the setting of growing concerns regarding dystocia, rather than regarding the protection of the viscera or drainage of the membrane.

The controversies in perinatal management of abdominal wall defects revolve primarily around the infant with gastroschisis. In the absence of complicating anomalies, such as intestinal atresia, improving the quality of the eviscerated bowel usually improves outcome. Potential interventions include earlier delivery, avoidance of labor and vaginal delivery, and intrauterine, rather than postnatal, transfer to tertiary-level care centers. No prospective, randomized study has provided a definitive answer to these issues. Most centers have concluded that cesarean section is not indicated except for obstetric concerns. There has been no significant benefit in terms of the outcome variables for infants with gastroschisis delivered by cesarean section. Good results can be achieved with early, immediate delivery room surgical intervention. The factors affecting outcome with postnatal transfer of patients are more directly related to resuscitation and attention to the appropriate handling of the intestine during transport to the surgeon.

NEWBORN PREOPERATIVE MANAGEMENT

Common principles of newborn resuscitation and preoperative management apply to these defects. Specific considerations for omphalocele relate to a close examination of the newborn for the integrity of the defect and an appreciation of any associated pulmonary disease that might accompany giant omphalocele. Procedures for endotracheal intubation, ventilation, and arterial and venous access are performed, based on an initial survey that identifies other severe cardiac or urologic anomalies. If transport is anticipated, the membrane should be covered with sterile saline-soaked gauze, and a protective barrier to prevent heat loss should be applied. Plastic wrap is ideal for omphalocele coverage and protection. Broad-spectrum antibiotics should be started.

Consideration of associated anomalies should have priority over the concern for surgical repair. An exception to this might occur with disruption of the membrane and evisceration. Most disruptions are minor, however, and can usually be sealed with sterile petrolatum-impregnated gauze while secondary evaluations are underway. The standard evaluation should include neonatal examination, plain chest films, echocardiography in the presence of a murmur, and subsequent abdominal ultrasound for urologic abnormalities.

The initial approach to gastroschisis is critical, as inappropriate or careless coverage of the eviscerated bowel may induce torsion of the vascular pedicle containing the mesenteric vessels. If this is covered with nontransparent dressings, progressive intestinal ischemia may develop. The use of transparent surgical bowel bags along with manual stabilization during transport should be emphasized. Nasogastric decompression is essential and should begin immediately after birth.

The optimal goals of surgical treatment of both defects is skin, fascia, and muscle coverage, which ultimately restore anterior abdominal wall. Only an omphalocele might qualify for nonoperative management when a covered ventral hernia can be established by the use of agents that initially provide a bacteriostatic eschar, followed by progressive epithelialization. Current practices include the application of silver nitrate, silver sulfadiazine cream, povidone-iodine (Betadine) solution, and triiodomethane petrolatum (iodoform) gauze. Any prolonged use of iodinated compounds is accompanied by the risk of thyroid suppression. Nonoperative management of giant omphalocele does not preclude reduction of viscera into the abdomen. Significant success has been achieved by repeated wrapping of the omphalocele in a figure-of-eight fashion with the use of semielastic gauze dressing. This material, when changed daily with increased tension, has allowed for progressive reduction of liver and bowel in the setting of resolving pulmonary disease or cardiac stabilization.

INTRAOPERATIVE MANAGEMENT

Omphalocele

Small and medium-sized defects can usually be handled with primary fascial closure while intra-abdominal pressure is monitored (Fig. 144–1). Elevation of abdominal pressure at abdominal wall closure results in decreased venous return, decreased cardiac output, decreased pulmonary compliance, decreased ventilation, and decreased splanchnic perfusion. Pressure monitoring may be aided by arterial and central venous lines, along with nasogastric tubes and Foley catheters. When transduced manometrically, the latter two give excellent indicators of elevated intra-abdominal pressure. Both intragastric pressures of less than 20 mm Hg and increases in central venous pressure of less than 20 mm Hg have been parameters that have successfully guided staged repair of both omphalocele and gastroschisis. With these guidelines, there appear to be no complications of increased intra-abdominal pressure.

Patients should be uniformly intubated for anesthesia and assisted ventilation during paralysis. Antibiotics are

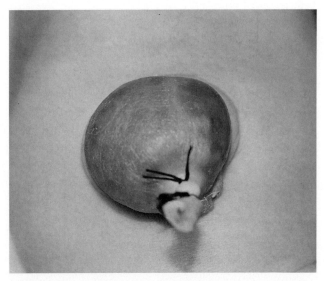

Figure 144–1. A small central omphalocele presents in a full-term newborn. The umbilical vessels have been ligated, and the cord transected. This simple lesion can be closed with primary fascial closure.

administered. Controversy has sometimes arisen over whether the sac should be removed, and many reports and experiences have presented both sides. Generally, the smaller the defect, the easier the removal of the sac before fascial closure. As the size of the defect increases, the sac remains attached to larger areas of the liver. The improved benefits of the removal of the portion of amnion and peritoneum is overshadowed by the risks of laceration of the newborn liver and hemorrhage.

If the sac is removed, the umbilical vessels must be identified and ligated. No specific intra-abdominal maneuvers are necessary. Slight stretching of the abdominal wall has been advocated by some but probably best serves to increase abdominal wall edema and to jeopardize the fascial closure.

If approximation can be accomplished within specific pressure limits, skin flaps are created by sharp dissection away from the fascia. Interrupted sutures are then placed in the fascia longitudinally from the superior portion of the defect to the inferior edge. These are sequentially tied while intra-abdominal pressure is monitored and care is taken to prevent extensive compression or decreased ventilation. Creative methods for skin closure of smaller defects have been described to enable formation of a false umbilicus. Subcuticular absorbable sutures placed in a pursestring fashion have yielded excellent results. Very small defects, known as "hernias of the cord," can be closed transversely.

Considerable experience, judgment, and art are required in the management of larger defects and giant omphaloceles (Fig. 144–2). Treatment options can lead to the following: (1) short-term (up to 14 days) silo reduction, followed by closure with the use of fascia or prosthetic materials when adequate skin coverage for both is available; (2) long-term (2 to 6 weeks) silo reduction, followed by the same maneuvers; or (3) a staged reduction closing skin flaps over the amnion, followed by delayed (6 to 12 months) closure of the ventral hernia.

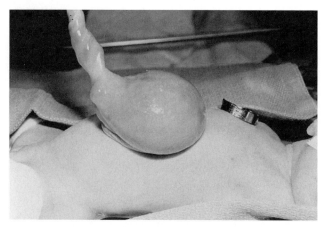

Figure 144–2. Large upper abdominal omphalocele with liver and bowel enclosed underneath the amnion. This type of omphalocele requires gradual closure and fascial advancement.

If short-term reduction is attempted, the surgeon attaches a Dacron-reinforced Silastic membrane to the right and left edges of the fascia after raising a minimal edge of skin (Fig. 144–3). Aggressive skin flap formation should not be performed because it leads to skin retraction that is detrimental to subsequent closure. The Silastic sheets are sutured at the superior and inferior margins of the defect, with closure in the middle creating a closed "silo." Alternatively pre-made silos are available with variable rig

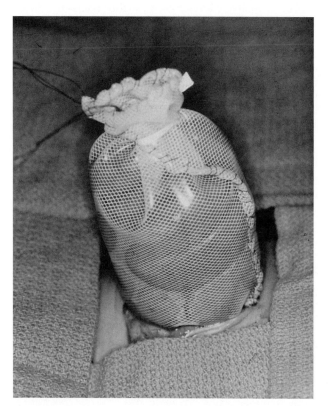

Figure 144–3. This is a completed silo formed from Dacron-reinforced Silastic. The cut edges of the Silastic have been sewn with a running Prolene, and the base has been fixed to the underlying fascia. Within it, intestinal contents can be viewed for both omphalocele and gastroschisis closure.

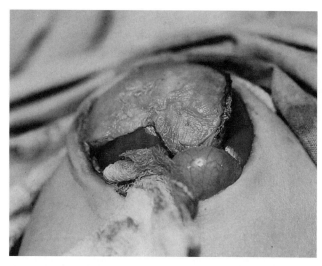

Figure 144–4. The amniotic membrane is left applied to the liver. Separation of this would result in significant bleeding and injury to the liver capsule. The amnion should be maintained whether primary closure is performed or prosthetic material is applied.

structures at the base for fixation under the fascia once the amniotic membrane is removed. Progressive closure for both systems will be accomplished by progressive tightening and closure at the center of the elevated silo. Numerous materials and devices have been described for this purpose; the most cost-effective methods are sutures and umbilical tape. For surgeons experienced with the use of Dacron-reinforced Silastic, there is no need to remove the amniotic membrane because this is a perfect bacteriostatic peritoneal layer over which the Silastic sheets can be applied (Figs. 144–4 and 144–5).

Gastroschisis

Three major concerns dominate the operative management of gastroschisis. The first is the recognition of sig-

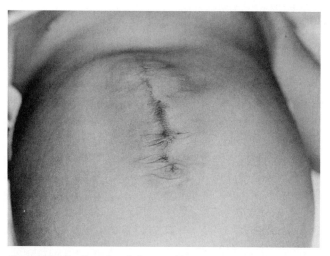

Figure 144–5. Completed closure of large supraumbilical omphalocele. Excellent cosmesis can be obtained when the appropriate fascial advancement and skin flaps have been planned and applied during the course of reduction.

nificant in utero complications, which include growth retardation, midgut volvulus, segmental bowel infarction, and intestinal perforation. The surgeon should examine the eviscerated abdominal contents after establishing mechanical support and maintaining vascular integrity in order to identify any of the complications listed previously. No attempt should be made to decompress the bowel or to remove the reactive peel.

Second, with heightened concerns for fluid replacement appropriate for increased losses, venous lines are placed, and at least 125 to 175 mL/kg per day of fluid is administered. Antibiotics, ampicillin 100 mg/kg per day and gentamicin 5 to 7 mg/kg per day, are administered intravenously. Appropriate conductive (water blanket) or convective (BAIR-Hugger, Augustine Medical, Eden Prairie, MN) warming is mandatory during the procedure.

After the abdomen has been prepared, the umbilicus is identified and preserved for reconstruction (Fig. 144–6). In as many as 75% of infants, the eviscerated contents can be reduced into the abdomen. Extension of the defect should continue superiorly for several centimeters to open a narrow defect and allow for reduction. Excessive manipulation of the bowel is not necessary and will lead to disruption of the fragile mesentery or bowel perforation. Any sustained pressure to achieve reduction indicates the need for silo reduction, as described later.

The third major challenge is the management of infarcted bowel, which should be carefully resected, with the open bowel ends oversewn. Interrupted sutures may be placed in areas of perforation, and no attempt should be made for primary anastomosis in areas of segmental infarction or identified atresia. Marginal or questionable bowel is best observed during silo reduction.

The intraoperative management of atresia has frequently been an area of concern, based on earlier unsuccessful attempts to establish continuity (Fig. 144–7). It has been argued that proximal decompression by an enterostomy could then be followed by delayed anastomosis

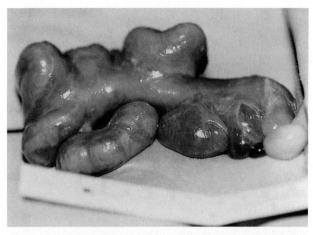

Figure 144–7. Significant peel and inflammation present on the serosa of the eviscerated bowel in gastroschisis. Two atretic segments of intestine are seen at the center. These should not be repaired at the same time as a reduction. The anastomosis will be tenuous and prone to disruption.

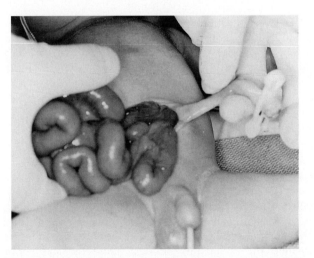

Figure 144–6. Gastroschisis with minimal peel and clear evisceration of intestine from the right side of the umbilicus. Reduction can take place through the defect itself or through a defect by an enlarged superior and inferior incision of the fascia on the midline. Note the Foley catheter in place for transduction of intra-abdominal pressure during decompression.

2 to 6 weeks after intestinal coverage and resolution of the inflammatory peel. Recent experience indicates that decompressive ostomies are not required. However, an area of in utero, postnatal, or intraoperative perforation should be exteriorized without disrupting the mesentery, adjacent to the silo. Bowel atresia can be successfully managed by nasogastric decompression for 2 to 4 weeks after abdominal wall closure, allowing for precise anastomosis of even multiple atretic segments with ancillary tapering enteroplasties. Delays in reanastomosis for 2 weeks result in resolution of the peel, but extension to 4 weeks may be necessary to allow for nutritional optimization. This may occur at the expense of further bowel dilation; however, tapering maneuvers should eliminate any further negative impact.

Once the abdominal contents, which may include small and large bowel, stomach, bladder, ovaries, uterine tubes, and testes, have been reduced, interrupted absorbable sutures are placed in the fascia (Fig. 144–8). Closure is then accomplished, with monitoring of intra-abdominal pressure, as for omphalocele. The skin is then closed over the defect, allowing the umbilicus to come to its normal central position.

The inability to accomplish complete reduction, questionable bowel perfusion, or elevated intra-abdominal pressure should prompt consideration of the use of skin flaps for coverage or, more appropriately, the use of Dacron-reinforced Silastic sheeting as a silo. The fascial defect is enlarged as for primary repair, and the Silastic sheeting is sewn with nonabsorbable sutures in a running fashion to either edge. The remaining edges of this silo are also closed with sutures. Progressive reduction without vascular compromise or perforation due to pressure can be accomplished by various means; the most simple and accessible is umbilical tape and heavy suture. Reduction to fascial approximation is usually reached in several days but may necessarily extend up to 2 weeks later.

In the setting of a large defect that allows for reduction but difficult closure of the fascia, Gore-Tex patches are an alternative if skin flaps can then be brought over the

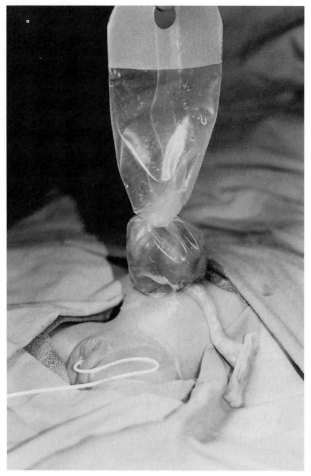

Figure 144–8. Reduction of abdominal contents in gastroschisis. The silo is supported by a subfascial ring. Gradual reduction occurs by simply sequentially tying the bag closer to the abdominal surface. Note the Foley catheter to allow for continuous monitoring of intra-abdominal pressure.

Gore-Tex. A durable closure is provided, which may or may not require further operative revision, owing to excellent regrowth of fibrous tissue into the patch. Long-term follow-up of patients who have undergone this method of repair has shown that many of these patches are extruded as the infant grows.

POSTOPERATIVE MANAGEMENT

The major immediate postoperative concerns are for respiratory insufficiency, nutritional support, and wound care. For both omphalocele and gastroschisis, total parenteral nutrition (TPN) via a central line should be initiated immediately. Paralysis and heavy sedation may be necessary to aid ventilatory support initially, but prolonged use is at the cost of increased peripheral and abdominal wall edema. Flaps should be examined for evidence of ischemia, cellulitis, or fasciitis. After repair of both defects, significant erythema of the abdominal wall can appear through the first 72 hours postoperatively. Surgeons must carefully examine the wound to differentiate the response from early wound infection. Oral or nasogastric decompression is maintained.

For both gastroschisis and omphalocele, the duration of mechanical ventilation postoperatively may be directly related to the degree of pulmonary compromise created by the repair. Although several methods of intraoperative intra-abdominal pressure monitoring have been described, only recently have real-time flow-volume curves been found to be helpful in postoperative respiratory management. Closure of the abdominal defect resulted in decreases to 50% of normal for forced vital capacity and respiratory system compliance. Forced vital capacity approaches normal 4 weeks after operation, while compliance remains 50% lower than that of control infants. Severe ventral defects may therefore result in impaired lung growth.

COMPLICATIONS

An association of gastroschisis with necrotizing enterocolitis (NEC) has been identified after repair. The presentation of NEC is by peritonitis due to delayed perforation, new-onset ileus, or other evidence of intra-abdominal sepsis. Pneumatosis with or without portal vein air will be present on abdominal films. Perforation rates may be lower in this group of patients. Episodes of NEC have occasionally occurred very late in the hospital course or in patients who have been readmitted with NEC. TPN-associated cholestasis, delayed enteral feedings, and other intestinal anomalies had a positive correlation with NEC. This high incidence of a relatively benign atypical form of NEC should not, therefore, preclude initiation of the enteral feedings as soon as possible. There is no direct evidence that earlier feeding is protective against postoperative NEC.

In the absence of any evidence of NEC, sepsis through the imperfect barrier of a silo is a real possibility for both groups of patients. The same is true for the newborns with giant omphalocele who have undergone conservative management with an intact amniotic membrane. A thorough search for any disruption of the membrane must be done, and a barrier re-established.

Delayed intestinal motility has been one of the central postoperative concerns in patients with gastroschisis. Patients who undergo primary reduction and closure have an advantage with respect to earlier institution of enteral feedings and discharge. Infants with primary repair performed either immediately or in the delivery room, earlier enteral feeding, shorter ventilator dependency, and more rapid discharge were observed.

OUTCOME AND THE NEED FOR SECONDARY SURGICAL REPAIR

Most secondary reconstructions are required for patients with giant omphaloceles. Ideally, eventual fascial repair is the goal. Fascial substitutes that have been described include Marlex and Prolene mesh, Gore-Tex, and lyophilized dura mater. The latter material was used as an adjunct for abdominal wall closing in three children without complications.

Experimentally, one of the most attractive options has been the use of an inner Gore-Tex patch reinforced

Pearls and Pitfalls

PEARLS

- In utero diagnosis requires karyotypic diagnosis for omphalocele.
- Gastroschisis associated with intestinal atresia, and growth retardation.
- C-section is not necessary to protect bowel.

PITFALLS

- Inadequate temperature protection from heat loss
- Inadequate fluid resuscitation
- Forcing a primary closure that results in abdominal compartment syndrome and ventilatory compromise
- Improper stabilization and bowel protection resulting in mesenteric ischemia
- Minimal bowel handling in gastroschisis
- Limited undermining of skin flaps in placing silo
- Gradual silo reduction through extended ring
- Early TPN
- Delayed repair of atresia

externally by Prolene or Marlex mesh. Few adhesions to the inner Gore-Tex were found, whereas dense fibrinous tissue readily infiltrated the external mesh.

Several reports of primary fascial closure after abdominal placement of tissue expanders show good long-term results. Another successive technique of tissue expansion involves placement of saline-filled expanders within the rectus sheath. If this technique provides enough fascial coverage, skin coverage can be provided by the use of subcutaneous tissue expanders. Excessive intra-abdominal pressure during tissue expansion, however, must be avoided.

The long-term results of patients with repaired gastroschisis and omphalocele appear to be good, but late surgical problems should be anticipated. When followed for a mean of 5 years, postoperative ventral hernia developed in 25% of patients with omphalocele and in an equal percentage of gastroschisis patients. Intestinal obstruction was more common after omphalocele repair. Complications occurred whether closure was primary or delayed.

In most cases of omphalocele, early termination of pregnancy owing to chromosomal abnormalities or early newborn death are the major sources of mortality. Morbidity for the remaining 20% to 50% of newborns rests in ongoing problems with associated malformations or

secondary reconstructions. Evidence of prolonged pulmonary compromise has been provided. Secondary infection of synthetic prosthetic materials may be anticipated and may require removal before final attempts at fascial closure. Recurrent small bowel obstructions due to adhesion and gastric outlet obstruction from excessive splenic or hepatic compression have been reported. Inguinal hernias and gastroesophageal reflux appear with greater frequency in these patients.

In a review of patients with gastroschisis, the ability to perform primary fascial closure ranged from 31% to 81% of patients. A critical review of patient parameters showed no differences with respect to patient weight, gestational age, and associated fetal complications and abnormalities. Survival is expected for infants with gastroschisis or omphalocele who do not have other anomalies. When one considers all patients, gastroschisis patients have a surgical closure rate of approximately 85% and omphalocele patients somewhat less, depending on the nature of other problems.

Life-long concerns of short gut syndrome, respiratory compromise, and developmental delay in nearly 20% of children require continued attention. Although improved clinical management has significantly diminished newborn morbidity and mortality rates, the potential remains to ameliorate earlier fetal injury and associated problems.

SELECTED READINGS

Coughlin JP, Drucker DE, Jewell MR, et al: Delivery room repair of gastroschisis. Surgery 1993;l14:822.

deVries PA: The pathogenesis of gastroschisis and omphalocele. J Pediatr Surg 1980;15:245.

Langer JC, Khanna J, Caco C, et al: Prenatal diagnosis of gastroschisis: Development of objective sonographic criteria for predicting outcome. Obstet Gynecol 1993;81:53.

Lewis DF, Towers CV, Garite TJ, et al: Fetal gastroschisis and omphalocele: Is cesarean section the best mode of delivery? Am J Obstet Gynecol 1990;163:773.

Moretti M, Khoury A, Rodriquez J, et al: The effect of mode of delivery on the perinatal outcome in fetuses with abdominal wall defects. Am J Obstet Gynecol 1990;163:833.

Nicholls U, Upadhyaya V, Gornall P, et al: Is specialist centre delivery of gastroschisis beneficial? Arch Dis Child 1993;69:71.

Novotny DA, Klein RL, Boeckman CR: Gastroschisis: An 18-year review. J Pediatr Surg 1993;28:650.

Schuster SR: A new method for the staged repair of large omphaloceles. Surg Gynecol Obstet 1967;125:837.

Schwartz MZ, Tyson KR, Milliorn K, et al: Staged reduction using a Silastic sac is the treatment of choice for large congenital abdominal wall defects. J Pediatr Surg 1983;18:713.

Wesley JR, Drongowski R, Coran AG: Intragastric pressure measurement: A guide for reduction and closure of the Silastic chimney in omphalocele and gastroschisis. J Pediatr Surg 1981;16:264.

Chapter 145
Pyloric Stenosis
François I. Luks

The first complete description of hypertrophic pyloric stenosis was published more than a century ago by Harald Hirschsprung, the Danish pediatrician who is also credited with the first patient series of esophageal atresia, the treatment of intussusception by hydrostatic enema reduction, and the description of congenital megacolon (Hirschsprung's disease). The disease course is well known, and its surgical treatment, as devised by Fredet and Ramstedt in the early 1900s, is straightforward. The etiology of pyloric stenosis, however, remains unknown.

Many investigators have, in recent years, searched for molecular and cellular causes of pyloric stenosis. Several mediators of vascular tone and intestinal motility (most notably nitric oxide) have been shown to be differentially expressed in the disease. However, pyloric stenosis is almost never associated with other conditions in which these mediators are implicated, and a true causative relationship has yet to be established.

Hypertrophic pyloric stenosis is one of the most common surgical conditions in infancy, occurring in 1 in 250 children. It is usually not present at birth, but typically develops in the first few weeks of life. There appears to be a slight familial incidence, although no clear pattern of inheritance is seen, and sporadic cases are much more common than familial ones. There is a strong male preponderance, and first-born infants tend to be more often affected. If pyloric stenosis occurs in a girl, her children are at a significantly increased risk for contracting stenosis also. Epidemiologic studies have failed to identify environmental, genetic, or dietary (breast milk versus formula) factors. Pyloric stenosis is more common in full-term infants; if preterm infants are affected, they are typically several weeks older than their term counterparts.

CLINICAL PRESENTATION

Pyloric stenosis appears to be a progressive process of pyloric muscular hypertrophy. It is now well documented that the full-blown syndrome, in which pyloric obstruction is complete, is often preceded by a period of intermittent pyloric spasm. The infant first vomits formula (but not water or Pedialyte), and this may be interpreted as intolerance to a particular type of formula. Not uncommonly, formula changes have been tried before pyloric stenosis is suspected. Nevertheless, there appears to be an increased awareness among pediatricians and primary care physicians, and pyloric stenosis is often suspected earlier in the disease course. As a result, the condition is now diagnosed several weeks earlier, on average, than 20 years ago.

The hallmark of pyloric stenosis is projectile, nonbilious vomiting. The mean age at onset is 2 to 3 weeks of life, but vomiting may still be intermittent for another week or two. The absence of bile helps exclude other, more distal, causes of intestinal obstruction, such as midgut volvulus or Hirschsprung's disease. The appearance of coffee ground vomiting suggests associated gastritis and is often a later finding. Other, nonsurgical conditions, such as sepsis, gastroenteritis, hepatitis, and metabolic disorders, are easily eliminated because the child with pyloric stenosis appears otherwise well and extremely hungry, and does not present with associated signs, such as diarrhea and abdominal tenderness. Mild jaundice is not uncommon in pyloric stenosis, and is believed to be secondary to glucuronyltransferase deficiency.

If the condition is allowed to progress untreated, the infant will become dehydrated, lethargic, and shocky. In severe cases, there may be signs of severe malnutrition, constipation, oliguria, and profound alkalosis. The latter is a pathognomonic sign of pyloric obstruction. As the child vomits chloride- and hydrogen-rich gastric contents, hypochloremic alkalosis sets in. Hypokalemia is the result of an intracellular shift of potassium ions (in exchange for hydrogen ions) and renal loss as the body attempts to conserve sodium. As potassium is depleted, sodium is exchanged for hydrogen ions in the proximal tubules, giving rise to paradoxic aciduria. The latter hastens systemic alkalosis and, ultimately, cardiovascular collapse.

Today, the full syndrome is very seldom seen. However, most large pediatric surgical centers treat at least one or two patients each year with profound shock and electrolyte imbalance due to longstanding, undiagnosed pyloric stenosis.

CLINICAL EXAMINATION

It is often said that pyloric stenosis can—and should—be diagnosed clinically in the vast majority of cases. However, palpation of the hypertrophic pylorus (the so-called olive or tumor) is sometimes difficult, and requires patience. Having the child in a parent's lap, in a quiet environment, and calmed with either a pacifier or a few sips of clear fluid (5% dextrose in water or Pedialyte) can be useful. If the stomach is full, one-time nasogastric aspiration facilitates the examination. In advanced cases, strong gastric peristaltic waves can be seen in the left upper quadrant, which may be all the more visible if the child is chronically malnourished and emaciated. This late presentation is much less common today.

The examiner stands on the child's left side, and the examining fingers gently palpate the abdomen from the right to the left upper quadrants. It is useful to first recognize the contour of the structures most likely to be confused with an enlarged pylorus: the right kidney, the spine, and the right and left rectus muscles. The pylorus is then gently teased from under the liver edge, and rolled between the examining fingers and the infant's spine.

LABORATORY TESTS AND IMAGING

If pyloric stenosis is suspected, few laboratory tests need to be obtained. A simple urinalysis may confirm mild or moderate dehydration and, less commonly, aciduria. A complete blood count is useful preoperatively, since 3- to 4-week-old infants have a physiologic anemia. The most important test, however, is a serum electrolyte panel. Hypokalemia, hypochloremia, alkalosis, and dehydration can be confirmed, and need to be corrected before surgical correction is entertained. If at all possible, blood should be drawn carefully (no heelstick) to avoid hemolysis and an erroneously elevated serum potassium value.

In general, no other laboratory tests are needed, unless other diagnoses are entertained. Imaging studies are theoretically superfluous if a clinical diagnosis was made. In reality, radiographs or an ultrasound will often have been obtained before the child is referred to a surgeon. In cases where the clinical diagnosis is uncertain, these tests are very helpful. Until the late 1980s, an upper gastrointestinal series was the radiographic examination of choice (Fig. 145–1). Typical radiographic signs are the mushroom impression of the antrum and protruding pyloric mucosa, the track sign caused by an elongated pyloric channel with straight, parallel mucosal folds, and the number 3 or umbrella sign formed by contrast medium in the first portion of the duodenum. A contrast-enhanced radiograph also helps exclude gastroesophageal reflux, which is the most common differential diagnosis.

Since its first description in 1982, the ultrasonographic examination of the pylorus has become the most accepted imaging test, supplanting the contrast-enhanced radiograph, with its radiation and risk of barium aspiration. The ultrasound signs of hypertrophic pyloric stenosis are well established: normally, the pyloric channel should be less than 16 mm in length, the total thickness (from serosa to serosa) of the pylorus should be less than 14 mm, and the muscular thickness (from serosa to mucosa

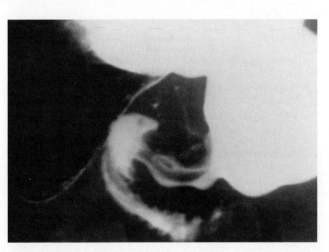

Figure 145–1. Contrast-enhanced radiograph in pyloric stenosis. Note the elongated pyloric channel with thickened, parallel mucosal folds ("mushroom" sign).

on either side of the lumen) should be less than 4 mm. With pyloric stenosis, any or all of the aforementioned values are increased. In addition, an experienced ultrasonographer will be able to see propulsive peristaltic waves of the antrum, the pyloric spasm, and, if present, gastroesophageal reflux.

PREOPERATIVE MANAGEMENT

Surgical correction of pyloric stenosis is the only sensible form of treatment (prolonged intravenous hydration and nutrition have been proposed in the past, and the self-limited nature of the disease has thus been demonstrated). However, the operation for pyloric stenosis is not considered an emergency. Rather, the infant should be well hydrated and the electrolyte anomalies mentioned earlier should be completely corrected. In severe cases, this may take 1 to 2 days, although today fewer than 10% of all infants with pyloric stenosis present with any electrolyte abnormality warranting delay of surgical intervention. A nasogastric tube is not routinely used, unless the child continues to vomit after feedings have been withheld. Intravenous hydration should take into account the source of fluid and electrolyte losses: 0.45 N saline or, in severe cases, 0.9 N saline solution should be used, supplemented with potassium chloride (10 to 30 mEq/L) after urine output has been documented. If electrolyte anomalies are present, they should be corrected gradually.

INTRAOPERATIVE MANAGEMENT

At the time of operation, any infant with pyloric obstruction is considered to have a full stomach. Studies have demonstrated that the risk of aspiration on induction is not reduced by nasogastric suctioning, even if performed immediately before anesthesia. Therefore, rapid sequence or awake intubation, with cricoid pressure, are the preferred methods of induction.

The technique of pyloromyotomy has not changed since its initial description. However, many approaches and incisions have been tried. Today, the vertical midline and Robertson incisions (a right upper quadrant muscle-splitting incision, in an attempt to prevent dehiscence in severely malnourished infants) are rarely used. A laparoscopic approach has been well described, but is not widely embraced by pediatric surgeons, because it offers only marginal cosmetic and no functional advantages over the open technique.

The classic approach is a horizontal incision over the right rectus muscle, halfway between the umbilicus and the xyphoid process. The anterior rectus sheath is divided, and the rectus muscle fibers can be retracted laterally or separated in the midportion of the rectus. Because of the newborn's physiologic diastasis and wide linea alba, a generous incision into the posterior rectus sheath and peritoneum can be made without the need to divide either rectus muscle or extend the incision into oblique muscles.

The pylorus can be grasped carefully with an eyed forceps (Singli or Tuttle), or the greater curvature of the stomach can be exteriorized first, before the pylorus is delivered into the wound. To identify the stomach through a relatively small incision, it is helpful to introduce the corner of a dry sponge into the abdomen, thereby catching omentum. Omentum will lead to transverse colon, which will lead to stomach.

More recently, the umbilical approach has become popular. It is a cosmetically gratifying, but anatomically awkward incision, and delivering the pylorus is more difficult. A semicircular, full 180-degree line is drawn just outside the most peripheral umbilical fold, to maximize the length of the incision. Once the wound is deepened down to the fascia, a superior flap is created to expose the linea alba over 2 to 3 cm. The peritoneum is entered through a vertical midline incision in the fascia, staying to the left of the umbilical vein (round ligament). The pylorus is delivered as above. One should not hesitate to extend the fascial or skin incision a little, if necessary.

The pylorus is grasped between the thumb and the index finger of the nondominant hand, inserting the digits in the gastric and duodenal "lumens" (Fig. 145–2). A very superficial incision is made anterosuperiorly, in an avascular field, over the entire length of the pylorus, and extending onto gastric serosa. The knife handle or one blade of the Benson pyloric spreader is gently inserted in the incision, and the longitudinal muscle fibers are carefully pried open. Once the pyloric incision is sufficiently widened, both blades of the spreader are inserted and gradual pressure is exerted on the two walls of the incision. Care must be taken not to insert the instrument too deeply, or to spread it too forcefully, in order to avoid tearing the pyloric mucosa.

The muscle fibers are eventually split down to the submucosa, which pops out into the pyloric wound (see Fig. 145–2). Muscle fibers should be split from the gastric to the duodenal end. Completeness of the pyloromyotomy is confirmed by the ability to move each half of the pyloric muscle independently. Finally, gastric content (fluid and/or air, administered through a nasogastric tube if necessary) is squeezed through the pylorus and into the duodenum, to search for mucosal leaks.

Should a mucosal tear occur, it is repaired with an absorbable suture (4-0 or 5-0 polyglycolic acid or similar material). Omentum can be placed over the pylorus in Graham patch fashion. In the unlikely event that the repair compromises the results of the pyloromyotomy, the pylorus can be rotated 180 degrees along its axis, exposing

its inferoposteror surface, and a second pyloromyotomy can be performed.

It is not uncommon to encounter some bleeding from pyloric capillaries; no attempt should be made at hemostasis, unless a larger vessel has been injured. Most often, the bleeding appears excessive because of venous congestion caused by the exteriorization of the pylorus. Bleeding will stop promptly once the pylorus is returned into the peritoneal cavity.

The fascia is closed with absorbable sutures (3-0 polyglycolic acid or equivalent). If the umbilical incision is used, it is important to recognize that the linea alba in infants may be weak and the superior corner of the fascial incision may be attenuated. Not recognizing this may lead to fascial dehiscence. A helpful technique is to place a stay suture at the upper corner of the fascial incision before the peritoneal cavity is entered.

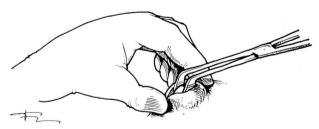

Figure 145–2. Pyloromyotomy. Once the pylorus is exteriorized, it is stabilized between the thumb and the index finger of the nondominant hand (one fingertip on each side of the pyloric channel). The pyloric spreader (with serrations on the outside) gently splits the hypertrophied muscle fibers until the mucosa and submucosa are seen protruding through the gap.

Pearls and Pitfalls

PEARLS

- When one examines an infant for pyloric stenosis, it is helpful to identify normal structures first: right kidney, rectus muscles, liver edge, and spine.
- Standing on the infant's left, the examiner should be able to gently roll the pylorus from under the liver and over the spine.
- The definitive treatment of pyloric stenosis is pyloromyotomy, but it is not considered an emergency; rehydration and correction of the electrolyte imbalance is.
- The classic approach is a transverse incision over the right rectus muscle, whereby the muscle is retracted laterally, rather than divided. A cosmetically attractive alternative is the umbilical incision.
- To facilitate exteriorization of the pylorus, a "push-pull" technique can be helpful, with gentle downward pressure on the abdominal wall. Once exteriorized, the pylorus is best stabilized between the thumb and the index finger of the nondominant hand.
- Completeness of pyloromyotomy is confirmed by the ability to move each half of the pyloric muscle independently.

PITFALLS

- Difficulties in establishing a clinical diagnosis: perseverance is key (may take 20 minutes).
- Difficulties in delivering the pylorus intraoperatively: incision (skin and fascia) should be large enough, but too wide an incision makes it difficult to maintain the pylorus in an exteriorized position.
- Initial pyloric incision should be shallow (serosa only); avoid forceful spreading of the pyloric walls; isometric pressure is safer.
- Most mucosal perforations occur on the duodenal side, where the mucosa folds on itself.
- Avoiding intraoperative complications: mucosal perforation and peritonitis are serious complications best avoided by meticulous technique and vigilance. When one uses the umbilical incision, the upper edge of the linea alba incision is best identified with a stay suture, to facilitate adequate fascial closure.

POSTOPERATIVE MANAGEMENT

A nasogastric tube is not usually necessary. Feedings are resumed within 6 hours, and advanced gradually from 15 to 30 mL of an electrolyte solution (Pedialyte) to full formula or breast milk. This will typically take 5 or 6 feedings, each 3 hours part. Many different feeding regimens exist, and differences may not be relevant. A few principles should be observed: some vomiting is still expected postoperatively, either from gastric spasms if the child has been ill for a prolonged period of time or, more commonly, because of coexisting gastroesophageal reflux. If this happens, feedings can be held, but should be resumed 3 hours later. As feedings are advanced, it is important to introduce formula or breast milk (full- or half-strength) early on, before increasing the volume. Clear fluids alone are not enough to keep the pylorus open, and recurrent pyloric stenosis may occur if curds are not allowed to stimulate the pyloric channel. The infant is discharged home once a full feeding schedule is attained, usually within 24 of 36 hours.

COMPLICATIONS AND OUTCOMES

Major complications are very rare, unless the infant was severely malnourished preoperatively. Wound infection may occur, and appears to be slightly more common than with comparable, clean operations (e.g., inguinal herniorrhaphy). The incidence of wound complications may be as high as 4% to 5%, according to some series.

Skin, or rarely fascial dehiscence may occur as well. Treatment is conservative, unless fascial dehiscence or evisceration is present. Antibiotic prophylaxis has been advocated by some, but has not been shown to alter the risk of infectious complications.

Recurrent pyloric stenosis is well described and requires a repeat pyloromyotomy (see earlier). However, it is a very unusual event today, and most instances of postoperative vomiting are due to reflux. Unrecognized mucosal perforation (usually on the duodenal side) and peritonitis are serious complications that can be avoided by meticulous technique and vigilance. The success rate of pyloromyotomy for infantile pyloric stenosis should approach 100%, and late recurrence does not occur.

SELECTED READINGS

Chen EA, Luks FI, Gilchrist BF, et al: Pyloric stenosis in the age of ultrasonography: Fading skills, better patients? J Pediatr Surg 1996;31:829.

Fredet P: La cure de la sténose hypertrophique du pylore chez les nourrissons par la pyloromyotomie extra-muqueuse. J Chir 1927;29:385.

Hirschsprung H: Fälle von angeborener Pylorusstenose, beobachtet bei Sauglingen. Jahrb Kinderheilk 1888;27:61.

Hulka F, Harrison MW, Campbell TJ, et al: Complications of pyloromyotomy for infantile hypertrophic pyloric stenosis. Am J Surg 1997;173:450.

Leinwand MJ, Shaul DB, Anderson KD: The umbilical fold approach to pyloromyotomy: Is it a safe alternative to the right upper-quadrant approach? J Am Coll Surg 1999;189:362.

Ramsted C: Zur Operation der angeborenen Pylorusstenose. Med Klin 1912;8:1702.

Teele RL, Smith EH: Ultrasound in the diagnosis of idiopathic hypertrophic pyloric stenosis. N Engl J Med 1977;296:1149.

Vanderwinden JM, Mailleux P, Schiffmann SN, et al: Nitric oxide synthase activity in infantile hypertrophic pyloric stenosis. N Engl J Med 1992;327:511.

Chapter 146
Intussusception
Arlet G. Kurkchubasche

Intussusception is the most common abdominal emergency seen in the early childhood years (3 months to 6 years), exceeding even appendicitis in this age group. In contrast with the older child and adult, 80% to 90% of patients younger than 3 years of age experience idiopathic ileocolic intussusception, for which, in the absence of peritonitis, nonsurgical management is the mainstay of therapy.

Intussusception occurs when one segment of intestine (intussusceptum) is circumferentially invaginated and propulsed into the adjacent distal segment (intussuscipiens), resulting in luminal obstruction with progressive venous, lymphatic, and, eventually, arterial compromise. The explanations proposed for this form of intestinal obstruction are manifold and have no established scientific basis. The most widely held theory is that the submucosal lymphoid aggregates (Peyer's patches), the source of secretory immunoglobulins, enlarge in response to antigenic stimulation from newly introduced food substances or viral infections (suggested by seasonal variation coincident with viral gastroenteritis and respiratory infections). The Peyer's patches project into the lumen of the intestine, presenting a transient and pseudopolypoid lead point. Alternative theories include the differential size and motility of adjacent segments of intestine. This theory may be relevant in viral enteritis, but also in the postoperative intussusception, which usually involves the proximal jejunum, devoid of Peyer's patches.

Although intussusception has been recognized since the mid-1700s, successful operative management was not reported until the mid-nineteenth century, when infants and children continued to have a high rate of mortality related to sepsis and dehydration. In 1878, when Harold Hirschsprung first proposed hydrostatic reduction, the survival rates of 50% with hydrostatic reduction were superior to those achieved with operative reduction. In the United States, William Ladd was a proponent for the use of the contrast-enhanced enema for diagnosis in 1913, but only in 1948 was it accepted for therapeutic intervention. Air reduction techniques were first reported from China, where there is an inordinate incidence of intussusception, and were introduced to the United States as an alternative to the contrast-enhanced enema in the 1990s. Ultrasonographic evaluation of the abdomen has become established as an alternative, less invasive tool for the diagnosis of intussusception. Doppler imaging provides the advantage of being able to assess intestinal blood flow when used in (and thus identifying) patients who would not benefit from attempts at hydrostatic reduction. In some centers, it has been used to monitor saline enema reductions.

CLINICAL PRESENTATION

Other than age, demographic features are rarely helpful in the differential diagnosis. Boys and girls, and various ethnic and racial groups, appear to be equally affected. The typical history is that of a child, 6 months to 2 years of age (two thirds occur before age 1 year), waking with the abrupt onset of abdominal pain, causing the child to double over and draw their legs to the abdomen. This episode resolves with the child either returning to sleep or resuming normal activity, only to be interrupted again by a wave of colicky abdominal pain, that may be followed by emesis and passage of a normal stool. The child frequently is diaphoretic and pale during these episodes and with time becomes progressively more apathetic and lethargic. As the bowel obstruction persists, emesis progresses to bilious emesis, and the child may pass a bloody, mucous stool (currant jelly stool). Diagnosis rests on a high level of clinical suspicion based on the history provided by a parent or caretaker. Depending on the duration of symptoms, the physical signs may vary. By the time a surgeon is typically asked to see the patient, the child may be quite lethargic and apathetic from dehydration. During a relaxed phase, between episodes, it is possible to palpate the abdomen and identify the essentially pathognomonic features of an empty right lower quadrant (sign of Dance) with a sausage-like mass in the right upper quadrant. Occasionally, a mass in the rectum or even a protrusion analogous to rectal prolapse can be encountered. Gross or occult blood is often detected at this stage. During acute episodes of colic, no reliable abdominal examination can be performed and may lead to the false conclusion of an acute abdomen, prompting potentially unnecessary laparotomy. Consideration of this diagnosis and patience exercised during the examination are thus necessary.

PREOPERATIVE MANAGEMENT

In the patient with a high index of suspicion for intussusception, intravenous access should be promptly established and fluid repletion in the form of isotonic fluid should be administered to correct the estimated deficit. This assessment relies on the adequacy of peripheral perfusion (measured as either capillary refill or a difference in core and peripheral temperatures), the presence of lethargy, electrolyte derangements, or metabolic acidosis. Fluid resuscitation usually requires 10 to 20 mL/kg of either normal saline (NS) or lactated Ringer's (LR) solution, with subsequent provision of dextrose-containing fluids (either D_5NS or D_5LR) at rates of maintenance and a half. The use of antibiotics (i.e., ampicillin and gentamicin), although routine in the past, has now been reserved for patients who require operative intervention.

Radiographic studies useful in establishing the diagnosis of intussusception include supine and left lateral views of the abdomen, which may delineate a paucity of gas in the right lower quadrant with a density in the right upper quadrant, perhaps even delineating the intussusceptum outlined by air (Fig. 146–1). In advanced cases, features of a small bowel obstruction will be apparent. The abdominal x-ray film can, however, be completely unremarkable, and this should not exclude the diagnosis in a patient with a strong clinical history. If expert ultrasonographic evaluation is available, this can be used as an alternative means for diagnosis. The intussusception appears as a target-shaped lesion (Fig. 146–2). When confirmed by sonogram or suspected by radiograph or physical examination, the next intervention both from a diagnostic and, most often, therapeutic standpoint is the contrast-enhanced or pneumatic enema. This intervention is performed only after ascertaining that there are no peritoneal signs. Although not essential, some radiologists request that the child be sedated to facilitate the reduction. The child's ability to maintain the airway when already in a lethargic state with intestinal obstruction, must be taken into consideration. Obviously, the presence of a physician capable of managing the airway in a critical situation is mandatory. General anesthesia is not warranted.

The method of choice for hydrostatic or pneumostatic reduction varies with institutions. Barium, iso-osmolar water-soluble agents, and air reduction all have their proponents. In any form of hydrostatic reduction, the catheter inserted into the rectum must be secured so as to ensure an airtight seal. Most radiologists use a catheter

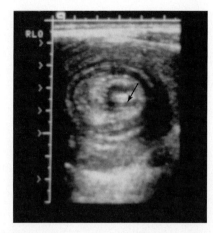

Figure 146–2. Sonogram of intussusception with appendix *(arrow)* as lead point in patient with cystic fibrosis.

with a bulbous tip and tape the buttocks together, rather than using a Foley catheter with insufflation of the balloon to avoid rectal trauma. Guidelines for the height of the contrast column or pressure generated by air insufflation are followed so as to minimize the risk of perforation. When present, the intussusceptum can be seen outlined as it moves retrograde toward the ileocecal valve (Fig. 146–3). It is critical to visualize the complete reduction of the intussusception, evidenced by free reflux of contrast material or air into the distal small intestine. Multiple attempts at reduction in the hemodynamically stable patient may be required before complete reduction is achieved. Hydrostatic reduction should involve the most experienced personnel before a decision is made to go to operative intervention. Once the intussusception is reduced, the child immediately acts as if he or she feels better and typically falls into a sound sleep. Patients are admitted for continued hydration and are observed for the recurrence of the intussusception, which may occur with an incidence of between 5% to 8% within 24 hours of reduction. If asymptomatic the following morning, the child is offered liquids and is advanced to a diet appropriate for age, in anticipation of probable discharge to home. The surgeon treats recurrent symptoms with repeat hydrostatic reduction, again ensuring that a complete reduction is achieved. Older children with recurrences at greater intervals must be suspected of having a pathologic lead point.

OPERATIVE MANAGEMENT

Surgical intervention becomes necessary when a patient presents with unequivocal peritonitis. This usually follows a history of abdominal pain in excess of 48 hours and suggests the presence of intestinal gangrene. Other indices of severe ischemia or gangrene include ultrasonographic findings documenting an absence of mural blood flow or the inability to reduce the intussusception with optimal technique. In the latter circumstance, it is acceptable in some institutions with the appropriate personnel to proceed with one final attempt at hydrostatic reduction in the operating room with the patient under general

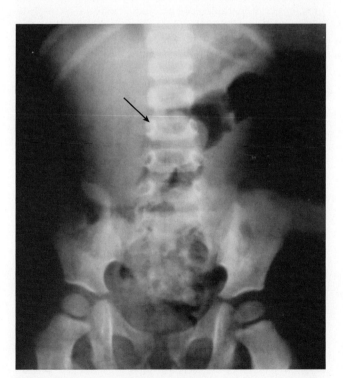

Figure 146–1. Abdominal film demonstrating a mass *(arrow)* within cecum extending into midtransverse colon.

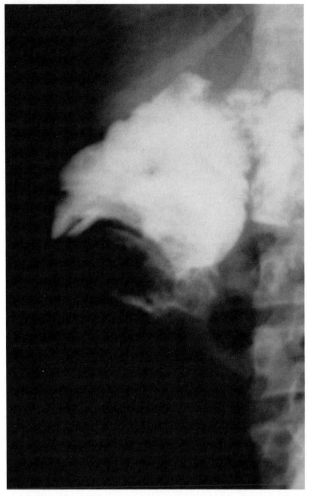

Figure 146–3. Hydrostatic reduction of intussuscipiens by retrograde movement of contrast material.

anesthesia. The inability to reduce the intussusception may also indicate a pathologic lead point.

Operative management consists of either a supraumbilical right transverse laparotomy or, more commonly, a standard muscle-splitting McBurney incision. It is not uncommon to encounter chylous fluid from chronic lymphatic obstruction. The intussusception often cannot be eviscerated, owing to the foreshortened mesentery, and the initial reduction is performed intra-abdominally. Manual reduction is performed by milking the intracolonic mass bimanually in a retrograde fashion, analogous to the hydrostatic reduction. Once the ileocecum alone is involved, the residual intussusception may be brought to the abdominal wall surface, where the complete reduction is accomplished again with the use of a technique of retrograde compression of the leading edge, rather than attempting to pull the ends apart (Fig. 146–4). If serosal tears are encountered in this phase, this usually suggests that resection will be the safest alternative. If reduction is achieved, the congested intestine is wrapped in warm laparotomy pads to maximize perfusion and even returned to the abdomen to minimize venous congestion. After reinspection to verify the absence of necrosis or perfora-

tion, and for repair of potential small serosal tears, the intestine is returned to the abdomen. A standard appendectomy is performed if the McBurney incision was used. Inversion appendectomy is not considered to be optimal in this instance, since it may encourage reintussusception.

When the intussusception cannot be reduced manually, this generally implies necrosis, and a resection with primary anastomosis is typically performed (Fig. 146–5). Only in the event of established perforation with shock would a temporary stoma be considered. Ileocecal resection in this instance is associated with a high potential for injury to the main superior mesenteric vessel axis. These vessels are deceivingly close to the line of mesenteric division, since a portion of the mesentery is involved in the intussusception. Division and ligation of mesenteric vessels must therefore occur as close to the intestine as possible to avoid a devastating loss of midgut. Typically, an end-to-end anastomosis in one or two layers is performed.

POSTOPERATIVE MANAGEMENT

Postoperative management requires ongoing fluid resuscitation and perioperative antibiotic therapy. Recurrent intussusception encountered after operative reduction without resection, should be managed with attempted hydrostatic reduction.

Special Considerations in Pediatric Intussusception

Only 2% to 8% of children younger than 2 years of age with intussusception have a pathologic lead point. This most commonly consists of a Meckel's diverticulum. The prevalence of pathologic lead points may be as high as 57% after age 4 years, but is still markedly less than that in the adult (97%). These atypical causes often result in ileal-ileal, rather than ileocolic intussusception, and thus they are not as easily diagnosed and are not amenable to hydrostatic reduction. Ultrasonography plays a major role in diagnosis here. Other lead points may be provided by

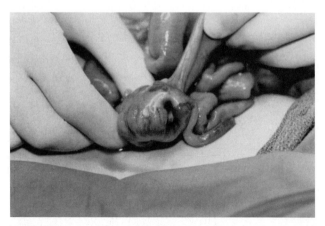

Figure 146–4. Operative reduction of ileocecal intussusception. Note compression of the cecum to squeeze intraluminal intestine retrograde.

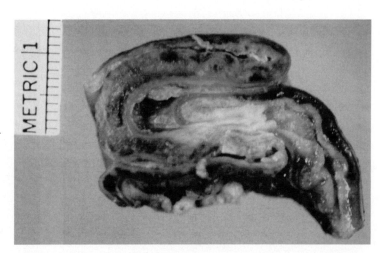

Figure 146–5. Pathology specimen of irreducible intussusception.

hamartomas associated with Peutz-Jeghers syndrome, or mural lesions such as heterotopic pancreatic nodules, enteric cysts, adenoma, acute lymphoblastic leukemia, neurofibroma, or hemangioma. Conditions resulting in mucosal and submucosal hemorrhage, such as Henoch-Schönlein purpura, disseminated intravascular coagulation, hemophilia, and even trauma, have been associated with intussusception. Although mucoviscidosis (cystic fibrosis) may present with intestinal pseudo-obstruction in the later childhood years, one must consider the possibility of intussusception, which in these cases is most often associated with an enlarged, congested appendix.

Idiopathic intussusception occasionally can occur after unrelated upper abdominal or even thoracic procedures. The heralding features include an early postoperative bowel obstruction with high nasogastric outputs despite a decompressed-appearing distal intestine as seen on plain radiograph. Diagnosis is established by either ultrasound or upper intestinal series.

COMPLICATIONS

The primary complications related to intussusception occur as the result of delayed diagnosis, and consequent dehydration acidosis and potential sepsis, and account for a fatality rate of about 1%. The most serious complications related to the hydrostatic reduction are intestinal perforations either in the rectum related to the catheter or, more proximally, related to intraluminal distention against a fixed obstruction. Rates of perforation are reported to be 0.18% with hydrostatic reduction, in contrast with rates between 1% and 2% with pneumatic reduction. With successful hydrostatic reduction, parents must be warned of the potential for recurrence, which is suspected on the basis of recurrent abdominal pain and is again treated with hydrostatic reduction.

OUTCOMES

The vast majority of children who experience idiopathic intussusception are managed with hydrostatic or pneumatic reduction. The rate of successful reduction with

barium enema is approximately 85% within 12 hours of onset of symptoms and decreases to 70% after 24 hours, with an overall success rate of 80%. This rate of success, despite prolonged symptoms, supports an attempt at hydrostatic or pneumatic reduction, in the absence of peri-

---

Pearls and Pitfalls

PEARLS

- Remember to consider the diagnosis in young children with abdominal pain.
- A child who is quiet and does not object to examination is not a "good" patient, but potentially a very sick patient.
- Unequivocal peritonitis or small bowel obstruction as seen on radiograph should prompt urgent laparotomy.

PITFALLS

- Assuming that competency of the ileocecal valve accounts for the lack of free reflux of contrast material or air into the distal ileum—this usually indicates incomplete reduction.
- Excluding this diagnosis on the basis of normal-appearing plain abdominal films.
- Mistaking lethargy or vomiting for meningitis.

Anatomic Considerations

PEARLS

- When performing a resection, be aware of the proximity of the superior mesenteric vessels due to the shortened mesentery.
- Serosal tears indicate excess force in surgical reduction and should prompt resection.

Pathology Change

PEARLS

- Do not mistake the swollen ileocecal valve for a polyp.
- Look for pathologic lead points in older children, and consider cystic fibrosis if the appendix is the lead point.

toneal signs or definite evidence of a small bowel obstruction. The rate of successful reduction was found to be improved with repeated attempts at either barium enema or air reduction after a rest period of variable duration (30 minutes to several hours) only if there was some retrograde movement of the intussusception with consecutive attempts. Of the patients requiring surgery, approximately 60% to 80% can be managed without resection. A total of 10% of intussusceptions are found to have spontaneously reduced at operation. Recurrent intussusception occurs in 4% to 8% of patients, and the majority of cases are treated with repeated attempts at hydrostatic or pneumatic reduction.

SELECTED READINGS

DiFiore JW: Intussusception. Semin Pediatr Surg 1999;8:214.

Guo J-Z, Ma X-Y, Zhou Q-H: Results of air pressure enema reduction of intussusception: 6396 cases in 13 years. J Pediatr Surg 1986;21:1201.

Ravitch MM: Intussusception in infancy and childhood: An analysis of seventy-seven cases treated by barium enema. N Engl J Med 1958;22:1058.

West KW, Stephens B, Rescorla FJ, et al: Postoperative intussusception: Experience with 36 cases in children. Surgery 1988;104:781.

Chapter 147

Meckel's Diverticulum

Donald L. Sorrells, Christopher K. Breuer, and Thomas F. Tracy, Jr.

INTRODUCTION

HISTORY. The first written description of a Meckel's diverticulum has been attributed to Fabricus Hildanus in 1598. Meckel's diverticulum derives its name from Johann Friedrich Meckel, professor of anatomy, whose 1809 account of the origin of this diverticular structure was so clear that his name has been eponymously attached to it ever since.

EMBRYOLOGY. Meckel's diverticulum is a vestigial structure, which results from failure of the omphalomesenteric (vitelline) duct to involute. The yolk sac is connected by the omphalomesenteric duct to the primitive gut. This duct attenuates, involutes, and separates from the intestine between the fifth and seventh weeks of gestation. Failure of the yolk sac to involute results in a persistent omphalomesenteric duct remnant whose anatomy is determined by the stage at which arrest of involution occurs. In a small proportion of diverticula there is an omphalomesenteric duct remnant extending from the apex of the diverticulum to the undersurface of the umbilicus. The omphalomesenteric duct remnant may be a patent mucosa-lined fistula, cystic mass, or fibrous band. Most often there is no connection between the diverticulum and the undersurface of the umbilicus. Instead, a band representing the remnants of the vitelline vessels joins the diverticulum to the mesentery of the small bowel.

ANATOMY AND HISTOLOGY. Meckel's diverticulum is a true diverticulum arising from the antimesenteric border of the ileum. As such it contains all layers of the intestinal wall. The mucosa of the diverticulum can be heterotopic, with either gastric or pancreatic mucosa. Grossly, the diverticulum is usually several centimeters long, although occasional cases of giant Meckel's diverticulum have been described (Fig. 147–1). The diverticulum may have either a broad or a narrow base. The blood supply of the Meckel's diverticulum is usually the same as that of the ileum. The vitelline artery can also persist and act as the primary blood supply to the diverticulum. Occasionally, the blood supply can arise from the abdominal wall. Meckel's diverticulum is usually located within 100 cm of the ileocecal valve.

INCIDENCE. Meckel's diverticulum is the most common congenital anomaly of the gastrointestinal tract. It occurs in between 1.3% and 2.2% of the population, based on autopsy studies. The ratio of males to females in asymptomatic patients is nearly equal, whereas the incidence in symptomatic patients is three to one.

ASSOCIATED ANOMALIES. Meckel's diverticulum is associated with several other congenital and acquired disorders. The incidence of Meckel's diverticulum is increased sixfold in patients with esophageal atresia and fivefold in patients with imperforate anus. Some studies point to an increase in Meckel's diverticulum in patients with cardiac or neurologic abnormalities. Exomphalos also increases the likelihood of a patient's having a Meckel's diverticulum. It is interesting that Crohn's disease is associated with a higher incidence of Meckel's diverticulum, with a threefold increase noted in patients who required surgery for Crohn's disease.

NATURAL HISTORY. Mayo stated that "Meckel's diverticulum is frequently suspected, often looked for, and seldom found." Most Meckel's diverticula are clinically silent. Clinically significant Meckel's diverticulum includes those that are symptomatic (40%) and those discovered incidentally (60%). Symptomatic Meckel's diverticulum presents in a variety of ways depending on the pathophysiology involved. Complications of Meckel's diverticulum include obstruction, inflammation, or bleeding. The original descriptions of Meckel's diverticulum assumed a complication rate of 25%; however, a review of a baseline population of over one million people over a 15-year period determined the chance of a Meckel's diverticulum being a cause of disease to be 6% over one's lifetime. Symptomatic lesions are age dependent, accounting for 85% of the cases in children less than 1 month of age and 77% of those between 1 month and 2 years of age. In contrast, symptomatic lesions were found in only 15% of cases of children over 4 years of age. More than 50% of patients with symptoms referable to Meckel's diverticulum will be identified before 2 years of life.

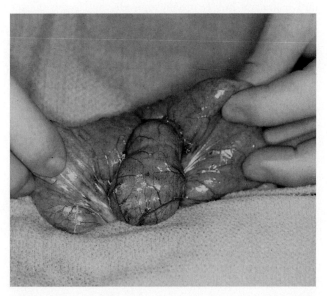

Figure 147–1. Meckel's diverticulum after reduction of intussusception in a 6-year-old patient.

CLINICAL PRESENTATION

Pathophysiology

The clinical presentations arising from a Meckel's diverticulum can arise from one of four basic pathophysiologic causes: hemorrhage, inflammation, obstruction, or congenital ductal persistence. Hemorrhagic complications of Meckel's diverticulum arise from heterotopic gastric mucosa that results in peptic ulceration of the surrounding or opposing ileal mucosa, causing lower gastrointestinal bleeding. Inflammatory clinical manifestations result from diverticular obstruction or perforation secondary to either peptic ulceration or penetration by a foreign body, both leading to Meckel's diverticulitis. Obstructive causes of pathophysiology include intussusception in which the Meckel's diverticulum acts as a lead point, volvulus around a persistent omphalomesenteric remnant, internal herniation through a mesodermal band (vitelline artery remnant), incarceration of a Littre's hernia, external compression by a omphalomesenteric cyst, or segmental intestinal fibrosis from peptic stricture secondary to heterotopic gastric mucosa in a Meckel's diverticulum. Congenital abnormalities leading to pathophysiology include umbilical fistula secondary to patent omphalomesenteric duct or paraumbilical cysts or cords caused by omphalomesenteric duct remnants.

Hemorrhage

Bleeding is the most common clinical presentation of Meckel's diverticulum. Bleeding accounts for between 25% and 56% of patients who present with symptomatic lesions. Usually the patient presents with painless gastrointestinal bleeding before 5 years of age. The lower gastrointestinal bleeding can produce either melena or hematochezia. The bleeding varies considerably in quantity and character but is usually episodic and often causes anemia requiring transfusion. Occult bleeding with anemia is an infrequent presentation of Meckel's diverticulum.

DIAGNOSIS OF HEMORRHAGE. When bleeding is the presenting symptom for a Meckel's diverticulum, gastric mucosa is nearly always present. Scintigraphy can be used to detect this gastric mucosa. This study is based on the uptake and excretion of pertechnetate isotope by gastric mucosa. Normally the stomach and urinary bladder demonstrate a dense uptake of the radionuclide whereas the duodenal loop and proximal jejunum demonstrate accumulation. A positive study shows an abnormal accumulation of radionuclide in the right lower quadrant, but it may be anywhere or move from one location to another. The sensitivity of this study is 85%, the specificity is 95%, and the accuracy is 90%. Pentagastrin, histamine blockers, and glucagon can be used to increase the accuracy of scanning. During active episodes of bleeding, arteriography or bleeding scans can also be used to help localize the source of bleeding.

Obstruction

Meckel's diverticulum may cause intestinal obstruction through many mechanisms. Intussusception and volvulus are the most frequent causes of obstruction secondary to Meckel's diverticulum. In a combined series of over 1000 patients, intussusception accounted for 46% of the obstructions and volvulus, 24%. Typically intestinal obstructions present with crampy abdominal pain and vomiting that can become bilious. If an obstruction persists and progresses from a partial to a complete blockage, the intestine will become ischemic and can eventually become gangrenous and perforate. At this point peritoneal signs will develop and the pain will become constant. Associated symptoms can include fever, dehydration, lethargy, diarrhea, or hematochezia.

DIAGNOSIS OF OBSTRUCTION. The diagnosis of intestinal obstruction is a clinical diagnosis. Plain abdominal radiographs, including a flat and upright or a decubitus view, are also essential in making the correct diagnosis. Meckel's diverticulum is rarely diagnosed preoperatively as the cause of the bowel obstruction. If intussusception is suspected, the diagnosis can be confirmed using ultrasound, or the patient can proceed directly to fluoroscopy at which either a barium enema or air contrast enema can be performed to make the diagnosis and possibly reduce the intussusception. If a Meckel's diverticulum is the lead point of the intussusception, the chance of reducing the intussusception nonoperatively is unlikely.

Inflammation and Diverticulitis

Meckel's diverticulitis is a common cause of a complication of a Meckel's diverticulum, but it is unusual in children. Typically patients present with vague abdominal pain that localizes to the right lower quadrant. Associated symptoms include anorexia, nausea, vomiting, and fever. Meckel's diverticulitis is usually misdiagnosed as acute suppurative appendicitis for it closely simulates the clinical features of appendicitis and its complications. Meckel's diverticulitis should be suspected in all operations for suspected appendicitis in which the appendix is normal.

DIAGNOSIS OF MECKEL'S DIVERTICULITIS. The diagnosis of Meckel's diverticulitis is usually made during laparotomy. The indications for surgery are the same as those of appendicitis and typically are based on clinical findings. Computed tomography and ultrasound occasionally can be valuable adjuncts to making the diagnosis.

Fistula

A fistula connecting the ileum to the umbilicus as the result of a persistent omphalomesenteric duct usually presents during the newborn period and should be suspected in all infants with umbilical polyps or granulation tissue, especially if there is an associated sinus tract. A history of discharge of ileal contents or passage of flatus through the fistula is pathognomonic for a patent omphalomesenteric duct. In the case of a complete omphalomesenteric duct, there can be varying degrees of prolapse based on the diameter of the fistula. When the fistula is short and broad, the ileum may intussuscept through it onto the surface of the umbilicus, producing a double-horned segment of bowel, inside out, with the lumen evident on each horn. When the fistula is incomplete, there is either an associated cyst that typically presents after the newborn period when it gets secondarily infected or a cord that may act as the source of intestinal obstruction.

DIAGNOSIS. The diagnosis of a fistula can be confirmed by performing a sinogram, which should demonstrate a communication between the umbilicus and ileum in the case of a complete fistula. Ultrasound is another useful radiologic adjunct, particularly for diagnosing incomplete, cystic omphalomesenteric duct remnants.

PREOPERATIVE AND INTRAOPERATIVE MANAGEMENT

Each of the four clinical consequences of a Meckel's diverticulum possesses its own special considerations for preoperative preparation. Resection of diverticulum is common to all presentations.

Because the bleeding from a Meckel's diverticulum can be episodic and frequently stops spontaneously, elective surgery usually can be deferred until the diagnosis is confirmed and the patient is stabilized. Frequently the hemorrhage has been extensive and discovered late. Blood transfusion and rehydration are usually necessary. Emergency exploratory surgery is usually not required, however.

A transverse right lower quadrant or McBurney[1] incision is used. The diverticulum is located by tracing the ileum back from its junction with the cecum. Dark blood can be noted downstream from the Meckel's diverticulum. Appropriate treatment is resection of all heterotopic gastric mucosa through either diverticulectomy or segmental ileal resection. Areas of bleeding or ulceration should be carefully sought out and resected. Incidental appendectomy is also performed to prevent confusion with respect to the right lower quadrant incision. The bleeding should not recur after surgery; if it does, a retained portion of gastric mucosa should be ruled out. Overall results for diverticulectomy or segmental ileal resection are excellent.

Standard preoperative preparation for bowel obstruction consists of intravenous hydration, correction of electrolyte abnormalities, nasogastric decompression, and antibiotic administration. After adequate resuscitation, the patient is taken urgently to the operating room and, when intussusception is suspected, a right lower quadrant transverse abdominal incision is used. The point of obstruction is identified and relieved either through reducing the internal hernia, manual retrograde reduction of intussusception, or derotation of the volvulus. Once the obstruction is relieved, the obstructed or strangulated bowel is allowed adequate time to recover. Any gangrenous segments are resected and the primary cause of the obstruction surgically addressed. This may include resection of the diverticulum at the lead point of an intussusception or division of an omphalomesenteric band

as the source of a volvulus. If bowel is resected, primary anastomosis is almost universally accomplished. Rarely is it necessary to bring out an ostomy. The long-term outcome is determined by the amount of bowel resected.

The acutely inflamed Meckel's diverticulum can proceed to perforation, with either formation of a localized abscess or generalized peritonitis. When the diagnosis is known or suspected before operation, a small, transverse, right infraumbilical incision can be used. If the diagnosis is made during operation at the time of exploration for appendicitis, the inflamed diverticulum and adjacent ileum can be delivered easily through the appendectomy incision and the diverticulectomy performed outside the abdomen. If severe inflammation of the Meckel's diverticulum is causing edema and induration of the surrounding ileum or if the base of the diverticulum is very broad, it is appropriate to excise the adjacent inflamed ileum and perform an end-to-end small bowel anastomosis. On only rare occasions is exteriorization or temporary stoma required.

Surgical management of umbilical sinus or fistula anomalies is best approached through the same incision previously described. Dissection is facilitated by placing a catheter or feeding tube in the tract. The umbilical end of the tract is transected or circumscribed, detached, and removed in continuity with any persistent abnormal structures. Any connection with the intestine is either excised primarily or excised with a small bowel resection if primary closure would result in a significant narrowing of the intestinal lumen. Long-term results of surgery are excellent.

INCIDENTALLY DISCOVERED MECKEL'S DIVERTICULUM. The surgical management of incidentally discovered Meckel's diverticulum has been controversial. Accurately assessing the lifetime probability of complications arising from an incidentally discovered Meckel's diverticulum was previously difficult. Most current studies estimate the risk to be strongly age dependent at around 5%. This is far less than the original estimate of a 25% incidence of complications arising from an asymptomatic, incidentally discovered diverticulum. Factors associated with an increased likelihood of complications arising from Meckel's diverticulum include diverticular length greater than 2 cm, age less than 40 years, and heterotopic mucosa.

In some situations there is some degree of unanimity. For instance, resection appears to be clearly indicated in patients with palpable thickening in the diverticulum that is consistent with heterotopic mucosa, with a history of unexplained abdominal pain, or in patients with omphalomesenteric duct remnants or attachments to the abdominal wall. However, in other patient populations the indications for resection of an asymptomatic, incidentally discovered Meckel's diverticulum are less clear, are debatable, and present an unacceptable risk-benefit ratio.

COMPLICATIONS OF MECKEL'S DIVERTICULUM

Neoplasms can occur in Meckel's diverticulum. These rare tumors can be either benign or malignant. Meckel's

Pearls and Pitfalls

PEARLS

- Meckel's diverticulum is the most common congenital anomaly of the GI tract.
- Pathophysiologic problems resulting from Meckel's diverticulum can arise from four basic causes: hemorrhagic, inflammatory diverticulitis, obstruction due to intussusception, or a congenital tract associated with an omphalomesenteric duct.
- Meckel's scans, CT, and ultrasound are valuable diagnostic adjuncts.

PITFALLS

- False-negative scans with intense lower GI bleeding should NOT delay exploration.
- Meckel's diverticulum is often misdiagnosed as acute appendicitis, whose clinical features it closely resembles.
- Surgical management of incidentally discovered Meckel's diverticulum has been controversial. In most older patient populations, indication for resection of asymptomatic Meckel's diverticulum is debatable.

diverticulum is not predisposed to neoplasm formation; instead, the diverticula are susceptible to any pathologic process that can affect the ileum. Malignant tumors occur more frequently than benign tumors. The most common malignancies are sarcomas, followed by carcinoids, and finally adenocarcinomas. The great majorities of malignancies arising in a Meckel's diverticulum are metasta-

sized at the time of diagnosis. Benign neoplasms include leiomyoma, fibromatous hemangioendotheliomas, and lipoma. Diagnosis, staging, and treatment of these diverse tumors are the same as if they arose in the ileum.

SELECTED READINGS

Ashcraft KW, Holder TM: Pediatric Surgery. Philadelphia, WB Saunders, 1993, pp 435–439.

Harkins H: Intussusceptions due to invaginated Meckel's diverticulum: Report of two cases with a study of 160 cases collected from the literature. Ann Surg 1933;98:1070.

Kusumoto H, Yoshida M, Takahashi I, et al: Complications and diagnosis of Meckel's diverticulum in 776 patients. Am J Surg 1992;164:382.

Matsagas MI, Fatouros M, Koulouras B, Gannoukos AD: Incidence, complications, and management of Meckel's diverticulum. Arch Surg 1995;130:143.

Mayo C: Meckel's diverticulum. Proc Mayo Clin 1933;8:230.

Meckel JF: Bey trage zur Vergleichenden Anatomie. Leipzig: Karl Heinrich Reclam, 1808.

Neis C, Zielke A, Hasse C, et al: Carcinoid tumors of Meckel's diverticula. Dis Colon Rectum 1992;35:589.

O'Neill JA, Rowe MI, Grosfeld JL, et al: Pediatric Surgery. Boston, CV Mosby, 1998, pp 1173–1184.

Simms M, Corkery J: Meckel's diverticulum: Its association with congenital malformation and the significance of atypical morphology. Br J Surg 1980;67:216.

Soderlund S: Meckel's diverticulum; A clinical and histologic study. Acta Chir Scand 1959;248 (suppl):1.

Soltero MJ, Bill AH: The natural history of Meckel's diverticulum and its relation to incidental removal: A study of 202 cases of diseased Meckel's diverticulum found in King County, Washington, over a fifteen-year period. Am J Surg 1976;132:168.

Spitz L, Coran AG: Rob & Smith's Operative Surgery: Pediatric Surgery. New York, Chapman & Hall, 1995, pp 372–382.

Vane DW, West KW, Grosfeld JL: Vitelline duct anomalies: Experience with 217 childhood cases. Arch Surg 1987;122:542.

Zinner MJ, Schwartz SI, Ellis H: Maingot's Abdominal Operations. Stamford, CT, Appleton & Lange, 1997, pp 1131–1140.

ONCOLOGY

Breast

Chapter 148
Diagnosis and Assessment of Benign and Malignant Breast Diseases
LaNette F. Smith and V. Suzanne Klimberg

CLINICAL ASSESSMENT AND EVALUATION

The definitive diagnosis of breast cancer requires histologic examination of breast tissue to confirm or exclude the presence of malignant cells. However, many signs and symptoms must be evaluated in patients who are concerned about breast complaints or nodules. It is the clinical presentation along with diagnostic tests that leads to biopsy and subsequent determination of benign versus malignant disease. Therefore, a thorough understanding of the complete assessment and evaluation of the breast "lump" is imperative.

The assessment of a patient with a breast complaint typically begins with a thorough history and physical examination, with special attention paid to the presence of possible risk factors for breast cancer. Attention should be directed to the patient's complaint of lumps, pain, or discharge from the breast, along with information about her menstrual cycle. The duration of symptoms, their persistence over time, and their fluctuation with menses should also be considered.

Breast cancer has many risk factors that are known to pose an increased risk for each patient. Gender is the greatest risk factor. For every 100 women who develop breast cancer, only 1 man will. Age is the second greatest risk factor. As age progresses, there is a sixfold increase in the risk of breast cancer between the ages of 35 and 65. However, 66% of women with breast cancer have no known risk factors, and so every woman's complaint should be taken seriously and thoroughly evaluated regardless of age or family history.

Other risk factors may be related to hormonal influences. As a general rule, uninterrupted menstrual cycling for prolonged periods increases a woman's risk of breast cancer. Therefore, women with early menarche, and later menopause, may be at increased risk. The reproductive history of the patient is also valuable in her risk assessment. Nulliparity increases a woman's risk by nearly 30%. Patients should be questioned regarding their use of exogenous estrogens and oral contraceptives. Although hormone replacement carries many benefits, such as a possible decreased risk of Alzheimer's disease, coronary artery disease, and osteoporosis, studies suggest that taking hormone replacements for more than 5 years may increase a woman's risk of breast cancer compared with women who do not take any hormone replacement. Therefore, the individual risks and benefits of hormone replacement therapy should be weighed for each patient. The possible increased risk of breast cancer with long-term oral contraceptive use has been widely debated. However, after 10 years of discontinuation, the risk of past users appears to be equal to that of nonusers.

Although a breast mass is the most common physical presentation for cancer, complaints of breast pain, nipple discharge, or a change in the appearance of the breast may be potential warning signs. In a series of 240 patients with operable breast cancer, Preece and colleagues reported breast pain as a presenting symptom for breast cancer in 15% of patients and as the only symptom in 7%. Therefore, it is important not to disregard either diffuse or particularly well-localized breast pain.

Nipple discharge that is unilateral, from a single duct orifice, and spontaneous is considered suspicious. The consistency of the discharge should be ascertained. Serous, serosanguineous, bloody, or clear discharge requires further investigation to exclude cancer by mammography, ultrasound, galactography, or surgical excision of the retroareolar ducts. Benign-appearing nipple discharge is usually milky or thick and yellow or green. Typically, it is bilateral, nonspontaneous, and from multiple ducts.

Physical examination involves inspection of both breasts in the sitting and the supine position. Breasts should be compared for differences in size and shape, although small size differences are normal. Evidence of bulging, dimpling, or retraction of overlying skin may indicate a malignant process. This can result from tumors involving Cooper's ligaments. Edema or peau d'orange may indicate obstruction of dermal lymphatics with tumor cells. Irradiation may also make it difficult to differentiate benign from malignant breast edema. Abscesses may present with erythema and warmth. However, one must be careful to exclude an inflammatory cancer with this presentation. The nipples and areola should be assessed for retraction, ulceration, and eczema. Crusting and ulceration of the nipple may indicate Paget's disease, which presents with 1% to 4% of all breast cancers.

The breast itself is best palpated with the patient in the supine position with the ipsilateral arm above the patient's head. Some examiners prefer a particular pattern of examination of the breast (radial, concentric, or iron grid). However, the key is to examine all aspects of the breast within its anatomic boundaries; that is, from the clavicle superiorly, the sternum medially, the rectus inferiorly, to the midaxillary line laterally. The upper outer quadrant and inframammary ridge are more often difficult to evaluate with physical examination because these areas are naturally more nodular in consistency. Comparison between the two breasts is usually helpful. If the patient has a particular area of concern, special attention should be given to that area. Difficult examinations may need to be repeated at a different stage of the menstrual cycle when the breasts are less nodular and less tender. The best time is typically 1 week after menses begins, when hormonal levels are at a nadir. Any dominant mass requires additional evaluation with imaging studies and/or biopsy, regardless of presentation.

Any palpable masses that are appreciated on physical examination deserve further investigation. Although a mass may appear consistent with a cyst on physical examination, cysts cannot reliably be distinguished from solid masses on physical examination. Figure 148–1 reviews the evaluation of a nonsuspicious palpable mass. Needle aspiration can be performed quickly and easily in the office and distinguishes cysts from solid masses. This may be performed under ultrasound guidance. Fluid should be sent for cytology if it appears bloody. If a palpable mass or ultrasound density remains after aspiration, the mass should be excised. Also recurrence of the cyst after a second aspiration mandates excision. Figure 148–2 reviews the evaluation of a suspicious palpable mass.

Palpation of the supraclavicular and axillary lymph nodes should be performed from behind, with the patient in the upright position. Any palpable adenopathy should be characterized with regard to location, consistency, and fixation. Palpable adenopathy may preclude certain treatment options, such as sentinel lymph node biopsy. However, clinical assessment of the axilla is correct only approximately 50% of the time.

IMAGING STUDIES

Mammography is the only technique with proven efficacy for breast cancer screening and has been found to reduce mortality rates by 20% to 30% in women younger than 40 years of age and by 29% in women 50 to 69 years of age. However, a meta-analysis taken from only the Swedish trials showed a decrease in mortality from breast cancer as the result of screening since 1985, but an increase in overall mortality. Currently, mammography is thought to be the best tool available for breast cancer screening. The American College of Radiology, the National Cancer Institute, and other organizations recommend a baseline bilateral mammogram and physical examination by age 40 years, with repeat examinations every 1 to 2 years between the ages of 40 and 49 years, and yearly thereafter. Although mammography is very good for screening purposes, it does have a false-negative rate of 10% to 30%, and therefore any palpable lesion should be biopsied even in the setting of a negative mammogram.

There are two major types of mammography: screening mammography and diagnostic mammography. Screening mammography is used for the detection of breast cancer in asymptomatic patients. Patients with specific symptoms, such as a lump, localized pain, or nipple discharge, are best evaluated with diagnostic mammography, which allows for specialized views. With the goal of visualization of all breast tissue, there are standard mammographic views. Each patient will have a craniocaudal (CC) and a mediolateral oblique (MLO) view of each breast. The CC view is used to visualize the central and medial portions of the breast, along with the subareolar tissue. The MLO view images the posterior aspect of the breast as well as the upper outer quadrant, or tail of Spence. Adequacy of the MLO view is determined by visualizing the pectoralis muscle at least to the level of the nipple. An exaggerated craniocaudal (XCC) view is taken with the patient rotated medially and is performed if a lesion in the axillary portion of the breast is inadequately visualized on the standard CC view. A 90-degree mediolateral view is best for localizing lesions at the twelve and six o'clock positions in the central portion of the breast and is most often used for needle-localization procedures. Compression views are used to isolate a small portion of breast tissue regarding which there is concern in the standard mammographic views. This view can help differentiate benign or sharply marginated lesions from malignant masses and evaluate architectural distortions. Magnification views allow better characterization of calcifications.

The lack of uniformity in mammographic reporting and then subsequent confusion regarding therapeutic options has resulted in the American College of Radiology establishing a standardized reporting system for mammography. The BI-RADS (Breast Imaging Reporting and Data System) is a concise, organized format that describes the reason for the examination and provides a description

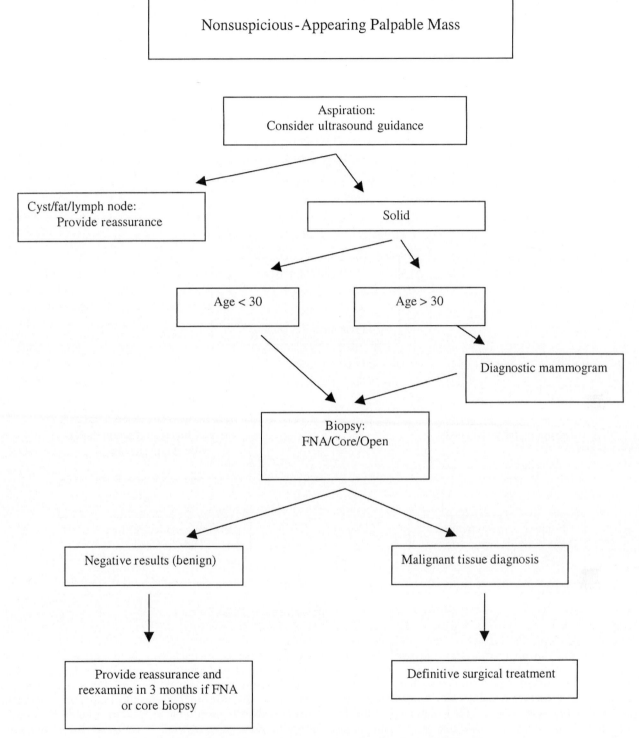

Figure 148–1. Algorithm for non–suspicious-appearing palpable mass.

of the overall breast composition and a description of findings using standardized terms; then, an overall impression and recommendations for follow-up and/or treatment is given a category number from 0 to 5 (Table 148–1).

A description of the mammographic findings commonly involves a description of any masses or calcifications encountered. The shape and margins of any masses give a clue to their likelihood of malignancy. In general, irregular and spiculated masses are considered more suspicious for malignancy. Figure 148–3 reviews the evaluation of a mammographic lesion. Calcifications are also evaluated based on their morphologic characteristics. Calcifications greater than five in number that are clustered in distribution and/or more pleomorphic or heterogeneous in shape have a higher probability of malignancy.

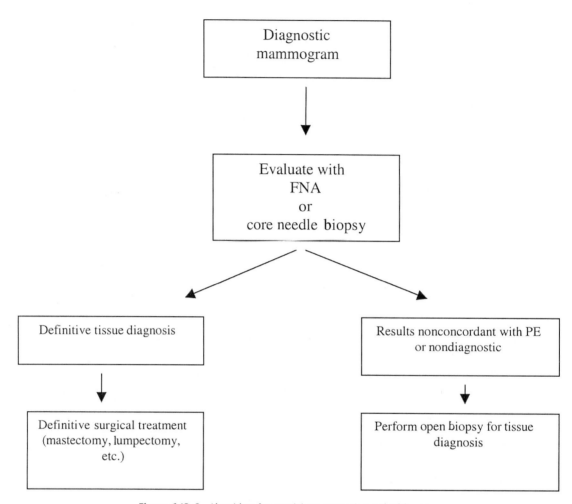

Figure 148–2. Algorithm for suspicious-appearing palpable mass.

Fine, linear, or branching calcifications may also be more worrisome. Any of these findings on mammogram may lead one to perform additional studies, such as ultrasound and magnetic resonance imaging (MRI), or possibly proceed directly to biopsy. Figure 148–4 shows a plan for the work-up of a patient with calcifications on mammography.

Ultrasound is recognized as being an important adjunct to mammography in the evaluations of breast lesions. At present, it is not used for screening purposes but is of much greater benefit in the evaluation of palpable lesions or mammographic abnormalities. Originally, ultrasound was used to differentiate cystic from solid lesions and thus subvert the need for approximately 20% of biopsies performed prior to its development. Today, there are many clinical uses for breast ultrasound. It can be used for both diagnostic and interventional purposes. It is of particular benefit in patients with young, dense breasts,

which are not as amenable to mammography. In pregnant women, ultrasound allows evaluation of the breast without any exposure to radiation. One of the more common uses is as a guide for core-needle biopsy in the office. Frequently, the ultrasound is used as a guide for needle or wire placement in needle-localization breast biopsies. Novel uses include ultrasound as a guide for excisional biopsy of nonpalpable breast lesions in the operating room without the need for a localizing needle or wire. Ultrasound, currently, is not recommended for the evaluation of calcifications in the breast.

Most breast ultrasonographers agree that high-quality breast ultrasound requires the use of a high-frequency, real-time, linear array transducer of at least 7.5 MHz. Frequently, a radial scanning technique is utilized and limited to a focused area of the breast, rather than complete breast examination with ultrasound. The radial tech-

Table 148–1	**BI-RADS Assessment of Mammographic Findings**

	CATEGORY	ASSESSMENT	DESCRIPTION AND MANAGEMENT RECOMMENDATION
Incomplete category	0	Needs additional imaging	Finding for which additional imaging evaluation is needed. This is almost always used in a screening situation and should rarely be used after a full imaging work-up. A recommendation for additional imaging evaluation includes the use of spot compression views, magnification, special mammographic views, ultrasound, and so forth. The radiologist should use judgment in how vigorously to pursue previous studies.
Final categories	1	Negative	There is nothing to comment on. Routine screening.
	2	Benign finding	This is also a negative mammogram, but the interpreter may wish to describe a finding. Routine screening.
	3	Probably benign finding	A finding placed in this category should have a very high probability of being benign. It is not expected to change over the follow-up interval, but the radiologist would prefer to establish its stability. Short interval follow-up suggested (usually 6 mo).
	4	Suspicious abnormality	These are lesions that do not have the characteristic morphologies of breast cancer but have a definite probability of being malignant. The radiologist has sufficient concern to urge a biopsy. If possible, the relevant probabilities should be cited so that the patient and her physician can make the decision on the ultimate course of action. Biopsy should be considered.
	5	Highly suggestive of malignancy	These lesions have a high probability of being cancer. Appropriate action should be taken.

American College of Radiology (ACR): Breast imaging reporting and data system (BI-RADS™). 3rd ed. Reston, VA, American College of Radiology, 1998, with permission.

nique allows the examiner to view the full extent of the breast architecture. The major structures evaluated in ultrasound of the breast include the skin, subcutaneous tissues, glandular tissue, underlying retromammary fat, pectoralis muscle, and the ribs. Any lesion identified should be viewed in both the transverse and the longitudinal planes.

As with mammography, lesions on ultrasound are characterized as being more likely malignant or benign based on their morphologic and ultrasonographic characteristics. In general, lesions that are irregular and jagged along their margins and have strong irregular retrotumoral shadowing are more likely to be malignant. Also, lesions that are taller than they are wide and thus grow against normal tissue planes are more suspicious.

Breast MRI produces detailed information regarding the character and extent of breast lesions. However, at its current availability, it is considerably more expensive than mammography or ultrasound. When used appropriately in the management of breast disease, MRI may result in overall reduced costs for breast cancer management by avoiding some unnecessary biopsies and allowing earlier detection of breast cancer. The overall sensitivity has been reported as high as 100%, with a specificity that ranges from 37% to 100%, based on the particular series and MRI technique utilized.

Breast MRI methods may be quite varied. The International Working Group for Breast MRI has been instrumental in establishing practice guidelines for MRI indications, techniques, and interpretation. Our institution utilizes both pre– and post–contrast-enhanced fat-suppressed images with gadolinium as a contrast agent. This process works under the premise that cancers take up contrast material much earlier and more readily than does breast parenchyma. Since most breasts are composed of a significant proportion of fat, many techniques utilize fat suppression. Current clinical applications for breast MRI may include determination of the extent of residual disease prior to surgical treatment and evaluation of the success of induction chemotherapy; MRI has also been shown to be helpful in detecting multicentric disease and for lobular carcinoma where physical examination and ultrasound may not be as valuable. After lumpectomy, MRI may be indicated for evaluating patients with close or positive margins to evaluate for residual disease. MRI also has a definite indication in patients with axillary adenopathy and no known primary lesion. A further indication includes patients with silicone augmentation whose mammograms may be less than adequate to exclude cancer. MRI can also be used to evaluate the extent of chest wall involvement prior to surgery and therefore to assist in surgical planning.

Other less-proven imaging modalities are being evaluated for the breast. These include scintimammography and positron emission tomography (PET) scanning. Scintimammography involves the use of radiopharmaceuticals to image the breast, most commonly technetium 99m sestamibi. Some centers propose that its usefulness in breast cancer is that it improves on the sensitivity and specificity of mammography. At present, this technique remains largely investigational.

Like scintimammography, PET scanning utilizes a radioisotope, F 18 fluorodeoxyglucose (FDG), to evaluate the breast. The scan assesses the biochemical activity

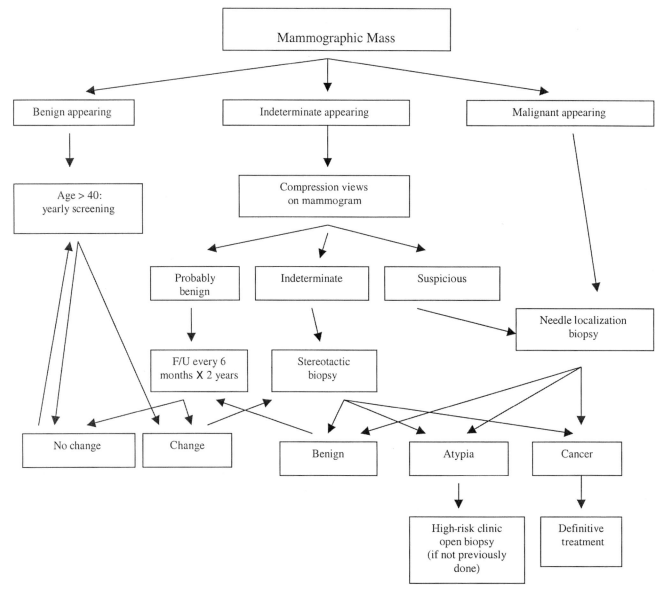

Figure 148–3. Algorithm for mammographic mass.

within the breast tissue. Studies have shown that tumor cells have increased uptake of F 18-FDG compared with that of normal breast tissue. This method's sensitivity for the detection of breast cancer is reported between 68% and 94%, with a specificity between 84% and 97%. Proponents claim that it has possible usefulness in detecting primary breast cancer, discovering axillary lymph node metastases, and detecting distant metastases. PET scanners are not widely available throughout the country, and therefore this technique also has limited application.

BIOPSY TECHNIQUES

The method of biopsy depends on the individual patient, the palpability of the mass, and the imaging modality by which the lesion is detected. Choices include fine-needle aspiration (FNA) cytology, core-needle biopsy, image-guided biopsy, and open excisional biopsy.

Breast FNA is rapid and highly cost-effective, compared with other biopsy methods. It is easily performed with very little discomfort to the patient. Results can be obtained in the office in a matter of minutes. This procedure should not be confused with large-core-needle biopsy, which obtains a larger tissue sample for histologic evaluation instead of cellular material for cytologic evaluation. Either method can provide enough material to obtain estrogen and progesterone receptors.

In this procedure, a very small gauge needle, usually 22 gauge, is inserted into the lesion of question after suction is placed on the syringe. One advantage of the method is that several passes through several different areas of the targeted lesion can be accomplished. The suction is then released, and the needle withdrawn. The cellular contents should be visible in the hub of the needle. These contents are expressed onto a glass slide. The slide is then fixed and best examined by an experienced cytopathologist. The results may be reported as

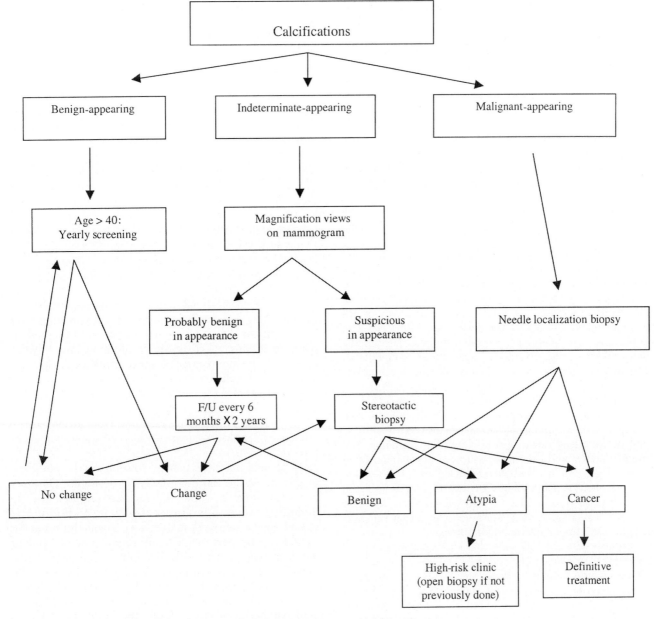

Figure 148–4. Algorithm for calcifications.

benign, proliferative, suspicious for carcinoma, malignant, or inadequate. Benign findings should be correlated with clinical and mammographic results, whereas malignant findings necessitate definitive therapy. Reports of proliferative changes dictate repeat FNA in 2 weeks, and reports suspicious for carcinoma require that an excisional biopsy be performed. The combination of physical examination, mammography, and FNA may produce a diagnostic accuracy approaching 100%, a sensitivity of 100%, and a specificity of 49%.

Large-core-needle biopsies can be performed on palpable masses or with image-guidance for nonpalpable lesions. Like FNA, these biopsies too can be performed in the office with minimal local anesthetic and similar sensitivity and specificity. Both manual and automatic gun devices are available. This size biopsy, which is commonly

14 gauge, provides information regarding the histology of the specimen and therefore can be used to differentiate invasive versus intraductal cancer. A pathology report of atypical hyperplasia or carcinoma in situ requires further investigation with some type of open excisional biopsy.

Ultrasound guidance adds a great deal to large-core-needle biopsy. In 1993, Parker reported on a large series of patients with 181 ultrasound-guided core-needle biopsies. In Parker's series, there was 100% correlation between the core biopsy diagnosis and the excisional biopsy results with no reported complications. The average procedure time was reported to be approximately 20 minutes. Liberman and colleagues have looked at the cost-effectiveness of ultrasound-guided core breast biopsy and found it to be 56% less expensive than open excisional biopsy. Additional benefits, versus other biopsy modalities, include the following: no radiation exposure, all areas of the breast and axilla are accessible, and no need for breast compression.

Mammographically guided biopsy techniques are available for biopsying lesions that are nonpalpable and are clusters of microcalcifications, solid nodular densities, or areas of architectural distortion. There are many devices included under this heading of mammographically guided, or stereotactic core-needle biopsy. These include 14-gauge core-needle biopsy, 11- or 14-gauge suction-assisted core biopsy (Mammotome [Biopsys Medical Instruments, Inc., San Juan Capistrano, CA]) or stereotactic-coring excisional biopsy (Advanced Breast Biopsy Instrument [ABBI, United States Surgical Corporation]), along with several other devices of differing brands. Wire-localized breast biopsy does involve stereotactic principles, but this is addressed later in the chapter.

All of these procedures require a specialized table and computerized technology to provide the digital images and coordinates of the targeted lesion. After the patient is placed on the table in a prone position and the breast has been compressed, an initial image and a pair of 15-degree angled images of the lesion are obtained. The depth and coordinates are also determined. The needle biopsy device utilized varies as listed earlier, generally an 11-gauge device is used and several passes are made through the lesion. These devices take samples from suspect lesions and are not intended for the complete excision of a lesion. The Mammotome device is an automatic multiple core-sampling device, which uses a vacuum to pull breast tissue down into a trough for sampling. The trough rotates, and therefore tissue can be sampled from a 360-degree radius without removing the device from the breast. Mammographic films are obtained after the procedure to ensure that the intended lesion has been removed or sampled. The Mammotome device can now also be used under ultrasound guidance.

Patients with the following characteristics are not ideal candidates for stereotactic core-needle biopsy procedures. These include patients with lesions not clearly visualized in the stereotactic unit (usually lesions deep in the breast along the chest wall), lesions found in small breasts (which compress to less than 2 cm in the stereotactic unit), and asymmetrically dense breast tissue. Patients who are unable to lie prone for 30 minutes or have arm movement limitations are also not acceptable candidates for this procedure.

Velanovich and associates compared the various mammographically guided breast biopsy techniques in a recent article in the *Annals of Surgery* and found that technical success was achieved in 94.3% of stereotactic core-needle biopsies, 96.4% of Mammotome biopsies, and 92.5% of ABBI biopsies. The ABBI device takes samples from 5 mm to 2 cm in size. Therefore, the possibility of obtaining margins with this device is being investigated. The large size of tissue taken with this device has prompted its opponents to liken it to an open surgical procedure with all of the inherent risks of surgical complications. While the ABBI method had the least number of cases requiring repeat biopsy (7.5%), 63.6% of the ABBI cases had positive surgical margins and required open excisional biopsy. Furthermore, ABBI biopsy has not been approved for surgical excision by the U.S. Food and Drug Administration (FDA).

Stereotactic MRI biopsy is a relatively new endeavor that is performed only in a few centers. At the University of Arkansas, Harms and colleagues have found that approximately 70% of MRI-detected occult lesions can be successfully biopsied by ultrasound with the use of the MR coordinates for localization, thus reserving MRI guidance for lesions that cannot be otherwise identified and localized. MRI stereotactic biopsy also requires the patient to lie prone with minimal movement for up to an hour for completion of the biopsy. In addition, patients who are claustrophobic are not candidates for this procedure. A compression device is used to immobilize the breast, and coordinates are obtained and plotted with laser guidance after a series of images are produced. Percutaneous core-needle biopsies are then obtained in a fashion similar to the other previously mentioned stereotactic methods using needles and instruments that do not interfere with the magnet.

Both open excisional biopsy and needle-localization breast biopsy are usually performed in an operating room by a surgeon. Open excisional biopsy is attempted on palpable lesions, while needle-localization breast biopsy is reserved for nonpalpable lesions or microcalcifications. The anesthetic choices for either of these procedures can vary from pure local anesthetic to a complete general anesthetic. This choice is usually determined on the basis of the patient's preference and level of anxiety and is influenced by the size and location of the lesion to be removed.

In general, incisions parallel to or along the periphery of the areola are more cosmetically desirable. However, one must keep in mind the incision required for the definitive cancer operation subsequent to the biopsy, should one be required. A significant amount of tunneling should not be performed to remove a more peripheral lesion through a periareolar incision. An incision placed directly over the lesion is preferred, while the possibility of a future mastectomy incision should be kept in mind.

Wire- or needle-localization breast biopsy has been the gold standard against which all other methods of image-guided biopsies are compared. Failure rates up to 22% have been reported with this method but, more commonly, range from 3% to 5%. There are various wire-localizing devices available. The individual device chosen depends largely on the familiarity and preferences of the radiologist and surgeon involved in the patient's care. However, a nontransectable wire is preferred. All the wires must be placed under some type of image guidance, usually mammographic or ultrasound, depending on how the lesion is best viewed. Some surgeons prefer the needle to be left in place over the wire to allow traction during the procedure. Complications associated with this method include vasovagal reactions when the wire is inserted in up to 10% and the possibility of the wire breaking, migrating, or falling out before the procedure is completed. Furthermore, it requires coordination between the radiologist and the surgeon on the day of surgery to efficiently localize the lesion and then remove it in the operating room. A specimen mammogram should

Pearls and Pitfalls

PEARLS

- The best treatment for mastalgia is to exclude breast cancer.
- A suspicious breast mass should be biopsied even if imaging studies are normal.
- Preoperative knowledge that a mass is cancer, either by ultrasound-guided or stereotactic biopsy, may improve breast conservation rates.
- Positive margins may have direct impact on recurrence and survival; therefore, the margins of any excisional breast biopsy should be marked with ink.
- Intraoperative frozen sections should not be utilized in breast surgery to abrogate the possibility of technical destruction of cancers and micrometastases in sentinel lymph node biopsies.
- Positive surgical margins indicate the need for tumor re-excision to clear the area, in the same way that local regional tumor control is the raison d'être of surgical therapy.

always be obtained at the completion of the procedure to prove the lesion in question was indeed removed.

PATHOLOGIC ASSESSMENT

Tissue should be sent fresh for evaluation of pathology and hormone receptor status. Sending small lesions for frozen section may not reserve any specimen for hormone receptor analysis. This may have significant therapeutic implications for the patient. With the increased use of mammography and other imaging modalities, a very small lesion could be lost entirely if frozen section is performed.

Once a specimen is sent to pathology, the six margins should be inked and identified for later reference. The ink should not contaminate the interior aspect of the specimen, and the specimen should not be cut into prior to the inking process. Random frozen sections of the margins are not indicated as stated previously and may actually be detrimental.

Newer techniques are being evaluated for pathologic

assessment of breast lesions. One of these is touch prep. This technique involves touching a specimen onto a glass slide, similar to pressing a rubber stamp onto a paper. The theory is that tumor cells adhere to the glass slide. Imprints are taken of all six margins of the specimen and the lesion in question. The sensitivity of this method has been reported at 96.3% with 100% specificity. In assessing margins, touch prep has a reported sensitivity and specificity of 100%, while studies evaluating the accuracy of frozen section for the intraoperative diagnosis of nonpalpable lesions demonstrate a positive predictive value ranging from 68% to 97.7%. With minimally invasive cancers, the false-negative rate for frozen section is reported at 8.8%. Since the best cosmetic results are usually achieved when negative margins are obtained at the initial surgery, accurate and thorough pathologic assessment is essential.

SELECTED READINGS

American College of Radiology (ACR): Breast imaging reporting and data system (BI-RADS™). 3rd ed. Reston, VA, American College of Radiology, 1998.

Bland KI, Copeland EM: The Breast Comprehensive Management of Benign and Malignant Diseases, 2nd ed. 1998.

Collaborative Group on Hormonal Factors in Breast Cancer: Breast cancer and hormonal contraceptives. Collaborative reanalysis of individual data on 53,297 women with breast cancer and 100,239 women without breast cancer from 54 epidemiologic studies. Lancet 1996;347:1713.

Gotzsche PC, Olsen O: Is screening for breast cancer with mammography justifiable? Lancet 2000;355:129.

Harms SE: Integration of breast magnetic resonance imaging with breast cancer treatment. Top Magn Reson Imaging 1998;9:79.

Hermansen C, Poulsen HS, Jensen J, et al: Palpable breast tumours: "Triple diagnosis" and operative strategy. Acta Chir Scand 1984;150:625.

Klimberg VS, Westbrook KC, Korourian S: Use of touch preps for diagnosis and surgical margins in breast cancer. Ann Surg Oncol 1998;5:220.

Liberman L, Feng TL, Dershaw DD, et al: US-guided core breast biopsy: Use and cost-effectiveness. Radiology 1998;208:717.

Nystrom L, Rutqvist LE, Walls S, et al: Breast cancer screening with mammography: Overview of Swedish randomised trials. Lancet 1993;341:973.

Parker S, Job W, Dennis M, et al: US-guided automated large-core breast biopsy. Radiology 1993;187:507.

Preece PE, Baum M, Mansel RE, et al: The importance of mastalgia in operable breast cancer. BMJ 1982;284:1299.

Silva OE, Zurrida S: Breast cancer: A guide for fellows, 1999.

Smith LF, Rubio IT, Henry-Tillman R, et al: Intraoperative ultrasound-guided breast biopsy: For presentation Southwest Surgical Congress, April 2000.

Staren ED, O'Neill TP: Surgeon-performed ultrasound. Surg Clin North Am 1998;78:219.

Velanovich V, Lewis FR, Nathanson SD, et al: Comparison of mammographically guided breast biopsy techniques. Ann Surg 1999;229:625.

Chapter 149

High-Risk Indicators: Microscopic Lesions, Personal and Family History, Assessment, and Management

Susan W. Caro and David L. Page

The identification of individuals, or groups, at increased risk for developing breast cancer provides the opportunity for education and counseling, the institution of increased screening regimens, and possibly the opportunity for evaluation or utilization of interventions for decreasing risk. This chapter reviews the concepts of risk, risk assessment, high-risk lesions, and management options for women at increased risk.

CONCEPTS OF RISK

Health care providers must take care in discussing the concepts of risk in relation to breast cancer so that their patients will understand the complex issues associated with breast cancer risk. Breast cancer risk is a difficult subject to discuss, what with the rapidly growing body of new data that must be considered in the context of the existing knowledge base. Breast cancer is also very commonly discussed in the lay press, and not always precisely. Significant misconceptions may occur.

For a discussion of the concept of risk to have value, one must consider the simple question, Risk of what? The risk of developing breast cancer, the risk of dying of breast cancer, or the risk of having an inherited predisposition to breast cancer? There are different types and levels of risk. Of these, the least significant for any given individual woman is the risk over a lifetime. Although this number is often quoted, it is useful only as an indicator of the societal burden of the disease, not as an indicator of individual risk. It is essential to understand how risk operates over a finite time from the age of assessment. Time periods of 10 to 15 years have actually been verified for similar women of similar ages; comparisons do not include risks in the distant future. For example, for a woman in her forties, the risk of cancer in her seventies is not a current, realistic concern.

LIFETIME RISK. The lifetime risk of breast cancer for a given population is the risk of developing breast cancer during one's lifetime. This estimate is 1 in 8 for women in the United States. The lifetime risk of dying of breast cancer is 1 in 28.

RELATIVE RISK. Relative risk (RR) is a measure of the strength of a risk factor or condition and its association with cancer. Relative risk compares the risk of cancer in

one group with the risk in a reference population, which is usually the general population, or a group without the specific risk factor. A relative risk of 1.0 means no difference between the two groups. A relative risk of 2 means that the risk of one group is twofold, or two times, the risk in the reference population. This can also be expressed as a 100% increase in risk. Risks of this nature, when reported in the media, without an adequate explanation of what the terms mean, can be confusing and frightening for women. Relative risk and lifetime risk cannot be multiplied in an attempt to come up with an accurate risk assessment for the individual. It is possible, however, to take a relative risk and use age-adjusted risks to determine risk estimates over specific time periods. For example: If one considers the relative risk (RR) of developing breast cancer to be 1.7 for women with a first-degree relative with breast cancer, the risk of developing breast cancer for a woman aged 40 years during her 40th year might increase from approximately 1 in 1000 that year to 1.7 per 1000. An abstract risk or comparative risk is not very useful clinically unless it can be placed in context for the individual woman.

ABSOLUTE RISK. Absolute risk is the risk of developing cancer over a specified time period. Estimates of absolute risk are based on age-adjusted risk. From the viewpoints of both patient and clinician, however, a more meaningful statistic is absolute risk (AR). That is, it is far more useful for a patient to know her own risk of developing breast cancer than to know how much more likely she is to develop breast cancer than some other woman. Dupont and Plummer have developed software to help clinicians to translate relative risks into absolute risks for their individual patients (see http://www.mc.vanderbilt.edu/prevmed/absrisk.htm) and graphs demonstrating 15-year absolute risks that can be used to aid in applying RR information to the individual woman.

It is also important to consider what degree of risk is of clinical importance. What degree of risk might alter screening practices or identify women appropriate for consideration of interventions for decreasing risk? In the authors' view, only a relative risk of 2 (Table 149–1), or risk reliably determined to be at least double that of the general population, qualifies as a clinically meaningful elevated risk.

Breast cancer is a common cancer in women, account-

Table 149–1	Classification of Breast Cancer Risk by Magnitude

Slight or mild risk elevation	1.5–2 times comparison group
Moderate risk elevation	4–5 times comparison group
High elevation	9–11 times comparison group

Note: The major reason for this approach is to indicate that 10 times is about as great an elevation of risk as has been demonstrated to be reliably predicted in any group of women over a 10- to 15-year interval (the range often chosen for counseling).

ing for approximately 30% of new cancer diagnoses each year in American women. The probability of developing cancer of any site for women in the United States from birth to death is 1 in 3. The often-quoted "lifetime risk" of developing breast cancer for women in the U.S. is 1 in 8, or approximately 12%. This is the risk for all women in this country, including those at very high risk and those without identifiable risk factors. It is also important to note that because breast cancer is a common disease the majority of women diagnosed have no significant identifiable risk factors. This is why screening of all women is so important.

RISK FACTORS FOR BREAST CANCER

Female gender and advanced age are the most important elements in the risk of breast cancer. Breast cancer does occur in men, although it is much less common. Often-cited hormonal factors that may be associated with an increased risk of breast cancer include early menarche, late menopause, nulliparity, and first childbirth after the age of 30 years. Lactation, early childbirth, and early menopause are associated with decreased risk. However, none of these factors alter risk by a significant amount, with less than a 50% alteration of risk associated with any given factor in most reports.

We have little knowledge of the interactions among specific risk factors except where such interactions have been studied specifically. Some of these have included the tissue-based assessment of risk, particularly the atypical hyperplasias (discussed later), and family history and post-menopausal hormone replacement.

Age

Advanced age is a significant risk factor for breast cancer. Table 149–2 provides some age-adjusted risk estimates that are helpful in putting risk in perspective for the individual woman. Another way of evaluating this parameter is by assessing the risk of developing breast cancer during specific age intervals, as shown in Table 149–3.

Family History

Family history has long been known to be associated with breast cancer risk. Women with a family history of breast or ovarian cancer may be at significantly increased risk

Table 149–2	Approximate Age-Adjusted Risk per Year, U.S. Women, all Races

AGE IN YEARS	RISK OF BREAST CANCER THAT YEAR
30	1 in 5000
40	1 in 1000
50	1 in 500
60	1 in 350
70	1 in 270
80	1 in 250

Adapted from SEER Cancer Statistics Review 1973–1996, National Cancer Institute, and Henderson IC: Risk factors for breast cancer development. Cancer 1993;(suppl):2127–2140.

for developing breast cancer. The family history is most important when it includes multiple family members, cancers diagnosed at younger ages, and bilateral cancer or multiple cancer sites. Women who have a prior personal history of breast or ovarian cancer are also at increased risk.

RISK ASSESSMENT MODELS. There are various models available in the medical literature to assist in providing risk estimates for women based on family history. For example, Claus and others developed age-specific risk estimates for individuals based on a family history of breast cancer, including consideration of maternal and paternal cancers in the family, age at onset of breast cancer, and incidence of cancer in first- and second-degree relatives. There are many other models as well.

The Gail model is used to estimate the chance that a woman of a specific age will develop breast cancer over a specific time interval. The model has been used in the National Surgical Adjuvant Breast Project (NSABP) breast cancer prevention trials. Factors such as age at menarche, age at first birth, number of previous breast biopsies, and number of first-degree relatives with breast cancer are used to calculate risk. The Gail model initially did not include specific pathologic indicators associated

Table 149–3	Age-Specific Probability of Developing Invasive Breast Carcinoma in 10-Year Intervals

CURRENT AGE IN YEARS	NO INCREASED RISK	2× INCREASED RISK	4× INCREASED RISK
20	1 in 2000	1 in 1000	1 in 500
30	1 in 256	1 in 128	1 in 64
40	1 in 67	1 in 34	1 in 17
50	1 in 39	1 in 20	1 in 10
60	1 in 29	1 in 15	1 in 7

Note: These ranges of risk indicate the chance that a woman who is cancer free at her current age will develop breast carcinoma in the subsequent 10 years. The risk that an individual woman will develop breast carcinoma during any single year varies according to age, but it is considerably lower than the cumulative risk that she will develop carcinoma during an entire lifetime.

Modified from Ries LAG, Kosary CL, Hankey BF, et al (eds): SEER Cancer Statistics Review: 1973–1975. Bethesda, MD, National Cancer Institute; 1998.

with increased risk; it used the number of prior breast biopsies as an indicator of risk. It has now been adapted to include atypical hyperplasias as a risk factor. Also, because the Gail model considers only first-degree relatives, it does not consider paternal family history of breast cancer, in the absence of a father with breast cancer, or second-degree relatives.

The Gail model is now available as a computer program from the National Cancer Institute. The program produces a risk estimate over the 5 years subsequent to the time of assessment and over the lifetime of the person. It should be stressed that these are only "risk estimates" and there are always some limitations to applying information or models from the literature to individuals. The specificity of the risk estimate increases when the estimate is applied to groups of women, and is obviously imprecise when the estimate is applied to an individual woman—becoming truly a "likelihood."

The last decade has seen incredible advances in our understanding of inherited breast cancer. The identification of two breast cancer predisposition genes, *BRCA1* (for BReast CAncer gene No. 1; on chromosome 17 described in 1990 and isolated in 1994) and *BRCA2* (on chromosome 13, identified in late 1994), and the commercial availability of the testing for mutations of these genes have greatly altered the clinician's ability to evaluate risk in women with significant family histories. The majority of breast and ovarian cancers are not due to inherited syndromes. In the general population, an estimated 5% to 10% of breast cancer cases are associated with one of the breast-ovarian cancer genes. There are now risk models available to aid the clinician in predicting the likelihood of carrying a mutation in the *BRCA1* or *BRCA2* genes.

TESTING FOR PREDISPOSITION GENES

Testing for genetic mutations that predispose to cancer is a complex process that necessitates considerable education and counseling to aid women and their families in making the decision to proceed with testing. Professional expertise and experience are needed to integrate complex clinical situations and provide risk assessment and counseling to appropriate patients and families. Several medical specialties may be involved, including pathologists, medical, surgical, or gynecologic oncologists, and geneticists. Adequate counseling and education are time-consuming; thus, in many settings they become the domain of advanced-practice nurses or genetic counselors with specialized expertise and training in cancer risk assessment, in consultation with other medical specialists. The risk consultation process may include the following: pedigree documentation, review of pathology from affected family members or prior breast biopsies, review of the basic concepts of cancer and genetics, and review of the concepts of risk and risk factors, along with information about the limitations of testing, risks and benefits of testing, costs, and implications of a positive, negative, or inconclusive result for those considering testing.

Consideration of which families and women to test is

not straightforward, and is likely to be very personal for the patient and family members and will involve individual perceptions. Table 149–4 lists conditions that make an individual appropriate for consideration of testing. The ideal is to test an affected family member. If that individual is found to have a mutation, one can test unaffected members for the same specific mutation (at a reduced cost). Testing unaffected family members after identifying the mutation in the family provides specific and often valuable information. If there are no affected family members to test (all of them are deceased or unavailable), testing the unaffected individual is possible but less ideal. Finding a mutation in such an individual provides valuable information about his or her cancer risk and makes testing others possible. Not finding a mutation in that person does not exclude the possibility of significant inherited risk. In this situation, risk estimates may be based on empirical data.

Women who are found to carry a mutation in *BRCA1* or *BRCA2* have significantly increased risks of breast and ovarian cancers (Table 149–5). Concerns exist that the initial risk estimates are too high, as the families studied to determine these numbers were those with the most significant family histories. *BRCA1* carriers may face a risk of breast cancer of up to 73% by age 50 and 87% by age 70. Those previously diagnosed with breast cancer may have a 60% risk of a second primary breast cancer. The ovarian cancer risk in *BRCA1* carriers may be 16% to 44% by age 50 and 18% to 56% by age 70. The risks for *BRCA2* carriers of breast cancer are, overall, similar, but they may occur slightly later, with an estimated risk of 28% by age 50 and 84% by age 70, and a 5% to 10% lifetime risk for men. The risk of a second breast primary appears to be similar to that in carriers of *BRCA1*. Other studies have shown less penetrance for breast and ovarian cancers in certain subgroups of patients, specifically those of Ashkenazi Jewish heritage. Great care must be taken in interpreting results and sharing risk estimates in the context of what is known at the present time about the genes and about the particular mutation found in the individual.

The goals of cancer risk assessment and counseling are to (1) provide information about cancer risk and, when appropriate, the likelihood of having an inherited cancer

Table 149–4	**Individuals Appropriate for Consideration for Genetic Testing for *BRCA1* and *BRCA2* Mutations**

A strong family history of personal history of breast and/or ovarian cancer
Family or personal history of bilateral cancers of the breast or ovary
Cancers diagnosed at earlier-than-expected ages
Multiple affected family members, autosomal dominant pattern of inheritance on pedigree
Family or personal history of breast and/or ovarian cancer and Ashkenazi Jewish (Eastern Euorpean) heritage
Family history of males with breast cancer
Diagnosis of more than one cancer, e.g., breast and ovarian

Table 149–5	**Risks of Cancer Associated with *BRCA1* and *BRCA2* Mutations**

Breast cancer risk by age (women)	*BRCA1 (%)*	*BRCA2 (%)*
40	19	12
50	50	28
60	64	48
70	85	84
Contralateral breast cancer by age		
70	60	52
Ovarian cancer by age		
40	0.6	
50	22	0.4
60	30	7.4
70	63	27
Breast cancer in men		6

Risk of Ashkenazi individuals with mutation in *BRCA1* or *BRAC2* (185delAG, 5382insC, 6174delT) not selected for family history:

Breast cancer by age	
50	33%
70	56%
Ovarian cancer	
70	16%
Prostate cancer	
70	16%
80	39%

Easton DF, Ford D, Bishop T, and the Breast Cancer Linkage Consortium: Breast and ovarian cancer incidence in *BRCA1*-mutation carriers. Am J Hum Genet 1995;56:265.

Easton D, et al, and The Breast Cancer Linkage Consortium. Cancer risks in *BRCA2* mutation carriers. J Natl Cancer Inst 1999;91:1310.

Ford D, Easton DF, Stratton M, et al: Genetic heterogeneity and penetrance analysis of the *BRCA1* and *BRCA2* genes in breast cancer families. Am J Hum Genet 1998;62:676.

Struewing JP, Hartge P, Wacholder S, et al: The risk of cancer associated with specific mutations of *BRCA1* and *BRCA2* among Ashkenazi Jews. N Eng J Med 1997;336:1401.

Ford D, Easton DF, Bishop DT, Narod SA, Goldgar DE, and the Breast Cancer Linkage Consortium: Risks of cancer in *BRCA1*-mutation carriers. Lancet 1994;343:692.

predisposition gene; (2) offer recommendations for screening, and discuss medical and/or surgical options for decreasing risk; (3) provide access to genetic testing, with informed consent; (4) facilitate access to a network of health care providers who may assist in cancer surveillance or other options to decrease risk, including clinical trials; (5) serve as an ongoing resource for clients, to address concerns when new information becomes available or new questions or issues arise.

PATHOLOGIC INDICATORS OF RISK

In the 1970s, it was widely believed that women who had multiple biopsies had a greater risk of breast cancer, and this risk was held to be in the range of two to five times. Many studies since that time have defined the lesions within such biopsies that are associated with increased risk, and have determined a fairly large group of women who may have benign breast biopsies and not have an increased risk because they lack these lesions (Table 149–6; see Table 149–1).

It is extremely important to recognize that risk is not a simple "yes or no" determination. Rather than being dichotomous, it is extremely complex, with a broad range of magnitudes and a range of weaker and stronger certainties. Most of the risks that are discussed in the popular press involve minor risk and are not discussed further here. For clinical purposes, the authors believe that the risk should be at least double that of otherwise comparable women over the same number of years, with a risk of lesser amount not considered of great importance, although even minor risk alterations may have a part in encouraging women to get yearly mammograms.

With regard to the lesions presented in Table 149–6, it can be noted that we have come a very long way from the time when fibrocystic changes were thought to have some intrinsic meaning. While fibrocystic changes may be of some general importance in being different between populations of high and low geographic incidence of breast cancer, these are not reliable indicators of risk for high-risk areas such as North America and most of Europe. There is some evidence that recurrent very large cysts in the immediate premenopausal period may indicate an increased risk of a magnitude similar to that of the atypical hyperplasias.

Sclerosing adenosis is a special concern here because well-developed sclerosing adenosis carries a risk of subsequent breast cancer that is slightly higher than that of the other elements that have been associated with the

Table 149–6	**Relative Risk of Invasive Breast Carcinoma Based on Microscopic Examination of Otherwise Benign Breast Tissue, Usually at Biopsy**

Slightly increased risk (1.5–2.0 times)

Women with the following lesions have a slightly increased risk of invasive breast carcinoma compared with women who have not had a breast biopsy as well as women with breast biopsies who lack these lesions on microscopic examination:

Moderate or florid hyperplasia without atypia	Common
Fibroadenoma with complex features	Uncommon
Sclerosing adenosis	Relatively common
Solitary papilloma without coexistent atypical hyperplasia	Relatively common

Moderately increased risk (4.0–5.9 times)

Women with the following lesions have a moderately increased risk of invasive breast carcinoma compared with women who have not had a breast biopsy:

Atypical ductal hyperplasia (ADH)
Atypical lobular hyperplasia (ALH)
Focal ductal pattern atypia in papillomas

Markedly increased risk (8.0–10.0 times)

Women with the following lesions have a high risk of invasive breast carcinoma compared with women who have not had a breast biopsy:

Ductal carcinoma in situ (DCIS), incompletely resected, according to strict criteria
Lobular carcinoma in situ (LCIS), according to strict criteria, uncommon compared with ALH (see above)

Each of these histologic diagnoses has its own associations with clinical presentation, detectability, and precision of diagnosis. For example, sclerosing adenosis may be diagnosed with little histologic change, but the indication of increased risk demands specific criteria that have been linked to increased cancer risk after prolonged follow-up.

ADH, atypical ductal hyperplasia; ALH, atypical lobular hyperplasia.

fibrocystic complex. By itself, it approaches a risk of two times, but this has not been confirmed in very many studies and demands precise histologic confirmation of enlarged lobular units and other features. These special considerations are referenced in detail in recent publications of Page and colleagues and Fitzgibbons and co-workers.

Fitzgibbons and others clearly discuss that some associations are found only in solitary studies, and have not been verified by others in follow-up studies of different sets of patients. This repeated verification is a constant requirement, as situations and conditions evolve with time.

Many studies have indicated the importance of hyperplasia without atypia as a mild indicator of increased risk (Fig. 149–1; see Table 149–1). Indeed, this group of women may be more important than the much smaller group of women with the atypical hyperplasias. Approximately 25% of women who were biopsied in both the premammographic and the current mammographic era have hyperplasia without atypia, while the atypias are found in 4% to 5%. Moreover, there may be ways of substratifying their risk by ascertaining hormonal markers in these women.

The specifically defined atypical hyperplasias have been verified in several studies, and are beginning to be recognized as having separate risk indications. Atypical lobular hyperplasia (ALH) has a slightly greater risk of later breast cancer than that of atypical ductal hyperplasia (ADH), but the diagnosis of ALH in a woman after the age of 55 has lesser significance. The graph presented as Figure 149–1 presents this information from the group of women followed by Dupont and Page in Nashville, Tennessee. Much of the indication of cancer risk after 10 to 15 years depends on the cumulative effect of the cancer developed in those first 10 to 15 years, with rate per year staying about the same or falling compared with age-matched control subjects. The authors have presented the graph as restricted to women younger than age 55 because this particular cohort does not have a large number of women older than that, and the relevance of the information is most informative and validated for the majority of women from this group who are aged 40 to 55 years at the time of biopsy.

The specifically defined atypical hyperplasias, certainly atypical lobular hyperplasia and lobular carcinoma in situ, have attained greater practical interest recently because of the National Surgical Adjuvant Breast Project prevention trial. This study indicated that women who had identified themselves as having atypical hyperplasia or lobular carcinoma in situ had a much greater reduction of later cancer as a result of taking tamoxifen than did other women. There is a good indication that lobular carcinoma in situ should be diagnosed rarely. Most of the cases of atypical hyperplasia of the lobular type from the Nurses Study at Harvard as well as the Nashville Cohort are called atypical lobular hyperplasia, rather than any other term. Lobular carcinoma in situ is a very uncommon diagnosis of very advanced changes in which there is evidence that the risk is slightly higher than that given in Figure 149–1 for atypical lobular hyperplasia. Both types, however, are risk factors for later development of cancer, which is certainly bilateral but may somewhat favor the breast in which the original biopsy identified the atypical hyperplasia. Note also in Figure 149–1 that the risk associated with ADH is somewhat less than that associated with ALH.

MEDICATIONS

Much attention has been given to hormonal medications and breast cancer risk. Every new research finding is met with significant media attention and significant fear generated for women struggling with the decision to take hormonal medications. This fear is fed by the medical recommendation to stop hormonal medications once breast cancer is diagnosed. Many women diagnosed with breast cancer believe that the hormones were responsible for their cancer. There is a large volume of research studying the risk of breast cancer associated with menopausal hormonal medication. The majority of these have not shown a significant increase (RR >2) in breast cancer risk associated with hormone therapy. Comparison of studies is hampered by differing types, dosages, and regimens of hormone therapy used. A reanalysis of the worldwide literature on menopausal hormone therapy and breast cancer risk found that current users, or those who stopped using hormones within the past 1 to 4 years prior

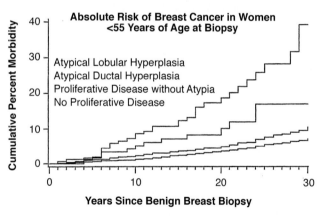

Figure 149–1. Cumulative morbidity of the development of invasive breast cancer with prolonged follow-up from the Nashville Cohort for 2000 (preliminary data of extended follow-up courtesy of WD Dupont and DL Page). The analysis of maximal likelihood estimates gives risk ratios compared with women without proliferative disease of 4.4 for ALH (95% confidence interval 3.1 to 6.3), 2.9 for ADH (95% CI 1.9 to 4.5), and 1.4 for PDWA (95% CI 1.2 to 1.7). The P value for all of these values is less than 0.001 for the atypical hyperplasias and approximately 0.0003 for the larger group of women with proliferative disease without atypia. *Note:* The present restriction to women younger than 55 years of age at the time of biopsy is made in order to make very clear that the majority of women from this particular cohort were less than 55 at the time of biopsy and that these numbers, at least with regard to ALH, are more important before the age of 55. There is good evidence that this risk of ALH falls after the age of 55. ALH, atypical lobular hyperplasia; ADH, atypical ductal hyperplasia; PDWA, proliferative disease without atypia.

and had undergone hormone therapy for 5 years or longer (average length of use 11 years), had a relative risk of 1.35 when compared with newer users. At a point of five years or more after stopping hormone therapy, there was no significant increase in breast cancer risk. Cancers diagnosed in women who had used hormone therapy tended to be less advanced clinically than those diagnosed in women who had never used hormone therapy. Regimens of hormone therapy administration have varied over time. Progestins are given to women who have an intact uterus to prevent the increased risk of endometrial cancer associated with unopposed estrogen use; however, this risk has not been shown to have any effect on survival because the endometrial carcinomas in this setting are overwhelmingly confined to the uterus. Recent evidence suggests that estrogen-progestin regimens may be associated with an increase in risk over estrogen-only regimens, and this was most evident in thin women. Again, the magnitude of this risk is small.

The relationship between oral contraceptives and breast cancer risk has been reviewed recently with a reanalysis of the worldwide data, including 54 studies in 25 countries. The main conclusion was that there was a slightly increased risk of breast cancer in women taking oral contraceptives and in the 10 years following cessation of such medication. For current users, the RR was 1.24; for those who stopped 1 to 4 years ago, the RR was 1.16; and for those who had stopped 5 to 9 years previously, the risk was 1.07. There was no appreciable increase in risk 10 years after stopping. Thus, this often-cited concern with regard to breast cancer risk is actually of small magnitude.

RECOMMENDATIONS FOR SCREENING OF WOMEN AT HIGH RISK

The American Cancer Society has established guidelines for breast cancer screening for women in the general population. These include the following:

- Monthly breast self-examination after age 20
- Clinical breast examination every 3 years from ages 20 to 39, yearly after age 40
- Mammogram yearly after age 40

By definition, these recommendations are for women without specific breast problems or complaints. The recommendations for the evaluation of specific breast problems or for screening of women at increased risk should be considered more specifically.

Women identified as at high risk for breast cancer should be offered a more intensive screening, and initiation of mammography screening should occur at an earlier age in these patients. Instruction for and encouragement of breast self-examination should be given, or more frequent clinical breast examination should be performed in patients who are uncomfortable or too anxious to do monthly breast self-examination; clinical breast examination may be offered every 6 months, and mammograms yearly, starting at an earlier age than in the general population. The recommendations for screening women with an inherited *BRCA1* or *BRCA2* mutation (or for those

who have a significant likelihood of a mutation) have been developed by a panel of experts, although the effectiveness of such screening has yet to be established. These recommendations include monthly breast self-examination, annual or semiannual (every 6 months) clinical breast examination beginning at ages 25 to 35, and annual mammography beginning at ages 25 to 35.

INTERVENTIONS FOR DECREASING THE RISK OF BREAST CANCER

The first breast cancer prevention trial in the United States, called NSABP P-1, was an NCI-sponsored trial that began in May 1992. The trial was designed to study the effectiveness of tamoxifen versus placebo in decreasing the risk of breast cancer. Tamoxifen is a selective estrogen receptor modulator (SERM); in other words, it has estrogenic effects on some tissues and antiestrogenic effects on others. It has been used in the treatment of breast cancer for many years. The P-1 trial followed more than 13,000 women older than 35 years of age. The women were identified as appropriate for inclusion in the study if they were at a risk equal to that of a 65-year-old woman. The Gail model was used to assess risk in women for inclusion in the trial. The trial was stopped in March 1998 because the women receiving tamoxifen were found to be 44% less likely to develop breast cancer than the women receiving placebo, including particularly strong evidence of breast cancer reduction in women with atypia and lobular carcinoma in situ. Other trials are forthcoming.

Another SERM medication, raloxifene, has been noted to decrease breast cancer in a study designed to evaluate its use in the treatment of osteoporosis. A new prevention trial, NSABP P-2, is currently underway to study the effectiveness of these two medications (tamoxifen and raloxifene, STAR Trial) in lowering the risk of breast cancer in postmenopausal women.

Prophylactic mastectomy is clearly controversial, but it may be considered by some women. A recent study demonstrated a 90% reduction in the incidence of breast cancer in women with a family history of breast cancer. It is clear that there may be many different ways of accomplishing the reduction of breast cancer risk by the removal of breast tissue mass. In any case, this is never an emergency as a prophylactic procedure, even in the presence of a high risk with atypical hyperplasia and family history. The authors suggest that the clinician encourage even the most anxious woman to wait 6 months before committing to this irreversible procedure.

CONCLUSION

Health care providers in all clinical settings make judgments about risk and discuss the concepts of risk with patients every day. If the clinician tailors the medical history to include identification of individuals at increased risk for breast and other cancers, he or she may identify those women who have special concerns about breast and other cancer risk. Specifically asking about cancers in the family, age of onset of the cancer, site of the primary

Pearls and Pitfalls

PEARLS

- When one discusses risks with patients, concepts of risk need to be carefully defined to avoid confusion. Types of risk include lifetime risk, absolute risk, and relative risk.
- Risk assessment models should be used with care in application to the individual patients, with an appreciation of the limitations of the particular model and its applicability to the clinical situation.
- The most important risk factors for breast cancer are female gender, advanced age, family history, and pathologic indicators of increased risk.
- Breast cancer predisposition genes *BRCA1* and *BRCA2* have been identified, and testing is commercially available.
- Neither menopausal hormone replacement therapy nor oral contraceptive use significantly alters breast cancer risk.
- Interventions for decreasing the risk of breast cancer include medications and prophylactic surgery. More intensive screening is indicated in high-risk populations with the hope of finding cancer at an earlier, more treatable stage.

PITFALLS

- Discussion of breast cancer risk is often imprecise. If definitions of terms, context, age groups, and other important topics are not carefully delineated, such discussion can contribute to undue fears and anxieties on the part of the patient and the family.
- Likewise, cancer risk counseling and genetic predisposition testing are not always a matter of hard-and-fast rules. Personal experience and knowledge of the patient and her family play an important role in the decision to proceed to predisposition testing.
- An understanding of the limitations of cancer genetic predisposition testing is essential. For example, a negative test result in an unaffected individual with no known mutation previously identified in the family provides no information about her cancer risk.
- Professional nurses and genetic counselors may be important adjuncts to other health care providers in educating women about breast cancer risk.

cancer, bilaterality, and cause of and age at death may help identify those at risk for an inherited cancer syndrome. The discussion of prior breast procedures and the review of benign biopsy results may also identify women at increased risk. Because of the significant fear of breast cancer and the complex issues surrounding cancer risk assessment as well as the availability of gene tests for cancer predisposition, consultation with specialists committed to educating and counseling patients and providing risk assessment may be a valuable adjunct in selected patients.

SELECTED READINGS

American Cancer Society: Cancer Facts and Figures. Atlanta, GA, 2000.

Armstrong K, Eisen A, Weber B: Assessing the risk of breast cancer. N Engl J Med 2000;342:564.

Benichou J, Gail MH, Mulvihill JJ: Graphs to estimate an individualized risk of breast cancer. J Clin Oncol 1996;14:103.

Burke W, Daly M, Garber J, et al: Recommendations for follow-up care of individuals with an inherited predisposition to cancer. II. *BRCA1* and *BRCA2*. Cancer Genetics Studies Consortium. JAMA 1997;277:997.

Chlebowski RT, Collyar DE, Somerfield MR, Pfister DG: American Society of Clinical Oncology technology assessment on breast cancer risk reduction strategies: Tamoxifen and raloxifene. J Clin Oncol 1999;17:1939.

Claus EB, Risch NJ, Thompson WD: Age at onset as an indicator of familial risk of breast cancer. Am J Epidemiol 1990;131:961.

Collaborative Group on Hormonal Factors in Breast Cancer: Breast cancer and hormone replacement therapy: Collaborative reanalysis of data from 51 epidemiological studies of 52,705 women with breast cancer and 108,411 women without breast cancer. Lancet 1997;350:1047.

Dupont WD, Plummer WD Jr: Understanding the relationship between relative and absolute risk. Cancer 1996;77:2193.

Dupont WD, Page DL, Parl FF, et al: Estrogen replacement therapy in women with a history of proliferative breast disease. Cancer 1999;85:1277.

Egan KM, Stampfer MJ, Rosner BA, et al: Risk factors for breast cancer in women with a breast cancer family history. Cancer Epidemiol Biomarkers Prev 1998;7:359.

Feuer EJ, Wun LM, Boring CC, et al: The lifetime risk of developing breast cancer. J Natl Cancer Inst 1993;85:892.

Fisher B, Costantino JP, Wickerham DL, et al: Tamoxifen for prevention of breast cancer: Report of the National Surgical Adjuvant Breast and Bowel Project P-1 Study. J Natl Cancer Inst 1998;90:1371.

Fitzgibbons PL, Henson DE, Hutter RV: Benign breast changes and the risk for subsequent breast cancer: An update of the 1985 consensus statement. Cancer Committee of the College of American Pathologists. Arch Pathol Lab Med 1998;122:1053.

Gail MH, Brinton LA, Byar DP, et al: Projecting individualized probabilities of developing breast cancer for white females who are being examined annually. J Natl Cancer Inst 1989;81:1879.

Hartmann LC, Schaid DJ, Woods JE, et al: Efficacy of bilateral prophylactic mastectomy in women with a family history of breast cancer. N Engl J Med 1999;340:77.

Jacobs TW, Byrne C, Colditz G, et al: Radial scars in benign breast-biopsy specimens and the risk of breast cancer. N Engl J Med 1999;340:430.

Kelsey JL: Breast cancer epidemiology: Summary and future directions. Epidemiol Rev 1993;15:256.

Marshall LM, Hunter DJ, Connolly JL, et al: Risk of breast cancer associated with atypical hyperplasia of lobular and ductal types. Cancer Epidemiol Biomarkers Prev 1997;6:297.

Offit K: Clinical Cancer Genetics: Risk Counseling and Management. New York, Wiley-Liss, 1998, p 2.

Page DL, Caro SW, Dupont WD: Management of the patient at high risk. In Bland KI, Copeland EM (ed): The Breast: Comprehensive Management of Benign and Malignant Diseases. Philadelphia, WB Saunders, 1998, pp 1453–1459.

Page DL, Jensen RA, Simpson JF: Premalignant and malignant disease of the breast: The roles of the pathologist. Mod Pathol 1998;11:120.

Schairer C, Lubin J, Troisi R, et al: Menopausal estrogen and estrogen-progestin replacement therapy and breast cancer risk [see comments]. JAMA 2000;283:485.

Shattuck-Eidens D, McClure M, Simard J, et al: A collaborative survey of 80 mutations in the *BRCA1* breast and ovarian cancer susceptibility gene: Implications for presymptomatic testing and screening. JAMA 1995;273:535.

Chapter 150

In Situ Carcinoma of the Breast: Ductal and Lobular Origin

Theresa A. Graves and Kirby I. Bland

DUCTAL CARCINOMA IN SITU (DCIS)

Introduction

The optimal management of ductal carcinoma in situ (DCIS) is one of the most controversial topics in the treatment of breast disease. The widespread availability of high-resolution screening mammography has increased the diagnosis of DCIS from 2% to 14% of all breast cancer diagnoses and from 20% to 40% of mammographically detected breast malignancies. As mammographic screening has become a national health priority, this trend is expected to continue. Historically, this poorly understood breast cancer was predominantly treated with mastectomy. The increase in breast-conserving therapy (BCT) for invasive cancer has spurred a movement toward a similar management for DCIS; however, limited information exists about the natural history of DCIS to use as a basis for treatment decisions. Critical to the management of DCIS is the recognition that it represents a heterogeneous group of lesions with diverse malignant potentials. As an in situ disease, it does not express the full malignant phenotype, lacking invasion and metastatic potential. Mastectomy is considered curative, with a 0 to 1% disease-specific mortality. Therefore, an invasive local recurrence following BCT carries the risk of increased breast cancer mortality. Each patient must be considered individually, with her unique presentation and clinical, radiographic, and pathologic features weighed carefully in the management process.

Clinical Presentation

Prior to expanded screening with high-resolution mammography, DCIS typically presented with a palpable mass, bloody or serous nipple discharge, or Paget's disease. Today, most DCIS lesions are detected mammographically as clustered microcalcifications, although 10% may present as an uncalcified mass and only occasionally are diagnosed without mammographic findings. Routine as well as 90-degree lateral magnification views should be obtained in order to characterize the microcalcifications. Classically, high-grade DCIS demonstrates a linear branching pattern following a ductal distribution. These microcalcifications tend to represent the comedo necrosis often seen in grade III lesions. Indeterminate or pleomorphic calcifications may also indicate DCIS. Microcalcifications may also represent benign fibrocystic changes, such as sclerosing adenosis, with DCIS identified only incidentally and not associated with the microcalcifica-

tions. Consequently, it is critical that the specimen of biopsied tissue, either open or core, undergo specimen radiography and that the pathologists specify whether the DCIS is associated with the microcalcifications. While mammography is an excellent diagnostic tool, its specificity in distinguishing benign lesions from malignant ones is only 50% to 60% and it may frequently underestimate the extent of disease.

Preoperative Management

Diagnosis

The diagnosis of DCIS requires histopathologic evaluation. Image-directed procedures are needed for both diagnosis and treatment. Stereotactic core-needle biopsy of the breast may be the initial step in diagnosing nonpalpable mammographic abnormalities. Not all lesions are amenable to stereotactic biopsy, owing to the technical limitations of low-volume breasts or very superficial or deep lesions. When stereotactic biopsy is employed, multiple cores (11- or 14-gauge) should be obtained to ensure adequate sampling of the microcalcifications. If all microcalcifications are removed, a wire clip should be left as a marker for future localization and excision. Percutaneous core biopsy may reveal a diagnosis of atypical ductal hyperplasia (ADH) or DCIS. Complete surgical excision of these lesions often results in upstaging of ADH to carcinoma (both DCIS and infiltrating ductal carcinoma) in 20% to 40% of cases and of DCIS to an invasive carcinoma in 20% of cases. When stereotactic biopsy is not possible or returns a pathologic diagnosis of ADH or DCIS, a wire localization open biopsy is necessary. This will allow a complete diagnosis and may achieve therapeutic breast conservation for the patient with DCIS only. Initial diagnosis by stereotactic core biopsy may reduce the volume of tissue removed in order to achieve margin-negative lumpectomies for breast conservation.

Pathology

The histologic classification of DCIS has evolved slowly; traditionally it has been based on an architectural pattern with two main categories: comedo and noncomedo (cribriform, micropapillary, papillary, and solid). Comedo lesions demonstrate prominent necrosis and tumor cells with pleomorphic nuclei and higher mitotic rates. Noncomedo types typically are of low nuclear grade without prominent necrosis. Comedo lesions more frequently demonstrate microinvasion, a greater degree of angiogenesis, and higher proliferative rate. Overexpression of *her-2-neu*, cyclin D-1, and p53 oncogenes and the absence of ER and *Bcl-2* expression are also more common with comedo than noncomedo lesions. Lesions may display a wide range of architectural patterns, however, with or without necrosis. Recently, pathologists have proposed new classifications based on nuclear grade and the presence or absence of necrosis, which may represent better prognostic factors in guiding optimal therapy.

Imaging

Careful correlation of the pathologic findings with the mammographic examination is important in determining the extent and distribution of disease. Standard mammographic views may underestimate the volume of disease, and magnification views are critical in the evaluation of microcalcifications. Multifocality (foci in proximity to the index lesion) may be treated with breast conservation, whereas multicentric lesions (those located in a separate quadrant) have a negative impact on the success of breast conservation. Holland has reported that the majority of lesions demonstrate multifocal, and not multicentric, patterns. The well-differentiated DCIS lesion is more likely to demonstrate a multifocal pattern than is the poorly differentiated tumor (70% versus 10%). Magnetic resonance imaging (MRI) with contrast enhancement has shown promise in better defining the extent and distribution of DCIS in the breast and may assist in surgical decision making.

Surgical Options

Initial surgical decision making for DCIS is usually based on the histopathologic sampling of a stereotactic biopsy, breast imaging, and patient factors. It is less common to have an excisional specimen that provides complete histologic details, volume of disease, and margin status. Surgical options include mastectomy with or without immediate reconstruction, or excision with negative margins to be followed by observation or adjuvant breast radiation. Mastectomy remains the most aggressive surgical therapy for DCIS and the standard by which the outcomes of all other therapies are measured. Clear indications for mastectomy include multicentric disease with two or more foci, diffuse malignant-appearing (or proven) microcalcifications, and cases with persistent positive margins after surgical re-excision. Certain patient factors that may preclude the use of radiation constitute a relative indication for mastectomy, but alternatively, if clinically appropriate, they may be an indication for excision alone. These factors include a history of collagen vascular disease, previous irradiation to the breast or chest, and pregnancy. Prognostic factors based on recurrence data may also be utilized in predicting which lesions will have such a high rate of local recurrence regardless of the addition of radiation that mastectomy would be the preferred initial treatment. Unfortunately, many of these factors become known only following excisional biopsy; therefore, they are discussed in the section on postoperative management. Mastectomy provides maximal risk reduction but

may represent overtreatment for the majority of patients with small mammographically detected lesions.

Indications for breast-conserving surgery include DCIS detected mammographically or a localized palpable lesion without multicentricity or diffuse microcalcifications. The decision for the addition of radiation to BCT is also based on the prognostic factors that influence local recurrence and may be affected by radiation therapy.

A critical factor in preoperative management is assessing the patient's needs and expectations regarding breast preservation. Treatment should be tailored to patient preference and to the understanding of risk management in the treatment of DCIS.

Intraoperative Management

Mastectomy

Mastectomy may be performed with or without immediate reconstruction. The most significant recent advance in breast reconstruction has been the use of skin-sparing mastectomy, in which a total mastectomy, including the nipple and areola complex, is performed through a periareolar incision. Large retrospective studies have shown no increase in the local breast cancer recurrence rates. Axillary resection is not necessary for the management of most patients with DCIS, as the incidence of nodal metastasis in pure DCIS is 0 to 1%. Although the use of sentinel node biopsy has been proposed, it should be considered only in the context of clinical trials. Following the diagnosis of DCIS by stereotactic core biopsy and in cases with extensive DCIS of high nuclear grade, unsuspected invasive or microinvasive disease may be identified pathologically in the mastectomy specimen. Lagios and colleagues noted a relationship between the extent of disease and the likelihood of finding stromal invasion. DCIS lesions smaller than 25 mm showed no evidence of invasion on pathologic review, whereas 48% of lesions larger than 55 mm demonstrated stromal invasion. Consequently, for patients with large lesions undergoing mastectomy, a sentinel lymph node biopsy may be performed in conjunction with axillary sampling, which is achieved during resection of the tail of Spence. If a clinically suspicious node is identified, touch-prep or frozen section should be performed, and if a positive lymph node is identified a level I to II lymph node dissection should be completed. This may avoid a second operative procedure in the event that an invasive focus is identified in the mastectomy specimen. This is particularly advantageous when immediate reconstruction has occurred.

Breast-Conserving Therapy (BCT)

Critical to BCT is the successful excision of the lesion, with careful attention to margin status as well as the maintenance of an acceptable cosmetic outcome. Nonpalpable, mammographically detected lesions are excised following presurgical localization of the abnormality with a guide wire placed under radiographic assistance. More accurate excision may be achieved with multiple wires bracketing the abnormality. The exact location of the wire tip is assessed by triangulation using the post-wire, two-view mammograms, which should accompany the patient to the operating room. A curvilinear skin incision is made closest to the wire tip, and extensive tunneling should be avoided. Careful attention is paid to margin status, although this is hampered by an inability to distinguish nonpalpable intraductal lesions from surrounding normal breast tissue. The specimen is preferably removed in one piece, with precise anatomic orientation through clips, ties, or a six-color margin inking scheme. Such marking is critical for correctly identifying the location of any positive margins and will greatly facilitate any subsequent re-excision. Additional shave margins have been advocated to avoid false-positive margins identified in inking systems. Intraoperative touch-preps have also been suggested as a means of avoiding re-excision for positive margins. The rate of re-excision for positive or close (<1 mm) margins is estimated to be as high as 55% and re-excision generally detracts from the overall cosmetic result. Meticulous hemostasis avoids hematoma formation, which may create an unnecessary delay in adjuvant radiation therapy as well as difficulty in interpreting follow-up mammography. Under some circumstances, reapproximation of the biopsy cavity affords a better cosmetic outcome and closure is accomplished with a subcuticular technique.

An intraoperative specimen radiograph should be obtained and correlated with the perioperative mammogram. While specimen radiography is not adequate for determining the completeness of excision, two views in magnification increase resolution and may assist in identifying microcalcifications (or mass) extending to the margins of the specimen, and further resection may then be accomplished. The absence of the radiographic abnormality within the specimen radiograph usually indicates that it has not been removed. The specimen radiograph should accompany the specimen to pathology to assist in accurately sampling the abnormality. Frozen-section examination of image-guided excision specimens is discouraged as ADH or DCIS may be indistinguishable from each other and small foci of microinvasion may be missed. Metallic clips should be placed in the operative site to assist with precise localization of the tumor bed for adjuvant radiation therapy to the breast.

Postoperative Management

Technical Aspects

Total-mastectomy patients who will not undergo immediate reconstruction are managed with a single closed suction drain, which is removed when the volume of output diminishes to less than 30 mL/day. BCT rarely requires drainage. Management following immediate reconstruction is based on the form of reconstruction with tissue transfer techniques requiring closer monitoring for viability of the transferred tissue.

Anesthetic and Hospital Stay Considerations

Under ideal circumstances, total mastectomy without reconstruction may be performed as an outpatient procedure following general anesthesia. However, 24-hour observation is more common. Breast-conserving surgery is performed with local anesthesia and sedation. At the patient's preference, a general anesthetic may be utilized. Larger segmental mastectomies are often better tolerated with a general anesthetic. Excisions and partial mastectomies are performed as outpatient procedures.

Assessment of Risk Factors for Local Recurrence

The recurrence rate following mastectomy is 0 to 2%, whereas for BCT the reported rates range from 3% to greater than 46%. The most critical issue in the optimal management of the patient pursuing BCT is minimizing the risk of local relapse. Events leading to local relapse are multifactorial, with technical, tumor-related, and patient-related factors playing roles in local recurrence following BCT.

Resection Margins

The main technical consideration in local control is achieving adequate resection margins, which represent the distance between the DCIS and the edge of the excised specimen and reflect the adequacy of excision. Routine postoperative mammograms with magnification should be obtained as soon as the patient can tolerate compression to evaluate for residual calcifications and ensure complete resection of the mammographic abnormality. Postoperative mammogram and margin status are complementary in assessing the completeness of excision. As DCIS lacks invasive and metastatic potential, complete excision should produce a cure. Standardized methods of assessing histologic margins did not exist until the late 1980s and early 1990s, and, consequently, earlier studies failed to demonstrate margin status as a significant factor in local control. Silverstein reported on the most recent analysis of the influence of margin width on local recurrence in DCIS. Patients were stratified by margin width (>10 mm, 1 to 9 mm, and <1 mm). In patients with margins greater than 10 mm, the addition of irradiation did not lower the recurrence rate, with an estimated 4% probability of recurrence at 8 years. The statistical power to depict a difference in this group, however, is low. In the 1- to 9-mm group, a 20% local recurrence risk was noted at 8 years without adjuvant radiation, and 12% with radiation. While this difference was not statistically significant, the number of patients and events preclude a clear conclusion. In addition, the irradiated lesions were significantly larger and more likely to have comedo necrosis and were followed for 20 months longer than were the nonirradiated group. The addition of irradiation to DCIS resected with margins less than 1 mm resulted in a statistically significant improvement from 58% to 30% local recurrence rate; however, both rates are prohibitively high. Work by Holland and colleagues demonstrated that DCIS may have gaps or skipped lesions measuring up to 10 mm or more, which raises the question of the adequacy of 1- to 2-mm margins. Patients are currently being enrolled in prospective protocols evaluating the use of excision alone in selected patients, and these data, obtained with the use of modern techniques of margin measurement and tumor characterization, may better define the influence of margins on local recurrence.

Tumor Factors

The presence of necrosis in DCIS has long been associated with poor prognosis and higher recurrence rates. It has recently been determined that cellular architecture and nuclear grade influence local recurrence more predictably than does comedo necrosis alone. Recurrences in high-grade groups occurred within a much shorter interval than those in the low-grade or intermediate groups. Solin reported a 5-year recurrence rate of 12% versus 3% for high-grade compared with low-grade lesions, respectively, but by 10 years the recurrence rates were not statistically different, at 18% and 15%, respectively, again supporting a difference in time to progression rather than potential to recur. Tumor size, like margin width, reflects the distribution of the disease and the ability of the surgeon to adequately excise the DCIS. Making an accurate determination of the true size of a DCIS lesion is a challenge. A useful pathologic technique for size estimation is recording both the extent of disease in a single slide and the total number of blocks involved with disease. Submitting the entire specimen for microscopic examination in sequential sections of uniform thickness may also more accurately reflect the size and extent of disease.

Van Nuys Prognostic Index (VNPI)

With the use of the prognostic factors of nuclear grade and comedo necrosis in combination with tumor size and margin width, the VNPI was developed to select subgroups of patients who do not require irradiation if BCT is chosen. In addition, the VNPI may be used to select patients whose recurrence risk is prohibitively high regardless of additional irradiation, so that mastectomy is indicated. Table 150–1 shows the VNPI scoring system with the total of three scores—ranging from 3 to 9—from each of the predictors. The scores are translated into a treatment recommendation. This numerical algorithm is based on the outcome of 461 patients with DCIS treated with breast preservation. With patients divided into three

subgroups by score (3 to 4; 5, 6, or 7; or 8 to 9), the probability of local recurrence was significantly different for each subgroup (Fig. 150–1). The patients in the lowest subgroup demonstrated no difference in recurrence-free survival at 8 years, regardless of irradiation, and could be considered for excision alone. The intermediate group demonstrated a statistically significant reduction in recurrence with radiation therapy. An unacceptably high rate of recurrence was seen in the highest subgroup when the patients were treated with BCT, and these should be considered for mastectomy. A number of caveats limit the use of the VNPI. The VNPI subgroups are based on retrospective subset analysis and on retrospective comparison of patients treated with different diagnostic, pathologic, and therapeutic techniques. In addition, reproduction of meticulous pathologic handling is necessary for accurately reflecting tumor size and margin status. Therefore, outside validation and longer follow-up will better establish the VNPI as a guide to treatment planning.

Patient Factors

Family history has been analyzed as a predictor of local recurrence following treatment for DCIS. Two reports indicate that family history may have a measurable effect, one study indicating a 37% recurrence rate for women with positive family history versus 9% for those without a family history of breast carcinoma. Younger women appear to have a more aggressive tumor biology as well as longer periods during which they are at risk for recurrence. Van Zee and co-workers reported a significantly lower risk of recurrence with increasing age, comparing women older than 70, women aged 40 to 69, and women younger than 40 years of age. Actuarial 6-year local relapse rates were 10.8%, 14%, and 47.2%, respectively. The impact of youth and family history on recurrence risk is controversial and will require further evaluation and possible prospective analysis. Genetic factors, specifically *BRCA1* and *BRCA2*, and their role in local recurrence, incidence of a second primary, or contralateral breast disease have not been sufficiently documented as supporting a particular management algorithm. Finally, the concerns and wishes of the patient and her ability to handle the risks of local recurrence must be considered when one discusses treatment options.

Adjunctive Breast Radiation

The role of radiation continues to evolve in the management of DCIS patients treated with BCT. Further clarifi-

Table 150–1	Van Nuys Prognostic Index (VNPI) Scoring System		
	SCORE		
	1	**2**	**3**
Size (mm)	≤15	16–40	≥41
Margins (mm)	≥10	1–9	<1
Pathologic classification	Non–high-grade without necrosis (nuclear grades 1, 2)	Non–high-grade with necrosis (nuclear grades 1, 2)	High-grade with or without necrosis (nuclear grade 3)

From Silverstein MJ, Masetti R: Hypothesis and practice: Are there several types of treatment for ductal carcinoma in situ of the breast? Recent Results Cancer Res 1998;152:105–122.

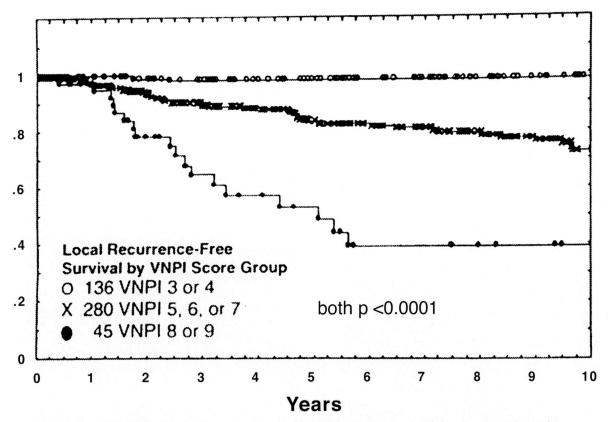

Figure 150–1. Probability of local recurrence-free survival for DCIS patients treated with breast conservation and grouped by Van Nuys Prognostic Index score. (From Silverstein MJ, Masetti R: Hypothesis and practice: Are there several types of treatment for ductal carcinoma in situ of the breast? Recent Results Cancer Res 1998;152:105.)

cation of an appropriate role for radiation therapy may be achieved by identifying the DCIS characteristics that, in combination or alone, differentiate the patients who will not benefit from the addition of radiation. One prospective and several retrospective randomized trials have demonstrated an approximately 50% reduction in local recurrence with the addition of radiation. The largest retrospective trial by Solin reported a 19%, 15-year actuarial local failure rate in 270 DCIS patients treated with BCT plus radiation therapy. Half of the recurrences were invasive disease and the cause of specific mortality was 4%. In 1993, the National Surgical Adjuvant Breast and Bowel Project (NSABP) reported on the B-17 trial, which represents the first prospective randomized trial testing the benefit of radiation therapy in BCT. A total of 790 patients were randomized to excision or excision with radiation with a 5-year actuarial recurrence rate of 16.4% versus 7%, respectively. Recurrent DCIS was reduced from 10.4% to 7.5% ($P = 0.055$), and the cumulative incidence of locally recurrent invasive cancer was reduced from 10.5% to 2.9% ($P < 0.001$). The 8-year update with a mean follow-up of 90 months has shown a consistent significant reduction in ipsilateral breast DCIS recurrence from 13.4% to 8.2% ($P = 0.007$), with a reduction in invasive ipsilateral breast tumor recurrence from 13.4% to 3.9% ($P < 0.0001$). The results of the B-17 trial remain controversial, as it suggests that all DCIS patients treated with BCT should receive radiation. The trial, however, was not designed to determine whether there is a subset

that might be selected to forego radiation. The recent Silverstein report evaluated margin width alone as a potential discriminator for which DCIS patients treated with BCT may require radiation therapy to significantly reduce local recurrence. The limitations of this study have already been described. Clearly, factors of favorable tumor characteristics, excellent margin width, and small size have demonstrated promise as factors limiting local recurrence. The Radiation Therapy Oncology Group (RTOG) is accruing patients with this favorable profile to randomize to excision or excision with radiation therapy. In addition, all patients will receive tamoxifen. Analysis of these factors with modern pathologic and radiographic techniques in this randomized prospective fashion with additional stratification for pertinent patient factors will allow clarification of radiation's role in the treatment of DCIS.

Role of Chemoprevention: Tamoxifen and Selective Estrogen Receptor Modulators (SERM)

Tamoxifen is a nonsteroidal selective estrogen receptor compound with both estrogenic and antiestrogenic effects that has demonstrated effectiveness in reducing ipsilateral breast cancer (IBC) and systemic recurrence in estrogen receptor–positive invasive breast cancer patients. The recent NSABP meta-analysis has also demonstrated the reduction of DCIS or invasive contralateral breast cancer

(CBC) from 5.1% to 1.9% at 5 years in patients taking tamoxifen. Such observations led to the initiation of tamoxifen-based prevention trials. The largest study (NSABP P-1) randomized more than 13,300 high-risk patients to tamoxifen or placebo and demonstrated a 50% reduction in the incidence of both DCIS and invasive ductal carcinoma at 43 months of follow-up. A possible role for tamoxifen in DCIS has been established through the NSABP B-24 trial, which randomized DCIS patients treated with BCT and radiation therapy to tamoxifen or placebo. Tamoxifen therapy resulted in a consistent reduction in both IBC and CBC. In fact, the incidence of CBC was similar to IBC recurrence after treatment with radiation therapy, with accumulated 5-year risk with an invasive CBC of 2.3% and 4.2% for IBC. This was reduced to 1.8% and 2.1%, respectively, with the use of tamoxifen. Tamoxifen did not significantly reduce the incidence of ipsilateral DCIS recurrence, with a cumulative 5-year incidence of 5.1% versus 3.9%. The contralateral breast DCIS incidence was reduced from 1.1% to 0.2% with tamoxifen. Neither negative margin status or unicentric disease was required for trial entry, and this may influence the rate of ipsilateral breast DCIS recurrence in this trial. With the accumulated tamoxifen data demonstrating an average relative risk reduction of 50% in both ipsilateral recurrence and second primary disease, the RTOG and others have initiated trials in which tamoxifen alone is offered as a treatment arm in BCT for DCIS. Tamoxifen use is not without risk, given its potential adverse side effects, especially in postmenopausal women, with at least a two-fold increase in endometrial cancer, from a cumulative risk of 5.4 per thousand to 13 per thousand in patients taking tamoxifen. In addition, thromboembolic events are increased two-fold with tamoxifen use compared with control subjects. Premenopausal women were not as significantly affected; however, the vasomotor and psychological effects of tamoxifen-induced menopausal symptoms are more notable in pre- and perimenopausal patients. Favorable end-organ effects of the maintenance of bone mineral density and reduction in lipid profiles with the use of tamoxifen were also noted. The adverse effects of tamoxifen have provided the impetus for developing new compounds with antiestrogenic effects on both the breast and the uterus while maintaining the more favorable estrogenic qualities. Raloxifene (Evista) is a second-generation SERM developed specifically to promote bone mineralization and prevent osteoporosis. Its use promotes a favorable lipid profile and does not stimulate endometrial hyperplasia, although the thromboembolic events and menopausal symptoms were similar to those experienced with tamoxifen use. The Multiple Outcomes of Raloxifene Evaluation study (MORE trial) and larger retrospective meta-analyses of more than 10,575 women randomized to raloxifene in osteoporosis trials demonstrated a 55% reduction in the relative risk of developing invasive breast cancer, compared with placebo control after only 40 months of follow-up. This has prompted the initiation of the second chemoprevention trial (NSABP P-2) comparing tamoxifen and raloxifene in high-risk, postmenopausal women. At this time, there are no data that support the use of raloxifene in invasive or noninvasive breast cancer. A clinical trial to test the newest SERM—LY353381 HCl—is being considered for patients with DCIS treated with BCT and randomized to radiation or no radiation therapy.

Complications

The specific surgical complications of breast hematoma, chronic seroma, wound dehiscence, and infection may be limited by the use of meticulous hemostasis. Recent data marginally supported the use of preoperative prophylactic antibiotics to reduce the incidence of wound infections. Closed suction drains utilized with mastectomy reduce hematoma and chronic seroma, but prolonged duration of an indwelling drain increases the incidence of infection.

IBC recurrence in patients treated with BCT may be considered a complication whose incidence should be limited, as the consequences of an invasive cancer include disease-specific mortality. Approximately 50% of all local failures are invasive disease, and the median time frame of invasive recurrence is nearly 5 years, with many invasive recurrences identified at more than 10 years of follow-up. Most noninvasive recurrences occur within the first 5 years. The treatment of recurrent disease if BCT was performed with adjunctive radiation therapy is an ipsilateral mastectomy with or without axillary dissection, depending on the presence of invasion. If BCT without radiation therapy was the primary treatment, re-excision with adjunctive radiation therapy could be considered, depending on the patient's desires and the availability of breast volume. Patients initially treated with mastectomy generally require local excision, chest wall irradiation, and chemotherapy.

Radiation therapy may be complicated by cardiac and pulmonary side effects in a small percentage of patients. Radiation fibrosis of the breast, a more common side effect, changes the texture of the breast and skin and makes radiographic follow-up more difficult, thus potentially delaying the diagnosis of a local recurrence. More modern radiation techniques, however, are limiting these complications.

The potential deleterious effects of tamoxifen must be considered when this chemopreventive agent is used to further reduce the incidence of recurrence, particularly when the incidence may be already substantially lowered by surgical resection or radiation therapy, or both. Specifically, in postmenopausal women who have retained their uterus, the greater than two-fold incidence of endometrial carcinoma and thromboembolic events is a significant complication potential. In patients who are at increased risk for thromboembolic events (atrial fibrillation, history of deep venous thrombosis, history of pulmonary embolus, and relative contraindications of extreme age associated with limited mobility), tamoxifen use is contraindicated.

Outcomes

Mastectomy remains the most aggressive and successful surgical treatment for DCIS and the standard against which the outcomes of all other therapies are compared. Long-term follow-up of mastectomy has shown a recurrence rate of 0 to 2% and disease-specific mortality of 0 to 1%. Disease-specific mortality is a reflection of unrecognized foci of invasive disease in patients with DCIS. An attempt at risk prediction should be made for the patient pursuing BCT, given the absence of clinical trials comparing mastectomy with BCT. A reasonable estimate of local recurrence with BCT is 10% at 10 years, with 50% of recurrences presenting as invasive disease. When one uses an estimated mortality of 30% to 40% for invasive breast cancer, an absolute mortality risk of 2% exists for women choosing breast conservation. Silverstein evaluated the outcomes of invasive local recurrence after BCT for patients with DCIS. The 8-year probability of local invasive cancer in a cohort of 707 patients was 9.3%, and the probability of breast cancer–specific mortality was 2.1%. For patients who developed an invasive recurrence, the disease-specific mortality rate was 14.1%, with a distant recurrence rate of 27.1%. The median time to noninvasive cancer recurrence was 22 months and 58 months for invasive local recurrence. A total of 51% of patients presented with a stage I invasive breast carcinoma. The remainder demonstrated a more advanced stage at the time of recurrence, with an average stage of IIA.

Further perspective is gained by considering the risk of developing a contralateral breast cancer, with a 5% to 10% risk of contralateral breast cancer at 5 to 10 years. Bilateral prophylactic mastectomy would, therefore, be the choice of treatment that would produce the least IBC or CBC recurrence but would substantially overtreat the majority of women. Consideration of the risk of developing ipsilateral and contralateral breast cancer allows a rational algorithm for management of DCIS with relative

and absolute risk reductions in calculated outcomes (Fig. 150–2).

LOBULAR CARCINOMA IN SITU (LCIS)

Introduction

Lobular carcinoma in situ (LCIS), or lobular neoplasia, is a noninvasive breast lesion arising from the lobules and terminal ducts of the breast. The true incidence of LCIS is unknown because of the lack of clinical and radiographic signs. A rise in the frequency of LCIS has been attributed to both greater recognition of the pathologic entity and the increasing use of screening mammography. LCIS represents 10% of diagnoses noted incidentally from mammographically directed biopsies. Historically, total mastectomy, modified radical mastectomy, and bilateral mastectomy have been used for the management of LCIS. With a greater understanding of the natural history of this process, clinicians now recognize LCIS as a risk factor, rather than a precursor for the development of breast cancer. A nonoperative approach, therefore, has been adopted, with lifelong surveillance as the consensus for treatment. Recent results of the NSABP P-1 trial demonstrate a significant reduction in breast cancer incidence with the use of tamoxifen in high-risk patients, including those with LCIS. This has allowed an effective alternative to either observation or bilateral mastectomy.

Natural History

The critical issue in the management of LCIS is the risk of subsequent development of an invasive cancer,

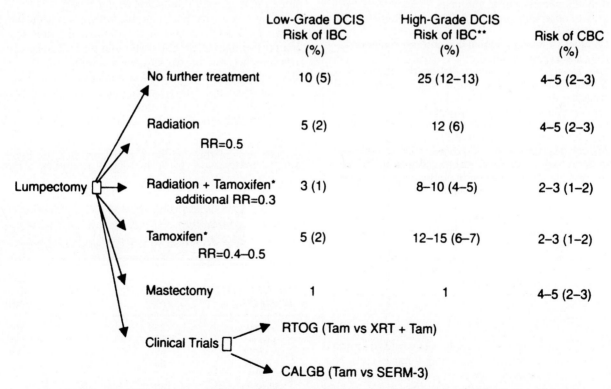

	Low-Grade DCIS Risk of IBC (%)	High-Grade DCIS Risk of IBC** (%)	Risk of CBC (%)
No further treatment	10 (5)	25 (12–13)	4–5 (2–3)
Radiation RR=0.5	5 (2)	12 (6)	4–5 (2–3)
Radiation + Tamoxifen* additional RR=0.3	3 (1)	8–10 (4–5)	2–3 (1–2)
Tamoxifen* RR=0.4–0.5	5 (2)	12–15 (6–7)	2–3 (1–2)
Mastectomy	1	1	4–5 (2–3)

Lumpectomy

Clinical Trials → RTOG (Tam vs XRT + Tam)
→ CALGB (Tam vs SERM-3)

Figure 150–2. Algorithm for the management of DCIS with relative and absolute risk reductions for the development of ipsilateral (recurrent) and contralateral breast cancer stratified by low and high-grade DCIS. (From Hwang ES, Esserman LJ: Management of ductal carcinoma in situ. Surg Clin North Am 1999;79:1007.)

Pearls and Pitfalls

LCIS

PEARLS

- LCIS represents a risk factor for the development of bilateral breast cancer.
- Clinical follow-up with lifelong surveillance represents the consensus for treatment.
- The risk of developing breast cancer is approximately 1% per year and persists indefinitely.
- Bilateral mastectomy may be considered an alternative approach to surveillance, specifically where hereditary factors may influence choice of treatment. There is no role for unilateral mastectomy in LCIS.
- Chemoprevention with tamoxifen may reduce the incidence of breast cancer development by 50% or more.
- There is no evidence that radiation therapy or cytotoxic chemotherapy offers any reduction in the potential risk of subsequent breast cancer development.
- Consider clinical prevention trial (NSABP P-2) for postmenopausal women.

DCIS

PEARLS

- The majority of DCIS lesions are detected mammographically as clustered microcalcifications; however, the microcalcifications may underestimate the extent of disease.
- Stereotactic core-needle biopsy is the preferred diagnostic procedure for nonpalpable mammographic abnormalities.
- Total mastectomy (TM) is considered curative, with a 0 to 1% disease-specific mortality.
- Breast-conserving surgery (BCS) is an alternative for localized DCIS.
- Complete resection should be ensured radiographically and pathologically.
- The addition of adjuvant radiation therapy to BCS is based on prognostic factors that influence local recurrence.
- Excision alone may be appropriate for selected women with small, low-grade lesions and excellent margins (consider clinical trial).
- Axillary dissection is not indicated in DCIS; however, in large high-grade DCIS lesions proceeding to mastectomy, sentinel lymph node biopsy with low axillary sampling may avoid reoperation if invasion is identified.
- Approximately 50% of all local recurrences present as invasive disease with a disease-specific mortality of 2% to 4%.
- Tamoxifen may be considered an adjunctive treatment for reduction in both ipsilateral recurrence and contralateral breast cancer.

cer and DCIS still represent the majority of subsequent breast cancers identified. The occurrence of infiltrating ductal cancer and the bilateral equality of risk combined with the observation that the majority of patients diagnosed with LCIS do not develop invasive breast cancer support the hypothesis that LCIS represents a risk factor for, rather than a precursor of, breast cancer. The estimated relative risk for the development of invasive breast cancer ranges from 5.9 to 12 times the baseline risk of the index population. The Haagensen Research Foundation provides 18 years of median follow-up for LCIS patients treated with observation. The cumulative incidence of breast cancer following diagnosis of LCIS was 13% at 10 years, 26% at 20 years, and 35% at 35 years after the LCIS diagnosis. Long-term follow-up has shown that the risk of subsequent cancer development is equal bilaterally. The risk of developing a cancer is also dependent on the age of the patient at the time of the initial LCIS diagnosis, with a higher risk in patients younger than age 40 (Table 150–2). The incidence of subsequent ILCA in this update of the Haagensen data was 27%, with infiltrating ductal cancer representing 41% and pure DCIS 22% of subsequent cancers.

Treatment

Given the hypothesis that LCIS represents a risk factor for breast cancer development, careful observation with lifelong surveillance is the management option that has become the most widely accepted. Surveillance includes annual screening mammography, monthly breast self-examination, at least twice-yearly clinical breast examination, and diagnostic evaluation as necessary.

Clearance of surgical margins with re-excision has no rationale, as LCIS is known as a multifocal lesion disseminated throughout both breasts. Margin clearance cannot resolve the risk of subsequent bilateral breast cancer development. Similarly, blind contralateral breast biopsies are not indicated without radiographic or clinical criteria for biopsy. Axillary dissection is not warranted, as the risk of transmission to the axillary lymph nodes is less than 1%.

Operative management, if elected, involves bilateral simple mastectomy with or without immediate recon-

Table 150–2	Relative Risk of Developing Cancer by Age at Initial Diagnosis of Lobular Carcinoma in Situ

AGE AT INITIAL LCIS (YEARS)	PATIENTS (n)	CANCER (n)	RELATIVE RISK (%)
<40	23	7	10.5
40–44	53	17	6.6
45–49	89	21	5.0
50–54	36	11	5.4
≥55	35	6	3.2
All patients	236	62	5.4

From Bodian CA, Perzin KH, Lattes R: Lobular neoplasia: Long-term risk of breast cancer and relation to other factors. Cancer 1996;78:1024–1034.

allowing for cancer-specific mortality. The subsequent malignancies may be either infiltrating lobular or ductal. There is proportionately a greater incidence of infiltrating lobular cancer (ILCA) identified following a diagnosis of LCIS than the 5% to 10% incidence of ILCA found in the general population. However, infiltrating ductal can-struction. Both breasts are considered a single field of risk and, therefore, unilateral mastectomy has no role. Patients at additional risk—such as those with genetic patterns of *BRCA1* and *BRCA2*, those unwilling to accept the 1% per year risk of developing a subsequent cancer, or those who will be unable to maintain a close surveillance—may choose this surgical option.

Data from the NSABP P-1 prevention trial included 826 women with LCIS. Over the median follow-up of approximately 55 months, a 56% reduction in the incidence of invasive breast cancer was noted among women taking tamoxifen, compared with those receiving placebo. This chemoprevention management strategy offers a therapeutic alternative that lies between the management extremes of observation and bilateral mastectomy.

Patients may be considered for randomization in the ongoing NSABP P-2 trial randomizing high-risk postmenopausal women, including patients with LCIS, to receive either tamoxifen or raloxifene as a chemopreventive agent.

Outcomes

Observational studies providing the longest follow-up have demonstrated up to a 7% lifetime cancer-specific mortality associated with observation alone. This is concomitant with the approximate 1% per year risk of developing a subsequent cancer. Newer studies, however, have indicated a substantially lower mortality. With the emergence of tamoxifen as a major potential component of observation, the incidence of mortality may be significantly altered. Bilateral prophylactic mastectomy reduces the risk of future breast cancer to 0 to 2% with negligible cancer-specific mortality but will overtreat the majority of women who would never progress to an invasive cancer.

SELECTED READINGS

Bodian CA, Perzin KH, Lattes R: Lobular neoplasia: Long-term risk of breast cancer and relation to other factors. Cancer 1996;78:1024.

Fisher B, Dignam J, Wolmark N, et al: Lumpectomy and radiation therapy for the treatment of intraductal breast cancer: Findings from National Surgical Adjuvant Breast and Bowel Project B-17. J Clin Oncol 1998;16:441.

Fisher B, Dignam J, Wolmark N, et al: Tamoxifen in treatment of intraductal breast cancer: National Surgical Adjuvant Breast and Bowel Project B-24 randomised controlled trial. Lancet 1999;353:1993.

Fisher ER, Dignam J, Tan-Chiu E, et al: Pathologic findings from the National Surgical Adjuvant Breast Project (NSABP) eight-year update of protocol B-17: Intraductal carcinoma. Cancer 1999;86:429.

Hiramatsu H, Bornstein BA, Recht A, et al: Local recurrence after conservative surgery and radiation therapy for ductal carcinoma in situ. Cancer J Sci Am 1995;1:55.

Holland PA, Gandhi A, Knox WF, et al: The importance of complete excision in the prevention of local recurrence of ductal carcinoma in situ. Br J Cancer 1998;77:110.

Hwang ES, Esserman LJ: Management of ductal carcinoma in situ. Surg Clin North Am 1999;79:1007.

Lagios MD: Ductal carcinoma in situ: Pathology and treatment. Surg Clin North Am 1990;70:853.

Newman LA, Kuerer HM, Hunt KK, et al: Presentation, treatment and outcome of local recurrence after skin sparing mastectomy and immediate breast reconstruction. Ann Surg Oncol 1998;5:620.

Silverstein MJ, Lagios MD, Groshen S, et al: The influence of margin width on local control of ductal carcinoma in situ of the breast. N Engl J Med 1999;340:1455.

Silverstein MJ, Lagios MD, Martino S, et al: Outcome after invasive local recurrence in patients with ductal carcinoma in situ of the breast. J Clin Oncol 1998;16:1367.

Silverstein MJ, Masetti R: Hypothesis and practice: Are there several types of treatment for ductal carcinoma in situ of the breast? Recent Results Cancer Res 1998;152:105.

Solin LJ, Kurtz J, Fourquet A, et al: Fifteen-year results of breast conserving surgery and definitive breast irradiation for the treatment of ductal carcinoma in situ of the breast. J Clin Oncol 1996;14:754.

Taghian AG, Powell SN: The role of radiation therapy for primary breast cancer. Surg Clin North Am 1999;79:1091.

Van Zee KJ, Liberman L, Samli B, et al: Long-term follow-up of women with ductal carcinoma in situ treated with breast-conserving surgery: The effect of age. Cancer 1999;86:1757.

Winchester DP, Strom EA: Standards for diagnosis and management of ductal carcinoma in situ (DCIS) of the breast. American College of Radiology, American College of Surgeons, College of American Pathologists, Society of Surgical Oncology. CA: Cancer J Clin 1998;48:108.

Chapter 151
Breast Carcinoma: Stages I and II

Scott R. Schell and Edward M. Copeland, III

During the past decade, the lifetime risk of breast cancer for American women has increased from less than 10% to over 12%, rendering it the most frequently diagnosed form of cancer for American women. While the frequency of breast cancer diagnoses has continued to rise during the past 20 years, the risk of death from breast cancer has remained relatively constant at approximately 3.6%. Invasive breast cancers represent a heterogeneous population of tumors, with the consequence that more than half of the patients with this diagnosis will survive their cancers, and die from other causes. Thus, while the absolute and relative incidence of breast cancer has risen, it appears that earlier diagnosis and surgical intervention, combined with effective chemotherapy and radiotherapy treatments may be responsible for maintaining the risk of death at constant levels.

Following the introduction and confirmation of the therapeutic efficacy of surgical techniques for breast conservation, application of this procedure to early breast cancers has risen dramatically. While some controversies remain regarding application of sentinel lymph node biopsy, extent of axillary dissection, and other issues related to postoperative radiotherapy, breast conservation surgery has become standardized, well accepted by surgeons, and highly sought after by patients.

This chapter reviews the current standards for diagnosis and treatment of stage I and II breast cancers and discusses the technical issues involving mastectomy and breast conservation surgery, problems and pitfalls dealing with the care of these patients, and current controversies regarding their management. Table 151–1 summarizes the TNM classifications defining stage I and II breast cancers, as well as crude 5-year survivals for patients with these diagnoses.

CLINICAL PRESENTATION

Numerous risk factors have been associated with an increased risk of breast cancer. These factors include family history in first-degree female relatives and, more recently, genetic history, especially as predicted by the BRCA cluster of genetic mutations. A previous history of benign or malignant breast disease, particularly with multiple previous biopsy procedures, is correlated with an increased risk of breast cancer. Finally, hormonal, dietary, and environmental factors have each been proposed as additional risk factors.

Most breast cancers are detected during physical examination by the patient's performing breast self-examination (BSE) or by the health care provider. BSE should be performed monthly, after the menses, beginning when the patient is in her early twenties. This allows the patient to learn the character and texture of her breasts, making her better able to detect changes. Unfortunately, physical examination is only 20% to 30% specific for the detection of suspicious breast lesions, and many lesions become palpable only when they exceed 2 cm. The application of annual screening mammography has increased the sensitivity and specificity of detecting lesions before they become palpable, and it is invaluable for detecting microcalcifications and other radiologic findings suspicious for malignancy. The current recommendations are that women undergo baseline mammograms at age 35, and annual mammograms beginning at age 40. Women with higher risks, as discussed earlier, may begin with baseline and annual screening mammograms at an earlier age, as dictated by their specific risk.

The majority of patients with stage I and II breast cancers have no lymph node metastases from their tumors. However, the risk of nodal metastases increases with the increasing size of the tumor, and this risk is summarized, stratified by tumor histologic subtype, in Table 151–2. Past surgical practice, as mandated by the super-radical mastectomy, included dissection and examination of the internal mammary lymph nodes. However, a number of studies have shown that this morbid procedure

Table 151–1	TNM Classification and 5-Year Survival for Stage I and II Breast Cancers				
STAGE	TUMOR	NODAL STATUS	METASTASES	5-YEAR SURVIVAL (%)
I	T1	N0		85
IIa	T0	N1		
	T1	N1	M0	
	T2	N0		66
IIb	T2	N1		
	T3	N0		

Primary tumor: T1 ≤2 cm; T2 2–5 cm; T3 ≥5 cm.
Regional lymph nodes: N0, No regional lymph node metastasis; N1, metastasis to moveable ipsilateral axillary lymph node.
Distant metastasis: M0, no distant metastasis.

Table 151–2	Incidence of Positive Lymph Nodes in T1 and T2 Breast Cancers					
STAGE	**TUBULAR**	**COLLOID**	**MEDULLARY**	**DUCTAL**	**LOBULAR**	**TOTAL**
T1a	3.1	1.5	24	8.6	10.0	8.3
b	4.6	2.2	24	14.0	13.1	13.3
c	13.7	5.1	25	28.5	23.7	27.2
T2	21.1	13.6	31	46.5	41.6	44.8

Percent positive per category.

From Winchester D, et al: National Cancer Data Bank, Commission on Cancer. Chicago, IL, American College of Surgeons, 1997. Presented at the Society for Surgical Oncology.

provides no clinical advantage for patients, and it has been abandoned. The role of careful pathologic examination of the axillary lymph nodes, however, remains clear, as the evaluation of these lymph nodes provides valuable prognostic information, dictating subsequent adjuvant chemotherapy and regional lymph node irradiation, and reducing the subsequent risk of disease recurrence in the axilla.

During the patient's initial clinical presentation, the authors' practice includes a comprehensive family and social history, complete medical history and review of symptoms, and meticulous physical examination of both breasts and axillae. The authors' review of the patient's history involves consideration of any past history of chest wall or axillary irradiation, as well as any history of scleroderma or similar connective tissue disorders that may impact on patient suitability for breast conservation or reconstruction. Patients with strong histories of early or pervasive breast or ovarian cancers in their siblings or relatives are referred to the authors' oncologic geneticists for evaluation for BRCA gene mutation testing for themselves, and possible testing of these other family members. In families with strong histories of breast and ovarian cancers, this genetic testing is most beneficial for identifying the patient's susceptible siblings and children. These other relatives, once identified as having the same genetic mutation, can be provided disease-specific counseling for close monitoring or prophylactic surgical treatment.

PREOPERATIVE MANAGEMENT

In the authors' practice, all patients with palpable breast lesions undergo bilateral mammography prior to surgical intervention. Preoperative bilateral mammography provides a baseline examination for subsequent follow-up, examines the affected breast for indications of multicentric disease and microcalcifications, and examines the contralateral breast. Outside mammograms are routinely reviewed by the surgical and radiology staff at the authors' institution. If the mammographer detects additional suspicious nonpalpable lesions or microcalcifications in either the ipsilateral or the contralateral breast, stereotactic core-needle biopsy of these lesions can often be accomplished at the same time as mammography, providing prompt tissue diagnosis. The addition of ultrasound to mammography has been very useful for characterization and biopsy of lesions difficult to visualize with the use of mammography alone, and allows for aspiration and pathologic evaluation of complex or recurrent cysts.

All patients in the authors' practice undergo core-needle or fine-needle aspiration (FNA) biopsies of palpable lesions prior to any other surgical intervention, typically as part of their initial clinical evaluation. Patients with small, or difficult to palpate, lesions and those with suspicious microcalcifications are scheduled to undergo either stereotactic core biopsy, or a needle-localized biopsy procedure, depending on the size and anatomic location of the lesion within the breast. Patients with skin or nipple changes suggestive of inflammatory breast cancer undergo punch-biopsy of the affected region, for pathologic review. Our pathology staff routinely reviews biopsy specimens obtained outside the authors' institution, providing confirmation of tumor diagnosis, histologic characteristics, and specimen margins.

Preoperative evaluation includes routine laboratory and radiology studies, including serum alkaline phosphatase measurement and chest radiograph. Preoperative chest and abdominal computed tomography scans are reserved for patients with symptoms that generate much concern, primary lesions approaching the upper limit of T3 size, or clinically positive axillary lymph node examination. Patients who present with a history of bone pain or elevated alkaline phosphatase also undergo preoperative bone scan.

The option of breast conservation is discussed with all patients preoperatively. Patients who have contraindications to breast conservation are those in whom lumpectomy cannot be performed with suitable margins of disease-free tissue, based on breast size or tumor location, and patients in whom the risk of recurrence is high because of multiple primary lesions or extensive ductal carcinoma in situ (DCIS), which impairs the surgeon's ability to obtain accurate negative margins with certainty. Relative contraindications to breast conservation include breasts that are difficult to evaluate mammographically or by physical examination, owing to significant fibrosis of the breast tissue or cosmetic implants. Cosmetic implants may also be a contraindication to breast conservation because of an inability to adequately field postoperative radiotherapy. The relative contraindications to breast conservation followed by the authors are summarized in Table 151–3.

During the past 5 years, numerous studies have qualified sentinel lymph node dissection (SLND) as an appropriate diagnostic tool for minimally invasive evaluation of the axillary lymph nodes in early-stage breast cancers. The authors' institution has experienced excellent results with the sensitivity, specificity, and safety of SLND in its

Table 151–3	**Contraindications to Breast Conservation**

Inability to achieve adequate disease-free margins due to breast size and tumor size or location

Multifocal disease, including invasive cancers, DCIS, and other high-risk lesions

Previous chest or axillary radiotherapy

Mammographically inapparent lesions

Breasts on which it is difficult to perform a physical examination or mammography

Breast tissue factors, including significant fibrosis, cosmetic implants, and connective tissue disorders

patients with breast cancers. This success relies on the surgical staff's having undergone a rigorous series of training and evaluation cycles, including performance of SLND on 30 patients who immediately underwent subsequent level I and II axillary dissection, before performing SLND as a definitive diagnostic procedure. Based on the authors' institutional experience, and review of the continuously forthcoming data on SLND, they believe that it is appropriate to routinely offer this procedure to all patients with T1a lesions, to patients with T1b lesions exhibiting favorable histologic markers, and to patients with extensive DCIS. The average incidence of axillary metastases in these patients is 10%. If the false-negative rate for SLND were to be 10%, then only 1 in 100 patients would have an incorrectly staged axilla.

Patients who elect treatment with modified radical mastectomy (MRM), or who are not candidates for breast conservation, are offered the option of immediate reconstruction following mastectomy, unless they are candidates for postoperative radiotherapy. The authors' institution favors the use of a transverse rectus abdominis myocutaneous (TRAM) flap or lattissimus dorsi reconstruction, based on the superior cosmetic results obtained after reconstruction, and for carefully selected tumors its staff perform a skin-sparing mastectomy to accommodate the mobilized flap. Postoperative chemotherapy and radiotherapy have been shown to increase survival for patients with lymph node metastases. Thus, the authors prefer to delay reconstruction until radiotherapy is completed, rather than to irradiate reconstructed tissue.

INTRAOPERATIVE MANAGEMENT

Patients undergoing either mastectomy or breast conservation with axillary lymph node dissection (ALND) are prepped to include the ipsilateral arm. This allows abduction of the arm across the chest wall for easy movement of the chest wall muscles to expose the axillary contents for optimal exposure and minimal risk of injury to contained neurovascular structures.

Lumpectomy

The authors' approach to lumpectomy is based first on sound oncologic principles, and second on the desire to provide optimal cosmetic results. Curvilinear incisions,

placed along the Langer lines immediately overlying lesions, are used in the breast quadrants (Fig. 151–1), although radial incisions are also acceptable. Previous biopsy scars are excised as part of the lumpectomy incision, and great care is taken to avoid development of large skin flaps or tangential tunneling toward the lesions. All specimens are excised, along with surrounding normal breast tissue measuring approximately 20% of the tumor diameter. Lesions with significant associated calcifications are excised with more generous margins, owing to the multifocal nature of DCIS. Small and difficult to palpate lesions are excised following needle localization in mammography, and the specimens from these lesions as well as any associated microcalcifications undergo specimen radiography to confirm the presence of the lesion or calcifications of interest following removal.

Following excision, the authors prefer either to mark the specimen using suture or to ink the specimen while the patient is in the operating room to provide the pathologist with proper orientation of the specimen for accurate margin determination. A suggested marking and inking algorithm is listed in Figure 151–2. Additional tissue margins obtained from the borders of the biopsy cavity may be helpful in ascertaining disease-free margins, can be quickly examined using frozen section while the patient is in the operating room, and do not require dissection of the principal specimen. If all borders of the biopsy cavity are examined by this method, pathologic evaluation of the resection specimen during the biopsy procedure is unnecessary. Personally reviewing and orienting the gross specimen with the pathologist prior to dissection and fixation is the best method of addressing irregularly shaped and unusually situated lesions, and will often obviate any confusion regarding orientation and margins.

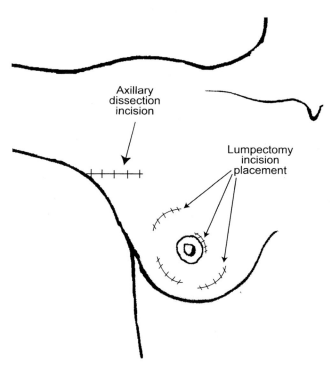

Figure 151–1. Incision location for breast conservation surgery and axillary dissection.

Specimen Marking

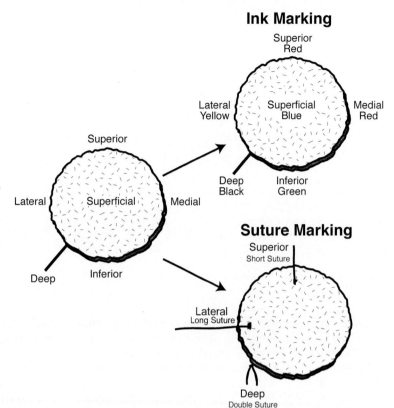

Figure 151–2. Marking algorithm for breast conservation pathology specimens.

Following excision, the biopsy cavity is carefully inspected to ensure perfect hemostasis, and copiously irrigated to remove any fragments of fat or tissue. Small titanium hemoclips are useful for marking the margins of the biopsy cavity as a guide for radiotherapists to direct postoperative radiotherapy. The authors routinely obliterate the biopsy cavity using interrupted absorbable sutures, as they find that this provides superior cosmesis and hemostasis. However, if closing the deep tissues compromises cosmesis, only the subcutaneous tissues and skin are closed. The biopsy cavity is not drained routinely.

Axillary Lymph Node Dissection

Patients with clinically negative axillary lymph nodes undergo level I and II lymph node dissection. Axillary anatomy is depicted in Figure 151–3. Level III lymph nodes are not included in this dissection, based on the very low risk, 0.5% to 3% in most studies, of skip lymph node metastases beyond negative level I and II nodes. If pathologically positive lymph nodes are encountered during the level I and II axillary dissection, level III lymph nodes should be dissected only if they are positive. If, however, the level III lymph nodes are clinically negative, they are not dissected, as complete (ALND) increases the risk of ipsilateral arm lymphedema. Additionally, radiotherapy to the axilla may subsequently be indicated, and the level III lymph nodes may be included in the radiation field. Complete axillary dissection combined with axillary radio-

therapy triples the incidence of arm lymphedema, and leaving the level III lymph nodes undisturbed in these patients greatly reduces this risk.

Dissection is ideally completed sharply, with care taken to ligate all vessels and lymphatics. Electrocautery dissection is minimized in order to avoid injury to adjacent nerves, and to minimize the risk of postoperative lymph leak and seroma. Meticulous care is taken to identify the long thoracic, thoracodorsal, and intercostobrachial nerves and carefully protect these from the field of dissection. In the situation in which it is necessary to sacrifice any of the lateral cutaneous nerves for complete axillary dissection, preinjection of the nerve sheath with local anesthetic prior to division has been shown in some studies to decrease the risk of the neurapraxia and chronic pain syndromes that occasionally result.

Following axillary dissection, copious irrigation and meticulous attention to hemostasis precede placement of a single large-bore closed-suction drain, and closure of the wound in layers.

Sentinel Lymph Node Dissection

The authors perform SLND using technetium sulfurcolloid alone. The injection of blue dye added to the authors' SLND technique has not improved their ability to identify the sentinel lymph node, and thus it is not included routinely. The authors' practice includes preoperative lymphoscintigraphy to identify the lymph node

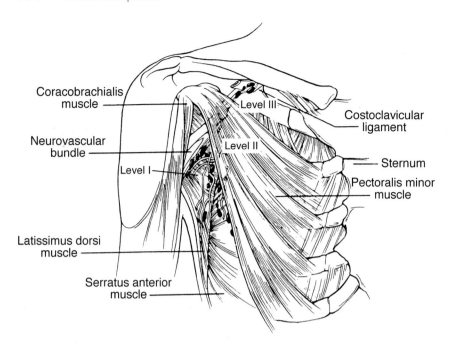

Coracobrachialis muscle

Level III

Neurovascular bundle

Level II

Level I

Costoclavicular ligament

Sternum

Pectoralis minor muscle

Latissimus dorsi muscle

Serratus anterior muscle

Figure 151–3. Axillary anatomy and landmarks. (From Bland KI, Copeland EM III [eds]: The Breast: Comprehensive Management of Benign and Malignant Diseases. Philadelphia, WB Saunders, 1991, p 574.)

number and drainage pattern, following subdermal radiotracer injection overlying the lesion or previous biopsy site. Lymphoscintigraphy is equally effective when it is performed the day prior to, or on the morning of, surgery, and at the time of this procedure the radiologist marks the skin overlying the sentinel lymph node or nodes in the x and y axes. The authors find lymphoscintigraphy very useful for mapping the drainage pattern of the sentinel lymph node or nodes, especially when a sentinel lymph node is positive for tumor only by immunohistochemical (IHC) staining. In this situation, if the only IHC-positive lymph node is the first in a chain of lymph nodes identified during lymphoscintigraphy, completion ALND for these patients may possibly be unnecessary.

Dissection begins with an incision placed in the usual position for full axillary dissection (see Fig. 151–1). Careful palpation is done to exclude the presence of clinically positive lymph nodes. The Gamma probe is oriented to minimize readings from the injection site, and a background count level is ascertained. The sentinel lymph node is judged to be the lymph node or nodes with counts at least 10-fold above background. If no sentinel lymph node can be identified, the patient undergoes standard level I and II axillary dissection, as described previously. After the sentinel lymph node is identified, it is carefully dissected free from the surrounding tissue, with the use of the same meticulous technique described earlier for full axillary dissection. Following removal, the remainder of the axilla should return only background levels of counts, while the removed lymph node continues to emit readings between 8- and 10-fold over background. If additional "hot" lymph nodes are identified, they are removed and are submitted in decreasing order of radioactivity.

Following identification and removal of the sentinel lymph node, frozen-section pathologic examination of the sentinel lymph node or nodes is undertaken to determine the presence of any metastases. If no metastases are found, the node or nodes are submitted for serial thin sectioning and examination using both traditional hematoxylin and eosin (H&E) microscopy, and staining for cytokeratin to examine for micrometastases. If metastases are found on light microscopy during frozen section, or subsequent serial sectioning of the permanent sections, the patient undergoes standard level I and II axillary dissection as described previously.

Following completion of SLND, meticulous hemostasis and copious irrigation are obtained. Closed-suction drains are placed only if the dissection involved in identifying and removing the sentinel lymph node or nodes has been extensive. The majority of patients who undergo SNLD are treated as outpatients and are discharged home on the day of surgery.

The number of sentinel lymph node biopsies combined with axillary dissection required for demonstrating proficiency in SLND is dependent on the combined expertise of the surgeon, nuclear medicine physician, and pathologist making up the team who perform this procedure. At least 20 combined procedures should be completed prior to relying on the sentinel lymph node to accurately reflect the pathology of the remaining axillary lymph nodes.

Modified Radical Mastectomy

The purpose of MRM is to remove virtually all of the breast tissue, including the breast mound, nipple-areola complex, and the axillary tail of Spence, and to perform dissection of level I and II lymph nodes. Modified radical mastectomy is performed through an elliptical incision, which is oriented to include the nipple and areola and any previous biopsy scar (Fig. 151–4). If the skin overlying the lesion is tethered, the incision must include this skin, with a margin large enough to remove the dermal lymphatics that may be grossly infiltrated with tumor. Also, postoperative radiotherapy to at least the skin flaps should

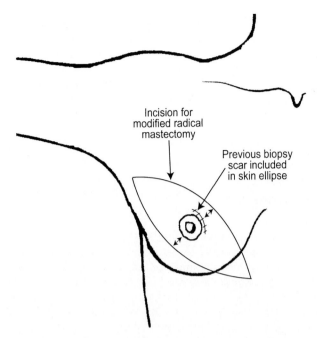

Figure 151–4. Incision design and location for MRM.

Incision for
modified radical
mastectomy

Previous biopsy
scar included
in skin ellipse

be considered in these patients to eliminate any residual microscopic disease remaining in the flaps.

The margins needed for MRM range from the inferior border of the clavicle superiorly to the inframammary crease inferiorly, lateral sternal border medially to include the entire axillary tail of Spence with an adequate margin of fat laterally, and Camper's fascia superficially to the pectoralis major fascia at the deep layer. Skin flaps are fashioned to remove the breast tissue, but not to devascularize the skin flaps, and these flaps can be accomplished by dissecting the plane immediately superficial to Camper's fascia. Sharp dissection is preferred, but electrocautery dissection is acceptable if one recognizes the potential hazards associated with thrombosis of the dermal vasculature. Following MRM, large-bore closed-suction drains are placed beneath the mastectomy flaps, and in the axilla. During dissection, the authors meticulously attempt to avoid entry into any previous biopsy cavity owing to the theoretical risk of tumor cell spillage into the mastectomy wound from this cavity.

The basis of these extensive margins is to reduce the risk of local recurrence, which is particularly important in patients with multifocal invasive cancer or DCIS. During the past 20 years, attention at the authors' institution to maximal excision of all identified breast tissue, combined with the application of postoperative radiotherapy, has yielded a 10-year actuarial local control rate of 96% for stage I lesions, and 95% for stage II lesions.

Patients who are candidates for immediate reconstruction who do not have peripherally located biopsy scars or involvement of skin overlying their lesions are candidates for a skin-sparing mastectomy. Dissection begins with liberal infiltration of the subcutaneous tissues with dilute local anesthetic, as this allows for easier separation of the breast tissue from Camper's fascia. A circumareolar incision is created, and flaps are developed radially outward from this incision with the use of sharp dissection.

Centrally located biopsy scars are incorporated into this radial extension. As the operation continues, the full extent of dissection proposed previously for MRM can be achieved by retracting the skin flaps toward the margin of interest. After the breast is reflected off the pectoralis major fascia, the axillary dissection may be completed through this incision, or via a separately placed incision in the axilla. Following dissection, the appropriate reconstruction can be completed, with the use of the newly created skin flaps, and nipple reconstruction may possibly be completed during the same operation.

Patients who are unable to undergo autologous tissue reconstruction, owing to previous abdominal surgery, or other factors, may have immediate reconstruction using saline implants, through standard or skin-sparing approaches, with acceptable cosmetic results as well.

Postoperative Management

Axillary and mastectomy flap drains are left in place until drainage is 20 mL or less daily, or for a maximum of 10 days, whichever comes first. Any evidence of infection surrounding a drain insertion site is an indication for early removal. Prior to discharge, patients and their families are instructed in the management of their drains, and provided a chart for recording drain output for review on their first postoperative clinic visit.

After operation, patients undergoing ALND, as part of breast conservation or MRM, are instructed in a regimen of arm and shoulder exercises. Patients who demonstrate proficiency in these exercises seldom need formal physical therapy. Early arm and shoulder mobilization has been very helpful in minimizing postoperative pain and range-of-motion limitations. Seromas occur in as many as 25% of patients, and require subsequent aspiration.

Most patients remain in the hospital overnight as "23-hour" stay patients, and are discharged the morning after surgery. Older patients who require MRM may stay for up to 48 hours postoperatively. Patients treated with SLND, who do not require formal axillary dissection, may be discharged on the day of surgery.

Following treatment, breast cancer patients at the authors' institution are presented in a weekly multidisciplinary breast cancer conference. Patient presentation includes a comprehensive review of the clinical history, imaging studies, pathologic review of all surgical specimens, and a detailed discussion of relevant operative findings. The surgical, radiology, pathology, medical, and radiation oncology staff then formulates a comprehensive plan for subsequent additional metastatic evaluation, chemotherapy, and radiotherapy. Patients are referred for adjuvant therapy immediately on removal of their drains. Hormonal therapy recommendations are based on hormone receptor status, age, and the patient's reproductive plans.

COMPLICATIONS

Complications observed following treatment of stage I and II breast cancers relate principally to complications arising from axillary dissection, the most common of

Table 151–4	Patient-Reported Complications Following Axillary Dissection	
SYMPTOM		**FREQUENCY (%)**
Pain		50
Swelling		38
Numbness		34
Decreased motor function		17

From Lind, D.S., Department of Surgery, University of Florida, 1998.

which are lymphedema, chronic pain and neurapraxia, and seroma formation. The frequency of morbidity following axillary dissection is proportional to the extent of dissection and the addition of postoperative radiotherapy. Table 151–4 summarizes the patient-reported complications following axillary dissection at our institution.

Lymphedema

In the past, radical dissection of axillary levels I, II, and III was associated with a risk of permanent lymphedema approaching 30%. With more moderate axillary dissections, this risk has fallen to approximately 5% in most large series. Patients who develop lymphedema often have mild arm swelling that is not debilitating. However, some patients develop severe lymphedema requiring upper-extremity compression stockings and other interventions for control. Predicting which patients are likely to develop significant postoperative lymphedema is difficult.

Neurapraxia

Injuries to the lateral cutaneous, intercostobrachial, long thoracic, and thoracodorsal nerves may occur following axillary dissection. Most injuries to the long thoracic and thoracodorsal nerves are avoidable by meticulous dissection, clear identification of these structures, and avoidance of electrocautery.

Many women experience a small area of numbness or paresthesia on the medial upper arm following axillary dissection, resulting from injury to or division of the cutaneous nerves. In most cases, these symptoms become less noticeable in the weeks and months following surgery.

Arm and shoulder pain may result from injury to the intercostobrachial nerves, but it is more likely secondary to the failure to obtain full range of motion of the shoulder via appropriate postoperative exercises. These symptoms may become quite debilitating, and require evaluation and treatment by physical and occupational therapists, or pain specialists. The authors follow our postoperative patients carefully, to ensure that they are progressing properly with range-of-motion exercises.

Seroma

Seroma represents a potentially serious complication, as it may delay the start of postoperative radiotherapy. The authors practice is to remove mastectomy flap and axillary

drains when total drain volumes are below 20 mL daily. Occasionally, after drain removal, patients will reaccumulate fluid beneath their mastectomy flaps or in their axillae. If this occurs, the fluid collection is aspirated in the clinic, and followed for 2 weeks. If the fluid collection cannot be eliminated by frequent aspirations, a drain is reinserted to resolve the problem. Patients who begin radiotherapy with a seroma present are at risk for a fibrosis of the cavity surrounding the seroma, preventing future resorption.

OUTCOMES

Patient survivals following both MRM or breast conservation for stage I and II breast cancers have been reported in numerous previous studies. Comparison of disease-free survival and overall survival from NSABP B06, with data stratified to 12 years, in patients treated with MRM or breast conservation and radiotherapy confirms equivalent survivals with these two treatments.

Pearls and Pitfalls

PEARLS

- Breast conservation can be offered to most patients.
- Immediate reconstruction following MRM, particularly utilizing TRAM and skin-sparing mastectomy, provides superb cosmetic results and should be considered when it does not impair postoperative radiotherapy.
- SLND is evolving as an accurate technique for minimally invasive axillary lymph node biopsy. However, the technique must be applied by surgeons with significant experience and success with the technique.
- Early arm mobilization is important for reducing postoperative pain, and improving range of motion of the arm.

PITFALLS

- Failure to radically remove all identifiable breast tissue during MRM.
- Failure to adequately excise biopsy scars or involved skin overlying lesions to ensure negative margins during breast conservation therapy.
- Incomplete or inaccurate marking of breast conservation specimens that interferes with the accurate determination of margin by the pathologist.
- Failure to identify long thoracic, thoracodorsal, and intercostobrachial nerves during ALND.
- Failure to aggressively drain axillary seromas following ALND.
- Inadequate lymph node sampling during level I and II axillary dissection.

Anatomic Considerations

PEARLS

- Anatomic margins of MRM.
- Anatomy of axilla during ALND and SLND.
- Adequate margins during breast conservation.

Indications and Timing of Adjuvant Therapy

There are two principal uses for adjuvant radiation therapy. *First,* radiotherapy is indicated in virtually all patients who undergo breast conservation, and in patients undergoing MRM who predictably may have disease left behind on the chest wall following operation. Examples are patients who have large hematomas after a biopsy procedure, and residual disease in their mastectomy specimen. The hematoma may be contaminated with breast cancer cells, increasing the risk of residual disease left behind in the skin flaps, since usually it is not possible to remove all residual ecchymosis with the specimen. *Second,* patients with medial primary lesions and positive axillary lymph nodes benefit from postoperative radiotherapy that includes the internal mammary chain.

Chemotherapy is valuable when cancer cells predictably have spread to areas outside the operative field. The size of the lesion (>1 cm), its pathologic characteristics (nuclear grade and differentiation), biologic markers (estrogen and progesterone receptors, *her2-neu* oncogene expression, S-phase, and ploidy), and patient age are important in determining candidacy for chemotherapy in axillary node–negative patients. Positive axillary nodes take precedence over all other tumor characteristics as an indication for chemotherapy. Hormonal therapy is based on hormone receptor activity and the need for prophylaxis for the opposite breast.

The sequencing of adjuvant therapy is important, since some chemotherapeutic agents, including Adriamycin (doxorubicin HCl), sensitize the skin to radiation, and these combinations can result in a severe burn to the chest wall. As a rule, if the implication of distant metastases outweighs the implications for local recurrence, chemotherapy is given first. For example, in a patient who undergoes breast conservation and is found to have positive lymph nodes, radiation therapy to the intact breast is often delayed until chemotherapy is begun.

SELECTED READINGS

Axelson CK, Mouridsen HT, Zedeler K, et al: Axillary dissection of level I and II lymph nodes is important in breast cancer classification. The Danish Breast Cancer Cooperative Group (DBCG). Eur J Cancer 1992;28A:1415.

Fisher B, Anderson S, Redmond CK, et al: Reanalysis and results after 12 years of follow-up in a randomized clinical trial comparing total mastectomy with lumpectomy with or without irradiation in the treatment of breast cancer. N Engl J Med 1995;333:1455.

Fowble B: The significance of resection margin status in patients with early-stage invasive cancer treated with breast-conservation therapy. Breast J 1998;4:126.

Guiliano AE, Kirgan DM, Guenther JM, et al: Lymphatic mapping and sentinel lymphadenectomy for breast cancer. Ann Surg 1994;220:391.

Harris JR, Connolly JL, Schnitt SJ, et al: The use of pathologic features in selecting the extent of surgical resection necessary for breast cancer patients treated by primary radiation therapy. Ann Surg 1998;201:164.

Krag D, Weaver D, Ashikaga T, et al: The sentinel node in breast cancer: A multicenter validation study. N Engl J Med 1998;339:941.

Orr RK: The impact of prophylactic axillary node dissection on breast cancer survival: A Bayesian meta-analysis. Ann Surg Oncol 1999;6:109.

Overgaard M, Hansen PS, Overgaard J, et al: Post-operative radiotherapy in high-risk premenopausal women with breast cancer who receive adjuvant chemotherapy. N Engl J Med 1997;337:949.

Recht A, Come SE, Henderson C, et al: The sequencing of chemotherapy and radiation therapy after conservative surgery for early-state breast cancer. N Engl J Med 1995;334:1356.

Recht A, Houlihan MJ: Axillary lymph nodes and breast cancer. Cancer 1995;76:1491.

Turne RR, Ollila DW, Krasne DL, Guiliano AE: Histopathic validation of the sentinel lymph node hypothesis for breast carcinoma. Ann Surg 1997;226:271.

White RE, Vezeridis MP, Konstadoulakis M, et al: Therapeutic options and results for the management of minimally invasive carcinoma of the breast: Influence of axillary dissection for treatment of T1a and T1b lesions. J Am Coll Surg 1996;183:575.

Chapter 152

Advanced Breast Carcinoma (Stages IIIa and IIIb)

Samuel W. Beenken, Marshall M. Urist, and Kirby I. Bland

Patients with stage IIIa and stage IIIb breast carcinoma have advanced local and/or regional disease, but have no clinically detected distant metastases. Surgery plays a crucial role in the treatment of such disease. It is the quickest and most effective single treatment modality for establishing local and regional disease control. There are, however, significant limitations to the long-term efficacy of surgery alone in this setting. It fails to treat the distant micrometastases that are present in almost all patients and also fails locally in a significant number of those patients who survive for 2 or more years following surgery.

In an effort to improve local and regional disease-free survival, as well as distant disease-free survival, in stage IIIa and IIIb breast carcinoma, surgery has been integrated with radiotherapy, chemotherapy, and hormonal therapy. For operable disease, primary (neoadjuvant) chemotherapy can reduce the size of the primary cancer and permit conservation surgery. For inoperable disease, neoadjuvant chemotherapy can decrease the local and regional tumor burden and permit subsequent surgery to establish local and regional control of disease. Postoperative (adjuvant) chemotherapy is used to maximize distant disease-free survival. To maximize local and regional disease-free survivals, adjuvant external-beam radiotherapy is applied to the supraclavicular lymph nodes and chest wall following modified radical mastectomy, or to the supraclavicular lymph nodes and breast when neoadjuvant chemotherapy permits conservation surgery. Figure 152–1 summarizes current treatment recommendations.

CLINICAL PRESENTATION

Haagensen's "grave signs" concerning the clinical presentation of breast carcinoma included edema of the skin of the breast, skin ulceration, chest wall fixation, an axillary lymph node greater than 2.5 cm in diameter, and fixed axillary lymph nodes (Haagensen and Stout, 1943). Patients with two or more signs had a 42% local recurrence rate and a 2% 5-year disease-free survival. Today, these grave signs have been incorporated into the American Joint Committee for Cancer (AJCC) TNM staging system for breast cancer. Stage groupings are summarized in Table 152–1. Stage IIIa breast carcinoma includes (1) primary cancers that are 5 cm or larger with associated ipsilateral axillary lymph node metastases and (2) primary cancers of any size (or undetectable) with associated ipsilateral axillary lymph node metastases that are fixed to one another or to surrounding structures. Stage IIIb breast carcinoma includes (1) primary cancers that extend directly to the chest wall or skin (edema, ulceration, satellite

skin nodules) with associated axillary or internal mammary lymph node metastases, (2) inflammatory breast carcinoma, and (3) any primary cancer with associated internal mammary lymph node metastases.

Denial on the part of a patient can result in the late presentation of a primary breast cancer. Occasionally, a woman with large pendulous breasts will be unaware of an enlarging cancer. Eventually, however, the cancer will distort, infiltrate, or ulcerate the overlying skin. In the absence of an obvious primary breast cancer, axillary lymphadenopathy may be recognized late in the course of disease. While axillary lymph node metastases usually present as a mobile mass or vague fullness in the axilla, undetected disease may present with pain, decreased range of motion in the shoulder, or the new onset of arm edema. The isolated clinical presentation of internal mammary lymphadenopathy is rare, but enlarged internal mammary lymph nodes can present as a painless, subcutaneous parasternal mass with or without skin involvement.

Inflammatory Breast Carcinoma

Inflammatory breast carcinoma is a clinicopathologic entity characterized by diffuse brawny induration and the presence of erythema and edema (peau d'orange) of the skin of the breast with a raised edge reminiscent of erysipelas. There may or may not be an associated breast mass. Dermal lymphatic invasion can be seen in skin biopsy tissues. The clinical differentiation of inflammatory breast carcinoma from noninflammatory advanced breast cancer can be extremely difficult. Table 152–2 summarizes the differences. Inflammatory breast carcinoma can also be mistaken for a bacterial infection of the breast, but mastitis and abscess are usually seen only in lactating breasts. In addition, inflammatory breast carcinoma is very infrequently associated with fever and leucocytosis.

PREOPERATIVE MANAGEMENT

Work-Up

All patients with a suspicious palpable breast mass require a thorough physical examination (especially the ipsilateral axillary and supraclavicular lymph nodes and the contralateral breast), bilateral mammography, and fine-needle or core biopsy. A suspicious axillary mass requires a thorough physical examination (especially the ipsilateral breast and supraclavicular lymph nodes) and fine-needle or core biopsy. If metastatic disease in an axillary lymph node is found that is consistent with a breast primary carcinoma,

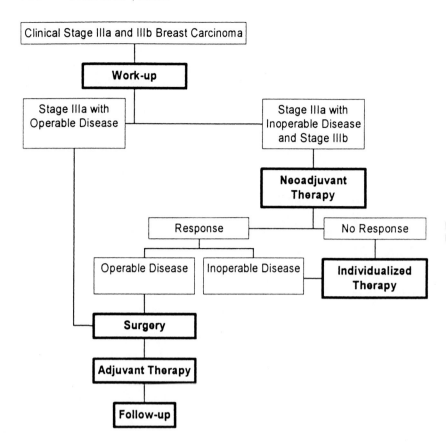

Figure 152–1. Treatment pathways for stage IIIa and stage IIIb breast carcinoma.

bilateral mammography is indicated. In this setting, stereotactic or ultrasound-guided breast biopsy may be indicated. The importance of thorough and competent pathology review of all biopsy specimens cannot be overemphasized.

Almost all patients with stage IIIa and IIIb breast carcinoma have macroscopic or microscopic distant metastatic disease, and a search for these metastases is an important part of the preoperative evaluation. This includes chest radiograph, complete blood count (CBC), and liver function studies. Most surgeons include abdominal ultrasound, computed tomography (CT), or magnetic resonance imaging (MRI) and a bone scan in their evaluation. Tumor estrogen and progesterone receptor status also provides information critical to the development of an appropriate treatment strategy.

Neoadjuvant Chemotherapy

In the early 1970s, systemic chemotherapy became an integral part of the strategy for the management of locally

| Table 152–1 | American Joint Committee on Cancer (AJCC) Staging for Breast Cancer* |

STAGE GROUPING			
0	Tis	N0	M0
I	T1	N0	M0
IIa	T0	N1	M0
	T1	N1	M0
	T2	N0	M0
IIb	T2	N1	M0
	T3	N0	M0
IIIa	T0	N2	M0
	T1	N2	M0
	T2	N2	M0
	T3	N1	M0
	T3	N2	M0
IIIb	T4	Any N	M0
	Any T	N3	M0
IV	Any T	Any N	M1

*American Joint Committee on Cancer: Manual for Staging of Cancer, 5th ed. Philadelphia, Lippincott-Raven, 1997.

| Table 152–2 | Characteristics of Inflammatory Breast Cancer |

INFLAMMATORY	NONINFLAMMATORY
Dermal lymphatic invasion is present with or without inflammatory changes.	Inflammatory changes are present without dermal lymphatic invasion.
Tumor is not sharply delineated.	Tumor is better delineated.
Erythema and edema frequently involve more than one third of the skin over the breast.	Erythema is usually confined to the lesion, and edema is less extensive.
Extensive lymph node involvement is usually present.	Lymph nodes are involved in about 50% of the cases.
Distant metastases are more common at initial presentation.	Distant metastases are less common at presentation.

Adapted from Chitloor SR, Swain SM: Locally advanced breast cancer: Role of medical oncology. In Bland KI, Copeland EM (eds): The Breast: Comprehensive Management of Benign and Malignant Diseases. Philadelphia, W.B. Saunders, 1998.

advanced breast carcinoma. During that period, The National Cancer Institute in Milan, Italy, initiated two prospective, randomized, multimodality clinical trials for patients with T3b or T4 breast carcinoma. Both trials incorporated repeated cycles of combination chemotherapy (doxorubicin and vincristine) as initial treatment. In the first trial (1974), patients also received radiotherapy as part of the initial treatment and then were randomized to (1) no treatment or (2) additional chemotherapy, if they showed no evidence of residual disease (complete response; DeLena et al, 1978). Chemotherapy alone produced some response in 89% of patients. The addition of radiotherapy produced a complete response in 83% of these patients. In the second trial (1975), after initial combination chemotherapy, patients were randomized to radiotherapy or surgery (radical or modified radical mastectomy). After these treatments, the patients then received additional combination chemotherapy (Valagussa et al, 1983). The best results were achieved when surgery was interposed between chemotherapy courses, with 82% complete local control and a 25% 5-year disease-free survival.

Noninflammatory Breast Carcinoma

The National Surgical Adjuvant Breast and Bowel Project (NSABP) has evaluated the role of neoadjuvant chemotherapy in women with operable breast carcinoma (B-18). Patients entered into this study were randomized to surgery followed by chemotherapy or primary chemotherapy followed by surgery. There was no significant difference in estimated 5-year disease-free survival among patients in either group (Fisher et al, 1990). Before randomization, lumpectomy was proposed for 3% of women with tumors larger than 5.0 cm. After neoadjuvant chemotherapy, there was a 175% increase in lumpectomies performed in that group of women. It was suggested that neoadjuvant chemotherapy be considered for the initial management of breast tumors judged too large for lumpectomy.

Current recommendations for inoperable stage IIIa disease and for noninflammatory stage IIIb disease are neoadjuvant chemotherapy with an anthracycline-containing regimen (i.e., doxorubicin), followed by a modified radical mastectomy if possible, followed by adjuvant radiotherapy, followed by additional chemotherapy (National Comprehensive Cancer Network). Some oncologists recommend that tamoxifen be added to the neoadjuvant therapy regimen, especially for patients with estrogen receptor–positive tumors.

Inflammatory Breast Carcinoma

Surgery alone and surgery with adjuvant radiotherapy have produced disappointing results in patients with inflammatory breast carcinoma. Current treatment recommendations for inflammatory breast carcinoma are neoadjuvant chemotherapy with an anthracycline-containing regimen (i.e., doxorubicin), followed by a modified radical mastectomy if possible, followed by adjuvant radiother-

apy, followed by additional chemotherapy (National Comprehensive Cancer Network).

INTRAOPERATIVE MANAGEMENT

The role of radical surgery in advanced breast carcinoma has historically been a matter of considerable controversy. Based on a review of breast cancer patients treated with radical mastectomy, Haagensen and Stout recognized that patient's with "grave signs" were beyond cure by radical surgery. Patey advocated a modified radical mastectomy for the management of breast carcinoma, explaining, "Until an effective general agent for treatment of carcinoma of the breast is developed, a high proportion of cases are doomed to die . . ." (Patey and Dyson, 1967). Maddox, in his analysis of findings from the Alabama Breast Cancer Project, found that stage III patients treated with modified radical mastectomy accounted for 6% of the total study population, but 20% of the total local recurrences, while stage III patients treated with radical mastectomy accounted for 5% of the total study population and only 6% of the total local recurrences (Maddox et al, 1987). Today, stage IIIa patients are divided into those who have operable disease and those who have inoperable disease (see Fig. 152–1). Current treatment recommendations for patients with operable stage IIIa disease are surgery, usually a modified radical mastectomy, followed by adjuvant chemotherapy with an anthracycline-containing regimen (i.e., doxorubicin), followed by radiotherapy (National Comprehensive Cancer Network).

Ablative Surgery

Modified Radical Mastectomy

The most commonly performed procedure for stage IIIa and stage IIIb breast carcinoma is the modified radical mastectomy. The limits of the resection are delineated *laterally* by the inferior margin of the latissimus dorsi muscle, *medially* by the midline of the sternum, *superiorly* by the subclavius muscle, and *inferiorly* by the caudal extension of the breast inferior to the inframammary fold (Bland et al, 1998). Skin flap thickness varies with patient habitus; but, ideally, flap thickness should be 7 to 8 mm, inclusive of skin and tela subcutanea. Once the skin flaps are fully developed, the pectoralis major fascia and overlying breast tissue are elevated off the underlying pectoralis musculature.

An axillary dissection is then performed. The loose areolar tissue of the lateral axillary space is elevated with identification of the lateral-most extent of the axillary vein. The vein is sharply exposed on its anterior and ventral surfaces in a lateral-to-medial direction. Caudal to the vein, the loose areolar tissue at the juncture of the axillary vein with the anterior margin of the latissimus dorsi is swept inferomedially to include the *lateral and subscapular nodal groups (level I)* of the axilla. Care is taken to preserve the thoracodorsal neurovascular bundle, which is fully invested with the loose areolar tissue and nodes of the lateral group. The dissection then continues medially, with extirpation of the *central nodal group (level*

2). The long thoracic nerve (respiratory nerve of Bell) is identified and preserved as it travels in the deep investing (serratus) fascia of the axillary space along the lateral chest wall. If there is palpable lymphadenopathy in the *apical (subclavicular) nodal group (level 3)*, the tendinous portion of the pectoralis minor muscle is divided near its insertion on the coracoid process (Patey procedure), allowing dissection of the axillary vein medially to the costoclavicular (Halsted's) ligament. Finally, the breast and axillary contents are removed from the wound as one specimen and sent to pathology.

Halsted Radical Mastectomy

The Halsted radical mastectomy, which originated in 1882 at the Roosevelt Hospital in New York City and was popularized at Johns Hopkins Hospital in Baltimore, entailed en bloc resection of the breast with the pectoralis major and pectoralis minor muscles and the regional lymphatics. The intervening century has seen the integration of radiotherapy, chemotherapy, hormonal therapy, and surgery into multimodality treatment strategies for breast carcinoma, resulting in the utilization of less radical surgical procedures. However, in patients with disease that is refractory to chemotherapy, but with no evidence of distant metastases, a radical procedure may be necessary for achieving local and regional control of disease. If required, the procedure can be extended to include resection of a portion of the bony chest wall.

Reconstructive Surgery

The goals of reconstructive surgery following ablative surgery for stage IIIa and IIIb breast carcinoma are (1) wound closure and (2) breast reconstruction. Immediate breast reconstruction is not recommended for this group of patients. Instead, breast reconstruction is delayed until the patient has successfully completed adjuvant therapy and has been free from local and regional recurrence of disease for 3 to 6 months.

In many patients, removal of local and regional disease can be accomplished with a modified radical mastectomy and primary approximation of the wound edges. However, when skin invasion or fixation to the chest wall is present, a more radical ablative procedure may be necessary. If the resultant defect involves only skin and subcutaneous tissue, a skin graft provides functional coverage that will tolerate postoperative radiotherapy. More extensive soft tissue defects are best reconstructed with myocutaneous flaps (Bostwick et al, 1978). Many different types of flaps can be used, but the latissimus dorsi and the rectus abdominis myocutaneous flaps are most commonly employed.

The latissimus dorsi myocutaneous flap consists of a skin paddle based on the underlying latissimus dorsi muscle and is supplied by the thoracodorsal artery with contributions from the posterior intercostal arteries. The TRAM (transverse rectus abdominis myocutaneous) flap consists of a skin paddle based on the underlying rectus abdominis muscle and is supplied by vessels from the deep inferior epigastric artery. The free TRAM flap uses microvascular

anastomoses to establish blood supply to the flap (Grotting et al, 1989).

When surgery for stage IIIa or IIIb breast carcinoma requires resection of one or two ribs, reconstruction of the bony defect is usually not necessary. If good flap coverage is provided, sufficient scar tissue will form to stabilize the chest wall. If more than two ribs are sacrificed, it is advisable to stabilize the chest wall with Marlex mesh, which is completely covered externally with viable tissue utilizing a latissimus dorsi or TRAM flap.

POSTOPERATIVE MANAGEMENT

Adjuvant Chemotherapy

Current treatment recommendations for operable stage IIIa disease are surgery followed by adjuvant chemotherapy with an anthracycline-containing regimen (i.e., doxorubicin), followed by radiotherapy (National Comprehensive Cancer Network, 1999). These recommendations are based in part on results of NSABP B-15, in which positive-node breast cancer patients with tamoxifen-nonresponsive tumors were randomized to 2 months of therapy with doxorubicin and cyclophosphamide (AC) versus 6 months of conventional cyclophosphamide, methotrexate, and fluorouracil (CMF) if they were either 49 years of age or younger or were 50 to 59 years of age with a progesterone receptor level less than 10 fmol/mg (Fisher et al, 1990). There was no significant difference in relapse-free survival or overall survival, and patients preferred the shorter regimen.

Adjuvant Hormonal Therapy

Some oncologists recommend that tamoxifen be added to the adjuvant therapy regimen, especially for patients with estrogen receptor–positive tumors. This recommendation is based on a 1992 overview analysis of 40 randomized trials that compared adjuvant treatment with tamoxifen versus the same adjuvant treatment without tamoxifen (Early Breast Cancer Trialists' Collaborative Group). Almost without exception, these trials demonstrated a significant improvement in relapse-free survival for women randomized to tamoxifen.

Adjuvant Radiotherapy

For women with breast carcinoma who are at high risk for local and/or regional recurrence of disease following surgical therapy, adjuvant radiotherapy given in combination with chemotherapy reduces recurrence rates (Fig. 152–2). Current recommendations for stage IIIa and stage IIIb breast carcinoma are (1) radiotherapy to the breast and supraclavicular lymph nodes following neoadjuvant chemotherapy and lumpectomy, (2) radiotherapy to the chest wall and supraclavicular lymph nodes following neoadjuvant chemotherapy and modified radical mastectomy, and (3) radiotherapy to the chest wall and supraclavicular lymph nodes following primary modified radical mastectomy and adjuvant chemotherapy (National Comprehensive Cancer Network).

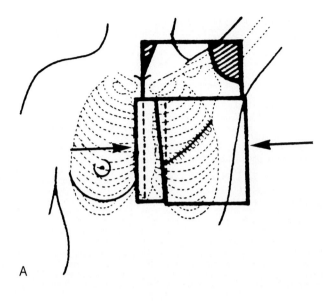

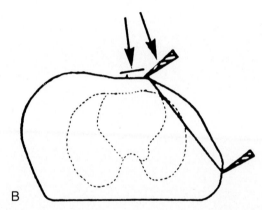

Figure 152–2. Radiotherapy for stage IIIa and stage IIIb breast carcinoma. *A,* Comprehensive chest wall and nodal radiotherapy, anterior view. *B,* Cross-sectional view showing tangential field.

COMPLICATIONS OF MASTECTOMY

Surgical Complications (Table 152–3)

Postoperative Complications

Seromas in the axillary dead space or beneath the skin flaps have represented the most frequent complication of mastectomy, reportedly occurring in as many as 25% to 30% of cases. During the past two decades, use of closed-system suction drainage has resulted in a reduction in the incidence of this complication. Wound catheters are retained postoperatively until drainage diminishes to less than 30 mL/day. Wound infections occur infrequently after mastectomy, the majority occurring secondary to skin flap ischemia and necrosis. Culture of the wound for aerobic and anaerobic organisms, débridement, and appropriate antibiotic therapy provide for effective management. Moderate to severe hemorrhage in the immediate postoperative period is rare and is best managed with early wound exploration for control of hemorrhage and re-establishment of closed-system suction drainage.

The incidence of lymphedema after modified radical

Pearls and Pitfalls

PEARLS

- Treat stage IIIa breast carcinoma patients with modified radical mastectomy followed by adjuvant therapy, but treat stage IIIb patients initially with neoadjuvant chemotherapy.
- The Patey modified radical mastectomy is employed, when necessary, to encompass nodal disease at level III of the axilla.
- Primary breast reconstruction is contraindicated in patients with advanced-stage breast carcinoma. Perform breast reconstruction 3 to 6 months following adjuvant therapy if the patient remains disease free.
- Modified radical mastectomy following neoadjuvant chemotherapy in patients with inflammatory breast carcinoma provides important information about the histologic response to chemotherapy and allows a lower dose of radiotherapy to be delivered to the chest wall.
- If inflammatory skin changes do not completely resolve following neoadjuvant chemotherapy in patients with inflammatory breast carcinoma, beware of a high probability of microscopic disease at the skin margins following modified radical mastectomy. In this situation, consider radiotherapy prior to surgery.
- The Halsted radical mastectomy is employed, when necessary, to encompass residual disease after neoadjuvant chemotherapy. Chest wall resection is advisable in some circumstances.
- The precise role, if any, for high-dose chemotherapy with autologous bone marrow transplantation in advanced-stage breast carcinoma remains to be established. Encourage patients to enroll in clinical trials.

mastectomy is approximately 10%. Extensive axillary node dissection, axillary radiotherapy, and the presence of pathologic nodes and obesity are predisposing factors. Most patients have mild lymphedema that is functionally insignificant. For more severe cases, individually fitted compressive sleeves and intermittent compression devices are helpful.

OUTCOMES

Relative survival rates for patients diagnosed with breast carcinoma between 1983 and 1987 have been calculated

Table 152–3	Surgical Complications

Vascular Injury
The first and second perforating vessels are too large for cautery. They should be ligated.
The axillary vein, if torn, should be repaired.
Ligation may cause chronic edema.
Nerve Injury
Thoracodorsal Nerve
If cut, medial rotation and adduction of the humerus will be weakened.

Long Thoracic Nerve
If cut, a "winged scapula" deformity will result.

Medial and Lateral Thoracic Nerves
If cut, the pectoralis muscles will atrophy.

based on Surveillance, Epidemiology, and End Results (SEER) Program data. For stage IIIa patients, 5-year survival was 52%. For stage IIIb patients, 5-year survival was 48%. By comparison, survival for stage I was 94%, stage IIa was 85%, stage IIb was 70%, and stage IV was 18%.

SELECTED READINGS

American Joint Committee on Cancer: Manual for Staging of Cancer, 5th ed. Philadelphia, Lippincott-Raven, 1997.

Bland KI, Chang HR, Copeland EM: Modified radical mastectomy and total (simple) mastectomy. In Bland KI, Copeland EM (eds): The Breast: Comprehensive Management of Benign and Malignant Diseases. Philadelphia, WB Saunders, 1998, pp 881–912.

Bostwick J, Vasconez LO, Jurkiewicz MJ: Breast reconstruction after a radical mastectomy. Plast Reconstr Surg 1978;61:682.

DeLena M, Zucali R, Viganotti G: Combined chemotherapy-radiotherapy approach in locally advanced (T₃ᵦ-T₄) breast cancer. Cancer Chemother Pharmacol 1978;1:53.

Early Breast Cancer Trialists' Collaborative Group: Systemic treatment of early breast cancer by hormonal, cytotoxic, or immune therapy: 133 randomised trials involving 31,000 recurrences and 24,000 deaths among 75,000 women. Lancet 1992;339:1.

Fisher B, Brown AM, Dimitrov NV, et al: Two months of doxorubicin-cyclophosphamide with or without interval reinduction therapy compared with 6 months of cyclophosphamide, methotrexate, and fluorouracil in positive-node breast cancer patients with tamoxifen non-responsive tumors: Results from the National Adjuvant Breast and Bowel Project B-15. J Clin Oncol 1990;8:1483.

Fisher B, Bryant J, Wolmark N, et al: Effect of preoperative chemotherapy on the outcome of women with operable breast cancer. J Clin Oncol 1998;16:2672.

Grotting JC, Urist MM, Maddox WA, Vasconez LO: Conventional TRAM flap versus free microsurgical TRAM flap for immediate breast reconstruction. Plast Reconstr Surg 1989;83:842.

Haagensen CD, Stout AP: Carcinoma of the breast: II. Criteria of operability. Ann Surg 1943;118:859–870, 1032–1051.

Maddox WA, Carpenter JT, Laws HT: Does radical mastectomy still have a place in the treatment of primary operable breast cancer? Arch Surg 1987;122:1317.

National Comprehensive Cancer Network: Oncology Practice Guidelines, vol. 6. Oncology 1999;13:187.

Patey DH, Dyson WH: The prognosis of carcinoma of the breast in relation to the type of operation performed. Br J Cancer 1967;21:260.

Valagussa P, Zambetti M, Bignami P: T₃ᵦ-T₄ breast cancer: Factors affecting results in combined modality treatments. Clin Exp Metastasis 1983;1:191.

Chapter 153

Metastatic Carcinoma of the Breast (Stage IV)

Nuhad K. Ibrahim and Gabriel N. Hortobagyi

We have witnessed significant strides in the management of breast cancer over the past four decades. While early diagnosis and the multidisciplinary approach to the treatment of primary breast cancer have made a significant impact on the natural history of the disease, metastatic breast cancer remains a significant source of morbidity and mortality for patients. In the United States, from 3% to 6% of patients have clinical evidence of distant metastasis at the time of initial diagnosis. In addition, approximately 20% to 80% of patients diagnosed with stage I to III disease will develop metastatic disease. The majority of the recurrences occur within the first 3 to 5 years. This incidence declines gradually with time, but the risk of developing metastatic breast cancer never reaches zero; it drops significantly after 10 years, and it is a rare event beyond 20 years. Bone is the most common site of metastatic involvement with breast cancer. It is the first manifestation of metastatic breast cancer in 30% to 40% of the patients, and 80% to 90% of the patients who die of metastatic breast cancer demonstrate evidence of bone invasion. Other sites of metastasis, in descending order of frequency, are the soft tissues, lymph nodes, lungs, pleura, liver, and brain. Certain subtypes of breast cancer, such as invasive lobular carcinoma, show a preference toward abdominal carcinomatosis. In addition, rapidly growing (high-grade, aneuploid) and hormone receptor–negative tumors are more likely to metastasize to visceral organs, such as the liver, lungs, and brain. Conversely, tumors that are well differentiated, express hormone receptors, and have a slower growth rate are more likely to develop metastases to bone and soft tissues and are less likely to develop life-threatening manifestations, such as lymphangitic lung metastasis, fulminant liver metastasis, or brain metastasis. The main objective of the treatment of patients with metastatic breast cancer, however, remains optimal palliation and prolongation of life.

Recurrent or metastatic breast cancer is often responsive to systemic therapy, although it is rarely cured (Greenberg et al, 1996). Therefore, it is important to define the phenotypic characteristics of the disease and the sites of spread (complete staging work-up; Fig. 153–1) to select the optimal treatment intervention for each patient. Systemic therapy (hormonal therapy and/or chemotherapy) is the mainstay of the treatment of metastatic breast cancer (Fig. 153–2), whereas radiation therapy and surgery play an adjunctive palliative role with no significant impact on survival.

HORMONAL THERAPY

About two thirds of breast cancers express estrogen receptors and, to a lesser extent, progesterone receptors. In general, hormone receptor–positive tumors have a 50% probability of objective response (complete or partial remission) to a hormonal agent. The response rate is higher if both receptors are expressed, but less than 10% of receptor-negative tumors respond to hormonal therapy. Until recently, the selection of first-line hormonal therapy was usually based on the safety profile of the agent; that is, the hormonal agent with fewer side effects is used first. This is based on the assumption that all hormonal therapies, whether ablative or additive, achieve similar response rates in untreated metastatic breast cancer. Therefore, for the past 25 years, the least toxic hormonal intervention has consisted of antiestrogens (tamoxifen) and, more recently, anastrozole, which may prove to be less toxic and probably offers a longer duration of response.

For premenopausal women, an alternative to the use of tamoxifen as front-line or second-line treatment after progression of the disease while the patient was taking tamoxifen is ovarian ablation, which can take the form of surgical intervention or, preferably, medical therapy with the use of luteinizing hormone–releasing hormone (LH-RH) agonists, such as goserelin and leuprolide. The combination of an LH-RH agonist or tamoxifen has been shown to be more effective and probably results in longer duration of response than either agent alone (Jonat et al, 1995). In addition to the hormone receptor status, the antihormonal agents may be utilized in patients whose receptors are unknown but who have a prolonged disease-free interval. The selection of hormonal agents is also

Complete physical examination
Blood work: complete blood count (CBC), differential, platelet count, serum glutamate pyruvate transaminase (SGPT), lactate dehydrogenase (LDH), total bilirubin, alkaline phosphatase, calcium, total proteins, creatinine, and blood urea nitrogen (BUN)
Estrogen receptor, progesterone receptor, and HER2 status of the primary tumor or, preferably, of the biopsy of a metastatic lesion
Radiologic studies
    Chest radiograph
    CT scan or ultrasound of abdomen
    Bone scan and plain films and/or MRI or CT scans of areas of suspicious increased uptake
    MRI of brain if clinically suspicious for metastasis
    MRI of spine if cord compression is suspected
    CT scan of chest if solitary lung lesion by chest radiograph or lymphangitic spread is suspected
    Ultrasound of local or regional recurrence if it is the only site of disease
Biopsy of a solitary lesion to confirm its metastatic nature

Figure 153–1. Recommended staging work-up for patients with metastatic breast cancer.

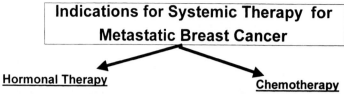

Indications for Systemic Therapy for Metastatic Breast Cancer

Hormonal Therapy

1. Hormone-receptor positive

2. Prolonged disease-free interval (>2 years*)

3. No life-threatening or bulky visceral disease

4. No significant symptomatology from metastatic disease

5. Response to prior hormonal therapy

Chemotherapy

1. Hormone-receptor negative

2. Short disease-free interval†

3. Life-threatening or bulky visceral disease

4. Significant symptomatology

5. No response to prior hormonal therapy‡

Figure 153–2. Indications for the selection of hormonal or chemotherapy options for patients with metastatic breast cancer. *If hormone receptor is negative or unknown; †if hormone receptor is negative or unknown; ‡hormone-resistant tumor.

influenced by the menopausal status of the patient. Aromatase inhibitors are considered the second line of therapy of choice after tamoxifen for postmenopausal, but not for premenopausal, women. Aromatase is the enzyme responsible for converting androgenic precursors to estrogens. This enzyme is particularly critical in postmenopausal women, for whom the bulk of estrogen is produced in peripheral fatty tissue and muscles; thus, its inhibition can virtually halt estrogen production in the host.

The duration of response to front-line hormonal therapy is critical to the subsequent implementation of additional hormonal therapies. Disease that has been stable for longer than 6 months is considered equivalent to a partial response. A patient's response to a chosen hormonal therapy is predictive of response to another subsequent line of therapy. The sequential use of endocrine therapies, therefore, is an appropriate strategy for min-

imizing toxicity of treatment and maintaining an acceptable quality of life. An outline of hormonal intervention in metastatic breast cancer is shown in Figure 153–3.

Tamoxifen, due to its dual agonist and antagonist estrogen activity, may rarely result in significant side effects, including uterine cancer, subcapsular cataracts, and thromboembolic disease. More common side effects include vasomotor changes (urogenital, hot flushes, and mood changes) and cognitive derangement. The development of pure antiestrogens or selective estrogen receptor modulators may substantially improve the therapeutic index and the long-term effect of such agents (Ibrahim and Hortobagyi, 1999). Aromatase inhibition with aminoglutethimide also may result in significant side effects and may require steroidal replacement therapy owing to its nonselective inhibition. The last 5 years have witnessed the development of many new selective aromatase inhibi-

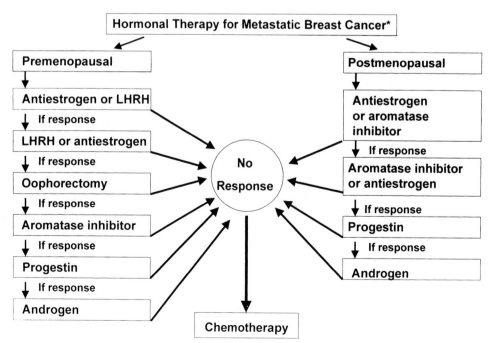

Figure 153–3. Optimal sequence of hormonal therapy in premenopausal and postmenopausal patients with metastatic breast cancer.

*Research phase I-III studies should be considered at every step, if available.

tors. Selective aromatase inhibition allows the administration of such agents without the need for steroidal replacement therapy. Several compounds have been developed clinically as second- or third-line therapy for metastatic breast cancer after tamoxifen failure. Randomized prospective studies have demonstrated that they are at least equivalent to, and probably are more effective and better tolerated than, progestins (megestrol acetate). These agents are currently considered as the second-line therapy of choice after tamoxifen for postmenopausal women. Owing to the relative lack of cross-resistance between the various hormonal agents, progestins (megestrol acetate) are currently used as the third line of hormonal therapy.

CYTOTOXIC MONOTHERAPY IN METASTATIC BREAST CANCER

Systemic chemotherapy for metastatic breast cancer is indicated in patients who are hormone receptor negative, who have bulky visceral involvement (hepatic, lymphangitic spread) that results in significant organ dysfunction or morbidity, whose tumors are not responsive to hormonal therapy, or who choose to be treated with chemotherapy instead of hormonal therapy (see Fig. 153–2). More than 60 chemotherapeutic agents have been tested in the treatment of breast cancer, with responses ranging from 0 to 71%. The most active single agents, however, belong to the taxanes (paclitaxel and docetaxel), the anthracycline family, particularly doxorubicin, the vinca alkaloids (vinblastine, vindesine, and vinorelbine), cyclophosphamide, fluorouracil, methotrexate, and mitomycin C. Doxorubicin is among the most active agents in breast cancer. Cardiomyopathy limits its use to 400 to 500 mg/m^2 IV by bolus administration and up to 700 to 800 mg/m^2 IV by 48- to 96-hour continuous infusion. Epirubicin, a semisynthetic doxorubicin analogue, is probably equally effective (in equivalent myelosuppressive doses), but it can also result in cardiomyopathy. Mitoxantrone, an anthraquinone derivative of doxorubicin, is less effective than either doxorubicin or epirubicin; however, mitoxantrone poses a smaller risk of cardiomyopathy.

Taxanes (paclitaxel, docetaxel) have proved to be substantially active single agents in the treatment of metastatic breast cancer, both as front-line and salvage therapies. Both agents are administered intravenously every 3 weeks. As a single agent, the response to paclitaxel in patients with metastatic breast cancer can reach 60% as front-line and 32% as second-line therapy; the response rates are largely dose-dependent. Single-agent docetaxel given as front-line chemotherapy for metastatic breast cancer produces response rates ranging from 40% to 68% (Antoine et al, 1997). As salvage therapy, particularly for anthracycline-resistant tumors, the response rates were 20% to 50% (Antoine et al, 1997). Finally, weekly administration of taxanes is very well tolerated with significant activity as front-line or salvage therapy (Hainsworth et al, 1999; Seidman, 1999).

COMBINATION CHEMOTHERAPY IN METASTATIC BREAST CANCER

Chemotherapy for metastatic breast cancer was developed in the 1960s. In the 1970s, the combination of cyclophosphamide, methotrexate, and 5-fluorouracil (CMF) dominated the clinical practice of treating metastatic disease and adjuvant disease as well. An anthracycline-based regimen such as fluorouracil, Adriamycin (doxorubicin), and Cytoxan (cyclophosphamide) (FAC) provided additional options and therapeutic advantages to the patients. In his meta-analysis of randomized clinical trials for metastatic breast cancer, Fossati (1998) has shown that anthracycline-based chemotherapy regimens yield significantly higher response rates than regimens that do not have anthracycline, although with an increased incidence of side effects. The overall survival, however, did not seem to be affected by the use of anthracycline. On the other hand, Greenberg and colleagues (1996) have demonstrated the impact of an anthracycline-based regimen (FAC) in metastatic breast cancer. In a series of 1581 patients treated with FAC front-line therapy at M.D. Anderson Cancer Center, 263 (17%) patients achieved complete remission, 766 (48%) patients had partial remission, and only 141 (9%) patients had progression of disease; the remaining 374 patients had stable disease. Over a follow-up period of 20 years, about 3% of the patients (17% of those in complete remission) maintained complete remission. The factors that may have influenced this prolonged disease-free survival include the following: small tumor burden, better performance status, and younger age. Tomiak and associates (1996) further characterized the determinants of long-term survival of 75 complete responders (CR) to chemotherapy. At a median follow-up of 61 months, 24% of the patients who achieved complete remission were alive with no evidence of disease. The median overall survival for the whole group was 32.5 months. Twenty-two variables were considered for their effect on survival in a multivariate analysis. Anthracycline-based chemotherapy and World Health Organization (WHO) performance status were the only significant prognostic factors affecting survival in complete responders.

Many concepts that dominated the management of metastatic breast cancer during the 1970s and 1980s, however, are widely challenged. First, it was widely accepted that pre-taxane polychemotherapy resulted in better responses and survival (Fossati et al, 1998), yet taxane single agents, or taxane in combination with doxorubicin, proved to be more effective. Secondly, lower doses of traditional polychemotherapy are less effective than standard doses (FAC, CMF), implying a threshold effect. Such threshold effect also occurs with the taxanes. However, higher doses of chemotherapy, even with cytokine support, do not necessarily translate into better response or survival. Finally, the appearance of newer and more effective agents opened the controversy about the relative benefits and risks of combination therapy versus single-agent sequential chemotherapy, since patients treated with standard combination chemotherapies, on the one hand, or single-agent chemotherapy, on the other hand, failed to show differences in survival. Although the newer doxorubicin-taxane combinations are promising, until these controversies are resolved the standard combination chemotherapies are FAC, AC, and, perhaps, the judicious use of an anthracycline-taxane combination.

TAXANE COMBINATIONS

Paclitaxel Combinations

Paclitaxel and doxorubicin in combination have been extensively studied in phase II trials as first-line treatment for metastatic breast cancer. Pharmacokinetic studies have shown that doxorubicin may have a higher Cmax and lower clearance if it was preceded by paclitaxel, resulting in more toxicity. Using the proper sequence, Gianni and co-workers (1996) gave doxorubicin, 60 mg/m² as an IV bolus, followed by paclitaxel, 200 mg/m² IV as a 3-hour infusion, as a front-line regimen. The overall response rate (OR) was 94% (CR 38%), while the primary toxicities were neutropenia and stomatitis. The incidence of congestive heart failure resulting from such a combination was particularly high (18% to 21%). The 3-year follow-up data showed that congestive heart failure is markedly reduced whenever the cumulative dose of doxorubicin is limited to less than 360 mg/m². The superiority of the doxorubicin-paclitaxel combination over the doxorubicin + cyclophosphamide–based regimen has been shown in two recent randomized clinical trials. Non–anthracycline-based paclitaxel combinations proved to be very efficacious (Perez, 1999).

Paclitaxel, combined with cisplatin as front-line therapy for metastatic breast cancer, resulted in an OR of 23% to 85%, with a CR of 0 to 12%. The addition of 5-fluorouracil and folinic acid to the paclitaxel-cisplatin combination resulted in an OR of 83% and a CR of 29%. In previously treated patients, the paclitaxel and fluorouracil–folinic acid combination showed an OR of 51% to 54% (CR, 3% to 6%). Paclitaxel was also combined with carboplatin as first-line therapy, resulting in an OR of 53% to 62% and a CR of 12% to 16%.

Docetaxel Combinations

Docetaxel, 100 mg/m², was found to be associated with a higher response rate than doxorubicin, 75 mg/m², when both agents were compared as single agents in a randomized clinical trial (Crown, 1999). Phase I to II studies combining docetaxel and doxorubicin have shown this combination to be well tolerated and effective: it does not seem to be associated with increased congestive heart failure and has an OR of 67%. When cyclophosphamide was added to this doublet, the OR was 73%.

The combination of docetaxel and doxorubicin (AT) was compared with doxorubicin and cyclophosphamide (AC) as first-line therapy for metastatic breast cancer in a randomized trial. There was a statistically significant difference in the response rates (65% versus 50%) in favor of the AT arm; however, there was a higher incidence of toxicity (neutropenic fever). Moreover, the AT arm proved to be better in terms of the time to progression (*P* = .01) and the time to treatment failure (*P* = .04). Longer follow-up is needed to evaluate any survival advantage.

A randomized trial comparing single-agent docetaxel with mitomycin C and vinblastine in anthracycline-resis-

tant metastatic breast cancer patients showed the superiority of docetaxel in terms of response, time to progression, and survival benefits; however, there was increased hematologic and nonhematologic toxicity. Docetaxel was also compared with a methotrexate and fluorouracil combination in a phase III randomized trial in anthracycline-resistant patients. Response rate and time to progression were in favor of docetaxel; however, with more hematologic toxicity. Finally, docetaxel was compared with vinorelbine and fluorouracil as second-line therapy in a phase III randomized trial. Docetaxel appeared to be as effective, yet less toxic, than the combination arm.

VINORELBINE

Single-agent vinorelbine is active in patients who relapsed after anthracycline-based therapy and has been active as a first- and second-line therapy (Weber et al, 1995). When vinorelbine was combined with doxorubicin as front-line therapy for metastatic breast cancer, the overall response rate ranged from 34% to 82% and the complete remission rate ranged from 12% to 21%. No cardiotoxicity was seen in patients receiving this combination. Vinorelbine has also demonstrated significant antitumor activity against metastatic breast cancer when combined with epirubicin, 5-fluorouracil, mitomycin C, cisplatin, docetaxel, and paclitaxel. Several studies that evaluate various vinorelbine combinations are currently underway.

CAPECITABINE (XELODA)

Capecitabine is a 5-fluorouracil prodrug that is administered orally. It is absorbed unchanged and is transformed both in the liver and in mammary tumors, which are rich in the enzyme dThdPase, to 5-fluorouracil (FU). The resultant high tumor concentration of FU (tumor/plasma FU ratio is 5 to 10) produces results somewhat similar to those achieved with the inconvenient continuous FU infusion schedules. Capecitabine was evaluated in an open-label, single-arm, multicentric phase II study (Blum et al, 1999). A total of 162 patients received 2510 mg/m² per day in two divided doses of capecitabine. All were paclitaxel-resistant. The response rate was 20%. The major toxicities included diarrhea and hand-foot syndrome, affecting 14% and 10% of the patients, respectively. Many studies are underway to define the exact role of capecitabine regimens in the management of advanced breast cancer. Figure 153–4 is an algorithm for the selection of chemotherapy options for the treatment of metastatic breast cancer.

Trastuzumab Combinations

HER2 is a member of the epidermal growth factor receptor family that is overexpressed in approximately 30% of invasive breast cancers. Trastuzumab (Herceptin) is a humanized monoclonal antibody that recognizes the external domain of HER2 protein with a high affinity and specificity. To corroborate the synergy between trastuzu-

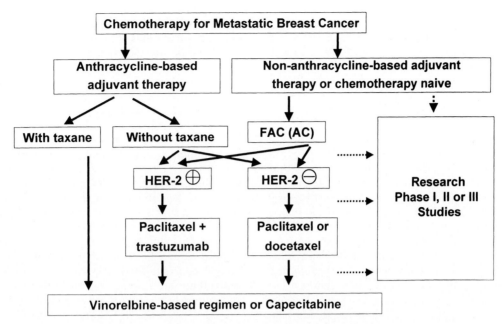

Figure 153–4. Optimal sequence of chemotherapy regimens in patients with metastatic breast cancer.

mab and chemotherapy, a multicenter, randomized phase III study was done involving 469 women with HER2-overexpressing stage IV breast cancer. Patients had significant improvement of response rates with the combinations of trastuzumab and paclitaxel or doxorubicin and cyclophosphamide. In addition, the trastuzumab-paclitaxel arm proved to produce less cardiac toxicity and was associated with improved survival (Norton et al, 1999).

The efficacy of a weekly schedule of paclitaxel and Herceptin was determined. The majority of the patients (70%) in this study had failed front-line therapy for metastatic breast cancer. The dose of paclitaxel was 90 mg/m², and the dose of Herceptin was 2 mg/kg weekly. The combination was given for patients with positive or negative HER2 tumors, by immunohistochemistry. Among patients with HER2-positive tumors, 62% responded, and among 42 HER2-negative tumors 44% responded. The combination was very well tolerated; febrile neutropenia and cardiotoxicity were rare events. The regimen's good response and tolerance, however, do not imply that it is better than the 3-weekly paclitaxel and weekly Herceptin regimen, nor do they justify its use in patients with HER2-negative tumors. The combination of docetaxel and trastuzumab trials is ongoing.

A combination of vinorelbine and Herceptin in patients with HER2-positive metastatic breast cancer who had three or fewer chemotherapy regimens proved to be effective with a partial response of 71% (95% confidence interval [CI]: 53% to 85%) and median time to progression of 31 weeks (Burstien et al, 1999). A confirmatory randomized trial at M.D. Anderson Cancer Center is underway.

MALE BREAST CANCER

Male breast cancer tends to behave like breast cancer in women and, more often than not, like breast cancer in postmenopausal women (Jaiyesimi et al, 1992). Male breast cancer tends to be predominantly hormone receptor positive (80% to 90% of patients have estrogen receptor–positive and progesterone receptor–positive tumors), and therefore sequential hormonal interventions are likely to be more effective in the palliation of the disease than in women with hormone-responsive disease. The same sequence of hormonal ablation as that detailed for postmenopausal women should be adopted for male patients with metastatic breast cancer. By the same token, the same cytotoxic regimen described earlier can be similarly used in the management of male breast cancer.

MANAGEMENT OF BONE METASTASES IN ADVANCED BREAST CANCER

Bone metastases are present to 6% to 8% of patients with advanced breast cancer, and it is the first manifestation of the metastatic disease in 30% to 40% of the patients. The median survival of patients with bone-only metastatic disease is 5 years. Bone metastases are a source of significant morbidity to the patients, including pain, pathologic fractures, hypercalcemia, and spinal cord compression. Systemic therapy for advanced breast cancer can alleviate or prevent some of these complications; however, surgical or radiation therapy intervention may prove vital to the preservation of the quality of life of the patient. Pain management secondary to bony metastases can be achieved in many instances with nonsteroidal anti-inflammatory medications, various analgesics, narcotics, and occasionally anticonvulsant medications for neuropathic pain. Refractory pain or progressive pain despite antitumor systemic therapy should be further investigated, since it may be due to failure of that therapy. Recent onset or worsening of vertebral pain, whether or not associated with tenderness or neurologic deficit, should raise the suspicion of cord compression, and a magnetic resonance imaging (MRI) scan is indicated. Radiation therapy is indicated for the palliation of bone lesions and for the prevention or treatment of cord compression. In many instances, this should be accompanied by a change of the systemic therapy regimen. Surgical intervention followed by radiation therapy is also indicated for acute-onset cord compression in which the stability of the vertebral column is compromised or immediate decompression of the spinal cord is believed to be necessary for the prevention of further neurologic compromise.

Bisphosphonates are pyrophosphate analogues that bind tightly to bone hydroxyapatite. They are believed to limit bone resorption and modulate cytokines that may interfere with cell motility in bone metastases. Their major function, therefore, is to inhibit tumor-induced bone resorption, correct hypercalcemia, reduce pain, and reduce the chances of pathologic fractures and related morbidity. Currently, they are considered the therapeutic agents of choice for the treatment of tumor-induced hypercalcemia. Several bisphosphonates have been clinically developed that vary in order of potency: pamidronate ($1\times$), clodronate ($10\times$), alendronate (100 to $<1000\times$), risedronate (1000 to $10,000\times$), and zoledronate ($>10,000\times$). Currently, pamidronate is approved for patients with lytic bone disease. Hortobagyi and colleagues evaluated the long-term effectiveness and safety of intravenous pamidronate for up to 2 years in combination with systemic therapy. In this randomized, double-blind parallel-group trial, the degree of skeletal complications was significantly better in the pamidronate arm, and such benefits proved to extend beyond 24 months after study entry and to decrease the need for bone radiation and the morbidity resulting from bone metastases. In addition, there are several therapeutic advantages of pamidronate with regard to a number of endpoints, including ameliorating pain and decreasing bone turnover. Currently, pamidronate is used only in patients with lytic bone disease. More data are needed to support its use in patients with blastic metastatic disease.

Bisphosphonates are also investigated to study their role in preventing the development of bone metastases and therefore their use in adjuvant therapy settings. A phase III multicentric study of zoledronate began during the year 2000, as well as a study planned by the National Surgical Adjuvant Breast and Bowel Project to investigate clodronate, as agents that may help prevent the development of bone metastasis.

CENTRAL NERVOUS SYSTEM METASTASES

Central nervous system metastases usually represent a second or third relapse. They more often represent a preterminal stage. However, they seldom present at the time of first relapse or initial diagnosis. The management of such late developments varies among patients, depending on the general prognosis of the patient, life expectancy, prior exposure to systemic therapies, and quality of life. Surgical resection followed by total brain radiation is recommended for solitary or resectable lesions. Multiple brain lesions or deep-seated unresectable lesions are candidates for total brain radiation or Gamma

knife treatment. In addition, Gamma knife therapy is indicated for limited second brain relapse. Brain relapse should not be considered as a sign of failure of concurrent systemic therapy, since most of the systemic agents used for the treatment of metastatic breast cancer have no proven ability to cross the blood-brain or the tumor-brain barrier. Finally, treatment of brain metastases should be considered largely palliative because it is associated with very poor prognoses and limited survival.

Leptomeningeal carcinomatosis is another form of central nervous system metastasis. Single-agent intrathecal or preferably intraventricular chemotherapy (using the Omaya intraventricular shunt) with methotrexate, thiotepa, or cytosine arabinoside has limited short-term therapeutic benefits; however, these benefits supersede the benefits achieved with neural-axis radiation. Such interventions should be weighed against the prognosis, morbidity, inconvenience, and costs of such procedures. Currently, there are efforts to investigate oral temozolomide compounds in the treatment of metastatic brain disease.

Summary

Doxorubicin- and cyclophosphamide-based regimens remain the gold standard, front-line therapy for metastatic breast cancer. More patients, however, are receiving doxorubicin, with or without a taxane, as adjuvant therapy; thus, the need for a new front-line therapy for metastatic breast cancer that takes into account such prior exposure to doxorubicin and taxanes. Therefore, all patients with metastatic breast cancer should be considered candidates for clinical trials that test new chemotherapeutic and biologic agents. Development of newer agents and/or combinations that are not cross-resistant with anthracycline and taxanes may help improve the survival and quality of life of patients with metastatic breast cancer.

A detailed list of suggested readings can be obtained from authors at this e-mail address: nibrahim@mdanderson.org.

SELECTED READINGS

Antoine EC, Rixe O, Auclerc G, et al: Docetaxel: A review of its role in breast cancer treatment. Am J Clin Oncol 1997;20:429.

Blum JL, Jones SE, Buzdar AU, et al: Multicenter phase II study of capecitabine in paclitaxel-refractory metastatic breast cancer. J Clin Oncol 1999;17:485.

Burstien HJ, Kuter I, Richardson PG, et al: Herceptin (H) and vinorelbine (V) as a second-line therapy for HER-2–positive (HER 2+) metastatic breast cancer (MBC): A phase II study. Abstract 18, 22nd Annual San Antonio Breast Cancer Symposium, 1999.

Crown J: Phase III randomized trials of docetaxel in patients with metastatic breast cancer. Semin Oncol 1999;26(Suppl 8):33.

Fossati R, Confalonieri C, Torri V, et al: Cytotoxic and hormonal treatment for metastatic breast cancer: A systematic review of published randomized trials involving 31,510 women. J Clin Oncol 1998;16:3439.

Gianni L, Capri G, Tarenzi E, et al: Efficacy and cardiac effects of 3-h paclitaxel (P) plus bolus doxorubicin (DOX) in women with untreated metastatic breast carcinoma. Proc Am Soc Clin Oncol 1996;15:116. Abstract 128.

Greenberg PA, Hortobagyi GN, Smith TL, et al: Long-term follow-up of patients with complete remission following combination chemotherapy for metastatic breast cancer. J Clin Oncol 1996;14:2197.

Hainsworth JD, Burris HA 3rd, Greco FA: Weekly administration of docetaxel (Taxotere): Summary of clinical data. Semin Oncol 1999;26:19.

Hortobagyi GN, Theriault RL, Lipton A, et al: Long-term prevention of skeletal complications of metastatic breast cancer with pamidronate. Protocol 19 Aredia Breast Cancer Study Group. J Clin Oncol 1998;16:2038.

Ibrahim NK, Hortobagyi GN: The evolving role of specific estrogen receptor modulators (SERMs). Surg Oncol 1999;8:103.

Jaiyesimi IA, Buzdar AU, Sahin AA, et al: Carcinoma of the male breast. Ann Intern Med 1992;117:771.

Jonat W, Kaufmann M, Blamey RW, et al: A randomised study to compare the effect of the luteinising hormone releasing hormone (LHRH) analogue goserelin with or without tamoxifen in pre- and perimenopausal patients with advanced breast cancer. Eur J Cancer 1995;31A:137.

Norton L, Slamon D, Loyland-Jones B, et al: Overall survival (OS) advantage to simultaneous chemotherapy (Crx) plus the humanized anti-HER2 monoclonal antibody Herceptin (H) in HER2-overexpressing (HER2+) metastatic breast cancer. Proc Am Soc Clin Oncol 1999;18:127a. Abstract 483.

Perez EA: Paclitaxel plus nonanthracycline combinations in metastatic breast cancer. Semin Oncol 1999;26:21.

Seidman AD: Single-agent paclitaxel in the treatment of breast cancer: Phase I and II development. Semin Oncol 1999;26:14.

Tomiak E, Piccart M, Mignolet F, et al: Characterisation of complete responders to combination chemotherapy for advanced breast cancer: A retrospective EORTC Breast Group study. Eur J Cancer 1996;32A:1876.

Weber BL, Vogel C, Jones S, et al: Intravenous vinorelbine as first-line and second-line therapy in advanced breast cancer. J Clin Oncol 1995;13:2722.

Chapter 154

Breast Reconstruction

Paul M. Gardner and Luis O. Vasconez

Breast reconstruction following mastectomy has evolved from the creation of a breast mound to artistic results closely matching the normal breast. Data now show that it is safe from an oncologic perspective, and does not interfere significantly with cancer surveillance. Recent legislation mandating third-party payers to cover the procedure facilitates the provision of breast cancer patients with the emotional and physical benefits of breast reconstruction.

CLINICAL PRESENTATION

The breast cancer patient's concern over dealing with a malignancy is greatly increased by the emotionally devastating prospect of losing her breast. Part of a woman's perceived femininity and wholeness involves having breasts. The fear of lost sexuality, coupled with the high premium society places on appearance, compounds the emotional distress. Prosthetics are a poor substitute. Although advances have augmented comfort and usability, even the best prosthetics can result in embarrassing moments. Finally, the patient and her partner must still deal with the mutilated appearance of the absent breast.

Treatment of the patient's cancer should never be compromised by reconstruction. The mastectomy must be performed according to sound oncologic principles. The implementation of adjuvant therapy should proceed without interference. Finally, postoperative surveillance must not be obscured.

There is no increased risk of local recurrence in reconstructed patients. In fact, superior aesthetic results are obtained with the skin-sparing technique, which preserves much of the breast skin. The thicker, more abundant skin overcomes the thin, tight flaps left behind from the standard mastectomy incision. When the mastectomy incisions are planned properly, there is no increase in native skin flap necrosis.

The administration of adjuvant therapy is not affected by reconstruction. Preoperative and postoperative chemotherapy can be given, although the reconstructive procedure should be delayed for several weeks after preoperative administration. Radiotherapy may result in delay of the reconstruction, affect the final aesthetic result, and increase the incidence of complications. However, breast reconstruction does not interfere with its administration.

Monitoring for local and regional recurrence is an important consideration. Almost all recurrences occur at the level of the skin, between the native breast skin and the reconstructed tissue. No delay in the diagnosis of local or regional recurrence after reconstruction has been noted. In fact, mammography of the reconstructed breast is considered by many to be unwarranted, since physical examination alone effectively detects recurrence.

PREOPERATIVE MANAGEMENT

The preoperative consultation allows the plastic surgeon to determine whether the patient is a candidate for breast reconstruction. The next decision is whether an immediate or delayed procedure is done. The history and physical examination guide the surgeon in deciding which type of reconstruction is most suitable.

Almost any patient who is healthy enough to undergo mastectomy is a candidate for reconstruction. Advanced age and bilaterality are not contraindications, although they have a bearing on which type of reconstruction is done. Tumor stage is a consideration. Generally, any patient with preoperative stage I or II disease is an acceptable candidate. Higher stages are controversial. However, if both the oncologic and the plastic surgeon are comfortable with the plan, reconstruction can be performed.

The timing of reconstruction must be addressed. Immediate reconstruction offers a number of advantages and is now favored by most plastic surgeons. There are a number of advantages to accomplishing most of the reconstruction in one procedure. The final aesthetic result is improved, since the skin flaps are soft and pliable, the inframammary fold can be preserved, and scarring is avoided. Psychologically, the patient is spared waking up from surgery without a breast. Delay of reconstruction may be chosen if the patient is known to need postoperative radiation and wishes to avoid the complications that can occur, such as fat necrosis in autogenous tissue reconstruction, and capsular contracture in implant reconstruction. Other reasons for delay include inflammatory carcinoma, mastectomy for recurrence, and patients who may not be able to psychologically cope with the entire experience.

The next step is to choose which type of reconstruction is appropriate. A number of factors must be considered in this decision, including health issues, age, weight, bilaterality, smoking history, breast size, body habitus, and desired results. The patient's tolerance for scars on other parts of the body and the magnitude of the operative procedure must also be determined. All of these factors are taken into account.

Alloplastic (implant) and autogenous breast reconstruction are the two general methods currently available. Which method is used depends on the factors described earlier, as well as the plastic surgeon's preferences and abilities. Each procedure has distinct advantages and disadvantages.

Alloplastic reconstruction utilizes either saline or silicone gel implants to create a breast mound. In delayed reconstruction, a tissue expander or expandable implant is usually necessary for the creation of adequate skin coverage. This is usually not an issue with immediate reconstruction if a skin-sparing mastectomy is used. The advantages include less operative and recovery time, no other scars, and less expense. The main disadvantage is capsular contracture, which can form a thick scar around the implant. This can lead to firmness, distortion, and even pain. Another disadvantage is the inability to assist in dealing with infection, which usually requires removal of the implant until the infection clears. Finally, the cosmetic result of an implant reconstruction seldom equals that of autogenous tissue.

The types of implants currently available for breast reconstruction are saline and silicone gel. Saline implants have a solid grade silicone shell and are filled with normal saline. They are generally considered safe, but do not feel like normal breast tissue, have a significant deflation rate, and may have a wrinkled or rippled appearance. In recent years, the use of silicone implants was quite controversial. However, they have recently been cleared of association with systemic disease and are being used with more frequency. They provide a more natural look and feel, although they have the same problems with contracture as do other implants.

Alloplastic reconstruction is often accompanied by some sort of muscle coverage. The pectoralis muscle is commonly used to cover the superior pole of the implant. The latissimus muscle transposed as a flap, or the serratus muscle, can be used to cover the inferior pole (Figs. 154–1 and 154–2).

An autogenous breast reconstruction creates a breast that feels and looks natural since it utilizes the patient's own tissue. It gives superior aesthetic results, provides living tissue that fights off infection, and has the capacity to help the entire mastectomy wound heal. Its disadvantages include longer operation time, longer recovery time, scars on parts of the body other than the mastectomy site, and added expense.

The main type of flap used in autogenous reconstruction is the transverse rectus myocutaneous (TRAM) flap. The conventional TRAM flap is based on the superior epigastric vessels and is useful in most patients (Figs. 154–3 and 154–4). For obese patients, and those with a history of smoking, the free TRAM flap is indicated. This involves a microvascular anastomosis of the deep inferior epigastric vessels and provides better blood supply to the flap (Fig. 154–5).

Other sources of tissue for autogenous reconstruction include the latissimus myocutaneous flap, thoracoepigastric flap, lateral thigh free flap, free gluteal flap, and

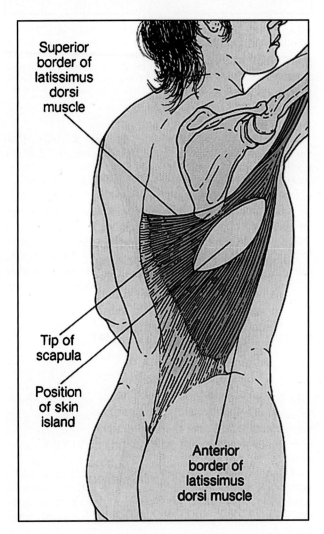

Figure 154–1. The latissimus dorsi muscle is outlined with a skin island oriented obliquely or transversely. The musculocutaneous unit is completely freed up, leaving it attached to its insertion at the humerus. (From Vasconez LO, Lejour M, Gamboa M: Atlas of Breast Reconstruction. Philadelphia, JB Lippincott, 1991.)

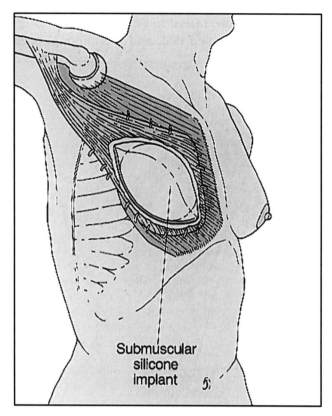

Figure 154–2. The latissimus dorsi musculocutaneous unit has been transposed anteriorly to the chest. The unit moves as a pendulum to avoid an axillary bulge. Note that the transversely oriented skin island takes an oblique orientation on the chest. (From Vasconez LO, Lejour M, Gamboa M: Atlas of Breast Reconstruction. Philadelphia, JB Lippincott, 1991.)

"Rubin's flap," a free flap based on the circumflex iliac vessels. These are generally used in patients who are not candidates for a TRAM flap.

Once the type of reconstruction is selected, the remainder of the preoperative work-up is similar to that of a mastectomy. A detailed history should screen for coagulation disorders, smoking history, and medications that may influence flap survival. Physical examination looking for scars on the breast and abdomen may change the type of reconstruction considered. Laboratory studies include a complete blood count, platelet count, and coagulation factors.

INTRAOPERATIVE MANAGEMENT

The patient is marked in the standing position just prior to the procedure. The marking for the mastectomy incision is made with both oncologic and plastic surgeons present. If a skin-sparing incision is used, any biopsy scars are included. Often the skin between the areolar complex and the biopsy scar must be included to prevent skin necrosis.

The positioning of the patient is similar in both delayed and immediate breast reconstruction. In the immediate reconstruction, the plastic surgeon and oncologic surgeon should be present. The TRAM flap can be raised while

the oncologic surgeon is doing the mastectomy. Other types of reconstruction require coordination between surgeons. For example, if the latissimus muscle is used, the patient must be in the prone or in the lateral decubitus position for flap harvest. The mastectomy is done either before or after the harvest. The arms should be padded and secured, to allow the patient to be sat up during the procedure. Wide exposure during draping to include both breasts is essential. Care is taken not to erase the preoperative marks during the prep. They can be tattooed with methylene blue and a 22-gauge needle to preserve them.

Antiembolic devices are generally used for longer cases and are activated prior to induction. Prophylactic antibiotics are given. If a TRAM flap is done, it is helpful to minimize the use of nitrous oxide to facilitate closure. Separate instruments are used for the mastectomy and reconstruction.

After the mastectomy is completed, the skin flaps are evaluated for viability. Any questionable skin is excised. The inframammary fold and anterior axillary folds are reconstructed to help shape the reconstructed breast. If implants are used, the pectoralis muscle is raised to cover

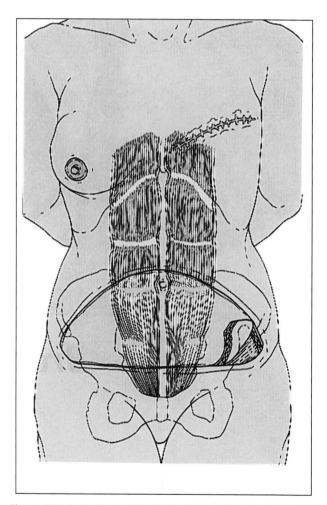

Figure 154–3. Outline of the TRAM flap on the lower abdomen. The most important point is to make the upper incision at the level of the umbilicus. The authors prefer an ipsilateral design for unilateral reconstruction. (From Vasconez LO, Lejour M, Gamboa M: Atlas of Breast Reconstruction. Philadelphia, JB Lippincott, 1991.)

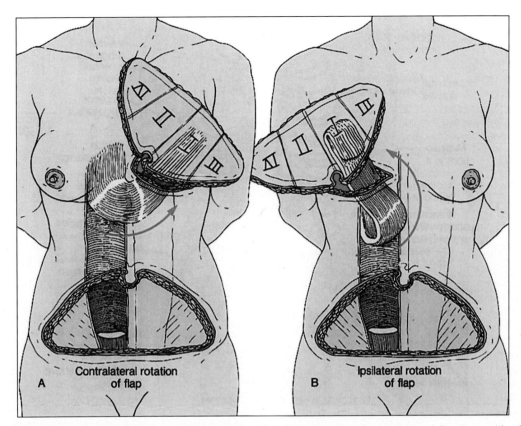

Figure 154–4. The elevated TRAM flap can be rotated in either the ipsilateral or the contralateral direction—with relative safety. One always discards zone IV and, if possible, also zone II. (From Vasconez LO, Lejour M, Gamboa M: Atlas of Breast Reconstruction. Philadelphia, JB Lippincott, 1991.)

the superior pole. If a free flap is planned, the thoracodorsal or internal mammary vessels are dissected.

When the reconstructed breast is near completion, the patient is sat up to check for symmetry. Often, a procedure is planned on the opposite breast to obtain symmetry, such as reduction or mastopexy. On completion of the procedure, the patient is placed in a mammary support dressing.

POSTOPERATIVE MANAGEMENT

The same postoperative care given to mastectomy patients applies to patients with implant reconstruction, since the magnitude of the procedure is not significantly increased. Antibiotics may be continued for several days, depending on the physician's preference. The length of stay in the hospital with the combined procedure is equivalent to that of mastectomy alone.

Patients with flap reconstruction should have their hematocrit checked. Significant changes in hematocrit should be treated with transfusion, to provide better blood flow. Free tissue transfer patients have their flaps closely monitored. They receive supplemental oxygen and a caffeine-free diet for 2 weeks. Patients with a TRAM flap reconstruction are given a clear liquid diet initially, and are advanced as tolerated. Drains are left in place until output drops below a predetermined level.

Patients who undergo extensive procedures are sat in a chair on the first postoperative day, followed by ambulation on the second. Vigorous pulmonary toilet is essential, especially in TRAM flap patients. Showers are permitted on the third day. They are usually discharged from 3 to 7 days postoperatively.

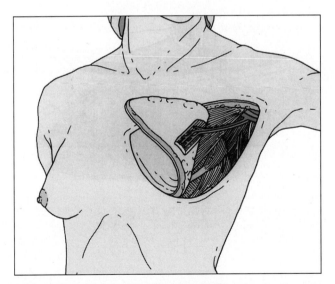

Figure 154–5. Diagram of a "free TRAM." The microvascular anastomosis is most often made to the thoracodorsal vessels. Note the relatively small amount of rectus muscle that is sacrificed. (With permission from Vasconez LO, Lejour M, Gamboa M: Atlas of Breast Reconstruction. Philadelphia, JB Lippincott, 1991.)

COMPLICATIONS

Complications with alloplastic reconstruction can occur shortly after surgery or months postoperatively. Large hematomas can form in the breast implant pocket requiring evacuation. Necrosis of skin flaps leads to skin slough and exposure. Dehiscence of the incision can result in extrusion. Infection rarely occurs, but it usually requires removal of the implant. Seroma formation may require drainage. Deflation of saline implants requires replacement. Rupture of silicone implants can lead to silicone granulomas if the gel leaks outside the capsule. Lesser problems include asymmetry and wrinkling of the implant.

The most common problem with alloplastic reconstruction is capsular contracture. All implants develop a scar, or capsule, around them. If the capsule hardens, it can lead to firmness of the reconstructed breast, distortion, displacement, and even pain. The treatment is often simple capsulotomy. Severe contracture may require removal of the implant and replacement with autogenous tissue.

Autogenous tissue reconstruction complications can affect the reconstructed breast as well as the donor site. They vary from intraoperative to late postoperative problems. Vascular compromise is the biggest intraoperative challenge. Injury to the blood vessels supplying the flap (pedicle) can result in impaired blood supply and flap loss. Excessive tension, twisting of the pedicle, and folding of the flap all can impair vascularity.

Aside from complete flap loss, partial flap loss can occur and is often manifested later as fat necrosis, and/or skin slough. Patients undergoing TRAM flap can develop an abdominal hernia at the donor site. Contour irregularities can also be bothersome at the donor site in all flap patients. Seroma, hematoma, asymmetry, and severe scarring can occur at the reconstructed and donor sites.

OUTCOMES

Most breast reconstruction is successful, although several procedures may be required to obtain a satisfactory result. The majority of patients have one extensive procedure, followed by one or more revisions. A nipple is usually reconstructed at one of these revisions.

Failures occur when a flap is lost, or capsular contracture is so severe that it results in removal of an implant. Reported failure rates approximate 21% after tissue expansion, 3% in TRAM flaps, and 9% in latissimus flaps.

Failures are often corrected with a different kind of reconstruction. For example, a patient with a severe cap-

---

Pearls and Pitfalls
Breast Reconstruction
PEARLS

- Immediate breast reconstruction with skin-sparing mastectomy provides the best opportunity for obtaining a satisfactory result owing to the suppleness of the skin flaps and lack of scar.
- Making the flaps a bit thicker to preserve the subcutaneous plexus can reduce complications with skin flap necrosis in skin-sparing mastectomies.
- Previously radiated breasts require special consideration because of the increased potential for complications:

  1. Incisions for biopsy or completion mastectomy should be planned with a plastic surgeon to avoid skin flap necrosis.
  2. The use of implant or expanders for reconstruction should be avoided.
  3. Autogenous tissue, TRAM, or latissimus myocutaneous flap should be used, since it brings in a nonradiated blood supply.

- Strong consideration should be given for free tissue transfer or reduction of the opposite breast in patients with obesity or those with large breasts.
- Exposure of a saline or silicone implant usually necessitates removal, although salvage may sometimes be accomplished with coverage using a latissimus myocutaneous flap.

---

sular contracture may opt to have the implant removed followed by some type of flap. The latissimus myocutaneous flap is often used as a salvage procedure for a failed TRAM flap. Overall, the patient is almost always provided some type of reconstruction despite initial failures.

SELECTED READINGS

Brody GS: Safety and effectiveness in breast implants. In Spear SL (ed): Surgery of the Breast: Principles and Art. Philadelphia, Lippincott-Raven, 1998, pp 335–343.

Carlson GW, Bostwick J III, Styblo TM, et al: Skin-sparing mastectomy: Oncologic and reconstructive considerations. Ann Surg 1997;225:570.

Dowden RV: Selection criteria for successful immediate breast reconstruction. Plast Reconstr Surg 1991;88:628.

Elliot LF: Options for donor sites for autogenous tissue breast reconstruction. Clin Plast Surg 1994;21:177.

Kroll SS, Baldwin BB: A comparison of outcomes using three different methods of breast reconstruction. Plast Reconstr Surg 1992;90:455.

Moyer A, Salovey P: Psychosocial sequelae of breast cancer and its treatment. Ann Behav Med 1996;18:10.

Vasconez LO, Lejour M, Gamboa M: Atlas of Breast Reconstruction. Philadelphia, JB Lippincott, 1991.

Webster DJT, Mansel RE, Hughes LE: Immediate reconstruction of the breast after mastectomy. Is it safe? Cancer 1984;53:1416.

Yule GJ, Concannon MJ, Croll GH, Puckett CL: Is there liability with chemotherapy following immediate breast reconstruction? Plast Reconstr Surg 1996;97:969.

Skin and Soft Tissues

Chapter 155
General Evaluation and Biopsy of Cutaneous Lesions

David L. Brown and David J. Smith, Jr.

INTRODUCTION

The ability to evaluate and treat a variety of cutaneous lesions is essential to the armamentarium of the general surgeon. The simple skin biopsy is the foundation of the evaluation of cutaneous lesions and can be mastered with the understanding of a few basic principles.

CLINICAL PRESENTATION

Criteria for Biopsy of Skin Lesions

It has been well documented that clinical evaluation of cutaneous lesions, even among the most experienced practitioners, is inconsistent. In general, biopsy and pathologic examination of suspicious lesions is warranted to exclude malignancy, to establish a tissue diagnosis even for benign-appearing tumors, to allay patient concerns, to correlate the clinical evaluation of a dermatologic condition with a histologic diagnosis, and to evaluate the effect of treatment.

Pigmented lesions are particularly difficult to identify with absolute confidence clinically. To that end, common dictum states, "Any suspicious pigmented lesion should be presumed a melanoma until proven otherwise." Biopsy should be strongly considered for any newly developed pigmented lesion and for existing pigmented lesions that show evidence of the "ABCDs" (Asymmetry, irregular Borders, variegated Color, or Diameter greater than 6 mm). Additional factors raising suspicion include itching, bleeding, or nonhealing and recurrent ulcerative lesions. Because the Breslow depth, or tumor thickness in millimeters, is the single most important factor for predicting prognosis and guiding therapy options in the treatment of melanoma, any pigmented lesion should be diagnosed with an excisional or incisional full-thickness biopsy. Margins of 1 to 2 mm on the initial biopsy are usually adequate.

Nonpigmented lesions probably represent less aggressive malignancies (basal cell or squamous cell carcinomas) or benign processes (benign masses, inflammatory and vascular lesions). Their biopsy should be guided by correlation with clinical evaluation. Standard margins of excision for basal cell and squamous cell carcinomas are 5 and 10 mm, respectively. The morphea variant of basal cell carcinoma may require Mohs' chemosurgery excision.

PREOPERATIVE MANAGEMENT

Despite the minimally invasive and seemingly trivial nature of skin biopsy, a focused pertinent history should be elicited from the patient. Such relevant information includes a history of abnormal wound healing or bleeding tendency, diabetes mellitus, coronary artery and peripheral vascular disease, and hypertension. The need for prophylactic antibiotics due to mitral valve prolapse, rheumatic valve disease, or the presence of artificial joints, valves, and grafts should be addressed. Perioperative oral antibiotic therapy may be indicated in these conditions.

A thorough medication history is essential. A history of administration of anticoagulants, nonsteroidal anti-inflammatory drugs (NSAIDs), aspirin, and aspirin-containing products should be obtained. In most cases, minor cutaneous biopsy can be performed without discontinuation of these medications, provided that appropriate precautions are taken to ensure operative hemostasis.

Preoperative physical examination can often be focused but should include pulse and blood pressure measurements. Routine laboratory evaluation is superfluous, but in cases of thrombocytopenia with platelet counts less than 10,000/mm³ biopsy should be postponed.

INTRAOPERATIVE MANAGEMENT

Skin Preparation

Resident cutaneous flora consist mainly of gram-positive aerobes, anaerobes, and fungi. Less often, gram-negative microbes (*Klebsiella, Proteus,* and *Enterobacter* spp.) are present. A significant percentage of bacteria are located within hair follicles. If desired, electric hair clippers should be used around the operative site. The use of razors for shaving results in a higher incidence of postoperative wound infection.

Anesthesia

Lidocaine, in either 1% or 0.5% concentration, is widely utilized in cutaneous biopsy procedures. It is a member of the amide group of local anesthetics and exhibits an extremely low incidence of sensitization reactions. True allergic reactions are seen only with the ester group of local anesthetics, and most sensitizations to amides are due to the preservative found in multiple-use vials.

Administration of toxic levels must be avoided. Recommended maximal dosing of plain lidocaine is 4 mg/kg (7 mg/kg with epinephrine). A 1% solution contains 10 mg/mL; therefore, the maximal dose of 1% lidocaine with epinephrine is 50 mL in a 70-kg patient. The effects of lidocaine toxicity are seen mainly in the cardiac and central nervous systems. Patients should be counseled to alert the physician for the central nervous system symptoms of perioral numbness and tingling, lightheadedness, and tinnitus, which often preclude slurred speech, nystagmus, hallucinations, and seizures. Cardiac manifestations include atrioventricular block, ventricular arrhythmias, myocardial depression, and hypotension. Vigilance in looking for the manifestations of lidocaine toxicity is paramount.

Marcaine (bupivacaine HCl; epinephrine bitartrate) may be used, either in place of or in addition to lidocaine administration. It has a slower onset of anesthesia, but a significantly longer duration of effect. A mixture of lidocaine and Marcaine has the combined effect of rapid onset with long-lasting postoperative pain control and is quite useful in cutaneous biopsy surgery.

Epinephrine is typically added to stock solutions of 1% lidocaine in concentrations of 1:100,000. It can be extremely useful when one performs small, cutaneous procedures, particularly in highly vascular areas such as the face and scalp. In addition to providing a nearly bloodless operative field, it doubles the 90-minute effective duration of plain lidocaine. Classic teaching dictates that 5 to 7 minutes be allowed for an adequate vasoconstrictive effect prior to incision. Many physicians caution against the use of epinephrine in vascular end-organs, such as the fingers, toes, and penis. However, the safe use of epinephrine has been reported in these locations.

Pregnancy, acute-angle closure glaucoma, and hyperthyroidism are also relative contraindications to its use.

The main side effects of epinephrine include tachycardia and tachyarrhythmias; therefore, its use must be guarded in patients with hypertension and/or significant cardiovascular disease. One potentially dangerous combination is the induction of severe, uncontrollable hypertension and reflex bradycardia that can occur when epinephrine is used in patients taking a beta blocker (e.g., propranolol).

One should remember to *outline* the lesion to be excised *prior* to the infiltration of an epinephrine-containing solution, as blanching of the lesion and the surrounding skin tends to obscure margins.

Several techniques can be utilized to minimize the inherent discomfort of local anesthetic administration. A 27- or 30-gauge needle should be used, with the bevel oriented upward. Pinching the area of the skin to be injected augments slow injection speed. Stimulation of sensory pain fibers in the area by pinching partially blocks transmission of other painful stimuli (i.e., the needle stick and injection). In order to keep epinephrine stable in solution, the pH is lowered in the mixture with lidocaine. Bicarbonate can be added just prior to injection, in the ratio of 1:10, thereby increasing the pH of the solution and decreasing the pain of injection. Finally, EMLA cream (eutectic mixture of local anesthetic—a combination of lidocaine and prilocaine) can be applied to intact skin, and the skin covered with an occlusive dressing 60 to 90 minutes prior to injection. This maneuver is particularly useful in children.

General Biopsy Considerations

ORIENTATION OF BIOPSY. The orientation of the biopsy should be governed most by the factors that will maximize the available diagnostic information and optimize future treatment. Functional and aesthetic aspects are considered secondarily. Specific site considerations include potential distortion of nearby critical structures, particularly on the face, and contraction of underlying joints. A thorough knowledge of anatomy is paramount in performing a safe, effective biopsy.

Aesthetic concerns should also govern biopsy orientation, such as following relaxed skin tension lines (RSTLs), or Kraissl's lines (Fig. 155–1). Facial animation and joint movement can be used to demonstrate RSTLs. Often, it is practical to simply excise the lesion as a circle and observe the resulting orientation of the wound. The oval configuration can then be converted to a fusiform ellipse for would closure. Frequently, this minimizes the length of the resulting scar and maximizes the aesthetic orientation of the incision in the RSTLs.

BIOPSY LOCATION RELATIVE TO LESION. For representative sampling of inflammatory lesions, a mature lesion should be selected. Incisional biopsy specimens should include a portion of adjacent normal skin, the advancing margin, and the central zone. Subcutaneous fatty tissue should be included, as the lower dermis and upper fatty layer frequently show important histologic characteristics in dermatoses.

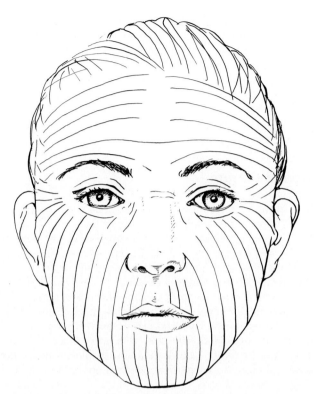

Figure 155–1. If possible, biopsies should be oriented along relaxed skin tension lines (RSTLs), or Kraissl's lines. Potential oncologic concerns should, of course, take precedence. Facial animation and joint movement can be used to demonstrate RSTLs.

Several methods of simple skin biopsy should be a part of any general surgeon's armamentarium. In choosing the most appropriate technique, a number of factors must be weighed, including lesion location, lesion morphology, and differential diagnostic possibilities.

Punch Biopsy

The punch biopsy is best utilized for the evaluation of inflammatory and neoplastic processes. The most commonly used punch sizes are 4 and 6 mm (diameter), and many sizes are available in reusable and disposable forms. One major limitation inherent in this technique is the possibility of sampling error due to the small specimen size. For example, punch biopsy of a cutaneous melanoma may yield inaccurate information regarding the most critical aspect of the diagnosis, the Breslow depth.

Several technical points warrant emphasis. Care should be taken not to crush the specimen when removing it from surrounding skin. "Spearing" the dermis with the small-bore needle used for the anesthetic is a useful maneuver. In many locations, such as the tip of the nose and the medial canthus, the wound can be left to heal secondarily without increased scarring, and without "dog-ears" or distortion of structures resulting from primary closure. When one closes the incision, *layered* closure is important, with both deep dermal and epidermal approximation, to avoid scar widening and dermal thinning. Typically, with single-layer closure, the resultant widening of the scar is equal to the width of the wound prior to epidermal closure. Both of these consequences of single-layer cutaneous closure have obvious aesthetic limitations.

Shave Biopsy

The shave biopsy is a controversial technique for routine use in a surgical practice. Its use demands precise clinical insight regarding the preoperative differential. It can be useful for evaluation of raised, superficial, or pedunculated nonpigmented lesions (i.e., verrucae, seborrheic keratoses, actinic keratoses). Shave biopsy is contraindicated, however, for inflammatory conditions and pigmented lesions in which there is even the faintest possibility of melanoma. This technique is best reserved for the dermatologist, who may be seeing a wider clinical array of cutaneous lesions, a higher percentage of which may be amenable to this type of diagnostic modality.

Fusiform Incisional and Excisional Biopsy

The term *fusiform,* rather than *elliptical,* is a better descriptor of the most commonly used and time-honored technique of cutaneous biopsy. It is the most widely applicable and diagnostically sound method for evaluation of skin lesions. Classically, a football-shaped excision is planned, with a length-to-width ratio of approximately 3:1, although tissue laxity in the area of the biopsy often permits shorter lengths. When designed with angles of 30 degrees at the ends, dog-ears are avoided (Fig. 155–2). Typical use involves excisional biopsy. When complete excision is not possible or preferred, however, the most suspicious section of the lesion should be sampled. In pigmented lesions, this is often the darkest and/or most elevated region.

The design can be altered, depending on site-specific needs (see Fig. 155–2). An **S**-plasty modification has the advantage of increasing the length of the scar between the two ends, making it particularly useful over convexities (i.e., the cheek or an extremity). Contraction of a straight-line scar in these areas may produce a depression, which creates undesirable highlights and shadowing, thereby drawing attention to the scar. An **S**-shaped scar is straightened by contraction and usually does not cause depression.

Meticulous attention to the standard principles of good surgical technique will ensure diagnostically accurate biopsy specimens, minimization of scarring potential, and

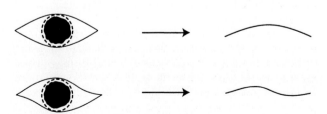

Figure 155–2. *A,* Fusiform excision. A 3:1 length-to-width ratio, with angles of 30 degrees at the ends, will typically avoid "dog-ears." *B,* For use over convexities, the design can be altered, creating an "S-plasty." The resulting scar is straightened by contracture, and it usually does not cause depression.

distortion of aesthetic and functional parameters. This includes minimizing the number of passes of the knife used to penetrate the dermis, avoiding pass-pointing, or cross-hatching, of the ends of the proposed excision and ensuring an even thickness of the excision. Undermining of the wound edges just beneath the dermis is rarely needed. When undermining is performed, it is essential to undermine the entire perimeter of the defect, or the ends may rise up over time as the result of scar contraction. As emphasized earlier, a *layered closure* is vital to adequate full-thickness reapproximation of the dermis, thus avoiding the consequences of scar widening and dermal thinning.

Hemostasis

Proper preoperative infiltration of the skin and subcutaneous tissues surrounding the biopsy site with an epinephrine-containing solution, as outlined earlier, will provide adequate hemostasis under most circumstances. Adjunctive control methods abound, and it is important to have several available.

PRESSURE. Direct application of pressure is the easiest and least destructive means of obtaining hemostasis in small cutaneous wounds. The temporary, mechanical occlusion of small bleeding vessels allows time for the mechanisms of clotting to take place. Firm, directed pressure should be applied for 5 to 10 minutes, and it can be incorporated into the design of the dressing.

ELECTROCOAGULATION. Electrocoagulation should be used sparingly in the routine of minor cutaneous biopsy. The process results in the destruction of local tissues and creates nonviable debris within the wound. Electrocautery is not a solution for oozing from dermal vessels, which is efficiently controlled by suture approximation of wound edges. It can, however, be indispensable when used for spot application to gain control of a larger vessel. Disposable battery-powered heat cauterizing units ("ophthalmic cauterizers") are not as efficacious but may prove useful in the ambulatory office setting. Hyfrecators are another alternative but provide poor assistance with coagulation of subcutaneous vessels compared with electrocautery.

TOPICAL AGENTS. Silver nitrate is useful as a chemical cauterizing agent, owing to its protein-denaturing effect. By its nature, it is also destructive to adjacent tissues. Patients should be alerted to its pain-provoking potential, often realized after leaving the office. Applicator sticks make spot-directed application simple. Ferric sulfate (Monsel's solution) also acts to denature protein. A significant drawback to its use is its deposition of pigment in the wound. Aluminum chloride (Drysol) causes protein precipitation and therefore also causes damage to nearby tissues, increasing risks of delayed wound healing. These agents can be quite useful in certain specific situations, such as curettage and shave biopsy. Their utility in excisional biopsy is limited.

Flap Closure

Flap closure of cutaneous defects following excisional biopsy permits removal of larger areas of skin, while reducing the complications of excessive wound tension and distortion of surrounding structures. The surgeon can raise small cutaneous flaps and use them to close defects, with a modest amount of knowledge of the concepts of flap dynamics and perfusion. A thorough description of cutaneous flap reconstruction is beyond the scope of this chapter. The application of cutaneous flaps should be performed only by surgeons comfortable with their design and technique.

Wound Closure

Skin closure preferences are as varied as surgeons themselves. The key to a solid cutaneous wound closure, aside from ensuring tension-free approximation of the wound edges, is a *layered closure* with *deep dermal approximation* (Fig. 155–3). Simple, superficial dermal or epidermal suture closure of wounds is problematic, as stated earlier. This method provides for a closure that is less strong and is prone to dehiscence, scar widening, and dermal thinning. An example of an adequate closure that promotes wound strength and favorable scar appearance involves 4-0 or 5-0 inverted deep dermal absorbable sutures. This should then be followed by epidermal approximation.

POSTOPERATIVE MANAGEMENT

Dressing

For the most part, the specific type of dressing used for cutaneous biopsy sites has little impact on the overall result. Dressings can be varied according to site and epidermal closure method. For example, closures performed with a "pull-out" stitch are conveniently dressed

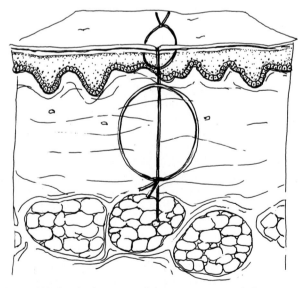

Figure 155–3. The key to a solid cutaneous wound closure, aside from ensuring tension-free approximation of the wound edges, is a *layered closure* with *deep dermal approximation*. An example of an adequate closure that promotes wound strength and favorable scar cosmesis involves inverted deep dermal absorbable sutures, followed by epidermal approximation.

with Steri-Strips. This keeps the exposed ends of the sutures protected and provides additional strength to the wound in the early healing period. Steri-Strips come in flesh tones for use on the face. Patients are instructed that they may get the strips wet, but they should not soak them. On the other hand, closures performed with interrupted epidermal sutures are expediently covered with antibiotic ointment, with or without a gauze dressing. Patients are instructed to wait 24 hours prior to getting the incision wet.

Suture Removal

The timing of suture removal strikes a balance between adequate healing for wound strength, and the creation of permanent stitch marks owing to suture track epithelialization. Classically, sutures on the face are removed by postoperative day 5. The intradermal closure permits early removal of surface sutures. The early removal time is based on the desire to avoid suture marks on this highly visible area, as well as the fact that the highly vascular tissues of the face heal rapidly.

Specimen Handling

The standard fixative and transport medium for specimens that will be submitted for permanent sectioning is 10% formalin, adjusted with phosphate buffer to pH 7.0. Container size should be relative to the size of the biopsy specimen, allowing for an approximately 20:1 fixative-to-specimen volume ratio. Preoperative suspicion regarding the need for specific pathologic procedures will avoid errors in processing technique. For example, if immuno-histochemistry, electron microscopy, special stains, or cultures are to be required on a specimen, individualized processing procedures must be followed when one submits samples to pathology. In these instances, preoperative consultation with a pathologist is recommended.

COMPLICATIONS

The most prevalent complications common to cutaneous biopsy include hematoma, infection, and dehiscence. Hematoma usually presents within the first 2 to 3 days postoperatively. Depending on the size and location, hematomas should usually be drained, through an opening in the incision. This will prevent distortion of adjacent structures, limit subcutaneous scar formation, eliminate a potential haven for bacterial seeding, and avoid hematoma-induced necrosis of overlying tissues. Generally, the incision can be reclosed after hematoma evacuation.

Infection is a rare occurrence following cutaneous biopsy. Its treatment is one of clinical discretion, ranging from observation to drainage and antibiotic therapy. Meticulous attention to proper surgical practices and sterile technique will significantly lower the incidence of biopsy-associated postoperative infections.

Wound dehiscence is also rare and is typically the result of infection or hematoma. Many uncomplicated wound dehiscences can be reclosed within 2 to 3 days of the original biopsy closure.

OUTCOMES

Most cutaneous lesions can be easily and safely biopsied according to the aforementioned guidelines. Meticulous adherence to standard surgical principles will maximize the benefit from the biopsy. Attention to details, such as orienting incisions within resting skin tension lines, and intradermal wound closure, will maximize the appearance of the resulting scar. Good results in each of these areas will improve patient care and satisfaction.

Pearls and Pitfalls

COMMON PROBLEMS AND PITFALLS

- Aesthetic and functional concerns should be considered secondarily to factors that will maximize diagnostic information and allow for optimal future therapy.
- Allow adequate time (7 minutes) for maximal hemostatic effect of epinephrine prior to making an incision.
- Use a *layered closure*. Single-layer closure, even of simple biopsy sites, results in undesirable scar formation.

PEARLS

- Add bicarbonate to local anesthetic in a 1:10 mixture and use a 27- or 30-gauge needle to minimize patient discomfort.
- Outline the lesion to be excised prior to the infiltration of an epinephrine-containing solution.
- Excise small lesions as circles, first. Remove "dog-ears" after ascertaining the direction in which the surrounding tissues tend to pull the defect. The resulting orientation (in RSTLs) and length of the scar will often be improved.
- Remove epidermal sutures on the face in 4 to 5 days to avoid excessive scarring.

COMMON ERRORS OF PRACTICE

- Beware of the inherent sampling error of the punch biopsy technique when diagnosing a lesion that is potentially a melanoma.
- The shave biopsy is an unacceptable technique for the diagnosis of a lesion that may have the faintest possibility of being a melanoma.

ANATOMIC CONSIDERATIONS, DANGER POINTS, ANATOMY

- Eyelids—fine iris scissors can often be used for excising lesions.
- Nose—a punch biopsy defect of as much as 4 mm can often be closed, with good cosmesis.
- Scalp—the incision should be angled in the direction of hair shafts, to avoid alopecia.
- Fingers—understanding the anatomy, particularly of neurovascular structures, is critical. The use of epinephrine is controversial.
- Face—a thorough knowledge of the anatomy of the facial nerve branches and superficial arterial arcade is essential.

SELECTED READINGS

Arca MJ, Bierman S, Johnson TM, Chang AE: Biopsy techniques for skin, soft-tissue, and bone neoplasms. Surg Clin North Am 1995;4:157.

Chang AE, Johnson TM, Rees RS: Cutaneous neoplasms. In Greenfield LJ (ed): Surgery: Scientific Principles and Practice. Philadelphia, Lippincott-Raven, 1997, pp 2231–2246.

Fisher J, Gingrass MK: Basic principles of skin flaps. In Georgiade GS (ed): Plastic, Maxillofacial, and Reconstructive Surgery. Baltimore, Williams & Wilkins, 1997, pp 19–28.

Marks MW: Basic principles of surgical techniques. In Georgiade GS (ed): Plastic, Maxillofacial, and Reconstructive Surgery. Baltimore, Williams & Wilkins, 1997, pp 10–12.

Smith DJ Jr, Chung KC, Robson MC: Wounds and wound healing. In Lawrence PF (ed): Essentials of General Surgery. Philadelphia, Lippincott–Williams & Wilkins, 2000, pp 113–122.

Chapter 156

Staging and Selection of Treatment Options for Melanoma

Julie R. Lange, Jeffrey E. Gershenwald, and Charles M. Balch

The incidence of melanoma has increased dramatically over the past four decades. Approximately 47,700 patients are diagnosed with invasive melanoma, and approximately 7700 patients die of melanoma each year in the United States. At the time of diagnosis, 80% to 85% of patients have stage I or II disease (localized disease only), 10% to 13% have stage III disease (regional disease), and 2% to 5% have stage IV disease (distant metastasis). All patients with stage I, II, or III melanoma require surgery. The goals of surgery in melanoma patients are local and regional control, nodal staging, and, in most cases, cure.

Knowing the prognostic factors and staging criteria that predict the risk of metastatic disease is crucial for determining the goals of surgery (cure, palliation, and staging) before one selects from among treatment options. Outcome for patients with melanoma is related to the stage. Fortunately, most melanoma patients are diagnosed at an early stage today and are usually curable with surgery alone. The type and extent of surgery required is determined by the stage at diagnosis. All patients with newly diagnosed primary melanoma require a wide excision of the surrounding skin for local control. With adequate wide local excision, local recurrence rates can be minimized. Patients with primary melanoma should also be considered for nodal staging. Sentinel node biopsy may be considered for many patients with newly diagnosed melanoma as a diagnostic procedure. This chapter reviews the diagnosis and evaluation of patients with melanoma, the current staging system, and the rationale for selecting treatment options.

CLINICAL PRESENTATION AND BIOPSY TECHNIQUES

Cutaneous melanoma can arise anywhere on the body. The most common site in women is the lower extremity, and the most common site in men is the back. Clinical features typical of melanoma include variegated color, irregular borders, and a history of a change in such a skin lesion. Some melanomas do not have typical features; some are nonpigmented and may resemble other dermatologic entities, such as basal cell carcinoma, squamous cell carcinoma, dermatofibroma, or seborrheic keratosis. The indications for biopsy of a suspicious skin lesion include the following: the presence of features considered to be typical for melanoma; a history of a change in a pre-existing skin lesion, such as an increase in size, change in color (often darkening), development of variegation; and a history of itching or bleeding. Individuals at particularly increased risk for melanoma are those with a prior

history of melanoma, a family history of melanoma, a high number (more than 20) of benign moles, atypical moles, or congenital nevi.

Proper biopsy of a suspicious lesion is critical to proper staging. The surgeon should perform a full-thickness biopsy on suspicious lesions in order to accurately interpret the maximal tumor thickness, the presence or absence of ulceration, and the level of invasion. Excisional biopsy with a narrow margin of normal-appearing skin for small lesions is preferred; this can be performed on most lesions up to 2 cm in diameter. Orientation of an excisional biopsy should be carefully considered. The biopsy scar should be oriented to be compatible with a subsequent wide local excision, should the lesion prove to be melanoma. On the extremities, a longitudinal or oblique incision is preferred. On the trunk or the head and neck, the biopsy should be oriented parallel to the skin lines.

Incisional biopsy—usually a punch biopsy—is appropriate for lesions that are large or that are at a vital anatomic site where one would want to know the diagnosis before removing the entire lesion. Patient survival and the risk of metastasis are not influenced by the type of biopsy. Incision into a melanoma does not promote dissemination. Incisional biopsy should be performed at the most raised area, but since it removes only part of a tumor, a repeat biopsy may be necessary if the histologic diagnosis does not agree with the clinical impression. Final determination of the tumor thickness cannot be made until the entire lesion has been excised and examined by the pathologist. Although punch biopsy is often appropriate, a shave biopsy of lesions suspicious for melanoma must be avoided because it may compromise the histologic interpretation and proper measurement of thickness.

At the time of diagnosis of primary melanoma, a number of clinical features and pathologic features are associated with prognosis. Some anatomic sites of the melanoma are associated with an increased risk of recurrence, especially those on the head and neck. Next in frequency of recurrence are trunk melanomas, and least common are extremity melanomas. Age is associated with a risk of recurrence, with patients older than 60 years of age at a greater risk than patients younger than 60. Tumor thickness remains the single most important prognostic feature of the primary melanoma. The presence of ulceration signifies a locally advanced tumor with a greatly increased risk of local, regional, and distant recurrence. The level of invasion into the dermis and the histologic growth pattern of the primary lesion have some prognostic significance. The most common types of cutaneous melanoma are the superficial spreading and nodular types,

Table 156–1	**Clinical and Pathologic Features of Primary Melanoma Associated with Risk of Metastasis**

CLINICAL FEATURES	METASTATIC RISK	COMMENT
Anatomic site		
Extremities	+	Except ALM°
Trunk	+ +	
Head and Neck	+ + +	Except LMM°
Age		
<60 years	+	Continuous variable of risk
>60 years	+ +	

PATHOLOGIC FEATURES	METASTATIC RISK	COMMENT
Tumor thickness	+/+ + +	Continuous variable of risk
Ulceration	+ + +	Locally advanced or poorly differentiated tumor
Level of invasion	+/+ + +	Especially important when deeply invasive, in thin lesions
Growth pattern°	+/+ + +	SSM and NM have the same prognosis, LMM lesions have a better prognosis, ALM and DM have a worse one
Number of metastatic nodes	+ +/+ + +	More than 3+ nodes have high risk

°ALM, acral lentiginous melanoma; DM, desmoplastic melanoma; LMM, lentigo maligna melanoma; NM, nodular melanoma; SSM, superficial spreading melanoma.

constituting more than 85% to 90% of all melanomas; these two types have approximately the same prognostic significance when they are matched for tumor thickness. Lentigo maligna melanoma has a better prognosis, whereas acral lentiginous melanoma and desmoplastic melanoma have a worse prognosis. Among all pathologic features, the status of the regional lymph nodes is the single most important prognostic feature. Table 156–1 summarizes the clinical and pathologic features associated with prognosis in patients with newly diagnosed melanoma.

NEW MELANOMA STAGING SYSTEM

Staging of melanoma combines the clinical and pathologic features of melanoma that best predict the survival outcome of the patient. Patients with a localized melanoma are categorized as stage I or II (depending on the thickness), those with regional metastases as stage III, and those with distant metastases as stage IV. New insights about the biology and natural history of melanoma have resulted in major revisions of the melanoma staging criteria. The value of knowing the staging system is that it enables the surgeon to group patients according to the risks of local and distant recurrences. Understanding how to predict outcome is vital for the surgeon when he or she is deciding on the extent of the initial evaluation and on appropriate treatment options, and interpreting results of clinical trials published in the literature.

The Melanoma Task Force of the American Joint Committee on Cancer (AJCC) has recently revised the melanoma staging system. These changes will be employed in 2002, and include the following: (1) melanoma thickness and ulceration, but not level of invasion (except for T1 melanomas), are to be used in the T classification; (2) the number of metastatic lymph nodes (rather than their largest dimension), and the delineation of microscopic versus macroscopic nodal metastases, are to be used in the N classification; (3) the site of distant metastases and elevated levels of serum lactate dehydrogenase (LDH) are included in the M classification; (4) all patients with stage I, II, or III disease should have their staging increased when the primary melanoma is ulcerated; (5) combining satellite metastases around a primary melanoma and in transit metastases into a single staging entity that is grouped into stage III disease; and (6) the physician should take into account the staging information gained from intraoperative lymphatic mapping and sentinel node biopsy.

Tumor thickness and ulceration are the two dominant prognostic factors of the primary lesion that best predict the risk of occult (microscopic) nodal and distant metastases.

The thickness of a melanoma (Breslow thickness, as measured with an ocular micrometer) is probably related to the rate of growth and/or the duration of a melanoma. The presence of ulceration (microscopic interruption of the surface epithelium by tumor) in a melanoma probably reflects a more aggressive biology of that melanoma. The risk of nodal and distant metastases increases linearly with the tumor thickness and is greater in all thickness groupings when the primary melanoma is ulcerated. In a prognostic factor analysis from the University of Texas M.D. Anderson Cancer Center and the Moffitt Cancer Center, thickness and ulceration were the two most powerful predictors of microscopic nodal metastasis detected by sentinel lymphadenectomy. The presence or absence of nodal metastasis was the most powerful predictor of survival.

For patients with stage III melanoma, the number of involved lymph nodes is the strongest predictor of outcome, regardless of whether the patient has macroscopic or microscopic nodal metastases. In all studies that have examined prognosis based on the number of metastatic nodes, patients with one metastatic node did better than did patients with two or more metastatic nodes. The secondary criterion for determining the N classification relates to tumor burden, as reflected by whether the nodal metastases are clinically detectable ("macroscopic") or clinically occult ("microscopic"). With the increased use of nodal staging with intraoperative lymphatic mapping and selective lymphadenectomy, a substantial number of patients are identified with clinically occult nodal disease. Patients with microscopic nodal involvement fare better than do those who have a therapeutic node dissection for clinically evident nodal metastases. Among patients with positive regional lymph nodes, ulceration of the primary lesion provides additional prognostic value and is incorporated in the new staging system. The TNM classification is displayed in Table 156–2. Stage groupings are in Table 156–3.

Table 156–2	Melanoma TNM Classification

T CLASSIFICATION	THICKNESS (mm)	ULCERATION STATUS
T1	1.0	a: w/o ulceration and level II/III b: with ulceration or level IV/V
T2	1.01–2.0	a: w/o ulceration b: with ulceration
T3	2.01–4.0	a: w/o ulceration b: with ulceration
T4	>4.0	a: w/o ulceration b: with ulceration

N CLASSIFICATION	NO. OF METASTATIC NODES	NODAL METASTATIC MASS
N1	1 node	a: micrometastasis° b: macrometastasis†
N2	2–3 nodes	a: micrometastasis° b: macrometastasis† c: in-transit metastasis(es)/satellite(s) without metastatic nodes
N3	Four or more metastatic nodes or matted nodes, or in-transit metastasis(es)/satellite(s), and metastatic node(s)	

M CLASSIFICATION	SITE	SERUM LDH
M1	Distant skin, SC or nodal metastases	Normal
M2	Lung metastases	Normal
M3	All other visceral metastases	Normal
	Or any distant metastases	Elevated

°Micrometastases are diagnosed after elective or sentinel lymphadenectomy.

†Macrometastases are defined as clinically detectable nodal metastases confirmed by therapeutic lymphadenectomy or when nodal metastases exhibit gross extracapsular extension.

From the AJCC website: *www.cancerstaging.org/initiatives/html*

Table 156–3	Stage Groupings for Cutaneous Melanoma

	*CLINICAL STAGING				†PATHOLOGIC STAGING		
0	Tis	N0	M0	0	Tis	N0	M0
IA	T1a	N0	M0	IA	T1a	N0	M0
IB	T1b	N0	M0	IB	T1b	N0	M0
	T2a	N0	M0		T2a	N0	M0
IIA	T2b	N0	M0	IIA	T2b	N0	M0
	T3a	N0	M0		T3a	N0	M0
IIB	T3b	N0	M0	IIB	T3b	N0	M0
	T4a	N0	M0		T4a	N0	M0
IIC	T4b	N0	M0	IIC	T4b	N0	M0
III	Any T	N1	M0	IIIA	T1–4a	N1a	M0
		N2			T1–4a	N2a	M0
		N3					
				IIIB	T1–4b	N1a	M0
					T1–4b	N2a	M0
					T1–4a	N1b	M0
					T1–4a	N2b	M0
					T1–4a/b	N2c	M0
				IIIC	T1–4b	N1b	M0
					T1–4b	N2b	M0
					Any T	N3	M0
IV	Any T	Any N	M1	IV	Any T	Any N	M1

*Clinical staging includes microstaging of the primary melanoma and clinical and/or radiologic evaluation for metastases. By convention, it should be used after complete excision of the primary melanoma with clinical assessment for regional and distant metastases.

†Pathologic staging includes microstaging of the primary melanoma and pathologic information about the regional lymph nodes after partial or complete lymphadenectomy. Pathologic stage 0 or stage 1A patients are the exception; they do not need pathologic evaluation of their lymph nodes.

From the AJCC website: *www.cancerstaging.org/initiatives/html*

PREOPERATIVE EVALUATION

Evaluation of the patient with newly diagnosed primary cutaneous melanoma should focus on a careful physical examination with attention toward the skin, regional nodal basins, and subcutaneous tissues. The primary site should be evaluated for the presence or absence of satellite lesions, and the biopsy scar should be inspected with planning of the subsequent surgical excision in mind. Subcutaneous tissues between the primary site and the draining node basins should be inspected and palpated for any evidence of in-transit lesions. The regional nodal basin should be palpated carefully for evidence of regional metastatic disease. Additionally, a thorough dermatologic evaluation is essential, since as many as 5% of patients with newly diagnosed melanoma will be found to have another dermatologic malignancy on careful inspection, which may be a second melanoma or a basal cell carcinoma or a squamous cell carcinoma.

In the absence of any physical findings or complaints suggestive of regional or distant metastatic disease, the initial evaluation should be limited to standard chest radiograph and liver function tests, including LDH. If these are normal, no further preoperative testing is warranted. Computed tomography (CT) scans, bone scans, and positron emission (PET) scans may be used selectively to evaluate patients with advanced melanoma (stage III or IV), but they are discouraged for patients with early-stage melanoma, as the diagnostic yield in these studies is extremely low. If results of the chest radiograph or blood tests are abnormal in patients with stage I or II melanoma, further studies, including CT scans, bone scan, magnetic resonance imaging (MRI), and PET scan, can be pursued as specifically indicated. For patients with questionable palpable adenopathy, ultrasound has been found to be of some value. Ultrasound can define the size and texture of regional lymph nodes and provide an imaging method for targeting with fine-needle aspiration.

The primary lesion should be reviewed by an experienced dermatopathologist to confirm the diagnosis and the microstaging. Microstaging with an ocular micrometer is routine in the measurement of maximal tumor thickness. The presence or absence of ulceration should be documented. Other features of the primary tumor worth noting include level of invasion, mitotic rate, degree of regression (if any), and presence of tumor-infiltrating lymphocytes. The pathologic report of the primary melanoma is the main document from which clinical decisions are made.

INDICATIONS FOR SENTINEL NODE BIOPSY

A rational alternative to elective lymph node dissection (ELND) in patients with clinically negative regional lymph node basins at the time of presentation has emerged over the past decade, and has already significantly altered the surgical approach to primary melanoma in most centers. Initially described by Morton and colleagues, this approach, termed *sentinel lymphadenectomy,* includes lymphatic mapping and sentinel lymph node biopsy. It is a highly accurate, minimally invasive method of identifying patients with primary melanoma who may have clinically occult nodal metastases. The technique is based on the now well-supported hypothesis that lymphatic metastases of melanoma follow an orderly progression through afferent lymphatic channels to sentinel lymph nodes before spreading into other regional, nonsentinel lymph nodes. Although initially sentinel lymph nodes were identified in approximately 80% of the patients who underwent the procedure, current rates approach 100% because of improvements in preoperative lymphoscintigraphy and intraoperative mapping techniques, including combined-modality intraoperative sentinel lymph node localization, which uses both dye and radiolabeled colloid.

Most experts recommend lymphatic mapping and sentinel lymphadenectomy as a staging procedure for patients with clinical stage I or II melanoma if their primary tumor is at least 1 mm thick, or, if it is less than 1 mm thick, when the tumor is ulcerated or is Clark's level IV or V. The lymph node status has important prognostic and clinical implications. Patients found to be node positive are then classified as having stage III melanoma and will require a therapeutic complete lymphadenectomy of that nodal basin and will be considered for systemic adjuvant therapy. Knowledge of the nodal status is also important for appropriate stratification of patients who are being considered for entry into a clinical trial.

It is essential that the decision to perform a sentinel node biopsy be made prior to the wide excision of the primary site, as the wide excision itself may make subsequent attempts at sentinel node biopsy unreliable. The accuracy of the sentinel node procedure has been documented only for patients who have not yet undergone wide excision. Sentinel node biopsy can potentially provide even more accurate staging information than that achievable by elective lymph node dissection because the limited pathologic specimen permits more complete assessment of these select lymph nodes, which are most likely to contain metastases, using more specialized pathologic techniques. In general, lymphatic mapping and sentinel node biopsy are used for most patients with T2, T3, or T4 melanomas (using the new staging criteria) and a clinically negative regional node basin because the morbidity is low and the information gained is valuable. In the event that sentinel node biopsy is unavailable or not technically feasible (e.g., because of prior wide excision), elective lymph node dissection may be considered in some patients with intermediate-thickness, nonulcerated melanoma.

RATIONALE FOR SURGICAL TREATMENT OPTIONS

Every primary melanoma requires a wide excision for local control. The magnitude of the surgical margin must be tailored to the tumor thickness and the anatomic location of the melanoma. While the main goal of wide excision is to decrease the risk of local recurrence, issues of cosmesis and function should also be considered. Decades ago, all melanomas were excised with a 4- to 5-cm margin. A series of prospective, randomized surgical trials have clearly shown that a reduced surgical excision is safe and appropriate for all primary melanomas. The World Health Organization (WHO) Melanoma Programme randomized 612 patients with primary melanoma less than 2 mm in thickness to be treated with either 1-cm or 3-cm margins. The two randomized groups did not differ significantly in either local recurrence rate or in 10-year survival rate. Only four local recurrences were reported, all of which were from primary melanomas between 1 and 2 mm that had been excised with a 1-cm margin. Thus, a 1-cm margin is recognized as an appropriate margin for all T1 (<1 mm) melanomas.

The Intergroup Melanoma Surgical Trial randomized 740 patients with intermediate-thickness melanomas (1.0 to 4.0 mm) in order to prospectively determine whether a 2-cm radial margin of excision is equivalent to a 4-cm radial margin with respect to survival and local recurrence rates. Patients with melanomas located on a trunk or a proximal extremity (N = 468) were randomized to receive either a 2- or 4-cm excision margin. A separate group of patients (N = 272) with head and neck or distal extremity primaries were treated with 2-cm excision margins.

Patients assigned to 2-cm margin were much less likely to require a skin graft and experienced no diminution in overall survival or local recurrence rates compared with patients who had a 4-cm surgical excision. Ulceration of the primary lesion was associated with a dramatic increase in local recurrence rates. Among all the patients randomized, the recurrence rates were 6.6% for ulcerated melanomas versus 1.1% for nonulcerated melanomas. Thus, for intermediate-thickness melanoma (T2 and T3), wide excision with 2-cm margin is appropriate.

No randomized studies have ever been done to evaluate appropriate margins for T4 (>4 mm) melanomas. A retrospective study at the University of Texas M.D. Anderson Cancer Center showed no difference in local recurrence rates or survival in patients with T4 melanoma who had excision with a radial margin less than or equal to 2 cm compared with those who underwent excision with a radial margin wider than 2 cm. Thus, there appears to be no advantage in margins wider than 2 cm for patients with thick melanoma.

Most wide local excisions can be performed as an elliptical excision with primary closure. Excision is carried down to—but not through—the underlying muscle fascia in most patients. In extremely obese patients, the depth need not be all the way to the muscular fascia, but it should be at least to the superficial fascia. Primary closure is often facilitated by a length-to-width ratio approximately 3:1. The closure is usually accomplished by a standard advancement flap, although occasionally either rotational flaps or a split-thickness skin graft may be necessary for coverage of the defect. On the trunk and the head and neck, the direction of the long axis of the wide local excision usually should be parallel to the skin lines. On an extremity, the orientation should be either longitudinal or somewhat oblique in order to facilitate closure and cosmesis. When a split-thickness skin graft is used to cover the defect, the skin graft donor site should be preferentially chosen outside the area of any potential

Table 156–4	**Recommended Surgical Margins for Primary Melanoma**

THICKNESS OF PRIMARY TUMOR	RADIAL EXCISION MARGIN
Melanoma in situ	5 mm
<1 mm	1 cm
1–2 mm	1 or 2 cm*
2–4 mm	2 cm
≥4 mm	≥2 cm

*A 2-cm margin is preferable, but 1 cm may be acceptable in anatomically restricted areas.

in-transit metastases. Guidelines for wide local excision of a primary melanoma are summarized in Table 156–4. These guidelines may sometimes need to be modified, based on specific clinical situations such as the location of the primary lesion. Table 156–5 displays a decision tree for the surgical management of stage I and II melanoma.

In all patients with resectable regional disease (positive regional nodes or limited in-transit lesions), surgical resection should be pursued for regional control and possible cure. Those with positive nodes should have a formal, anatomic lymphadenectomy; limited in-transit lesions should be excised to a negative margin. For patients with stage IV disease, surgery is usually limited to palliation of specific, symptomatic lesions, although there are rare reports in the literature of prolonged survival following resection of solitary metastatic lesions. Clinical trials of systemic therapy are encouraged for patients with stage III and stage IV disease. Table 156–6 displays a decision tree for the management of stage III and IV melanoma.

FOLLOW-UP

The risk of recurrence in patients with surgically treated melanoma is related to the pathologic features of the melanoma at its presentation, especially tumor thickness, presence of ulceration, and presence of nodal metastases. Common sites of melanoma recurrence are near the primary excision site and the regional nodal basin. Common sites of distant recurrences include cutaneous and subcutaneous sites distant from the primary, distant lymph nodes, and the lung. Less commonly, first relapses may involve the liver, brain, or bone. Melanoma can have an unpredictable metastatic pattern and can spread to unusual sites, such as the gastrointestinal tract and thyroid gland. For most patients with surgically treated stage I, II, or III disease, recommended follow-up is primarily with periodic history taking and physical examination. It has not been documented that routine radiologic tests and screening blood tests improve survival, but they may be ordered at the discretion of the treating physician.

While most recurrences occur within the first 2 to 3 years after diagnosis, late recurrences (even after 10 years) can occur. There is no clear evidence that structured follow-up of patients with treated melanoma will change outcome. However, routine surveillance may allow earlier detection of disease recurrence, when it is more

| Table 156–5 | **Surgical Options for Clinically Localized (Stage I and II) Melanoma** |

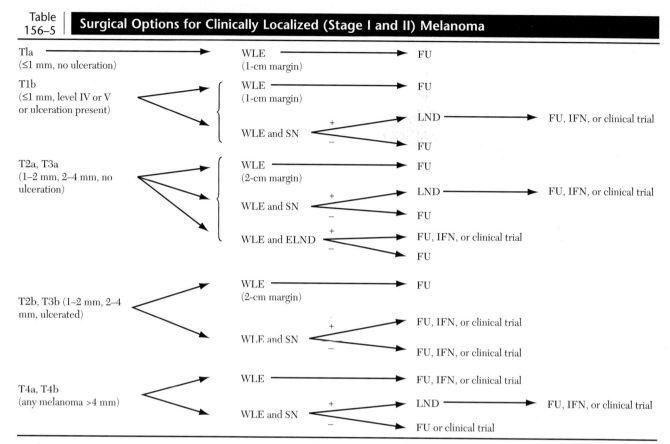

Clinical trial, adjuvant systematic therapy in a prospective clinical trail; ELND, elective lymph node dissection; FU, routine folllow-up for metastatic melanoma; IFN, interferon–alfa-2B; LND, lymph node dissection; SN, sentinel node lymphadenectomy after lymphatic mapping; WLE, wide local excision of primary melanoma.

| Table 156–6 | **Surgical Options for Metastatic Melanoma (Stage III or IV)** |

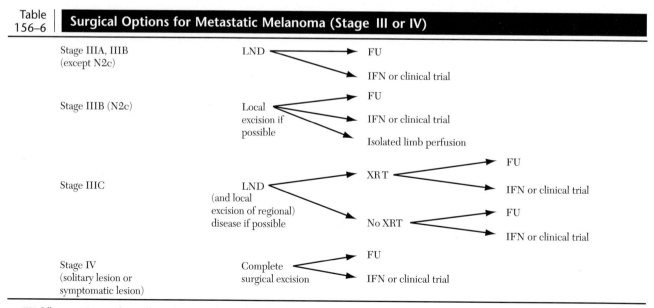

FU, follow-up; IFN, interferon–alfa-2B; LND, lymph node dissection; XRT, radiation therapy.

Pearls and Pitfalls

PEARLS

- Biopsy of lesions suspicious for melanoma must be full-thickness.
- In the absence of symptoms or signs of metastatic disease, the preoperative evaluation of a patient newly diagnosed with melanoma should be limited to physical examination, chest radiograph, and serum liver function tests, including lactate dehydrogenase.
- The measured tumor thickness, the presence or absence of ulceration on histologic review, and the number of metastatic lymph nodes are the most important prognostic features of melanoma.
- Indications for sentinel node biopsy include primary invasive melanoma at least 1 mm in thickness, with no evidence of regional or distant metastases, or primary melanoma less than 1 mm with ulceration or level IV or V.
- Sentinel node biopsy should always be done before the wide local excision.
- The margin of excision around a primary melanoma should be a 1-cm radial margin for melanomas less than 1 mm, and a 2-cm margin for all thicker melanomas whenever anatomically feasible.

likely to be surgically resectable. Appropriate follow-up schedules for patients who have surgically resected disease are based on the initial staging. One reasonable schedule is the following: for patients with a thin primary melanoma and negative nodes, clinical examination for evidence of recurrence every 6 to 12 months for the first 2 years, and then annually; for patients with intermediate or thick melanomas and negative regional nodes, follow-up examination should be every 4 to 6 months for the first 2 to 3 years and every 6 to 12 months for the next 2 to 3 years, then annually; and for patients with resected regional disease, follow-up should be every 3 to 4 months for the first 2 years, and then every 6 months up to year 5, and then yearly. All patients need routine lifelong dermatologic screening. Patients with a history of melanoma remain at higher than average risk for a second primary melanoma and are also at risk for other cutaneous malignancies.

SELECTED READINGS

Albertini J, Cruse C, Rappaport D, et al: Intraoperative radiolymphoscintigraphy improves sentinel lymph node identification for patients with melanoma. Ann Surg 1996;223:217.

Balch CM: Cutaneous melanoma: Prognosis and treatment results worldwide. Semin Surg Oncol 1992;8:400.

Balch CM: Randomized surgical trials involving elective node dissection for melanoma. Adv Surg 1999;32:255.

Balch CM, Buzaid AC, Soong SJ, et al: Final version of the AJCC staging system for cutaneous melanoma. J Clin Oncol 2001. In press.

Balch CM, Houghton AN, Sober AJ, Soong S: Cutaneous Melanoma. St. Louis, Quality Medical Publishing, 1998.

Balch CM, Soong S: Long-term results of a multi-institutional randomized trial comparing prognostic factors and surgical results for intermediate thickness melanomas (1.0 to 4.0 mm). Intergroup Melanoma Surgical Trial. Ann Surg Oncol 2000;7:87.

Gershenwald JE, Colome MI, Lee JE, et al: Patterns of recurrence following a negative sentinel lymph node biopsy in 243 patients with stage I or II melanoma. J Clin Oncol 1998;16:2253.

Gershenwald JE, Thompson W, Mansfield PF, et al: Multi-institutional melanoma lymphatic mapping experience: The prognostic value of sentinel lymph node status in 612 stage I or II melanoma patients. J Clin Oncol 1999;17:976.

Gershenwald J, Tseng C-H, Thompson W, et al: Improved sentinel lymph node localization in primary melanoma patients with the use of radiolabeled colloid. Surgery 1997;124:203.

Heaton KM, Sussman JJ, Gershenwald JE, et al: Surgical margins and prognostic factors in patients with thick (>4 mm) primary melanoma. Ann Surg Oncol 1998;5:322.

Krag D, Meijer S, Weaver D, et al: Minimal-access surgery for staging of malignant melanoma. Arch Surg 1995;130:654.

Morton D, Wen D, Wong J, et al: Technical details of intraoperative lymphatic mapping for early stage melanoma. Arch Surg 1992;127:392.

POO-HWU WJ, Ariyan S, Lamb L, et al: Follow-up recommendations for patients with American Joint Committee on Cancer Stages I–III malignant melanoma. Cancer 1999;86:2252.

Veronesi U, Cascinelli N: Narrow excision (1-cm margin): A safe procedure for thin cutaneous melanoma. Arch Surg 1991;126:438.

Technique and Application of Sentinel Lymph Node Biopsy in Melanoma and Breast Cancer

Douglas Reintgen, Rosemary Giuliano, Ni Ni Ku, Claudia Berman, and Charles Cox

An epidemic of melanoma exists in the United States, and breast cancer is one of the most common malignancies that makes up a large part of most surgeons' practices. Melanoma is a tumor that affects individuals who are young and in the most productive years of their lives, constituting a major public health problem. The numbers for breast cancer show that 186,000 new cases are diagnosed each year in the United States.

The care of patients with melanoma has changed in the last 5 years with the development of new lymphatic mapping techniques that reduce the cost and morbidity of nodal staging, the emergence of more sensitive assays for occult melanoma metastases, and the identification of interferon alfa-2b as an effective adjuvant therapy for the treatment of patients with melanoma who are at high risk for recurrence.

Breast cancer was one of the first tumors for which adjuvant therapy was found to be beneficial and nodal staging was considered to be important. However, complete axillary node dissection has significant morbidity, and physical complaints due to the dissection are what women voice most often after undergoing breast cancer surgery.

Lymphatic mapping and sentinel node biopsy for melanoma and breast cancer have the potential to be a more conservative operation that will produce less morbidity but also will provide a mechanism for more accurate staging. This chapter explores the technical points of this new technology.

LYMPHATIC MAPPING AND SENTINEL LYMPH NODE BIOPSY FOR MELANOMA

A new procedure has been developed to assess the status of the regional lymph nodes more accurately and decrease patient morbidity and the cost to the health care system of a complete elective lymph node dissection (ELND). The technique, termed *intraoperative lymphatic mapping and selective lymphadenectomy*, relies on the concept that regions of the skin have specific patterns of lymphatic drainage not only to the regional lymphatic basin but also to a specific lymph node (sentinel lymph node, SLN) in the basin. Morton initially proposed the technique (*Archives of Surgery*, and *Surgical Oncology Clinics of North America*) using a vital blue dye method and showed that in animals and initial human trials, the SLN is the first node in the lymphatic basin into which the primary melanoma consistently drains. With the blue dye method, the surgeon gets a visual clue as to where these first nodes in the chain of lymphatics are located. Morton hypothesized that defined patterns of lymphatic drainage allow determination of the first node in the basin that receives lymphatic flow from the primary site. He went on to state that the absence of metastatic melanoma in the SLN will accurately reflect the absence of metastatic melanoma in the remaining regional lymph nodes. Complete nodal staging could be obtained with an SLN biopsy.

Results of Melanoma Mapping

In Morton's initial report, he and his colleagues identified the SLN in 194 of 237 lymphatic basins and found that 40 specimens (21%) contained metastatic melanoma detectable by routine histologic examination with hematoxylin and eosin (H&E) stains (12%) or only by immunohistochemical staining (9%). Metastases were present in 47 of 259 (18%) SLNs, while non-SLNs were the exclusive site of metastases in only 2 of 3079 nodes from 194 dissections, a false-negative rate of 1%. Only 1 SLN drained a particular primary site in 72% of basins. Two SLNs were found in 20% of the basins, and 8% of the basins contained 3 or more SLNs. The success rate in SLN identification ranged from 72% to 96%, depending on where the surgeon was on the "learning curve." This new technique accurately identified patients with occult lymph node metastases who might have benefited from radical lymphadenectomy (Morton et al, 1992a, 1992b).

These data have been confirmed by numerous other institutions, including the Moffitt Cancer Center (MCC) (Reintgen et al, 1994), M.D. Anderson Cancer Center (Ross et al, 1993), the Sidney Melanoma Unit (SMU) (Thompson et al, 1995), and the University of Vermont (Krag et al, 1995, 1995). These studies have confirmed an orderly progression of melanoma nodal metastases. The data from these surgical trials for patients with melanoma demonstrated that the pattern of nodal metastases from cutaneous primary sites is not random. The SLNs in the lymphatic basins can be individually identified, and they reflect the presence or absence of melanoma metastases in the remainder of the nodal basin.

With the addition of intraoperative radiolymphoscintigraphy to vital blue dye lymphatic mapping (Krag et al,

1995; Albertini et al, 1996; Essner et al, 1994), the SLN localization becomes easier and more widely applicable. In the initial study from MCC that combined the vital blue dye and radiocolloid mapping technique, 450 μCi of technetium-labeled sulfur colloid was used with the standard isosulfan blue and injected at the site of the primary cutaneous melanoma. A nuclear probe (Navigator, USSC, Norwalk, CT) was used to trace lymphatic channels from the primary site to lymph nodes in the regional lymphatic basin.

This study consisted of 106 consecutive patients with cutaneous melanoma larger than 0.76 mm at all primary site locations. A total of 200 SLNs and 142 neighboring nonsentinel nodes (non-SLN) were harvested from 129 basins in 106 patients. When the sentinel lymph node biopsy was correlated with the vital blue dye mapping, 70% of the SLNs demonstrated blue dye staining while 84% of SLNs were defined as being "hot" by radioisotope localization. With the use of both intraoperative mapping techniques, identification of the SLN was possible in 96% of the nodal basins sampled. Micrometastases were identified in SLNs in 15% of the patients by routine histology, while 2 patients had micrometastatic disease in "hot," but not blue-stained, nodes. These data suggest that the radiocolloid localization identifies more SLNs, some of which are clinically important because they contain micrometastatic disease. MCC has the experience of doing more than 2000 mappings in patients with melanoma and has achieved a success rate of identification of the SLN in 99%. With a mean follow-up of 3 years, the risk of nodal recurrence after a negative SLN biopsy is less than 1%.

A National Cancer Institute (NCI)–sponsored prospective trial is currently being performed that randomizes patients to receive either wide local excision (WLE) of the primary melanoma site versus WLE and SLN biopsy of the regional lymphatic basins at risk for metastases. The end-point of the study is whether this surgical strategy can extend the survival of the melanoma patient. The study is different from the previous randomized trials that addressed the efficacy of ELND because only a percentage of the patients with melanomas larger than 1.0 mm received a complete node dissection. Survival data from this trial are not expected to be available until 2001.

The other national trial examining the role of this new procedure is the industry-sponsored Sunbelt Melanoma Trial (SBMT). Sixty institutions across the country are participating, equally divided between university centers and community hospitals. Again, patients with melanomas at least as thick as 1.0 mm are undergoing lymphatic mapping and SLN harvest. The SLN are examined with routine histology, serial sections, and immunohistochemical staining. If the SLN is negative on initial screening, a more sensitive reverse transcriptase–polymerase change reaction (RT-PCR) assay based on a panel of four melanoma-specific markers is performed. This study evaluates in a multicenter setting the clinical relevance of the up-staging that can occur with more sensitive methods of identifying occult metastatic disease. In addition, the role of interferon alfa-2b in patients with microscopic nodal disease is being investigated.

Technical Details

Lymphoscintigraphy has been shown to be of assistance in predicting lymphatic basins at risk for the development of metastatic disease in patients with cutaneous malignant melanoma (Norman et al, 1991). The preoperative lymphoscintigraphy serves as a road map for the surgeon and is used for four distinct reasons in the planning of the surgical procedure. These include the following:

1. To identify all nodal basins at risk for metastatic disease (Fig. 157–1)
2. To identify any in-transit nodes that can be tattooed by the nuclear medicine colleague for later harvesting (in-transit metastases occur in 5% of the melanoma population and may, by definition, be considered the SLN)
3. To identify the location of the SLN in relation to the rest of the nodes in the basin (Godellas et al, 1995)
4. To estimate the number of SLNs in the regional basin that will need to be harvested

The timing of the injection of the mapping reagents is critical to the success of the procedure. Some compounds like the vital blue dye travel to the regional basin very quickly within a matter of minutes, while most radiocolloids are concentrated over hours in the SLN. Localization ratios for technetium 99m sulfur colloid are greatest 2 to 24 hours after injection, accomplishing three points that are helpful to the surgeon. The increased ratios (hot spot/background ratio, SLN versus neighboring non-SLN) allow for easier localization. The prolonged retention in the SLN or SLNs permits the radiocolloid to be injected by a nuclear radiologist hours prior to the actual operation. Accordingly, the actual injection can be performed in the nuclear medicine area, and surgeons do not need special licenses for handling of radioactive material. Finally, scheduling of cases becomes more convenient, as

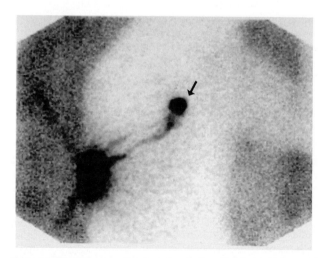

Figure 157–1. Preoperative lymphoscintigraphy in a patient with an "intermediate-thickness" melanoma of the back. A total of 450 μCi of technetium 99m sulfur colloid in injected into the skin around the primary melanoma. The colloid is taken up by the cutaneous lymphatics and deposited and concentrated in the SLN (arrow). If this node is negative for metastases, the basin should be staged node negative.

there is a period of time (2 to 24 hours after injection of the radiocolloid) in which the intraoperative mapping can be easily accomplished.

All lymphatic basins at risk for metastatic spread, in-transit nodes, and the SLNs in the regional basin are identified and marked for harvesting. The patient is then taken to the operating room 4 to 24 hours later and 1 mL (per direction of drainage) of 1% Lymphazurin is injected around the primary site. After prepping and draping the primary site and regional basin and allowing 10 minutes for the vital blue dye to travel to the SLN, attention is directed initially to the regional basin. With the hand-held Gamma probe, the hot spot in the regional basin is identified and the hot spot/background ratio is noted. If "shine-through" from the primary site is a problem, WLE of the primary may be performed first. Surgical dissection is aided both by visualization of the stained afferent lymphatic down to the blue-stained node and by a directed dissection with the use of the hand-held Gamma probe down to the SLN. The SLN is identified and removed with sharp or electrocautery dissection. The entire SLN is removed, and afferent and efferent lymphatics from the SLN, some of which are identified with blue staining, are controlled with hemoclips (Fig. 157–2), since the electrocautery does not seal lymphatics. This technique decreases the chance of postoperative wound seroma.

The excised SLN is checked with the Gamma probe (Fig. 157–3) to ascertain whether it is radioactive in order to correctly identify it as the SLN. The radioactivity in the basin is checked with the Gamma probe after removal of the SLN to ensure that all SLNs have been removed. If radioactivity has not decreased to the level of the background, the use of the hand-held Gamma probe to direct additional dissection minimizes unnecessary flaps that are created when one is looking for additional blue-stained afferent lymphatics.

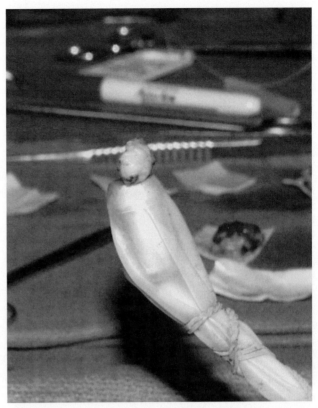

Figure 157–3. Ex vivo, the SLN is checked for counts of radioactivity to ensure that the correct node has been removed.

Lymphatic mapping and SLN biopsy is routinely performed for melanomas larger than 0.76 mm in thickness.

LYMPHATIC MAPPING IN BREAST CANCER

For most solid tumors, the most powerful and predictive prognostic factor is the status of the regional nodes. For breast cancer, the presence of regional metastases decreases 5-year survival approximately 28% to 40% (Haagensen, 1977; Bonadonna, 1989). Many prognostic factors for breast cancer have been defined on the basis of the primary tumor, and yet in regression analysis they add very little to prognostic models once lymph node status is considered.

The ability to limit the full axillary lymph node dissection to only women with documented nodal metastases would be a major advance in the surgical treatment of women with breast cancer.

Technique of Lymphatic Mapping for Breast Cancer

Lymphoscintigraphy is performed in women with breast cancer in a fashion similar to that with melanoma, except for the fact that the radiocolloid is injected into the breast parenchyma around the primary tumor. Larger volumes of radiocolloid are used, with the same amount of radioactivity as that used for melanoma (450 μCi in 6-mL vol-

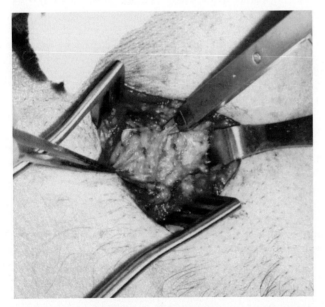

Figure 157–2. A blue-stained afferent lymphatic is identified draining into a blue-stained node. Afferent lymphatics are being clipped to prevent postoperative seroma formation.

ume), owing to the fact that the breast lymphatics are not as rich as the cutaneous lymphatics. Massage is used to drive the mapping agents into the lymphatics by increasing interstitial pressure.

What occurs in nuclear medicine directly influences the success rate of the surgeon in finding the axillary SLN. The radiocolloid injection needs to be diffuse enough around the tumor so that the mapping agent has a chance of being taken up by the breast lymphatics. For patients with mammographically detected tumors, localization wires (either mammographically or ultrasound directed) are placed, and with mammograms available so that the surgeon can judge the depth of the injection or with ultrasound guidance the radiocolloid is injected around the wire and the tumor. No injection is performed through the localization needle, since the needle will act as a wick for the radiocolloid to come back and possibly contaminate the skin. For women with palpable tumors, the injection is straightforward and placed tightly around the circumference of the tumor. Patients who have had an excisional biopsy are injected with ultrasound direction so that the radiocolloid is placed in the breast parenchyma around the biopsy cavity. If the radiocolloid is placed in the tumor or biopsy cavity, it will not migrate. The timing of the injection of the radiocolloid is not as critical, as long as a period of time is allowed between the injection and the SLN harvest for the mapping agent to migrate into the SLN (2 to 24 hours).

Lymphoscintigraphy in women with breast cancer can be used to identify women who show drainage from their primary tumors bidirectionally into the axilla and internal mammary nodes. In this circumstance, one may select these women for inclusion of the internal mammary nodes in their radiation ports after the lumpectomy, or the SLNs in this location can be harvested.

The technique followed for intraoperative lymphatic mapping and SLN identification in breast cancer patients is similar to that previously reported for melanoma patients. Patients come to the operating room 2 to 24 hours after the injection of the radiocolloid in the nuclear medicine suite. The technique involves a peritumor injection of an average 450 μCi of filtered (0.2-μm filter) technetium sulfur colloid. For palpable tumors, isosulfan blue 1% dye (Lymphazurin, 5 mL) is injected around the circumference of the primary tumor in the operating room 10 to 15 minutes prior to the surgical procedure. For nonpalpable cancers, the tumor is localized in radiology with a wire, the radiocolloid injected around the localization wire, and the wire left in place for guidance for the subsequent vital blue dye injection. After the vital blue dye is injected, the breast is massaged for 5 minutes to facilitate migration of the mapping agents.

A hand-held, Gamma-detection probe is used to assist in SLN detection. The probe is used prior to making a skin incision to identify the area of greatest activity in the axilla in counts per second. Isobar levels of radioactivity are drawn emanating from the primary site, and hot spots of radioactivity are marked along each one of these isobars. This is possible if there is good separation in space between the primary site and the regional basin. If possible, the afferent lymphatic is mapped leading to a hot spot in the axilla where the SLN is located. A small axillary incision (2 to 4 cm) is made over the hot spot, the dissection is directed with the hand-held Gamma probe through the axillary fat, and the SLN is identified. Ideally, this SLN should be hot and blue. If a cluster of nodes is encountered, the vital blue dye facilitates the determination of which one in the cluster is the SLN. It is reasonable to remove a neighboring non-SLN in order to have an internal control for radioactive counts. Ratios of activity (SLN/background in vivo, SLN/neighboring non-SLN ex vivo) are generated to ensure that the node removed fulfills the criteria of an SLN. Careful dissection is used to identify the blue-stained afferent lymphatics, and these lymphatics can be followed to the SLN or SLNs that stained a pale blue. Surgeons take advantage of the fact that the afferent lymphatics may be visualized by clipping or tying them, since the Bovie knife does not seal lymphatics.

The SLN is defined if it meets one of the following three criteria: the node is blue, the node has a blue-stained afferent lymphatic leading to it, or the node has an appropriate ratio of radioactivity. Occasionally, the SLN may be full of tumor, and one will see a dilated blue-stained lymphatic leading to such a node, but the node may not take up the dye or the radiocolloid readily. The mean number of axillary SLNs removed for breast lymphatic mapping is 2.0 per patient.

Results of Lymphatic Mapping for Breast Cancer from MCC

Over the last 5 years, lymphatic mapping and SLN harvest has been performed on 1356 women with breast cancer at MCC. With the use of a combination radiocolloid and vital blue dye technique, the success rate of finding an axillary SLN is 96.0%. The incidence of positive SLNs is 28.6%. On completion lymph node dissection (CLND) after a positive SLN, 39.9% of the patients had higher nodes involved with tumor. A total of 9.2% of the so-called histologic negative population is found to have micrometastatic disease with more sections of the SLN and cytokeratin staining. In the initial part of the trial when a concomitant CLND was being performed with a SLN harvest, there was one skip metastasis, in a patient who had a previous excisional biopsy. With a mean follow-up of 20 months and following 809 patients who had a negative SLN biopsy without a CLND, there has been no axillary recurrences. More follow-up is needed, but the initial results of the series are encouraging. Armando Giuliano, (personal communication), from the John Wayne Cancer Center, has had a similar experience with more than 500 women being followed after a negative SLN biopsy without a single axillary recurrence.

A number of national multicenter protocols are examining the role of SLN biopsy in the care of the woman with breast cancer. The American College of Surgeons (ACS) has instituted a trial in which women with invasive breast cancers undergo lymphatic mapping and SLN biopsy. If the SLN is negative, patients are observed and a blinded cytokeratin analysis is performed. If the SLN is positive, patients are randomized to receive either CLND or observation of their regional basin. It is assumed that

Pearls and Pitfalls

PEARLS

- Use the proper vital blue dye (1% isosulfan blue solution)—it has the correct particle size to be taken up by the lymphatics, does not diffuse passively through the tissues to a great extent, and is trapped in the first node in the basin.
- Use the proper radiocolloid—an unfiltered or filtered radiocolloid (technetium sulfur colloid) is key, since it is trapped and concentrated by the reticulum and dendritic cells of the SLN.
- For breast lymphatic mapping, make sure of a diffuse injection into the breast parenchyma around the tumor. Follow this with 5 minutes of intense massage to increase interstitial pressure and drive the mapping agents into the lymphatics. The timing is critical.
- A detailed pathology examination of the SLN should include serial sections and immunohistochemical staining.

all these women will receive appropriate radiation therapy to the breast and postoperative adjuvant therapy. The end-points of this trial are to define the role of CLND in women with invasive breast cancer and to begin to examine the clinical relevance of upstaging with IHC.

The NSABP and Dr. David Krag of the University of Vermont have started a trial that will randomize patients with invasive breast cancers who are undergoing breast preservation to either SLN biopsy versus SLN biopsy with concomitant CLND.

Summary

- Lymphatic mapping and SLN biopsy requires good collaboration between practitioners of nuclear medicine, surgery, and pathology.
- The true advantage of SLN biopsy is the ability of the surgeon to give the pathologist the nodes from the

basin most likely to contain disease. The pathologist can perform a more detailed examination of the SLN, resulting in more accurate staging.

- SLN biopsy identifies metastatic disease in patients who are determined to be node negative with routine methods. The clinical relevance of this upstaging is being determined in clinical trials.

SELECTED READINGS

Albertini J, Cruse CW, Rapaport D, et al: Intraoperative radiolymphoscintigraphy improves sentinel lymph node identification in melanoma patients. Ann Surg 1996;223:217.

Bonadonna G: Karnofsky Memorial Lecture. Conceptual and practical advances in the management of breast cancer. J Clin Oncol 1989;7:1380.

Essner R, Foshag L, Morton D: Intraoperative Radiolymphoscintigraphy: A Useful Adjunct to Intraoperative Lymphatic Mapping and Selective Lymphadenectomy in Patients with Clinical Stage 1 Melanoma. 48th Cancer Symposium, Society of Surgical Oncology, Houston, 1994. [Abstract.]

Godellas CV, Berman C, Lyman G, et al: The identification and mapping of melanoma regional nodal metastases: Minimally invasive surgery for the diagnosis of nodal metastases. Am Surg 1995;61:97.

Haagensen CD: Treatment of curable carcinoma of the breast. Int J Radiat Oncol Biol Phys 1977;2:975.

Krag DN, Meijer SJ, Weaver DL, et al: Minimal-access surgery for staging of melanoma. Arch Surg 1995;130:654.

Krag D, Meijer S, Weaver D, et al: Minimal Access Surgery for Staging Regional Nodes in Malignant Melanoma. 48th Cancer Symposium, Society of Surgical Oncology, Boston, 1995. [Abstract.]

Morton DL, Wen DR, Wong JH, et al: Technical details of intraoperative lymphatic mapping for early stage melanoma. Arch Surg 1992a;127:392.

Morton DL, Wen DR, Cochran AJ: Management of early-stage melanoma by intraoperative lymphatic mapping and selective lymphadenectomy or "watch and wait." Surg Oncol Clin North Am 1992b;1:247.

Multicenter Selective Lymphadenectomy Trial: National Cancer Institute Grant No. PO1 CA29605–12.

Norman J, Cruse CW, Wells K, et al: A re-definition of skin lymphatic drainage by lymphoscintigraphy for malignant melanoma. Am J Surg 1991;162:432.

Reintgen DS, Albertini J, Berman C, et al: Accurate nodal staging of malignant melanoma. Cancer Control: Journal of the Moffitt Cancer Center 1995;2:405.

Reintgen DS, Cruse CW, Berman C, et al: An orderly progression of melanoma nodal metastases. Ann Surg 1994;220:759.

Ross M, Reintgen DS, Balch C: Selective lymphadenectomy: Emerging role of lymphatic mapping and sentinel node biopsy in the management of early stage melanoma. Semin Surg Oncol 1993;9:219.

Thompson JF, McCarthy WH, Balch C, et al: Sentinel lymph node status as an indicator of the presence of metastatic melanoma in regional lymph nodes. Melanoma Res 1995;5:255.

Chapter 158
Surgical Treatment of Malignant Melanoma

Constantine P. Karakousis

Malignant melanoma is no longer a rare neoplasm. There are more than 38,000 new cases of invasive melanoma diagnosed annually in the United States, and about 30,000 to 50,000 of in situ cases. The lifetime risk for white males is 1/70 (Rigel, 1996). The major known etiologic factor in the causation of malignant melanoma is exposure to ultraviolet radiation. About 10% of melanomas occur within families, constituting the so-called familial melanoma. The incidence of melanoma in the white population is 10 times that of the black population. Melanoma arises primarily from melanocytes of the skin; however, a small percentage of cases represent melanomas arising in the mucous membranes or the choroid of the eye. There is a special clinical entity, that of dysplastic nevus syndrome, in which patients have numerous, often hundreds of, atypical moles. Histologically, these moles present disordered proliferation of atypical melanocytes in a lentiginous epidermal pattern. Patients with sporadic dysplastic nevus syndrome have a 6% lifetime risk of developing melanoma, while those with an additional history of familial melanoma have an incidence close to 100%.

The two most important measures for curbing the incidence of and mortality from malignant melanoma are prevention and early diagnosis. Prevention consists of avoidance of exposure to sunlight, and the use of sunscreen products during the summer. Early diagnosis is facilitated by increased awareness, by both the public and physicians, of the existence of this condition and recognition of its early features. Melanomas typically show irregularity of their borders and coloration. A mnemonic for melanoma characteristics may be called AB-CDE: A = asymmetry; B = border irregularity; C = color variegation; D = diameter greater than 6 mm; and E = evolution over a short period of time. Ulceration of the lesion is also a suspicious sign. There are four major growth patterns that have been recognized: superficial spreading melanoma (70% of the cases), nodular melanoma (15% to 30%), lentigo melanoma (4% to 10%), and acral lentiginous melanoma (2% to 8%) of the cases. Subungual melanoma is a rare form of melanoma presenting with a brownish-black discoloration of the nail bed. A small percentage of nodular and subungual melanomas may lack pigment (5% to 10%). About 4% of melanomas arise in a subcutaneous site, a nodal basin or other site, without any known primary skin site and no history of a prior lesion that regressed spontaneously or was cauterized without the benefit of pathologic evaluation.

DIAGNOSIS

If the mole is suspicious, it should be biopsied to determine its nature. This can be done through an incisional or punch biopsy of the most suspicious area of the mole. However, the most effective and preferred technique is an excisional biopsy of the entire lesion, which provides the full lesion for pathologic evaluation to determine its nature, in addition to permitting exact microstaging of the lesion if the latter turns out to be a melanoma. The excisional biopsy should be performed with the use of an elliptical incision with the longitudinal axis pointing toward the regional nodal basin. Thus, for extremity melanomas, the ellipse should be longitudinal on the skin of the extremity, being thus in line with the lymphatic flow and facilitating easier primary closure after wide excision. Transverse incisions in the extremities should be avoided. In the trunk, the elliptical incision should usually have its longest axis pointing toward the nodal basin, since the surgical margin is thus greater in the direction of lymphatic flow.

The growth patterns of malignant melanoma have prognostic indications, nodular melanomas having a generally worse prognosis than that of superficial spreading melanomas, while lentiginous melanomas have a better prognosis. The microstaging of the primary lesions, which was developed by Clark and Breslow, has allowed a far more accurate prognostication. The method developed by Clark in 1969 classifies melanomas according to the level of the skin layer involved. Thus, melanomas restricted to the epidermis (in situ) are level I, those penetrating through the basement membrane into the papillary dermis are level II, those reaching the interface between the papillary and the reticular dermis are level III, those extending into the reticular dermis are level IV, and those penetrating into the subcutaneous fat are level V (Clark et al, 1969).

The method reported by Breslow in 1970 is based on measuring the greatest vertical thickness of the lesion on cross-section, with the use of an ocular micrometer from the granular layer of the epidermis to the point of deepest penetration (Breslow, 1970). This method is considered to provide more accurate prognostication than Clark's method. Ulceration is also an important prognostic parameter, ulcerated lesions having a worse prognosis. Other prognostic, but less dominant, indicators in localized melanoma are (1) the gender of the patient, women having a better outlook than men; (2) the anatomic location of the lesion, extremity locations having better prognoses than those of trunk locations; and (3) the age of the patient, younger patients having a better prognosis than older ones.

STAGING OF THE DISEASE

The AJCC staging system involves the tumor, node, metastasis (TNM) concept and correlates well with prognosis. In the latest staging system, Tis is melanoma in situ; T1 is a primary lesion ≤1 mm (T1a is a lesion without ulceration, T1b is a lesion with ulceration of level IV or V); T2 is a primary melanoma 1.01 to 2 mm thick; T3 is a primary lesion 2.01 to 4 mm thick; and T4 is a lesion more than 4 mm thick. Each T category is subdivided into the following: a, without ulceration; and b, with ulceration. The classification of the nodal basin is N0 for negative regional nodes; N1 for one positive lymph node; N2 for two to three positive lymph nodes; and N3 for four or more metastatic lymph nodes or a combination of in-transit metastases, satellites, or ulcerated melanoma and metastatic lymph nodes. N1a is involvement of one lymph node, with micrometastasis; N1b is involvement with macrometastasis; N2a is involvement of two to three lymph nodes with micrometastases; N2b is involvement with macrometastases; and N2c is in-transit metastases or satellites without metastatic lymph nodes. Regional nodal micrometastases are diagnosed after elective or sentinel lymphadenectomy; macrometastases are clinically detectable nodal metastases confirmed by lymphadenectomy or lymph node metastasis with gross extracapsular extension. M is the stage of metastatic hematogenous dissemination and is subdivided into M1, involving distant skin, subcutaneous, or lymph node metastases with a normal LDH; M2, pulmonary metastases, with normal LDH; and M3, all other visceral or distant metastases with normal or elevated LDH. The stages are depicted in Table 158–1 (Balch et al, 2000). In summary, compared with the previous staging system, the new staging system proposes the following: (1) thickness and ulceration, but not level of invasion, in the T classification; (2) the number of metastatic regional lymph nodes and delineation of microscopic versus macroscopic status, but not the diameter of palpable nodes; and (3) merging of satellite and in-transit metastases into a single entity in stage III.

TREATMENT OF PRIMARY MELANOMA

The recommended margin for melanomas less than 1 mm thick is 1 cm. In a prospective randomized trial, it was found that for lesions 1 to 4 mm thick, the 2-cm margin provides as good local surgical control as does a 4-cm margin; therefore, it is the recommended margin for providing the surgeon with the frequent opportunity for primary closure and for achieving a decrease in patient morbidity and cosmetic disfiguration (Karakousis et al, 1996). For melanomas greater than 4 mm in thickness, a wide, usually 2- to 3-cm margin is recommended whenever that can be obtained; although for these lesions, which tend to metastasize through the lymphatics but also and predominantly hematogenously, the major concern is that of distant recurrence. When the surgeon performs wide excision, the margin is measured from the center of the previous biopsy excision. Usually, a longitudinal ellipse is made (at least for extremities) with the lateral margin being the minimum recommended margin for the particular thickness of the lesion. With the use of the longitudinal ellipse, one actually has a wider margin in the direction of the lymphatic flow and the ellipse also facilitates the closure of the wide excision site. After the ellipse is made through the skin, the dissection is carried vertically through the subcutaneous fat to the fascia. The fascia may or may not be removed at the discretion of the surgeon. The specimen is oriented for the pathologist so that in the event of microscopic extension close to one of the margins, it will be known on which side of the wide excision additional margin should be procured. The flaps of the wide excision are undermined, and layer closure is effected by approximating the subcutaneous fat and then the skin. If, due to tension, the absorbable subcutaneous sutures, as they are tied, cut through the fat, one should include in the suture bites the cutis reticularis (deep dermis) with the knot on the inside, since the dermis has tensile strength. In the latter situation, one places essentially a deep subcuticular layer of interrupted absorbable sutures, on which may be superimposed the usual subcuticular closure with a running suture (at a more superficial layer of the dermis), or skin sutures or skin staples. When it is expected that a skin graft will be needed, after the skin incision is made one dissects obliquely through the subcutaneous fat in a direction away from the site of the biopsy so as to obtain a wider excision of the subcutaneous fat layer at the level of the fascia compared with the excision margin at the level of the skin. After the excision, the skin edges are approximated to the underlying fascia or muscle, and then a skin graft is applied directly to the fascia or muscle layer. Suturing the skin edge of the defect to the fascia or underlying muscle stabilizes the edge to which the skin graft will be attached. Having removed a greater diameter of the subcutaneous fat from that of the skin excision, the transition from the level of the surrounding skin to that of the skin graft area becomes smooth, rather than an abrupt precipice. After the skin graft is obtained, usually from the contralateral side, it is applied to the area of the skin defect directly over the underlying fascia or muscle. It is attached to the surrounding skin with staples or other sutures. Nonadherent gauze is applied on the skin graft and the donor site. The skin graft itself may be tacked to the underlying tissues if there is a tendency to lift from its bed. Wet cotton balls are applied to the nonadhering gauze, and several silk sutures are placed on either side

Table 158–1	AJCC Staging for Cutaneous Melanoma		
0	Tis	N0	M0
IA	T1a	N0	M0
IB	T1b	N0	M0
	T2a	N0	M0
IIA	T2b	N0	M0
	T3a	N0	M0
IIB	T3b	N0	M0
	T4a	N0	M0
IIC	T4b	N0	M0
IIIA	T1-4a	N1b(C), N1a(P)	M0
IIIB	T1-4a	N2b(C), N1b(P)	M0
	T1-4a	N2a(P)	M0
IIIC	any T	N2c(C), N2b, N2c(P)	M0
	any T	N3	M0
IV	any T	any N	any M

(C) = Clinical staging includes microstaging of the primary melanoma and clinical or radiologic evaluation for metastases.

(P) = Pathologic staging includes clinical staging and pathologic information about the regional lymph nodes after partial or complete lymphadenectomy.

From AJCC Cancer Staging Manual, 5th ed. Philadelphia, Lippincott-Raven, 1998, p 158.

of the skin graft and tied over the bolster so as to exert compressive force, through the cotton balls and nonadhering gauze, and push the skin graft against the underlying tissues. The bolster remains in place for about 5 days, and then it is removed. Nonadhering gauze is applied to the skin graft for the next couple of weeks until the skin graft is firmly adherent.

In the case of an unknown primary melanoma located in the subcutaneous tissue or a nodal basin, the surgeon should use wide excision or node dissection, respectively, because the ensuing survival is similar, stage for stage, to that of melanoma with a known and controlled primary site.

REGIONAL NODES

Elective Dissection

In the past, many surgeons believed that elective dissection improved the overall survival of the patients by eliminating the microscopic disease that is present in about 20% of the patients with intermediate-thickness melanomas. Retrospective studies tended to show about 25% improvement in survival, since the 5-year survival with therapeutic node dissection was around 25% and that of patients with elective dissection and microscopically involved nodes was about 50% (Morton et al, 1992). However, this was not accepted universally, and some of the retrospective studies did not show a survival difference between elective dissection and observation with regard to the regional nodal basin. Two prospective randomized studies in the past showed no difference in survival between patients having wide excision only of the primary lesion and those treated with wide excision plus elective node dissection (Sim et al, 1978; Veronesi et al, 1977). The most recent and largest prospective randomized study showed no overall improvement in survival with elective node dissection, but there was a significant improvement in the subset of patients younger than 60 years of age who had melanomas 1 to 2 mm thick (Figs. 158–1 and 158–2) (Balch et al, 1996). In the latest analysis of this trial, it was concluded that, overall, patients with nonulcerated melanomas may benefit from elective dissection (Balch et al, 2000).

Sentinel Node Biopsy

The drawback of elective node dissection is that the majority (80%) of patients who undergo elective node dissection do not have microscopic disease in the regional lymph nodes and, therefore, have an unnecessary operation. In addition, a complete lymphadenectomy is associated with some morbidity, which is usually temporary, but in the case of groin dissection permanent lymphedema of the ipsilateral lower extremity may result. The pioneering work of Morton and colleagues, with the use of intraoperative lymphatic mapping or sentinel node biopsy, provided a way of determining the histologic status of the regional nodal basin through the biopsy of a single lymph node or, occasionally, two lymph nodes, which are the first node or nodes to receive the lymphatic drainage from the

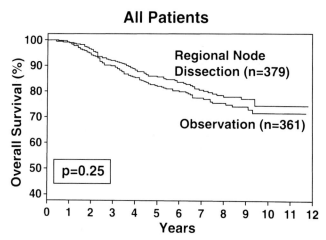

All Patients

Figure 158–1. Survival curves of patients who either underwent dissection or were followed with observation. There is no significant difference in survival. (From Balch CM, Soong S-J, Bartolucci AA, et al: Efficacy of an elective regional lymph node dissection of 1 to 4 mm thick melanomas for patients 60 years of age and younger. Ann Surg 1996;224[3]:258, with permission of Lippincott-Raven.)

primary skin site (Morton et al, 1992). The original technique involved the use of a dye only, but the modified technique includes the combination of prior injection of a radiocolloid (technetium 99m sulfur colloid) and a blue dye; that is, isosulfan blue (Lymphazurin). The radiocolloid is injected intradermally at four sites around the biopsy incision 3 to 4 hours before the operation. The regional nodal basins are then scanned, and one can determine the nodal basin or basins that drain the particular skin site with a degree of accuracy that far exceeds the clinical impression of drainage based on Sappey's lines. At the time of surgery on the operating table, with the aid of a Gamma probe, one can find and mark at the level of the skin the "hottest" area over the nodal basin. One also injects 3 mL of a blue dye (isosulfan blue)

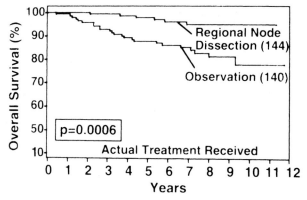

Without Ulceration & Thickness 1.0-2.0mm, Age ≤60

Figure 158–2. Survival curves of patients without ulceration and who had melanoma thickness of 1 to 2 mm and age up to 60 years, and were treated with elective dissection or observation. There is a highly significant improvement in survival with elective dissection. (From Balch CM, Soong S-J, Bartolucci AA, et al: Efficacy of an elective regional lymph node dissection of 1 to 4 mm thick melanomas for patients 60 years of age and younger. Ann Surg 1996;224[3]:260, with permission of Lippincott-Raven.)

intradermally on the side of the biopsy incision facing the nodal basin (Fig. 158–3). The intradermal injection of a large bolus (3 mL) of dye initially, although some of the dye diffuses in the subcutaneous fat, may be preferable to injection of 0.5 to 1.0 mL of the dye, repeated every 20 minutes until the sentinel node is found as originally suggested (Morton et al, 1992). This preference is based on the fact that in the latter technique there is a distinct possibility the afferent lymphatics may be interrupted during the initial dissection at the nodal basin, in which case additional dye injections at the primary site will not be helpful. The primary site is elevated if anatomically feasible (as in the case of the extremities and by tilting the table for trunk lesions) for 5 minutes, and then an incision is made in the nodal basin in the same way that one would make it for the node dissection, except a shorter incision is made, centered over the hottest spot. The incision is then carried vertically through the subcutaneous fat toward the lymph nodes with the use of a scalpel or light cautery, with the surgeon observing intently for any blue-stained lymphatic channels. There is no reason to insist on identifying first a blue-stained lymphatic channel in the subcutaneous fat (which can be traced to the sentinel node) by raising a flap toward the primary site, as originally suggested (Morton et al, 1992). This approach is more tedious, is less likely to be successful, and may contaminate planes that should be reserved for node dissection should the sentinel node prove to be positive. With a direct vertical approach toward the nodal basin, one should be able to identify, within 15 minutes, a stained lymphatic channel or the sentinel node and then demonstrate the continuity between the two (Fig. 158–4).

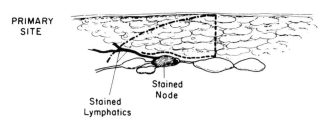

PRIMARY SITE

Stained Node

Stained Lymphatics

Figure 158–4. The surgeon carries the incision for sentinel node biopsy vertically through the subcutaneous fat toward the nodal basin (– – –), observing intently for a blue-lymphatic channel or blue-stained node, in preference to raising a flap toward the primary site and insisting on first identifying the lymphatic channel (• – • – •). (From Karakousis CP, Grigoropoulos P: Sentinel node biopsy before and after wide excision of the primary melanoma. Ann Surg Oncol 1999;6: 786, with permission of Lippincott–Williams & Wilkins.)

After the first layer of subcutaneous fat is traversed, one checks again with the probe as to the direction of highest radioactivity so as to direct further dissection toward that area. One may identify blue-stained lymphatic channels, which are traced to the sentinel node or, first, the blue-stained node, and then the afferent lymphatics. Usually, the node is partially blue-stained at the pole at which the blue-stained lymphatic channels (usually one to three) are entering. The sentinel node should be the spot of highest radioactivity in the entire basin. After the node is removed, the radioactivity of the sentinel node is checked ex vivo. The level of radioactivity should be at least two times higher, better still four times higher, than the background radioactivity in the nodal basin after removal of the sentinel node. If this is indeed the case, one can be assured that the sentinel node has been removed on the basis of both the blue dye coloration and the highest radioactivity count, and one can also be assured that there is no second sentinel node. If the residual radioactivity count in the nodal basin is more than one half that of the ex vivo sentinel node, further searching is done for a second sentinel node. The second sentinel node may be identified with the combination of blue coloration and high radioactivity count or high radioactivity alone. The gold standard is the blue dye staining of the sentinel node, as it more discretely delineates this node and because the radiocolloid tends to migrate along the lymphatic chain during the waiting period to higher nodes that are not sentinel nodes. The dye, on the contrary, colors only the first lymph node or nodes encountered and dissipates as it migrates farther. The radiocolloid, however, is extremely useful in (1) orienting the surgeon toward the sentinel node, facilitating and corroborating the latter's identification; (2) avoiding unnecessary dissection for a second sentinel node if there is a clear drop in radioactivity count at the nodal basin after removal of the first sentinel node; and (3) being the only method of identifying the sentinel node whenever insufficient migration of blue dye prevents coloration of the sentinel node, as is more likely to happen in the head and neck and trunk locations of the primary melanoma. The probe has its highest utility in the head and neck area, where there are several groups of nodes. The lymphoscintigram for a melanoma of the forehead shows the hot area at the primary site, a radioac-

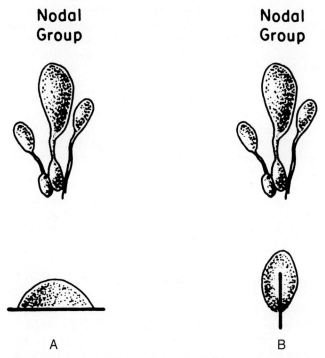

Nodal Group

Nodal Group

A

B

Figure 158–3. The dye is injected intradermally on the side (A) or at the apex of the biopsy incision (B) facing the nodal basin. (From Karakousis CP, Grigoropoulos P: Sentinel node biopsy before and after wide excision of the primary melanoma. Ann Surg Oncol 1999;6: 786, with permission of Lippincott–Williams & Wilkins.)

tive node at some distance and then farther down the neck one or two additional cervical nodes. The first hot node should be the sentinel node, while the others represent activity as the radiocolloid migrates along the lymphatic chain. By looking at the lymphoscintigram, one often cannot tell whether the first node "lighting" is preauricular, postauricular, or just below the parotid gland. By placing the probe on the skin of the primary site and then traveling the possible lymphatic pathways and maintaining skin contact, the radioactivity declines as one moves away from the primary site but there is a jump in radioactivity over the sentinel node, pinpointing its location. Beyond this point, the radioactivity drops, but further jumps in radioactivity may be noted over higher echelons of nodes that pick up radioactivity, which are not sentinel nodes and need not be dissected. Sentinel node biopsy is done before the wide excision because after wide excision one may inject the radiocolloid and/or the blue dye at a site sufficiently far from the primary site to be received by a node other than the true sentinel node draining the original primary site. There can also be distortion of the lymphatic flow leading to the same result. Wide excision of the primary site is done immediately after sentinel node biopsy in the same sitting.

However, some patients are referred for sentinel node biopsy after wide excision. In the author's experience, it seems that even after wide excision, as long as no flap rotation was used, one can reliably identify the same sentinel node as would be identified after excisional biopsy, provided again that no flap rotation was used to cover the defect of the wide excision (Karakousis and Grigoropoulos, 1999).

The method by Morton and co-workers (1999) has been found to be reliable in the hands of other surgeons, in terms of both its staging value and its success in identifying the sentinel node. Sentinel node biopsy provides staging more accurate than that of elective dissection, because in the former the single lymph node provided can be examined in detail by both routine hematoxylin and eosin (H&E) staining and by immunohistochemistry. There is a prospective randomized trial by Morton and colleagues in which patients are randomized to wide excision alone or wide excision plus sentinel node biopsy, which will provide us with information as to whether sentinel node biopsy has an impact on the survival of these patients. If the sentinel node is negative, the chance of later development of a palpable positive node in the nodal basin is about 3% (Karakousis and Grigoropoulos, 1999). If the sentinel node is positive, a complete lymphadenectomy should be performed because about 20% of such patients have additional positive nodes in the specimen of node dissection (Morton et al, 1992). In patients with localized melanoma and clinically negative regional nodes, the histologic status of the sentinel node is the most important prognostic indicator.

REGIONAL RECURRENCE

Local Recurrence

Local recurrence has been defined in the past variously as a recurrence within 5 cm or 2 cm of the surgical scar

of the primary site. Lately, the 2-cm distance definition of a local recurrence has prevailed. Lesions occurring beyond the 2-cm margin are called in-transit lesions. In a trial, the incidence of local recurrence for intermediate-thickness lesions with either 2- or 4-cm margins was about 4% (Karakousis et al, 1996). The prognosis of patients with local recurrence is dismal, given that in this study 80% of the patients with local recurrence succumbed to their disease. However, the location of the local recurrence may be of critical prognostic importance. Thus, patients with local recurrence within the surgical scar of the primary excision apparently have a much better survival, about 80% at 5 years, with wide resection of the local recurrence site (Dzewiecki and Andersson, 1995). This discrepancy in survival between various types of local recurrence may be due to the fact that the local recurrence within the surgical scar may be true local recurrence from residual melanoma cells at the primary site, while "local" recurrences appearing at some distance, separate from the surgical scar, even though at a 2-cm distance, may represent biologically in-transit lesions due to melanoma cells traveling along the lymphatics adjacent to the primary site. Wide resection is the simplest form of treatment of local recurrence, whether this is a single or multiple lesions around the primary site, the latter representing an instance of satellitosis.

In-Transit Lesions

In-transit lesions are lesions that appear in the skin or subcutaneous tissue between the primary site and the regional nodal basin after melanoma cells have been trapped within subdermal lymphatics as they were in transit to the nodal basin. When the number of these lesions is limited, and they are close together, wide excision may be sufficient. Patients with multiple in-transit lesions, particularly when they occupy a large area of an extremity, may not be practically treated with surgical therapy; for these patients, hyperthermic perfusion is considered the most effective treatment modality. With this treatment, particularly when one uses interferon gamma and tumor necrosis factor in addition to melphalan, the complete response rate is high, approximately 90% (Lienard et al, 1991), although later recurrences in the extremity are frequent. In-transit lesions occur infrequently; they are more likely to appear after a regional node dissection, particularly in the lower extremities, where the trapping of melanoma cells in transit to the nodal basin within subdermal lymphatics may be facilitated by gravity through stasis.

Therapeutic Node Dissections

When the regional nodes become palpable at the time of follow-up or are palpable at the time of diagnosis of the primary lesion, therapeutic lymphadenectomy is indicated, provided that there is no evidence of distant metastatic disease. Involvement by metastatic melanoma causes a lymph node to become firm, with roughly a spherical shape, while a hyperplastic node, although enlarged, retains its fusiform shape and is flat and soft on palpation. Percutaneous needle aspiration is advisable to confirm the diagnosis prior to therapeutic lymphadenectomy. When excisional biopsy of the palpable node is employed, it should also be followed with complete lymphadenectomy, since 60% to 75% of these patients have additional positive nodes.

In lymph node dissections of any nodal basin with positive lymph nodes, the number of tumor-containing lymph nodes is the most significant prognostic parameter, although characteristics of the primary lesion such as thickness continue to exert an effect.

In the literature, there is a wide variation in the rates of local recurrence within the nodal basin after a therapeutic node dissection (from 4% to 50%), which suggests that the thoroughness with which this procedure is performed is critically important.

Groin Dissection

In this area, when the inguinal nodes are palpable, as the result of regional spread by malignant melanoma, the chance of the deep (iliac or obturator) nodes being positive is approximately 40% (Karakousis and Bland, 1995). A slightly oblique but nearly vertical incision is employed from about two fingerbreadths superomedial from the anterosuperior iliac spine to the apex of the femoral triangle (Karakousis and Bland, 1995). This type of incision is preferable because it centers over the course of the lymphatics and the array of the lymph nodes in the groin and facilitates their complete excision, reducing the amount of lymphedema by preserving some of the subcutaneous lymphatics, compared with a transverse incision. This incision also allows the in-continuity dissection of the iliac and obturator nodes by dividing the inguinal ligament lateral to the femoral artery and the anterolateral abdominal wall muscles medial to the iliac crest and by ligating and dividing the inferior epigastric vessels, creating one continuous field between the deep (iliac and obturator) and the inguinal nodes (Fig. 158–5). This type of continuous exposure not only improves the exposure but also facilitates the dissection and complete removal of all the deep nodes. In the repair that follows the dissection, the anterolateral abdominal wall muscles are approximated and the inguinal ligament is sutured to the iliac fascia lateral to the vessels and to Cooper's ligament medial to the vessels, thus effectively precluding a postoperative incisional hernia.

In the author's practice, given the appreciable rate of involvement of the deep nodes when the inguinal nodes

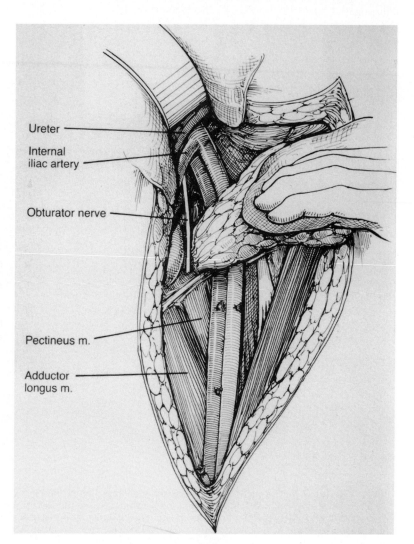

Figure 158–5. Operative field in an ilioinguinal dissection following division of the inguinal ligament, showing in-continuity exposure and dissection of the inguinal and deep nodes. (From Karakousis CP, Bland KI: Surgery of the primary lesion and nodal dissections in malignant melanoma. In Bland KI, Karakousis CP, Copeland EM [eds]: Atlas of Surgical Oncology. Philadelphia, WB Saunders, 1995, p 115, with permission.)

Ureter

Internal iliac artery

Obturator nerve

Pectineus m.

Adductor longus m.

are palpable, and that the 5-year survival rate of patients with positive deep nodes is about 35% (10-year survival rate 25%) (Karakousis and Bland, 1995), it seems worthwhile to remove the deep nodes in continuity with the inguinal group of nodes whenever the latter are palpably involved. Some authors, however, report a 5-year survival rate of 0 to 9% following dissection of positive deep nodes and, considering the slightly increased incidence of lymphedema with deep node dissection, advocate dissection of the lymph nodes only when Cloquet's node (at the lower end of the femoral canal) is positive on frozen section and/or there are four or more positive nodes in the inguinal group specimen.

Patients who have only superficial groin dissection for palpable nodes should be followed up with periodic computed tomography (CT) scans of the pelvis to exclude relapse in the deep group of nodes.

Popliteal Node Dissection

The popliteal nodes are infrequently involved by malignant melanoma, since these nodes drain only a small area of the posterior calf and perhaps their filtering capacity may be low. However, when these nodes become palpable, popliteal node dissection should be performed (Karakousis and Bland, 1995). Usually, these patients have a concomitant involvement of the inguinal nodes, and it

becomes necessary to do a node dissection of both nodal areas.

Axillary Node Dissection

A transverse incision is usually employed between the border of the pectoralis major and that of the latissimus dorsi, approximately two fingerbreadths below the axillary crease. Since effective adjuvant modalities are lacking at the present time for melanoma, a thorough node dissection should be performed, including nodes above the axillary vein and level III nodes, in order to eliminate disease in the entire basin and thus, by avoiding local recurrence within the nodal basin, realize the highest potential 5-year survival in patients who do not have distant occult disease. Nodes above the axillary vein are also included in the specimen, since occasionally they are involved, as well as the lymph nodes between the pectoralis major and the pectoralis minor muscles (Rotter's nodes), with the dissection continuing behind the pectoralis minor to the apex of the axilla (Fig. 158–6). If there are large lymph nodes at level II behind the pectoralis minor, one has to divide the pectoralis minor at its origin and near the insertion to the coracoid process (for its en bloc removal) and incise the lateral edge of the pectoralis major for approximately 2 inches into the muscle in order to allow better retraction and exposure for the level III

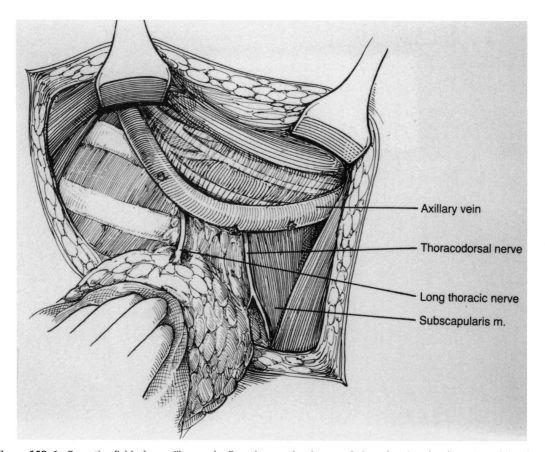

Figure 158–6. Operative field of an axillary node dissection nearing its completion, showing the dissection of the thoracodorsal and long thoracic nerves and the skeletonization of the axillary vein all the way to level 3. (From Karakousis CP, Bland KI: Surgery of the primary lesion and nodal dissections in malignant melanoma. In Bland KI, Karakousis CP, Copeland EM [eds]: Atlas of Surgical Oncology. Philadelphia, WB Saunders, 1995, p 101, with permission.)

lymph nodes. The incised border of the pectoralis major after the node dissection is reapproximated with the use of absorbable sutures. This type of dissection—removing the supra-axillary nodes, the fat pad and nodes above the axillary vein, thus exposing the brachial plexus; removal of all nodes to level III; and/or removal of the pectoralis minor—does not cause any significant increase in the expected lymphedema of the ipsilateral upper extremity, which is about 4% and usually moderate in degree (Karakousis and Bland, 1995). If the axillary vein is involved, it can be resected with the adherent lymph nodes. In this case, one can expect some degree of edema, although it is not pronounced and can be ameliorated with periodic elevation of the upper extremity. A small percentage (15%) of patients with such extensive axillary involvement (of the vein, muscles, or nodes above the vein) attain 5-year survival (Karakousis and Bland, 1995). Patients who have simultaneous involvement of the axillary and cervical nodes and have no distant disease, along with other favorable characteristics such as a long disease-free survival, may have dissection of the axillary and cervical nodes in continuity, if necessary, by removing the central portion of the clavicle (Karakousis and Bland, 1995).

Neck Dissection

This is usually a modified radical neck dissection. However, when the clinical involvement of the nodes justifies a more extended procedure, a radical neck dissection may be advisable. The dissection is carried underneath the platysma, since this provides a sturdier flap with better blood supply. Removal of the platysma may increase the incidence of edge necrosis, particularly when the flaps are wide. In the upper neck, resection of the platysma or the cervical branch of the facial nerve may interfere with the downward retraction and eversion of the lower lip on the same side when the patient grins or laughs. However, when the involved lymph nodes are close to the skin, the platysma may have to be removed en bloc with the underlying lymph nodes.

ADJUVANT THERAPY

In the past, numerous attempts were made to improve the survival of patients with metastases to the regional lymph nodes with the use of various therapeutic agents; but, at least in prospective randomized studies, there was no detectable survival benefit. The first report that adjuvant therapy might have some effect came out of a multicenter prospective randomized study employing interferon alfa-2β in patients with positive regional nodes and/or melanomas thicker than 4 mm. In this study, it appeared that adjuvant interferon alfa-2β improved the disease-free and overall survivals by about 11%, compared with surgical controls. However, in an interim analysis of a follow-up study, although the disease-free benefit continued to exist, overall survival was not significantly different between the treated and the control groups. More recently, there has been intense interest in the use of tumor vaccines in stimulating an immune response in the host and thereby improving the disease-free and overall survivals of patients who are at a high risk for recurrence.

STAGE IV DISEASE

Patients with stage IV disease have hematogenous dissemination of their melanoma, although patients with heavy involvement of the regional lymph nodes such as large, fixed, or matted lymph nodes are also included in this stage. Involvement of distant nodal basins is also considered stage IV disease. For patients with fixed, large lymph nodes in the regional nodal basin, there is no question that an attempt at surgical resection should be made, as it provides the best palliative and therapeutic results. The same is true of patients with involvement of two nodal basins or a distant nodal basin.

Prognostic factors for stage IV melanoma are the number of metastatic lesions, their locations (superficial, i.e., subcutaneous or nodal, versus visceral metastases), the stage of the disease preceding distant metastases, and the prior disease-free interval. Thus, patients with a small number of metastatic lesions (up to 4), metastases that are superficial, those with stage I or stage II disease prior to distant disease (rather than stage III), and patients with disease-free intervals longer than 18 months have a better long-term survival with metastasectomy than do patients without these characteristics. In patients with these characteristics, metastasectomy provides a 5-year survival rate in the range of about 20%, a survival rate that is not attainable with other nonsurgical treatments. Patients with stage IV disease should be treated preferably in the context of a protocol and in combination with other adjuvant modalities, such as vaccine therapy, following metastasectomy.

Patients with solitary brain metastasis usually have resection of this metastasis followed by radiation, although systemic therapies are also required. Patients with symptomatic gastrointestinal metastases (e.g., bleeding and obstructing lesions) may benefit from resection of these metastases, whenever the clinical condition permits, in terms of improved palliation and occasional long-term survival.

SYSTEMIC THERAPY

Chemotherapy for malignant melanomas historically has produced modest results, with an overall response rate of about 20%. The main drug has been dacarbazine, which as a single agent produces a response rate in about 20% of patients. Combinations of other drugs have not conclusively demonstrated an improved response rate or survival. Biologic therapies such as high-dose interleukin 2 with or without LAK cells have occasionally produced complete regressions. However, the overall response rate is not significantly better than that after chemotherapy, and there is also substantial toxicity. Combinations of chemotherapy and biologic therapy have also been evaluated and may be slightly more effective. Active specific immunotherapy in the form of tumor vaccines is currently being actively pursued after resection of hematogenous metastases. However, these immunotherapeutic approaches are undergoing an evolution, since at the present time it is not known how to optimally immunize the patient's immune system against the melanoma.

Pearls and Pitfalls

	PEARLS	PITFALLS
• Biopsy incision in the extremities	A longitudinal biopsy incision makes for easier primary closure after resection.	A transverse incision often requires a skin graft after wide excision
• Melanoma 1 to 4 mm thick	Wide excision with 2-cm margin	Wide excision with a 4-cm margin—a 2-cm margin is as effective and produces less morbidity
• Unknown primary melanoma after excisional biopsy	Wide excision, including node dissection if primary is in a node basin	Observation
• Positive sentinel node	Complete lymphadenectomy—20% to 30% of patients have additional positive nodes	Observation is not recommended at present
• Status after excisional biopsy of a palpable positive node	Complete lymphadenectomy—60% to 75% of patients have additional positive nodes	Observation
• Palpable positive (cytology) node in the axilla	Radical axillary node dissection—dissection of level 1 to 3 nodes for eradication of all disease	Level 1 dissection—adjuvant therapy not as effective as in breast cancer
• Computed tomography evidence of enlarged inguinal and deep nodes, no other disease	Radical groin dissection—35% of patients with positive deep nodes attain 5-yr survival	Systemic therapy—at present, it is not effective for measurable disease

SELECTED READINGS

Balch CM, Soong S-J, Bartolucci AA, et al: Efficacy of an elective regional lymph node dissection of 1 to 4 mm thick melanomas for patients 60 years of age and younger. Ann Surg 1996;224:255.

Balch CM, Buzaid AC, Atkins MB, et al: A new American Joint Committee on Cancer staging system for cutaneous melanoma. Cancer 2000;88:1484.

Balch CM, Soong S-J, Ross MI, et al: Long-term results of multi-institutional randomized trial comparing prognostic factors and surgical results for intermediate thickness melanomas (1.0 to 4.0 mm). Ann Surg Oncol 2000;7:89.

Breslow A: Thickness, cross-sectional areas and depth of invasion in the prognosis of cutaneous melanoma. Ann Surg 1970;172:901.

Clark WH Jr, From L, Bernardino EA, Mihm MD: The histogenesis and biologic behavior of primary human malignant melanomas of the skin. Cancer Res 1969;29:705.

Dzewiecki KT, Andersson AP: Local melanoma recurrences in the scar after limited surgery for primary tumor. World J Surg 1995;19:346.

Karakousis CP, Balch CM, Urist MM, et al: Local recurrence in malignant melanoma: Long-term results of the multi-institutional randomized surgical trial. Ann Surg Oncol 1996;3:446.

Karakousis CP, Bland KI: Surgery of the primary lesion and nodal dissections in malignant melanoma. In Bland KI, Karakousis CP, Copeland EM (eds): Atlas of Surgical Oncology. Philadelphia, WB Saunders, 1995, pp 93–128.

Karakousis CP, Grigoropoulos P: Sentinel node biopsy before and after wide excision of the primary melanoma. Ann Surg Oncol 1999;6:785.

Kirkwood JM, Strawderman MH, Ernstoff MS, et al: Interferon alfa-2β adjuvant therapy of high-risk resected cutaneous melanoma: The Eastern Cooperative Oncology Group Trial EST 1684. J Clin Oncol 1996;14:7.

Lienard D, Lejeune FJ, Delmotte JJ, et al: High dose of rTNF-α in combination with IFN-gamma and melphalan in isolated perfusion of the limbs for melanoma and sarcoma. J Clin Oncol 1991;122:52.

Morton DL, Wen D-R, Wong JH, et al: Technical details of intraoperative mapping for early stage melanoma. Arch Surg 1992;127:392.

Morton DL, Thompson JF, Essner R, et al: Validation of the accuracy of intraoperative lymphatic mapping and sentinel lymphadenectomy for early-stage melanoma: A multicenter trial. Ann Surg 1999; 230:453.

Rigel DS: Malignant melanoma: Perspectives on incidence and its effects on awareness, diagnosis, and treatment. CA Cancer J Clin 1996;46:195.

Sim FH, Taylor WF, Ivins JC, et al: A prospective randomized study of the efficacy of routine elective lymphadenectomy in management of malignant melanoma. Cancer 1978;41:948.

Veronesi U, Adamus J, Bandiera DC, et al: Inefficacy of immediate node dissection in stage I melanoma of the limbs. N Engl J Med 1977;297:627.

Chapter 159

Management of Regional and Systemic Metastases of Melanoma

George Tsioulias and Donald L. Morton

The incidence of malignant melanoma is increasing faster than that of all other cancers except lung cancer in women. Approximately 51,400 new cases and 7,800 deaths from the disease are estimated for 2001, with a person's lifetime risk of developing melanoma being 1 in 75. Mounting evidence suggests that increased exposure to sunlight and the thinning of the ozone layer are critical factors in the development of melanoma. When diagnosed early in the biologic course of the disease, melanoma is readily cured with simple wide surgical excision. However, this neoplasm has the relatively unusual ability to spread to almost any organ site, and no treatment currently available reliably affects its course. At the John Wayne Cancer Institute (JWCI), the overall survival rate in patients with regional metastatic melanoma is 46% at 5 years, 41% at 10 years, and 38% at 15 years. Once melanoma metastasizes to distant sites, the estimated 5-year survival rate is 5.5% and the median survival is only 7.5 months.

CLINICAL PRESENTATION AND PREOPERATIVE MANAGEMENT

Regional Metastasis

Regional lymph nodes are the most common site of metastatic melanoma. Metastases may be discovered when a patient presents with palpable but usually painless nodes in one or more lymph node basins. Any adenopathy suspected of harboring metastatic disease should be investigated. Either fine-needle aspiration or open biopsy is warranted to verify the clinical diagnosis. Lymph node metastasis may also be discovered when pathologic examination of nodes removed during elective lymph node dissection reveals clinically occult tumor deposits.

Regional metastasis can occur at the time of diagnosis of the primary melanoma or at a later date. It may also be diagnosed without a known primary lesion. The prognosis in all three cases is essentially the same, but the number of tumor-involved lymph nodes has an inverse correlation with survival. Patients with clinically occult lymph node involvement are generally considered to have a better prognosis than those with palpable lymph nodes. Data from the JWCI indicate that long-term survival of patients with subclinical regional node metastases is 16% better than that of patients with clinically positive nodes. The overall survival rate of patients with tumor-positive nodes is 46% at 5 years, 41% at 10 years, and 38% at 15 years.

The propensity of malignant melanoma to spread via lymphogenous and hematogenous routes indicates careful examination of the regional lymph nodes as well as the liver, the spleen, and all other accessible lymph node basins. A total-body skin examination conducted in a well-illuminated environment, with detailed description of all suspicious lesions, is of critical importance in identifying local recurrence around the primary site, satellitosis, in-transit metastases, or new primary melanoma. Serial photography or newer systems of computerized skin charting, illumination with the Wood lamp, and magnification of lesions with epiluminescence microscopy are useful tools for this examination.

The preoperative work-up for all patients scheduled to undergo lymphadenectomy should include a complete blood count (CBC); liver function tests, including lactate dehydrogenase (LDH); and chest radiography. For patients with palpable lymphadenopathy, the higher risk of concurrent distant metastases justifies computed tomography (CT) of the chest, abdomen, and pelvis as well as magnetic resonance imaging (MRI) of the brain. Patients with specific signs and symptoms, and/or abnormal laboratory or chest radiograph findings, should undergo a thorough work-up to rule out metastatic disease. The authors have found positron emission tomography (PET) to be more sensitive than CT for the detection of occult metastases.

Systemic Metastasis

Melanoma can metastasize to almost every major organ and tissue. Systemic metastases can be visceral or nonvisceral. Nonvisceral metastases, such as those of the distant skin, soft tissue, or lymph node basin, are slightly more common than are visceral metastases. The single most common site of isolated visceral metastasis is the lung. Patients with isolated pulmonary metastases have a median survival of 11 months, compared with 4 to 6 months for patients with isolated metastases in the brain, liver, or bone. Most isolated visceral or nonvisceral metastases eventually spread to multiple organs.

In 12% to 20% of patients, the brain is the first site of metastasis, and 50% to 70% of patients dying with melanoma develop cerebral metastasis at some point during their clinical course. Signs and symptoms may be due to mass effect and include headache, double vision, and seizures as well as symptoms associated with the location of the lesion in the brain.

The lungs represent one of the most frequent sites of metastatic involvement by melanoma. They are usually asymptomatic at the time of detection by abnormal chest radiograph. Eventually, the patient develops persistent cough, hemoptysis, shortness of breath, and/or chest pain. Evaluation of lung nodules in patients with a history of melanoma should include chest CT, complemented as necessary by needle biopsy. Approximately 30% of biopsied nodules are found to harbor a new primary neoplasm or benign disease.

Gastrointestinal metastasis is frequent and usually asymptomatic or associated with vague and nonspecific signs and symptoms, such as epigastric distress, nausea, anorexia, and weight loss. Occasionally, the patient may present with massive bleeding or an acute abdomen. Most gastrointestinal metastases are diagnosed in conjunction with occult blood loss or as obstructing lesions at the lead point of an intussuscepting segment of small bowel. Ten to twenty percent of patients with metastatic melanoma have hepatic involvement, which usually remains asymptomatic until it is far advanced, at which point the patient can develop anorexia with weight loss, fever, sweating spells, and jaundice. Patients with hepatic metastases generally have disseminated disease, and their prognosis is poor.

Bone metastases are usually osteolytic, present in 10% to 20% of patients with metastatic disease, and commonly found in the spine. They can result in compression fractures, leading to neurologic signs and symptoms, such as radicular pain, paresthesia or paresis of the legs, or urinary retention.

The work-up for a patient with suspected systemic metastasis should include a CBC, liver function tests including lactate dehydrogenase, chest radiography, and CT of the chest, abdomen, and pelvis. In addition, MRI of the brain is indicated to accurately assess the extent of metastatic disease. Other imaging studies, such as bone scan, should be ordered to clarify specific symptoms.

CT or ultrasound-guided biopsy confirmation of the suspected lesion should be considered if it will provide information that may have an impact on patient management. PET may be useful in confirming the metastatic nature of questionable lesions or lesions that are difficult to biopsy, or during routine follow-up after resection of metastatic disease.

INTRAOPERATIVE MANAGEMENT

Elective Versus Therapeutic Lymphadenectomy

The only effective treatment currently available for melanoma patients with lymph node metastasis is surgical excision of the involved lymph nodes. Lymphadenectomy performed for palpable lymph node disease is referred to as *therapeutic*. When lymphadenectomy is performed in the patient without palpable metastases but because there is sufficient risk of nodal involvement, it is referred to as immediate or *elective*. There is little argument about the utility of therapeutic lymphadenectomy because surgical excision is the only effective modality for both local control and potential cure.

The efficacy of elective lymphadenectomy in the management of clinically uninvolved lymph nodes remains controversial. If melanomas metastasize sequentially to regional lymph nodes and subsequently to distant sites, patients treated earlier in the natural history of the disease, prior to the dissemination of tumor cells to distant sites, should have a survival advantage compared with patients treated for clinically palpable disease. Several studies have shown a significantly longer survival for patients with clinically negative but histopathologically positive lymph nodes than that for patients with clinically and histopathologically positive nodes. However, approximately 80% of patients with clinically normal regional lymph nodes have no regional disease. Elective lymphadenectomy subjects these patients to an operation with little or no likely therapeutic benefit and not inconsiderable morbidity.

Several studies have examined whether early lymph node dissection in patients with clinically negative lymph nodes offers any therapeutic advantage over dissection after the patient has developed palpable lymph node metastases. Most retrospective, single-institution studies have demonstrated a small but consistent therapeutic benefit for patients who have intermediate-to-thick melanomas and undergo immediate lymph node dissection. Prospective, multicenter studies, such as the World Health Organization (WHO) study, the Mayo Clinic study, and the Intergroup Melanoma Surgical Trial, suggest that any value achieved by immediate lymphadenectomy may, at best, be confined to a subgroup of patients with lesions of intermediate thickness.

Intraoperative Lymphatic Mapping and Sentinel Lymphadenectomy

In 1990, Donald L. Morton introduced a minimally invasive surgical technique for accurately assessing the status of clinically normal regional lymph nodes without subjecting the patient to the morbidity of complete lymph node dissection. The technique of intraoperative lymphatic mapping and sentinel lymphadenectomy (LM/SL) is based on the concept that the efferent lymphatic channel draining a primary tumor will lead directly to the first—"sentinel"—lymph node (SN) in the regional lymphatic basin. This lymphatic channel can carry malignant cells from the primary tumor to the SN. The tumor cells can then lodge in the subcapsular sinus of the lymph node and proliferate into a nodal metastasis. Thus, the SN is the lymph node most likely to harbor metastatic disease if a regional nodal metastasis is present.

Successful LM/SL is preceded by preoperative lymphoscintigraphy to identify the regional lymphatic drainage basins. Lymphoscintigraphy is particularly important when the primary lesion is on an area of ambiguous drainage, such as the head or neck or the trunk. Intraoperative LM/SL is usually performed within a few hours of, or on the day after, preoperative lymphoscintigraphy. Isosulfan blue dye is injected intradermally around the primary melanoma. An incision is made in the regional lymphatic basin and the efferent lymphatic channel is followed through the fatty subcutaneous tissue of the lymph basin to the first blue-staining lymph node or nodes—that is, the SN—in that basin. It is imperative to identify the blue-stained lymphatic channel first and follow it to the blue-stained SN; otherwise, more proximal blue nodes may be overlooked.

Dye-directed LM/SL should be complemented by intraoperative radiolymphoscintigraphy. In this case, a handheld gamma probe is used to track the lymphatic path of the radiopharmaceutical injected at the time of preoperative lymphoscintigraphy. A radioactive ("hot") SN is defined by a radioactive count at least twofold higher than that of the background site. A skin incision is made, and all hot nodes are excised.

Much has been written comparing dye-directed and probe-directed mapping techniques. At present, the dye must remain the gold standard, since approximately 8% of blue nodes are not hot, and some of these will be the only site of metastasis. However, concurrent use of both the dye and a radiopharmaceutical can increase the intraoperative accuracy of SN identification. In the authors' most recent series, they identified the SN in 98% of lymphatic basins mapped using both blue dye and radiocolloid.

Although the therapeutic value of LM/SL has not yet been determined, the data suggest that it is the same as that of elective node dissection. Moreover, because the SN specimen is much smaller than the nodal specimen removed during a standard elective lymphadenectomy, it can be examined in a cost-effective manner with the use of serial sectioning and immunohistochemical techniques. Thus, LM/SL has superior staging accuracy. A multicenter trial is currently underway to evaluate the survival of patients with early-stage primary melanoma following wide excision alone, versus wide excision plus LM/SL, with complete lymph node dissection if the SN is tumor-positive (Multicenter Selective Lymphadenectomy Trial Group [MSLT], principal investigator D.L. Morton).

Technical Details of Site-Specific Regional Lymph Node Dissections

Neck Dissection

Although lymphatic drainage of head and neck melanomas generally follows a predictable pattern, there are notable deviations, especially for midline or scalp lesions. It is therefore advisable to use preoperative lymphoscintigraphy whenever possible. Melanomas located in the anterior scalp and face usually metastasize to the lymph nodes of the parotid gland and upper cervical region, whereas those in the posterior scalp usually drain to the occipital, postauricular, and posterior triangle lymph nodes.

In patients with nonpalpable cervical lymph nodes, LM/SL should be employed whenever technically feasible. If the SN contains metastatic disease, a completion modified radical neck dissection should be performed. If elective node dissection is indicated but the surgeon is not familiar with LM/SL, the extent of the lymphadenectomy is dictated by the location of the primary melanoma. For melanomas of the ear, anterior scalp, face and/or neck, a level I to IV lymphadenectomy with ipsilateral parotidectomy should be performed. Patients whose mel-

anomas are in the posterior scalp and neck should undergo a level II to V lymphadenectomy that includes the occipital lymph nodes.

Palpable metastatic lymph nodes should be excised during a modified radical neck dissection that preserves the spinal accessory nerve, the sternocleidomastoid muscle, and the internal jugular vein—assuming that these structures are free from tumor. Clinical involvement of the parotid gland or suspected subclinical metastatic disease is an indication for superficial parotidectomy that includes adjacent lymph nodes but avoids the facial nerve. Potential microscopic disease of the deep lobe is handled preferably by surgical resection, but radiotherapy is also an option. In patients with advanced disease, en-bloc resection of the metastatic lesion and the tumor-involved anatomic structure should be performed as necessary to achieve clear margins.

In terms of local control, modified radical neck dissection with preservation of the internal jugular vein, spinal accessory nerve, and sternocleidomastoid muscle, unless they are directly involved, appears to be equivalent to radical neck dissection, but without the latter procedure's associated morbidity.

Axillary and Epitrochlear Dissection

Upper-extremity melanomas routinely drain to the axillary lymph node basin, which is also a common site of lymphatic drainage from truncal melanomas. Axillary lymph node dissection is indicated for all patients with palpable metastatic axillary lymph nodes, as well as for those who have a positive SN. Axillary lymphadenectomy must include level III nodes medial to the pectoralis minor muscle.

The patient is placed in the supine position with the ipsilateral arm positioned on an arm board. The arm, shoulder, axilla, and anterior chest wall are prepped into the surgical field. A transverse incision is made from the superior border of the pectoralis major muscle to the edge of the latissimus dorsi muscle, approximately two finger-breaths inferior to the axillary crease. Skin flaps are raised superiorly to the pectoralis major muscle, medially over the pectoralis fascia to the midclavicular line, laterally to the anterior border of the latissimus dorsi muscle, and inferiorly to the sixth rib. The specimen is dissected free from the lateral border of the latissimus dorsi and the thoracodorsal nerve, and vessels are identified and preserved. The dissection proceeds cephalad beneath the axillary vein and brachial plexus. Exposure of the upper axilla is achieved by adduction and internal rotation of the arm. If the tumor has invaded the axillary vein, the involved segment can be resected and the proximal and distal stumps ligated, or a vein graft can be used. If the brachial plexus is circumferentially encased by tumor, sensory nerves can be sacrificed with relative impunity; however, motor nerves should be spared and postoperative radiation therapy used if it is necessary to resect gross tumor off these nerves.

The pectoralis minor muscle is divided at its origin, if necessary, to facilitate the exposure and dissection of the apical lymph nodes. The dissection continues inferiorly along the anterior aspect of the pectoralis minor, with preservation of the medial pectoral nerve, and over the pectoralis major. If supraclavicular lymph nodes are palpable, en-bloc resection of the two nodal basins is accompanied by resection of the lymphatics passing beneath the clavicle.

The dissection is completed at the level of the sixth rib by sweeping the specimen from the underlying subscapularis and anterior serratus muscle, after identifying the long thoracic nerve. Two 10-mm closed-suction catheters are placed percutaneously in the axilla through a dependent area, and the wound is closed in two layers with absorbable sutures.

Patients with distal upper-extremity melanoma occasionally present with an enlarged epitrochlear lymph node on the medial portion of the volar aspect of the elbow, superficial to the fascia. A small incision of the skin overlying the epitrochlear lymph node parallel to the elbow crease is performed, and thin skin flaps are raised around the node. The deep fascia is incised and the brachial artery and median nerve are exposed. The dissection includes a portion of the deep fascia and the overlying lymph nodes, and the basilic vein and medial cutaneous nerve of the forearm if involved.

Inguinal (Superficial and Deep) and Popliteal Dissection

Lower-extremity melanomas and, occasionally, lower trunk and anorectal melanomas drain to the inguinal lymph nodes. Patients with palpable or suspicious groin lymph nodes should undergo a superficial dissection of all lymph nodes within the femoral triangle, including Cloquet's node; that is, the most superior of the superficial lymph nodes located at the femoral triangle. Patients with at least four positive lymph nodes or a positive Cloquet's node, or patients whose preoperative images suggest deep inguinal node involvement, should undergo dissection of all iliac and obturator nodes.

The patient is placed in the supine position with the lower extremity flexed at the knee and externally rotated. If general anesthesia is contraindicated, epidural or spinal anesthesia can be used. Muscle paralysis is avoided to help identify the motor branches of the femoral nerve. The lower extremity, the lower abdomen, and the genitals are prepped in the standard fashion, and a Foley catheter is inserted.

A "lazy S"–shaped incision that includes all prior biopsy scars is performed, and medial and lateral flaps are raised just above Scarpa's fascia. The dissection proceeds medially to the level of the medial border of the gracilis muscle, superiorly 3 to 4 cm above the inguinal ligament and down to the fascia of the external oblique muscle, and laterally to the medial border of the sartorius muscle. The dissection continues posteriorly until the femoral ring and Cloquet's node are identified and marked with a suture. The saphenous vein and its tributaries are ligated at the saphenofemoral junction. The dissection is continued distally until the apex of the femoral triangle is reached, and the saphenous vein is ligated and divided. Two self-suction drains are placed through separate stab

wounds superior to the incision, and the skin is closed in two layers with absorbable sutures.

For deep groin dissection, the inguinal ligament and the anterolateral abdominal wall are divided lateral to the femoral vessels. The inferior epigastric vessels are ligated, and the retroperitoneal space is developed by blunt dissection. Fatty tissue extending up to the common iliac vessels laterally and to the bladder medially is gently swept off the underlying structures after the ureter is identified. The dissection ends by removing the hypogastric and obturator nodes down to the obturator foramen and identifying and preserving the obturator nerve. The transversalis fascia, internal oblique muscle, and external oblique aponeurosis are reapproximated. The inguinal ligament is repaired and approximated to the Cooper ligament medial to the femoral vessels. The sartorius muscle should be transposed over the vessels in a tension-free fashion by detaching its proximal attachment at the anterior superior iliac spine.

The popliteal lymph nodes drain the posterior surface of the calf and do not often contain tumor. However, if they are clinically involved, they should be excised, even when the inguinal lymph nodes harbor metastases. The patient is placed in the prone position, and a lazy S–shaped incision is made, with its transverse portion over the popliteal crease. Cutaneous flaps are developed superiorly to the hamstring muscles and inferiorly to the gastrocnemius. The muscle-investing fascia is incised, and the adipose tissue and lymph nodes within the popliteal fossa are dissected, with division of the short saphenous vein. The sciatic nerve proximally, the tibial nerve medially, and the common peroneal nerve laterally are identified and preserved, and the dissection is completed by removing the tissue off the surface of the popliteal vessels.

POSTOPERATIVE MANAGEMENT

Patients usually recover fairly quickly from these procedures unless there are aggravating comorbid factors. Postoperative laboratory tests are not routine. Patients undergoing groin lymphadenectomy are allowed to ambulate the next day, and are encouraged to use thigh-high compression stockings (20 to 30 mm Hg pressure gradient) during the daytime and to keep the leg elevated when not ambulating for at least 6 months. Patients with persistent lymphedema should continue to use compression stockings. Drains are kept in place until the output drops below 20 mL per day. The incision site is inspected daily for early signs of skin necrosis or wound infection. The average length of stay is 2 to 3 days. Mobilization of the extremity is enhanced by an exercise program that starts a week after surgery. Vigorous exercise is discouraged for at least 4 to 6 weeks.

COMPLICATIONS

The most common complications associated with lymph node dissection are those related to the wound itself. The severity and type of the complication vary with the site of node dissection. Wound hematoma, seroma, and infection, along with wound breakdown and skin necrosis, are among the most frequently encountered postoperative complications. The morbidity associated with axillary and neck dissections generally is minimal. Wound hematoma, seroma, infection, and brachial plexus injury are relatively infrequent after axillary dissection, and significant arm edema occurs in only 1% to 2% of patients. Similarly, long-term complications associated with neck dissection are infrequent and usually do not involve significant functional deficits. Chyle leak from injury of the thoracic duct is rare (1% to 2%), usually occurring after modified radical dissections of the left neck, and can be managed successfully with conservative measures. Accessory nerve impairment due to direct trauma or ischemia is an infrequent complication; recovery of nerve function usually occurs within the first year. Paresis or paralysis of the facial nerve, salivary fistulas, and gustatory sweating (Frey's syndrome) are uncommon and preventable complications after parotidectomy.

Radical inguinal node dissection, on the other hand, may be associated with significant edema, particularly if the iliac and obturator nodes are removed with the superficial inguinal nodes. In approximately 3% to 10% of patients, this can be particularly debilitating. The rate of edema formation can be minimized by careful surgical handling of the skin flaps, with excision of a 1- to 2-cm margin of skin prior to skin closure, and by prophylactic measures following inguinal node dissection, such as leg elevation and application of elastic compression stockings.

INTRAOPERATIVE MANAGEMENT OF DISTANT METASTASES

Traditionally, melanoma metastatic to distant sites has been managed with single-drug or multiple-drug chemotherapy regimens. However, complete response rates have been less than 5%, and the increase in median survival is minimal. Several investigators have re-examined the role of complete surgical metastasectomy for patients with stage IV melanoma according to the American Joint Committee on Cancer (AJCC) criteria. Recent series have demonstrated 5-year survival rates of 20% to 27% following pulmonary metastasectomy and 28% to 41% following complete resection of gastrointestinal metastases. In all of these reports, patients rendered disease-free by surgical resection fared significantly better than those undergoing incomplete surgical resection or nonoperative management. Thus, surgical excision of metastases can provide excellent palliation and sometimes long-term survival in selected patients.

Only 14% of melanoma patients have synchronous metastases at multiple distant organ sites. A total of 86% initially present with metastases confined to a single organ site, such as the lung, and many months later develop asynchronous metastases at other organ sites. The authors have found that most patients with melanoma have only 1 to 3 initial synchronous metastases at a single organ site, and 80% to 90% of these initial metastases can be completely removed by surgery. The most important prognostic indicators are the initial site of distant metastasis, the disease-free interval before distant metastases, and the stage of disease preceding distant metastases.

Although the lungs, liver, brain, and lymph nodes are the most common sites of metastatic melanoma, essentially every visceral site may be involved. Patients with AJCC stage IV melanoma can be divided into three distinct prognostic groups based on their initial site of metastases: (1) cutaneous, nodal, or gastrointestinal metastases (median survival, 12.5 months; estimated 5-year survival rate, 13.5%), (2) lung metastases (median survival, 11 months; estimated 5-year survival rate, 3.6%), and (3) liver, brain, or bone metastases (median survival, 4.4 months; estimated 5-year survival rate, 2.5%). The number of metastatic sites also is an important prognostic variable. Median survival is 7 to 12 months for patients with one metastatic site, but only 2 to 8 months for patients with multiple metastatic sites.

Nonsurgical treatment options include chemotherapy, radiotherapy, immunotherapy, and combination therapies. Observation should be considered if curative treatment is not possible and palliative approaches would impair quality of life without significantly prolonging survival. Asymptomatic patients with stable disease who are not surgical candidates can be observed until they develop symptoms or progression of disease is noted. Elderly, debilitated, or terminally ill patients are unlikely to benefit from aggressive treatment of their metastatic disease, and the risks usually outweigh the benefits.

Brain Metastases

The frequency with which melanoma spreads to the brain and causes dramatic symptoms makes treatment of cerebral metastases challenging. Symptomatic short-term relief can be achieved with steroids. Some brain metastases appear to be solitary, in which case surgical resection may relieve associated symptoms and occasionally allow long-term survival. Several retrospective analyses have suggested that excision of a solitary brain metastasis results in improved survival and an 87% rate of neurologic improvement. Prospective randomized studies also indicate the value of surgical resection of solitary brain metastases. Postoperative cranial radiotherapy is generally considered because the patient may have other occult lesions. Stereotactic radiosurgery (gamma knife) is a relatively safe, noninvasive palliative alternative, with results matching those of surgery and other forms of radiation in patients whose brain lesions are less than 3 cm in greatest diameter.

Lung Metastases

The treatment strategy for pulmonary metastasis is determined by the site and number of nodules, resectability, presence or absence of metastasis in other organs, and adequate residual pulmonary function. Bilateral lung metastasis is not a contraindication for surgical resection. Among patients who do not fulfill these criteria, surgery should be undertaken only if it is likely to provide good palliation, such as in cases of bronchial obstruction and distal pulmonary suppuration.

Patients are initially evaluated according to the tumor doubling time. Patients with a tumor doubling time of more than 60 days are considered for thoracotomy. Although the best candidates for resection are patients with a solitary pulmonary lesion, no evidence of extrapulmonary intrathoracic metastases, and a tumor doubling time longer than 60 days, patients with multiple metastases and no extrapulmonary intrathoracic disease can still have a 5-year survival rate of 19% and therefore should be considered for resection.

Gastrointestinal and Liver Metastases

Indications for surgery are most frequently associated with acute bowel obstruction from intussuscepting small bowel or chronic gastrointestinal bleeding. Exploration usually reveals multiple sites of involvement. Operative intervention, whether for curative or palliative intent, can be performed with minimal morbidity and mortality. A JWCI study reported a 5-year survival rate of 41% for 46 patients undergoing curative resection of gastrointestinal tract metastases. Patients with liver metastasis usually have other sites of metastasis and are not usually candidates for surgical resection. Resection is a good palliative treatment option, even for the rare patient with solitary liver metastasis, since occasional long-term survival is observed.

Bone Metastases

The mean survival of patients with bone metastases is 4 to 6 months. Such metastases are rather infrequent but can cause severe symptoms that significantly impair the patient's quality of life. Symptomatic relief is usually achieved with external-beam radiation. Impending fracture of weight-bearing bones may be treated with surgical stabilization, especially if radiation has not contained the progression of disease and the expected survival is at least 2 months. For vertebral metastases causing spinal cord compression, decompressive laminectomy followed by radiation therapy can dramatically improve symptoms.

NONSURGICAL TREATMENT MODALITIES FOR METASTATIC MELANOMA

Radiotherapy

Although the adjuvant role of radiotherapy has not been well established, recent reports suggest that it might be useful following surgical resection in the axillary, vaginal, and head and neck regions. In these sites, where microscopic disease is often present following surgical resection, radiation may enhance local control and/or disease-free survival. Radiation has also been widely used, often with excellent results, for the palliation of symptoms from metastatic melanoma. Metastatic sites where radiation has been of great palliative benefit include the lungs, lymph nodes, subcutaneous nodules, bone, spinal cord, and abdomen. Whole-brain radiotherapy has proved efficacious for palliating symptoms of brain metastases. The response rates depend on the dose of radiation that can be safely delivered to the involved region, as well as the volume of disease and intrinsic radiosensitivity of the tumor cells. Gamma knife radiosurgery for brain metastases less than 3 cm in diameter has emerged as a safer, less morbid alternative to surgical resection and whole-brain radiation.

Chemotherapy

Chemotherapy, both as adjuvant therapy and for the treatment of metastatic disease, remains unsatisfactory. A National Cancer Institute (NCI) review of 30 drugs used for the treatment of metastatic melanoma revealed that only two of them produced response rates greater than 10%. Dacarbazine (DTIC) remains the most active single agent, with response rates between 10% and 20%. Responses are observed most frequently in patients with cutaneous and subcutaneous lesions, or lymph node and lung metastasis; there is little response among patients with liver, bone, or brain involvement. The Dartmouth regimen, which comprises DTIC, carmustine, cisplatin, and tamoxifen, was reported to have a response rate of about 50%, but in a randomized trial it was no better than DTIC alone in prolonging survival, and it had more toxicity.

The most recent advance in multiple-drug chemotherapy for melanoma is the combination of chemotherapy with the biologic agents interleukin-2 (IL-2) and interferon-alfa (IFN-α). Initial reports from single-institution trials have demonstrated response rates as high as 60% and short-term complete remission rates of 12% to 15%. The toxicity of high-dose IL-2 limits its use in younger patients with high performance levels, a group that traditionally responds to dacarbazine alone. Investigators at the JWCI have shown that concurrent biochemotherapy with the use of decrescendo dosing of IL-2, post-treatment granulocyte colony-stimulating factor (G-CSF), and low-dose tamoxifen produced a 57% overall response rate in patients with poor-prognosis metastatic melanoma. This modified regimen was associated with significantly lower toxicity levels than those with standard concurrent biochemotherapy. Several institutions are currently comparing the efficacy of these newer biochemotherapy regimens with that of dacarbazine-based combination therapy.

Immunotherapy

Many investigators have examined recombinant cytokines, particularly interferons and IL-2, and melanoma vaccines for immunotherapy for melanoma. Adjuvant IFN-α has been used in patients at high risk for recurrence. Despite initial promising results from an early Eastern Cooperative Oncology Group (ECOG) study, a larger randomized trial conducted by the same group failed to demonstrate any statistically significant survival advantage. Although disease-free survival was prolonged, there was significant treatment-related toxicity. At present, adjuvant IFN-α therapy should be considered an option among other ongoing clinical trials for adjuvant therapy.

In the metastatic melanoma trials using IFN-α, the overall objective response rate was 15%, with a fraction of durable complete responses. Smaller tumor masses appear to respond more frequently to IFN-α than do larger masses. This response follows a time course that may be more characteristic of hormonal therapy than of chemotherapy, with some responses observed after protracted periods of treatment. The optimal dosage for therapy, however, has not been rigorously determined, nor have in vitro correlates of response been defined among the multiple mechanisms known to be influenced by IFN-α and its subspecies.

IL-2 has produced objective responses in 20% of patients with metastatic melanoma, with a small fraction of these patients achieving sustainable remissions. The multisystem toxicities associated with this regimen restrict its application to the fittest of patients. Nevertheless, high-dose IL-2 represents an evolving area of research in biologic therapy and forms the basis of the only systemic biologic therapy for disseminated melanoma that has been approved by the U.S. Food and Drug Administration (FDA).

IL-2 has been combined with IFN-α and, more recently, with IFN-γ, tumor necrosis factor (TNF), low-dose cyclophosphamide, DTIC, and cisplatin and amifostine (WR2721). These combinations have not significantly elevated the response rate to IL-2. The experience to date with IL-2 and IFN-α has been the largest, and while the 17% to 20% response rates are somewhat above those for either IFN-α or IL-2 alone, there is no evidence of synergism or an additive survival benefit that might justify the toxicity of this combination.

Melanoma vaccines derived from allogeneic or autologous whole melanoma cells, purified melanoma antigens, or melanoma-cell oncolysates are at various stages of clinical development. Although low responses have been reported in patients with advanced disease, more promising results have been achieved in the adjuvant setting. Investigators from the JWCI have reported encouraging results for the adjuvant use of an allogeneic polyvalent melanoma cell vaccine (CancerVax) following complete surgical resection of AJCC stage III or IV melanoma. The median length of survival increased from 32 to 62 months ($P = 0.002$) for stage III, and from 7.5 to 23 months ($P = 0.0001$) for stage IV melanoma patients.

Although no phase III trial has demonstrated a statistically significant survival benefit associated with the use of a melanoma vaccine, all have shown dramatic improvement in the survival of patients who had a positive immune response to vaccine therapy. Recently, JWCI investigators initiated two multicenter phase III trials of postoperative adjuvant CancerVax immunotherapy for patients with AJCC stage III or IV melanoma.

OUTCOMES

Regional Lymph Node Metastases

The overall survival of JWCI patients with tumor-positive lymph nodes is 46% at 5 years, 41% at 10 years, and 38% at 15 years, similar to that reported by other groups. The clinical status of the lymph nodes (palpable versus nonpalpable), the number of positive lymph nodes, the extracapsular extent of metastases, and synchronous versus metachronous metastases significantly affect survival.

Pearls and Pitfalls

PEARLS

- The most promising approach to metastases in the regional nodes or distant sites is more aggressive surgery in combination with postsurgical adjuvant therapy.
- Phase II studies with melanoma vaccines have been promising, and the results of multicenter phase III trials should become available shortly.
- There has been no significant progress in extending the survival of patients with distant metastases, despite multiple trials of cytotoxic chemotherapy agents.
- When combined with biologic response modifiers such as interferons and interleukins, immunotherapy based on specific melanoma antigens, whether active or adoptive, probably holds the greatest promise for future progress.

The rate of local recurrence following regional lymphadenectomy is reportedly 2% to 30%, and appears to depend on the tumor burden in the lymph node basin, the extent of extranodal disease, the extent of the procedure performed, and the surgeon's experience. Wide excision with histologically negative margins and redissection of the entire nodal basin are recommended. About 10% to 15% of patients with regional lymph node recurrence following lymphadenectomy may experience long-term survival. Although a few studies support adjuvant radiotherapy for the enhancement of regional control, it should be considered investigational at present.

Distant Metastases

Several series have indicated that aggressive surgical resection of distant metastases is associated with prolonged survival. Surgical resection of melanoma metastases carries a median survival of 8 to 16 months and a 2-year survival rate of 15% to 30%. Favorable prognostic factors include a longer disease-free interval prior to the presentation of metastasis, a longer tumor doubling time, the presence of only a single site of disease versus multiple metastatic sites, the absence of visceral metastases, and complete resection of all metastases.

SUGGESTED READINGS

Balch CM, Soong SJ, Bartolucci AA, et al: Efficacy of an elective regional lymph node dissection of 1 to 4 mm thick melanomas for patients 60 years of age and younger. Ann Surg 1996;224:255.

Barth A, Wanek LA, Morton DL: Prognostic factors in 1521 melanoma patients with distant metastases. J Am Coll Surg 1995;181:193.

Cascinelli N, Morabito A, Santinami M, et al: Immediate or delayed dissection of regional nodes in patients with melanoma of the trunk: A randomised trial. WHO Melanoma Programme. Lancet 1998;351:793.

Chan AD, Morton DL: Active immunotherapy with allogeneic tumor cell vaccines: Present status. Semin Oncol 1998;25:611.

Essner R, Conforti A, Kelley MC, et al: Efficacy of lymphatic mapping, sentinel lymphadenectomy, and selective complete lymph node dissection as a therapeutic procedure for early-stage melanoma. Ann Surg Oncol 1999;6:442.

Hsueh EC, Gupta RK, Glass EC, et al: Positron emission tomography plus serum TA90 immune complex assay for detection of occult metastatic melanoma. J Am Coll Surg 1998;187:191.

Karakousis CP, Velez A, Driscoll DL, Takita H: Metastasectomy in malignant melanoma. Surgery 1994;115:295.

Morton DL, Wanek LA, Nizze JA, et al: Improved long-term survival after lymphadenectomy of melanoma metastatic to regional nodes. Ann Surg 1991;214:491.

Morton DL, Wen DR, Wong JH, et al: Technical details of intraoperative lymphatic mapping for early-stage melanoma. Arch Surg 1992;127:392.

Morton DL, Foshag LJ, Hoon DSB, et al: Prolongation of survival in metastatic melanoma after active specific immunotherapy with a new polyvalent melanoma vaccine. Ann Surg 1992;216:463.

Morton DL, Ollila DW, Hsueh EC, et al: Cytoreductive surgery and adjuvant immunotherapy: A new management paradigm for metastatic melanoma. CA Cancer J Clin 1999;49:101.

Morton DL, Thompson JF, Essner R, et al: Validation of the accuracy of intraoperative lymphatic mapping and sentinel lymphadenectomy for early-stage melanoma: A multicenter trial. Multicenter Selective Lymphadenectomy Trial Group. Ann Surg 1999;230:453.

O'Day SJ, Gammon G, Boasberg PD, et al: Advantages of concurrent biochemotherapy modified by decrescendo interleukin-2, granulocyte colony-stimulating factor, and tamoxifen for patients with metastatic melanoma. J Clin Oncol 1999;17:2752.

Patchell RA, Tibbs PA, Walsh JW, et al: A randomized trial of surgery in the treatment of single metastases to the brain. N Engl J Med 1990;322:494.

Schwimmer J, Essner R, Patel A, et al: A review of the literature of whole-body FDG PET in the management of patients with melanoma. Q J Nucl Med 2000;44:153.

Tafra L, Dale PS, Wanek LA, et al: Resection and adjuvant immunotherapy for melanoma metastatic to the lung and thorax. J Thorac Cardiovasc Surg 1995;110:119.

Thompson JF, McCarthy WH, Bosch CM, et al: Sentinel lymph node status as an indicator of the presence of melanoma in the regional lymph nodes. Melanoma Res 1995;5:255.

Chapter 160

Management of Soft Tissue Sarcomas: Extremity and Chest Wall

Ana M. Grau and Raphael E. Pollock

Soft tissue sarcomas are rare tumors of mesodermal origin that account for fewer than 1% of all newly diagnosed adult cancers and 7% of all malignancies diagnosed in the pediatric population in the United States. Tumors of the peripheral nervous system and some tumors of uncertain histogenesis are included as soft tissue tumors, even though they do not arise from mesoderm.

This disease includes more than 20 histologically distinct sarcoma subtypes of variable grade, categorized according to the normal tissue that they putatively resemble. The histologic subtypes most commonly found are malignant fibrous histiocytoma (MFH), liposarcoma, synovial sarcoma, fibrosarcoma, leiomyosarcoma, and rhabdomyosarcoma; their biologic behavior is best predicted by the histologic grade and the size of the lesion. Because of the ubiquity of connective tissue, soft tissue sarcomas are found throughout the body. Approximately 60% of sarcomas occur in the extremities, 15% in the trunk (of which 9% occur in the thorax), 15% in the retroperitoneum, and 10% in head and neck sites. The thigh is the most common area affected by this tumor. Known risk factors for soft tissue sarcomas include the following: exposure to herbicides, Thorotrast, vinyl chloride, and arsenic, previous radiation therapy, chronic lymphedema, genetic predisposition (Gardner's syndrome and desmoid tumors, Li-Fraumeni syndrome, von Recklinghausen's disease), and inactivation of tumor suppressor genes, such as the $p53$ and Rb genes.

DIAGNOSIS AND STAGING EVALUATION

The work-up of patients with suspected soft tissue sarcoma includes biopsy of the primary lesion as well as imaging to evaluate the extent of both local and distant disease. The history and physical examination should include assessment of the size and depth of the mass, mobility of the mass and fixation to deep structures, involvement of skin or regional lymph nodes, motor and sensory nerve function, and distal swelling in the case of an extremity sarcoma. Although pain can be present in as many as a third of cases, most patients present with a painless mass that has been growing for a variable length of time, or a mass noted after an injury that does not rapidly resolve. Any of these presentations should prompt biopsy, especially if the soft tissue mass is larger than 5 cm or has persisted for more than 4 weeks. There are no clinical signs that will reliably differentiate benign from malignant soft tissue masses.

Diagnostic Modalities

Diagnostic maneuvers should be carefully planned so as to avoid compromising future therapeutic options. For this reason, it is essential that the surgeon who performs the biopsy be aware of all possible operative and reconstructive options appropriate to the location of a specific tumor (Fig. 160–1).

Core-needle biopsy permits satisfactory tissue diagnosis in most centers, with an overall accuracy of 95%. Image-guidance by ultrasonography or computed tomography (CT) may be needed for deep-seated sarcomas. If core-needle biopsy is not feasible or is nondiagnostic, an open biopsy may be required. Excisional biopsy is reserved for small superficial sarcomas (T1a) located in sites remote from the joints and neurovascular bundles so as to permit a 2-cm circumferential negative margin.

It is important to orient the biopsy incision parallel to the long axis of the extremity, centered over the mass at its most superficial point. In this way, the biopsy site can be excised en bloc and in continuity with the underlying tumor at the time of definitive resection. The incision for a chest wall tumor biopsy or resection should generally follow the longitudinal axis of the tumor if the lesion is elongated to prevent the creation of unnecessarily large closure flaps. Alternatively, if the tumor is not elongated, the incision can be oriented parallel to the course of the ribs. Meticulous hemostasis should be obtained to avoid dissemination of tumor cells into tissue planes that might be dissected by an expanding hematoma, thereby remarkably increasing the total body area requiring radiation therapy or surgical excision. Biopsy specimens should be oriented by the surgeon for pathologic analysis. Fine-needle aspiration is an appropriate diagnostic modality for soft tissue sarcoma in centers that have superlative expertise in cytologic diagnosis. However, this capacity is usually found only in major sarcoma centers.

Staging Modalities

Evaluation of the extent of disease should include imaging studies of both the primary lesion and the potential sites of distant disease. The primary lesion can be studied with magnetic resonance imaging (MRI) or CT. MRI is favored for extremity sarcomas because it can provide both sagittal and coronal views with high-resolution definition of muscle groups, neurovascular structures, and the tumor–normal tissue interface.

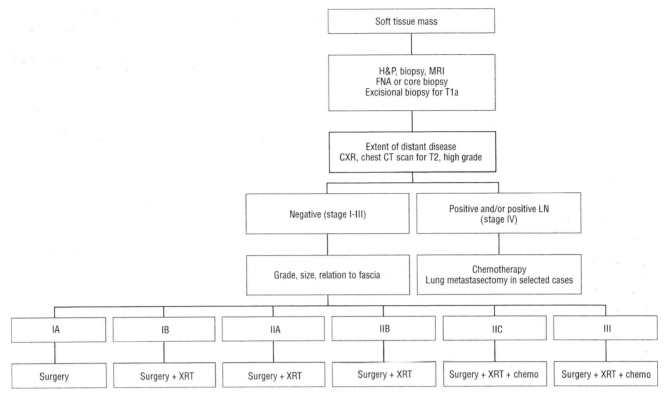

Figure 160–1. Diagnosis, staging, and management of soft tissue sarcomas of the extremity and chest. (Modified from Pisters PWT: Combined modality treatment of extremity soft tissue sarcomas. Annals of Surgical Oncology 1998; 5(5):464–472. With permission.)

The most frequent site of metastatic disease for both extremity and chest wall sarcomas is the lung. Chest radiography is recommended for patients with small (T1 tumors) or low-grade extremity primaries because of the less than 5% risk of pulmonary metastasis in this subset of patients. CT scanning of the chest is recommended for patients with T2 or high-grade lesions because of a 30% to 50% ultimate incidence of pulmonary metastasis for such lesions.

UICC/AJCC Staging System

The revised staging system for soft tissue sarcoma of the International Union Against Cancer/American Joint Committee on Cancer (UICC/AJCC; Table 160–1) is based on tumor size, lymph node status, presence of distant disease, and histologic tumor grade. Tumors are further divided according to their relationship to the investing fascia, where "a" is a superficial tumor located above the superficial fascia without invasion of the fascia, and "b" is a deep tumor located either beneath the superficial fascia or invading through the fascia. Histologic grade, size, and depth of the lesion are the major determinants of prognosis. The criteria used to determine grade vary from center to center and include considerations such as cellularity, vascularity, degree of necrosis, cellular pleomorphism, and mitosis per high-power field. Unfortunately, grading is imprecise, with high discordance rates observed among expert sarcoma pathologists.

Except for some specific histologic subtypes, such as

epithelioid sarcoma (40%), embryonal rhabdomyosarcoma (15%), and synovial sarcoma (20%), the vast majority of soft tissue sarcomas do not metastasize to regional lymph nodes, and an overall incidence of nodal involvement of less than 3% is noted. Nodally metastatic sarcomas are classified as N1 stage IV disease, and disease-specific survival appears to be the same for these patients as for patients with other sites of metastasis with or without LN involvement. Five-year disease-free survival rates and overall survival correlate well with the stage of disease (stage I: 78% and 99%; stage II: 64% and 82%; stage III: 36% and 52%, respectively).

MANAGEMENT OF LOCAL DISEASE

Wide Local Excision

A sarcoma grows as an expansile mass that compresses peritumoral normal tissue, thereby creating a pseudocapsule. Frequently, microscopic trabeculations penetrate through the pseudocapsule and extend beyond this rim of tissue. Simple enucleation of the sarcoma by removing it from the surrounding pseudocapsule is associated with unacceptably high local recurrence rates. To resect the primary tumor with attached microscopic extensions, a 2-cm margin of normal tissue should also be resected, although a smaller margin with use of radiotherapy may be acceptable if needed to preserve critical neurovascular structures, provided that they are not infiltrated by tumor. En-bloc resection is performed with an elliptical incision

Table 160–1	Staging UICC/AJCC Staging System for Soft Tissue Sarcomas

Primary Tumor (T)	
TX	Primary tumor cannot be assessed
T0	No evidence of primary tumor
T1	Tumor 5 cm or less in greatest dimension
T1a	Superficial tumor°
T1b	Deep tumor°
T2	Tumor more than 5 cm in greatest dimension
T2a	Superficial tumor°
T2b	Deep tumor°
Regional Lymph Nodes (N)	
NX	Regional lymph nodes cannot be assessed
N0	No regional lymph node metastasis
N1	Regional lymph node metastasis
Distant metastasis (M)	
MX	Presence of distant metastasis cannot be assessed
M0	No distant metastasis
M1	Distant metastasis
Histopathologic Grade (G)	
GX	Grade of differentiation cannot be assessed
G1	Well differentiated
G2	Moderately differentiated
G3	Poorly differentiated
G4	Undifferentiated
Stage IA	G1, 2, T1a, b, N0, M0
Stage IB	G1, 2, T2a, N0, M0
Stage IIA	G1, 2, T2b, N0, M0
Stage IIB	G3, 4, T1a, b, N0, M0
Stage IIC	G3, 4, T2a, N0, M0
Stage III	G3, 4, T2b, N0, M0
Stage IV	Any G, Any T, N1, M0
	Any G, Any T, Any N, M1

°See text.

Used with permission of the American Joint Committee on Cancer (AJCC), Chicago, Illinois. From AJCC Cancer Staging Manual, 5th ed. Philadelphia, Lippincott-Raven, 1997.

incorporating the previous biopsy site; hence, the necessity of longitudinal biopsy scar orientation. The incision can be extended proximally or distally as needed. A current MRI or CT scan should be available to precisely locate the tumor, thereby avoiding unnecessary violation of uninvolved tissue planes. Imaging studies also help to define rib involvement in chest wall sarcomas. Involved muscles are divided proximally and distally to create 2-cm margins. Proximal and distal control of major vessels must be obtained. Depending on the proximity of the lesion, the sheath of the vessels and nerves abutting the tumor can be resected en bloc, provided that there is no infiltration of the vessel. In that latter scenario, resection en bloc with vascular graft reconstruction is indicated. En-bloc resection of peripheral underlying lung may be necessary to completely resect chest wall sarcomas if there is adherence to pulmonary parenchyma. Before closing the incision, meticulous hemostasis must be obtained, devitalized edges of the wound resected, and the incision coapted over closed-suction drains. Drains should be exteriorized no more than 1.5 cm from the edge of the incision so as to avoid creating an unnecessarily large area of tissue requiring radiation therapy. Wound healing in a previously irradiated field is a potential problem; rotational or free flap microvascular reconstruction to provide a bridge of autologous healing tissue should be considered in a previously irradiated patient.

Reconstruction after chest wall resection may not be needed if fewer than two ribs have been resected or if the defect is deep to the scapula. Absorbable mesh closure is needed for larger defects. Alternatively, methylmethacrylate interposed between mesh may be needed.

Amputation

Amputation for extremity sarcoma is indicated for extensive tumors that have major osseous or neurovascular involvement not amenable to cytoreduction by preoperative chemoradiation. Generally, amputation should be performed one joint above the tumor. Hip disarticulation may be required for proximal thigh sarcomas and is feasible when the tumor does not involve pelvic bony structures. Posterior flap (gluteus muscles) hemipelvectomy may be required for the management of anterior and medial proximal thigh and groin sarcomas. Anterior flap hemipelvectomy is indicated for posterior lesions not amenable to wide local excision, such as sarcomas with extensive gluteal or sciatic nerve involvement. The anterior flap is created from the quadriceps femoris muscle pedicled on the superficial femoral vessels. Forequarter amputation may be indicated in the management of sarcomas of the proximal arm and shoulder region, when the brachial plexus is involved with tumor.

Hyperthermic Isolated Limb Perfusion (HILP)

This experimental technique is indicated mainly for the management of unresectable locally advanced primary or recurrent extremity soft tissue sarcomas that would otherwise require amputation. Delivery of drug concentrations 20 to 50 times higher than is possible by systemic administration can be achieved with the use of this technique. In some patients, the reduction of tumor burden is sufficient to render limb salvage feasible. Combinations of melphalan and tumor necrosis factor have provided the best responses, and have resulted in limb salvage rates of 70% to 80%, with minimal to moderate systemic toxicity.

COMBINED-MODALITY APPROACH

The use of combined-modality approaches to soft tissue sarcoma of the extremities has allowed for limb preservation with improved functional outcomes while achieving complete tumor extirpation. As a result, the rate of amputation for extremity soft tissue sarcoma has decreased to less than 10% in the United States, where primary amputation rates of less than 3% are consistently achieved in most major sarcoma centers. In a prospective randomized study performed at the National Cancer Institute (NCI), the outcomes were compared for patients with extremity soft tissue sarcomas treated with limb-sparing surgery plus radiation therapy versus primary amputation. No significant differences in overall survival and disease-free survival were observed between the treatment groups. Furthermore, the addition of radiation therapy to limb-sparing resection has significantly decreased the risk of local recurrence from 30% to 50% when local surgical excision is utilized as the sole therapy, compared to less than 10% when radiation therapy is added to the treatment regimen. Limb-sparing resection without radiation therapy is generally inadequate as treatment for soft tissue sarcomas that are T2 lesions; that is, larger than 5 cm in diameter. Surgery as the only modality of treatment should be reserved only for patients with superficial T1 lesions in which 2-cm negative surgical margins can be obtained circumferentially. In this latter subset of patients treated with surgery alone, the local recurrence rate is less than 10%. The remainder of stage I patients should generally be treated with limb-sparing resection combined with radiation therapy.

Stage II and III patients may require limb-sparing resection with radiation therapy as well as systemic chemotherapy.

Radiation Therapy

Radiation therapy modalities include external-beam radiation therapy (EBRT), given either preoperatively or postoperatively, and brachytherapy. Available evidence suggests that there may be no major difference in local control between these treatment modalities, although definitive prospective randomized studies directly comparing these techniques are not available. The theoretical advantages of preoperative radiotherapy include the presence of well-oxygenated tissue that is devoid of surgical scarring, resulting in a smaller dose required for achieving comparable tumor control (50 Gy compared with 65 Gy for postoperative radiation therapy), and smaller radiation fields, in that postoperative treatment mandates a radiation field that extends beyond the area of surgical resection.

Interstitial irradiation (brachytherapy) involves much smaller total treatment volume fields and less total cost than those of conventional external-beam radiotherapy. This radiotherapy approach results in minimal scatter radiation and has the convenience of combining surgery and radiation treatment that can be delivered over the course of a 10-day hospitalization. Prospectively generated data demonstrate that adjuvant brachytherapy improves local control for patients with completely resected high-grade soft tissue sarcomas (9% local failure rate), compared with nonirradiated control subjects (30% local failure rate).

Chemotherapy

The role of adjuvant postoperative chemotherapy in the treatment of extremity soft tissue sarcomas remains controversial. Prospective randomized adjuvant chemotherapy trials have failed to consistently show an improvement in overall survival. A recent meta-analysis of all 14 randomized adjuvant trials has demonstrated that doxorubicin-based chemotherapy significantly improved recurrence-free survival and disease-free survival. However, although there was a trend toward improved overall survival (absolute benefit of 4% at 10 years), this was not statistically significant. The use of chemotherapy is reserved for patients with adverse prognostic factors, such as large tumor size, deep tumor location, high histologic grade, and/or recurrent tumor. Doxorubicin and ifosfamide have the greatest activity in soft tissue sarcoma, with reported response rates ranging from 40% to 80%. However, there are significant chemotherapy-associated toxicities, including permanent cardiac damage, the possibility of transient urothelial hemorrhage, and temporary severe myelosuppression. Because of these toxicities, systemic chemotherapy should be administered only in the context of clinical trials.

MANAGEMENT OF LOCALLY RECURRENT DISEASE

Locally recurrent soft tissue sarcoma is not necessarily a harbinger of distant disease. Therefore, attempts should be made to treat local recurrences by re-resection, with consideration for chemotherapy or radiation if the patient is naïve to these modalities. Surgical treatment depends on the anatomic location of the tumor and the ability to re-resect versus amputation, and also on the prior therapy that has been administered. For patients who have already received radiation, the use of further radiotherapy is controversial. Re-resection with brachytherapy boost may be an option in some patients, depending on previous treatments. Chemotherapy should be considered in locally recurrent high-grade tumors with adverse prognostic significance and in lower grade lesions whose location would otherwise require amputation for extirpation. A recent University of Texas M.D. Anderson Cancer Center analysis of the patients presenting with locally recurrent soft tissue sarcoma of the extremities treated with combined modalities demonstrated that limb-sparing conservative surgery was possible in 75% of patients; and of those, 44% experienced no further recurrence after a median follow-up of 5 years. The 5-year actuarial local recurrence-free, recurrence-free, and overall survival rates in that series were 72%, 45%, and 77%, respectively.

MANAGEMENT OF METASTATIC DISEASE

Treatment of stage IV disease (regional or distant disease) is usually based on chemotherapy. In these clinical contexts, surgery and radiotherapy are usually reserved for palliative purposes. Pulmonary metastases represent an exception to this generalization. In this situation, patients are selected for treatment based on the following criteria: (1) complete resection of the primary tumor can be accomplished; (2) there are no extrathoracic metastases; and (3) there is sufficient pulmonary reserve to allow complete resection of the metastases. In these patients, thoracotomy and metastasectomy can result in a 30% to 50% 3-year survival rate. Favorable prognostic factors include a long disease-free interval prior to the development of metastases as well as complete resection of lung metastases with negative microscopic margins. Bilateral disease and multiple lesions do not appear to influence prognosis, provided that a complete resection can be achieved, although the presence of more than four metas-

Pearls and Pitfalls

PEARLS

- Biopsy should be performed in patients with a mass that has been growing over time, or a mass noted after injury that does not resolve rapidly (especially if the mass is more than 5 cm in diameter or has persisted for more than 4 weeks).
- Core-needle biopsy permits satisfactory tissue diagnosis in most centers and may be performed under ultrasonography or CT guidance for deep-seated sarcomas.
- Excisional biopsy is reserved for small, superficial sarcomas in which a 2-cm negative margin can be obtained.
- The biopsy incision should be oriented parallel to the long axis of the extremity; for chest wall lesions, the incision should follow the longitudinal axis of the tumor.
- Staging of soft tissue sarcomas is based on tumor size, relationship to the investing fascia, histologic grade, lymph node status, and the presence of distant disease.
- The primary lesion can be studied by MRI or CT; the former being favored as more accurate for extremity sarcomas.
- Pulmonary metastatic disease should be studied with chest radiography in patients with T1 or low-grade tumors, and with CT scan of the chest in patients with T2 or high-grade lesions.
- The surgeon should obtain 2-cm margins of resection, although a smaller margin with the use of radiation therapy may be needed to preserve critical neurovascular structures, provided that they are not infiltrated by tumor.
- Simple enucleation of the tumor is associated with unacceptably high recurrence rates and should not be performed.
- En-bloc resection is performed with an elliptical incision incorporating the previous biopsy site; hence, the ne-cessity of longitudinal scar orientation. Unnecessary flaps should be avoided, meticulous hemostasis must be obtained, and drains should be exteriorized no more than 1.5 cm from the edge of the incision.
- Amputation is indicated only for extensive tumors that have major osseous or neurovascular involvement not amenable to cytoreduction by preoperative chemoradiation.
- The use of combined-modality approaches to soft tissue sarcoma of the extremities has allowed for limb preservation with improved functional outcomes while achieving complete tumor extirpation, and has reduced the rate of amputation to less than 10%.
- Radiation therapy (EBRT or brachytherapy) has decreased the risk of local recurrence from 30% to 50% to less than 10% when combined with limb-sparing resection, and it has produced the same overall survival as well as disease-free survival as that achieved with amputation.
- Surgery as the sole modality of treatment should be reserved only for patients with superficial T1 lesions in which 2-cm negative surgical margins can be obtained circumferentially.
- The role of adjuvant postoperative chemotherapy is controversial, and this therapy should be administered only in the context of clinical trials.
- Local recurrence may be treated with re-resection; chemotherapy or radiation should be considered, particularly if the patient has not been previously treated with these modalities.
- Treatment of metastatic disease is based on chemotherapy, although in selected cases pulmonary metastases may be resected with curative intent.

tases has been associated with worse prognosis in some studies.

SURVEILLANCE

Surveillance should be tailored to the risk and most likely site or sites of recurrence as defined by standard prognostic factors, such as size, histologic grade, and depth of the lesion. Approximately 80% of all recurrences will become evident during the first 2 years after therapy. Follow-up during this period should include a history and physical examination every 3 months and a chest radiograph every 3 months, and a CT scan or (preferably) MRI of the tumor site, which should be performed every 6 months after obtaining a baseline study 3 months after definitive therapy. Alternatively, ultrasonography can be performed every 3 months, and any abnormality should prompt an MRI or CT scan. For the next 3 years, patients should be examined every 6 to 8 months with chest radiography and imaging of the primary tumor site. After 5 years,

a physical examination and chest radiograph should be performed annually for at least the next 10 years.

SUGGESTED READINGS

AJCC Cancer Staging Manual. Soft Tissue Sarcoma, 5th ed. Philadelphia, Lippincott-Raven, 1997, pp 149–155.

Beech DJ, Pollock RE: Surgical management of primary soft tissue sarcoma. Hematol Oncol Clin North Am 1995;9:707.

Bland KI, Karakousis CP, Copeland EM: Atlas of Surgical Oncology. Philadelphia, WB Saunders, 1995, pp 283–400.

Pisters PWT: Combined modality treatment of extremity soft tissue sarcoma. Ann Surg Oncol 1998;5:464.

Pisters PW, Pollock RE: Staging and prognostic factors in soft tissue sarcoma. Semin Radiat Oncol 1999;9:307.

Pollock R, Brennan M, Lawrence W: Society of Surgical Oncology Practice guidelines: Soft tissue sarcoma. Oncology 1997;11:1327.

Pollock RE, Karnell LH, Menck HR, Winchester DP: The National Cancer Data Base report on soft tissue sarcoma. Cancer 1996;78:2247.

Pollack A, Zagars GK, Goswitz MS, et al: Preoperative vs. postoperative radiotherapy in the treatment of soft tissue sarcomas: A matter of presentation. Int J Radiat Oncol Biol Phys 1998;42:563.

Tierney JF: Adjuvant chemotherapy for localized resectable soft-tissue sarcoma of adults: Meta-analysis of individual data. Lancet 1997;350:1647.

Yang JC, Chang AE, Baker AR, et al: Randomized prospective study of the benefit of adjuvant radiation therapy in the treatment of soft tissue sarcomas of the extremity. J Clin Oncol 1998;16:197.

ENDOCRINE

Chapter 161

Goiter and Nontoxic Benign Thyroid Conditions

Christopher R. McHenry

The term *goiter* refers to enlargement of the thyroid gland. It is the most common endocrine problem worldwide, affecting an estimated 5% to 12% of the world's population. Goiter is classified as endemic when it occurs in more than 10% of the population in a specific geographic area. Endemic goiter is most commonly caused by iodine deficiency. Iodine deficiency may occur as a consequence of a low iodine diet. Ingestion of goitrogens also inhibits iodine transport and results in goiter.

Nonendemic or sporadic goiter is the predominant type seen in the iodine-sufficient United States. Sporadic goiter may be diffuse or nodular, unilateral or bilateral, toxic or nontoxic, confined to the neck, or substernal in location. The etiology of nontoxic, sporadic goiter is unknown. Familial defects in the synthesis, release, or metabolism of thyroid hormone, autoimmune disease, exposure to goitrogens including thyroid blocking agents, such as lithium and amiodarone, are factors that have been associated with the development of nontoxic, sporadic goiter. In most patients with sporadic goiter, the etiology remains obscure. The purpose of this chapter is to review the clinical manifestations, diagnosis, and management of sporadic goiter and the nontoxic benign thyroid conditions that give rise to it. The principal conditions that are reviewed include the solitary thyroid nodule, diffuse and multinodular goiter, and chronic lymphocytic thyroiditis (CLT).

SOLITARY THYROID NODULE

Nodular thyroid disease is a common clinical problem occurring in 4% to 7% of the population. The prevalence of thyroid nodules has been shown to vary with the method of detection. Ultrasound studies and autopsy series have revealed thyroid nodules in as many as 50% of patients 50 years of age or older. At least half of the patients with nodular thyroid disease present with a solitary thyroid nodule, which is defined as a discrete mass in an otherwise normal thyroid gland. Solitary thyroid nodules occur four times more commonly in women, and the incidence increases with age, exposure to ionizing radiation, and iodine deficiency.

A solitary thyroid nodule is benign in 90% to 95% of patients (Table 161–1). The challenge in the evaluation and management of patients with a solitary thyroid nodule is to distinguish between patients at high risk for cancer who will benefit from surgical therapy, and patients with benign disease who can be followed clinically. This is accomplished with a routine history and physical examination, screening thyrotropin (TSH) level, fine-needle aspiration biopsy (FNAB), and the selective use of iodine-123 thyroid scintigraphy (Fig. 161–1).

Most patients with a nontoxic, solitary thyroid nodule seek medical attention because of a recent discovery of a new lump or swelling in the neck. Patients are usually asymptomatic. All patients are questioned about the following: symptoms of hyperthyroidism or hypothyroidism; neck pain; compressive symptoms such as dyspnea, choking spells, hoarseness, or dysphagia; rapid growth of the nodule; a prior history of head or neck irradiation; and a family history of thyroid cancer or other endocrinopathies seen in the multiple endocrine neoplasia syndromes (Table 161–2). Symptoms of hyperthyroidism are often seen in patients with a functioning follicular adenoma. Neck pain and signs and symptoms of hypothyroidism or hyperthyroidism can be present in patients with thyroiditis. A prior history of head and neck irradiation, a family history of thyroid cancer, rapid nodule growth, and significant compressive symptoms should increase the physician's suspicion regarding the existence of a carcinoma.

The physical examination should include an assessment of the following: the size and character of the nodule, the position of the trachea, and whether there is associated cervical lymphadenopathy. Laryngoscopic examination should be performed in patients with hoarseness, and prior to reoperative thyroid surgery. A hard, fixed nodule, associated cervical lymphadenopathy, and vocal cord paralysis are physical findings that are highly suggestive of a diagnosis of carcinoma. Neck tenderness may be present in patients with thyroiditis.

The diagnostic evaluation of patients with a solitary nontoxic thyroid nodule, should include a routine FNAB (see Fig. 161–1). The results of cytologic analysis of a FNAB specimen can be divided into one of four diagnostic categories: malignant, cellular, nondiagnostic, or benign. A cellular result refers to an FNAB specimen with cytologic features consistent with either a follicular or a Hürthle cell neoplasm. FNAB is unable to distinguish a benign follicular or Hürthle cell adenoma from its malignant counterpart. A diagnosis of follicular or Hürthle cell

Table 161–1	Benign Conditions Manifesting as a Solitary Nontoxic Thyroid Nodule

Colloid nodule
Adenomatous hyperplasia
Follicular adenoma
Hürthle cell adenoma
Thyroiditis
Cyst

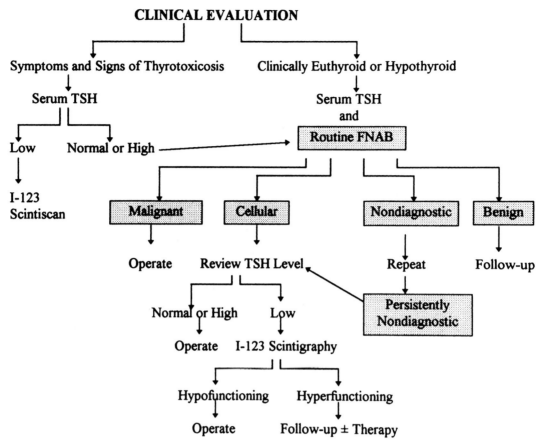

Figure 161–1. Algorithm for the evaluation of patients with a dominant thyroid nodule. (From McHenry CR, Slusarczyk SJ, Askari AT, et al: Refined use of scintigraphy in evaluation of nodular thyroid disease. Surgery 1998;124:656–662, with permission.)

carcinoma is made by demonstration of capsular or vascular invasion, which requires tissue examination. FNAB is associated with a 1% incidence of false-positive and a 2.5% to 5% incidence of false-negative results. The overall accuracy of FNAB is 95%. Ultrasound-guided FNAB is useful for evaluating clinically significant nodules (≥1.5 cm) that are difficult to palpate or are nonpalpable.

Table 161–2	Multiple Endocrine Neoplasia (MEN) Syndromes

MEN I
Pituitary adenoma
Hyperparathyroidism
Islet cell tumors of the pancreas
Rarely, adrenal, thyroid, or carcinoid tumors and multiple lipomas

MEN IIA
Medullary thyroid carcinoma
Pheochromocytoma
Hyperparathyroidism
Lichen planus amyloidosis
Hirschsprung's disease

MEN IIB
Medullary thyroid carcinoma
Pheochromocytoma
Marfanoid habitus
Mucosal neuromas
Ganglioneuromatosis of the gastrointestinal tract

Cystic nodules account for approximately 20% of all thyroid nodules. The term *cystic thyroid nodule* refers to any fluid-filled thyroid nodule, most of which occur as the result of cystic degeneration of some underlying thyroid pathology. A cystic nodule can be distinguished from a solid nodule, based on the presence of fluid retrieved from a FNAB, obviating the need for routine ultrasonography. All cystic thyroid nodules should be completely aspirated. A repeat FNAB should be performed when a residual mass is palpable. FNAB specimens and cyst fluid are submitted for cytologic analysis. The management of patients with a cystic thyroid nodule is based on the results of FNAB (see Fig. 161–1). The accuracy of FNAB is the same for cystic and solid thyroid nodules, although patients with cystic nodules are known to have a higher incidence of nondiagnostic FNAB. In patients with complex cystic-solid tumors, the solid area should be biopsied after removal of the cyst fluid, as the cells in the solid area have not undergone degeneration. FNAB of cystic thyroid nodules may also be therapeutic, with cyst resolution occurring in approximately 15% of patients.

A screening TSH level should be obtained in all patients with a solitary thyroid nodule. The third-generation TSH assay is the most sensitive test of thyroid function and, for screening purposes, is the only thyroid function test necessary. A solitary thyroid nodule in a patient with a normal or increased serum TSH level is almost uniformly hypofunctioning. However, it is important to recognize that a solitary hypofunctioning nodule may also occur in patients with underlying thyrotoxicosis and, as a result, the serum TSH level will be low. The serum TSH level is low in approximately 90% of patients with a hyperfunctioning nodule. Clinically significant carcinoma has been reported in fewer than 1% of patients with hyperfunctioning nodules, compared with about 20% of patients with hypofunctioning nodules.

An iodine-123 thyroid scan is reserved for selected patients with a solitary thyroid nodule. Thyroid scintigraphy is unnecessary in patients with a solitary thyroid nodule who have a benign or malignant FNAB result because the findings do not alter subsequent management. An iodine-123 thyroid scan is obtained in patients with a cellular or persistently nondiagnostic FNAB and a low serum TSH level to distinguish a hyperfunctioning nodule (Fig. 161–2), which can be managed nonoperatively, from a hypofunctioning nodule (Fig. 161–3) occurring in a patient with underlying thyrotoxicosis, which should be treated surgically. Patients with a solitary hypofunctioning thyroid nodule and a cellular FNAB, consistent with either a follicular or a Hürthle cell neoplasm, have a 20% to 30% incidence of carcinoma. Patients with a solitary hypofunctioning nodule and a persistently nondiagnostic FNAB have a 9% incidence of carcinoma.

Thyroidectomy is recommended for patients with a solitary thyroid nodule who have the following: a prior history of head or neck irradiation; compressive symptoms; a malignant FNAB result; and either a cellular FNAB consistent with a follicular or Hürthle cell neoplasm or a persistently nondiagnostic FNAB when the serum TSH level is normal or high or when a hypofunctioning nodule is demonstrated on thyroid scintigraphy. Patients with a solitary thyroid nodule and a benign FNAB result are re-evaluated in 3 months to ensure that

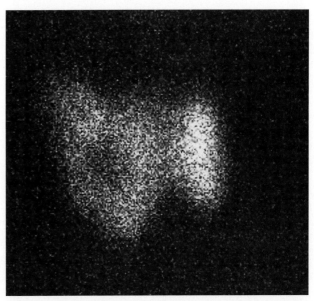

Figure 161–3. Iodine-123 thyroid scan demonstrating a solitary hypofunctioning nodule in the right lobe of the thyroid gland.

there is no rapid increase in nodule size. If the patient is asymptomatic and there is no change in nodule size, they are seen at yearly intervals for a routine history and physical examination and a screening serum TSH level. A yearly ultrasound examination of the thyroid gland may be useful in following a nonpalpable or palpable thyroid nodule. Thyroidectomy is recommended for patients with a solitary thyroid nodule and a benign FNAB result when there are associated compressive symptoms or there is a progressive increase in nodule size.

Patients with a solitary nontoxic thyroid nodule and a prior history of low-dose head or neck irradiation have an approximately 40% incidence of carcinoma. It is not infrequent that radiation-associated carcinoma will involve the thyroid gland at a site other than the index nodule. As a result, patients with radiation-associated nodular thyroid disease are treated with total thyroidectomy. Patients with a solitary nontoxic thyroid nodule and a malignant FNAB are preferably treated with a total thyroidectomy when it can be performed safely. However, it is acceptable to treat patients with "low-risk" malignancy with a thyroid lobectomy.

Patients with a solitary benign nontoxic thyroid nodule that is growing or causing compressive symptoms are treated with a thyroid lobectomy and isthmectomy. The isthmus of the thyroid gland is always removed to prevent potential recurrent disease from occurring directly over the trachea. The opposite lobe of the thyroid gland is palpated at surgery and a near-total or total thyroidectomy is performed when there is nodular disease discovered in the opposite lobe of the thyroid gland.

The most conservative therapeutic approach in patients with a solid nontoxic thyroid nodule and a cellular FNAB, consistent with either a follicular or a Hürthle cell neoplasm, is a thyroid lobectomy and isthmectomy. The pathology in patients with a FNAB consistent with a follicular neoplasm is most commonly a benign follicular adenoma and, less frequently, adenomatous hyperplasia,

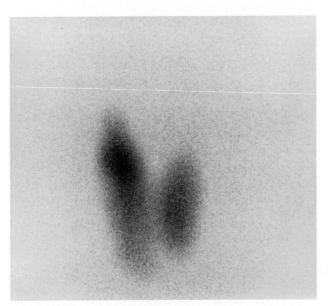

Figure 161–2. Iodine-123 thyroid scan demonstrating a solitary hyperfunctioning nodule in the superior pole of the right lobe of the thyroid gland, without suppression of the remaining thyroid gland. (From McHenry CR, Sandoval BA: Management of follicular and Hürthle cell neoplasms of the thyroid gland. Surg Oncol Clin North Am 1998;7:893, with permission.)

follicular carcinoma, or a follicular variant of papillary carcinoma. In patients with a Hürthle cell neoplasm, the pathology is most commonly a benign Hürthle cell adenoma and, less commonly, multinodular goiter, thyroiditis, or Hürthle cell carcinoma. Patients are informed of the potential need for a completion thyroidectomy for clinically significant carcinoma that is diagnosed postoperatively. In patients with an adequate FNAB, frozen-section examination rarely provides any additional information and, as a result, is not routinely performed. Because of the known 20% to 30% risk of carcinoma in patients with a cellular FNAB, some patients opt to proceed with a definitive near-total or total thyroidectomy to avoid the possibility of a second operation.

Patients with a solitary nontoxic thyroid nodule, and a persistently nondiagnostic FNAB, are treated with a thyroid lobectomy and isthmectomy. A frozen-section examination of a nodule in a patient with a nondiagnostic FNAB is of value because the results affect intraoperative decision making. When frozen-section examination identifies a colloid nodule, adenomatous hyperplasia, thyroiditis, or a follicular or Hürthle cell neoplasm, no additional surgery is performed, whereas a definitive total thyroidectomy is performed for patients with a frozen-section diagnosis of carcinoma.

Postoperatively, most patients who have undergone thyroidectomy are observed for 23 hours or less prior to discharge. A serum calcium level is obtained the morning after surgery only in patients who have undergone bilateral or completion thyroidectomy. Symptomatic hypocal-

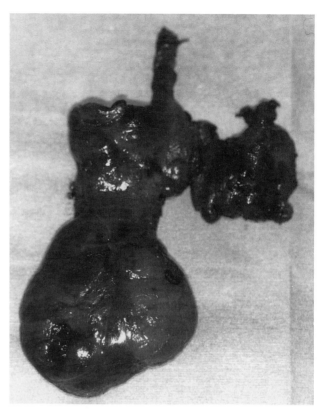

Figure 161–5. A secondary substernal goiter arising from the inferior pole of the right lobe of the thyroid gland.

cemia is treated with oral calcium carbonate as an outpatient. 1,25-Dihydroxyvitamin D_3 is started for patients with persistent symptoms of hypocalcemia despite oral calcium carbonate. Laryngoscopy is performed selectively in patients with persistent postoperative hoarseness. A serum TSH level is drawn 4 to 6 weeks postoperatively to determine whether thyroid hormone replacement is necessary in patients who have undergone thyroid lobectomy. A replacement dose (1.6 μg/kg) of thyroxine is started postoperatively in patients with benign disease who have undergone total thyroidectomy.

DIFFUSE OR MULTINODULAR GOITER

In the early phase of goitrogenesis, the thyroid gland is diffusely enlarged. As goitrogenesis progresses, the thyroid gland becomes nodular in character (Fig. 161–4). This occurs as the result of variability in iodine turnover, colloid accumulation, growth, and function among individual thyroid follicles. With time, some follicles become larger than others. Progressive colloid accumulation, degeneration, hemorrhage, and fibrosis contribute to nodule formation. The end result is a morphologically and functionally heterogeneous multinodular thyroid gland.

Substernal goiter, defined as the presence of more than 50% of the enlarged thyroid gland below the sternal notch, can be primary or secondary and occurs in 3 to 16% of patients with euthyroid goiter. Most substernal goiters are secondary to the inferior extension of a cervical goiter (Fig. 161–5). Mediastinal extension is the path of

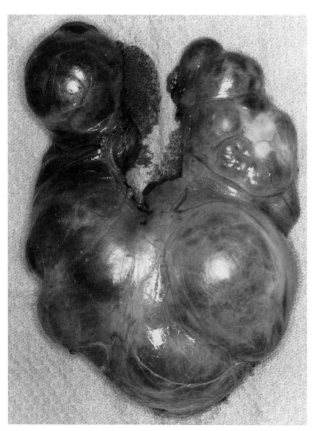

Figure 161–4. A large resected multinodular goiter.

least resistance for an enlarging thyroid gland. Inferior extension is facilitated by swallowing, the force of gravity, and negative mediastinal pressure. Substernal goiters are located primarily in the anterior mediastinum in front of the subclavian and innominate vessels, although 10% to 15% of patients have a posterior mediastinal goiter (Fig. 161–6). Secondary substernal goiters derive their blood supply from the inferior thyroid artery in the neck. Primary substernal goiters, which accounts for fewer than 1% of all substernal goiters, arise from aberrant thyroid tissue and have no anatomic connection with the cervical thyroid gland. Primary substernal goiters derive their blood supply from the intrathoracic vessels, usually the internal mammary artery.

Most patients with diffuse or multinodular goiter seek medical advice because of visible thyroid enlargement (Fig. 161–7). Initially, patients may be asymptomatic, and they are usually euthyroid. The clinical course of most patients with euthyroid goiter is characterized by a slow progressive increase in size of the thyroid gland, with transition from a diffuse to nodular goiter. Patients may remain asymptomatic for many years despite progressive increase in goiter size. However, many patients develop compressive symptoms as well as symptoms of hypothyroidism or hyperthyroidism.

Compressive signs and symptoms are more likely to occur in patients with substernal goiter. This is because substernal thyroid tissue is confined between the sternum and the vertebral bodies and, therefore, may displace or impinge on the trachea, esophagus, recurrent laryngeal nerve, and, rarely, the superior vena cava or the cervical sympathetic chain. As a result, patients may experience difficulty in breathing or a choking sensation, particularly when they are recumbent; dysphagia; hoarseness; or facial swelling with the development of prominent venous collaterals in the neck or chest wall, or Horner's syndrome. A sudden rapid increase in goiter size, especially in a

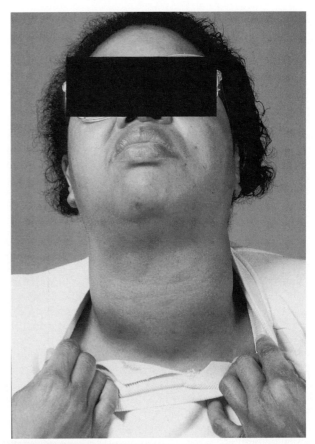

Figure 161–7. A patient presenting with an easily visible multinodular goiter.

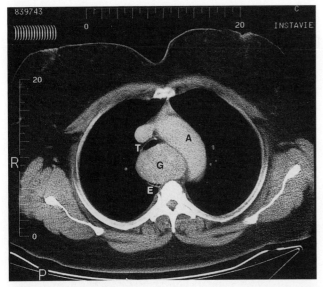

Figure 161–6. A large posterior mediastinal substernal goiter (G) in the posterior mediastinum extending below the level of the arch of the aorta (A), with impingement and anterior displacement of the trachea (T) and compression of the esophagus (E).

patient with a long history of goiter, should suggest the possibility of poorly differentiated carcinoma, anaplastic carcinoma, or lymphoma. However, rapid growth of a goiter may also occur as the result of hemorrhage or cyst fluid accumulation.

Physical examination of the neck reveals thyromegaly, which can involve one or both lobes of the thyroid gland and can be either smooth or nodular in character. Tracheal deviation may be present. Dilated veins of the neck and chest wall may be seen in patients with superior vena cava obstruction. Substernal extension is diagnosed when the inferior portion of the goiter cannot be felt at the thoracic inlet. The inferior extent of the goiter may become palpable with the patient recumbent and the neck hyperextended, a maneuver that helps to elevate the intrathoracic goiter. Patients with a large substernal goiter may have a Pemberton's sign, which denotes the occurrence of airway obstruction, facial flushing, or dilatation of the veins of the neck or chest wall when the patient's arms are raised straight above the head.

All patients with a goiter should have a screening serum TSH level to confirm the functional status of the thyroid gland. Patients with an abnormal TSH level should also have a free thyroxine (T_4) and total triiodothyronine (T_3) level measured. An antimicrosomal and antithyroglobulin antibody titer should be obtained when a diagnosis of CLT is suspected. Although Graves' and Plummer's' diseases are not covered in this review, it should be recognized that patients with Graves' disease present with a diffuse goiter and thyrotoxicosis and patients with Plummer's disease present with a solitary nodule or a multinodular goiter and thyrotoxicosis.

Patients with one or more dominant nodules in a multinodular goiter should have a FNAB of all dominant nodules to exclude the possibility of carcinoma. Subsequent management is based on the results of cytologic analysis of the FNAB specimen, identical to the management of the patient with a solitary thyroid nodule (see Fig. 161–1). The incidence of carcinoma in a dominant nodule within a multinodular goiter is similar to a solitary thyroid nodule.

Patients who complain of hoarseness should be evaluated with laryngoscopy to document the function of the vocal cords. The finding of vocal cord paralysis should raise the physician's suspicion regarding malignancy. A plain radiograph of the neck and chest is obtained to evaluate the patient for tracheal displacement or impingement, particularly in the patient with marked thyroid enlargement (Fig. 161–8). Computed tomography (CT) of the neck and chest is obtained selectively. It is primarily of value in the diagnosis of substernal goiter in the rare patient with an anterior mediastinal mass detected on a chest radiograph without palpable enlargement of the cervical thyroid gland. CT is of value in determining the inferior extent of a goiter when this cannot be appreciated on physical examination, although this rarely affects subsequent management (see Fig. 161–6). CT is also the best modality for documentation of tracheal impingement and for determining the diameter of the tracheal lumen (Fig. 161–9; see Fig. 161–6).

In patients whose symptoms seem out of proportion to the size of their goiter, additional testing may be appropriate to exclude other pathologic entities. For example, a barium esophagram may be indicated to exclude primary esophageal pathology in a patient with dysphagia. Pulmonary function testing with a flow volume loop is of

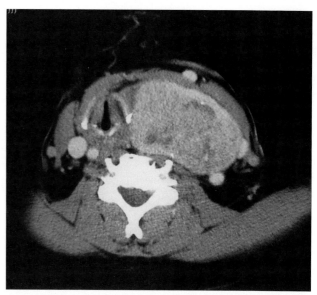

Figure 161–9. Massive left-sided thyroid enlargement with impingement of the trachea at the level of the thyroid cartilage.

value in distinguishing dyspnea related to primary lung disease from extrinsic tracheal obstruction. Patients with tracheal compression from a euthyroid goiter have reduced forced inspiratory flow rates (Fig. 161–10). A peak inspiratory flow rate of less than 1.5 L/sec has been reported to be an indication of urgent thyroidectomy in patients with goiter because of a high risk of acute respiratory failure.

Measurements of radioiodine uptake and thyroid scintigraphy are often obtained to evaluate patients with euthyroid goiter, but they are rarely of any clinical value. Radioiodine uptake is usually normal, and thyroid scanning typically reveals diffuse patchy uptake of isotope with areas of hypofunction and hyperfunction. Occasionally, substernal thyroid tissue may be identified on scintigraphy; however, most substernal goiters do not trap radioiodine.

Similarly, ultrasound is not of value in the routine evaluation of patients with euthyroid goiter. It has been replaced by FNAB, which distinguishes cystic nodules from solid ones. Ultrasound-guided FNAB is indicated for the evaluation of an incidentally discovered, nonpalpable dominant nodule that is 1.5 cm or greater in size. Ultrasound may also have a role in the follow-up of some patients with a nonpalpable or palpable dominant nodule.

Patients with an asymptomatic euthyroid goiter that is confined to the neck, require no additional evaluation. They can be followed yearly with a history and physical examination and a screening serum TSH level. Routine monitoring of serum TSH levels is important because patients may develop a change in their thyroid functional status. It should be recognized that patients with euthyroid goiter have areas of autonomous function dispersed throughout the thyroid gland. As the areas of autonomous function grow, patients may become hyperthyroid. Also, patients with euthyroid goiter secondary to CLT may develop hypothyroidism, emphasizing the importance of long-term follow-up.

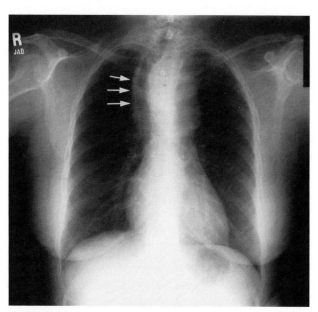

Figure 161–8. A large, left substernal goiter displacing the trachea to the right (*arrows* demonstrate trachea with goiter on the left).

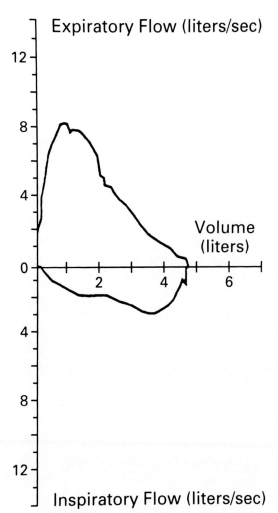

Figure 161–10. Flow volume loop from a patient with a large goiter demonstrating marked reduction in inspiratory flow rate. (From Hermus ADR, Huysmans DA: Treatment of benign nodular thyroid disease. N Engl J Med 1998;338:1438–1447, with permission.)

Surgical therapy is indicated for patients with diffuse or multinodular goiter when there is suspected carcinoma, associated compressive symptoms, or radiographic evidence of tracheal impingement. Surgical therapy should also be considered in the asymptomatic patient when there is a progressive increase in goiter size, especially with a substernal component.

Surgical treatment of multinodular goiter should consist of removal of all abnormal tissue. When nodular goiter is confined to one lobe of the thyroid gland, a lobectomy and isthmectomy is adequate treatment. When nodular goiter involves both lobes of the thyroid gland, a bilateral subtotal thyroidectomy is the minimum procedure that should be performed. Sometimes, a total thyroidectomy has to be performed in order to remove all diseased thyroid tissue. The problem with bilateral subtotal thyroidectomy is the potential for development of recurrent goiter, which is reported to occur in approximately 10% to 20% of patients after 10 years and 40% of patients at 30 years, and may even be higher, depending on the amount and character of the thyroid tissue left

behind. This, coupled with the marked increase in morbidity associated with reoperation for patients with recurrent goiter, makes near-total or total thyroidectomy a better operation if it can be performed safely.

Nearly all secondary substernal goiters can be removed through a standard collar incision. This can usually be accomplished by dividing the superior thyroid artery and mobilizing the lateral part of the cervical goiter first. Division of the strap muscles may facilitate lateral dissection in patients with marked thyroid enlargement. With upward traction on the thyroid gland, the index finger can be used to elevate the inferior-most portion of the goiter into the operative field. When the caudal-most portion of the gland cannot be reached with a finger, a soup spoon can be used to relieve the negative mediastinal pressure so that the substernal goiter can be delivered into the neck. Primary intrathoracic goiters are resected through a thoracotomy or a median sternotomy incision.

Other therapeutic options for patients with euthyroid goiter include the use of TSH suppressive doses of thyroid hormone and radioiodine. With the possible exception of patients with CLT, thyroxine administration has not been effective in reducing the size of a nodular goiter, and it may reduce bone mineral density and exacerbate ischemic heart disease, especially in the elderly. High-dose radioiodine has been used primarily in elderly patients who are poor surgical risks in an attempt to destroy enough functioning thyroid tissue to reduce or ameliorate compressive symptoms. The results of a radioiodine treatment are variable, and large doses are required. Radioiodine is taken up by the functioning areas in the thyroid gland, and it may reduce the mean thyroid volume by as much as 40% after 1 year. However, in patients with predominant areas of hypofunction, corresponding to extensive colloid nodular disease and degeneration, radioiodine is not effective. The early side effects of radioiodine administration include thyroiditis, neck pain, exacerbation of compressive symptoms, and esophagitis.

CHRONIC LYMPHOCYTIC THYROIDITIS (CLT)

CLT, also known as Hashimoto's disease, is the most common cause of euthyroid goiter in developed countries. It is also the most common cause of acquired spontaneous hypothyroidism in Western countries. The highest prevalence of CLT is seen in countries with the highest iodine intake, such as the United States, where it has been reported to affect as many as 2% of the population. CLT is a familial autoimmune condition that occurs predominantly in middle-aged women, often in association with other autoimmune diseases. Affected patients frequently have a family history of CLT, and comprehensive evaluation reveals some autoimmune or functional thyroid condition in as many as half of first-degree relatives.

Patients with CLT usually present with an asymptomatic, incidentally discovered euthyroid goiter. Approximately 25% of patients with CLT present with hypothyroidism. Rarely, patients may be hyperthyroid (hashitoxicosis) as the result of both stimulating and inhibiting antibodies or immunoglobulins increasing thyroid hormone production. An additional 10% to 20% of patients with euthyroid goiter will eventually develop hypothyroidism, but the condition can take many years to manifest itself.

The thyroid gland in most patients with CLT is diffusely enlarged, firm, and bosselated, usually without a distinct nodule. The diagnosis of CLT can be made by documenting elevated serum antimicrosomal or antithyroglobulin antibody titers or by demonstrating the typical cytologic features on a FNAB specimen, which include the following: a predominance of lymphocytes in association with plasma cells, histiocytes, and/or Hürthle cells. A dominant nodule in the patient with CLT, although infrequent, always needs to be evaluated with FNAB.

Patients with euthyroid goiter secondary to CLT can be observed without specific treatment. They are followed with a yearly history and physical examination and a serum TSH level. It should be recognized that CLT is often associated with a defect in intrathyroidal organification of iodine. As a result, patients with euthyroid goiter secondary to CLT may develop hypothyroidism after receiving a large iodine load, which occurs after administration of intravenous contrast material or iodine-containing drugs.

Euthyroid patients with a large symptomatic goiter may be treated with thyroid hormone in an attempt to reduce the goiter size and relieve compressive symptoms. Thyroid hormone treatment has been reported to be successful in reducing goiter size by up to 30% in 50% to 90% of patients with CLT. Surgical therapy is rarely required for CLT and should be reserved for patients with a large, symptomatic goiter that is causing compressive symptoms that are not relieved by thyroid hormone therapy.

Patients with CLT are at higher risk for developing thyroid lymphoma. It is most commonly an intermediate- or high-grade, B-cell variant of non-Hodgkin's lymphoma. In as many as 80% of patients with thyroid lymphoma, the residual, non-neoplastic gland is affected by CLT. CLT may be a predisposing factor for the development of thyroid lymphoma. It is also possible that thyroid lymphoma and CLT have a common etiologic factor. Nevertheless, patients with CLT require long-term follow-up. FNAB should be performed in patients with CLT when there is a sudden, rapid increase in goiter size, or when a discrete nodule develops. FNAB specimens should be obtained for both microscopic examination and flow cytometry.

SELECTED READINGS

Dayan CM, Daniels GH: Chronic autoimmune thyroiditis. N Engl J Med 1996;335:99.

Pearls and Pitfalls

PEARLS

- A solitary thyroid nodule is benign in 90% to 95% of patients.
- The evaluation of a dominant thyroid nodule consists of a routine FNAB and a serum TSH level and selective iodine-123 thyroid scintigraphy.
- A nondiagnostic FNAB should not be equated with benign disease.
- Thyroidectomy is recommended for patients with a solitary thyroid nodule who have the following: a prior history of head and neck irradiation; compressive signs and symptoms; a malignant FNAB result; a cellular or persistently nondiagnostic FNAB result when the serum TSH is normal or high; and a nodule that is progressively increasing in size.
- Compressive symptoms are more likely to occur in patients with substernal goiter.
- In patients with compressive signs and symptoms that are out of proportion to thyroid enlargement, other pathologic entities should be considered.
- Surgical therapy for multinodular goiter should consist of removal of all abnormal thyroid tissue.
- Almost all secondary substernal goiters can be resected through a collar incision.
- Primary substernal goiters are resected through a median sternotomy or a thoracotomy.
- CLT is the most common cause of euthyroid goiter in developed countries.
- Patients with CLT are at higher risk for lymphoma and should be followed for the development of rapid thyroid enlargement or a discrete nodule.

Delbridge L, Guinea AI, Reeve TS: Total thyroidectomy for bilateral benign multi-nodular goiter: Effect of changing practice. Arch Surg 1999;134:1389.

Hermus ADR, Huysmans DA: Treatment of benign nodular thyroid disease. N Engl J of Med 1998;338:1438.

Liu Q, Djuricin G, Prinz R: Total thyroidectomy for benign thyroid disease. Surgery 1998;123:2.

Mack E: Management of patients with substernal goiters. Surg Clin North Am 1995;75:377.

McHenry CR, Piotrowski JJ: Thyroidectomy in patients with marked thyroid enlargement, airway management, morbidity and outcome. Am Surg 1994;60:586.

McHenry CR, Sandoval BA: Management of follicular and Hürthle cell neoplasms of the thyroid gland. Surg Oncol Clin North Am 1998;7:893.

McHenry CR, Slusarczyk SJ, Askari AT, et al: Refined use of scintigraphy in evaluation of nodular thyroid disease. Surgery 1998;124:656.

McHenry CR, Slusarczyk SJ, Khiyami A: Recommendations for management of cystic thyroid disease. Surgery 1999;126:1167.

Mittendorf EA, McHenry CR: Follow-up evaluation and clinical course of patients with benign nodular thyroid disease. Am Surg 1999;6:653.

Rojmark J, Jarhult J: High long-term recurrence rate after subtotal thyroidectomy for nodular goiter. Eur J Surg 1995;161:725.

Chapter 162

Papillary Thyroid Cancer
Peter Angelos

Thyroid carcinomas make up approximately 1% of all human malignancies. Despite this low number, thyroid cancer is the most common endocrine malignancy and accounts for approximately 90% of all endocrine cancers. More than 75% of thyroid cancers occur in women. Papillary thyroid cancers make up approximately 80% of all thyroid cancers in iodine-sufficient areas.

The best treatment of papillary thyroid cancer is controversial. The optimal extent of surgical resection has been debated, as has been the question of whether to use radioactive iodine for these patients. Similarly, the question of whether a lymph node dissection is beneficial to patients has been raised. Most patients with papillary thyroid cancers will do very well regardless of how the physicians caring for the patient proceed with treatment. Since most patients have such an excellent prognosis, only a large study with several decades of follow-up would be able to detect advantages among the treatment options just presented. To date, there have been no randomized studies to evaluate the benefits of the different treatment modalities. In the following pages, the author presents an approach to the surgical management of patients with papillary thyroid carcinoma, along with the rationale for using this approach over the alternatives.

CLINICAL PRESENTATION

Most patients with papillary thyroid cancer present with a painless thyroid nodule or mass. Occasionally, hoarseness is present. Difficulty in swallowing or breathing is uncommon unless the tumor is quite large at the time of presentation. A history of radiation exposure to the head, neck, or chest, or a family history of thyroid cancer significantly increases the risk of papillary thyroid cancer.

Several different types of studies are available to aid in distinguishing benign thyroid nodules from malignant ones. Thyroid scanning can distinguish hot, warm, and cold nodules, but, in so doing, only estimates the risks of cancer in a nodule. Ultrasonography can be helpful in assessing the entire thyroid and the characteristics of the nodule in question as well as whether enlarged lymph nodes are present in the neck. Cystic nodules are uncommonly malignant. The presence of microcalcifications within a solid thyroid nodule raises the concern for papillary thyroid carcinoma, as these microcalcifications may be psammoma bodies. Computed tomography (CT) and magnetic resonance imaging (MRI) may be useful in selected situations in patients with very large or invasive tumors but are unnecessary for most patients with thyroid nodules.

Fine-needle aspiration (FNA) biopsy with experienced cytologic evaluation is usually the most helpful study for making the diagnosis of papillary thyroid cancer. FNA may be done with or without ultrasonographic guidance. The latter is usually necessary only for small nodules or for multiple nodules. Four cytologic categories are possible: inadequate, benign, indeterminate, or malignant. When an inadequate result is obtained, the FNA should be repeated. A benign result usually means that the patient can be safely followed for changes in the nodule, since about 96% of such nodules are benign on permanent histology. An indeterminate result is most commonly encountered with follicular and Hürthle cell neoplasms. A benign follicular adenoma and a benign Hürthle cell adenoma can be distinguished from a malignant follicular or Hürthle cell carcinoma only on the basis of capsular or vascular invasion. Capsular invasion cannot be determined on the basis of cytology, since the entire capsule must be examined. An indeterminate finding on FNA usually warrants at least an ipsilateral thyroid lobectomy. A finding of malignancy usually requires a total thyroidectomy, as will be detailed later, because approximately 99% are found to be cancer on permanent histology.

PREOPERATIVE MANAGEMENT

A detailed history should be taken for all patients, and all patients should undergo a careful physical examination. The surgeon must ensure that the patient is euthyroid by obtaining a blood thyroid-stimulating hormone (TSH) level. Attention should be directed to the possible presence of enlarged cervical or supraclavicular lymph nodes. If lymphadenopathy is identified in the anterior cervical chain contralateral to the thyroid nodule, in the posterior cervical chain, or in the supraclavicular region, consideration should be given to additional evaluation with CT or ultrasound to try to identify involved lymph nodes that may be present outside the central compartment where nodes would be routinely assessed intraoperatively. In patients with very large or fixed masses or who have significant tracheal deviation, CT or MRI scanning might be warranted to assess possible tracheal narrowing or tracheal or esophageal invasion. In patients who present with hoarseness or after previous neck surgery, preoperative vocal cord evaluation to exclude cord paralysis is essential. Patients should also have a serum calcium level preoperatively so that if abnormalities in parathyroid size or consistency are noted intraoperatively, these findings can be appropriately interpreted and treated. Perioperative antibiotics are not routinely necessary in patients undergoing thyroidectomy because of the low risk of infection in this clean operation.

INTRAOPERATIVE MANAGEMENT

As noted in the introduction to this chapter, the extent of surgery for the optimal treatment of papillary thyroid cancer is controversial. For papillary thyroid carcinomas larger than 1.0 cm in diameter or with extension outside the thyroid capsule, or with angioinvasion, or with involvement of lymph nodes, the author favors total thyroidectomy with removal of any involved lymph nodes. Papillary thyroid cancers smaller than 1.0 cm in diameter and with no extension beyond the thyroid capsule meet the criteria of "minimal papillary carcinoma" and carry a very low risk of progression or spread. Such minimal papillary carcinomas, when confined to the thyroid gland, may be effectively treated with an ipsilateral thyroid lobectomy (Fig. 162–1).

Although other authors have argued in favor of a lobectomy for patients with larger than minimal papillary carcinomas, this author believes that a more extensive surgical approach has several esssential benefits. Most importantly, if a total (or even near-total) thyroidectomy has been done, radioactive iodine can be used to ablate any residual thyroid cells or thyroid cancer cells in lymph nodes or elsewhere in the body. Several studies have shown decreased recurrence rates and increased survival rates among patients treated with total thyroidectomy and postoperative [131]iodine therapy. In addition, once the thyroid has been successfully ablated, thyroglobulin levels can be used to closely follow patients for recurrence of papillary thyroid cancer. Furthermore, total thyroidectomy eliminates the risk of leaving a focus of papillary carcinoma in the remaining lobe. The risk of bilateral lobar involvement of papillary thyroid cancer was 19% in a large series from the Mayo Clinic and more than 80% in patients treated at the M.D. Anderson Cancer Center. Part of this difference was due to a more thorough study of the remnant tissue in Texas. Finally, once a total thyroidectomy has been performed, the development of distant metastases at any time can usually be identified and treated with [131]iodine.

Patients are prepared for thyroid operations as for other operations. All patients who have had previous neck operations, or any patient with a change in voice or hoarseness, needs to have preoperative direct laryngoscopy. In the operating room after induction of anesthetic and intubation, the author routinely positions the patient with a beanbag behind the shoulders to extend the neck. The patient is placed in semi-Fowler's position to decompress neck veins, and a flexible ether screen is attached to the bed extending over the patient's face (Fig. 162–2). Once the endotracheal tube is attached to the ether screen, the table is turned 90 degrees so that the anesthesiologist has access to the patient only at the right hand. After sterile draping, this positioning allows the surgeon and assistant to move around the entire head of the table and facilitates retraction so that the entire superior pole of the thyroid lobes can be readily exposed and completely removed.

The technical aspects of the thyroidectomy involve

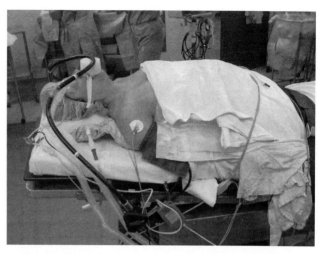

Figure 162–2. Intraoperative positioning for thyroidectomy.

dissection on the side of the dominant nodule first. The strap muscles are separated in the midline from the suprasternal notch to the thyroid cartilage. They are then retracted laterally and rarely need to be divided. After mobilizing the tissue lateral to the thyroid gland with the use of blunt dissection, the middle thyroid vein or veins are identified, ligated, and divided. The superior and inferior pole vessels are individually ligated at the level of the thyroid capsule. All tissue on the lateral aspect of the thyroid gland is carefully dissected off the thyroid capsule with the use of sharp and blunt dissection so that the parathyroid glands remain with their blood supply intact. The tubercle of Zuckerkandl is elevated from its position anterior to the recurrent laryngeal nerve by pulling up on the lobe and medially rotating it (Fig. 162–3). Branches of the inferior thyroid artery are individually ligated and divided, with the surgeon taking care to identify and preserve the recurrent laryngeal nerve. No electrocautery is used in proximity to the nerve. The pyramidal lobe is identified and traced to its most cranial point. During this portion of the dissection, delphian lymph nodes situated in the cricothyroid membrane should be identified and removed. The same approach is then used on the remaining lobe. If the surgeon is ever concerned that the recurrent laryngeal nerve (RLN) or parathyroids cannot be safely preserved, a near-total lobectomy on the contralateral side from the dominant nodule may be performed to decrease the risk of hypoparathyroidism or bilateral nerve injury. This approach leaves the posterior capsule of the thyroid, along with a small remnant of

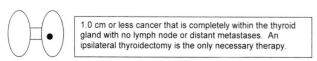

1.0 cm or less cancer that is completely within the thyroid gland with no lymph node or distant metastases. An ipsilateral thyroidectomy is the only necessary therapy.

Figure 162–1. Minimal papillary carcinoma.

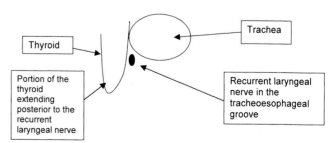

Thyroid

Trachea

Portion of the thyroid extending posterior to the recurrent laryngeal nerve

Recurrent laryngeal nerve in the tracheoesophageal groove

Figure 162–3. Tubercle of Zuckerkandl.

thyroid tissue (usually less than 1.0 g), in the region of the nerve and parathyroid glands.

In the unusual case in which a papillary thyroid cancer encases the recurrent laryngeal nerve, the surgeon will be faced with the question of whether to sacrifice the nerve in order to perform a more complete resection or to leave the nerve intact and in so doing leave the thyroid cancer in place. Previous experience suggests that because small amounts of papillary thyroid cancer are readily ablated with radioactive iodine, there is little indication to knowingly sacrifice the nerve in the treatment of papillary thyroid carcinoma. However, should it be necessary to sacrifice the recurrent laryngeal nerve, consideration should be given to performing an immediate microsurgical reanastomosis of the nerve.

After the thyroid gland has been removed, nodes in the central and lateral compartments should be carefully assessed for enlargement. In any location where abnormal lymph nodes are found, that group of lymph nodes should be removed. Radical lymph node dissection is not indicated in the treatment of papillary thyroid cancer. The role of prophylactic lymph node dissection in the management of papillary thyroid cancer has been controversial. The author believes that all enlarged lymph nodes should be removed, but as long as [131]iodine ablation is used postoperatively, there does not appear to be a role for prophylactic lymph node dissection.

Drains are not commonly necessary unless a very large tumor has been removed or an extensive lymph node dissection has been necessary. Prior to closing the wound, the parathyroids should be reinspected to ensure that they are viable. Any nonviable parathyroid glands should be minced into 1-mm pieces and autotransplanted into a pocket in the sternocleidomastoid muscle. A minimal dressing should be used on the neck so that any hematoma, which should only rarely occur, will be readily evident.

POSTOPERATIVE MANAGEMENT

After a total thyroidectomy, patients can be given liquids immediately and advanced to solid food as soon as tolerated. Calcium levels should be checked during the first 24 hours, as a small percentage of patients will require calcium supplementation. It is generally not necessary to check calcium levels prior to approximately 8 to 16 hours after surgery. Although a few surgeons are recommending same-day surgery, the author believes that most patients should not be discharged on the day after surgery. The author is concerned that if a rare patient developed a neck hematoma at home, it could be life-threatening.

Generally, patients are not started on thyroid hormone replacement so that they might develop hypothyroidism in anticipation of radioactive iodine scanning. Different protocols of thyroid hormone replacement can be used in order to allow hypothyroidism to develop. The simplest approach is not to start levothyroxine after total thyroidectomy. Usually, within 4 to 6 weeks, TSH levels will rise to concentrations greater than 30 µIU/mL, which is considered adequate for the stimulation of radioiodine uptake in metastatic lesions. Another approach is to treat the condition with approximately 50 µg of triiodothyronine

(25 µg bid PO) for 4 to 6 weeks and then discontinue for 2 weeks. This method of treatment subjects the patient to a shorter period of hypothyroidism that not only is uncomfortable for most patients but also may stimulate some thyroid cancer to grow. Patients should also receive an iodine-deficient diet for 2 weeks prior to scanning and have a blood TSH level, thyroglobulin (TG) level, and a pregnancy test prior to the administration of any radioiodine. An outpatient diagnostic scan can be used to determine the amount of uptake in the neck or elsewhere. On the basis of this diagnostic scan, or the risk group of the patient, a therapeutic dose (usually requiring an inpatient stay) is decided on and given. Generally, approximately 30 millicuries (mCi) is given for low-risk patients with uptake only in the thyroid bed and 100 to 200 mCi is administed to high-risk patients or to those with tumor outside the thyroid bed.

After radioactive iodine ablation, patients should be started on levothyroxine with the goal of treatment being suppression of TSH to less than 0.1 µIU/mL without associated hyperthyroidism. Cytomel (T_3) is also often given for several days with levothyroxine to return the patient to the euthyroid state more quickly. TSH levels can be checked approximately 6 weeks after initiating treatment, and modifications in dosing made as needed.

COMPLICATIONS

The complications of thyroid surgery are well known and include the following: hematoma, recurrent laryngeal nerve injury, and hypoparathyroidism. The development of a postoperative neck hematoma occurs in about 1 in 200 patients. If a hematoma develops, it is best managed with early identification and evacuation. Patients should be brought back to the operating room for neck exploration as rapidly as possible. If intubation is not possible, the incision should be immediately opened to release the hematoma prior to intubation and reexploration.

Recurrent laryngeal nerve injury should be a rare occurrence in the hands of an experienced thyroid surgeon. In most large series, the incidence of permanent RLN injury is about 1%. In patients who have had previous thyroid or parathyroid surgery, the incidence of nerve injury is increased to less than 4%. The risks of temporary RLN injury are higher, but they can be minimized by avoiding excessive manipulation to the nerve.

The risk of permanent hypoparathyroidism after total thyroidectomy for papillary thyroid cancer is about 1% when the operation is done by an experienced thyroid surgeon. As with recurrent laryngeal nerve injury, the risk is significantly higher if the patient has had previous neck surgery (<4%). Complications are also more likely in patients who have large or invasive tumors with extensive lymphadenopathy. The incidence of parathyroid injury or removal during thyroidectomy can be minimized by meticulous technique in dissecting the parathyroids off the thyroid capsule. Some surgeons advocate routine autotransplantation of one parathyroid gland into the sternocleidomastoid muscle. Certainly, any devascularized parathyroid gland should be biopsied to confirm that it is a parathyroid and then autotransplanted.

OUTCOME

The vast majority of patients diagnosed with papillary thyroid cancer have an excellent prognosis. In order to try to predict which patients are at higher risk for a poor prognosis, several classification systems have been proposed for patients diagnosed with well-differentiated (papillary and follicular) thyroid carcinoma.

The most basic risk group classification can be made on the basis of age and gender. All patients younger than 45 years of age at the time of diagnosis of papillary thyroid carcinoma are considered low risk unless distant metastases are present. All older patients are considered high risk. Subsequent more complex postoperative risk classification systems have been proposed: AGES (age, grade, extent, size), AMES (age, metastases, extent, size), and MACIS (metastases, age, completeness of surgery, invasion of cancer, size). The most complex of these systems, the MACIS system, defines a prognostic score as follows:

MACIS = 3.1 (if age <39 years) or 0.08 × age (if age >40 years), + 0.3 × tumor size (in centimeters), + 1 (if incompletely resected), + 1 (if extrathyroidal invasion), + 3 (if distant metastases present)

Four risk groups are defined on the basis of MACIS score: <6.0, 6.0 to 6.9, 7.0 to 7.9, and 8.0+. Patients with a score of less than 6.0 are in the low-risk group. Hay and colleagues (1993) reported that approximately 84% of papillary thyroid carcinomas from the Mayo Clinic series fall into this low-risk group. The 20-year cause-specific survival rates for patients with MACIS less than 6, 6 to 6.99, 7 to 7.99, and 8 and over were 99%, 89%, 56%, and 24%, respectively. The recurrence rate was significantly lower in patients who had bilateral operations in both low- and high-risk groups, and survival was better in high-risk patients who had bilateral procedures.

With the increasing use of thyroglobulin levels to follow patients for recurrence, a dilemma arises when the thyroglobulin level suggests recurrent disease but the diagnostic scans are negative. Recent evidence suggests that the majority of such patients with a negative diagnostic [131]iodine scan will have a positive scan after being given a therapeutic dose of [131]iodine. Ultrasound studies of the neck or PET scanning of the body may reveal the site of the recurrent tumor. One should also be certain that thyroglobulin-positive, radioiodine uptake–negative patients are not iodine-loaded, as this loading suppresses iodine uptake.

Some subtypes of papillary thyroid cancer portend a worse prognosis than usual. Tall cell, columnar cell, and insular cell variants of carcinoma all seem to be associated with a poorer prognosis.

A small number of patients treated as described previously will develop recurrent papillary thyroid cancer. In most of these patients, it is due to lymph node metastases or, less commonly, recurrence in the thyroid bed or contralateral lobe. In general, palpable disease should be resected and nonpalpable disease or patients with no tumor on ultrasound treated with [131]iodine. A very small number of patients with recurrent papillary thyroid carcinoma will have a recurrence that is inoperable. Approximately a quarter of these patients with recurrent inopera-

ble papillary thyroid carcinoma will be found not to concentrate [131]iodine. In this subset of patients, Tsang and coauthors have recently shown success with external-beam radiation in a limited number of patients.

Pearls and Pitfalls

PEARLS

- By using large subplatysmal flaps, excellent exposure can be obtained by moving the incision around on the patient
- Avoid the use of any electrocautery in proximity to the nerves; if cautery is needed in these locations, consider bipolar cautery
- Use needle-tip cautery pencil on a low setting for increased precision
- Follow superior pole all the way up to the end of the gland prior to ligating vessels; elevate the tubercle of Zuckerkandl to lift the thyroid out of the neck; follow the pyramidal lobe all the way up to its end prior to ligating and dividing it

PITFALLS

- Making a large skin incision to gain adequate exposure to remove a normal-sized thyroid gland
- Transient RLN injury even when the nerve is seen to be intact
- Excess tissue damage from electrocautery
- Significant uptake in the thyroid bed after scanning for presumed "total" thyroidectomy

---

SELECTED READINGS

Bai J, Sherrod AE, Raghavan D: Uncommon cancers of the thyroid. In Raghavan D, Brecher ML, Johnson DH, et al (eds): Textbook of Uncommon Cancer, 2nd ed. New York, John Wiley & Sons, 1999, pp 259–68.

Cady B, Rossi R: An expanded view of risk-group definition in differentiated thyroid carcinoma. Surgery 1988;104:947.

Clark OH, Hoelting T: Management of patients with differentiated thyroid cancer who have positive serum thyroglobulin levels and negative radioiodine scans. Thyroid 1994;4:501.

DeGroot LJ, Kaplan EL, McCormick M, Straus FH: Natural history, treatment, and course of papillary thyroid carcinoma. J Clin Endocrinol Metab 1990;71:414.

Grant CS, Hay ID, Gough IR, et al: Local recurrence in papillary thyroid carcinoma: Is extent of surgical resection important? Surgery 1988;104:954.

Harness JK, Fung L, Thompson NW, et al: Total thyroidectomy: Complications and technique. World J Surg 1986;10:781.

Hay ID, Bergstralh EJ, Goellner JR, et al: Predicting outcome in papillary thyroid carcinoma: Development of a reliable prognostic scoring system in a cohort of 1779 patients surgically treated at one institution during 1940 through 1989. Surgery 1993;114:1050.

Hay ID, Grant CS, Taylor WF, McConahey WM: Ipsilateral lobectomy versus bilateral lobar resection in papillary thyroid carcinoma: A retrospective analysis of surgical outcome using a novel prognostic scoring system. Surgery 1987;102:1088.

Hay ID: Papillary thyroid carcinoma. Endocrinol Metab Clin North Am 1990;19:545.

Jossart GH, Clark OH: Well-differentiated thyroid cancer. Curr Probl Surg 1994;31:933.

Mazzaferri EL, Jhiang SM: Long-term impact of initial surgical and medical therapy on papillary and follicular thyroid cancer [see comments] [published erratum appears in Am J Med 1995;98:215]. Am J Med 1994;97:418.

Pacini F, Lippi F, Formica N, et al: Therapeutic doses of iodine-131 reveal undiagnosed metastases in thyroid cancer patients with detectable serum thyroglobulin levels. J Nucl Med 1987;28:1888.

Schlumberger MJ: Papillary and follicular thyroid carcinoma. N Engl J Med 1998;338:297.

Tsang RW, Brierley JD, Simpson WJ, et al: The effects of surgery, radioiodine, and external radiation therapy on the clinical outcome of patients with differentiated thyroid carcinoma. Cancer 1998;82:375.

Chapter 163

Follicular, Hürthle Cell, and Anaplastic Thyroid Cancer

Herbert Chen and Robert Udelsman

INTRODUCTION

Thyroid cancer is the most common endocrine malignancy, accounting for more than 18,000 estimated new cases in 1999. Approximately 1200 people die of thyroid cancer each year in the United States. Papillary thyroid cancer is the most common thyroid malignancy with the best overall prognosis. Follicular, Hürthle cell, and anaplastic carcinomas constitute about 15% of cases and are more aggressive. However, among these three tumors, follicular cancers tend to be more differentiated and less aggressive, followed by Hürthle cell cancers, and then anaplastic cancers, which are usually poorly differentiated and extremely aggressive. Follicular carcinoma is the second most common thyroid malignancy and is often grouped together with papillary thyroid cancer as "well-differentiated thyroid cancers." Follicular carcinomas tend to be solitary tumors. They metastasize hematogenously to bone, lung, brain, and liver. About 20% of patients with follicular cancers present with or develop metastases. Lymph node metastases are less common than in patients with papillary thyroid cancer. Hürthle cell carcinomas are less common than follicular cancer, making up 1% to 3% of all thyroid cancers. Hürthle cell carcinomas have been reported to behave in a more aggressive fashion than follicular cancers, as evidenced by a higher incidence of metastases and a lower survival rate. Hürthle cell carcinomas metastasize to lung, lymph nodes, bone, and brain in about 30% of patients. Anaplastic thyroid carcinomas tend to present in older patients with long-standing goiters or previous well-differentiated thyroid cancers, or both. Anaplastic or undifferentiated thyroid cancers account for fewer than 1% of thyroid cancers. They are the most aggressive thyroid tumors, which, fortunately, have been decreasing in frequency over the last few decades.

CLINICAL PRESENTATION

Patients with follicular or Hürthle cell cancer typically present with an otherwise asymptomatic thyroid nodule. The prevalence of thyroid nodules in the U.S. population ranges from 4% to 7%. Although the vast majority are benign, 5% eventually prove to be malignant. The surgeon's dilemma is distinguishing nodules that are suspicious for malignancy and need operative management. Patients with anaplastic carcinoma usually present with an enlarging mass (mean size >8 cm) or symptoms resulting from compression or invasion of adjacent structures.

Routine evaluation includes a careful history focusing on signs and symptoms associated with the thyroid lesion, such as shortness of breath, dysphagia, and hoarseness. Duration of the nodule and an interval change in its size are also important. A newly detected, rapidly growing nodule is more likely to be cancer. Questions regarding hyperthyroidism or hypothyroidism should be included, such as temperature intolerance and changes in weight and energy level. Two important questions asked during the evaluation focus on the risk factors for thyroid cancer. A family history of thyroid cancer and other endocrinopathies could suggest an inherited form of thyroid cancer; namely, medullary thyroid cancer and papillary thyroid cancer. Previous exposure to head and/or neck irradiation, more commonly utilized 15 to 20 years ago, is the most important risk factor for subsequent thyroid carcinoma.

A thorough physical evaluation should be performed. Temperature elevation may suggest an inflammatory or infectious process, such as thyroiditis. Tachycardia could be due to hyperthyroidism. Respiratory signs, including stridor or tachypnea, may be present in patients with obstructive thyroid lesions. The physical examination includes a detailed inspection of the neck. Having the patient drink water and swallow often aids in the visualization of the thyroid gland as well as in determining the mobility of a nodule. Palpation of the thyroid gland is frequently easier when the physician stands behind the patient and palpates the gland with both hands and fingers simultaneously. Again, having the patient swallow water helps with palpation of the thyroid. One should note the presence of a dominant nodule as well as other thyroid nodules. The neck is then palpated for any signs of adenopathy. Finally, indirect or direct laryngoscopy is performed to assess vocal cord function preoperatively in all patients with hoarseness or change in voice, or who have had previous neck operations.

In addition to a complete history and physical examination, thyroid-stimulating hormone (TSH) is measured, and the authors perform a fine-needle aspiration (FNA) of the dominant and other significant thyroid nodules or masses, or suspicious lymph nodes. FNA has revolutionized the management of thyroid nodules, providing an extremely sensitive and cost-effective method for detecting malignancy. This entire evaluation is routinely conducted during a single outpatient visit.

Imaging studies are not routinely utilized in the evaluation of thyroid nodules. Ultrasonography is occasionally useful for guiding FNA biopsies and localizing other thyroid nodules. In the past, thyroid scintiscanning was commonly employed to distinguish "hot" from "cold" nodules. A "hot" nodule is a hyperfunctioning nodule relative to normal thyroid gland, and, rarely, hot nodules are malignant. "Cold," or hypofunctioning, nodules have about a 20% risk of malignancy. It is important to remember that although malignant lesions tend to be "cold," the vast majority of cold nodules are benign. The authors reserve thyroid scintiscanning during the initial evaluation for patients who are hyperthyroid by history and/or TSH level. In cases of large thyroid masses, computed tomography (CT) scans or magnetic resonance imaging (MRI) can be helpful in determining the extent of involvement of surrounding structures, or in localizing recurrent disease, especially when there is evidence of local fixation, vocal cord paresis, or substernal extension.

PREOPERATIVE MANAGEMENT

FINE-NEEDLE ASPIRATION. FNA is the first-line diagnostic tool in the preoperative work-up of a patient with a thyroid nodule. The overall sensitivity and specificity of FNA for malignancy have ranged from 68% to 98% and 56% to 100%, respectively. The most common cause of FNA failure is an inadequate or insufficient sample. It is therefore useful to have onsite cytologic review to ensure that an adequate sample is obtained. FNA is performed with the patient in a supine position, with a pillow placed behind the shoulders to extend the neck. The skin is cleansed with 70% isopropyl alcohol. Local anesthetics are rarely required and tend to distort the anatomy and often result in more discomfort. The thyroid nodule is localized between the fingertips of the nondominant hand. With the surgeon using the dominant hand, a 25- or 27-gauge, 1.5-inch needle with an attached 10-mL syringe is advanced into the lesion. Nonaspiration techniques are often the most successful, as they result in less blood contamination. On entering the lesion, the needle is rapidly moved back and forth several times until material is seen within the hub of the needle. Three to six separate passes at different angles are often required for adequate sampling. If fluid is encountered (i.e., a cyst), it is completely aspirated and sent for cytologic analysis. The region of the cyst is then re-examined, and the FNA is repeated if a residual mass is palpated. Once sampling is completed, the needle is detached from the syringe, the syringe is filled with air and re-attached, and 1 or 2 drops of the material is expressed onto a glass microscope slide with the needle bevel pointing downward. A second microscope slide is placed on top of the first slide, and the material is smeared by pulling the slides apart in a horizontal direction. Slides are either wet- or dry-fixed. The remaining tissue samples are harvested by rinsing the needle with phosphate-buffered saline and are saved as a block pellet.

FOLLICULAR NEOPLASMS. About 20% of thyroid nodules are follicular neoplasms by FNA biopsy. They are characterized by a predominance of follicular epithelial cells forming microfollicles with a paucity of colloid. Cytologic features include follicular cells with nuclear atypia and minimal cytoplasm with overlapping nuclei (Fig. 163–1). Follicular neoplasms can be either follicular adenomas (benign) or follicular carcinomas. Follicular carcinomas constitute about 20% of follicular neoplasms. Therefore,

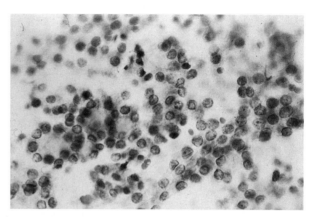

Figure 163–1. Follicular neoplasm, cytology. Hypercellularity, paucity of colloid, and microacinar pattern in a follicular neoplasm.

the majority of follicular neoplasms are benign adenomas. The sine qua non for determining malignancy in follicular neoplasms is the presence of capsular or vascular invasion on permanent histology. Cytology alone cannot reliably distinguish a benign follicular adenoma from a carcinoma. Frequently, a significant degree of nuclear atypia is seen in follicular adenomas. Conversely, follicular carcinomas may have relatively benign cytologic features. Because malignancy cannot be reliably determined without permanent histology, patients with follicular neoplasms generally undergo thyroid lobectomy.

HÜRTHLE CELL NEOPLASMS. Hürthle cell neoplasms are encapsulated collections of Hürthle cells, large polygonal eosinophilic cells with pleomorphic hyperchromatic nuclei and fine granular acidophilic cytoplasm, representing an abundance of mitochondria. The individual cells are 10 to 15 μm in diameter and vary in shape and size from small dumbbells to bizarre giant cells. Because Hürthle cells are commonly associated with Graves' disease, Hashimoto's thyroiditis, and nodular goiters, as well as with well-differentiated thyroid cancers, multiple needle passes containing predominantly Hürthle cells are required to reliably diagnose a Hürthle cell neoplasm. Hürthle cell neoplasms appear as nests of Hürthle cells in a microfollicular pattern, often intermixed with follicular cells (Fig. 163–2). Hürthle cell neoplasms are often classified as a subset of follicular neoplasms. Hürthle cell neoplasms will prove to be carcinomas in about 25% of cases. As with follicular neoplasms, the diagnosis of a Hürthle cell carcinoma cannot be reliably made cytologically. Malignant criteria require histologic evidence of vascular and capsular invasion. However, since Hürthle cell carcinomas generally behave in a more aggressive manner than that of follicular carcinomas, metastasizing more frequently and less likely to respond to radioactive iodine, they are categorized as a distinct subset of follicular thyroid carcinomas. Similar to follicular neoplasms, patients with Hürthle cell neoplasms generally undergo thyroid lobectomy.

ANAPLASTIC CARCINOMA. The three types of anaplastic carcinoma are squamoid, giant cell, and spindle cell. The most common variant is the giant cell type. Thus, the cytologic findings of anaplastic carcinoma reflect the

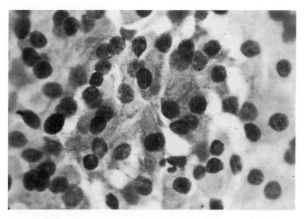

Figure 163–2. Hürthle cell neoplasm, cytology. Larger polygonal cells with granular cytoplasm and increased pleomorphism in a Hürthle cell neoplasm.

particular cell types, including polygonal cells, giant cells, and mesenchymal spindle cells (Fig. 163–3). These cells are frequently bizarre in appearance, with irregular nuclei and prominent nucleoli. Anaplastic carcinomas may be difficult to distinguish from poorly differentiated medullary thyroid carcinoma, metastatic carcinoma, or thyroid lymphoma based on morphologic findings alone. Therefore, negative immunohistochemical stains for calcitonin, CEA, chromogranin A, T-cell antigens, and B-cell immunoglobulins effectively rule out medullary thyroid cancer and lymphoma and, by exclusion, are suggestive of anaplastic carcinoma. Occasionally, the features of a preexisting well-differentiated tumor of origin can be seen on cytologic review.

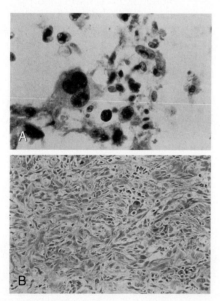

Figure 163–3. Anaplastic carcinoma, cytology *(A)* and histology *(B)*. Extremely hypercellular, bizarre pleomorphism, coarse irregular chromatin, multiple macronucleoli, and sarcomatoid features. (From Chen H, Nicol TL, Rosenthal DL, et al: The role of fine-needle aspiration in the evaluation of thyroid nodules. In Norton JA (ed): Problems in General Surgery: Surgery of the Thyroid Gland. New York, Lippincott-Raven, 1997, with permission.)

INTRAOPERATIVE MANAGEMENT

FOLLICULAR NEOPLASMS. Patients with follicular neoplasms generally undergo operative exploration. Prior to surgery, a complete discussion with the patient should emphasize that there is approximately a 20% chance of malignancy. The minimal operation for a patient with a follicular neoplasm is a thorough neck exploration, an ipsilateral thyroid lobectomy and isthmectomy, and palpation of the contralateral gland. This is adequate treatment for a follicular adenoma. However, if the lesion turns out to be a follicular carcinoma, the authors' belief is that total thyroidectomy is the treatment of choice. As previously mentioned, the only way of distinguishing a follicular adenoma from a carcinoma is the presence of vascular and/or capsular invasion (Fig. 163–4). Often, this diagnosis cannot be made intraoperatively. However, at exploration, if evidence of malignancy, such as invasion of adjacent structures or lymph node metastases, is present, the authors confirm malignancy by obtaining a guided frozen section and, if it is malignant, perform a total thyroidectomy. The authors would also perform an initial total thyroidectomy for a follicular neoplasm if the patient had a history of head and neck irradiation or if bilateral nodular thyroid disease is present at neck exploration. Radiation therapy is associated with an increase risk of thyroid cancer as well as multifocal disease. Furthermore, some patients, after learning about the 20% risk of carci-

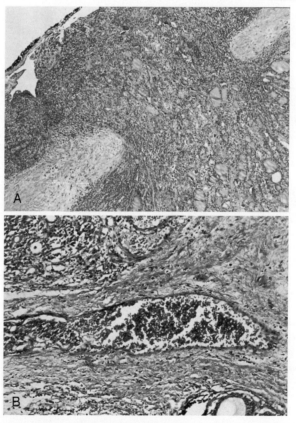

Figure 163–4. Follicular-Hürthle carcinoma, histology. *(A),* Full-thickness, transcapsular penetration by tumor. *(B),* Well-defined, medium-sized blood vessel invasion by tumor.

noma with follicular neoplasms, may elect to have an initial total or near-total thryoidectomy, rather than having to undergo a potentially staged completion thryoidectomy should cancer be found.

In the past, intraoperative frozen-section analysis had been advocated as a guide for surgical management. These surgeons would perform an ipsilateral thyroid lobectomy and isthmectomy, employ frozen section on the nodule, and proceed with a total thryoidectomy if the frozen section revealed vascular or capsular invasion. However, the authors and others have shown that frozen-section evaluation of follicular thyroid neoplasms is of minimal diagnostic value, renders no additional information in the vast majority of cases, and can actually mislead the surgeon. In a series of 125 patients with follicular neoplasms, frozen section did not provide any additional information 87% of the time. Furthermore, frozen-section analysis misled the surgeon as frequently as it correctly modified the surgical procedure. Therefore, for the management of follicular neoplasms, the authors recommend that routine frozen-section analysis be omitted, resection of the lobe with the nodule be performed, and the surgeon and pathologist examine the gross specimen for evidence of gross invasion. If there is a suspicious region, a guided frozen section can be diagnostic of malignancy. However, in the majority of cases, definitive operative management is based on permanent histology. If permanent histology is diagnostic of carcinoma, a completion thyroidectomy is recommended for the majority of patients.

The authors believe that total thyroidectomy is the treatment of choice for most follicular carcinomas of the thyroid. One of the most controversial issues in endocrine surgery focuses on the extent of thyroidectomy for differentiated thyroid cancer, including follicular carcinomas. The most commonly recommended options range from thyroid lobectomy–isthmectomy for all but the most aggressive cases to a total extracapsular thyroidectomy for virtually all cases of clinically significant follicular thyroid cancer. There are no randomized, prospective trials comparing the results of different operative treatments of well-differentiated thyroid malignancies. It is unlikely that such a study will be undertaken because to complete a prospective trial, between 3000 to 12,000 individuals with thyroid cancer would have to be randomized to analyze the end points of recurrence, treatment-related complications, and tumor-specific mortality. However, based on several large retrospective reports that have addressed the extent of thyroidectomy, it appears that total thyroidectomy is the treatment of choice for clinically significant, follicular thyroid cancer.

Total thyroidectomy improves the ability to use radioactive iodine (^{131}I) therapy postoperatively, which has been shown to prolong survival and reduce recurrence rates in patients with follicular thyroid cancer. Since ^{131}I ablation is highly dependent on the amount of residual thyroid tissue remaining after surgery, total thyroidectomy lowers the dose of ^{131}I needed. Following thyroid remnant ablation, serum thyroglobulin measurements have been shown to be the most sensitive marker for tumor recurrence. Furthermore, ^{131}I scans can be utilized to diagnose

and localize recurrent disease. This is of significance because the probability of living with persistent disease or of dying after the treatment of recurrent thyroid cancer is less for ^{131}I-detected recurrence compared with clinically diagnosed recurrence (9.5% versus 54%). Most importantly, several studies have suggested that total or near-total thyroidectomy plus ^{131}I improves survival in patients with well-differentiated thyroid cancer. Clark reported that total thyroidectomy reduced the cancer death rate from 5% to 2% to 3%. In the largest series to date, Mazzaferri and colleagues reported a lower 30-year mortality rate for patients with stage 2 or 3 disease who had total or near-total thyroidectomy versus subtotal thyroidectomy (9% versus 6%; $P < 0.02$). In their series of more than 1300 patients, not a single individual with a tumor less than 1.5 cm confined to the thyroid gland who underwent total or near-total thyroidectomy died. The data clearly suggest that in high-risk patients, total or near-total thyroidectomy plus ^{131}I improves survival. The significance of this survival advantage has been put in perspective by Wong and associates; the benefits of total thyroidectomy plus ^{131}I are similar to those obtained by the patient not smoking or by the performance of coronary artery bypass surgery in patients with three-vessel coronary artery disease.

Similar studies have shown that total or near-total thyroidectomy reduces the cancer-recurrence rate in patients with well-differentiated thyroid cancer. Preventing tumor recurrence is important because 50% of patients who have recurrences in the central neck ultimately die of thyroid cancer. Total thyroidectomy plus ^{131}I also reduces the risk of developing pulmonary metastases. In one study, the prevalence of pulmonary metastases was 1.3% in patients who had total thyroidectomy plus ^{131}I, 5% in those who had subtotal thyroidectomy plus ^{131}I, and 11% in those who had only partial thyroidectomies (lobectomies). Several authors have reported that total thyroidectomy performed by an experienced thyroid surgeon can result in morbidity and mortality rates similar to those of thyroid lobectomy in the treatment of well-differentiated thyroid cancer. There should be less than a 2% rate of recurrent laryngeal nerve injury or permanent hypoparathyroidism. Anaplastic thyroid cancer has a dismal prognosis and, in some cases, is thought to arise from a focus of well-differentiated thyroid cancer. Total thyroidectomy, in theory, would prevent the occurrence of anaplastic carcinoma in a gland that already has evidence of malignant potential.

HÜRTHLE CELL NEOPLASMS. Fine-needle aspiration biopsy cannot reliably distinguish a Hürthle cell adenoma from a carcinoma. Hürthle cell carcinomas make up about 25% of Hürthle cell neoplasms. Because malignancy cannot be reliably determined without permanent histology, patients with Hürthle cell neoplasms generally undergo operative exploration. Earlier studies suggested that the clinical behavior of these neoplasms was unpredictable. Therefore, in the past, total thyroidectomy was recommended by some authors for all Hürthle cell neoplasms. However, subsequent investigators have shown that the distinction between Hürthle cell adenomas and carcinomas can be made on the basis of permanent histology, relying on the presence of capsular and/or vascular invasion exclusively in carcinomas. Hürthle cell carcinomas behave in a more aggressive fashion than that of other well-differentiated thyroid cancers, as evidenced by a higher incidence of metastases and a lower survival rate. In addition, they have decreased avidity for ^{131}I. Accordingly, most experienced surgeons recommend aggressive surgical treatment of Hürthle cell carcinomas, usually in the form of a total thyroidectomy with removal of involved lymph nodes. In contrast, Hürthle cell adenomas are generally treated with a thyroid lobectomy.

Thus, the minimal operation for a patient with a Hürthle cell neoplasm is a thorough neck exploration, an ipsilateral thyroid lobectomy and isthmectomy, and palpation of the contralateral gland. This is adequate treatment for a Hürthle cell adenoma. However, if the lesion proves to be a Hürthle cell carcinoma, the authors' belief is that total thyroidectomy is the treatment of choice. Carcangiu and associates have shown that local recurrence of Hürthle cell carcinoma is correlated with the extent of surgery, with recurrence rates for nodulectomy, thyroid lobectomy, and total thyroidectomy of 75%, 40%, and 15%, respectively. As previously noted, the only way of distinguishing a Hürthle cell adenoma from a carcinoma is the presence of vascular and/or capsular invasion. In the vast majority of patients, this delineation cannot be made preoperatively. However, at exploration, if evidence of malignancy, such as invasion of adjacent structures or lymph node metastases, is present, the authors would obtain a guided frozen section to establish the diagnosis, and perform a total thyroidectomy. The authors would also perform an initial total thyroidectomy for a Hürthle cell neoplasm if the patient had a history of head and neck irradiation or bilateral nodular thyroid disease at neck exploration. Radiation therapy is associated with an increased risk of subsequent cancer as well as multifocal disease. Furthermore, some patients, knowing the 25% risk of carcinoma, may elect to have an initial total thyroidectomy, rather than having a completion thyroidectomy should cancer be found. Finally, the size of a Hürthle cell neoplasm correlates with its malignant potential. In a series of 57 consecutive Hürthle cell neoplasms, tumors 1 cm or less in size were found to be malignant in 17% of cases. However, 65% of tumors at least 4 cm in diameter proved to be malignant. Therefore, size should be considered when one decides on operative management (Fig. 163–5). Thus, if the tumor is 4 cm or larger in diameter on intraoperative gross inspection, the authors consider performing a total thyroidectomy because of the high risk of cancer. Intraoperatively, if there is no evidence of malignant disease and the tumor is less than 4 cm in diameter, the authors perform an ipsilateral thyroid lobectomy-isthmectomy and await permanent histologic analysis. Routine intraoperative frozen sections are often performed in patients with Hürthle cell neoplasms but are of minimal value. If permanent histology is diagnostic of carcinoma, a completion thyroidectomy is performed for the majority of patients.

ANAPLASTIC THYROID CANCER. Primary treatment of anaplastic thyroid carcinoma involves chemotherapy, often in combination with radiotherapy. Some patients are candidates for surgical resection. The diagnosis can usually be made by history, physical examination, and FNA biopsy. However, occasionally, a Tru-Cut or open biopsy is required to make a definitive tissue diagnosis. Once the diagnosis is made, chemotherapy with or without irradiation can be initiated. Most reports of single-modality treatment have been dismal. Surgery is occasionally required for palliation to relieve airway obstruction and/or dysphagia. Increasingly, surgical extirpation can be part of aggressive combined-modality protocols. There are some reports that multiple-modality treatment with radiation, doxorubicin, Taxol (paclitaxel), and/or surgical debulking has resulted in better local control.

POSTOPERATIVE MANAGEMENT

Patients are generally admitted for observation overnight. The authors monitor for physical signs of a neck hematoma or hypocalcemia, and check a serum ionized calcium the morning after surgery.

ROLE OF RADIOACTIVE IODINE (^{131}I). Total thyroidectomy and ^{131}I ablation reduces the recurrence rate and death from follicular cancers. Only about 7% of Hürthle cell cancers respond to ^{131}I, and most anaplastic thyroid tumors fail to respond. In the authors' practice, after total thyroidectomy for follicular or Hürthle cell cancer, patients are placed on Cytomel (T_3) for 4 weeks. Cytomel is then stopped for an additional 2 weeks to allow the TSH level to rise to more than 50 mIU/L. Patients are also placed on a low-iodine diet. The authors then check the serum thyroglobulin and perform a 2 to 5 mCi ^{131}I scan. If the scan is positive for a thyroid remnant, an ablation dose of ^{131}I is administered. Occasionally, patients with follicular carcinoma have evidence of lung or bone metastases on the diagnostic scan. A therapeutic dose of ^{131}I is administered in these patients.

The role of ^{131}I therapy in the treatment of Hürthle cell carcinoma is less compelling. The authors selectively treat patients with Hürthle cell carcinoma after total thyroidectomy with ^{131}I therapy to ablate residual thyroid bed uptake, if present. Some metastases from Hürthle cell carcinomas have been reported to be ^{131}I-responsive (7%). In these rare cases, almost exclusively pulmonary metastases, Hürthle cell carcinoma metastases are treated with ^{131}I. With the utilization of recombinant TSH testing, which is likely to replace thyroid hormone withdrawal, patients will not have to experience the side effects of hypothyroidism associated with traditional ^{131}I scans. After ablation of the thyroid remnant, serum thyroglobulin levels can be used to monitor for recurrence in patients with follicular or Hürthle cell carcinoma.

L-THYROXINE SUPPRESSIVE THERAPY. Patients with follicular or Hürthle cell carcinoma are placed on thyroid hormone suppression therapy after total thyroidectomy. Suppression of TSH by administration of thyroid hormone (L-thyroxine) improves survival and reduces recurrence rates after thyroidectomy. However, high doses of thyroid hormone may have adverse effects on the bone

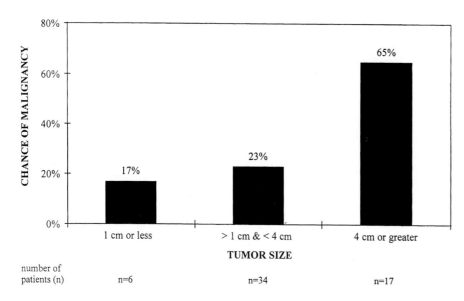

Figure 163–5. Hürthle cell neoplasms—tumor size is predictive of malignancy. With increasing tumor size, the chance of malignancy increases. (From Chen H, Nicol TL, Zeiger MA, et al: Hürthle cell neoplasms of the thyroid: Are there factors predictive of malignancy? Ann Surg 1998;227:542–546, with permission.)

and heart. Ideally, the lowest dose of thyroid hormone that suppresses tumor recurrence should be used.

MANAGEMENT OF LYMPH NODE METASTASES. Follicular and Hürthle cell cancers occasionally metastasize to cervical lymph nodes. Generally, prophylactic resection of occult cancer in cervical lymph nodes is not necessary. In rare cases, patients who present with follicular and Hürthle cell carcinomas and palpable lymphadenopathy preoperatively undergo cytologic confirmation of metastases and a modified radical neck dissection, as described by Bocca, is performed at the time of total thyroidectomy. This technique spares the sternocleidomastoid muscle, internal jugular vein, and accessory nerve. Routine nodal dissection in the absence of gross nodal disease is not advocated, as there are no data demonstrating the benefit of prophylactic nodal dissection. If enlarged lymph nodes are not palpable preoperatively but are found during neck exploration, suspicious nodes are sampled and intraoperative frozen-section analysis is obtained. If the lateral compartment lymph nodes are positive, the authors perform a modified radical neck dissection. Modified neck dissections provide control of lymph node disease equivalent to that with radical neck dissections, but are associated with less morbidity. In general, a unilateral neck dissection is performed, but if clinically significant nodal disease is present bilaterally, bilateral neck dissections are indicated.

RECURRENT DISEASE IN THE NECK. If recurrent disease is detected by an ^{131}I scan and/or an elevated thyroglobulin, the authors first-line imaging study is ultrasonography, but they will often include CT or MRI scans. If any of these studies localize recurrent disease, surgical resection is considered. If these imaging studies do not show enlarged lymph nodes or thyroid bed recurrence, therapeutic doses of ^{131}I are usually administered for follicular cancers and, occasionally, for Hürthle cell cancers. For recurrent nodal disease, modified radical neck dissection is performed. If a subsequent gross recurrence occurs, repeat neck dissections are considered. Following resection, repeat ^{131}I scanning and treatment are generally recommended. A subset of patients will develop recurrent follicular cancer, manifested by a rising serum thyroglobulin level, but will have negative ^{131}I scans. The management of these patients is controversial. The authors image these patients with additional techniques, including ultrasonography, CT, MRI, and, occasionally, positron emission tomography (PET) scans. If any of these studies demonstrate local resectable disease, surgical intervention is considered. If these studies are negative, therapeutic doses of ^{131}I are administered, since some will respond in the setting of a negative ^{131}I test dose.

COMPLICATIONS

RECURRENT LARYNGEAL NERVE INJURY. It is paramount that thyroid surgery be performed safely. The recurrent laryngeal nerves must be protected. In experienced hands, the incidence of laryngeal nerve damage should be rare. A unilateral nerve injury usually results in hoarseness, although it may be asymptomatic. Bilateral nerve injury usually causes severe airway compromise and may necessitate tracheostomy. Recurrent laryngeal nerve injury is diagnosed by assessment of the vocal cords with direct or indirect laryngoscopy. The ipsilateral vocal cord will be in the midline or paramedian position if an injury has occurred. More commonly, the injury is transient in nature. If the surgeon is unable to resect the thyroid gland without compromising the nerve, then a near-total thyroidectomy, leaving less than 2 g of normal thyroid tissue adjacent to these structures, is an acceptable alternative. The residual thyroid tissue can easily be ablated with [131]I. It is important for all surgeons to remember that it is far better, if necessary, to leave a little bit of normal thyroid in situ than it is to have a little bit of normal recurrent nerve ex vivo. In some circumstances, the authors consider performing a thyroid lobectomy, rather than total thyroidectomy. In addition, for the noncompliant patient who will not take thyroid hormone or for patients in areas of the world without access to thyroid hormone, a thyroid lobectomy may be appropriate.

SUPERIOR LARYNGEAL NERVE INJURY (EXTERNAL BRANCH). Injury to this nerve occurs during mobilization of the superior thyroid lobe. It manifests as the inability to make high-pitched sounds, or the impaired ability to project the voice. Often, this complication is unrecognized.

HYPOPARATHYROIDISM. Hypoparathyroidism after thyroidectomy usually is secondary to devascularization of the parathyroid glands. This can be transient or permanent. The parathyroid glands are usually supplied by both the inferior and the superior thyroid arteries. To avoid this complication, when the surgeon mobilizes the thyroid, the inferior thyroid artery must be ligated close to the capsule of the thyroid gland. The parathyroids must be identified, and their blood supply preserved. When an adequate blood supply cannot be preserved to a parathyroid gland, it should be biopsied and autotransplanted. The incidence of permanent hypoparathyroidism should be less than 2% in experienced hands.

POSTOPERATIVE BLEEDING. Bleeding into the neck after thyroidectomy can be a life-threatening situation. The neck is a small, closed space. An expanding hematoma can quickly cause obstruction of the airway. If an expanding hematoma develops postoperatively, the wound should be opened quickly at the bedside (if necessary) through the strap muscles in order to remove pressure on the airway. Afterward, the patient is taken emergently to the operating room for neck exploration and ligation of bleeding vessels. This complication can be minimized by meticulous hemostasis during thyroidectomy.

OUTCOMES

SURVIVAL. Follicular thyroid cancers tend to present in older patients. Hematogenous spread not uncommonly occurs and may cause bone metastases. The estimated 10-year survival for patients with follicular thyroid cancer is about 75%. Patients who undergo total thyroidectomy and radioactive iodine treatment have improved survival and decreased recurrence rates. Hürthle cell carcinomas also occur in older patients. Similar to follicular cancers, Hürthle cell tumors metastasize hematogenously, but they may also involve the regional lymph nodes. The estimated 10-year survival for patients with Hürthle cell cancer is approximately 70%. The vast majority of Hürthle cell carcinomas (93%) are resistant to radioactive iodine, and surgical resection is the only curative treatment. Anaplastic thyroid cancers generally present in much older patients. These tumors grow rapidly and are associated with local, nodal, and hematogenous metastases. The estimated 10-year survival for patients with anaplastic carcinoma is less than 2%. The mean survival is 3 to 6 months.

MORBIDITY. A recent study has shown that surgeon experience is significantly associated with clinical and economic outcomes for patients who underwent thyroidectomy in Maryland between 1991 and 1996. High-volume surgeons (those who have performed more than 100 thyroid procedures per year) had a significantly shorter hospital length of stay and lower complication rates compared with low- or moderate-volume surgeons. Furthermore, the differences in outcomes were especially true for patients with thyroid cancer; high-volume surgeons had more than 60% fewer complications. Thus, surgical experience appears to play an important role in morbidity rates after thyroidectomy.

Summary

Thyroid cancer constitutes 1% of solid organ malignancies, and is the most common endocrine tumor. Follicular, Hürthle cell, and anaplastic thyroid cancer account for about 15% of all thyroid malignancies. Thyroidectomy is the mainstay of therapy for follicular and Hürthle cell cancers, while chemotherapy and radiation are used to treat most patients with anaplastic thyroid cancer. Patients with follicular and Hürthle cell cancers generally have a favorable prognosis and enjoy a long-term survival. Unfortunately, patients with anaplastic thyroid cancer have a dismal prognosis.

Pearls and Pitfalls

Follicular Thyroid Cancer

PEARLS

- Follicular thyroid cancer constitutes 10% to 15% of thyroid cancers.
- These cancers hematogenously metastasize to bone, lung, brain, and liver.
- FNA yields follicular neoplasm; it cannot determine malignancy (20% malignancy).
- Frozen-section analysis is rarely useful.
- Treatment is total thyroidectomy plus ^{131}I ablation.
- 10-year survival is 75%.

Hürthle Cell Cancer

PEARLS

- Hürthle cell cancers make up 1% to 3% of thyroid cancers.
- They hematogenously metastasize to bone, lung, brain, and lymph nodes.
- FNA yields Hürthle cell neoplasm; it cannot determine malignancy (25% malignancy).
- Frozen-section analysis is rarely useful.
- Treatment is total thyroidectomy plus ^{131}I ablation.
- 10-year survival is 70%.

Anaplastic Thyroid Cancer

PEARLS

- Anaplastic thyroid cancers constitute fewer than 1% of thyroid cancers.
- These cancers are very aggressive.
- FNA biopsy is diagnostic, yielding bizarre, irregular nuclei.
- Treatment is primary chemotherapy with or without radiation therapy.
- 10-year survival is less than 2%.

SELECTED READINGS

Chen H, Nicol TL, Rosenthal DL, Udelsman R: The role of fine-needle aspiration in the evaluation of thyroid nodules. In Norton JA (ed): Problems in General Surgery: Surgery of the Thyroid Gland. New York, Lippincott-Raven, 1997, pp 1–44.

Chen H, Nicol TL, Udelsman R: Follicular lesions of the thyroid: Does frozen-section evaluation alter operative management? Ann Surg 1995;222:101.

Chen H, Nicol TL, Zeiger MA, et al: Hürthle cell neoplasms of the thyroid: Are there factors predictive of malignancy? Ann Surg 1998;227:542.

Chen H, Udelsman R: Hürthle cell adenoma and carcinoma. In Clark OH, Duh QY (eds): Textbook of Endocrine Surgery. Philadelphia, WB Saunders, 1997, pp 101–106.

Clark OH: Total thyroidectomy: The treatment of choice for patients with differentiated thyroid cancer. Ann Surg 1982;196:361.

Mazzaferri EL, Jhiang SM: Long-term impact of initial surgical and medical therapy on papillary and follicular thyroid cancer. Am J Med 1994;97:418.

Sosa JA, Bowman HM, Tielsch JM, et al: The importance of surgeon experience for clinical and economic outcomes from thyroidectomy. Ann Surg 1998;228:320.

Tennvall J, Lundell G, Hallquist A, et al: Combined doxorubicin, hyperfractionated radiotherapy, and surgery in anaplastic thyroid carcinoma. Cancer 1994;74:1348.

Udelsman R, Lakatos E, Ladenson P: Optimal surgery for papillary carcinoma. World J Surg 1996;20:88.

Chapter 164

Medullary Thyroid Carcinoma

Geoffrey B. Thompson

Medullary thyroid carcinoma (MTC) accounts for fewer than 10% of all primary thyroid malignancies. It was first described, as an entity separate from anaplastic thyroid carcinoma, by Hazard and colleagues at the Cleveland Clinic in 1959. MTC arises from the parafollicular C-cells of the thyroid, making calcitonin (immunoreactive calcitonin, or iCT) a useful clinical marker for tumor progression and recurrence. The biologic behavior of MTC ranks between that of differentiated thyroid cancer and anaplastic carcinoma. About 25% of medullary thyroid cancers are hereditary, and their ultimate occurrence can be predicted prior to the development of MTC by neonatal screening of DNA from circulating lymphocytes. The presence of specific mutations in the *RET* proto-oncogene (Fig. 164–1), a known tumor suppressor gene located within the long arm of chromosome 10, band q11.2, results in the development of MTC in all affected kindred members and less often results in the development of pheochromocytomas, hyperparathyroidism (HPT), or the classic phenotypic picture of multiple endocrine neoplasia type 2B (MEN 2B) patients. Patients who have tested positive for any of these mutations can be selected early for prophylactic thyroidectomy; unaffected members can be reassured and will avoid lifetime fears and frequent biochemical testing.

CLINICAL PRESENTATION

The clinical presentation of MTC is varied and protean. The types, frequency, and clinical presentations of MTC syndromes are summarized in Table 164–1. Eighty percent of cases are sporadic or nonhereditary, presenting in older adults, typically with a thyroid mass, cervical lymphadenopathy, or local cervical symptomatology.

Hereditary forms (25%) of MTC present at a younger age and include MEN 2A (MTC, pheochromocytomas, HPT), MEN 2B (MTC, pheochromocytomas, mucosal and ganglioneuromas, marfanoid phenotype), or FMTC (MTC alone in at least two family members).

MEN 2B patients can be detected early by an astute pediatrician as the result of their characteristic phenotype (Figs. 164–2 and 164–3). MEN 2B patients have the most aggressive form of MTC and can present with metastases during infancy.

Most hereditary cases are now diagnosed in the preclinical, asymptomatic, period because of appropriate genetic testing of affected kindred members. All patients, however, presenting with MTC should be screened for *RET* mutations, as they may represent the index case for a new kindred. MEN 2A patients with mutations in codon 634 are at higher risk for developing pheochromocytomas and HPT. Mutations in codon 918 are associated with MEN 2B and confer a worse prognosis. More than 20% of sporadic MTC patients have somatic mutations in codon 768 and codon 918. Mutations in MEN 2A, 2B, and FMTC convert *RET* into a dominant transforming gene with oncogenic activity.

RET Proto-Oncogene

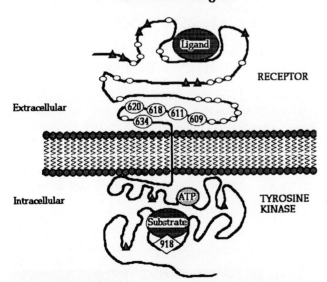

Figure 164–1. Diagrammatic representation of *RET* proto-oncogene. Missense mutations associated with MEN 2A and familial non-MEN medullary thyroid cancer have been found in codons encoding extracellular cysteine residues (codons 609, 611, 618, 620, and 634). Missense mutation associated with MEN 2B has been found in tyrosine kinase (codon 918). (ATP, adenosine triphosphate). (From Clark OH, Duh Q-Y [eds]: Textbook of Endocrine Surgery. Philadelphia, WB Saunders, 1997, with permission.)

Table 164–1	Types, Frequency, and Clinical Presentation of MTC Syndromes	
PHENOTYPES	**FREQUENCY**	**CLINICAL PRESENTATION**
Sporadic MTC	80%	MTC
MEN 2A:		
MEN 2A (1)	4%	MTC, pheochromocytoma, hyperparathyroidism
MEN 2A (2)	4%	MTC, pheochromocytoma
MEN 2A (3)	1%	MTC, hyperparathyroidism
MEN 2B	3%	MTC, pheochromocytoma, ganglioneuromatosis, marfanoid habitus
FMTC	1%	MTC (in at least 4 family members)
Other FMTC	7%	MTC (in 2 or 3 family members)

MTC, medullary thyroid carcinoma; MEN 2A, multiple endocrine neoplasia type 2A; MEN 2B, multiple endocrine neoplasia type 2B; FMTC, familial MTC.

From Heshmati HM, Gharib H, van Heerden JA, Sizemore G: Advances and controversies in the diagnosis and management of medullary thyroid carcinoma. Am J Med 1997;103:60–69; with permission.

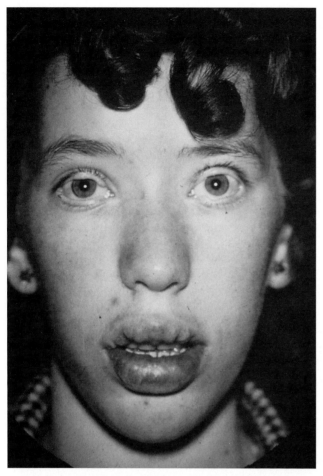

Figure 164–2. Characteristic facies in a girl with MEN 2B. Features include elongated face; thick, lumpy lips caused by mucosal neuromas; and thick eyelids with marked eversion. (From Heshmati HM, Gharib H, van Heerden JA, Sizemore G: Advances and controversies in the diagnosis and management of medullary thyroid carcinoma. Am J Med 1997;103:60–69, with permission.)

Thirty to fifty percent of patients with MEN 2 develop pheochromocytomas. The disease is usually bilateral, multicentric, and rarely malignant. Adrenal medullary hyperplasia is the precursor lesion. Clinical manifestations are often subtle and may include nervousness and palpitations. In younger patients, only 50% may have detectable hypertension (sustained or paroxysmal). Sudden death can occur because of hypertensive crisis, and these tumors must be ruled out and an adrenalectomy or adrenalectomies performed after alpha-blockade and hydration prior to other operative procedures or pregnancies.

HPT occurs in 10% to 20% of MEN 2A patients. Sequelae are less severe than those in sporadic or MEN I HPT patients. Hyperplasia occurs, but it is often strikingly asymmetric.

In MEN 2B patients, the ganglioneuromatosis can affect not only the tongue, lips, and eyelids but also the gastrointestinal (GI) tract. GI involvement can lead to chronic constipation, diarrhea, abdominal pain, megacolon, obstruction, and volvulus. The marfanoid habitus occurs without cardiac manifestations in MEN 2B patients and is characterized by long, thin extremities and digits, hyperextensible joints, and epiphyseal abnormali-

ties. In addition to iCT, MTC can elaborate a variety of peptides and amines, occasionally giving rise to unique clinical syndromes. These include carcinoembryonic antigen (CEA), histaminase, neuron-specific enolase, calcitonin gene–related peptide, somatostatin, thyroglobulin, thyroid-stimulating hormone (TSH), adrenocorticotropic hormone (ACTH) (the *Cushing syndrome*), gastrin-related peptide, serotonin or substance P *(flushing and diarrhea)*, and chromogranin. Levels of iCT appear to correlate with the bulk of disease, whereas higher CEA levels correlate with more aggressive biologic behavior. MTC associated with MEN 2B appears to have the most aggressive behavior, whereas MTC associated with MEN 2A and FMTC appears to have the least aggressive behavior. Sporadic MTC demonstrates variable behavior among the various subsets.

The unique histopathology and immunostaining characteristics of MTC are described in Figure 164–4. In more than 80% of sporadic cases, the tumor is solitary, compared with familial cases in which MTC is bilateral, multifocal, and associated with C-cell hyperplasia in more than 90% of patients.

PREOPERATIVE MANAGEMENT

The majority of MTC cases are diagnosed preoperatively by fine-needle aspiration (FNA) biopsy of a palpable thyroid mass or associated lymphadenopathy. If a cytologic diagnosis is suspected but is not certain, and amyloid is not clearly present on the smear, immunostaining for iCT can be performed on cytologic slides. Open excisional nodal biopsies are to be discouraged unless FNA biopsy is suggestive of lymphoma. In all other cases, such open biopsies should be avoided so as to prevent unnecessary scars in a patient about to undergo thyroidectomy and lymph node dissection.

MTC has a propensity to spread, first to locoregional lymph nodes (Fig. 164–5A), followed by lung, liver, and bone. More than 50% of MTC patients with a thyroid mass larger than 2 cm have nodal metastases (clinically apparent or occult). As many as 12% of such patients harbor stage IV disease (Table 164–2). In patients with MTC, pTNM stage is one of the most important risk factors for survival (Table 164–3; Fig. 164–6). Preoperative imaging is imperative for proper staging, which allows for appropriate patient counseling and planning of operative strategy. Patients with obvious nodal metastases must understand preoperatively that the likelihood for cure is low, but that effective palliative surgery can result in long-term survival. All MTC patients should be screened for *RET* proto-oncogene mutations, because familial patients

Table 164–2	pTNM Staging for MTC	
Stage I	Disease confined to thyroid	
Stage II	Intrathyroidal	
	Mobile regional nodes	
Stage III	Invasion of local structures	
	Fixed regional nodes	
Stage IV	Distant metastases	

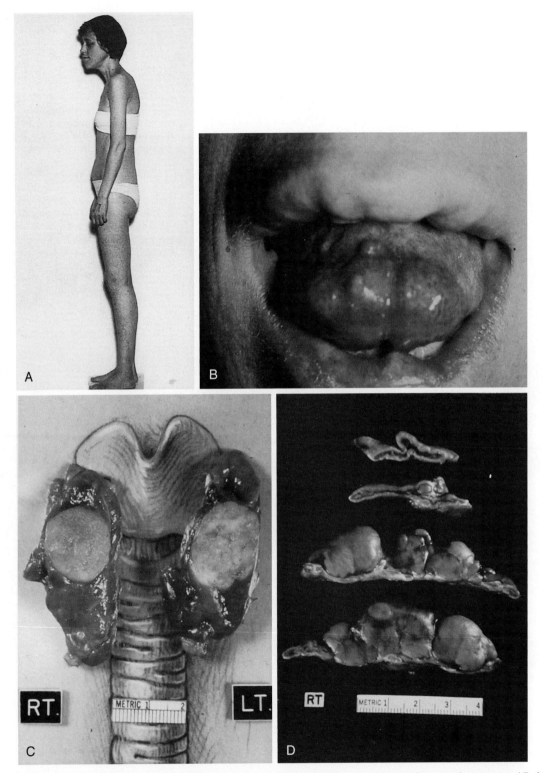

Figure 164–3. MEN 2B patient demonstrating (*A*) marfanoid body habitus, (*B*) tongue with mucosal neuromas, (*C*) thyroid with bilateral upper pole cancers, and (*D*) adrenals with pheochromocytomas and bilateral adrenomedullary hyperplasia.

can present with a solitary thyroid nodule in adulthood and because a seemingly sporadic case can represent an index case for a new hereditary kindred. Fewer than 3% of hereditary cases today are *RET* negative. False-positive and -negative cases should not result unless sample mix-

up occurs. Reassurance can be obtained with repeat testing. Testing of the potential proband is critical for family members as well.

Blood should be drawn to obtain basal and stimulated calcitonin levels (Table 164–4) on induction of anesthesia,

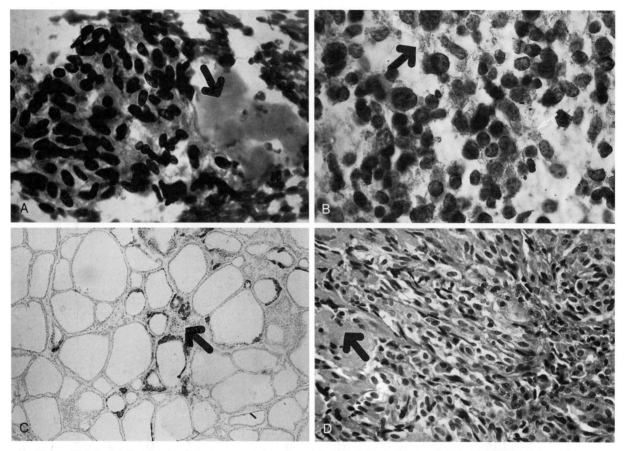

Figure 164–4. Cytologic and histologic presentation of medullary thyroid carcinoma. Fine-needle aspiration biopsy shows spindle-shaped cytoplasmic processes and elongated nuclei; amyloid is also identified (*arrow; upper left*). Fine-needle aspiration biopsy specimen on immunoperoxidase staining for calcitonin (*arrow*) is consistent with medullary thyroid carcinoma (*upper right*). Specimen from patients with familial medullary thyroid carcinoma shows foci of C-cell hyperplasia (*arrow*) identified by positive immunostaining for calcitonin (*lower left*). Medullary thyroid carcinoma tumor containing large amounts of amyloid deposits (*arrow*) in the stroma (*lower right*). (From Heshmati HM, Gharib H, van Heerden JA, Sizemore G: Advances and controversies in the diagnosis and management of medullary thyroid carcinoma. Am J Med 1997;103:60–69, with permission.)

Table 164-3	Prognostic Factors in MTC		
FACTORS	**GOOD PROGNOSIS**	**POOR PROGNOSIS**
RET mutations	Codons 609, 611, 618, 620, 634, 768, 804	Codon 918
Sex	Female	Male
Plasma iCT	Low	High
Plasma iCT/CGRP	High	Low
Plasma CEA	Low	High
Age at surgery	Young	Older
Surgical resection	Complete	Incomplete
Tumor size	Small	Large
DNA ploidy	Diploid	Nondiploid
iCT immunoreactivity	High	Low
Amyloid staining	Positive	Negative
pTNM staging		
Extrathyroidal invasion	Absent	Present
Nodal metastasis	Absent	Present
Distant metastasis	Absent	Present

MTC, medullary thyroid carcinoma; iCT, calcitonin; CGRP, calcitonin gene–related peptide; CEA, carcinoembryonic antigen; DNA, deoxyribonucleic acid.

to avoid the patient's having to experience the unpleasant side effects associated with pentagastrin stimulation (metallic taste, esophageal spasm, nausea, flushing, warmth, and urinary urgency). Pentagastrin is no longer readily available, and calcium stimulation alone (perhaps less accurate) has become the secretagogue of choice. It is essential to obtain values prior to resection that serve as a baseline marker for persistent or recurrent MTC postoperatively. Basal iCT levels greater than 10,000 pg/mL may indicate distant disease. False-negative and -positive tests may be observed in 5% to 20% of cases. When a prophylactic thyroidectomy is performed, elevated iCT levels can be seen with C-cell hyperplasia alone, contrary to the beliefs of some authors.

Routine cervical ultrasonography should be performed preoperatively. It is very sensitive in detecting lymph node involvement, which may not be apparent grossly at the time of surgery. Indeterminate lymph nodes can be biopsied with FNA techniques, under ultrasound guidance. Vascular involvement can also be detected with the use of this technology.

Computed tomography (CT) and magnetic resonance imaging (MRI) are useful tools for screening the mediastinum, lungs, and liver. All MTC patients should have 24-

Table 164-4	Differences in Basal and Pentagastrin-Stimulated* Plasma CT Levels in Normal Subjects	
SEX	**BASAL iCT (pg/mL)**	**STIMULATED iCT (pg/mL)**
Male	0–19	≤110
Female	0–14	≤30

*Pentagastrin (0.5 μg/kg of body weight) by a bolus injection with blood sampling at 0, 1.5, and 5 minutes.
iCT, calcitonin
Data from Gharib et al, 1987.

hour urinary catecholamines and metanephrines checked. Positive studies, in the absence of interfering substances, should be followed with either iodine 123 MIBG (metaiodobenzylguanidine) scanning or whole-body MRI with the goal of locating bilateral and extra-adrenal disease (paragangliomas). If serum calcium levels are elevated, PTH levels should be obtained with the use of an ICMA assay.

All members of known MEN 2A, MEN 2B, and FMTC families (*RET*-positive) should be screened for *RET* mutations soon after birth. Genetic testing for these germline mutations has simplified the process, obviating the need for yearly stimulated calcitonin testing, which is quite unnerving for parents, as well as very unpleasant for their children. Prophylactic operations, in *RET*-positive patients, should be performed during their first year of life in MEN 2B children, before the age of 5 or 6 in MEN 2A patients, and by the age of 5 or 6 in FMTC patients. These recommendations are based on knowledge of the biologic behavior of MTC in each of these hereditary MTC syndromes. Screening for pheochromocytoma should ensue annually after age 6 until the sixth decade of life. Serum calcium levels should be checked every 2 years for a similar period of time.

In *RET*-negative families with hereditary MTC, linkage analysis may identify gene carriers. However, such analysis is not as accurate as *RET* mutation analysis; therefore, if the results are negative, yearly biochemical testing must continue.

Preoperative vocal cord examination should be performed routinely, as recurrent nerve infiltration is not uncommon with MTC. Hemoptysis, dysphagia, and hoarseness should be evaluated with neck CT and/or laryngoscopy, bronchoscopy, and esophagoscopy, looking for a direct invasion of these structures that would alter the surgical plan.

Prior to surgery, complete blood count, electrolytes, liver function tests, creatinine, chest radiograph, and electrocardiogram should be obtained, as a general health profile prior to anesthesia.

The author has seen patients with intrahepatic cholestasis reversible after MTC tumor debulking. In patients with elevated liver function tests and negative imaging, this diagnosis should be considered. More likely, however, is miliary seeding of the liver, which is best seen with laparoscopy. Hypercoagulability is also a potential problem in MTC patients. Sequential lower extremity compression devices should be instituted preoperatively as deep vein thrombosis (DVT) prophylaxis. Higher risk patients should also receive subcutaneous heparin administrated perioperatively. Patients with known DVT and pulmonary emboli should be considered for preoperative inferior vena caval (IVC) filter placement.

Aspirin therapy, especially when combined with vitamin E, should be stopped 7 to 10 days prior to surgery, to reduce the risk of bleeding complications.

INTRAOPERATIVE MANAGEMENT

The operative procedure is carried out with the patient under general endotracheal anesthesia. The patient is

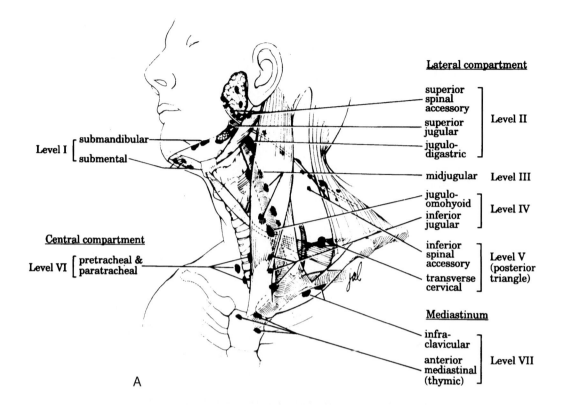

Lateral compartment

superior
spinal
accessory

superior
jugular   Level II

jugulo-
digastric

midjugular   Level III

jugulo-
omohyoid
inferior   Level IV
jugular

inferior
spinal
accessory   Level V
                        (posterior
transverse   triangle)
cervical

Mediastinum

infra-
clavicular

anterior
mediastinal   Level VII
(thymic)

Level I ⎡ submandibular
         ⎣ submental

Central compartment

Level VI ⎡ pretracheal &
          ⎣ paratracheal

A

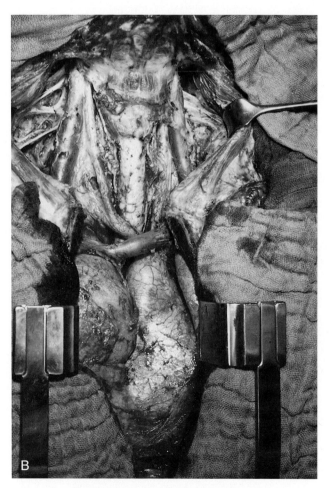

B

Figure 164–5 *See legend on opposite page*

positioned supine with arms tucked at the side. A blanket is placed beneath the shoulders, and the neck is extended to facilitate exposure of the thyroid gland. Care must be taken to avoid cervical hyperextension, especially in older patients with cervical osteophytes. The endotracheal tube should be securely positioned above the ears. The patient is prepped from the chin and pinnae to below the umbilicus, providing adequate exposure for bilateral modified neck dissections and median sternotomy, if necessary. With extensive nodal disease and upper mediastinal involvement, a urinary catheter, radial arterial line, and two large-bore peripheral intravenous lines are placed.

A 6- to 8-cm primary collar incision is made, and superior and inferior subplatysmal flaps are fashioned. The strap muscles are retracted laterally. If extensive lateral disease is known preoperatively, the collar incision is extended superiorly along the anterior border of the sternocleidomastoid muscle or muscles, to the level of the hyoid bone. In children, modified neck dissections can often be performed with lateral, rather than superior, extensions of the collar incision. Because of the potential for bilateral and multifocal disease in patients with MTC, a total thyroidectomy should be performed. C-cells do not take up I^{131}, and therefore the only way of eliminating localized MTC and the C-cell mass is with complete extirpation of the thyroid gland. Care must be taken to identify and protect the recurrent laryngeal nerves throughout their course in the neck and upper mediastinum; 0.3% of right laryngeal nerves are nonrecurrent, often traveling directly toward the cricothyroid muscle with the inferior thyroid artery. This anomaly is associated with an aberrant right subclavian artery. The right subclavian artery can be palpated behind the esophagus. The best way of avoiding injury to the external branch of the superior laryngeal nerve (tensor of the vocal cord) is to individually ligate the superior pole vessels on the thyroid capsule. Only the terminal branches of the inferior thyroid artery should be divided. Ligation of the main arterial trunk can lead to unnecessary hypoparathyroidism. Although some authors favor total parathyroidectomy with autotransplantation to facilitate a more complete central compartment node dissection, the author prefers vascular preservation, whenever possible, to limit the occurrence of postoperative hypoparathyroidism. Attempts should be made to identify all four parathyroid glands, especially in MEN 2A patients. Devascularized normal parathyroid glands should be minced into 1-mm cubes and transplanted into the sternocleidomastoid muscle, marking the site with metal clips or nonabsorbable suture for future reference. In MEN 2A patients, only enlarged glands need be removed, unlike the case of primary hyperplasia in MEN 1 patients who require subtotal parathyroidectomy (3 to 3.5 glands) and transcervical thymectomy for maintenance of eucalcemia. When normal-appearing MEN 2A parathyroids are devascularized, they should be transplanted immediately into either a subcutaneous chest wall pocket or the forearm musculature (brachioradialis muscle) on the nondominant side, so as to facilitate volume reduction in the future should the transplant hyperfunction. Cryopreservations of abnormal parathyroid tissue can, when autotransplanted successfully, treat hypoparathyroidism in 50% to 60% of patients.

Central compartment lymph node dissections (CCND-levels VI and VII) are routinely performed in conjunction with therapeutic thyroidectomies (see Fig. 164–5A). The necessity of CCND in patients undergoing prophylactic thyroidectomy, based on RET mutation analysis, is still uncertain. If gross thyroid or central node disease is discovered during the course of a prophylactic thyroidectomy, a CCND should be performed that would include a transcervical thymectomy; otherwise, central node sampling alone seems appropriate for minimizing the risk of postoperative hypoparathyroidism.

When primary tumors exceed 2 cm in diameter, central nodes are positive, or lateral nodes are positive grossly or by preoperative or intraoperative ultrasonography, a formal modified or functional neck dissection should be performed, sparing the spinal accessory nerve, the sternocleidomastoid muscle, and, in most instances, the internal jugular vein. The lateral nodes include those cited in Figure 164–5, levels II, III, IV, and V (posterior triangle), and the infraclavicular portion of level VII. Care must be taken to avoid injury to the contents of the carotid sheath, thoracic duct, and innominate vein, as well as the marginal mandibular branch of the facial nerve, hypoglossal, spinal accessory, vagus, and phrenic nerves, as well as the cervical and brachial plexuses. The best way of avoiding injury to these structures is by exposing them completely as part of the dissection. Nerves, including the recurrent laryngeal nerve, that are directly infiltrated by MTC should be sacrificed as part of a potentially curative operation, because of the aggressive nature of the disease and

Figure 164–5. *A,* The anatomic landmarks and lymph node compartments in the neck and upper mediastinum encountered in surgical reinterventions in medullary thyroid carcinoma. The central compartment is delimited inferiorly by the innominate vein, superiorly by the hyoid bone, laterally by the carotid sheaths, and dorsally by the prevertebral fascia. It comprises lymphatic and soft tissue around the esophagus and pretracheal and paratracheal lymph nodes that drain the thyroid bed (level VI). The submandibular nodal group (level I) is subsumed in the central compartment by some classifications. The lateral compartments span the area between the carotid sheath, the sternocleidomastoid muscle, and the trapezius muscle. The inferior border is defined by the subclavian vein, and the hypoglossal nerve determines the superior boundary. The lymph node chain adjacent to the jugular vein is divided cranially to caudally in superior jugular nodes (level II), midjugular nodes (level III), and inferior jugular nodes (level IV). Lymph nodes situated in the posterior triangle between the dorsolateral sternocleidomastoid muscle, the trapezius muscle, and the subclavian vein are classified as level V nodes. Mediastinal lymphatic tissue is referred to as level VII lymph nodes. (From Musholt TJ, Moley JF: Management of recurrent medullary thyroid carcinoma after total thyroidectomy. Prob Gen Surg 1997;14:89–110, with permission.) *B,* Neck and mediastinal microdissection (e) as performed by Professor H. Dralle, Germany.

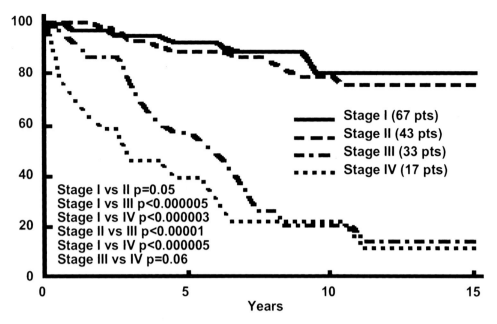

Figure 164–6. Survival by stage (pTNM) for MTC. (From Saad MF, Ordonez NG, Rashid RK, et al: Medullary carcinoma of the thyroid: A study of the clinical features and prognostic factors in 161 patients. Medicine 1984;63: 319–342, with permission.)

the lack of effective adjuvant therapy (chemotherapy, I^{131}, external-beam radiotherapy). When the internal jugular vein is invaded by matted jugular nodes, it is best to perform an en bloc resection with the vein, rather than risk spillage of tumor cells into the surrounding soft tissues. Direct invasion of the trachea, esophagus, or larynx should be managed aggressively with resection, as would any primary tumor confined to this region, in order to avoid subsequent asphyxiation, hemorrhage, and obstruction.

Any lymphatic leakage noted at the completion of the dissection should be sought, and the offending lymphatic or lymphatics should be ligated. This holds true for the main (left-sided) thoracic duct, as well. Closed-suction drainage and intravenous cephalosporins are routinely continued for a few days after modified neck dissection.

POSTOPERATIVE MANAGEMENT

Despite the magnitude of some of these operations, recovery is rapid, with discharge taking place within 2 to 3 days. Stridor occurring immediately post extubation should be evaluated with flexible fiberoptic laryngoscopy in the operating room. An inadequate glottic opening (bilateral cord paralyses) mandates immediate reintubation or tracheostomy. The use of steroids in this setting is controversial. Patients can normally return to a regular hospital bed unless the operation has involved the upper aerodigestive tract or the great vessels and their major branches (e.g., the carotid artery).

The author prefers that patients have the head of their bed elevated 30 to 45 degrees. Humidification of room air can be helpful. When nausea subsides, oral intake can be resumed rapidly and intravenous lines discontinued. Patients with recurrent laryngeal nerve palsy may temporarily choke with the intake of clear liquids. These patients often do better with solids. Serum calcium levels are monitored twice daily until stabilization has occurred, usually within the first 24 to 72 hours. The author does

not treat hypocalcemia unless the patient is symptomatic or the total serum calcium level is below 7.5 mg/dL (see section on complications). Patients are started on a replacement dose of thyroxine (T_4) and are instructed to have a total T_4 and sensitive thyroid-stimulating hormone (sTSH) level checked in 8 weeks. Adjustments are made according to sTSH levels. Drains are removed when outputs are low (usually less than 50 mL per day) and the character of the output is nonchylous.

Rarely is intravenous calcium gluconate required in treating postoperative symptoms of hypocalcemia. Most patients can be weaned off oral calcium and vitamin D supplements during the initial 8-week postoperative period.

Blood is drawn for basal iCT, CEA, calcium, phosphorus, T_4, and sTSH at the 8-week recheck. Persistent hoarseness is evaluated by direct laryngoscopy.

COMPLICATIONS

Permanent complications occur in fewer than 1% to 2% of all patients (both children and adults) undergoing total thyroidectomy with or without a modified neck dissection. When permanent recurrent laryngeal nerve injuries are apparent and contralateral cord compensation has not occurred, a type I thyroplasty can improve phonation considerably. At least 6 months should pass before the physician assumes that the hoarseness is permanent.

Permanent hypoparathyroidism is rare; however, it may be difficult for the physician to treat it, with the goal of alleviating the patient's symptoms (numbness, tingling, twitching, and irritability) and yet avoiding the development of kidney stones. Oral calcium agents, 1,25-dihydroxyvitamin D, phosphate binders, and thiazide diuretics all play a role in the chronic management of hypoparathyroidism.

Chylous fistulas can be a difficult problem after neck dissection, leading to lymphopenia and hypoproteinemia. Low-output fistulas often close with closed-suction drainage, low-fat, medium-chain triglyceride diets, and time. Early return to the operating room for high-output fistulas is warranted, in the hopes of finding and ligating a large leaking vessel. If this surgical intervention fails, ligation of the thoracic duct at the level of the diaphragm, via a limited right thoracotomy, is the next step. Eight ounces of cream should be given 8 hours preoperatively to distend the thoracic duct at the time of surgery.

Bleeding is a rare but dreaded complication soon after neck surgery. Patients with expanding hematomas should be returned to the operating room immediately, with reintubation, evacuation of the hematoma, and ligation of bleeding points. Either a slipped ligature off the superior thyroid artery or a branch of the inferior thyroid artery is the most likely source. When patients are in extremis on the floor, the wound should be opened at the bedside, to immediately relieve airway obstruction.

Most nerve injuries encountered are stretch-related neurapraxias, and most of these will resolve with time. The best way of avoiding nerve injury is to have a thorough understanding of neck anatomy and to routinely expose nerves prior to any sharp dissection. Motor nerves can be reapproximated with fine, monofilament, nonabsorbable sutures with the use of magnification. Nerve autografting and innervated muscle transfers can be attempted when deficits are debilitating to the patient. The results are highly variable at best.

Infections are exceedingly rare in the neck but must be managed like any other surgical wound infection. Prophylactic antibiotics for thyroidectomy alone do not appear warranted.

OUTCOMES

Cure rates are highest for FMTC and MEN 2A patients and lowest for sporadic and MEN 2B patients; pTNM stage is a major prognostic indicator (see Fig. 164–6). Other prognostic factors for survival in MTC are outlined in Table 164–3. Early diagnosis and treatment are critical to the survival of patients with MTC. Thus, patients who are screened for *RET* mutations shortly after birth, followed by total thyroidectomy (prophylactic) at a young age, are unlikely to die from MTC. The overwhelming majority of these patients have stage I disease or C-cell hyperplasia alone. Long-term follow-up studies should demonstrate a near-zero cause-specific mortality rate in these patients. Most sporadic patients as well as MEN 2A/FMTC index cases, however, present with a palpable thyroid mass or cervical adenopathy, or both. Locally advanced disease occurs in more than 50%, and distant micrometastases (occult) are found in nearly 15% of patients, often negating the chance of cure from the time of diagnosis. In fact, persistent hypercalcitoninemia is the most likely postoperative scenario in this subgroup of patients.

These findings have led to two schools of thought. The first, a more conservative postoperative approach, and the second, an aggressive form of surgical re-intervention termed *microdissection*. The latter approach has been championed by Tisell and Dralle in Europe and the team at Washington University in St. Louis. A meticulous four-

Pearls and Pitfalls

PEARLS

- When fine-needle aspiration biopsy is indeterminate for medullary thyroid carcinoma, immunostain for iCT.
- Preoperative evaluation for MTC includes basal and stimulated iCT, CEA, *RET* mutation analysis, neck ultrasonography, CT or MRI of the chest or abdomen, measurement of Ca^{2+} (PTH if increased), and 24-hour urinary level of catecholamines and metabolites.
- In most cases, therapeutic surgery includes total thyroidectomy, CCND, and lateral neck dissection.
- Prophylactic surgery includes total thyroidectomy and central node sampling or complete nodal removal.
- Operative complications can be minimized by doing the following:
  1. Identifying and preserving vascularized parathyroid tissue; devitalized parathyroid glands should be autotransplanted
  2. Identifying and tracing out the nerves in the operative field: the RLN; the external branch of the SLN; the vagus, phrenic, spinal accessory, and hypoglossal nerves; the marginal mandibular branch of VII; and the cervical and brachial plexuses
  3. Identifying and ligating the thoracic duct if injured
- For persistent or recurrent hypercalcitoninemia, perform a four-compartment microdissection; or reoperate, based on imaging studies. Long-term follow-up studies are needed.
- Prophylactic thyroidectomy is performed in (1) all *RET*-positive patients; (2) all patients with hereditary *RET* with a positive linkage analysis; (3) patients with MEN 2B during the first year of life; (4) patients with MEN 2A from age 5 to 6; and (5) patients with FMTC by age 5 to 6.

compartment (right and left lateral, central, and upper mediastinal via a median sternotomy) nodal dissection is performed, regardless of negative localizing studies, in patients without evidence of distant metastases (see Fig. 164–5B). Laparoscopy is frequently utilized to exclude miliary liver metastases prior to microdissection. Overall, studies show that approximately one third of patients normalize stimulated calcitonin levels, one third have some decrease in iCT levels, and in one third the iCT levels remain unchanged. Exactly how this correlates with improved survival will need to be determined with long-term follow-up studies. The morbidity resulting from this procedure, in experienced hands, is quite acceptable.

The more *conservative approach* awaits evidence of recurrent or persistent disease based on localizing studies performed at regular intervals (6 to 12 months), including neck ultrasonography, abdominal or chest CT or MRI, nuclear imaging using thallium 201 thallous chloride, technetium 99m pentavalent dimercaptosuccinic acid, I^{123}-MIBG, or indium 111 pentetreotide. Nuclear imaging has, at best, a 50% accuracy rate. Again, laparoscopy should be utilized prior to any repeat neck operation that carries with it an increased operative morbidity. In patients with very high iCT levels and radiographically occult disease, selective venous catheterization techniques with iCT stimulation can be employed to help regionalize this disease. In a series of patients managed conservatively at the Mayo Clinic, none had normalization of iCT levels following removal of radiographically detectable disease, yet the 10-year survival rates in these patients approached 86%, making a strong argument for this approach.

Radioguided surgery utilizing hand-held Gamma probes and preoperatively administered anti-CEA monoclonal antibodies is under investigation for localization of occult disease.

SELECTED READINGS

Chi DD, Moley JF: Medullary thyroid carcinoma: Genetic advances, treatment recommendations, and the approach to the patient with persistent hypercalcitoninemia. Surg Oncol Clin North Am 1998;7:681.

Gimm O, Dralle H: Reoperation in metastasizing medullary thyroid carcinoma: Is a tumor stage–oriented approach justified? Surgery 1997;122:1124.

Heshmati HM, Gharib H, van Heerden JA, Sizemore GW: Advances and controversies in the diagnosis and management of medullary thyroid carcinoma. Am J Med 1997;103:60.

Juweid M, Sharkey RM, Swayne LC, Goldenberg DM: Improved selection of patients for reoperation for medullary thyroid cancer by imaging with radiolabeled anticarcinoembryonic antigen antibodies. Surgery 1997;122:1156.

Modigliani E, Cohens R, Campos J-M, et al, GETC Study Group: Prognostic factors for survival and for biochemical cure in medullary thyroid carcinoma: Results in 899 patients. Clin Endocrinol 1998;48:265.

Moley JF, DeBenadetti MK: Patterns of nodal metastases in palpable medullary thyroid carcinoma: Recommendations for extent of node dissection. Ann Surg 1999;229:880.

Moley JF, DeBenedetti MK, Dilley WG, et al: Surgical management of patients with persistent or recurrent medullary thyroid carcinoma. J Intern Med 1998;243:521.

O'Riordain DS, O'Brien T, Crotty TB, et al: Multiple endocrine neoplasia type 2B: More than an endocrine disorder. Surgery 1995;118:936.

O'Riordain DS, O'Brien T, Weaver AL, et al: Medullary thyroid carcinoma in multiple endocrine neoplasia types 2A and 2B. Surgery 1994;116:1017.

Pyke CM, Hay ID, Goellner JR, et al: Prognostic significance of calcitonin immunoreactivity, amyloid staining, and flow cytometric DNA measurements in medullary thyroid carcinoma. Surgery 1991;110:964.

Tiede DJ, Tefferi A, Kochhar R, et al: Paraneoplastic cholestasis and hypercoagulability associated with medullary thyroid carcinoma. Cancer 1994;73:702.

Tisell LE, Dilley WG, Wells SA Jr: Progression of postoperative residual medullary thyroid carcinoma as monitored by plasma calcitonin levels. Surgery 1996;119:34.

van Heerden JA, Grant CS, Gharib H, et al: Long-term course of patients with persistent hypercalcitoninemia after apparent curative primary surgery for medullary thyroid carcinoma. Ann Surg 1990;212:395.

Wells SA Jr, Skinner MA: Prophylactic thyroidectomy, based on direct genetic testing, in patients at risk for the multiple endocrine neoplasia type 2 syndromes. Exp Clin Endocrinol Diabetes 1998;106:29.

Chapter 165

Hyperparathyroidism

Nancy D. Perrier and Orlo H. Clark

The Swedish anatomist Ivor Sanstrom first described the parathyroid glands both grossly and microscopically in 1880. He and others reported that most individuals have four parathyroid glands and they are typically situated on the posterior lateral surface of the thyroid gland. Their principal secretory product, parathyroid hormone (PTH), is involved in a direct feedback loop, which tightly regulates the serum calcium concentration. PTH hormone secretion is inhibited by calcium via calcium sensors on the parathyroid cell surface. The hormone acts on specific receptors in the peripheral target tissues.

The ability to make the diagnosis of overactivity of these glands, or hyperparathyroidism (HPT), has improved substantially since the introduction of sensitive and specific assays for the intact 84 amino acid peptide. Such immunoradiometric or immunochemoluminescence assays accurately differentiate HPT from almost all other causes of hypercalcemia. Most cases of hyperparathyroidism are primarily caused by parathyroid abnormalities (primary HPT, or PHPT), whereas other cases are caused by secondary or external factors that stimulate the parathyroid glands to increase production of parathyroid hormone (secondary HPT). The most common cause of secondary HPT, stimulation of the parathyroid glands to grow abnormally, is chronic renal failure. If this situation persists after successful kidney transplantation, the term "tertiary HPT" is often used. This chapter primarily deals with PHPT.

CLINICAL PRESENTATION

PHPT is a common disorder occurring in at least 1 in every 500 women older than 40 years and in 1 in every 2000 men. It is estimated that PHPT develops in 100,000 patients every year in the United States. PHPT is usually sporadic in nature, but it also occurs in patients with multiple endocrine neoplasia (MEN) types 1, 2A, and, rarely, 2B. Fibrous jaw tumor syndrome is a distinct familial entity that occurs in association with PHPT but without other associated endocrinopathies. Neonatal hyperparathyroidism occurs in members of families with benign familial hypocalciuric hypercalcemia (BFHH) who have a homozygous mutation on chromosome 3.

Three different pathologic lesions can produce primary HPT: adenoma, hyperplasia, and carcinoma. Adenomas are composed of chief, oncocytic, water-clear, transitional, or a mixture of cell types. Stromal fat is scant. Approximately 85% of all patients with HPT have a solitary parathyroid adenoma. Patients with primary parathyroid hyperplasia have an absolute increase in chief, oncocytic, or transitional cells in the parathyroid glands. This disorder is usually distinguished from adenomas based on the combination of gross features and histologic parameters.

By definition, hyperplasia involves all parathyroid glands, whereas multiple adenomas may occur in two or more glands but at least one gland is histologically normal. Carcinoma is responsible for 1% of cases. It is usually distinguishable from the aforementioned conditions by its invasive character and adherence to surrounding structures. Other rare conditions that can cause HPT are lipoadenoma and carcinosarcoma.

Most patients given the diagnosis of PHPT do not have the classic clinical manifestations, such as osteitis fibrosa cystica, nephrolithiasis, nephrocalcinosis, peptic ulcer disease, gout, or pseudogout. The pentad of painful bones, kidney stones, abdominal groans, psychic moans, and fatigue overtones is more common. Symptoms range from mild to severe. Clinical manifestations of PHPT are listed in Table 165–1. These symptoms, associated conditions, and long-term survival outlook appear to improve in most patients after successful parathyroidectomy.

MAKING THE DIAGNOSIS

The development of intact PTH assay has made the diagnosis of PHPT considerably easier. PHPT is the most common cause of hypercalcemia in outpatients, whereas malignancy remains the most common cause of hypercalcemia in hospitalized patients. Table 165–2 lists the differential diagnoses for hypercalcemia. Patients with documented hypercalcemia for more than 6 months do not have malignancy-associated hypercalcemia because these patients do not live that long. Patients with hypercalcemia, an elevated or inappropriately high PTH level, and absence of hypocalciuria virtually all have PHPT. Therefore extensive testing is not needed to make an accurate diagnosis. A rare nonparathyroid tumor may secrete pure PTH and cause PHPT.

Table 165–1	Symptoms and Conditions of Hyperparathyroidism	
SYMPTOMS	**ASSOCIATED CONDITIONS**	
Bone pain/joint pain	Hypertension	
Hypertension	Nephrolithiasis	
Renal colic	Hematuria	
Hematuria	Nephrocalcinosis	
Constipation	Osteitis fibrosa cystica	
Dyspepsia	Gout/pseudogout	
Fatigue	Peptic ulcer disease	
Exhaustion	Joint swelling	
Depression	Weight loss	
Weakness	Pancreatitis	
Polydipsia	Polyuria	
Pruritus	Nocturia	

Table 165–2	**Differential Diagnosis of Hypercalcemia**

Cancer, especially breast, squamous cell lung, multiple myeloma, and lymphoma
Endocrinopathies
    Hyperparathyroidism
    Hyperthyroidism
    Hypothyroidism
    Vipoma
    Addison's disease
    Pheochromocytoma
Granulomatous disease (especially sarcoidosis)
Increased consumption of calcium, vitamin D, vitamin A, alkali, and thiazides
Immobilization
High turnover bone disease (Paget's)
Acute renal failure with rhabdomyolysis
Benign familial hypocalciuric hypercalcemia

IMAGING

Preoperative localization studies are not considered to be cost effective in patients before initial operations if a bilateral standard parathyroid exploration is to be used. In these cases, the experienced surgeon can identify all glands and remove those that are abnormal. Preoperative imaging with sestamibi scanning or ultrasonography is essential in patients with PHPT if a limited, minimally invasive procedure is planned. Such noninvasive localization studies are approximately 85% to 90% accurate in patients with solitary adenomas but are only 35% accurate in patients with multiple abnormal glands or hyperplasia. Proper selection of patients who are unlikely to have multiple gland disease, such as those without familial disease, is essential in making decisions regarding imaging and limited exploration. Results of localization studies are highly dependent on the expertise of the radiologist or nuclear medicine physician. Limitations of sestamibi scanning include increased uptake by thyroid nodules, leading to false-positive studies; limitations of ultrasound include the inability to detect adenomas behind the upper part of the sternum or the mediastinum or deeply situated parathyroid glands in the neck. One or both of these tests, when combined with intraoperative PTH testing, allow a limited exploration with an excellent outcome. Magnetic resonance imaging and computed tomography (CT) scanning are helpful before reoperations but are not cost effective if done in patients before initial parathyroid operations. Highly selective venous catheterization for PTH assay is useful for patients with persistent or recurrent HPT when the noninvasive studies are negative or equivocal, or suggest different sites for the elusive parathyroid tumor or tumors.

PREOPERATIVE MANAGEMENT

Optimization of success of parathyroid surgery requires an experienced surgeon. Studies have shown that the success rate of experienced surgeons in treating PHPT is greater than 95% and complications are less than 1%, compared with operations performed by less experienced surgeons who have a success rate of 70% and more frequent complications. Documentation of renal function, serum phosphorous, serum chloride, alkaline phosphatase, and uric acid can be helpful (Table 165–3). Elevation of bone serum alkaline phosphatase preoperatively identifies those patients who will probably require calcium replacement in the postoperative period because of "bone-hunger" and a sometimes longer period of hospitalization. Likewise, identification of subperiosteal resorption on industrial-grade hand films in patients with an elevated alkaline phosphatase study clarifies the diagnosis and expedites therapy before PTH values return.

Completing the preoperative workup for PHPT includes obtaining a 24-hour urine test for calcium and creatinine to rule out BFHH. Documenting the urinary calcium to rule out BFHH is not necessary in patients who were previously documented to be normocalcemic. BFHH is the metabolic condition that can mimic PHPT from a laboratory point of view with increased blood calcium and increased PTH. These patients have a low urinary calcium, less than 100 mg per 24 hours, and have family members younger than 10 years old with hypercalcemia. Other preoperative tests are obtained selectively, such as an electrocardiogram, chest radiograph, or platelet count.

INTRAOPERATIVE MANAGEMENT

Treatment for patients with sporadic disease and a preoperative study highly suggestive of a solitary adenoma can be by a bilateral approach or by a limited parathyroidectomy in conjunction with use of an intraoperative parathyroid hormone assay. The latter is particularly beneficial for patients who are at increased surgical risk owing to respiratory or cardiovascular disease, because it can be done under local anesthesia. The incision should be approximately 2 to 3 cm in length and placed directly over the suspected adenoma as identified on preoperative imaging. It should be made in a normal skin line so that it can be extended in case the PTH level does not decrease appropriately. The gamma probe, after sestamibi injection, has been recommended to place the incision directly over the tumor, although we have not found this test to be worthwhile.

The patient is placed in a supine position with a cervical roll behind the neck and shoulders to allow for slight neck hyperextension. The entire neck, from chin to midsternum, is prepped into the operative field. For bilateral explorations, the head is directly straight forward, whereas for a focused approach the head is turned slightly to the opposite side, but not so much so as to preclude extension of the incision across the midline. The cricoid cartilage is palpated; one fingerbreadth below this prominence

Table 165–3	**Biochemical Testing in Patients with Primary Hyperparathyroidism**

90% have a chloride/phosphorous ratio >33
75% in "hypercalcemic crisis" have elevated alkaline phosphatase and subperiosteal resorption
50% have a low phosphorus level
33% have elevated uric acid level
10% have elevated alkaline phosphatase level

consistently marks the location of the thyroid isthmus. For bilateral operations, a 3- to 5-cm incision is made, depending on the girth of the neck and the position of the cricoid cartilage. For a focused operation, a 2- to 3-cm incision is made laterally on the side of the suspected adenoma. The subcutaneous tissues and platysma are divided. The sternocleidomastoid muscle is retracted laterally and the carotid sheath and its contents are gently deviated laterally. The middle thyroid vein is identified and usually is divided. The lower parathyroid is almost always anterior to the recurrent laryngeal nerve, whereas the upper parathyroid is deeper in the neck and just posterior to the recurrent laryngeal nerve at the level of the cricoid cartilage (Fig. 165–1). Thorough knowledge of the embryology and anatomy of parathyroid glands is essential to know ectopic sites where parathyroid glands are situated. Normal parathyroid glands should rarely be removed. They should be biopsied when there is a question of whether one normal or hyperplastic gland exists or whether a lesion is truly a parathyroid gland when a focused operation is being performed.

During a focused operation, the suspected adenoma is identified (Fig. 165–2). When an intraoperative PTH assay is being performed, a 5-mL syringe and 23-gauge needle are used to obtain blood from the internal jugular vein or the blood is obtained from the arm vein. The blood is placed in an EDTA purple top tube and iced in the operating theater. The abnormal-appearing gland is excised. Ten minutes after adenoma removal, a second blood sample is obtained from the same vein. During this time, the neck tissue and other presumably normal parathyroid glands should not be manipulated. The "before" and "after" removal blood specimens are analyzed

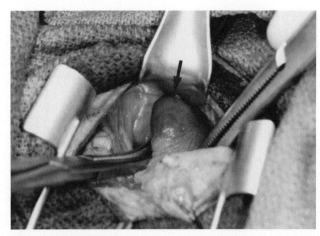

Figure 165–2. A parathyroid adenoma identified as the thyroid is retracted medially.

by a quick intact assay technique. A greater than 50% decrease in value of the second serum sample suggests that the operation is successful. If less than a 50% decrease in PTH is noted this PTH level should be repeated, as it occasionally falls slowly. If it still has not fallen by 50% or an adenoma is not identified, or both glands appear normal or abnormal, the incision should be extended to allow complete exploration of both the ipsilateral and contralateral sides of the neck. When all glands are abnormal, the most normal parathyroid that is not immediately adjacent to the recurrent laryngeal nerve is biopsied or a subtotal resection is performed. The other abnormal parathyroid glands are then removed.

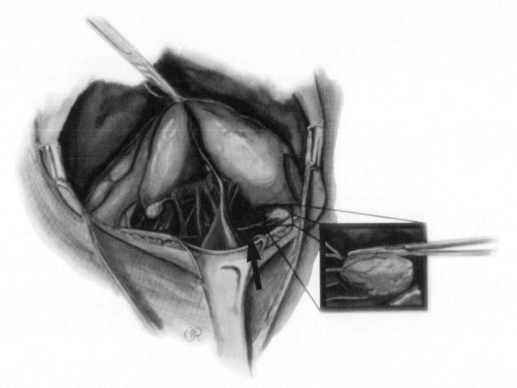

Figure 165–1. Normal anatomic position of the parathyroid glands. (Redrawn from Al-Sobhi S, Clark OH: Parathyroid hyperplasia: parathyroidectomy. In Clark OH, Duh Q-Y [eds]: Textbook of Endocrine Surgery. Philadelphia, WB Saunders, 1997, p 372.)

Hemostasis is assured, the muscle layers are approximated with interrupted absorbable suture, and the skin is closed.

For patients with sporadic disease and preoperative localization studies that either do not document abnormal parathyroid glands or document more than one parathyroid gland (no uptake or multiple areas of increased uptake), we recommend a standard bilateral exploration. We encourage identification of four parathyroid glands and removal of the adenoma with or without biopsy of one normal parathyroid gland. During this operation, the thyroid lobe is retracted medially and the carotid structures laterally. Care is taken not to fracture a parathyroid gland because this might result in parathyroidomatosis.

In patients with sporadic hyperplasia, we recommend biopsy of the most normal of the hyperplastic glands, histologic confirmation to confirm that it is a parathyroid gland, removal of the other abnormal glands, and removal of the upper thymus bilaterally. The latter is done because approximately 15% of such patients may have more than four parathyroid glands and the most common site is in the thymus or the perithymic fat.

Although most patients with familial HPT have more than one abnormal parathyroid gland, in those with a solitary tumor, we recommend removal of the solitary tumor, removal of the normal parathyroid gland and fibrofatty tissue on that same side of the neck, marking of the other normal-appearing parathyroid glands with a clip or stitch, and removal of the thymus bilaterally. This approach is necessary in case recurrent disease occurs; in this situation, only one side of the neck would require re-exploration. Reasons for removal of the thymus and parathymic fat in patients with MEN-I are twofold: (1) these are often sites for ectopic parathyroid glands, (2) malignant carcinoid tumors in the thymus develop in approximately 8% of patients with MEN-I.

For patients with MEN-I or familial HPT and multiple abnormal glands, subtotal parathyroidectomy leaving a 60-mg remnant of parathyroid tissue from the most "normal-appearing" gland, bilateral thymectomy, and parathyroid cryopreservation is recommended. Cryopreservation decreases the risk of permanent hypoparathyroidism, although autotransplantation and cryopreservation of parathyroid tissue function adequately in only approximately 60% of patients when reimplanted. Immediately autotransplanted parathyroid tissue appears to function in approximately 95% of patients. If one cannot be sure that the biopsied parathyroid remnant is viable during a parathyroid operation, this gland should be removed and autotransplanted, usually into the forearm of the nondominant arm, or another hyperplastic gland should be biopsied and marked before removing all other hyperplastic glands.

In patients with parathyroid hyperplasia resulting from secondary or tertiary hyperparathyroidism, we recommend subtotal parathyroidectomy with bilateral thymectomy. All glands should be identified and the gland closest in size to normal and not situated on the recurrent nerve should undergo subtotal resection. The remnant should be the size of a normal parathyroid gland, 60 mg. If viability of the remnant is in question, another gland should be selected and the biopsied gland removed. We recommend parathyroid cryopreservation for all patients

Table 165–4	**Indications for Total Parathyroidectomy with Autotransplantation**

Patients with secondary hyperparathyroidism (HPT) who are noncompliant and will not take medications to suppress parathyroid stimulation (e.g., 1,25-dihydroxyvitamin D, phosphate binders)
Agonal patients who would not tolerate general anesthesia in a reoperation
Technical reasons that make it difficult to preserve viable parathyroid
Neonatal HPT

having subtotal or total parathyroidectomy with autotransplantation. Total parathyroidectomy should be performed in a select set of circumstances as noted in Table 165–4. When total parathyroidectomy is planned, all parathyroid glands are first identified, as is the thymus. The parathyroid tissue that is to be autotransplanted should be from one of the least abnormal parathyroid glands. Its identity should be confirmed by frozen section. Most of the parathyroid gland to be used should be immediately placed in iced physiologic saline for autotransplantation. Twelve to fifteen 1-mm pieces of hyperplastic parathyroid tissue are autotransplanted into separate pockets in the forearm muscles via one skin incision. The advantage of this site of autotransplantation is that hyperplastic parathyroid graft can be excised under local anesthesia and if it overfunctions it can be identified by documenting a twofold increase in intact PTH at the level of the basilic vein proximal to the autotransplant.

POSTOPERATIVE MANAGEMENT

Following successful parathyroidectomy, the serum calcium decreases and usually reaches its nadir at 36 to 48

Table 165–5	**Possible Complications and Treatments Following Parathyroid Surgery**

COMPLICATION	CIRCUMSTANCES	TREATMENT
Hypocalcemia	Hungry bone syndrome Aparathyroid Hypoparathyroid	**Acute:** 1–2 g calcium (Ca) carbonate q4h orally or 10% Ca gluconate in 100 mL normal saline, intravenously or Rocaltrol (vit D) 0.25–1.0 µg q12 h orally **Chronic:** 1–2 g Ca carbonate with meals to bind phosphorus in the gastrointestinal tract or aluminum hydroxide to bind phosphorus
Hematoma	Bilateral exploration Less likely, unilateral exploration	Emergency airway problem: open wound at bedside or operating room and evacuate blood
Recurrent laryngeal nerve injury	Unilateral injury	Weak voice, adequate airway
	Bilateral injury	Voice OK but inadequate airway, which may require tracheostomy

hours after the operation. Postoperative hypocalcemia is common in patients who have an elevated blood alkaline phosphatase level and severe skeletal depletion of calcium with osteitis fibrosa cystica, commonly referred to as "bone hunger." Manifestations of low calcium are perioral numbness, tingling of the fingers, muscle cramps, anxiety, trembling of the masseter muscle with facial nerve stimulation anterior to the ear (Chvostek's sign), and carpopedal spasm (Trousseau's sign). When left untreated, convulsions and opisthotonos may occur. If mild symptoms appear, calcium supplementation should be given orally with calcium carbonate (500 to 1000 mg by mouth three times a day). If symptoms are moderate, the calcium dose can be increased or calcitriol (Rocaltrol) at (1,25-dihydroxyvitamin D, 0.25µg to 1.0 µg by mouth twice daily) should be prescribed. This treatment with 1,25-dihydroxyvitamin D facilitates gastrointestinal absorption of calcium and mobilization of calcium from the skeleton. If symptoms are severe, one ampule of 10% calcium gluconate (90 mg elemental calcium) dissolved in 100 mL of normal saline should be administered intravenously over 15 minutes, followed by a constant infusion of calcium (10 ampules of 10% calcium gluconate in 1000 mL of normal saline) at 20 to 100 mL/hr. One must be certain that the intrave-

nous line is intact because subcutaneous infusions can result in full-thickness tissue necrosis. Hyperventilation and vomiting should be addressed because alkalosis aggravates symptoms. Serum calcium should be checked frequently until symptoms decrease and the patient's calcium level increases. Treatment with vitamin D or intravenous calcium is rarely necessary unless the patient suffers severe osteitis fibrosis cystica. Following limited focused unilateral operations, same-day discharge is recommended by some surgeons, whereas 23 hours of observation remains the standard for bilateral exploration.

COMPLICATIONS

Prolonged symptomatic hypocalcemia (hypoparathyroidism), hematoma formation, and recurrent laryngeal nerve injury are uncommon but possible complications. Treatment is outlined in Table 165–5. We have not seen permanent hypoparathyroidism or recurrent laryngeal nerve injury after an initial parathyroid operation in more than 1500 patients having parathyroid operations using a bilateral approach.

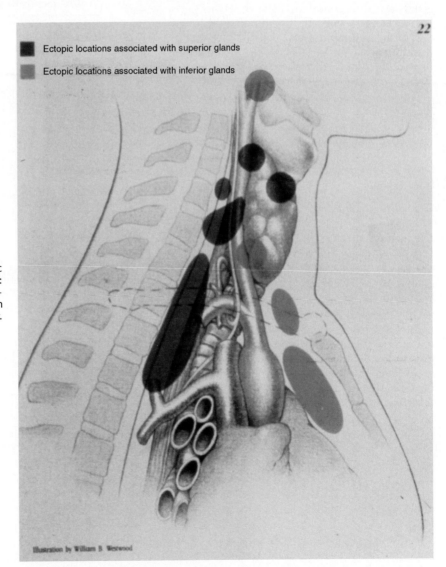

Figure 165–3. A common location of ectopic parathyroid glands. (Redrawn from Duh Q-Y: Surgical approach to primary hyperparathyroidism (bilateral approach). In Clark OH, Duh Q-Y [eds]: Textbook of Endocrine Surgery. Philadelphia, WB Saunders, 1997, p 360.)

OUTCOME

More than 95% of hyperparathyroid patients can be cured when treated by an experienced endocrine surgeon using a bilateral exploration. This approach remains the standard operation because it is safe and it avoids missing a second adenoma or other abnormal glands in patients with asymmetric hyperplasia. It also does not require intraoperative PTH assays or gamma probe localization. A unilateral, focused approach is acceptable if the prevalence of a double adenoma and hyperplasia is low. Most noninvasive studies are, at best, 80% sensitive for single adenomas and less so for double adenomas or hyperplasia. However, the addition of IOPTH can improve the success of surgery when relying on these techniques to about 93%.

The most common reasons for persistent HPT are an ectopically situated parathyroid tumor or multiple abnormal parathyroid glands. Inexperienced surgeons are often unfamiliar with the locations where these glands may be situated (Fig. 165–3). The inferior parathyroid glands and thymus develop from the third brachial pouch and descend to the lower thyroid area and the anterior mediastinum, respectively. Approximately 85% of parathyroid glands are situated within 1 cm of where the recurrent laryngeal nerve and the inferior thyroidal artery cross. Ectopically situated lower parathyroid glands are frequently within or adjacent to the thymus in the perithymic fat. Rarely, the lower gland may fail to descend and may be situated at the level of the carotid bulb.

The superior parathyroid glands develop from the fourth brachial pouch. They migrate a shorter distance and therefore have less variation in position. They are most commonly located superior-posterior to the junction of the inferior thyroid artery and recurrent laryngeal nerve at the level of the cricoid cartilage. Ectopic locations include (1) the tracheoesophageal groove posteriorly, (2) along the esophagus in the posterior mediastinum, (3) intrathyroidal, or (4) within the carotid sheath.

Unsuccessful operations may result from failure to identify one or more other abnormal parathyroid glands. Use of intraoperative PTH should help with intraoperative management of this problem because successful adenomectomy would be anticipated with a decline in PTH level of greater than 50% at 10 minutes after excision and an unsuccessful operation can be expected when PTH fails to decline. Reasons for unsuccessful subtotal parathyroidectomy include persistent disease resulting from the presence of a fifth supernumerary gland or subtotal resection of one or more of the hypercellular glands. As mentioned earlier, approximately 15% of patients have more than four parathyroid glands.

Pearls and Pitfalls

PEARLS

- The diagnosis of PHPT is confirmed with an inappropriately elevated PTH value in the setting of normal or elevated calcium.
- A solitary adenoma is the most common cause of HPT (85%).
- The half-life of parathyroid hormone is 3 minutes.
- The most common cause of secondary HPT is chronic renal failure.
- Ninety percent of patients with PHPT have a chloride to phosphorus ratio greater than 33.

PITFALLS

- BFHH can mimic PHPT. The differentiating aspect is a normal 24-hour urine study.
- Patients with familial disease are more likely to have multiple gland involvement.
- Cancer (breast, squamous cell, lung, multiple myeloma, and lymphoma) is a common cause of hypercalcemia.
- Transient hypocalcemia can occur in the postoperative period as a result of hungry bone syndrome.
- Ninety percent of patients with MEN I syndrome are first seen with HPT.

Summary

Primary hyperparathyroidism can be diagnosed precisely. Clinical manifestations improve in most patients after successful surgery. Preoperative localization testing is helpful but not essential and the success rate of parathyroidectomy is greater than 95% when the operation is performed by an experienced surgeon. Patients with familial primary hyperparathyroidism need more aggressive treatment than do patients with sporadic disease because they are more prone to both persistent and recurrent disease. Even so, most cases can be successfully treated with surgery.

SELECTED READINGS

Clark O, Duh Q-Y: Textbook of Endocrine Surgery. Philadelphia, WB Saunders, 1997.

Edis AJ, Grant C, Egdahl R: Manual of Endocrine Surgery, 2nd ed. New York, Springer-Verlag, 1984.

Greenfield LJ, Mulholland M, Oldham K, et al: Essentials of Surgery: Scientific Principles and Practice. Philadelphia, Lippincott-Raven, 1997.

Carty SE, Norton JA: Management of patients with primary hyperparathyroidism. World J Surg 1991;15:716.

Udelsman R (ed): Operative Techniques in General Surgery: Surgical Exploration for Hyperparathyroidism. Philadelphia, WB Saunders, 1999.

Chapter 166

Functioning and Nonfunctioning Adrenal Tumors

Quan-Yang Duh

The most common indications for adrenalectomy are for hormonal hypersecretion and for concern of possible cancer. This chapter reviews the diagnosis and treatment of various functioning and nonfunctioning tumors of the adrenal gland. Adrenal tumors can be diagnosed as the result of (1) clinical suspicion leading to tumor-directed imaging studies, (2) known risk factors, such as family history or other associated conditions, leading to genetic, biochemical, or imaging screening, or (3) an incidentally discovered adrenal mass detected on imaging studies done for other reasons (incidentaloma). In general, whenever a patient is found to have an adrenal tumor, the physician should ask two questions: Does it produce adrenal hormones? Is it a cancer? With few exceptions, adrenal tumors that secrete hormones and those that are high risk for cancer need to be resected.

HORMONE-SECRETING ADRENAL TUMORS

Aldosteronoma

Patients with an aldosteronoma are invariably hypertensive and most are also hypokalemic. Primary hyperaldosteronism is clinically suspected when hypertension is difficult to control, even with multiple medications. The diagnosis of primary hyperaldosteronism is made when the serum aldosterone level is elevated and there is concurrent low plasma renin activity (aldosterone/renin ratio greater than 25 to 30).

Approximately one third of patients with primary hyperaldosteronism have bilateral disease (hyperplasia) and the hypertension and hypokalemia fail to respond to unilateral adrenalectomy. This needs to be distinguished from unilateral disease (adenoma or rarely unilateral primary hyperplasia) in which the hypertension improves in approximately 75% of patients and the hypokalemia resolves in almost all patients. In the past, saline loading, postural studies, or both were used to distinguish unilateral or adenomatous disease from bilateral or hyperplastic disease. The former patients benefited from adrenalectomy, whereas the latter underwent medical treatment. These tests, however, are only approximately 80% to 85% accurate and have, in general, been replaced by thin-cut computed tomography (CT) (3-mm cuts or spiral) scans that identify the aldosteronoma in 90% to 95% of patients.

When the patient has a definitive clinical and biochemical diagnosis of primary hyperaldosteronism and the CT scan shows a 0.5- to 2-cm adrenal tumor with a normal contralateral adrenal gland, the diagnosis and localization of the aldosteronoma are complete, no further study is needed, and an adrenalectomy is indicated (Fig. 166–1).

If the CT scan shows a bilateral abnormality (bilateral hyperplasia versus unilateral aldosteronoma and a contralateral nonsecreting adenoma) or bilateral normal adrenal glands (bilateral hyperplasia versus aldosteronoma too small to see), then selective venous catheterization is indicated. Selective venous catheterization measuring aldosterone/cortisol ratio can identify the side of hypersecreting adenoma. Adrenalectomy is indicated if there is a unilateral increase of aldosterone/cortisol ratio. The cortisol level is determined to be sure that the catheter is properly positioned in the adrenal vein. The level is higher when the catheter is closer to the adrenal gland. Catheterization of the left adrenal gland is almost always successful, whereas only approximately 90% of the right adrenal veins can be successfully cannulated.

Iodomethylnorcholesterol (Np-59) adrenal cortical scanning has been advocated by some to identify the hyperfunctioning tumor. It is accurate for larger tumors, which are usually identifiable on CT scan, but frequently negative for very small tumors, when it is needed most. We occasionally use Np-59 scanning to determine whether a tumor found on CT scan is functioning. Normal adrenal function should be suppressed with dexamethasone for this test.

Potassium-sparing diuretics, such as spironolactone,

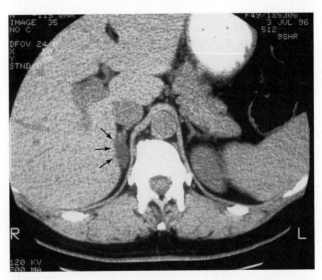

Figure 166–1. Abdominal computed tomography scan showing a 1.5-cm right adrenal aldosteronoma in a 49-year-old woman who has chronic severe hypertension and hypokalemia. The tumor is characteristically hypodense. The left adrenal gland is normal.

are used to normalize the serum potassium level and to confirm the diagnosis of primary hyperaldosteronism. Patients who respond well to spironolactone are also likely to be cured by adrenalectomy. They may not tolerate long-term treatment with spironolactone because of side effects, such as gynecomastia and impotence.

Currently, aldosteronomas are routinely resected by laparoscopic adrenalectomy. The standard operation is complete resection of the entire adrenal gland including the tumor. Although subtotal adrenalectomy, leaving the normal-appearing part of the gland, is advocated by some surgeons, we believe that saving the ipsilateral cortical tissue is unnecessary and may risk recurrence by leaving residual tumor. The contralateral adrenal gland in patients with an aldosteronoma is at low risk for development of another tumor.

More than 95% of patients with aldosteronoma benefit from adrenalectomy because the hypokalemia almost always resolves, and blood pressure becomes normal (75%) or easier to control with fewer drugs. Spironolactone should be stopped after adrenalectomy. Older men, especially those with a long-standing history of hypertension, are at higher risk for persistent hypertension. If hypertension persists, serum aldosterone and renin activity levels should be measured to determine whether it is due to persistent disease or to residual essential hypertension.

Pheochromocytoma

Almost all patients with pheochromocytoma have hypertension, half have chronic persistent hypertension, and the others have intermittent spikes of high blood pressure. The classic triad of headache, diaphoresis, and palpitations is present in only approximately one third of these patients. Because of the increasing use of abdominal imaging studies—CT, magnetic resonance imaging (MRI), and ultrasound—currently approximately half of the pheochromocytomas are found incidentally on abdominal imaging studies. Most of these patients also have hypertension, but it is usually not severe enough for the clinician to have suspected the presence of a pheochromocytoma. The most sensitive (98%) biochemical diagnostic test is 24-hour urinary excretion of metanephrine and normetanephrine. Twenty-four–hour urinary excretion of vanilmandelic acid and catecholamines are slightly less sensitive. Plasma levels of catecholamines are less useful for diagnosis because they may be falsely elevated by stress and falsely normal in intermittently secreting tumors.

Pheochromocytoma is called the "ten-percent" tumor, which refers to the likelihood of familial disease, bilateral disease, extra-adrenal tumor, multiple tumors, or malignancy. Once the biochemical diagnosis is made, the tumor should be localized. General abdominal exploration for possible tumors, in both adrenal glands and along the aorta down to the bifurcation, was once considered the standard of care; this is no longer routine. Excellent localization studies have enabled a focused, imaging-directed resection for patients with pheochromocytoma.

Thin-cut or spiral CT scanning, including both adrenal

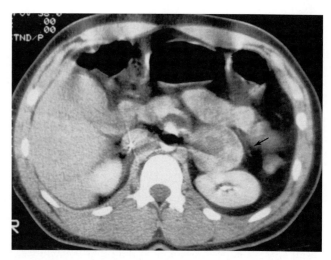

Figure 166–2. Abdominal computed tomography scan showing a 7-cm left adrenal pheochromocytoma in a 32-year-old man with "pheo-crisis" with multisystem failure. The tumor shows characteristic heterogeneity owing to hemorrhage.

glands and down to the aortic bifurcation, is the best localization study (Fig. 166–2). CT provides good anatomic details to guide the operation. Symptomatic pheochromocytomas are almost always larger than 2 to 3 cm. MRI is useful when the diagnosis is less certain, and 90% of pheochromocytomas characteristically enhance on T2-weighted MRI scans or after injection of gadolinium. Metaiodobenzylguanidine (MIBG) scanning is indicated when the tumor is not located in the adrenal gland, when metastases are suspected, or when multiple tumors are likely, such as in patients with familial disease. We routinely obtain MIBG scans in young patients and in those with multiple endocrine neoplasia type II or other syndromes (von Hippel-Lindau, neurofibromatosis, or Osler-Weber-Rendu syndrome), in those with persistent or recurrent disease after a prior adrenalectomy, in those with an extra-adrenal tumor, or when CT scanning shows possible metastases.

Adrenalectomy for pheochromocytoma is safe when the patient is well prepared preoperatively. The patient should be given α-adrenergic blocker phenoxybenzamine for at least 1 to 3 weeks preoperatively. Blood pressure should be controlled and intravascular volume is restored gradually by oral hydration. With effective therapy, the patients gain weight, have orthostatic hypotension, do not perspire, and may be uncomfortable with a stuffy nose. Adequate α-adrenergic blockade dampens intraoperative fluctuation of blood pressure and, in patients who have been rehydrated, it prevents hypotension and vascular collapse when the adrenal vein is ligated and the tumor is removed. Prazosin, a less specific α-blocker, and calcium channel blockers have also been used to prepare patients with pheochromocytomas, but these are associated with more fluctuation of blood pressure intraoperatively and postoperatively.

Laparoscopic adrenalectomy for pheochromocytoma has a higher risk of hemorrhage because of the abundant blood supply and numerous large thin-walled veins. Early ligation of the adrenal vein is not necessary and can cause venous congestion, making the subsequent dissection bloodier. A strong nylon bag should be used to extract the tumor and the adrenal gland to avoid breakage that can cause serious hypertension and risk seeding of tumor and recurrence. For patients with bilateral adrenal pheochromocytomas, subtotal adrenalectomy, leaving part of the normal cortex of one adrenal gland, is an option. It may prevent addisonian crisis, but risks recurrent pheochromocytoma from remaining microscopic foci of medullary tissue. For patients with pheochromocytomas suspected to be malignant, an open operation is recommended. Patients with malignant pheochromocytomas may live for years and usually benefit from surgical debulking of recurrent tumors to provide symptomatic relief.

Intraoperative hypertension can be controlled by nitroprusside or phentolamine. With adequate preoperative α-blockade, postoperative problems are rare, but cardiovascular collapse and hypotension can occur and require treatment with epinephrine or Neo-Synephrine. Postoperative hypoglycemia can be a problem, especially in children.

Cushing's Syndrome

Adrenalectomy is indicated for almost all patients with adrenocorticotropic hormone (ACTH)-independent Cushing's syndrome and for some patients with ACTH-dependent Cushing's syndrome who have failed surgical treatment or whose primary tumor cannot be found. ACTH-independent Cushing's syndrome is caused by adrenal cortical adenoma, adrenal cortical carcinoma, or primary adrenal hyperplasia (macronodular or micronodular). ACTH-dependent Cushing's syndrome is most commonly caused by ACTH-secreting pituitary tumors (Cushing's disease) and rarely by ectopic ACTH-secreting tumors (cancers or carcinoids).

Hypercortisolism (Cushing's syndrome) causes a characteristic syndrome of central obesity, moon facies, purple striae, easy bruising, muscle wasting, hypertension, hyperglycemia, weakness, and mood changes. The diagnosis is made by demonstrating that plasma cortisol level has lost its normal diurnal variation or that it cannot be suppressed by low-dose (1 mg) dexamethasone, or that 24-hour urinary free cortisol level is elevated. Once the diagnosis of hypercortisolism is made, ACTH measurement then determines whether the patient has ACTH-dependent Cushing's syndrome (high level of ACTH as the primary problem) or ACTH-independent Cushing's syndrome (low level of ACTH because the pituitary is suppressed).

The definitive treatment for ACTH-dependent Cushing's syndrome is to resect the ACTH-secreting primary tumor. Transsphenoidal resection of a pituitary adenoma has a high success rate, especially for microadenomas. Persistent or recurrent disease after resection can also be treated with irradiation. Approximately 10% of patients with Cushing's disease require bilateral adrenalectomy to control recurrent or persistent hypercortisolism. Adrenal-

ectomy for an ectopic ACTH syndrome is indicated if the source is occult (most likely small carcinoid tumors that are commonly in the chest and rarely in the abdomen) or if the primary tumor cannot be resected but life expectancy is long (e.g., disseminated medullary thyroid cancer that secretes ACTH).

ACTH-independent Cushing's syndrome is most commonly caused by an adrenal cortical adenoma (Fig. 166-3). Adrenal cortical carcinomas can usually be distinguished from adenomas because the cancers are larger, more heterogeneous and irregular, or they have metastases or are locally invasive. At times, however, it is difficult to know whether a tumor is benign or malignant even after resection and pathologic examination. In general, carcinomas are larger than adenomas, but size alone is not a reliable criterion. Carcinomas are also more likely than adenomas to also secrete intermediate products of cortisol synthesis in addition to other steroid hormones such as androgens. Other rare causes of Cushing's syndrome are primary bilateral hyperplasia. Macronodular hyperplasia is diagnosed on CT scan, whereas the rarest micronodular hyperplasia may have only minimal abnormal adrenal findings on CT scans.

Laparoscopic adrenalectomy is the procedure of choice for patients with Cushing's syndrome resulting from bilateral adrenal disease, because these cases are almost always benign. The laparoscopic surgeon should understand the disease process as well as the technical aspects of laparoscopic surgery. Complete resection of all adrenal tissue is crucial because any remaining tissue can cause persistent or recurrent disease. Subtotal adrenalectomy is not a good option because all of the cortical tissue is at risk for continuing growth and cortisol secretion. Autotransplantation of cortical tissue has been attempted but has been rarely successful.

Laparoscopic adrenalectomy is more controversial for Cushing's syndrome because the adrenal tumor is unilat-

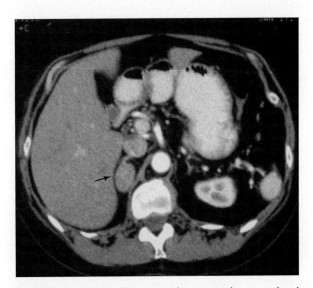

Figure 166–3. Abdominal computed tomography scan showing a 3.5-cm right adrenal cortical tumor in a 51-year-old woman who has adrenocorticotropic hormone–independent Cushing's syndrome. The left adrenal gland is normal.

eral. Because of the risk of tumor breakage and seeding, laparoscopic adrenalectomy may increase the risk of local recurrence for cancer. We recommend open resection for better tumor control if the CT scan shows obvious local invasion or if the tumor is larger than 10 cm and technically more difficult to manipulate laparoscopically. Others have recommended open resection for all Cushing's adrenal tumors larger than 3 to 5 cm, or for any tumors that are possible cancers.

Cushing's patients are at higher risk for wound infection than those who have adrenalectomy for other reasons, and a single dose of perioperative antibiotics is recommended. Cushing's patients also recover more slowly postoperatively, primarily because of muscle weakness but also because of mood changes. Stress dose glucocorticoid supplementation (usually 100 mg hydrocortisone intravenously every 8 hours) is required in Cushing's patients undergoing adrenalectomy and is tapered postoperatively. After unilateral adrenalectomy for Cushing's syndrome, it may take many months to taper off glucocorticoid because of suppression of the contralateral gland and the pituitary. After bilateral adrenalectomy, glucocorticoid replacement (usually hydrocortisone 20 mg in the morning and 10 mg in the evening) is essential for life. The patient is at risk for addisonian crisis and needs extra glucocorticoid in times of stress or trauma. Mineralocorticoid supplement (usually Florinef [fludrocortisone acetate] 0.1 mg once a day) is usually required in these patients.

CANCERS

Adrenal Cortical Carcinoma

Approximately two thirds of patients with adrenal cortical carcinomas have either systemic symptoms from increased hormonal secretion or local symptoms from the large size of the cancer or local invasion. Cortisol oversecretion results in Cushing's syndrome, androgen or estrogen oversecretion leads to masculinization or feminization, and aldosterone oversecretion causes hyperaldosteronism and hypertension. Tumors that secrete multiple hormones such as cortisol and aldosterone are likely malignant.

Adrenocortical carcinomas are usually heterogeneous, with areas of focal necrosis and irregular margins; occasionally, they have regional nodal involvement and liver metastases. They have high Hounsfield units on CT scanning and enhanced T2-weighted imaging on MRI, and they are cold on Np-59 scanning.

Surgical resection is the only potentially curative treatment. Radical resection including regional lymph nodes and adjacent organs such as the kidney may be necessary. Thus, open adrenalectomy is usually indicated. Laparoscopic adrenalectomy for large invasive adrenal cortical carcinomas is difficult and risks inadequate resection with tumor capsular rupture and possible seeding. Chemotherapy with mitotane or cis-platinum is only occasionally effective and is associated with significant side effects. Re-resection of local recurrence is indicated if technically feasible.

Metastatic Cancer to the Adrenal Gland

Solitary metastasis to the adrenal gland is resectable and potentially curable. The most common cancers that metastasize to the adrenal gland are lung cancer, breast cancer, colon cancer, and, less commonly, renal cell carcinoma and melanoma. The patient is more likely to be cured if the solitary adrenal metastasis is metachronous, especially years after the initial curative treatment, and less likely cured if synchronous, presenting at the same time of the extra-adrenal primary cancer. An adrenal tumor larger than 2 cm in a patient with a prior history of cancer is likely to be a metastasis.

Laparoscopic resection of a solitary adrenal metastasis appears to be safe if the CT scan does not show obvious invasion, because metastatic tumors tend to be less fragile than primary adrenal cortical carcinoma and thus are less likely to be fractured. As in all adrenalectomies, however, periadrenal fat should be resected with the adrenal gland and the tumor to decrease the risk of local recurrence.

Metastatic adrenal tumors may rarely be resected to alleviate symptoms, even in the presence of an unresectable or incurable primary cancer if the patient has a reasonable life expectancy.

INCIDENTALOMAS

In 1% to 4% of imaging studies of the abdomen, an unexpected adrenal tumor may be seen. Ninety percent of these are smaller than 2 cm. Most of these tumors, especially the smaller ones, are most likely to be nonfunctioning adrenal cortical adenomas. Some, however, may have clinically unapparent hormonal secretion, and others may be metastases or primary adrenal cortical cancers. A logical approach must be used in patients with incidentalomas to determine whether the tumor needs to be observed or resected.

Simple cysts and myelolipomas are benign adrenal lesions that can be definitively diagnosed by evaluating the CT scan. They do not need to be resected unless they cause local symptoms, usually when larger than 8 to 10 cm. For other adrenal incidentalomas, however, it is necessary to appropriately rule out hormonal hypersecretion and metastatic disease. A complete history and physical examination with screening chest radiograph, mammogram, and laboratory studies should identify most patients with extra-adrenal primary cancers. Occult extra-adrenal primary cancers are rare. If an extra-adrenal primary cancer is discovered, it is treated, and if no other metastases are found, the adrenal metastasis can then be resected for possible cure. Screening tests for hormonal hypersecretion should include a 24-hour urinary cortisol and 24-hour urinary total metanephrine excretion test to rule out subclinical Cushing's syndrome and pheochromocytoma, respectively. Patients with hypertension and smaller incidentalomas should also be screened for aldosteronoma by serum potassium, aldosterone, and renin activity. Patients with masculinization and feminization need to be screened with androgen and estrogen levels. All hormonal secreting tumors should be resected, most commonly by laparoscopic adrenalectomy.

The remaining nonsecreting tumors are either nonfunctioning adenomas or nonfunctioning carcinomas. In these patients, the risk of adrenalectomy needs to be balanced against the risk of unresected adrenal cortical carcinoma. Size and appearance of the tumor on CT or MRI, and age and comorbidity of the patients are important variables in the decision. In general, we recommend observation and follow-up for tumors less than 3 cm and resection for tumors larger than 5 cm. For tumors between 3 and 5 cm, we recommend resection for young healthy patients who have low surgical risk and observation for older patients who are more likely to have nonfunctioning adenomas.

Fine-needle aspiration may be useful in patients with suspected metastatic disease, but it is almost never useful and may be dangerous in the workup of patients with primary adrenal tumors. Cytologic examination cannot definitively distinguish between benign and malignant pheochromocytomas or between adrenal cortical adenomas and carcinomas. Fine-needle aspiration should never be performed until after pheochromocytoma has been ruled out and only when the cytologic findings will alter clinical management of the patient, such as whether or not to resect the primary nonadrenal cancer.

SURGERY FOR ADRENAL TUMORS

Open Adrenalectomy

The classic approach to adrenalectomy is the open anterior approach via a midline or bilateral subcostal incision. It gives exposure to both adrenal glands if needed. When performing a right adrenalectomy, a Kocher maneuver helps move the duodenum and pancreatic head medially. The liver is retracted upward and medially. The inferior vena cava is identified and the usually short right adrenal vein is ligated as it drains into the vena cava. For a larger or higher positioned right adrenal gland, the liver is mobilized by incising the triangular ligament and retracting medially. When performing a left adrenalectomy, the gastrocolic ligament is open, the peritoneum over the inferior edge of the pancreas is incised, and the pancreas is lifted superiorly. The left adrenal vein is identified, usually as the left inferior phrenic vein joins it, before draining into the left renal vein. For a larger or higher positioned left adrenal gland, the splenic flexure of the colon, the spleen, and the tail of the pancreas are mobilized medially (medial visceral rotation).

The posterior open approach was also formerly used for the removal of small tumors. It resulted in a more rapid recovery because of less ileus and fewer complications than the anterior open approach. A "hockey-stick" incision is made curving onto the 12th rib, which is resected. The retroperitoneal space is small and dissection is more limited. This approach has mostly been replaced by laparoscopic adrenalectomy.

The lateral retroperitoneal approach is done with the patient in the decubitus position and resecting the 10th or 11th rib. The retroperitoneal space is entered laterally and provides more room for dissection than the posterior approach and is therefore used for larger unilateral tumors. A thoracoabdominal approach may be useful for removing very large or invasive adrenal cancers and makes it easier to resect adjacent involved organs or tissues. It is associated with a longer recovery time.

Laparoscopic Adrenalectomy

Laparoscopic adrenalectomy is currently the standard operation for removing most adrenal tumors, except for the very large (greater than 10 to 12 cm) or invasive cancers. These are relative contraindications, mainly because of the technical limitations, and may possibly be overcome by hand-assisted laparoscopic adrenalectomy. Nonrandomized studies have shown conclusively that patients who undergo laparoscopic adrenalectomy suffer less pain and complications and recover faster than those who undergo open adrenalectomy. The difference is even more dramatic than that between laparoscopic and open cholecystectomy.

The most commonly used laparoscopic approach is the lateral transabdominal approach. The patient is placed in the lateral decubitus position; gravity helps retract the viscera away from the adrenal gland. Four trocars are inserted below the costal margin evenly spaced from midclavicular to the midaxillary line. For right adrenalectomy, the triangular ligament is incised and the liver rotated medially to expose the right adrenal gland. For left adrenalectomy, the spleen and the tail of the pancreas are mobilized and retracted medially to expose the left adrenal gland. Once resected, the adrenal gland with the tumor should be placed in a strong bag and extracted either whole or morcellated.

A retroperitoneal approach, either posteriorly or later-

Pearls and Pitfalls

PEARLS

- Localize the adrenal tumor preoperatively, usually with a thin-cut CT scan, to avoid the need for a generalized abdominal exploration.
- Work-up for hormonal hyperfunction or presence of extra-adrenal primary cancer in patients with adrenal incidentalomas.
- Prepare the patient medically (e.g., α-blockade for pheochromocytoma, spironolactone for aldosteronoma) before adrenalectomy.
- Give stress dose glucocorticoids perioperatively and taper it slowly after adrenalectomy if the patients have hypercortisolism resulting from adenoma, carcinoma, or hyperplasia.

PITFALLS

- Do not needle biopsy adrenal tumors routinely. Do it only if the result will change patient management and if it is not a pheochromocytoma.
- Do not perform laparoscopic adrenalectomy for a very large tumor, obviously invasive tumors, or if technical expertise is not available.

ally, has also been successfully used, but the space is more limited and resection of larger tumors is more difficult.

Most patients can be discharged after laparoscopic adrenalectomy within 1 or 2 days and require less pain medication and recovery time than those after an open adrenalectomy. They also return to work more quickly.

Summary

All functioning tumors of the adrenal gland need to be resected, whereas nonfunctioning tumors are removed selectively. Localization of the adrenal tumors preoperatively allows for focused resection, most commonly by laparoscopic adrenalectomy. The preoperative diagnosis of adrenal cortical carcinoma may be difficult and one must balance the risk of delay in removal with the risk of the operation.

SELECTED READINGS

Barresi RV, Prinz RA: Laparoscopic adrenalectomy. Arch Surg 1999;134:212.

Duh QY, Siperstein AE, Clark OH, et al: Laparoscopic adrenalectomy. Comparison of the lateral and posterior approaches. Arch Surg 1996;131:870.

Harrison LE, Gaudin PB, Brennan MF: Pathologic features of prognostic significance for adrenocortical carcinoma after curative resection. Arch Surg 1999;134:181.

Kebebew E, Duh QY: Benign and malignant pheochromocytoma: Diagnosis, treatment, and follow-up. Surg Oncol Clin North Am 1998;7:765.

Kim SH, Brennan MF, Russo P, et al: The role of surgery in the treatment of clinically isolated adrenal metastasis. Cancer 1998;82:389.

Lee JE, Curley SA, Gagel RF, et al: Cortical-sparing adrenalectomy for patients with bilateral pheochromocytoma. Surgery 1996;120:1064.

Loh KC, Koay ES, Khaw MC, et al: Prevalence of primary aldosteronism among Asian hypertensive patients in Singapore. J Clin Endocrinol Metab 2000;85:2854.

Rossi R, Tauchmanova L, Luciano A, et al: Subclinical Cushing's syndrome in patients with adrenal incidentaloma: Clinical and biochemical features. J Clin Endocrinol Metab 2000;85:1440.

Shen WT, Lim RC, Siperstein AE, et al: Laparoscopic vs open adrenalectomy for the treatment of primary hyperaldosteronism. Arch Surg 1999;134:628.

Chapter 167

Neuroendocrine Tumors of the Pancreas

Joseph F. Buell, Ronald Witteles, Maha Lakshmana Rao Koka, Sonia L. Sugg, and Edwin L. Kaplan

Because of the physiologic effects of their hormonal secretions, islet cell tumors of the pancreas present some of the most interesting syndromes in clinical medicine. This chapter discusses the syndromes and their treatment as well as the surgical treatments and other therapy for functional and nonfunctional islet cell neoplasms.

CLINICAL PRESENTATION

Insulinoma

Insulinoma is the most common neoplasm of the endocrine pancreas, accounting for 60% of all islet cell tumors, with an incidence of approximately one case per 1 million population per year. Insulinomas have a 2:1 female predominance, 87% to 90% are solitary, 84% to 90% are benign, and 4% are associated with multiple endocrine neoplasia type I. When MEN-I is present, multiple tumors may secrete insulin and/or other hormones.

The most common clinical presentations are one or more temporary nonfocal neurologic symptoms (apathy, dizziness, clouded sensorium, behavioral disturbance, coma, seizures). At least one of these symptoms can be found in 92% of patients with an insulinoma. Even though focal neurologic deficits unilaterally (e.g., paralysis, sensory loss, diplopia) can occur, these are much less common, occurring in only 5% of patients. Patients also have palpitations, pallor, precordial pain, weight gain, hunger, and nausea or vomiting.

Symptomatic hypoglycemic attacks usually occur with *fasting* or *exercise*, and are most common before breakfast and in the late afternoon. The severity of the clinical presentation does not predict either the size or the malignant potential of an insulinoma.

The *differential diagnosis* of an insulinoma includes other causes of fasting hypoglycemia, which can be due to inhibition of glucose production in the liver (hormone deficiencies, enzyme defects, substrate deficiency, liver disease, alcohol, drugs) or to stimulation of glucose utilization by adipose and muscle cells (hyperinsulinism, extrapancreatic tumors). It is important to differentiate fasting hypoglycemia from postprandial (reactive) hypoglycemia, which is a much more common problem that occurs in normal individuals and in patients who have had gastric surgery. In addition to the patient's history, a differentiation between postprandial and fasting hypoglycemia can be made clinically by the amount of glucose that must be infused intravenously to prevent hypoglycemia. If more than 200 g of glucose is required per day, a

diagnosis of fasting hypoglycemia resulting from hyperinsulinism can be made with confidence.

If a diagnosis of hyperinsulinism is made, the differential diagnosis includes insulinoma, exogenous insulin, infections, sulfonylureas, immune disease with insulin antibodies, and nesidioblastosis or islet cell hyperplasia. Nesidioblastosis is an uncommon cause of adult hyperinsulinemia (only 32 cases have been reported), but it is important to keep in the differential because of its identical clinical presentation to insulinoma.

In 1935, Whipple and Frantz described what has come to be known as "Whipple's triad" as criteria for the diagnosis of an insulinoma: (1) the signs and symptoms of hypoglycemia occur during periods of fasting or exertion, (2) at the time of symptoms, the blood sugar levels must be less than 45 mg/dL, and (3) the symptoms are ameliorated by the administration of oral or intravenous glucose. Even though the criteria of Whipple's triad still apply, most authors believe that a 72-hour fast should be the standard diagnostic test for insulinoma, diagnosing an insulinoma in more than 95% of cases. A serum insulin (μU/mL) to glucose (mg/dL) ratio of greater than 0.3 is found in almost all patients with insulinomas, and a glucose level of less than 40 mg/dL with concomitant insulin levels of greater than 6 μU/mL is confirmatory of insulinoma (Fig. 167–1). C-peptide levels (also secreted from the islet cells with insulin) should also be elevated; other-

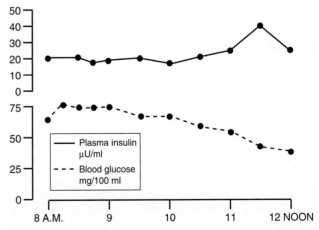

Figure 167–1. Levels of plasma insulin and blood glucose during the last 4 hours of a 12-hour fast in a patient with an insulinoma. Note that, despite severe hypoglycemia, the secretion of insulin continues unabated. (From Kaplan EL, Arganini M, Kang S-J: Diagnosis and treatment of hypoglycemic disorder. Surg Clin North Am 1987;67:395, with permission.)

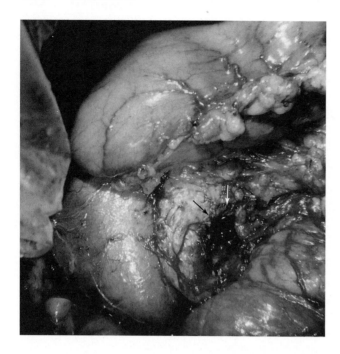

Figure 167–2. Insulinoma of the head of the pancreas. These lesions can almost always be enucleated. During enucleation, careful blunt dissection should be used immediately on the capsule of the insulinoma to prevent damage to the common bile duct or to the pancreatic duct, which could result in a fistula.

wise, the possibility of exogenous insulin administration must be pursued. Measurement of the proinsulin level is also important because this is usually increased in patients with an insulinoma. Levels are generally highest with less-differentiated tumors.

In severely hypoglycemic patients, it is important to always draw an insulin level as well as C-peptide and proinsulin levels if possible before giving glucose. Also, urinary testing for oral hypoglycemic agents should be done.

For patients in whom the diagnosis is strongly suspected but not proven by previous testing, a variety of provocative tests can be used to cause release of insulin and concomitant hypoglycemia. These include the tolbutamide test (80% sensitivity), the glucagon test (72% sensitivity), the L-leucine test (50% sensitivity), and a calcium infusion test. A glucose tolerance test can also be performed, showing an exaggerated hypoglycemic phase in 60% of insulinoma patients.

Insulinomas occur with equal frequency in the head, body, (Figs. 167–2 and 167–3), and tail of the pancreas and are generally small tumors that can sometimes be difficult to find. Therefore, once the diagnosis of insulinoma has been made, most authors recommend preoperative localization studies or procedures. Standard radiographic tests (ultrasound, computed tomography [CT], and magnetic resonance imaging [MRI]) can be used but are relatively insensitive given the frequently small size of insulinomas (90% less than 2 cm in diameter; 40% less than 1 cm). Angiography has historically been used to localize insulinomas by the demonstration of the characteristic tumor "blush," with sensitivities ranging from 50% to 80% (Fig. 167–4).

Transgastric ultrasound has been used effectively to localize the insulinomas. We have found this technique to be the most successful localization technique. Percutaneous transhepatic portal venous sampling (PTPVS) involves insulin levels being measured along the splenic

vein and from the other major pancreatic draining veins. Whereas the sensitivity of PTPVS is 70% to 95%, it is an invasive procedure that has a morbidity associated with percutaneously cannulating the portal vein through the liver.

A more recent preoperative method that has been increasingly used is arterial stimulation and venous sampling (ASVS), in which calcium is injected selectively into the major pancreatic arteries—the gastroduodenal, splenic, and superior mesenteric arteries—and the insulin levels are measured from a hepatic vein before and after stimulation (Fig. 167–5). This technique allows correct regionalization, in most cases, of the insulinoma to the area of the pancreas supplied by a given artery, and is associated with much less morbidity than PTPVS. We use this technique when transgastric ultrasound is negative.

Gastrinoma and the Zollinger-Ellison Syndrome

The Zollinger-Ellison (ZE) syndrome is characterized by severe peptic ulcer disease and gastric hyperacidity resulting from an excessive secretion of gastrin from a pancreatic or duodenal gastrinoma. Whereas it was originally thought that a pancreatic gastrinoma was the most important cause, in recent years the importance of a duodenal gastrinoma (Fig. 167–6) as a cause of ZE syndrome has been emphasized. More than half of all gastrinomas are malignant. Clinical presentation is most common as a duodenal ulcer in the usual anatomic position, followed by a postbulbar ulcer, although ectopic ulcers further down the gastrointestinal tract and in the stomach and distal esophagus may also occur. Diarrhea occurs in up to 50% of patients and up to 10% have diarrhea as the sole manifestation of the disease. The diarrhea is due to gastric hypersecretion of acid, which results in gut irritation and inhibition of pancreatic lipase

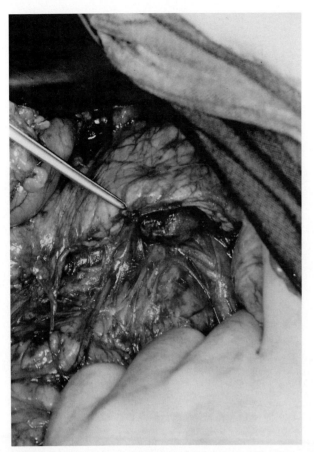

Figure 167–3. An insulinoma of the inferior surface of the body of the pancreas is seen (the forceps points to the tumor). This was easily enucleated.

and which disappears with nasogastric suction of the gastric juice or treatment with H₂ blockers or proton-pump inhibitors. Gastrinoma must be differentiated from ordinary ulcer disease. It is estimated that 0.1% of patients with duodenal ulcer and 2% of patients with recurrent ulcers have a gastrinoma as a cause.

The diagnosis of gastrinoma is made by documenting *an elevated fasting serum gastrin level in the presence of severe gastric hypersecretion of acid.* The presence of gastric hyperacidity documented by an elevated basal acid output (BAO) greater than 15 mEq per hour (normal, less than 10 mEq per hour) or a basal acid output to maximally stimulated (BAO/MAO) ratio of 0.6 or greater can be diagnostic when an elevated serum gastrin level is present. In the presence of gastric hyperchlorhydria, a serum gastrin level of 1000 pg/mL (normal less than 100 pg/mL) is virtually diagnostic of a gastrinoma. With lower basal gastrin levels, stimulation with calcium, secretin, or both may be important. A paradoxical elevation of serum gastrin of 200 pg/mL or greater soon after secretin injection is diagnostic of a gastrinoma.

Not all patients with an elevated serum gastrin and hypersecretion of acid have a gastrinoma, however. It is important to rule out gastric outlet obstruction and a retained antrum of the stomach following a gastrectomy and a Billroth 2 operation. Both can be accompanied by gastric hypersecretion and an elevated serum gastrin

level. Less commonly, these findings can occur following a substantial small bowel resection.

An elevated serum gastrin level accompanies achlorhydria or hypochlorhydria, which is present in pernicious anemia, chronic or atrophic gastritis, postvagotomy, or following H₂ blockers or proton-pump inhibitors of gastric acid. Thus, one must know that gastric hyperacidity is present before diagnosing a gastrinoma.

Antral G-cell hyperplasia also results in hypersecretion of gastric acid and hypergastrinemia but does so especially after eating. The diagnosis can be made by an exaggerated response of these parameters to a standard test meal.

Gastrinomas are often small, especially when they arise from the duodenum. Hence, conventional imaging techniques (CT, MRI) often are not diagnostic except to rule out liver metastases. Endoscopic examination of the duodenum and transgastric ultrasound can often be helpful in localizing these small duodenal and pancreatic tumors. Octreotide scan is helpful, especially for gastrinomas (Fig. 167–7) and can image the primary tumor or metastatic disease. The selective injection of secretin individually into the gastroduodenal, splenic, and superior mesenteric arteries, with measurement of gastrin from a hepatic vein (the Imamura test), can "regionalize" the site of a gastrinoma with considerable accuracy and appears to have less morbidity than percutaneous transhepatic sampling of gastrin from the pancreatic veins.

Gastrinomas are sporadic in 75% of cases but approximately one fourth of these are part of the MEN-I syndrome. As such, they are frequently associated with hy-

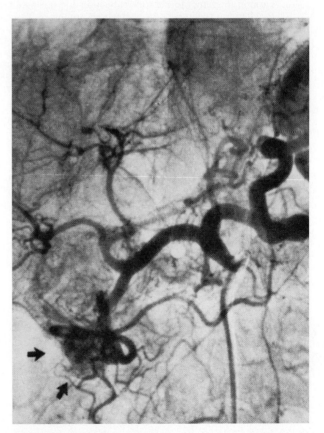

Figure 167–4. Insulinoma of the head of the pancreas (*arrows*) demonstrated by arteriography.

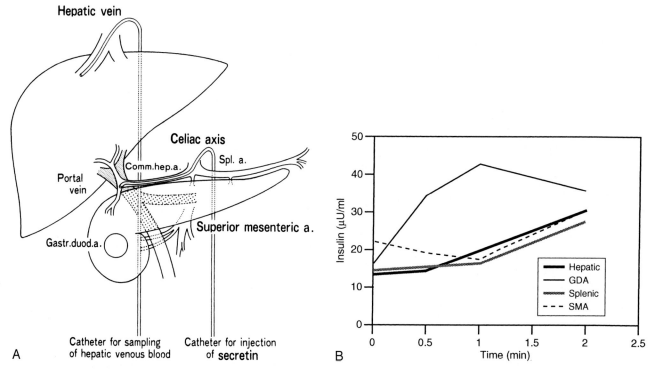

Figure 167–5. *A,* A schema for selective arterial stimulation and venous sampling (ASVS). Standard pancreatic arteriography includes selective injections of contrast material into the gastroduodenal artery (Gastroduod.a.), proximal splenic artery (Spl. a.), superior mesenteric artery (a.), and common hepatic artery (Comm. hep.a.). After each selective arteriogram, calcium gluconate (0.025 mEq Ca²⁺/kg) diluted in saline to a 5-mL bolus is injected rapidly through the catheter in each selectively catheterized artery. Five-milliliter samples of blood are obtained from the right hepatic vein before calcium injection and at 30, 60, and 120 seconds after calcium injection. Each plasma sample is frozen until assayed for insulin. A twofold increase in insulin levels after injection of the gastroduodenal or superior mesenteric arteries localizes the tumor to the pancreatic head and uncinate process; a twofold increase after injection into the splenic artery localizes the insulinoma to the body and tail. *B,* Results of selective intra-arterial calcium stimulation test (ASVS) in a patient with an insulinoma of the pancreatic head. Note that when calcium was injected into the gastroduodenal artery (GDA), a rapid elevation of circulating insulin occurred (within 30 seconds). No elevation in insulin values followed injections of calcium into the superior mesenteric artery (SMA), splenic artery, or hepatic artery. (*A* modified with permission from Imamura M, Takahashi K, Adachi H, et al: Usefulness of selective arterial secretion injection test for localization of gastrinoma in the Zollinger-Ellison syndrome. Ann Surg 1987;205:230. *B* from Doppman JL, Miller DL, Chang R, et al: Intraarterial calcium stimulation test for detection of insulinomas. World J Surg 1993;17:439, with permission.)

perparathyroidism and pituitary tumors. When gastrinomas are part of the MEN-I syndrome, multiple islet tumors of the pancreas and in the duodenum are the rule. However, the gastrinomas are still usually in the duodenal submucosa or head of the pancreas and the other pancreatic tumors are frequently nonfunctional.

Glucagonoma

Glucagonomas are pancreatic islet cell tumors of alpha cell origin that produce an excess of glucagon. Glucagon

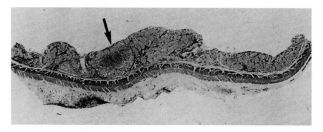

Figure 167–6. Small gastrinoma in duodenal submucosa (*arrow*).

is a catabolic hormone that breaks down protein to sugar. Thus, even though a few patients may be asymptomatic, most have a distinctive clinical syndrome consisting of a constellation of symptoms, including diabetes mellitus (or glucose intolerance), a very characteristic rash known as *necrolytic migratory erythema* (Fig. 167–8), glossitis and stomatitis, weight loss, and weakness. Less common components of this disease process are vascular thromboses, anemia, bowel habit alterations, and neurologic changes, including depression.

The most frequent but not universal presentation of glucagonoma is with diabetes mellitus or glucose intolerance. The migratory rash can vary from mild to severe with associated glossitis, stomatitis, cheilosis, and dystrophic fingernails and toenails. This rash (see Fig. 167–8) follows a typical cycle, with lesions arising over 7 to 14 days, forming a blister, oozing, and then healing over the next 2 to 3 weeks (see Fig. 167–8). Biopsy of the lesion at the margin can be diagnostic by demonstrating superficial necrosis of the epithelium. Significant weight loss is also a constant finding in most patients with glucagonomas. A high incidence of thromboembolic disease is related to "factor X" elevation produced by pancreatic alpha cells.

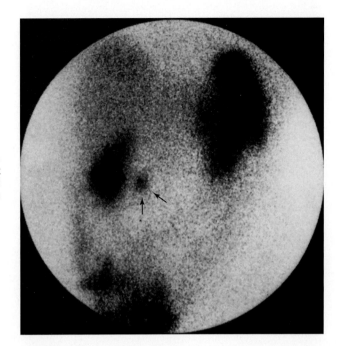

Figure 167–7. An octreotide scan can be useful in localizing insulinomas and gastrinomas. The tumor is represented by a hot spot just medial to the right kidney. (From van Eyck CHJ, Bruining HA, Reubi J-C, et al: Use of isotope labeled somatostatin analogs for visualization of islet cell tumors. World J Surg 1993;17:444, with permission.)

These can be either deep venous thrombosis or arterial thromboses involving the renal, cerebral, or mesenteric vessels.

Laboratory features include normochromic anemia, hypocholesterolemia, hypoproteinemia, hypoaminoacidemia. Plasma glucagon levels should be obtained in all diabetic patients with an unexplained skin rash. Normal glucagon levels range between 25 and 250 pg/mL, whereas patients with glucagonomas have levels between 500 and 1000 pg/mL or more. There are no provocative tests to confirm the diagnosis in patients with marginal glucagon levels. Other causes of hyperglucagonemia in-

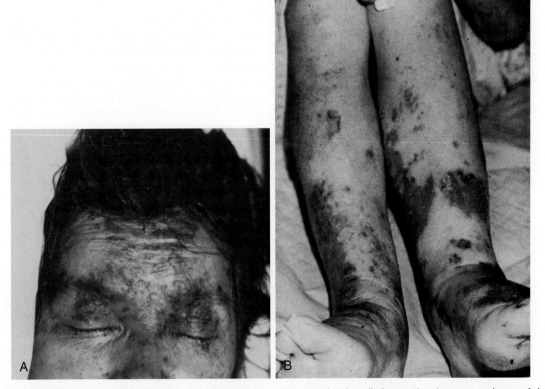

Figure 167–8. A patient with a glucagonoma demonstrating the typical rash, called necrotic migratory erythema of the face and legs. (From Kaplan EL, Michclassi F: Endocrine tumors of the pancreas and their clinical syndromes. In Nyhus LM (ed): Surgery annual, vol. 18. East Norwalk, CT, Appleton & Lange, 1986, pp 181–223.)

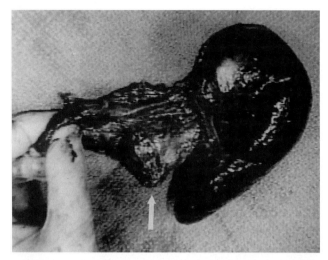

Figure 167–9. A large glucagonoma of the pancreatic tail (*arrow*). A distal pancreatectomy was performed. (From Findley A, Arenas RB, Kaplan EL: Insulinoma. In Percopo V, Kaplan EL [eds]: GEP and multiple endocrine tumors. Padova, Italy: Piccin Nuova Libreria SpA, 1996:314.)

clude steroid usage, renal failure, burns, septicemia, Cushing's syndrome, hypoglycemia, hepatic failure, and severe stress.

Most glucagonomas are fairly large, so localization can be performed by abdominal CT. Furthermore, most glucagonomas are malignant and involve the body or tail of the pancreas (Fig. 167–9). Some are calcified. Liver metastases are frequently present and can be readily imaged preoperatively in most cases. In few instances, small metastatic deposits are not identified before exploration.

VIPoma

VIPomas secrete excessive amounts of vasoactive intestinal polypeptide, or VIP, causing a syndrome of large volume *w*atery *d*iarrhea, severe *h*ypokalemia, and *a*chlorhydria or hypochlorhydria (hence, the name WDHA was used in the past). First described in 1958, VIPoma was also called the Verner-Morrison or watery diarrhea syndrome. VIP is found in pancreatic D_1 cells and enteric neurons, and plays a role in modulating intestinal secretion under normal circumstances. All patients with the syndrome have secretory diarrhea, often excreting more than 3 L per day, causing hypokalemia and resultant muscle weakness from potassium losses in the stool. Hypochlorhydria, which is found in 75% of patients, results from inhibition of gastrin and gastric acid secretion by VIP. VIP is a glycogenolytic hormone, and hyperglycemia also occurs in 25% to 50% of patients. It also has vasodilatory properties, but flushing occurs in a minority of patients. Most VIPomas occur in the pancreas (85%) and most of these (80%) are in the body and tail. Extrapancreatic sites include duodenum, along the autonomic chain, especially in the retroperitoneum, and in the adrenal glands. Forty percent of VIPomas are malignant, and 1% are associated with the MEN-I syndrome.

The differential diagnosis includes infectious diarrhea, inflammatory bowel disease, malabsorptive diseases such as celiac sprue, carcinoid syndrome, thyrotoxicosis, medullary cancer of the thyroid, ZE syndrome, villous adenoma of the rectum, and laxative abuse.

The diagnosis of VIPoma requires severe secretory diarrhea (>700 mL per day), an elevated fasting serum VIP (>200 pg/mL), and the presence of a tumor, typically imaged on CT scan. An angiogram or Octreoscan (indium In 111 pentetreotide) may be helpful. Ultrasound or MRI examinations have also been used.

Somatostatinoma

A somatostatinoma is a rare and usually malignant neuroendocrine tumor that develops from the D cells in the pancreas. More recently, the tumor has been shown to be polysecretory, sometimes involving adrenocorticotropic hormone (ACTH), calcitonin, VIP, pancreatic polypeptide (PP), gastrin, insulin, glucagon, or serotonin secretion as well, which results in altered clinical pictures. After the initial report of the syndrome in 1977, fewer than 200 cases have been described in the literature. Somatostatin is "the great inhibitor" of hormone secretion and motility.

The somatostatinoma syndrome, or inhibitory syndrome, encompasses diabetes mellitus (60%), cholelithiasis (50%), steatorrhea (50%), and hypochromic anemia (35%). Because of the frequency of these findings in the general populations and the vagueness of these symptoms, many clinicians do not find the use of this "syndrome" helpful as an early diagnostic tool. The diagnosis is not usually made until the tumor has grown to a substantial size and large hepatic metastases are often present.

The differential diagnosis of a somatostatinoma is extensive. Diarrhea and diabetes are the most frequent presentation for neuroendocrine tumors, so other diarrheogenic tumors (gastrinoma, VIPoma, carcinoid, and glucagonoma) and diabetogenic tumors (glucagonoma, enteroglucagonoma, and oat cell tumor) must be excluded. Finally, a workup of each patient who has diabetes associated with gallbladder disease would be inefficient. A retrospective analysis of such patients demonstrated an incidence of somatostatinoma of 2% or less.

Laboratory testing can be preformed to confirm the presence of somatostatin-like immunoreactivity (SLI). Normal values are 136 ± 8 pg/mL, whereas patients with tumors may have levels of 9000 to 13,000 pg/mL. Elevated levels of other hormones may also be present.

The majority of tumors are localized to the duodenum, especially in the periampullary region (50%), whereas (40%) of tumors are found in the pancreas. Within the pancreas, the head is the principal site (>50%). Duodenal tumors are usually diagnosed at an earlier interval and smaller size (2 to 3 cm) because of obstructive symptoms, whereas pancreatic tumors are larger (5 to 6 cm) and most commonly associated with hepatic metastases. Localization usually requires endoscopy as well as some form of conventional abdominal imaging. More than 80% of lesions can be diagnosed by ultrasonography, CT, or MRI. In patients with small tumors, selective angiography or venous sampling may be beneficial.

A syndrome consisting of a somatostatinoma of the ampulla of Vater with a pheochromocytoma in a patient with neurofibromatosis has been described.

Other Rare Functional Tumors

GRFomas secrete excessive amounts of GRF (growth hormone–releasing factor) and present with acromegaly and a pancreatic mass. Thirty percent of patients are first seen with metastatic disease, 50% have associated gastrinomas, and one third have MEN-I. *Corticotropin-producing tumors* are typically malignant pancreatic islet cell tumors that secrete ectopic ACTH in association with another peptide such as gastrin. The resulting hypercortisolism (Cushing's syndrome) is often difficult to control by tumor resection or medically, and bilateral adrenalectomy may be required to control the effects of severe hypercortisolism. *PTHrP (parathyroid hormone–related protein) producing tumors* of the pancreas are rare and cause severe hypercalcemia. Most are malignant.

Nonfunctional Endocrine Pancreatic Tumors

"Nonfunctioning" pancreatic endocrine tumors (NFPETs) constitute 15% to 20% of all pancreatic islet cell tumors. Although NFPETs are called "nonfunctional," radioimmunoassay and immunohistochemistry studies have shown that most of these tumors secrete hormones; some are even multihormonal. Most tumors (up to 90%) stain positive with immunohistochemical testing for one or more peptide hormones (insulin, glucagon, somatostatin, VIP, pancreatic polypeptide). Identification of progesterone and somatostatin receptors often imply a benign lesion. The lack of detectable biologic activity of these tumors may be due to insufficient hormone production or release, insufficient or defective receptors, secretion of antagonistic hormones, episodic secretion, and synthesis of psychologically inactive hormones or hormone precursors. Many of these tumors secrete pancreatic polypeptide (called PPomas) for example.

Most studies find an equal prevalence of the tumors among male and female patients, with the highest incidence occurring in the sixth decade of life. Clinical signs and symptoms are usually nonspecific and are related to the pancreatic mass, including abdominal mass effect, abdominal pain, nausea, vomiting, anorexia, fever, jaundice, weight loss, steatorrhea, and gastrointestinal bleeding. Causes of bleeding include direct invasion of blood vessels by tumor and from gastric and esophageal varices resulting from portal hypertension caused by thrombosis of the splenic vein from compression by the tumor. NFPETs have a strong predilection to present in the pancreatic head, which accounts for the fact that jaundice constitutes one of the most common symptoms. Because of the nonspecificity in presentation, many authors believe NFPETs tend to present at a later time than functioning tumors, with resultant larger sizes and a higher risk of malignancy ranging from 44% to 92%. Both of these points are controversial, however, and some reports find no increased size or risk of malignancy when comparing the two types of tumors.

The most common disease in the differential diagnosis is an exocrine tumor of the pancreas. Several criteria should increase suspicion for diagnosing an NFPET. These include a clinical history of a pancreatic neoplasm with unexpected survival in a patient affected by the MEN-I syndrome, a high degree of vascularity of the tumor, presence of a large tumor in the head of the pancreas, presence of calcification within the tumor, and high density on injecting contrast medium compared with surrounding parenchyma in the absence of a clinical endocrine syndrome. Calcification occurs in 10% to 23% of NFPETs.

NFPETs were originally believed to develop from nonsecretory cells. With the development of radioimmunoassay and immunohistochemistry, many peptide hormones and nonspecific neuroendocrine markers have been identified. Serum levels of such markers are frequently elevated in patients with NFPETs. The best known marker is neuron-specific enolase (NSE), and serum values greater than 12 ng/mL are generally considered to be above normal. NFPETs stain positive for NSE in more than 90% of cases in some studies. Because NSE levels are higher in malignant tumors, it is a useful indicator for radical surgery and an indicator of persistence or recurrence of disease. Other markers include synaptophysin, protein S-100, 7B2, PGP 9.5, and α- and β-human chorionic gonadotropin.

Unlike for insulinomas and gastrinomas, conventional radiologic tools (ultrasound, CT, MRI) are very sensitive for identifying NFPETs because of their relatively large size at presentation. The only exception is in patients with MEN-I, who can have multiple small tumors below the threshold of the imaging studies. CT scans can identify the tumors in 85% to 96% of cases, and can evaluate resectability of the tumor and detect metastases, most commonly found in the liver and regional lymph nodes.

PREOPERATIVE MANAGEMENT

Preoperative management of neuroendocrine tumors of the pancreas includes controlling excess hormone secretion, which means, in effect, controlling the syndrome that results from the excess hormone. The mainstay of therapy in *insulinoma* is the prevention of hypoglycemia. Frequent meals and minimizing prolonged exercise may be sufficient. Diazoxide is the most frequent medication used, although most authors recommend discontinuing it at least 1 week before surgery because it interferes with the ability to monitor changes in blood glucose during the operation. Other medications that have been used with some success for hypoglycemia include octreotide, calcium channel blockers, propranolol, glucagon, and glucocorticoids.

The hypersecretion of acid caused by *gastrinomas* can be controlled in almost every patient by the use of H_2-receptor blocking agents including cimetidine, ranitidine, and famotidine, and by proton pump inhibitors such as omeprazole and lansoprazole. In patients with *glucagonoma*, improvement of hyperglycemia, migratory rash, and nutritional status should be obtained before exploration. Nutritional status can be improved by administration of total parenteral nutrition. The somatostatin analogue octreotide reduces secretion of glucagon and is of considerable help in treating patients with the glucagonoma syndrome. On this medication, the rash clears rapidly, nutrition improves, and the threat of thromboembolic events is lessened. Perioperative anticoagulation is advised in these patients. Octreotide is the most effective method of reducing the secretory diarrhea in *VIPoma* and has made a very substantial impact in the preoperative therapy of these patients; with its use, the severe electrolyte disorders can be normalized. Octreotide may also aid in the preoperative management of patients with gastrinoma by helping to reduce diarrhea and gastric hypersecretion. Finally, patients who may undergo a subtotal or distal pancreatectomy should also receive the pneumococcal vaccine, because splenectomy is sometimes necessary.

INTRAOPERATIVE MANAGEMENT

Operative exposure for removal of pancreatic neuroendocrine tumors is best achieved through a bilateral subcostal or an upper transverse incision. A thorough and meticulous examination should be carried out of the entire abdominal cavity for suspicious nodules in the liver, lesser omentum, greater omentum, small bowel mesentery, small intestine, stomach, and pelvis (including the ovaries in females). Intraoperative ultrasound (IOUS) is a useful tool to evaluate for hepatic metastases and is useful to aid in detection of gastrinomas and insulinomas in the pancreas, because of their small size (Fig. 167–10). A generous Kocher maneuver allows careful palpation of the head and neck of the pancreas (Fig. 167–11). The lesser omental sac is then entered, either through the greater omentum below the curvature of the stomach or by reflecting the omentum off of the transverse colon and its mesocolon. The body and tail of the pancreas is mobilized by incising the peritoneum along the inferior edge and this area is then carefully inspected and palpated. The spleen is sometimes mobilized to aid in this inspection. All lymph nodes in the upper abdomen should be inspected and palpated, and suspicious lymph nodes and nodules should be removed for histologic examination by frozen section.

For tumors not imaged preoperatively, such as insulinomas or gastrinomas, IOUS of the pancreas is usually employed at this point in the operation (Fig. 167–12). Eighty-four percent to 86% of solitary insulinomas are detected by this method, and lesions as small as 4 mm can be seen (see Fig. 167–12). In addition, IOUS can provide valuable information about the relationship of the

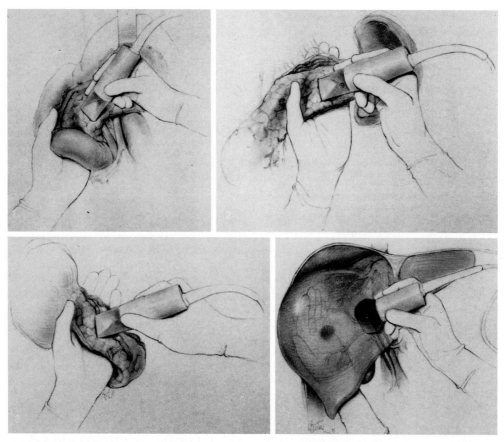

Figure 167–10. Use of intraoperative ultrasonography can be helpful to localize gastrinomas and insulinomas in the head (*upper left*), body (*upper right*), and tail (*lower left*) of the pancreas. This technique can also be useful in identifying liver metastases (*lower right*). (From Zeiger MA, Shawker TH, Norton JA: Use of intraoperative ultrasonography to localize islet cell tumors. World J Surg 1993;17:448 with permission.)

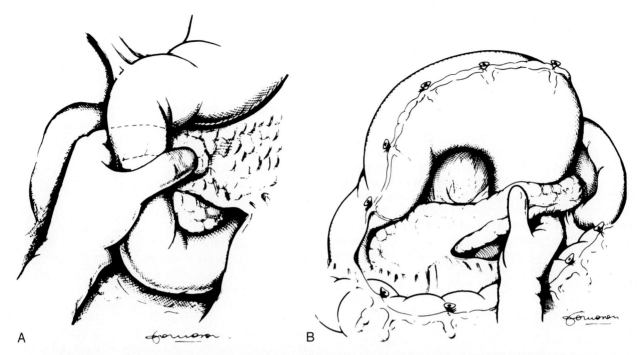

A   B

Figure 167–11. Technique of exploration. A generous Kocher maneuver is made and the head of the pancreas is inspected and palpated (*left*). After mobilizing the body and tail of the pancreas, this also is inspected and carefully palpated. (From Findley A, Arenas RB, Kaplan EL: Insulinoma. In Percopo V, Kaplan EL [eds]: GEP and multiple neuroendocrine tumors. Padova, Italy: Piccin Nuova Libreria SpA, 1996:314.)

tumor to structures such as the pancreatic duct, the portal vein, the common bile duct, and the superior mesenteric vessels. For insulinomas, the entire pancreas should be carefully palpated and evaluated by IOUS, because these tumors are evenly distributed throughout the pancreas.

For gastrinomas, an extensive evaluation must be made for tumors within the *gastrinoma triangle* involving the

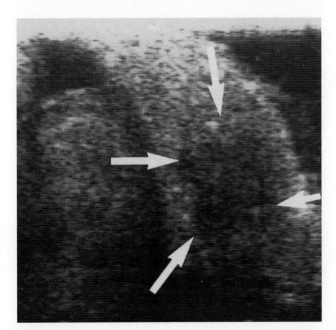

Figure 167–12. An insulinoma of the tail of the pancreas (*arrows*) is recognized by intraoperative ultrasonography because it is hypoechoic relative to the remaining pancreatic tissue.

duodenum, head of the pancreas and peripancreatic lymph nodes. Endoscopic transillumination of the duodenum may identify small duodenal tumors, but longitudinal duodenotomy is the most sensitive means of detecting these tiny submucosal tumors and should be routinely done. Forty percent or more of all gastrinomas are not in the pancreas but are found in the duodenal submucosa. This is especially true in patients with MEN-I and gastrinoma.

When a single pancreatic neuroendocrine tumor (most commonly an insulinoma or gastrinoma) is detected, enucleation is the preferred method for its removal if it can be done safely. If the tumor is in the head of the pancreas, care must be taken to avoid damage to the pancreatic duct and to the common bile duct, sometimes necessitating cannulation of the bile duct in order to prevent its damage. Always enucleate these lesions carefully and meticulously to avoid a fistula. Distal pancreatectomy is the treatment of choice if multiple lesions are found within the body or tail, if the lesion is large, or if the mass is adjacent to the pancreatic duct (where enucleation could lead to a fistula or pseudocyst).

If no lesion can be detected by palpation or by IOUS, treatment is controversial. For *insulinoma*, some authors recommend stopping the operation at this point if limited preoperative localization studies were performed. Others recommend a "blind" distal pancreatic resection at this point if extensive preoperative testing was performed and if one is certain that the lesion is not in the pancreatic head or uncinate process. A blind distal pancreatectomy performed after extensive preoperative localization is successful in controlling hypoglycemia in approximately two thirds of cases. Subtotal pancreatectomy is also recommended as the treatment of choice for patients with *adult onset nesidioblastosis or islet cell hyperplasia* (accounting for up to 10% of adult hyperinsulinemic hypoglycemia). This condition is diagnosed as the cause of hypoglycemia only after permanent histologic analysis and by the failure to find an insulinoma grossly or microscopically. In patients with sporadic gastrinomas, there is no role for a blind resection of the pancreas because symptoms can be controlled medically in most cases. The role for total gastrectomy is reserved for patients who will not or cannot take their proton-pump inhibitors or H_2 blockers.

The role of surgery in patients with MEN-I and the ZE syndrome is controversial. The most common symptomatic pancreatic tumor in MEN-I is *gastrinoma*. These tumors are most frequently found in the duodenum, but other neuroendocrine tumors, some functional and some nonfunctional, are usually scattered throughout the entire pancreas. Some authors recommend early exploration to promote a cure and to prevent later metastatic spread. Thompson advocates distal pancreatic resection with enucleation of all other lesions of the head of the pancreas, duodenotomy with removal of single or multiple tumors, and regional nodal resections. Others have found that early exploration rarely results in a cure and they advocate operation only when the tumor is large enough to be imaged. They treat nonoperative patients with MEN-I syndrome with acid inhibitors.

Whereas 90% of *insulinomas* are single, multiplicity is the rule when an insulinoma is part of the MEN-I syndrome. Such patients also usually require distal pancreatic resection with enucleation of lesions of the head of the pancreas.

In both gastrinoma and insulinoma patients with the MEN-I syndrome, parathyroidectomy is done first if primary hyperparathyroidism is present. Parathyroid hyperplasia is the rule. Most investigators recommend subtotal parathyroidectomy with thymectomy. However, others favor total parathyroidectomy with autotransplantation of parathyroid tissue into the arm. In both instances, recurrent hyperparathyroidism is common.

Glucagonomas, VIPomas, somatostatinomas, and nonfunctional pancreatic neuroendocrine tumors generally typically present as large tumors (>5 cm), often with associated lymph node or hepatic metastases. If feasible, complete resection should be attempted, because prognosis for neuroendocrine tumors of the pancreas is relatively good, especially when compared with the usual exocrine pancreatic carcinomas. Functional metastatic tumors are often poorly controlled by medical therapy and patients might benefit symptom-wise for substantial periods of time from surgical tumor debulking. Hepatic disease can be managed by segmental or nonanatomic resection when margins can be obtained. Recently, cryoablation and/or radiofrequency ablation have been performed on hepatic metastases of neuroendocrine tumors as well.

POSTOPERATIVE MANAGEMENT

The postoperative management of these patients is similar to that for any patient undergoing pancreatic or duodenal surgery. Closed suction drains are placed near the sites of pancreatic enucleation or resection and the patient takes nothing by mouth (remains NPO) with a nasogastric tube until gastrointestinal function returns. Drains are removed after the patient is maintained on a regular diet and the absence of a pancreatic leak is confirmed. If a duodenotomy was performed, some surgeons favor a Gastrografin swallow to confirm the integrity of the duodenal wall before feeding. The routine prophylactic use of octreotide to prevent postoperative leaks or fistulas has not been proved by some studies but is used by many surgeons postoperatively.

COMPLICATIONS

Routine perioperative complications that occur include bleeding, wound infection, dehiscence, deep venous thrombosis, pulmonary embolus, and pneumonia. Specific to these operations are the complications of a pancreatic leak or duodenal suture dehiscence. A pancreatic or duodenal leak is managed by stopping oral intake, total parenteral nutrition, and octreotide to decrease the fistula output. Most pancreatic leaks will stop if enough time is given. A high-volume duodenal leak may present a considerable problem and require further operative intervention. After a successful operation for insulinoma, a short period of hyperglycemia occurs but usually resolves spontaneously after several days to a week. Insulin is sometimes needed. With extensive pancreatic resections (≤85%), however, the incidence of diabetes mellitus increases.

OUTCOMES

Insulinomas

Most (95% or more) patients with sporadic insulinoma are cured with surgical exploration when performed by an experienced surgeon. The risk of diabetes mellitus increases with greater than 85% resection of the pancreas. Persistent hypoglycemia in the case of a benign insulinoma or unresectable malignant disease can be treated by medical therapy including diazoxide, octreotide, calcium channel blockers, or adrenocortical steroids.

Gastrinomas

In a recent study by Norton and colleagues of 151 patients who underwent surgical exploration, 34% of patients with sporadic gastrinomas were disease-free at 10 years, whereas none of the patients with MEN-I were cured. The 10-year survival rate was 94%. The most frequent location of the gastrinoma was the duodenum. Furthermore, duodenal gastrinomas offer the best opportunity for surgical cure. In patients with sporadic gastrinomas, duodenal gastrinomas were 3.4 times more common than pancreatic gastrinomas, whereas in MEN-I patients duodenal gastrinomas were 2.7 times more common than pancreatic lesions. With the success of medical control of acid secretion, the progression of metastatic disease has become the main determinant of long-term survival. The presence of liver metastases predicts the worst prognosis.

Pearls and Pitfalls

PREOPERATIVE

- A convincing diagnosis must be obtained before surgery for a gastrinoma. Avoid operating for hypergastrinemia alone, because this is frequently due to achlorhydria and not the ZE syndrome.
- Detailed patient studies and family histories should be obtained to detect syndromes of multiple endocrine neoplasia (MEN-I).
- Symptoms and signs of hormonal excess should be treated before operation.
- Gastrinomas and insulinomas frequently cannot be localized using conventional imaging studies because they are usually small.
- Endoscopic ultrasound, somatostatin receptor scintigraphy, and selective angiograms with rapid calcium or secretin infusion, followed by hormone sampling from the hepatic veins are very useful studies to localize insulinomas and gastrinomas, respectively.
- A CT scan is useful for detection of metastatic disease as well as for visualization of large islet cell tumors, which are usually found in glucagonomas, VIPomas, and somatostatinomas and often in nonfunctional tumors.

INTRAOPERATIVE

- Intraoperative ultrasonography is useful for intraoperative detection of small pancreatic tumors or metastases, especially for gastrinomas and insulinomas. Explore all

parts of the pancreas even if localization tests suggest that one area is involved.
- For islet cell tumors, exploration and resection of abnormal regional lymph nodes are mandatory.
- A duodenotomy should always be performed in operations for a gastrinoma. Enucleate all insulinomas or gastrinomas of the head of the pancreas and elsewhere when possible if lesions are not adjacent to the pancreatic duct. A distal resection is appropriate if enucleation cannot be safely done.
- A blind resection of the pancreas should not be done for insulinoma if the patient has not been studied extensively preoperatively.
- Curative resections should be performed even in the setting of advanced disease, if morbidity is not prohibitive.
- Debulking of unresectable disease may alleviate symptoms of hormonal excess for considerable periods of time.
- Always drain the pancreatic bed when an enucleation or distal resection has been performed.

POSTOPERATIVE

- After removal of an insulinoma, transient hyperglycemia usually occurs. Avoid treatment with insulin unless it is necessary.
- Octreotide is usually helpful in the treatment of pancreatic fistulas.

Other Pancreatic Neuroendocrine Tumors

Seventy percent of patients with glucagonomas and 30% to 40% of those with VIPomas, somatostatinomas, and GRFomas are diagnosed with metastatic disease at the time of presentation. Nonfunctional pancreatic islet tumors are malignant 60% of the time. However, the metastatic disease typically progresses slowly and patients may live many years.

Management of Unresectable Metastases in Functional and Nonfunctional Pancreatic Neuroendocrine Tumors

The somatostatin analogue octreotide, may ameliorate the symptoms of hormonal excess and occasionally may result in partial tumor regression or tumor stabilization. Hepatic metastases often benefit from hepatic artery chemoembolization. Tumor necrosis can lead to hormone release, so appropriate blocking agents should be used before this is done. When diffuse disease is present, systemic chemotherapy should be administered. Typical agents include 5-flourouracil, streptozotocin, doxorubicin, and dimethyl-triazeno-imidazole-carboxamide (DTIC). Administration of α-interferon has produced some responses.

ACKNOWLEDGMENTS

This study was supported, in part, by a grant from the Nathan and Frances Goldblatt Society for Cancer Research. We thank Ms. Kim Maddy for her assistance in the preparation of this manuscript.

SELECTED READINGS

Arnold R, Neuhaus C, Benning R, et al: Somatostatin analogue sandostatin and inhibition of tumor growth in patients with metastatic endocrine gastroenteropancreatic tumors. World J Surg 1993;17:511.

Carty SE, Jensen RT, Norton JA: Prospective study of aggressive resection of metastatic pancreatic endocrine tumors. Surgery 1992;112:1024.

Imamura M, Takahashi K: Use of selective arterial secretin injection test to guide surgery in patients with Zollinger-Ellison syndrome. World J Surg 1993;17:433.

Kadowaki M, Kaplan EL: Pancreatic islet cell tumors. In Cameron JL (ed): Current Surgical Therapy, 3rd ed. Toronto, BC Decker, 1989, pp 341–351.

Norton JA, Fraker DL, Alexander HR, et al: Surgery to cure the Zollinger-Ellison syndrome. N Engl J Med 1999;341:635.

Norton JA, Jensen RT: Unresolved surgical issues in the management of patients with Zollinger-Ellison syndrome. World J Surg 1991;15:151.

Percopo V, Kaplan EL (eds): GEP and multiple neuroendocrine tumors. Padova, Italy. Piccin Nuova Libreria, 1996.

Sugg SL, Norton JA, Fraker DL, et al: A prospective study of intraoperative methods to find and resect duodenal gastrinomas. Ann Surg 1993; 218:138.

Thompson NW. Pancreatic surgery for endocrine tumors. In Clark OH, Duh Q-Y (eds): Textbook of Endocrine Surgery. Philadelphia, WB Saunders, 1997, pp 599–606.

Wayne JD, Tanaka R, Kaplan EL: Insulinomas. In Clark OH, Duh Q-Y, Siperstein A (eds): Textbook of Endocrine Surgery. Philadelphia, WB Saunders, 1997, pp 577–591.

Zeiger MA, Shawker TH, Norton JA: Use of intraoperative ultrasonography to localize islet cell tumors. World J Surg 1993;17:488.

Chapter 168

Carcinoid Tumors

Rose B. Ganim and Jeffrey A. Norton

Carcinoid tumors are derived from cells of the diffuse neuroendocrine system, known as Kulchitsky cells. They are traditionally classified along the lines of their presumed origin from the three divisions of the embryonic gut. *Carcinoid* is a term coined to reflect the mostly indolent nature of these tumors and has been used historically to set them apart from gastrointestinal adenocarcinomas. There are believed to be at least 19 normal neuroendocrine cell types in the human gut, modulating digestive function by endocrine, paracrine, and neurocrine mechanisms. The ability to take up aromatic amines or their precursors and decarboxylate them classifies carcinoid tumors among the Apudomas. As such, they share cytochemical and histopathologic features with other neuroendocrine tumors, medullary thyroid carcinoma, melanoma, pheochromocytoma, and in their most undifferentiated form, small cell carcinoma. As endocrine tumors, carcinoids are capable of producing the carcinoid syndrome if sufficient hormone products are released into the systemic circulation.

HISTOPATHOLOGY

By ordinary light microscopy, these tumors appear as regular small round cells with relatively few mitotic figures, and cannot be distinguished from other neuroendocrine tumors. An early technique for distinguishing carcinoid cells is based on silver staining. Some carcinoid cells have the property of taking up and reducing silver salts and are termed *argentaffin cells*. Others may take up silver but are unable to reduce it without the addition of exogenous reducing agents and are termed *argyrophilic cells*. These differences are due to the heterogeneity of the biogenic amine products within the secretory granules of the cell. On the whole, tumors that are argentaffin positive are more aggressive than those that are argyrophilic.

Histologic patterns of growth include insular, trabecular, glandular, undifferentiated, and mixed. Malignancy often cannot be determined histologically and must be established by the identification of metastases. Foregut tumors commonly have a trabecular or mixed pattern and are argyrophilic or nonreactive. Midgut tumors have the most typical histology and are often insular with surrounding fibrosis. Most tumors in this location are both argentaffin positive and argyrophilic. Carcinoids of the hindgut are usually trabecular or mixed architecture and have variable silver staining. Undifferentiated tumors may be distinguished from other neuroendocrine tumors by silver staining as well. Atypical histology is characterized by pleomorphism, increased frequency of mitoses, and areas of necrosis. Atypical histology is associated with a poorer prognosis than tumors with typical histology.

Within carcinoid cells are granules containing hormones that are identified by immunohistochemistry. The pathognomonic finding for carcinoid tumor is the ability to synthesize serotonin (5-hydroxytryptamine [5-HT]) from dietary tryptophan. Serotonin is not, however, the only hormone produced. Carcinoids may release any one or combination of tachykinins, histamine, prostaglandins, gastrin, substance P, neuron-specific enolase, synaptophysin, chromogranin A and C, insulin, growth hormone, growth hormone–releasing hormone, neurotensin, adrenocorticotropic hormone, pancreatic polypeptide, bombesin, and various growth factors.

DISTRIBUTION

Most carcinoid tumors are found within the organs derived from the embryonic foregut (including the bronchopulmonary system, stomach, and duodenum), midgut (jejunoileum to appendix), and hindgut (colorectum) (Table 168–1). Three fourths of carcinoid tumors are found in the gastrointestinal tract, with the remaining one fourth found in the bronchopulmonary system. Occasional reports of more unusual locations exist.

Within the gastrointestinal tract, approximately 30% of tumors occur in the small bowel, increasing in frequency distally, with half found in the ileum. Twenty percent occur in the hindgut, increasing in frequency distally also, with half presenting in the rectum.

Understanding the incidence and distribution of carcinoids, especially those of the appendix, has been complicated by differing reporting criteria over time and the often asymptomatic nature of these tumors. Early databases included both benign and malignant tumors, whereas the more recent Surveillance, Epidemiology, and End Results program database excluded benign tumors from 1973 to 1986. Because the vast majority of appendiceal carcinoids are benign, their proportion appears to have decreased dramatically from 45% (1950 to 1969) to 7.6% (1973 to 1991). This apparent decrease has been exacerbated by the decline in the rate of both incidental and primary appendectomy for presumed appendicitis. The result is that an asymptomatic lesion is found much less frequently, perhaps because it is sought much less frequently, and for a period, not even reported. Autopsy studies report carcinoid incidence as high as 1% (inclusive of all locations), whereas carcinoid is diagnosed in only 2 per 100,000 living patients.

Small bowel carcinoids account for one third of all cases, and they are metastatic 70% of the time. These tumors are also among the most likely to produce the carcinoid syndrome. Bronchopulmonary carcinoids tend to be less invasive than those in the gastrointestinal tract. They are usually small but are easier to detect through

Table 168–1	**Distribution of Carcinoid Tumors**					
		N (% OF TOTAL)		**% WITH METASTASIS**		**5-YEAR SURVIVAL**
GROUP	**LOCATION**	**1950–1971**	**1973–1991**	**1950–1971**	**1973–1991**	**1950–1971**	**1973–1991**
Foregut	Trachea, bronchi, lung	190 (10.4)	1756 (32.7)	21	27.2	87	76.6
	Stomach	41 (2.2)	204 (3.8)	55	30.9	52	48.6
	Pancreas		46 (0.9)		76.1		34.1
Midgut	Duodenum		114 (2.1)				
	Jejunum		123 (2.3)				
	Ileum		945 (17.6)				
	Small Intestine NOS	366 (20.1)	564 (8.7)	60	70.7	54	55.4
	Appendix	820 (44.9)	410 (7.6)	5	35.4	99	85.9
Hindgut	Colon	112 (6.1)	607 (11.3)	71	71.2	52	41.6
	Rectum	295 (16.2)	545 (10.1)	15	14.2	83	72.2
All sites		1824 (100)	5468 (100)	25	45.3	82	50.4

NOS, not otherwise specified.
Adapted from Modlin IM, Sandor, A. An analysis of 8305 cases of carcinoid tumors. *Cancer 1997;* 79(4):813–829.

clear symptoms, flexible bronchoscopy, and magnetic resonance imaging using T_1 and T_2 imaging. In contrast, ileal, colonic, and pancreatic tumors tend to have obscure symptoms, are difficult to localize, and are more likely to be metastatic at diagnosis.

The most common site of metastasis is to the regional lymph nodes (90%) followed by the liver (45%). Other less common sites of metastatic spread include the peritoneum, pancreas, lungs, bone, and brain.

EPIDEMIOLOGY

Age at presentation ranges widely from 8 to 93 years, with a mean of 55 years, which is slightly lower than for other cancers. Mean age for appendiceal carcinoid is 42 years. Overall, carcinoid tumors are slightly more common in women.

Approximately 10% of patients with carcinoid disease have multiple endocrine neoplasia type I (MEN-I). In 13% of patients with MEN-I and Zollinger-Ellison syndrome, carcinoid tumor of the stomach develops. Carcinoid tumors are also associated with chronic atrophic gastritis type A (CAG-A). The elevated gastrin levels characteristic of both Zollinger-Ellison syndrome and CAG-A have been postulated to cause hyperplasia of antral enterochromaffin-like (ECL) cells. These tumors are often multifocal and arise from surrounding ECL hyperplasia. In contrast, sporadic gastric carcinoid is usually solitary and is surrounded by normal gastric tissue. Hypergastrinemia induced by chronic omeprazole use in a rat model has been associated with gastric carcinoid; however, a clear human correlate has not been made in the absence of MEN or CAG. Sporadic gastrinoma (in the absence of MEN-I) is not associated with carcinoid tumors, and, similarly, sporadic gastric carcinoid (in the absence of MEN-I or CAG-A) is not associated with hypergastrinemia.

CLINICAL PRESENTATION

The symptoms caused by carcinoid tumors are related to location of the primary tumor and extent of metastases.

Appendiceal carcinoids are most commonly found at appendectomy for appendicitis. The most common presenting complaint for jejunoileal carcinoid is abdominal pain consistent with partial small bowel obstruction. The nonspecificity of this complaint translates into a median 2-year delay in diagnosis. Pain may be caused by mesenteric fibrosis, bowel kinking, venous ischemia, and intussusception. Bronchial and thymic carcinoid may be found incidentally on chest radiograph or may present as asthma, pneumonia, cough, hemoptysis, or carcinoid syndrome. Most gastric and duodenal carcinoids are found incidentally at endoscopy, and almost three fourths of these patients have anemia. Rectal carcinoids are most often found incidentally at endoscopy as well, but large tumors may cause obstruction.

CARCINOID SYNDROME

Twenty-five percent of patients with carcinoid tumors have the carcinoid syndrome at presentation. Symptoms associated with carcinoid syndrome include flushing, diarrhea, wheezing, valvular heart disease, and pellagra (Table 168–2). "Typical" flushing, resulting from fore or midgut tumors, occurs with a sudden onset of a violaceous erythema of the face, neck, and upper body. Early in the course of the disease, these episodes may last only a

Table 168–2	**Carcinoid Syndromes and Mediators**	
SYMPTOM	**FREQUENCY WITH SYNDROME (%)**	**PROPOSED MEDIATOR**
Flushing	90	5-HT, histamine, kallikrein, substance P, prostaglandins
Diarrhea	70	5-HT, histamine, vasoactive intestinal peptide, prostaglandins, gastrin
Heart disease	40	5-HT, neurokinin A, substance P
Wheezing	15	5-HT, histamine
Pellagra	5	Niacin deficiency

couple of minutes, but they can progress to lasting hours. A flush may be accompanied by the sensation of warmth, itching, lacrimation, facial edema, or palpitations. Flushing caused by "atypical" bronchial carcinoids tends to be more diffuse and, with repeated episodes, can cause persistent red or cyanotic discoloration of the skin. These flushes are more prolonged and may cause hypotension as well as the other symptoms. Gastric tumors lead to a more patchy distribution and are more often pruritic. The differential diagnosis for flushing includes menopause, reaction to alcohol or glutamate, medications (chlorpropamide, calcium-channel blocker, nicotinic acid), chronic myelogenous leukemia, and systemic mastocytosis.

Diarrhea is secretory, persists despite being given nothing by mouth, and can range from 2 to 30 stools daily. Most often, diarrhea occurs with episodes of flushing. Valvular heart disease is due to patchy endocardial fibrosis, which affects primarily the tricuspid and pulmonary leaflets and chordae. Carcinoid tumors may steal tryptophan for serotonin production to such an extent that pellagra results from an inability to synthesize nicotinic acid.

For these symptoms to occur, sufficient quantities of hormones must be released into the general circulation. Most often this occurs after substantial metastases to the liver. For gastrointestinal tumors, hormone products are released into the portal circulation and are inactivated by the liver. The preponderance of right- over left-sided heart lesions implicates the release of vasoactive and fibrotic substances from liver metastases into the hepatic veins. With tumors in locations outside the gastrointestinal tract (e.g., ovary and lung), mediators of carcinoid syndrome are released directly into systemic circulation and can cause symptoms before metastases to the liver.

BIOCHEMICAL EVALUATION

Pathophysiology of Serotonin Metabolism and Effect on Serology

Ninety percent of dietary tryptophan is converted to 5-hydroxytryptophan (5-HTP). In a "typical" carcinoid tumor, this 5-HTP is converted to serotonin (5-HT) and released into the blood (Fig. 168–1). "Atypical" carcinoids lack the dopa-decarboxylase necessary for this conversion and therefore release 5-HTP instead. This makes for a different serologic profile. For typical carcinoids, 5-HT is taken up by platelets and some remains in the serum where monoamine oxidase and aldehyde dehydrogenase convert it to 5-hydroxy indoleacetic acid (5-HIAA). As a result, urinary levels of 5-HT and 5-HIAA are elevated. In the atypical case, some 5-HTP is decarboxylated by the kidney, causing elevated urinary levels of 5-HT with low levels in the serum. 5-HIAA may be slightly elevated in the urine.

The standard initial biochemical test in the workup of a patient with possible carcinoid syndrome is measurement of 24-hour urinary 5-HIAA. Elevation of urinary 5-HIAA levels is 100% specific for carcinoid, with sensitivities ranging from 92% for midgut, 29% for foregut, and 0% for hindgut. Urinary 5-HIAA levels can also be falsely

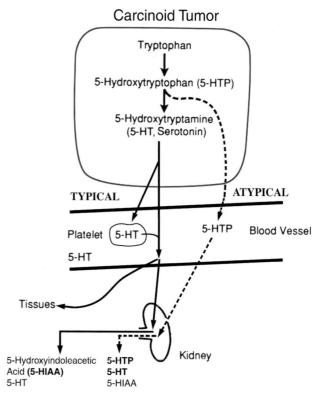

Figure 168–1. Typical and atypical tryptophan metabolism in carcinoid cells. Atypical tryptophan metabolism occurs in some tumors as a result of the lack of the dopa decarboxylase necessary to convert 5-hydroxytryptamine (5-HT) to 5-hydroxytryptophan. This is not the same as having atypical histology, and these terms should not be confused. Atypical metabolism produces a distinctive flush and lacks the elevated serum and platelet 5-HT and urinary 5-hydroxyindoleacetic acid levels that are more customary for carcinoid syndrome.

elevated with the ingestion of serotonin-rich foods such as bananas, pineapples, kiwi, avocados, pecans, hickory, and walnuts. Medications causing false-positive results include guaifenesin, acetaminophen, salicylates, and L-dopa. Measurements of platelet levels of serotonin are not affected by diet and have a better sensitivity profile with 100% for midgut, 50% for foregut, and 20% for hindgut. Carcinoids of the foregut are often atypical and may result in elevated plasma 5-HTP instead of 5-HT.

Chromogranin A is a glycoprotein found within neuroendocrine cells and the serum levels of chromogranin A are elevated in 80% to 100% of patients with neuroendocrine tumors, in general. In one series, plasma levels of chromogranin A were found to be elevated in 79% of patients with foregut carcinoid tumors, 87% with midgut tumors, and 100% with hindgut tumors. This test is especially useful in the diagnosis of rectal carcinoids where there are no more reliable serum markers.

LOCALIZATION AND IMAGING

Somatostatin Receptor Scintigraphy

For localization of carcinoid tumors, somatostatin receptor scintigraphy (SRS) has become the study of choice

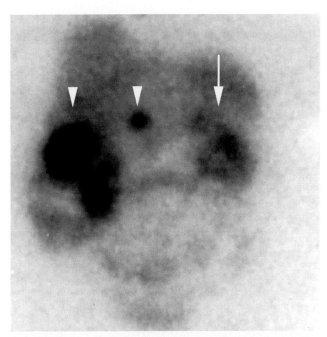

Figure 168–2. Abdominal somatostatin receptor scintigraphy (SRS) revealing liver metastases (*arrowheads*) as well as the small bowel primary tumor (*arrow*).

(Fig. 168–2). This nuclear medicine scan takes advantage of the fact that close to 90% of carcinoid tumors express somatostatin receptors with a moderate to high affinity for somatostatin analogues. Indium In 111 pentetreotide scans have a specificity of 100% and sensitivity reported up to 95% when used as a first line test. The sensitivity of this technique is not only dependent on tumor size, which may be small, but also on the target-to-background receptor ratio. The study should be done with single-photon emission computed tomography imaging. Furthermore, a positive imaging study predicts response to medical therapy with somatostatin analogues.

Computed Tomography

Computed tomography is poor at localizing carcinoid tumors, especially those in the small bowel. Reported localization rates range from 2% to 82%. If visualized, a mesenteric mass with a stellate configuration and dense mesenteric stranding is considered virtually pathognomonic for carcinoid (Fig. 168–3). Furthermore, thickening of the bowel wall is also seen. Liver metastases are hypervascular and better seen during the arterial dominant phase of contrast. Large metastatic liver lesions may have pseudocysts.

Endoscopy

An endoscopic approach to diagnosis and therapy for small tumors can be used for bronchopulmonary, gastric, and colorectal sites. Gastric carcinoid may appear as a small ulcerating mass on endoscopy.

Gastrointestinal Series

Overall, gastrointestinal contrast studies are poor at visualizing carcinoids. A gastric carcinoid may appear as an ulceration on upper gastrointestinal imaging. Some cecal and ascending colon lesions may be seen with contrast enema, but descending colon and rectal tumors are poorly identified.

Ultrasound

Transabdominal ultrasound is only able to image approximately one third of small bowel tumors and two thirds of liver metastases. Ultrasound may be most useful as guidance for liver biopsy. Endoscopic ultrasound is a superior approach and has been found to be 75% to 90% accurate at determining local involvement of colorectal carcinoids.

Chest Roentgenography

Routine chest radiographs are most responsible for detecting bronchopulmonary tumors. They often appear as a notched mass associated with atelectasis or pneumonia.

Other Nuclear Scans

Metaiodobenzylguanidine (MIBG) is concentrated by carcinoids and pheochromocytomas via an Na^+-dependent pump. ^{123}I-MIBG scanning is less sensitive and specific than SRS for carcinoid, but may be useful for detection of metastatic disease. Technetium bone scans may also still be superior for identification of bony metastases.

SURGICAL RESECTION

Guidelines for surgical resection of carcinoid tumors varies with primary site.

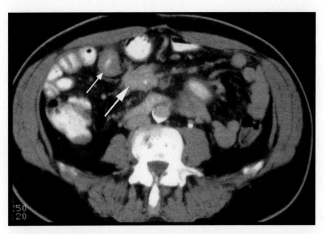

Figure 168–3. Abdominal computed tomography showing the classic finding of a carcinoid stellate mass (*large arrow*) and thickened adjacent small bowel (*small arrow*).

Appendix

For tumors less than 1 cm in diameter, a simple appendectomy is considered curative. Tumors greater than 2 cm require a right hemicolectomy with regional lymph node excision. For the treatment of tumors between 1 and 2 cm in diameter, involvement of the mesoappendix or the base of the appendix is an indication for a cecectomy or right hemicolectomy. In the absence of these features, a simple appendectomy with surveillance is appropriate.

Jejunum and Ileum

Malignant potential of these tumors may be independent of size, with reports of metastatic spread from primaries of less than 1 cm in diameter ranging between 15% and 70%. Between 10% and 30% of tumors have multiple primary sites, so wide excision is essential (Fig. 168–4). Any tumor less than 2 cm in diameter may be treated with a wide resection, including mesenteric lymph nodes. Tumors 2 cm and greater require an extended resection.

Rectum

Carcinoids less than 1 cm in diameter may be treated with local excision. In carcinoids between 1 and 2 cm, however, metastatic spread occurs in approximately 10%. An approach in this instance is to first perform a local full-thickness excision. If there is invasion of the muscularis propria, then one should proceed to a low anterior resection. Tumors greater than 2 cm should be treated with either low anterior or abdominoperineal resection.

Stomach

Malignant behavior of these carcinoids is dependent on not only size but also histology and the presence or absence of hypergastrinemia. Tumors smaller than 2 cm in diameter with typical histology and/or associated with

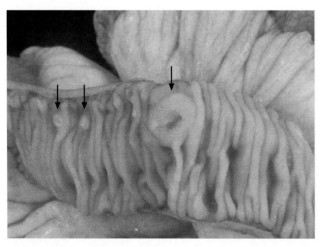

Figure 168–4. Multiple carcinoid primaries in a small bowel surgical specimen.

hypergastrinemia can be treated with endoscopic resection and surveillance. Tumors larger than 2 cm or with atypical histology, regardless of gastrin levels, require a partial or total gastrectomy with regional lymph node excision.

Metastatic Disease

The average survival expectation for patients with hepatic metastases is 5 years, and the 5-year survival rate is approximately 20% to 40%. This indicates a relatively indolent course or slow progression of disease. For this reason, surgery or other therapy should not be life threatening. Cytoreductive liver surgery has been recommended in cases in which 90% of the tumor burden can be relieved with retention of hepatic function. However, patients may have extensive bilobar metastases with limited benefit from debulking. When carcinoid tumor is localized, resection of the primary and lymph node metastases may still offer cure in some cases. Similarly, excision or debulking of hepatic metastasis plus extensive locoregional disease can improve symptoms of carcinoid syndrome and extend both quantity and quality of life. Recurrent disease after radical excision occurs in 80% of patients; however, these recurrences may not become clinically apparent for many years.

Liver transplantation has been performed in a small number of patients with unresectable liver disease and no evidence of extrahepatic disease with a 5-year actuarial survival of nearly 70%.

MEDICAL MANAGEMENT

Somatostatin Analogues

The somatostatin analogues are the mainstay of symptomatic medical treatment of carcinoid syndrome (Fig. 168–5). These medications are effective at relieving flushing, diarrhea, and wheezing, and show some antiproliferative effects in vitro. Somatostatin is a peptide hormone that binds specific receptors on the tumor cell surface and inhibits the secretion of a broad range of hormones. Its half-life is extremely brief and longer lasting analogues have been developed. Octreotide is the most widely studied somatostatin analogue and the dose ranges from 50 to 200 μg subcutaneously three times daily. Symptomatic improvement is reported in approximately 90% of patients, biochemical response (reflected as >50% reduction in urinary 5-HIAA levels) in approximately 70%, and temporary stabilization of tumor growth in as many as 85%. Recently, two much longer lasting versions, Sandostatin-LAR and lanreotide-PR, have become available. These are polymer microsphere preparations of octreotide and lanreotide, which are dosed 20 mg intramuscularly every 4 weeks and 30 mg intramuscularly every 2 weeks, respectively. Studies of lanreotide-PR have found subjective improvement in 40% to 75% of patients, biochemical response in 40% to 55%, and stabilization of tumor growth in 0% to 80%. The most substantial adverse reactions to these agents are development of cholelithiasis (likely caused by reduced cholecystokinin release) and

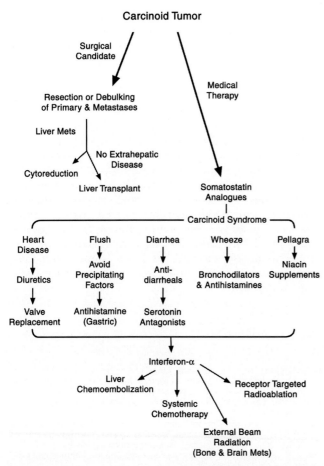

Figure 168–5. Flow diagram for the treatment of carcinoid tumors. Treatment with octreotide is necessary to prevent perioperative carcinoid crisis.

tachyphylaxis. Patients with extensive or metastatic carcinoid tumor should undergo prophylactic cholecystectomy at the time of any surgery. Other side effects include pain from the injection, diarrhea, steatorrhea, nausea, vomiting, and mild hyperglycemia.

Perioperative medical management of patients with carcinoid syndrome, including cytoreductive surgery and chemoembolization of liver metastases, must include vigorous hydration and high-dose intravenous octreotide (100 to 200 μg every 8 hours × 1 day) to prevent carcinoid crisis. This life-threatening complication occurs during anesthesia induction or tumor resection. It includes severe bronchoconstriction and hemodynamic instability, and can be completely ameliorated by intravenous octreotide.

Serotonin Antagonists

Serotonin receptor blockade with agents such as cyproheptadine, methysergide, and p-chlorophenylalanine, is most effective at relieving diarrhea. These agents have no beneficial effect with flushing or carcinoid heart disease.

Interferon-α

Interferon-α therapy provides significant symptomatic and antitumor responses. Evidence exists for three anti-proliferative mechanisms, including cell cycle blockade, augmentation of an antitumor immune response, and induction of apoptosis. It is believed that apoptosis followed by intratumoral fibrosis accounts for the finding that radiographic tumor size often does not change after therapy. Studies have shown symptomatic improvement in 40% to 70% of patients, a biochemical response in 40% to 50%, tumor regression in 10% to 15%, and tumor stabilization in 25% to 40%. Median response durations are 16 to 20 months. In at least one center, patients have been treated three times weekly for more than 10 years with significant survival benefit. In patients who have become resistant to octreotide therapy alone, the addition of interferon-α may be synergistic, providing a biochemical response in up to 80% of patients studied.

Adverse reactions include a flulike syndrome during the beginning of treatment, a chronic fatigue syndrome in up to half the patients, development of antinuclear or antithyroid autoantibodies, development of antibodies to the recombinant interferon, and anemia.

Locoregional Control of Hepatic Metastases

The first attempts at locoregional control of hepatic metastases consisted of operative ligation or proximal embo-

---

Pearls and Pitfalls

PEARLS

- As with any malignancy, delay in diagnosis can adversely affect patient outcome.
- SRS is a superior diagnostic study.
- Include plasma chromogranin A and platelet 5-HT levels in the workup.
- Formation of gallstones is a significant adverse effect of long-term and high-dose octreotide therapy. Gangrenous cholecystitis may occur after chemoembolization therapy.
- Appendicitis is the most common presentation for appendiceal carcinoid tumor.
- Carcinoid crisis can be fatal and is easily avoided.
- Because of the indolent growth pattern of most carcinoid tumors, significant improvement in quality and quantity of life can be achieved in many patients.

PITFALLS

- Failure to consider the diagnosis of carcinoid in a patient with chronic abdominal pain, partial small bowel obstruction, recurrent pneumonia, or rectal complaints.
- Use of abdominal CT to "rule out" carcinoid tumor.
- Use of urinary 5-HIAA levels to "rule out" carcinoid tumor.
- Failure to perform a cholecystectomy in a patient undergoing an operation for extensive or metastatic carcinoid.
- Failure to perform an interval appendectomy in a patient with resolved appendicitis.
- Failure to use intravenous octreotide to prevent perioperative carcinoid crisis.
- Failure to consider aggressive medical and surgical therapy in a patient with metastatic disease.

lization of the hepatic artery. These strategies were based on the fact that carcinoid metastases are hypervascular, are sensitive to ischemia, and derive their blood supply from hepatic artery radicals. Undue morbidity and mortality were associated with these procedures, and tumor revascularization was rapid in many patients.

Minimally invasive transcatheter distal hepatic artery embolization has provided better antitumor responses with much diminished morbidity and mortality rates. A further improvement in this technique involves the combination of distal hepatic artery delivery of chemotherapeutic agents (5-fluorouracil, doxorubicin, streptozotocin, or dacarbazine as oil emulsions, and/or interferon-α) with Gelfoam embolization. Because of its success, this technique has become the next stage in therapy for patients who are not surgical candidates and who fail octreotide and interferon therapy. In this population, studies have seen reduction in tumor size as well as biochemical and symptomatic response in 35% to 100% of patients. In one group, chemoembolization and embolization alone had similar initial results; however, their duration of response was 18 and 4 months, respectively. It is not clear that survival is increased, however, and there is an approximately 3% mortality rate as well as 10% adverse responses including nausea, pain, fever, abscess, and ileus.

Systemic Chemotherapy

Systemic chemotherapy for treatment of carcinoid tumor has been disappointing with single, double, triple, and quadruple drug therapy all providing tumor response in 0% to 30% of patients.

Radiation

^{131}I-MIBG or ^{111}In-octreotide for targeted radioablation may be used in patients with positive MIBG or SRS scans with response rates up to 60%. External beam radiation therapy is reserved for patients with bony metastases.

PROGNOSIS

Poor prognostic indicators are ill-defined for carcinoid tumors, and a guarded outlook has been taken for patients with advanced metastases or carcinoid syndrome. With aggressive medical and surgical therapy, however, a median survival expectation of 7 years in patients with liver metastases and carcinoid syndrome has been found in several series. The most discouraging prognostic findings seem to be carcinoid heart failure, with a median survival time of 2.5 years and of 1 year in cases of extra-abdominal metastasis. Nearly one half of patients who die of their carcinoid disease succumb to heart failure. One third succumb to cachexia resulting from mesenteric and intestinal entrapment.

SELECTED READINGS

Dolan J, Norton JA: Neuroendocrine tumors of the pancreas and gastrointestinal tract and carcinoid disease. In: Norton JA (ed): Surgery: Scientific Basis and Evidence-Based Practice. New York, Springer-Verlag, 2000.

Godwin JD: Carcinoid tumors: An analysis of 2837 cases. Cancer 1975; 36:560.

Jensen RT, Norton JA: Carcinoid tumors and the carcinoid syndrome. In: DeVita VT, Hellman S, Rosenberg SA (eds): Cancer: Principles and Practice of Oncology, 5th ed. Philadelphia, Lippincott-Raven, 1997.

Loftus JP, van Heerden JA: Surgical management of gastrointestinal carcinoid tumors. Adv Surg 1995;28:317.

Modlin IM, Sandor A: An analysis of 8305 cases of carcinoid tumors. Cancer 1997;79:813.

Moertel CG: Treatment of the carcinoid tumor and the malignant carcinoid syndrome. J Clin Oncol 1983;11:727.

Moertel CG: Karnofsky memorial lecture. An odyssey in the land of small tumors. J Clin Oncol 1987;10:1502.

GYNECOLOGY

Chapter 169

Surgical Management of Pelvic Inflammatory Disease

Holly E. Richter, Robert L. Holley, Seine Chiang, and R. Edward Varner

Pelvic inflammatory disease (PID) affects women worldwide in epidemic proportions.

In the United States, a recent national survey indicated that almost 8% of all women and 11% of African-American women reported that they have received treatment for PID at some time in their reproductive lives. It has been estimated that more than 1 million American women seek treatment for PID annually. The acute infection may result in tubal scarring and adhesions with the potential long-term sequelae of tubal infertility and chronic pelvic pain resulting from the formation of adhesions. In one study, 1 in 10 patients had an ectopic pregnancy in their first pregnancy after having PID as compared with 1 in 66 patients without a history of PID. The estimated cost of PID was approximately $4.2 billion in 1990, including both the direct and indirect costs of acute treatment as well as the costs from infertility and ectopic pregnancy resulting from PID.

Ascent of *Chlamydia trachomatis* and *Neisseria gonorrhoeae* from the lower to the upper genital tract is thought to be the most common antecedent of PID. These two pathogens can be isolated from the cervix or upper genital tract in approximately two thirds of PID cases. Anaerobic gram-negative rods (*Bacteroides, Prevotella*) as well as genital mycoplasmas and *Gardnerella vaginalis* frequently accompany the presence of *C. trachomatis* and *N. gonorrhoeae* in the upper genital tract. It is not known whether anaerobes and facultative bacteria cause PID directly, or whether they ascend from the lower genital tract into the upper tract as a consequence of *N. gonorrhoeae* or *C. trachomatis*. Bacteria found in the upper genital tract of women with PID are the same bacteria associated with bacterial vaginosis, the most common infectious cause of vaginitis. There is evidence that bacterial vaginosis–associated bacteria in the upper genital tract are associated with salpingitis and endometritis independent of *N. gonorrhoeae* and *C. trachomatis* infections.

Several risk factors have been consistently related to enhanced risk for sexually transmitted diseases and PID. These include multiple sexual partners, early age at first intercourse, frequent acquisition of new sexual partners, black race, and lower socioeconomic status. Also, younger individuals, primarily adolescents, are more likely to contract sexually transmitted diseases because of their patterns of sexual activity as well as their larger area of cervical ectopy and greater permeability of cervical mucus.

CLINICAL PRESENTATION AND NONSURGICAL PRIMARY TREATMENT

PID presents a difficult diagnostic challenge in many patients. PID should be highly suspected in patients with fever, leukocytosis, lower abdominal pain, vaginal discharge, and uterine and adnexal tenderness on pelvic examination. However, patients infected with *C. trachomatis* may be asymptomatic and others are undiagnosed because the patient or the health care provider fails to recognize mild or nonspecific symptoms or signs (abnormal uterine bleeding, dyspareunia, vaginal discharge). There is no established, accurate test that predicts the development of reproductive complications. Although the severity of inflammation upon direct inspection of the pelvic organs at laparoscopy is predictive of the development of infertility, laparoscopy is invasive and infrequently used for diagnosing PID in the United States. Indeed, PID associated with *C. trachomatis* infection has a generally less dramatic presentation than that associated with *N. gonorrhoeae*, yet *C. trachomatis* infection paradoxically results in a higher rate of infertility. For these reasons, health care providers should maintain a low threshold for the diagnosis of PID.

The variable presentations of PID prompted the establishment of formal diagnostic criteria that include physical findings, laboratory values, and the results of other diagnostic tests such as ultrasonography (Table 169–1).

Empirical treatment of PID should be initiated in sexually active young women with lower abdominal tenderness, adnexal tenderness, and cervical motion tenderness. Diagnosis and management of other common causes of lower abdominal pain (ectopic pregnancy, acute appendicitis, and functional abdominal pain) are unlikely to be impaired by initiating empirical antibiotic therapy for PID. Treatment guidelines for oral and parenteral regi-

Table 169–1	Diagnostic Criteria for Pelvic Inflammatory Disease

All of the following:
Lower abdominal pain with tenderness on examination
Adnexal tenderness
Cervical motion tenderness

PLUS

One or more of the following:
Temperature greater than 38°C (100.4°F)
Leukocytosis (white blood cell count >10,500/mm³)
Culdocentesis with leukocytes and bacteria
Inflammatory mass on pelvic examination or ultrasound
Elevated erythrocyte sedimentation rate (ESR)
Evidence of *Neisseria gonorrhoeae* and/or *Chlamydia trachomatis* in the endocervix; that is, mucopurulent cervicitis, positive antigen test, culture, and/or Gram stain

Adapted from Hager WD, Eschenback DA, Spencer MR, Sweet RL: Criteria for diagnosis and grading of salpingitis. Obstet Gynecol 1983;61:113–114.

mens for uncomplicated PID are detailed in the 1998 Centers for Disease Control and Prevention (CDC) "Guidelines for Treatment of Sexually Transmitted Diseases." Uncomplicated PID is thought to be present in a patient with the aforementioned minimal criteria and without evidence of advanced peritonitis or a tubo-ovarian abscess (TOA).

Because the development of sequelae is unpredictable, some authorities have suggested that all women who desire future fertility be hospitalized. No current available data compare the efficacy of parenteral with oral therapy or inpatient with outpatient treatment settings with respect to differences in long-term sequelae. The CDC recommends hospitalization for patients who are suspected of having PID under the following conditions:

- Possible presence of surgical emergencies such as appendicitis
- Pregnancy
- Failure of the patient to respond clinically to oral antibiotic therapy
- Inability of the patient to follow or tolerate outpatient oral regimens
- Concomitant severe illness, nausea, and vomiting or high fever
- Presence of a TOA
- Presence of immunodeficiency (patient is infected with human immunodeficiency virus, has some other disease, or is undergoing immunosuppressive therapy)

Operative Management

In patients with worsening signs and symptoms despite conservative management, or in patients in whom a surgical emergency cannot be excluded, a surgical approach may be considered. Ultrasonographic or computed tomography (CT) evaluation should be performed to evaluate for the presence of a TOA (Fig. 169–1). TOAs cause more than 80% of medical therapy failures in PID. De-

Table 169–2	Characteristics of a Tubo-ovarian Abscess

Most severe form of pelvic inflammatory disease (PID) and may progress to sepsis and death with or without rupture
Occurs in 5%–30% of all patients with PID
Causes more than 80% of medical therapy failure in PID
May present with more severe pain
May present with ileus
Appears ultrasonographically as one or more (usually contiguous) relatively homogeneous, symmetrical, cystic, relatively thin-walled masses

pending on clinical presentation and practice pattern, a transvaginal ultrasound examination may be done at initial presentation; however, if the patient continues with fever and peritoneal signs after 48 to 72 hours of antibiotics, a transvaginal sonogram should be performed to rule out the presence of a TOA. Even with current antibiotic regimens, as many as 25% of women who have TOAs require surgery. Characteristics associated with a TOA are listed in Table 169–2.

More recently, the ultrasonographic distinction between TOA and tubo-ovarian complex (TOC) has become more fully appreciated. TOC presents as an inflammatory pelvic mass representative of adherent, edematous infected pelvic structures in PID. Sinus tracts containing pus are often present; however, no devitalized abscess wall or accumulation of large amounts of pus within a cavity occurs. As perfused, living tissue, a TOC responds to medical management in greater than 95% of cases. Because a TOC and TOA cannot be differentiated clinically, ultrasonographic evaluation is necessary.

The approach to the surgical management of PID and TOA has undergone a progressive change over the past 20 years from one of radical gynecologic surgery as primary management to a more conservative approach including hospitalization and intensive medical management with broad-spectrum antibiotics, including anaerobic coverage

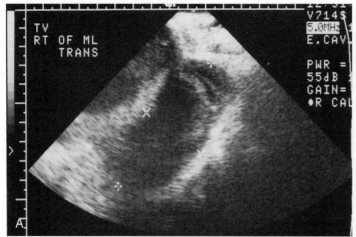
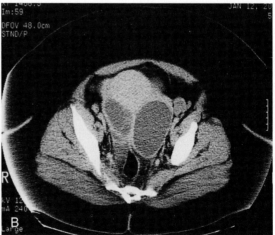

Figure 169–1. A 42-year-old female with a 2-day history of suprapubic pain and nausea that improved after antibiotics were initiated for cystitis/pyelonephritis. Her abdominal pain continued, with spiking fevers. A fluctuant mass was palpated in the lower abdomen-pelvis. *A,* Ultrasound shows a 9 × 8 × 10 cm, left pelvic mass with debris and septations. *B,* On CT, the large abscess was seen to displace the uterus to the right. Endovaginal drainage was performed with the return of 300 mL of purulent material.

(Table 169–3). If surgical intervention is indicated because of medical management failure (greater than 72 hours on intravenous antibiotics), with continued fevers and a worsening clinical condition, the approach continues to be conservative with abscess drainage and removal of devitalized tissue. In cases in which the whole adnexa is involved, removal may be necessary, but if the uterus and contralateral adnexa appear to be normal, particularly in women who desire future fertility, conservation should be considered. A ruptured TOA is a medical emergency requiring immediate exploratory laparotomy and removal of infected tissue and pus. Surgical management may also be indicated in patients with large pelvic abscesses that are easily accessible to endoscopic drainage. These patients should be started on intravenous antibiotics and drainage performed sooner rather than later to enhance clinical response.

The surgical management of TOA is discussed in the following paragraphs.

LAPAROSCOPY

Preoperative Management

Preoperative management for laparoscopy for TOA includes the following:

- Continuance of intravenous antibiotics
- Typing and screening of blood
- Performance of preoperative patient assessment
- Not giving the patient anything by mouth (NPO) for 6 to 8 hours before surgery
- Discussing with the patient the potential for exploratory laparotomy with adnexectomy, possible hysterectomy, and potential complications

Laparoscopic visualization of the pelvic structures in a clinical setting of PID allows definitive diagnosis of acute salpingitis in approximately 60% to 70% of suspected cases. It is the gold standard in the diagnosis of PID, allowing the collection of microbiological specimens and aiding in decision making regarding further treatment and management. Laparoscopy furthermore allows aspiration of a TOA, other purulent discharge including the subdiaphragmatic and subhepatic spaces, and lysis of adhesions. Individual surgical experience with laparoscopy

Table 169–3	**Reasons for Surgery in Pelvic Inflammatory Disease**

Ruptured pelvic abscess (surgical emergency)
Persistent or enlarging mass with continued symptoms
Failure to respond to 48 to 72 hr of intravenous antibiotics
Unsure diagnosis with continued pain; that is, exclude appendicitis, appendiceal abscess, diverticular abscess, uterine pyomyoma, pyometrium, degenerating myoma, ectopic pregnancy, endometriosis, ruptured ovarian cyst, adnexal torsion, pelvic neoplasms
Intraperitoneal bleeding caused by erosion of a major vessel
A "pointing" abscess that can be drained extraperitoneally
A large pelvic abscess or abscesses easily accessible to endoscopic (transvaginal) drainage

dictates whether a primary laparoscopic approach is performed versus exploratory laparotomy.

Intraoperative Management

Patients undergo general anesthesia and legs are placed in laparoscopy stirrups. A uterine manipulator is placed transvaginally, a Foley catheter is placed, and one or both of the patient's arms may be tucked. Single or double television monitors are appropriately positioned. A single monitor placed at the foot of the table is adequate and orients the operating surgeon well.

An infraumbilical incision is made, followed by placement of the Veress needle and creation of a pneumoperitoneum of CO_2 created at 1 L per minute with maximum pressure set at 15 mm Hg. A 10-mm trocar is placed in the infraumbilical site with verification of intra-abdominal placement, after which CO_2 insufflation is increased to 6 L per minute. A 5-mm suprapubic port is inserted under direct visualization and a generalized inspection of the upper abdomen and pelvis is performed with tilting of the table performed as necessary to facilitate inspection of each quadrant. Other trocar sites are placed as necessary. A thorough evaluation of the subhepatic and subdiaphragmatic spaces should be performed as well as inspection of bowel for intraloop abscesses. Laparoscopic treatment of a TOA will most likely involve adhesiolysis, aspiration of the abscess cavity with culture, dissection and excision of necrotic tissue, tubal lavage, and thorough irrigation of the abdomen and pelvis. Peritoneal cavity and cul-de-sac fluid should be aspirated and biopsy samples should be obtained from infected or inflamed tissue (fimbrial biopsy) for culture. When the tube and ovary cannot be separated, a unilateral salpingo-oophorectomy may be necessary. Where dense adhesions of bowel, omentum, uterus, and adnexa exist, conversion to laparotomy may be necessary. A Malecot or Jackson-Pratt drain may be placed through a posterior colpotomy.

Postoperative Management

Postoperative management may include use of nasogastric suction if the patient has had increasing symptoms consistent with ileus or findings of partial bowel obstruction. The patient is then kept NPO until flatus occurs, and diet is advanced slowly as tolerated. Intravenous antibiotics should be continued until the patient has been afebrile for 48 to 72 hours and is clinically improved. Laparoscopic management facilitates early ambulation; however, deep vein thrombosis (DVT) prophylaxis (intermittent compression hose) should be used as necessary. The incision sites should be inspected daily for signs of infection. At discharge, the patient should continue broad-spectrum oral antibiotics for a total length of 10 to 14 days.

Complications

Complications of laparoscopic surgery for the management of PID include those complications associated with all laparoscopies, including complications related to CO_2

insufflation and anesthesia, trocar site bleeding, injury to abdominal and pelvic vessels, bowel and bladder injury, wound infection, and recurrence of abscess.

Outcomes

Studies have shown that laparoscopic treatment of complications of PID, such as TOA, results in good clinical recovery, but is associated with up to 35% long-term outcome complications including chronic pelvic pain and adhesion formation.

EXPLORATORY LAPAROTOMY

Preoperative Management

The preoperative management for planned exploratory laparotomy is the same as that for laparoscopy, with inclusion of the following:

- Discuss the potential for definitive management with removal of all pelvic organs.
- Survey for *sepsis syndrome*, if evidence suggests acute abscess rupture (a surgical emergency).
- Obtain vital signs and perform physical examination, including mental status evaluation.
- Obtain blood cell counts, chemistry studies, and arterial blood gas measurements, as indicated.
- Perform coagulation studies.
- Obtain chest radiograph and electrocardiogram.
- Measure urine output.
- Ensure broad-spectrum antibiotic coverage.

Intraoperative Management

The patient is placed supine on the operating table in laparotomy stirrups and undergoes general endotracheal anesthesia. A vertical infraumbilical incision is indicated because this type of operation is often bloody; it may involve contiguous structures including bowel, bladder, and uterus; it is often hampered by distorted tissue planes; and it may involve abscesses that extend laterally to involve the pelvic sidewall, posteriorly to the rectum or even superiorly toward the umbilicus. A vertical incision also provides the advantages of adequate exposure and ease of extension because exploration of the upper abdomen for abscess pockets is necessary. After adequate exposure is ensured and abscess location verified, the extent of surgical intervention should be based on the patient's desire for future fertility and the extent of pelvic organ involvement. Any adhesions of bowel, bladder, and uterus should be freed from the pelvic abscess and other involved organs. This often requires careful dissection of markedly distorted tissue planes. If a hysterectomy is indicated, a supracervical hysterectomy may be chosen when pericervical tissue planes are distorted and significant bleeding is present. If a total hysterectomy is performed, the vaginal cuff should be left open with a running locking suture to secure the vaginal edges. Careful exploration of the upper abdomen for concealed accumu-

lations of pus is performed, after which copious irrigation of the abdomen and pelvis is carried out before closure. The use of Malecot or Jackson-Pratt drains has been advocated, exiting through the vaginal cuff if a total hysterectomy is performed or through a colpotomy incision if the uterus or cervix is left in situ. Placement of a subcutaneous drain brought through a separate stab incision may also be used. The drains may be removed 48 to 72 hours postoperatively, or when there is no further significant drainage.

A mass closure of peritoneum, muscle, and fascia with a monofilament suture is performed and a delayed closure of skin and subcutaneous tissue is advised. The wound is then packed wet to dry and a delayed primary wound closure performed as indicated.

Postoperative Management

In patients in whom there is evidence of septic shock (hypotension and dysfunction of two or more organ systems) or evidence of adult respiratory distress syndrome, postoperative management should be initiated in the intensive care unit setting. As in laparoscopic postoperative management, nasogastric suction may be indicated with slow advancement of diet. Deep vein thrombosis prophylaxis (intermittent compression hose) should be used until ad lib ambulation is ensured. Broad-spectrum antibiotic treatment should be continued for at least 10 to 14 days; after marked clinical improvement, part of this regimen may be oral agents taken on an outpatient basis. It has been suggested that patients be evaluated weekly with bimanual examination for 2 to 3 weeks after initial resolution.

Complications

Complications of exploratory laparotomy for the management of PID include those complications associated with all laparotomies: risk of significant blood loss; risks associated with anesthesia; recurrent infection; injury to bowel, bladder, and other organs; vesicovaginal fistula; risk of wound infection; abdominal wall abscess; septic pelvic thrombophlebitis; pneumonia; and deep vein thrombosis.

Outcomes

Aggressive surgical intervention with hysterectomy and bilateral oophorectomy for a ruptured TOA results in a greater than 95% recovery rate. More conservative surgical approaches have resulted in a higher rate of subsequent recurrence of the disease and subsequent repeat operative procedures. Long-term outcomes include pelvic pain and adhesion formation greater than that seen in the laparoscopic surgical approach; however, overall, more severe and extensive infections are generally treated by laparotomy.

POSTERIOR COLPOTOMY

Preoperative Management

The preoperative management for posterior colpotomy is the same as for laparoscopy and laparotomy, as well as the following:

- Discuss the potential for complications including bowel injury, bleeding, and need for exploratory laparotomy.
- Preoperatively, ensure that the abscess is midline, adherent to the cul-de-sac parietal peritoneum, and dissecting the upper one third of the rectovaginal septum to ensure extraperitoneal drainage.

Intraoperative Management

After adequate anesthesia, the patient is placed in dorsolithotomy position and examination under anesthesia is performed. The posterior lip of the cervix is then grasped with a tenaculum or Lahey clamp and drawn down and forward. A transverse incision at least 2 cm in length is made through the vaginal mucosa at the junction of the posterior vaginal fornix and cervix with heavy scissors. A Kelly clamp is used to puncture the peritoneum and abscess wall. Before blunt entry of the abscess cavity, an 18- or 20-gauge spinal needle with syringe may be used to localize the abscess cavity. The clamp is spread, facilitating drainage. Exploration for other loculations/abscesses may be performed with the surgeon's finger or the use of a clamp as necessary. A sample of purulent discharge is sent for aerobic and anaerobic culture and sensitivity. Penrose, Malecot, or closed suction drains are placed to facilitate drainage or irrigation for 48 to 72 hours.

Postoperative Management

Intravenous antibiotics are continued until clinical improvement is noted and a full 10- to 14-day course is completed, part of which may consist of oral antibiotic agents. The Penrose or closed suction drains may be left for several days; however, the Malecot catheter should be removed in 48 to 72 hours. Diet is usually quickly advanced because these patients infrequently have bowel symptoms. Early ambulation is encouraged.

Complications

Complications inherent in all surgeries, risk of bleeding, recurrent infection, and risks inherent in anesthesia are possible with this procedure. In the posterior colpotomy there is increased risk of bowel perforation and care must be taken when directing a long Kelly clamp into the pelvis to avoid injury to the iliac vessels and ureter. Where the strict requirements of posterior colpotomy are not met (abscess dissecting the upper one third of the rectovaginal septum), there is increased risk of diffuse peritoneal sepsis and death. Documented increased risk of definitive operations has been seen following posterior colpotomy.

Outcomes

In general, if the strict criteria for posterior colpotomy drainage is met and a unilocular cul-de-sac abscess is present, results are favorable. Because most cases of TOA do not meet the requirements for a posterior colpotomy

---

Pearls and Pitfalls

PEARLS

- Treatment of PID should involve broad-spectrum coverage as recommended by current Centers for Disease Control and Prevention guidelines; when a TOA is present, anaerobe coverage is mandatory.
- Anesthetic considerations for operative management of a TOA suggest the use of general endotracheal anesthesia, especially when bacteremia is a possibility.
- Consider aggressive definitive operative management (total abdominal hysterectomy with bilateral salpingo-oophorectomy) for PID/TOA refractory to medical management in women who are immunosuppressed or have significant medical comorbidities (e.g., diabetes).
- In the case of generalized pelvic cellulitis (ligneous pelvic cellulitis), or "woody or frozen pelvis," try to avoid surgery; if surgery is necessary, drain abscess only, as attempts to remove involved structures is associated with significant morbidity. In the case of fulminating, rapidly progressive sepsis, the patient should be stabilized and moved rapidly for surgical intervention.
- In patients with TOA and evidence of *Clostridium* on Gram stain or culture, initiate penicillin and plan surgical intervention.
- Many cases of PID result from inadequate outpatient treatment of *N. gonorrhoeae* and *C. trachomatis* cervicitis. The oral 1-g single-dose azithromycin regimen for *C. trachomatis* is preferable to the 7-day course of doxycycline when possible, particularly because of the estimated 30% to 50% lack of compliance with the latter regimen.
- Endometrial biopsy with a Pipelle or another aspiration device is a reliable method for diagnosing upper genital tract infection in equivocal cases. Although it involves a delay in specimen fixation and interpretation, the presence of plasma cells or polymorphonuclear neutrophils is strongly correlated with the presence of salpingitis.
- *Chlamydia trachomatis* is an intracellular bacterium that is cultured from the endocervix. Relying on cervical mucus alone may provide an inadequate specimen for culture. Bending the cotton-tipped swab and performing a minicurettage of the endocervical canal allows a more reliable sample of cells for culture.

---

vaginal approach and there is a high rate of complications, this procedure is infrequently performed.

INTERVENTIONAL RADIOLOGIC AND ULTRASONOGRAPHIC TECHNIQUES FOR TOA DRAINAGE INCLUDING PERCUTANEOUS AND TRANSVAGINAL TECHNIQUES

Surgeries necessitating general endotracheal anesthesia, as well as colpotomy drainage, have been primarily used for treatment of TOA associated with PID until the last 10 years. With a more conservative approach to pelvic organ-sparing procedures in the treatment of TOAs, less invasive procedures such as interventional radiologic techniques have been developed as effective alternatives to operative drainage. In a setting of a TOA resistant to medical management, interventional radiologic techniques are often used as first line therapy with excellent success rates.

The advantages of using these techniques include avoidance of the morbidity and mortality associated with anesthesia and major surgery, pelvic organ preservation, excellent visualization of intervening structures, and lower costs.

COMMENT

There currently exists no standard of care treatment for TOA, except in the presence of acute rupture. The various surgical and interventional radiologic techniques available for the diagnosis and treatment of PID with TOA allow individualization of therapy. For women who desire the most conservative treatment possible in the presence of a TOA resistant to conservative medical management with intravenous broad-spectrum antibiotics, surgical therapy may involve transvaginal drainage of the abscess under radiologic/ultrasonic or laparoscopic guidance, versus solely laparoscopic management. In the woman who has no desire for future fertility, definitive surgical management consisting of a total abdominal hysterectomy with bilateral salpingo-oophorectomy may be indicated. Furthermore, technical limitations may dictate the use of one procedure over another. For example, a transabdominal percutaneous drainage procedure may be limited by the retrouterine position of the abscess and intervening vascular structures or bowel.

The surgical treatment of pelvic abscesses associated with PID is performed only after a failed attempt at medical management with broad-spectrum antibiotics. The approach taken should first involve discussion with an interventional radiologist for possible endovaginal or transcutaneous drainage procedures. Depending on the surgeon's expertise, a laparoscopic versus exploratory laparotomy should be performed if other measures fail.

SUGGESTED READINGS

Centers for Disease Control and Prevention: 1998 Guidelines for Treatment of Sexually Transmitted Diseases, Centers for Disease Control Recommendations and Reports. Atlanta, GA, U.S. Department of Health and Human Services, Centers for Disease Control and Prevention (CDC). Adaptation printed March, 1998.

Ginsburg DS, Stern JL, Hamod KA, et al: Tubo-ovarian abscess: A retrospective review. Am J Obstet Gynecol 1980;138:1055.

Hager WD: Follow-up of patients with tubo-ovarian abscess(es) in association with salpingitis. Obstet Gynecol 1983;61:680.

Henry-Suchet J, Tesquier L: Role of laparoscopy in the management of pelvic adhesions and pelvic sepsis. Baillieres Clin Obstet Gynecol 1994;8:759.

Landers DV, Sweet RL: Tuboovarian abscess: Contemporary approach to management. Rev Infect Dis 1983;5:876.

Landers DV, Sweet RL: Current trends in the diagnosis and treatment of tuboovarian abscess. Am J Obstet Gynecol 1985;151:1098.

Livengood CH: In Mead PB, Hager WD, Faro S (eds): Tubo-ovarian Abscess in Protocols for Infectious Diseases in Obstetrics and Gynecology, 2nd ed. Malden, MA, Blackwell Science, 2000, p 412.

Mecké H, Semm K, Freys I, Gent HJ: Pelvic abscesses: Pelviscopy or laparotomy. Gynecol Obstet Invest 1991;31:231.

Nelson AL, Sinow RM, Renslo R, et al: Endovaginal ultrasonographically guided transvaginal drainage for treatment of pelvic abscess. Am J Obstet Gynecol 1995;172:1926.

Sweet RL, Gibbs RS (eds): Mixed Anaerobic-Aerobic Pelvic Infection and Pelvic Abscess in Infectious Diseases of the Female Genital Tract, 3rd ed. Baltimore, Williams & Wilkins, 1995, pp 189–230.

Chapter 170

Endometriosis

Rakesh K. Mangal and Robert R. Franklin

The growth of endometrial glands and stroma in areas outside the uterus is known as endometriosis. Many theories have been proposed to explain the pathogenesis of endometriosis; none have been proven. However, substantial scientific evidence supports either Sampson's theory of transplantation or the related theory of underlying induction of mesothelium as the mechanism for its development. Central to both theories is retrograde menstruation.

CLINICAL PRESENTATION

Endometriosis should be considered in the differential diagnosis of all women who have pelvic pain, dyspareunia, dysmenorrhea, or infertility. Specific questions should be asked to determine the character of the pain, exacerbating and relieving factors, and time of pain in the menstrual cycle. The review of symptoms should include a careful description of urinary or gastrointestinal symptoms, especially as they relate to the menses. The physician should perform a careful pelvic examination. Positive physical findings include lateral displacement of the cervix, tenderness or nodularity in the uterosacral ligament or cul-de-sac, uterine immobility, and adnexal masses (Table 170–1).

There are no available serologic or radiographic tests that are sufficiently sensitive and specific to be of much value in the definitive diagnosis of endometriosis. Ultrasonography is the most commonly used ancillary diagnostic measure for detecting ovarian endometrioma. Until a reliable noninvasive test for endometriosis is clinically available, laparoscopy remains the gold standard for the definitive diagnosis.

Table 170–1	Clinical Presentation

I. Symptoms that should raise a suspicion of endometriosis:
   A. Pain
      1. Chronic pelvic, low back, or rectal pain, often worse before or at time of menses
      2. Dysmenorrhea unresponsive to nonsteroidal anti-inflammatory drug treatment
      3. Dyspareunia
   B. Bowel or bladder symptoms
      Bladder or bowel symptoms synchronous with menstrual cycle
   C. Infertility
II. Signs that indicate suspicion of endometriosis
   A. Tender uterosacral ligaments or cul-de-sac nodularity
   B. Fixed, retroflexed uterus, laterally deviated cervix
   C. Tender pelvic mass, especially an enlarged ovary
   D. Colored lesions in umbilicus, surgical scars, vulva, vagina, or cervix

PREOPERATIVE MANAGEMENT

In preoperative assessment, an abstract of hysterosalpingogram, office hysteroscopy, pelvic ultrasound, and old operative reports provide indispensable information at surgery. Routine blood chemistries, chest radiograph, and electrocardiogram are obtained as deemed necessary. Consultations with colon rectal surgeons, urologists, or other specialists should be scheduled to help ensure that the surgery produces the maximum benefits for the patients.

When endometriosis is strongly suspected, we recommend preoperative medical suppression with gonadotropin-releasing hormone (GnRH) agonists for 3 months. This is based on the thinking that surgical therapy is, at best, a "debulking" operation. Therefore, GnRH agonist is considered as chemotherapy before the debulking surgery. Before bowel surgery, mechanical and antibiotic bowel preparation is essential to protect against planned or inadvertent entry into the bowel lumen.

INTRAOPERATIVE MANAGEMENT

The patient, because of her symptoms, helps decide the proper management of treatment. Although the medical management is of great value in some patients, it is only a temporary measure.

Strategies to Perform Operation

Conservative Surgery (Operative Laparoscopy or Laparotomy)

Laparoscopy is done with the patient in modified dorsolithotomy position and Trendelenburg under general anesthesia with endotracheal intubation as described by Nezhat and colleagues. Our operating room setup for laparoscopy is shown in Figure 170–1.

The pelvic organs should be inspected meticulously in a systematic fashion so that all areas are evaluated in the same way each time to avoid overlooking any lesions. It is important to place peritoneum on tension to help visualize otherwise not-so-obvious implants. Each surgeon must acquire laparoscopic experience in treating *minimal, mild, and moderate* endometriosis before advancing to more complex procedures. Before the surgeon makes a transition from laparoscopic "diagnostician" to surgical therapist, it is absolutely imperative that the surgeon is comfortable with the use of two, three, and four puncture techniques. Dissections that once were performed only by means of laparotomy now can be accomplished through therapeutic laparoscopic techniques using scissors, lasers

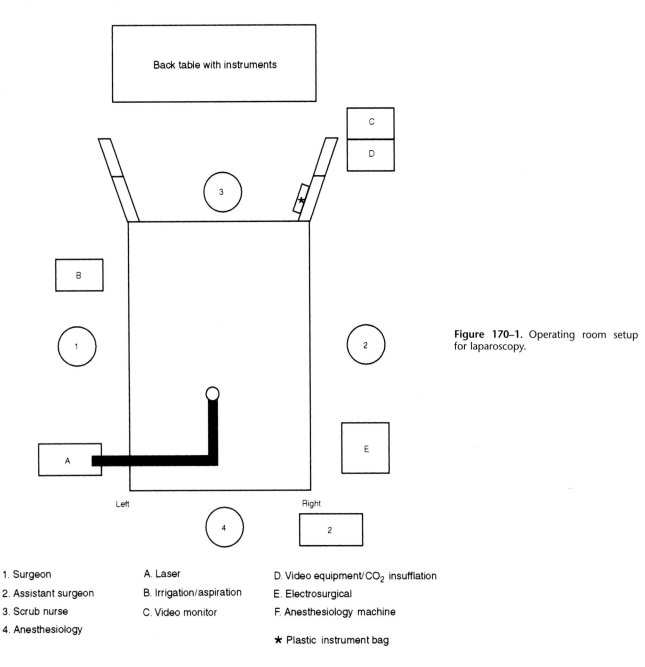

Figure 170–1. Operating room setup for laparoscopy.

1. Surgeon
2. Assistant surgeon
3. Scrub nurse
4. Anesthesiology

A. Laser
B. Irrigation/aspiration
C. Video monitor

D. Video equipment/CO_2 insufflation
E. Electrosurgical
F. Anesthesiology machine

★ Plastic instrument bag

(the authors prefer the CO_2 laser), hydrodissection, and electrosurgical instruments.

Pelvic surgery via laparoscopy or laparotomy may be viewed as a series of operations. By approaching each different pelvic location as a separate operation, some of the more complex disease patterns may be treated effectively. In selected cases of severe endometriosis, placement of *ureteral stents* helps with the identification of ureters during the pelvic surgery.

From start to finish, the surgery should proceed smoothly, with an easy rhythm. When a laparotomy is indicated, visualization being extremely important, a wide Pfannenstiel incision or, if necessary, a Maylard incision is made. For severe midline dysmenorrhea, a presacral neurectomy is indicated. Advanced endometriosis is frequently associated with significant pelvic adhesions. Therefore, it is particularly important in problems of

infertility to release any peritubal and periovarian adhesions that might interfere with the ovum transport.

Ovarian Endometriosis

Before working on the endometriomas, the ovary is completely mobilized by lysis of any adhesions to restore a normal anatomic relationship. Small superficial endometriotic implants (less than 1 cm in diameter) are vaporized or excised. Small endometriomas (less than 2 cm) often have a poorly developed fibrous capsule that does not strip from the ovary. These must be excised. Large endometriomas are old enough that a fibrotic host response has developed a fibrous capsule that can be peeled easily from the ovary. This sac should be removed (Fig. 170–2). The endometrioma is drained and irrigated to prevent

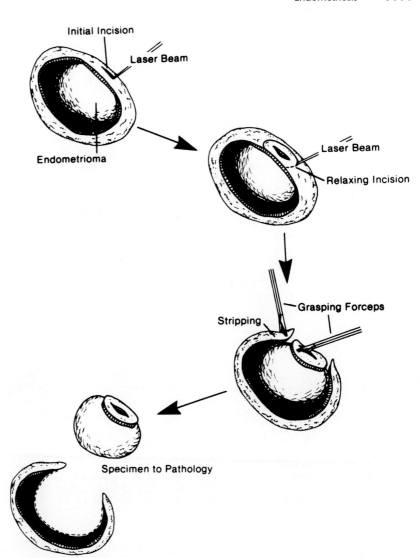

Initial Incision

Laser Beam

Endometrioma

Laser Beam

Relaxing Incision

Stripping   Grasping Forceps

Specimen to Pathology

Figure 170–2. Surgical technique in removing ovarian endometrioma. (From Martin DC [ed]: Intra-abdominal Laser Surgery, 2nd ed. Research Press City: Memphis, TN, 1986, Fertility Institute of Mid-South.)

spillage, then pushed toward the periphery with pitressin injected into the ovarian cortex. The endometrioma is stripped with grasping forceps and by placing traction on the sac (with a teasing, twisting motion) and countertraction on the ovary edge.

Cul-de-Sac Endometriosis

The cul-de-sac is opened by exaggerated anteflexion of the uterus. Frequent intraoperative rectovaginal examinations by the assistant surgeon to help determine pelvic anatomy allows one to distinguish between deep lesions in the anterior (vaginal) and posterior (rectal) halves of the cul-de-sac. The endometriosis can involve the *anterior rectal wall* and, at times, penetrate the mucosa of the posterior *vaginal vault*. If endometriosis penetrates into the posterior vaginal fornix, it can be removed by combined laparoscopic and transvaginal dissection. In such cases, the pneumoperitoneum is maintained with sponge on a ring forceps in the vagina.

Gastrointestinal Tract Endometriosis

Ten percent to 15% of patients with endometriosis harbor significant gastrointestinal foci of the disease. Up to 50%

of patients with severe endometriosis have gastrointestinal endometriosis. The most common sites of bowel endometriosis are the sigmoid and rectosigmoid (51%), the appendix (15%), the terminal ileum (14%), the rectum (14%), and the cecum and colon (5%). The potential for delayed small bowel perforation and peritonitis exists if endometriotic lesions are treated with coagulation or vaporization because of the thin wall of the bowel.

Laparoscopic management of bowel involvement is being done by expert laparoscopic surgeons with apparent good results. Our approach is still by laparotomy. At laparotomy, we place traction sutures in the uterus and the ovaries. The uterosacral ligament is then identified, transfixed, and elevated. An incision is made with hand-held CO_2 laser or scissors in the line of maximal fibrosis at the junction of the rectum and uterus. Once a plane of dissection is achieved, blunt finger dissection is used to sweep away the less dense tissue.

Most bowel lesions are superficial and may be destroyed by electrocautery or laser or sharply excised. Intramural nodules invading the bowel wall and causing significant bowel distortion must be excised by extraluminal resection when possible, or by wedge resection (Fig. 170–3). In the case of large or bulky, deep (intramural or

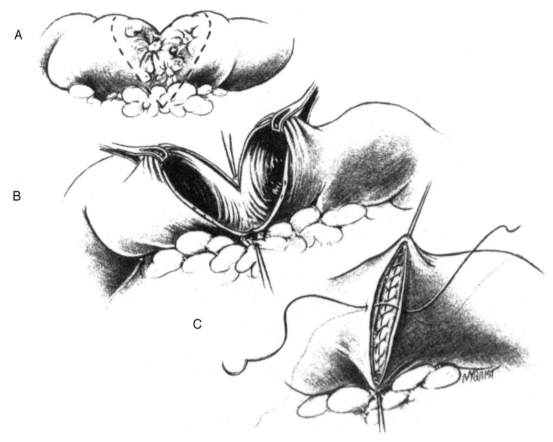

Figure 170–3. Surgical technique in removing deep bowel endometriosis. *A*, A stay suture is placed on either side to outline the extent of the endometriotic nodule. *B*, A full-thickness wedge resection is completed. *C*, The bowel wall is closed. (From Batt RE, Udagaw SM, Wheeler JM: Endometriosis: Microconservative surgery. In Hunt RB [ed]: Atlas of Female Infertility Surgery, 2nd ed. Chicago, Year Book Medical, 1992.)

transmural) lesions, the bowel disease is best treated by segmental resection and primary anastomosis. Long-term experience in dealing with patients with bowel endometriosis has led us to an increasingly aggressive approach to these lesions (Figs. 170–4 and 170–5). We irrigate with copious amounts of Ringer's lactate solution and ensure homeostasis. A Jackson-Pratt drain is placed in the perirectal space as necessary. A nasogastric suction tube is usually not necessary when operating on the colon.

When endometriosis involves, or is near, the ureter at laparoscopy, an opening is made with the CO_2 laser into the normal peritoneum lateral to the ureter. Hydrodissection is used to elevate the lesion. The lesion is circumscribed with the laser, then the edge of the lesion is grasped on tension by the assistant surgeon and excised with laser or scissors. Hemostasis is achieved by bipolar coagulation.

Definitive Surgery

In some cases, complete extirpation of endometriosis and reproductive organs may be necessary to preserve health and quality of life at the cost of fertility. Hysterectomy remains the most definitive chance for "cure" for endometriosis. However, even with hysterectomy, the disease

must be excised completely because often with hormone replacement therapy it can remain active. Hysterectomy for endometriosis may be a simple procedure for a benign disease or may be as difficult as radical pelvic surgery

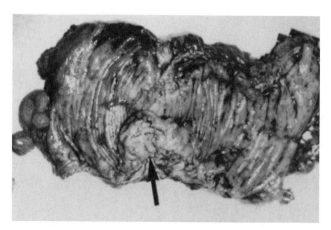

Figure 170–4. Surgical specimen obtained at segmental resection of rectosigmoid colon. Note nodular mass of endometriosis (*arrow*). This lesion was almost totally obstructive as evidenced by dilated proximal segment (*left*) with flattened mucusoal folds. (From Coronado C, Franklin R, Lotze EC, et al: Surgical treatment of symptomatic colorectal endometriosis. Fertil Steril 1990;53:411–416.)

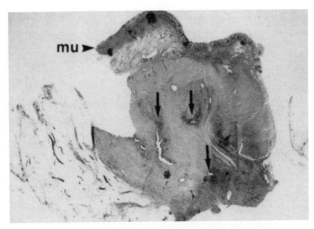

Figure 170–5. Photomicrograph of rectosigmoid wall showing endometrial glands and stroma (*arrows*) surrounded by markedly hyperplastic colonic muscularis. The interstitial mucosa (mu) is not involved (hematoxylin and eosin × 4). (From Coronado C, Franklin R, Lotze EC, et al: Surgical treatment of symptomatic colorectal endometriosis. Fertil Steril 1990;53:411–416.)

because of the fibrotic tissue, dense adhesions, and gross distortion of the pelvic anatomy.

Management of Unexpected Findings

Endometriomas that rupture during mobilization of the ovary at laparoscopy can be lavaged to prevent an inflammatory response, and the pelvic endoscopic surgery may be performed immediately, or in selected cases, delayed until after 3 months of GnRH agonists to suppress inflammatory host response.

POSTOPERATIVE MANAGEMENT

After operative laparoscopy, as compared to diagnostic laparoscopy, there is an increased chance of an overnight admission and increase in length of postoperative recovery. However, for hospitalized patients who undergo laparotomy, the recovery time is longer than for laparoscopy. Routine postoperative care with advancement of diet and pain control is achieved. The patient is discharged to home after tolerating a select diet, usually on day 3 or 4.

Long-term management plans are based on the surgical results, prognosis, and the patient's desires (e.g., pain relief, fertility, or health). For instance, if desiring pain relief, after her course of GnRH agonist, the patient is placed on oral contraceptive pills *continuously* for 3 months at a time to minimize the recurrence of endometriosis until pregnancy is desired. One should not hesitate to use estrogen replacement therapy for menopausal symptoms after complete removal of endometriosis.

POSTOPERATIVE COMPLICATIONS AND TREATMENT

Recurrence of symptoms of cyclic pain and mass (if examined at the proper time) following total abdominal hysterectomy–bilateral salpingo-oophorectomy (TAH/BSO)

Pearls and Pitfalls

PEARLS

- Endometriosis in the early stages (preinvasive) may be halted by medical therapy; in the late stages, surgery is the best treatment.
- The typical, or classic, appearance of endometriosis is a false concept because there is no single lesion that is typical of endometriosis appearance.
- Most mild endometriosis progresses; therefore, diagnosis and treatment as soon as possible is important in avoiding infertility and the worsening of pain.
- If the pain is unresponsive to oral contraceptive pills and nonsteroidal anti-inflammatory drugs, laparoscopy is indicated.
- Proper treatment of endometriosis may involve multiple modalities (medical, surgical) and multiple specialists (gynecologist, urologist, general surgeon, or colon rectal surgeon); endometriosis can humble even the most skilled surgeons.
- Laparoscopy is the procedure of choice because it allows for diagnosis and treatment during the same procedure.
- During endometrioma removal, one should be extremely careful to avoid injuring the ovarian blood supply. Otherwise, the ovary will malfunction because of its communication hormonally with the hypothalamic-pituitary axis.
- Usually, invasion of the bowel by endometriosis extends through the serosa to the muscularis, but the mucosa is not directly involved by the disease process; this is an important diagnostic point in the differentiation of endometriosis from carcinoma of the bowel because the carcinoma arises from the mucosa and extends toward the muscularis.
- An injudiously timid approach to surgery results in leaving residual disease behind.
- The ureter should be located and protected before one attempts to excise the endometriosis from the broad ligament and uterosacral ligament.
- In most cases of partial obliteration of the cul-de-sac, the rectum can be dissected free from the uterosacral ligament laterally, with minimal risk of entering the bowel lumen; the bulk of the endometriosis is usually located in the uterosacral ligament.
- The areas of greatest risk during peritoneal endometriosis surgery include the ureters (throughout their course), the internal iliac vein (near its bifurcation), the external iliac vessels (the superior aspect of the broad ligaments just beneath the ovary), and the uterine vessels and ureter (the cardinal and uterosacral ligaments).

---

should make one suspicious of the presence of residual functional ovarian tissue. Reoperation and removal is usually required. Endometriosis of the vaginal cuff is a complication of hysterectomy for endometriosis. This causes pelvic pain and deep dyspareunia. The treatment of choice is cuff excision along with the residual endometriosis. A patient with an unrecognized perforation of bowel at laparoscopy usually has symptoms of localized or generalized peritonitis within 12 to 36 hours after surgery. Prompt antibiotic coverage, exploration, and repair are mandatory. The primary resection and repair are usually possible as long as a *healthy bowel* can be approximated.

OUTCOMES

A recent Canadian study suggests that surgical ablation of even the *superficial endometriotic lesions* is associated with significant improvement in subsequent fecundity. Predictions about the outcome of any surgical treatment for endometriosis also must take into consideration the training, 1iu501skill, and experience of the surgeon. In regard to deep bowel endometriosis, we have shown that full-thickness resection of the colon (by either wedge or segmental resection with end-to-end anastomosis) is a safe procedure with low rates of associated morbidity, good postoperative relief of symptoms, and favorable pregnancy rates.

SELECTED READINGS

Batt RE, Udagaw SM, Wheeler JM: Endometriosis: Microconservative surgery. In Hunt RB (ed): Atlas of Female Infertility Surgery, 2nd ed. Chicago, Year Book Medical, 1992.

Coronado C, Franklin R, Lotze EC, et al: Surgical treatment of symptomatic colorectal endometriosis. Fertil Steril 1990;53:411.

Mangal RK, Taskin O, Nezhat C, Franklin R: Laparoscopic vaporization of diaphragmatic endometriosis in a woman with epigastric pain: A case report. J Reprod Med 1996;41:64.

Marcouse S, Matieux R, Berube S: Laparoscopic surgery in infertile women with minimal or mild endometriosis. Canadian Collaborative Group on Endometriosis. N Engl J Med 1997;337:217.

Martin DC (ed): Intra-abdominal Laser Surgery, 2nd ed. Research Press, Memphis, TN, 1986, Fertility Institute of Mid-South.

Nezhat C, Crowgey S, Nezhat F: Videolaserscopy for the treatment of endometriosis associated with infertility. Fertil Steril 1989;51:237.

Nezhat C, Nezhat F, Pennigton E: Laparoscopic treatment of lower colorectal and infiltrative rectovaginal septum endometriosis by the technique of video laparoscopy. Br J Obstet Gynecol 1992;99:664.

Prystowsky JB, Stryker SS, Ujiki GT, Poticha SM: Gastrointestinal endometriosis: Incidence and indications for resection. Arch Surg 1988;123:855.

Sampson JA: Peritoneal endometriosis, due to menstrual dissemination of endometrial tissue into the peritoneal cavity. Am J Obstet Gyncol 1927;14:22.

Chapter 171

Ovarian (Adnexal) Neoplasm, Benign

Mark Hiraoka and Matthew Borst

The surgical management of adnexal masses requires a broad understanding of female reproductive biology and a disciplined application of surgical judgment in order to perform the appropriate surgical intervention with the minimum disturbance of anatomy or reproductive function. The clinical significance of an adnexal mass may range from an asymptomatic functional ovarian cyst to a malignant ovarian neoplasm that has undergone torsion and has extension or metastases to the gastrointestinal tract. There are important guiding principles that can help determine the likelihood of malignancy and guide the preparation and performance of surgical care. This chapter outlines those principles in an organized framework to assist surgeons faced with evaluating adnexal masses and preparing for surgery.

DOES THE PATIENT NEED SURGERY?

The answer to this question emerges after careful analysis of the patient's symptoms and personal and family history (including reproductive history) as well considering the possibility of primary or metastatic cancer involving the adnexa. The potential consequences of inaction or surgical delay must also be considered.

IS THE MASS LIKELY TO BE MALIGNANT?

The likelihood of malignancy can be reasonably estimated by correlating the patient's history and physical examination with the results of imaging studies (ultrasound) and scrum markers (CA 125). For postmenopausal patients who have an adnexal mass in conjunction with an elevated CA 125 blood test, the positive predictive value for malignancy can approach 90% to 95%. For younger patients with no personal or family history of breast or ovary cancer who have simple cysts on ultrasound, no ascites, and normal CA 125 levels, the risk of malignancy can be as low as 1% to 3%. The thorough surgeon evaluates these parameters, discusses them with the patient and her family, and takes them into account during operative planning.

WHAT ARE THE PATIENT'S FUTURE FERTILITY PLANS?

Preservation of fertility capacity in accordance with the patient's wishes is an important goal of surgery. This consideration needs to be balanced with the need for the surgery to provide definitive management. In many cases, a benign adnexal mass can be excised and the ovary can be preserved. In other cases, the entire ovary and possibly entire adnexa must be removed. Most stages and histologic cell types of ovarian cancer require surgical removal of the entire internal pelvic organs. There are, however, specific presentations of germ cell ovarian cancers and well-differentiated epithelial ovarian cancers that can be surgically staged and treated, yet allow preservation of fertility capacity. The surgeon must be knowledgeable of up-to-date treatment strategies in order to counterbalance the need for disease treatment with the patient's fertility desires.

WHAT SURGICAL TECHNIQUE WILL MOST BENEFIT THE PATIENT?

For patients without symptoms and in whom the risk of malignancy is estimated to be very low, the best course of management may prove to be careful periodic surveillance or laparoscopic evaluation with biopsy or excision. For symptomatic patients or patients estimated to be at substantial risk of malignancy, a well-prepared laparotomy should be planned.

CLINICAL PRESENTATION

Natural History

It is important to assess whether the adnexal mass is likely to be a discrete adnexal lesion or a process that also involves the gastrointestinal or urologic systems. Symptoms of urinary frequency, hematuria, constipation, hematochezia, fever, pelvic pressure, back pain, or leg swelling may indicate extension of disease outside the adnexa. Historical factors such as previous colon or breast cancer, inflammatory bowel disease, or extensive prior surgery may also indicate a disease process that does not originate in the adnexa. Physical examination findings such as a fixed pelvic mass or nodularity involving the parametria or rectovaginal septum also would indicate the mass may not be a discrete gynecologic process. The presence of any of these factors would require consideration for a broad differential diagnosis and preoperative evaluation.

Differential Diagnosis

The age of the patient and her menstrual status can be an effective way to first consider a differential diagnosis

Table 171–1	Differential Diagnosis of Pelvic Mass Based on Age				
INFANCY	**PREPUBERTAL**	**ADOLESCENT**	**REPRODUCTIVE**	**PERIMENOPAUSAL**	**POSTMENOPAUSAL**
Functional cyst	Germ cell tumor	Functional cyst	Functional cyst	Leiomyoma	Ovarian tumor Benign

Germ cell tumor		Pregnancy	Pregnancy	Ovarian tumor
				  Benign
					Borderline
					  Invasive cancer

		Dermoid
		Other germ cell
		  tumors
			Leiomyoma	Borderline
				  Invasive cancer
					Bowel
					  Malignant

			Ovarian epithelial tumors Benign	Functional cysts	Inflammatory

		Obstructing
		  vaginal or uterine
		  anomalies
			Borderline
			  Invasive cancer
				Bowel
				  Malignant
				  Inflammatory
					Metastases

		Epithelial ovarian tumors			

for an adnexal mass and stratify the risk of malignancy (Table 171–1). Another way of considering the differential diagnosis of an adnexal mass is to use the historical factors and physical examination findings to estimate whether the mass is of gynecologic or nongynecologic origin (Table 171–2).

Diagnostic Studies

Adjunctive studies with ultrasound and tumor marker analysis with CA 125 can prove very useful in further characterizing an adnexal mass (Table 171–3).

Table 171–2	Differential Diagnosis of Adnexal Masses	
GYNECOLOGIC ORIGIN		**NONGYNECOLOGIC ORIGIN**

Non-neoplastic
  Ovarian
    Physiologic cysts
    Follicular
    Corpus luteum
    Theca luteum cyst
    Luteoma of pregnancy
    Polycystic ovaries
    Endometriosis
    Inflammatory cysts
  Nonovarian
    Ectopic pregnancy
    Congenital anomalies
    Embryologic remnants
    Tubal
      Pyosalpinx
      Hydrosalpinx
Neoplastic
  Ovarian
    Benign
    Borderline
    Invasive cancer
  Nonovarian
    Leiomyoma
    Paraovarian cyst
    Paratubal cyst
    Endometrial cancer
    Tubal carcinoma
    Sarcoma

Non-Neoplastic
    Appendiceal abscess
    Diverticulosis
    Adhesions (bowel or omentum)
    Peritoneal cyst
    Feces in rectosigmoid
    Urine in bladder
    Pelvic kidney
    Urachal cyst
    Anterior sacral meningocele

Neoplastic
  Carcinoma
    Sigmoid
    Cecum
    Appendix
    Bladder
    Lymphoma
    Carcinoid tumor
    Retroperitoneal neoplasm
    Presacral teratoma

PREOPERATIVE MANAGEMENT

Completion of Workup

The use of adjunctive studies can prove helpful after completing the history and physical examination.

For most patients, transvaginal ultrasound uses a better acoustic window and can more readily evaluate subtle features of adnexal masses. Doppler studies demonstrating decreased resistance and pulsatility indices are currently being evaluated as predictors of malignancy. The use of targeted studies should be based on clinical factors derived from the history and physical examination. Preoperative testing should be limited to studies that will directly affect operative considerations.

Optimization of Patient

Counseling

It is important to counsel the patient in detail regarding the broad differential diagnosis associated with adnexal masses. It is also important that the informed consent document explain the potential surgical procedures that may be required to manage the adnexal mass. The potential compromise of future fertility and the potential for surgical castration must be discussed.

Bowel Preparation

In nonemergent cases, a preoperative bowel preparation can make surgery technically easier and safer. This allows

Table 171–3	Ultrasound Features of Adnexal Masses	
MORE LIKELY BENIGN		**MORE LIKELY MALIGNANT**
Unilateral		Bilateral
Cystic		Solid or complex
Mobile		Fixed
Smooth surface		Irregular surface
Minimal or no internal septations		Complex internal septations
No ascites		Ascites

the surgeon to potentially work through a smaller incision and work with more confidence in proximity to the lower gastrointestinal tract.

Pathology

Reliable pathology services are a requirement for management of adnexal masses. Intraoperative frozen section analysis of the surgical specimen in major referral centers can distinguish benign from malignant masses with a 90% to 95% level of accuracy. This facilitates intraoperative decision making and early postoperative discussions.

INTRAOPERATIVE MANAGEMENT

Positioning

The lithotomy position is advantageous for adnexal mass surgery. The first advantage is that it allows for intraoperative bimanual rectovaginal examination. This can be critical for orientation of distorted anatomy. It can also allow for placement of vaginal or rectal obturators to help delineate anatomic relationships between the bladder, vagina, and rectum that may have been altered by the disease process or prior surgery. The second advantage is that the lithotomy position can allow the second assistant to be close enough to actively participate in surgery. These considerations are particularly important when performing adnexal mass surgery for a patient who has previously had a hysterectomy.

Types of Approaches

Laparoscopy

A growing body of literature is investigating the role of laparoscopy in the management of adnexal masses. Although advantages of laparoscopy include reduced cost, decreased risk of adhesions, shorter recovery time, and the ability to perform the surgery in an ambulatory setting, concerns do remain. When deciding between laparoscopy and laparotomy, it is clear that preoperative patient selection is critical. Patient history, age, family history, physical findings, ultrasound findings and tumor markers may aid in determining the risk of malignancy preoperatively. Herman was able to correctly predict benign masses in 177 of 185 patients (96%) using ultrasound findings. The combined use of ultrasound, clinical findings, and CA 125 values were used to correctly identify 25 of 25 masses as benign by Parker and Berek. However, despite careful selection, it is possible that a mass, initially thought to be benign, may subsequently prove to be malignant.

The inappropriate use of laparoscopy may result in a delay in therapy and improper cancer staging, and it may raise the concern of worsening the prognosis as a result of intraoperative rupture of the malignant mass. A great deal of attention has been focused on the importance of intraoperative rupture. In 1973, Webb et al. reported that tumor rupture worsened prognosis. More recently,

Dembo and colleagues found that rupture did not significantly influence relapse rates in 519 patients with stage I epithelial ovarian cancer. Still, by avoiding rupture of stage I tumors, additional chemotherapy may be prevented.

If there is any suspicion of malignancy, then laparotomy should be performed. However, if the ovarian mass is thought to be benign, then laparoscopy may be considered. When laparoscopy is performed, peritoneal washings should be obtained, the upper abdomen and pelvis explored for evidence of metastases, the ovaries inspected for surface abnormalities, and the specimen sent for frozen analysis. If there are any suspicious findings, then laparotomy should be performed. Cyst aspiration alone is not acceptable. Ovarian cyst aspirates carry a 10% to 66% false-negative rate and are thus not sufficient to establish a diagnosis.

Laparotomy

Pfannenstiel incisions may be very appropriate for management of small adnexal masses that are mobile and strongly suspected to be benign. If greater exposure is required the tendinous insertions of the abdominal recti muscles on the symphysis pubis can be cut to convert the incision to a *Cherney* incision. Enough tendon must be preserved on both the symphysis and the rectus muscle to allow re-approximation of tendon to tendon rather than sewing tendon directly to bone. A muscle splitting *Maylard* incision can give excellent pelvic sidewall exposure. It is applicable to cases in which upper abdominal dissection is not required. It is important to secure excellent hemostasis of the inferior epigastric vessels when doing a Maylard incision in order to avoid a postoperative subfascial hematoma.

Vertical Approach

A low vertical midline abdominal incision allows direct exposure to the pelvis and pelvic mass. This can facilitate a retroperitoneal exposure and enhance the prospect for an en bloc removal. It also allows the flexibility for extending the incision if necessary for radical surgery.

Retroperitoneal Approach

Incising the parietal peritoneum over the psoas muscle and developing the pararectal space is an important step in mobilizing an adnexal mass from the pelvic sidewall and identifying the ureter. This is a critical technique when operating upon a fixed adnexal mass or a very large adnexal mass. An intraperitoneal mass deviates the ureter laterally; a retroperitoneal mass deviates the ureter medially. It is not necessary to transect the round ligament of the uterus to access the retroperitoneal spaces. Identification of the ureter at the pelvic brim where it crosses the common iliac artery and tracing the ureter throughout its pelvic course is an important step that promotes safety and allows a definitive approach to en bloc removal of adnexal masses.

Techniques

Cystectomy

Open ovarian capsule with linear incision on side opposite hilum. Conduct fine dissection of cyst with traction and counteraction. Excise cyst. Close ovarian surface with fine (3-0 or 4-0) absorbable sutures using imbricating technique and meticulous hemostasis. Consider methylcellulose adhesion barrier to wrap residual ovary (Fig. 171–1).

Oophorectomy

Ligate ovarian artery and vein lateral to ovarian mass (after identifying ureter). Ligate ovarian ligament medial to ovary close to uterine cornua. Dissect posterior sheath of broad ligament to excise mass. Use meticulous hemostasis. Consider preservation of fallopian tube and methylcellulose adhesion barrier to cover residual fallopian tube and broad ligament. It is sometimes necessary to close the broad ligament sheaths with a running lock suture for hemostasis.

Unilateral Salpingo-oophorectomy

Procedure is the same as for oophorectomy except also ligate and excise the fallopian tube proximally at the uterine cornua (Fig. 171–2).

Special Considerations

Torsion

Ovarian torsion is best managed by unilateral salpingo-oophorectomy in perimenopausal or postmenopausal patients. For reproductive age patients, conservation of the adnexa can be considered. The prerequisites for conservation include (1) excision of any neoplastic pathology (the minimum procedure would be an excisional cyst wall biopsy), (2) intraoperative evaluation of the adnexa to assess viability of tissue (consider fluorescein dye study), and (3) ovarian resuspension using a triangulation technique to preclude a recurrent episode of torsion (Fig. 171–3).

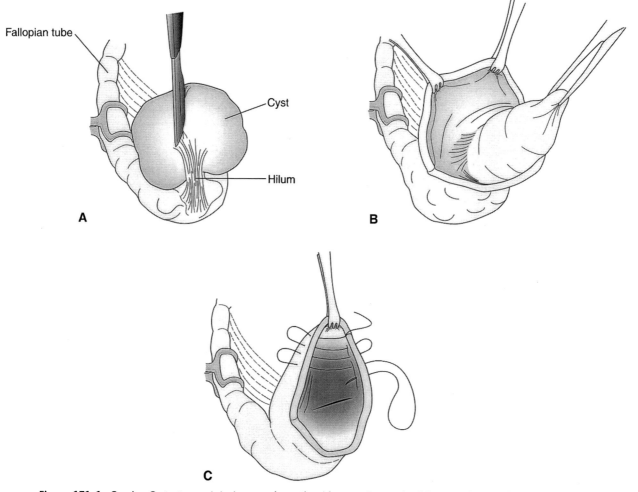

Figure 171–1. Ovarian Cystectomy. *A*, Incise capsule on the side opposite ovarian hilum. *B*, Blunt and sharp dissection to enucleate cyst. *C*, Close ovarian capsule with five absorbable sutures.

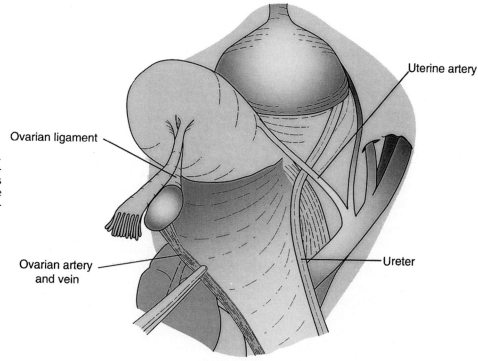

Figure 171–2. Oophorectomy. Open peritoneum over common iliac artery. Identify ovarian vessels and ureter. Clamp, cut, and ligate ovarian vessels and ovarian ligament.

Uterine artery

Ovarian ligament

Ovarian artery and vein

Ureter

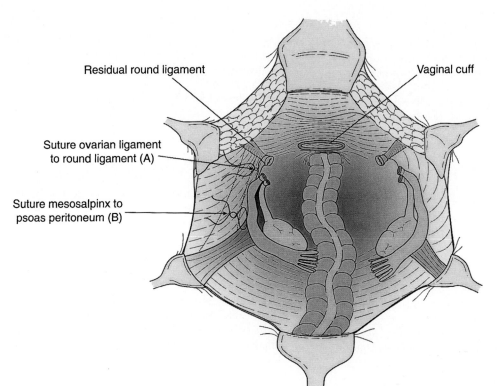

Residual round ligament

Vaginal cuff

Suture ovarian ligament to round ligament (A)

Suture mesosalpinx to psoas peritoneum (B)

Figure 171–3. Adnexal suspension by triangulation technique. A, Suture ovarian ligament to regional round ligament. B, Suture mesosalpinx to psoas peritoneum.

Adnexal Mass During Pregnancy

The risk of malignancy involving adnexal masses in this age group is low (approximately 1%). Indications for surgery include the risk of torsion (10% to 15%), risk of rupture, as well as management of pain and prevention of dystocia. Current perinatal guidelines recommend removal of any complex or solid adnexal mass that persists after 14 weeks' gestation. The ideal timing for surgery is between 15 and 19 weeks of gestational age when the major risk of spontaneous first trimester abortion has subsided but the uterus has not yet expanded to prevent exposure. Minimally traumatic surgery through a paramedian incision under regional anesthesia is recommended. Obstetric perioperative consultation is advised.

Adnexal Mass in a Posthysterectomy Patient

Anatomic distortion should be expected in these patients. The importance of a preoperative bowel preparation and lithotomy positioning cannot be overstated. The rectosigmoid colon and mesentery frequently overlie a mass involving a residual left ovary. If ovarian conservation is planned, then attempts at ovarian suspension outside the true pelvis should be made. One method of suspension is to suture the medial aspect of the ovarian ligament to the residual round ligament near the internal inguinal ring. The mesosalpinx of the fallopian tube can then be sutured to the parietal peritoneum over the psoas muscle to complete the triangulation resuspension (see Fig. 171–3).

Peripostmenopausal Patient

The American College of Obstetrics and Gynecology (ACOG) recommends that patients undergoing pelvic surgery after the age of 40 should consider undergoing bilateral salpingo-oophorectomy (BSO). BSO should also be considered at a younger age for patients whose personal or family history puts them at increased risk for ovarian cancer. The 1992 American College of Surgeons "Patterns of Care" study for ovarian cancer revealed 1 of 8 cases of ovarian cancer in the USA (more than 3000 per year) occurred in women who underwent hysterectomy after the age of 40 years but did not have BSO performed. It is believed this number can be substantially reduced by appropriately performing BSO for any peripostmenopausal woman undergoing pelvic surgery.

Fixed Pelvic Mass

A fixed pelvic mass found on examination must raise the possibility of involvement with the gastrointestinal or genitourinary tract. Preoperative colonoscopy, barium enema, or intravenous pyelography can further evaluate these concerns. Bowel preparation is imperative in these cases and consideration should be given for retrograde ureteral stent placement to facilitate surgery.

Mucinous Tumors and Dermoid Cysts

Mucinous tumors and dermoid cysts should be removed as en bloc specimens in order to avoid intraoperative spill that can cause reactive peritonitis. There is theoretical concern that this can lead to pseudomyxoma peritonei. Spill of these tumors should be followed by extensive abdominal pelvic irrigation with hypotonic solutions.

Malignancy

Two general principles underlie the surgical management of ovarian cancer: (1) surgical excision and debulking of all accessible macroscopic tumor (cytoreductive surgery) and (2) full surgical staging to detect occult sites of malignancy to allow accurate prognosis and guide adjuvant treatment planning. There are two circumstances in which these goals can be accomplished and fertility capacity can be preserved: (1) unilateral adnexal involvement of ovarian germ cell malignancies and (2) unilateral involvement of well-differentiated ovarian epithelial malignancies.

Surgical restraint should be used before extirpation of pelvic organs for patients of reproductive age. Intraoperative gynecology-oncology consultation can facilitate integration of operative findings and frozen section pathology results before embarking on surgical staging or tumor debulking. Operative management of malignancies metastatic to the adnexa is dependent on treatment principles that apply to the cancer site of origin.

POSTOPERATIVE MANAGEMENT

Strategies for Postoperative Care

Deep Venous Thrombosis Prophylaxis

Venous pooling and stasis can be a by-product of even minimally invasive surgery. Deep venous thrombosis prophylaxis with pneumatic compression stockings, heparin, or low-molecular-weight heparin should always be considered in conjunction with early postoperative ambulation.

Pulmonary

Preoperative teaching and postoperative utilization of incentive spirometry can reduce the rate of postoperative febrile morbidity and risk of pneumonia. The use of β_2-mimetic nebulizer treatments is recommended for patients with reactive airway disease.

Hematoma

Raw pelvic peritoneal surfaces can lead to adhesions or pelvic hematoma formation. Meticulous surgical techniques and possible use of biologic adjuncts for hemostasis (Gelfoam, Surgicel, NU-knit, thrombin spray) may reduce these risks.

Adhesions

The potential for adhesions can be reduced by atraumatic operative techniques and possible use of methylcellulose adhesion barriers at the conclusion of surgery.

Gastrointestinal Tract

Clinical judgment is required to determine when resumption of gastrointestinal intake should be started. Length of surgery, amount of packing, and extent of surgical dissection are important factors to be accounted for when making this decision.

MANAGEMENT OF COMPLICATIONS

Ovarian Failure

Even when ovarian tissue has been conserved, some patients experience postoperative ovarian failure. This is thought to be due to alteration of the ovarian microvasculature by surgery. This condition manifests with classic symptoms of the climacteric: hot flushes, insomnia, mood swings, and vaginal dryness. Serum follicle-stimulating hormone levels can be used to confirm ovarian failure. Follicle-stimulating hormone values greater than 40 are indicative of ovarian failure.

Postmenopausal Status

Surgical menopause can be a consequence of BSO or of failure of residual ovarian tissue. With few exceptions, these patients should be candidates for hormone replacement therapy. Direct benefits of hormone replacement therapy include reduced symptoms of climacteric and reduced risk of osteoporosis and cardiovascular disease.

Ileus and Small Bowel Obstruction

Serial physical examination in conjunction with selected laboratory tests and radiographic evaluations distinguish adynamic ileus from mechanical small bowel obstruction. Mature clinical judgment is required to monitor these patients and provide timely interventions.

Hematoma

Operative intervention is required for pelvic hematomas that obstruct the gastrointestinal or urologic tract. Stable hematomas without obstructive signs or symptoms can be monitored with serial surveillance and potentially be drained by percutaneous access.

Infection

Wound infections can be managed by antibiotic therapy and débridement based on classic surgical principles. Pelvic abscess can often be managed with antibiotics and percutaneous drainage, thereby avoiding surgery.

OUTCOMES

Fertility Preservation

Patients undergoing unilateral salpingo-oophorectomy can maintain fertility rates (85%) close to normal as long as the contralateral adnexa is normal.

Pearls and Pitfalls

PEARLS

- Always consider the possibility of concurrent pregnancy (test urine or serum human chorionic gonadotropin). Always consider future fertility capacity when operating for reproductive age women.
- Conservative surgery is the rule—do not perform extirpative pelvic surgery in reproductive-age women unless mandated by pelvic hemorrhage or gross anatomic or histologic abnormalities.
- Preoperative bowel preparation can set the stage for a thorough and safe pelvic dissection.
- Retroperitoneal masses deviate the ureter medially; intraperitoneal masses deviate the ureter laterally.
- Retroperitoneal dissection is the preferred method of surgery to promote safety of the ureter and facilitate en bloc resection of the adnexal mass.
- The possibility of cancer should be evaluated as carefully as possible when one chooses the surgical approach (scope versus open).
- Strongly consider BSO when doing pelvic surgery for patients who are perimenopausal or postmenopausal. This is believed to reduce the risk of reoperation and reduce the risk of ovarian cancer. It is also advisable to consider hysterectomy, which may serve to streamline long-term hormone replacement therapy regimens.
- Operative cases that involve an open vaginal cuff or management of pelvic abscesses require perioperative antibiotics.
- In the event of hemorrhage, there is no vein in the pelvis that cannot be ligated. The external iliac artery is the only artery that cannot be tied. Bilateral ligation of the anterior division of the internal iliac arteries can reduce the pelvic pulse pressure approximately 40% to 50%.
- The appropriate use of obstetric-gynecology specialty and subspecialty consultation can facilitate and streamline perioperative decision making.

Cosmesis

Patient satisfaction can be enhanced by meticulous surgical judgment and techniques. Judicious use of laparoscopy, minilaparotomy, and wound closure techniques can promote a patient's sense of well-being.

Failures

Treatment failures can be categorized into acts of commission and acts of omission. Treatment failure acts of commission include the unnecessary removal of the adnexa or entire reproductive tract. This can be avoided with cautious interpretation of intraoperative pathology results and with the timely use of intraoperative consultation with obstetric-gynecologic specialists or subspecialists (perinatal, endocrinology, oncology). Treatment failures based on acts of omission can include failure to consider a coexisting pregnancy, failure to consider the possibility of malignancy, and failure to excise and stage a malignancy properly.

SELECTED READINGS

American College of Obstetricians and Gynecologists: ACOG Technical Bulletin No. 111. Prophylactic oophorectomy. ACOG Technical Bulletin, 1987.

Averette HE, Nguyen HN: The role of prophylactic oophorectomy in cancer prevention. Gynecol Oncol 1994;55:S38.

Dembo AJ, Davy M, Stennig AE, et al: Prognostic factors in patients with stage I epithelial ovarian cancer. Obstet Gynecol 1990;75:263.

Hankins GD, Clark SL, Gilstrap L: Operative Obstetrics. Norwalk, Conn: Appleton & Lange, 1995:Chapter 22.

Herman U, Locher G, Goldhirsch A: Sonographic patterns of ovarian tumors: Prediction of malignancy. Obstet Gynecol 1987:69:777.

Malkasian GD Jr, Knapp RC, Lavin PT, et al: Preoperative evaluation of serum CA125 levels in premenopausal and postmenopausal patients: Discrimination of benign from malignant disease. Am J Obstet Gynecol 1988:159:341.

Parker WH, Berek JS: Management of selected cystic adnexal masses in postmenopausal women by operative laparoscopy. Am J Obstet Gynecol 1990;163:1574.

Vasilev S, Schlaerth J, Campeay J, Morrow P: Serum CA125 levels in preoperative evaluation of pelvic masses. Obstet Gynecol 1988:71:751.

Webb MJ, Decker DG, Mussey E, Williams TJ: Factors influencing survival in stage I ovarian cancer. Am J Obstet Gynecol 1973;116:222.

Chapter 172

Malignant Ovarian Neoplasms

Elvis S. Donaldson, Jr.

Malignant tumors of the ovary present many management problems for the pelvic surgeon. Even though progress has been made over the past 10 years with efforts at developing techniques for early diagnosis, more than 60% of ovarian cancer presents in advanced stages. Despite aggressive treatment, many patients still die of progressive small bowel obstruction and malnutrition. It is estimated that approximately 23,000 new cases of ovarian cancer are diagnosed annually and 14,000 deaths occur. Ovarian cancer will develop in 1 in 70 women during their lifetime.

Several factors have been implicated in the risk of development of ovarian cancer. Age and long periods of uninterrupted ovulation increase risk. The use of oral contraceptives is protective. If a patient has a cumulative use for greater than 10 years, her risk of ovarian cancer may be reduced as much as 80%. This protection persists after discontinuing use of birth control pills.

Five percent to 10% of ovarian cancers are familial. A woman with a single first-degree relative with ovarian cancer has a risk of 1 in 40 for development of an ovarian malignancy. If there are two first-degree relatives, her risk may increase to approximately 1 in 3.

Familial ovarian cancer tends to occur at a younger age than nonfamilial tumors. The familial syndromes are transmitted by autosomal dominance with varying penetrance. Three types are well described. The Lynch II syndrome (nonpolyposis colon cancer, breast, ovarian, or endometrial cancer), familial ovarian-breast cancer syndrome, and site-specific ovarian cancer (less common). Mutation in the *BRCA1* tumor suppressor gene is associated with familial ovarian cancer. This mutation is rarely found in sporadic tumors. Women with this mutation, however, may have a risk of ovarian cancer as high as 90% in their lifetime.

Tumors of the ovary can develop from any tissue within the ovarian structure; that is, germ cells, specialized gonadal stroma, supporting mesenchyme, and tumors from the surface coelomic epithelium covering the ovary (Table 172–1).

Malignant ovarian tumors in the young tend to be of the germ cell type and clinically can behave very aggressively. This type is therapy sensitive with high cure rates and can be managed for the most part with conservative surgery and aggressive adjunctive chemotherapy.

Approximately 5% to 10% of ovarian malignancies are sex cord–stromal tumors (specialized stroma). Surgical management depends on the age of the patient. Most of these tumors are unilateral and confined. With careful staging, conservative surgery can be performed in the young patient. When reproductive function is not a consideration, hysterectomy and bilateral salpingo-oophorectomy is standard treatment. Adjunctive therapy is usually not necessary with stage I stromal tumors.

Epithelial tumors are the most common, accounting for 85% to 90% of ovarian cancers (Table 172–2). Histologically, they can assume the form of any tissue derived embryologically from the coelomic epithelium. Because the majority of ovarian cancers are of epithelial origin, the author has directed this discussion primarily at their management, realizing that the surgical management of any advanced ovarian malignancy is similar.

CLINICAL PRESENTATION

An understanding of the likely anatomic spread of ovarian cancer is helpful in explaining some of the problems with diagnosis. The natural history of most ovarian malignancies probably includes a prolonged occult course with an asymptomatic lesion. Once the surface of the ovary is perforated, tumor cells are shed into the peritoneal cavity and implantation can occur, generally along the tract of flow of peritoneal fluid along the right pericolic gutter to the diaphragm, the omentum, and other surfaces that are bathed by peritoneal fluid.

The occasional occurrence of malignancies of the peritoneal surface histologically identical to ovarian cancer but following bilateral oophorectomy also suggests the potential of the coelomic epithelium (the peritoneum) to de novo malignant degeneration. This may be the case in individuals with advanced disease, when little or no tumor is demonstrated within the ovarian structure.

Penetration can occur through peritoneal lymphatics to iliac, hypogastric, obturator, and aortic lymph nodes. As many as 30% of tumors apparently confined to the ovary have occult peritoneal, omental, or lymphatic metastasis found only on pathologic examination, thus emphasizing the importance of surgical staging. Increasing peritoneal fluid progressing to ascites occurs with advancing disease and progressive peritoneal lymphatic obstruc-

Table 172–1	Classification of Ovarian Cancer
Epithelial Tumors	Sex Cord Stromal
Serous	Granulosa–thecal cell tumors
Mucinous	Sertoli-Leydig cell tumors
Endometrial	Gynandroblastoma
Mesonephroid (clear cell)	Lipid cell tumors
Brenner	Nonspecific Mesenchymal Tumors
Carcinosarcoma	Sarcoma
Cell Tumors	Lymphoma
Teratomas	Metastatic Tumors
Mature	Endometrium
Immature	Breast
Dysgerminoma	Gastrointestinal
Endodermal sinus tumor	
Gonadoblastoma	
Choriocarcinoma	

Table 172–2	Percentage of Ovarian Cancers by Histologic Class	
CLASS	**% OF OVARIAN CANCER**	
Epithelial	85–90	
Germ cell	10+	
Sex cord stromal	5+	
Mesenchymal	1	
Metastatic	1	

Table 172–4	Physical Findings Suggesting Malignancy	
Solid mass	Pelvic nodularity	
Irregular mass	Abdominal distention	
Fixed mass	Abdominal mass	
Bilateral mass		

tion. Hepatic parenchymal disease and lesions found outside the abdomen are generally late manifestations of advanced intraperitoneal disease.

As surface disease progresses, gastrointestinal function is compromised, producing vague abdominal symptoms such as pain, gaseous distention, anorexia, and nausea. A pleural effusion may occur resulting from increasing intra-abdominal pressure and diaphragmatic lymphatic obstruction. Advancing disease may include obstructive symptoms related to loss of small bowel function. Colonic dysfunction can occur when the disease process impinges the lumen or invades the muscularis.

DIAGNOSIS

Surprisingly, advanced disease may produce few symptoms. Most patients have increasing abdominal discomfort and bloating that result from abdominal or pelvic masses or ascites. Many patients give a history of a short period of discomfort. On further questioning, however, many admit to more long-term symptoms of "indigestion," gaseous bloating, or vague abdominal pain (Table 172–3). There is no clinically proven screening test for ovarian cancer; thus, most cases of early disease are diagnosed incidentally by palpation of a mass at the time of routine pelvic examination or at the time of abdominal or pelvic surgery for unrelated problems.

The importance of a careful history and physical assessment, including a complete abdominal and pelvic examination and digital rectal examination, cannot be overemphasized. A surprising number of advanced ovarian cancers are diagnosed by computed tomography following months to a year of abdominal symptoms during which no physical examination is documented. Physical findings suggesting malignancy are shown in Table 172–4. The use of transvaginal and pelvic ultrasound can help delineate the characteristics of a pelvic mass, assess possible spread, and determine the presence of ascites. Findings on ultra-

Table 172–3	Presenting Symptoms of Ovarian Cancer
Dyspepsia	
Bloating	
Vague abdominal pain	
Increased abdominal girth	
Loss of appetite and/or nausea	

sound studies that predict a higher risk of malignancy include multicystic lesions with thick septations, solid components within the tumor, internal or external excrescences, and ascites. The value of assessing Doppler blood flow of ovarian lesions has not been established. Ultrasound examination may be of particular help in the postmenopausal patient with a relatively small lesion. Unilocular cysts less than 10 cm in diameter in asymptomatic postmenopausal women have a minimal risk of ovarian cancer. In contrast, increased complexity of ovarian masses results in a higher, more significant risk for malignancy.

The differential in the risk of pelvic adnexal masses is age dependent as well. The highest risks are for the young premenarchal patients and for the postmenopausal patients. In the reproductive age, approximately 5% of the adnexal masses are malignant. Most are functional abnormalities related to the ovulatory cycle and resolve spontaneously in an otherwise normal reproductive age female. A rule of thumb is that any cystic mass less than 8 cm in diameter can be observed for one to two menstrual cycles for shrinkage or resolution before invasive evaluation is undertaken. A more aggressive approach is indicated with solid or mixed masses and in the very young or the postmenopausal patient.

The need for imaging studies is determined by the findings of the history and physical examination. In most cases, multiple studies can be avoided. Computed tomography may be helpful if the body composition prevents assessment of the character of the mass by palpation or ultrasound. However, if a large, fixed, irregular, multidense pelvic mass is easily palpable or apparent on ultrasound imaging, computed tomography can add little further information.

Patients with symptoms of constipation, cramping, diarrhea, or physical findings suggesting colon or rectal involvement should have a colonoscopy or sigmoidoscopy and biopsy. If the results are indeterminate as a result of stricture or fixation, a barium enema should be done to assist in differentiating intrinsic from extrinsic involvement of the colon by tumor.

Because some lesions may present as large encapsulated cysts, diagnostic paracentesis of ascites is discouraged. There is a possibility of rupture and leakage of tumor cells.

Serum CA 125 levels can be elevated by many conditions, such as endometriosis, pelvic inflammation, leiomyomata, liver disease, congestive heart failure, benign ovarian tumors, and malignancies other than ovarian cancer. However, a baseline level may be of help in determining malignant risk, particularly in the postmenopausal patient. Levels greater than 65 U/mL predict a malignancy (ovarian, endometrial, or other) approximately 75% of the time. Preoperative elevations predict its usefulness as a postoperative marker for follow-up. In the premenopausal woman, the preoperative CA 125 measurement is less helpful because of other conditions that may cause an elevated serum level, but again serial levels are helpful for follow-up.

PREOPERATIVE MANAGEMENT

Once a lesion has been detected and a significant risk of malignancy established, the standard management is primary surgical exploration, assessment of disease spread, and attempted optimal (complete) surgical removal of tumor masses.

Because most of these patients are postmenopausal, many have pre-existing medical conditions that can affect surgical outcome. Careful attention should be paid to the patient's past medical history and her list of current medications. Common medical problems that could result in adverse outcomes include diabetes and its secondary effect on multiple organ systems, heart disease, peripheral vascular disease, chronic lung disease or compromised pulmonary function, history of stroke or transient ischemia, obesity, and musculoskeletal joint disease that prevents or hinders postoperative mobilization. If any of these exist, they should be investigated and maximally stabilized preoperatively.

The patient should be fully informed of the surgical possibilities. These range from a simple or complicated resection of a benign lesion to an extensive radical surgical procedure requiring resection of the reproductive organs and large tumor masses in multiple areas throughout the abdominal cavity. The patient should be made aware of the possibility of fecal diversion or single or multiple bowel resections and reanastomoses. Women in their childbearing years should realize that reproductive function likely will be eliminated unless the disease is confined to one ovary and encapsulated. The patient should also be prepared for the possibility that no meaningful resection can be done because of disease extent and location. If adequate attention to detail is given to the patient's overall medical condition and she is informed regarding the goals and risks of the operative procedure, both the patient and the surgeon can approach treatment informed and secure that optimal care will be provided.

Basic preoperative assessment includes a complete blood count, metabolic panel, chest radiograph, and electrocardiogram. Any patient who demonstrates evidence of pulmonary disease should have preoperative pulmonary function tests and baseline arterial blood gas measurements. If there is a history of cardiac disease, a cardiology evaluation including an echocardiogram and stress testing may be indicated.

Care must be taken to predict and avoid intraoperative and postoperative complications. To achieve the goals of surgery, bowel resection and reanastomosis may be necessary. A mechanical bowel prep lowers the risk of intraperitoneal spillage. Antibiotic prophylaxis reduces the risk of postoperative infections. Patients with large ab-

dominal distention and ascites have tremendous fluid shifts intraoperatively and postoperatively. Utilization of a central line or right heart catheter assists in assessment of intravascular volume and facilitates management. Red blood cells should be available at the initiation of the surgical procedure because blood loss can be considerable.

Intravascular volume depletion and dehydration are not uncommon preoperatively, particularly if a mechanical bowel prep is done. Care must be taken that patients are well hydrated with an expanded vascular volume in order to avoid precipitous fluctuations in blood pressure with induction of anesthesia and when the abdomen is opened with a large volume of ascites.

If pulmonary function is compromised by massive abdominal distention from ascites, preoperative paracentesis can be done to allow adequate diaphragmatic excursion. Occasionally, large pleural effusions compromise oxygenation, necessitating preoperative thoracentesis. Chest tubes are rarely necessary because relief of abdominal pressure is adequate to prevent rapid recurrence.

Patients with a compromised nutritional status as a result of the effects of their disease may need nutritional support postoperatively. Preoperative planning should include provisions for initiating enteral or, as needed, parenteral feedings as soon as possible. The surgeon should be prepared for an extended procedure that could involve multiple organ systems.

INTRAOPERATIVE MANAGEMENT

When the patient is brought to the operating room, the attending surgeon should be present at the time the patient is positioned and all monitoring is placed. The lithotomy position should always be considered so that end to end anastomotic staples can be used for low anterior colon resections. If a large volume of ascites is present or an extended surgical procedure is expected, central venous access should be placed. Transverse incisions are avoided because upper abdominal examination is imperative for adequate exposure for staging and resection of extrapelvic tumor. The surgeon should be familiar with the staging of ovarian cancer (Table 172–5) and be able to perform all the required steps to accomplish complete surgical staging in apparent early stage disease (Table 172–6).

The importance of aggressive tumor removal in advanced stage disease and complete surgical staging in apparent early stage disease cannot be overemphasized. In patients inappropriately staged initially, up to 30% are upstaged by reoperation. Multiple studies demonstrate the survival advantage of optimal cytoreduction. Because dense, adherent disease may exist between the anterior abdominal wall and the intra-abdominal contents, care must be taken to avoid bowel injury upon entering the abdomen. Once the peritoneum is entered, peritoneal fluid is sent for cytology. The surgeon must then accurately assess the extent of the disease process. An orderly exploration should be carried out and, if necessary, adhesions taken down to allow palpation and visualization

Table 172–5	**International Federation of Gynecology and Obstetrics (FIGO) American Joint Committee on Cancer (AJCC) Staging of Primary Carcinoma of the Ovary**

TNM CATEGORIES	FIGO STAGES	
TX		Primary tumor cannot be assessed.
T0		No evidence of primary tumor.
T1	I	Tumor limited to ovaries (one or both).
T1a	IA	Tumor limited to one ovary; capsule intact, no tumor on ovarian surface. No malignant cells in ascites or peritoneal washings.°
T1b	IB	Tumor limited to both ovaries; capsules intact, no tumor on ovarian surface. No malignant cells in ascites or peritoneal washings.°
T1c	IC	Tumor limited to one or both ovaries with any of the following: capsule ruptured, tumor on ovarian surface, malignant cells in ascites or peritoneal washings.
T2	II	Tumor involves one or both ovaries with pelvic extension.
T2a	IIA	Extension and/or implants on uterus and/or tube(s). No malignant cells in ascites or peritoneal washings.
T2b	IIB	Extension to other pelvic tissues. No malignant cells in ascites or peritoneal washings.
T2c	IIC	Pelvic extension (2a or 2b) with malignant cells in ascites or peritoneal washings.
T3 and/or N1	III†	Tumor involves one or both ovaries with microscopically confirmed peritoneal metastasis outside the pelvis and/or regional lymph node metastasis.
T3a	IIIA	Microscopic peritoneal metastasis beyond pelvis.
T3b	IIIB	Macroscopic peritoneal metastasis beyond pelvis 2 cm or less in greatest dimension.
T3c and/or N1	IIIC	Peritoneal metastasis beyond pelvis more than 2 cm in greatest dimension and/or regional lymph node metastasis.
M1	IV†	Distant metastasis (excludes peritoneal metastasis).

°The presence of nonmalignant ascites is not classified. The presence of ascites does not affect staging unless malignant cells are present.

†Liver capsule metastases are T3/stage III; liver parenchymal metastasis, M1/stage IV. Pleural effusion must have positive cytology for M1/stage IV.

Used with permission of the American Joint Committee on Cancer (AJCC), Chicago, Illinois. Modified from AJCC Cancer Staging Manual, 5th ed. Philadelphia, Lippincott-Raven, 1997, p 66.

of all abdominal contents. The exploration includes the omentum, both sides of the diaphragm, the liver surface and parenchyma, the upper gastrointestinal tract and its mesentery, and the pericolic gutters. The retroperitoneal space, the pelvis, and the periaortic region are assessed for nodularity. In addition, all peritoneal surfaces are inspected. In the absence of obvious disease outside the pelvis, surgical staging as outlined in Table 172–6 is imperative.

In advanced cases, a large omental cake is often present and, because of its effect on exposure, is resected initially to allow better exposure. It may be necessary to dissect adherent loops of small bowel away from the omentum and occasionally a bowel resection and anastomosis is required. Separation of the transverse colon from the omentum may be difficult; however, it is rarely necessary to do a colon resection. Generally the vascular pedicles can be identified and ligated. The disease may extend along the greater curvature of the stomach into the left upper quadrant near or involving the surface of the spleen. On occasion, if complete debulking is otherwise possible, a splenectomy may be performed.

Many times, the initial inspection of the pelvic disease presents a daunting picture, suggesting the impossibility of resection. However, in the setting of extensive anatomic alteration, it is helpful to approach the pelvis laterally, opening the peritoneum along the lateral pelvic wall in a retroperitoneal approach. The ovarian blood supply is located, divided, and ligated. Care is taken to identify and isolate the ureters. The lateral dissections are continued inferiorly across the midline in order to develop the bladder flap, distal to any tumor implants. The round ligaments are identified and divided. The peritoneum is lifted superiorly and the bladder dissected off its underside down to the anterior uterine wall. A bladder reflection can then be extended to the upper third of the vagina. Posteriorly the peritoneum is peeled out of the cul-de-sac.

Once this is accomplished, traction can be applied medially, the ureter retracted laterally, and vessels identified and ligated. The rectovaginal space is then developed and the cardinal ligament divided. The dissection is continued inferiorly, below the peritoneal reflection to the vaginal angles, where they are then divided and an enbloc specimen removed.

Fecal diversion is avoided unless it is necessary to relieve obstruction or impending obstruction, or to accomplish complete gross surgical cytoreduction with minimal or no intraperitoneal disease. Colon resections for advanced ovarian cancer in which gross residual disease remains in the upper abdomen does not improve overall long-term survival. Low anterior resection and reanastomosis is appropriate when all gross disease can be removed.

Following resection of the pelvic disease, the pelvic and periaortic retroperitoneum is explored and bulky adenopathy is resected. Upper abdominal implants are removed if complete resection is possible.

Table 172–6	**Surgical Staging Procedure for Apparent Early-Stage Disease**

Remove primary tumor intact, send for frozen section if necessary. If apparently confined to ovaries or pelvis:

1. Thoroughly inspect pelvis and upper abdomen.
2. Submit any free fluid for cytology.
3. If no free fluid, peritoneal washings should be obtained.
4. Obtain biopsy tissue of any adhesions or suspicious areas. If none, sample multiple areas of the peritoneum.
5. Sample right diaphragm by biopsy or scraping sent for cytology.
6. Perform infracolic omentectomy.
7. Biopsy or remove pelvic and periaortic lymph nodes.

Even though some degree of debulking can be accomplished in almost every case, there are situations when resection is impossible. Examples include the following:

1. Perforation through the anterior abdominal wall in continuity with a large intraperitoneal omental cake with intrinsic, extensive involvement of upper gastrointestinal tract and the small bowel mesentery.
2. Extensive disease on the surface of the mesentery and in the mesenteric lymph nodes causing foreshortening, fixation, and extensive stricture of large segments of small bowel mesentery.

Pelvic disease rarely causes unresectability. Extensive upper abdominal disease, however, may make cytoreductive surgery prohibitive. In this case, a biopsy and description of the extent of disease is all that can reasonably be accomplished surgically.

The extent of the surgical procedure cannot be determined preoperatively. The operating surgeon should have experience and adequate time to allow the extensive dissections sometimes necessary. With care and persistence, significant cytoreduction can often be accomplished.

POSTOPERATIVE MANAGEMENT

Extensive dissection, particularly in the pelvis and in the retroperitoneum, increases the risk of pulmonary embolus, making antiembolic measures such as sequential compression hose important. Massive areas of deperitonealization, ascites, and malnutrition with low plasma oncotic pressure predispose the patient to fluid shifts, particularly depletion of intravascular volume into the extracellular third space. Thus, central venous monitoring should be considered. Gastrointestinal function may be delayed and nutritional support is an important consideration.

Because of the potential for volume shifts and electrolyte disorders, careful monitoring of blood chemistries is necessary, particularly in the first 48 hours postoperatively. Because of the extent of the surgical procedures, postoperative bleeding may occur and the blood counts should be monitored in the early postoperative period. Rapid resumption of physical activity with ambulation results in shorter hospital stays. Preadmission counseling and attitude are extremely important in encouraging patients to ambulate postoperatively and point toward earlier discharge.

In summary, postoperative management includes several important measures to prevent complications. These include early ambulation, thromboembolic prevention, fluid and electrolyte management, and early nutritional support. Care is also taken to ensure maintenance of pulmonary toilet and oxygenation to prevent atelectatic changes and pulmonary infections.

OUTCOMES

In the past 20 years, the overall 5-year survival rate for ovarian cancer has improved from approximately 30% to approximately 50%. Even though marked improvement in response rates to chemotherapy has been noted, the extent of residual disease is the significant indicator for long-term survival. If disease is localized, the 5-year survival rate is 90% as opposed to 28% if the tumor is stage III or IV. The majority of tumors, however, continue to be diagnosed in advanced stage. Efforts to improve prevention or early detection will hopefully result in a continued positive impact on survival.

Quality-of-life issues should be taken into consideration in each patient. An elderly patient who is compromised by antecedent medical conditions and who obviously has an advanced peritoneal carcinomatosis is probably better served by an initial trial of chemotherapy and an assessment of response.

Virtually every patient other than those with a stage IA, grade I ovarian cancer requires chemotherapy. The most active primary therapy is combined treatment with platinum compounds (carboplatin or cisplatin) plus paclitaxel given every 3 to 4 weeks for six courses or until there is disease progression.

Most patients do die of their disease. Efforts at extending useful life with symptom relief are important. Generally the patients have an extended course of dysfunctional gastrointestinal function with eventual mechanical obstruction and profound malnutrition. Sound judgment should be used when considering further surgery or chemotherapy as opposed to effective supportive palliative measures.

Interventions such as decompression gastrostomy, interval paracentesis, and thoracentesis with pleural sclerosis are useful on an individualized selective basis. Early involvement of hospice services is a tremendous resource for the patient and her family. The dying process can be

---

Pearls and Pitfalls

PEARLS

- A complete history and physical examination is generally more informative than a computed tomography scan.
- Most early-stage ovarian cancer is diagnosed serendipitously.
- There are conditions in the female pelvis other than ovarian cancer that cause masses.
- In unstaged cases of ovarian cancer that are clinically confined to the ovaries, a complete surgical staging procedure results in upstaging 30% to 40% of the time.
- Extensive disease in the pelvis alone is rarely, if ever, the reason that a patient cannot undergo cytoreduction.
- In medically compromised patients with obvious far advanced disease, neoadjuvant therapy with the goal of interval resection may offer the best quality of life.
- It is extremely important that physicians who provide ongoing care for patients with ovarian cancer are well trained and familiar with the disease. Even though ovarian malignancies are chemotherapy sensitive, resistance eventually develops and disease progresses. It is vital that those who provide care recognize the point at which further therapeutic intervention is fruitless and change the focus to quality-of-life measures.

prolonged and stressful. It is important that the attending surgeon maintain open proactive communication for support. These experiences can be most rewarding.

SELECTED READINGS

American College of Obstetrics and Gynecology Educational Bulletin. Washington, DC, American College of Obstetrics and Gynecology, August 1998, p 250.

Bailey CL, Ueland FR, Land GL, et al: The malignant potential of small cystic ovarian tumors in women over 50 years of age. Gynecol Oncol 1998;69:3.

Bridgewater JA, Nelstrop AE, Rustin GJS, et al: Comparison of standard and CA-125 response criteria in patients with epithelial ovarian cancer treated with platinum or paclitaxel. J Clin Oncol 1999;17:501.

Bristow RE, Lagasse LD, Karlan BY: Secondary surgical cytoreduction for advanced epithelial ovarian cancer. Cancer 1996;78:2049.

DiSaia PJ, Creasman WT: Epithelial ovarian cancer. In Clinical Gynecologic Oncology. St. Louis: Mosby–Year Book, 1997, pp 282–350.

Fleming ID, Cooper JS, Henson DE, et al (eds). AJCC Cancer Staging Handbook, From the AJCC Cancer Staging Manual, 5th ed. Philadelphia: Lippincott Williams & Wilkins, 1998, p 188.

Gershenson DM: Contemporary treatment of borderline ovarian tumors. Cancer Invest 1999;17:206.

Greenlee RT, Murray T, Bolden S, et al: Cancer statistics 2000. Cancer 2000;50:7.

Narod SA, Risch H, Moslehi R, et al: Oral contraceptives and the risk of hereditary ovarian cancer. N Engl J Med 1998;339:424.

Vergote I, De Wever I, Tjalma W, et al: Neoadjuvant chemotherapy or primary debulking surgery in advanced ovarian carcinoma: A retrospective analysis of 285 patients. Gynecol Oncol 1998;71:431.

Chapter 173

Endometrial Cancer

Terri B. Pustilnik

Endometrial cancer is the most common gynecologic malignancy and is the fourth most common cancer in women, preceded by breast, lung, and colorectal cancer. Approximately 36,000 new cases are diagnosed each year, with 6500 women dying from this disease (Cancer Facts and Figures, 2000). Most women with uterine cancers are diagnosed at an early stage, leading to an overall 5-year survival rate greater than 75% for patients with stage I disease. Although the incidence is higher among white women when compared with African American women, the mortality rate for this minority group is nearly double that of whites. This is likely due to the later stage of presentation and higher incidence of more aggressive tumor-type in this group. Surgery remains the treatment of choice for uterine carcinoma, since a clear survival advantage is seen when compared with treatment with other modalities alone. Surgical staging, adopted in 1988, includes a total abdominal hysterectomy, bilateral salpingo-oophorectomy, pelvic washings, and evaluation of the pelvic and periaortic lymph nodes, along with careful inspection of the abdomen and pelvis to assess for extrauterine spread (Benedet et al, 2000). These measures are important to determine the presence of extrauterine spread, which correlates with survival.

CLINICAL PRESENTATION

Initial Evaluation

The most common presentation for women with endometrial cancer is abnormal uterine bleeding, which generally causes women to seek medical care. Consequently, over 75% of all endometrial cancers are found at an early stage. The diagnosis is typically made in the office setting, with an endometrial biopsy by means of a narrow Pipelle endometrial suction curet. The sensitivity of this method approaches 97%, and it is easy to perform. For the rare patients unable to undergo an office evaluation because of an atrophic, stenotic endocervical canal or an inability to tolerate an office biopsy, or who have had a nondiagnostic endometrial biopsy with clinical factors highly suspicious for uterine cancer, a formal dilation and curettage is recommended. A pelvic ultrasound may also be useful in the evaluation of these patients. An endometrial stripe of greater than 5 mm delineates an abnormal value in the postmenopausal patient.

Risk Factors

Several risk factors are associated with the development of endometrial adencarcinoma (Table 173–1). These include obesity, postmenopausal status, family history, infer-

tility, and complex endometrial hyperplasia with atypia. Although the cause of endometrial carcinoma is unknown, the association of unopposed estrogen with well-differentiated adenocarcinoma is clearly documented. Postmenopausal women with an intact uterus who take estrogen therapy alone have a 4-fold to 15-fold risk of developing endometrial carcinoma. Therefore, the current practice recommendation when administering hormone replacement therapy is to prescribe both low-dose estrogen and progesterone. This combination regimen has been shown to decrease substantially the risk of developing uterine cancer when compared with estrogen alone. Other states associated with increased levels of estrogen, and therefore an increased risk of endometrial carcinoma, are in women with granulosa germ cell tumors of the ovary, and those with prolonged anovulation as in polycystic ovarian disease. Both pregnancy and oral contraceptive use provide protection against the development of endometrial cancer.

Tamoxifen, the antiestrogen agent used in the treatment and prevention of breast cancer, also appears to be associated with a twofold to threefold increased risk of endometrial carcinoma (American College of Obstetricians and Gynecologists, 1996), and it likely exerts a stimulatory effect on the endometrium. However, the true incidence of endometrial carcinoma due to tamoxifen use is difficult to assess, because of confounding factors and bias. Women who are taking tamoxifen have more physician visits than those who are not on tamoxifen. Additionally, since there is a known genetic association between breast, colon, and endometrial cancer, these women may be more predisposed to developing endometrial carcinoma compared with those who do not take tamoxifen.

The current recommendation for women on tamoxifen is yearly gynecologic examinations. Routine screening for endometrial cancer with ultrasound or endometrial biopsy is not advocated, but physician discretion may be used. It is most important that any abnormal uterine bleeding that develops in these patients should be promptly evaluated by endometrial sampling. An association between tamoxi-

Table 173–1	Risk Factors Associated with Endometrial Carcinoma

Unopposed estrogen
Obesity
Tamoxifen
Endometrial hyperplasia with atypia
Nulliparity
Late menopause
Genetic predisposition (e.g., hereditary nonpolyposis colon cancer)

Table 173–2	Corpus Cancer Surgical Staging, FIGO 1988		
Stage IA	Grade 1,2,3	Tumor limited to endometrium	
Stage IB	Grade 1,2,3	Invasion of less than one half the myometrium	
Stage IC	Grade 1,2,3	Invasion of more than one half the myometrium	
Stage IIA	Grade 1,2,3	Endocervical glandular involvement only	
Stage IIB	Grade 1,2,3	Cervical stromal invasion	
Stage IIIA	Grade 1,2,3	Tumor invades serosa and/or adnexa, and/or positive peritoneal cytology	
Stage IIIB	Grade 1,2,3	Vaginal metastases	
Stage IIIC	Grade 1,2,3	Metastases to pelvic and/or para-aortic lymph nodes	
Stage IVA	Grade 1,2,3	Tumor invasion of bladder and/or bowel mucosa	
Stage IVB	Grade 1,2,3	Distant metastases, including intra-abdominal and/or inguinal lymph nodes	
	Grade 1	5% or less of a nonsquamous or nonmorular solid growth pattern	
	Grade 2	6%–50% of a nonsquamous or nonmorular solid growth pattern	
	Grade 3	>50% of a nonsquamous or nonmorular solid growth pattern	

FIGO, International Federation of Gynecology and Obstetrics.

fen use and benign uterine pathology, such as endometrial polyps and cystic endometrial atrophy, has been noted.

PREOPERATIVE MANAGEMENT

Preoperative Evaluation

An initial evaluation consists of a thorough examination, including palpation of the supra-clavicular, inguinal, and pelvic lymph node regions. Careful attention should be directed to palpation of the cervix, vaginal wall, parametrium, pelvic sidewall, and cul de sac, as these are sites that may be involved with metastases. A chest radiograph is performed for staging purposes to rule out distant metastases, and routine blood specimens are drawn for examination, such as a hematocrit in preparation for surgery. Depending on other factors, such as age, underlying medical conditions, and anesthesia risks, other testing may include assessment of cardiac and renal function. Preoperative imaging studies such as a CT scan do not usually alter a treatment plan (Connor et al, 2000). CT scans have a limited ability to detect lymph node metastasis (particularly microscopic involvement) and to evaluate accurately the depth of myometrial invasion. Since most patients have disease confined to the uterus, preoperative radiographic testing is not routinely recommended unless examination or symptoms warrant evaluation.

The role of preoperative uterine irradiation has been evaluated extensively in clinical trials by the multi-institutional Gynecologic Oncology Group but has not been shown to have an impact on survival or to alter a clinical course or treatment plan. Consequently, radiation therapy is usually reserved for the postoperative patient with high-risk factors for recurrence.

Staging

In 1988, the International Federation of Gynecology and Obstetrics (FIGO) changed the staging of endometrial carcinoma from clinical to surgical (Benedet et al, 2000). This method has provided a more accurate assessment of the true extent of disease and is consequently a better reflection of prognosis. The current FIGO staging classification for uterine carcinoma is outlined in Table 173–2. Clinical staging is reserved for the rare patient who is not a surgical candidate (Table 173–3). Treatment in this setting usually consists of pelvic radiation therapy. An improved survival benefit is seen in patients with endometrial carcinoma who are treated surgically when compared with radiation therapy. Consequently, a surgical approach with proper staging is recommended if medically feasible.

INTRAOPERATIVE MANAGEMENT

An exploratory laparotomy is performed through a low midline incision, which allows for adequate visualization of the deep pelvis and pelvic vessels. Pelvic washings are then taken, followed by careful palpation of the abdomen and pelvis to evaluate for any evidence of extrauterine spread, such as peritoneal or adnexal implants. A total abdominal hysterectomy and bilateral salpingo-oophorectomy are then performed, followed by surgical removal of pelvic and periaortic lymph nodes. Neither reperitonealization of the retroperitoneal space nor placement of a drain is routinely necessary. Attempts at resection of gross disease outside the uterus are reasonable after consideration of the risks and benefits of the procedure.

Table 173–3	Corpus Cancer Clinical Staging, FIGO 1971
Stage I	The carcinoma is confined to the corpus
IA	The length of the uterine cavity is 8 cm or less
IB	The length of the uterine cavity is more than 8 cm
II	The carcinoma involves the corpus and cervix
III	The carcinoma extends outside the uterus but not outside the true pelvis
IV	The carcinoma extends outside the true pelvis or involves the bladder or rectum
G1	Highly differentiated adenomatous carcinoma
G2	Differentiated adenomatous carcinoma with partly solid areas
G3	Predominantly solid or entirely undifferentiated carcinoma

FIGO, International Federation of Gynecology and Obstetrics.

Table 173–4	**Risk Categories Following Surgical Staging**	
LOW RISK	**INTERMEDIATE RISK**	**HIGH RISK**
IA (grade 1,2)	IA (grade 3) IB, IC (grade 1,2,3) IIA, IIB (grade 1,2,3) Positive cytology only	IIIA, IIIB, IIIC (grade 1,2,3) IVA, IVB (grade 1,2,3)

Evaluation of Lymph Node Status

Pelvic and periaortic lymph node assessment is important for accurately staging patients, since it aids in determining prognosis and the need for adjuvant treatment. Based on the staging information, patients can be divided into high- and low-risk categories for tumor recurrence (Table 173–4). Lymph node metastases typically spread in a stepwise fashion, and periaortic lymph nodes are rarely involved if pelvic lymph nodes are negative. The risk for periaortic lymph node metastases has been associated with several factors, including deep myometrial invasion, adnexal involvement, and higher tumor grade. Detecting periaortic involvement in the high-risk patient is important, since long-term survival may be improved if adjuvant therapy with extended field radiation is used (Morrow et al, 1991).

Controversy over the extent of the lymph node evaluation still exists. Some researchers routinely recommend a complete pelvic and periaortic lymphadenectomy, while others recommend only a lymph node sampling. Roughly half of all lymph node metastases are less than 1 cm, making palpation and preoperative imaging techniques inadequate for detection. Additionally, a significant number of lymph nodes must be evaluated in order to detect the presence of metastases. Recently, an improvement in survival has been noted in patients who receive a complete lymphadenectomy. Kilgore and associates (1995) compared a group of patients with endometrial carcinoma who underwent extensive lymph node excision with a group that had limited or no lymph node sampling. Survival was significantly improved in those who had a complete surgical evaluation of the pelvic and periaortic sites. When further stratified into high- and low-risk groups based on whether the tumor appeared to be confined to the uterus, the low-risk group also demonstrated an improved survival. Limitations of this study, however, include the small number of patients and the retrospective nature of the report.

On the contrary, other investigators have concluded that surgical staging provides prognostic information only, with no associated survival benefit. Additionally, an increased complication rate of up to 19% has been reported when a thorough staging lymphadenectomy is performed (Morrow et al, 1991). Complications included gastrointestinal injury or obstruction, genitourinary injury or obstruction, thrombophlebitis, pulmonary embolism, wound abscess, hemorrhage, evisceration, death, lymphedema, and lymphocyst formation, all of which can result in longer hospital stays. The complication rate also increases with the addition of postoperative radiation therapy.

An intraoperative assessment based on frozen section of the uterus is used by some as a guide to determine the extent of lymph node dissection. If low-risk factors are present (such as less than 50% myometrial invasion, no cervical or lower uterine segment tumor involvement, and a well-differentiated tumor grade), a lymph node sampling may be deferred. However, since treatment is based on an intraoperative pathologic evaluation, the surgeon should be aware of the possible discrepancy of the frozen section with the final pathologic diagnosis.

The only patient in whom the risk/benefit ratio may be limited for a lymph node evaluation is the patient with a well-differentiated tumor with superficial or no myometrial invasion. In this subset of patients, the incidence of lymph node metastases is 0% to 3%. However, difficulty arises in identifying these patients preoperatively and intraoperatively, given the limitations in accuracy of preoperative screening and frozen section.

Surgical Cytoreduction

Prolonged survival for patients with gross disease extending beyond the uterus is variable and depends on the sites involved and tumor volume; therefore, the role of surgical tumor cytoreduction for women with advanced stage endometrial adenocarcinoma is not well defined. However, a few reports have documented an improved survival in patients who had successfully received an optimal tumor reduction with residual disease of less than 2 cm. In a retrospective review, Chi and colleagues (1997) evaluated the impact of surgical tumor cytoreduction and survival in patients with stage IV endometrial carcinoma and noted an improved survival in those who had an optimal tumor reduction. To date, no prospective randomized trials have been performed. Therefore the patient's underlying medical condition, prognosis, and feasibility of tumor resection should be taken into consideration when gross intra-abdominal metastases are found.

Laparoscopy

Laparoscopic staging of patients with endometrial carcinoma may play a role in the properly chosen patient. Limitations include operator skill and body habitus. Several preliminary nonrandomized studies have confirmed the feasibility and safety of this technique. An initial cost evaluation has demonstrated no difference between laparoscopy and laparotomy. Improvement in operator time and number of nodes recovered increases with the number of procedures done, and morbidity with this technique does appear acceptable. Currently, the role of laparoscopy-assisted vaginal hysterectomy and lymph node dissection is being evaluated in a randomized fashion by the Gynecologic Oncology Group in patients with stages I and IIA endometrial carcinoma.

POSTOPERATIVE MANAGEMENT

Since many patients with endometrial cancer are elderly and obese, postoperative care should include prophylactic measures to prevent pneumonia and thromboembolic disease. Therefore, the use of incentive spirometer is initiated early once the patient is awake. Because women who have an underlying malignancy and undergo pelvic surgery have an approximately 20% risk of developing a deep venous thrombosis, compression boots should be left in place until the patient is fully ambulatory. The Foley catheter is left in place until the first postoperative day to allow recovery of bladder function. Depending on the extent of surgery, clear liquids can be started on the first postoperative day and the diet advanced slowly. Most patients can be discharged on postoperative day 3 if the course has been unremarkable.

Prognostic Factors

Several studies have helped identify features that are important in determining the risk for tumor recurrence. These factors include stage, presence of lymph node metastases, depth of myometrial invasion, cervical involvement, histologic grade, aneuploidy, lymph-vascular space invasion (LVSI), and the number of risk factors present (Morrow et al, 1991; Creasman et al, 1987). In a large trial evaluating the surgical and pathologic risk factors associated with endometrial carcinoma, Morrow and associates (1991) identified a subgroup of patients with the greatest risk for treatment failure. These included patients with extrauterine spread, especially para-aortic lymph node metastasis, and those with multiple risk factors. Histologic grade was noted to be important for the patient with disease confined to the uterus. For example, when a grade 3 tumor is present, the risk of recurrence is fifteen. Additionally, the depth of invasion correlated with the risk for recurrence. A 5-year survival rate of 95% for patients with less than 50% myometrial invasion was reported, compared with 75% for those with greater than 50% invasion. Others have noted a poorer outcome when LVSI was present. For example, patients with LVSI had a 27% rate of disease recurrence or death, compared with 9% when LVSI was not present. Additionally, the Gynecologic Oncology Group (Creasman et al, 1987) demonstrated a 5-year survival of 61% vs. 86% in women with early-stage disease who had LVSI. The significance of isolated positive peritoneal cytology is less well established.

Several trials have attempted to evaluate the specific risks associated with these various prognostic factors. However, because of the large number of risk factors, the development of a risk profile for the individual patient is extremely difficult and not practical at present.

Adjuvant Therapy

Treatment with adjuvant therapy remains controversial, as few randomized trials have been performed to compare different treatment strategies. The most commonly used adjuvant therapy in the treatment of endometrial cancer is radiation, either external beam whole pelvic radiation, vaginal brachytherapy or both. Complications resulting from postoperative radiation therapy are not insignificant and range from minor bowel disturbances to serious gastrointestinal and genitourinary hemorrhage and bowel obstruction. External beam irradiation is often used if metastatic spread is found in the pelvic and periaortic regions, or for the patient with possible occult micrometastases.

Two studies have evaluated the utility of postoperative irradiation in a randomized fashion. The first study randomized patients with early-stage endometrial cancer following initial surgical treatment and vaginal brachytherapy to external beam radiation versus observation therapy and then compared outcomes (Aalders et al, 1980). Although fewer locoregional recurrences were found in the radiotherapy arm (1.9% vs. 6.9%), distant metastases were more common (9.9% vs. 5.4%). Overall 5-year survivals were similar between the two groups. When a subgroup analysis was performed, adjuvant therapy in patients with poorly differentiated tumors and deep myometrial invasion demonstrated a possible benefit. The second study randomized patients with stage I endometrial carcinoma to pelvic radiotherapy versus observation (Creutzberg, 2000). Actuarial 5-year survival rates were similar, and locoregional recurrences were higher in the control group than in the treated group (14% vs. 4%).

These two trials confirm a reduction in local recurrence with radiation therapy. However, no improvement in long-term survival has been shown. At present, many oncologists recommend adjuvant radiation therapy for the patients with early-stage disease who have higher risk factors for recurrence, such as extensive myometrial invasion or grade 3 disease or both (Naumann et al, 1999).

Various cytotoxic chemotherapies have been evaluated in the treatment of endometrial cancer, and the most active agents are cisplatin, carboplatin, doxorubicin (Adriamycin), and paclitaxol (Taxol). These agents are

---

Pearls and Pitfalls

PEARLS

- Perform endometrial evaluation (biopsy) on any postmenopausal patient with vaginal bleeding.
- Abnormal uterine bleeding in any patient taking tamoxifen requires an evaluation.
- Do not use unopposed estrogen in a patient with an intact uterus because of the increased risk of endometrial cancer
- Accurately stage the patient with endometrial adenocarcinoma in order to determine prognosis. This requires a surgical evaluation of the pelvic and periaortic lymph nodes when technically and medically possible.
- Consider postoperative therapy in patients with stage I disease with poor prognostic features, as well as in those with extrauterine spread.
- Use caution when ligating the infundibulopelvic ligament and uterine artery, as the most common site of ureteral injury during a hysterectomy is at the pelvic brim and the cardinal ligament.

Table 173–5	Overall 5-Year Survival of Patients with Carcinoma of the Uterus

SURGICAL STAGE	5-YEAR SURVIVAL (%)
I	87
II	71.9
III	50.8
IV	8.8

often reserved for the patient with advanced disease or in the salvage setting. Previous trials have used a combination of agents in patients with stage I disease with high-risk features, as well as single agents in conjunction with radiation therapy. However, the optimal role of chemotherapy in endometrial carcinoma has not yet been determined.

Hormonal agents such as progesterone have demonstrated some efficacy in the treatment of endometrial adenocarcinoma. Although variable, responses are mainly limited to patients with well-differentiated, progesterone receptor–positive tumors. In general, first-line therapy with these agents is reserved for the patient who is not a surgical or irradiation candidate. Routine use in the adjuvant setting for high-risk patients is not currently recommended, as reports have not demonstrated an improved survival when these agents are used, either alone or in conjunction with standard treatment.

OUTCOMES

Overall five-year survival varies with stage (Table 173–5), and patients with stage IA disease have the best prognosis, with a 5-year survival of over 90%. Of patients who ultimately undergo recurrence, approximately half are found to have locoregional disease. Treatment results are poor for patients with distant recurrences, with a reported long-term survival rate of only 4% (Aalders et al, 1980). Patients who have local recurrence and have not received previous pelvic radiotherapy may be treated with radiation therapy. It has been suggested that patients with local recurrence who have not received pelvic radiotherapy have an improved survival when compared with those who have received previous radiotherapy (Aalders et al, 1980; Creutzberg et al, 2000). Those who have previously received maximal radiation therapy to the pelvis may be treated with chemotherapy or hormonal agents. Rarely, recurrent disease will present as an isolated vaginal mass in a patient who has previously received pelvic irradiation. In this setting, after a thorough survey to rule out distant metastasis, a pelvic exenteration may be considered.

SELECTED READINGS

Aalders J, Abeler V, Kolstad P, Onsrud M: Postoperative external irradiation and prognostic parameters in stage I endometrial carcinoma: Clinical and histopathologic study of 540 patients. Obstet Gynecol 1980;56:419.

American College of Obstetricians and Gynecologists Committee on Gynecologic Practices: Tamoxifen and endometrial cancer: Committee opinion. Danvers, MA, Copyright Clearance Center, 1996, p 169.

American Cancer Society: Cancer Facts and Figures 2000. Dallas, TX, American Cancer Society; 2000, p 17.

Benedet JL, Bender H, Jones III H, et al: FIGO staging classifications and clinical practice guidelines in the management of gynecologic cancers. FIGO Committee on Gynecologic Oncology. Int J Gynecol Obstet 2000;20:209.

Chi DS, Welshinger M, Venkatraman ES, Barakat RR: The role of surgical cytoreduction in stage IV endometrial carcinoma. Gynecol Oncol 1997;67:56.

Connor JP, Andrews JI, Anderson B, Buller RE: Computed tomography in endometrial carcinoma. Obstet Gynecol 2000;95:692.

Creasman WT, Morrow CP, Bundy BM, et al: Surgical pathologic spread patterns of endometrial cancer: A Gynecologic Oncology Group Study. Cancer 1987;60:2035.

Creutzberg CL, van Putten WLJ, Koper PCM, et al: Surgery and postoperative radiotherapy versus surgery alone for patients with stage-1 endometrial carcinoma: Multicentre randomised trial. Lancet 2000;355:1404.

Kilgore LC, Partridge, EE, Alvarez RD, et al: Adenocarcinoma of the endometrium: Survival comparisons of patients with and without pelvic node sampling. Gynecol Oncol 1995;56:29.

Morrow CP, Bundy BM, Kurman RJ, et al: Relationship between surgical-pathological risk factors and outcome in clinical stage I and II carcinoma of the endometrium: A Gynecologic Oncology Group Study. Gynecol Oncol 1991;40:55.

Naumann RW, Higgins RV, Hall JB: The use of adjuvant radiation therapy by members of the Society of Gynecologic Oncologists. Gynecol Oncol 1999;75:4.

Chapter 174
Cervical Cancer

James W. Orr, Jr.

The incidence of invasive cervical malignancy began to decline in the United States in the 1940s and has continued to decrease following the introduction and routine incorporation of the Papanicolaou smear into well-woman health care. Regardless of this trend, cancer of the cervix is still regarded as an important women's health problem, ranking as the sixth most common cause of cancer deaths in the United States and the second most common cause of female cancer deaths worldwide. The false-negative rate of a single Papanicolaou screening test is reported to approach 50% in some clinical situations. This potential problem has resulted in the development and acceptance of new screening techniques (i.e., liquid-based cytology) as well as automated and other computerized technologies to evaluate the primary smear and to facilitate the process of mandatory re-screening of negative smears. While contributing to an increased number of diagnoses of intraepithelial lesions and perhaps a lessened need for "repeat" of unsatisfactory or atypical squamous cells of undetermined significance (ASCUS) smears, new Pap smear technologies have not been directly linked to an improved diagnosis of invasive cancer, lessening the risk of developing invasive cervix cancer, or favorably affecting the survival of women alternately diagnosed with cervix cancer. Despite the ready availability of screening and the development of new screening techniques and strategies, more than 50% of new diagnoses and the majority of cervical cancer deaths can be linked to a failure to obtain recent cervical cancer screening (e.g., patient failure to obtain cytology, physician failure to perform screening, or inappropriate evaluation of an abnormal or unsatisfactory cytologic smear).

Following diagnosis, management of cervical cancer may necessitate the need for a number of surgical procedures of varying complexity and risk, used alone or in combination, to establish a diagnosis, to define extent of disease (staging), or to treat primary or recurrent disease (Table 174–1).

DEMOGRAPHICS, RISK FACTORS, AND SYMPTOMS

Whereas premalignant disease (intraepithelial neoplasia) frequently occurs in the second and third decade of life, the average age of women with invasive cervix cancer is approximately 50 years. Many risk factors have been identified (Table 174–2) that qualify cervical malignancy as a sexually transmitted disease. The oncogenic subtypes of the human papillomavirus (HPV) are of particular known etiologic importance. Typically, women with cervix cancer are not obese (weighing approximately 150 pounds), but frequently abuse nicotine. The associated increased risk of coexisting pulmonary disease and predis-

position to perioperative pulmonary complications is of importance, both because of their relationship to development of perioperative pulmonary morbidity and because of their associated risk for development of a concurrent or subsequent second primary. Fewer than half (40%) of women with invasive disease have other significant coexisting medical disease that may increase the risk of surgical morbidity. Regardless of perceived patient risk, no definitive surgical treatment should be undertaken without a thorough preoperative clinical evaluation to exclude or detect the presence of existing comorbidity so as to prepare for pulmonary, cardiac, renal, gastrointestinal, or other perioperative morbidity.

Whereas intraepithelial neoplasia is usually asymptomatic, women with early and advanced invasive cervical disease may have a myriad of signs and symptoms, including abnormal bleeding, postcoital spotting, abnormal vaginal discharge, lower extremity edema, obstructive uropathy, or pelvic or back pain that prompts clinical investigation. Regardless of clinical findings, it would be unusual and perhaps inappropriate to complete definitive surgical therapy without obtaining histologic confirmation of the presence and extent of invasive disease.

DIAGNOSTIC AND STAGING SURGICAL PROCEDURES

Despite the incidence of false-negative results, Papanicolaou smears represent one of the few proven beneficial

Table 174–1	Cervix Cancer Surgical Procedures
DIAGNOSIS AND STAGING	**TREATMENT**
Colposcopy	Conization
Conization	LEEP
LEEP	Cold knife
Cold knife	Trachelectomy
Trachelectomy	Hysterectomy
Hysterectomy	Abdominal
Abdominal	Vaginal
Vaginal	Laparoscopic assisted
Laparoscopic assisted	Radical hysterectomy
Lymphadenectomy	Abdominal
Transperitoneal	Modified abdominal
Retroperitoneal	Vaginal
Laparoscopic	Laparoscopic assisted
Ovarian transposition	Radical trachelectomy
	Radical parametrectomy
	Lymphadenectomy
	Abdominal
	Laparoscopic
	Exenteration (partial or total)
	Urinary conduit
	Rectal reanastomosis
	Vaginal reconstruction

LEEP, loop electric excision procedure.

Table 174–2 | Cervix Cancer: Risk Factors

Human papillomavirus infection (oncogenic subtype)
Early intercourse (younger than 17 years of age)
Multiple sexual partners
Early pregnancy
Urban population
Low socioeconomic status
Immunocompromised state
Nicotine abuse
History of abnormal cytology
Failure to participate in screening
Nutritional deficits
Infertility (tubal damage)
Use of oral contraceptives
Intercourse with high-risk males
Diethylstilbestrol (DES) exposure

screening tests for cancer. All women with cytologic high-grade intraepithelial abnormalities and many with lesser smear abnormalities are customarily evaluated with a colposcopic (magnification) examination to establish a diagnosis before definitive treatment. The latter group is of particular importance because a significant proportion (≥60%) of patients with histologic evidence of high-grade preinvasive and invasive disease are initially evaluated during the investigation of low-grade cytologic abnormali-

ties. Many patients with high-grade intraepithelial neoplasia may be effectively evaluated and efficiently treated with local incision at the initial visit. However, colposcopic examination remains the gold standard of evaluation for patients with high-grade cytologic abnormalities and a significant proportion of all patients with any abnormal cervical cytology. This relatively painless, minor office procedure requires no anesthesia, carries little risk of significant bleeding or infection (≤1%), and allows targeted or directed biopsy of the most abnormal-appearing cervical epithelium. Colposcopy can be made simple and less painful using an appropriately sized vaginal speculum and sharp biopsy instruments.

In patients with clinically occult cervical disease, an office LEEP (loop electric excision procedure) cone or cold knife conization may be necessary to establish the presence or extent of invasive disease (Table 174–3). These diagnostic procedures are invaluable in that the histologic results obtained at conization have absolute implications for the prescription of surgery and other therapy. LEEP can typically be completed in the office setting using local (paracervical) anesthesia with a minimal risk of significant bleeding, infection, or other problems (≤5%). Even though LEEP is a minor surgical procedure, the results are highly operator dependent. Surgical methods to ensure complete resection of the

Table 174–3 | FIGO Staging for Carcinoma of the Cervix

STAGE	DESCRIPTION
Stage 0	Carcinoma in situ, intraepithelial carcinoma.
Stage I	The carcinoma is strictly confined to the cervix (disregard extension to corpus).
IA	Invasive cancer identified only microscopically. All gross lesions even with superficial invasion are stage IB cancers. Invasion is limited to measured stromal invasion with maximum depth of 5 mm and no wider than 7 mm°
IA1	Measured invasion of stroma no greater than 3 mm in depth and no wider than 7 mm.
IA2	Measured invasion of stroma greater than 3 mm and no greater than 5 mm in depth, and no wider than 7 mm.
IB	Clinical lesions confined to the cervix or preclinical lesions greater than stage IA.
IB1	Clinical lesions no greater than 4 cm in size.
IB2	Clinical lesions greater than 4 cm in size.
Stage II	The carcinoma extends beyond the cervix but has not extended to the pelvic wall. The carcinoma involves the vagina but not as far as the lower third.
IIA	No obvious parametrial involvement.
IIB	Obvious parametrial involvement.
Stage III	The carcinoma has extended to the pelvic wall. On rectal examination, there is no cancer-free space between the tumor and the pelvic wall.† The tumor involves the lower third of the vagina. All cases with a hydronephrosis or nonfunctioning kidney are included unless they are known to be due to other causes.‡
IIIA	No extension to the pelvic wall.
IIIB	Extension to the pelvic wall and/or hydronephrosis or nonfunctioning kidney.
Stage IV	The carcinoma has extended beyond the true pelvis or has clinically involved the mucosa of the bladder or rectum. A bullous edema as such does not permit a case to be allotted to stage IV.
IVA	Spread of the growth to adjacent organs.¶
IVB	Spread to distant organs.

°The depth of invasion should not be more than 5 mm taken from the base of the epithelium, either surface or glandular, from which it originates. Vascular space involvement, either venous or lymphatic, should not alter the staging.
†A patient with a growth fixed to the pelvic wall by a short and indurated but not nodular parametrium should be assigned to stage IIB. It is impossible, at clinical examination, to decide whether a smooth and indurated parametrium is truly cancerous or only inflammatory. Therefore, the case should be placed in stage III only if the parametrium is nodular on the pelvic wall or if the growth itself extends to the pelvic wall.
‡The presence of hydronephrosis or nonfunctioning kidney due to stenosis of the ureter by cancer permits a case to be assigned to stage III even if, according to the other findings, the case should be assigned to stage I or II.
¶The presence of bullous edema, as such, should not permit a case to be allocated to stage IV. Ridges and furrows in the bladder wall should be interpreted as signs of submucous involvement of the bladder if they remain fixed to the growth during palpation (i.e., examination from the vagina or the rectum during cystoscopy). A finding of malignant cells in cytologic washings from the urinary bladder requires further examination and biopsy from the wall of the bladder.
From FIGO, International Federation of Gynecology and Obstetrics.

ectocervical or endocervical lesion should be incorporated to improve outcome and lessen the need for additional evaluation or treatment. Although frequently adequate for the management of intraepithelial neoplasia, it has been suggested that the histologic specimens obtained at LEEP conization are less predictive than those from cold knife conization in establishing the correct diagnosis of early invasive cervical disease. This bias is likely related to repeated problems with tissue orientation and the frequent occurrence of coagulation artifact at the surgical margins. Given these potential problems, knowledge of direct or indirect procedural risks must be incorporated into every treatment or diagnostic decision. Cold knife conization carries the additional risk of requiring general or regional anesthesia and an increased risk of additional (unnecessary) cervical stroma resection, potentially predisposing women to difficulties with future fertility, premature delivery, or pregnancy loss. The selection of the "best" diagnostic procedure should be individualized and either LEEP or cold knife conization can be performed safely in most clinical situations. Both have significant diagnostic and therapeutic benefits and neither offers significant patient risk in the absence of pregnancy or early invasive adenocarcinoma. It is rarely necessary to perform conization during pregnancy. Invasive disease can usually be excluded during colposcopic evaluation and there is no *apparent* reason to treat premalignant cervical disease during pregnancy. In fact, many high-grade intraepithelial abnormalities undergo spontaneous regression after cervical dilatation and vaginal delivery. Residual postdelivery intraepithelial neoplasia can be safely treated in the postpartum state. The multifocal nature of cervical adenocarcinoma probably mandates the incorporation of cold knife conization as the diagnostic or therapeutic method of choice for women with in situ or early invasive adenocarcinoma. Like for other surgical procedures, the surgeon must decide clinically as to the potential risk–benefit ratio of the operative procedure, allowing rational, individualized selection of the most appropriate surgical approach. Adequate conization (negative margins) is diagnostic and usually therapeutic in women with intraepithelial disease. Hysterectomy is not necessary following conization with intraepithelial neoplasia and negative margins but may be required or used in women with other coexisting gynecologic problems or recurrent high-grade intraepithelial disease. The use of total hysterectomy (vaginal, abdominal, laparoscopic-assisted) as primary treatment of intraepithelial neoplasia increases surgical risks. Additionally, the presence of intraepithelial squamous cell disease and involved conization margins does not necessitate hysterectomy. At least 60% of women with involved margins have no residual disease at subsequent hysterectomy. However, if postconization hysterectomy is not performed, this population subset deserves close surveillance with frequent examinations. Repeat cervical cytologic sampling at 6-month intervals or sooner is recommended.

Adequate conization (negative margins) may also suffice as adequate treatment for those with stage IA1 squamous cell disease. Just as with intraepithelial disease, hysterectomy may be indicated for treatment of coexisting gynecologic disease. Although lacking extensive documentation, recent information suggests that early invasive adenocarcinoma can be successfully managed with the same treatment as early invasive squamous cell cancers. Additional postconization treatment (hysterectomy, radical hysterectomy) is usually recommended for women with early invasive disease and involved conization margins. Persistent invasive disease or more significant invasive disease is present in one of four women who have positive margins and early invasive disease on conization.

The technique of these minor surgical procedures as well as the appropriate histologic evaluation of excised tissues has been described elsewhere; however, attention to surgical technique designed to maximize the opportunity for establishing the correct diagnosis and offering cure while minimizing the amount of excised cervical stroma potentially lessens the adverse effect on later reproductive outcome.

STAGING

Cervical cancer remains a *clinically* staged disease. Specific studies (Table 174–4) are allowed by the International Federation of Gynecology and Obstetrics to complete clinical staging. Whereas findings from additional radiologic and endoscopic evaluation may dramatically alter actual treatment strategy and facilitate the delivery of directed therapy, results from these studies should not be used to assign clinical disease stage. Importantly, most radiologic and endoscopic procedures can be safely omitted in women with early disease (less than or equal to stage 1B1) who will undergo an attempt at surgical cure.

Gynecologic oncologists are the surgical subspecialists specifically trained in the surgical and nonsurgical management of cervical cancer, and consultation and referral could benefit any woman with an invasive cervical malignancy. This consult is of specific importance to patients because it effectively lessens the adverse effects associated with the long learning curve associated with performing gynecologic cancer surgery.

SURGICAL TREATMENT FOR EARLY-STAGE DISEASE

A majority (52%) of women with invasive cervix cancer are first seen with disease clinically confined to the

Table 174–4	**Staging Procedures Allowed by FIGO**

Physical examination. Palpate lymph nodes, examine vagina, bimanual rectovaginal examination.
Radiologic studies. Intravenous pyelogram, barium enema, chest radiograph, skeletal radiograph.
Procedures. Biopsy, conization, hysteroscopy, colposcopy, endocervical curettage, examination with patient under anesthesia, cystoscopy, proctoscopy.
Optional studies. The information from which the clinical stage cannot change include the following: computed axial tomography, lymphangiography, ultrasonography, magnetic resonance imaging, radionuclide scanning, positron emission tomography, and laparoscopy.

From FIGO, International Federation of Gynecology and Obstetrics.

cervix (stage I). Adequate treatment may vary dramatically depending on substage (see Table 174–3). Although not exact, clinical stage indicates the extent of disease (and necessity of treatment and evaluation) of the cervix, parametrium, and regional nodes. The need or benefit of pretreatment radiologic or endoscopic studies in these women to detect parametrial or extracervical involvement is unproved and considered to be of little clinical benefit.

Earliest stage invasive cervical disease (1A1) exhibits an extremely low risk of parametrial or nodal involvement and is adequately treated by conization alone, with an exceptionally low risk of recurrence (≤1%). When conization margins are negative and there is no evidence of lymph vascular space involvement, this low-risk procedure can be safely offered as definitive therapy to women who wish to maintain their fertility or to women not deemed to be candidates for a more extensive (total vaginal or abdominal hysterectomy) surgical procedure for other indications. When conization is the anticipated diagnostic and therapeutic approach, cold knife excision is the preferred method of management because it is most likely to result in the correct diagnosis and ensure margin adequacy. However, if the diagnosis is established after review of a specimen from a LEEP cone, re-excision may be unnecessary when the initial margins are deemed adequate.

In specific situations (desire to maintain fertility), conization alone may be considered adequate therapy for women with stage 1A2 disease. However, more extensive procedures should be considered the standard care for women with stage 1A2 disease (particularly with lymph vascular space involvement) because they have a risk of nodal disease (8%) and exhibit a low, but significant, risk of recurrence with less than "radical" therapy. Although controversial, the incidence of parametrial involvement is low (≤4%) and in most instances surgical resection at the cervical-parametrial interface (total hysterectomy) is safe. Whereas an abdominal operation allows adequate exposure and facilitates the completion of lymph node dissection, a vaginal operation combined with a laparoscopic lymphadenectomy represents an acceptable alternative for those women deemed candidates. Regardless of approach, adequate nodal dissection involves evaluation and dissection of the external, internal, common iliac, and lower para-aortic lymph nodes using the inferior mesenteric artery as the superior border, the mid psoas muscle as the lateral margin, the obturator nerve as the inferior margin, and the circumflex iliac vein as the distal margin. Even though operative time may be increased and it may be more expensive, laparoscopic nodal dissection when combined with total vaginal or laparoscopic-assisted vaginal hysterectomy offers the potential for less operative morbidity and improved quality of life. The latter results in a short hospital stay (2 days or less) and rapid return to full function (3 weeks or less). The laparoscopic node procedure is technically more difficult in women with high body mass index (>35). If parametrial resection is deemed necessary in this population subset, a modified resection to minimize acute and long-term morbidity is advisable. Cure should be the expected result in greater than or equal to 95% of women with stage IA2 disease.

With more advanced disease (IB1), curative surgical therapy is designed to resect the cervix, a portion of the parametrium (≥50%), 2 to 3 cm of the upper vagina, and regional lymph nodes. The classic Wertheim hysterectomy (technically described elsewhere) resects nearly the entire parametrium and is associated with a higher short-term and late complication rate than a total hysterectomy. Safe completion of the parametrial resection involves complete "unroofing" of the bladder from the distal pelvic ureter and is associated with an increased risk of urinary injury. In fact, estimated blood loss approaches 1000 mL, urinary injury occurs in approximately 3% of operations, and neurologic injury occurs in 1% of patients. Infection morbidity is relatively rare (≤5%). Bladder dysfunction after parametrial resection is common and nearly 50% of women void with straining. Additionally, parametrial resection increases the risk of rectal dysfunction.

Important modifications to the classic radical procedure include the development of modified radical hysterectomy that results in a lessened parametrial resection and decreased risk of perioperative complications. Acute complications of bleeding are also less and the risk of long-term bladder dysfunction is significantly reduced. Less radical resection of the parametrium is a safe alternative in that the majority of involved parametria are confined to the medial half.

Importantly, the risk of postradiation intestinal and other complications is significantly increased in women treated with pelvic radiation following completed radical hysterectomy. The treating physician should attempt to minimize these risks by incorporating protective procedures (omental J-flap, pelvic prosthesis) to facilitate the safe introduction of adjuvant radiation therapy, which may be needed in women with close or involved surgical margins, deep cervical invasion, parametrial involvement, nodal metastasis, or other high-risk factors. It seems prudent to offer chemotherapy as combined treatment in specific high-risk populations.

The recent introduction of laparoscopic nodal dissection with radical vaginal hysterectomy or laparoscopic-assisted radical hysterectomy has been associated with a prolonged operative time, lessened operative risk, less blood loss, and shorter hospital stay while producing initial excellent clinical results in terms of disease-free interval.

Regardless of surgical approach, perioperative attention must be directed to those manipulations that minimize specific thromboembolic, cardiovascular, pulmonary, or infectious complications (Table 174–5). Single-dose antibiotic prophylaxis, use of less traumatic transverse incisions, incorporating small-caliber, minimally reactive suture material, and minimizing the use of pelvic drains (which may increase complications) should be incorporated into the perioperative scheme. Patients with low-risk I_{B1} disease with negative nodes (>95% survival rate) are not likely to benefit from adjuvant therapy. Women with high-risk factors have a decreased survival rate (65% to 75% or less), even with the addition of radiation therapy.

Table 174–5	**Perioperative Care**

Preoperative
  Informed consent
  Single-dose antibiotic prophylaxis
  Mechanical bowel preparation
  Thromboembolic prophylaxis (pneumatic calf compression ± heparin)
Intraoperative
  Adequate incision (Pfannenstiel is acceptable)
    Inscribed boldly
    Minimal electrocautery
  Allen stirrup
  Intra-abdominal evaluation to exclude extracervical disease
  Adequate retraction (table stabilized)
  Small (2-0) polyglycolic acid sutures
  Cuff closure
  No drains
  Avoid subcutaneous sutures
Postoperative
  Thromboembolic prophylaxis
  Incentive spirometry

Pearls and Pitfalls

PEARLS

- Cervical cancer patients frequently abuse nicotine and therefore have an increased risk of perioperative pulmonary complications.
- Cold knife conization is rarely necessary during pregnancy.
- Positive margins on cold knife conization or LEEP do not necessitate further procedures such as repeat cone or hysterectomy because 60% to 80% of these women will not have persistent disease.
- Cold knife conization is the diagnostic procedure of choice in evaluating in situ or early invasive adenocarcinoma.
- A modified radical hysterectomy for stage IB lesions reduces complications with probably the same clinical benefit.
- The combination of radical hysterectomy and pelvic radiation significantly increases the risk of complications.
- Women with a diagnosis of invasive cervical cancer should be referred to a gynecologic oncologist.

SPECIAL SITUATIONS

Cervix Cancer (≥IA2) Found After Total Hysterectomy

Regardless of preoperative evaluation, it is inevitable that some women will be found to have invasive cervical cancer following hysterectomy for nonmalignant indications.

Even though early invasive lesions (IA1) may be cured by "simple" extirpative surgery, the pathology of any removed invasive cervix cancer should be reviewed to allow planning for or exclusion of additional therapy. Total hysterectomy is deemed inadequate therapy for women with IB disease or greater. Patients with an involved margin or cut-through following total hysterectomy should receive pelvic (or extended) radiation therapy after appropriate evaluation following an incomplete surgical approach. In women with stage IB1 disease who are deemed candidates, radical parametrectomy and lymph node dissection can be successfully completed with the same morbidity and survival expectations of those initially treated by radical hysterectomy. Although successful, this procedure should only be performed by those experienced in performing radical pelvic surgery. The initial early favorable experience with laparoscopic-assisted radical parametrectomy has been reported.

Cancer Diagnosed During Pregnancy

The anxieties associated with the diagnosis of cervix cancer diagnosed during pregnancy should not prevail over rational treatment planning. Careful consideration of the diagnostic procedures are necessary. Conization during pregnancy is associated with increased maternal and fetal morbidity and, if necessary, should be performed in the early second trimester. Current literature suggests that delayed radical surgery to allow and promote fetal viability (28 gestational weeks or more) results in little in-creased maternal risk. There appears to be little reason to rush to initiate treatment of stage 1A2 (or less) lesions. Perioperative morbidity and survival expectations of radical surgery are comparable to those associated with operations completed in the nonpregnant state. Even though there is controversy, there appears to be little adverse effect of vaginal delivery in women with occult invasive disease.

Recurrent Cervix Cancer

Although surgical procedures may be palliative in most women with recurrent cervix cancer, exenterative or ultra-radical extirpative surgery is a potentially curative option for select women with postradiation central pelvic recurrent cervix cancer. Even though numerous factors, including time to recurrence, affect outcome, preoperative preparation should focus on obtaining radiologic or clinical information in an attempt to eliminate the presence of clearly unresectable or extracervical disease. When the disease is thought to be resectable, operative intervention with partial (anterior, posterior) or total exenteration should be considered. These procedures result in significant perioperative morbidity and mortality. Incorporation of continent conduits, low rectal reanastomosis, and vaginal reconstruction improves quality of life. Importantly, 5-year survival rates approach 40% in patients with negative margins.

SELECTED READINGS

Altgassen C, Possover M, Krause N, et al: Establishing a new technique of laparoscopic pelvic and para-aortic lymphadenectomy. Obstet Gynecol 2000;95:348.

Azodi M, Chambers SK, Rutherford TJ, et al: Adenocarcinoma in situ of the cervix: Management and outcome. Gynecol Oncol 1999;73:348.

El-Bastawissi AY, Becker TM, Daling JR: Effect of cervical carcinoma in situ and its management on pregnancy outcome. Obstet Gynecol 1999;93:207.

Giacalone PL, Laffargue F, Alifier N, et al: Randomized study comparing two techniques of conization: cold knife versus loop excision. Gynecol Oncol 1999;75:356.

Linder J, Zahniser D: ThinPrep Papanicolaou testing to reduce false-negative cervical cytology. Arch Pathol Lab Med 1998;122:139.

Magrina JF, Goodrich MA, Lidner TK, et al: Modified radical hysterectomy in the treatment of early squamous cervical cancer. Gynecol Oncol 1999;72:183.

Morris M, Mitchell MF, Silva EG, et al: Cervical conization as definitive therapy for early invasive squamous carcinoma of the cervix. Gynecol Oncol 1993;51:193.

Orr JW Jr, Orr PJ, Bolen DD, Holimon JL: Radical hysterectomy: Does the type of incision matter? Am J Obstet Gynecol 1995;173:399.

Ostor AG: Early invasive adenocarcinoma of the uterine cervix. Int J Gynecol Pathol 2000;19:29.

Shingleton HM, Orr Jr JW: Cancer of the cervix: Diagnosis and management. Philadelphia, JB Lippincott, 1995.

Spitzer M: Cervical screening adjuncts: Recent advances. Am J Obstet Gynecol 1998;179:544.

Suris JC, Dexeus S, Lopes-Marin L: Epidemiology of preinvasive lesions. Eur J Gynaecol Oncol 1999;20:302.

Trombos JB, Hellebrekers BW, Kenter GG, et al: The long learning curve of gynaecological cancer surgery: An argument for centralization. Br J Obstet Gynaecol 2000;107:19.

VASCULAR

Chapter 175

Management of Cerebrovascular Disease

Fernando E. Kafie and Wesley S. Moore

Cerebrovascular disease is the third leading cause of death after heart disease and cancer in developed countries. It is also the leading cause of disability in patients with cardiovascular disease, and 5% of the population older than 65 years are affected by a stroke. The loss of these patients from the work force and the extended hospitalization they require during recovery make the economic impact of the disease one of the most devastating in medicine. Cerebrovascular disease is caused by one of several pathologic processes involving the blood vessels of the brain. The process may be intrinsic to the blood vessel (dissection), originate remotely (embolus), result from decreased perfusion pressure (stenosis) or increased blood viscosity (polycythemia) with inadequate cerebral blood flow, or result from a rupture of the blood vessel (hemorrhage). This chapter focuses on those disorders that lead to decreased cerebral blood flow through stenosis or embolization.

PATHOPHYSIOLOGY

Atherosclerotic lesions tend to occur at branching points along the vascular tree. These areas experience turbulent flow and possibly intimal damage with the resultant creation of plaques. These plaques, in turn, may have complex composition and surface configuration. Possible mechanisms of cerebral ischemia related to these plaques include superficial ulceration with distal embolization, spontaneous intraplaque hemorrhage with occlusion of the vessel, or progressive atherosclerotic narrowing with spontaneous thrombosis. Significant atherosclerotic plaque formation is a localized rather than a diffuse process, and it preferentially affects certain segments of the arterial tree such as the carotids. Arteriosclerotic plaques in the carotid circulation usually form at the origin of the common carotid artery as it arises from the aortic arch, at the bifurcation of the common carotid artery in the neck, or intracranially in the siphon portion of the internal carotid artery. Most clinically significant carotid plaques are localized in the carotid bifurcation, making surgical treatment by endarterectomy possible.

The correlation of plaque ulceration with ischemic neurologic symptoms and the need for surgery is difficult for several reasons. First, studies have shown poor interobserver agreement in the identification of carotid plaque ulceration, using either ultrasound or arteriographic examinations, and poor correlation between pathologic specimens and radiographically demonstrated plaque ulceration. Second, in symptomatic patients, deep ulceration is most commonly found in conjunction with sig-

nificant degrees of carotid stenosis and it becomes difficult to separate clinical symptoms between these two findings. However, the most recent data from the North American Symptomatic Carotid Endarterectomy Trial (NASCET) show that, in medically treated patients with 70% to 99% stenosis (proven to be unequivocal surgical candidates), the presence of plaque ulceration in conjunction with stenosis significantly increases the risk of stroke.

The significance of intraplaque hemorrhage as a predictor of ischemic symptoms is also unclear. Heterogeneous plaque morphology on duplex scanning (consistent with intraplaque hemorrhage) was a significant risk factor for subsequent neurologic events in one study, if the underlying stenosis was greater than 50%, but other studies have not found this relationship. Furthermore, lipid-filled lesions, demonstrated by low echogenicity, have a high tendency toward development of thrombosis, embolism, and ulceration, and low plaque echogenicity has been reported to be a better predictor of associated neurologic symptoms than the degree of carotid stenosis caused by the plaque. Therefore, accurate information about lesion echogenicity is important in planning therapeutic strategies for stenotic carotid lesions.

Risk Factors

Atherosclerosis is associated with a number of well-recognized systemic risk factors such as hyperlipidemia, hypertension, cigarette smoking, and diabetes mellitus. Modification of risk factors is a very important element in the long-term care of the vascular patient, and risk factor reduction can slow the progression of atherosclerotic disease and reduce the risk of stroke. Hypertension is the most important risk factor for stroke. Reducing the diastolic pressure in hypertensive patients by only 6 mm Hg reduces the risk of stroke by 42%. Cigarette smoking doubles the risk of stroke and stopping smoking promptly reduces that risk, whereas smoking cessation for 5 years returns the stroke risk to that of a nonsmoker. Diabetes mellitus increases the risk of ischemic stroke but it is unclear whether strict glucose control reduces the stroke risk in a patient with diabetes mellitus. Similarly, control of hyperlipidemia decreases the risk of coronary heart disease and serum lipids appear to correlate with carotid atherosclerosis, but the effect of blood lipids on stroke risk is unknown.

CLINICAL SYNDROMES

Clinical syndromes associated with cerebrovascular disease include ischemic stroke and transient ischemic attacks. An ischemic stroke is an acute neurologic injury that occurs as a result of one of the previously described pathologic processes (embolization or thrombosis). Normal brain function requires a continuous supply of oxygenated blood and the interruption of cerebral blood supply may lead to irreversible changes in brain matter (cerebral infarction) and subsequent loss of function. The treatment of stroke is intimately related to its cause. Thus, the evaluation of the patient with a stroke must include a clear understanding of the character and location of symptoms resulting from the stroke, the character of the cerebral lesion that is the likely cause of those symptoms as seen on imaging studies, and the possible cause of that lesion. Intervention by the vascular specialist in a patient with a completed stroke has three goals: to reduce the risk factors for subsequent stroke, to prevent recurrent stroke (by removing the underlying pathologic process), and to minimize secondary brain damage by optimizing perfusion to ischemic neurologic areas.

The term transient ischemic attack (TIA) has been applied to any sudden focal neurologic deficit that clears completely in less than 24 hours. However, ischemic symptoms that last for more than an hour are usually accompanied by tissue injury, even though it may not be visualized by current testing, because only 14% of TIAs that last longer than 1 hour resolve. TIAs may herald all types of strokes, but they are most common in infarcts resulting from large vessel atherosclerosis. The symptoms of a TIA may point to the particular cerebral territory involved. For example, repetitive, short-lived episodes of hand and arm weakness suggest transient focal ischemia in the contralateral motor cortex, whereas a single episode of speech difficulty, with or without motor deficit, suggests embolic TIA in the contralateral frontal lobe. Short-lived episodes of pure motor deficits occurring without dysphasia suggest transient ischemia in the internal capsule or corticospinal tract of the ventral pons (a "lacunar" TIA), and TIAs in the vertebrobasilar system often present with short-lived, repetitive episodes of dizziness, diplopia, and dysarthria.

TIAs are commonly atherothrombotic, occurring when enlarging atherosclerotic plaque involving the extracranial or intracranial carotid system leads to a severe compromise of the arterial lumen and artery-to-artery emboli or arterial thrombosis. However, up to 50% of patients with TIAs have minimal carotid atherosclerosis and TIAs may be caused by cardiac emboli, ulcerated lesions of the aortic arch, arteritis, hypercoagulable states, small vessel disease, and multiple nonvascular problems. Small platelet emboli from a stenotic or ulcerated atherosclerotic lesion at the origin of the internal carotid artery may occlude either only the ophthalmic artery or the very distal vessels of the middle cerebral artery, causing transient monocular blindness (amaurosis fugax) or small asymptomatic infarctions in the cerebral cortex. Larger emboli may lead to discrete and easily recognizable neurologic syndromes that suggest the area involved, as previously mentioned. Severe stenosis or occlusion of the internal carotid artery may also result in infarction or ischemia in the "watershed areas" in patients with inadequate collateral circulation through the circle of Willis so

that hypotension, cardiac arrhythmias, or increased blood viscosity may lead to TIA or stroke in these patients.

Screening for Asymptomatic Carotid Disease

The costs of screening the general population for asymptomatic carotid disease appear to negate any potential benefits of carotid artery surgery in asymptomatic carotid artery stenosis. However, because peripheral vascular disease (PVD) is associated with a high probability of carotid atherosclerosis, screening for carotid artery disease has been advocated in patients with PVD to identify patients at risk for stroke. With the use of noninvasive testing, it has become apparent that carotid artery lesions may be present in up to 33% of patients with peripheral atherosclerosis. In patients with at least moderate PVD, up to 25% of those with asymptomatic carotid disease were potential candidates for treatment (carotid stenosis greater than 60%). Risk factors for carotid artery disease that presents with PVD are increasing age, worsening severity of PVD, and the presence of a carotid bruit. The authors believe that all patients who seek medical attention for PVD should be screened for carotid artery disease. Hemodynamically significant atherosclerotic narrowing of the coronary and carotid circulation also frequently occurs simultaneously and the reported incidence of significant (>50%) carotid stenosis in patients with coronary heart disease is as low as 2.3% or as high as 54%. However, routine preoperative screening for carotid disease in all patients selected for coronary artery bypass graft (CABG) is not warranted and does not appear to be cost-effective. Rather, the authors believe that an adequate focused history (looking for risk factors of female sex, PVD, history of TIA or stroke, history of smoking) and physical examination (assessing for carotid bruits) identifies patients with coronary artery disease at risk for the presence of significant carotid disease.

MANAGEMENT OF CAROTID OCCLUSIVE DISEASE

Recent prospective, randomized studies have shown the benefits of carotid endarterectomy in selected patients with both symptomatic and asymptomatic carotid occlusive disease. The NASCET study demonstrated a 17% reduction in the overall stroke risk and an 11% reduction in the risk of major or fatal stroke at 24 months in patients with 70% to 99% symptomatic carotid stenosis undergoing carotid endarterectomy compared with medical therapy. Similarly, the MCR European Carotid Surgery Trial demonstrated an 11% reduction in the risk of major stroke or death at 3 years in patients with greater than 80% symptomatic carotid stenosis undergoing carotid endarterectomy compared with medical treatment. The NASCET study also demonstrated a 7% stroke risk reduction at 5 years in patients with 50% to 69% symptomatic carotid stenosis undergoing carotid endarterectomy, whereas patients with lesser degrees of stenosis did not benefit from the procedure in either trial. The

Asymptomatic Carotid Atherosclerosis Study (ACAS) study demonstrated a 6% stroke risk reduction (55% relative risk reduction) at 5 years in patients with 60% to 99% asymptomatic carotid stenosis undergoing carotid endarterectomy compared with those treated medically. In addition, the Veteran's Administration (VA) Cooperative Trial demonstrated a 12% reduction in the risk of stroke plus TIAs over a similar time frame in patients with greater than 50% asymptomatic carotid stenosis randomized to surgery. Surprisingly, in the ACAS trial, the reduction in stroke risk was not increased as the degree of stenosis between 60% and 99% increased because other studies of asymptomatic carotid stenosis and the NASCET trial demonstrate that the risk of stroke increases significantly when the percentage of carotid stenosis reaches 80%.

Several further important points can be made from these comparisons of carotid endarterectomy and medical therapy in patients with symptomatic and asymptomatic carotid disease. First, the risk of stroke and death with medical therapy is much greater in symptomatic patients than in asymptomatic patients. Second, because of the benign prognosis with medical therapy in patients with asymptomatic carotid stenosis, the benefits of carotid endarterectomy are likely realized only in those patients with severe stenosis (>80%, by duplex criteria) when the procedure is done with a perioperative disabling stroke or death rate less than 3%. "Symptomatic" refers to focal unilateral hemispheric or retinal deficits, and patients with nonfocal symptoms such as blurred vision, dizziness, and vertigo should be considered asymptomatic with respect to carotid disease. Thus, in summary, carotid endarterectomy in patients with severe *symptomatic* stenosis leads to a dramatic reduction in stroke risk, whereas in patients with moderate *symptomatic* stenosis, the benefits are realized only if the surgical results are superb (perioperative disabling stroke or death rate less than 2%). In addition, in patients with less than 50% *symptomatic* stenosis, carotid endarterectomy is of no benefit. In patients with *asymptomatic* carotid stenosis, the benefit of the procedure, although significant, is limited and seen only in patients with the most severe stenosis so that, again, surgical excellence is necessary to achieve benefit in these patients.

Patient Evaluation

A thorough history and physical examination should accompany the evaluation of any patient with known carotid disease. Particular attention should be focused on the risk factors for atherosclerosis and the symptoms of other commonly encountered atherosclerotic diseases such as coronary heart disease and PVD. Symptoms of diseases associated with the risk factors for atherosclerosis (e.g., pulmonary disease associated with cigarette smoking) should also be sought. On physical examination, auscultation of the carotid and the subclavian arteries may reveal bruits, and bilateral arm pressures indicate the hemodynamic significance of the subclavian bruits. The lower extremities should also be examined carefully because patients frequently have concomitant evidence of arterial occlusive disease in other locations.

Testing for Carotid Disease

Accurate evaluation of carotid bifurcation disease has become particularly important in view of recent studies indicating the benefits of carotid endarterectomy in subsets of patients based on the degree of carotid stenosis. Carotid arteriography has traditionally been thought to be the examination of choice for the assessment of extracranial carotid disease; this was the carotid imaging technique used in the previously discussed randomized trials that now form the basis for the management of patients with carotid occlusive disease. However, carotid contrast angiography is associated with small but significant risks. Estimates of the incidence of stroke during carotid arteriography in patients with carotid atherosclerosis range from 0.3% to 3%, and almost 25% of the strokes that occurred in the perioperative period in the ACAS study were associated with carotid arteriography. Besides neurologic complications, renal insufficiency, allergic reactions including anaphylactic shock, and puncture site complications (false aneurysm, hematoma) have been reported. These risks, as well as the cost of the procedure, have encouraged the development of alternative noninvasive modalities for imaging the extracranial carotid arteries, including duplex ultrasonography (US), magnetic resonance angiography (MRA), and computed tomography angiography (CTA). The use of these noninvasive testing techniques, potentially in combination (to maximize accuracy), likely will minimize the preoperative risk and maximize the benefits of carotid endarterectomy in the treatment of patients with cerebrovascular disease.

Duplex Ultrasonography

Duplex scanning, which combines real-time imaging with Doppler spectrum analysis, is considered the most complete, accurate, and reproducible noninvasive diagnostic modality for evaluation of carotid artery stenosis. It can provide information regarding arterial luminal caliber, flow characteristics, and plaque morphology. The degree of stenosis present at the carotid bifurcation is determined based on flow velocities (peak systolic, end diastolic) obtained from pulsed Doppler ultrasound samplings positioned within the common, internal, and external carotid arteries using B-mode ultrasound imaging. The accuracy of duplex ultrasonography when compared with contrast angiography in assessing the degree of stenosis at the carotid bifurcation has been quoted in the range of 69% to 97%, so that it is important to realize that the sensitivity and specificity of duplex ultrasonography vary between laboratories. Anatomic variations (e.g., high carotid bifurcation, large neck, scarring, tortuosity) can also make carotid duplex interrogation difficult, thereby reducing its accuracy. Severe stenosis or occlusion on the opposite side increases flow velocity (and therefore estimated degree of stenosis) in a variable manner. Differentiation of high-grade stenosis from total occlusion using carotid duplex ultrasonography has also been reported to be difficult, although the introduction of color flow duplex ultrasonography has significantly overcome this problem. Other information obtained from an angiogram, including the level of the carotid bifurcation, the length of the stenotic lesion, the presence of a significant ulcer, and the presence or absence of an adequate anterior communicating circle of Willis, is not available from a carotid duplex examination. However, ulceration alone was not demonstrated to be an indication for endarterectomy in the recent randomized trials that have defined the current indications for carotid endarterectomy. Furthermore, significant intracranial stenoses are rare and several studies have found the benefit of carotid endarterectomy to be unaffected when a tandem high-grade intracranial stenosis exists.

Criteria for defining the degree of carotid artery stenosis from carotid duplex examinations have been developed by comparative studies with carotid contrast arteriography. The most common form of determining angiographic carotid artery stenosis used in these studies has been measuring the ratio of residual lumen to the estimated normal bulb diameter, the method of the European Carotid Surgery Trial. This method results in a significant "overestimation" of carotid artery stenosis by comparison with the ACAS, NASCET, and VA Cooperative Trials in which carotid artery stenosis was determined by comparing the carotid minimal residual lumen (MRL) and the distal internal carotid lumen diameter. An 80% to 99% stenosis by the bulb estimated diameter reduction method correlates with an approximately 55% to 75% stenosis by the method that compares minimal residual bulb lumen with the distal cervical carotid. Thus, traditional duplex criteria for determining the degree of carotid artery stenosis cannot be used to select patients for carotid endarterectomy based on the results of NASCET and ACAS, particularly if the carotid duplex examination is the only preoperative imaging study. New duplex criteria have been developed since the publication of the NASCET and ACAS studies that correlate well with angiographic stenosis determined using the "NASCET" criteria. The accuracy of carotid stenosis determined using these criteria has led many surgeons to perform carotid endarterectomy without preoperative carotid contrast arteriography in selected patients. However, as previously noted, the accuracy of carotid duplex ultrasonography is variable and such an approach is only appropriate in an institution with an accredited vascular laboratory that documents a high degree of accuracy by routine quality assurance reviews.

Magnetic Resonance Arteriography

Magnetic resonance images are based on the behavior of proton magnetization when placed in a homogeneous magnetic field. Radiofrequency (RF) pulses of varying duration and amplitude are applied to the region of interest. Protons within the selected slice are then deflected into transverse alignment and brought into phase by the RF pulse. After the RF pulse, the affected protons begin to de-phase and realign along the longitudinal magnetization vector. These "realigning" protons produce currents that are then transformed via complex computer algorithms into a visual or gray-scale display of signal intensities. Most MR imaging techniques suppress images from

flowing blood (i.e., black) whereas MRA highlights flowing blood by doing the opposite: suppressing signals from stationary tissue and maximizing signals from flowing blood.

MRA is noninvasive, involves no exposure to ionizing radiation, and does not require intravenous contrast so that MRA is often the procedure of choice for patients who have contraindications to intravenous contrast. MRA is also a multiplanar imaging modality that can image directly in the axial, sagittal, coronal, or oblique planes and, unlike CTA, MRA is relatively unaffected by superimposed bone. Limitations of MRA include the time the examination generally takes to complete (approximately 15 to 45 minutes) and the fact that the patient must hold absolutely still for this time period because magnetic resonance, in general, is more susceptible to motion-induced artifact than CT or US. The bore of some magnets is also particularly narrow and, because of this, a small percentage of patients are claustrophobic or are too large to fit within the magnet bore. Unstable or critically ill patients are unsuitable for MRA because it is difficult to monitor patients within the magnet. Furthermore, patients with ferromagnetic implants (aneurysm clips, vascular clamps, intravascular coils, stents or filters, ocular or otologic implants, pacemakers, and heart valves) may experience problems when exposed to a strong magnetic field.

In a review of 12 studies, Bowen et al. found that, in patients with normal or near normal carotid MRA studies, significant (>70% luminal narrowing) carotid stenosis was unlikely. The same study also concluded that MRA is more sensitive than ultrasound for differentiating high-grade stenosis from occlusions. However, other studies have found that MRA tends to overestimate the degree of carotid stenosis compared with contrast angiography in patients with high-grade lesions and that signal dropout in such patients can result in the misinterpretation of a high-grade stenosis as an occlusion (similar to duplex ultrasound). In the assessment of lesions with 70% to 99% stenosis, three-dimensional time-of-flight (TOF) MRA has been reported to have a sensitivity of 94%, a specificity of 85%, and an accuracy of 88%. Furthermore, the combination of MRA and duplex ultrasonography has been shown to have an even higher sensitivity and specificity, so that with the use of both of the techniques, cerebral contrast arteriography can be reserved for patients with discordant results. MR imaging can be performed at the same time as MRA with little added effort so that ischemic disease, tumors, or vascular malformations, which could also account for the patient's symptoms, can be detected. However, studies of brain imaging by CT before carotid endarterectomy have shown such imaging to be of little value. Similarly, MRA visualization of ulceration at the carotid bulb is poor and MRA has limited ability to accurately image the intracranial circulation (i.e., tandem lesions), but as previously noted, these limitations do not appear to be of significant clinical importance.

Computed Tomography Angiography

Relatively long scan time and the resulting necessity for large doses of intravenous contrast have limited the evaluation of cerebrovascular disease using conventional CT. To obtain a CT arteriogram of the carotid bifurcation, the scan needs to be made within the narrow period, during which there is vascular enhancement. In contrast, CTA of carotid bifurcation disease is feasible using spiral CT scanning, which has no rotating x-ray tube, allowing extremely short scan times (50 to 500 msec). The technique involves continuous movement of the patient through the CT scanner as the x-ray tube rotates around the patient so that the scan is obtained quickly and with usually only a single breath. The accuracy of CTA for the carotids is dependent on technique, which has not yet been fully defined, but recent reports demonstrate a correlation between CTA of the carotids and cerebral angiography of 82% to 100%. Potential advantages of CTA over MRA include a superior ability to depict calcium within carotid plaques, a shorter time of acquisition, and a more favorable environment for claustrophobic patients. There is also no contraindication of CTA in patients that have implanted devices or pacemakers. CTA may more accurately demonstrate carotid stenosis and depict ulceration than MRA, and it may be more sensitive than MRA or US in differentiating high-grade stenosis from occlusion. Potential disadvantages of CTA are that short segment stenosis may be missed because of volume averaging or motion artifact and that CTA cannot be used when metallic clips are in the field because of excessive artifact. CTA also relies on the use of intravenous contrast and is therefore of limited use in patients with renal insufficiency.

OPERATIVE MANAGEMENT OF CAROTID OCCLUSIVE DISEASE

Carotid endarterectomy is essentially a prophylactic procedure, so that the patient takes the risk of the carotid endarterectomy to reduce the risk of future stroke. Therefore, the benefits of the procedure can only be realized if the complications are kept to a minimum and the patient survives long enough to achieve the benefit of the reduction in stroke risk provided by the procedure. Preoperative preparation, operative technique, and postoperative care influence the incidence of complications associated with carotid endarterectomy. The most critical part of patient management is the intraoperative care, and the technical details of the operation mandate perfection to minimize postoperative morbidity and mortality risks. However, proper patient selection and preoperative preparation can also limit complications after carotid endarterectomy.

Preoperative Cardiac Evaluation

It is well established that patients with extracranial carotid artery disease have a higher than normal incidence of coronary artery disease. Indeed, the risk of perioperative myocardial infarction exceeds the risk of perioperative stroke in many reported series of carotid endarterectomy. Several major questions arise when one plans treatment of a patient with carotid artery disease who likely also has coronary artery disease. First, what is the appropriate workup of the coronary circulation in patients with carotid artery disease? Second, what is the risk of coronary revascularization in a patient with a high-grade asymptomatic stenosis or a carotid bruit? Third, when significant coronary artery disease is identified in a patient with carotid artery disease (asymptomatic or symptomatic), what is the appropriate management (staged carotid and then coronary revascularization, combined procedure, or "reversed staged" coronary revascularization and then delayed carotid endarterectomy)?

Cardiac workup in patients with significant carotid artery disease is generally guided by the history and symptoms of the patient. In patients with a history of heart disease, abnormal resting electrocardiogram, or angina, a cardiology consultation should be obtained preoperatively and workup with an exercise or dipyridamole scan obtained. If there is evidence of significant myocardial ischemia, coronary angiography is performed. When the results of cardiac evaluation indicate the need for coronary revascularization, the question becomes one of timing of the surgical procedures. This then also raises the question of the risk of coronary revascularization in a patient with high-grade asymptomatic carotid stenosis. It is clear that patients with significant carotid disease have a higher incidence of stroke associated with CABG. It is also clear that carotid endarterectomy in such patients can reduce the long-term risk of stroke as demonstrated in the ACAS study. Whether endarterectomy also reduces the risk of perioperative stroke after coronary artery bypass grafting is unclear. Regardless, we recommend that patients with greater than 80% asymptomatic carotid stenosis undergo a combined carotid endarterectomy with coronary revascularization whenever possible. With careful hemodynamic monitoring and good anesthetic technique, we are able to routinely perform combined carotid endarterectomies with coronary revascularization and the senior author (W.S.M.) has observed good results using this approach. In contrast, when symptomatic carotid stenosis and significant myocardial ischemia are present, the authors' preference is to do a staged procedure whenever possible, proceeding first with the carotid endarterectomy.

Operative and Postoperative Care

At our institution, general anesthesia is preferred for carotid endarterectomy because it provides a calm operative field, excellent airway control, and reduced metabolic demands of the affected hemisphere. Cervical block anesthesia may be used in patients with contraindication to general anesthesia but these patients must be able to psychologically tolerate the procedure. Blood pressure monitoring is essential throughout the procedure and is accomplished with an arterial line. The patient is placed in a supine position with shoulder roll and neck rotated to the side opposite the incision. Hyperextension of the neck should be avoided. The operative field should be prepped to include the mastoid process, mandibula, sternal notch, clavicle, entire neck, and lower earlobe. The incision may be directed along the anterior border of the sternocleidomastoid muscle, centered at the bulb, and directed toward the mastoid process. If the incision is directed anterior to the earlobe, damage to the marginal branch of the facial nerve may ensue. An alternative incision can be placed along skin creases if these are found to lie on the surface of the carotid bulb. Incision is made and carried down to the medial border of the sternocleidomastoid muscle. The jugular vein is identified and the transverse facial vein is ligated. This usually lies superficial to the carotid bulb. Identification of the vagus nerve within the carotid sheath is made along with the hypoglossal nerve. Proximal control of the carotid artery is made first, followed by external and internal carotid control. Care should be taken to avoid undue manipulation of the carotid bulb. The carotid branches should be mobilized proximally and distally to points where they are circumferentially soft and pliable. Carotid control is made with either vessel loops or umbilical tape for shunting if needed. In lesions of the internal carotid that extend to the base of skull, styloid process resection or division of digastric muscle can be performed.

At our institution, we routinely use intraoperative electroencephalogram (EEG). Under general anesthesia, any changes in intraoperative EEG mandate use of a shunt. Patients with a previous infarct on the side of the operation also require routine shunting. In 1967, the senior author reported the use of intraoperative internal carotid artery back pressures as a means of quantifying the adequacy of collateral blood flow and predicting the need for shunting. In patients who have had no prior cerebral infarction, a mean internal carotid artery back pressure in excess of 25 mm Hg has been a reliable parameter against which to judge the adequacy of cerebral blood flow. If accurate EEG is not available, measurement of stump pressures, routine shunting, or endarterectomy under local/regional anesthesia should be performed. An awake patient allows the surgeon to appraise cerebral responses during carotid artery clamping by asking the patient to move the extremities opposite the side of operation and to make verbal responses to questioning. When an internal shunt is required, we prefer to use a Javid 10F shunt. The carotid artery should be opened at the most lateral aspect, thereby decreasing the risk of narrowing if primary closure is used. The superior end of the shunt is inserted into the normal internal carotid and allowed to back bleed. The shunt is clamped and inserted into the common carotid artery. The shunt is then secured and the translucent area is observed for bubbles or particulate matter before unclamping. If these are observed, the shunt is allowed to back bleed when taken out of the common carotid artery. The endarterectomy is then performed, with care being taken to obtain clean proximal and distal endpoints.

Although the authors currently routinely patch closures with prosthetic graft, primary closure may be performed on most carotid arteries. The decision to patch and what type of material to use is controversial. More importantly, it is vital that, no matter which closure is chosen, small accurate bites be performed on the arterial wall, with care being taken not to narrow the lumen of the internal carotid artery. Female patients tend to have smaller internal carotid arteries and may have better long-term results with routine patching. Although vein can be used for patching, the authors believe that the risk reduction from infection is negligible and only adds unnecessary time to the procedure. On completion of closure, flow is reestablished and the technical adequacy of the procedure must be verified carefully. The authors prefer completion angiography. A 20-gauge needle is bent at a 60-degree angle and placed in the common carotid artery. Contrast medium is then injected under fluoroscopic control. The internal, external, and intracranial carotid, as well as the middle cerebral, are inspected for tandem lesions and technical success of endarterectomy. If there are any technical imperfections, they are corrected before the patient leaves the operating room.

The authors routinely give their patients preoperative antibiotics and copiously irrigate the wound before closure with antibiotic irrigation. A small closed drain is used and taken out on postoperative day 1. The platysmal layer is closed and the skin is approximated with a subcuticular stitch. At the University of California at Los Angeles, patients routinely go to the floor after a short observation period in the recovery room. Intensive care monitoring is used for patients who are unstable hemodynamically. Most patients are discharged on the first postoperative day. Follow-up is scheduled for 1 week postoperatively and every 6 months thereafter (for surveillance duplex ultrasonography). At the first postoperative visit, a baseline duplex is obtained of the operated site.

Patients in whom recurrent significant stenosis develops less than 2 years postoperatively usually have neointimal hyperplasia. Those who are more than 2 years out usually have recurrent atherosclerosis. Recurrent atherosclerosis is amenable to endarterectomy, whereas intimal hyperplasia is best treated by performing patch angioplasty (with prosthetic material) or replacing the involved segment of artery with a vein or prosthetic graft. However, recurrent stenoses caused by intimal hyperplasia rarely become symptomatic and only those progressing to high-grade lesions should be considered for treatment.

VERTEBROBASILAR DISEASE

The management of vertebrobasilar disease can be challenging and rewarding. The first step in managing these patients is the recognition of their symptoms (dizziness, vertigo, ataxia, drop attacks). Once these symptoms are identified, other medical conditions that may cause these symptoms must be ruled out (arrhythmias, intracranial tumors, multiple sclerosis). Unlike the carotid artery, in which symptoms are believed to be predominantly due to thromboembolic disease from the bifurcation, vertebrobasilar insufficiency is believed to be mainly from inadequate blood flow to the tributaries of the distal vertebral and basilar arteries. Atherosclerosis is the most common cause of intrinsic disease to arteries of the posterior brain and the most frequent location of the plaque is in the subclavian artery, either impinging on the orifice of the vertebral artery or obstructing blood flow in the subclavian proximal to the vertebral artery. Other conditions that may involve the vertebral arteries include fibromuscular dysplasia, kinking, and arteritis. Diagnosis of lesions in the vertebral system is still heavily dependent on angiography because duplex scanning can only demonstrate the direction of flow and velocity in the middle portion of the vertebral arteries. There is little role for the treat-

Pearls and Pitfalls

PEARLS

- In evaluating asymptomatic patients for a possible diameter-reducing stenosis of 60% or greater, this percent stenosis will best correlate with a duplex scan stenosis category of 80% to 99%.
- Do not rely on MRA alone. Always have confirmation with either duplex or CTA and, if necessary, contrast-enhanced angiography.
- Always mobilize the internal carotid artery for a longer distance than is thought necessary. Assess the distal vessel for freedom from plaque by palpating the distal internal carotid artery in two planes against an angle clamp.
- Always assess the technical result of operation with an imaging study such as contrast angiography or duplex ultrasound before wound closure.
- Always place the skin incision along the theoretical line connecting the suprasternal notch with the mastoid process.
- Extend the arteriotomy as far distal as necessary to directly visualize the endpoint. The liberal use of patch closure of the arteriotomy eliminates the risk of producing a stenosis in an otherwise normal-diameter segment.
- Always place the distal portion of the shunt first, and allow backflow to fill the shunt and wash out any loose debris. Use a long shunt with a clamp on the shunt. After unclamping the carotid artery, open the clamp on the shunt slowly to look for trapped air bubbles or debris.

PITFALLS

- Percentage of stenosis as measured on carotid duplex scanning refers to stenosis of the bulb of the carotid artery, not a diameter-reducing stenosis of the internal carotid artery as measured by angiography.
- MRA frequently overestimates the percent of stenosis because turbulence causes signal dropout in the scan.
- Plaque in the internal carotid artery frequently extends more distally than anticipated and takes the form of a narrow tongue in the posteromedial aspect of the vessel.
- Most perioperative strokes are due to technical error.
- Cephalad extension of the skin incision anterior to the ear limits distal carotid artery exposure and risks injury to the marginal mandibular branch of the seventh cranial nerve.
- Most technical errors involve failure to visualize the distal endpoint of the endarterectomy in the internal carotid artery.
- Inadvertent embolization of air bubbles or atheromatous debris through an internal shunt may result in cerebral infarction.

---

ment of asymptomatic lesions identified incidentally on angiogram. For patients who have restrictive lesions and symptoms in the carotid and vertebral system, carotid endarterectomy is the procedure of choice. Vertebral reconstruction (through reimplantation, patch angioplasty, endarterectomy, bypasses, and balloon angioplasty) is reserved for the symptomatic patient without reconstructible carotid disease.

BALLOON ANGIOPLASTY

There have been multiple case reports of balloon angioplasty and stenting of the carotid system but no studies to date have compared this therapy with the more established treatments of carotid artery disease (carotid endarterectomy, antiplatelet therapy). The reported stroke rates in these preliminary series have also been higher than the rates generally reported for carotid endarterectomy. The authors await the results of the CREST (carotid revascularization endarterectomy versus stent trial) before making recommendations about this emerging form of therapy. Reports of vertebral artery balloon angioplasty are also preliminary and are largely based on the extrapolation of techniques from other sites in the body.

SELECTED READINGS

Ahn SS, Baker JD, Walden K, Moore WS: Which asymptomatic patients should undergo routine screening carotid duplex scan? Am J Surg 1991;162:180.

Anonymous: Endarterectomy for asymptomatic carotid artery stenosis. Executive Committee for the Asymptomatic Carotid Atherosclerosis Study. JAMA 1995;273:1421.

Barnett HJ, Taylor DW, Eliasziw M, et al: Benefit of carotid endarterectomy in patients with symptomatic moderate or severe stenosis. North American Symptomatic Carotid Endarterectomy Trial Collaborators. N Engl J Med 1998;339:1415.

Bowen BC, Quencer RM, Margosian P, Pattany PM: MR angiography of occlusive disease of the arteries in the head and neck: Current concepts [see comments]. AJR Am J Roentgenol 1994;162:9.

Cosgrove DM, Hertzer NR, Loop FD: Surgical management of synchronous carotid and coronary artery disease. J Vasc Surg 1986;3:690.

Dion JE, Gates PC, Fox AJ, et al: Clinical events following neuroangiography: A prospective study. Stroke 1987;18:997.

Eliasziw M, Streifler JY, Fox AJ, et al: Significance of plaque ulceration in symptomatic patients with high grade stenosis. Stroke 1994;25:304.

European Carotid Surgery Trialist's Collaborative Group: MRC European Carotid Surgery Trial: Interim results for symptomatic patients with severe (70% to 99%) or with mild (0% to 29%) carotid stenosis. Lancet 1991;337:1235.

Gomez CR: Carotid plaque morphology and risk for stroke. Stroke 1990;21:148.

Jones RH, Loftus CM, Sheldon WC, et al: Concomitant carotid and coronary disease. Patient Care 1992;15:49.

Marek J, Mills JL, Harvich J, et al: Utility of routine carotid duplex screening in patients who have claudication. J Vasc Surg 1996;24:572–577; discussion 577–579.

Moore WS, Barnett HJM, Beebe HG, et al: Guidelines for carotid endarterectomy: A multidisciplinary consensus statement from the Ad Hoc Committee, American Heart Association. Circulation 1995;91:566.

Ramsey DE, Miles RD, Lambeth A, Summer DS: Prevalence of extracranial carotid artery disease: A survey of an asymptomatic population with noninvasive techniques. J Vasc Surg 1987;5:584.

Veterans Administration Cooperative Trialists: Role of carotid endarterectomy in asymptomatic carotid stenosis. Stroke 1986;17:534.

Walker WA, Harvey WR, Gaschen JR, et al: Is routine carotid screening for coronary surgery needed? Am Surg 1996;62:308.

Chapter 176

Management of Thoracic, Abdominal, Peripheral, and Visceral Aneurysmal Disease

W. Anthony Lee and Christopher K. Zarins

Aneurysms are localized arterial enlargements that can occur almost anywhere in the arterial circulation. They are considered clinically significant if the diameter is at least twice that of the adjacent normal artery. True aneurysms involve degeneration and expansion of all three layers of the arterial wall, as distinguished from false or pseudoaneurysms, in which there is an absence of or defect in a normal arterial wall with containment of blood by the surrounding soft tissue. This chapter focuses on true aneurysms of the aorta and its major branches. Table 176–1 lists the approximate incidence and distribution of true aneurysms.

ABDOMINAL AORTIC ANEURYSMS

Abdominal aortic aneurysms (AAAs) are present in approximately 4% of the population. The incidence of AAA increases with age, and aneurysms are found in approximately 10% of men older than 75 years. Aortic aneurysms are more likely to develop in men, with a male-to-female ratio of 8:1. The natural history of untreated AAA is to enlarge and rupture. Approximately 50% of patients with AAAs, if untreated, die of aneurysm rupture. The risk of rupture increases with aneurysm size in accordance with Laplace's law, T (wall tension) $= P$ (pressure) $\times R$ (radius)/W (wall thickness). The mean rate of growth of aneurysms is approximately 3.2 mm per year; however, there is a wide variation among individuals with some aneurysms not increasing at all and some increasing at a much faster rate. Table 176–2 gives the estimated annual risk of rupture according to size. Approximately 50% of patients with AAA rupture die before they reach a hospital. Among those who reach a hospital and undergo emergency surgery, only 58% leave the hospital alive, for an overall mortality rate of 79%.

Clinical Presentation

Most AAAs are asymptomatic and are discovered incidentally during routine physical or radiologic examinations. Primary risk factors include family history (25% in first order relative), male sex, age, smoking, and hypertension. On physical examination, a prominent, widened aortic pulse is noted in the epigastrium. However, in obese patients, the aortic pulse cannot be palpated and even large aortic aneurysms often are not detected. The sensi-

tivity of physical examination is estimated to be approximately 60%.

A patient with a known AAA and sudden onset of abdominal or back pain, especially associated with hypotension, has a ruptured aneurysm until proven otherwise and should be taken immediately to the operating room. In a hemodynamically stable patient with no known aneurysm, an urgent computed tomography (CT) scan may be obtained to make certain of the diagnosis. CT evidence of an aneurysm with back pain, even without evidence of rupture, should prompt urgent operative repair.

Imaging studies are useful to diagnose the size and type of AAA and presence of associated intra-abdominal pathologies or anatomic variations. These include iliac aneurysms, which are present in approximately 20% to 25% of AAAs, occult tumors, metastatic disease, pancreatitis, or diverticular disease. Anatomic variations include an anomalous left renal vein (posterior or circumaortic), abnormal inferior vena cava (duplicated or right sided), and a horseshoe kidney (Fig. 176–1). The indications for repair of an asymptomatic AAA include an aneurysm with a transverse diameter of 5 cm, aneurysms 4 to 5 cm in diameter with evidence of recent enlargement more than 0.5 cm, and focal aneurysms that are more than twice the diameter of the adjacent normal aorta.

Preoperative Management

Patient selection for elective AAA repair starts with a complete history and physical examination. Particular attention is paid to a history of cerebrovascular events, chronic obstructive pulmonary disease, current and past smoking status, myocardial ischemic events, poor exercise tolerance, renal failure, and signs and symptoms of peripheral occlusive disease, as well as risk factors for car-

Table 176–1	Incidence of Aneurysms in Decreasing Order of Frequency	
ANEURYSM LOCATION	**INCIDENCE (%)**	
Abdominal aorta	90	
Thoracic aorta	5	
Popliteal artery	3	
Femoral artery	2	
Visceral arteries	<1	

Table 176–2	Estimated Annual Risk of Abdominal Aortic Aneurysm Rupture According to Size	

SIZE (cm)	RISK OF RUPTURE PER YEAR (%)
>4–5	3
>5–6	11
>6–7	25
>7	50

diovascular disease such as hypertension, diabetes mellitus, smoking, and hypercholesterolemia. Current quality of life and life expectancy should also be considered in the overall decision to offer a patient surgical repair. The risks of the operation must be weighed against the risk of rupture or death from other causes.

An abdominal ultrasound is the best initial diagnostic imaging modality. It can be used to determine the presence or absence of an aneurysm, document aneurysm size, and for follow-up examinations of small aneurysms. The most definitive aneurysm imaging modality is the spiral CT scan with intravenous timed-bolus contrast enhancement. Interval CT sections of 3 to 5 mm can delineate the locations of the visceral vessels, aneurysm type (perivisceral, pararenal, juxtarenal, or infrarenal), and involvement of the iliac arteries. Alternatively, if a patient has renal insufficiency or iodine-contrast allergy, magnetic resonance (MR) angiography may be used with gadolinium-contrast infusion, which is minimally nephrotoxic. Conventional aortography may be used to define aneurysm morphology and branch vessel disease but is increasingly being replaced by CT scanning or MR imaging. Indications for angiography include the presence of concomitant lower extremity occlusive disease, mesenteric or renal occlusive disease, or previous aortoiliofemoral bypass surgery.

Intraoperative Management

Intraoperative management requires general anesthesia and hemodynamic monitoring. Large bore intravenous catheters, a radial arterial line, and a urinary drainage catheter are used routinely. The patient is positioned for either a transperitoneal or retroperitoneal approach. A variety of incisions may be used including a vertical midline or a supraumbilical transverse incision for a transperitoneal approach, and a left-sided or right-sided supraumbilical flank incision for a retroperitoneal approach to the aorta.

The principles of open AAA repair include good exposure with meticulous dissection, secure proximal and distal vascular control, systemic anticoagulation, and suture anastomoses of a prosthetic graft to normal artery proximally and distally. The conduct of a standard infrarenal AAA repair proceeds as follows. After retraction of the viscera or the peritoneal sac to the right, the aortic neck proximal to the aneurysm just below the level of the renal arteries is exposed. Care is taken to avoid injury to the left renal vein as it is mobilized from the anterior aspect of the aorta. The inferior mesenteric artery, which arises from the anterior surface of the aneurysm, is exposed and controlled. The common iliac arteries are exposed distal to the aneurysm to allow safe placement of clamps. If the common iliac arteries are aneurysmal, the external and internal iliac arteries are controlled. The patient is given intravenous heparin for systemic anticoagulation and the aorta is clamped proximally and the iliac arteries are clamped distally. The aneurysm is opened on its anterior surface and the intraluminal mural thrombus is removed. Patent lumbar arteries, which back-bleed into the aneurysm sac, are oversewn (Fig. 176–2).

After transection of the infrarenal aortic neck at its junction with the aneurysm, a prosthetic polyester or ePTFE (expanded polytetrafluoroethylene) graft is anastomosed to the proximal aortic neck using monofilament polypropylene suture. A straight tube graft is used when the aneurysm is localized to the infrarenal aorta and a bifurcated graft is used if the aneurysm involves the iliac arteries. The distal anastomosis to either the terminal aorta or the iliac arteries is similarly performed with nonabsorbable, monofilament polypropylene sutures. After flushing the graft, clamps are removed and flow is restored to the lower extremities. Special attention should be paid to avoid injury to the ureters as they cross the iliac bifurcation and the iliac veins, which can be injured,

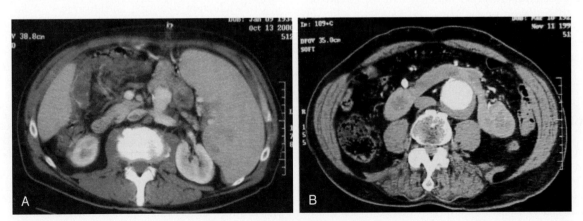

Figure 176–1. Spiral computed tomography scan demonstrating two renal abnormalities that may be encountered during treatment of abdominal aortic aneurysm: (A) retroaortic left renal vein and (B) horseshoe kidney.

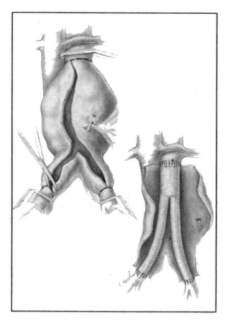

Figure 176-2. Open surgical abdominal aortic aneurysm repair. The aneurysm is opened after proximal and distal control, and a bifurcated graft is sewn directly to the aorta and the iliac arteries with the use of nonabsorbable, monofilament sutures.

resulting in significant hemorrhage. If the inferior mesenteric artery is patent and at least 3 mm in diameter, it is reimplanted into the prosthetic graft to reduce the risk of postoperative colonic ischemia. The residual aneurysm sac and the retroperitoneum are closed over the graft, and the abdomen is closed.

Postoperative Management

Postoperative management following open AAA repair requires careful fluid management to maintain stable hemodynamics and perfusion, optimization of cardiopulmonary mechanics (early extubation, incentive spirometry, mobilization), and perioperative nitrates and beta-blockade when indicated. Uncomplicated patients may usually be transferred to the general care floor on the first postoperative day. Early ambulation is encouraged and diet may be initiated once bowel function returns, usually on postoperative day 3 or 4. When the patient is able to tolerate solid food, passes stool, and ambulates without assistance, he or she may be discharged home. The usual length of stay following an uncomplicated AAA repair ranges from 5 to 8 days but may be prolonged in patients who are elderly with multiple comorbidities.

Complications

The range of complications after AAA repair can be divided into early and late events. In the immediate perioperative period, bleeding and cardiopulmonary events are the most significant. Although it is not unusual to require transfusion of one or two units of packed red blood cells in the first 12 to 24 hours, signs of ongoing

bleeding require aggressive correction of coagulopathy and rapid return to the operating room for exploration. Even if a point source of bleeding is not identified, simple evacuation of the hematoma and warm saline irrigation can result in remarkable improvements in respiratory mechanics and subsequent hemostasis.

Cardiopulmonary complications are usually the result of a prolonged and complicated intraoperative course, involving large amounts of transfusions and other fluids. As a general rule, active smokers should be discouraged from smoking at least 2 weeks before the date of operation. Close hemodynamic monitoring should be carried out to avoid overresuscitating these patients with excess fluids, and judicious use of early, gentle diuresis is helpful.

A dreaded but rare complication after AAA repair is colonic ischemia. Colonic ischemia may present as a maroon-colored, heme-positive stool on the third to fifth postoperative day with tachycardia and metabolic acidosis. The diagnosis is made at the bedside with flexible sigmoidoscopy. Most cases represent partial thickness sloughing of the mucosa and submucosa, which can be managed conservatively with antibiotics and bowel rest, but a small percentage involve patchy areas of full-thickness necrosis requiring a prompt colectomy and a colostomy with a Hartmann's pouch or a mucous fistula. The mortality rate of patients who suffer colonic ischemia is high and survivors face a risk of late graft infection.

Late complications of aortic aneurysm repair include graft thrombosis, pseudoaneurysm, graft infection, para-anastomotic aneurysmal degeneration, and aortoenteric fistula. Graft thrombosis is unusual and typically occurs in the setting of concomitant occlusive disease. Graft thrombosis may be treated with graft thrombectomy or thrombolysis with revision of the anastomosis or graft extension to the femoral or popliteal artery. Pseudoaneurysms may form as the result of infection or primary suture-tissue disruption at the anastomosis. These require surgical correction and repair. Operations for pseudoaneurysms may be quite challenging and can result in significant morbidity. Aortoenteric fistulas with erosion of the graft into the duodenum or small bowel may present as upper gastrointestinal bleeding. This is a life-threatening complication, which requires immediate reoperation to remove the infected graft, repair the bowel, and restore flow to the lower extremities.

Graft infection following aortic surgery is one of the most life-threatening late complications. Often, the presentation is subtle, and by the time a patient has systemic signs of sepsis or aortoenteric bleeding, mortality rate is very high. Once the diagnosis is established or strongly suspected, urgent surgery should be undertaken. The traditional approach has been to perform an extra-anatomic bypass followed by graft excision as a staged procedure. This, however, has been fraught with complications of its own involving late blowout of the aortic stump and secondary infection of the extra-anatomic bypass. Alternatively, construction of a "neoaorta" using superficial femoral veins is a reasonable option. This offers the benefit of an in-line, totally autogenous reconstruction that is infection resistant and eliminates the aortic stump problem.

Outcomes

Open AAA repair is a durable repair with nearly 5 decades of surgical experience behind it. Perioperative mortality rate for elective repairs ranges from 2% to 8%. Mortality rate for emergent operations is significantly higher. Urgent operations for symptomatic aneurysms that are not ruptured or leaking on exploration carry a mortality rate of 15% to 20%. In most cases, once a patient recovers from open surgical repair, he or she may be considered free from risk of aneurysm rupture. However, 5% to 10% of all patients may require some kind of reintervention related to their repair or require treatment of another aneurysm during their lifetime.

ENDOVASCULAR AAA REPAIR

Since the first reported endoluminal AAA repair by Juan Parodi in 1991, a number of endovascular devices to treat aortic aneurysms have been developed and are currently in various stages of the U.S. Food and Drug Administration (FDA) clinical investigation and trials or have been approved for clinical use. The fundamental design of most aortic stent grafts is similar and consists of a fabric graft joined to a self-expanding or balloon-expandable metallic stent, with or without hooks or barbs. Most have a bifurcated design, although straight tube devices are available. The devices are constructed of thin polyester or ePTFE graft material reinforced by a metallic endoskeleton-exoskeleton. Most devices are modular systems, although one approved device is a single-unit bifurcated construction (Fig. 176–3). A complete bifurcated repair consists of two or three modules joined together (bifurcation device plus one or two iliac devices). Separate extension cuffs are available to tailor the repair precisely to the individual anatomy. Currently, two endovascular devices have been FDA approved for use in AAA repair. They are the AneuRx device by Medtronics AVE (Santa Rosa, California) and the Ancure-EVT device by Guidant (Menlo Park, California). Both devices are deployed through femoral cutdowns and each requires special training and catheter and guidewire skills. The procedures may be performed in the operating room (OR) or in an OR-compatible angiographic suite (see Fig. 176–3).

Preoperative Management

Evaluation of patients for endovascular stent graft repair requires accurate determination of anatomic dimensions and morphology of the aortic aneurysm, infrarenal aortic neck, and iliac arteries, as well as an understanding between the surgeon and the patient about the potential risks and benefits of this type of repair compared with conventional open repair. Even though early results of endovascular repair are encouraging, long-term outcome data are not yet available.

The main anatomic criteria required for endovascular repair include the diameter and length of the infrarenal aortic neck, the length of aorta between the renal arteries and the hypogastric arteries, the diameters of the common iliac arteries, the diameter of the terminal aorta, and tortuosity of the proximal neck and the iliac arteries. The single most important imaging study is a thin-cut spiral CT scan. In many cases, this alone may allow determination of anatomic eligibility for stent graft repair. The CT scan may be complemented with angiography using graduated marker catheters to completely define aneurysm morphology. Depending on the endovascular device used, approximately 50% to 60% of all infrarenal AAAs are anatomically suitable for endovascular therapy.

Intraoperative Management

The anesthetic management of endovascular repair is simpler than open repair and the entire procedure may be performed under an epidural or a long-acting spinal

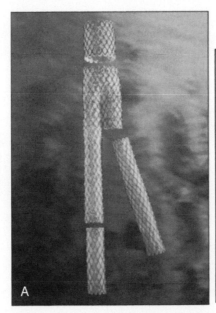
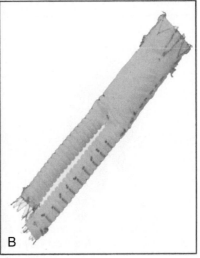

Figure 176–3. The two-stent graft devices currently approved by the U.S. Food and Drug Administration for endovascular abdominal aortic aneurysm repair. *A,* AneuRx device (Medtronic AVE, Santa Rosa, California). *B,* Ancure device (Guidant, Menlo Park, California).

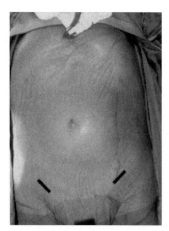

Figure 176–4. Location of incisions for bilateral common femoral artery exposures.

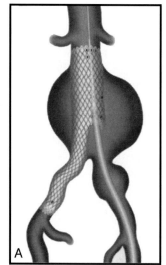
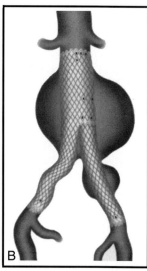

Figure 176–6. Endovascular abdominal aortic aneurysm repair using the AneuRx stent graft device. *A,* Insertion of contralateral iliac delivery catheter. *B,* Completed stent graft repair.

anesthetic. The lack of an abdominal incision, extensive dissection, and aortic cross-clamping significantly reduces the usual intraoperative cardiovascular and pulmonary stresses. Even patients with NYHA (New York Heart Association) class III angina or congestive heart failure, and oxygen-dependent chronic obstructive pulmonary disease can safely undergo the procedure with careful medical management.

The technique of endovascular aneurysm repair using a modular stent graft system is as follows. The patient is positioned supine and is prepped and draped as for a standard open aneurysm repair. Both common femoral arteries are exposed for a length of 2 to 3 cm through small transverse, oblique incisions (Fig. 176–4). Under fluoroscopic control, bilateral transfemoral guidewire access is obtained to the infrarenal aorta. Through one femoral artery, the larger of the two delivery catheters, which contains the bifurcated module, is advanced over a stiff guidewire to the level of the suprarenal aorta. On the contralateral side, an angiographic catheter is inserted for intraoperative aortography (Fig. 176–5A).

An aortogram is obtained to localize the renal arteries. The bifurcated device is deployed by retracting the covering sheath with the proximal end of the stent graft placed just below the origin of the most inferior renal artery (see Fig. 176–5B). The opening to the contralateral limb of the bifurcated device is then selectively cannulated using a wire and a guiding catheter. This wire is exchanged for a stiff guidewire, the contralateral limb delivery catheter is advanced into its opening, and the self-expanding stent graft is deployed by retracting its covering sheath (Fig. 176–6). A completion angiogram is obtained to assess the proximal and distal fixation and to look for extravasation into the aneurysm sac (endoleak). Following completion of the procedure, all sheaths and guidewires are removed from the femoral arteries and they are repaired with primary suture closure. An addi-

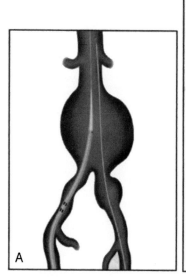
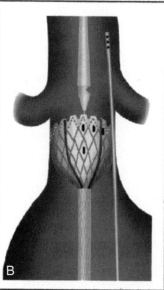

Figure 176–5. Endovascular abdominal aortic aneurysm repair using the AneuRx stent graft device. *A,* Insertion of main bifurcated delivery catheter (right femoral) and contralateral angiographic catheter (left femoral). *B,* Start of deployment of bifurcated stent graft device.

tional femoral closure procedure such as an endarterectomy or patch angioplasty is required in approximately 15% of the cases.

Postoperative Management

The postoperative morbidity rate following an endovascular AAA repair is minimal. Most patients may be recovered in the recovery room and transferred to a general care floor or a monitored telemetry unit. They may resume a regular diet that same day and ambulate as tolerated. Most are discharged home on the first or second postoperative day.

Complications

Although all of the current endovascular devices require at least one groin dissection (and most require two), there are surprisingly few groin-related complications (e.g., lymphoceles, seromas, hematomas, infections). This is largely attributable to the use of small, oblique transverse incisions with limited groin dissections and avoidance of the inguinal crease. Device-related complications include inability to advance the device through the iliac artery, inability to deploy the device, modular separation, torn fabrics or stent fractures, incomplete aneurysm exclusion and endoleak, aneurysm rupture, graft limb thrombosis, colonic ischemia, renal failure, and the need for conversion to open surgical repair. Most device-related complications are amenable to endovascular revision but a few require late, open conversions.

Outcomes

Review of data from multicenter clinical trials reveal significant advantages of endovascular AAA repair compared with open surgical repair. Although there was no difference in operative mortality rates, there was a significant reduction in morbidity rates of patients undergoing endovascular repair with reduced blood loss, reduced operative and anesthetic time, reduced intensive care unit time, reduced hospital stay, and earlier recovery and return to function. Accordingly, patients who would otherwise be denied conventional repairs based on their cardiopulmonary status could be offered endovascular repair. Some of the disadvantages of stent graft repair have also become apparent. They include the need for lifelong surveillance and the uncertainty, at least at the present time, of the long-term results of endovascular repair. Patients may have persistent flow in the aneurysm sac (endoleak) following endovascular repair and may experience continuing aneurysm enlargement and rupture. Although this is a rare event, follow-up times have been short. Thus, all patients with endovascular repair must undergo lifelong follow-up and postoperative imaging.

THORACIC AORTIC ANEURYSMS

Thoracic aortic aneurysms (TAAs) are much less common than abdominal aortic aneurysms and their treatment is more complex. The size criterion for repair is slightly larger, 6 cm, than for AAAs (5 cm), owing to the larger size of the normal thoracic aorta compared with the abdominal aorta and the greater risk of significant morbidity and mortality after surgery of the thoracic aorta. In addition, rupture of TAA of less than 6 cm in diameter appears uncommon. Management of aneurysms of the ascending aorta and the arch involves cardiopulmonary bypass and hypothermic circulatory arrest. This chapter is limited to the management of descending thoracic aortic aneurysms.

Clinical Presentation

Most descending TAAs are discovered incidentally on chest radiographic study or CT scan obtained for other indications. Patients may complain of vague, intermittent upper back pain, which leads to a workup. Unlike for the abdominal aorta, ultrasound is not useful. The imaging modality of choice is a timed-bolus contrast-enhanced spiral CT scan. CT scanning should include scanning from the base of the neck to the aortic bifurcation. This study provides dimensional and morphologic data sufficient to determine the need and the type of intervention possible. CT scanning may be complemented with aortography.

If a patient has a sudden onset of upper back pain and has a history of an untreated TAA, then treatment should be for a symptomatic or a ruptured aneurysm until proven otherwise. If the patient is hemodynamically stable and clearly not in shock, an urgent CT scan should be obtained to rule out a rupture. If a leak is not detected, preparations should be made for an urgent repair during the same admission.

Preoperative Management

The preoperative management of elective descending thoracic aneurysm repair should be focused on optimization of the patient's cardiopulmonary status. Many asymptomatic patients harbor occult coronary artery disease that may be addressed preoperatively either through pharmacologic optimization or coronary angioplasty, with or without a stent. Furthermore, most patients have a long history of smoking and some degree of chronic obstructive pulmonary disease. Delineation of baseline pulmonary function and initiation of bronchodilator therapy with chest physiotherapy is critical in maximizing postoperative ventilatory recovery.

Intraoperative Management

The intraoperative management of TAA depends on the proximal and distal extent of the aneurysm. The patient is placed in a left lateral decubitus position on a beanbag, with the hips partially rotated so that the femoral arteries are easily accessible. Intraoperative hemodynamic monitoring with arterial lines, Swan-Ganz catheter with or without transesophageal echocardiography is mandatory. A cell-saver is used if the operation is not performed on cardiopulmonary bypass. Proximal descending thoracic aneurysms may be approached through a fourth interspace posterolateral thoracotomy, whereas mid-descending thoracic aneurysms may be exposed through the seventh or eighth interspace. The distal end of the incision depends on the extent of the aneurysm. If the aneurysm is entirely in the chest, the incision may be limited to the thoracotomy, but with true Crawford type I to III thoracoabdominal aneurysms (TAAA), a left paramedian abdominal extension is performed with division of the seventh to tenth costal cartilages and the left hemidiaphragm.

Proximal and distal clamps are placed in a sequential fashion as each portion of the repair is completed to allow the earliest segmental reperfusion and minimize the total length of aortic occlusion at any given time. Any large intercostals are reimplanted as a patch using the inclusion technique. Frequently, an anatomic distal neck can be identified proximal to the celiac axis. If an infrarenal aneurysm is present, the repair should be staged, rather than undertaken as a single thoracoabdominal reconstruction.

Postoperative Management

Postoperative management is focused on maintaining cardiovascular volume and perfusion and the prevention and treatment of cardiopulmonary complications. Despite the routine use of thoracic epidural analgesia and intercostal nerve blocks, the pain from a large thoracotomy can be a significant impediment to proper pulmonary mechanics and successful weaning from the ventilator. The combination of fluid shifts, atrial distention, and myocardial edema frequently precipitate supraventricular tachyarrhythmias in the early postoperative period. These are generally well tolerated but almost always require pharmacologic intervention to slow down the ventricular rate and effect spontaneous cardioversion. Bleeding is a significant potential complication and should be treated with aggressive correction of hypothermia, underlying coagulopathy, and re-exploration if significant postoperative bleeding occurs.

Complications

One of the most dreaded complications of thoracic aortic surgery is paraplegia resulting from interruption of the blood supply to the spinal cord, which may arise from an intercostal artery arising from the thoracic aneurysm. Although spinal cord drainage, spinal cord cooling, and reimplantation of intercostal arteries have been used, no single method has consistently prevented this problem. Even in the most experienced hands, paraplegia rates for aneurysms involving the proximal segments of the descending thoracic aorta have ranged from 10% to 15%. These events, which result from irreversible spinal cord ischemia mainly affecting the descending fibers of the anterior motor horn, are usually permanent and sometimes associated with bladder and bowel dysfunction. Attempts to identify the so-called artery of Adamkiewicz or *arteria radicularis magna* through preoperative aortography and its reimplantation have not yielded significant improvements in outcome.

Outcomes

Perioperative mortality rates from thoracic aneurysm repair are higher than for abdominal aneurysm repair and range from 10% to 15%. Postoperative morbidity is significant and the incidence of severe, long-term disability and need for chronic institutional rehabilitation can be up to 30%. In the absence of significant complications, a successful repair of TAA results in a gratifying, long-term treatment of a potentially life-threatening problem.

ENDOVASCULAR THORACIC AORTIC ANEURYSM REPAIR

Endovascular repair of TAAs is particularly attractive because of the higher morbidity and mortality rates associated with open surgical repair. Patient selection requires demonstration of a localized aneurysm with at least 2 cm of nonaneurysmal aorta distal to the subclavian artery and proximal to the celiac artery. Careful assessment of preoperative CT scanning is necessary to determine the type of surgical therapy that can be offered to the patient. Shortly after the first abdominal aortic stent graft was placed, one of the earliest series of stent graft repairs of descending TAAs was reported by Dake et al. from Stanford University in 1994. Currently, several commercial endovascular devices are undergoing clinical investigation for thoracic aortic stent grafting. They include the Excluder device by W. L. Gore (Flagstaff, Arizona), the Talent device by Medtronic World-Medical (Sunrise, Florida), and the AneuRx device by Medtronic AVE (Santa Rosa, California). The Talent device may be able to overcome shorter landing zones by using a section of uncovered stent, which can be placed over distal branch vessels. Occasionally, limited proximal fixation sites can be overcome by a preoperative left subclavian to carotid transposition or bypass, which can yield an additional 1 to 2 cm of proximal neck length.

Intraoperative Management

The introducers and delivery systems for thoracic stent grafts are larger than abdominal devices. Thus, introduction may not be possible through the femoral arteries. Patients are approached in a manner similar to abdominal stent grafting but may require exposure of the iliac artery or abdominal aorta in order to introduce the device. Similar to the abdominal aortic stent grafts, these endografts are deployed under fluoroscopic guidance. They are technically easier to deploy, because all are single-lumen, unibody designs that are stacked to achieve the required length.

Postoperative Management

The management following stent graft repair of thoracic aneurysms is similar to that for abdominal aortic stent grafts. Patients are extubated in the operating room, observed in a monitored setting, started on a diet that same day, and discharged usually on the second postoperative day. A pre-discharge CT angiogram is obtained as a baseline for future follow-up and to ensure that the stent graft is in proper position and that the aneurysm is fully excluded from the circulation (no endoleak).

Complications

For reasons that are not quite understood, the incidence of paraplegia following endovascular repair of TAAs appears to be lower than following open surgical thoracic aneurysm repair. Patients who have previously had abdominal aneurysm repair or who are undergoing concomitant AAA repair are at increased risk for paraplegia, presumably because of the loss of lumbar collaterals. If paraplegia or paraparesis does occur following endovascular repair, early therapeutic spinal fluid drainage for 24 to 48 hours may be beneficial. Some clinicians have reported marked improvement and reversal of symptoms following such intrathecal decompression.

Outcomes

As with abdominal aortic stent grafts, patients who have undergone stent graft repairs of their descending thoracic aneurysms require careful, lifelong follow-up with CT scanning or MR imaging to determine aneurysm size and the presence or absence of endoleak. Even though some of the lessons learned from the abdominal aortic experience may be extrapolated to the thoracic aorta, the differences in anatomy, physiology, and the actual stent graft configurations preclude direct analogies from being made.

PERIPHERAL ARTERY ANEURYSMS

Isolated aneurysms of the peripheral vasculature have been described in nearly every major named artery, including the common carotid, internal carotid, subclavian, innominate, brachial, ulnar, common femoral, deep femoral, popliteal, and tibial arteries. Many are exceedingly rare and few studies report on more than a small group of patients. In general, when multiple rare aneurysms occur, one should be suspicious of either mycotic aneurysms or some underlying connective tissue disorder such as Marfan's or Ehlers-Danlos syndrome. The recommended management in most cases involves complete exclusion with or without resection of the aneurysm and a bypass procedure with autogenous or prosthetic conduit. The only exception is in the case of Ehlers-Danlos syndrome type IV in which simple ligation may be the only and the safest option. The remaining discussion is limited to the management of femoral and popliteal aneurysms.

Clinical Presentation

Like most aneurysms, femoral and popliteal aneurysms are usually asymptomatic. They are typically discovered during routine physical examination when an abnormally prominent pulse is palpated. Approximately 5% of patients with AAAs have femoral and popliteal aneurysms, but 60% to 80% of patients with popliteal or femoral aneurysms have AAAs. A duplex ultrasound scan in a vascular laboratory is the diagnostic modality of choice. Baseline size and distal pressure and waveform measurements may be obtained. Usual size criteria for repair are greater than 2.5 cm for femoral aneurysms and greater than 2 cm for popliteal aneurysms. Preoperative workup includes an angiogram in preparation for a bypass. Not infrequently, one or more of the tibial vessels are occluded as a result of chronic embolization.

Femoral and popliteal aneurysms may present acutely with life-threatening hemorrhage or limb-threatening occlusion. Femoral aneurysms can rupture and hemorrhage into the thigh, posing a significant threat to life and limb. More rarely, they present with distal embolization and acute thrombosis. In contrast, the usual acute presentation of popliteal aneurysms involves acute thrombosis or distal embolization, both with severe limb threat. Rarely, popliteal aneurysms may compress the popliteal vein, resulting in a deep vein thrombosis or tibial nerve compression resulting in pain. Although popliteal aneurysms may rupture, this is exceedingly uncommon.

Preoperative Management

Following a duplex ultrasound examination, further evaluation includes a lower extremity angiogram. Patients with a femoral or popliteal aneurysm should undergo an abdominal ultrasound or CT scan to evaluate for presence of an AAA, which may be present in 60% to 80% of cases. If a patient is found to have an AAA during a workup for a femoral or popliteal aneurysm, then the AAA should be addressed first if indicated by the usual criteria and if the distal aneurysms are asymptomatic.

Intraoperative Management

The patient is prepared in the usual manner for a lower extremity bypass procedure. Through a longitudinal incision, the femoral aneurysm is exposed directly. Proximal control is obtained of the distal external iliac artery, which may be easily exposed from the groin by firm upward retraction on the inguinal ligament. The lateral and medial femoral circumflex and inferior epigastric arteries should be preserved because they provide important pelvic-thigh collateral circulation. Distal control is obtained at the superficial femoral artery and the profunda femoris artery. Commonly, the first 1 to 2 cm of the superficial femoral artery can be aneurysmal and control should be obtained within the grossly normal-appearing segment. In contrast, the profunda femoris artery is rarely aneurysmal but control should be obtained at least at the level of the first segmental branch.

After systemic heparinization, the arteries are clamped and the aneurysm is opened longitudinally. Once the aneurysm is decompressed, it can be readily dissected away from the femoral vein and the surrounding femoral sheath and completely excised. If there is extensive inflammation, the adherent portions of the wall should be left intact and the excess trimmed. Reconstruction can be performed in a variety of ways using an 8- or 10-mm interposition tube graft from the external iliac artery to the femoral bifurcation. The proximal anastomosis is performed in an end-to-end fashion using monofilament polypropylene sutures. Distally, there are several options: (1) the distal end of the graft may be anastomosed to the superficial femoral artery and the profunda femoris artery reattached in a posterolateral location, (2) the orifices of the profunda femoris and superficial femoral arteries may be kept together for a beveled anastomosis, or (3) the bifurcation may be re-created by syndactylizing the two arteries and sewing the end of the graft to a single large orifice. Regardless of the nature of the reconstruction, it is important to revascularize the profunda femoris artery.

The repair of popliteal aneurysms follows similar principles. Frequently, the aneurysm extends to the infrageniculate popliteal artery or to the tibial trifurcation. The original description of a popliteal aneurysm repair involved the Matas' operation of endoaneurysmorrhaphy in which, after proximal and distal control, the popliteal aneurysm is opened, the intraluminal clot is evacuated, all the feeding geniculate arteries are ligated, and an interposition graft is anastomosed end-to-end proximally and distally. For focal popliteal aneurysms behind the knee joint, a posterior approach yields a good exposure with minimal musculoskeletal dissection. Alternatively, in the absence of compressive symptoms, a superficial femoral artery or suprageniculate popliteal artery to distal popliteal artery bypass can be performed with the use of autogenous greater saphenous vein. The intervening popliteal segment is ligated proximally and distally to exclude it from direct circulation and to prevent further distal embolization.

Finally, a few patients have ipsilateral synchronous femoral and popliteal aneurysms as part of a generalized arteriomegaly. These may be repaired simultaneously with an interposition iliofemoral bypass to the profunda femoris artery and reconstruction with a femoral-popliteal bypass.

Postoperative Management

The patient is monitored for graft patency and pulses postoperatively and mobilized as tolerated. Once able to ambulate without assistance, the patient is discharged. Follow-up is usually within 2 to 4 weeks, when a baseline graft flow duplex scan is obtained. When the patient is seen with bilateral aneurysmal disease, the two sides may be staged 4 to 6 weeks apart to allow for adequate interval rehabilitation.

Complications

Intraoperative and perioperative complications are similar to those in other lower extremity bypass procedures and include early graft thrombosis and wound problems. The groin incision may be complicated by seromas, lymphoceles, and superficial infections. The presence of prosthetic material warrants aggressive measures with intravenous antibiotics at the earliest sign of cellulitis or wound drainage.

In patients with an acutely ischemic leg from distal embolization or acutely thrombosed popliteal aneurysm, the management depends on the viability of the limb. Motor or sensory deficits signal imminent limb loss, and these patients should be immediately anticoagulated and taken to the operating room. Four-compartment fasciotomies are frequently required to avoid a postoperative compartment syndrome. Selective antegrade and retrograde tibial thrombectomies may sometimes be required. These are difficult cases when no suitable target vessel is identified and risk of amputation is significant. In contrast, when the limb is viable with early ischemic changes, the patient may be a candidate for catheter-guided thrombolysis. This not only restores flow but also allows identification of distal target vessels for a bypass procedure.

Outcomes

Surgical results following *elective* femoral and popliteal aneurysm repairs are excellent. Bypass patency and limb salvage rates for elective popliteal aneurysm repairs range from 80% to 90% and 90% to 100%, respectively, at 10 years. Graft surveillance and serial leg pressure measurements should be performed as part of routine follow-up. Endovascular or surgical therapies may be used to achieve durable secondary patencies.

VISCERAL ARTERY ANEURYSMS

Visceral artery aneurysms refer to, in decreasing order of frequency, aneurysms of the splenic, renal, hepatic, superior mesenteric, celiac, pancreaticoduodenal, and gastroduodenal arteries.

Clinical Presentation

Most visceral artery aneurysms are asymptomatic and are discovered as part of a workup for an unrelated condition. Infrequently, they can present with pain, gastrointestinal bleeding, or hematuria. Unlike aortic aneurysms, there is no widely accepted size criterion for elective repair of these aneurysms. In general, however, indications for surgical intervention include presence of symptoms, females of childbearing age, or lesion size greater than 2 cm in an otherwise good-risk patient. Pregnancy has been identified as a significant risk factor for aneurysm rupture, particularly of splenic artery aneurysms. Although the risk of rupture of most Bland splenic artery aneurysms is approximately 2%, more than 95% of aneurysms discovered during pregnancy have ruptured, with fetal and maternal mortality rates exceeding 75%. Thus, early elective repair should be performed for splenic artery aneurysms discovered during pregnancy or in women who anticipate future conception.

Preoperative Management

Preoperative management of these patients involves a diagnostic CT scan and a selective aortogram with visceral or renal angiography. This serves as a roadmap for any visceral arterial variations, assessment of the proximal and distal neck, presence of collaterals, and availability of suitable autogenous arterial conduits, such as the hypogastric arteries.

Intraoperative Management

Many options are available for visceral arterial reconstruction for aneurysmal disease. Regardless of what approach is used, however, the goal is to completely exclude or resect the aneurysm from the circulation. Restoration of arterial continuity is secondary owing to the rich collateral circulation of the splanchnic bed. The only exceptions to this are renal (RA) and superior mesenteric artery (SMA) aneurysms in which direct reconstruction is almost always necessary to preserve end-organ viability and function. For nearly all visceral artery aneurysms, the approach may be transperitoneal through a bilateral subcostal incision. At least one leg should be prepped for possible greater saphenous vein harvest for bypass.

Splenic artery aneurysms are approached directly through the lesser sac along the superior border of the pancreas. After proximal and distal ligation, the aneurysm may be opened and any small feeding branches oversewn directly, or these branches may be ligated externally and the aneurysm excised. Reconstruction of the splenic artery is usually not needed because the spleen is richly supplied by the short gastric arteries and branches from the left gastroepiploic artery. Care should be taken to avoid inadvertent injury to the splenic vein, which may be adherent to the aneurysm wall. In this case, it is best to leave the aneurysm in situ. In cases of distal splenic artery aneurysms, a splenectomy may be required. If this is anticipated, appropriate immune complex vaccines should be administered at least 2 weeks before the anticipated date of surgery. Endovascular therapy using coil occlusion of inflow and outflow branches and aneurysm thrombosis have also been successful. This may be an attractive option in a poor surgical candidate.

Celiac artery aneurysms may be approached anteriorly through the lesser sac with division of the left hepatic triangular ligament and the diaphragmatic crus. Distal control of the common hepatic and splenic arteries is obtained. The left gastric artery, which frequently comes off the aneurysm, is ligated and divided. The aneurysm is excised with preservation of the bifurcation if possible. Using a partially occluding aortic clamp, a prosthetic or saphenous vein graft is taken off the supraceliac aorta and anastomosed in an end-to-side fashion to the celiac bifurcation with the bevel extended on to the common hepatic artery. Under certain circumstances, the bifurcation may be preserved without a bypass or simply ligated, if the SMA and gastroduodenal-pancreaticoduodenal collaterals are patent on angiography.

SMA aneurysms frequently occur a few centimeters distal to their origins. The pulsation can be palpated through the transverse mesocolon or just along the inferior border of the pancreas. The SMA is approached anteriorly through the transverse mesocolon, along the path of the middle colic artery. The inferior border of the pancreas is lifted away from the anterior surface of the SMA aneurysm and dissection proceeds proximally until sufficient length of proximal neck is obtained. Small jejunal branches coming off the aneurysm may be ligated. The aneurysm wall is left in situ and an interposition graft is sewn in place. Arterial reconstruction is almost always necessary to prevent severe mesenteric ischemia.

Renal artery aneurysms may be approached transperitoneally, with or without medial visceral rotation, or retroperitoneally. For isolated main branch artery aneurysms, an aneurysmectomy may be performed with either a di-

---

Pearls and Pitfalls

PEARLS

- AAAs are lethal.
- There is no *medical* management of AAAs.
- Death from a ruptured AAA is not the worst outcome for a patient. A decision *not* to operate may be best for the patient and the most difficult for the surgeon.
- An AAA with back or abdominal pain is ruptured until proven otherwise.
- Endovascular AAA repair is neither experimental nor investigational. It is part of standard care. Clinicians should be prepared to discuss and offer this therapy if available.
- Aneurysms are systemic and genetic. Peripheral aneurysms should be sought in patients with AAA, and vice versa. First-degree relatives have a 25% risk of AAA.
- Elective repair of popliteal aneurysms may be done if the lesions are greater than 2 cm or if there is evidence of distal embolization. Prognosis is poor for limb salvage in acutely thrombosed popliteal aneurysms.
- Elective repair of splenic aneurysms should be done in pregnant women and women of childbearing age.

PITFALLS

- Diagnosis of AAA by physical examination alone is unreliable.
- Open surgical AAA repair carries a 5% to 10% risk of long-term complications, including graft infection, para-anastomotic recurrence, and aortoenteric fistula. All patients require infrequent, but definite, follow-up for life.
- "A patient is too sick for AAA repair; he should be offered repair if aneurysm enlarges." Either the patient should be offered repair or a decision should be made not to treat or follow the AAA at all.
- An angiogram is rarely necessary in the preoperative imaging of a patient with AAA. A spiral CT scan is the single most important diagnostic study.
- Endovascular therapy should not alter the indications for AAA repair (i.e., there still is no proven indication for routine repair of AAAs less than 4 cm in diameter).
- The long-term natural history of endovascular AAA repair is not known. Patients need to have lifelong follow-up to look for signs of ongoing risk of aneurysm rupture.
- Hypogastric (internal iliac) arteries should be preserved so that the patient will have no buttock pain.
- The inferior mesenteric artery should be reimplanted if patent and larger than 2 mm.

rect aortorenal bypass or hepatorenal or splenorenal bypass. For complex aneurysms involving multiple first or second order branches, ex vivo renal artery reconstruction may be preferred.

Management of other visceral aneurysms involves anatomic exposure, arterial control, and proximal and distal ligation. Arterial reconstruction is not necessary except for hepatic artery aneurysms, in which direct saphenous vein bypass is recommended. These aneurysms frequently present as ruptures and emergency surgery is accompanied by high morbidity and mortality rates.

Postoperative Management

The postoperative management is geared toward adequate fluid resuscitation and avoidance of hypotension. A central venous line can be helpful in guiding fluid management. Following mesenteric revascularization, a brief period of above-maintenance fluid requirements may be expected as a result of mesenteric reperfusion syndrome. Liver function tests, amylase, electrolytes, and acid-base status should be routinely monitored as indirect markers of graft function. If there is any question of graft patency, an abdominal duplex examination should be the initial imaging study obtained from an experienced vascular laboratory. Indeterminate or abnormal examinations should be followed with an angiogram to look for technical causes and aid in surgical revision.

Complications

Complications following visceral artery aneurysm repair include transient or permanent end-organ ischemic injury, visceral emboli, and early graft thrombosis. Visceral emboli may require segmental resection or may result in late stricture requiring stricturoplasty or elective bowel resection. Early graft thrombosis may be symptomatic or completely asymptomatic. If symptomatic, early reoperation is critical to avoid a catastrophic intestinal or hepatic ischemia or loss of a kidney. Like most early graft failures, the reason is usually technical. If asymptomatic, the patient may be managed expectantly.

Outcomes

Elective resection of visceral artery aneurysms may be successfully performed with a 1% to 2% mortality rate. The outcome for emergency surgery for ruptured visceral aneurysms is less encouraging. For ruptures of splenic aneurysms in pregnant women, maternal mortality rate exceeds 70% and fetal mortality rate is in excess of 75%. When these aneurysms are discovered in pregnant women, elective resection should be offered during the second trimester.

SELECTED READINGS

Carr SC, Pearce WH, Vogelzang RL, et al: Current management of visceral artery aneurysms. Surgery 1996;120:627–633; discussion 633–634.

Coselli JS, LeMaire SA, Miller CC 3rd, et al: Mortality and paraplegia after thoracoabdominal aortic aneurysm repair: A risk factor analysis. Ann Thorac Surg 2000;69:409.

Cronenwett JL, Johnston KW: The United Kingdom Small Aneurysm Trial: Implications for surgical treatment of abdominal aortic aneurysms. J Vasc Surg 1999;29:191.

Dake MD, Miller DC, Semba CP, et al: Transluminal placement of endovascular stent grafts for the treatment of descending thoracic aortic aneurysms. N Engl J Med 1994;331:1729.

Diwan A, Sarkar R, Stanley JC, et al: Incidence of femoral and popliteal artery aneurysms in patients with abdominal aortic aneurysms. J Vasc Surg 2000;31:863.

Finlayson SR, Birkmeyer JD, Fillinger MF, Cronenwett JL: Should endovascular surgery lower the threshold for repair of abdominal aortic aneurysms? J Vasc Surg 1999;29:973.

Hallett JW Jr: Management of abdominal aortic aneurysms [Review]. Mayo Clin Proc 2000;75:395.

Lipsitz EC, Ohki T, Veith FJ: Overview of techniques and devices for endovascular abdominal aortic aneurysm repair. Semin Interv Cardiol 2000;5:21.

Moore WS, Kashyap VS, Vescera CL, Quinones-Baldrich WJ: Abdominal aortic aneurysm: A 6-year comparison of endovascular versus transabdominal repair. Ann Surg 1999;230:298–306; discussion 306–308.

Wagner WH, Allins AD, Treiman RL, et al: Ruptured visceral artery aneurysms. Ann Vasc Surg 1997;11:342.

Webb TH, Williams GM: Thoracoabdominal aneurysm repair. [Review]. Cardiovasc Surg 1999;7:573.

Chapter 177

Diagnosis and Management of Chronic Peripheral Arterial Occlusive Disease

James M. Seeger

Chronic peripheral arterial occlusive disease is a common problem. As many as 10% of patients older than 65 years have been estimated to have intermittent claudication, and limb-threatening ischemia develops in as many as 1% to 2% of patients in the same age group. Intermittent claudication occurs when extremity blood flow is reduced to the point of being inadequate for metabolic needs during exercise, whereas limb-threatening ischemia develops when extremity perfusion is inadequate even for resting metabolic demands. Increased extremity perfusion resolves these symptoms if irreversible injury has not occurred, but the techniques available for correction of arterial occlusive disease are invasive and associated with significant risk in the elderly patients who have chronic peripheral arterial occlusive disease. This chapter reviews the pathophysiology of extremity ischemia, the symptoms and diagnostic techniques that allow accurate detection of chronic peripheral arterial occlusive disease, and the currently available therapies for this problem. In addition, the natural history of chronic peripheral arterial occlusive disease is presented to allow an understanding of the appropriate selection of patients for treatment of symptoms of this common problem.

PATHOPHYSIOLOGY

Demographics and Etiology of Chronic Peripheral Arterial Occlusive Disease

Atherosclerosis is the primary cause of chronic lower extremity arterial occlusive disease. Age is the primary risk factor for atherosclerosis, and it is uncommon to see a patient with symptomatic peripheral atherosclerosis younger than 40 years of age, although patients with severe type I diabetes mellitus can be the exception (Table 177–1). Atherosclerosis in the upper extremities is also uncommon at any age, except in the aortic arch. The origin of the subclavian arteries is the site most commonly involved, and 75% of atherosclerotic occlusions of subclavian arteries occur on the left. Other arteries of the upper extremities are usually spared, again except in patients with severe, long-standing diabetes mellitus. Thus, when a patient younger than 40 years of age without longstanding diabetes mellitus has symptoms of lower extremity peripheral arterial insufficiency, uncommon causes of chronic arterial occlusion must be considered: popliteal artery entrapment syndrome, adventitial cystic disease, fibromuscular dysplasia, Buerger's disease, homocystinemia, and early onset atherosclerosis. Similarly, when symptoms of upper extremity arterial insufficiency are encountered, particularly in younger patients or patients without diabetes mellitus, again other causes such as arterial complications of thoracic outlet syndrome, Buerger's disease, or immune arterial diseases such as Takayasu's or giant cell arteritis must be sought. Finally, depending on the patient's past medical history, hypercoagulable states, radiation-induced arterial damage, or previously unrecognized traumatic arterial injury should be considered.

Hemodynamic Changes

Surgical and nonsurgical treatment of symptomatic chronic extremity arterial insufficiency requires identification and treatment of arterial lesions associated with hemodynamic disturbances, which reduce arterial blood flow. Pressure and flow changes develop once an arterial stenosis reaches 50% diameter reduction, and the curves that illustrate the relationship between lumen size, flow

Table 177–1	Etiology of Chronic Arterial Occlusive Disease

Lower Extremity
>40 Years of age
  Atherosclerosis
  Occluded peripheral aneurysm
  Chronic atheroemboli
  Radiation vascular injury
<40 Years of age
  Early-onset atherosclerosis
  Atherosclerosis associated with diabetes mellitus
  Buerger's disease
  Hypercoagulable states
  Popliteal entrapment
  Adventitial cystic disease
  Previous vascular trauma

Upper Extremity
Any Age
  Arch atherosclerosis
  Buerger's disease
  Arterial thoracic outlet syndrome
  Vasculitis (e.g., giant cell arteritis, Takayasu's arteritis)
  Arm or forearm atherosclerosis associated with diabetes mellitus
  Hypercoagulation states
  Chronic atheroemboli
  Previous vascular trauma

velocity, and pressure decline have a single sharp bend, supporting the concept of a *critical* degree of stenosis. Viscous energy losses occur within the stenosis and depend primarily on the radius of the stenosis, whereas inertial energy losses occur at the entrance and exit of the stenosis and can be significant because of dissipation of kinetic energy in a zone of turbulence. Inertial energy losses across a stenosis are usually greater than viscous energy losses so that the length of the stenosis is unimportant. Inertial energy losses are also proportional to the square of the blood velocity and turbulence is more likely to develop as flow increases. Because of this, multiple short stenoses limit blood flow more than a single long stenosis and a stenosis that does not produce a significant pressure decrease during low flow may be associated with a hemodynamically significant pressure gradient during exercise.

Two processes maintain distal extremity perfusion in the presence of hemodynamically significant arterial occlusive disease. As atherosclerotic plaque accumulates, the overall diameter of the vessel increases to maintain a near normal luminal diameter and resistance to flow. Arterial enlargement to compensate for atherosclerotic plaque development is limited, however, and, as more disease accumulates within the arterial wall, hemodynamically significant arterial stenosis or arterial occlusion occurs and extremity perfusion then must be maintained through collateral arteries. Collateral arteries develop from the terminal distribution branches of large and medium-sized arteries and are not new vessels but preexisting pathways that enlarge when a stenosis or occlusion develops in a main artery. The stimulus for opening of preexisting collateral arteries is not entirely clear but is related to a change in the pressure gradient across the collateral network and increased blood velocity within the collateral vessels, which stimulates the release of nitric oxide and/or inflammatory cytokines in experimental animals. This process requires days to weeks to occur but collateral compensation for slowly developing chronic extremity ischemia is often at least partially successful in improving extremity perfusion. However, collateral blood flow cannot compensate completely as the degree of arterial occlusive disease increases because resistance of smaller, longer collateral vessels is higher than resistance in normal, unobstructed large arteries.

NATURAL HISTORY OF CHRONIC ARTERIAL OCCLUSIVE DISEASE

Older studies suggest that the natural history of patients with intermittent claudication is generally good, with 70% to 80% of patients remaining in stable condition or improving. In contrast, more recent studies in which objective testing was done to document the degree of peripheral arterial occlusive disease have shown progression to limb-threatening ischemia during 2.5 to 8 years of follow-up in 20% to 80% of such patients. Factors that predicted a poor outcome included continued cigarette smoking, diabetes mellitus, and, most important, the severity of the arterial occlusive disease when the patient entered the study. Patients with no pedal Doppler signals uniformly do poorly, whereas limb-threatening ischemia develops within 1 year in 25% of those with ankle-brachial systolic pressure indices less than 0.4. In contrast, patients with ankle-brachial indices greater than 0.8 seldom have progressive disease. Long-term survival rates also vary with the severity of lower extremity arterial disease, with an approximately 90% 5-year survival rate in patients with mild claudication, an 80% 5-year survival rate in patients with claudication requiring surgical therapy, a 50% 5-year survival rate in patients undergoing operations for limb-threatening ischemia, and a 12% 5-year survival rate in patients requiring reoperation for limb-threatening ischemia. The impact of arterial reconstruction on the natural history of arterial occlusive disease is not entirely clear. However, reconstructive failure may not return the patient to his or her "pre-reconstruction" symptoms and anatomy, and prosthetic graft failure in particular appears to be commonly associated with a worsening of the degree of ischemia present before treatment. Therefore, the usually benign course of mild arterial occlusive disease and the possibility of worsened ischemia from reconstructive failures are generally considered reasons to avoid arterial reconstruction in patients with mild intermittent claudication.

DIAGNOSIS

The diagnosis of chronic peripheral arterial occlusive disease can be made in most patients on the basis of symptoms and physical findings (Fig. 177–1). Vascular laboratory testing of extremity hemodynamics at rest and with exercise allows confirmation of the diagnosis and quantification of the degree to which extremity hemodynamics are disturbed. Angiography is reserved for patients whose symptoms are sufficiently severe to require therapy because arteriography provides only an anatomic image of the arterial tree, whereas diagnosis and therapy of arterial occlusive disease are based on detection and correction of abnormal hemodynamics.

Clinical Manifestations

Symptoms of chronic peripheral arterial occlusive disease range from intermittent claudication to continuous ischemic rest pain. Intermittent claudication is pain in a major muscle group of the extremity (calf, thigh or buttock for the lower extremity, forearm or shoulder for the upper extremity) with exercise, which is relieved by a short period of rest (usually less than 10 to 15 minutes). The pain is described as cramping although the discomfort in the extremity can also be described as fatigue, heaviness, or numbness. Additional characteristics that make the diagnosis of intermittent claudication more secure include pain that does not occur with the first step or arm movement. Rather, the pain occurs after a reproducible amount of exercise, and activities that increase extremity energy expenditure such as walking on uneven ground, walking uphill, climbing stairs, or arm activities above the head decrease the distance or time at which the pain with exercise begins. Walking distance or amount of exercise necessary to produce pain may vary from day to day, and

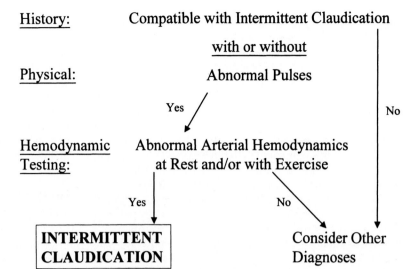

Figure 177–1. Algorithm for the diagnosis of intermittent claudication.

some patients can "walk through the pain," although this finding is unusual and must raise questions about whether the symptoms the patient is describing are due to exercise-induced extremity ischemia. Ischemic rest pain is typically described as foot pain, usually across the metatarsal heads. When it is intermittent, it almost always occurs at night, awakening the patient from sleep and often being associated with paresthesias, particularly numbness of the toes. Placing the extremity in a dependent position relieves or significantly reduces the pain. When the extremity ischemia is severe, elevation of the affected extremity increases the pain but dependence may not entirely relieve it and the pain is very difficult to control with pain medications.

Examination of the chronically ischemic extremity usually reveals minimal neurologic changes (primarily decreased light touch) even when ischemic rest pain is present. Muscular function is also intact unless an acute, profound reduction in blood flow has recently occurred. Pulses are diminished or absent, although normal pulses by palpation at rest can be observed in patients with intermittent claudication (Fig. 177–2). Trophic skin changes such as dry, scaling skin, subcutaneous atrophy, loss of hair, thickening of the nails, hyperpigmentation in blacks, pallor with elevation, and rubor with dependency document chronic extremity ischemia. Ischemic tissue loss is an obvious sign of severe extremity ischemia and both ischemic ulcers and gangrene may occur spontaneously or after trauma and infection. Ischemic ulcers are typically pale, "punched out" lesions that are very painful. Rubor around the ulcer is common and should not be considered a sign of adequate perfusion for healing. Ulcers are considered "nonhealing" when no evidence of healing is seen after 4 to 6 weeks of local therapy or when progressive necrosis occurs despite good local therapy, including control of infection. Gangrene is always due to ischemia and is usually a consequence of large vessel occlusion. Even in patients with diabetes mellitus, pedal ulceration or digital gangrene is due to arterial occlusive disease above the ankle at least 75% of the time, whereas occlusion of the pedal or digital arteries (which can be distinguished by the presence of normally palpable pulses in the affected foot) is the cause in the remainder. "Small vessel" disease affecting the arterioles is not a cause of

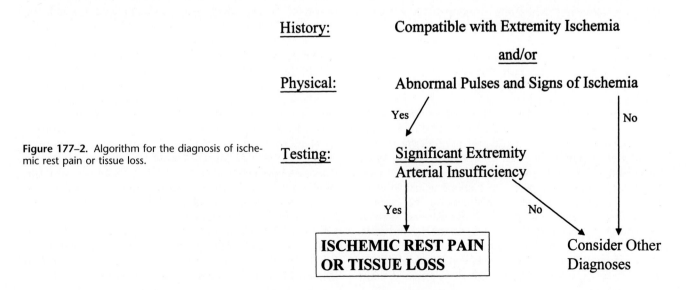

Figure 177–2. Algorithm for the diagnosis of ischemic rest pain or tissue loss.

pedal gangrene in patients with diabetes mellitus, as this type of disease has never been demonstrated in multiple, carefully done studies examining the arterial tree of amputated limbs from patients with diabetes mellitus.

Symptoms and physical findings often allow localization of the arterial occlusive disease responsible for the extremity ischemia. Exercise-induced ischemia resulting from significant occlusive disease in the aorta-iliac system is usually manifested as thigh or buttock pain in addition to calf pain, although many patients have calf claudication alone. Absent femoral pulses allows detection of hemodynamically significant aorta-iliac occlusive disease in such patients. Ischemic rest pain or tissue loss is uncommon in patients with isolated disease in the iliac or superficial femoral arteries and patients with ischemic rest pain and tissue loss usually have disease both above and below the inguinal ligament. In contrast, pedal and digital ischemia is common in patients with isolated severe disease in the infrapopliteal arteries where collateral pathways are poor. Resting digital ischemia can also be caused by atheroemboli from the aorta or iliac arteries. Differentiation of digital ischemia resulting from atheroemboli from digital ischemia caused by occlusive disease is usually simple because patients with "blue toe syndrome" essentially always have palpable pedal pulses demonstrating patent vessels to the foot, which serve as a conduit for the emboli.

Nonvascular Causes of Extremity Pain With Exercise and at Rest

Extremity pain with exercise may also be due to joint diseases such as arthritis. As opposed to intermittent claudication, extremity pain in patients with musculoskeletal disease usually occurs with the initiation of standing or walking and improves after the first few steps. Severely limited extremity venous outflow after iliofemoral venous thrombosis may also cause extremity pain with exercise and this "venous claudication" is typically described as a "bursting" pain that is slow to resolve with rest. Extremities of patients with venous claudication are also warm and swollen, with skin changes consistent with chronic venous insufficiency. Symptoms of neurospinal compression resulting from stenosis of the spinal canal may closely mimic the symptoms of intermittent claudication, but patients with this problem usually also complain of burning, numbness, and tingling in the extremities with walking, which is not relieved by cessation of walking alone. Furthermore, the pain begins in the back and radiates down both legs with standing or the first step of walking.

The pedal pain at rest that must be differentiated from ischemic rest pain is diabetic neuropathy. This is particularly important because patients with diabetes mellitus often also have significant arterial occlusive disease. The most common symptoms of diabetic neuropathy are sensory complaints including paresthesias such as spontaneous tingling (pins and needles), dysesthesias with an unpleasant, hypersensitive response to touch, and complaints of sensory deficits such as numbness and decreased light touch. However, some patients also have severe, burning distal foot pain, which is worse at night.

Association of foot pain with the other neurologic abnormalities seen in patients with diabetes mellitus and the observation that the pain is not relieved by dependency or increased by elevation may be helpful in differentiating painful diabetic neuropathy from ischemic rest pain. Absence of skin changes characteristic of chronic ischemia may also be helpful, although the autonomic neuropathy of diabetes may produce rubor. Hemodynamic testing may be necessary to differentiate ischemic rest pain from diabetic neuropathy.

Hemodynamic Testing

Determination of extremity arterial hemodynamics confirms the presence (or absence) of extremity arterial insufficiency, suggests the likely natural history of the disease, and allows objective follow-up for detection of disease progression. The most commonly used method of assessing extremity arterial hemodynamics is measurement of extremity blood pressures using continuous wave Doppler to detect arterial flow while specially designed pressure cuffs are inflated at various positions on the leg or arm. The simplest screening test for lower extremity arterial occlusive disease in most patients is the ankle-brachial systolic pressure index (the ABI). This is determined by measuring ankle pressures using both the dorsalis pedis and the posterior tibial artery Doppler signals and brachial artery pressures in both arms. The index is then calculated by dividing the highest of the ankle pressures from each side into the highest of the two brachial pressures. Normally, this index is 1 or greater, and values less than 0.95 are considered abnormal. Patients with intermittent claudication usually have ABIs between 0.4 and 0.95, those with rest pain between 0.2 and 0.5, and those with tissue loss less than 0.3. However, there is significant overlap between these three categories. Measurement of pressures at additional positions on the extremity allows localization of the segment of the arterial tree responsible for decreased arterial pressure at the ankle. Pressure cuffs are generally placed on the thigh and below the knee to allow determination of whether disease in the aorta-iliac segment, the femoral popliteal segment, or the tibial artery segment is responsible for the overall extremity pressure gradient determined by the ABI. Results of segmental pressure determinations compare well with results of arteriography in most patients, but severe stenosis or complete occlusion of the vessels in the aorta-iliac segment may obscure pressure gradients in the femoropopliteal or infrapopliteal regions. Furthermore, separation of aorta-iliac occlusive disease from femoropopliteal occlusive disease can be difficult, because to obtain an accurate measurement of thigh pressure, a wide cuff must be used to compensate for the increased diameter of the thigh. Use of such a cuff means that only a single thigh pressure measurement can be made and occlusion of the proximal portion of the superficial femoral artery cannot be separated from aorta-iliac or common femoral occlusion. This problem can be overcome using a specially designed narrow cuff that allows pressure measurement close to the groin, but an approximately 20-mm Hg increase in pressure resulting from the small cuff must be taken into account when this is done. Use of the small thigh cuff improves the accuracy of localization of aorta-iliac and femoral occlusive disease, but isolated profunda femoral artery disease still results in an apparent aorta-iliac pressure gradient. Discrimination between aorta-iliac and femoral occlusion and superficial femoral artery occlusion may still not be possible in up to 25% of cases. In addition, conditions associated with abnormal stiffening of the peripheral arteries, such as medial calcification resulting from diabetes mellitus, an abnormally large limb, or excessive local scarring, may invalidate pressure measurements at any position because the measured pressure reflects the pressure required to overcome the intraluminal arterial pressure plus the pressure required to collapse the arterial wall and surrounding tissue (which is usually negligible).

Techniques used to assess extremity hemodynamics that do not use blood pressure measurements include Doppler waveform analysis and plethysmography. Doppler detectors produce an analog signal that is proportional to the velocity of the blood in the vessel being studied, and the shape of the waveform reflects the status of the vessel proximal to the point at which the Doppler signal is recorded. Normal lower extremity velocity is triphasic during each cardiac cycle, with reversal of flow in early diastole caused by the high resistance of the extremity vascular tree and a second phase of forward flow resulting primarily from elastic recoil of the aorta. Increasing severity of occlusive disease proximal to the point of study initially eliminates the reversed flow phase followed by blunting of the systolic upstroke and increased flow during diastole. Doppler waveform analysis is most commonly used to aid in distinguishing aorta-iliac occlusive disease from femoropopliteal disease. The shape of the waveform, however, is also influenced by disease in the arteries distal to the point of study, which produces a high false-positive rate. Blood flow into the extremity also causes an increase in extremity volume during systole, which returns to baseline during diastole. Using a variety of plethysmographic recording devices, these changes can be recorded and abnormal extremity hemodynamics can be detected from qualitative evaluation of the plethysmographic waveform. Volume changes are measured at the thigh, calf, and ankle levels, and, based on waveform changes, significant areas of occlusive disease within an extremity can be localized. Serial measurements are reproducible so that progression of occlusive disease can be detected and plethysmographic waveforms can also be recorded from extremity digits, so that qualitative or quantitative (when used in combination with small blood pressure cuffs) assessment of digital hemodynamics is possible. Such measurements are important in determining whether digital or foot amputations will heal and in assessing blood flow in patients in whom more proximal measurements are invalid because of arterial stiffening (e.g., patients with diabetes mellitus), which uncommonly occurs in digital arteries.

Even though most patients with advanced arterial occlusive disease can be evaluated at rest, early lesions in patients with symptoms of intermittent claudication may produce significant hemodynamic disturbances only during the increased flow associated with exercise. Assessing hemodynamics during exercise can also allow differentiation of intermittent claudication from other causes of exercise-induced extremity pain. In the lower extremity, the simplest and most physiologic method of increasing extremity blood flow is to have the patient walk on a treadmill so that walking speed can be standardized. Ankle pressures are measured repeatedly after walking and compared with baseline pressures. The distance at which extremity pain with exercise begins is also determined and the reason the patient stops walking is assessed. Patients without arterial occlusive disease have no significant change (or an increase) in ankle pressure after walking, whereas those with flow-limiting arterial lesions will have at least a 15% decrease in ankle pressure that fails to return to baseline pressure within 2 minutes.

Arterial Imaging

Contrast arteriography using iodinated contrast agents is the principal technique for arterial imaging currently in use. Magnetic resonance arteriography is also being more commonly used in the assessment of arterial occlusive disease, and the overall accuracy of the arterial images produced by this technique is approaching that achieved using contrast arteriography. Regardless, using either technique for arterial imaging, only the lumen of the arteries being studied is visualized so that characteristics of the occlusive disease within the arterial wall must be inferred. Contrast arteriography has a limited role in the *diagnosis* of symptomatic peripheral arterial occlusive disease; rather it is used to visualize abnormal arterial *anatomy* responsible for previously defined areas of abnormal hemodynamics and to provide a "road map" to be used in planning therapy. Areas of arterial occlusion are usually easily identified, as are areas of severe arterial stenosis. Recent introduction of less toxic contrast agents such as the non-ionic monomers (iohexol, Hexabrix), improved imaging systems such as electronic digital enhancement (digital subtraction arteriography), which allow the use of less contrast, and techniques that use smaller catheters for contrast delivery have made contrast arteriography easier, more accurate, and much safer. In addition, development of CO_2 gas as a contrast agent has virtually eliminated the risk of renal failure associated with contrast arteriography using iodinated contrast agents. No hemodynamic information is obtained from contrast arteriography, although hemodynamic testing is possible during the procedure using direct intra-arterial pressure measurements through the catheters inserted for contrast injection. Pull-back pressures across arterial lesions can determine whether an area of stenosis seen during arteriography is responsible for a significant pressure gradient at rest (usually greater than 15 to 20 mm Hg). Similarly, femoral artery pressure measurement after injection of vasodilators is useful in determining which patients with both aorta-iliac and infrainguinal occlusive disease need correction of inflow disease before infrainguinal bypass and whether an iliac artery can provide adequate inflow for a femoral-femoral bypass.

The limitations of arterial imaging by contrast arteriography must be kept in mind if appropriate therapy is to be provided to the patient with arterial occlusive disease. First, whereas visualization of an artery usually confirms vessel patency, nonvisualization does not necessarily mean that the vessel is occluded. Demonstration of an artery by arteriography depends on a patent arterial lumen *and* delivery of contrast to that lumen. In the presence of occlusive disease, blood flow and, thus, contrast delivery into arteries distal to a point of severe stenosis or occlusion occur through collateral vessels. If these collateral vessels arise from segments of the arterial system into which contrast is not injected, the arteries that they supply will not be visualized. An example of this is seen when the femoral arteries are supplied by the inferior epigastric artery from the internal mammary artery after iliac artery occlusion. Injection of contrast into the aortic arch may be necessary to demonstrate these vessels, whereas arteriography done by injection of contrast into the infrarenal aorta may incorrectly demonstrate these vessels to be occluded. Second, contrast arteriography usually underestimates the amount of disease present in a patent artery. This is due to the imaging of the vessel lumen rather than the arterial wall and to the fact that imaging is usually only done in only one plane, an anteroposterior projection. Atherosclerotic plaque is commonly eccentric and a significant portion of plaque in peripheral arteries is in the posterior wall so that an image of the lumen in one projection may underestimate (or overestimate) the severity of the disease present. In addition, if the vessel is diffusely diseased, the degree of stenosis in an arterial segment may be underestimated because the apparently normal segment to which the lumen of the stenotic segment is compared may also be narrowed. Finally, opacifying the arterial lumen with dense, radiopaque contrast obscures luminal detail, making an irregular, diseased artery appear more normal.

Color flow duplex ultrasound imaging has recently been used as an alternative, indirect technique for obtaining information similar to that obtained from contrast arteriography, with the identification and localization of significant arterial occlusive lesions being based on changes in systolic and diastolic blood flow velocities and audio spectral analysis displays. Accuracy for detecting stenoses of greater than 50% ranges from 67% to 89% (popliteal to iliac arteries, respectively), and stenosis can be differentiated from occlusion in 98% of cases. Infrapopliteal arteries are visualized in 83% to 96% of cases (peroneal to posterior tibial arteries) and continuous patency to the ankle in these arteries is accurately assessed 80% to 90% of the time. Preliminary studies have also shown that accurate preoperative surgical planning based on arterial duplex mapping alone is possible in more than 83% of patients undergoing infrainguinal arterial bypass procedures (compared with 90% for contrast arteriography). Duplex ultrasound surveillance of patients who have undergone lower extremity vascular bypass grafting also significantly improves graft patency and limb salvage by detecting bypass graft stenoses prior to graft occlusions, and contrast arteriography before repair of these lesions may be unnecessary in most cases.

THERAPY FOR CHRONIC ARTERIAL OCCLUSIVE DISEASE

Indications for Treatment

Treatment of chronic peripheral arterial occlusive disease is clearly indicated in essentially all patients who have limb-threatening ischemia (Table 177–2) except those who will not benefit from such treatment. This includes patients with ischemic rest pain, gangrene or nonhealing tissue loss, *and* objective evidence of severe pedal ischemia, including the following: ABIs less than 0.4, ankle pressures less than or equal to 60 mm Hg, flat or barely pulsatile pulse volumes or Doppler velocity waveform recordings at the ankle or metatarsal level, and toe pressures less than 40 mm Hg. Ischemic ulceration should have been present for 4 to 6 weeks without evidence of healing or be severe or progressing despite local therapy for it to be considered "nonhealing." Such patients require therapy for limb salvage because, without improved extremity perfusion, the risk of amputation is high (>80%). Invasive treatment of patients with intermittent claudication should be more selective. Patients with economic or lifestyle-limiting symptoms can be considered for therapy, but the decision to treat such cases must always be balanced against the natural history of arterial occlusive disease in such patients. Certain subgroups of patients with intermittent claudication, including those with progressive symptoms, symptoms after walking less than 100 to 150 feet, ABIs less than 0.4, and significant dependent rubor, have a significant risk of progression to critical ischemia in a relatively short period of time (1 to 2 years). In contrast, limb-threatening ischemia is unlikely to develop in the near future in patients with stable symptoms that occur after walking long distances and ABIs greater than 0.5. Invasive therapy in such patients should be considered only after a trial of "medical therapy," including cessation of tobacco use, involvement in regular exercise, and, potentially, failure of drugs such as cilostazol to adequately control symptoms. Even in patients with the predictors of an unfavorable natural history of their claudication, medical therapy should be instituted while consideration is given to more invasive therapy.

Table 177–2	**Indications for Invasive Therapy for Chronic Arterial Occlusive Disease**

Limb-Threatening Ischemia
  Requirements: Gangrene or nonhealing tissue loss or ischemic rest pain *PLUS* ABI <0.3 or ankle pressure <40 mm Hg or toe pressure <40 mm Hg or flat PVR
Severe Intermittent Claudication
  Requirements: Rapidly progressive symptoms or walking distance <100–150 ft or significant dependent rubor *PLUS* ABI <0.4 or positive lower-extremity exercise study
Lifestyle-Limiting Intermittent Claudication
  Requirements: Good-risk patient and failure of "medical therapy" *PLUS* ABI <0.8 and a positive lower-extremity exercise study

ABI, ankle-brachial systolic index; PVR, peripheral vascular resistance.

Requirements for Successful Treatment of Chronic Arterial Occlusive Disease

Successful therapy for chronic arterial occlusive disease requires a number of factors (Table 177–3). *First*, the patient to be treated must be likely to benefit from improved extremity blood flow. Lower extremity arterial reconstruction is generally not indicated if the patient does not ambulate. Amputation may be more appropriate if limb-threatening ischemia is present, unless the patient uses the extremity for transfer and to live independently. In addition, arterial repair is not indicated in patients with intermittent claudication when other medical problems limit activity to an equal or greater degree than extremity arterial insufficiency. Arterial reconstruction may also seem contraindicated in patients with severe medical illness and limb-threatening ischemia, but once this problem develops, invasive therapy usually cannot be avoided unless the patient's life expectancy is very short. *Second*, the arterial lesion causing increased resistance to extremity blood flow must be identified. Reconstruction of the arterial system is possible because severe atherosclerosis causing critical arterial stenosis or occlusion is usually localized, and, in most cases, identification of the lesion or lesions that limit extremity blood flow is simple. However, in some patients, diffuse arterial disease without an obvious area of critical stenosis is seen. Therapy in these patients must be based on hemodynamic measurements rather than the angiographic appearance of the arterial disease. Similarly, management of patients with significant multilevel occlusive disease must be based on hemodynamic measurements because repair of hemodynamically significant lesions in the aorta and iliac arteries improves symptoms in approximately three fourths of such patients, and the addition of a procedure to correct infrainguinal occlusive disease increases the patient's risk. However, combined (preferably staged) procedures for correction of both aorta-iliac and infrainguinal occlusive lesions should be considered in those patients with severely diseased profunda femoris arteries or those with significant pedal tissue loss.

Requirements for a successful arterial reconstructive procedure also include absence of hemodynamically significant arterial lesions proximal to the area of the reconstruction (*adequate inflow*), vessels distal to the area of

arterial reconstruction that will deliver adequate nutrient blood flow for relief of ischemic symptoms and allow adequate flow through a bypass graft to maintain patency (*adequate runoff*), and *adequate conduit* if a surgical bypass procedure is required. Inflow can be assessed using segmental pressure testing or intra-arterial pressure monitoring after vasodilator injection. A normal palpable femoral pulse or arteriography showing widely patent vessels to the level of the required reconstruction can also be used to determine the adequacy of inflow, but confirmation of the arteriogram using hemodynamic testing should be done if there is any question. Unfortunately, outflow can only be assessed before reconstruction by the angiographic appearance of the arteries distal to the site of the reconstruction. A patent and minimally diseased profunda femoris artery is adequate outflow for an aorta-iliac reconstructive procedure, whereas at least one patent, minimally diseased artery connecting the area of the distal anastomosis to the foot is necessary for an infrainguinal bypass done for pedal ischemia. Patent pedal arteries (dorsal pedal, posterior tibial, tarsal) also are adequate targets for infrainguinal bypasses, and healing of pedal ischemic lesions can be achieved with bypasses to these arteries, regardless of the location of the ischemic lesion (forefoot versus heel lesions) or the absence of an intact pedal arch. Establishment of pulsatile flow to the foot as shown by continuous wave Doppler interrogation of pedal pulses at the end of the procedure is a good indicator of adequate outflow for an arterial bypass, whereas absence of audible pulses demonstrates inadequate outflow, which requires conversion to a different site for the anastomosis. Low flow rates through the bypass (less than 50 to 70 mL/min) at the completion of the procedure, measured using an electromagnetic flow meter, can also identify poor outflow and suggest the need for a different site for the distal anastomosis to maintain bypass graft patency. Venous conduit can be assessed before surgery using B-mode ultrasound imaging and intraoperatively using video angioscopy.

Choice of Type of Therapy

Once the arterial segment or segments responsible for the reduction in extremity blood flow have been identified, the type of therapy to be used to correct the lesion can be chosen. Options currently available for correction of chronic arterial occlusive lesions are generally grouped into surgical-arterial reconstruction and endovascular-arterial therapy. Surgical arterial reconstruction is the gold standard of therapy for chronic arterial occlusive disease because surgical procedures have been well studied over many years and results are predictable and generally durable (bypass graft patency rates ranging from 70% to 95% at 5 years). In addition, surgical arterial reconstruction is applicable to essentially all types and locations of arterial occlusive lesions. However, surgical arterial reconstructive procedures are associated with significant operative mortality (2% to 4%) and morbidity risks, and patients require up to 6 weeks for full recovery following the procedure. Successful endovascular procedures (balloon angioplasty, stent placement) are generally associated

Table 177–3	**Requirements for Successful Reconstruction in Chronic Arterial Occlusive Disease**

Patient who will benefit from the procedure
Identifiable area of arterial occlusive disease responsible for hemodynamic compromise
If surgical bypass is chosen:
    Adequate inflow to the area to be treated
    Adequate runoff below the area to be treated
    Adequate conduit
If endovascular therapy is chosen:
    Localized (<5–10 cm) area of disease in an artery demonstrated to respond well to endovascular therapy
    Adequate inflow and runoff, as described above

with less risk so that these procedures are attractive alternatives to surgical arterial reconstruction in patients with chronic arterial occlusive disease. However, the likelihood of successful treatment of chronic arterial occlusive disease using endovascular procedures is generally lower than with surgical arterial reconstruction and the type and location of arterial occlusive lesions that can be successfully treated are limited.

Endovascular therapy for treatment of chronic arterial occlusive disease is best suited for treatment of localized arterial lesions in patients without limb-threatening ischemia. Localized (<5 cm) stenotic lesions in the common iliac arteries are ideal for treatment using balloon angioplasty (Fig. 177–3). Continuing patency and clinical improvement can be expected to be 80% at 2 years and 60% at 5 years after successful angioplasty of such lesions. Routine use of endoluminal stents with iliac artery angioplasty does not improve the results of successful iliac angioplasty alone, although stents can be valuable in the salvage of hemodynamically unsuccessful procedures. Use of stents may also be associated with improved results in longer common iliac artery lesions but no comparative studies have been done to document this. Results of treatment of even localized stenosis in other arteries using balloon angioplasty are not as good, with continuing patency at 2 years after successful balloon angioplasty of only 50% to 70% for external iliac artery lesions and, at best, 50% for femoral or popliteal arterial lesions. Factors that predict the best results include patients treated for claudication, patients with stenoses, and patients with good runoff. In contrast, a less-than-15% continuing patency at 1 year is seen in patients with limb-threatening ischemia whose femoral or popliteal lesions are treated with balloon angioplasty. Even poorer results are seen when longer superficial femoral artery stenoses are treated using angioplasty (77% occlusion by 6 months, 100% failure by 30 months for lesions >7 cm). The use of endovascular stents in infrainguinal arteries does not appear to improve results and, in some series, has been associated with an increased risk of immediate arterial thrombosis. Other types of endovascular therapy for chronic arterial occlusive disease, including atherectomy and laser-assisted balloon angioplasty, have been abandoned because of unacceptable results, whereas thrombolysis appears to be most effective in the treatment of acute arterial or bypass graft occlusions. Endovascular placement of prosthetic grafts for aortoiliac and femoral popliteal bypasses is currently being investigated, but studies are too preliminary to demonstrate anything other than the feasibility of such procedures.

Management of Chronic Aorta-Iliac Arterial Occlusive Disease

Localized lesions, particularly in the common iliac arteries, are treated with balloon angioplasty and stenting because good initial and long-term results can be expected after such treatment. Similar lesions in the external iliac arteries can also be treated in this manner, although long-term results are not as good, and such therapy should only be used in selected patients who are poor surgical candidates. Aortofemoral bypass is the treatment of choice for aorta-iliac occlusive disease, which is inappropriate for treatment using balloon angioplasty, particularly when diffuse disease is present. Mortality rate from this procedure is less than 2%, initial graft patency approaches 100%, and graft patency at 5 years averages 80% and at 10 years 75%. Functional improvement occurs in 95% of patients. Of those patients employed before surgery, 85% return to work. Potential morbidity directly associated with the procedure includes renal failure, ischemic colitis, and distal embolization; however, the risk of these complications in modern series is 1% or less. In contrast, significant systemic morbidity such as cardiac or pulmonary complications may occur in up to 10% of patients undergoing aortofemoral bypass. An end-to-end aortic anastomosis is chosen when appropriate because of the superior hemodynamics of this type of anastomosis; however, if the patient will lose important flow to the

	Aorta/Iliac Disease	**Femoropopliteal Disease**	**Infrapopliteal Disease**
Indications for Therapy	• Limb-Threatening Ischemia • Significant Claudication	• Limb-Threatening Ischemia • Significant Claudication	• Limb-Threatening Ischemia • Claudication in "ideal" patients only

Therapy by Disease Type	Localized: Balloon Angioplasty
	+
	−
	Endoluminal Stent
	
	Diffuse: Good Risk ➔ ABF
	           Poor Risk ➔ Ax-Fm-Fm
	                or Fem-Fm
		Localized: ?Balloon Angioplasty
		           ?Endarterectomy
		
		Diffuse: Femoral Popliteal
		          Bypass
			Localized: Unlikely to Occur
			
			Diffuse: Femoral Infrapopliteal
			         or Pedal Bypass

Technical Points	1) ABF should extend over profunda femoris orifice 2) Extra-anatomic bypasses should use externally supported grafts 3) Multi-level disease treatment should be staged	1) Vein grafts to below knee popliteal artery 2) Prosthetic graft used for above knee popliteal bypass only when vein not available 3) Bypass to popliteal island of limited value	1) Vein graft essential 2) Inflow sources other than common femoral artery acceptable 3) Confirm ideal outflow artery (intraoperative angiogram)

Figure 177–3. Algorithm for the management of chronic arterial occlusive disease. ABF, aortobifemoral bypass; Ax-Fm-Fm, axillofemoral femoral bypass; Fem-Fm, femoral femoral bypass.

inferior mesenteric or hypogastric arteries, an end-to-side proximal anastomosis is done. Aortic dissection is limited in males to the area between the renal arteries and the inferior mesenteric artery in an attempt to avoid disturbing the anatomic nervus plexus, which controls the male sexual function. A knitted Dacron or expanded polytetrafluoroethylene (ePTFE) graft is used, matching the size of the aorta and femoral arteries as closely as possible. Graft limbs are anastomosed end-to-side to the femoral artery with the femoral anastomosis extended over the orifice of the profunda femoris artery to ensure an adequate outflow tract.

In patients at high risk for intra-abdominal surgery, an ileofemoral or a femorofemoral bypass is done if only one iliac artery is involved with disease; an axillobifemoral bypass is done when the aorta and both iliac arteries are diseased. Treatment of the inflow iliac artery with angioplasty and possibly stenting to correct a hemodynamically significant stenosis does not affect long-term femorofemoral bypass graft patency. The axillobifemoral bypass is usually from the right axillary artery (if the brachial artery pressures are equal) and use of grafts with external support appears to be associated with improved long-term graft patency. Unilateral axillofemoral bypass procedures are avoided because of a substantially decreased patency of such grafts compared to an axillobifemoral bypass. Primary patency for both of these "extra-anatomic" bypass grafts is less than for aortobifemoral bypass grafts (60% to 70% at 5 years), but with careful follow-up and revision, secondary graft patency approaches that achieved using aortobifemoral bypass. However, extra-anatomic bypasses should always be considered secondary procedures in a patient with aorta-iliac occlusive disease.

Management of Chronic Infrainguinal Arterial Occlusive Disease

As previously noted, balloon angioplasty has a very limited role in the treatment of infrainguinal arterial occlusive disease because of poor results. Therefore, arterial bypass surgery is the procedure of choice for treatment of the great majority of patients with infrainguinal chronic arterial occlusive disease, especially those with limb-threatening ischemia. Patients with either lifestyle-limiting claudication or limb-threatening ischemia can appropriately undergo femoropopliteal bypass for treatment of superficial femoral artery occlusive disease. In contrast, bypass procedures to infrapopliteal arteries are generally reserved for patients with limb-threatening ischemia, although selected patients with short distance claudication, low ankle brachial pressure indices, and very good runoff vessels can be treated with such bypasses. The common femoral artery has traditionally been used as the inflow vessel for infrainguinal bypass procedures, but the superficial femoral and popliteal arteries have been shown by arteriography to be appropriate inflow sites if occlusive disease proximal to this level is mild as shown by arteriography (no stenosis greater than 50%). Adequacy of such vessels for inflow can be confirmed using intraoperative papaverine testing. Shorter vein bypasses appear to have

superior patency. The popliteal artery can be used as an outflow vessel if at least one of the three infrapopliteal arteries is in continuity with the popliteal artery and is minimally diseased throughout its length. The above-knee segment of the popliteal artery is used for the site of the distal anastomosis if the middle portion of the popliteal artery is free of disease; if not, the below-knee site is preferred because progression of existing disease in the mid-popliteal artery will threaten the bypass. When the popliteal artery is severely diseased or occluded, or if no infrapopliteal vessel is in continuity with the popliteal artery, a femoral-to-tibial or peroneal artery bypass is required. A tibial artery (anterior tibial or posterior tibial), which is patent into the foot and has minimal occlusive disease, is chosen for the distal anastomosis, if possible; however, a large-caliber, disease-free peroneal artery with good collateral vessels to the foot is equally appropriate and preferred over a diseased tibial artery. Use of intraoperative pre-bypass arteriography confirms the quality of the artery distal to the point chosen as the site of the distal anastomosis from the preoperative arteriogram and is associated with a change in the distal bypass target approximately 20% of the time. Bypass to the ankle level or to the pedal arteries should be done when pedal tissue loss is present and no suitable vessel proximal to this level is seen. Such bypasses are effective in healing tissue loss and have adequate long-term patency for limb salvage.

Prospective evaluation has shown saphenous vein to have superior long-term patency to all types of synthetic grafts for infrainguinal bypass. Five-year patency of infrainguinal bypasses done using saphenous vein is 60% to 80% compared with 10% to 40% for prosthetic bypasses (infrapopliteal to popliteal bypasses, respectively). The in situ technique of infrainguinal saphenous vein bypass has been suggested to be associated with superior long-term graft patency but prospective comparisons of in situ and reversed vein grafts have failed to document this superiority. In contrast, vein size (<3 mm in diameter) and vein quality (sclerosis, thick vein wall, areas of recanalization) have been shown to negatively influence long-term vein graft patency. Whereas as many as 90% of patients have some type of venous conduit that can be used for infrainguinal bypass, as few as 50% have a good-quality ipsilateral saphenous vein. Use of prosthetic grafts for above-knee femoropopliteal bypass is acceptable in that prospective studies have not shown a statistically significant difference in patency at 4 years between autogenous saphenous vein and PTFE grafts (despite an overall patency difference of approximately 20%). However, failure of prosthetic femoral popliteal bypasses is associated with more severe limb ischemia compared with femoral popliteal vein graft failure. Below-knee femoropopliteal bypass using PTFE can also be considered when no adequate vein is available, because at least short-term patency of such bypasses is acceptable. However, patency of such bypasses done with alternative venous conduits (arm veins, lesser saphenous veins) is significantly higher (approximately 70% at 5 years). Venous conduits should be used if possible for infrapopliteal bypass because of the very poor results of prosthetic graft bypass to infrapopliteal arteries (approximately 20% 2-year patency), and alternative sources of veins such as arm veins or lesser saphenous veins should be sought when adequate greater saphenous vein is not available. Anticoagulation after prosthetic bypass to infrainguinal arteries improves long-term graft patency to as much as 37% at 4 years. However, these results are still inferior to those achieved with the use of venous conduits of any type, and prosthetic grafts should likely only be used when short-term graft patency will potentially allow limb salvage (e.g., healing of an ischemic ulcer).

Management of Upper Extremity Chronic Arterial Occlusive Disease

Proximal stenosis or occlusion of the subclavian artery associated with arm claudication is most successfully treated by ipsilateral common carotid to subclavian artery bypass using a prosthetic bypass graft. The risk of this procedure is minimal and graft patency at 10 to 20 years approaches 95%. Patency of this bypass is superior to that of an axillary artery to axillary artery bypass, and long-term results using PTFE grafts are better than those achieved using saphenous vein grafts. Balloon dilatation and endoluminal stenting of subclavian artery stenotic lesions is also possible in approximately 90% of cases (50% of occlusions), and long-term results appear acceptable (75% primary patency at 8 years). Treatment of other arterial occlusive lesions of the upper extremity should be based on the same principles as arterial bypass to infrapopliteal arteries. Because the arteries in the arm are of small caliber, venous conduit should be used for bypasses below the subclavian or proximal axillary artery level. Arterial complications of thoracic outlet syndrome are usually due to arterial embolization from subclavian artery aneurysms that form as a consequence of poststenotic turbulence; less commonly, arterial occlusion can occur. These problems are usually associated with bony abnormalities of the thoracic outlet such as cervical ribs or abnormal first ribs. Repair requires thoracic outlet decompression by resection of the cervical and/or abnormal first rib and replacement of the damaged portion of the subclavian artery, usually with a prosthetic graft. Balloon dilatation in the treatment of these problems should not be considered because of the risk of embolization and because the underlying structural abnormality of the thoracic outlet is not repaired.

Outcome and Follow-Up After Arterial Reconstruction

It is important for the patient and the treating physician to understand that the goal of therapy in patients with chronic arterial occlusive disease is palliation of symptoms and that "cure" is unlikely. Although patency of the arterial reconstructions and correction of hemodynamic abnormalities are important determinants of successful treatment of chronic arterial occlusive disease, restoration of function and maintenance of ambulation and independent living are also critical from the patient's point of view. Recent randomized studies have demonstrated that, despite improved hemodynamics after balloon angioplasty in patients with claudication, improvement in walking distance and health status is limited and no better than with medical therapy. Similarly, after surgical bypass for critical limb ischemia, only a small percentage (14%) of patients have an ideal result (an uncomplicated procedure with long-term symptom relief and no recurrence of ischemia), whereas more than half require a subsequent operative procedure for wound complications or limb ischemia, up to one fourth require amputation during follow-up, and only three fourths are still ambulatory

---

Pearls and Pitfalls

PEARLS

- Claudication *does not* occur with the patient's first step; rather, it is increased by walking fast, carrying a load, and climbing stairs.
- Exercise hemodynamic testing can identify patients with nonvascular causes of exercise-induced leg pain.
- Ischemic rest pain is always associated with severe arterial insufficiency by hemodynamic testing.
- Digital pressures or waveform and pulse volume recordings are usually unaffected by diabetes.
- Femoral pressure testing with vasodilatation reliably identifies hemodynamically significant aortoiliac occlusive disease.
- Arch contrast injection, arterial duplex, magnetic resonance angiography, and intraoperative arteriography can identify target arteries not seen on routine aortogram and runoff studies.
- Extremity hemodynamics predict natural history of disease and "medical therapy" can ameliorate symptoms of mild claudication.
- Long-term success (patency or limb salvage) of aortobifemoral and vein infrainguinal bypasses exceeds 70% to 85%.
- Bypass surgery is no riskier than amputation and is associated with better long-term outcome.

PITFALLS

- Exercise-induced leg pain is not always due to arterial insufficiency.
- Claudication can be present in patients with palpable pulses.
- Diabetic neuropathy alone is associated with foot numbness, pain, and rubor at rest that is worse at night.
- Extremity blood pressures are artifactually elevated by diabetes mellitus, scarring, and end-stage renal disease.
- Diffuse aortoiliac stenosis by arteriography may or may not be hemodynamically significant.
- Nonvisualization of infrainguinal arteries by arteriography does not confirm arterial occlusion.
- Invasive treatment of patients with mild claudication may not lead to long-term improvement and can result in worsened ischemia.
- Balloon angioplasty is ineffective in the treatment of diffuse iliac and essentially all infrainguinal arterial occlusive disease.
- Severe arterial occlusive disease commonly associated with significant medical problems appears to limit therapeutic options.

and living independently 5 years after the procedure. However, excellent patency of the reconstructive procedure is necessary to achieve even these results and follow-up, including duplex ultrasound graft surveillance, should be continued as long as the graft is patent. In addition, long-term anticoagulation should be used after infrainguinal bypasses, particularly in patients at high risk for graft failure (poor outflow, poor conduit, previous graft failure) where it has been shown to improve graft patency and limb salvage. Atherosclerotic risk factors (hypertension, elevated cholesterol, tobacco use) should also be actively treated, because patients requiring treatment for chronic arterial occlusive disease are at high risk for other life-threatening complications of atherosclerosis. Exercise therapy in the form of a regular walking program should be encouraged because this can decrease cardiac risk, improve walking distance in patients with intermittent claudication equivalent to successful infrainguinal angioplasty, and help maintain ambulation and independent living after bypass for critical ischemia.

Summary

Extremity ischemia caused by chronic peripheral arterial occlusion is a common problem. Fortunately, chronic arterial occlusion is usually well tolerated and limb loss is unlikely unless severe ischemia occurs. Reconstructive procedures are indicated in patients with limb-threatening ischemia and in carefully selected patients with functionally limiting intermittent claudication. Procedures must correct abnormal extremity hemodynamics documented to be the cause of the extremity symptoms to be successful. Arterial bypass remains the mainstay of therapy for chronic peripheral arterial occlusive disease, although balloon angioplasty and endoluminal stenting in selected patients with appropriate lesions can be an acceptable alternative. Finally, persistence in attempting to reestablish and maintain extremity perfusion will allow long-term limb salvage and maintenance of function in the majority of patients with symptomatic chronic arterial occlusive disease.

SELECTED READINGS

Bergamini TM, Towne JB, Bandyk DF, et al: Experience with in situ saphenous vein bypasses during 1981 to 1989: Determinant factors of long-term patency. J Vasc Surg 1991;13:137.

Bosch JL, Hunink MG: Meta-analysis of the results of percutaneous transluminal angioplasty and stent placement for aortoiliac occlusive disease. Radiology 1997;204:87.

Brewster DC, Perler BA, Robinson JG, Darling RC: Aortofemoral graft for multilevel occlusive disease: Predictors of success and need for distal bypass. Arch Surg 1982;117:1593.

Faries PL, Arora S, Poposelli FB, et al: The use of arm vein in lower-extremity revascularization: Results of 520 procedures performed in eight years. J Vasc Surg 2000;31:50.

Mattos MA, van Bemmelen PS, Hodgson KJ, et al: Does correction of stenoses identified with color duplex scanning improve infrainguinal graft patency? J Vasc Surg 1993;17:54.

McDaniel MD, Cronenwett JL: Basic data related to the natural history of intermittent claudication. Ann Vasc Surg 1989;3:273.

Nicoloff AD, Taylor LM, McLafferty RB, et al: Patient recovery after infrainguinal bypass grafting for limb salvage. J Vasc Surg 1998;27:256.

Parsons RE, Suggs WD, Lee JJ, et al: Percutaneous transluminal angioplasty for the treatment of limb threatening ischemia: Do the results justify an attempt before bypass grafting? J Vasc Surg 1998;28:1066.

Results of a prospective randomized trial evaluating surgery versus thrombolysis for ischemia of the lower extremity. The STILE trial. Ann Surg 1994;220:251.

Seeger JM, Pretus HA, Carlton LC, et al: Potential predictors of outcome in patients with tissue loss who undergo infrainguinal vein bypass grafting. J Vasc Surg 1999;30:427.

Tangelder MJD, Lawson JA, Algra A, Eikelboom BC: Systematic review of randomized controlled trials of aspirin and oral anticoagulants in the prevention of graft occlusion and ischemic events after infrainguinal bypass surgery. J Vasc Surg 1999;30:701.

Taylor LM, Edwards JM, Porter JM: Present status of reversed vein bypass grafting: Five-year results of a modern series. J Vasc Surg 1990;11:193.

Taylor LM, Moneta GL, McConnell D, et al: Axillofemoral grafting with externally supported polytetrafluoroethylene. Arch Surg 1994;129:588.

Veith FJ, Gupta SK, Ascer E, et al: Six-year prospective multicenter randomized comparison of autologous saphenous vein and expanded polytetrafluoroethylene grafts in infrainguinal arterial reconstructions. J Vasc Surg 1986;3:104.

Whyman MR, Fowkes FGR, Kerracher EMG, et al: Is intermittent claudication improved by percutaneous transluminal angioplasty? A randomized controlled trial. J Vasc Surg 1997;26:551.

Chapter 178

Visceral Artery Occlusive Disease

Thomas S. Huber

RENAL ARTERY OCCLUSIVE DISEASE

Significant renal artery occlusive disease can result in a decrease of blood flow to the kidney, with the development of hypertension and the loss of renal function. Renovascular hypertension is the most common cause of surgically correctable hypertension and accounts for 0.2% to 5% of all causes of hypertension. Although the incidence is relatively low, the absolute number of adults in the United States with renovascular hypertension has been estimated at 1 million. Similarly, ischemic nephropathy accounts for approximately 15% of all end-stage renal disease in the United States, and the incidence is increasing.

Renovascular Hypertension

Pathophysiology and Etiology

The pathophysiology of renovascular hypertension requires a brief review of the renin-angiotensin system. Renin is released by the granular cells of the juxtaglomerular apparatus in response to a variety of interrelated stimuli, including arterial pressure, plasma sodium concentration, sympathetic innervation, and angiotensin I. Renin catalyzes the conversion of the plasma protein angiotensinogen into the relatively inactive angiotensin I. Angiotensin I is subsequently broken down into angiotensin II by the angiotensin-converting enzyme (ACE) located in the vascular endothelium. Angiotensin II is both a potent vasoconstrictor and a stimulus for aldosterone secretion; the net effect of both actions is to increase arterial pressure. In the presence of a significant unilateral renal artery stenosis and a normal contralateral kidney (Goldblatt one-clip, two-kidney model), renin secretion is increased in the affected kidney and suppressed in the contralateral one. The normal contralateral kidney is usually able to partially compensate for the elevated renin through changes in the intravascular volume. The net result is renin-mediated hypertension and a normo- or hypovolemic state that is sensitive to ACE inhibitors.

In the presence of bilateral renal artery stenoses (Goldblatt one-clip, one-kidney model), the effects of the renin-angiotensin system are manifested primarily through the hyperaldosteronemia and increased intravascular volume. The hyperaldosteronemia leads to sodium retention that suppresses renin secretion. Patients experience hypertension and symptoms associated with increased intravascular volume, and the treatment with ACE inhibitors is effective only with sodium depletion. Unfortunately, this explanation of the pathophysiologic changes associated with single and bilateral renal artery stenoses is an oversimplification that is more relevant in animal models than the clinical scenario. The distinction between renin-mediated and aldosterone-mediated symptoms is blurred in the clinical setting.

The majority of renal artery stenoses are due to atherosclerosis. The plaque morphology of these lesions is identical to those found in other vascular beds and reflects the systemic nature of the process. The risk factors for atherosclerosis in the renal artery are the same for those elsewhere and include male gender, age, diabetes, hypertension, smoking, hypercholesterolemia, and family history. The presence of atherosclerotic lesions in the renal artery is relatively common, and significant lesions have been reported in approximately half of normotensive patients and three fourth of hypertensive patients in autopsy studies. These atherosclerotic lesions are found most commonly at the orifice or within the proximal one third of the main renal artery and are frequently bilateral (Fig. 178–1A). The orificial lesions are believed to represent a manifestation of aortic atherosclerosis and have been termed "aortic spillover" lesions.

Fibromuscular disease accounts for the second leading cause of renal artery stenosis, although it is far less common than atherosclerosis. This group of arterial fibrodysplasias is classified by pattern and extent of involvement and includes intimal, medial and perimedial varieties, with the medial type accounting for approximately 85% of the total. The etiology of these lesions is poorly defined. Medial fibroplasia occurs almost exclusively in women, with the most common age of presentation during the fourth decade of life. It has a characteristic "string of beads" appearance on arteriogram that results from a series of aneurysms alternating with stenoses (see Fig. 178–1B). These changes are seen most commonly within the distal main renal artery but may extend into the branch vessels. These changes are frequently bilateral and can also occur in the extracranial internal carotid artery and the external iliac artery. The histology of these fibrodysplastic arteries is characterized by the replacement of the smooth muscle cells within the media by fibrous tissue and the excessive deposition of ground substance within the same layer.

Clinical Presentation and Diagnosis

The diagnosis of renovascular hypertension requires a high index of suspicion. Unfortunately, there is no perfect diagnostic test, and the presence of renal artery stenosis does not necessarily confirm the diagnosis of renovascular hypertension because patients may have both a renal artery stenosis and underlying essential hypertension. It is impractical and cost ineffective to screen the general hypertensive population for a renal mechanism. However, several clinical presentations suggest a renovascular

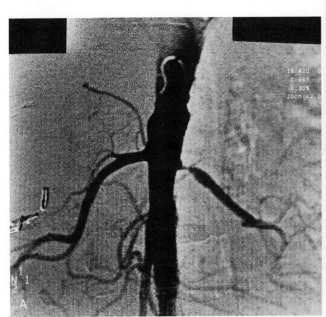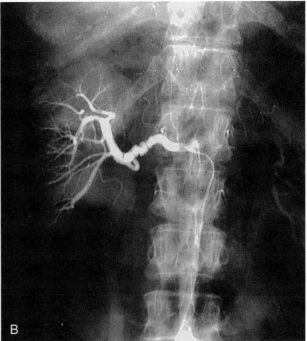

Figure 178–1. *A,* Renal artery stenosis from atherosclerosis. Note the orificial distribution of the disease from "aortic spillover." *B,* Renal artery stenosis from medial fibroplasia. Note the serial stenoses and dilatations characteristic of the "string-of-beads" appearance.

mechanism and merit further investigation. These include a diastolic blood pressure greater than 115 mm Hg (particularly in whites), worsening of mild to moderate essential hypertension, hypertension during childhood, rapid onset of hypertension in individuals over 50 years of age, deterioration of renal function on ACE inhibitors, normalization of blood pressure control on ACE inhibitors, and moderate hypertension with asymmetric kidney size.

A variety of screening tests for renovascular hypertension and renal artery stenosis have been reported, including renal artery duplex, peripheral renin levels, peripheral renin levels after captopril, and isotope renography. However, only renal artery duplex has received widespread use. The false-negative rates for both peripheral renin levels and isotope renography are too great to be used as effective screening tools. Peripheral renin levels after captopril have an acceptable false-negative rate, although the necessary preparation is cumbersome. In contrast, the sensitivity, specificity, and overall accuracy of renal artery duplex for detecting renal artery stenoses exceed 90% in experienced vascular laboratories. The examination allows interrogation of the main renal artery from the aorta to the hilum, although assessment of the branch and polar vessels is limited. Renal size may also be determined during the examination using standard ultrasound techniques. Unfortunately, renal artery duplex is technically challenging, operator dependent, and not available in all centers. Implementation requires validation with standard contrast arteriography, and its use requires ongoing quality control.

Standard contrast arteriography has been the traditional "gold standard" for imaging the renal arteries during the diagnostic evaluation of patients with presumed

renovascular hypertension and offers the potential for simultaneous therapeutic intervention. Furthermore, documentation of renal artery stenosis by arteriography and the appropriate clinical setting is usually sufficient to predict improvement after revascularization. The findings that suggest a hemodynamically significant renal artery stenosis include a greater than 75% reduction in the luminal diameter, the presence of collaterals, poststenotic dilatation, diminished ipsilateral renal artery size, and a pressure gradient across the stenosis greater than 20% of the systolic pressure. The absolute threshold that defines a significant pressure gradient, however, is somewhat controversial. Measuring the gradient requires placing a catheter across the stenosis and can artifactually lead to an increase in the gradient. It has been reported that a 10 mm Hg pressure gradient is sufficient to activate the renin-angiotensin mechanism and stimulate the development of collaterals. Arteriograms are indicated for patients with abnormal duplex studies and for the small subset of patients with equivocal duplex studies and strong clinical predictors of renovascular hypertension. However, the renal arteriogram should be viewed as a preinterventional study and not simply a diagnostic study, because it is expensive and associated with a small, yet finite, risk. Renal insufficiency is also a relative contraindication to standard arteriography due to the contrast-associated nephrotoxicity. However, this may be reduced or eliminated with the use of periprocedural renal dose dopamine infusion or non-nephrotoxic contrast agents such as carbon dioxide or gadolinium. A lateral aortogram should be routinely obtained as part of the evaluation of patients with renal artery stenosis to interrogate the origin of the celiac axis in case extra-anatomic renal artery bypasses from the splenic or hepatic arteries are considered.

The role of magnetic resonance arteriography and contrast-enhanced CT scans in the evaluation of patients with presumed renovascular hypertension remains unresolved. The image quality of the magnetic resonance arteriograms, particularly with gadolinium enhancement, continues to improve. Magnetic resonance arteriography offers many potential advantages over standard contrast arteriography and merits further investigation.

Isotope renography after captopril challenge and the measurement of renin in the direct venous effluent from the kidney have both proved beneficial in the small subset of patients in whom the diagnosis of renovascular hypertension is equivocal. The utility of isotope renography as a diagnostic test for renovascular hypertension is contingent on the fact that the glomerular filtration in the affected kidney depends on the vasoconstrictive effects of angiotensin on the efferent arterioles. Administration of the converting enzyme inhibitor captopril in this setting results in a decrease in both uptake and excretion of the isotope. The utility of the renal vein renin assay is contingent on the fact that renin secretion is increased in the affected kidney and suppressed in the contralateral normal one in the presence of unilateral stenosis, as noted earlier. A ratio of the renal vein renin levels between the affected kidney and the unaffected kidney that is 1.5 or more is considered positive and highly suggestive of renovascular hypertension. Accurate sampling requires a preparation similar to that noted for the peripheral renin assay. Specifically, patients should be placed on a 2-g sodium diet, all antihypertensives except diuretics should be held for 5 days prior to the study, 40 mg of furosemide should be administered orally the evening before the test, and the patients should remain flat at bed rest for 4 hours prior to and during the study. Unfortunately, the sampling of renal vein renin levels has limited application for patients with bilateral renal artery stenoses or a single kidney owing to the lack of compensatory response in the normal, contralateral kidney.

Treatment Strategies

The treatment indications for patients with renovascular hypertension include poor blood pressure control or recurrent congestive heart failure or both. The underlying objectives of the treatment options are to limit the systemic complications of the hypertension and preserve renal function. The various options include medical management alone, endovascular or operative revascularization, and nephrectomy. The choice is contingent on the underlying disease process, the status of the patient, and the various treatment outcomes, although it usually boils down to the decision between endovascular or operative revascularization. Medical management alone is rarely optimal and may be associated with deterioration in renal mass or function in the face of significant renal artery stenosis. Furthermore, failure of medical management is usually the impetus to look for a renovascular component for the hypertension. Similarly, primary nephrectomy should be reserved only for situations in which there is an insufficient quantity of renal mass; a kidney length of over 7 cm is commonly used as a criteria for a salvageable kidney.

Endovascular revascularization is currently the initial treatment of choice for most cases of renovascular hypertension. Angioplasty alone has proved a durable, long-term solution for medial fibrodysplasia of the main renal artery although it is relatively contraindicated in the presence of branch artery disease and aneurysms. Additionally, the use of renal artery stents in conjunction with angioplasty has significantly improved the long-term outcome for atherosclerotic lesions. Admittedly, the endovascular approach may not be as durable as operative revascularization for these atherosclerotic lesions, but the periprocedural complication rates, including mortality, are significantly less. The current mortality rate for renal artery angioplasty-stent for atherosclerotic lesions is less than 2%, and the restenosis rate is less than 20% at 1 year. Operative revascularization for renovascular hypertension should probably be reserved for lesions not amenable to endovascular treatment, recurrent stenoses after endovascular treatment, and patients with long life expectancy and low operative risk.

Operative Revascularization

The preoperative evaluation for patients undergoing renal revascularization is similar to that for any major vascular procedure. Patients should undergo a complete history and physical examination, with documentation of their peripheral pulse examination, including ankle brachial indices. An electrocardiogram, chest radiograph, and blood work should be obtained according to the usual routine. All active medical problems, including abnormalities identified on the preoperative evaluation, should be optimized. The optimal cardiac workup is controversial and somewhat institution-dependent, although several published algorithms are available, including one from the American Heart Association Task Force. All patients should undergo vein survey if bypass is planned and should be started on beta-blockers and aspirin. Imaging specific to the kidney should include an ultrasound to document size and an arteriogram to confirm the presence and document the extent of the stenosis.

Several different options exist for operative renal revascularization, including aortorenal bypass, renal endarterectomy, and extra-anatomic bypass. The choice is contingent on the extent of atherosclerosis within the aorta, the requirement for bilateral revascularization, the requirement for concomitant aortic procedures, and the experience of the surgeon. No procedure is ideal for every clinical scenario, and surgeons should be familiar with the different approaches. Aortorenal bypass is the most commonly performed procedure and probably the procedure of choice for most situations. Renal endarterectomy may be performed through a variety of approaches. The transected renal artery may be everted and reimplanted. The orifices of the renal arteries may be approached through a transaortic incision oriented either longitudinally or transversely, with the latter technique frequently employed during concomitant aortic reconstructions. Alternatively, the renal arteries may be approached through a transrenal incision. The endarterectomy technique is potentially less time consuming than aortorenal bypass and may be performed concomitant with mesenteric endarterectomy in patients with severe central aortic disease.

The disadvantages of endarterectomy are that it is technically more challenging and it is often difficult to obtain a suitable end-point. Remedial procedures are necessary when a suitable end-point cannot be achieved, potentially dramatically extending the duration of renal ischemia. Extra-anatomic bypass may be performed with the inflow source originating from the splenic artery, the hepatic artery, or less commonly, the common iliac arteries. The major advantage of the extra-anatomic bypass is that it obviates the need to apply a clamp to the infrarenal aorta and is useful for patients with severe aortic atherosclerotic disease, infrarenal aneurysms, and previous aortic reconstructions.

The technical conduct of an aortorenal bypass may be summarized (Fig. 178–2). Although the procedure may be performed through either a midline or transverse incision, the latter provides the most optimal exposure and is the incision of choice. A bilateral subcostal incision is used when bilateral revascularization is planned, whereas a unilateral incision with extension across the midline is used for unilateral cases. The kidney is exposed by reflecting the right or left colon for unilateral revascularization, with the dissection extending medially to the aorta. Exposure during bilateral renal revascularization may be obtained simply by incising the retroperitoneum over the juxtarenal aorta in the midline or, alternatively, by incising the retroperitoneum over the aorta and the peritoneal reflection of the right colon and completely mobilizing the right colon and small bowel superiorly. The renal vein is skeletonized to provide exposure to the underlying artery, and this frequently requires ligating the gonadal,

adrenal, and lumbar tributaries on the left side. The renal artery is dissected free from its origin to a point beyond the distal extent of the intraluminal disease to allow a suitable location for vascular clamp application. This frequently requires dissection out to the primary branches. Similarly, the infrarenal aorta is dissected free at a suitable location for vascular clamp application. Saphenous vein is harvested and prepared by means of standard technique. Although the studies comparing saphenous vein and prosthetic conduits for aortorenal bypass have been somewhat equivocal, saphenous vein is the recommended conduit, particularly when the bypass is performed to a relatively small kidney. Patients are administered heparin (100 units/kg), mannitol (25 g), and renal-dose dopamine (3 μg/kg per minute) prior to clamp application.

The proximal anastomosis is performed to the anterolateral aspect of the aorta in an end-side configuration, with the use of a partially occluding aortic clamp if possible. The renal artery is transected at its origin and flushed with 240 mL of iced heparinized saline. The renal artery anastomosis is performed in an end-end configuration. Bypasses to the right kidney may be tunneled either anterior or posterior to the vena cava, although the latter is preferred because the grafts tend to lie better and are less prone to kinking. The technical success of the procedure is confirmed with continuous wave Doppler or, ideally, duplex ultrasound.

The immediate postoperative course after renal revascularization is comparable to that after aortic reconstruction. Patients are transferred directly from the operating room to the intensive care unit and are usually extubated shortly thereafter. Patients are continued on aspirin and beta-blockers, but all preoperative antihypertensive medications are withheld with the exception of those that cannot be stopped abruptly. Blood pressure control in the immediate postoperative period is impacted on by multiple factors, including volume status and incisional pain in addition to the renin-mediated component. Indeed, the serum half-life of the plasma protein renin is in the range of minutes, and thus improvements may be expected from this component within a short period of time. Antihypertensives may be serially reintroduced throughout the postoperative period as necessary. Additional imaging of the reconstruction is usually obtained in the postoperative period to confirm again the technical result of the procedure. Renal duplex, standard contrast arteriography, and magnetic resonance arteriography all are appropriate, with the choice usually contingent on institutional expertise.

An acute, sustained increase in the blood pressure within the early postoperative period suggests thrombosis of the aortorenal graft or renal revascularization and merits investigation. Isotope renography is useful in this setting, since it is usually sufficient to determine whether the reconstruction is patent and does not require nephrotoxic contrast medium. Unfortunately, reconstructions that thrombose in the early postoperative period are not usually salvageable and often result in loss of the kidney due to the resultant warm ischemia. The overall postoperative length of stay after renal revascularization is comparable to that for most aortic reconstructions, with a median of 9 days in a recent nationwide series. Patients are seen at

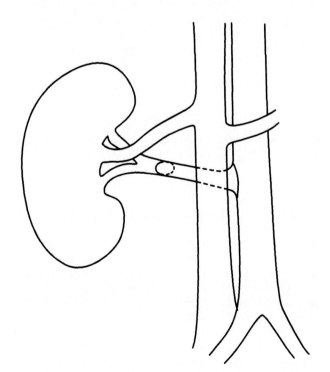

Figure 178–2. Aortorenal bypass originating from the infrarenal aorta using saphenous vein. Note that the graft is tunneled beneath the inferior vena cava.

6-month intervals as outpatients after recovery from the procedure, and the reconstruction is interrogated with a duplex examination. Abnormalities on duplex examination or deterioration in blood pressure control mandates additional imaging and potentially repeat intervention. Patients are continued on aspirin and encouraged to modify their risk factors for atherosclerosis.

The outcome after operative revascularization for renovascular hypertension is quite good. The reported operative mortality rate is less than 5% and is partially contingent on the nature of the report (single-institution versus multiple-institution). Notably, a recent nationwide series reported a 4.4% mortality rate for aortorenal bypass. The immediate technical success rate of operative revascularization is over 97%. Approximately 90% of the patients undergoing revascularization for atherosclerotic lesions experience improvement in their blood pressure control, although only roughly 20% are cured. Both graft patency and sustained blood pressure control are approximately 90% at 5 years after revascularization for atherosclerotic lesions. Outcome after operative revascularization for stenoses secondary to fibromuscular disease is even better, although the indications for operation are relatively few secondary to success of endovascular treatment.

The role of concomitant aortic reconstructions and renal revascularizations remains in question. The mortality and morbidity rates for the combined procedures are significantly greater than either individual procedure and were found to be approximately 8% in recent nationwide series. Combined aortic reconstruction and renal revascularization are mandatory during aneurysm repair when the aneurysm involves the orifice of the renal artery, and are probably justified during aortic reconstructions when the traditional indications for renal revascularization are satisfied. Proponents of the combined procedures for asymptomatic renal artery stenoses have contended that the lesions are preocclusive and merit intervention. However, a recent analysis of patients with renal artery stenoses who underwent aortic reconstruction alone found that the natural history of these lesions was fairly benign and associated with an increase only in the antihypertensive requirements.

Ischemic Nephropathy

Bilateral renal artery stenoses or unilateral stenosis in patients with a solitary kidney may lead to the development of ischemic nephropathy. As noted earlier, this potentially correctable cause of end-stage renal disease has been estimated to account for approximately 15% of all new cases. The diagnosis should be suspected in patients with rapid decline in their renal function, particularly if precipitated by the introduction of ACE inhibitors. The diagnostic approach is comparable to that outlined earlier for renovascular hypertension, although renal vein renin studies are not helpful because of the bilateral nature of the disease (absence of a normal kidney). The predictors of renal salvage with revascularization include bilateral occlusions, normal distal arteries, renal length over 8 cm, and a history of rapidly declining renal function with severe hypertension. Notably, operative revascularization

is associated with improved renal function in approximately 50% of patients despite the absence of function by isotope renography or the failure to visualize patent distal renal arteries on arteriography. In contrast, the likelihood of improved renal function and dialysis-free survival is minimal in patients with unilateral renal artery disease and those without hypertension.

The treatment options for patients with ischemic nephropathy are essentially the same as outlined earlier for renovascular hypertension. Medical management is appealing because it avoids the potential complications associated with intervention; however, the dialysis-free survival in patients with ischemic nephropathy is limited. Furthermore, the prognosis of patients with end-stage renal disease secondary to ischemic nephropathy is limited, with a reported median survival of 27 months and an annual mortality rate of 20%. Endovascular treatment in this setting remains poorly defined secondary to the limited experience. Operative revascularization is associated with a reported 9% mortality rate. However, operative revascularization is associated with improved long-term survival and a slowing of the gradual deterioration in renal function in properly selected patients.

MESENTERIC ARTERY OCCLUSIVE DISEASE

Mesenteric artery occlusive disease may present as either chronic or acute mesenteric ischemia. Although both problems represent an imbalance between the supply and demand of oxygen and nutrients, the clinical presentations, diagnostic approaches and treatments are different. Acute mesenteric ischemia may result from emboli, in situ thrombosis, nonocclusive mechanisms, and mesenteric venous thrombosis. Although the latter two mechanisms are not secondary to mesenteric artery occlusive disease, they will be discussed together for completeness.

Chronic Mesenteric Ischemia

Pathophysiology and Etiology

The underlying pathophysiology of chronic mesenteric ischemia is the inability to achieve postprandial hyperemic intestinal blood flow. Appreciation of the pathophysiologic changes requires an understanding of the determinants of intestinal blood flow and the visceral collateral network. Intestinal blood flow in the normal fasting state is fairly modest but increases markedly postprandially, with the magnitude contingent on the size and composition of the meal. The majority of the hyperemic changes occur in the pancreas and small bowel and peak within 30 to 60 minutes after eating. In the presence of significant arterial occlusive disease, this postprandial hyperemia is not possible, and patients develop ischemic pain similar to angina pectoris, appropriately termed *mesenteric angina*. The normal visceral circulation is fairly redundant and has a rich collateral network. The celiac artery communicates with the superior mesenteric artery through the superior and inferior pancreaticoduodenal arteries. The superior mesenteric artery communicates with the inferior mesenteric artery via the meandering mesenteric artery that runs within the proximal mesentery. This collateral has multiple eponyms but should be differentiated from the less significant collateral known as the marginal artery of Drummond that is located in the distal mesentery. Lastly, the inferior mesenteric artery communicates with the internal iliac artery via the superior and middle hemorrhoidal arteries. The symptoms of mesenteric ischemia usually do not occur unless two of the three visceral vessels are significantly diseased because of this rich collateral network. However, symptoms may occur with isolated disease in the superior mesenteric artery in the absence of well-developed collaterals.

The overwhelming majority of visceral artery stenoses are due to atherosclerosis. A variety of other etiologies have been reported, including neurofibromatosis, rheumatoid disorders, aortic dissection, radiation, Buerger's disease, and certain drugs, although these are collectively less common. Symptomatic visceral artery occlusive disease is relatively rare despite visceral artery stenoses being reported in 5% to 10% of the population at autopsy. The atherosclerotic process usually involves just the origin of the visceral vessels, and patients with occlusive disease in the celiac and superior mesenteric arteries frequently have renal artery stenoses and vice versa. The risk factors for visceral artery atherosclerosis are the same as those for the other vascular beds.

Clinical Presentation and Diagnosis

The appearance and presentation of patients with chronic mesenteric ischemia are fairly characteristic. The majority of patients are cachectic elderly women with strong smoking histories. Indeed, chronic mesenteric ischemia is one of the few cardiovascular problems that is more common in women, with a reported ratio of approximately 3:1. The mean age of patients undergoing repair in a recent national series was 66 years, although the disease process is not exclusive to elderly people and is frequently found in patients in their fourth and fifth decades of life. Abdominal pain is frequently the presenting symptom and initially occurs postprandially, but it may progress to a persistent nature in the latter stages of the disease process. Unfortunately, the pain has no specific characteristics. As a result of the pain, patients develop a fear of food and avoid eating. The net result is a predictable weight loss, with a mean of 35 pounds reported in a recent large clinical series. It should be noted that the cause of the weight loss is poor nutrition rather than an abnormality of intestinal absorption. Patients may develop nausea or vomiting, constipation, or diarrhea. Indeed, mesenteric ischemia is a fairly strong cathartic, and motility symptoms rather than pain may be the predominate symptom. Patients with chronic mesenteric ischemia frequently have evidence of systemic vascular disease although there are no characteristic physical findings.

The diagnostic approach to patients with presumed chronic mesenteric ischemia requires a stepwise approach, with evaluation of the more common problems first. Although the appearance and clinical presentation of patients with chronic mesenteric ischemia is fairly

characteristic, the differential diagnosis of patients with abdominal pain and weight loss is extensive and includes gastrointestinal malignancy foremost. Indeed, chronic mesenteric ischemia is usually not even considered in the initial differential diagnosis of abdominal pain and weight loss by most primary care providers, and this is reflected by the fact that the mean duration from presentation to diagnosis is approximately 9 months. The initial diagnostic workup for patients with abdominal pain and weight loss should include esophagogastroduodenoscopy, colonoscopy, abdominal ultrasound, and an abdominal or pelvic CT scan. Notably, gastric ulcers are relatively common in patients with chronic mesenteric ischemia and likely result from ischemia, since the gastric pH is slightly elevated. Additionally, a surprising number of patients are subjected to cholecystectomy as part of their workup before the definitive diagnosis of chronic mesenteric ischemia is made.

Mesenteric duplex is an excellent screening tool for visceral artery stenosis, with reported sensitivity and specificity rates of approximately 90%. As with renal duplex, the examination is technically challenging, operator dependent, and not available in all centers. A variety of criteria have been proposed to grade the severity of stenoses based on the systolic and diastolic velocities or frequency shifts. These various criteria are probably equivalent as far as their accuracy in grading the degree of stenosis. However, it is imperative that they be validated at each institution by comparison with the "gold standard" contrast arteriogram. A variety of provocative tests have been proposed to unmask clinically significant visceral artery stenoses, although their utility is unclear and they have not achieved widespread use.

Standard contrast mesenteric arteriography is the definitive diagnostic test for visceral artery stenosis. Arteriograms are indicated as the sole diagnostic test if mesenteric duplex imaging is not available or to confirm or refute the duplex findings. Despite the accuracy of mesenteric duplex imaging, arteriograms are obtained in all patients before surgery and may be indicated in the small subset of patients with normal or equivocal duplex findings and a compelling history for chronic mesenteric ischemia. A lateral arteriogram is mandatory as part of the examination to assess accurately the origins of the celiac and superior mesenteric arteries because of their anterior or posterior orientation. The significant findings on arteriogram include ostial stenoses of the celiac and superior mesenteric arteries, the presence of visceral collaterals, and the presence of central aortic atherosclerotic disease (Fig. 178–3A and B). Additionally, a small percentage of patients with chronic mesenteric ischemia may have visceral artery aneurysms, presumably from increased flow through the collateral vessels.

Treatment Strategies

All patients with chronic mesenteric ischemia require treatment. The natural history of the untreated disease process is lethal. Patients either waste away from inanition or their bowel infarcts. The potential treatment options include medical management with total parenteral nutri-

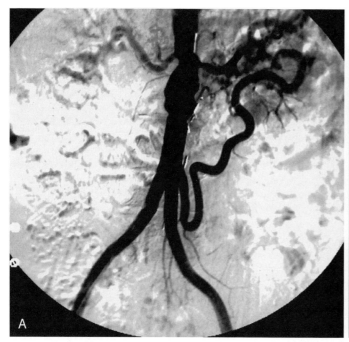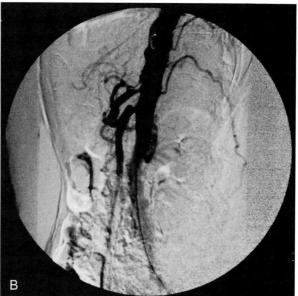

Figure 178–3. *A,* Anteroposterior view of a mesenteric arteriogram in a patient with chronic mesenteric ischemia. Note the large meandering mesenteric artery that serves as a major collateral between the superior and inferior mesenteric artery distributions. *B,* Lateral view of a mesenteric arteriogram in a patient with chronic mesenteric ischemia. Note the high-grade celiac and superior mesenteric artery stenoses.

tion or revascularization with either endovascular or operative techniques. However, operative revascularization is the cornerstone of treatment. The role of long-term parenteral nutrition is unclear, but it probably has only a very limited application. Chronic parenteral nutrition is associated with multiple complications, including those associated with the infusion catheters. Furthermore, patients with chronic mesenteric ischemia may not be able to metabolize the parenteral nutrition. Endovascular treatment (angioplasty with or without stenting) affords an attractive option in this group of high-risk patients, but the experience is very limited and the outcomes ill defined. The reported experience suggests that the initial success rate is quite good, and the periprocedural morbidity and mortality rates are comparable or better than those of operative revascularization. However, the long-term success rates are relatively poor despite stenting, and it appears that endovascular revascularization is currently appropriate only as a bridge to operative revascularization. In addition, embolization of visceral artery aneurysms that result from mesenteric artery occlusive disease without revascularization should be strongly discouraged because it may compromise a significant collateral pathway and precipitate acute mesenteric ischemia.

Operative Revascularization

The preoperative workup for patients undergoing mesenteric revascularization is identical to that outlined earlier for patients undergoing renal artery revascularization. An arteriogram is mandatory both to confirm the diagnosis and to plan the operative procedure. There is no clear-cut role for extended preoperative parenteral alimentation

to replete the nutritional stores, and some studies suggest that it is detrimental.

The optimal operative procedure remains unresolved. A variety of procedures have been reported and include antegrade aortoceliac or superior mesenteric bypass, retrograde aortosuperior mesenteric artery bypass, and visceral endarterectomy. Unfortunately, the relative infrequency of the problem has prevented the requisite randomized, controlled trials. The current outstanding issues include the configuration of the bypass (antegrade versus retrograde), conduit choice (autogenous versus prosthetic), and the number of vessels to be revascularized (1 versus 2 versus 3). The antegrade aortoceliac or superior mesenteric bypass using a bifurcated prosthetic graft appears to have the largest number of supporters and is probably the procedure of choice.

The antegrade aortoceliac-superior mesenteric artery bypass is performed using a bilateral subcostal incision with a midline extension up to the xiphoid process (Fig. 178–4). The left lobe of the liver is mobilized by taking down its peritoneal reflection, and it is reflected right laterally with the assistance of the Buckwalter retractor. The supraceliac aorta is exposed by incising the overlying crus of the diaphragm. The celiac axis is exposed by continuing the dissection on the anterior aspect of the aorta caudally. Distal control of the multiple celiac axis branches may be obtained by continuing the dissection caudally from the origin or cephalad from the takeoff of the gastroduodenal artery. The superior mesenteric artery is exposed through the lesser space immediately caudal to the pancreas. The bypass is performed using either a 12 × 6-mm or 12 × 7-mm bifurcated prosthetic graft, and the limb to the superior mesenteric artery is tunneled deep to the pancreas. It is notable that this is one of the

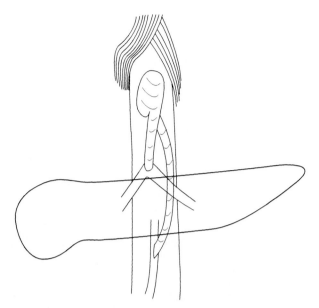

Figure 178–4. Aortoceliac or superior mesenteric artery bypass originating from the supraceliac aorta, using a bifurcated prosthetic graft. Note that the limb of the graft to the superior mesenteric artery is tunneled deep to the pancreas.

few locations in the peripheral circulation where a small-caliber prosthetic graft is preferable to saphenous vein.

Patients are administered heparin, mannitol, and renal-dose dopamine prior to clamp application, as outlined earlier. The proximal anastomosis is performed end to side to the supraceliac aorta, and the limbs of the graft are oriented on top of each other, with the superior limb used for the celiac anastomosis. Aortic control can usually be obtained with a partial occluding clamp. The celiac anastomosis is performed end to end, whereas the superior mesenteric artery anastomosis is performed end to side. Bypass to the inferior mesenteric artery with the use of saphenous vein in an aortoinferior mesenteric artery configuration is occasionally performed in conjunction with the antegrade bypass. Indeed, it has been reported that the recurrence of symptoms after mesenteric revascularization for chronic mesenteric ischemia was inversely related to the number of vessels bypassed (1 versus 2 versus 3).

The immediate postoperative care of patients after mesenteric revascularization for chronic mesenteric ischemia is similar to that after renal artery bypass, and patients should likewise undergo visceral imaging with either duplex or arteriography to confirm an adequate technical result. However, several additional concerns merit further comment. Mesenteric revascularization can initiate a profound inflammatory process likely due to ischemia-reperfusion injury that can lead to multiple organ dysfunction. The pulmonary injury is usually the most significant and is marked by the acute respiratory distress syndrome. This usually occurs on the second to third postoperative day and can persist from several days to a few weeks. Other common manifestations of the ischemia-reperfusion injury include thrombocytopenia and hepatic dysfunction, with prolongation of the prothrombin time and elevation of the transaminases. There are no

clinically approved therapies to prevent the ischemia-reperfusion injury, and the current treatment is simply supportive. This multiple organ dysfunction often translates into a prolonged hospital stay. The median length of stay across the country in a recent series was 18 days, and the mean length of stay in the author's institution was 36 days. Additionally, mesenteric revascularization usually results in a prolonged ileus that is treated most effectively with early initiation of parenteral nutrition. Patients are seen at 6-month intervals after recovery from the operative procedure, and the mesenteric reconstruction is interrogated with duplex. Any recurrent symptoms or abnormalities on duplex merit further investigation with arteriography. A small subset of patients experience prolonged diarrhea after mesenteric revascularization. The etiology of this is unclear although bacterial overgrowth has been postulated as one potential cause.

Mesenteric revascularization for chronic mesenteric ischemia is associated with a mortality rate of approximately 15% in a recent nationwide series. However, the long-term outcome among those who survive the procedure is quite good, with a 65% to 80% survival rate and an 80% graft patency rate at 5 years. The incidence of recurrent symptoms is less than the incidence of graft occlusion (20% at 5 years) and the majority of patients return to their presymptom weight.

Acute Mesenteric Ischemia

Acute mesenteric ischemia can result from an embolus, in situ thrombus, nonocclusive mesenteric ischemia, and venous thrombosis. The symptoms of acute mesenteric ischemia are similar among the groups although the treatments are different. Fortunately, the underlying mechanism can usually be determined from the history and clinical setting. Acute mesenteric ischemia results in bowel infarction, peritonitis, and death if untreated. The mortality rates associated with treatment are approximately 50% and have remained stable during the past few decades.

Embolus

An embolus is the most common cause of acute mesenteric ischemia. The embolus usually lodges in the superior mesenteric artery and originates from a cardiac source as a result of atrial fibrillation, an acute myocardial infarction, or a ventricular aneurysm. The extent of bowel ischemia or infarction is contingent on the extent of the collateral circulation, the pattern of the arterial occlusion, and the duration of the ischemia. In this setting, the bowel progresses from ischemia to infarction in a time-dependent fashion, although it may remain viable for 6 to 12 hours. Acute embolic occlusion of the superior mesenteric artery usually results in ischemia or infarction of the bowel from the proximal jejunum to the transverse colon. The duodenum and descending colon are spared because they are supplied by branches of the celiac and inferior mesenteric arteries, respectively.

Patients with acute mesenteric ischemia from an embolus present with diffuse abdominal pain. The classic description of the pain secondary to acute mesenteric ischemia is pain out of proportion to the physical findings although this scenario is not always present. Peritoneal signs occur late in the disease process and are suggestive of bowel infarction. Patients often experience vomiting or diarrhea or both because mesenteric ischemia is a potent cathartic, as noted earlier. The hemodynamic status of the patients spans the spectrum from normovolemia to profound hypovolemic shock with acidosis and is contingent on the status of the bowel and the duration of symptoms.

The diagnosis of acute mesenteric ischemia from an embolus may be difficult. The differential diagnosis includes the more common causes of acute abdominal pain. Furthermore, patients are often critically ill in the intensive care setting, and their history and physical examination findings may not be reliable. Diagnosis requires a high index of suspicion and an aggressive approach, since delays in diagnosis adversely affect outcome. Abdominal radiographs and CT scans are nondiagnostic for acute mesenteric ischemia although they are helpful to rule out other causes of the acute abdomen. Bowel wall thickening is a nonspecific CT finding suggestive of bowel ischemia, whereas pneumatosis intestinalis and portal vein air are later, ominous findings. Standard contrast arteriography is the definitive test, and the finding of a superior mesenteric artery occlusion in the appropriate clinical setting is diagnostic (Fig. 178–5). However, arteriography is not mandatory and may delay rather than expedite the ultimate operative intervention. Mesenteric duplex imaging, although an excellent screening test for chronic mesenteric ischemia, is not usually helpful in patients with acute mesenteric ischemia.

Patients should be taken emergently to the operating room once the diagnosis of acute mesenteric ischemia is made. They should be systemically anticoagulated with heparin and started on broad-spectrum antibiotics against enteric organisms. An extensive preoperative evaluation is unnecessary and potentially harmful in light of the narrow window for salvaging the bowel. Patients are frequently hypovolemic but can usually be sufficiently resuscitated during transfer to the operating room and prior to the induction of anesthesia. Both midline and transverse incisions provide adequate exposure, and the choice is usually based on surgeon preference. The diagnosis is usually confirmed by the distribution of the ischemic and/or infarcted bowel from the proximal jejunum to the transverse colon. However, the diagnosis should be further substantiated by interrogating the visceral vessels with continuous wave Doppler imaging. The embolus may be extracted from the superior mesenteric artery using a Fogarty thromboembolectomy catheter.

The superior mesenteric artery may be approached in several different ways. Access may be obtained by incising the retroperitoneum immediately caudal to the pancreas after entering the lesser space through the avascular plane between the stomach and transverse colon. It may also be obtained by incising the ligament of Treitz and reflecting the duodenum right laterally. Alternatively, the superior mesenteric artery may be exposed by incising the mesocolon at the base of the transverse colon after retracting the transverse colon caudally. This approach is preferred for an embolectomy because of its simplicity, although it is less than optimal if a bypass is required. The arteriotomy in the superior mesenteric artery may be performed in either a longitudinal or transverse orientation. The longitudinal arteriotomy requires a patch closure to prevent narrowing the lumen of the vessel, although it is probably the approach of choice because it affords greater flexibility in case a bypass procedure is necessary.

The management of the bowel for patients with acute mesenteric ischemia merits further comment. All obviously dead bowel should be resected. Intestinal anastomosis to restore bowel continuity has been advocated in this setting, although the creation of proximal and distal ostomies is safer and most likely the optimal approach. This mandates a second procedure to restore bowel continuity but it allows the bowel (i.e., mucosa) to be examined during the postoperative period, and it does not require an anastomosis using ischemic or borderline ischemic tissues. Bowel that is ischemic yet not frankly necrotic should be revascularized and then re-examined before any final decision about resection is made. A conservative approach toward bowel resection should be adopted because many of the borderline areas will remain viable. Admittedly, the differentiation between viable and nonviable bowel may be difficult. Adjuncts to visual inspection and the presence of peristalsis include continuous wave Doppler imaging and intravenous fluorescein in combination with a Wood lamp. Additionally, the decision to perform a second-look operation to reassess the viability of the bowel should be made at the initial procedure. This is routinely performed 24 to 48 hours after the first procedure.

The postoperative course after embolectomy for acute mesenteric ischemia is similar to that after revasculariza-

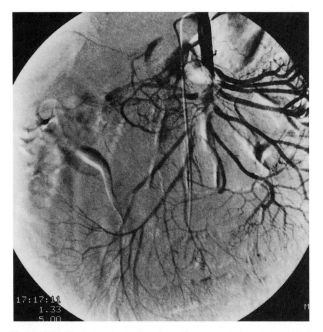

Figure 178–5. Anteroposterior view of a mesenteric arteriogram in a patient with acute mesenteric ischemia. Note the embolus in the superior mesenteric artery.

tion for chronic mesenteric ischemia, although the incidence of postoperative complications and multiple organ dysfunction is greater. Patients should be continued on broad-spectrum antibiotics throughout the initial postoperative period and require long-term anticoagulation owing to the underlying pathology that precipitated the event.

In Situ Thrombosis

Patients with chronic visceral artery occlusive disease may also present with acute mesenteric ischemia secondary to thrombosis. The presentation is usually superimposed on the symptoms of chronic mesenteric ischemia and can usually be differentiated from the other causes of acute mesenteric ischemia. However, patients may present with bowel ischemia or infarction, or both, as the initial symptom of their visceral occlusive disease. The clinical presentation, diagnostic approach, and immediate postoperative care of patients with acute mesenteric ischemia secondary to thrombosis is similar to that outlined earlier for emboli, although the operative approach is somewhat different.

Patients with acute mesenteric ischemia secondary to thrombosis of stenotic visceral vessels require mesenteric bypass. Although antegrade aortoceliac or superior mesenteric artery bypass is probably the optimal bypass for chronic mesenteric ischemia, the objectives and treatment are somewhat different in the acute setting. The main objective is to restore blood flow to the ischemic vascular bed as safely and expeditiously as possible. This usually requires only bypass to the superior mesenteric artery. Patients with isolated celiac artery stenosis rarely develop acute mesenteric ischemia because the collateral blood flow to the foregut is so good, and the liver may be sustained on portal blood flow alone. A variety of bypass configurations may be used, including antegrade bypass from the supraceliac aorta or retrograde bypass from the infrarenal aorta or common iliac arteries. The main requirements are a relatively disease-free site for the anastomosis and the absence of any hemodynamically significant proximal stenoses. The major advantage of the retrograde bypass is the ease of exposure for the inflow source; the major disadvantage is the orientation of the graft and its potential to kink.

The superior mesenteric artery may be exposed as described earlier, although the approach immediately caudal to the pancreas is optimal if a retrograde bypass is planned. A longitudinal arteriotomy in the superior mesenteric artery should be performed. Occasionally it may be difficult to determine whether the acute mesenteric ischemia is secondary to an embolus or thrombosis, and it is tempting to perform a transverse arteriotomy. However, this temptation should be resisted because of the added flexibility provided by the longitudinal arteriotomy. Prosthetic conduits are relatively contraindicated in the setting of acute mesenteric ischemia owing to the potential for bowel infarction or perforation and graft infection. Autogenous conduits with either saphenous or superficial femoral vein are suitable, although the latter may be more durable.

Occasionally patients will undergo bowel resection for infarction by a nonvascular surgeon, and the diagnosis of mesenteric ischemia will be missed both preoperatively and intraoperatively. The bowel infarction is usually due to thrombosis of chronically diseased visceral vessels in this setting. It is imperative that the etiology of all bowel infarctions be established in an attempt to prevent recurrences. A mesenteric arteriogram should be obtained in the early postoperative period and the necessary treatment, including anticoagulation and revascularization, implemented in a timely fashion.

Nonocclusive Mesenteric Ischemia

Nonocclusive mesenteric ischemia may develop in critically ill patients in the intensive care unit. There are multiple potential etiologies, including cardiogenic shock, septic shock, major burns, or trauma. The common precipitating cause among these diverse conditions is a decrease in cardiac output, a decrease in systemic perfusion, and an increase in portal venous pressure. These result in a paradoxic splanchnic vasoconstriction with loss of autoregulation, and this may be exacerbated by exogenous catecholamines or digoxin, or both.

The diagnosis of nonocclusive mesenteric ischemia requires a high index of suspicion and the proper clinical setting. Patients may develop abdominal pain. Their physical examinations are frequently unreliable because of multiple active medical problems and unreliable sensorium. Similarly, a variety of laboratory abnormalities are common, including acidosis, leukocytosis, elevated lactate levels, and hyperamylasemia, but these are all relatively nonspecific markers of the underlying shock state. Mesenteric arteriography is diagnostic and potentially therapeutic. The arteriographic findings of nonocclusive mesenteric ischemia include narrowing or irregularity and segmental spasm of the superior mesenteric artery and its branches. Additionally, arteriography is helpful to rule out the other potential causes of acute mesenteric ischemia.

The initial treatment of patients with nonocclusive mesenteric ischemia is nonoperative and directed at the underlying condition. Patients should be resuscitated in an attempt to improve their cardiac output and systemic perfusion. Vasoactive drugs should be stopped if at all possible, and patients should be started on broad-spectrum antibiotics directed against enteric organisms. Systemic anticoagulation with heparin should be started unless there are strong contraindications. Despite these efforts, the characteristic mesenteric vasoconstriction may persist. Continuous intra-arterial papaverine administered through a catheter placed into the superior mesenteric artery may reverse the vasoconstriction and should be considered. A 45-mg test dose of papaverine should be given over 15 minutes, and a continuous infusion of 30 to 60 mg/hr should be started if no adverse reactions are encountered. Serial mesenteric arteriograms should be performed to monitor the response to the papaverine, with the first one performed 1 hour after initiating therapy. The intra-arterial infusion may be continued up to 24 hours. Note that the infusion will reverse the mesenteric vasoconstriction only if the underlying hemodynamic instability is corrected. Operative treatment of nonocclusive mesenteric ischemia should be reserved only for the clinical scenario when bowel infarction is suspected, because resection is the only treatment.

Mesenteric Venous Thrombosis

Mesenteric venous thrombosis may also result in acute mesenteric ischemia, although the degree of ischemia is usually less than with arterial occlusion. The pathophysiology is similar to that of venous thrombosis in other vascular beds and may be explained in terms of Virchow's classic triad of stasis, intimal injury, and hypercoagulable states. Mesenteric venous stasis may result from congestive heart failure or portal hypertension, whereas intimal injury may result from general anesthesia or any number of intra-abdominal infectious processes. A hypercoagulable state is perhaps the strongest of the contributory factors and has been identified in up to 90% of patients with mesenteric venous thrombosis.

Mesenteric venous thrombosis results in edema in the bowel and mesentery, with significant third-space fluid losses. This may result in bloody ascites, and, indeed, a bloody tap at the time of paracentesis may be diagnostic. The venous thrombosis has been reported to cause bowel infarction in up to 40% of the cases despite therapy. Progression to bowel infarction depends on the magnitude of the clot load and its distribution. Clot localized to the portal or superior mesenteric vein usually does not lead to bowel infarction because of the collateral channels, whereas clot in the peripheral mesenteric veins is more likely to result in infarction. The natural history of untreated mesenteric venous thrombosis is poor and almost universally progresses from bowel infarction to perforation and death.

Patients with mesenteric venous thrombosis usually present with vague, mild abdominal pain. The pain is usually insidious in onset and frequently present for some time before the patients seek medical attention. Furthermore, the pain is usually not localized to any specific quadrant. Physical examination is notable only for mild, diffuse abdominal pain. Peritoneal signs are suggestive of bowel infarction but are only found late in the disease

---

Pearls and Pitfalls

Renal Artery Occlusive Disease

PEARLS

- Renovascular mechanisms should be considered in hypertensive patients with very poor blood pressure controls and those at the extremes of age.
- Deterioration in renal function with ACE inhibitors suggests significant renal artery stenosis.
- A lateral arteriogram should be obtained during the diagnostic workup to assess the orifice of the celiac axis for extra-anatomic bypass.
- Renal artery stenosis in the appropriate clinical scenario is sufficient indication for revascularization without additional diagnostic or function studies.
- Ischemic nephropathy should be considered in patients with rapid deterioration in renal function and sufficient renal mass (kidney length greater than 7 cm by ultrasound).

PITFALLS

- Not all patients with renal artery stenosis have renovascular hypertension.
- Renal vein renin studies are not reliable in patients with bilateral renal artery stenoses.
- Revascularization for ischemic nephropathy is unsuccessful in patients with unilateral stenosis and those without hypertension.
- The mortality rate for combined aortic procedures and renal artery bypass is significantly greater than the individual procedures and should be avoided unless there are compelling reasons.

Mesenteric Artery Occlusive Disease

PEARLS

- Chronic mesenteric ischemia should be considered early in the diagnosis of chronic abdominal pain and weight loss.
- Gastric ulcers in conjunction with chronic abdominal pain and weight loss suggest chronic mesenteric ischemia.
- The presence of a prominent meandering mesenteric artery suggests significant visceral artery occlusive disease.
- Prosthetic bypass conduits are preferable to autogenous vein for patients undergoing mesenteric revascularization for chronic ischemia.
- Revascularization for mesenteric ischemia is associated with a high incidence of multiple organ dysfunction.
- Mesenteric venous thrombosis is associated with a high incidence of hypercoagulable states and merits long-term anticoagulation even in the absence of an identifiable condition.

PITFALLS

- Chronic mesenteric ischemia does not usually occur unless two thirds of the visceral vessels are stenotic, although isolated superior mesenteric artery stenosis may occasionally be symptomatic.
- Embolization of visceral artery aneurysms in patients with visceral occlusive disease may precipitate acute mesenteric ischemia.
- The superior mesenteric artery should be exposed caudal to the pancreas and a longitudinal arteriotomy performed if the diagnosis of embolus is uncertain, and a mesenteric bypass may be required.
- Intra-arterial vasodilators will not reverse the splanchnic vasoconstriction in patients with nonocclusive mesenteric ischemia without the appropriate resuscitation.

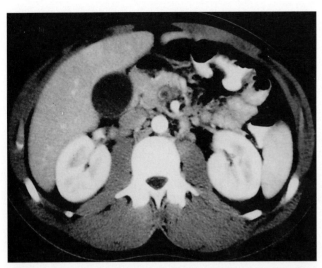

Figure 178–6. Abdominal computed tomography scan of a patient with acute mesenteric ischemia from mesenteric venous thrombosis. Note the thrombus within the superior mesenteric artery, with the surrounding inflammation.

process. Abdominal CT scanning is the diagnostic study of choice. The significant findings include bowel edema and thrombus within the mesenteric veins with inflammation of the vessel wall (Fig. 178–6). Plain abdominal radiographs may suggest abdominal wall edema and are helpful in ruling out other causes of the abdominal pain. Mesenteric arteriography may be helpful, but it is inferior to CT scanning. The arteriographic findings that suggest mesenteric venous thrombosis include arterial spasm with a prolonged arterial phase, opacification of the bowel wall, extravasation of the contrast material into the bowel lumen, and visualization of the venous thrombus.

The primary treatment of patients with mesenteric venous thrombosis is anticoagulation. Patients should be aggressively anticoagulated with heparin when the diagnosis is made and should be maintained on long-term anticoagulation with warfarin. A hypercoagulable workup should be performed prior to initiation of anticoagulation. However, long-term anticoagulation should be continued even in the absence of an identifiable hypercoagulable state. Patients frequently require fluid resuscitation at the time of diagnosis because of significant third-space losses from the bowel edema. Exploratory laparotomy should be reserved for cases in which bowel infarction is suspected. The intraoperative findings include edematous or rubbery bowel, bloody ascites, and thrombus within the mesentery. A wide resection of the bowel should be performed in the presence of infarction. Primary enteric anastomosis is probably safe if the margins of resection are free from thrombus within the mesentery. Proximal and distal stomas are advisable if the viability of the bowel at the margins of resection is questionable. Recurrent venous thrombosis has been reported in up to one third of cases, with the site of recurrence at the anastomosis in the majority of these. Attempts at venous thrombectomy are not advocated.

SELECTED READINGS

Benjamin ME, Hansen KJ, Craven TE, et al: Combined aortic and renal artery surgery: A contemporary experience. Ann Surg 1996;223:555.

Caps MT, Perissinotto C, Zierler RE, et al: Prospective study of atherosclerotic disease progression in the renal artery. Circulation 1998;98:2866.

Dean RH, Englund R, Dupont WD, et al: Retrieval of renal function by revascularization. Ann Surg 1985;202:367.

Dean RH, Tribble RW, Hansen KJ, et al: Evolution of renal insufficiency in ischemic nephropathy. Ann Surg 1991;213:446.

Dorros G, Jaff M, Mathiak L, et al: Four-year follow-up of Palmaz-Schatz stent revascularization as treatment for atherosclerotic renal artery stenosis. Circulation 1998;98:642.

Gentile AT, Moneta GL, Taylor LM, et al: Isolated bypass to the superior mesenteric artery for intestinal ischemia. Arch Surg 1994;129:926.

Harward TRS, Brooks DL, Flynn TC, Seeger JM: Multiple organ dysfunction after mesenteric artery revascularization. J Vasc Surg 1993;18:459.

Harward TRS, Green D, Bergan JJ, et al: Mesenteric venous thrombosis. J Vasc Surg 1989;9:328.

Mateo RB, O'Hara PJ, Hertzer NR, et al: Elective surgical treatment of symptomatic chronic mesenteric occlusive disease: Early results and late outcomes. J Vasc Surg 1999;29:821.

McAfee MK, Cherry KJ, Naessens JM, et al: Influence of complete revascularization on chronic mesenteric ischemia. Am J Surg 1992;164:220.

McMillan WD, McCarthy WJ, Bresticker MR, et al: Mesenteric artery bypass: Objective patency determination. J Vasc Surg 1995;21:729.

Moawad J, McKinsey JF, Wyble CW, et al: Current results of surgical therapy for chronic mesenteric ischemia. Arch Surg 1997;132:613.

Moneta GL, Lee RW, Yeager RA, et al: Mesenteric duplex scanning: A blinded prospective study. J Vasc Surg 1993;17:79.

Rodriguez-Lopez JA, Werner A, Ray LI, et al: Renal artery stenosis treated with stent deployment: Indications, technique, and outcome for 108 patients. J Vasc Surg 1999;29:617.

Sachs SM, Morton JH, Schwartz SI: Acute mesenteric ischemia. Surgery 1982;92:646.

Van de Ven PJ, Kaatee R, Beutler JJ, et al: Arterial stenting and balloon angioplasty in ostial atherosclerotic renovascular disease: A randomised trial. Lancet 1999;353:282.

Williamson WK, Abou-Zamzam AM, Moneta GL, et al: Prophylactic repair of renal artery stenosis is not justified in patients who require infrarenal aortic reconstruction. J Vasc Surg 1998;28:14.

Chapter 179

Management of Acute Arterial Occlusions

Timur P. Sarac and Kenneth Ouriel

The treatment and management of acute arterial occlusion remains a challenge to vascular surgeons as well as to the broad spectrum of practitioners involved in treating this problem. Before the 1900s, there was little to offer in terms of therapy and primary amputation was the only alternative. However, the pioneering work by Dos Santos on femoral thromboendarterectomy provided the opportunity to improve arterial perfusion and effect limb salvage. Thereafter, improvement in anesthetic techniques and the widespread availability of heparin led to an increased number of surgical alternatives. Most recently, the advent of devices such as percutaneously delivered mechanical thrombectomy catheters have been investigated in the treatment of acute peripheral arterial occlusion.

In 1963, Thomas Fogarty reported his early work with balloon catheters to remove thromboemboli from the peripheral circulation. Although traditional surgical teaching advocated immediate operation with rapid exploration and revascularization for patients with acute arterial occlusion, prior to the Fogarty catheter the technical aspects of treating thromboemboli were cumbersome, and the results unrewarding. Thrombectomy procedures with a balloon catheter revolutionized the treatment of embolic arterial occlusion by making it simple to remove the thrombus from the occluded native artery or bypass graft. If an underlying lesion responsible for the occlusion were then identified, it could be addressed with a variety of techniques, such as patch angioplasty or placement of a "jump graft" around the lesion. However, the ability to accurately identify a culprit lesion was compromised in the operating room, because there were no efficient imaging modalities. For this reason, it was standard practice to routinely assume that femoropopliteal bypass grafts failed as a result of distal anastomotic stenotic lesions. Following balloon catheter thrombectomy, distal anastomotic patch angioplasty was performed, sometimes regardless of whether the patient needed it or not (in other words, regardless of whether a tightly stenotic lesion could be accurately identified). If this failed, a new distal bypass was performed.

Even with the Fogarty catheter, the mortality rate of operative treatment for acute arterial occlusions remained high. Only in the past decade have less invasive and innovative techniques been investigated in a controlled fashion. The outcome of the traditional surgical approach to acute limb ischemia has been quite unsatisfactory. In a modified meta-analysis of more than 30 surgical series performed in the era following the advent of the balloon thromboembolectomy catheter, Blaisdell documented in-hospital death in more than 25% of the cases, with limb loss in a similar percentage of the survivors. This observation prompted Blaisdell to recommend an initial *nonoperative* approach with high-dose intravenous heparin therapy, delaying surgical revascularization until the patient had been fully stabilized and prepared. This strategy never gained popularity among vascular surgeons, because most clinicians were unwilling to delay definitive revascularization for fear of increasing the risk of limb loss. Despite improvements in anesthesia and intensive postoperative care, the 1990s saw little improvement in the mortality rate. In fact, overall patient survival did not change dramatically since the report of Blaisdell more than 20 years ago. The discordance of limb salvage and patient survival is explained by the specific factors controlling the two events. Whereas *mortality* occurs as a result of concurrent medical comorbidities and the fragile baseline medical state of patients presenting acute limb ischemia, *limb loss* is related to an unsuccessful revascularization procedure. As such, the rate of amputation has diminished over the decades with improvements in surgical technique, but the ability to rapidly restore arterial flow to the extremity with an operative procedure continues to represent a significant insult to medically compromised individuals—one that all too frequently culminates in death of the patient.

Recently, a push to employ preoperative and intraoperative angiographic assessment of the patient with acute limb ischemia has altered traditional teaching. Many surgeons have realized that the time required to perform preoperative angiographic evaluation is well worth the information obtained, information that is essential to the operative plan. In addition, there has been a push toward the placement of a new bypass graft as opposed to thrombectomy of an old graft or diseased native arterial segment. For instance, a thrombosed femoropopliteal bypass graft that was routinely treated by an immediate trip to the operating room for thrombectomy and distal patch angioplasty might now be managed with preoperative angiographic assessment and placement of a new autogenous vein bypass graft around the blocked arterial segment.

The search for less invasive revascularization strategies has been ongoing, seeking to lessen the morbidity of the procedures without compromising the satisfactory rate of limb salvage that has been achieved with contemporary surgical procedures. Pharmacologic thrombolysis and, recently, percutaneous mechanical thrombectomy hold potential in this regard. Both techniques can effect clearance of the occluding thrombus from a peripheral artery in a minimally invasive fashion, restoring blood flow to the extremity and allowing the identification of any underlying lesion that was responsible for the occlusive event. The unmasked culprit lesion can then be addressed in a directed fashion with angioplasty, stenting, or a limited operative procedure performed electively, in a well-prepared patient.

PATHOPHYSIOLOGY, ETIOLOGY, AND NATURAL HISTORY

It is essential to respond rapidly when evaluating an acutely ischemic limb, because the ischemic process can quickly progress and eventually lead to an unsalvageable limb. Ischemia for longer than 6 hours has classically been promoted as the longest time one can go without blood flow before permanent damage occurs, based on animal studies in dogs with normal circulation. In reality, the time interval in which a limb can be maintained depends on the patient's preocclusive state (i.e., collateral circulation) and chronicity of arterial occlusive disease. Therefore, a thorough and expedient history and physical examination is the most important determinant of the urgency.

The most common etiology of acute limb ischemia is from thromboemboli from the heart followed by thrombosis of a chronically ischemic limb. Occluded bypass grafts, atherosclerotic emboli, emboli from aortic aneurysms, trauma, aortic dissections, venous gangrene, and compartment syndrome lag behind (Table 179–1). Rheumatic heart disease was formerly the most common event accounting for the source of emboli, but its decreased incidence accounts for a change to acute myocardial infarction and atrial fibrillation as the most frequent etiology.

The typical location of emboli is usually at arterial branch points, where the caliber of the vessels abruptly changes in diameter. Elliot reported that 84% of an acutely ischemic process occurs in the aortofemoral circulation with the remaining 16% occurring in the carotid-visceral distribution. He also found that, if these patients had simultaneous multiple emboli to the peripheral and carotid-visceral distribution, their mortality rate increased from 35% to 100%. However, patients maintained on long-term anticoagulation survived twice as long. The 5-year recurrence rate of an acute arterial occlusion is reported to be as high as 40% in patients not anticoagulated; this is reduced by one half if chronic anticoagulation is initiated. Conservative management without intervention in the acutely ischemic limb ultimately leads to limb loss in up to 50% of patients. Even so, in 1982 Abbott reported that, although limb salvage could be

Table 179–1	Etiologies of Acute Arterial Occlusion
	Thromboemboli of cardiac origin
	Arterial thrombosis of an atherosclerotic artery
	Bypass graft occlusion
	Aortic dissection
	Atheroemboli
	Compartment syndrome
	Venous gangrene

increased to 86% with appropriate surgical therapy, the mortality rate remained at 20%.

CLINICAL PRESENTATION AND DIAGNOSIS

The classic symptoms of acute limb ischemia have been categorized into the six "p's": pain, pulselessness, pallor, paresthesia, paralysis, and poikilothermia (coolness). Patients with acute limb ischemia usually have pain and sensory loss, because neural tissue is the most sensitive to loss of circulation. The pain is sequentially followed by mottling of the skin and then loss of muscle function. For example, loss of sensation in the first and second lower extremity digit web space is a subtle first sign of ischemia, manifesting ischemia to the peroneal nerve.

The location of lodgment of emboli can usually be surmised from clinical observation. The involved extremity is cool up to the proximal branch point; for example, an emboli lodging at the superficial femoral and deep femoral arterial junction produces ischemic changes of pulselessness and cool mottling up to the mid-thigh level. Symptoms from acute thrombosis of a diseased profunda femoral artery or thrombosis of a bypass graft usually present as pain in the foot or calf.

Whereas bedside continuous wave Doppler examination of the extremity is a useful adjunct to determine the patency of specific vessels, hearing audible signals over a pedal pulse is not a reliable sign to guide the urgency for revascularizing an acutely ischemic limb. A patient may have no detectable signals in an extremity, but the chronicity of the occlusion may afford the luxury of obtaining preoperative imaging studies in an elective setting. On the other hand, in a young patient with no preformed collaterals, a faint signal may be detected over a vessel, but urgent revascularization should not be delayed. The most reliable sign of the urgency of the clinical scenario is whether the patient has neuromotor changes to that extremity. In the presence of severe pain, immediate revascularization should be performed promptly before the loss of motor function.

PERIOPERATIVE MANAGEMENT

The initial management always includes a complete history and physical examination, which can often give valuable diagnostic clues to the etiology. If a patient gives a history of claudication or previous bypass grafting, then the ischemia likely results from thrombosis. If a patient has a history of atrial fibrillation or recent myocardial infarction, then embolism is usually the cause. Whether the inciting event is thrombosis or embolism, prompt fluid resuscitation and cardiopulmonary stabilization are imperative to minimize early complications.

Although the location of the occluded segment can frequently be made at the bedside, an arteriogram can be useful in planning the operative procedure in the absence of neuromotor changes. The decision whether to obtain an arteriogram should be based on three concepts:

1. Are the patient's symptoms severe enough that the extra time to acquire an arteriogram places the limb

in jeopardy? In this case, an expeditious trip to the operating room with preparation for intraoperative imaging studies may be in the patient's best interest.

2. Is the diagnosis of acute arterial occlusion in doubt? If one is unsure, additional diagnostic studies are necessary.

3. Is a percutaneous interventional procedure planned? If so, a diagnostic arteriogram can be followed by a definitive endovascular procedure.

Regardless of these considerations, immediate anticoagulation with 100 units/kg of heparin and institution of a heparin drip at 20 units/kg per hour can prevent propagation of the thrombus. Laboratory tests seldom shed light on the preoperative differentiation of embolus from thrombosis, but electrolyte and acid base abnormalities are common and should be corrected before reperfusion.

If the patient's condition warrants immediate surgical intervention, preoperative planning of the incision can expedite intervention. The patient should be prepped from chin to toes, because the axillary artery may be needed as an inflow source. For lower extremity ischemia, exposure of the femoral vessels with an arteriotomy made over the bifurcation of the common femoral artery into the superficial and deep femoral arteries allows easy access to both the iliac and popliteal arteries with a balloon catheter. If a thrombus *cannot* be extracted with an embolectomy catheter, it is likely the diagnosis is not thromboembolism, so this incision then allows for convenient placement of the distal limb of an axillofemoral or femoral-femoral bypass. Thromboemboli to the tibial vessels cannot be adequately addressed through a groin incision. Thus, in cases in which the popliteal pulse is palpable, one should direct initial efforts with an infragenicular popliteal exposure and isolation of the take-off of the three tibial vessels. For upper extremity symptoms, one should make an incision just distal to the antecubital fossa to allow exposure of the brachial bifurcation.

Once the limb is revascularized, if there is any question or concern about reperfusion and edema of the revascularized limb that would further compromise perfusion, a four-compartment fasciotomy in the leg and a two-compartment fasciotomy in the arm should be performed without hesitation.

PHARMACOLOGIC THROMBOLYSIS

Thrombolytic agents are in widespread use for the dissolution of arterial and venous pathologic thrombi. Clinical settings where thrombolysis has played an important role include the acute coronary syndromes, peripheral arterial occlusion, stroke, pulmonary embolism, and deep venous thrombosis. Thrombolytic agents have been successfully employed in each of these areas, achieving dissolution of the occluding thrombus, reconstitution of blood flow, and improvement in the status of the tissue bed supplied or drained by the involved vascular segment.

In the setting of peripheral arterial occlusion, catheter-directed thrombolytic treatment strategies were popularized in the 1970s by Dotter, who suggested that fibrinolytic dissolution would occur more rapidly and with less systemic side effects if the agent were delivered directly

into the thrombus through an indwelling arterial catheter. In the 1980s, McNamara developed a protocol of graded intra-arterial urokinase administration, which, with minor modifications, remains in widespread use. Despite excellent studies by well-established clinicians, the validation of the safety and efficacy of thrombolysis in acute limb ischemia awaited the completion of prospective, randomized trials comparing it with open surgical intervention.

Pharmacology of Fibrinolytic Agents

All thrombolytic agents in clinical use are actually *plasminogen activators*. As such, they do not *directly* degrade fibrinogen. Rather, they are trypsin-like serine proteases that have high specific activity directed at the cleavage of a single peptide bond in the plasminogen zymogen, converting it to plasmin. Plasmin is the active molecule that cleaves fibrin polymer to cause the dissolution of thrombus. Effective thrombolysis can only be achieved when *fibrin-bound* plasminogen is converted to its active form plasmin at the site of the thrombus.

We have found it most useful to classify thrombolytic agents into groups based on the origin of the parent compound. It is most efficient to divide the agents into four groups: the streptokinase compounds, the urokinase compounds, the tissue plasminogen activators, and an additional, miscellaneous group consisting of novel agents distinct from agents in the three other groups.

Outcome Studies of Thrombolysis Versus Primary Operation

Three multicenter, randomized trials were published in the 1990s comparing thrombolysis with operation for arterial occlusion (Table 179–2). The purpose of the first trial, the Rochester Study, was to compare urokinase to immediate operation in patients with peripheral arterial occlusion. The primary endpoint was amputation-free survival. It was reasoned that if thrombolytic agents were effective, the subgroup with the highest chance of success would be those with the most severe ischemia. It was in this population that operative therapy had a poor track record, with a high rate of both amputation and death. Patients with acute limb-threatening ischemia were randomly assigned to thrombolysis with urokinase (N = 57) or to immediate operation (N = 57). At 1 year, the *amputation free survival rates* were 75% and 52% respectively, a statistically significant difference. A closer analysis revealed this finding to be the result of a higher rate of death in the operative group, deaths that occurred in association with perioperative cardiopulmonary complications. It appeared that the need to take patients with severe ischemia directly to operation without the opportunity for preparation resulted in a high frequency of complications that culminated in patient death. Thrombolysis produced rapid initiation of enough antegrade blood flow to convert the limb to a viable state, despite requiring more than 24 hours for completion. Adjuvant operation, when required to repair an unmasked lesion, could then be performed on an elective basis in a well-prepared patient. Despite the requirement for supplementary oper-

Table 179–2	**Thrombolytic Trials**						
			THROMBOLYTIC THERAPY		PRIMARY OPERATION		
TRIAL	**PATIENTS**	**TIME PERIOD (mo)**	**Amputation* (%)**	**Death (%)**	**Amputation* (%)**	**Death (%)**	
Rochester	114	12	18	16	18	42	
STILE	393	1	5	4	6	5	
TOPAS-II°	544	12	35	20	30	17	

°Amputation figures represent amputation-free survival, because amputation alone was not tabulated in this trial.

ation following thrombolysis in approximately two thirds of patients, the duration of hospitalization and hospital costs were similar in the two treatment groups.

The second large, multicenter evaluation of thrombolysis versus surgery was entitled the trial of Surgery versus Thrombolysis for Ischemia of the Lower Extremity, or STILE. In this multicenter trial, two different thrombolytic agents, recombinant tissue plasminogen activator (rt-PA) and urokinase, were compared with immediate operation in patients with lower extremity ischemic symptoms of less than 6 months' duration. The primary endpoint was a composite outcome index that included ongoing or recurrent ischemia, death or major amputation, life-threatening hemorrhage, and a variety of perioperative complications. Amputation and death were not in themselves primary endpoints. At the completion of the trial, 393 patients were randomly assigned to surgery or to thrombolysis with either rt-PA or urokinase. Clinical outcomes for both thrombolysis groups were similar, so their data were combined for the overall comparison of thrombolysis with surgery. Post hoc stratification of patients into two subgroups on the basis of the duration of symptoms before enrollment (more than 14 days versus less than 14 days) showed that, among patients with symptoms of longer duration, the surgical group had lower amputation rates than the thrombolysis group at 6 months (3% versus 12%, $P = 0.01$). In contrast, among patients with symptoms of shorter duration, patients assigned to thrombolysis had lower amputation rates than surgical patients (11% versus 30%, $P = 0.02$). Nevertheless, some pitfalls of STILE were that randomization occurred before attempting to place the infusion catheter into the thrombus, and appropriate thrombus cannulation was not possible in 28% of patients in the thrombolytic group. Also, successful catheter placement was not possible in 39% of patients with bypass graft occlusion.

The third and largest multicenter trial, designed after evaluation of the results of the Rochester trial, was the Thrombolysis or Peripheral Arterial Surgery trial (TOPAS). Recombinant Urokinase (r-UK) was compared with primary operation in 757 patients with lower extremity native artery or bypass graft occlusions of *14 days' duration or less*. The primary endpoint of the dose-ranging trial (213 patients) was arteriographic (the extent of clot lysis on the 4-hour arteriogram). *Amputation-free survival rates* 6 months after randomization (phase II, 544 patients) were 71.8% in the r-UK and 74.8% in the operative group ($P = 0.43$; 95% confidence interval for

the difference between treatments 10.5% to 4.5%). There was also no significant difference in the rates of amputation-free survival at discharge from the hospital or in the rate of mortality at the time of discharge. At the end of 6 months, Kaplan-Meier analyses showed that 31.5% of the thrombolytic patients were alive and had avoided amputation or open surgical procedures. When the rate of open surgical procedures was tabulated over 6 months of follow-up, the thrombolytic patients had significantly fewer open interventions (315 versus 551). Thus, intra-arterial r-UK thrombolysis achieved a similar rate of amputation-free survival, with a lower requirement for open surgical procedures when compared with primary operation. By contrast, the vast majority of the patients randomized to primary operation underwent open surgery (94.2%), a rate that was not unexpected because of the design of the trial. The median length of hospitalization was 10 days in both treatment groups for patients who survived to discharge. Among patients who were assigned to thrombolysis, those with occlusions in bypass grafts had better clinical outcomes and rates of clot dissolution compared with those patients with native artery occlusions.

Major hemorrhagic complications occurred in 32 patients (12.5%) in the r-UK group as compared with 14 patients (5.5%) in the surgery group ($P = 0.005$). Patient's age, duration of infusion, and activated partial thromboplastin times at baseline were unrelated to the risk of bleeding. The risk of bleeding was significantly greater when *therapeutic heparin* was used as compared to when it was not ($P = 0.02$ by Fisher's exact test). Use of therapeutic heparin accounted for an increase in the risk of bleeding with a relative risk ratio of 2.19 (95% confidence interval = 1.13 to 4.24, $P = 0.02$).

The major conclusions of the TOPAS trial were as follows:

1. Similar rates of limb salvage and patient survival were achieved with r-UK when compared with primary operation, concurrent with a lower requirement for open surgical procedures of 12 months' follow-up.
2. Concomitant full heparin therapy was associated with a significant increase in the risk of hemorrhagic complications.

Comparison of the Agents in Studies of Peripheral Vascular Disease

To date, there have been few well-designed clinical comparisons of various thrombolytic agents in the peripheral vasculature. Of the variety of retrospective studies, most point to improved efficacy and safety of UK and rt-PA over streptokinase (SK).

There have been two prospective, randomized comparisons of UK and rt-PA. Neither was blinded. Meyerovitz and associates from the Brigham and Women's Hospital randomized 32 patients with peripheral arterial or bypass graft occlusions of less than 90 days' duration to rt-PA or UK. There was significantly greater systemic fibrinogen degradation in the rt-PA group ($P = 0.01$), indicating that the theoretical fibrin-specificity of rt-PA was lost at this dosing regimen. rt-PA patients achieved more rapid initial thrombolysis, but efficacy was identical in the two groups by 24 hours. The trade-off to more rapid thrombolysis was a trend toward a higher rate of bleeding complications in the rt-PA treated patients ($P = 0.39$)

The second randomized comparison of UK and rt-PA was STILE, a three-armed multicenter comparison of UK, rt-PA, and primary operation. There was one intracranial hemorrhage in the UK group (0.9%) and two in the rt-PA group (1.5%), a difference that did not attain statistical significance. Although actual rates of overall bleeding complications and efficacy were not reported for the two thrombolytic groups, the authors remarked that there were no significant differences detected in any of the outcome variables. In a subsequent "reanalysis" of the data, the frequency of complete clot lysis was similar with UK and rt-PA at the time of the early arteriographic study. This recent information suggests that the rate of thrombolysis may be quite similar, in direct contradistinction to the popularly held view that rt-PA is a much more rapidly acting agent.

Newer Agents for Peripheral Thrombolysis

Reteplase (Retavase, Centocor) was developed with the goal of avoiding the necessity of a continuous intravenous infusion in the setting of acute myocardial infarction, thereby simplifying ease of administration. Reteplase, produced in *Escherichia coli* cells, is non-glycosylated, demonstrating a lower fibrin-binding activity and a diminished affinity to hepatocytes when compared with rt-PA. This latter property accounts for a longer half-life than rt-PA, potentially enabling bolus injection versus prolonged infusion. The fibrin affinity of reteplase was only 30% of that exhibited with t-PA, similar to UK. The decrease in fibrin affinity was hypothesized to reduce the incidence of distant bleeding complications, in a manner similar to that of SK over rt-PA. In fact, several properties of reteplase may account for its decreased risk of hemorrhage, including poor lysis of platelet-rich, older clots. To date, reteplase has been extensively studied in the coronary setting and has demonstrated some benefit over rt-PA in the RAPID 1 and RAPID 2 studies, but was equivalent to rt-PA in GUSTO III.

There are many other novel thrombolytic agents, all of which have undergone extensive preclinical study, but few have been adequately evaluated in patients. Vampire bat plasminogen activator ("Bat PA," DSPA$_{\forall 1}$), was cloned and expressed from the saliva of the vampire bat *Desmo-*

dus rotundus. This agent manifests extraordinary fibrin specificity, in that the plasminogenolytic activity is more than 100,000 times greater in the presence of fibrin. The half-life of DSPA$_{\forall 1}$ is five to nine times longer than that of rt-PA, offering some potential advantages with respect to ease of administration. To date, clinical trials have been limited to phase I study in healthy volunteers.

POSTOPERATIVE TREATMENT

The postoperative care of patients who have had an acutely ischemic limb revascularized can be challenging. Subsequent reperfusion of an ischemic limb poses several management problems for the involved limb as well as life-threatening systemic sequelae. Reperfusion of muscle fibers that have necrosed releases large stores of intracellular potassium from the nonviable cells, which can rapidly lead to myocardial instability. Additionally, the ischemic muscle accumulates large stores of lactic acid from anaerobic metabolism, further complicating treatment. Necrotic muscle cells also release myoglobin, which can precipitate in the kidney and lead to renal failure. Finally, prolonged ischemia can cause capillary leak at the cell membrane level, which increases extremity swelling and edema. This can result in the "no reflow" phenomenon, with arteriolar occlusion resulting from increased swelling at the cellular level and compartment syndrome at the tissue level. Treatment includes aggressive fluid administration with correction of acid-base and electrolyte abnormalities. Prompt four-compartment fasciotomy should be performed for neurologic deficit or if measured compartment pressures exceed 25 to 30 mm Hg. Finally, diuresis and alkalinization of the urine (pH 5.5 to 7) can prevent the precipitation of myoglobin in the tubules.

PROMISING NEW THERAPIES

Recently, percutaneous mechanical thrombectomy devices have been employed in an effort to rapidly extract intravascular thrombus and restore blood flow. The Food and Drug Administration originally approved each device for use in dialysis access graft occlusion. The devices have, however, been employed "off-label" for the treatment of acute lower extremity arterial occlusions. The potential benefits of mechanical thrombectomy devices include the ability to establish more rapid reperfusion of the ischemic extremity, shorten the duration and lessen the dose of pharmacologic thrombolysis by debulking the thrombus, and, in some cases, avoid the use of thrombolytic administration altogether when contraindications to thrombolysis are present.

Hydrodynamic Thrombectomy Catheters

Several percutaneously delivered devices can remove thrombus from peripheral arteries using a rapid stream of fluid and hydrodynamic forces to extract material from the lumen. The devices differ in the method of fluid instillation: one uses a dedicated fluid delivery machine to achieve rapid flow rates, and the other devices use a standard angiographic injector.

The available devices have a number of limitations. Each device carries the potential to induce distal embolization as it is passed through the thrombus. Also, arterial wall damage may be induced. The efficacy of the device is limited by the diameter of the cylindrical core of thrombus that can be extracted with each pass of the catheter (this property is dependent on the size of the device). However, this limitation must be balanced by the convenience of placing the device through a relatively small-bore sheath, as well as the increased safety associated with use of a smaller device in the tibial vessels. Another limitation of the currently available devices is the amount of red blood cell damage that can occur. Hemolysis with hemoglobinemia and hemoglobinuria may occur, especially after protracted use of the devices. Lastly, fluid overload can develop if one is not careful to monitor the amount of irrigation instilled intravascularly during use.

Despite these potential limitations, the ability of the percutaneous thrombectomy devices to rapidly restore arterial perfusion is an attractive advantage. In patients with significant ischemia that precludes the obligatory delay associated with pharmacologic thrombolysis, the percutaneous thrombectomy devices may rapidly clear a channel through the occluded segment. Partial reperfusion of the extremity may provide enough improvement in ischemia to allow complete removal of thrombus with thrombolytic infusions over the subsequent 12- to 24-hour period. As well, the devices may be employed as sole therapy in patients with contraindications to thrombolytic administration, for instance, in those patients who have recently undergone a major surgical procedure.

Recommended Treatment Plan for Acute Limb Ischemia

Recently, a rational treatment plan was initiated by the Trans Atlantic Inter-Society Consensus based on the clinical data presented for patients with arterial occlusion of the lower extremities. Patients must be individually assessed to determine the degree of ischemia and the suitability of the various therapeutic options. Patients with arterial occlusions of *greater than 2 weeks' duration* appear best treated with operative intervention. In particular, vein grafts are unlikely to undergo successful clot dissolution following prolonged occlusion because of sclerosis, contraction, organization of thrombus, and endothelial necrosis. The thrombus within prosthetic grafts is less dependent on the duration of the process, in that the prosthetic material delays organization of the clot and the artificial conduit does not undergo changes related to thrombosis. Therefore, we frequently waive the somewhat arbitrary cutoff of 2 weeks in occluded prosthetic grafts. One must keep in mind, however, that available data suggest superior limb salvage may be achieved in patients with chronic occlusions treated with insertion of a new bypass graft. Patients with acute embolic occlusions and neuromotor changes are best treated surgically in the absence of extensive proximal or distal propagation of the clot. This is particularly true when dealing with a localized common femoral embolus that can be surgically removed under local anesthesia.

Pearls and Pitfalls

- Do not observe patient if neuromotor changes occur.
- Physical examination determines whether the patient should go directly to the operating room.
- Heparinize all patients with acute ischemia early in this course.
- Consider thrombolysis or percutaneous mechanical thrombectomy if time allows.
- Perform arteriotomy at branch points of major vessels (e.g., common femoral, superficial femoral, profunda femoral arteries).
- Perform fasciotomy in operating room if indicated.
- Investigate etiology of ischemia (thrombosis versus embolism).

These factors notwithstanding, it may be advantageous to consider thrombolytic therapy in any *viable* limb with an acute arterial occlusion. Thrombolysis can restore arterial perfusion, providing the opportunity to address the unmasked causative lesion through a directed, elective approach. An open surgical procedure such as a patch angioplasty, interposition of a segment of autogenous graft, or an endovascular procedure can then be employed to correct the underlying lesion.

Summary

The treatment of patients with acute limb ischemia must involve multiple modalities, each of which should be tailored to the individual clinical presentation. Open surgical revascularization remains the standard with which all newer therapies must be compared. Surgical revascularization is associated with satisfactory results in most patients, but data suggest that an increased rate of complications is associated with immediate operative intervention in medically compromised patients with severe ischemia. Thrombolytic therapy has emerged as a less invasive modality in these patients, with the potential to lower morbidity and mortality risks, using catheter-directed infusions of thrombolytic agents to dissolve the occluding thrombus. In a similar fashion, percutaneous mechanical thrombectomy devices have recently been evaluated, with or without adjuvant thrombolytic infusions. Whether pharmacologic thrombolysis, mechanical thrombectomy, or both are used, removal of the thrombus is followed by an endovascular procedure (angioplasty or stenting) or open surgical procedure directed at remediation of the culprit lesion deemed responsible for the occlusive event. It is hoped that less invasive treatment strategies such as these may culminate in improved outcome in patients with acute lower extremity ischemia.

SELECTED READINGS

Abbott WM, Maloney RD, McCabe CC: Arterial embolism: A 44 year perspective. Am J Surg 1982;143:460.

Anonymous: Results of a prospective randomized trial evaluating surgery versus thrombolysis for ischemia of the lower extremity. The STILE trial. Ann Surg 1994;220:251.

Ascer E, Collier P, Gupta SK, Veith FJ: Reoperation for polytetrafluoroethylene bypass failure: The importance of distal outflow site and operative technique in determining outcome. J Vasc Surg 1987;5:298.

Blaisdell FW, Steele M, Allen RE: Management of acute lower extremity arterial ischemia due to embolism and thrombosis. Surgery 1978;84:822.

Edwards JE, Taylor LM Jr, Porter JM: Treatment of failed lower extremity bypass grafts with new autogenous vein bypass grafting. J Vasc Surg 1990;11:136.

Elliott JP, Hageman JH, Szilagyi DE: Arterial embolization: Problems of source, multiplicity, recurrence and delayed treatment. Surgery 1980;88:833.

Fogarty TJ, Cranley JJ, Krause RJ: A method for extraction of arterial emboli and thrombi. Surg Gynecol Obstet 1963;116:241.

Jivegård L, Holm J, Scherstén T: Acute limb ischemia due to arterial embolism or thrombosis: Influence of limb ischemia versus pre-existing cardiac disease on postoperative mortality rate. J Cardiovasc Surg 1988;29:32.

McNamara TO, Fischer JR: Thrombolysis of peripheral arterial and graft occlusions: Improved results using high-dose urokinase. AJR Am J Roentgenol 1985;144:769.

Meyerovitz M, Goldhaber SZ, Reagan K, et al: Recombinant tissue-type plasminogen activator versus urokinase in peripheral arterial and graft occlusions: A randomized trial. Radiology 1990;175:75.

Ouriel K, Shortell CK, DeWeese JA, et al: A comparison of thrombolytic therapy with operative revascularization in the initial treatment of acute peripheral arterial ischemia. J Vasc Surg 1994;19:1021.

Ouriel K, Veith FJ, Sasahara AA: Thrombolysis or peripheral arterial surgery: Phase I results. TOPAS Investigators. J Vasc Surg 1996;23:64.

Ouriel K, Veith FJ, Sasahara AA: A comparison of recombinant urokinase with vascular surgery as initial treatment for acute arterial occlusion of the legs. N Engl J Med 1998;338:1105.

Perry MO, Shires TG, Albert SA: Cellular changes with graded limb ischemia and reperfusion. J Vasc Surg 1984;1:536.

Yeager RA, Moneta GL, Taylor LM Jr, et al: Surgical management of severe acute lower extremity ischemia. J Vasc Surg 1992;15:385.

Chapter 180
Management of Vascular Trauma

James W. Dennis

Vascular trauma has both frightened and excited physicians for centuries. The early accounts of Paré or Fleming, who first treated hemorrhaging wounds, have documented some of the first recorded attempts to manage injuries to major arteries or veins. Up until the second half of the twentieth century, most of all medical knowledge on vascular trauma came from military experience. Urban violence is currently the dominant source of most penetrating vascular injuries, and motor vehicle crashes are the source of most blunt injuries. This chapter outlines current concepts in the management of vascular trauma (both penetrating and blunt) to the extremities, neck, and torso, focusing on the common problems encountered by the practicing general surgeon.

PATHOPHYSIOLOGY

The largest series published of more than 5000 cases of vascular trauma by Mattox and colleagues gives important demographic information. Penetrating wounds causing vascular injury are predominantly caused by gunshot wounds, accounting for approximately half of all injuries. Stab wounds are the second most common etiology at 30% to 35%, followed by shotgun blasts at 5%. Blunt trauma represents the mechanism of injury in the remaining 10% to 15%. Injuries to blood vessels can cause several types of morphologic changes. Lacerations and transections are the most common pattern, together representing 80% to 85% of the injuries seen. If an artery is transected, active hemorrhage initially occurs, often followed by acute occlusion, especially in young people whose arteries intensely spasm and retract. Lacerations are more likely to cause persistent hemorrhage. Smooth luminal narrowing seen on arteriography (AG) occurs secondary to arterial wall hematomas, extrinsic compression, and spasm. Other morphologic appearances include intimal irregularities or flaps, false or pseudoaneurysms, and arteriovenous (AV) fistulas. The kinetic energy absorbed by the tissue influences the type of pathophysiologic injury seen. Large, high-velocity bullets cause a large surrounding blast effect to the vessel wall many times the size of the bullet, resulting in larger segments injured.

The distribution of 211 consecutive arterial injuries at one institution is shown in Table 180–1. The femoral artery is the most commonly injured (35%), followed by the brachial artery (30%), then the popliteal artery (20%). The brachial artery is the most likely to be injured with penetrating trauma in proximity to it, probably because of the small amount of soft tissue surrounding the artery. In the neck, the common carotid artery is by far the most common site of injury, accounting for 70% to 90% of the cervical arterial trauma.

Blunt trauma can cause blood vessel injury by either direct force disrupting the wall, by indirect tension on the vessel wall by surrounding structures, or by bony fragments acting as penetrating agents. Five specific orthopedic injuries have been shown to have a high association with vascular trauma and mandate an extremely high index of suspicion. They are first rib fracture, supracondylar femur fracture, pelvic fracture, mid or distal humerus fracture, and posterior knee dislocation. In addition, acute deceleration motor vehicle crashes can lead to descending aortic disruption, and hyperextension of the neck can lead to carotid dissection. Blunt injuries tend to involve longer segments of blood vessels, thus requiring more extensive repairs, often with interposition grafts.

NATURAL HISTORY

The natural history of the acute vascular lesions caused by trauma has been well documented over the years. Actively bleeding lacerations usually lead to shock, which can be fatal if not addressed quickly. If the extravasation of blood is contained by the surrounding tissue, then a pseudoaneurysm results. These pseudoaneurysms usually

Table 180–1	Distribution of 211 Consecutive Arterial Injuries
Thoracic	
Innominate	5 (2.4%)
Pulmonary	2 (0.9%)
Thoracic aortia	2 (0.9%)
Upper Extremity	
Subclavian	4 (1.9%)
Axillary	3 (1.4%)
Brachial	26 (12.3%)
Radial	13 (6.2%)
Ulnar	10 (4.7%)
Neck	
Carotid	6 (2.5%)
Abdominal	
Hepatic	1 (0.4%)
Renal	5 (2.4%)
Abdominal aorta	12 (5.7%)
Inferior mesenteric	1 (0.4%)
Iliac	19 (9.9%)
Lower Extremity	
Common femoral	11 (5.2%)
Deep femoral	9 (4.3%)
Superficial femoral	37 (17.5%)
Popliteal	22 (10.4%)
Tibioperoneal trunk	3 (1.4%)
Anterior tibial	7 (3.3%)
Posterior tibial	4 (1.9%)
Peroneal	3 (1.4%)

From Sharma PV, Babu SC, Shah PM, et al: Changing patterns in civilian injuries. J Cardiovasc Surg 1985;26:7–11.

enlarge over time and produce local symptoms of pain, nerve compression, or thrombosis or embolization in the affected artery. Small pseudoaneurysms (less than 2 cm) occasionally resolve or improve without treatment. Acute arterial occlusions usually result in profound ischemia to the involved extremity or an ipsilateral stroke if in the neck. Acutely ischemic extremities usually demonstrate the five "p's" of acute ischemia on physical examination (PX) including pulselessness, pallor, pain, paresthesias (or paralysis), and poikilothermia. The risk of a major amputation following acute untreated occlusion of specific arteries is listed in Table 180–2.

AV fistulas develop when adjacent lacerations to both an artery and vein occur. These typically enlarge over time and cause localized edema in the extremity and chronic venous stasis changes. Occasionally, diminished distal perfusion leads to claudication-like symptoms of the affected extremity. If an AV fistula is large and centrally located, over time the heart will enlarge, become tachycardic, and even precipitate congestive heart failure. Direct compression occluding these AV fistulas results in an immediate decrease in the heart rate, a maneuver known as the Branham-Nicoladoni sign. For decades, any abnormality seen on AG was thought to require operative intervention and repair, even if clinically occult. Recent evidence indicates that certain "minimal injuries" (injuries seen on AG but with no physical findings) do not require operative intervention in the majority of cases. Smooth arterial narrowings caused by external compression, intramural thrombus, or spasm almost always resolve without any intervention (Fig. 180–1). Intimal irregularities or flaps also have a benign natural history in that almost 90% resolve on their own (Fig. 180–2). The morphology or direction of the flap does not have any predictive value in determining which ones are likely to deteriorate. Small pseudoaneurysms and AV fistulas also resolve spontaneously, but they have to be watched over time, because they are more likely to deteriorate and require operative repair. Those that do worsen, do so in the first 3 months after trauma. In close to 10 years of follow-up, no evidence of late complications has been seen in observation of these "minimal injuries" after 3 months post injury.

CLINICAL PRESENTATION AND DIAGNOSIS

General Principles

The cornerstone of management for all vascular trauma is the findings of a close PX performed by an experienced surgeon. In the 1960s, the presence of "hard" signs signifying vascular injury that necessitated immediate intervention (usually operative repair) was first demonstrated.

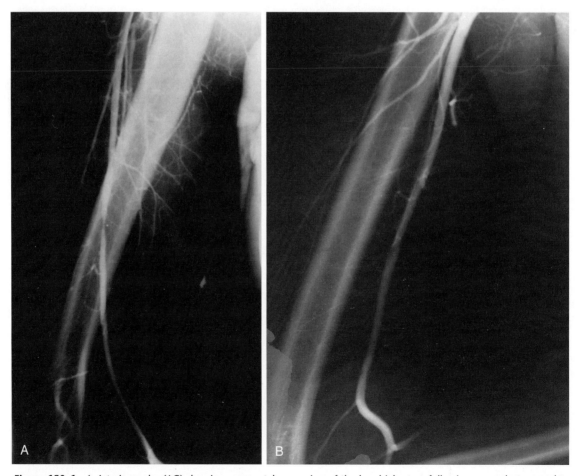

Figure 180–1. *A,* Arteriography (AG) showing segmental narrowing of the brachial artery following a gunshot wound to the upper arm. *B,* Complete resolution seen on repeat AG 2 weeks later.

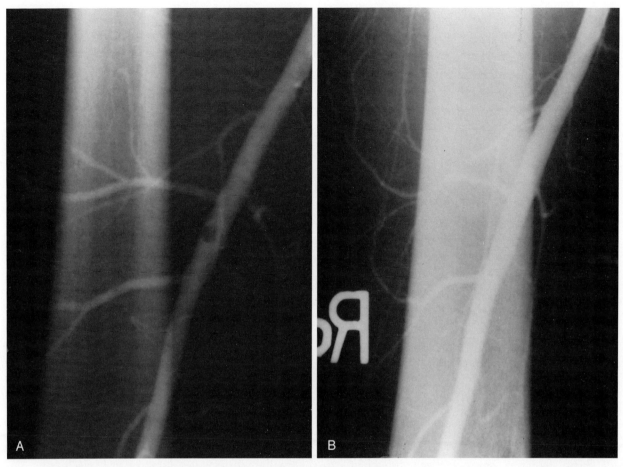

Figure 180–2. *A,* Arteriography (AG) showing an intimal irregularity or defect following a through-and-through gunshot wound to the thigh. *B,* Repeat AG 4 weeks later shows complete resolution.

In the extremities, these hard signs include active hemorrhage, expanding hematoma, distal ischemia, pulse deficit, and bruit or thrill over the wound. Similar findings are sought in the neck with a central neurologic deficit indicating distal ischemia. Significant vascular injuries in the chest often manifest decreased breath sounds on the affected side and evidence of respiratory distress and shock. PX of the abdomen is somewhat unreliable following trauma. Additional testing (ultrasound [US], diagnostic lavage, or computed tomography [CT] scan) must generally be done in the stable patient, and operative exploration in the unstable patient.

Extremity Injuries

General agreement exists that formal AG is no longer needed in penetrating extremity injuries to confirm or exclude vascular trauma requiring operative repair. Multiple studies have shown that, if hard signs are present on PX, then operative repair is warranted, and, if not, observation is indicated (Fig. 180–3). Some centers continue to obtain a single-shot, hand-injected AG performed by the traumatologists either in the emergency department or operating room (if there for associated injuries). Even though this imaging has been shown to be highly accurate, the risk for local complications becomes increased and the overall limited need for any type of imaging makes this technique seldom useful. Other centers have advocated the use of duplex US to further confirm the results found on PX. Although duplex US is as accurate as AG and noninvasive, no study to date has

Table 180–2	Risk of Amputation Following Acute Occlusion of Extremity Arteries

ARTERY INVOLVED	RISK OF AMPUTATION (%)
Upper Extremity	
Subclavian	28
Axillary	43
Brachial	26
Radial	5
Ulnar	1
Radial and ulnar	39
Lower Extremity	
Common iliac	54
External iliac	47
Common femoral	81
Superficial femoral	55
Popliteal	72
Anterior tibial	8
Posterior tibial	13
Peroneal	14
Both anterior and posterior tibial	65

From DeBakey ME, Simeone FA: Battle injuries of the arteries in World War II: An analysis of 2,471 cases. Ann Surg 1946;123:534–579; and Rich NM, Spencer FC: Vascular Trauma. Philadelphia, WB Saunders, 1978.

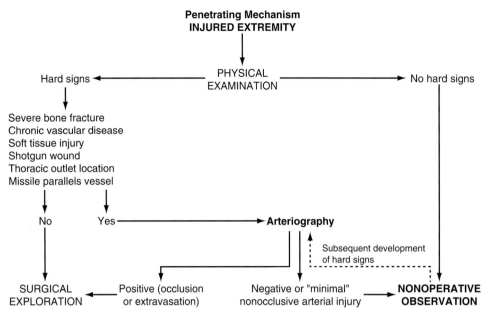

Figure 180–3. Algorithm of the current management of penetrating extremity vascular trauma.

shown it to be more accurate than PX alone in managing these patients. One study showed a sensitivity of only 50% as well as difficulty imaging the axillary artery, bifurcated arteries, and any unusual anatomy.

Blunt extremity trauma is less likely to cause vascular injury but is more difficult to diagnose because of the damage to surrounding muscle, bone, and nerves. The absence of any hard signs reliably excludes significant arterial injury requiring repair. Patients with blunt extremity trauma and hard or equivocal signs of vascular injury usually require AG to identify the location and extent of the injury. Severely displaced limbs should be straightened and splinted as much as possible before AG to minimize kinking and torsion on the vessels. Patients taken directly to the operating room for life-threatening associated injuries can undergo limited AG there by either percutaneous or direct cut-down techniques.

Cervical Injuries

AG is widely used to evaluate penetrating injuries to zone 1 (below the cricoid cartilage), which is poorly amenable to PX and US. Zone 3 (angle of mandible to base of skull) penetrating injuries are the least common and most difficult to repair of all cervical injuries. Some surgeons suggest that PX alone is adequate to confirm or exclude significant vascular injuries requiring repair, although most centers still liberally use AG. With advancements in endovascular treatments, the role of AG appears to be shifting from one of diagnosis to one of treatment.

The ideal management of zone 2 (between the cricoid and mandible) penetrating neck trauma remains somewhat controversial. Few trauma centers still advocate routine exploration of wounds deep to the platysma, an approach only applicable in military situations. The current predominant approach, termed "selective" management, is used to determine whether surgery is needed. This involves operative exploration if hard signs are present, and the routine use of either AG or duplex US to identify

occult injuries. Missed injury rates using the selective approach are 1% or less. A third school of thought has also developed, which states that PX alone is safe and accurate in evaluating neck wounds for surgically significant vascular trauma. Missed injury rates are reported to be equal to those of selective management using AG and US, with much less expense. AG still best evaluates blunt injuries because of the limitations of PX and US in evaluating the proximal and distal cervical vessels.

Thoracic Injuries

Evaluation of penetrating trauma to the thorax begins with a close PX to identify the entrance and exit wounds and any hard signs of vascular injury. Special attention should be given in determining differences in the upper extremity pulses, the presence of a periclavicular hematoma, or the absence of normal bilateral breath sounds. A chest radiograph (CXR) is important to identify the location of any retained bullet, a hemothorax, or widened mediastinum. Patients in stable condition with any evidence of vascular injury or with proximity of the missile path to the great vessels should undergo thoracic AG, which remains the gold standard of diagnostic techniques in the thorax. Patients in unstable condition should be taken immediately to the operating room if a response to resuscitation is observed. Patients in refractory shock or in cardiac arrest should have an emergency center thoracotomy performed for rapid control of the injured vessel. Severe blunt thoracic trauma, particularly following rapid deceleration and in those wearing seat belts, may result in a disruption of the descending thoracic aorta, usually just distal to the takeoff of the left subclavian artery. Patients not wearing seat belts or those suffering from vertical trauma commonly demonstrate disruption of the ascending aorta. The innominate artery is the second most common artery to be injured following blunt thoracic trauma, usually at its origin. Physical findings such as sternal contusions, systolic murmurs, and decreased femoral pulses occur in the minority of patients. Abnormalities seen on CXR should raise the suspicion of a possible aortic disruption. The three most sensitive findings are loss of aortic knob outline, loss of descending aorta, and widened mediastinum (defined as greater than 8 cm at the level of the aortic knob on a 100-cm CXR or a mediastinal width/chest width ratio greater than 25%).

Multiple modalities can be used to confirm the diagnosis of a suspected vascular injury of the thorax following blunt trauma. AG is widely available, highly accurate, and can evaluate the aorta and all four great vessels. Some centers advocate the use of digital subtraction AG as a faster but equally accurate means to identify vascular injuries. More recently, advances in CT scanning and transesophageal echocardiography have resulted in their use in diagnosing these injuries. Studies have shown all these methods to be 95% to 100% accurate in finding significant arterial injuries. Which approach is used depends on the local availability and experience of the institution. Patients with pelvic fractures, particularly if secondary to anterior-posterior compression, have a fourfold to ninefold increased risk of thoracic aortic dissection than patients with similar histories and no pelvic fractures.

Abdominal Injuries

Currently, most trauma centers perform exploratory celiotomies on all penetrating wounds to the abdomen (defined as between the nipples and upper thighs). The presence of shock should alert the surgeon that a vascular injury may be present and any delays should be avoided. Abdominal US or peritoneal lavage is used to identify free blood in the peritoneal cavity to help determine whether surgery or other intervention is needed in patients in stable condition suffering from blunt trauma. Patients in unstable condition are usually taken directly to the operating room for definitive care. Patients with pelvic fractures and persistent hypotension in the face of a normal US or lavage should warrant AG to treat bleeding of the pelvis.

PREOPERATIVE MANAGEMENT

As a general rule, very little in the way of preoperative workup or any type of procedure is needed before definitive treatment of penetrating vascular trauma of the extremities, neck, or abdomen. Securing an airway and ensuring adequate breathing is the first priority in any penetrating neck or thoracic trauma, and a CXR should be obtained if possible. AG is recommended in stable patients with thoracic trauma as discussed earlier. Most patients should have blood typed and cross-matched for packed red blood cells once a vascular injury is detected.

Patients with multisystem blunt trauma may require a CT scan of the head before operative repair of vascular injuries if the patient is clinically stable. AG is indicated in suspected arterial injuries of the extremities, neck, and thorax. Studies consistently show optimal limb salvage if restoration of flow can be accomplished within 6 to 8 hours. Any excessive delays for unnecessary testing or in transporting the patient to the operating room often results in additional morbidity.

OPERATIVE MANAGEMENT

General Principles

Some simple lacerations (10% to 15% of arterial injuries) can be repaired primarily with lateral suture following minimal débridement of the arterial wall. When more extensive damage occurs, all visibly injured tissue should be resected and a primary end-to-end anastomosis performed (30% to 40% of cases). Care must be taken to avoid any excessive tension on the suture line. The anastomosis can be triangulated as originally described by Carrel; however, most surgeons simply bevel the ends and use two running monofilament sutures. If required, mobilization of the arterial ends may be performed to relieve tension on the anastomosis. This works best in the superficial femoral arteries, where up to 2 cm of a blood vessel can usually be resected without having to use an interposition graft. Most other extremity, neck, or torso vessels can only withstand 1 cm of resection before grafting is needed. Autogenous saphenous or cephalic veins are usually the preferred conduits for interposition grafting for vessels on the extremity proper, for the internal carotid artery, and for other major branch vessels. Major arterial injuries within the torso requiring interposition grafting are generally performed with prosthetic graft material for optimal size matching. Occasionally, a bullet or missile may enter a blood vessel and embolize to a remote location. If no exit wound exists and the bullet is not identified on plain radiograph, a search must be undertaken to find the missing bullet, a process often including AG and venography.

Extremity Vascular Injuries

For repair of lower extremity vascular injuries, both legs should be prepped and draped from the umbilicus to toes. If the injury is to the upper extremity, both the entire arm and a leg should be included in the operative field. A generous incision is made parallel and directly over the site of the penetrating injury to get proximal and distal control of the injured vessel. Usually no anticoagulation is necessary and only local heparinized saline is infused, unless an extended, complex reconstruction is anticipated. Depending on the extent of the injury, either primary repair or an interposition graft is used. Most surgeons prefer reversed saphenous vein from the contralateral leg if a graft is needed; however, polytetrafluoroethylene (PTFE) material may also be used in wounds with little or no contamination with satisfactory results. Simple ligation of a single forearm or tibial artery may be undertaken only if distal perfusion of the involved arch can be demonstrated through another uninjured artery.

When both the artery and vein are injured, most authors recommend repairing the vein first to relieve outflow obstruction and to enhance arterial flow once the artery is fixed. Arterial injuries associated with bony fractures indicate severe tissue damage, carrying an overall worse prognosis. In these patients, there is general agreement that the arterial injury should be first addressed to restore blood flow into the extremity. This usually involves definitive repair. The exception to this rule is in patients whose extremities are in grossly unstable condition. In these cases, a temporary shunt may be placed first, followed by the orthopedic stabilization and then the definitive arterial repair. The operating surgeon should do a final examination of the vascular repair after all orthopedic manipulations are completed.

An intraoperative AG should always be done to ensure technical adequacy of the repair. The need for fasciotomies should be considered in the operating room at the time of the vascular repair and the immediate postoperative period. In cases of a delayed diagnosis of an arterial injury, consideration should be given to performing fasciotomies before the vascular repair.

Cervical Vascular Injuries

Vascular injuries to zone 1 of the neck usually require a median sternotomy to obtain proximal control. The one exception is an injury to the proximal left subclavian artery, which can better be handled through a left lateral thoracotomy incision because of the posterior location of this vessel. Injuries to the larger diameter vessels in this zone usually require an interposition graft with prosthetic material unless gross contamination from the aerodigestive tract is also present. In these cases, autogenous vein from any site (jugular, superficial femoral, paneled reversed saphenous vein) may be used.

Zone 2 vascular injuries are approached with an incision along the anterior border of the sternocleidomastoid muscle and dissection carried down onto the chest and up to the ear as needed for proximal and distal control. Common carotid injuries can be repaired primarily or with prosthetic grafts. Internal carotid artery injuries, unable to be closed primarily without undue tension or narrowing, should have RSV interposition grafts placed or have the external carotid artery transposed over to make up short length deficits of the proximal internal carotid. Shunting is not required in most cases, unless a prolonged, complex repair is anticipated. Internal carotid dissections as a result of blunt trauma usually do not require surgery and are treated medically with anticoagulation. These are usually seen as a tapered narrowing of the internal carotid artery (called "dunce's cap" or "string sign") 1 or 2 cm above the bifurcation.

The distal zone 3 vascular injuries are the most difficult to repair from a technical standpoint. Maneuvers available to assist high exposure include nasotracheal intubation, division of the digastric (posterior belly), styloglossus, stylopharyngeus, and stylohyoid muscles, along with mandibular subluxation. Injuries near the base of the skull should be considered for endovascular treatment. If direct or endovascular repair is not feasible, the internal carotid artery may be ligated without risk of stroke if the mean back pressure is greater that 70 mm Hg. An acutely thrombosed internal carotid artery does not need to be ligated in that no documented case of delayed bleeding

has ever been reported in the literature. Consideration should be given to anticoagulation if no other significant associated injuries exist because propagation of thrombus distal to the internal carotid artery can occur, resulting in a stroke or extension of an established stroke.

Thoracic Vascular Injuries

Although only 15% of thoracic trauma requires major operative intervention, most of these are from major vascular or cardiac life-threatening injuries. In hemodynamically unstable patients with penetrating injuries to the chest and suspected vascular injuries, a left anterior thoracotomy with extension across the sternum provides immediate exposure to most vessels. Preoperative evaluation of stable patients allows a more defined approach to specific injury locations. Similar to zone 1 of the neck, common carotid and subclavian injuries in the thorax are best approached through a median sternotomy incision. The aortic arch, pulmonary vessels, and major thoracic veins are also well visualized by this approach. The one exception remains the proximal left subclavian artery, which is better visualized through a posterior-lateral thoracotomy between the second and third interspace. Intrathoracic injuries of the descending aorta are also approached via thoracotomy incisions, depending on the location of the injury.

Penetrating wounds lateral to the mid-clavicle can usually be approached by obtaining proximal control at the supraclavicular level and distally near the upper extremity proper, thus avoiding a thoracotomy. Partial claviculectomy may be required for injuries directly posterior to the bone.

In all cases, the goal of the surgeon is to stop ongoing hemorrhage, repair the damaged vessel, and restore continuity if possible. Prosthetic grafts are usually required when extensive vessel damage is found. Adjunctive measures, including partial cardiopulmonary bypass or heparin-bonded shunts, should be performed only by surgeons familiar with their use. The ideal technique for repairing descending aortic injuries in the acute situation (clamp and go, cardiopulmonary bypass, shunt) is still debated. In most cases, the experience of the surgeon should dictate the method of repair. Several reports have described operating on a delayed basis on patients with stable descending aortic disruptions. Strict medical management with afterload-reducing agents to lower the dP/dT and blood pressure is used in much the same way as for spontaneous descending aortic dissections. Once the patient is stabilized from any associated injuries, elective repair is undertaken.

Abdominal Vascular Injuries

Intra-abdominal vascular injuries are approached through a generous midline incision from the xiphoid to the pubis. Vascular injuries above the level of the renal arteries are exposed via medial mobilization of the abdominal viscera from the left side. Difficult injuries to the celiac axis can be treated with ligation; however, superior mesenteric artery injuries should be repaired even if an interposition graft is required. Infrarenal aortic and iliac vessel injuries are approached by elevation of the transverse colon cephalad and retraction of the small bowel laterally in a manner similar to elective aneurysm repair. Standard practice dictates obtaining proximal and distal control with vascular clamps, primary repair, or placement of a Dacron or PTFE interposition graft. If a concomitant bowel injury with extensive contamination is encountered, unilateral iliac injuries can be oversewn and a femoral-femoral bypass completed upon closure of the abdomen. Superficial femoral vein is probably the best replacement conduit of an injured aortic segment when extensive contamination also exists. Renal artery trauma can be approached using either of these maneuvers, depending on the side and exact location of the injury. As in most vascular trauma, systemic heparin is usually not needed and only localized heparinized saline in infused. Routine passage of Fogarty catheters proximally and distally is also useful if there is any delay in restoring flow through the repair.

Inferior vena cava injuries are exposed by an extended Kocher maneuver and right-sided medial visceral mobilization with the kidney left in place. Venous injuries are initially controlled with sponge stick compression followed by carefully placed vascular clamps. Primary repair of all venous injuries is preferable if possible. Extensive tissue loss of the vena cava or iliac veins often results in massive blood loss and an unstable condition. Ligation of the injured vein in this situation is acceptable. If the patient's condition remains stable, however, patch repair using saphenous or superficial femoral vein can be undertaken. Contained, stable, retrohepatic hematomas should be packed and the patient closed to allow thrombosis to occur. Actively bleeding or rapidly expanding retrohepatic hematomas represent a formidable challenge. Infrahepatic and right atrial control of the vena cava is accomplished by the addition of a median sternotomy. If needed, an atriocaval shunt can then be placed to further divert the venous return before directly repairing or ligating the involved veins.

ENDOVASCULAR MANAGEMENT

At the current state-of-the-art, endovascular management has only small role in the treatment of most acute trauma with hard signs of vascular injury. The long delays, the extensive amount of equipment and personnel needed, and the lack of readily available stented grafts for each specific situation often make this approach unfeasible. As this field develops, experience and new devices will dictate which injuries will be treated best using endovascular techniques. The main advantages to endovascular therapy are as follows: access is from a remote, nontraumatized location, the magnitude of the operation is less, and entering the abdominal or thoracic cavity is avoided.

The initial appeal for the use of stents, stented grafts, or embolization has been, for acute vascular injuries, very difficult to approach openly. Embolization of pelvic arterial bleeding has been described for many years and is a mainstay in treating these vascular injuries. Emboliza-

tion of nonessential end arteries to stop persistent bleeding has also been shown to be safe and effective. More recently, the availability of a broad spectrum of stents and prefabricated stented grafts has naturally led investigators into using these devices to treat certain vascular injuries. Stents have been reported to be used successfully in the treatment of renal artery, internal carotid artery, and descending aortic dissections secondary to blunt trauma. Vertebral artery injuries are probably better treated with endovascular techniques than open procedures because of their poorly accessible location.

In less acute situations, the role of endovascular therapy is just now being defined. Traumatic pseudoaneurysms and AV fistulas in large arteries have been successfully treated with stented grafts, particularly when they present in a delayed fashion. Delayed injuries presenting on the extremities or zone 2 are still best handled by standard open procedures until further development of smaller stented grafts occurs and their short-term effectiveness and long-term patency is proven.

POSTOPERATIVE MANAGEMENT

Anticoagulation is seldom required following either primary arterial repair or interposition graft placement. Patients requiring major venous reconstruction may be benefited by short-term anticoagulation to prevent early thrombosis. Traumatic injuries to the iliofemoral veins or inferior vena cava result in a high risk of subsequent deep venous thrombosis, and prophylactic placement of Greenfield filters should be considered in these situations. Careful serial PXs should be performed in the immediate postoperative period. Generally, most young trauma patients have normal palpable pulses after successful arterial repair and loss of distal pulses warrants immediate attention. The possibility of delayed development of compartment syndrome must be monitored by PX and compartment pressure measurements. Normal extremity compartment pressures are approximately 5 to 10 mm Hg. If pressures greater than 30 to 40 mm Hg or approaching diastolic blood pressure is found, immediate fasciotomies should be performed to prevent tissue loss. If pulses are lost, the patient should be returned to the operating room for revision of the repair if compartment syndrome is not found. AG is usually not required unless a long time interval has elapsed between repair and subsequent thrombosis; this can be done in the operating room as needed.

OUTCOMES

Relatively speaking, there is little information on the long-term follow-up of patients with arterial injuries in that only 2% to 3% of all articles concerning vascular injuries deal with long-term outcome. Much of the problem in obtaining this information stems from the difficulty in getting this group of often transient and unsophisticated patients to return for follow-up. One study using mailings, telephone contacts, vascular clinic records, and a paid

Pearls and Pitfalls

PEARLS

- Consider compartment syndrome with every vascular injury in the extremity.
- If a pulse feels decreased on one side, compare it with the opposite side (built-in control).
- Try to repair the popliteal vein as well as the artery if both are injured.
- The brachial artery is more difficult to repair primarily than the superficial femoral artery because less mobilization is possible, thereby requiring a vein graft more often.
- It is safe to ligate the internal carotid artery if the back pressure is 70 mm Hg or more.

PITFALLS

- Do not depend on a Doppler study to determine whether there is an arterial injury in the extremity.
- Do not obtain arteriograms in the face of hard signs of vascular injury following penetrating trauma.
- Avoid prolonged procedures to repair the vertebral artery, which is better treated by endovascular techniques.
- Never remove one kidney following a vascular injury without checking for a functioning contralateral kidney.
- Obtain a CXR with all penetrating neck trauma.

social worker resulted in only a 33% follow-up of patients.

Approximately 1% to 2% of patients will have a missed injury no matter what type of approach is used for diagnosis (PX, AG, exploration). The vast majority (>90%) are usually seen within 10 days and almost all are seen within 3 months. Those patients seen after a delay most commonly have a pseudoaneurysm or AV fistula, which can usually be repaired electively without complication. Follow-up of patients having undergone arterial repair show an approximately 75% patency rate with PTFE grafts with a mean follow-up of 5.1 years, and 90% to 95% patency after 5 years with vein grafts and primary repair. The exception to these excellent results occurs in the distal forearm and calf arteries, which have approximately a 50% patency rate after 2 years of follow-up following repair. The actual rate of limb loss is less, approximately 15% overall, but is higher in blunt injuries, shotgun wounds, and when all three arteries are injured. The use of PX alone in the management of proximity arterial injuries of the extremities has recently been reported for up to 10 years. This study demonstrated the safety and accuracy of using PX alone to confirm or exclude the presence of a significant arterial injury following penetrating proximity trauma. Also, minimal injuries (smooth narrowings, intimal irregularities) were shown not to dete-

riorate over the long term and, in most cases, to resolve.

SELECTED READINGS

Attebery LR, Dennis JW, Menawat SS, et al: Physical examination alone is safe and accurate for evaluation of vascular injuries in penetrating zone II neck trauma. J Am Coll Surg 1994;179:657.

Biffl WL, Moore EE, Rehse DH, et al: Selective management of penetrating neck trauma based on cervical level of injury. Am J Surg 1997;174:678.

Bishara RA, Pasch AR, Lim LT, et al: Improved results in the treatment of civilian vascular injuries associated with fractures and dislocations. J Vasc Surg 1986;3:707.

Bynoe RP, Miles WS, Bell RM, et al: Noninvasive diagnosis of vascular trauma by duplex ultrasonography. J Vasc Surg 1991;14:346.

Dean RH: Management of renal artery trauma. J Vasc Surg 1988;8:89.

DeBakey ME, Simeone FA: Battle injuries of the arteries in World War II: An analysis of 2,471 cases. Ann Surg 1946;123:534.

Dennis JW, Frykberg ER, Crump JM, et al: New perspectives on the management of penetrating trauma in proximity to major limb arteries. J Vasc Surg 1990;11:84.

Dennis JW, Frykberg ER, Veldenz HC, et al: Validation of nonoperative management of occult vascular injuries and accuracy of physical examination alone in penetrating extremity trauma: 5- to 10-year follow-up. J Trauma 1998;44:243.

Duke BJ, Ryu RK, Coldwell DM, et al: Treatment of blunt injury to the carotid artery by using endovascular stents: An early experience. J Neurosurg 1997;87:825.

Duhaylongsod FG, Glower DD, Wolfe WG: Acute traumatic aortic aneurysm: The Duke experience from 1970 to 1990. J Vasc Surg 1992;15:331.

Fabian TC, Patton JH, Croce MA, et al: Blunt carotid injury: Importance of early diagnosis and anticoagulation therapy. Ann Surg 1996;223:513.

Feliciano DV: Abdominal vascular injuries. Surg Clin North Am 1988;68:441.

Feliciano DV: Management of traumatic retroperitoneal hematoma. Ann Surg 1990;211:109.

Flint LM, Snyder WH, Perry MO, et al: Management of major vascular injuries in the base of the neck. An 11-year experience with 146 cases. Arch Surg 1973;106:407.

Fry WR, Fry RE, Fry WJ: Operative exposure of the abdominal arteries for trauma. Arch Surg 1991;126:289.

Frykberg ER, Crump JM, Dennis JW, et al: Nonoperative observation of clinically occult arterial injuries: A prospective evaluation. Surgery 1991;109:85.

Itani KMF, Burch BH, Spjut-Patrinely V, et al: Emergency center arteriography. J Trauma 1992;32:302.

Marin ML, Veith FJ, Panetta TF, et al: Transluminally placed endovascular stented graft repair for arterial trauma. J Vasc Surg 1994;20:455.

Mattox KL, Feliciano DV, Burch J, et al: Five thousand seven hundred and sixty cardiovascular injuries in 4459 patients: Epidemiologic evolution 1958 to 1987. Ann Surg 1989;209:698.

Merion RM, Harness AK, Ramsburgh SR, et al: Selective management of penetrating neck trauma. Arch Surg 1981;116:691.

Mirvis SE, Bidswell JK, Buddemeyer EU, et al: Value of chest radiography in excluding traumatic aortic rupture. Radiology 1987;163:487.

Ordog GJ, Albin D, Wassenberger J, et al: 110 bullet wounds to the neck. J Trauma 1985;25:238.

Perry MO: Compartment syndromes and reperfusion injury. Surg Clin North Am 1988;68:853.

Rich NM, Baugh JH, Hughes CW: Acute arterial injuries in Vietnam: 1,000 cases. J Trauma 1970;10:359.

Rich NM, Spencer FC: Vascular Trauma. Philadelphia, WB Saunders, 1978.

Rozycki GS, Ochsner MG, Jaffin JH, et al: Prospective evaluation of surgeon's use of ultrasound in the evaluation of trauma patients. J Trauma 1993;34:516.

Sclafani SJA, Panetta T, Goldstein AS, et al: The management of arterial injuries caused by penetration of zone III of the neck. J Trauma 1985;25:871.

Sharma PV, Babu SC, Shah PM, et al: Changing patterns in civilian injuries. J Cardiovasc Surg 1985;26:7.

Veith FJ, Abbott WM, Yao JS: Endovascular Graft Committee. Guidelines for development and use of transluminally placed endovascular prosthetic grafts in the arterial system. J Vasc Surg 1995;21:670.

Von Oppell UO, Dunne TT, De Groot MK, et al: Traumatic aortic rupture: Twenty year metaanalysis of mortality and risk of paraplegia. Ann Thorac Surg 1994;58:585.

Chapter 181

Management of Venous and Lymphatic Disease

Anthony J. Comerota, Lori I. Cindrick, and Steven A. Kagan

PHYSIOLOGY OF THE VENOUS SYSTEM

Most veins are thin-walled, collapsible structures that accommodate large changes in volume with minimal changes in pressure (large venous capacitance). Changes in core body temperature, exercise, sleep, pain, and emotional stimuli can alter venous tone, although temperature regulation is mostly a cutaneous venous response to local stimuli. Adrenergic receptors are present in the walls of most veins, although they are most concentrated in the cutaneous veins, and these receptors are important in controlling the cutaneous venous tone and are responsible for the central temperature regulation integrated with the brainstem.

The venous system contains approximately two thirds of the blood volume in the resting state, and approximately 500 mL of blood is shifted to the legs when an individual assumes a standing position. On reaching a circular configuration, venous capacitance is maximized and further increases in venous volume are accompanied by increased intraluminal pressure. Obstruction to venous flow changes the pressure-volume relationship, and subsequent reflux into the superficial femoral veins may lead to a pathologic increase in venous pressure. In the supine position, resting foot venous pressure is the sum of the residual kinetic energy of the heart minus the resistance in the capillaries and arterioles. This resting pressure (which measures approximately 15 mm Hg) creates a pressure gradient to the right atrium, which has a pressure of 2 to 3 mm Hg. In the upright position, resting foot venous pressure includes the hydrostatic pressure from the column of blood extending from the right atrium to the foot, measuring approximately 100 mm Hg in a 72-inch individual.

Blood normally flows from the superficial to the deep venous system, although in the foot blood flows from the deep to the superficial veins. Normal lower extremity venous flow fluctuates with respiration as a result of changes in intra-abdominal pressure, and a reverse flow velocity of at least 30 cm/sec is required for venous valve closure. During ambulation, the leg muscles, particularly the calf muscles, augment venous return by functioning as a pump that is primed by the deep veins so that during muscle contraction, the blood is propelled cephalad. In the presence of competent venous valves, the exercising pressure recorded at the foot is less than 50% of the standing venous pressure. In contrast, in the presence of valvular incompetence or venous obstruction, the exercising venous pressure increases, and this high pressure is often transmitted through incompetent perforating veins

to the skin and subcutaneous tissues, leading to the clinical manifestations of venous hypertension.

ACUTE VENOUS THROMBOSIS

The etiology of venous thrombosis includes stasis, a hypercoagulable state, and vein wall injury (Virchow's triad). Although stasis alone has not been shown to be causally related to deep venous thrombosis (DVT), combined with an underlying hypercoagulable state or vein wall injury, stasis becomes an important etiologic factor. Increases in procoagulant activities in plasma, including increases in platelet counts and adhesiveness, changes in the coagulation cascade, and changes in endogenous fibrinolytic activity all contribute to the hypercoagulability of blood. Known thrombophilic states include deficiencies of antithrombin III, protein C, and protein S, the presence of a lupus anticoagulant, anticardiolipin and antiphospholipid antibodies, activated protein C resistance, Factor V Leiden mutation, and prothrombin gene mutation. Venous endothelial injury provides a potent stimulus to thrombosis, because of the exposure of subendothelial collagen. Whereas direct injury obviously leads to venous endothelial damage, there is strong evidence suggesting that venous endothelium is also indirectly injured by remote trauma. The hypothesis is that products of tissue injury are produced by operative trauma and released at the operative site, gaining entry into the bloodstream through capillaries and lymphatics. Such substances may have an effect on platelets and leukocytes as well as altering the function of endothelium and having a direct effect (or indirect through mediators) on vascular smooth muscle.

Diagnosis

It is well established that an objective diagnosis of DVT is necessary because clinical evaluation frequently is inaccurate. However, clinical features can be used to classify symptomatic patients with suspected DVT and improve diagnostic strategies. Venous duplex imaging has excellent sensitivity and specificity in patients with clinically suspected DVT. Some centers have also reported good results in high-risk asymptomatic patients. In addition, magnetic resonance venography (MRV) has demonstrated good sensitivity for the diagnosis of proximal venous thrombosis when compared with ascending phlebography, although its availability and cost and the limitations caused by metallic implants and claustrophobia limit its application. The D-dimer blood test has also been found to be useful in the diagnosis of acute DVT. Although D-dimer levels are elevated in postoperative and acutely ill patients, a negative D-dimer test in patients with suspected proximal venous thrombosis has a high negative predictive value.

In patients suspected of having acute DVT, venous duplex imaging is the initial test (Fig. 181–1). If the results are positive, patients are treated for DVT. If negative, patients should be stratified according to the degree of clinical suspicion before venous duplex imaging. A low clinical suspicion accompanied by a negative duplex study effectively excludes DVT, and no further evaluation is necessary. If moderate clinical suspicion exists, a negative duplex study should be followed by a repeat examination in 3 to 5 days, or a D-dimer test and a negative D-dimer offers good assurance that the patient does not have DVT. A positive D-dimer assay following a normal venous duplex imaging requires further evaluation with MRV or ascending phlebography. Patients in whom a high clinical suspicion exists despite a negative venous duplex study should have additional investigation with MRV, ascending phlebography, or a repeat duplex study.

Treatment

Anticoagulation with unfractionated heparin followed by oral warfarin compounds has been the mainstay of therapy for acute DVT. These agents interrupt thrombus formation but do not actively dissolve the thrombus; however, effective anticoagulation prevents clot propagation and allows the body's endogenous fibrinolytic system the opportunity to reduce thrombus burden and recanalize occluded veins. Prospective trials have shown a 15-fold

increase in recurrent DVT when early anticoagulation goes below therapeutic levels. Early aggressive anticoagulation, maintaining the activated partial thromboplastin time greater than 100 sec, is associated with fewer recurrent thromboembolic complications without an increased risk of bleeding (in the absence of associated comorbidities for bleeding). In addition, natural history studies of acute DVT have shown that vein segments undergoing early clot lysis (within 3 months) have a higher likelihood of preserved valvular function than segments that have delayed or no clot lysis.

Investigators have repeatedly confirmed that a prescriptive approach to heparin administration (Table 181–1) is more effective than the subjective, individual approach attempted by many clinicians. Therefore, it is reasonable to adopt a titration nomogram using the activated partial thromboplastin time in patients receiving unfractionated heparin for venous thromboembolic disease. Furthermore, low-molecular-weight heparins (LMWH), which function by inhibiting Factor Xa activity and Factor IIa activity, with relatively more anti-Xa activity (2:1 to 4:1), recently have been developed for clinical use. Compared with unfractionated heparin, LMWH preparations have a longer plasma half-life and substantially higher plasma levels following subcutaneous injection (89%). As a result, they have less variability in anticoagulant response to a fixed dose compared with unfractionated heparin, and they can obtain a stable and sustained anticoagulant effect when administered subcutaneously once or twice daily. In addition, laboratory monitoring is not necessary and there is less risk of heparin-induced thrombocytopenia (HIT) and osteoporosis with prolonged administration. Many randomized studies have demonstrated equivalent and some superiority of the

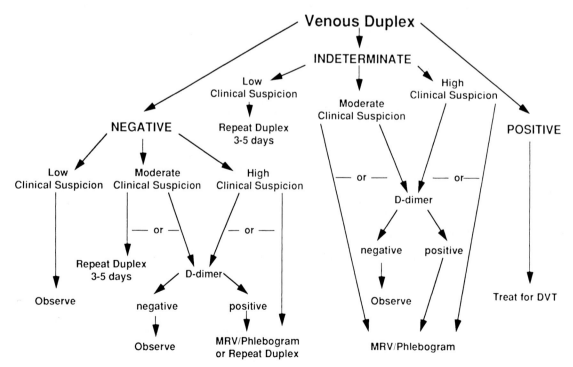

Figure 181–1. Algorithm for the diagnosis of deep vein thrombosis (DVT) according to clinical suspicion. MRV, magnetic resonance venography.

Table 181–1	**A Prescriptive Approach to Intravenous Heparin Therapy: A Titration Nomogram for Activated Thromboplastin Time**		

| | INTRAVENOUS INFUSION | | |
aPTT*	Rate Change (mL/hr)	Dose Change (units/24 hr)†	ADDITIONAL ACTION
≤45	+6	+5760	Repeat aPTT‡ in 4–6 hr
46–54	+3	+2880	Repeat aPPT in 4–6 hr
55–85	0	0	None§
86–110	−3	−2280	Stop heparin for 1 hr; repeat aPTT 4–6 hr after restarting heparin
>110	−6	−5760	Stop heparin sodium for 1 hr; repeat aPTT 4–6 hr after restarting heparin

°Activated partial thromboplastin time.
†Heparin sodium concentration, 20,000 units/500 mL = 40 units/mL.
‡With the use of Actin-Fs thromboplastin reagent (Dade, Mississauga, Ontario).
§During the first 24 hr, repeat aPTT in 4–6 hr. Thereafter, the aPTT will be determined once daily, unless subtherapeutic.

LMWH compounds when compared with intravenous unfractionated heparin for treatment of DVT. Patients with proximal vein thrombosis who have a contraindication to anticoagulation, as well as those who have had pulmonary emboli while being therapeutically anticoagulated, are treated with vena caval filtration (Table 181–2). If the indication for caval filtration is failure rather than a contraindication to anticoagulation, anticoagulation should be continued following filter placement in order to treat the primary process—DVT.

Oral anticoagulants (warfarin compounds) inhibit the vitamin K–dependent clotting factors II, VII, IX, and X and also inhibit vitamin K–dependent carboxylation of proteins C and S, naturally occurring anticoagulants that function by inhibiting Factors Va and VIIIa. Warfarin compounds do not have an immediate effect on the coagulation system, in that the normal vitamin K–dependent clotting factors present in the circulation must be cleared (4 to 5 days). Furthermore, any vitamin K antagonist can potentially produce a transient hypercoagulable state before achieving its anticoagulant effect, because the half-lives of proteins C and S are substantially shorter than the half-lives of the targeted clotting factors. Therefore, patients should be given heparin during this time. The appropriate intensity of oral anticoagulation has been well studied, and an International Normalized Ratio (INR) of 2.0 to 3.0 is recommended for preventing recurrent thromboembolic events. The appropriate duration of oral anticoagulation has been a topic of debate; however, a minimum of 6 to 12 months is recommended following an initial episode of DVT. Warfarin compounds cross the placenta and have been associated with teratogenic effects when given during the first trimester of pregnancy. There are similar concerns in the second trimester as well as the risk of fetal bleeding during and after delivery, so that warfarin compounds should be avoided when treating a pregnant woman, and all women of childbearing potential taking warfarin compounds must avoid pregnancy. If anticoagulation is indicated during pregnancy, subcutaneous heparin or LMWH is recommended.

Treatment Strategies

Superficial venous thrombosis, commonly known as superficial phlebitis, usually presents as a painful swelling along the length of a vein beneath the skin, often associated with erythema. Superficial phlebitis of the greater saphenous vein that extends to the proximal thigh and is not associated with a marked inflammatory response can be expediently treated by ligation and stripping. If there is an associated inflammatory response, stripping is difficult, if not impossible, and treatment is a nonsteroidal anti-inflammatory agent, topical moist heat, and compression. If the thrombus extends to the proximal thigh, ligation of the saphenofemoral junction is recommended to prevent extension into the deep system. If operative intervention is not performed, 6 to 12 weeks of anticoagulation should be considered to prevent extension into the deep veins. Treatment of recurrent superficial thrombophlebitis should be directed at resolving the inflammation and then removing the involved vein once the surrounding inflammation has subsided.

Treatment of venous thrombosis limited to the calf veins remains controversial. Although calf vein thrombi usually do not cause major sequelae and do not place the patient at high risk for pulmonary emboli, studies have shown that up to 30% will propagate. Accumulated evidence indicates that symptomatic isolated calf vein thrombosis should be treated with anticoagulation for at least 3 months and asymptomatic isolated calf vein thrombosis in patients at risk for propagation should be treated similarly. If anticoagulation cannot be given, serial noninvasive studies should be performed to assess for proximal extension of the thrombus during the next 7 to 14 days.

Anticoagulation is the standard treatment for DVT

Table 181–2	**Indications for Vena Caval Filter**

Traditional Indications
Pulmonary embolism while patient is therapeutically anticoagulated
Proximal DVT or PE and a contraindication to anticoagulation
Complications of anticoagulation
Pulmonary embolectomy

Evolving Indications
Pelvic or long bone fracture
Recurrent PE
DVT in patient with poor cardiopulmonary function

DVT, deep venous thrombosis; PE, pulmonary embolism.

involving the superficial femoral and popliteal veins. If intravenous unfractionated heparin is chosen, supratherapeutic anticoagulation early in the course of therapy is suggested in preference to adjusting the partial thromboplastin time within a targeted range (in patients without a comorbidity for bleeding). Oral anticoagulation is started immediately and continued over the long term, maintaining an INR of 2.0 to 3.0. Patients are allowed to ambulate normally throughout therapy. Oral anticoagulation is continued for 6 to 12 months following an initial venous thrombotic episode, whereas recurrent DVT is treated indefinitely. LMWH is becoming the preferred initial therapy for most patients with DVT, and a weight-adjusted subcutaneous injection of enoxaparin of 1 mg/kg twice daily or 1.5 mg/kg per day is the recommended dose. LMWH is continued until the patient has received oral anticoagulants for 4 or more days and the INR is therapeutic. Hospitalization is not mandatory for safe and effective therapy, but an initial hospitalization of 24 hours for patient instruction and education and for planning the logistics of ongoing care is beneficial for many patients, and is covered by most health insurance programs.

Although anticoagulation is also used for the treatment of iliofemoral venous thrombosis, eliminating the thrombus from the iliofemoral venous system improves short- and long-term venous function, reduces morbidity, and improves the patient's quality of life (Fig. 181–2). A large randomized trial of venous thrombectomy versus anticoagulation for acute DVT also demonstrated successful clearing of thrombus from the deep venous system to be associated with improved valvular function and reduced post-thrombotic symptoms. In patients without contraindications to thrombolytic therapy, intrathrombus infusion of plasminogen activators via catheter delivery is preferred. Recombinant tissue plasminogen activator (rt-PA) is used, delivering a 2- to 8-mg bolus into the clot followed by 2 to 4 mg per hour. Concurrent heparin is infused at 500 to 1000 units/hr. With appropriate catheter positioning, lysis is achieved in 80% to 90% of patients if treatment is initiated within 3 weeks of thrombosis. An underlying lesion in the iliac vein is commonly observed and should be corrected, usually with balloon angioplasty and occasionally with the addition of a stent. Patients who have free-floating thrombus in their vena cava should have caval filters placed before catheter-directed thrombolysis. If catheters cannot be positioned into the occluded iliofemoral venous system or if contraindications to thrombolysis exist, a venous thrombectomy with an adjunctive arteriovenous fistula is recommended. The steps of a contemporary venous thrombectomy are listed in Table 181–3. If unobstructed ipsilateral venous drainage cannot be established, a cross-pubic venous bypass with a 10-mm externally supported polytetrafluoroethylene graft combined with an arteriovenous fistula is recommended. However, endoluminal repair with venoplasty and stenting can usually be accomplished and is the preferred method of correcting a short, segmental residual lesion in the ipsilateral iliac vein following thrombectomy. Therapeutic intraoperative anticoagulation and long-term postoperative anticoagulation is suggested to avoid recurrent thrombosis.

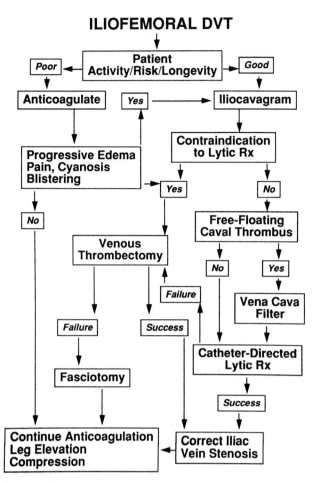

Figure 181–2. Algorithm for the treatment of acute iliofemoral deep vein thrombosis.

CHRONIC VENOUS INSUFFICIENCY

The underlying pathophysiology of chronic venous insufficiency is ambulatory venous hypertension. The elevated venous pressures are due to reflux of blood through incompetent valves, obstruction of the deep venous system, or both. Patients can have "primary" venous insufficiency, in which there is an inherent weakness in the vein wall, leading to pure valvular reflux, or "secondary" venous insufficiency, which is usually the result of DVT with the resultant valvular dysfunction and residual venous obstruction. "Congenital" venous insufficiency is the result of both anatomic and physiologic venous abnormalities present at birth. If the patient has primary venous insufficiency located in the superficial veins (greater saphenous or lesser saphenous), it is potentially curable. Perforating vein incompetence is also curable if those perforators are interrupted. Deep venous insufficiency may be curable as well, especially if the patient has primary valvular incompetence without a scarred or obstructed deep venous system, whereas secondary deep venous insufficiency is controllable with good compression but is difficult to "cure."

Diagnosis

The diagnosis of chronic venous insufficiency begins with the appropriate placement of the patient into one of six

Table 181-3	**Technical Considerations for Venous Thrombectomy**

1. Visualize proximal extent of thrombus; include contralateral iliofemoral phlebography and venacavagram.
2. Full anticoagulation throughout procedure and postoperatively.
3. Prepare OR for fluoroscopy and radiograph.
4. Preferentially use general anesthesia with positive end-expiratory pressure during thrombectomy.
5. Type and cross-match 2 to 3 units of blood.
6. Use an autotransfusion device during the procedure.
7. Use inguinal incision to expose and control common femoral, saphenous, superficial femoral, and profunda femoris veins.
8. Obtain right retroperitoneal caval control and caval venotomy for removal of caval thrombus.
9. If a caval filter is in place, use fluoroscopy during thrombectomy, with contrast material used to inflate the venous thrombectomy catheter balloon.
10. Pass venous thrombectomy catheter part way into iliac vein for several passes before advancing into vena cava (use No. 8 or No. 10 venous thrombectomy catheter).
11. Consider intraoperative infusion of plasminogen activators after thrombectomy, with balloon occlusion of the iliac vein.
12. Evaluate and exsanguinate leg with rubber bandage to expel infrainguinal clot.
13. If lower leg extrusion maneuver does not clear infrainguinal clot, consider infrainguinal balloon catheter thrombectomy. Cut-down to posterior tibial vein and advance No. 3 Fogarty catheter to femoral venotomy. Attach and guide No. 4 Fogarty catheter retrograde in leg to allow balloon cathether thrombectomy in selected patients (especially patients with thrombus in or inadequate drainage from profunda) and repeat as needed. Flush leg with high-volume or high-pressure heparin-saline solution and infuse rtPA 4–8 mg in 50 mL saline before ligating posterior tibial vein (consider leave catheter in posterior tibial vein for heparin infusion).
14. After completing thrombectomy, evaluate iliofemoral system with completion phlebogram or fluoroscopy.
15. If iliac system has residual stenosis or small segment occlusion, balloon dilation with stenting (if necessary) is performed under fluoroscopic guidance. If the iliac system has persistent long segment occlusion, a cross-pubic pubic venous bypass with a 10-mm externally supported PTFE graft and associated AVF is performed.
16. Construct a small-diameter AVF (4 mm) with the saphenous vein or one of its large proximal branches to the proximal superficial femoral artery (AVF is considered permanent). Encircle saphenous AVF with PTFE or Silastic and loop with O-Prolene and leave in subcutaneous wound in case closure of AVF becomes necessary.
17. Measure femoral vein pressure before and after AVF is opened. If pressure increases, either the AVF is too large or a proximal iliac vein stenosis persists. Re-evaluate iliac venous system, and correct lesion or band AVF to decrease flow and normalize pressure.
18. Apply external pneumatic compression devices in the recovery room.
19. Continue heparin throughout the postoperative period, converting the patient to oral anticoagulation.
20. Maintain the patient on good elastic compression hose, using a minimum of 3 to 40 mm Hg ankle gradient compression.

OR, operating room; PTFE, polytetrafluoroethylene; AVF, arteriovenous fistula.

clinical categories using the CEAP classification (Table 181–4). The patient is examined for varicose veins and their location, and the skin is examined for dermatitis, eczema, and skin breakdown (Fig. 181–3). Lymphedema is a common consequence of chronic venous insufficiency and should be documented. A hand-held venous Doppler examination is done and phasic respiratory venous return and normal augmentation should be observed in the non-obstructed venous system with the patient in the supine position. Sites of interrogation include the common femoral, superficial femoral, popliteal, and posterior tibial veins. The patient is then examined in the standing position for valvular incompetence by manually compressing the thigh and calf muscle and rapidly releasing while auscultating in the same positions. A prolonged retrograde velocity signal of greater than 0.5 second is abnormal and suggests valvular incompetence.

Venous duplex examination is a valuable addition to the diagnostic evaluation of patients with chronic venous insufficiency and, coupled with air plethysmography, is all that is required for the preoperative evaluation of many patients, especially those who will only be considered for procedures on their superficial and perforating veins. Air plethysmography assesses venous valvular function by measuring the rate of venous refill when the patient assumes a standing position from the supine leg raised position, and the calf muscle pump function is evaluated with single and then repetitive tiptoe exercises. Results of air plethysmography correlate well with ambulatory venous pressure measurements (the gold standard venous function test) done by inserting a needle into a dorsal vein of the foot and measuring the pressure at rest and after exercise. Factors contributing to the final pressure reading include the efficiency of the calf muscle pump, mobility of the ankle joint, the degree of valvular reflux, overall venous volume, degree of venous outflow obstruction, relative competence of the perforating and connecting veins, and vein wall compliance. Ascending phlebograms also provide information regarding incompetent perforating veins and their relative location, the number and locations of deep venous valves, and the location of deep venous obstruction. However the importance of these anatomic features must be evaluated with physiologic testing and descending phlebography, which demonstrates valvular incompetence, the site of valves, and the potential for their direct repair.

Table 181-4	**Classification of Chronic Venous Disease ("CEAP" Classification)**

Clinical Class
0—No visible signs
1—Telangiectasias or reticular veins
2—Varicose veins
3—Edema
4—Pigmentation, venous eczema, lipodermatosclerosis
5—Skin changes with healed ulceration
6—Skin changes with active ulcer

Etiologic Class
C—Congenital
P—Primary
S—Secondary

Anatomic Class
S—Superficial
D—Deep
P—Perforating

Pathophysiologic Class
R—Reflux
O—Obstruction
RO—Reflux and obstruction

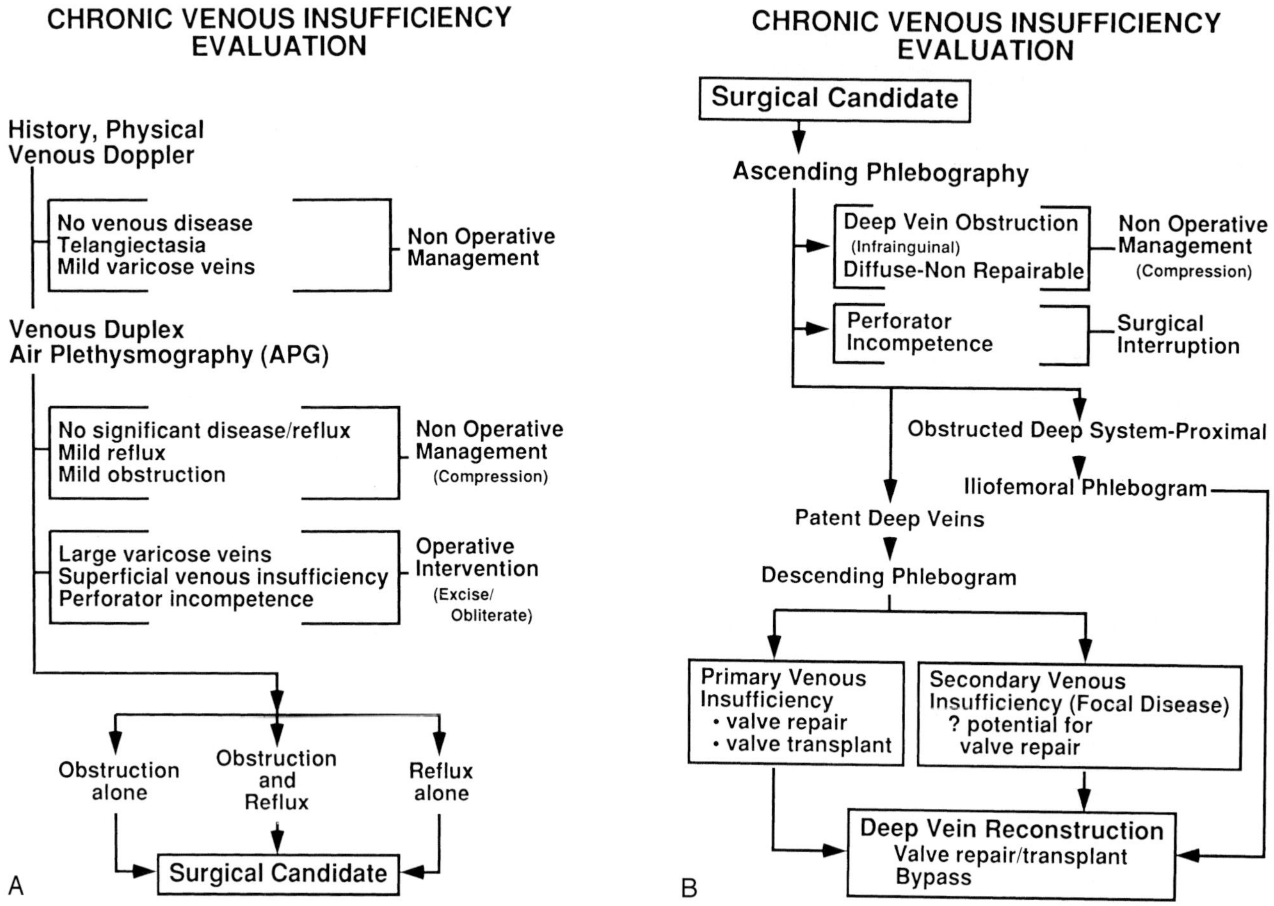

CHRONIC VENOUS INSUFFICIENCY EVALUATION

**History, Physical
Venous Doppler**

| No venous disease
Telangiectasia
Mild varicose veins | Non Operative
Management |

**Venous Duplex
Air Plethysmography (APG)**

| No significant disease/reflux
Mild reflux
Mild obstruction | Non Operative
Management
(Compression) |

| Large varicose veins
Superficial venous insufficiency
Perforator incompetence | Operative
Intervention
(Excise/
Obliterate) |

Obstruction
alone

Obstruction
and
Reflux

Reflux
alone

A

Surgical Candidate

CHRONIC VENOUS INSUFFICIENCY EVALUATION

Surgical Candidate

Ascending Phlebography

| Deep Vein Obstruction
(Infrainguinal)
Diffuse-Non Repairable | Non Operative
Management
(Compression) |

| Perforator
Incompetence | Surgical
Interruption |

Obstructed Deep System-Proximal

Iliofemoral Phlebogram

Patent Deep Veins

Descending Phlebogram

| Primary Venous
Insufficiency
• valve repair
• valve transplant | Secondary Venous
Insufficiency (Focal Disease)
? potential for
valve repair |

Deep Vein Reconstruction
Valve repair/transplant
Bypass

B

Figure 181–3. *A* and *B*, Evaluation of patients with chronic venous insufficiency.

Nonoperative Treatment

The majority of patients with chronic venous insufficiency are treated nonoperatively. The cornerstone of therapy is external compression. Compression that relieves leg edema generally controls the chronic venous insufficiency problem. Although the exact mechanism of benefit of compression is not entirely known, a number of physiologic alterations, including reduction of ambulatory venous pressure, improvement in skin microcirculation, and increased subcutaneous pressure, which counters transcapillary fluid leakage, have been observed. Most patients require compression only to the knee, because thigh swelling is infrequent. When it does occur, it is associated with minimal morbidity. Mild venous insufficiency is treated with 20 to 30 mm Hg ankle gradient stockings. However, most patients with swelling, stasis dermatitis, and brown discoloration require at least a 30 to 40 mm Hg ankle gradient compression stockings, whereas patients with the post-thrombotic syndrome who have residual venous obstruction require a 50 mm Hg ankle gradient stocking, or perhaps more. Stockings should be worn from the time the patient awakens in the morning until he or she goes to sleep at night. If patients cannot apply any stocking because of arthritis or other physical limitation, an elastic bandage firmly applied daily from the base of the toes to the knee is an effective alternative. Nonelas-

tic compression in the form of a Velcro wrap (Circaid) from the foot to the knee is also an effective means of controlling swelling. Most cases of severe chronic venous insufficiency and of venous ulceration are treated with an initial period of bed rest with leg elevation to reduce serious swelling and control erythema. Antibiotics treat associated cellulitis. Mild corticosteroid ointment is applied in areas of stasis dermatitis that may surround the ulcer. Elastic compression is used to further reduce edema, protect the ulcers, and speed healing, and pneumatic compression pumps may be added to relieve edema and speed ulcer healing. Our personal preference is to apply a triple-layer compression dressing to manage patients with venous ulceration and intractable leg edema. The gauze wrap in contact with the skin is impregnated with zinc oxide and dressings are applied from the base of the toes to the anterior tibial tubercle with snug, graded pressure. A plain gauze wrap followed by a self-adhering elastic wrap or Coban is the final layer. These dressings can usually be left in place from several days to 3 weeks, depending on patient hygiene. The pneumatic compression garment can be applied over the triple-layer compression dressing or over graded compression stockings. Once ulcers are healed, edema is controlled with graded compression stockings as described earlier. Patients are then fully evaluated for potential correction of their chronic venous insufficiency.

Operative Management of Chronic Venous Insufficiency

Surgical correction of superficial venous insufficiency is indicated for a variety of conditions, including pain, thrombophlebitis, leg heaviness, easy leg fatigue, bleeding, or advanced changes of chronic venous insufficiency including hyperpigmentation, lipodermatosclerosis, or venous ulcers. Patients with signs and symptoms of chronic venous insufficiency, superficial varicosities, and incompetence of the greater saphenous or lesser saphenous veins usually respond well to ligation and stripping of the greater or lesser saphenous veins. When patients have associated perforating vein incompetence, interruption of the incompetent perforators performed with the new technique of subfascial endoscopic perforator surgery is recommended. The essentials of a good operation are flush ligation of the greater saphenous at the common femoral vein, division of all associated branches, stripping of the greater saphenous vein to just below the knee, and stab avulsion of all remaining visible varicosities in the leg.

Relatively few patients require deep venous reconstruction. However, those who do, should have a complete anatomic and physiologic evaluation of the deep venous system, resulting in specific recommendations for deep vein repair (see Fig. 181–3). Direct deep vein valve repair has been successful, especially in patients with primary valvular insufficiency. Both open and closed techniques have been developed to resuspend the floppy venous valve, and both are associated with reasonable results (65% to 80% normal venous competence on long-term follow-up). Axillary vein transfer (to the distal superficial femoral vein or popliteal vein) is used when direct valve techniques are inadequate or a repairable valve is not present. Alternatively, the transfer of an incompetent distal vein to an adjacent but competent proximal venous segment, usually the incompetent superficial femoral vein to the proximal greater saphenous vein or to the profunda femoris vein, below a competent valve can be done. However, the long-term success rates are disappointing at 17% to 50%. Venous bypasses are effective in a highly selective group of patients with severe veno-occlusive disease who are incapacitated by their symptoms and whose lesions have the potential to be bypassed. A cross-pubic venous bypass is the most common, which bypasses an occluded iliofemoral system. A small arteriovenous fistula is usually constructed as an adjunctive procedure to improve patency. Saphenopopliteal bypasses, popliteal-femoral bypasses, and other procedures can also be devised depending upon the individual needs of the patient.

LYMPHATIC DISEASE

Physiology and Pathophysiology

The lymphatic system transports intercellular fluid from the periphery to the central venous circulation. Lymphatic dysfunction leads to the abnormal accumulation of protein-rich interstitial fluid within the skin and subcutaneous tissue and lymphedema is the clinical syndrome of limb swelling, which results from lymphatic dysfunction.

Primary lymphedema is the result of a congenitally malformed or hypoplastic lymphatic system, whereas secondary lymphedema is the result of exposure to noxious stimuli known to damage the lymphatic system, such as infection, surgery, or radiation therapy. The goals of treatment of lymphedema are the reduction of lymph fluid production, improvement of lymph fluid return, preservation of existing lymphatics, and, in highly selected cases, operative removal of severely diseased soft tissue.

The lymphatic system has three main functions: (1) to clear the interstitial space of macromolecules, including protein and the accompanying fluid loss from capillaries, (2) to clear foreign material and infectious agents, and (3) to absorb substances (mainly fat) from the gastrointestinal tract. Interstitial fluid, an ultrafiltrate of plasma, is formed by capillary filtration and the rate of its formation is determined by differences in the hydrostatic and colloid osmotic pressures between the intravascular (capillary) space and the interstitial space. Lymph is formed by the absorption of this excess interstitial fluid into the terminal lymphatic vessels in which the basement membrane is absent (or loosely organized), which allows fluid and macromolecules (greater than 1000 kd) to traverse open junctions. Under physiologic conditions, the capillaries allow 40% to 80% of intravascular protein to enter the interstitial space with lymphatic recirculation occurring within 24 hours. Lymph flow is facilitated by muscular contractions and arterial pulsations and by respiration. Furthermore, it is hypothesized that an intrinsic lymph pump exists that is mediated by smooth muscle fibers contracting spontaneously and rhythmically.

Lymph flow can be impeded by many factors, including abnormalities in lymphatic anatomy or an elevated central venous pressure, which also increases the amount of fluid filtered into the interstitial space. A normal lymphatic system has a capacity to increase its rate of lymph return by tenfold but significant increases in the amount of fluid formation may even overwhelm the compensatory mechanisms of a normal lymphatic system. This protein-poor interstitial fluid is usually confined to the subcutaneous compartment and initially produces a soft pitting edema. With time, the protein concentration in this ultrafiltrated fluid increases, leading to subcutaneous inflammation and fibrosis that worsens lymphatic obstruction, reduces lymph return, and increases lymphedema.

Primary lymphedema is due to a congenital abnormality of the lymphatic system and accounts for 10% to 15% of reported cases. *Congenital lymphedema* is diagnosed shortly after birth or during childhood. *Milroy's disease*, an X-linked form of congenital lymphedema, presents as extremity edema and is caused by aplasia of the lymphatic trunks. *Lymphedema praecox* accounts for 80% of cases of primary lymphedema and has an onset during adolescence. *Lymphedema tarda* presents after age 35 years and accounts for up to 15% of cases. Primary lymphedema can be further subdivided into hypoplastic and hyperplastic subtypes based on lymphangiographic findings with the majority of cases (90%) showing a hypoplastic pattern. Secondary lymphedema develops in response to injury to a previously normal lymphatic system. Infestation of lymph nodes by the parasite *Wuchereria bancrofti* (filariasis) is the most common cause of acquired lymphedema worldwide. Other causes include surgery, trauma, radiation, tumor invasion (late), infection, lymphogranuloma, actinomycosis, and chronic inflammation. Radical mastectomy may lead to severe lymphedema in up to 15% of patients and lower extremity revascularization (especially with harvesting of the greater saphenous vein) may lead to secondary lymphedema because of interruption of regional lymphatics.

Diagnosis

The diagnosis of lymphedema is usually made with an adequate history and physical examination. Typically, there is gradual onset of pitting edema that begins distally (usually in the foot and ankle) and progresses proximally over a period of several months. The involved extremity increases in size, with the patient complaining of swelling and fatigue. If the edema is not controlled, subcutaneous fibrosis develops and progresses, with the limb becoming indurated with the characteristic nonpitting spongy edema. The skin may become hyperkeratotic and ulcerated. Eosinophilia is commonly seen with filariasis. Other important laboratory tests include serum albumin, total protein, electrolytes, and renal and liver function tests. Contrast lymphangiography is rarely performed because of the risk of additional lymphatic damage and infection but, used selectively, can provide valuable information in the evaluation of patients with lymphangiectasia, abdominal or thoracic lymphatic fistulas, and anomalies of the thoracic duct. Lymphoscintigraphy is the preferred test in patients with lymphedema. Although it is essentially a functional study of lymphatic clearance (lymph flow), improved imaging techniques can offer important anatomic information.

Lymphedema can be differentiated from other causes of limb swelling on a clinical basis. The most common causes of bilateral lower extremity edema include congestive heart failure, renal failure, and hepatic insufficiency. Unilateral edema is most commonly caused by venous obstruction or insufficiency. Chronic venous insufficiency can lead to skin atrophy, with characteristic brawny edema and ulcer formation. Limb swelling caused by venous disease usually improves within hours of leg elevation, whereas swelling caused by chronic lymphedema may require several days of elevation, often combined with aggressive external compression.

Treatment

Limb elevation and compression, which mobilize excess interstitial fluid, are the keys to controlling lymphedema. The earlier lymphatic drainage is reestablished, the better the treatment outcome. Patients must also maintain good hygiene and skin care to limit the risk of infection. A lanolin-based skin lotion may prevent desiccation of the skin. Infections are treated aggressively with antibiotics that are specific for staphylococcal and streptococcal (and occasionally antifungal) agents, and the patient should always have antibiotics available to take at the earliest sign of soft-tissue infection. Effective compression ther-

apy improves limb function and appearance, removes protein-rich fluid that leads to subcutaneous fibrosis and, by reducing soft-tissue fluid volume, reduces recurrent infections. Pneumatic compression pumps substantially reduce limb volume by sequentially compressing the extremity to propel the edema fluid proximally. Compressive garments (e.g., support stockings, sleeves, or gloves) are worn continuously between treatment sessions and should be custom fitted with a 30- to 40-mm Hg ankle gradient for early lymphedema and 50 to 60 mm Hg ankle gradient for more advanced lymphedema. Massage therapy (manual lymphatic drainage and complex decongestive therapy) is also effective if properly performed and is becoming increasingly available. The central lymphatics are massaged to empty them to receive the peripheral lymph fluid from subsequent limb massage and multiple sessions may be required per day with the limb tightly wrapped with bandages between sessions to prevent fluid reaccumulation. Pharmacotherapy may also reduce interstitial protein content (e.g., benzopyrones can reduce the amount of interstitial protein by increasing the number of macrophages), decreasing excessive limb volume by 15% to 20%.

Surgical treatment of lymphedema is generally reserved for patients with severe, uncontrolled symptoms. The goal of surgical therapy is to drain (physiologic procedures) or remove (excisional procedures) the edematous skin and subcutaneous tissues to improve function and appearance of the limb and to reduce the incidence of recurrent infections. Microsurgical lymphatic reconstruc-

---

Pearls and Pitfalls

PEARLS

- Supratherapeutic partial thromboplastin time (>100 seconds) during heparin (unfractionated) anticoagulation for DVT is not associated with increased bleeding in patients without comorbidities for bleeding.
- Compression is the key to the control of chronic venous insufficiency. "Control swelling and control the problem."
- Clearing the iliofemoral venous system of clot (in patients with iliofemoral DVT) reduces post-thrombotic symptoms and improves quality of life.
- A negative D-dimer test reliably excludes proximal DVT.
- Correcting primary superficial venous insufficiency (saphenofemoral incompetence) can improve associated deep venous insufficiency.

PITFALLS

- Allowing partial thromboplastin time to go below therapeutic values during heparin anticoagulation for acute DVT significantly increases rate of recurrent DVT.
- Inadequate compression for chronic venous insufficiency.
- Treating all DVT as a single entity.
- Assuming that a positive D-dimer test is diagnostic for acute DVT.
- Not correcting primary superficial venous insufficiency if there is associated deep venous insufficiency.

tions (physiologic procedures) include lymphonodal-venous and lymphovenous shunts. A lymphonodal-venous shunt entails transplanting a lymph node (usually femoral) to a neighboring vein (usually the femoral or saphenous) while a lymphovenous shunt is an anastomosis between a patent, functional lymphatic vessel in the proximal medial thigh and a branch of the saphenous vein. Lympholymphatic shunts involve the use of a functional, autologous lymphatic vessel (harvested from a healthy extremity) to bypass a segmental lymphatic obstruction. Lymphangioplasty is the surgical implantation of a prosthetic material into a lymphedematous limb in order to promote the formation of fibrous channels and increase lymph flow by capillary action.

The Charles procedure (an excisional procedure mentioned primarily for historical interest) includes excision of all the skin and subcutaneous tissue from the tibial tuberosity to the malleoli and may include fascial excision as well. A split- or full-thickness skin graft (from the excised tissue) covers the resultant defect. The Thompsons buried dermal flap procedure (also mentioned for interest) involves excising a portion of the edematous subcutaneous tissue beneath a flap, and burying the deepithelized leading edge into the underlying muscle compartment, theoretically to improve lymphatic drainage to the normal muscle lymphatics. A more current and perhaps a more reasonable surgical approach to the patient with severe uncontrollable lymphedema is a staged subcutaneous excision underneath skin flaps because the goal of this procedure is to achieve improvement in edema while minimizing postoperative complications. This operation removes as much subcutaneous tissue and skin as possible while maintaining a viable flap to achieve a primary closure. Regardless, all of the surgical procedu... for treatment of lymphedema are only palliative.

SELECTED READINGS

Allen E: Lymphedema of the extremities. Classification, etiology, and differential diagnosis: Study of 300 cases. Arch Intern Med 1934;54:606.

Casley-Smith JR: The pathophysiology of lymphedema and the action of benzopyrones in reducing it. Lymphology 1988;21:190l.

Comerota AJ, Throm RC, Mathias S, et al: Catheter-directed thrombolysis for iliofemoral DVT improves health-related quality of life. J Vasc Surg 2000;32:130.

Conti S, Daschbach M, Blaisdell FW: A comparison of high dose versus conventional dose heparin therapy for deep venous thrombosis. Surgery 1982;92:972.

Criado E, Passman MA: Physiologic assessment of the venous system. In Rutherford RB (ed): Vascular Surgery, 5th ed. Philadelphia, WB Saunders, 2000:165.

Ginsberg JS, Kearon C, Douketis J, et al: The use of D-dimer testing and impedance plethysmographic examination in patients with clinical indications of deep venous thrombosis. Arch Intern Med 1997;157:1077.

Hull RD, Raskob GE, Hirsh J, et al: Continuous intravenous heparin compared with intermittent subcutaneous heparin in the initial treatment of proximal-vein thrombosis. N Engl J Med 1986;315:1109.

Kistner RL, Masuda EM: A practical approach to the diagnosis and classification of chronic venous disease. In Rutherford RD (ed): Vascular Surgery, 5th ed. Philadelphia, WB Saunders, 2000, pp 1990–1998.

Meissner MH, Manzo RA, Bergelin RO, Strandness DE: Deep venous insufficiency: The relationship between lysis and subsequent reflux. J Vasc Surg 1993;18:596.

Mewissen MW, Seabrook GR, Meissner MH, et al: Catheter directed thrombolysis for lower extremity deep venous thrombosis: Report of a national multicenter registry. Radiology 1999;211:39.

Plate G, Akesson H, Einarsson E, et al: Long-term results of venous thrombectomy combined with a temporary arteriovenous fistula. Eur J Vasc Surg 1990;4:483.

Raju S: Surgical treatment of deep venous vascular incompetence. In Rutherford RB (ed): Vascular Surgery, 5th ed. Philadelphia, WB Saunders, 2000:2037.

Richman DM, O'Donnell TF, Zelikovski A: Sequential pneumatic compression for lymphedema. Arch Surg 1985;120:1116.

Servelle M: Surgical treatment of lymphedema. A report on 652 cases. Surgery 1987;101:484.

Chapter 182
Vascular Access for Hemodialysis

C. Keith Ozaki

More than 300,000 people were being treated for end-stage renal disease (ESRD) in the United States at the end of 1997. Almost 80,000 new patients started ESRD treatment that year, and a recent estimated rate of growth of new ESRD cases is 6% per year. The condition is costly—total ESRD spending by all payers in 1997 was more than $15 billion, with an estimated Medicare spending per patient per year of $44,764.

ESRD patients have three therapeutic options: hemodialysis, peritoneal dialysis, or transplantation. Hemodialysis is used in more than 80% of all patients who undergo dialysis in the United States, and almost 85% of all ESRD patients use hemodialysis as their initial treatment modality. This chapter is limited to establishment of standard permanent hemodialysis access by way of arteriovenous fistulas (AVFs) and prosthetic (or bridge) grafts, although another hemodialysis access modality deserves mention. Percutaneous temporary and permanent (tunneled under the skin) catheters offer the advantages of immediate access under local anesthesia, and they can be placed by qualified nonsurgical clinicians outside of the operating room. They are an excellent choice when only short-term access is needed. However, for long-term access, these catheters hold significant drawbacks of patient inconvenience, frequent thrombosis, insertion-related events, infection risk, and contribution to central venous pathologies. In general, hemodialysis catheters are best reserved for patients with limited life expectancies, as a bridge to more permanent access or transplant, or when short-term access only is needed, as in reversible causes of acute renal failure. Children weighing less than 30 kg who cannot undergo peritoneal dialysis should also have catheter-based angioaccess while they await transplantation.

PREOPERATIVE MANAGEMENT

Before placing permanent hemodialysis access, the surgeon should ensure that consideration has been given to other management modalities (peritoneal dialysis and transplantation). Thoughtful preoperative planning probably stands as the primary determinant of long-term success of permanent hemodialysis access (Table 182–1). Discussions with the referring nephrologist should include projected time to dialysis initiation and life expectancy. Once need for hemodialysis is anticipated, upper extremity veins must be preserved for later constructions. Placement of an autogenous access is appropriate several months before anticipated dialysis initiation. If a prosthetic graft will be needed, placement of these limited durability grafts should be, at most, 1 month before need for dialysis, although this can be difficult to predict.

Patient evaluation should continue by documenting which of the patient's hands is dominant. Preference is given to placing access in the nondominant hand (all other factors being equal) to allow dominant hand activity during dialysis and to minimize risk of procedural complications to the dominant hand. Blood pressures in both arms (gradient greater than 15 mm Hg suggests proximal arterial occlusive disease), a full pulse examination, and an Allen test to screen for arterial inflow problems are performed. Abnormalities should be investigated by way of vascular laboratory arterial studies and contrast angiography. A frequent cause of early radiocephalic AVF failure is atherosclerotic disease of the forearm arteries, a common finding in elderly diabetic patients.

The venous anatomy is evaluated using a tourniquet. Patency can be confirmed by percussion of the distal vein with palpation of the proximal vein for a transmitted wave. Venous duplex examinations using a tourniquet or contrast venography may also be useful if physical examination does not locate a target autogenous vein. Histories of failed previous access attempts or indwelling central catheters should prompt imaging studies to rule out central vein pathologies. The author and colleagues employ CO_2 angiography in patients not yet on dialysis. Magnetic resonance venography holds promise as a means to interrogate central veins. Lower extremity duplex examinations can ensure that the saphenous and superficial femoral veins are suitable for conduit.

ESRD patients usually have multiple comorbid conditions that increase perioperative risk. Thirty-five percent of patients are reported to have congestive heart failure and 25% have documented coronary artery disease. Optimization of cardiac, metabolic, nutritional, and volume status, and treatment of active infections should be carried out before elective access placement.

OPERATIVE MANAGEMENT

Primary Graft Placement

Early discussions with the anesthesiology team assist in selection of the optimal anesthetic technique. Anatomi-

Table 182–1	Vital Information for Planning Hemodialysis Access Placement

√ Projected patient lifespan, time to initiation of dialysis
√ Dominant hand
√ History of previous access attempts, indwelling central venous lines
√ Allen's test
√ Upper-extremity blood pressures, arterial pulse examination → if abnormal, obtain segmental arm pressures, plethysmography → if abnormal, obtain angiography
√ Venous examination with tourniquet → if no clear conduit, perform duplex imaging → if no clear conduit, perform contrast venography. Once conduit has been selected, protect that vein from puncture or trauma
√ If history of failed ipsilateral access or central venous lines, consider contrast venography to rule out central venous pathologies
√ Ensure that patient is optimized for operation (cardiac, metabolic, and volume status; nutritional and infectious issues resolved)

cally straightforward radial-cephalic AVFs can be performed using local anesthesia (without epinephrine to minimize vasoconstriction) in the cooperative patient. Regional techniques are used for more complex constructions if the likelihood of needing to operate on another extremity is low. Complicated cases in which the operative strategy depends on the quality of the vein at exploration or composite conduits are best performed under the controlled circumstances of general anesthesia.

The clinician should prepare and drape a wide sterile field in case the second- or third-choice constructions are needed intraoperatively. Similarly, groin and thigh should be prepared in case extra length of vein (saphenous or superficial femoral vein) is needed for an upper extremity AVF. Perioperative antibiotics should be given before skin incision and dosed appropriately for the patient's creatinine clearance. A prospective randomized study demonstrated that 750 mg of intravenous vancomycin preoperatively reduced the risk of postoperative dialysis graft infection from 6% to 1%.

A well-functioning access demands adequate arterial inflow, low resistance to outflow, and sufficient length for punctures. The access should be constructed to facilitate easy cannulation and patient comfort during the dialysis run. Attempts should be made to avoid the need for excessive arm supination during cannulation.

Table 182–2 offers a suggested sequence for permanent hemodialysis access placement. The radiocephalic autogenous AVF remains the best form of long-term hemodialysis access. It also allows preservation and sometimes maturation of more proximal access vessels. Current community practice is, for the most part, placing a forearm prosthetic bridge graft before upper arm AVF, especially basilic vein AVF. However, the technically more challenging basilic vein AVF is probably superior to the bridge graft. Our current practice is to avoid prosthetic materials as long as a vein greater than 2.5 mm in diameter is available for AVF construction. Occasionally, unusual constructions such as ulnar-basilic, axillary-axillary, or superficial femoral vein loops provide durable access.

Several technical considerations deserve mention. Use of two padded arm boards placed side by side allows for

Table 182–2	**Suggested Sequence for Permanent (Noncatheter) Hemodialysis Access***

1. Radial-cephalic AVF in nondominant hand
2. Radial-cephalic AVF in dominant hand
3. Cephalic or brachial forearm transposition to radial or ulnar artery AVF
4. Brachial-cephalic upper arm AVF
5. Brachial-basilic upper arm AVF
6. Forearm prosthetic bridge graft
7. Upper arm prosthetic bridge graft
8. Thigh saphenous or superficial femoral vein transposition AVF
9. Upper-arm loop using translocated superficial femoral vein
10. Thigh prosthetic graft
11. Central configurations, such as axillary artery to contralateral axillary vein, subclavian artery to subclavian vein

*The decision to exhaust options on a single extremity versus keeping strictly with this sequence and using nondominant, then dominant, arm should be individualized, depending on patient circumstances.
AVF, arteriovenous fistula.

a firm, adjustable operating surface that moves with the patient's bed. Patients should be comfortably positioned as close as possible to the ipsilateral side of the table to facilitate access to the upper arm. When the patient is under general anesthesia, the endotracheal tube and associated hardware must be positioned contralateral to the arm of interest in order to optimize exposure.

The author usually gives 20 units/kg of intravenous heparin sulfate before construction of tunnels or vein division, although many clinicians perform limited access procedures without such low-dose anticoagulation or with regional heparin alone. An end-of-vein to side-of-artery construction usually results in the highest flow rates, with minimized distal venous hypertension. Rigid tubular tunnelers are useful for ensuring that grafts are not twisted or kinked and that they lie with evenly distributed tension. Making a line along the top of a vein before harvest from its bed can also help ensure that it does not twist when translocated. The conduit for access should be superficial enough that dialysis nurses can access it easily. Care must be taken when making incisions that cross joints in order to avoid a flexion scar contracture. Usually, these can be made while leaving a small skin bridge.

Performance of an AVF is similar to the distal anastomosis for a lower extremity tibial bypass and requires equivalent meticulous attention to standard vascular surgery details. In some ways, the anastomosis can be more challenging, because the lower pressure of the AVF can be less forgiving and make an overly angulated anastomosis prone to twists and kinks. Ideally, vein size should be greater than 3 mm, although we will attempt constructions with a 2.5-mm vein. Papaverine (30 mg/mL) injected into perivascular tissues and applied topically helps to limit vasospasm. Any AVF or graft construction that fails to achieve expected results in the operating room demands intraoperative angiographic evaluation for technical problems.

Most bridge grafts are constructed using expanded polytetrafluoroethylene. Usually a graft 6 mm in diameter is selected for hemodialysis access. Commercial vendors have developed several innovations such as multilayer wall grafts for immediate cannulation, large hoods to facilitate completion of a wide venous anastomosis, externally supported devices, and grafts that taper from 4 to 7 mm. None has been proved to be clearly superior. If the radial artery is of large caliber, then a straight configuration to the antecubital veins may be constructed. When the radial artery is small, a loop graft from the brachial artery to the antecubital veins may be used, and a distal counterincision aids in tunneling.

Bulky postoperative dressings may impede wound evaluations for patency and bleeding. Tight circumferential dressings that may impede flow through the conduit should be avoided. Heavy adhesive tape must be avoided on the often fragile skin of the chronic renal failure patient.

The Failing or Failed Conduit

High recirculation rates and venous pressures, or low flow rates despite a patent access conduit, all suggest a failing

AVF or graft. Close communication with the dialysis technicians who have been using the site can provide valuable information. The workup should begin with a fistulogram to interrogate the anatomy of the anastomoses and the central veins. Some centers report that duplex ultrasonography is useful in conduit surveillance, although there are no widely accepted standards for velocity waveform analysis and this evolving test remains highly operator dependent. Revision of a failing AVF or graft yields a more durable access than resurrecting one that has already thrombosed.

The failed hemodialysis access should be managed expeditiously, but does not constitute a surgical emergency. Our practice is to work these patients into the regular operating room schedule within 2 days of failure using the standard vascular surgery team. We prefer surgical thrombectomy under at least axillary block by dissecting out both the arterial and venous anastomoses and by using various thrombectomy catheters. Adherent clot, graft thrombectomy, and abrasive catheters may be used for mature, adherent debris in grafts, but they should never be used in native vessels. Usually revision of the venous anastomosis is required, either by patch angioplasty or jump graft. If a prosthetic graft is extended across a joint such as the elbow, then medial placement away from the crease and the use of an externally supported prosthesis may prevent kinking when the arm is flexed. For failing bridge grafts, segments of the prosthesis that remain palpably thickened with wall degeneration and pseudoaneurysms should be replaced.

Because site options for hemodialysis access remain finite, each site should be revised until it no longer remains an option. An unsalvageable access demands replacement with the most optimal configuration (see Table 182–2). Even when faced with a failing or failed conduit, all autogenous configurations remain preferable. Appropriate operative time and field of anesthesia must be allotted for construction of a new access when exploring the failing or failed access.

Endovascular Management

Open surgical repair of the failing or failed conduit currently stands as the established standard of care. No widely accepted protocol exists regarding the role of catheter-based thrombolytic and endovascular therapy (balloon angioplasty, stents). Such nonoperative approaches are probably more expensive than standard surgical revision, and they suffer limited durability. A contemporary prospective, randomized comparison of surgical versus endovascular management of thrombosed dialysis access grafts found significantly longer primary patency in the surgical group. Primary endovascular therapy for a failed conduit should be reserved for situations in which central venous pathologies are suspected, and in patients with limited access options wherein anatomic information is needed for planning future procedures. Occasionally, we move straight to thrombolytic therapy in the access that was working well (good flow rates, low recirculation rates) but thromboses when excessive pressure is applied for hemostasis.

POSTOPERATIVE MANAGEMENT

Several potential postoperative complications necessitate diligent early observation and patient education, the latter being vital because many of these procedures are being completed in a same-day surgery setting (Table 182–3). Early recognition of AVF or graft failure permits further planning. Post–anesthesia care nurses should be given a specific endpoint to follow for patency (e.g., line on the skin where there is a palpable thrill), and patients should also be instructed to follow patency. Mild edema usually responds to elevation. Massive edema, however, should prompt investigation for central venous occlusive pathologies. As with all surgical wounds, patients should be instructed regarding the signs and symptoms of bleeding and infection.

Patience and clear communication with the dialysis team is required to avoid complications (bleeding, thrombosis) from premature cannulation. Prosthetic grafts should be healing well with minimal edema before being used (usually at least 2 weeks). Signs suggestive of perigraft seromas or poor incorporation demand evaluation by the surgeon before use of the access. At least 1 month, and usually more, should be allowed for maturation (vein dilation and thickening) of AVFs.

Probably the most debilitating and potentially limb-threatening complication is distal extremity ischemia, with the usual culprit being limited inflow. The median nerve can be affected (mimicking carpal tunnel syndrome), often while the patient is undergoing dialysis and arterial inflow demands are maximal. Temporary bedside finger occlusion of the AVF or graft can assist in determining whether there is an inflow problem, or whether the arterial flow distal to the arterial anastomosis has been interrupted. For instance, if hand arterial perfusion returns to baseline with AVF compression, then inflow is inadequate to maintain flow to the hand and the AVF. If the extremity remains ischemic, then there may be a problem with the arterial anastomosis that occludes outflow or there may

Table 182–3	**Complications of Permanent (Noncatheter) Hemodialysis Access**
COMPLICATION	**ETIOLOGIC FACTORS**
Early thrombosis	Technical errors, premature cannulation
Late thrombosis	Venous outflow neointimal hyperplasia
Failure to mature	Technical errors, inadequate inflow, vein pathologies
Edema	Venous hypertension, central venous occlusive pathologies
Infection	Immunocompromised patient, foreign body prosthetic graft
Extremity ischemia	Limited arterial inflow caused by occlusive pathologies, anastomotic technical errors, thromboemboli
Pseudoaneurysms	Conduit deterioration caused by multiple cannulations
Aneurysms	Conduit degeneration
Congestive heart failure	High-volume arteriovenous fistula or graft, occasionally ischemic cardiomyopathy caused by arch occlusive disease and retrograde flow in mammary cardiac bypass graft

be thromboembolic complications. The diagnosis is confirmed by segmental arm and finger pressures, followed by repeated examination while the access is occluded. If inflow is inadequate, then improvement of distal pressures and symptoms should occur while the AVF or graft is compressed. Attempts at banding the conduit are rarely effective because of their imprecision. Arterial ligation distal to origin of the AVF can eliminate the steal physiology while arterial bypass grafting from above to below the AVF revascularizes the extremity (distal revascularization-interval ligation procedure).

Postoperative infections occur in up to 10% of access placement wounds, usually from *Staphylococcus* species. Cellulitis generally requires antibiotics and close observation. Infected AVFs not involving the anastomosis can be salvaged by local wound care and antibiotics. Care must be taken to avoid desiccation of any exposed conduit. Aggressive infections with expanding necrosis require AVF ligation. Under most circumstances, infected grafts require excision and resolution of the infection before construction of alternative access. Other rare access complications include aneurysms, pseudoaneurysms, high-output congestive heart failure resulting from high flow through the conduit, and perigraft seromas.

OUTCOMES

Few operative procedures rival hemodialysis access placement for high failure rates and limited durability. Even contemporary series indicate that three of four hemodialysis patients suffer access thrombosis each year. Primary patency rates at 1 year for autogenous AVFs range from 43% to 90%, although some may be patent but not usable for dialysis. One- to two-year primary patency for hemodialysis bridge grafts stands at 20% to 50%. Venous outflow stenosis (usually caused by anastomotic neointimal hyperplasia) with resulting thrombosis remains the primary cause of access failures. Finally, yearly mortality rates of up to 20% for patients on hemodialysis limit the usual personal rewards associated with other types of surgical patient care. Life expectancies of ESRD patients are between 16% and 38% of the U.S. population matched for age, sex, and race.

Maintenance of adequate access for dialysis currently stands as the leading cause of hospitalization for this patient population. In some series, ESRD patients spend more than 3 days of every 3-month period in the hospital, and their perceived overall quality of life satisfaction is significantly lower than that of age-matched control patients or transplant recipients.

In addition to this quality-of-life toll, maintenance of adequate dialysis access extorts a significant financial burden. The average patient charge for attempted salvage of a failed hemodialysis access graft in 1994 was $4350. Estimated Medicare expenditures for dialysis access complications stood at a staggering $150 million in 1993. Between 1993 and 1997, spending on vascular surgery and diagnostic and therapeutic radiology grew at rates of 7.3% and 8.3% annually, respectively. These higher than average rates have been attributed to an increasing incidence of vascular access complications, perhaps related

---

Pearls and Pitfalls

PEARLS

- Ensure that consideration has been given to peritoneal dialysis, transplantation, or long-term catheters (patients with limited lifespan).
- Thoughtful preoperative planning and imaging increase likelihood of autogenous access.
- Use standard vascular surgery techniques; pay meticulous attention to detail.
- Under most circumstances, failed grafts are best managed by open surgical exploration, thrombectomy, and revision.
- Act early on extremity ischemia after hemodialysis procedures.

PITFALLS

- Maintenance of permanent hemodialysis access when other ESRD therapies would have been more appropriate can negatively affect costs and quality of life.
- Prosthetic grafts have limited durability and should be avoided when autogenous constructions are possible.
- Overly angulated anastomoses are prone to twists and kinks.
- Contemporary endovascular approaches are expensive and suffer limited durability.
- Delay in recognition and therapy can result in upper extremity disability or limb loss.

---

to a strong trend from autogenous AVFs to prosthetic grafts, which are associated with higher complication rates.

In summary, surgical placement of permanent hemodialysis access requires thoughtful planning and attention to detail. With the exception of an occasional autogenous AVF that survives for decades, the endeavor remains expensive because of limited durability and numerous potential complications. Current endovascular technologies have not economically extended the lifespan of these conduits. The aging population, the expanding number of ESRD patients, and the continued pressure for health care cost containment make vascular access for hemodialysis a procedure in dire need of improvement.

SELECTED READINGS

Berman SS, Gentile AT, Glickman MH, et al: Distal revascularization-interval ligation for limb salvage and maintenance of dialysis access in ischemic steal syndrome. J Vasc Surg 1997;26:393.

Brotman DN, Fandos L, Faust GR, et al: Hemodialysis graft salvage. J Am Coll Surg 1994;178:431.

Coburn MC, Carney WIJ: Comparison of basilic vein and polytetrafluoroethylene for brachial arteriovenous fistula. J Vasc Surg 1994;20:896.

Cull DL, Taylor SM, Russell HE, et al: The impact of a community-wide vascular access program on the management of graft thromboses in a dialysis population of 495 patients. Am J Surg 1999;178:113.

Dougherty MJ, Calligaro KD, Schindler N, et al: Endovascular versus surgical treatment for thrombosed hemodialysis grafts: A prospective, randomized study. J Vasc Surg 1999;30:1016.

Feldman HI, Held PJ, Hutchinson JT, et al: Hemodialysis vascular access morbidity in the United States. Kidney Int 1993;43:1091.

Hodges TC, Fillinger MF, Zwolak RM, et al: Longitudinal comparison of dialysis access methods: Risk factors for failure. J Vasc Surg 1997;26:1009.

Huber TS, Ozaki CK, Flynn TC, et al: Case report: Use of superficial femoral vein for hemodialysis arteriovenous shunt. J Vasc Surg 2000;31:1038.

Kalman PG, Pope M, Bhola C, et al: A practical approach to vascular access for hemodialysis and predictors of success. J Vasc Surg 1999;30:727.

Marston WA, Criado E, Jaques PF, et al: Prospective randomized comparison of surgical versus endovascular management of thrombosed dialysis access grafts. J Vasc Surg 1997;26:373.

Matsuura JH, Rosenthal D, Clark M, et al: Transposed basilic vein versus polytetrafluorethylene for brachial-axillary arteriovenous fistulas. Am J Surg 1998;176:219.

Shinde TS, Lee VS, Rofsky NM, et al: Three-dimensional gadolinium-enhanced MR venographic evaluation of patency of central veins in the thorax: Initial experience. Radiology 1999;213:555.

Simmons RG, Abress L: Quality-of-life issues for end-stage renal disease patients. Am J Kidney Dis 1990;15:201.

U.S. Renal Data System, USRDS 1999 Annual Data Report, National Institute of Health, National Institute of Diabetes and Digestive and Kidney Diseases, Bethesda, MD, April 1999.

Zibari GB, Gadallah MF, Landreneau M, et al: Preoperative vancomycin prophylaxis decreases incidence of postoperative hemodialysis vascular access infections. Am J Kidney Dis 1997;30:343.

Chapter 183

Amputations

Timothy C. Flynn

The removal of a body part is one of the most ancient of surgical procedures. Surviving medical texts from India report on amputations and the fashioning of prostheses as early as 2000 BCE, and the writings of Hippocrates from 400 BCE describe the latest in surgical techniques for amputations. In the first century, Celsus described thigh amputations in detail, noting the need to cut the soft parts above the junction of the viable and nonviable tissue and that the bone was to be transected at the point where the healthy tissue began to adhere to it. The techniques of amputation were further developed on the battlefield, and Napoleon's surgeon, Dominic Jean Larrey, wrote of refinements in amputation technique that were widely applied. The introduction of firearms increased the amputation rate; during the American Civil War, 30,000 amputations were reported by the Union Army alone. Advances in surgical care and, in particular, the recognition of the need to repair vascular structures have reduced the number of amputations necessitated by trauma.

In civilian practice, amputations are usually done in patients with congenital abnormalities, tumors, trauma, or vascular diseases. In 1996, there were 159,000 amputations of the lower extremity done in the United States for a rate of 25 amputations per 100,000 population. More than 80% of these cases were done for complications of vascular insufficiency or diabetes. Indeed, more than half of the nontraumatic lower extremity amputations are in patients with diabetes, even though patients with diabetes make up only 3% of the total population. Of the 159,000 lower extremity amputations done in 1996, 59,000 were toe amputations, 18,000 foot amputations, 42,000 below-knee amputations, and 36,000 above-knee amputations. In 1993, the mean hospital charge for an amputation was $24,359 with an average length of stay of 15.7 days, excluding the subsequent rehabilitation and prosthesis cost. Only 54% of patients with an amputation were discharged home and 40% were transferred to another facility, including long-term care. In comparison, for patients who underwent bypass surgery, the average charge was $29,926, the average length of stay was 11.5 days, 85% of patients were discharged to home, and only 12% were discharged to another facility or to long-term care. Mortality rate was 6% for amputation, whereas it was 3.6% for revascularization procedures.

CLINICAL PRESENTATION

Multiple factors are known to be associated with an increased incidence of amputation including diabetes mellitus, end-stage renal disease (ESRD), and peripheral arterial occlusive disease. In a 14-year study from Wisconsin, patients with diabetes had an incidence of amputation of between 0.5% and 0.7% per year; the rate was higher for men and smokers, less for patients who reported daily aspirin use. However, as many as 40% to 50% of amputations in diabetic patients may be preventable. Peripheral neuropathy has been implicated in 80% of amputations in patients with diabetes. One of the most common ways of identifying the neuropathy in the diabetic patient is to use the Semmes Weinstein monofilament test. A study from Seattle showed that insensitivity to the 5.07-mm monofilament used in this test and foot deformities were associated with a higher rate of amputation. Amputations in diabetic patients are also associated with an ABI (ankle brachial systolic pressure index) of less than 0.35, retinopathy, neuropathy, higher levels of HgA1c, and renal insufficiency. In contrast, an organized system of foot care may reduce the incidence of amputation in this population.

Patients with ESRD are also at high risk for amputation. In 1994, the rate of lower limb amputation in this population was 6.2 per 100 person-years. If renal failure was due to diabetes, the rate was 13.8, and the rate of amputation in patients with diabetes and ESRD was 10 times the rate in patients with diabetes alone. Furthermore, two thirds of patients with ESRD who underwent amputation were dead within 2 years.

Many patients with chronic arterial occlusive disease manifested as claudication fear amputation because they know someone else who started with claudication and ended up with an amputation. However, amputation is a relatively rare outcome for the patient with claudication alone. Only 1% to 3% of patients with claudication require amputation over 5 years, and only 20% to 25% of patients deteriorate to limb-threatening ischemia during that time. Deterioration is most frequent during the first year after diagnosis (6% to 9% in the first year and only 2% to 3% per year thereafter), and smoking, diabetes, male gender, hypertension, ABI less than 0.35 at presentation, and walking distance of less than 100 yards are risk factors for progressive disease.

In contrast, the risk of amputation for untreated limb-threatening ischemia is approximately 80%. Chronic limb ischemia is estimated to affect 40 to 50 persons per 100,000 per year. For patients with rest pain, gangrene, or nonhealing ulcers, limb salvage is obtained in 75% to 80% in most series, 60% in patients with diabetes. In an audit in Great Britain, 16% of patients admitted to hospital with chronic limb ischemia underwent primary amputation, 66% had revascularization, and 18% conservative care. Poor runoff may predict those with a poor chance for long-term limb salvage and thus identify individuals who may benefit from primary amputation, although this remains to be demonstrated conclusively. Surprisingly, with a few exceptions, it has been difficult to show decreased rates of amputation in population studies in light of modern vascular surgical techniques. However, few vascular surgeons would argue primary amputation is a reasonable approach in the face of reconstructible vascular disease.

Acute limb ischemia is estimated to affect 13 persons per 100,000 population and the 30-day amputation rate in patients with acute limb ischemia ranges between 10% and 30%, whereas the mortality rate is up to 15%. The risk of death is greater when the acute limb ischemia is due to embolus from cardiac disease, whereas the risk of limb loss is greater in thrombosis caused by the extensive underlying vascular disease present in the extremity. Surprisingly, overall mortality rate for this presentation of limb-threatening ischemia has changed little over the past 20 years.

Interestingly, more amputations seem to be done in the southern states, with the highest incidence in southwestern Texas. This perhaps reflects an increased minority population or incidence of diabetes in the population in this area. Minorities tend to have a higher incidence of diabetes and are reported to be more likely to undergo amputation than revascularization. Data from Florida from 1992 to 1995 show the incidence of amputation as 50 per 100,000 for African Americans versus 25 per 100,000 in the white population. In addition, the incidence of revascularization was 30 per 100,000 in the African American population versus 71 per 100,000 in the white population. Although these differences might not be related as cause and effect with regard to the amputation rate, the precise factors responsible for this increased risk of amputation in some populations remain to be determined.

PREOPERATIVE MANAGEMENT

Clearly, optimal care is to prevent amputation. Care for patients at risk for lower extremity amputation should include a multidisciplinary team with a focus on limb salvage. Once intractable rest pain or tissue loss develops, the decision to pursue vascular reconstruction or to offer primary amputation must be made. The factors to be considered include the reconstructive potential of the patient, the functional status of the patient before the acute situation, and the desires of the patient, especially as they pertain to the patient's willingness to accept the possibility of a failed reconstruction. Although most vascular surgeons view amputation as a failure of their therapy, amputation is yet another arm of surgical care and, for the patient, the goal is to cure the presenting problem. This generally means removing the source of infection or pain, achieving primary healing without prolonged hospitalization or disability, and returning as much functional status as possible.

In our practice, the functional status of the patient has a significant role to play in determining the level of amputation. For the patient who has no rehabilitation potential because of preoperative status, we would most commonly offer the amputation most likely to heal, which, in most cases, is above the knee. Patients who have impaired neurologic function or severe motor deficits, patients with knee contractures greater than 15% to 20%, and patients with a contralateral amputation who do not use the currently affected limb for transport or pivoting are usually not good candidates for revascularization or conservative amputations. However, for the patient with any chance for rehabilitation, every effort is made to salvage a below-knee or more distal amputation.

The determination of amputation healing at any given level is not an exact science. Numerous preoperative tests have been devised, none of which is 100% sensitive in predicting healing. Furthermore, clinical experience remains an important part of the decision-making process and most centers accept a rate of failed distal amputations to ensure that every patient is given the opportunity to have an amputation that spares the foot or knee joint. Centers that adopt a policy of below-knee amputations for all patients with any chance of rehabilitation achieve a 70% to 80% success rate for healing amputations below the knee. A below-knee to an above-knee amputation ratio of 2.5 is generally considered ideal; however, national statistics show that almost as many people have an above-knee amputation as have a below-knee amputation.

Physical examination is important to delineate the degree of gangrene and to determine pulse status. In a series of 203 below-knee amputations, 79% failed when the femoral pulse was absent, 29% failed if there was a femoral pulse but no popliteal pulse, and only 10% failed if both pulses were palpable. In general, we are reluctant to perform an amputation in patients who have absent femoral pulses, because failure to heal an above-knee amputation frequently necessitates a hip disarticulation, which carries a very high mortality rate. Consideration should be given to revascularization of the profunda femoris in patients who need amputation and have no femoral pulse.

Multiple objective tests have been proposed as aids in the appropriate selection of amputation levels. Extremity arterial Doppler pressure measurements are commonly and easily performed; however, there is no single value that should be used to deny a patient a distal amputation. Patients with a pressure of at least 60 to 70 mm Hg at the ankle have been shown to have a 90% chance of healing a below-knee amputation; however, even patients with zero pressure at the ankle heal a below-knee amputation almost 50% of the time. Similarly, although toe pressures of 50 to 60 mm Hg are thought to be needed to heal toe or forefoot amputations, no single number accurately predicts which of these amputations will or will not heal. Transcutaneous oxygen tension measurements have also been evaluated in numerous amputation studies and have been shown to have a high predictive value. However, this technique requires adherence to fairly stringent criteria in performing the test in order to have any value in predicting amputation healing and has not received widespread acceptance. Xenon-133 studies that measure the rate of xenon washout as an indication of skin blood flow have also been investigated in the selection of appropriate amputation level. Again, this is a study that has had some research implications but little wide clinical application. Skin fluorescence, laser Doppler flow measurements, thermography, and pulse-volume recordings have all been used in selected studies to predict amputation healing with variable rates of accuracy and sensitivity. Finally, arteriography is seldom helpful in determining level of amputation and should be reserved for those patients who are being considered for reconstruction. As previously noted, the one area where we find arteriography helpful is in the patient with no femoral pulse in whom we would consider reconstruction before amputation.

The elderly patient with vascular disease who requires amputation brings numerous risk factors for surgery. These are primarily cardiac and pulmonary. Even though it is desirable to correct acute problems such as congestive heart failure or volume depletion, an extensive workup is seldom indicated. As with any other vascular patient, we would optimize volume status, treat acute pulmonary problems, use beta-blockers and aspirin, and appropriately use invasive intraoperative monitoring. Many of these patients are also malnourished and, although nutritional screening may not help in the selection of the site of amputation, evidence suggests that severely malnourished patients have a lower rate of wound healing at every level. Efforts should be made to restore nutritional levels of severely malnourished patients preoperatively if possible. As many as 30% of patients who come to amputation, especially younger patients, may also have a hypercoagulable state. In patients younger than 50 years of age, consideration should be given to working up the patient for a recognized syndrome that might lead to long-term anticoagulation.

Many of these patients also have sites of infection and even overt sepsis that should be controlled before definitive amputation. Cellulitis and local foot infections can usually be treated with antibiotics and drainage, whereas ankle or knee disarticulation may be needed before definitive amputation in patients with no chance for reconstruction of the foot and signs and symptoms of sepsis. Control of sepsis reduces the incidence of infection in the subsequent amputation. In addition, although it seems somewhat arcane, some patients may benefit from cryoamputation to prevent myoglobin release while they are being prepared for surgical amputation. Blood glucose should also be aggressively controlled because it contributes to control of infection. Preoperative antibiotics include coverage for gram-positive and -negative organisms as well as anaerobes, especially in the diabetic patient. All patients should receive prophylaxis for deep venous thrombosis, because the incidence of deep venous thrombosis in patients undergoing amputation is 10% to 15% and pulmonary embolus is a common cause of death after amputation.

The rehabilitation specialist should be involved in all cases in which patients have any potential for rehabilitation, and, if there is time, it is optimal to have the patient evaluated by rehabilitation services before amputation. In addition, we have found it helpful to have individuals who have successfully undergone rehabilitation after amputation to talk to patients preoperatively. Patients who have an idea about what to expect before amputation and what might be offered to them in terms of rehabilitation are generally more accepting of the need for amputation and more optimistic about their own care and future. Physical conditioning may also be valuable preoperatively to increase the patient's upper body strength and general level of physical strength. The author encourages quadriceps exercises because this is the muscle necessary to effec-

tively use a below-knee prosthesis. Care should also be taken to preserve the contralateral extremity during the preoperative period and to provide exercises for that extremity, which may have increasing demands placed upon it after amputation.

INTRAOPERATIVE MANAGEMENT

Anesthesia should be given by the same team that does anesthesia for vascular reconstructive procedures because the patients bring the same set of morbidities to amputation as they do to arterial reconstruction. We do not use a proximal tourniquet; therefore, hemostasis is important to prevent hematomas that inhibit wound healing. However, a drain should be used infrequently, if at all. All nerve transections result in a formation of a neuroma that could be painful if it is at a pressure point or becomes involved in the scar. Clean transection and retraction of the nerve is the best way of avoiding symptomatic neuroma. Care should be taken to be sure that excessive bone length does not put too much tension on the skin closure. Periosteum should be elevated to a point where the bone is divided and not any farther proximally so as not to leave a segment of bone without periosteum. Flaps should be kept thick, and dissection between the fascial planes and the subcutaneous tissue should be avoided, because this compromises blood flow to the skin. Open amputation or guillotine amputation for sepsis is best done through the joint space to prevent retraction of the cut muscle and development of edema. If there is potential for any undrained pus at the more proximal part of the limb, it is best to make a longitudinal incision in the affected compartment. This should be done in such a way as to preserve the posterior flap for patients in whom it is possible to salvage a below-knee amputation.

For below-knee amputation, preservation of the soleus muscle is not necessary, but preservation of at least some of the gastrocnemius is advised. In addition, muscles atrophy without an attachment to pull against. Thus, particularly in the younger patient who is expected to be active, there may be some value in attaching the muscle to the bone by drilling a hole in the bone and attaching the muscular fascia directly to the bone. This is seldom done in the elderly vascular patient, but we do close muscle and periosteum over the cut end of the bone in an attempt to prevent bursa formation between the muscle and the bone. In patients with previous prosthetic bypass grafts, we recommend removal of all the prosthetic material through a proximal incision so that there is no prosthetic material left at the amputation site that may form a nidus of infection or poor healing.

A number of procedures have been designed for amputation of specific body parts and, although there may be occasions for creative surgical procedures, it is usually optimal for rehabilitation to perform one of the standard, described amputation procedures. Toe amputations are the most common of the amputations performed, usually requiring little by way of rehabilitation. Nevertheless, toe amputations, especially first toe amputations, can profoundly affect pressure distribution of the foot, and patients need to be cognizant of this. Toe amputations can be done with a circular, or fishmouth, incision in the mid-portion of the toe if the amputation is through the proximal phalanx or through the classic racket incision with an extension on to the dorsal aspect of the foot for resection of the metatarsal head. As a general rule, the author would not recommend disarticulation at the metatarsal-phalangeal joint without removal of the metatarsal head itself because this creates a pressure point on ambulation and the relative avascular cartilage surface may inhibit healing. The racket incision should be created with a circular incision along the base of the toe and then a perpendicular incision from this down on the metatarsal itself. A wide "V" incision along the base of the toe may compromise blood flow to the other toes. We find it useful to use the oscillating saw when dividing bones because of the tendency of bone cutters to crush these small bones and lead to fragmentation. Tendons should be drawn into the wound, divided, and allowed to retract because these are avascular and may inhibit healing of the wound. Enough bone needs to be removed in order to be sure that the closure can be accomplished without tension.

With loss of the big toe and one other toe, it is frequently advisable to consider transmetatarsal amputation. Transmetatarsal amputation (Fig. 183–1) provides a functional amputation that can be weight bearing, usually without prosthesis. Although some authors have noted a 50% failure rate with this amputation, particularly in patients with diabetes, it remains a useful procedure for many patients. The procedure involves removal of the toes and metatarsal heads through the mid-shaft of the tarsal bones. A posterior flap is created and the sesamoid bones are removed below the great toe. As much plantar surface skin should be preserved as possible. The skin must be closed with no tension and the scar remains on the dorsum of the foot. Presence of a pedal pulse is usually a good indication for healing, although its absence may not preclude healing of this very functional amputation. A variety of other more proximal amputations in the foot have also been described. These include the Lisfranc amputation, which is through the tarsal-metatarsal joint,

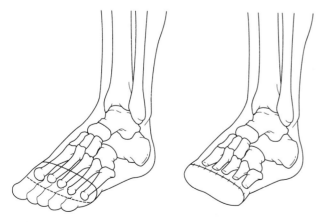

Figure 183–1. Transmetatarsal amputation showing line of incision. Note that plantar incision is made over the distal metatarsal heads. (From Flynn T: Amputations. In Levine BA, Copeland EM III, Howard RJ, et al [eds]: Current Practice of Surgery, vol 2. New York, Churchill Livingstone, 1993.)

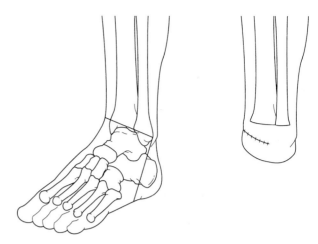

Figure 183–2. Syme amputation. The calcaneus is carefully removed to preserve the heel pad as a weight-bearing surface. (From Flynn T: Amputations. In Levine BA, Copeland EM III, Howard RJ, et al [eds]: Current Practice of Surgery, vol 2. New York, Churchill Livingstone, 1993.)

the Chopart amputation, which is between the talonavicular and calcaneocuboid joints, and the Syme amputation with its modifications, the Pirogoff and Boyd amputations. All provide for weight bearing on the distal stump (Fig. 183–2). Although some authors have suggested that these operations can be successful in patients with vascular disease, particularly after reconstruction, our experience is that these amputations have seldom resulted in foot salvage. For patients with other reasons for amputations, such as frostbite or traumatic injury, these may be quite useful.

When the foot cannot be salvaged, the below-knee amputation is the most desirable amputation level. The healing potential is good, and the chances of rehabilitation and ambulation are better than with an above-knee amputation, particularly in those patients who were previous ambulators. The most common method of performing below-knee amputations in the United States is the Burgess type procedure, which involves a long posterior flap. The skin is divided at approximately 10 to 12 cm below the tibial tuberosity (Fig. 183–3), carried down to mid-calf level with a slight superior fishmouth, and then carried parallel to the bones for a distance of 12 to 15 cm or one and a half times the diameter of the calf at that level. The posterior flap should be handled very gently and, as stated previously, it is unnecessary to preserve the soleus, but there should be no dissection between the fascial layers and the subcutaneous tissue. However, the posterior flap should not be so bulky as to create tension on the skin line when the posterior flap is sutured to the anterior facial layer. Some authors recommend a skew flap where the incision is essentially a fishmouth that runs anterior to posterior. This is positioned slightly lateral to the prominence of the tibia and performed approximately at 10 to 12 cm below the joint line. The gastrocnemius is preserved and then brought up as a flap to be sutured to the anterior fascia and periosteum. The skin is closed, leaving a vertical wound. Randomized studies have not shown superiority of this type of closure over the Burgess closure and, although some authors are enthusiastic about

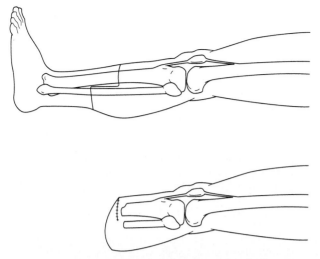

Figure 183–3. Below-knee amputation showing the long posterior flap incision. The skin incision should begin 10 to 12 cm below the tibial tuberosity. Note the anterior bevel of the tibia. (From Flynn T: Amputations. In Levine BA, Copeland EM III, Howard RJ, et al [eds]: Current Practice of Surgery, vol 2. New York, Churchill Livingstone, 1993.)

the skew flaps, it depends on the individual surgeon's experience and expertise as to which of these incisions would be best for any given patient.

The above-knee amputation (Fig. 183–4) is performed by creating either a circular or fishmouth incision over the middle of the femoral shaft and dividing the bone at a level that allows good closure without tension, most

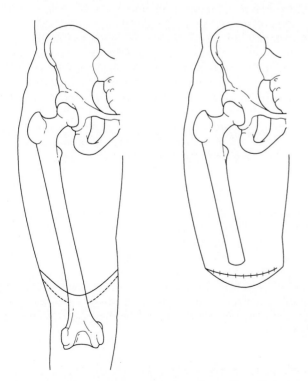

Figure 183–4. Above-knee amputation. (From Flynn T: Amputations. In Levine BA, Copeland EM III, Howard RJ, et al [eds]: Current Practice of Surgery, vol 2. New York, Churchill Livingstone, 1993.)

commonly at the apex of the proximal aspect of the fishmouth incision. Muscle stabilization may be important in this amputation, particularly for the younger and more active patient. Alternatively, some authors, particularly in the United Kingdom, have advocated a through the knee amputation or a Gritti Stokes amputation, which is through the femoral condyles. These amputations preserve length and can be easily fitted with a prosthesis, but there is little to indicate that these have any great advantage over the standard above-knee amputations. Most above-knee amputations heal; however, occasionally it is necessary to proceed with a hip disarticulation, which is associated with high morbidity and mortality rates. The rehabilitation opportunities are almost nil after this amputation in the elderly population, with vascular disease and frequent wound problems necessitating long hospitalizations after these procedures.

POSTOPERATIVE MANAGEMENT

The patient may be placed in a soft dressing or a rigid dressing with a fitted cast. Most rehabilitation specialists recommend a rigid cast, and some studies indicate that it may facilitate healing. A rigid dressing provides good protection for the residual limb that prevents contracture and potentially allows early ambulation. Some specialized centers may also fit the rigid dressing with a pylon for ambulation even within the first 2 or 3 days after amputation. Special expertise is needed to prevent pressure points when applying the rigid dressing, and complaints by the patient of pain should result in early removal if there is any concern about the wound or areas of potential pressure necrosis. A posterior splint may be helpful in patients in whom there is some concern about the placement of rigid dressing. Although edema is of some concern, tight-fitting or elastic dressing may not be appropriate for the dysvascular patient in the first 3 to 5 days after amputation. However, after that, aggressive efforts should be made to control edema and allow for shrinkage and remodeling of the residual limb for early fitting of a prosthesis. Early and aggressive physical therapy by the rehabilitation team is also indicated.

COMPLICATIONS

Assuming adequate technique, failure to heal as a result of poor blood supply is the most common complication after amputations. Wound breakdown, necessitating a more proximal amputation in 5% to 15% of amputations, occurs even in the most specialized centers. Higher healing rates can be accomplished by adopting a policy of only doing proximal amputations, but this deprives too many people of the functional advantage for more distal amputation. Minor skin separation should be treated conservatively but, for breakdown much greater than a centimeter or two, more extensive débridement with or without bone shortening may be necessary. The bone must be covered, which can be accomplished by closing the wound in the central area and leaving the medial and lateral aspects open to pack. Infection of amputation wounds should be treated with local drainage and packing and, assuming adequate blood supply, such infections should not result in more proximal amputations. Full-contact dressings may decrease the time to healing compared with standard wet to dry and elastic compression dressings. Occasionally, a skin graft may be needed, if it can be done in an area where the prosthetist can still fit a prosthesis without applying direct pressure to that area of skin graft. Similar treatment applies to the patient who falls in the early postoperative period and dehisces the wound. These individuals should be taken back to the operating room for irrigation and reclosure.

The sensation that the amputated limb is still present occurs in 80% to 90% of patients with an amputation. This sensation is frequently episodic and is usually not bothersome to the patient. Some patients report the phenomenon of telescoping, wherein they feel the phantom limb moving proximally into the residual limb until it disappears. Phantom limb pain is also common, but is usually not disabling. However, incapacitating phantom pain occurs in up to 10% of patients. There is some indication that this type of pain may be centrally mediated, although most therapies for this problem are directed locally toward the residual portion of the limb. These therapies include massage, compression, and the use of transcutaneous electrical nerve stimulation, but success with use of these modalities in patients with disabling phantom limb pain has been variable. Some authors have suggested that the perioperative use of local or regional anesthetics may reduce the incidence of phantom pain but this has not been proved. Others have tried electroconvulsive therapy and have reported some success, suggesting that the pain is a centrally mediated phenomenon.

Edema is a common problem in the amputation stump that interferes with wound healing and rehabilitation. Proper wrapping and use of rigid dressings can potentially prevent this. Joint contractures are also common, particularly in debilitated patients and, in above-knee amputations, the forces result in flexion and abduction of the stump. This can be prevented by not allowing the patient to prop the residual limb on a pillow and by having the patient prone for part of the day in order to extend the hip. In below-knee amputations, the problem is knee flexion. Rigid dressing, posterior splints, and early physical therapy to strengthen the quadriceps are indicated to prevent this problem. Skin problems in the residual limb are also not uncommon. Pressure points can develop calluses and breakdown with use of a prosthesis. Verrucous hyperplasia is a wartlike growth that can occur in the end of the stump and can potentially be accompanied by fissuring and infection. Folliculitis and sebaceous cysts can also occur and be troubling.

OUTCOMES

Unfortunately, amputation for vascular disease is associated with a high in-hospital mortality rate and poor long-term prognosis. Above-knee amputations still have a 9% to 15% mortality rate and below-knee amputations have a 2% to 5% mortality rate. Wound complications are seen in as many as 25% of patients and revisions are necessary

---

Pitfalls and Pearls

PEARLS

- Many amputations are avoidable. At-risk patients need education and monitoring to prevent tissue loss. Patients with ischemic lesions should be assessed for their suitability for bypass or treatment by a multispecialty wound care team.
- Always perform the most distal amputation possible. Accept some degree of wound failure in patients who are rehabilitation candidates. By the same token, do not subject patients who have no hope of rehabilitation to multiple procedures.
- Attention to technical detail is important. This is not the operation for the most junior member of the team to do alone.
- Rigid dressings probably do work, and your institution should develop the expertise to do this.
- Personnel from rehabilitation medicine, physical therapy, and prosthetics should be involved early. Clinicians should follow up by talking with the rehabilitation team about surgical results.
- Clinicians should remember that an amputation is a major event in the psychosocial life of the patient and the family.

---

in 8% to 15% of patients. Mortality rate at 2 years after amputation is 30% to 40% and at 5 years is 50% to 60%. In addition, as many as 25% to 40% of patients previously living independently become institutionalized after limb loss, and contralateral amputation becomes necessary in as many as 25% to 50% of patients within 5 years. Rehabilitation specialists believe that patients who were ambulatory before amputation should have an 80% to 90% chance of some degree of independent ambulation after amputation but this varies widely depending on the level of amputation, comorbidities, and the effectiveness of the rehabilitation system. In addition, walking requires 15% to 30% more energy after a below-knee amputation and 40% to 60% more energy after an above-knee amputation, even at velocities that are 40% to 50% less than that of the nonamputee. Community-based studies report that the actual rate of ambulation 5 years after amputation is only 20% to 30% in vascular patients.

The implications of amputation for the patient's emotional state should not be ignored. No one can lose a limb and not experience profound grief, significant alteration in body image, and great fear about the implications for future life. Patients worry about their loss of mobility, the impact of their disability on their families, and their own sense of dependency. The health care team should be honest about expected rehabilitation goals but be as positive as possible. Acknowledging the patient's fears and emotional turmoil can help in the patient's recovery. Some patients need intensive counseling along with their rehabilitation.

SELECTED READINGS

Barnes RW, Cox B: Amputations: An Illustrated Manual. Philadelphia, Hanley and Belfus, 2000.
Bohne WHO: Atlas of Amputation Surgery. New York, Thieme Medical, 1987.

Dormandy J, Heeck L, Vig S: Major amputations: Clinical patterns and predictors. Semin Vasc Surg 1999;12:154.

Ger R, Angus G, Scott P: Transmetatarsal amputation of the toe: An analytic study of ischemic complications. Clin Anat 1999;12:407.

Holstein PE, Sorensen S: Limb salvage in a multidisciplinary diabetic foot unit. Diabetes Care 1999;22(Suppl 2):B97.

Huber TS, Wang JG, Wheeler KG, et al: Impact of race on the treatment for peripheral arterial occlusive disease. J Vasc Surg 1999;30:417.

O'Dwyer KJ, Edwards MH: The association between lowest palpable pulse and wound healing in below-knee amputation. Ann R Coll Surg Engl 1985;67:232.

Termansen NB: Below-knee amputation for ischemic gangrene. Prospective, randomized comparison of a transverse and a sagittal operative technique. Acta Orthop Scand 1977;48:311.

Weinstein SM: Phantom limb pain and related disorders. Neurol Clin 1998;16:919.

Chapter 184

Management of Complications of Vascular Surgery: Infected Vascular Grafts, Aortoenteric Fistulas, and Pseudoaneurysms

Dennis F. Bandyk and Martin R. Back

The use of vascular grafts has permitted palliation of otherwise fatal or disabling vascular conditions. Morbidity owing to biomaterial failure (dilatation, rupture) or allergic foreign body reaction is rare, but implant failure as the result of infection, the development of aortoenteric fistula, or pseudoaneurysm formation is the most serious sequela of prosthetic graft usage. These complications require surgical intervention because antibiotics alone will not eradicate an established infection. Delay in intervention is associated with increased mortality risk and morbidity caused by sepsis, life-threatening hemorrhage, or graft thrombosis.

INFECTED VASCULAR GRAFTS

Vascular graft infection can present with a spectrum of clinical signs depending on graft location and virulence of the infecting organism. The incidence of infection involving a vascular graft varies, occurring after 0.4% to 5% of operations, and is influenced by anatomic site, indication for intervention, and patient comorbidities (Table 184–1). Approximately 20% of aortic graft infections are complicated by the development of graft-enteric erosion or fistula (GEE/GEF). Graft infection is more common after emergency procedures (e.g., for ruptured abdominal aortic aneurysm, acute arterial ischemia) and when the prosthesis is anastomosed to the femoral artery or placed in a subcutaneous tunnel (e.g., with axillofemoral or femorofemoral bypass). By comparison, infection involving autogenous vein bypass grafts and endovascular stent-grafts is uncommon (<1% incidence).

Vascular graft infections are classified by two schemes: the Szilagyi classification and the Bunt classification.

The Szilagyi classification is applicable to immediate postoperative infections:

Grade I—cellulitis involving wound
Grade II—infection involving subcutaneous tissue
Grade III—infection involving the vascular prosthesis

The Bunt classification encompasses terminology for the spectrum of graft infection:

Perigraft infection—early (<4 months) postoperative or
  late-appearing (>4 months) postoperative
Graft-enteric erosion or fistula (GEE/GEF)
Aortic stump sepsis

Surgical management is individualized to the type of graft infection with the primary goals of eradicating infection and maintaining circulation to the limbs and perfused organs. Treatment options are influenced by several important factors, including clinical presentation, anatomic location, extent of infection, type of graft material, virulence of infecting organism, signs of invasive infection, and overall status of the patient. Mortality rate is highest with aortic graft infection complicated by graft-enteric fistulas, whereas the risk of limb loss is greatest with lower limb graft infections. Sepsis and rupture of a mycotic pseudoaneurysm are grave clinical signs, requiring emergent intervention and total graft excision. For less virulent infections, in situ replacement with autogenous venous conduits, allografts, or antibiotic-impregnated grafts can be considered if specific principles are adhered to. Successful outcome requires accurate diagnostics, administration of culture-specific antibiotics, and surgical intervention to totally excise or replace the infected biomaterial.

Pathophysiology

A vascular prosthesis can be exposed to microorganisms (bacteria, fungi) and be colonized by one of three mechanisms: perioperative contamination, bacteremia (hematogenous) seeding, and mechanical erosion to skin, bowel, or genitourinary tract. Microorganisms can adhere to graft surfaces by direct contact during implantation or via the

Table 184–1	Incidence of Prosthetic Vascular Graft Infections Relative to Implant Site	
GRAFT SITE	**INCIDENCE (%)**	
Descending thoracic aorta	0.7–3	
Aortoiliac	0.4–1.3	
Aortofemoral	0.5–3	
Femorofemoral	1.3–3.6	
Axillofemoral	5–8	
Femoropopliteal	0.9–4.6	
Femorotibial	2–3.4	
Carotid patch	0–0.2	
Carotid-subclavian	0.5–1.2	
Axillary-axillary	1–4.1	
Iliac stent	<0.5	

surgical wound from disrupted lymphatic draining sites of remote infection or lower limb ulceration. Important sources of operative contamination include breaks in aseptic operative technique and contact with the patient's endogenous flora harbored within sweat glands, lymphatics, or openings of the gastrointestinal, biliary, or genitourinary tracts. If a fibrin seal does not develop in the surgical wound and heal promptly following operation, the underlying vascular prosthesis is susceptible to colonization from superficial wound problems (e.g., cellulitis, dermal necrosis, and lymphocele formation). A septic focus can develop in ischemic or injured tissues of the surgical wound and, with deep extension, can involve the prosthesis (Szilagyi—grade II infection). Diseased artery walls (atherosclerotic plaque, aneurysm thrombus) and reoperative wounds are another common source of bacteria, especially coagulase-negative staphylococci. Occult *Staphylococcus epidermidis* graft infection has been implicated in 60% of repaired femoral anastomotic pseudoaneurysms associated with prosthetic aortofemoral grafts.

Bacterial seeding of the prosthesis via a hematogenous route is an uncommon but important mechanism of graft infection. Experimentally, intravenous infusion of 10^7 colony-forming units of *Staphylococcus aureus* produces a clinical graft infection in nearly 100% of animals during the immediate postimplantation period. Bacteremia from sources such as intravascular catheters, an infected urinary tract, or remote tissue infection is common in elderly vascular patients. Parenteral antibiotic therapy can decrease the risk of graft colonization associated with direct contact and bacteremia, and is the basis for culture-specific antibiotic therapy in patients with known remote infection. The prosthesis becomes less susceptible to colonization as the luminal pseudointimal lining develops and matures over time, but vulnerability to infection from bacteremia has been documented beyond 1 year after implantation.

Vascular biomaterials and bacteria act together to produce co-inflammatory stimuli to activate the immune system. The resulting inflammatory process attempts to localize the infection, but produces adjacent tissue-damaging effects. Inflammation develops via the humeral and cellular immune systems with secretion of cytokines and recruitment of polymorphonuclear granulocytes. The prosthetic graft itself also invokes an immune foreign body reaction that causes an acidic, ischemic microenvironment conducive to bacterial colonization. Unlike autogenous grafts, implanted prosthetic grafts do not develop rich vascular connections with surrounding tissue, which prevents host immune defenses and antibiotics from exerting maximal effect on colonized bacteria. The natural history of graft infection, regardless of location, is tissue autolysis, vessel wall or anastomotic disruption, and hemorrhage. Perigraft tissue destruction leads to the formation of a perigraft cavity or abscess, spread of the infectious process along the graft, and involvement of adjacent structures (artery, skin, bowel). This pathobiology of graft infection can manifest clinically as a spectrum, from graft sepsis to a localized perigraft abscess, anastomotic pseudoaneurysm, graft cutaneous sinus tract, or graft-enteric erosion or fistula (GEE/GEF).

The pathogenesis of GEE/GEF has been attributed to mechanical erosion of the pulsatile prosthetic graft into adherent bowel. Theoretically, this should be avoidable by good soft-tissue coverage of the graft by either the aneurysm wall after abdominal aortic aneurysm repair or the retroperitoneal tissue. Nearly 50% of GEEs are associated with pseudoaneurysm of the proximal aortic anastomosis. Whether infection develops as a primary cause of GEF or secondarily after communication with the gastrointestinal tract is unclear, but in many GEFs, gram-positive bacteria rather than intestinal flora are cultured remote from the fistula, suggesting an underlying graft infection was initially present.

Predisposing Factors

Multiple risk factors for infection can be documented in patients in whom a vascular graft infection develops (Table 184–2). Early graft infections are usually the result of wound sepsis, reoperation for hematoma, concomitant remote infection, and impaired immunocompetence. Patients with late-appearing graft infections often have a history of multiple operations for graft thrombosis or false aneurysm. Gram-positive cocci, especially coagulase-negative staphylococci, are primary opportunists infecting vascular grafts and injured perigraft tissues. Altered immune function associated with malignancy, leukopenia, lymphoproliferative disorders, and drug administration (e.g., steroids or chemotherapy) can predispose patients to graft infection despite low numbers of contaminating bacteria.

Prevention of graft infection is an important concept, and the surgical team must be cognizant of preoperative, operative, and postoperative prophylactic measures. A prolonged preoperative hospital stay should be avoided to minimize the development of skin flora resistant to commonly used antibiotics (i.e., hospital-acquired strains).

Table 184–2	**Risk Factors Predisposing to Graft Infection: Bacterial Contamination of the Graft**

Faulty sterile technique
Prolonged preoperative hospital stay
Emergency surgery
Extended operating time
Reoperative vascular procedure
Simultaneous gastrointestinal procedure
Remote infection
Postoperative superficial wound infection

Altered Host Defenses
  Local factors
    Biomaterial
    Slime production
  Systemic factors
    Malnutrition
    Leukopenia
    Malignancy
    Corticosteroid administration
    Chemotherapy
    Diabetes mellitus
    Chronic renal failure
    Autoimmune disease

Prophylactic antibiotics are recommended for vascular prosthetic implantation because this has been shown to decrease the occurrence of both wound and graft infections. Recommended antibiotic prophylaxis in adults undergoing prosthetic grafting is as follows:

- Cefazolin 1 g intravenously (IV) before anesthesia induction and repeated every 8 hours for 24 hours.
- When methicillin-resistant *S. aureus* (MRSA) is cultured on body surfaces or is a known important pathogen in hospitalized patients, add vancomycin 1 g IV infused over 1 hour.
- If the patient has a cephalosporin allergy, give aztreonam 1 g IV every 8 hours.
- If the patient has a vancomycin allergy, give clindamycin 900 mg IV over 20 to 30 minutes.

Antibiotics should be administered before the skin incision and at regular intervals during the procedure to maintain tissue levels above the minimal bactericidal concentration for expected pathogens. Additional dosing may be needed in patients with prolonged procedures (>4 hours) or excessive changes in blood volume, fluid administration, or renal blood flow during the procedure. Vancomycin as antibiotic prophylaxis should be considered when hospital infection control indicates a higher prevalence of MRSA. Culture-specific antibiotics should be prescribed to patients undergoing vascular graft implantation with active soft-tissue infections.

Bacteriology

Although virtually any microorganism can infect a vascular prosthesis, gram-positive cocci (*S. aureus*, *S. epidermidis*) are prevalent pathogens (Table 184–3). Since the early 1970s, graft infections with *S. epidermidis* and other gram-negative bacteria have increased in frequency. Surgeons have become cognizant of microbiologic sampling error when low numbers of bacteria are present, despite clinical and anatomic signs of perigraft infection. Late-appearing graft infections caused by *S. epidermidis* and other coagulase-negative staphylococci are typically associated with negative cultures of perigraft fluid or tissue. Infections caused by gram-negative bacteria such as *Escherichia coli* and *Pseudomonas*, *Klebsiella*, *Enterobacter*, and *Proteus* species are particularly virulent. The incidence of anastomotic dehiscence and artery rupture is high, resulting from the ability of the organism to produce destructive endotoxins (e.g., elastase and alkaline protease) that act to compromise vessel wall structural integrity. Fungal infections of grafts (e.g., with *Candida*, *Mycobacterium*, and *Aspergillus* species) are rare, and most patients in whom these infections develop are either severely immunosuppressed or have an established fungal infection elsewhere.

Graft infection occurring within 4 months of graft implantation is associated with virulent pathogens, with *S. aureus* predominating. Recently, an increase in MRSA infections has been observed. These strains can produce hemolysis and toxins to leukocytes that provoke an intense local and systemic host response and permit early recognition of the infectious complications, but they complicate treatment by precipitating an increased incidence of anastomotic breakdown or vein rupture. Gram-negative organisms such as *E. coli*, *Proteus*, *Pseudomonas*, *Klebsiella*, and *Enterobacter* species can also be involved in early postoperative graft infections, with anastomotic bleeding associated with *Pseudomonas aeruginosa* infection. Graft healing complications, such as GEE/GEF, typically involve infection with gram-negative enteric bacteria.

Late-appearing graft infections (i.e., occurring more than 4 months after graft implantation) are commonly associated with less virulent bacteria, especially *S. epidermidis* and other coagulase-negative staphylococci. These organisms are a component of normal skin flora but have the ability to adhere to and colonize biomaterial surfaces and to grow within an adherent biofilm, resulting in an indolent infection. The bacteria-laden biofilm is eventu-

| Table 184–3 | Bacteriology of Prosthetic Vascular Graft Infections: Incidence from Collected Cases (n = 1258) |

MICROORGANISM	INCIDENCE (%)					
	AEF	AI	AF	FD	TA	ICS
Staphylococcus aureus	4	3	27	28	22	50
Staphylococcus epidermidis	2	3	26	11	25	20
Streptococcus species	9	3	10	11	2	—
Escherichia coli	18	30	12	7	2	—
Pseudomonas species	3	7	6	16	14	—
Klebsiella species	5	10	5	2	2	10
Enterobacter species	5	13	2	2	—	—
Enterococcus species	8	10	2	7	4	—
Bacteroides species	8	3	3	2	—	—
Proteus species	4	—	4	7	2	—
Candida species	3	—	1	1	4	—
Serratia species	1	—	1	2	—	—
Other species	3	2	4	6	0	—
No growth culture	18	13	2	2	16	20

AEF, aortoenteric fistula or erosion (n = 397); AI, aortoiliac or aortic tube graft (n = 39); AF, aortobifemoral or iliofemoral graft (n = 460); FD, femoropopliteal, femorotibial, axillofemoral, or femorofemoral graft (n = 251); TA, thoracic aorta graft (n = 55); ICS, innominate, carotid, or subclavian bypass graft or carotid patch following endarterectomy (n = 56).

ally recognized by host defense mechanisms, leading to inflammation of the perigraft tissue and adjacent artery and to the subsequent clinical manifestations of a late graft infection.

DIAGNOSTICS

Prompt diagnosis and treatment of prosthetic graft infections are essential to avoid complications (e.g., sepsis and hemorrhage) and death. The majority (>80%) of graft infections are diagnosed more than 4 months after graft implantation. Clinical signs are varied and may be subtle, particularly for grafts confined to the abdomen or thorax. Operative exploration is the most accurate method of excluding infection of a vascular prosthesis and may be required when clinical suspicion of GEE exists. Any gastrointestinal bleeding in a patient with an aortic graft should be considered to have GEE/GEF until another source of bleeding is conclusively identified or no graft-bowel communication is verified at operation.

Clinical Manifestations

History

Because graft infections can have subtle presenting signs, the vascular surgeon must have a low threshold for diagnostic testing when symptoms or signs suggest graft infection. Infection of intracavity (aortic, thoracic) grafts can manifest as unexplained sepsis, development of ileus and anorexia, or abdominal distention and tenderness. The classic triad of GEF symptoms (gastrointestinal hemorrhage, sepsis, abdominal pain) occurs in less than 30% of affected patients. If the infection involves a superficial graft segment (i.e., groin, limb, or neck), local signs of graft infection are usually apparent by findings of an inflammatory perigraft mass, cellulitis, a drainage sinus tract, or palpable anastomotic pseudoaneurysm.

Physical Examination

In the physical examination, the clinician should closely scrutinize the sites of graft implantation for signs of inflammation. Surgical wounds should be carefully inspected for erythema, tenderness, or drainage. Masses juxtaposed to anastomotic sites can represent perigraft abscesses or anastomotic pseudoaneurysms. The extremities should be examined for signs of septic embolization (e.g., clusters of petechiae downstream from the infected graft).

Laboratory Studies

An elevated white blood cell count (15,000 to 18,000 cells/mm^3) with left-shifted differential and an increased erythrocyte sedimentation rate (>20 mm per minute) are common but nonspecific findings associated with graft infection. Routine testing should also include a complete blood count, coagulation studies, urinalysis, blood cul-

tures, and cultures of any other potential sources of infection, such as foot and surgical wound drainage. Bacteremia is an uncommon sign (<5%), indicating advanced artery wall or mural thrombus infection, or the development of endocarditis. A stool guaiac test for blood is indicated in patients with suspected GEE/GEF, but findings are positive in only approximately two thirds of patients with documented lesions. All laboratory testing may be normal in patients with late-appearing perigraft infections caused by S. epidermidis.

Vascular Imaging

Vascular imaging is essential for the diagnosis and treatment of graft infection and its sequelae (Fig. 184–1). Anatomic signs of graft infection, such as perigraft abscess, anastomotic aneurysm, and GEE/GEF can be accurately (90% sensitivity) identified by a combination of ultrasonography, computed tomography (CT), magnetic resonance imaging (MRI), arteriography, and endoscopy. Functional radionuclide imaging (gallium-67 or indium-111–labeled leukocyte, technetium-99m hexametazime-labeled leukocyte) can confirm the presence of a clinically suspected graft infection when anatomic signs of perigraft abscess are equivocal. The combination of anatomic and functional vascular imaging techniques is highly accurate for confirming the presence of infection, planning management, and assessing operative sites for residual or recurrent infection. Arteriography is used to develop an operative strategy and should be routine.

Contrast-Enhanced Computed Tomography

- Contrast-enhanced CT is the preferred initial imaging technique for patients with suspected infection of aorto-femoral, abdominal aorta, or thoracic aorta grafts.
- Diagnostic criteria suggestive of infection include the loss of normal tissue planes of the retroperitoneal structures, indicative of inflammation; abnormal collections of fluid or gas around the graft; false aneurysm formation; hydronephrosis; adjacent vertebral osteomyelitis; and juxta-aortic retroperitoneal abscess
- Presence of fluid and air surrounding a vascular prosthesis is normal in the early postoperative period, thus limiting the diagnostic accuracy of CT. However, any gas in the periprosthetic tissues on CT scan is abnormal beyond 6 weeks after implantation.
- Perform contrast-enhanced CT with intravenous and oral contrast to better identify the lumen of the graft, delineate periprosthetic abscess, and define the relationship of the duodenum and small bowel to the aortic prosthesis.
- Contrast-enhanced CT can be performed with sufficient speed to be useful in evaluating symptomatic but hemodynamically stable patients with suspected GEE/GEF.

Ultrasonography

- Ultrasonography is a readily available imaging technique that is suited for portable examination.

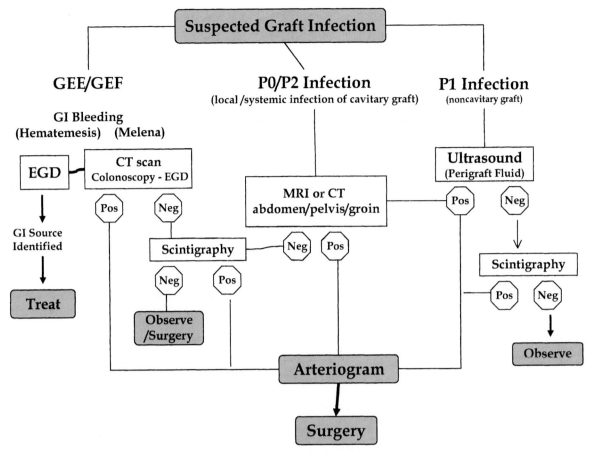

Figure 184–1. Algorithm for the evaluation of an infected vascular graft. GEE, graft-enteric erosion; GEF, graft-enteric fistula; EGD, esophagogastroduodenoscopy; CT, computed tomography; MRI, magnetic resonance imaging; GI, gastrointestinal; Pos, positive; Neg, negative.

- Color duplex scanning can reliably differentiate perigraft fluid collection from anastomotic pseudoaneurysm or hematoma and is thus useful in the evaluation of pulsatile masses.
- Diagnostic accuracy depends on the skill of the examiner and the ability to adequately image the graft, which can be obscured by abdominal distention as a result of large amounts of intestinal gas or obesity.
- Ultrasonography is the most useful initial imaging technique for verifying vessel or graft patency and assessing pulsatile masses adjacent to grafts in the groin and limbs.

Magnetic Resonance Imaging

- MRI is the preferred method by some vascular groups because of its superior imaging over CT.
- MRI is useful in differentiating between perigraft fluid collection and inflammation of the perigraft tissues.
- MRI has increased diagnostic accuracy compared with CT.

White Blood Cell Scanning

- This functional radionuclide imaging technique demonstrates sites of leukocyte accumulation.

- It is not useful during the early postoperative course because of nonspecific radionuclide take-up in the perigraft tissues. False-negative scan findings are unusual, so exclusion of early graft infection is possible.
- Normal findings have been reported in late-appearing aortic graft infection complicated by GEE.
- Accuracy of the functional imaging scans, especially indium-111–labeled white blood cell scans, approaches 90% in the detection of graft infection. Positive scan findings are associated with a positive predictive value of 80%.
- IgG scans are preferred over leukocyte scans because of the ease of preparation, the lack of staff exposure to the patient's blood, the absence of concomitant red blood cell and platelet imaging, and the long shelf-life.
- MRI and CT can be used in conjunction to delineate accurately the extent of graft involvement.

Endoscopy

- Endoscopy is an important diagnostic modality in patients with suspected GEE/GEF.
- It is essential that the entire upper gastrointestinal tract be inspected, including the third and fourth portions of the duodenum, which are the most common sites of GEF.

- Patients with recent massive gastrointestinal hemorrhage should be examined *in the operating room*, with preparation for operation in case exsanguination from the fistula is induced.
- Endoscopy can sometimes (<20%) visualize the graft eroded through the bowel mucosa, but the main purpose is to rule out other sources of bleeding, such as gastritis or ulcer disease.
- Negative examination findings do *not* exclude the possibility of an aortoduodenal fistula.

Arteriography

- Arteriography is not used to make a diagnosis of graft infection.
- Arteriography can accurately identify infection-associated complications, such as graft rupture and anastomotic aneurysm.
- Biplanar angiography with lower limb is recommended to assess the patency of the visceral or renal vessels and to evaluate the status of the proximal and distal vessels as potential sites for extra-anatomic bypass grafts.

Microbiologic Testing

Identification of the bacteria causing the graft infection is necessary to confirm the diagnosis and to select appropriate antibiotic therapy. Routine techniques for culture of graft surfaces and perigraft fluid are adequate in patients with invasive graft infections associated with fever and leukocytosis. Virulent organisms, such as *S. aureus*, streptococci, and gram-negative bacteria are typically isolated. More sensitive microbiologic techniques should be used to identify the causative organism when organisms are not seen on Gram stain of the perigraft fluid or tissues and when patients show no signs of graft sepsis (no fever or leukocytosis) or a graft biofilm infection is suspected. Mechanical disruption of the bacteria from the graft surface, either by tissue grinding or by ultrasonic disruption, and culture in broth media increase the identification of the bacteria, and are especially useful in recovery of coagulase-negative staphylococci such as *S. epidermidis*, compared with routine culture methods. These techniques overcome the sampling errors of routine culturing methods by isolating slow-growing microorganisms that reside in low numbers on the biomaterial surfaces.

Operative Findings

The most accurate method to determine graft infection is operative exploration. Graft exploration permits the surgeon to assess graft incorporation with surrounding tissue, the presence and characteristics of perigraft fluid, anastomotic integrity, and presence of GEE/GEF. Culture of explanted graft material in a broth culture is the only reliable method of confirming a bacterial biofilm infection. Operative exploration is mandatory in patients with prior aortic surgery and gastrointestinal bleeding in whom all other sources of bleeding have been excluded. Thorough mobilization and exploration of the duodenum, the

small bowel, and the aortic graft and proximal anastomoses will identify GEF in approximately 80% of cases.

MANAGEMENT OF GRAFT INFECTIONS

Treatment of vascular graft infections, GEE/GEF, and infected pseudo- or mycotic aneurysms requires adherence to the general principles of surgery, clinical presentation, and microbiology (Table 184–4).

Preparing the Patient for Surgery

Patients in septic shock or hypovolemia as a result of anastomotic bleeding secondary to a graft infection allow little time for preparation. Adequate blood and fluid volume resuscitation, perioperative cardiopulmonary monitoring, administration of broad-spectrum high-dose antibiotics, and planning an appropriate surgical approach form the essential elements of urgent preoperative treatment of these critically ill patients. Most patients with graft infection allow time for adequate preoperative preparation, identification of the infecting pathogen, and assessment of the extent of graft infection. Patients should be prepared physiologically and psychologically, including optimization of cardiac and renal function, assessment of pulmonary status, and, if nutritional reserves are depleted, supplemental enteral or parenteral nutrition. Arterial circulation to the upper and lower extremities should be assessed by Doppler-derived pressure measurements and arteriography for adequate determination of appropriate revascularization alternatives to maintain limb perfusion after graft excision. If autogenous vein replacement is planned, duplex ultrasonography of the lower limb deep veins should be done to assess caliber and absence of

Table 184–4	**Patient Selection Criteria for Excision Alone, In Situ Replacement, or Ex Situ Bypass and Total Graft Excision in the Treatment of Prosthetic Vascular Graft Infection**	
TREATMENT OPTION	**CLINICAL PRESENTATION**	**MICROBIOLOGY**
Excision Alone	Graft thrombosis and adequate collaterals	+ cultures
In Situ Replacement		
Autogenous vein	Invasive graft infections without sepsis or GEE/GEF	+ cultures
Prosthetic	Localized biofilm graft infections	*Staphylococcus epidermidis*
Excision and Ex Situ Bypass		
Simultaneous	Unstable patient with GEE/GEF	No excluding criteria
Preliminary staged	Stable patient with aortic infection ± GEE/GEF	No excluding criteria

GEE/GEF, graft-enteric erosion or fistula.

chronic venous thrombosis. Systemic antibiotics should be selected according to isolated or suspected pathogens.

Determining the Extent of Graft Infection

Because persistent infection of a retained graft segment or the arterial graft bed is the major reason for treatment failure, accurate assessment of the extent of graft infection is critical. In situ prosthetic replacement can be considered only when there is a bacterial biofilm infection and the intracavity graft segments are not involved. Computed tomography scanning, MRI, and white blood cell radionuclide scans are helpful in localizing the infected portion of the graft, but surgical exploration is the most reliable method of determining extent of graft infection. Hydronephrosis indicates advanced retroperitoneal inflammation and denotes diffuse aortic graft infection.

Graft Excision

Total graft excision is essential to eradicate the infectious process in patients with sepsis or in those with anastomotic bleeding. Attempts at graft preservation with antibiotics and local antibacterial irrigation have been reported, but the persistence of infection is common and patients remain at risk for exsanguination from anastomotic rupture.

When infection is localized to only a portion of the vascular graft, the surgeon should develop a patient-specific treatment plan. In situ replacement using lower limb deep vein is the preferred option for infected aortic and short segment ex situ (femorofemoral) grafts. In highly selected cases, amputation and mortality rates may be decreased by excising only the infected portion of the graft, with distal revascularization via remote bypass through tissues not involved with infection. In sites of graft replacement, antibacterials (Clorpactin [oxychlorosene sodium]) should be instilled via wound irrigation systems to cleanse perigraft tissues, and implantation of antibiotic-impregnated beads may also help sterilize the surgical wound.

Débridement of the Arterial Wall and Perigraft Tissues, and Drainage

After graft excision, débridement of all inflamed tissues and drainage of the graft bed are important principles for avoiding persistence of the infectious process. The artery wall and perigraft tissues should be excised to normal-appearing tissues, especially in the presence of purulence or false aneurysm. It is essential to use monofilament permanent sutures to perform artery ligation and aorta stump closure. Closed suction drainage should be positioned in the infected graft bed when gross purulence is present. Coverage of the arterial closures with viable, noninfected tissue, such as an omental pedicle or rotational muscle flaps, lessens the risk of artery infection and rupture.

Antibiotic Therapy

If the pathogens can be identified before operation, bactericidal-level antibiotics should be administered before operation and perioperatively. If the infecting organism has not been identified, broad-spectrum antibiotics (e.g., an aminoglycoside plus semisynthetic penicillin), a second-generation cephalosporin, or ampicillin plus sulbactam should be given. If *S. aureus* or *S. epidermidis* is suspected, an intravenous first- or second-generation cephalosporin and vancomycin would be appropriate. Once operative cultures have isolated the infecting organism, antibiotic coverage should be modified according to antibiotic susceptibility testing of the recovered strains. The duration of antibiotic administration after treatment by graft excision is empirical, but at least 2 weeks of systemic antibiotics is recommended. Patients who received long-term antibiotics (parenteral antibiotics for 6 weeks, followed by oral antibiotics for 6 months) had significantly better results than patients given short-term therapy (2 weeks). The incidences of recurrent infection and aortic stump blowout may be decreased with long-term antibiotic administration, especially in the presence of positive arterial wall culture findings.

Revascularization of Organs and Limbs

Graft excision, without revascularization, is possible in some patients with an infected prosthetic graft. Occluded grafts and grafts implanted to alleviate symptoms of claudication may be treated by total graft excision without revascularization or in combination with endovascular angioplasty. If a phasic Doppler arterial signal is present at the ankle after temporary graft clamping or if arterial systolic pressure is greater than 40 mm Hg, delayed reconstruction is an option. In the presence of critical limb ischemia (i.e., no audible Doppler signal at the ankle), arterial revascularization should not be delayed because of the associated increased morbidity and risk of limb loss.

It is preferable to perform limb revascularization before the infected graft is removed, but in the presence of a GEE/GEF with anastomotic bleeding and shock, control of hemorrhage takes precedence. Autogenous vein grafts (superficial femoral, greater saphenous vein) or endarterectomized iliac or superficial femoral artery, if available, can be used for lower limb or organ revascularization. If a prosthetic graft is used for an ex situ bypass, polytetrafluoroethylene (PTFE) conduits are preferred to Dacron grafts, although antibacterial-impregnated (rifampin-soaked [60 mg/mL], silver) grafts may eventually be the conduits of choice for the treatment of established graft infections by either in situ replacement or extra-anatomic bypass grafting. Several vascular groups have confirmed a decreased morbidity and mortality rate with staged or sequential treatment as compared with traditional treatment (i.e., total graft excision followed by immediate extra-anatomic bypass). Sequential treatment (i.e., preliminary revascularization followed by graft excision) prevents lower limb ischemia and avoids the necessity of keeping the patient heparinized during total graft excision and artery or aorta stump closure.

Graft preservation and in situ prosthetic replacement can be attempted in patients meeting specific criteria (Table 184–5). When infection involves the thoracic aorta, in situ prosthetic replacement may be the only practical approach. The perigraft infectious process should be low-grade, not associated with anastomotic hemorrhage, and cultures should be sterile, or the anatomic and microbiologic characteristics of the graft infection should suggest infection with *S. epidermidis*. In situ replacement appears to be a safe option for patients with graft infections secondary to *S. epidermidis*, but because of the indolent nature of this type of biomaterial infection, subsequent infection of retained graft segments may occur.

Treatment for Specific Graft Infections

Aortoiliac or Aortic Interposition Graft Infection

Aortoiliac or aortic interposition graft infections are best treated by preliminary (right-sided) axillobifemoral bypass grafting through clean, uninfected tissues, followed in 1 to 2 days by total graft excision of the infected aortic graft (Fig. 184–2). Extra-anatomic bypass grafting should be

Table 184–5	Selection Criteria and Treatment Adjuncts for Graft Preservation and In Situ Prosthetic Graft Replacement for Biofilm Graft Infection

Graft Preservation
Selection Criteria
  Patent graft that is not constructed of polyester (Dacron).
  Anastomoses are intact and not involved with infection.
  Patient has no clinical signs of sepsis.
Treatment Adjuncts
  Repeated and aggressive wound débridement in the operating room
  Daily wound dressing change at 8-hour intervals using dilute povidone-iodine (1 mL of 1% povidone-iodine in 1 L normal saline)
  Administration of culture-specific antibiotics
  Rotational muscle coverage of the exposed prosthetic graft segment

In Situ Prosthetic Graft Replacement
Selection Criteria
  Late-appearing graft infection without systemic signs of infection
  Biofilm graft infection with Gram stain of perigraft fluid showing no organisms
  Perigraft fluid culture showing no growth
  Graft biofilm infection demonstrates coagulase-negative staphylococci—*Staphylococcus epidermidis*
Treatment Adjuncts
  Perioperative administration of vancomycin—beginning 3 days before replacement
  Wide débridement of inflamed, abnormal perigraft tissue—sinus tracts
  Excision of anastomotic sites
  Cleansing perigraft tissues, retained graft with wound irrigation system
  Replace with rifampin-soaked (60 mg/mL) polyester gelatin- or collagen-impregnated polyester vascular prosthesis
  Muscle flap coverage of graft segment in groin
  Prolonged (6-week) parenteral administration of culture-specific antibiotics

performed without entry into the contaminated abdomen or retroperitoneum. Because the aortic graft is confined to the abdomen, the distal axillofemoral anastomoses can usually be performed to the common femoral arteries bilaterally. Systemic heparinization is used to maintain ex situ graft patency.

A retroperitoneal or transperitoneal approach can be used for excision of the infected aortic graft. Heparinization can be discontinued when proximal aortic control is achieved. In situ autogenous reconstruction using lower limb deep veins (superficial femoral-popliteal vein [SFPV]) can be considered as an option in the absence of GEE/GEF (Fig. 184–3). The entire infected abdominal aortic graft should be excised. Achieving proximal control at the supraceliac aorta before approaching the proximal anastomosis is recommended via a retroperitoneal approach in patients with a proximal anastomotic aneurysm or juxtarenal anastomosis. If necessary, the aorta can be excised to above the level of the renal arteries, with renal revascularization achieved via bypasses originating from the splenic or hepatic arteries.

After infrarenal aorta ligation, pelvic circulation can be adequately maintained via retrograde blood flow from the extra-anatomic femoral bypass through the external and internal iliac arteries. With excision of an infected aorta–external iliac graft, salvage of perfusion to one iliac artery via autogenous reconstruction should be considered. Inflow to a single internal iliac artery is usually sufficient to maintain adequate pelvic perfusion.

Aortobifemoral Graft Infections

Aortobifemoral graft infections are more difficult to treat because of groin involvement, mandating distal anastomoses of the ex situ bypass to the deep femoral, superficial femoral, or popliteal arteries. Preoperative vascular imaging studies can identify patients with localized aortofemoral graft limb infection, thus permitting partial aortofemoral graft limb excision. Patients should have no anatomic evidence of infection involving the proximal aorta and an intact aorta-graft anastomosis. In situ prosthetic graft replacement is appropriate in elderly patients with biofilm infections who are not good candidates for SFPV reconstruction. Muscle flap coverage of the exposed graft facilitates graft coverage and wound healing. Treatment without graft excision is appropriate only in carefully selected patients and is not recommended when patients are septic, the prosthetic graft is occluded, anatomic signs of arterial infection are present, or the infecting organism is a *Pseudomonas* species.

Infection localized to the femoral region of a single aortofemoral graft limb in a septic patient or anastomotic involvement should be treated by graft excision. A retroperitoneal exposure of proximal graft limb through an oblique, suprainguinal incision is recommended to obtain proximal control and assess extent of graft infection. If the graft limb is well incorporated, partial graft limb excision and SFPV bypass via the obturator canal is an option. Salvage of the common femoral artery is important in maintaining retrograde flow into the pelvis. If the superficial femoral artery is open, an alternative

Aortic Stump Closure

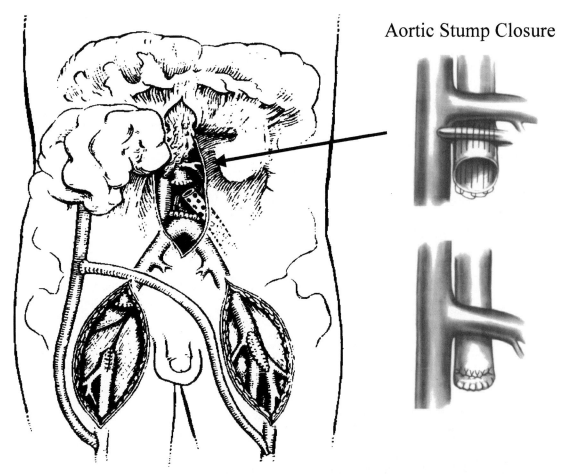

Figure 184–2. Excision of an infected aortobifemoral graft with extra-anatomic right axillobifemoral polytetrafluoroethylene bypass. Note techniques (femoral artery vein patch angioplasty, deep femoral–to–superficial femoral anastomosis, iliac artery anastomosis) available to maintain pelvic circulation.

method is to anastomose the superficial femoral artery to the deep femoral artery end to end in order to maintain pelvic flow via collaterals from the deep femoral system. After graft excision, all arterial ligation sites or anastomoses should be covered with viable tissue. A rotational sartorius muscle flap is particularly useful for groin infections. The groin wound should be left open and treated with topical 0.1% povidone-iodine or antibiotic dressings. Revascularization of the limb should be performed as necessary to maintain limb viability. Alternatives to revascularization depend on the patency of the distal circulation and can be performed to the deep femoral artery, the superficial femoral artery, or the popliteal artery. Revascularization should be accomplished via noninfected tissue planes using crossover femorofemoral grafts with medial tunneling or tunneling in the retropubic or suprapubic space, or lateral tunneling through the psoas tunnel to course diagonally distal to the distal outflow artery.

When the aortofemoral graft limb infection is localized to the groin region, presents more than 4 months after implantation, and is the result of *S. epidermidis* infection, then graft excision and in situ prosthetic replacement is an option. Wide débridement of all inflamed perigraft tissues, including the inflamed adjacent artery wall, is essential. In situ replacement with a PTFE or rifampin-soaked (60 mg/mL) gelatin- or collagen-impregnated–bonded prosthesis is recommended.

Aortoenteric Fistulas

In hemodynamically stable patients, the standard operative procedure is extra-anatomic bypass, preferably right axillofemoral ringed–PTFE bypass followed in 1 to 2 days (staged) with infected graft removal. When infection involves the graft at the femoral level and autogenous vein, cross-femoral graft is recommended. Bilateral axillofemoral or axillopopliteal grafts are not used because of limited runoff that affects patency and limb salvage. In situ replacement has been used successfully to treat secondary aortoduodenal fistula, with an operative mortality rate as low as 19%. Patients with GEE and minimal retroperitoneal infection fared best.

Complete graft excision is recommended and closure of the aorta should be performed at a site where it appears healthy and free of infection. The area of disrupted bowel should be débrided or excised, followed by a tension-free closure of normal-appearing bowel. The aortic stump should be covered by omentum or anterior spinal ligament and a closed suction drain placed if a retroperitoneal abscess was encountered.

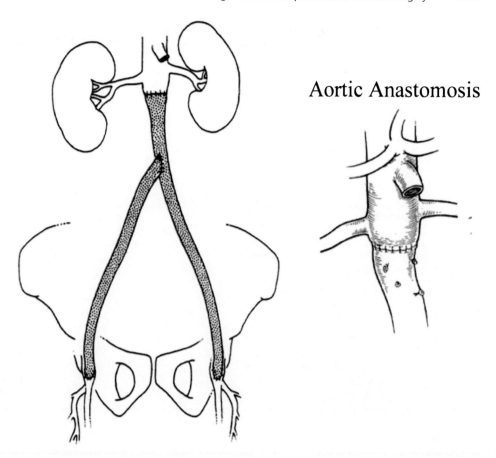

Aortic Anastomosis

Figure 184–3. Aortoiliac-femoral reconstructions using superficial femoral-popliteal deep lower limb veins (SFPV).

In the hemodynamically unstable patient, immediate celiotomy is required to control bleeding. If the condition of the aorta allows primary aortorrhaphy to control the bleeding, the procedure can be terminated, and once the patient is resuscitated, the staged approach to treatment of the infected aortic graft can be performed. Definitive treatment should be delayed more than 24 to 48 hours.

Results of Treatment of Aortic Graft Infections

Treatment of aortic graft infections with extra-anatomic bypass and excision of the entire graft is associated with a higher operative mortality and amputation rate than SFPV reconstruction (Table 184–6). The persistence of sepsis and aortic stump blowout are the major causes of early and late mortality. Lower extremity amputation caused by thrombosis and infection of the extra-anatomic bypass are major causes of late morbidity. The risk of major amputation of the extremity and of failure of extra-anatomic bypass grafts is higher for aortic grafts with groin infections than for infected aortoiliac grafts. The morbidity and mortality rates of extra-anatomic bypass grafting and total graft excision have prompted increased use of in situ replacement procedures using lower limb deep veins and antibiotic-bonded prosthetic grafts. In patients selected for in situ replacement, the operative mortality rate is in the range of 0% to 17% and the amputation rate is less than 10%. Successful treatment by either autogenous SFPV reconstruction or standard ex situ bypass followed by graft excision is associated with long-term survival in more than 70% of patients.

Early aortofemoral graft limb infections limited to the groin, without sepsis and an intact distal anastomosis, have been treated with local operative débridement, antibiotic therapy, and muscle flap coverage. Calligaro and associates achieved complete graft preservation and wound healing in 16 of 22 cases (73%) of graft infection resulting from gram-negative bacteria and in 23 of 33 cases (70%) of graft infection caused by gram-positive bacteria. However, the potential for treatment failure exists, and patients must be carefully monitored. All four deaths (10% mortality rate) in this series were due to graft sepsis; nine patients ultimately required total graft excision, and, in seven patients, surgical wounds never healed. *Pseudomonas* was a particularly virulent pathogen and was associated with nonhealing wounds, anastomotic disruption, and arterial bed hemorrhage. Treatment of bacterial biofilm graft infections by in situ prosthetic replacement appears to be safe and is associated with a low (9%) incidence of recurrent infection, but selection criteria must be adhered to.

In situ replacement following prosthetic graft infections has been reported sporadically, with initial reports describing high (25% to 40%) mortality rate in patients with GEE/GEF. More recent reports indicate a mortality rate of less than 20%, and long-term survival in 70% of patients when this procedure was limited to low-grade infections or allograft replacement was used.

Femoral, Popliteal, and Tibial Graft Infections

Once the diagnosis of infrainguinal prosthetic bypass graft infection is made, excision of the entire graft is recom-

Table 184–6	**Results of Treatment of Aortic Graft Infections**

EX SITU BYPASS AND TOTAL GRAFT EXCISION

Reference	No. Cases	Mortality Rate (%)	Early Amputation (%)	Stump Blowout (%)	Survival >1 Yr (%)	Infection of EAB (%)
Bandyk et al, 1984	18	11	11	0	66	17
O'Hara et al, 1986	84	18	27	22	58	25
Reilly et al, 1987	92	14	25	13	73	20
Schmitt et al, 1990	20	15	5	6	75	6
Yeager et al, 1999	60	13	7	4	74	10
Quinones-Baldrich et al, 1991	45	24	11	0	63	20
Seeger et al, 2000	36	11	11	3	86	6

IN SITU REPLACEMENT

Reference	No. Cases	Mortality Rate (%)	Early Amputation (%)	Graft Patency at 1 yr (%)	Survival >1 Yr (%)	Recurrent Infection (%)
Prosthetic: (biofilm infection)						
Towne et al., 1994	28	0	0	100	94	9
GEE/GEF:						
Jacobs et al., 1991	27	25	0	—	70	20
Bahnini, 1997	32	40	0	—	55	10
NAIS:						
Clagett et al., 1997	31	10	10	85	85	0
Nevelsteen, 1997	35	17	6	76	82	0
Allograft:						
Kieffer et al., 1992	103	19	5	70	82	7

EAB, extra-anatomic bypass.

mended in patients who have anastomotic disruption or graft sepsis. The same principles that apply to aortic graft infection should be followed, including removal of the entire graft. In situ autogenous venous reconstruction can be performed in the majority (80%) of patients. The treatment of peripheral graft infections is associated with a low mortality rate but the amputation rate is higher than with the treatment of aortic graft infections (Table 184–7). Patients who had prosthetic grafts inserted for claudication may be treated with graft excision alone. Patients with limb-threatening ischemia resulting from excision of the infected bypass should have revascularization, preferably with autogenous tissue. When autogenous tissue is not available, reconstruction with an allograft or prosthetic graft via remote, noninfected planes should be performed.

The local treatment of infrainguinal graft infections by aggressive perigraft tissue débridement, antibiotic use, and muscle flap coverage, without graft excision, has been successful in patients without graft sepsis or anastomotic disruption. Multiple authors have reported in small series of patients that this alternative treatment method can result in healing in approximately 70% of cases and may not be harmful to the patient as long as early aggressive management by graft excision is undertaken if sepsis or anastomotic disruption or bleeding occurs. If local

Table 184–7	**Results of Treatment of Femoropopliteal or Tibial Prosthetic Graft Infections**

Reference	No. Cases	Mortality Rate (%)	Amputation Rate (%)
Szilagyi et al., 1972	10	0	50
Liekweg and Greenfield, 1977	55	9	33
Yashar et al., 1978	3	0	67
Durham et al., 1986	3	0	67

COLLECTED SERIES OF TREATMENT OF THORACIC, INNOMINATE, CAROTID, OR SUBCLAVIAN PROSTHETIC GRAFT INFECTIONS

Graft Site	No. Cases	Operative Deaths	Perioperative Strokes	Survival >1 Yr†
Thoracic	50	6	0	42
Innominate, carotid, or subclavian bypass graft	33°	9	3	14
Carotid patch	11	3	2	5

°All patients with strokes were treated by carotid ligation without reconstruction, which resulted in four operative deaths and one late death.
†Late follow-up was not reported for 13 patients with an innominate, a carotid, or a subclavian bypass graft and for one patient with a carotid patch.

treatment is successful, it may result in a decreased rate of limb amputation resulting from infrainguinal graft infection; however, there is no conclusive evidence to support this treatment in favor of the more conventional therapy of total graft excision and remote revascularization.

Thoracic Aorta Graft Infections

The principles of graft excision and extra-anatomic bypass are not applicable to most cases of ascending, transverse aortic arch or of thoracic aorta graft infection. The principle of in situ maintenance of circulation must be followed. The operative approach to this severe infection should include wide débridement of the infected tissues, graft excision and replacement if anastomotic areas are involved or disrupted because of the infection, and coverage of the graft with viable, noninfected tissues. Pericardial fat pads, adjacent muscle (including the pectoralis major, the rectus abdominis, and the latissimus dorsi), and the greater omentum pedicle have been used for graft coverage. Using these principles of treatment, Coselli reported treatment of 40 patients with five operative deaths resulting from coagulopathy and hemorrhage (n = 2) or cardiopulmonary and renal complications (n = 3). Twenty-eight patients (70%) were alive and without evidence of recurrent graft infection during a follow-up of 4 months to 6.5 years. Infections of descending thoracic aorta grafts may be amenable to graft excision and revascularization through clean, uninfected planes of SFPV replacement. A remote bypass graft can be placed through a median sternotomy from the ascending aorta to the abdominal aorta, tunneling through the diaphragm through clean, uninfected tissue. This graft should be placed before excision of the descending thoracic graft. After placement of this graft, the patient should undergo graft excision via left thoracotomy.

Innominate, Subclavian, and Carotid Graft Infections

Management of infection of a bypass or patch graft of the innominate, subclavian, or carotid arteries is based on the same principles used for lower extremity graft infections. The treatment sequelae at these graft sites include not only persistent infections and hemorrhage but also stroke (see Table 184–7). The surgical approach to a patient with prosthetic infection of a transthoracic bypass graft often requires a median sternotomy and preparation for cardiopulmonary bypass and total circulatory arrest if needed for proximal control. Treatment should include total graft excision, administration of parenteral and topical antibiotics, and remote bypass, preferably with autogenous tissue, if needed. There have been reports of successful treatment of infected prostheses with local irrigation, but this is not recommended because graft excision and remote revascularization are usually possible.

An infected transthoracic or extrathoracic bypass graft for upper extremity ischemia can often be removed without the need for immediate revascularization. Ligation of the proximal innominate or subclavian arteries, unlike ligation of the iliac or common femoral arteries, is often tolerated without the onset of extremity ischemia. A subsequent bypass, if needed, can be performed after the infection is cleared. Only one case of upper extremity amputation following removal of a subclavian bypass graft for infection has been reported. If upper extremity ischemia results from graft excision, bypass with autogenous tissue through remote planes is preferred. Patients with transthoracic bypass grafts to the innominate and subclavian arteries often have multivessel disease of the aortic arch, necessitating that remote bypasses use the femoral artery, the descending thoracic aorta, or the supraceliac abdominal aorta as the inflow vessel. Remote bypass following excision of an infected carotid-subclavian bypass can be performed with a carotid-carotid bypass using saphenous vein or an axilloaxillary bypass using saphenous vein or SFPV. Blood flow after excision of an infected axilloaxillary graft can be successfully reestablished with a supraclavicular subclavian-subclavian bypass, a carotid-carotid bypass, or a femoral-axillary bypass.

Patients with infections of carotid artery bypasses or prosthetic patch infection after endarterectomy frequently do not tolerate ligation. Simple ligation of the common or internal carotid artery may be safely performed in patients with stump pressures of more than 70 mm Hg, but reconstruction of the artery to maintain cerebral blood flow and prevent stroke should be performed if possible. After graft excision, revascularization is preferably done with autogenous vein grafts. The anatomy of the extracranial carotid artery does not permit remote bypass through noninfected, uninflamed tissues, thus autogenous reconstruction is mandatory. Coverage of the bypass with muscle can be of value in this situation in preventing the recurrence of infection. Treatment of carotid prosthetic patch infections is usually best achieved by excision of the patch and reconstruction with vein bypass. Carotid shunts have been successfully and safely used to maintain cerebral perfusion during these difficult, challenging procedures. Stroke, recurrent infection, and carotid pseudoaneurysm formation are late complications in 12% of cases.

Pseudoaneurysms

Pseudoaneurysms result from several mechanisms, including infection, native artery degeneration, suture defect, and trauma. Anastomotic aneurysms after prosthetic grafting involve 0.4% (aorta) to 3% (femoral) of arterial anastomoses and represent a separation of the graft from the native artery with an enveloping fibrous capsule. Femoral pseudoaneurysms account for 75% of lesions requiring intervention. The treatment of a mycotic pseudoaneurysm is similar to that of an infected graft and, in most cases, in situ autogenous reconstruction is possible. In the absence of infection, resection of the aneurysm, graft, and adjacent weakened artery, followed by replacement with an antibiotic-bonded graft, is recommended because graft culture yields coagulase-negative staphylococci in many patients. In these circumstances, long-term antibiotic therapy should be prescribed.

Iatrogenic pseudoaneurysm after percutaneous arterial

Pearls and Pitfalls

PEARLS

- Use CT scanning, endoscopy, and, if necessary, operative exploration for diagnosis of GEE/GEF.
- Negative cultures associated with "sterile" pus indicate a low-grade graft infection—typically caused by *S. epidermidis*.
- If treating an invasive perigraft infection, all prosthetic grafts should be excised. Autogenous in situ reconstruction should be limited to patients without GEE/GEF.
- Preliminary axillofemoral bypass followed in 1 to 2 days with aortic graft excision is associated with less morbidity.

PITFALLS

- Failure to consider GEE/GEF in patients with gastrointestinal hemorrhage.
- Failure to diagnose graft infection when unincorporated graft is encountered.
- Failure to excise graft involved with infection.
- Prolonged limb ischemia associated with excision of an infected aortic graft.

---

access or endovascular intervention can be successfully treated by several techniques including ultrasound-guided compression (femoral artery), ultrasound-guided thrombin injection, or open surgical repair. For small (<3 cm) false aneurysms with an ultrasound-visualized "neck," direct injection of 0.5 to 2 mL of thrombin (1000 IU/mL) into the aneurysm cavity is successful in greater than 90% of cases.

Summary

Dissatisfaction with the morbidity and mortality results of treating graft infections, regardless of location, by total graft excision and remote bypass has been an impetus to the investigation of selective graft retention or in situ reconstruction. Selection criteria for these less aggressive treatment options have not been clinically verified, but experimental models have shown that treatment outcome depends on the virulence of the infecting organism, the extent of graft-artery infection, and the immune status of the patient. Use of lower limb deep veins is the preferred option for replacement of large-caliber prosthetic grafts, but, in many patients, standard therapy by staged ex situ bypass and total graft excision is a safer and more appropriate approach. Infection-resistant arterial conduits, including cadaveric arterial or venous homografts and antibacterial-impregnated prosthetic grafts, are treatment options in selected patients. Clinical safety efficacy has been demonstrated for various types of graft infection

but best results can be expected in the treatment of low-grade infections not complicated by GEE/GEF. Prophylactic use of an antibiotic-bonded graft would be of most clinical benefit in patients judged to be at increased risk for infection. Other adjuncts to sterilize the surgical wound (e.g., degradable antibiotic beads) may improve the efficacy of in situ replacement procedures.

SELECTED READINGS

Bandyk DF, Berni GA, Thiele BL, et al: Aortofemoral graft infection due to *Staphylococcus epidermidis*. Arch Surg 1984;119:102.

Bandyk DF, Bergamini TM, Kinney EV, et al: In situ replacement of vascular prostheses infected by bacterial biofilms. J Vasc Surg 1991;13:575.

Calligaro KD, Westcott CJ, Buckley RM, et al: Infrainguinal anastomotic arterial graft infections treated by selective graft preservation. Ann Surg 1993;216:74.

Clagett GP, Valentine RJ, Hagino RT: Autogenous aortoiliac/femoral reconstruction from superficial femoral-popliteal veins: Feasibility and durability. J Vasc Surg 1997;25:255.

Durham JR, Rubin JR, Malone JM: Management of infected infrainguinal bypass grafts. In Bergan JJ, Yao JST (eds): Reoperative Arterial Surgery. Orlando, Fla: Grune & Stratton, 1986, pp 359–373.

Fichelle JM, Tabet G, Cormier P, et al: Infected infrarenal aortic aneurysms: When is in situ reconstruction safe? J Vasc Surg 1993;17:635.

Geary KJ, Tomkiewicz ZM, Harrison HN, et al: Differential effects of a gram-negative and a gram-positive infection on autogenous and prosthetic grafts. J Vasc Surg 1990;11:339.

Hayes PD, Nasim A, London NJ, et al: In situ replacement of infected aortic grafts with rifampicin-bonded prostheses: The Leicester experience (1992–1998). J Vasc Surg 1999;30:920.

Jacobs MJHM, Reul GJ, Gregoric I, et al: In situ replacement and extra-anatomic bypass for the treatment of infected abdominal aortic grafts. Eur J Vasc Surg 1991;5:83.

Kieffer E, Bahnini A, Koskas F, et al: In situ allograft replacement of infected infrarenal aortic prosthetic grafts: Results in 43 patients. J Vasc Surg 1993;17:349.

Kitka MJ, Goodson SF, Rishara RA, et al: Mortality and limb loss with infected infrainguinal bypass grafts. J Vasc Surg 1987;5:566.

Liekweg WG Jr, Greenfield LJ: Vascular prosthetic infections: Collected experience and results of treatment. Surgery 1977;81:335.

Lorentzen JE, Nielsen OM, Arendrup H, et al: Vascular graft infection: An analysis of sixty-two graft infections in 2411 consecutively implanted synthetic vascular grafts. Surgery 1985;98:81.

O'Hara PJ, Hertzer NR, Beven EG, et al: Surgical management of infected abdominal aortic grafts: Review of a 25-year experience. J Vasc Surg 1986;3:725.

Quinones-Baldrich WJ, Hernandez JJ, Moore WS: Long-term results following surgical management of aortic graft infection. Arch Surg 1991;126:507.

Reilly LM, Stoney RJ, Goldstone J, et al: Improved management of aortic graft infection: The influence of operation sequence and staging. J Vasc Surg 1987;5:421.

Reilly LM, Altman H, Lusby RJ, et al: Late results following surgical management of vascular graft infection. J Vasc Surg 1984;1:36.

Robinson JA, Johansen K: Aortic sepsis: Is there a role for in situ graft reconstruction? J Vasc Surg 1991;13:677.

Seeger JM, Pretus HA, Welborn B, et al: Long-term outcome after treatment of aortic graft infection with staged extra-anatomic bypass grafting and aortic graft removal. J Vasc Surg 2000;32:451.

Towne JB, Seabrook GR, Bandyk DF, et al: In situ replacement of arterial prosthesis infected by bacterial biofilms: Long-term follow-up. J Vasc Surg 1994;19:226.

Trout HH, Kozloff L, Giordano JM: Priority of revascularization in patients with graft enteric fistulas, infected arteries, or infected arterial prostheses. Ann Surg 1984;199:669.

Walker WE, Cooley DA, Duncan JM, et al: The management of aortoduodenal fistula by in situ replacement of the infected abdominal aortic graft. Ann Surg 1987;205:727.

Yeager RA, Taylor LM Jr, Moneta GL, et al: Improved results with conventional management of infrarenal aortic infection. J Vasc Surg 1999;30:76.

Young RM, Cherry KJ Jr, Davis MP, et al: The results of in situ prosthetic replacement for infected aortic grafts. Am J Surg 1999;178:136.

Index

Note: Page numbers followed by the letter f refer to figures and those followed by t refer to tables.

ISBN 0-7216-8476-9

90038

9 780721 684765